Adapted from Jones MK, Castillo LA, Hopkins CA, Aaron WS (eds): St. Anthony's ICD-9-CM Code Book for Physician Payment, Vols 1 and 2, 5th ed. Reston, VA, St. Anthony Publishing, 1996.

LATEST APPROVED METHODS OF TREATMENT FOR THE PRACTICING PHYSICIAN

Edited by

ROBERT E. RAKEL, M.D.

Professor, Department of Family and Community Medicine
Baylor College of Medicine, Houston, Texas

W.B. SAUNDERS COMPANY
A Division of Harcourt Brace & Company
Philadelphia   London   Toronto   Montreal   Sydney   Tokyo

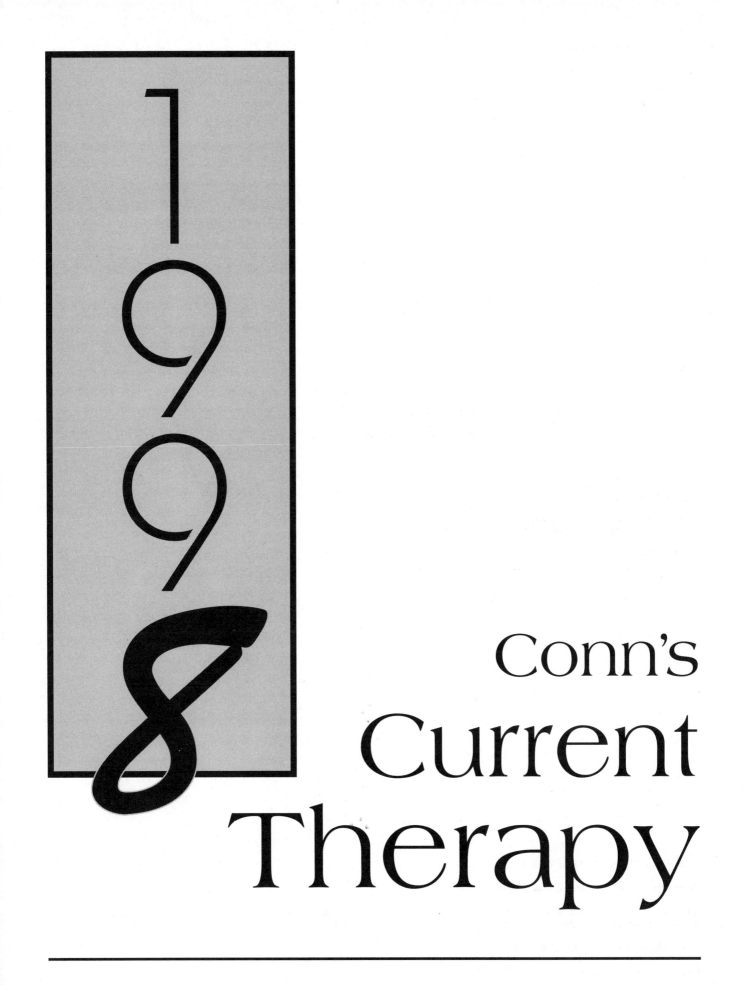

1998

Conn's
Current
Therapy

W.B. SAUNDERS COMPANY
A Division of Harcourt Brace & Company

The Curtis Center
Independence Square West
Philadelphia, Pennsylvania 19106

Library of Congress Cataloging-in-Publication Data

Current therapy; latest approved methods of treatment for the practicing physician.

Editors: H. F. Conn and others

v. 28 cm. annual.

ISBN 0–7216–7223–X

1. Therapeutics.   2. Therapeutics, Surgical.   3. Medicine—Practice.
  I. Conn, Howard Franklin, 1908–1982 ed.

RM101.C87   616.058   49–8328 rev*

CONN'S CURRENT THERAPY 1998   ISBN 0–7216–7223–X

Printed in the United States of America.

Last digit is the print number: 9   8   7   6   5   4   3   2   1

Contributors

ALLAN V. ABBOTT, M.D.

Professor of Clinical Family Medicine and Vice Chairman of Academic Affairs, Department of Family Medicine, University of Southern California School of Medicine, Los Angeles, California
Common Sports Injuries

ANTHONY ALBRIGHT, M.D.

St. Tammay Parish Medical Society and Affiliated Hospitals, St. Tammay Parish, Louisiana
Diverticula of the Alimentary Tract

DAVID H. ALPERS, M.D.

Professor of Medicine, Division of Gastroenterology, Washington University School of Medicine; Physician, Barnes-Jewish Hospital, and Consultant, John Cochrane Veterans Affairs Hospital, St. Louis, Missouri
Malabsorption

ROBERT J. ANDERSON, M.D.

Professor of Medicine, Creighton University School of Medicine; Chief, Section of Endocrinology, Diabetes and Metabolism, VA Medical Center, Omaha, Nebraska
Adrenocortical Insufficiency

STANLEY H. APPEL, M.D.

Professor and Chairman, Department of Neurology, Baylor College of Medicine; Chief of Neurology Service, The Methodist Hospital, Houston, Texas
Myasthenia Gravis

BAHA M. ARAFAH, M.D.

Associate Professor of Medicine, Case Western Reserve University; Director of Clinical Program, Division of Endocrinology, and Physician, University Hospitals of Cleveland, Cleveland, Ohio
Hypopituitarism

FRANK C. ARNETT, M.D.

Professor of Internal Medicine and Professor of Pathology and Laboratory Medicine, The University of Texas–Houston Health Science Center; Chief, Rheumatology, Hermann Hospital and Lyndon B. Johnson Hospital, Houston, Texas
Ankylosing Spondylitis and Other Spondyloarthropathies

PAUL S. AUERBACH, M.D., M.S.

Clinical Professor, Division of Emergency Medicine, Department of Surgery, Stanford University School of Medicine; Attending Physician, Emergency Medicine, Stanford University Hospital, Stanford, California
Hazardous Marine Animals

MATT H. BACKER, JR., M.D.

Professor and Chairman Emeritus, Department of Obstetrics and Gynecology, St. Louis University School of Medicine, St. Louis, Missouri; Clinical Professor of Obstetrics and Gynecology, Uniformed Services University of the Health Sciences, Bethesda, Maryland; Physician, St. Mary's Health Center, St. Louis, and Naval Medical Center, San Diego, California
Vaginal Bleeding in Late Pregnancy

HOWARD P. BADEN, M.D.

Professor of Dermatology, Harvard Medical School; Dermatologist, Massachusetts General Hospital, Boston, Massachusetts
Diseases of the Nails

ROBERT L. BAEHNER, M.D.

Professor of Pediatrics, Department of Pediatrics, University of Southern California School of Medicine; Staff Pediatric Hematologist/Oncologist, USC/LAC Women's and Children's Hospital, Los Angeles, California
Neutropenia

PHILIP L. BAILIN, M.D.

Professor of Medicine (Dermatology), Ohio State University School of Medicine; Chairman, Department of Dermatology, Cleveland Clinic Foundation, Cleveland, Ohio
Cancer of the Skin

ROBERT W. BALOH, M.D.

Professor of Neurology and Surgery (Head and Neck), University of California, Los Angeles, Medical School and Hospital, Los Angeles, California
Episodic Vertigo

J. RICHARD BARINGER, M.D.

H. A. and Edna Benning Professor and Chairman, Department of Neurology, University of Utah School of Medicine; Chief of Neurology, University of Utah Hospital, Salt Lake City, Utah
Viral Meningitis and Encephalitis

JOHN G. BARTLETT, M.D.

Professor of Medicine, The Johns Hopkins University School of Medicine; Chief, Infectious Diseases, The Johns Hopkins Hospital, Baltimore, Maryland
Primary Lung Abscess

JAMES W. BASS, M.D., M.P.H.

Professor, Department of Pediatrics, Uniformed Services University of the Health Sciences, Bethesda, Maryland; Clinical Professor, Department of Pediatrics, University of Hawaii School of Medicine; Senior Clinical Consultant, Pediatrics/Pediatric Infectious Diseases, Department of Pediatrics, Tripler Army Medical Center, Honolulu, Hawaii
Pertussis (Whooping Cough)

THOMAS H. BELHORN, M.D., PH.D.

Assistant Professor of Pediatrics, Division of Infectious Diseases, University of Texas–Houston Health Science Center; Physician, Hermann Hospital and M.D. Anderson Cancer Center, Houston, Texas
Varicella (Chickenpox)

ROBERT M. BENNETT, M.D.

Professor of Medicine and Chairman, Division of Arthritis and Rheumatic Diseases, Oregon Health Sciences University, Portland, Oregon
Bursitis, Tendinitis, Myofascial Pain, and Fibromyalgia

EDWARD J. BENZ, Jr., M.D.

Physician-in-Chief, The Johns Hopkins Hospital, Baltimore, Maryland
Thalassemia

ANDREW BERCHUCK, M.D.

Professor, Department of Obstetrics and Gynecology, Division of Gynecologic Oncology, Duke University School of Medicine and Medical Center, Durham, North Carolina
Cancer of the Endometrium

CHARLES S. BERENSON, M.D.

Associate Professor of Medicine, State University of New York at Buffalo; Physician, Department of Veterans Affairs Western New York Healthcare System, Buffalo, New York
Tularemia

WILMA F. BERGFELD, M.D.

Head, Clinical Research, Department of Dermatology; Head, Dermatopathology, Department of Pathology, The Cleveland Clinic, Cleveland, Ohio
Hair Disorders

JEFFREY D. BERNHARD, M.D.

Professor of Medicine and Director, Division of Dermatology, University of Massachusetts Medical School; Director, Division of Dermatology, University of Massachusetts Medical Center, Worcester, Massachusetts
Pruritus (Itching)

KARL R. BEUTNER, M.D., Ph.D.

Associate Clinical Professor of Dermatology, University of California, San Francisco, School of Medicine, San Francisco, California
Warts

RICHARD P. BILLINGHAM, M.D.

Clinical Associate Professor, Department of Surgery, University of Washington; Attending Surgeon, Northwest Hospital and Swedish Hospital Medical Center, Seattle, Washington
Hemorrhoids, Anal Fissure, and Anorectal Abscess and Fistula

JACOB D. BITRAN, M.D.

Professor of Medicine, University of Illinois, Chicago; Physician, Lutheran General Hospital and Cancer Care Center, Park Ridge, Illinois
Primary Lung Cancer

W. KLINE BOLTON, M.D.

Professor of Internal Medicine and Chief of Nephrology, University of Virginia School of Medicine and Health Sciences Center, Charlottesville, Virginia
Primary Glomerular Diseases

WILLIAM Z. BORER, M.D.

Associate Professor of Pathology, Thomas Jefferson University; Physician, Thomas Jefferson University Hospital, Philadelphia, Pennsylvania
Reference Intervals for the Interpretation of Laboratory Tests

MICHAEL C. BOYARS, M.D.

Associate Professor, Department of Internal Medicine, University of Texas Medical Branch, Galveston, Texas
Acute Respiratory Failure

PETER E. BRAVERMAN, M.D.

Instructor, Department of Medicine, The Johns Hopkins School of Medicine, Baltimore, Maryland
Disseminated Intravascular Coagulation

MAYER BREZIS, M.D.

Professor of Medicine, Hadassah–Hebrew University Medical School; Chief Physician, Department of Medicine, Hadassah University Hospital Mount Scopus, Jerusalem, Israel
Acute Renal Failure

JONATHAN R. BROOME, M.B., B.S.

Institute of Naval Medicine, Alverstoke, Hampshire, United Kingdom
Mountain Sickness

JON M. BURCH, M.D.

Professor of Surgery, University of Colorado Health Sciences Center; Chief, General Surgery, Denver Health Medical Center, Denver, Colorado
Acute Pancreatitis

KIM J. BURCHIEL, M.D.

John Raaf Professor and Head, Division of Neurosurgery, Oregon Health Sciences University; Attending Neurosurgeon, Section of Neurosurgery, Portland Veterans Affairs Medical Center and Shriner's Hospital, Portland, Oregon
Trigeminal Neuralgia

BRUCE M. CAMITTA, M.D.

Professor of Pediatrics, Medical College of Wisconsin, and Director, Midwest Children's Cancer Center; Director of Hematology-Oncology, Children's Hospital of Wisconsin, Milwaukee, Wisconsin
Acute Leukemia in Children

G. DOUGLAS CAMPBELL, Jr., M.D.

Professor of Medicine and Chief, Division of Pulmonary and Critical Care Medicine, Louisiana State University School of Medicine and Medical Center, Shreveport, Louisiana
Blastomycosis

GEORGE P. CANELLOS, M.D.

William Rosenberg Professor of Medicine, Harvard Medical School; Physician, Dana Farber Cancer Institute and Brigham and Women's Hospital, Boston, Massachusetts
Hodgkin's Disease: Chemotherapy

THOMAS R. CARACCIO, Pharm.D.

Assistant Professor of Emergency Medicine, State University of New York at Stony Brook; Assistant Professor of Pharmacology/Toxicology, New York College of Osteopathic Medicine, Old Westbury; Assistant Professor of Clinical Pharmacy, St. John's University College of Pharmacy, Jamaica; Clinical Manager of Long Island Regional Poison Control Center, Winthrop-University Hospital, Mineola, New York
Acute Poisonings

WILLIAM A. CARO, M.D.

Professor of Clinical Dermatology, Northwestern University Medical School; Attending Physician, Northwestern Memorial Hospital; Consulting Dermatopathologist, Children's Memorial Hospital, Chicago, Illinois
Melanocytic Nevi (Moles)

PAUL C. CARPENTER, M.D.

Associate Professor of Medicine, Mayo Graduate School of Medicine; Physician, Mayo Clinic and Mayo Foundation, Rochester, Minnesota
Cushing's Syndrome

VAL A. CATANZARITE, M.D., Ph.D.

Director of Perinatal Imaging, Sharp Perinatal Center; Associate Director, Maternal-Fetal Medicine, Sharp/Mary Birch Hospital for Women; Physician, Grossmont Hospital, San Diego, California
Antepartum Care

THOMAS R. CATE, M.D.

Professor of Medicine and Microbiology/Immunology, Baylor College of Medicine; Attending Physician, Ben Taub General Hospital, Houston, Texas
Influenza

BERNARD R. CHAITMAN, M.D.

Professor of Medicine, St. Louis University School of Medicine; Chief of Cardiology, St. Louis University Health Sciences Center, St. Louis, Missouri
Care After Myocardial Infarction

HENRY F. CHAMBERS, M.D.

Professor of Medicine, University of California, San Francisco; Chief, Division of Infectious Diseases, San Francisco General Hospital, San Francisco, California
Infective Endocarditis

P. JOAN CHESNEY, M.D.

Professor of Pediatrics, University of Tennessee, Memphis, College of Medicine; Physician, Le Bonheur Children's Medical Center and The Regional Medical Center at Memphis, Memphis, Tennessee
Toxic Shock Syndrome

INDER J. CHOPRA, M.D.

Professor of Medicine, Division of Endocrinology, University of California, Los Angeles, School of Medicine; Staff Physician, UCLA Center for Health Sciences, Los Angeles, California
Hypothyroidism

G. PATRICK CLAGETT, M.D.

Professor of Surgery, University of Texas Southwestern Medical Center; Attending Staff, Parkland Memorial Hospital and Zale Lipshy University Hospital, Dallas, Texas
Deep Venous Thrombosis of the Lower Extremities

RAY E. CLOUSE, M.D.

Professor of Medicine, Division of Gastroenterology, Washington University School of Medicine; Physician, Barnes-Jewish Hospital, St. Louis, Missouri
Irritable Bowel Syndrome

LAWRENCE S. COHEN, M.D.

The Ebenezer K. Hunt Professor, Yale University School of Medicine; Physician, Yale–New Haven Hospital, New Haven, Connecticut
Hypertrophic Cardiomyopathy

ROBERT E. CONDON, M.D., M.S.

Ausman Foundation Professor and Chairman Emeritus of Surgery, The Medical College of Wisconsin, Milwaukee, Wisconsin
Necrotizing Skin and Soft Tissue Infections

CATHY CONRY-CANTILENA, M.D.

Medical Officer, Department of Transfusion Medicine, National Institutes of Health; Physician, Warren G. Magnuson Clinical Center, Bethesda, Maryland
Therapeutic Use of Blood Components

JAMES D. COOK, M.D.

Phillips Professor of Medicine, Kansas University Medical Center; Attending Physician, University Hospital, Kansas City, Kansas
Iron Deficiency Anemia

JAMES J. CORRIGAN, JR., M.D.

Professor of Pediatrics and Internal Medicine, Tulane University School of Medicine; Physician, Tulane University Hospital and Medical Center of Louisiana, New Orleans, Louisiana
Vitamin K Deficiency

ROBERT B. COUCH, M.D.

Chairman and Professor of Microbiology and Immunology, Baylor College of Medicine; Physician, Ben Taub General Hospital and The Methodist Hospital, Houston, Texas
Viral Respiratory Infections

GILBERT H. DANIELS, M.D.

Associate Professor of Medicine, Harvard Medical School; Co-Director, Thyroid Associates, Massachusetts General Hospital, Boston, Massachusetts
Hyperthyroidism

DANIEL F. DANZL, M.D.

Professor and Chair, Department of Emergency Medicine, University of Louisville School of Medicine and Hospital, Louisville, Kentucky
Disturbances due to Cold

ROBERT N. DAVIDSON, M.D.

Senior Lecturer, Imperial College School of Medicine, London; Consultant, Department of Infectious and Tropical Diseases, Northwick Park Hospital, Harrow, England
Leishmaniasis

TERRY F. DAVIES, M.D.

Florence and Theodore Baumritter Professor of Medicine and Director, Division of Endocrinology and Metabolism, Mount Sinai School of Medicine; Attending Physician, The Mount Sinai Hospital, New York, New York
Thyroiditis

MICHAEL E. DeBAKEY, M.D.

Olga Keith Wiess Professor of Surgery, Distinguished Service Professor of Surgery, Director of the DeBakey Heart Center, Baylor College of Medicine; Senior Attending Surgeon, The Methodist Hospital; Consultant in Surgery, Veterans Administration Hospital, Houston, Texas
Acquired Diseases of the Aorta

ANTONIO V. DELGADO-ESCUETA, M.D.

Professor of Neurology, University of California, Los Angeles, School of Medicine; Staff Neurologist and Director, Epilepsy Program, West Los Angeles VA Medical Center; Attending Private Neurologist, UCLA Health Sciences Center, Los Angeles, California
Seizures and Epilepsies in Adolescents and Adults

TOM R. DeMEESTER, M.D.

Professor and Chairman, Department of Surgery, University of Southern California School of Medicine, Los Angeles, California
Gastroesophageal Reflux Disease

RICHARD D. DeSHAZO, M.D.

Professor of Medicine and Pediatrics, Director, Division of Allergy and Immunology, and Chair, Department of Internal Medicine, College of Medicine, University of South Alabama, Mobile, Alabama
Anaphylaxis and Serum Sickness

SEYMOUR DIAMOND, M.D.

Adjunct Professor of Pharmacology and Molecular Biology, Finch University of Health Sciences/The Chicago Medical School, North Chicago; Attending Staff, Columbus Hospital, Chicago, Illinois
Headache

SEAN F. DINNEEN, M.D. M.Sc.

Assistant Professor of Medicine, Mayo Medical School; Consultant, Divisions of Endocrinology and Health Services Evaluation, Mayo Clinic, Rochester, Minnesota
Diabetic Ketoacidosis

JOSÉ DOS SANTOS, JR., D.D.S., M.S.

Full Professor, Department of Restorative Dentistry (Division of Occlusion), University of Texas Health Science Center at San Antonio, School of Dentistry, San Antonio, Texas
Temporomandibular Disorders

ELIZABETH T. DOUGLASS, M.D.

Clinical Instructor, University of Texas Medical School at Houston; Staff Physician, Hermann Hospital, Houston, Texas
Acute Infectious Diarrhea

MARGARET C. DOUGLASS, M.D.

Attending Physician, Henry Ford Hospital, Detroit, Michigan
Donovanosis (Granuloma Inguinale); Lymphogranuloma Venereum

JAN EDWIN DRUTZ, M.D.

Associate Professor, Department of Pediatrics, Baylor College of Medicine; Active Staff, Texas Children's Hospital and Ben Taub General Hospital, Houston, Texas
Immunization Practices

DAVID L. DUNNER, M.D.

Professor and Vice Chairman and Co-Director, Center for Anxiety and Depression, Department of Psychiatry and Behavioral Sciences, University of Washington, Seattle, Washington
Mood Disorders

HERBERT L. DuPONT, M.D.

H. Irving Schweppe, Jr., M.D., Chair in Internal Medicine, Baylor College of Medicine, and Mary W. Kelsey Professor, University of Texas–Houston; Chief, Internal Medicine, St. Luke's Episcopal Hospital, Houston, Texas
Acute Infectious Diarrhea

PETER JAMES DYCK, M.D.

Professor of Neurology, Mayo Medical School, Rochester, Minnesota
Peripheral Neuropathy

LIBBY EDWARDS, M.D.

Clinical Associate Professor, Bowman Gray School of Medicine of Wake Forest University, Winston-Salem; Chief of Dermatology, Carolinas Medical Center, Charlotte, North Carolina
Condylomata Acuminata

JOHN H. EPSTEIN, M.D.

Clinical Professor of Dermatology, University of California, San Francisco, School of Medicine; Physician, University of California Hospital and Ralf K. Davies Hospital, San Francisco, California
Sunburn

STEPHEN I. ESSES, M.D.

Brodsky Professor and Director of Residency Program, Department of Orthopedic Surgery, Baylor College of Medicine, Houston, Texas
Low Back Pain

STANLEY FAHN, M.D.

H. Houston Merritt Professor of Neurology, Columbia University College of Physicians and Surgeons; Attending Neurologist, Presbyterian Hospital, New York, New York
Parkinsonism

SEBASTIAN FARO, M.D., PH.D.

John M. Simpson Professor and Chairman, Department of Obstetrics and Gynecology, Rush Medical College and Rush-Presbyterian–St. Luke's Medical Center, Chicago, Illinois
Vulvovaginitis; Chlamydia trachomatis

GEOFFREY C. FARRELL, M.D.

Robert W. Storr Professor of Hepatic Medicine, University of Sydney at Westmead Hospital, Westmead, New South Wales, Australia
Acute and Chronic Viral Hepatitis

NICHOLAS J. FIUMARA, M.D., M.P.H.

Clinical Professor of Dermatology, Tufts University School of Medicine, Boston; Associate Staff, Department of Dermatology, and Director, STD Clinic, New England Medical Center, Boston; Consulting Staff, Dermatology Department, Whidden Memorial Hospital, Everett, Massachusetts
Syphilis

MALCOLM T. FOSTER, JR., M.D.

Professor of Internal Medicine, University of Florida College of Medicine; Chief of Infectious Diseases, University Medical Center, Jacksonville, Florida
Relapsing Fever

RICHARD S. FOSTER, M.D.

Associate Professor of Urology, University of Indiana School of Medicine and Indiana University Hospitals, Indianapolis, Indiana
Malignant Tumors of the Urogenital Tract

ROGER S. FOSTER, JR., M.D.

Glenn Professor of Surgery, Emory University School of Medicine, and Chief of Surgical Services, Crawford Long Hospital of Emory University, Atlanta, Georgia
Diseases of the Breast

JACKSON E. FOWLER, JR., M.D.

Professor of Surgery, University of Mississippi School of Medicine; Chief of Urology, University of Mississippi Hospital and Clinics; Physician, Veterans Affairs Medical Center, Jackson, Mississippi
Nongonococcal Urethritis in Men

GARY S. FRANCIS, M.D.

Professor of Medicine, University of Minnesota School of Medicine; Physician, Fairview–University of Minnesota Hospital, Minneapolis, Minnesota
Congestive Heart Failure

EUGENE P. FRENKEL, M.D.

Professor of Internal Medicine and Radiology; Patsy R. and Raymond D. Nasher Distinguished Chair in Cancer Research; A. Kenneth Pye Professorship in Cancer Research, University of Texas Southwestern Medical Center; Attending Physician, Zale Lipshy University Hospital and Parkland Memorial Hospital, Dallas, Texas
Pernicious Anemia and Other Megaloblastic Anemias

STEVEN M. FRUCHTMAN, M.D.

Clinical Associate Professor of Medicine, Mount Sinai School of Medicine; Director, Bone Marrow Transplant Service, Mount Sinai Hospital, New York, New York
Polycythemia Vera

WILLIAM H. GEERTS, M.D.

Associate Professor of Medicine, University of Toronto; Director, Thromboembolism Program, Sunnybrook Health Science Centre, Toronto, Ontario, Canada
Pulmonary Embolism

LAYNE O. GENTRY, M.D.

Clinical Professor of Medicine, Microbiology, and Immunology, Baylor College of Medicine; Chief, Infectious Disease Section, and Medical Director, Infection Control, St. Luke's Episcopal Hospital, Houston, Texas
Osteomyelitis

RONALD B. GEORGE, M.D.

Professor and Chairman, Department of Medicine, Louisiana State University Medical School, Shreveport, Louisiana
Chronic Obstructive Pulmonary Disease

MICHAEL A. GERBER, M.D.

Professor of Pediatrics, University of Connecticut School of Medicine; Director of Pediatric Infectious Diseases, Connecticut Children's Medical Center, Hartford, Connecticut
Streptococcal Pharyngitis

ALFRED L. GEST, M.D.

Assistant Professor of Pediatrics, Newborn Section, Baylor College of Medicine, Houston, Texas
Resuscitation of the Newborn

RICHARD GLECKMAN, M.D.

Professor of Medicine, Boston University School of Medicine; Senior Lecturer on Medicine, Tufts University School of Medicine; Director of Medicine, Carney Hospital, Boston, Massachusetts
Acute Bronchitis

ANDREW W. GODDARD, M.D.

Associate Professor of Psychiatry, Yale University School of Medicine; Physician, Connecticut Mental Health Center, New Haven, Connecticut
Anxiety

MARK S. GOLD, M.D.

Professor, University of Florida Brain Institute, Departments of Neuroscience, Psychiatry, Community Health, and Family Medicine, College of Medicine; Physician, Shands Hospital at the University of Florida, Gainesville, Florida
Drug Abuse

EDMOND T. GONZALES, Jr., M.D.

Professor of Urology, Scott Department of Urology, Baylor College of Medicine; Head, Department of Surgery, and Chief, Urology Service, Texas Children's Hospital, Houston, Texas
Childhood Enuresis

JACK M. GORMAN, M.D.

Professor of Psychiatry, College of Physicians and Surgeons of Columbia University; Deputy Director, New York State Psychiatric Institute, New York, New York
Panic Disorder

CHRISTOPHER J. GOSTOUT, M.D.

Associate Professor of Medicine, Mayo Medical School and Clinic; Physician, St. Mary's Hospital of Rochester and Rochester Methodist Hospital, Rochester, Minnesota
Bleeding Esophageal Varices

ANTONIO M. GOTTO, Jr., M.D., D.Phil.

Professor of Medicine, Cornell University Medical College, New York, New York
Hyperlipidemia

STEPHEN B. GREENBERG, M.D.

Professor and Vice-Chairman, Department of Medicine, Baylor College of Medicine; Associate Chief of Staff and Chief, Medicine Service, Ben Taub General Hospital, Houston, Texas
Bacterial Pneumonia

RALPH G. GREENLEE, Jr., M.D.

Professor, Departments of Neurology and Neurosurgery, University of Texas Southwestern Medical College; Staff, Parkland Memorial Hospital and Zale Lipshy University Hospital, Dallas, Texas
Primary Intracerebral Hemorrhage

JOSEPH GREENSHER, M.D.

Professor of Pediatrics, State University of New York at Stony Brook; Medical Director and Associate Chairman, Department of Pediatrics, Winthrop-University Hospital; Associate Director, Long Island Regional Poison Control Center, Winthrop-University Hospital, Mineola, New York
Acute Poisonings

RONALD L. GROSS, M.D.

Associate Professor of Ophthalmology, Cullen Eye Institute, Baylor College of Medicine; Active Staff, The Methodist Hospital of Houston and Ben Taub General Hospital, Houston, Texas
Glaucoma

HANS W. GRÜNWALD, M.D.

Associate Professor of Medicine, Mount Sinai School of Medicine; Chief, Division of Hematology-Oncology, Department of Medicine, Queens Hospital Center, Jamaica; Attending, Department of Medicine, Mount Sinai Medical Center, New York, New York
Acute Leukemia in Adults

DAVID S. GUZICK, M.D., Ph.D.

Professor and Chair, Department of Obstetrics and Gynecology, University of Rochester; Physician, Strong Memorial Hospital, Rochester, Minnesota
Amenorrhea

LISA A. HAGLUND, M.D.

Assistant Professor of Clinical Medicine, Infectious Diseases Division, University of Cincinnati; Director of Infection Control, Good Samaritan Hospital; Acting Hospital Epidemiologist, University Hospital, Cincinnati, Ohio
Histoplasmosis

ANN E. HALLSTONE, M.D.

Assistant Clinical Professor of Medicine and Surgery, University of California, Davis; Staff Gastroenterologist, VA Northern California System of Clinics, Martinez, California
Nausea and Vomiting

BRUCE H. HAMORY, M.D.

Professor of Medicine, Pennsylvania State University College of Medicine; Milton S. Hershey Medical Center, Hershey, Pennsylvania
Typhus Fever

STEPHEN B. HANAUER, M.D.

Professor of Medicine and Clinical Pharmacology, University of Chicago Pritzker School of Medicine, Chicago, Illinois
Ulcerative Colitis

JAMES BARRY HANSHAW, M.D.

Professor of Pediatrics, University of Massachusetts Medical School; Chair, Department of Pediatrics, Memorial Hospital and Interim Chair, Pediatrics, University of Massachusetts Medical Center, Worcester, Massachusetts
Measles

PETER HANSON, M.Sc., M.D.

Professor of Medicine, Cardiology Section, University of Wisconsin Medical School; Physician, University of Wisconsin Hospital and Clinics, Madison, Wisconsin
Disturbances due to Heat

JOHN T. HARRINGTON, M.D.

Professor of Medicine and Dean, Tufts University School of Medicine; Senior Nephrologist, Tuft's–New England Medical Center, Boston, Massachusetts
Chronic Renal Failure

LOUIS A. HEALEY, M.D.

Clinical Professor, University of Washington School of Medicine, Seattle, Washington
Polymyalgia Rheumatica and Giant Cell Arteritis

ANDREA E. HERBERT, M.D.

Resident Physician, Department of Neurosurgery, University of Florida College of Medicine, Shands Hospital at the University of Florida, and Gainesville Veterans Administration Hospital, Gainesville, Florida
Acute Head Injuries in Children

DAVID N. HERNDON, M.D.

Professor of Surgery, University of Texas Medical Branch at Galveston; Chief of Staff, Shriners Burn Unit; Jesse H. Jones Distinguished Chair in Burn Surgery, University of Texas Medical Branch at Galveston, Texas
Burns

CHARLES B. HICKS, M.D.

Assistant Professor of Medicine, Division of Infectious Diseases, Duke University School of Medicine and Medical Center, Durham, North Carolina
Gonorrhea

DAVID R. HILL, M.D.

Associate Professor of Medicine, Division of Infectious Diseases, and Director, International Traveler's Medical Service, University of Connecticut, School of Medicine and Health Center, Farmington, Connecticut
Salmonellosis (Excluding Typhoid Fever)

HARRY R. HILL, M.D.

Professor of Pathology, Pediatrics and Medicine and Head, Division of Clinical Immunology, University of Utah School of Medicine, Salt Lake City, Utah
Rheumatic Fever

L. LEIGHTON HILL, M.D.

Professor of Pediatrics, Renal Section, and Assistant Dean of Admissions, Baylor College of Medicine; Active Staff, Texas Children's Hospital and Harris County Hospital District Hospitals, Houston, Texas
Intravenous Fluid Therapy in Infants and Children

THOMAS G. HILL, M.D.

Clinical Assistant Professor of Dermatology, Emory University School of Medicine; Physician, DeKalb Medical Center, Decatur, and Grady Memorial Hospital, Atlanta, Georgia
Premalignant Lesions

PAULA J. ADAMS HILLARD, M.D.

Associate Professor, Department of Obstetrics and Gynecology and Department of Pediatrics, University of Cincinnati College of Medicine; Physician, University Hospital and Children's Hospital Medical Center, Cincinnati, Ohio
Contraception

LOREN F. HIRATZKA, M.D.

Physician, The Jewish Hospital and The Christ Hospital, Cincinnati, Ohio
Atelectasis

KAREN A. HOLBROOK, M.D.

Assistant Professor of Medicine, Division of Infectious Diseases, Albert Einstein College of Medicine; Attending Physician, Montefiore Medical Center, Bronx, New York
Rat-Bite Fever

G. ALLEN HOLLOWAY, Jr., M.D.

Adjunct Professor, Department of Chemical, Bio and Materials Engineering, Arizona State University; Faculty and Attending Physician, Maricopa Medical Center; Attending Physician, Phoenix Indian Medical Center, Phoenix, Arizona
Pressure Ulcers

W. KEITH HOOTS, M.D.

Professor of Pediatrics, University of Texas M.D. Anderson Cancer Center; Pediatrician, Hermann Children's Hospital and M.D. Anderson Cancer Center, Houston, Texas
Hemophilia and Related Conditions

RICHARD B. HORNICK, M.D.

Adjunct Professor of Medicine, University of Florida School of Medicine; Vice President for Medical Education, Orlando Regional Healthcare System, Orlando, Florida
Typhoid Fever

PETER M. HORVATH, M.D.

Associate Professor, Obstetrics and Gynecology, and Head, Division of Reproductive Endocrinology, Albany Medical College; Physician, Albany Medical Center Hospital and St. Peter's Hospital, Albany, New York
Ectopic Pregnancy

JOHN W. HOUSE, M.D.

Clinical Professor, Department of Otolaryngology–Head and Neck Surgery, University of Southern California School of Medicine, Los Angeles; Associate Clinical Professor, Division of Otolaryngology–Head and Neck Surgery, University of California, Irvine; President, House Ear Institute, Los Angeles, California
Tinnitus

GORDON B. HUGHES, M.D.

Program Director, Department of Otolaryngology and Communicative Disorders, The Cleveland Clinic Foundation, Cleveland, Ohio
Acute Peripheral Facial Paralysis (Bell's Palsy)

ADRIAN P. IRELAND, M.D.

Research Fellow, Department of Surgery, University of Southern California, Los Angeles, California
Gastroesophageal Reflux Disease

C. GARY JACKSON, M.D.

Clinical Professor, Department of Otolaryngology/Head and Neck Surgery, Vanderbilt University; Clinical Professor of Otolaryngology/Head and Neck Surgery, Georgetown University Medical Center, Washington, D.C.; Clinical Professor, Department of Surgery, University of North Carolina, Chapel Hill, North Carolina; Physician, Baptist Hospital and Columbia Centennial Medical Center, Nashville; The Otology Group, Nashville, Tennessee
Meniere's Disease

JOSEPH JANKOVIC, M.D.

Professor of Neurology and Director, Parkinson's Disease Center and Movement Disorders Clinic, Baylor College of Medicine; Physician, The Methodist Hospital, Houston, Texas
Gilles de la Tourette Syndrome

MAUREEN A. JARRELL, M.D.

Physician, Moses H. Cone Health Systems, Greensboro, North Carolina
Carcinoma of the Uterine Cervix

SUZANNE R. JENKINS, V.M.D., M.P.H.

Assistant State Epidemiologist, Office of Epidemiology, Virginia Department of Health, Richmond, Virginia
Rabies

ROYCE H. JOHNSON, M.D.

Professor of Medicine, University of California, Los Angeles; Vice Chair, Medicine, and Chief, Infectious Diseases, Kern Medical Center, Bakersfield, California
Coccidioidomycosis

GERALD H. JORDAN, M.D.

Professor of Urology, Eastern Virginia Medical School; Physician, Sentara Norfolk General Hospital and Children's Hospital of the King's Daughters', Norfolk, Virginia
Anterior Urethral Stricture

ROBERT E. JORDON, M.D.

Professor and Chairman, Department of Dermatology, The University of Texas–Houston Medical School; Chief of Dermatology, Hermann Hospital and Lyndon B. Johnson General Hospital, Houston, Texas
Bullous Skin Diseases

JOSEPH L. JORIZZO, M.D.

Professor and Chair, Department of Dermatology, Bowman Gray School of Medicine of Wake Forest University; Physician, North Carolina Baptist Hospital, Winston-Salem Veterans Administration Clinic, and Salisbury VA Hospital, Winston-Salem, North Carolina
Cutaneous Vasculitis

STEPHEN M. JURD, M.B., B.S.

Clinical Senior Lecturer, Department of Psychological Medicine, University of Sydney; Drug and Alcohol Services, Royal North Shore Hospital, St. Leonard's, New South Wales; Program Director, Palm Beach—Currumbin Clinic, Currumbin, Queensland, Australia
Alcoholism

PETER J. KAHRILAS, M.D.

Professor, Departments of Medicine and Communication Sciences and Disorders, Northwestern University Medical School; Medical Director, Gastrointestinal Diagnostic Laboratory, and Staff Physician, Northwestern Memorial Hospital, Chicago, Illinois
Dysphagia and Esophageal Obstruction

H. BENFER KALTREIDER, M.D.

Professor of Medicine, University of California, San Francisco; Chief, Pulmonary and Critical Care Medicine Section, VA Medical Center, San Francisco, California
Hypersensitivity Pneumonitis (Allergic Alveolitis)

NORMAN M. KAPLAN, M.D.

Professor of Internal Medicine, University of Texas Southwestern Medical Center; Head, Hypertension Division, Parkland Memorial Hospital, Dallas, Texas
Hypertension

LISA G. KAPLOWITZ, M.D.

Associate Professor, Division of Infectious Diseases, Department of Medicine, Medical College of Virginia; Faculty, Medical College of Virginia Hospitals; Director, HIV/AIDS Center, Virginia Commonwealth University, Richmond, Virginia
Rocky Mountain Spotted Fever

RAYMOND H. KAUFMAN, M.D.

Professor, Department of Obstetrics-Gynecology and Pathology, Baylor College of Medicine, Houston, Texas
Tumors of the Vulva

A. PAUL KELLY, M.D.

Professor of Medicine (Dermatology), Charles R. Drew University of Medicine and Science; Clinical Professor of Medicine, University of California, Los Angeles; Chief, Division of Dermatology, King/Drew Medical Center, Los Angeles, California
Keloids

JAMES W. KENDIG, M.D.

Associate Professor of Pediatrics, University of Rochester School of Medicine and Dentistry; Physician, Children's Hospital at Strong and Rochester General Hospital, Rochester, New York
Hemolytic Disease of the Newborn (Red Cell Alloimmunization)

CHARLES D. KENNARD, M.D.

Physician, Department of Surgery (Dermatologic), Arlington Memorial Hospital, Arlington, Texas
Urticaria

JAY S. KEYSTONE, M.D.

Professor of Medicine, University of Toronto; Staff Physician, Centre for Travel and Tropical Medicine, The Toronto Hospital, Toronto, Ontario, Canada
Trichinosis

SUNDEEP KHOSLA, M.D.

Associate Professor of Medicine, Mayo Medical School; Physician, Division of Endocrinology, Metabolism, and Nutrition, Mayo Clinic, Rochester, Minnesota
Osteoporosis

ROBERT C. KIMBROUGH, III, M.D.

Professor, Department of Internal Medicine, Division of Infectious Disease, Texas Tech University Health Sciences Center and University Medical Center, Lubbock, Texas
Q Fever

CHARLES P. KIMMELMAN, M.D.

Director of Medical Education, Department of Otolaryngology, Manhattan Eye, Ear and Throat Hospital; Associate Professor of Otolaryngology, Cornell Medical College; Attending Otolaryngologist, New York Hospital, New York, New York
External Otitis

MICHAEL B. KIMMEY, M.D.

Professor of Medicine, University of Washington School of Medicine; Section Chief for Gastroenterology and Director, Gastrointestinal Endoscopy, University of Washington Medical Center, Seattle, Washington
Gastritis and Peptic Ulcer Disease

LOWELL R. KING, M.D.

Professor of Urology and Associate Professor of Pediatrics, Duke University Medical School; Head, Section on Pediatric Urology, Duke University Medical Center, Durham, North Carolina
Bacterial Infections of the Urinary Tract in Girls

WILLIAM J. KLISH, M.D.

Professor of Pediatrics, Baylor College of Medicine; Head, Pediatric Gastroenterology and Nutrition, Texas Children's Hospital, Houston, Texas
Normal Infant Feeding

ANTHONY L. KOMAROFF, M.D.

Professor of Medicine, Harvard Medical School; Senior Physician, Brigham and Women's Hospital, Boston, Massachusetts
Chronic Fatigue Syndrome

MARK J. KORUDA, M.D.

Associate Professor, Departments of Nutrition and Surgery, University of North Carolina; Associate Director, Nutrition Support Service, University of North Carolina Hospital, Chapel Hill, North Carolina
Parenteral Nutrition in Adults

THEODORE A. KOTCHEN, M.D.

Professor and Chairman, Department of Medicine, Medical College of Wisconsin, Milwaukee, Wisconsin
Primary Aldosteronism

MICHAEL S. KRAMER, M.D.

Professor, Departments of Pediatrics and Epidemiology and Biostatistics, McGill University Faculty of Medicine; Attending Pediatrician, Montreal Children's Hospital, Quebec, Canada
Fever

JOHN N. KRIEGER, M.D.

Professor, Department of Urology, University of Washington School of Medicine; Attending Surgeon, University of Washington Medical Center and Seattle Veterans Administration Medical Center, Seattle, Washington
Epididymitis

ROBERT A. KYLE, M.D.

Professor of Medicine and of Laboratory Medicine, Mayo Medical School; Consultant, Division of Hematology and Internal Medicine, Mayo Clinic and Mayo Foundation, Rochester, Minnesota
Multiple Myeloma

CHARLES R. LAMBERT, M.D., PH.D.

Professor of Medicine, Division of Cardiovascular Medicine, University of Florida School of Medicine; Director, Health First Heart Institute, Melbourne, Florida
Angina Pectoris

LEWIS LANDSBERG, M.D.

Professor, Northwestern University Medical School; Physician-in-Chief, Northwestern Memorial Hospital, Chicago, Illinois
Pheochromocytoma

RICHARD G. B. LANGLEY, M.D.

Instructor, Harvard Medical School; Dermatologist, Massachusetts General Hospital, Boston, Massachusetts
Cutaneous Melanoma

FRANK L. LANZA, M.D.

Clinical Professor of Medicine, Section of Gastroenterology, Baylor College of Medicine; Senior Attending Physician, GI Endoscopy Laboratory, Ben Taub General Hospital; Attending Physician, Memorial Hospital, Houston, Texas
Tumors of the Stomach

HAROLD E. LEBOVITZ, M.D.

Professor of Medicine and Chief, Section of Endocrinology, State University of New York Health Science Center at Brooklyn; Physician, University Hospital of Brooklyn and Kings County Hospital Center, Brooklyn, New York
Diabetes Mellitus in Adults

JAMES LEGGETT, M.D.

Associate Professor, Department of Internal Medicine, Oregon Health Sciences University; Assistant Director, Department of Medical Education, Providence Portland Medical Center, Portland, Oregon
Bacteremia and Septicemia

NORMAN LEVINE, M.D.

Professor, University of Arizona College of Medicine; Chief of Dermatology, University Medical Center, Tucson, Arizona
Pigmentary Disorders

N. SCOTT LITOFSKY, M.D.

Associate Professor, University of Massachusetts Medical School, Division of Neurosurgery, Worcester, Massachusetts
Brain Tumors

RICHARD F. LOCKEY, M.D.

Professor of Medicine, Pediatrics, and Public Health; The Joy McCann Culver House Professorship in Allergy-Immunology; Director, Division of Allergy and Immunology, University of South Florida College of Medicine and James H. Haley Veterans Hospital, Tampa, Florida
Allergic Reactions to Insect Stings

GERALD L. LOGUE, M.D.

Professor of Medicine, State University of New York at Buffalo; Physician, Buffalo VA Medical Center, Buffalo, New York
Adverse Reactions to Blood Transfusions

CHRISTINA LUEDKE, M.D., PH.D.

Instructor, Harvard Medical School; Assistant in Medicine, Children's Hospital; Clinical Associate in Pediatrics, Massachusetts General Hospital, Boston, Massachusetts
Diabetes Mellitus in Children and Adolescents

SHERWOOD C. LYNN, JR., M.D.

Associate Professor and Chief of Gynecology, University of South Alabama, College of Medicine; Physician, University of South Alabama Hospitals: Children and Women's, Medical Center, and Knollwood Park, Mobile, Alabama
Pelvic Inflammatory Disease

LAWRENCE E. MALLETTE, M.D., PH.D.

Associate Professor of Medicine, Baylor College of Medicine; Acting Chief of Endocrinology, Veterans Affairs Medical Center, Houston, Texas
Hyperparathyroidism and Hypoparathyroidism

STEPHEN R. MARDER, M.D.

Professor and Vice Chair, Department of Psychiatry and Biobehavioral Science, University of California, Los Angeles, School of Medicine; Director of Mental Health Services and Chief, Psychiatry Department, West Los Angeles VA Medical Center, Los Angeles, California
Schizophrenia

DONALD W. MARION, M.D.

Associate Professor of Neurological Surgery, University of Pittsburgh, School of Medicine; Director, Brain Trauma Research Center, and Attending Neurosurgeon, University of Pittsburgh Medical Center, Pittsburgh, Pennsylvania
Acute Head Injuries in Adults

DAVID H. MARTIN, M.D.

Harry E. Dascomb, M.D., Professor of Medicine, Professor of Microbiology, and Chief, Section of Infectious Diseases, Louisiana State University Medical School, New Orleans, Louisiana
Chancroid

JOHN A. MATA, M.D.

Associate Professor of Urology, Louisiana State University Medical Center; Physician, University Hospital and Shriner's Hospital for Children, Shreveport, Louisiana
Bacterial Infections of the Urinary Tract in Females

ALEXANDER MAUSKOP, M.D.

Associate Professor of Clinical Neurology, State University of New York—Health Science Center Brooklyn; Director, New York Headache Center, New York; Attending Neurologist, Long Island College Hospital, Brooklyn, New York
Pain

JOHN H. McANULTY, M.D.

Professor of Medicine, Oregon Health Sciences University, Portland, Oregon
Tachyarrhythmias

CHARLES H. McCOLLUM, M.D.

Professor of Surgery, Baylor College of Medicine; Senior Attending, Surgical Service, The Methodist Hospital; Active Staff and Associate Attending, General and Thoracic Surgery Service, Ben Taub General Hospital, Houston, Texas
Acquired Diseases of the Aorta

JOHN D. McCONNELL, M.D.

Professor and Chairman, Department of Urology, The University of Texas Southwestern Medical Center, Dallas, Texas
Benign Prostatic Hyperplasia

EDWARD J. McGUIRE, M.D.

Professor and Director, Department of Urology, The University of Texas–Houston; Physician, Hermann Hospital and M.D. Anderson Cancer Center, Houston, Texas
Urinary Incontinence

MARILYNNE McKAY, M.D.

Professor of Dermatology and Gynecology-Obstetrics, Emory University School of Medicine; Executive Director, Continuing Medical Education and Biomedical Media, The Emory Clinic, Emory University Hospital, Atlanta, Georgia
Pruritus Ani and Vulvae

ROBIN McKENZIE, M.D.

Assistant Professor of Medicine, The Johns Hopkins University School of Medicine; Physician, Division of Chemical Dependence, Department of Medicine, The Johns Hopkins Bayview Hospital, Baltimore, Maryland
Psittacosis

ROBERT McMILLAN, M.D.

Professor, The Scripps Research Institute, La Jolla, California
Platelet-Mediated Bleeding Disorders

SHLOMO MELMED, M.D.

Professor of Medicine, Cedars-Sinai Research Institute, University of California, Los Angeles, School of Medicine; Director, Endocrinology and Metabolism, Cedars-Sinai Medical Center, Los Angeles, California
Acromegaly

NANCY PRICE MENDENHALL, M.D.

Professor and Chairman, Department of Radiation Oncology, University of Florida College of Medicine, Gainesville, Florida
Hodgkin's Disease: Radiation Therapy

DEBORAH A. METZGER, PH.D., M.D.

Associate Clinical Professor of Obstetrics and Gynecology, Yale University School of Medicine, New Haven; Director, Reproductive Medicine Institute of Connecticut, Hartford, Connecticut
Endometriosis

DON R. MILLER, M.D.

Professor of Surgery Emeritus, University of California, Irvine, College of Medicine; Physician, University of California–Irvine Medical Center, Orange, California
Pleural Effusion and Empyema Thoracis

NEIL R. MILLER, M.D.

Professor, NeuroOphthalmology, The Johns Hopkins Medical Institutions, Baltimore, Maryland
Optic Neuritis

DANIEL R. MISHELL, JR., M.D.

The Lyle G. McNeil Professor and Chairman, Department of Obstetrics/Gynecology, University of Southern California School of Medicine; Chief of Professional Services, Los Angeles County–USC Medical Center, Women's and Children's Hospital, Los Angeles, California
Menopause

HOWARD C. MOFENSON, M.D.

Professor of Pediatrics and Emergency Medicine, State University of New York at Stony Brook; Professor of Pharmacology and Toxicology, New York School of Osteopathy, Westbury; St. John's University College of Pharmacy, Jamaica; Director, Long Island Regional Poison Control Center, Winthrop-University Hospital, Mineola; Attending Senior, Nassau County Medical Center, East Meadow, New York
Acute Poisonings

MARK E. MOLITCH, M.D.

Professor of Medicine, Center for Endocrinology, Metabolism and Molecular Medicine, Northwestern University Medical School; Attending Physician, Northwestern Memorial Hospital; Consultant, Lakeside VA Medical Center, Chicago, Illinois
Hyperprolactinemia

MALCOLM MOLYNEUX, M.D.

Professor of Tropical Medicine, College of Medicine, University of Malawi, and School of Tropical Medicine, University of Liverpool, United Kingdom; Physician, Queen Elizabeth Central Hospital, Blantyre, Malawi
Malaria

PETER MORGAN-CAPNER, M.B., B.S.

Consultant Virologist, Public Health Laboratory Service, Royal Preston Hospital, Preston, United Kingdom
Rubella and Congenital Rubella

JOSEPH F. MORTOLA, M.D.

Director, Division of Reproductive Endocrinology, Cook County Hospital, Chicago, Illinois
Premenstrual Syndrome

ARNOLD M. MOSES, M.D.

Professor of Medicine, State University of New York, Health Science Center; Attending Physician, University Hospital, Syracuse, New York
Diabetes Insipidus

ROBERT R. MUDER, M.D.

Associate Professor of Medicine, University of Pittsburgh School of Medicine; Physician, Pittsburgh VA Medical Center and University of Pittsburgh Medical Center, Pittsburgh, Pennsylvania
Legionellosis (Legionnaires' Disease and Pontiac Fever)

GERALD V. NACCARELLI, M.D.

Professor of Medicine, Chief of Cardiology, and Director, Penn State Cardiovascular Center, Penn State University, College of Medicine; Physician, University Hospital and M.S. Hershey Medical Center, Hershey, Pennsylvania
Heart Block

AUAYPORN NADEMANEE, M.D.

Associate Clinical Director, Department of Hematology and Bone Marrow Transplantation, City of Hope National Medical Center, Duarte, California
Non-Hodgkin's Lymphoma

DAVID L. NAHRWOLD, M.D.

Loyal and Edith Davis Professor and Chairman, Department of Surgery, Northwestern University Medical School; Surgeon-in-Chief, Northwestern Memorial Hospital, Chicago, Illinois
Cholelithiasis and Cholecystitis

RONALD M. NELSON, M.D.

Professor of Obstetrics and Gynecology, Loma Linda University; Physician, White Memorial Medical Center, Los Angeles, California
Dysmenorrhea

DAVID H. NEUSTADT, M.D.

Clinical Professor of Medicine, University of Louisville School of Medicine; Active Medical Staff, Jewish Hospital; Consulting Medical Staff, Alliant Medical Systems, Louisville, Kentucky
Osteoarthritis

S. K. NOORDEEN, M.B., B.S., D.P.H., M.P.H.

Director, Action Programme for the Elimination of Leprosy, World Health Organization, Geneva, Switzerland
Leprosy (Hansen's Disease)

TERRENCE P. O'BRIEN, M.D.

Assistant Professor of Ophthalmology, Johns Hopkins University School of Medicine, Baltimore, Maryland
Conjunctivitis

GARY D. OVERTURF, M.D.

Professor of Pediatrics, University of New Mexico; Director, Pediatric Infectious Diseases, University of New Mexico Health Science Center, Albuquerque, New Mexico
Diphtheria

CHARLES H. PACKMAN, M.D.

Professor of Medicine, University of Rochester School of Medicine and Dentistry; Attending Physician, Strong Memorial Hospital, Rochester, New York
Autoimmune Hemolytic Anemia

JOHN E. PARKER, M.D.

Adjunct Associate Professor, Pulmonary and Critical Care Medicine, West Virginia University School of Medicine; Attending Physician, Ruby Memorial Hospital, West Virginia University Health Sciences Center, and Mountain View Rehabilitation Hospital, Morgantown, West Virginia
Silicosis

RICHARD D. PEARSON, M.D.

Professor of Medicine and Pathology, Division of Geographic and International Medicine, Departments of Medicine and Pathology, University of Virginia School of Medicine; Physician, University of Virginia Health Sciences Center, Charlottesville, Virginia
Intestinal Parasites

MARK A. PEPPERCORN, M.D.

Professor of Medicine, Harvard Medical School; Director, Center for Inflammatory Bowel Disease, Beth Israel–Deaconess Medical Center, Boston, Massachusetts
Crohn's Disease

EDITH A. PEREZ, M.D.

Associate Professor of Medicine, Mayo Medical School; Consultant, Division of Hematology and Oncology, Mayo Clinic Jacksonville, Jacksonville, Florida
Nausea and Vomiting

PAUL C. PETERS, M.D.

Ashbel-Smith Professor Emeritus, The University of Texas Southwestern Medical School; Retired Chief of Urology, Parkland Memorial Hospital, Dallas, Texas
Trauma to the Genitourinary Tract

JOSEPH G. PHANEUF, M.D.

Clinical Instructor (Dermatology), University of California, San Francisco, San Francisco; Dermatologist, Kaiser Permanente Medical Center, Hayward, California
Spider Bites and Scorpion Stings

WILLIAM R. PHIPPS, M.D.

Associate Professor of Obstetrics-Gynecology, University of Rochester School of Medicine and Dentistry; Attending Physician, Strong Memorial Hospital, Rochester, Minnesota
Dysfunctional Uterine Bleeding

CLAUS A. PIERACH, M.D.

Associate Professor of Medicine, University of Minnesota Medical School; Attending Physician, Abbott Northwestern Hospital, Minneapolis, Minnesota
The Porphyrias

PAULA PIETRUCHA-DILANCHIAN, Pharm.D.

Clinical Coordinator, National Institutional Pharmacy Services, Inc., Houston, Texas
Drugs Approved in 1996

F. XAVIER PI-SUNYER, M.D.

Professor of Medicine, Columbia University College of Physicians and Surgeons; Director, Division of Endocrinology, Diabetes and Nutrition, and Director, Obesity Research Center, St. Luke's–Roosevelt Hospital Center, New York, New York
Obesity

BRUCE POLSKY, M.D.

Associate Professor of Medicine, Cornell University Medical College; Associate Attending Physician and Director, Retrovirology Laboratory, Infectious Disease Service, Memorial Sloan-Kettering Cancer Center, New York, New York
Human Immunodeficiency Virus Infection and Its Complications

JACOB RAJFER, M.D.

Professor of Urology, University of California, Los Angeles, School of Medicine; Chief of Urology, Harbor–UCLA Medical Center, Los Angeles, California
Impotence

JAMES E. RASMUSSEN, M.D.

Professor of Dermatology and Pediatrics, University of Michigan School of Medicine; Physician, University of Michigan Medical Center and Ann Arbor Veterans Affairs Hospital, Ann Arbor, Michigan
Bacterial Infections of the Skin

JONATHAN I. RAVDIN, M.D.

Nesbitt Professor and Chair, Department of Medicine, University of Minnesota; Chief of Staff, Fairview University Medical Center, Minneapolis, Minnesota
Amebiasis

LAWRENCE D. RECHT, M.D.

Professor of Neurology and Surgery (Neurosurgery), University of Massachusetts School of Medicine and Medical Center, Worcester, Massachusetts
Brain Tumors

WILLIAM P. REED, M.D.

Professor, University of New Mexico School of Medicine; Physician, Albuquerque VA Medical Center and University of New Mexico Hospital, Albuquerque, New Mexico
Plague

JIM REICHMAN, M.D.

Chief Resident, Department of Medicine, Hadassah University Hospital Mount Scopus, Jerusalem, Israel
Acute Renal Failure

ALEXANDER A. REITER, M.D.

Clinical Assistant Professor of Obstetrics-Gynecology, Baylor College of Medicine; Physician, St. Luke's Episcopal Hospital and the Woman's Hospital of Texas, Houston, Texas
Postpartum Care

TELFER B. REYNOLDS, M.D.

Clayton G. Loosli-Hastings Foundation Professor of Medicine, University of Southern California; Physician, Los Angeles County–USC Medical Center, Los Angeles, California
Cirrhosis

LAWRENCE RICE, M.D.

Associate Professor of Medicine and Program Director of Hematology, Baylor College of Medicine; Physician, Methodist Hospital, Houston, Texas
Hemochromatosis

JAMES P. RICHARDSON, M.D., M.P.H.

Associate Professor, Departments of Family Medicine and Epidemiology and Preventive Medicine, University of Maryland School of Medicine; Attending Physician, University of Maryland Medical System, Baltimore, Maryland
Tetanus

RICHARD S. RIVLIN, M.D.

Professor of Medicine, Cornell University Medical College; Program Director, Clinical Nutrition Research Unit, GI-Nutrition Service, Memorial Sloan-Kettering Cancer Center; Chief, Nutrition Division, New York Hospital–Cornell Medical Center, New York, New York
Vitamin Deficiency

W. NEAL ROBERTS, M.D.

Charles W. Thomas Associate Professor of Medicine and Director of Rheumatology Training Program, Medical College of Virginia, Virginia Commonwealth University; Physician, Medical College of Virginia Hospital, Richmond, Virginia
Hyperuricemia and Gout

JOHN A. ROCK, M.D.

James Robert McCord Professor and Chairman, Department of Gynecology and Obstetrics, Emory University School of Medicine; Chief, Gynecology and Obstetrics, Emory University Hospital, Atlanta, Georgia
Uterine Leiomyomas

ROY S. ROGERS, III, M.D.

Professor of Dermatology, Mayo Medical School/Mayo Foundation; Attending Physician, Rochester Methodist Hospital and St. Mary's Hospital; Consultant, Mayo Clinic, Rochester, Minnesota
Diseases of the Mouth

RICARDO L. ROSSI, M.D.

Professor of Surgery, Catholic University of Chile, Santiago, Chile
Chronic Pancreatitis

ELLIOT J. ROTH, M.D.

Professor and Chairman, Department of Physical Medicine and Rehabilitation, Northwestern University Medical School; Medical Director, Rehabilitation Institute of Chicago; Chairman, Department of Rehabilitation Medicine, Northwestern Memorial Hospital, Chicago, Illinois
Rehabilitation of the Stroke Patient

HARRY LEO ROTH, M.D.

Clinical Professor of Dermatology and Director, Atopic Dermatitis Clinic, University of California, San Francisco, School of Medicine; Consultant, St. Luke's Hospital, San Francisco; Provisional Staff, Seton Hospital, Daly City, California
Atopic Dermatitis

PAUL ROUSSEAU, M.D.

Adjunct Professor, Adult Development and Aging, Arizona State University, Tempe; Physician, VA Medical Center, Phoenix, Arizona
Hiccups

FINDLAY E. RUSSELL, M.D., PH.D.

Professor of Pharmacology and Toxicology, Health Sciences University of Arizona, Tucson, Arizona; Adjunct Professor, Department of Neurology, University of Southern California School of Medicine, Los Angeles, California
Snake Venom Poisoning

WILL G. RYAN, M.D.

Professor of Medicine, Rush Medical College; Physician, Rush Presbyterian–St. Luke's Medical Center, Chicago, Illinois
Paget's Disease of Bone

BIJAN SAFAI, M.D., D.Sc.

Professor and Chairman, Department of Dermatology, New York Medical College, Valhalla; Physician, Westchester County Medical Center, Valhalla, and Our Lady of Mercy Medical Center, Bronx, New York
Cutaneous T Cell Lymphoma

MARK H. SANDERS, M.D.

Professor of Medicine and Anesthesiology, University of Pittsburgh School of Medicine; Chief, Pulmonary Sleep Disorders Program, University of Pittsburgh Medical Center; Assistant Chief, Pulmonary Service, Veterans Affairs Medical Center, Pittsburgh, Pennsylvania
Sleep Apnea and Hypopnea

ARTHUR SAWITSKY, M.D.

Professor of Medicine—Emeritus, Albert Einstein College of Medicine; Director—Emeritus, Cancer Program, Long Island Jewish Medical Center, New Hyde Park, New York
Chronic Leukemias

ANTHONY J. SCHAEFFER, M.D.

Professor and Chairman, Department of Urology, Northwestern University Medical School; Physician, Northwestern Memorial Hospital, Chicago, Illinois
Prostatitis

W. MICHAEL SCHELD, M.D.

Professor of Medicine and Associate Chair for Residency Programs, University of Virginia School of Medicine; Physician, University of Virginia Health Sciences Center, Charlottesville, Virginia
Bacterial Meningitis

ALAN R. SEAY, M.D.

Professor of Pediatrics and Neurology, University of Colorado School of Medicine; Head, Division of Child Neurology, The Children's Hospital, Denver, Colorado
Reye's Syndrome

JOSEPH W. SEGURA, M.D.

Carl Rosen Professor of Urology, Mayo Medical School; Consultant, Mayo Clinic, Rochester Methodist Hospital, and St. Mary's Hospital of Rochester, Rochester, Minnesota
Renal Calculi

LYLE L. SENSENBRENNER, M.D.

Professor of Internal Medicine and Pediatrics, University of Maryland School of Medicine; Director, Bone Marrow/Stem Cell Transplantation Program, University of Maryland Medical System, Baltimore, Maryland
Aplastic Anemia

GRAHAM R. SERJEANT, M.D.

Professor in Faculty of Medical Science and Director, MRC Laboratories, University of the West Indies; Physician, University Hospital of the West Indies, Kingston, Jamaica
Sickle Cell Disease

PREDIMAN K. SHAH, M.D.

Professor of Medicine, University of California, Los Angeles, School of Medicine; Director, Division of Cardiology, and Shapell and Webb Chair in Cardiology, UCLA Center for the Health Sciences, Los Angeles, California
Acute Evolving Myocardial Infarction

GAIL G. SHAPIRO, M.D.

Clinical Professor of Pediatrics, University of Washington School of Medicine; Physician, Children's Hospital and Northwest Hospital, Seattle, Washington
Allergic Rhinitis Caused by Inhalant Factors

OM P. SHARMA, M.D.

Professor of Medicine, University of Southern California School of Medicine; Senior Physician and Director, Sarcoidosis Clinics, USC University Hospital and Los Angeles County–USC Medical Center, Los Angeles, California
Sarcoidosis

JOHN T. SHARP, M.D.

Clinical Professor of Medicine, Emory University School of Medicine; Emeritus, Tifton Medical Clinic, Atlanta, Georgia
Rheumatoid Arthritis

BENNETT A. SHAYWITZ, M.D.

Professor of Pediatrics and Neurology, Yale University School of Medicine, New Haven, Connecticut
Attention-Deficit / Hyperactivity Disorder

ALAN H. SHIKANI, M.D.

Assistant Professor, The Johns Hopkins Medical Institutions; Chief of Otolaryngology–Head and Neck Surgery, Good Samaritan Hospital, Baltimore, Maryland
Sinusitis

BAHA M. SIBAI, M.D.

Professor, University of Tennessee School of Medicine; Chief, Division of Maternal-Fetal Medicine, Crump Women's Hospital, Memphis, Tennessee
Hypertensive Disorders of Pregnancy

DONALD H. SILBERBERG, M.D.

Professor, Department of Neurology, University of Pennsylvania School of Medicine; Physician, Hospital of the University of Pennsylvania, Philadelphia, Pennsylvania
Multiple Sclerosis

FREDRIC J. SILVERBLATT, M.D.

Professor of Medicine, Brown University; Physician, Providence Veterans Medical Center, Providence, Rhode Island
Bacterial Infections of the Urinary Tract in Males

GARY L. SIMON, M.D., PH.D.

Professor of Medicine, Biochemistry and Molecular Biology, George Washington University School of Medicine; Director, Division of Infectious Diseases, and Associate Chairman, Department of Medicine, George Washington University Hospital, Washington, DC
Food-Borne Illness

BRADLEY E. SMITH, M.D.

Professor of Anesthesiology, Vanderbilt University; Attending Anesthesiologist, Vanderbilt University Hospital, Nashville, Tennessee
Obstetric Anesthesia

EDGAR B. SMITH, M.D.

Professor and Chairman of Dermatology, University of Texas Medical Branch and University of Texas Medical Branch Hospitals, Galveston, Texas
Fungal Diseases of the Skin

WILLIAM J. SNAPE, JR., M.D.

Clinical Professor of Medicine, University of California, Irvine; Director, Motility Center, Long Beach Memorial Medical Center, Long Beach, California
Gaseousness and Indigestion

ARTHUR J. SOBER, M.D.

Professor of Dermatology, Harvard Medical School; Associate Chief of Dermatology, Massachusetts General Hospital, Boston, Massachusetts
Cutaneous Melanoma

DOUGLAS W. SODERDAHL, M.D.

Chief Resident, Department of Surgery (Urology), Madigan Army Medical Center, Tacoma, Washington
Acute Pyelonephritis

RICHARD D. SONTHEIMER, M.D.

Professor of Dermatology and Internal Medicine and Vice-Chairman, Department of Dermatology, University of Texas Southwestern School of Medicine and Medical Center; Attending Staff, Parkland Memorial Hospital and Zale Lipshy University Hospital, Dallas, Texas
Autoimmune Connective Tissue Disorders

SHELDON L. SPECTOR, M.D.

Clinical Professor of Medicine, University of California, Los Angeles, School of Medicine; Physician, UCLA Medical Center, Los Angeles, and St. John's Hospital, Santa Monica, California
Asthma in Adolescents and Adults

MICHAEL E. SPEER, M.D.

Associate Professor of Pediatrics, Baylor College of Medicine; Active Staff, Texas Children's Hospital; Senior Attending, The Methodist Hospital, Houston, Texas
Care of the High-Risk Neonate

DAVID H. SPODICK, M.D., D.Sc.

Professor of Medicine, University of Massachusetts Medical School; Director of Clinical Cardiology and Director of Cardiovascular Fellowship Training, St. Vincent Hospital, Worcester, Massachusetts
Pericarditis

JAMES C. STANLEY, M.D.

Professor of Surgery, University of Michigan Medical School; Head, Section of Vascular Surgery, University Hospital, Ann Arbor, Michigan
Peripheral Arterial Disease

MARSHALL S. STANTON, M.D.

Associate Professor of Medicine, Mayo Medical School; Physician, Division of Cardiovascular Diseases, Mayo Clinic, Rochester, Minnesota
Atrial Fibrillation

ALLEN C. STEERE, M.D.

Professor of Medicine, Tufts University School of Medicine; Chief, Rheumatology/Immunology, New England Medical Center, Boston, Massachusetts
Lyme Disease

W. P. DANIEL SU, M.D.

Professor of Dermatology, Mayo Medical School; Consultant, Department of Dermatology, Mayo Clinic and Mayo Foundation, Rochester, Minnesota
Parasitic Diseases of the Skin

CIRO V. SUMAYA, M.D., M.P.H.T.M.

Professor of Pediatrics, Division of Infectious Diseases, and Associate Medical Dean, University of Texas Health Science Center at San Antonio; Attending Physician, Medical Center Hospital and Santa Rosa Children's Hospital, San Antonio, Texas
Infectious Mononucleosis

MORTON N. SWARTZ, M.D.

Professor of Medicine, Harvard Medical School; Chief, James Jackson Firm of Medical Services, and Chief, Emeritus, Infectious Disease Unit, Massachusetts General Hospital, Boston, Massachusetts
Brain Abscess

KOUICHI R. TANAKA, M.D.

Professor of Medicine, University of California, Los Angeles, School of Medicine, Los Angeles; Chief, Division of Hematology, and Associate Chairman, Department of Medicine, Harbor–UCLA Medical Center, Torrance, California
Nonimmune Hemolytic Anemia

LEON J. THAL, M.D.

Professor of Neurosciences, University of California, San Diego, School of Medicine; Physician, UCSD Medical Center and VA Medical Center, San Diego, California
Alzheimer's Disease

BARRY R. THARP, M.D.

Professor of Pediatrics and Neurology, Baylor College of Medicine, and Director, Blue Bird Clinic for Pediatric Neurology; Physician, The Methodist Hospital and Texas Children's Hospital, Houston, Texas
Epilepsy in Infants and Children

COLIN G. THOMAS, JR., M.D.

Byah Thomason Doxey–Sanford Doxey Professor of Surgery, University of North Carolina School of Medicine; Attending Surgeon, University of North Carolina Hospitals, Chapel Hill, North Carolina
Thyroid Cancer

MARCIA G. TONNESEN, M.D.

Associate Professor of Medicine and Dermatology, State University of New York at Stony Brook School of Medicine and Hospital; Chief of Dermatology, Northport VA Medical Center, Northport, New York
Erythema Multiforme

JEFFREY A. TOWBIN, M.D.

Associate Professor, Pediatrics (Cardiology) and Molecular and Human Genetics, Baylor College of Medicine; Director, Heart Failure Clinic, and Director, Phoebe Willingham Muzzy Molecular Cardiology Laboratory, Texas Children's Hospital, Houston, Texas
Congenital Heart Disease

STEPHEN K. TYRING, M.D., PH.D.

Professor of Dermatology, Microbiology/Immunology, and Internal Medicine, University of Texas Medical Branch; Physician, University of Texas Medical Branch Hospitals, Galveston, Texas
Viral Diseases of the Skin

RODRIGO L. VALDERRAMA, M.D.

Professor of Medicine, University of Chile, Santiago, Chile
Chronic Pancreatitis

FREDERIK P. L. VAN LOON, M.D., PH.D., M.P.H., M.B.A.

Visiting Scientist, Centers for Disease Control and Prevention, Atlanta, Georgia
Cholera

ARNOLD WALD, M.D.

Professor of Medicine, University of Pittsburgh School of Medicine; Associate Chief, Division of Gastroenterology and Hepatology, University of Pittsburgh Medical Center, Presbyterian University Hospital, Pittsburgh, Pennsylvania
Constipation

ELLEN R. WALD, M.D.

Professor of Pediatrics and Otolaryngology, University of Pittsburgh School of Medicine; Chief, Division of Allergy, Immunology, and Infectious Disease, Children's Hospital of Pittsburgh, Pittsburgh, Pennsylvania
Otitis Media

B. TIMOTHY WALSH, M.D.

William and Joy Professor of Clinical Psychiatry, College of Physicians and Surgeons, Columbia University; Attending Psychiatrist, Columbia-Presbyterian Medical Center; Director, Eating Disorders Research Unit, New York State Psychiatric Institute, New York, New York
Bulimia Nervosa

THEODORE E. WARKENTIN, M.D.

Associate Professor of Pathology and Medicine, McMaster University; Hematologist, Service of Clinical Hematology, and Head, Transfusion Medicine and Hemostasis, Hamilton Health Sciences Corporation, Hamilton, Ontario, Canada
Platelet-Mediated Thrombosis: Heparin-Induced Thrombocytopenia and Thrombotic Thrombocytopenic Purpura

ROBERT W. WARREN, M.D., PH.D., M.P.H.

Associate Professor of Pediatrics, Baylor College of Medicine; Chief, Rheumatology Service, Texas Children's Hospital; Attending Physician, Ben Taub General Hospital, Houston, Texas
Juvenile Rheumatoid Arthritis

GUILLERMO S. WATKINS, M.D.

Pontificia Catholic University of Chile, Santiago, Chile
Chronic Pancreatitis

GUY F. WEBSTER, M.D., PH.D.

Associate Professor, Departments of Dermatology and Internal Medicine, Thomas Jefferson University, Philadelphia, Pennsylvania; Physician, Thomas Jefferson University Hospital Medical Center of Delaware, Wilmington, Delaware
Acne Vulgaris and Rosacea

JOHN G. WEG, M.D.

Professor of Internal Medicine, University of Michigan Medical Center; Medical Director, Critical Care Medicine Support Services, University of Michigan Medical Center; Physician, Ann Arbor Veterans Administration Medical Center, Ann Arbor, Michigan
Tuberculosis and Other Mycobacterial Diseases

LOUIS M. WEISS, M.D., M.P.H.

Associate Professor of Medicine, Division of Infectious Diseases; Associate Professor of Pathology, Division of Parasitology and Tropical Medicine, Albert Einstein College of Medicine; Physician, Jack D. Weiler Hospital of Montefiore Medical Center and Bronx Municipal Hospital, Bronx, New York
Toxoplasmosis

ROBERT C. WELLIVER, M.D.

Professor of Pediatrics, State University of New York at Buffalo; Attending Physician, Children's Hospital of Buffalo, Buffalo, New York
Viral and Mycoplasmal Pneumonias

MARTHA V. WHITE, M.D.

Director of Research, Institute for Asthma and Allergy, Washington Hospital; Director of Research, Division of Asthma and Allergy, Department of Medicine, Washington Hospital Center, Washington, D.C.
Asthma in Children

ROGER D. WHITE, M.D.

Professor of Anesthesiology, Mayo Medical School; Physician, Mayo Clinic, Rochester, Minnesota
Cardiac Arrest: Sudden Cardiac Death

H. DAVID WILSON, M.D.

Dean and Professor of Pediatrics, University of North Dakota School of Medicine and Health Sciences; Consultant Physician, Altru Health Systems and Hospital, Grand Forks, North Dakota
Mumps

SIDNEY J. WINAWER, M.D.

Professor of Medicine, Cornell University Medical College; Chief of Gastroenterology and Nutrition, Memorial Sloan-Kettering Cancer Center, New York, New York
Tumors of the Colon and Rectum

ANDREW WINOKUR, M.D., Ph.D.

Professor, Departments of Psychiatry and Pharmacology, Dartmouth Medical School, Hanover; Director of Psychopharmacology, Dartmouth-Hitchcock Medical Center, Lebanon, New Hampshire
Insomnia

JOHN E. WOLF, Jr., M.D.

Professor and Chairman, Department of Dermatology, Baylor College of Medicine; Chief of Service, Dermatology, The Methodist Hospital and Ben Taub General Hospital, Houston, Texas
Contact Dermatitis

MARTIN S. WOLFE, M.D.

Clinical Professor of Medicine, George Washington University Medical School; Clinical Professor of Medicine, Georgetown University Medical School; Attending Physician, George Washington University Hospital and Georgetown University Hospital, Washington, DC
Giardiasis

JOSEPH I. WOLFSDORF, M.B., B.Ch.

Associate Professor of Pediatrics, Harvard Medical School; Clinical Director of Endocrinology, Children's Hospital; Chief of Pediatrics, Joslin Diabetes Center, Boston, Massachusetts
Diabetes Mellitus in Children and Adolescents

STEPHEN E. WOLVERTON, M.D.

Clinical Associate Professor, Department of Dermatology, Indiana University School of Medicine; Physician, Indiana University Hospitals and Roudebush VA Medical Center, Indianapolis, Indiana
Allergic Reactions to Drugs

GAYLE E. WOODSON, M.D.

Professor of Otolaryngology, University of Tennessee, Memphis; Active Staff, University of Tennessee Bowld Hospital and Le Bonheur Children's Medical Center, Memphis, Tennessee
Hoarseness and Laryngitis

CHARLES F. WOOLEY, M.D.

Professor of Medicine, Ohio State University College of Medicine and Medical Center, Columbus, Ohio
Mitral Valve Prolapse

KIM B. YANCEY, M.D.

Senior Investigator, Dermatology Branch, National Cancer Institute, National Institutes of Health; Adjunct Associate Professor of Dermatology, Uniformed Services University of the Health Sciences, Bethesda, Maryland
Skin Diseases of Pregnancy

FRANK M. YATSU, M.D.

Professor of Neurology, University of Texas–Houston Medical School; Staff Neurologist, Hermann Hospital, Houston, Texas
Ischemic Cerebrovascular Disease

JOHN A. YEUNG-LAI-WAH, M.B., Ch.B.

Clinical Associate Professor, University of British Columbia; Director of Electrophysiology Laboratory, St. Paul's Hospital, Vancouver, British Columbia, Canada
Premature Beats

EDWARD J. YOUNG, M.D.

Professor of Medicine and Professor of Microbiology and Immunology, Baylor College of Medicine; Chief of Staff, Veterans Affairs Medical Center, Houston, Texas
Brucellosis

JESS R. YOUNG, M.D.

Acting Chairman, Department of Vascular Medicine, The Cleveland Clinic Foundation, Cleveland, Ohio
Stasis Ulcers

STUART C. YUDOFSKY, M.D.

Professor and Chairman, Department of Psychiatry and Behavioral Sciences, Baylor College of Medicine; Physician, The Methodist Hospital and Ben Taub General Hospital, Houston, Texas
Delirium

MICHAEL ZANOLLI, M.D.

Associate Professor, Department of Medicine, Division of Dermatology, Vanderbilt University School of Medicine; Physician, Vanderbilt University Medical Center and St. Thomas Hospital, Nashville, Tennessee
Papulosquamous Diseases

IRWIN ZIMENT, M.D.

Professor of Medicine, University of California, Los Angeles, School of Medicine, Los Angeles; Chief of Medicine, Olive View–UCLA Medical Center, Sylmar, California
Cough

Preface

Our golden anniversary issue: this is the 50th edition of *Current Therapy,* which was conceived by the late Howard Conn, with the first edition being published in 1949. Great pains have been taken to make this edition special. A greater effort than usual was taken to select authors who are the foremost authorities in their field to write for this edition. They were asked to be sole authors and to avoid the temptation to ask a junior faculty member to write the piece as a co-author. As a result, 288 of the 298 chapters have only one author. In addition, 180 of the 310 authors for this edition are full professors and 64 are department chairs, section chiefs, or deans.

A few examples of the outstanding authorities contributing to this edition are Michael DeBakey, Acquired Diseases of the Aorta; Telfer Reynolds (one of the distinguished emeritus professors), Cirrhosis; Sidney Winawer, Tumors of the Colon and Rectum; Tony Gotto, Hyperlipidemia; Dan Mishell, Menopause; Geoffrey Farrell (Professor of Hepatic Medicine, Sydney, Australia), Acute and Chronic Viral Hepatitis; M. Molyneux (Professor at the University of Malawi), Malaria; Norman Kaplan, Hypertension; Herbert DuPont, Acute Infectious Diarrhea; Om Sharma, Sarcoidosis; Stanley Appel, Myasthenia Gravis; Findlay Russell, Snake Venom Poisoning; Charles Wooley, Mitral Valve Prolapse; Gerald Naccarelli, Heart Block; Stuart Yudofsky, Delirium; and the list goes on and on.

Our goal is the same as that established by Howard Conn 50 years ago: to provide the practicing physician with concise, authoritative information regarding the most up-to-date treatment of problems frequently encountered in practice. Each year a new authority is selected who often approaches the problem differently from the previous year's author, giving the reader a variety of options. These are physicians who see the problem frequently and are on the leading edge of new developments, often having conducted research leading to changes in therapy.

Sixteen chapters are written by authors from other countries who have expertise in diseases seen more commonly outside the United States.

Much of the credit for the success of this book for 50 years is the consistency and dependable quality of the editorial staff at W.B. Saunders. Those currently responsible are Ray Kersey, Senior Medical Editor, and Dave Kilmer, Senior Developmental Editor. Special thanks to my editorial assistant Caroline Kosnik, who manages the flow of manuscripts and galleys, ensuring that 95% of the material in each edition is entirely new. All drug dosages are checked by Paula Pietrucha-Dilanchian, Pharm.D., to ensure accuracy and appropriateness. My appreciation also goes to the physicians committed to ongoing quality care for their patients who have supported this book for the past 50 years.

ROBERT E. RAKEL, M.D.

NOTICE

Medicine is an ever-changing field. Standard safety precautions must be followed, but as new research and clinical experience broaden our knowledge, changes in treatment and drug therapy become necessary or appropriate. Readers are advised to check the product information currently provided by the manufacturer of each drug to be administered to verify the recommended dose, the method and duration of administration, and contraindications. It is the responsibility of the treating physician relying on experience and knowledge of the patient to determine dosages and the best treatment for the patient. Neither the publisher nor the editor assumes any responsibility for any injury and/or damage to persons or property.

THE PUBLISHER

SECTION 3. THE RESPIRATORY SYSTEM

SECTION 4. THE CARDIOVASCULAR SYSTEM

SECTION 5. THE BLOOD AND SPLEEN

SECTION 6. THE DIGESTIVE SYSTEM

SECTION 7. METABOLIC DISORDERS

SECTION 8. THE ENDOCRINE SYSTEM

SECTION 9. THE UROGENITAL TRACT

SECTION 10. THE SEXUALLY TRANSMITTED DISEASES

SECTION 11. DISEASES OF ALLERGY

SECTION 12. DISEASES OF THE SKIN

SECTION 13. THE NERVOUS SYSTEM

SECTION 14. THE LOCOMOTOR SYSTEM

SECTION 15. OBSTETRICS AND GYNECOLOGY

SECTION 16. PSYCHIATRIC DISORDERS

SECTION 17. PHYSICAL AND CHEMICAL INJURIES

SECTION 18. APPENDICES AND INDEX

Symptomatic Care Pending Diagnosis

PAIN

method of
ALEXANDER MAUSKOP, M.D.
New York Headache Center
New York

PHARMACOTHERAPY

Major advances are being made in the development of new drugs for pain, and several are being approved by the Food and Drug Administration each year. Pharmacologic management remains the mainstay of treatment of many pain syndromes. The three major groups of drugs used in pain management are nonsteroidal anti-inflammatory drugs (NSAIDs), opioids, and adjuvant medications.

Nonsteroidal Anti-inflammatory Drugs

Aspirin, ibuprofen (Advil, Motrin), and ketoprofen (Orudis) are sold over-the-counter, and many patients try them before seeking medical care. It is necessary to establish that the dosage and the frequency of self-administered medication were sufficient before giving up on this group of drugs. Failure of one NSAID to relieve pain does not mean that another one will not be effective. Side effects can also be idiosyncratic. For example, naproxen (Naprosyn) and indomethacin (Indocin) can produce gastrointestinal side effects in a particular patient, whereas naproxen sodium (Anaprox) and diclofenac (Voltaren) do not.

NSAIDs can be surprisingly effective in the relief of pain from metastatic bone disease. Opioids and NSAIDs have a different mechanism of action and together can have a synergistic effect. This combination may reduce the dose requirement of an opioid with reduction in the number and severity of its side effects. Longer acting NSAIDs, such as naproxen (Naprelan), 500 mg twice daily; piroxicam (Feldene), 20 mg once a day; diflunisal (Dolobid), 500 mg twice a day; choline magnesium trisalicylate (Trilisate), 1500 mg twice a day; nabumetone (Relafen), 1000 mg once a day; and sustained-release indomethacin (Indocin SR), 75 mg once a day, are preferred in patients with continuous pain. Short-acting NSAIDs include ibuprofen (Motrin, Advil), 400 to 600 mg every 4 hours; aspirin, 650 to 1000 mg every 3 to 4 hours; and ketoprofen (Orudis), 50 mg four times a day. Ketorolac (Toradol) is the only NSAID that is available in a parenteral form. The efficacy of a 30-mg intramuscular injection is comparable to an injection of 10 mg of morphine. Ketorolac (30 mg intravenously) has replaced dihydroergotamine (D.H.E. 45) as my second-line drug after sumatriptan (Imitrex) for office management of an acute migraine attack. I sometimes inject ketorolac in the office to relieve acute low back pain or other pains.

Opioids

Important characteristics of opioid drugs and their relative potencies are shown in Table 1. Unlike NSAIDs, opioid drugs do not have a ceiling effect. This means that with the development of tolerance, the dose of an opioid can be escalated indefinitely to regain pain relief. The development of side effects usually limits such escalation, although some patients can tolerate an equivalent of up to several grams of morphine a day given parenterally. These patients remain functional because of a gradual escalation of the dose, which leads to the development of tolerance not only to pain relief but also to side effects. The development of tolerance to an opioid is usually manifested by a shorter duration of action. Because cross-tolerance between different opioids is incomplete, switching to a different opioid may forestall escalation of the dose. Combining NSAIDs and adjuvant analgesics with opioids is another useful approach. Development of tolerance and physical dependence is often mistakenly equated with addiction. In a tolerant patient receiving a high dose of an opioid drug, symptoms of withdrawal can appear within a few hours of the last dose. Addiction, on the other hand, is characterized by craving for the drug, taking the drug despite its harmful effects, and not following a physician's directions regarding use.

Both physicians and patients often have a fear of opioids because of their potential for addiction. A survey of 10,000 patients in burn units across the country looked at patients receiving large doses of opioid drugs on a daily basis for periods of up to several months. With the exception of patients with a history of addiction, not a single patient became addicted. Sometimes the use of an opioid in a cancer patient is equated with imminent death. I always

1

TABLE 1. **Dosing Data for Opioid Analgesics**

Drug	Approximate Equianalgesic Oral Dose	Approximate Equianalgesic Parenteral Dose
Opioid Agonist		
Morphine	30 mg q 3–4 h (around-the-clock dosing) 60 mg q 3–4 (single dose or intermittent dosing)	10 mg q 3–4 h
Codeine	130 mg q 3–4 h	75 mg q 3–4 h
Hydromorphone (Dilaudid)	7.5 mg q 3–4 h	1.5 mg q 3–4 h
Hydrocodone (in Lorcet, Lortab, Vicodin, others)	30 mg q 3–4	Not available
Levorphanol (Levo-Dromoran)	4 mg q 6–8 h	2 mg q 6–8 h
Meperidine (Demerol)	300 mg q 2–3 h	100 mg q 3 h
Methadone (Dolophine, others)	20 mg q 6–8 h	10 mg q 6–8 h
Oxycodone (Roxicodone, also in Percocet, Percodan, Tylox, others)	30 mg q 3–4 h	Not available
Oxymorphone (Numorphan)	Not available	1 mg q 3–4 h
Opioid Agonist-Antagonist and Partial Agonist		
Buprenorphine (Buprenex)	Not available	0.3–0.4 mg q 6–8 h
Butorphanol (Stadol)	Not available	2 mg q 3–4 h
Nalbuphine (Nubain)	Not available	10 mg q 3–4 h
Pentazocine (Talwin, others)	150 mg q 3–4 h	60 mg q 3–4 h

Adapted from Agency for Health Care Policy and Research: Acute Pain Management in Adults: Operative Procedures. Washington, DC, Public Health Service, U.S. Department of Health and Human Services, 1992. Publication 92-0032.

bring up this topic because many patients do not verbalize their fears and, if not reassured, are reluctant to take sufficient amounts, if any, of the drug. Another obstacle to the proper use of opioids is an exaggerated concern about respiratory and central nervous system (CNS) depression. Tolerance to these side effects of opioids develops quickly. Patients do not become oversedated or stop breathing while in pain. When a patient receiving a steady dose of an opioid suddenly becomes drowsy or develops respiratory depression, the most likely cause is a new systemic problem, such as an infection or liver or kidney failure. When pain can be controlled only with some degree of sedation, a stimulant, such as dextroamphetamine (Dexedrine)* given at 5 mg twice a day, may not only improve the alertness but also provide additional analgesia. Dextroamphetamine and other stimulants have mild analgesic properties synergistic with opioid analgesia.

The major side effect of opioids that must be anticipated is constipation. Senna concentrate (Senokot) is an anecdotal favorite to combat this problem. Transdermal fentanyl (Duragesic) tends to produce less constipation than do oral opioids.

Meperidine (Demerol) is a popular drug, but it is the only opioid that should not be used with frequency for more than a few days. Meperidine is metabolized into normeperidine, which is a CNS stimulant. With long-term administration, meperidine can cause irritability, tremor, and generalized seizures.

In the past, the oral route of administration of medications had been preferred. With the introduction of transdermal fentanyl (Duragesic), I have found that many patients do better with the fentanyl patch. This product provides a steady level of an opioid drug with practical and psychologic benefits. Each patch lasts for about 3 days and comes in four strengths (25, 50, 75, and 100 μg per hour). Because of the long half-life of the drug, the process of determining the optimal dose of the patch may take up to a few weeks. While this adjustment is being made, patients should be given a short-acting opioid such as oxycodone (Percocet, Percodan, Tylox, Roxicet), morphine sulfate (Roxanol, MSIR), or hydromorphone (Dilaudid) as a rescue medication for breakthrough pain. This also applies to the titration phase of other long-acting oral opioids, including sustained-release morphine (MS Contin, Oramorph SR, Kadian), sustained-release oxycodone (Oxycontin), methadone (Dolophine), and levorphanol (Levo-Dromoran). Methadone is an excellent analgesic with good absorption and, in my experience, fewer side effects than other opioids. It is also one of the most inexpensive opioids, although it can be difficult to obtain from some pharmacies.

Rectal suppositories of morphine (Roxanol, RMS), hydromorphone (Dilaudid), and oxymorphone (Numorphan) are useful for patients who cannot take oral preparations. The rectal route is not practical for long-term management and when high doses are needed.

Intranasal administration of butorphanol (Stadol NS) offers a rapid onset of action. The limitation of this drug in current formulation is that each spray contains a dose that is excessive for many patients. This results in a high frequency of CNS side effects. Reformulation at a lower dose may improve the utility of this drug. Butorphanol is a partial agonist-antagonist drug with a lower potential for addiction. It should not be given to patients who are maintained with opioids that are pure agonists (see Table 1) because the antagonist properties can induce a with-

*Not FDA approved for this indication.

drawal reaction. Patients receiving long-term opioid maintenance become quite sensitive to all opioid antagonists. Should a need arise to reverse the effect of an opioid in such a patient, naloxone (Narcan) must be diluted with saline and infused gradually.

When a patient with continuous pain cannot take oral medications, subcutaneous (SC) infusion of opioids is an alternative to the transdermal route that has many advantages over the intravenous infusion. The patch should be tried first, but when it is ineffective at a high dose (e.g., 2 patches of 100-µg Duragesic) or causes side effects, SC infusion is the method of choice. SC infusion is administered by use of a programmable, portable pump that can be filled with a solution of any opioid, including morphine, hydromorphone, methadone, and levorphanol. The pump is connected to a 25-gauge butterfly needle that can be inserted subcutaneously by the patient or a family member. An intravenous infusion of an opioid may be necessary only if a patient requires a large volume of an opioid or if other routes are not tolerated.

The use of opioid analgesics has been limited mostly to cancer patients. Their prolonged use in noncancer pain patients remains controversial. Many anecdotal reports and my experience suggest that under strict supervision, selected noncancer pain patients can derive great benefits from long-term opioid therapy. Such patients are usually those who do not develop significant tolerance and remain on a steady dose for long periods with few side effects. I obtain a verbal informed consent from such patients warning them about the risk for addiction, see them at least once a month, and try to make opioids only a part of the pain management program.

Adjuvant Analgesics

This is a diverse group of medications that were not known to have analgesic properties when they were first introduced. The most useful drugs for chronic pain and headache management are tricyclic antidepressants (TCA).*

Among the TCAs, amitriptyline (Elavil) has been studied most extensively, but nortriptyline (Pamelor), imipramine (Tofranil), and desipramine (Norpramin) are also effective and may produce fewer anticholinergic side effects. If one TCA is ineffective or produces unacceptable side effects, another TCA should be tried.

The starting dose for any TCA is 25 mg in young or middle-aged patients and 10 mg in elderly or debilitated persons. The average effective dose is 50 to 75 mg taken once a day in the evening. Some patients may require and tolerate antidepressant doses of up to 300 mg a day or more to achieve pain or headache relief. Blood levels should be monitored when the dose of a TCA exceeds 100 mg per day. Patients must be told that these medications are antidepressants but that they are also used for chronic painful conditions, even if there is no associated depression. If patients discover from other sources that they were given an antidepressant drug, they often become angry and noncompliant; they may think that their complaints were interpreted as depressive symptoms and not real pain. Warning patients about possible side effects such as dryness of the mouth, drowsiness, and constipation also improves compliance. Some of the contraindications for the use of TCAs include concomitant use of monoamine oxidase inhibitors, recent myocardial infarction, cardiac arrhythmias, glaucoma, and urinary retention. An electrocardiogram should be obtained before the initiation of treatment in all elderly patients.

Other antidepressants including selective serotonin reuptake inhibitors (SSRIs),* fluoxetine (Prozac), sertraline (Zoloft), and paroxetine (Paxil) as well as the non-SSRI antidepressants* bupropion (Wellbutrin SR) and nefazodone (Serzone) may have some utility in pain management. No large trials of these drugs have been conducted in pain patients to show any benefits beyond their antidepressant effect. I frequently start with these antidepressants before resorting to TCAs because of their favorable side effect profile. SSRIs do not cause weight gain, drowsiness, or anticholinergic side effects, all of which can occur with TCAs. Nefazodone (Serzone) and bupropion (Wellbutrin SR) do not cause sexual dysfunction, which can occur with SSRI drugs.

Anticonvulsants* that are commonly used for pain relief are carbamazepine (Tegretol-XR) and phenytoin (Dilantin). It has been suggested that anticonvulsants are more effective for sharp, lancinating pain, whereas TCAs are better for burning, dysesthetic pain. Newer anticonvulsants, lamotrigine (Lamictal) and gabapentin (Neurontin), are being studied for their potential analgesic efficacy as well.

Dextromethorphan,* which is in wide use as an antitussive agent, has been found to have analgesic properties and possibly to delay the development of opioid tolerance. This drug produces analgesia through its blocking effect on the N-methyl-D-aspartate receptor. A gradual escalation of the dose up to 60 mg four times daily or more is often necessary to achieve an analgesic effect.

Hydroxyzine (Vistaril, Atarax)* may have some mild analgesic properties, but what makes it a useful adjuvant analgesic is its reduction of anxiety and nausea.

Caffeine* has been shown to enhance the effect of other analgesics and to have mild analgesic properties of its own. It is useful in a variety of pain syndromes, but it is most commonly used for headaches. Overuse of caffeine in drinks (coffee, tea, colas) and medications (Excedrin, Anacin, Fiorinal, Esgic, Norgesic) can lead to severe withdrawal or rebound headaches and other symptoms. As little as 3 cups of coffee a day can induce a withdrawal syndrome.

Corticosteroids can be effective in relieving pain from various causes. Long-term side effects and loss

---

*Not FDA approved for this indication.

*Not FDA approved for this indication.

of efficacy limit their use to treatment of acute pain syndromes, such as spinal cord, plexus, or nerve compression or severe migraine or back pain.

Benzodiazepines usually have little utility in pain management, except for acute pain of muscle spasm, such as in acute low back or neck pain or in an anxious patient. A short course (up to a few weeks) of diazepam (Valium) or clonazepam (Klonopin) in those circumstances carries little risk for addiction and may be of significant help.

PSYCHOLOGIC METHODS

These methods are indispensable in the management of patients with chronic pain. Pain affects all aspects of chronic pain patients' lives and the lives of people who surround them. For this reason, the psychologist is a crucial member of the pain management team. Chronic pain of long duration is unlikely to respond to a single treatment modality. Patients should not be allowed to pick and choose their treatment. I explain to such patients that pain control can be achieved only by attacking the problem with several methods at the same time. Psychologic methods may include behavior modification, cognitive psychotherapy, biofeedback, and relaxation training. On occasion, in an anxious patient with acute or cancer pain, simple reassurance may reduce the need for opioid analgesics. In some patients, music therapy can have beneficial effects.

ANESTHETIC APPROACHES

Muscle spasm is a common primary cause of pain, and it often accompanies pain of other types. Trigger point injections are effective in the management of acute pain due to muscle spasm. These injections can use a 1% lidocaine solution and must be combined with active physical therapy (by active, I imply an emphasis on strengthening exercises rather than passive modalities, such as heat, ultrasound, or massage).

Nerve blocks can provide temporary relief of pain in patients with local pain. Some use it to predict possible efficacy of a nerve ablation. Instead of a local anesthetic, which tends to have a brief effect, I usually inject a corticosteroid such as betamethasone (Celestone Soluspan) or methylprednisolone (Depo-Medrol) into an area around the nerve. Although such an injection cannot be considered a nerve block, similar techniques are used for both procedures. Examples of conditions that benefit from corticosteroid injections include carpal tunnel syndrome, meralgia paresthetica, and occipital neuralgia.

Sympathetic block is the most effective procedure for the treatment of reflex sympathetic dystrophy (now called "complex regional pain syndrome"), especially when blocks are combined with vigorous physical therapy and, if necessary, pharmacotherapy and psychologic methods. This combined treatment works best if it is started early in the course of the disease.

Epidural and spinal infusions of opioids and local anesthetics are useful in some cancer patients and in a few selected patients with a "failed back syndrome."

NEUROSURGICAL METHODS

In attempting to stop transmission of pain signals along the nervous system, neurosurgeons have tried placing lesions anywhere from the peripheral nerves all the way to the frontal cortex. Nerve section can be effective in patients with meralgia paresthetica, occipital neuralgia, and some other focal neuropathic pains. It is not effective, however, in patients with postherpetic neuralgia. Some patients with trigeminal neuralgia find temporary relief when the nerve leading to the trigger area is sectioned. A dorsal root entry zone lesion can sometimes relieve pain due to brachial plexus avulsion and anesthesia dolorosa. Section of half of the spinal cord (cordotomy) is effective in patients with cancer who have unilateral pain below the waist. Bilateral cordotomy usually leads to loss of sphincter control and should be reserved for cancer patients who already lost such control. Hypophysectomy should be considered in women with hormonal cancers (breast or ovarian) whose pain is resistant to other modalities.

PHYSICAL METHODS

Physical therapy is the main treatment modality for most patients with low back and neck pain. It is also essential in the management of complex regional pain syndrome (reflex sympathetic dystrophy). Patients with almost any pain syndrome benefit from regular exercise. Improved cardiovascular and pulmonary function from aerobic exercise is of significant benefit in itself, but it also provides important psychologic benefits. Patients feel that they are regaining some control over their bodies and feel less helpless and hopeless. Regular exercise helps to alleviate stress, which is a major contributing factor in chronic headaches, back pain, and other pain syndromes.

Other physical methods include transcutaneous electrical nerve stimulation and acupuncture. Neither method has been scientifically proved to be effective; however, a large body of anecdotal evidence indicates that they can be helpful in some patients. Results of experiments detailing opioid and nonopioid mechanisms of acupuncture analgesia in animals as well as the successful use of acupuncture in veterinary medicine suggest that the effect of acupuncture is superior to that of placebo. I usually use acupuncture in the elderly or other patients who do not tolerate any medications and in patients who have tried a variety of therapies without relief. In patients with chronic pain, acupuncture should be used as a part of the multidisciplinary approach.

Chiropractic, osteopathic, and other methods of manipulation are in wide use for a variety of painful conditions. With the exception of vigorous neck manipulation, these methods are generally safe. These therapies can provide lasting relief for some acute pain syndromes, such as low back pain, especially when they are used together with active physical therapy. Prolonged use of these methods should be avoided because they divert patients from obtaining more effective treatments and because of the cost.

NAUSEA AND VOMITING

method of
EDITH A. PEREZ, M.D.
Mayo Clinic Jacksonville
Jacksonville, Florida

and

ANN E. HALLSTONE, M.D.
Lafayette, California

Nausea and vomiting are among the most common symptoms in medicine. They are associated with a wide variety of disorders, some of which are relatively trivial, others of which may be serious and debilitating. Nausea and vomiting may be evoked by disorders of the gastrointestinal tract, but they also may reflect neurologic, psychogenic, endocrine, metabolic, iatrogenic, or toxic conditions and are common manifestations of pediatric illness (Table 1). Serious consequences of nausea and vomiting include electrolyte depletion, acid-base disorders, malnutrition, Mallory-Weiss syndrome, aspiration pneumonia, and esophageal rupture (Boerhaave's syndrome). Three recognized components of vomiting are nausea, retching, and emesis. Nausea refers to the urge to vomit. Retching is the rhythmic movement of vomiting without effect. Emesis is the forceful expulsion of gastric contents from the mouth. Nausea and its physical signs of pallor, flushing, tachycardia, diaphoresis, decreased gastric and pyloric tone, and increased duodenogastric reflux are under autonomic nervous system control, whereas retching and vomiting require coordinated effort of the somatic nervous system.

Control of vomiting involves two anatomically and functionally distinct components: a vomiting center (VC) and a chemoreceptor trigger zone (CTZ). The exact location of the VC in humans has not been identified, but current evidence suggests that it lies within the lateral reticular formation adjacent to medulla oblongata areas involved in respiration, salivation, cardiovascular response, and cranial nerves VIII and X. This area is directly excited by visceral afferent nerve impulses in the gastrointestinal tract and elsewhere. The CTZ, located in the area postrema of the fourth ventricle, is responsive to blood- and cerebrospinal fluid–borne chemical agents. Although direct stimulation of the CTZ does not result in vomiting, the CTZ is responsive to chemical stimuli via the circulatory system and an emetic response requires an intact VC.

Once the VC is stimulated directly or via the CTZ, efferent pathways bring about vomiting via somatic phrenic, vagus, and spinal nerves to the respiratory and abdominal musculature and organs. Changes in stomach tone and motility during vomiting are mediated by visceral vagal efferent nerves. Somatic efferent nerves coordinate muscles of respiration responsible for retching and expulsion of gastric contents. The areas of the brain controlling nau-

TABLE 1. **Differential Diagnosis of Nausea and Vomiting**

Central Nervous System	Iatrogenic
Abscess	Chemotherapy
Epilepsy	Radiation therapy
Head injury	Surgery
Labyrinthitis	Medications (narcotics,
Malignancy	aminophylline, analgesics,
Meniere's disease	antibiotics, cardiac glycosides,
Meningitis	copper, mercury, ammonium
Migraine	chloride)
Motion sickness	
Pseudotumors	**Miscellaneous**
Vestibular disorder	Alcoholism
Endocrine	Asthma
	Graft-versus-host disease
Adrenal insufficiency	Myocardial infarction
Diabetic acidosis	
Hypercalcemia	**Pediatric**
Hyperparathyroidism	Atresia
Pregnancy	Feeding disorder
Thyrotoxicosis	Foreign body
	Gastroenteritis
Gastrointestinal	Gastroesophageal reflux
Adhesions	Hirschsprung's disease
Appendicitis	Intussusception
Biliary tract disease	Meconium-ileus
Carcinoid tumor	Meningitis
Cholecystitis	Necrotizing enterocolitis
Constipation, fecal	Pancreatitis
impaction, obstipation	Peritonitis
Food poisoning (toxins)	Pyloric stenosis
Gallstone ileus	Reye's syndrome
Gastroparesis	Subdural hematoma
Hepatitis	Tracheoesophageal fistula
Hernias	Volvulus or malrotation of gut
Infectious gastroenteritis	
(Norwalk agent, Hawaii	**Psychogenic**
agent, salmonella)	Anorexia nervosa
Inflammatory bowel	Anticipatory
disease	Anxiety
Intussusception	Bulimia nervosa
Malignancy	Cyclical vomiting
Meckel's diverticulum	Depression
Motility disorders	Eating disorders (self-induced)
Pancreatitis	
Parasitosis	
Peritonitis	
Pseudo-obstruction	
Peptic ulcer disease	
Superior mesenteric artery	
syndrome	
Visceral pain	
Zollinger-Ellison syndrome	

sea and vomiting, as well as the gastrointestinal tract, contain neurotransmitters such as serotonin, dopamine, histamine, acetylcholine, and endorphins. The evaluation of the patient with nausea and vomiting and the pharmacologic approach to treatment must take into consideration the etiology of symptoms. A thorough physical examination and medical history are essential. The history should include the character of the emesis; relation to meals; association with pain, fever, diarrhea, constipation, or vertigo; acute or chronic nature; whether there has been exposure to anyone else with a similar illness; emotional state; weight loss; history of biliary, pancreatic, or renal disease; possibility of pregnancy; surgical history; and medications. Laboratory studies should include serum electrolytes, glucose, calcium, amylase, lipase, creatinine, liver panel, and β-human chorionic gonadotropin if the patient is female and of childbearing age. Depending on the findings, radiologic imaging with chest radiographs or abdominal flat plates or brain computed tomography or magnetic resonance imaging may be helpful.

GENERAL MANAGEMENT

Supportive measures, such as correction of electrolyte or acid-base imbalance, hydration, and appropriate medications, should be offered, preferably tailored to the etiology of vomiting.

The clinical management of emesis includes pharmacologic mediation, support of the patient, and behavioral or psychologic mediation. Improved understanding of the neurochemistry of the emetic reflex has been instrumental in the development and applicability of newer antiemetic agents. Table 2 describes some commonly used antiemetic agents, their proposed mechanisms of action, appropriate doses, and types of emesis, for which they are used. Anticholinergic medications, such as scopolamine, are centrally acting and do not work on the CTZ. They are the most effective medications for motion sickness. Antihistamines, such as hydroxyzine (Atarax),* meclizine (Antivert), and diphenhydramine (Benadryl), also do not work on the CTZ but are effective in treating motion sickness and vestibular disturbances. Δ⁹-Tetracannabinate (dronabinol [Marinol]) inhibits intestinal motility and may be effective in some cases of chemotherapy-induced emesis. Prokinetic agents, such as cisapride (Propulsid)* and metoclopramide (Reglan), increase intestinal contractile force and accelerate transit, increase acetylcholine, and, in the case of metoclopramide, inhibit dopamine receptors; these agents may be useful in chemotherapy-induced emesis, as well as in intestinal pseudo-obstruction and functional or diabetic gastroparesis. Neuroleptic agents, such as chlorpromazine (Thorazine), prochlorperazine (Compazine), perphenazine (Trilafon), promethazine (Phenergan), and thiethylperazine (Torecan), inhibit the central dopamine receptors and affect the CTZ and are therefore effective in uremia, drug-induced emesis, carcinomatosis, and radiation sickness. The nausea and vomiting of pregnancy usually abate after the first trimester, although hyperemesis gravidarum may require supportive care. There are no currently approved drugs for treatment of nausea and vomiting during pregnancy.

Patients with malignancies require special consideration because their treatment as well as complications of their diseases may contribute to development of nausea and vomiting. Specifically, brain metastases, surgery, pain medications, bowel stasis, and abdominal distention, in addition to chemotherapy or radiotherapy, may all contribute to nausea and vomiting.

CHEMOTHERAPY-INDUCED EMESIS

Control of chemotherapy-induced nausea and vomiting is an important component in the overall treatment of patients with neoplastic disease.

---

*Not FDA approved for this indication.

Chemotherapy-induced emesis is a complicated multifactorial event. There are numerous neurotransmitters (histamine, acetylcholine, dopamine, serotonin) involved in the emetic reflex. Receptors for these neurotransmitters have been identified in the area postrema, in the CTZ, in other areas of the brain, and in gastrointestinal mucosa. A proposed mechanism of chemotherapy-induced emesis involves the rapid release of serotonin from enterochromaffin cells in the small intestinal mucosa. Serotonin may stimulate 5-hydroxytryptamine (5-HT₃) receptors on vagal afferent neurons in the gut and in the nucleus tractus solitarius of the VC in the brain. The VC is activated by afferent impulses from the CTZ, vestibular apparatus, midbrain, limbic system, or periphery (pharynx or gastrointestinal tract). After integration of the afferent impulses that can potentially result in vomiting, output to the nearby medullary control centers occurs, with subsequent activation of somatic and visceral efferent impulses to the effector organs.

Phases

Chemotherapy-induced emesis is generally categorized as anticipatory, acute (early and late onset), or delayed (Table 3). These categories of emesis are unique pathophysiologic events and give rise to different therapeutic problems. Failure to control acute emesis can lead to the activation of anticipatory and delayed emesis and to worsening of subsequent acute emesis.

Whereas acute phase emesis is mediated through the release of serotonin, the pathophysiology and pharmacology of delayed emesis are still unclear. Although delayed emesis is usually less severe in the frequency of emetic episodes, delayed emesis continues to result in significant morbidity.

The most important aspect of treatment in patients who are at risk for delayed emesis is clearly to achieve optimal control during the first 24 hours; poor control during the acute phase is the primary risk factor for delayed emesis.

Factors Affecting Emesis Control

Antiemetic therapy may fail in some patients due to the psychologic effects of antineoplastic therapy, previous emetic experiences, disease factors, or additional, unknown mechanisms.

Three risk factors have been identified that influence the ability of the clinician to control chemotherapy-induced emesis: patient-related characteristics, chemotherapy regimen, and antiemetic regimen. Of the various types of patients, women and children usually achieve poorer control of emesis than men and older patients on a regular basis; regular alcohol intake has been shown to decrease the risk of chemotherapy-induced emesis; and patients with poor control of emesis during previous chemotherapy are at increased risk for anticipatory and acute emesis during subsequent chemotherapy cycles. Chemotherapeutic agents are classified according to their poten-

TABLE 2. **Antiemetic Agents**

Agent	Mechanism of Action	Standard Doses and Schedule of Administration	Type of Emesis Used for
5-HT₃ Antagonists			
Ondansetron (Zofran)	5-HT₃ receptor blockade	32 mg IV × 1 *or* 0.15 mg/kg × 3 8 mg PO tid	Chemotherapy Radiation
Granisetron (Kytril)		10 µg IV *or* 1 mg PO bid	Postoperative
Substituted Benzamides			
Metoclopramide (Reglan)	Dopamine receptor blockade, 5-HT₃ receptor blockade	1–2 mg/kg IV q 2 h × 2–4 doses *or* 10 mg PO 30 min ac and hs	Chemotherapy Gastroparesis Gastroesophageal reflux
Phenothiazines			
Prochlorperazine (Compazine)	Dopamine receptor blockade	2.5–10 mg PO IM *or* IV q 3–4 h *or* 25 mg bid rectally	Carcinomatosis Uremia Radiation
Perphenazine (Trilafon) Promethazine (Phenergan) Thiethylperazine (Torecan) Chlorpromazine (Thorazine)		8–24 mg PO daily 12.5–25 mg PO *or* IM q 4–6 h 10 mg PO, IM, *or* rectally bid *or* tid 50–100 mg q 6–8 h	Drug induced Postoperative
Corticosteroids			
Dexamethasone*	Unclear	10–20 mg IV × 1 dose	Chemotherapy
Benzodiazepines			
Lorazepam (Ativan)*	Anxiolytic amnesic	0.5–1 mg IV q 4 h *or* 30 min before chemotherapy	Chemotherapy
Butyrophenones			
Haloperidol (Haldol)*	Dopamine receptor blockade	1–3 mg IV *or* 5 mg PO q 2–6 h	Chemotherapy
Droperidol (Inapsine)		0.5–2 mg IV q 4 h *or* 1–2 mg PO *or* IM q 8 h	
Cannabinoids			
Dronabinol (Marinol) Nabilone†	Central psychotropic action	5–10 mg PO q 3–4 h 2 mg PO q 6–12 h	Chemotherapy
Anticholinergics			
Scopolamine (Transderm Scōp)	Cholinergic blockade	1 patch behind ear 4 h before travel	Motion sickness Postoperative
Antihistamines			
Diphenhydramine (Benadryl) Hydroxyzine (Atarax)* Meclizine (Antivert)	H₁ receptor antagonism	50 mg PO q 4–6 h 25–100 mg PO *or* IM q 6–8 h 20–50 mg PO 1 h before travel	Motion sickness
Prokinetic Agents			
Cisapride (Propulsid)*	Increase postganglionic acetylcholine release	10 mg PO 30 min ac and hs	Gastroparesis

*Not FDA approved for this indication.
†Not yet approved for use in the United States.
Abbreviation: 5-HT₃ = 5-hydroxytryptamine.

TABLE 3. **Phases of Chemotherapy-Induced Emesis**

Type of Emesis	Time of Occurrence	Mechanism	Best Therapy
Anticipatory	Prechemotherapy	Learned response	Benzodiazepines
Acute—early onset	1–6 h after chemotherapy	Rapid release of serotonin	5-HT₃ receptor antagonism plus dexamethasone
Acute—late onset	7–24 h after chemotherapy	Gradual release of serotonin	Unknown, probably 5-HT₃ receptor antagonism plus dexamethasone
Delayed	16 h–6 d after chemotherapy	Undefined	Prevention of acute and late-onset acute emesis

tial to induce emesis (Table 4). In general, the potential for acute nausea and vomiting increases as doses of chemotherapy are increased. In addition, combination chemotherapy treatments are more likely to cause nausea and vomiting than are single drugs.

Management of Chemotherapy-Induced Emesis

In view of the undesirable consequences of poor antiemetic management, choosing an effective antiemetic agent and determining the optimal dosing regimen are critical. Antiemetic regimens should be tailored to the specific population of patients and emetogenicity of the chemotherapy to be administered (Table 5).

Antiemetic prophylaxis with intravenous 5-HT$_3$ receptor antagonists during chemotherapy has now become well established. The discovery and clinical application of the 5-HT$_3$ receptor antagonists have transformed the treatment of emesis induced by anticancer therapies and as a result have dramatically improved the quality of life of a significant proportion of those patients. The currently available 5-HT$_3$ receptor antagonists, granisetron (Kytril) and ondansetron (Zofran), have been shown to be as effective as or more effective than other antiemetic regimens in preventing chemotherapy-induced nausea and vomiting; they also have an improved therapeutic ratio. Another 5-HT$_3$ receptor antagonist (dolasetron [Anzemet-HMR]) will soon become available in the United States. Comparative clinical trials of granisetron and ondansetron given intravenously demonstrated similar efficacy and safety in patients receiving cisplatin- or cyclophosphamide-containing regimens. Owing to the relatively high cost of 5-HT$_3$

receptor antagonists, appropriate dosing and schedules have been investigated. The Food and Drug Administration–approved doses for intravenous ondansetron are 32 mg × 1 or 0.15 mg/kg every 4 hours × 3 for cisplatin (Platinol) and 32 mg intravenously × 1 for moderately emetogenic regimens, but doses lower than 32 mg in the last-named subgroup have been utilized (in combination with dexamethasone) with good efficacy. The Food and Drug Administration–approved dose of intravenous granisetron is 10 μg/kg × 1, on the day of either cisplatin or moderately emetogenic chemotherapy; doses less than 10 μg/kg intravenously are not recommended.

Although chemotherapy-induced emesis can be effectively controlled with intravenous antiemetic agents, oral therapy may be more convenient and acceptable to patients. An effective oral 5-HT$_3$ receptor antagonist would allow administration in ambulatory and outpatient settings, which is particularly important for patients in whom the onset of emesis may be delayed, such as women with breast cancer receiving treatment with cyclophosphamide. Outpatient administration would also reduce the requirement for medical resources, and the convenience of the dose form would benefit both patients and staff, translating into a reduction in the overall cost of chemotherapy and associated treatments. The oral antiemetics approved by regulatory agencies for chemotherapy-induced emesis include 3-day ondansetron (at a dose of 8 mg three times daily) treatment for patients receiving moderately emetogenic chemotherapy and granisetron (at a dose of 1 mg twice daily) on the day of either moderately or highly emetogenic chemotherapy. Studies have also demonstrated that a single daily dose of 2 mg of oral granisetron is as effective as the divided dose given on the day of chemotherapy. Of note is that oral granisetron

TABLE 4. **Emetogenicity of Commonly Used Chemotherapeutic Agents**

Low (<30%)	Moderate (30–60%)	Moderately High (60–90%)	High (>90%)
Bleomycin	Altretamine	Actinomycin D	Cisplatin
Busulfan	Asparaginase	Carmustine ≥100 mg/m²	Cytarabine >500 mg/m²
Chlorambucil	Azacitidine	Cyclophosphamide ≥600 mg/m²	Dacarbazine
Cladribine	Carboplatin	Dactinomycin >50 mg/m²	Ifosfamide >1.5 gm/m²
Corticosteroids	Carmustine <100 mg/m²	Doxorubicin >50 mg/m²	Mechlorethamine
Cytarabine ≤500 mg/m²	Cyclophosphamide <600 mg/m²	Lomustine	Streptozocin
Docetaxel	Daunorubicin <50 mg/m²	Methotrexate >200 mg/m²	
Etoposide	Doxorubicin ≤50 mg/m²	Procarbazine	
Fludarabine	Fluorouracil	Semustine	
Gemcitabine	Idarubicin		
Hydroxyurea	Ifosfamide ≤1.5 gm/m²		
Melphalan	Methotrexate >500 mg/m²		
Mercaptopurine	Mitomycin C		
Methotrexate	Mitoxantrone		
Paclitaxel			
Pentostatin			
Plicamycin			
Thioguanine			
Thiotepa			
Topotecan			
Vinblastine			
Vincristine			
Vinorelbine			

Table 5. **Guidelines for Selecting Antiemetic Treatment Before Chemotherapy**

1. Determine the relative emetogenic potential of the antineoplastic drugs (high, moderate, low). For moderate to highly emetogenic chemotherapy, a combination regimen of a 5-HT$_3$ receptor antagonist and a corticosteroid is generally effective in controlling emesis; for low-emetogenic chemotherapy, either corticosteroids or phenothiazines such as prochlorperazine therapy are recommended.
2. Determine ease of administration (duration of intravenous injection, oral versus intravenous availability and efficacy). The ease and convenience of using the particular antiemetic are important selection considerations, allowing patients to continue their normal daily activities and thus maintain their quality of life.
3. Efficacy, duration of action, and absolute and relative cost should also be considered.
4. Understanding of potential adverse reactions. It is sometimes difficult to evaluate the safety profile of an antiemetic in cancer patients, because cancer patients are generally polysymptomatic. The adverse events may be a result of the cancer rather than the treatment. Of importance to cancer patients, the 5-HT$_3$ receptor antagonists are not associated with the dystonia and akathisia observed with use of dopaminergic antagonists such as metoclopramide. The most common side effects observed with the 5-HT$_3$ antagonists are mild constipation, headache, asthenias, or diarrhea.
5. The 5-HT$_3$ receptor antagonists have clearly altered the choices available to oncologists, due to their excellent safety profile, flexibility, and efficacy. In an effort to reduce the cost of a particular antiemetic regimen, antiemetic agents should be used only for proven indications. Physicians need to identify and target those patients for whom clinical benefits of receiving 5-HT$_3$ antagonists are legitimate and explain the additional expenses arising from 5-HT$_3$ antagonist therapy. The significant health gain and low incremental cost incurred by 5-HT$_3$ receptor antagonist therapy clearly indicate its use for acute phase emesis in patients receiving moderately high to highly emetogenic chemotherapy. The physiologic basis for the use of serotonin antagonists in the prevention of acute phase emesis appears confirmed, but their role in delayed emesis is not clear.

is the only oral 5-HT$_3$ receptor antagonist approved for emetic prophylaxis in patients receiving cisplatin-based chemotherapy. The oral form of ondansetron is used for prophylaxis only in patients receiving moderately emetogenic chemotherapy. Double-blind randomized studies have shown that a 2-mg oral dose of granisetron is equivalent to 32 mg of intravenous ondansetron in patients receiving either cisplatin or moderately emetogenic chemotherapy.

Corticosteroids have not been approved by regulatory agencies for use as antiemetic agents; however, their efficacy (primarily that of dexamethasone*), has been extensively documented. Although effective as a single agent, dexamethasone, 10 to 20 mg intravenously, has been shown to increase the efficacy of conventional antiemetics, such as metoclopramide, and the 5-HT$_3$ receptor antagonists ondansetron and granisetron.

The mechanisms by which dexamethasone inhibits chemotherapy-induced emesis are not clearly understood, although several have been proposed. These include reduction of prostanoid turnover by inhibi-

tion of arachidonic acid release, modulation of substances derived from arachidonic acid metabolism (e.g., lipoxygenase products), reduction of the amount of available serotonin by activation of tryptophan pyrrolase (shunting metabolism away from serotonergic synthetic pathways), and modulation of vagal depolarization. Further studies to elucidate the pathophysiologic mechanisms of dexamethasone are warranted.

Compared with the excellent control of acute nausea and vomiting achieved in most patients receiving chemotherapy ($\geq 60\%$), the treatment of delayed emesis remains a significant problem. Delayed emesis may occur in 30 to 70% of patients receiving cisplatin-based chemotherapy. Recommended treatments include prochlorperazine plus dexamethasone or metoclopramide plus dexamethasone; the role of 5-HT$_3$ receptor antagonists in the management of delayed emesis has not been established.

Radiotherapy and High-Dose Chemotherapy–Induced Emesis

Serotonin is released from the gastrointestinal tract in response to various insults, including radiation therapy to the abdomen. The onset, incidence, and severity of radiation-induced emesis vary with the dose per fraction, field size, and site irradiated. Many studies have shown that 5-HT$_3$ receptor antagonists are active in preventing radiotherapy-induced emesis. However, their superiority over conventional antiemetics has not been proved, as the comparators have never reached an accepted standard, such as has been reached in chemotherapy-induced nausea and vomiting. In view of this problem and the cost of these agents, combined with the lack of adequate data on their superiority over conventional agents, it is not yet possible to recommend first-line use of 5-HT$_3$ receptor antagonists for the prevention of emesis in patients receiving radiation therapy.

Treatment with high-dose alkylating agents requiring stem cell rescue by peripheral blood stem cell transplants or bone marrow transplantation administered for 3 to 5 consecutive days and the use of total body irradiation lead to marked nausea and vomiting. Vomiting in this setting has been particularly difficult to manage, due to both the simultaneous use of potent emetogenic chemotherapeutic agents and the high radiation dose (8 to 11 Gy). The antiemetic failure rate in this group is greater than 50% in the first week of treatment; the use of oral granisetron plus dexamethasone appears to be as effective as the intravenous use of 5-HT$_3$ receptor antagonists in this setting.

*Not FDA approved for this indication.

GASEOUSNESS AND INDIGESTION

method of
WILLIAM J. SNAPE, JR., M.D.

*University of California, Irvine and Long Beach
Memorial Hospital
Long Beach, California*

GASEOUSNESS

A patient's complaint of gaseousness can reflect one or all of the following symptoms: increased belching, abdominal bloating, or increased flatus. The physician must determine whether these symptoms result from a pathologic alteration or are an excessive sensitivity to normal bowel function.

Belching is almost always caused by aerophagia, just as in the childhood prank. The aerophagia is often unrealized by the patient. It is a nervous habit that occurs during periods of stress or is associated with increased anxiety. The belching can often be eliminated by educating the patient about aerophagia, so that he or she can recognize and stop the behavior. Patients should also be advised to stop drinking carbonated beverages and not to drink with a straw. Some patients need further assistance with managing their anxiety. Tranquilizers or limited psychotherapy may help reduce symptomatic belching in these patients.

It is common for a patient with reflux esophagitis to also complain of excessive belching. These patients swallow multiple times during the day to expel acid from the esophagus with peristalsis or to neutralize the esophagus with the more alkaline saliva. Treatment in these patients involves decreasing acid production with H_2 antagonists or proton pump inhibitors.

Increased production of gas is a rare cause of belching. Patients with bacterial overgrowth in a large duodenal diverticulum can produce an increased amount of gas that may reflux into the stomach for eructation. Reflux of alkaline pancreatic secretions into an acidified stomach can release increased carbon dioxide and cause belching.

In some patients, a feeling of abdominal fullness is caused by ascites or an intra-abdominal mass. Impaired gastric emptying may also present as abdominal fullness. The increased gastric residual can be caused by either a blockage of the gastric outlet or poor or uncoordinated gastroduodenal contractions. These conditions must be identified and then treated accordingly. The delayed gastric emptying often responds to prokinetic therapy. Cisapride is most often used (Table 1). Several studies support the use of erythromycin, which stimulates the stomach through the motilin receptor.

Abdominal fullness or bloating is a common symptom in functional bowel disease, either nonulcer dyspepsia or irritable bowel syndrome. Studies showed that psychologic stimuli increase the visceral sensation of gas when the bowel is distended. Because several studies demonstrated no increased intra-abdominal gas, the increased sensation of fullness may be due to increased sensitivity in the visceral afferent nerves or in alterations in the tone of bowel wall. Standard therapy for functional bowel disease involves antispasmodic drugs. Prokinetic drugs may benefit some patients if hypomotility or uncoordinated motility is the underlying cause of the bowel dysfunction. Increased sensitivity of the visceral nervous system may cause the feeling of abdominal fullness. The tricyclic antidepressants, in low doses, decrease the sensitivity of the visceral nerves and often provide relief (Table 2).

Increased intestinal gas production can cause symptomatic bloating in many patients. The most common dietary cause of bloating is lactose intolerance. Milk products that have intact lactose cause symptoms through bacterial digestion of the sugar to volatile fatty acids and hydrogen. Hard cheeses and yogurt may not cause symptoms because of enzymatic or bacterial destruction of the lactose that occurs during production of the food. The symptoms are often relieved by decreasing, not eliminating, the intake of milk products, because the enzyme lactase may only be reduced. Taking lactase supplements (LactAid) before milk products are eaten or using lactose-free milk products can eliminate symptoms.

Flatus, in contrast to belching, is generally due to increased production of gas. Bacterial breakdown of undigested carbohydrate is the source of hydrogen, carbon dioxide, and methane production. Gas-producing foods (e.g., bran products, beans, onions, broccoli) should be reduced in the diet, or patients should pretreat themselves with α-D-galactosidase (Beano). A restriction diet is often needed to identify the major contributor to the gas. One study identified white bread as a cause of the flatus.

Gaseousness is generally a benign symptom. However, if the patient has alarm symptoms such as weight loss, fever, or blood in the stool, further evaluation is necessary to identify anatomic causes, such

TABLE 1. **Prokinetic Drugs**

Agent	Dosage
Cisapride (Propulsid)	10–20 mg bid to qid
Metoclopramide (Reglan)	10 mg bid to qid
Domperidone (Motilium)*	10–20 mg tid
Erythromycin†	250 mg tid
Bethanechol (Urecholine)†	10 mg tid

* Investigational drug in the United States.
† Not FDA approved for this indication.

TABLE 2. **Antinociceptive Drugs**

Agent	Dosage
Amitriptyline (Elavil)*	20–100 mg/24 h
Imipramine (Tofranil)*	20–100 mg/24 h
Doxepin (Sinequan)*	20–100 mg/24 h
Desipramine (Norpramin)*	20–100 mg/24 h

* Not FDA approved for this indication.

as neoplasia. The majority of patients can be treated with dietary manipulation or drugs.

INDIGESTION

Indigestion is a general term for a gastrointestinal upset consisting of upper abdominal pain, bloating, nausea, and occasionally vomiting. The pain is generally burning, but it can be cramping. It is no surprise that such nonspecific symptoms suggest a multiplicity of disease states. Most often, indigestion is transient and of little significance. Dyspepsia has been separated into three varieties: (1) esophagitis type, (2) peptic ulcer type, and (3) dysmotility type.

Those patients with symptoms similar to reflux disease rarely need endoscopy because their symptoms respond quickly to therapy. If endoscopy is performed, the mucosa usually appears normal. The patients can be treated with acid reduction by H_2 antagonists or prokinetic drugs. These patients rarely need proton pump inhibitors.

The patients with symptoms suggesting peptic ulcer disease often show improvement after acid reduction therapy. Many of these patients have infection of the gastric mucosa with *Helicobacter pylori*. Recent advances allow identification of this bacterium by use of serologic as well as breath tests. If no duodenal ulcer is found, the significance of *H. pylori* is uncertain. The recommendation of a National Advisory Panel is not to treat *H. pylori* infection unless a duodenal ulcer is identified. However, some patients' symptoms do improve with eradication of the organism.

Chronic indigestion is commonly seen in nonulcer dyspepsia. A variety of motility disorders have been identified in these patients. It is unclear which aspect of the abnormal motility is most responsible for symptoms. Patients with a delay in gastric emptying measured by a radionuclide scan often have postprandial antral hypomotility and respond to a prokinetic drug. Patients with normal or rapid gastric emptying may have uncoordinated contractions and may respond to antispasmodic drugs. Visceral hypersensitivity in these patients can be treated with low-dose tricyclic antidepressants.

There is no specific therapy for indigestion; this symptom complex encompasses a large number of disorders. The preceding suggestions are a guide to the empirical treatment of the patient's symptoms.

HICCUPS

method of
PAUL ROUSSEAU, M.D.
Carl T. Hayden VA Medical Center
Phoenix, Arizona
Arizona State University
Tempe, Arizona

Hiccups are ubiquitous annoyances that affect nearly everyone but serve no known physiologic function. The origin of the word hiccup is unknown, but it is thought to be an onomatopoetic derivation of the sound resulting from the act of hiccuping. The proper medical vernacular for hiccups is singultus, thought to be derived from the Latin *singult,* which means a sob, speech broken by sobs, or the act of catching one's breath while sobbing. Although frequently benign and of limited duration, hiccups can be debilitating when they become prolonged, particularly in chronically ill and frail patients.

Terminology defining the duration and severity of hiccups has been confusing, but three categories have been suggested: (1) hiccup bouts, episodes comprising several hiccups and persisting as long as 48 hours; (2) persistent hiccups, episodes lasting longer than 48 hours but less than 1 month; and (3) intractable hiccups, episodes lasting longer than a month. Interestingly, hiccups tend to occur in quantities of less than 7 or more than 63, with an average frequency of 4 to 60 per minute. Moreover, the frequency of hiccups can be increased with a fall in arterial P_{CO_2} and decreased with a rise in P_{CO_2}. Although a distinct male or female predominance is lacking, persistent and intractable hiccups occur more frequently in men. In addition, a circadian variation is discernible, with hiccups occurring more frequently during evening hours.

ANATOMIC CHARACTERISTICS

The anatomic mechanism precipitating hiccups remains unknown, although various reflexes have been described in the literature. In 1833, an English physician recognized the relationship between phrenic nerve irritation and hiccups, but it was not until 1943 that the existence of a hiccup reflex arc was suggested. Since then, a hiccup reflex pathway has been characterized, although confirmation remains elusive. The afferent portion of the reflex arc comprises the phrenic and vagus nerves and the sympathetic chain arising from thoracic segments T-6 to T-12. The primary efferent reflex branch is the phrenic nerve, although the glottis and accessory muscles of respiration nerves have also been implicated as efferents. The central connection between the afferent and efferent limbs of the reflex pathways has been attributed to a nonspecific anatomic location in the spinal cord between segments C-3 and C-5. More recently, it has been proposed that the central connection for hiccups involves an intricate association between the brain stem and midbrain areas, including the respiratory center, phrenic nerve nuclei, medullary reticular formation, and hypothalamus. This further confounds the anatomic specificity and supports the postulate that the phrenic nerve is not the sole efferent limb.

PATHOPHYSIOLOGY

The pathophysiology of hiccups is emerging as more is learned about this enigmatic malady. Several classification strategies have been proposed to categorize the numerous causes of hiccups; however, it is best to consider separately the sources of (1) benign and self-limited hiccup bouts and (2) persistent and intractable cases.

Benign Hiccup Bouts

Benign, self-limited hiccup bouts are often caused by gastric distention that arises from numerous causes, including aerophagia, excessive food and alcohol ingestion, and gastric insufflation secondary to endoscopy. Other causes include sudden changes in ambient or gastrointestinal temperatures (e.g., moving from a hot or cold area to one of contrasting temperature, drinking hot or cold beverages), sudden excitement or emotional stress, and tobacco use.

Persistent and Intractable Hiccups

The etiology of persistent and intractable hiccups encompasses more than 100 causes and can be broadly classified into three categories: organic, psychogenic, and idiopathic. To preclude misdiagnosis, hiccups should be classified as psychogenic or idiopathic only after an organic cause has been discounted.

Persistent and in particular intractable hiccups are not without significant adverse effects, especially in debilitated elders. Side effects include fatigue, exhaustion, insomnia, malnutrition and weight loss, dehydration, cardiac dysrhythmias, reflux esophagitis, aspiration pneumonia, and death.

EVALUATION OF PERSISTENT AND INTRACTABLE HICCUPS

A focused history and physical examination, coupled with select laboratory studies, assist in guiding therapeutic intervention of persistent and intractable hiccups. The history should ascertain the severity, duration, and characteristics of the hiccup episode as well as the use of tobacco, alcohol, and medication. Physical assessment should focus on the head and neck and the cardiopulmonary, abdominal, and neurologic systems. Suggested laboratory studies include a complete blood count and renal and electrolyte measurements. Clinical findings may dictate other studies, including liver function tests, serum calcium determination, toxicology screen, arterial blood gas analysis, electrocardiogram, lumbar puncture, chest radiography, computed tomography of the head and chest, and magnetic resonance imaging. Other more invasive studies that may be clinically indicated include endoscopy, esophageal manometry, and bronchoscopy.

TREATMENT

The numerous therapeutic approaches to hiccups are largely anecdotal, which emphasizes the ineffectiveness of any one intervention. As noted by the revered physician Mayo in 1932, "the amount of knowledge on any subject such as this can be considered as being in inverse proportion to the number of different treatments suggested and tried for it."

If a cause for hiccups is established, treatment should be directed at the underlying malady. However, if the cause is unknown, treatment is often empirical and involves nonpharmacologic and pharmacologic modalities.

Nonpharmacologic Treatment

Nonpharmacologic therapies are based on antediluvian and dubious remedies but nevertheless are occasionally effective (Table 1). Several treatments entail stimulation of the nasopharynx, which ostensibly interrupts the vagal afferent limb of the hiccup reflex arc. Methods that disrupt phrenic nerve transmission may also abort an episode of hiccups, as may interruption of normal respiratory function. Counter-

TABLE 1. Nonpharmacologic Treatment of Hiccups

Stimulation of the Nasopharynx

Forcible traction of the tongue
Lifting the uvula with a spoon
Cotton-tipped swab or catheter stimulation
Gargling with water
Sipping ice water
Sucking on hard candy
Swallowing granulated sugar
Swallowing hard bread
Drinking water from the far side of a glass
Biting on a lemon
Inhaling noxious irritants

Counterirritation of the Vagus Nerve

Carotid massage
Supraorbital pressure
Irritating tympanic membrane
Valsalva's maneuver
Digital rectal massage

Phrenic Nerve Disruption

Vapocoolant sprays
Ice packs
Electrical stimulation
Alcohol or bupivacaine injection
Phrenic nerve crushing, avulsing, or transection

Counterirritation of the Diaphragm

Pulling knees to chest
Leaning forward to compress chest
Applying pressure at points of diaphragmatic insertion

Interruption of Respiratory Function

Sneezing or coughing
Valsalva's maneuver
Hyperventilation
Use of continuous positive airway pressure
Breath holding
Gasping induced by noxious odors or fright
Rebreathing into a paper bag

Relief of Gastric Distention

Induced vomiting
Nasogastric aspiration
Gastric lavage
Reduction of rate of flow of tube feeding

Miscellaneous

Hypnosis
Behavior modification
Diaphragmatic pacing electrodes
Acupuncture
Prayer

irritation of the diaphragm has also been advocated to alleviate hiccups, as have several other miscellaneous nonpharmacologic approaches.

Pharmacologic Treatment

The success of various pharmacologic agents, similar to that of nonpharmacologic treatments, is largely anecdotal. Although numerous medications have been suggested, three categories of drugs are described: antipsychotics, anticonvulsants, and miscellaneous agents (Table 2).

Antipsychotics

Chlorpromazine (Thorazine) is the most widely used antipsychotic for the treatment of hiccups, al-

TABLE 2. **Pharmacologic Treatment of Hiccups***

Antipsychotics

Chlorpromazine 25–50 mg IV q 6 h prn; if effective, may change
  to oral formulation at same dose
Haloperidol 2–5 mg IM 1 time, then 1–4 mg PO 3 times/d

Anticonvulsants

Phenytoin 200 mg IV 1 time, then 300 mg/d PO with dose
  titrated to clinical effectiveness and blood levels
Carbamazepine 200 mg PO 4 times/d
Valproic acid 15 mg/kg/d PO with increases of 250 mg/d every 2
  wk as needed

Miscellaneous Agents

Metoclopramide 5–10 mg PO, IM, or IV 4 times/d
Baclofen 5–10 mg 3 or 4 times/d†
Amitriptyline 10–25 mg 1 to 3 times/d
Nifedipine 10 mg 3 times/d

*Most common medications with suggested initial dosages.
†Should not be discontinued abruptly.

though its success rate has varied from 0 to 80%.
Chlorpromazine is reportedly more effective when
it is administered intravenously, although postural
hypotension can be severe. Haloperidol (Haldol),* a
butyrophenone, is also efficacious in terminating hiccups, particularly in patients unable to tolerate
chlorpromazine.

Anticonvulsants

Several anticonvulsants have been used to treat
hiccups, including phenytoin (Dilantin),* carbamazepine (Tegretol),* and valproic acid (Depakene).*
Phenytoin is the preferred agent and is reportedly
efficacious for hiccups with a central nervous system
etiology. Carbamazepine has terminated hiccups in
patients with multiple sclerosis; valproic acid has
controlled hiccups for up to 1 year in cases of diverse
etiology.

The benzodiazepines have not been successful in
treating hiccups and in fact may encourage or worsen
episodes of hiccups.

Miscellaneous Agents

Metoclopramide (Reglan)* has been successful in
abating hiccups of diverse causes, particularly when
they are secondary to gastroparesis. Baclofen (Lioresal)* is also efficacious and is considered the pharmacologic agent of choice by many clinicians. Amitriptyline (Elavil)* has reportedly relieved hiccups,
although side effects limit its use in the elderly. Several other medications have also been recommended,
but most lack evidence of efficacy. Such agents include orphenadrine (Norflex),* ondansetron (Zofran),* methylphenidate (Ritalin),* ketamine (Ketalar),* amantadine (Symmetrel),* chloral hydrate
(numerous trade names),* nifedipine (Procardia),*
pentazocine (Talwin),* and morphine (Roxanol).*

*Not FDA approved for this indication.

ACUTE INFECTIOUS DIARRHEA
method of
ELIZABETH T. DOUGLASS, M.D.
*University of Texas Medical School at Houston
Houston, Texas*

and

HERBERT L. DuPONT, M.D.
*Baylor College of Medicine and University of Texas
  Medical School at Houston
Houston, Texas*

Diarrheal illness is one of the most common disorders
seen in clinical medicine. Enteric infection is frequently
self-limited, but appropriate specific therapy can shorten
the duration of illness in some cases and can be lifesaving
in some instances.

In developing countries, infectious diarrhea causes more
than 4 million deaths each year in children 5 years old
and younger. It is also the major cause of protein-calorie
malnutrition in the world. In the United States, children
suffer an average of two episodes of diarrhea per year, and
500 deaths per year are attributed to infectious diarrhea.
When fatality results from diarrhea in the United States,
it is primarily seen in the elderly. In the United States,
acute infectious diarrhea leads to 250,000 hospital admissions, 8 million visits to physicians resulting in multiple
days away from work, and an expense of approximately
$23 billion per year.

Diarrhea is a term that is difficult to define because the
pattern of bowel habits for each individual is different.
Therefore, diarrhea always implies a change in bowel habits. Mild diarrhea can be defined as the passage of one or
two unformed stools per day; moderate and severe, as
passing three to five and more than six unformed stools
during a 24-hour period, respectively.

ETIOLOGY

The causes of acute infectious diarrhea are numerous.
Bacterial, viral, and protozoan agents vary according to
the setting in which the diarrhea occurs.

Bacteria

Geographic location and season of the year play an important role in bacterial causes. In industrialized nations,
bacteria are responsible for approximately 30% of cases of
diarrhea. In developing tropical and subtropical nations,
approximately 50% of the cases are caused by bacterial
pathogens. Invasive bacteria such as *Shigella, Salmonella,*
and *Campylobacter jejuni* cause approximately 15% of diarrhea cases. *Vibrio cholerae* causes profuse watery and life-
threatening diarrhea in countries where the organism is
endemic. Enterohemorrhagic *Escherichia coli* O157:H7
causes outbreaks of bloody diarrhea that have been associated with the consumption of hamburgers and less commonly other food items. Enteropathogenic *E. coli* strains
have been implicated in outbreaks of diarrhea in newborn
nurseries on a worldwide basis. Other bacterial causes of
diarrhea include the noncholera vibrios, *Aeromonas* species, and *Plesiomonas shigelloides.*

Viruses

Viruses are responsible for most of the diarrheal illnesses in infants younger than 1 year. Rotavirus, which is

responsible for 1 million cases of fatal illness worldwide per year, may be the most important viral cause. It causes both vomiting and diarrhea, which lead to profound dehydration and mortality. Other viruses are enteric adenovirus, small round viral particles (i.e., Norwalk and Norwalk-like viruses), and caliciviruses. Norwalk virus is a major cause of food-borne and water-borne disease that affects primarily infants and children in developing nations and individuals of all ages in the United States.

Parasites

The three major parasites are *Giardia lamblia, Entamoeba histolytica,* and *Cryptosporidium parvum.*

G. lamblia causes diarrhea with the initial infection; after that, symptomatic infection is rare, especially in areas of high endemnicity. There is an increased frequency of *G. lamblia* infection in children attending day care centers. Persons during their initial exposure to *G. lamblia* and patients with IgA deficiency may experience a protracted clinical course.

E. histolytica causes diarrhea in tropical developing countries, affecting mostly patients of a low socioeconomic status. It is an important cause of hepatic abscess.

C. parvum, an important water-borne pathogen that is present in untreated and processed water throughout the world, has caused large water-borne outbreaks in the United States. There is a higher frequency of *C. parvum* infection in children attending day care centers. *C. parvum* usually causes a self-limited illness; however, in patients with acquired immune deficiency syndrome (AIDS), it may cause a chronic debilitating infection.

Outbreaks of *Cyclospora cayetanensis* have been reported during the summer months in the United States and Canada. *C. cayetanensis* causes explosive diarrhea lasting approximately 1 week and has been associated with the consumption of raspberries imported from Central America.

Other parasites that can lead to diarrhea are *Strongyloides stercoralis, Blastocystis hominis,* and *Dientamoeba fragilis.* In AIDS patients, in addition to *C. parvum,* microsporidians and *Isospora belli* can lead to protracted diarrhea.

DIAGNOSIS

In evaluating a patient with acute diarrhea, the history and the laboratory findings are the most essential features. Questions related to the individual's epidemiologic factors and clinical features may uncover the cause of the illness.

Epidemiologic Factors

Travel. Travel in general is associated with diarrhea. Patients traveling to an area of low risk have a 2 to 4% chance of developing diarrhea, presumably from the change in eating habits, stress, and increased alcohol consumption. In travel to an area of moderate risk, such as the northern Mediterranean, China, and countries of the former Soviet Union, the risk increases to about 10%. Individuals traveling to Latin America, South Asia, and Africa have as high as a 40% risk of developing traveler's diarrhea. The season of the year and geographic area play an important role in the cause and frequency of traveler's diarrhea. In high-risk areas, the diarrhea is mostly caused by bacterial pathogens. Our studies in Mexico among U.S. travelers have found an average frequency of occurrence for enteropathogens as follows: enterotoxigenic *E. coli,*

40%; *Shigella,* 10%; *Aeromonas* or *Plesiomonas,* 10%; *Salmonella,* 4%; *Campylobacter,* 3%; viruses, 10%; parasites, 2%; and in 20%, no pathogen was detected.

Antibiotic Treatment. Prior administration of antimicrobials up to 2 months before the development of diarrhea raises the possibility of pseudomembranous colitis, which is caused by overgrowth of cytotoxigenic *Clostridium difficile.* Previous treatment with clindamycin (Cleocin) is associated with an increased risk, as is colonization with *C. difficile.*

Homosexual Men. Homosexual men have a higher frequency of fecal-oral contamination and a higher occurrence of proctitis as a result of receptive anal intercourse. The pathogens implicated in proctitis are *Neisseria gonorrhoeae, Chlamydia trachomatis,* herpes simplex virus, and *Treponema pallidum.*

AIDS. Patients with AIDS have a higher frequency of gastrointestinal infection. Important bacterial pathogens are *Shigella, Salmonella,* and mycobacteria (especially *Mycobacterium avium* complex). Parasites such as *C. parvum, G. lamblia, I. belli,* microsporidians, and *Cyclospora* can lead to protracted diarrhea. Finally, patients with AIDS may have diarrhea caused by viral pathogens such as cytomegalovirus, herpes simplex virus, or the human immunodeficiency virus itself.

Case Clusters. Multiple individuals becoming ill during a similar time raises the possibility of a food-borne outbreak. When the incubation period is less than 4 hours, food intoxication is suspected; the common agents are *Staphylococcus aureus* and *Bacillus cereus.* If the incubation is greater than 8 hours, an enteric infection secondary to *Clostridium perfringens, Shigella, Salmonella,* or other pathogens is implicated.

Clinical Features

Dehydration, fever, vomiting, dysentery (bloody, mucoid stools), and duration and severity of illness are important clinical features that aid in the diagnosis of diarrhea.

Laboratory Evaluation

Mild cases of diarrhea are generally self-limited and do not merit further laboratory evaluation. In general, one should evaluate moderate to severe cases of diarrhea.

Fecal Leukocytes. This important test is performed by staining a strand of mucus or fresh stool with dilute methylene blue and examining under oil for the presence of leukocytes, which imply diffuse colonic inflammation. Fecal leukocytes are present in enteric infection caused by *Shigella, Salmonella, C. jejuni, Aeromonas, Yersinia enterocolitica, Vibrio parahaemolyticus,* and *C. difficile,* and in inflammatory bowel disease.

Stool Culture. The five indications to perform a stool culture are (1) severe diarrhea causing disability, (2) fever (temperature ≥102°F), (3) persistent diarrhea (≥2 weeks), (4) hamburger-associated diarrhea when *E. coli* O157:H7 is suspected, and (5) presence of fecal leukocytes.

Parasitic Examination. The five indications to perform parasitic examinations of the stool are (1) persistent diarrhea (≥2 weeks), (2) diarrhea in homosexual men, (3) diarrhea in areas endemic for *G. lamblia* (Russia and mountainous areas of North America), (4) regular exposure to day care centers, and (5) diarrhea in patients with AIDS.

Special Tests. Enzyme-linked immunosorbent assays for *C. difficile* toxin are available but occasionally have a false-negative result and should be followed up with a cytotoxic tissue culture assay if suspicion is high. Nylon string attached to a gelatin capsule (Entero-Test) is used to sample bowel mucus when *G. lamblia* or *Strongyloides* infection is suspected. Rotavirus antigen detection kits are available and useful to rapidly detect infection primarily in infants.

Flexible Sigmoidoscopy. In homosexual men, this tool is useful to differentiate proctitis (involvement confined to the distal 15 cm of colon), proctocolitis (involvement beyond 15 cm), and enteritis (no colitis) and to obtain adequate samples for diagnosis.

MANAGEMENT

Fluid Replacement

The most important part of the evaluation of an individual with acute infectious diarrhea is to accurately assess the volume status. Fluid replacement is essential for infants with rotavirus illness and any patient with cholera or cholera-like illness. The optimal electrolyte composition of oral rehydration solution contains 90 mmol per liter of sodium; it is recommended in dehydrating forms of diarrhea in developing countries and should be alternated with water or other low-sodium liquids. In industrialized nations where cholera is rare, the recommended solutions contain 30 to 60 mmol per liter of sodium.

Many children in developing countries become rapidly undernourished during the diarrheal illness. They may benefit from a cereal-based oral rehydration solution that can be made in nearly all regions

and is associated with both increased calorie intake and decrease in frequency of stooling.

Diet Alteration

The intestinal tract is unable to process complex carbohydrates during acute enteric infection, and therefore simple starches are recommended (rice, potato, and wheat). Breast-feeding should continue for infants, but other dairy products should be discontinued. In adults, the form of the stool dictates the recommended diet. When the stool is watery, soups, yogurt, vegetables, fresh fruit, and soft drinks are recommended. When they begin to show form, rice, baked potatoes, and broiled fish or chicken can be added. Once stools are normal, the diet may return to normal.

Nonspecific Therapy

The majority of cases of diarrhea can be managed without prescribing antimicrobial treatment. The three main categories of drugs that have been shown to improve the clinical course of diarrhea are (1) adsorbent drugs, (2) antisecretory agents, and (3) antimotility drugs. The classic adsorbent drug (Table 1) is a combination of kaolin and pectin. This combination drug and the more active drug attapulgite (Donnagel, Kaopectate) lead to an improvement in stool form and minimal shortening of the diarrheal episode.

TABLE 1. **Nonspecific Therapy for Acute Diarrhea**

Agent	Setting	Adults	Children
Attapulgite (Donnagel, Kaopectate)	When safety is paramount	1.2 gm (2 tbsp) initially, repeated after each unformed stool Maximal allowed dose, 8.4 gm (14 tbsp)	3–6 y: 300 mg (½ tbsp) repeated after unformed stools; maximum, 2.1 gm (3.5 tbsp) 6–12 y: 600 mg (1 tbsp) repeated after unformed stools; maximum, 4.2 gm (7 tbsp)
Loperamide (Imodium)	Most cases of diarrhea Effective in combination with antimicrobials for traveler's diarrhea Contraindicated when fever and dysentery are present	4 mg initially, repeated after unformed stool Not to exceed 8 mg/d (over-the-counter) or 16 mg/d (prescription), no longer than 48 h	>2 y, 11–21 kg: 1 tsp repeated after unformed stools; maximum, 3 tsp/d 22–26 kg: 2 tsp (1 caplet) followed by 1 tsp (½ caplet) after unformed stool; maximum, 4 tsp (2 caplets)/d 27–43 kg: 2 tsp (1 caplet) followed by 1 tsp (½ caplet) after each unformed stool; maximum, 6 tsp (3 caplets)/d
Diphenoxylate HCl with atropine (Lomotil)	Same indication as for loperamide Less expensive	5 mg qid prn Duration not to exceed 48 h	>2 y, 11–14 kg: 1.5–3.0 mL 12–16 kg: 2.0–3.0 mL 14–20 kg: 2.5–4.5 mL 17–32 kg: 2.5–5.0 mL 23–55 kg: 3.5–5.0 mL Doses qid prn; maximal duration, 48 h
Bismuth subsalicylate (Pepto-Bismol)	May be single therapy for many cases of acute diarrhea	30 mL (2 caplets) every 30 min not to exceed 8 doses/d May repeat on day 2	3–6 y: 5 mL (⅓ caplet) 6–9 y: 10 mL (⅔ caplet) 9–12 y: 15 mL (1 caplet) May repeat q 30 min; maximum, 8 doses/d

Bismuth subsalicylate (Pepto-Bismol) is an antisecretory compound whose salicylate portion blocks the effect of enterotoxins on the intestinal mucosa. It reduces the number of stools and duration of illness by 50% and has an antimicrobial effect, which explains the value of the drug when it is used to prevent traveler's diarrhea. Zaldaride,* an intestinal calmodulin inhibitor, has been shown to decrease the severity and duration of traveler's diarrhea.

The most important antimotility drug is loperamide (Imodium), which improves diarrhea by facilitating intestinal fluid absorption. It also has mild antisecretory effects by inhibiting calmodulin. It has been shown to be more effective than bismuth subsalicylate, and it reduced the number of stools and duration of illness by 80% compared with placebo. Another antimotility drug is diphenoxylate hydrochloride with atropine (Lomotil); however, because of the atropine, it can have unpleasant anticholinergic effects. Both antimotility drugs can worsen the clinical course of infection by an invasive bacterial pathogen and therefore should not be used in patients with fever and dysentery.

Antimicrobial Agents

Empirical Treatment

Most patients do not require treatment with antimicrobial drugs.

Antimicrobial treatment is indicated when fever and dysentery are present where *Shigella* and *C. jejuni* are the major etiologic agents. In these cases, a fluoroquinolone is advised for adults and trimethoprim-sulfamethoxazole (TMP-SMZ, Bactrim, Septra), for children.

Antibiotics are recommended in the therapy for traveler's diarrhea. In tropical and subtropical areas during the summer months, enterotoxigenic *E. coli* is the most common etiologic agent; in many areas, such as the interior of Mexico, TMP-SMZ can be used effectively in this setting. In the cooler months, in other dryer areas, and in most areas of the developing tropical and semitropical areas, trimethoprim-resistant bacterial pathogens including *Campylobacter* may be encountered; therefore, fluoroquinolones are advised for adults and TMP-SMZ plus erythromycin for children.

Bacterial Infection

Table 2 outlines the recommended antimicrobial agents, dosage, and duration of therapy for different bacterial pathogens.

Cholera should be treated with antimicrobials as well as aggressive rehydration. The recommended antimicrobials are tetracycline or fluoroquinolones for adults and furazolidone (Furoxone) for children.

Shigellosis should be treated under all circumstances. It can develop into a public health problem because only a few organisms are necessary to cause infection among contacts. The treatment of choice in the United States is TMP-SMZ for both children and adults.

The decision to treat *Salmonella* infection is more difficult. In immunocompetent patients with no fever, antimicrobial treatment is generally not recommended because it has been shown to prolong excretion of the organism. In the case of febrile disease, blood cultures should be performed because of the likelihood of bacteremia, and therapy should be initiated with a fluoroquinolone for adults and TMP-SMZ for children. If *Salmonella typhi* or *Salmonella paratyphi* is isolated, treatment should continue for 10 to 14 days. Patients with immunosuppression and infants younger than 3 months should be treated to prevent systemic complications.

Antimicrobial treatment is recommended for antibiotic-associated colitis secondary to *C. difficile* infection. The most effective treatment is oral vancomycin (Vancocin); however, oral metronidazole is also effective and is the treatment of choice, particularly in less severe cases because of the significantly lower cost and lower frequency of inducing vancomycin-resistant enterococci. Treatment usually lasts 10 days, but relapses are common (10 to 20%) and should be treated with 2 weeks of therapy followed by cholestyramine, which binds the toxin for 3 to 4 weeks. Patients with profound ileus, recent surgery, or other contraindication to oral therapy may be treated with intravenous metronidazole. Enteric precautions and discontinuation of the implicated antibiotic are also recommended.

Enteropathogenic *E. coli* and HEp-2 cell–adherent *E. coli* have been noted to have an increased in vitro resistance pattern to multiple antibiotics. Therefore, susceptibility testing is recommended when these pathogens are involved.

Parasitic Infection

Table 3 outlines the recommended drugs and duration of therapy for different parasites.

G. lamblia infection is at times treated empirically when diarrhea is persistent and no bacterial pathogen has been isolated. The recommended empirical treatment is metronidazole (Flagyl). When *G. lamblia* is confirmed, the treatment of choice is metronidazole for adults and furazolidone for infants unable to take solid medication.

Patients with symptomatic disease from *E. histolytica* should be treated with metronidazole for 5 days and iodoquinol (Yodoxin) for 20 days to prevent relapsing disease. Patients with asymptomatic infection should be treated with iodoquinol or diloxanide furoate (available from the Centers for Disease Control and Prevention) to prevent later enteric infection or liver abscess formation.

Infection with *C. parvum* is generally self-limited and does not require treatment. However, in AIDS patients, paromomycin (Humatin) has been shown to decrease the amount of stools per day, but relapses are common.

I. belli infections in AIDS patients should be

---

*Not available in the United States.

TABLE 2. **Antibacterial Therapy for Diarrhea**

Diagnosis	Recommendations for Adults	Recommendations for Children
Empirical Therapy		
Traveler's diarrhea		
Interior Mexico (summertime)	TMP-SMZ (Bactrim DS, Septra DS): TMP 160 mg, SMZ 800 mg bid for 3 d	TMP 10 mg/kg/d, SMZ 50 mg/kg/d in 2 divided doses for 3 d
Other times and places	Norfloxacin (Noroxin)† 400 mg bid, ciprofloxacin (Cipro) 500 mg bid, ofloxacin (Floxin)† 300 mg bid, or fleroxacin* 400 mg qd for 3 d	TMP-SMZ (same as above) plus eythromycin (see dose below) or furazolidone 7.5 mg/kg/d in 4 divided doses for 5 d
Febrile dysenteric illness	Ciprofloxacin 500 mg bid, fleroxacin* 400 mg qd, norfloxacin† 400 mg bid, or ofloxacin† 300 mg bid for 3 d	TMP-SMZ (same as above) plus erythromycin (see below) or furazolidone (same as above)
Persistent diarrhea (14 d or more)	Metronidazole (Flagyl) 250 mg qid for 7–10 d	Metronidazole 20 mg/kg/d in 4 divided doses for 7–10 d
Organism-Specific Therapy		
Cholera	Tetracycline 250 mg qid for 2 d	Furazolidone 7.5 mg/kg/d in 4 divided doses for 3 d

Campylobacteriosis	Erythromycin 250 mg qid for 5 d	Erythromycin
		  <12 kg: 250 mg/d
		  11–18 kg: 375 mg/d
		  18.5–25 kg: 500 mg/d
		  25.5–36 kg: 750 mg/d
		  >36 kg, 1 gm divided in 4 doses for 5 d

Shigellosis	TMP 160 mg, SMZ 800 mg bid for 3 d	TMP-SMZ (same as above) for 3–5 d
Salmonellosis without systemic toxic effects	No antimicrobial treatment	No antimicrobial treatment
Salmonellosis with systemic toxic effects	Ciprofloxacin 500 mg bid, fleroxacin* 400 mg qd, norfloxacin 400 mg bid, or ofloxacin 300 mg bid for 5–7 d	TMP-SMZ (same as above) for 5–7 d
Enteropathogenic *Escherichia coli*	Susceptibility testing necessary	
Yersiniosis	TMP 160 mg, SMZ 800 mg bid for 5–7 d	TMP-SMZ (same as above) for 5–7 d
Aeromonas or *Plesiomonas* diarrhea	TMP 160 mg, SMZ 800 mg bid for 3 d	TMP-SMZ (same as above) for 3–5 d
Clostridium difficile colitis	Metronidazole 250 mg qid or vancomycin 125 mg PO qid for 10 d	Doses not established

* Not available in the United States.
† Not FDA approved for this indication.
Abbreviation: TMP-SMZ = trimethoprim-sulfamethoxazole.

TABLE 3. **Antiparasitic Therapy**

Etiologic Agent	Recommendations for Adults	Recommendations for Children
Entamoeba histolytica asymptomatic excretion	Iodoquinol (Yodoxin) 650 mg tid for 20 d or paromomycin (Humatin) 500 mg tid for 7 d	Iodoquinol 40 mg/kg/d in 3 divided doses for 20 d
Entamoeba histolytica diarrhea	Metronidazole 750 mg tid for 5 d plus iodoquinol 650 mg tid for 20 d	Metronidazole 50 mg/kg/d in 3 divided doses for 10 d plus iodoquinol
Giardia lamblia diarrhea	Metronidazole 250 mg tid for 7 d; where available, tinidazole* 1.5–2.0 gm as a single dose	Metronidazole (same as above) for 5 d or furazolidone 5 mg/kg/d in 4 doses for 7 d
Cryptosporidiosis	No drug recommended, but in severe cases consider paromomycin 500 mg qid for 5–7 d, in AIDS for at least 2 wk	
Isosporiasis in HIV-positive patients	TMP-SMZ†: 160 mg, SMZ 800 mg qid for 10 d then qd 3 times/wk	
Cyclospora diarrhea	TMP 160 mg, SMZ 800 mg bid for 3–7 d	TMP 5 mg/kg, SMZ 25 mg/kg bid for 3–7 d
Microsporidiosis (*Encephalitozoon intestinalis*)	Albendazole† 400 mg bid for 2 wk may be helpful	

* Not available in the United States.
† Not FDA approved for this indication.
Abbreviations: AIDS = acquired immune deficiency syndrome; HIV = human immunodeficiency virus; TMP-SMZ = trimethoprim-sulfamethoxazole.

treated with TMP-SMZ for 10 days and then three times per week for prophylaxis or suppression.

C. cayetanensis infections can be treated with TMP-SMZ for 3 to 7 days.

Microsporidiosis caused by *Encephalitozoon intestinalis* has been shown to benefit from therapy with albendazole* and should be treated for at least 2 weeks.

---

*Not FDA approved for this indication.

CONSTIPATION

method of
ARNOLD WALD, M.D.
University of Pittsburgh Medical Center
Pittsburgh, Pennsylvania

CLINICAL CONSIDERATIONS

Constipation is a symptom rather than a disease and therefore represents a subjective interpretation of a real or imaginary disturbance of bowel function. Although it has been defined as a frequency of defecation of twice weekly or less on the basis of large population surveys in Western countries, frequency alone is not a sufficient criterion. Many constipated patients complain of excessive straining or discomfort at defecation, with or without small or hard stools, although frequency of defecation is within the normal range. For clinical purposes, the physician must use a combination of subjective and objective criteria in assessing such complaints. These include a frequency of defecation less than three times weekly, alone or in conjunction with other subjective complaints, especially if there has also been a distinct change in regular bowel habits. Understanding what the patient's perceptions are and attempting to correct misconceptions are a critical aspect of the initial evaluation.

PATHOPHYSIOLOGY

Constipation may be conceptually regarded as disordered movement through the colon and/or anorectum because, with few exceptions, transit through the proximal gastrointestinal tract is normal. Slowing of colonic transit occurs as a primary motor disorder in association with many diseases, or as a side effect of many drugs (Table 1). Diseases associated with constipation include neurologic, metabolic, and endocrine disorders and obstructing lesions of the gastrointestinal tract. Other abnormalities lead to impairment of defecation, such as congenital aganglionosis (Hirschsprung's disease) and acquired functional outlet disorder (pelvic floor dyssynergia). Finally, colonic transit is normal in many patients who complain of constipation, and various factors influence colorectal function or an individual's perception that constipation exists. These include dietary fiber, calorie and fluid intake, physical activity, level of education, psychologic makeup, and emotional factors. These should be considered when a patient is initially evaluated for chronic constipation or a recent alteration in bowel habits.

INITIAL EVALUATION

The initial evaluation incorporates a careful history with particular attention to identifying potential risk factors.

TABLE 1. Drugs Associated with Constipation

Analgesics
Anticholinergics
Anticonvulsants
Antidepressants and psychotherapeutic drugs
Antihypertensives
Antiparkinsonian drugs
Calcium channel blockers
Diuretics
Opiates
Cation-containing agents
    Aluminum (antacids, sucralfate)
    Bismuth
    Calcium (antacids, supplements)
    Iron supplements
    Metallic intoxicants (arsenic, lead, mercury)

This includes defining the nature and duration of the complaint and determining whether such complaints arise from misconceptions of the patient about normal bowel habits. If not associated with a readily definable cause of constipation (e.g., medications), a recent and persistent change in bowel habits should prompt an evaluation to exclude structural bowel changes or organic diseases. This is especially important in older adults who complain of excessive straining or a sense of incomplete evacuation or who also exhibit anemia or occult gastrointestinal bleeding. Only after such diseases have been excluded should a diagnosis of functional constipation be considered.

Flexible sigmoidoscopy and colonoscopy are superior techniques for identifying lesions that narrow or occlude the bowel. They also detect melanosis coli, a brown-black discoloration of the bowel mucosa associated with chronic use of anthraquinone laxatives.

Barium radiographs complement sigmoidoscopy in detecting organic causes and are also useful for diagnosing megacolon and megarectum. Barium radiographs show the aganglionic distal bowel with proximal dilatation of the colon in classic Hirschsprung's disease and should be obtained in children or young adults if this disorder is suspected. In such patients, bowel cleansing should not be ordered so that the characteristic changes are accentuated, and the insertion catheter should be removed to identify a short aganglionic segment. However, barium enema provides limited information about colonic transit and motor function in most patients with chronic constipation. Plain films of the abdomen can detect significant stool retention in the colon, suggest the diagnosis of megacolon, and be used to monitor bowel cleansing in patients with fecal retention.

Rectal biopsies are useful in patients with suspected Hirschsprung's disease. Suction biopsies should be obtained from the nondilated rectum at least 3 cm above the internal anal sphincter for appropriate testing.

INITIAL MANAGEMENT

The initial management of functional chronic constipation includes education of the patient, behavior modification, dietary changes, and judicious use of laxatives or enemas.

Education of the patient may include reassurance and an explanation of normal bowel habits. Efforts are made to have the patient reduce excessive use of laxatives and cathartics, increase fluid and fiber intake, exercise moderately, and use postprandial increases in colonic motility after being instructed to defecate after meals, particularly in the morning when colonic motor activity is highest. Dietary fiber and bulk laxatives such as psyllium or methylcellulose together with adequate fluids are the safest and most physiologic approach in most patients with constipation. In general, the use of stimulant laxatives should be restricted to those who do not respond to initial measures.

Dietary fiber is that portion of plant food that escapes digestion and is composed of both insoluble and soluble components. Cereal fibers generally possess cell walls that resist digestion and retain water within their cellular structures, whereas fiber found in citrus fruits and legumes stimulates the growth of colonic flora, which increases fecal mass. Wheat bran is one of the most effective fiber laxatives, and there is a clear dose-response effect for fiber with respect to fecal output. Particle size appears to be crucially important, and the large particle size of cereal products appears to enhance fecal bulking effects.

Patients with poor dietary habits may add raw bran (2 to 6 tablespoons with each meal) followed by a glass of water or another beverage. A significant laxative effect may not be observed for 3 to 5 days, and up to several weeks may be required to relieve chronic constipation. Raw vegetables and fruits contain soluble fiber and are often not adequate substitutes for raw bran. Patients should be warned that consuming large amounts of bran can cause abdominal bloating or flatulence. This effect can be modulated by starting with small amounts and slowly increasing to tolerance and efficacy.

Psyllium (Metamucil), calcium polycarbophil (FiberCon), and methylcellulose (Citrucel) are more refined and concentrated than bran, but they are also considerably more expensive. These agents should be well diluted to ensure adequate mixing with food and are generally consumed before meals or at bedtime. They increase the water content and bulk volume of the stool to decrease colonic transit time. There is some evidence that mechanical stimulation of nerves in the bowel wall also contributes to the action of dietary fiber and bulk-forming agents.

Sorbitol and lactulose (Chronulac, Cephulac) are often useful in patients with chronic constipation who do not tolerate or respond to dietary fiber or bulk-forming agents. These poorly absorbed sugars are hydrolyzed, in part, to lactic, acetic, and formic acids by coliform bacteria. Accumulation of fluid in the colon is stimulated by the osmotic effect of these acid metabolites, which usually produces soft, formed stools. In one well-controlled study in elderly patients with chronic constipation, sorbitol 70% administered at bedtime was as effective as lactulose and was well tolerated. Thus, sorbitol can be used as a low-cost alternative to lactulose. Patients should also be advised that these agents can cause abdominal bloating and flatulence.

Docusates (Colace, Surfak) soften the feces by reducing surface tension, thus permitting penetration of the fecal mass by intestinal fluids. However, the efficacy of docusates is highly questionable, and they are of marginal use for chronic constipation.

Mineral oil softens stool because of its emollient action and is particularly effective in enemas to soften fecal impactions. However, aspiration resulting in lipoid pneumonia is a recognized hazard of oral mineral oil, especially in elderly patients and in those with impaired swallowing, and anal seepage may also occur. It is an unattractive agent in view of the availability of effective bulk and osmotic laxatives.

When patients fail to respond to initial measures, stimulant laxatives may be considered for relatively short periods (weeks to months). These agents include cascara, senna, bisacodyl, phenolphthalein, and castor oil. Although the precise mechanism of action of each drug is not established, all produce a net accumulation of fluid and electrolytes in the lumen.

As stimulant laxatives are often abused, some clinicians recommend that they should be taken for no longer than 1 week, but this seems unduly restrictive. The continuous use of stimulant laxatives may produce diarrhea that is severe enough to cause hyponatremia, hypokalemia, dehydration, hyperaldosteronism, protein-losing gastroenteropathy, and steatorrhea. Subtle mucosal and myenteric nerve alterations have been seen with long-term use of stimulant laxatives, as have changes in the radiologic appearance of the colon, known as the "cathartic colon."

The anthraquinone-containing laxatives (i.e., senna, cascara sagrada) are widely used and abused. Their onset of activity is within 6 to 12 hours. Cascara (Nature's Remedy) has the mildest action and produces a soft or formed stool with little or no colic. Senna (Senokot) may be particularly helpful in patients with severe constipation and is apparently safe even in large doses. When combined with psyllium or other bulk-forming agents, smaller amounts of senna may be employed. Aloe-containing preparations (Nature's Remedy) are the most potent of the anthraquinone-containing laxatives and are best avoided because they almost always produce colic. Although most anthraquinone-containing laxatives discolor the colonic mucosa (melanosis coli), this effect is presumed to be innocuous and is reversible.

Bisacodyl (Dulcolax) and phenolphthalein (Ex-Lax, Feen-A-Mint) both stimulate peristalsis and alter active electrolyte transport to affect fluid movement. Bisacodyl produces a soft to formed stool, usually with little or no colic, whereas phenolphthalein is more likely to produce a semifluid stool. Because of phenolphthalein's enterohepatic circulation, its duration of action may be prolonged (3 to 4 days) in sensitive patients.

Patients who do not respond to oral laxatives can self-administer tap-water enemas every 3 to 4 days. The addition of other substances to an enema solution is of uncertain therapeutic value. However, the small-volume prepackaged sodium phosphate-biphosphate enema kits (Fleet Enema) are convenient and safe to administer.

Isotonic sodium chloride enema (1 level teaspoonful per pint of water) should be used cautiously in patients with sodium and fluid retention. Some enema solutions irritate the mucosa and can simulate early changes of ulcerative proctosigmoiditis. Hot water, peroxide, household detergents, and strong hypertonic salt solutions are most irritating and should not be used.

Weakness, shock, convulsions, and/or coma may result from water intoxication and dilutional hyponatremia in children and elderly patients and in patients with megacolon who are given a tap-water enema. Severe hypokalemia may also follow the use of a tap-water enema, especially in patients also receiving diuretics. Convulsions with hypocalcemia and hyperphosphatemia have occurred in children or adults with renal dysfunction who absorbed large amounts of the phosphate present in sodium phosphate-biphosphate enemas.

THERAPY FOR SEVERE CONSTIPATION

Ideally, therapy for patients with severe chronic constipation should be based on the nature of the complaint and presumed pathophysiologic mechanisms. More rational choices and consistent therapeutic outcomes require further understanding of both the psychologic and physiologic characteristics of this diverse group of patients.

Behavioral Approaches

Habit training has been successfully employed in children with severe constipation. The goal of such an approach is to achieve regular evacuation to prevent build-up of stool. A modified program may also be effective in many adults with neurogenic constipation, patients with dementia, and those with physical impairments.

Initially, patients should be disimpacted and the colon evacuated effectively. This can be accomplished with twice-daily enemas for up to 3 days. An alternative approach is to have the patient drink 4 liters (occasionally more) of a balanced electrolyte solution containing polyethylene glycol (Colyte, GoLYTELY) until cleansing is complete.

After bowel cleansing, sorbitol or lactulose is given to produce one stool per day or every other day. The patient is instructed to use the bathroom after eating breakfast to take advantage of meal-stimulated increases in colonic motility (the gastrocolonic response). An enema is administered if there is no defecation after 2 days, to prevent recurrence of fecal impaction. Once defecation occurs regularly for several months, gradual weaning from laxatives may be attempted. Positive reinforcement is given for successful toileting, and punishment for failure is prohibited. Office visits should be maintained regularly.

Such behavioral approaches have achieved success rates of up to 78% in children with idiopathic constipation, although relapses are not uncommon. Treatment failures have been attributed to behavioral disturbances and noncompliance of the patient and family, but underlying disturbances of bowel function may also play a role in some children.

A modified program may be used in demented or bedridden patients of all ages with fecal impaction. Initially, mineral oil enemas (Fleet Mineral Oil Enema) may be used to soften hard impactions and permit rectal evacuation. After disimpaction, bowel cleansing with enemas or polyethylene glycol–containing solutions should be performed. In demented patients or those with neurogenic bowel disorders, a fiber-restricted diet together with cleansing enemas once or twice per week assists nursing management by decreasing build-up of stool and recurrence of fecal impaction.

Another behavioral approach is biofeedback to correct inappropriate contraction of the pelvic floor muscles and external anal sphincter during defecation in patients with pelvic floor dyssynergia. Various techniques have been used to record defecation dynamics, including anal plugs and anorectal manometers that monitor external anal sphincter pressures during attempted expulsion of the apparatus. The patient watches the recordings of electromyographic activity or sphincter pressure responses and is asked to modify inappropriate responses through trial-and-error efforts. Clinical improvement has been reported in both children and adults who have received biofeedback for pelvic floor dyssynergia.

Pharmacologic Approaches

The use of drugs to promote colonic transit by increasing colonic motor activity has generally proved disappointing. Cholinergic agents such as bethanechol (Urecholine)* and neostigmine* have been tried with little success and may be associated with side effects. Prokinetic agents such as metoclopramide (Reglan)* and cisapride (Propulsid)* appear to be ineffective in most severely constipated patients. Some patients with severe constipation have been treated successfully with misoprostol (Cytotec),* a prostaglandin used to prevent nonsteroidal anti-inflammatory drug–associated peptic ulcers. Further studies are needed to assess the possible efficacy of this agent in severely constipated individuals.

Surgical Approaches

For severe slow transit constipation, subtotal colectomy with ileorectal anastomosis can dramatically ameliorate incapacitating constipation in carefully selected patients, although this is somewhat controversial. If surgery is undertaken, at least four criteria should be met: (1) the patient has chronic, severe, and disabling symptoms from constipation that are unresponsive to medical therapy; (2) the patient has

---

*Not FDA approved for this indication.

slow colonic transit of the inertia pattern; (3) the patient does *not* have intestinal pseudo-obstruction, as demonstrated by radiologic or manometric studies; and (4) anorectal function is normal. Potential complications of surgery include persistent abdominal pain and bloating, diarrhea, small intestinal obstruction, and postoperative infections. Recent studies have documented that greater than 90% of carefully studied patients have satisfactory long-term results.

Rectoceles and rectal intussusceptions are common in older nonconstipated women, and caution must be used when attributing defecatory difficulties to these entities. Indeed, surgical repairs frequently do not alleviate symptoms of difficult defecation. Optimally, one should demonstrate improved rectal evacuation when pressure is placed on the posterior wall of the vagina during defecation before a rectocele repair should be entertained.

Surgery is the treatment of choice for Hirschsprung's disease and varies according to the length of the aganglionic segment. In patients with short-segment or ultra-short-segment disease, anal myotomy, in which the internal sphincter and a varied length of rectal smooth muscle are incised, is often effective. With larger segments, bypassing or removing the aganglionic bowel is necessary to overcome the obstructing effect of the denervated segment. The choice of surgical technique depends on the surgeon, but excellent results have been reported for all of them.

ACKNOWLEDGMENT

The author thanks Ms. Helen Gibson for the expert preparation of this manuscript.

FEVER

method of
MICHAEL S. KRAMER, M.D.
McGill University Faculty of Medicine
Montreal, Quebec, Canada

The anterior hypothalamus normally regulates the set point for core body temperature at $37 \pm 1°C$ and responds to an increase or decrease in environmental temperature by neural impulses that lead to heat loss (vasodilatation and sweating) or conservation (vasoconstriction and shivering), respectively. If the body is unable to compensate for a gain of heat, the core temperature rises above the set point, a condition called hyperthermia. Fever is defined as an upward adjustment of the set point. Unlike hyperthermia, fever does not represent a loss of temperature regulation; rather, it is an upward shift of the temperature regulated. In the absence of hyperthermia, fever can therefore be considered present if the rectal temperature is 38°C or higher; approximately equivalent oral and axillary temperatures are 37.5°C or higher and 37.2°C or higher, respectively. Despite prevailing "wisdom" to the contrary, most mothers are able to subjectively (i.e., by touch) determine the absence of fever in their children. Moreover, the mothers' subjective assessments are sensitive for detecting high fevers ($\geq 39°C$).

A considerable body of research has demonstrated that vertebrates and even many invertebrates are capable of developing a febrile response. Ectotherms, such as fishes, amphibians, and reptiles, lack the capacity to adjust body heat by intrinsic physiologic mechanisms. Instead, they rely on behavioral adaptation; they seek appropriate environmental temperatures and assume optimal heat-conserving positions. In humans, shivering, peripheral vasoconstriction, and increased metabolic rate result in an increase of the core temperature to between 38 and 41°C. In clinical fevers, the hypothalamus carefully modulates the rise in set point so that temperatures rarely exceed 41°C, even in children.

Fever has been recognized as a cardinal sign of disease since the beginning of recorded history. Opinions have changed substantially, however, as to whether ill patients are better off with or without it. For Hippocrates and other ancients, fever was the body's defense mechanism for "cooking off" an excess of one of the four body humors: blood, phlegm, yellow bile, and black bile. The view that fever is beneficial persisted for more than 2 millennia; according to the noted 17th century English physician Thomas Sydenham, "Fever is Nature's engine which she brings into the field to remove her enemy." A change in this view occurred after experiments by Claude Bernard, the great 19th century French physiologist, demonstrated that animals died when their body temperature was experimentally raised to 5 or 6°C above normal. Although Bernard's experiments concerned hyperthermia rather than fever, fever became regarded as injurious to health.

Fever occurs as a result of the body's exposure to infecting microorganisms, immune complexes, or other sources of inflammation. The major pathophysiologic mechanism for its development involves the release of cytokines from circulating monocytes and lymphocytes and fixed tissue macrophages; these cytokines, which include interleukin-1 (IL-1), interleukin-6, tumor necrosis factor, and interferons, function as endogenous pyrogens. They stimulate prostaglandin E_2 production in the preoptic area of the anterior hypothalamus, which then brings about a rise in the temperature set point by the physiologic and/or behavioral mechanisms mentioned earlier. IL-1 and other cytokines have a number of direct effects on the immune response, including release and production of neutrophils from the bone marrow, increase of neutrophil oxidative activity, lactoferrin release, B cell proliferation and antibody production, and T cell activation. The lactoferrin release leads to a decrease in serum iron concentration, which inhibits the growth of many microorganisms. But the fever induced by endogenous pyrogens has additional immunologic benefits above and beyond these direct effects, including helper T cell proliferation; enhanced T cell cytotoxicity, B cell activity, and antibody synthesis; and interferon production and function. Moreover, the growth of some organisms (including poliovirus, pneumococcus, gonococcus, and syphilis treponeme) is inhibited at febrile temperatures.

In otherwise healthy children or adults, there is no evidence that temperatures below 42°C are harmful. However, the fever-induced increase in oxygen consumption and cardiac output could compromise the status of debilitated elderly persons or patients with severe pulmonary or cardiovascular disease. Children younger than 5 years, and especially those younger than 3 years, are at risk for febrile convulsions, particularly at temperatures of 40°C or higher, although many such convulsions occur early in the course of the febrile illness while the temperature is rising and in many cases before the parents are even aware of the presence of the fever. Unfortunately, there is no convincing evidence that antipyretic treatment is effective in preventing febrile seizures. Febrile illnesses are often accompanied by other symptoms of the acute phase response, including headache, anorexia, malaise, fatigue, and myalgias. It is not clear, however, to what extent these symptoms are a consequence of fever, because many of them appear to be mediated by IL-1 and other endogenous pyrogens.

TREATMENT

The first therapeutic decision concerning fever is whether or not to treat it. In patients with significant pulmonary or cardiovascular compromise or in severely debilitated elderly persons, lowering the hypothalamic set point should be beneficial in reducing oxygen consumption and cardiac output. Even in the absence of evidence of prophylactic efficacy, it also seems reasonable to treat fevers in children younger than 5 years with a history of febrile convulsions or in patients of any age who experience convulsions without fever.

In otherwise healthy children and adults, the decision to administer antipyretic therapy should be based on balancing the likely risks and benefits of treatment. The risks of treatment remain largely theoretical and relate to the improved immune responses (see earlier) observed at febrile temperatures. Nonetheless, therapeutic blood levels of commonly used antipyretic medications do not reduce the production of IL-1 or other endogenous pyrogens. In fact, few adverse effects have been documented with therapeutic doses of antipyretic drugs in the intact human host. In particular, antipyresis does not appear to prolong the duration of fever or other symptoms in young children with viral illness. Such children appear more alert and active when they are treated, although it is not clear whether such improvement is due to the antipyretic or analgesic properties of these drugs.

Because many patients, and especially young children, often appear comfortable despite febrile temperatures, the best policy, given existing evidence, is to treat fevers associated with significant discomfort. Although this is a natural policy to adopt for adults who elect to treat themselves, it is in marked contrast to the policy of many parents, who seem more focused on treating the thermometer rather than the child.

Once a decision has been made to treat a fever, the next decision involves the choice of therapy, which has traditionally comprised both pharmacologic and nonpharmacologic approaches. The major nonpharmacologic approach has been external cooling by removing clothing and/or bathing or sponging in cold or tepid water or application of isopropyl alcohol. Such measures are not very effective; moreover, they run counter to the physiologic mechanisms discussed earlier. Unless the hypothalamic set point is lowered pharmacologically, the evaporation induced by application of water or alcohol to the skin leads only to shivering (and therefore discomfort) as the body attempts to maintain the core temperature at the regulated set point. The discomfort induced by cold water or alcohol bathing or sponging can be considerable. Isopropyl alcohol can also be absorbed through the skin, with appreciable blood levels and risk for systemic toxic effects; its use should therefore be discouraged.

The safe and effective mainstays of treatment are pharmacologic and include acetaminophen, aspirin, and other nonsteroidal anti-inflammatory drugs (NSAIDs). All appear to work by inhibiting production of prostaglandin E_2 in the anterior hypothalamus in response to IL-1 and other endogenous pyrogens.

When an antipyretic effect alone is desired, acetaminophen is usually the drug of choice. The dosage of acetaminophen is 10 to 20 mg per kg per dose, up to the maximal adult dose of 650 to 1000 mg administered every 4 hours. Table 1 indicates acetaminophen dosages by age and weight (in kilograms). A variety of dosage forms are available. The adult tablets contain either 325 mg (regular strength) or 500 mg (extra strength). For young children, the usual dosage forms are drops (80 mg per mL), syrup (80 or 160 mg per 5 mL), chewable tablets (80 or 160 mg each), and swallowable junior tablets (160 mg each). Acetaminophen is conjugated in the liver to form sulfate and glucuronide derivatives. A small amount is metabolized to a toxic intermediate by a cytochrome P-450–mediated pathway; this metabolite is hepatotoxic when it is present in quantities greater than the capacity of the liver to conjugate it with glutathione or other sulfhydryl donors. Adult dosage forms therefore represent a major hazard for accidental or intentional overdose.

Aspirin is a gastric irritant that increases the risk for gastric ulcer, hemorrhage, and perforation. Its inhibition of cyclooxygenase also interferes with platelet function and may increase the risk for bleeding; this is of particular importance in the postoperative patient. Aspirin is also associated with a risk for asthma exacerbation and even serious anaphylactic reactions, particularly in adults with a pre-existing

TABLE 1. **Recommended Dosages of Acetaminophen by Age and Weight***

Age	Weight (kg)	Dose (mg q 4 h)
<1 mo	2.5–3.9	40
1–6 mo	4.0–7.9	80
7–18 mo	8.0–10.9	120
19 mo–3 y	11.0–14.9	160
4–5 y	15.0–20.9	240
6–7 y	21.0–27.9	320
8–9 y	28.0–35.9	400
10–11 y	36.0–44.9	480
12–13 y	45.0–59.9	650
14 y–adult	≥60	650–1000

* When age and weight categories do not coincide, base dosage on weight. Do not exceed 4 or 5 doses per day.

history of asthma and nasal polyps. The adult form of aspirin can be the vehicle for accidental poisonings in infants and toddlers and for suicide attempts in adolescents and adults. Overdose leads to a syndrome called salicylism, which is characterized by hyperventilation, depressed level of consciousness, and severe metabolic acidosis. Finally, there is unequivocal evidence linking the use of aspirin by children with influenza, varicella, and other viral infections to the subsequent development of Reye's syndrome, a rare disease manifested by liver dysfunction and severe encephalopathy. As use of aspirin as an antipyretic has become progressively rarer in children since the first reports of the aspirin–Reye's syndrome association in the early 1980s, so too has the frequency of, and mortality from, Reye's syndrome. In adults without a history of asthma or other allergic disease or peptic ulcer disease, and particularly those in need of aspirin's anti-inflammatory action (an action not shared by acetaminophen), the usual recommended dose is 650 mg (two 325-mg tablets) every 4 hours.

Other NSAIDs have also been used as antipyretic agents in children and adults, the most common being ibuprofen. Current evidence indicates that in doses of 5 to 10 mg per kg (up to a maximal adult dose of 400 mg), three or four times per day, ibuprofen is comparable in antipyretic efficacy with therapeutically equivalent doses of aspirin or acetaminophen. In acute overdoses, ibuprofen appears to be much safer than acetaminophen or aspirin. To a lesser extent than aspirin, ibuprofen can lead to gastric ulceration, perforation, and hemorrhage, particularly in the elderly, and exacerbate asthma or lead to anaphylactic reactions in asthmatics. Although there are no data linking ibuprofen to Reye's syndrome, the mechanism by which aspirin interacts with viruses to produce Reye's syndrome is not understood. To the extent that such a mechanism may be shared by ibuprofen or other NSAIDs, one might suspect (at least on theoretical grounds) such a link with these medications. Because ibuprofen is also more expensive than aspirin or acetaminophen, and because it does not appear to carry any unique therapeutic benefits, it is difficult to recommend it as a drug of first choice, even in adults.

COUGH

method of
IRWIN ZIMENT, M.D.
UCLA School of Medicine
Los Angeles, California
Olive View–UCLA Medical Center
Sylmar, California

Almost everybody is aware of the symptom of annoying cough that recurs in repeated bouts throughout the day for several days before the problem gradually abates. The common cough, which is usually accounted for by a viral upper respiratory tract infection (URI), does not require medical intervention. Nevertheless, at certain times of the year, a significant proportion of the afflicted population decides to seek the help of medical professionals, although it would be better for coughers to avoid the risk of spreading their infection in clinic waiting rooms. Only a minority of coughs necessitate detailed evaluation and specific therapy because most coughs are self-limited or require nonspecific management. Thus, it is appropriate to consider a cough as being simple, or more annoying, or complex with severe and persistent features; the physician must adapt the evaluation and therapy accordingly (Table 1).

SIMPLE COUGH

A cough that has been present for only hours or days can usually be regarded as simple, requiring only general supportive measures or nonspecific cough medication. Most patients treat themselves or are treated by their parents—even beyond childhood. If the cough appears not to be related to a URI, other considerations may need to be given attention.

General Management

Provocative exacerbating factors should be avoided. The use of angiotensin-converting enzyme (ACE) inhibitors can lead to a chronic cough in a significant number of patients, and alternative drug therapy is needed if this complication is suspected. Smoking and exposure to secondhand smoke or other inhaled irritants can cause coughing and are likely to exacerbate any acute cough. Breathing cold air or being in a draft may induce an annoying exacerbation of a new-onset cough, and many patients feel better if they remain in a warm but adequately humidified room or if they stay in bed. Warm drinks are of symptomatic benefit; these include teas, tisanes, soups, and syrupy drinks containing alcohol. Peppery drinks or hot-tasting foods may induce more coughing, and their therapeutic properties are likely to be appreciated mostly by those who are habituated to a diet containing pungent, spicy flavors. On the other hand, some coughs appear to be controlled by sucking strong mint or menthol preparations. Throat lozenges and cough candies of various types are popular, although their value is difficult to determine; nevertheless, local anesthetic preparations offering topical therapy for the throat and the popular germicidal agents are used in large amounts as tablets or candies or as gargles in the self-management of cough. A humidifier or steam inhaler may help, as may a hot shower or sitting in a steam room. Aromatic vapors delivered in steam from boiling water are extremely popular and have resulted in enormous sales, over many years, of proprietary products containing menthol, eucalyptus, camphor, storax, aloes, and other traditional agents. Many patients with coughs like to use esoteric folk remedies of unproven values, such as echinacea (to stimulate immu-

TABLE 1. **Management of Different Types of Cough**

Type of Cough	Causes	Management
Simple or temporary	Upper respiratory tract infection	General measures, aromatic inhalants
	Viral	Warmth, drinks, analgesics, antitussives
	Bacterial	Add antibiotics in selected cases
	Sinusitis, postnasal drip	Decongestants, steroids, (?) antibiotics
	Allergy	Antihistamines, steroids, cromolyn, nedocromil
	Postinhalation injury	Bronchodilators, antitussives
	Throat clearing, nervous tic	Drinks, cough tablets, counseling, biofeedback
	Secondary to angiotensin-converting enzyme inhibitor	Stop drug, or try nedocromil or indomethacin
Annoying or serious	Asthma or cough-variant asthma	Bronchodilators, steroids, antitussives
	Chronic obstructive pulmonary disease	Stop smoking, avoid inhaled irritants
	Bronchitis	Bronchodilators, mucokinetics, antibiotics
	Bronchiectasis	Bronchodilators, antibiotics, surgery
	Cystic fibrosis	Physical therapy, dornase, antibiotics
	After viral infection	Antitussives, antibiotics, local anesthetics
	Acute infection	Antibiotics, mucokinetics, antitussives, antihistamines
Severe or persistent	Complications of immunodeficiency	Appropriate antimicrobial regimen
	Pulmonary fibrosis	Antitussives, oxygen, lung transplantation
	Active mycobacterial infection	Antituberculosis regimen
	Tracheobronchial tumor	Surgery, radiotherapy, chemotherapy
	Malignant tumors	Antitussives, opioids
	Benign tumor or granuloma	Antitussives, local anesthetics
	Foreign body	Bronchoscopic or surgical removal
	Idiopathic	Antitussives, sedatives, acupuncture, homeopathy
	Sarcoidosis	Steroids, immunosuppressives, antitussives
	Other lung diseases	Specific therapy, antitussives
	Heart failure	Diuretics, cardiotonic drugs
	Gastroesophageal reflux	H_2 blockers, medical regimen, surgery
	Swallowing disorders	Aspiration precautions, surgery

nity) or coltsfoot, mullein, and hyssop (which are traditional antitussives). Fashionable food products such as vitamin C, other vitamins and minerals, fish oil, ginseng, and garlic are now in favor for their reputed powers as cold and cough preventers and relievers.

ANNOYING COUGH

When a cough persists in spite of adequate general measures, more active treatment is usually appropriate. Patients may complain of chest soreness or pain that is exacerbated by coughing, or the problem may interfere with eating, talking, exercise, sleep, or social interactions. Severe coughing may cause more annoying complications such as vomiting, incontinence, or syncope, and it may be impossible for the patient to remain at work or to live a normal life.

Such patients require thoughtful questioning about the history of the illness and a careful physical examination. The clinician must ask the patient to demonstrate the cough to enable an assessment of its characteristics (such as wheezing, whooping, or stridor) and its productivity; any sputum that is produced must be evaluated for odor, color, and the possible presence of blood and for its rheologic properties, such as viscosity and stickiness. If there is a suspicion of underlying lung disease, chest radiographs are needed. Any suspicion of heart failure, which can cause coughing, necessitates in addition an electrocardiogram and possibly an echocardio-

gram. Particular consideration must be given to the possible presence of sinusitis with postnasal drip; swallowing disorders that may cause aspiration; and gastroesophageal (GE) reflux that may induce reflex coughing, often with bronchospasm, even in the absence of overt aspiration. The possibility of psychogenic cough, which may be habitual, or of malingering must be given consideration if there is no other evident cause.

It is not always worth pursuing expensive work-ups, such as inhalational provocation tests to detect latent asthma; sinus radiographs or scans to evaluate the possibility of sinobronchial disease; or radiographic, endoscopic, or pH meter studies of the lower esophagus in an attempt to prove the presence of GE reflux. In most cases, if one diagnostic possibility stands out, it is appropriate and cost-effective to embark on specific therapy and to evaluate the outcome, because a clear therapeutic benefit may be considered as serving as a positive diagnostic test result. Thus, suspected sinusitis should be treated with a decongestant or a corticosteroid, with use of oral medications for more severe symptoms and topical aerosols or inhalants for less severe problems; an antibiotic is needed if bacterial infection is suggested by the presence of colored secretions. In all cases, 7 to 20 days of treatment may be required to produce significant control of the cough; simple inexpensive antibiotics should be used for the first week, and a more potent agent used subsequently if there is no improvement.

Suspected obstruction of the airways may require a variety of approaches: beta agonists or ipratropium may relieve bronchospasm and decrease cough in so-called cough-variant asthma; corticosteroids, nedocromil, or possibly cromolyn is required if there is chronic asthma or bronchospasm in association with atopy or airway hyper-reactivity. In some patients in whom the asthmatic condition appears to be a reaction to allergic rhinitis, the cough may respond particularly well to an antihistamine; diphenhydramine appears to have the most effective antitussive properties. An asthmatic cough may not clear up immediately with appropriate therapy, and regular treatment may be needed for a prolonged period to keep the cough under control, whereas the airway obstructive findings may respond more readily. If an aerosol steroid is used to treat cough in a subject with asthmatic airways, the patient should be instructed to exhale the aerosol from the lungs through the nose to provide some therapy for the nasal passages, because these often have inflammatory cell infiltration in those atopic patients who present with a chronic cough.

Swallowing disorders as a cause of cough should first be treated with drugs and may require physical therapy. GE reflux may respond to an H_2 blocker, a proton pump inhibitor, or a gastric motility stimulator. The patient should avoid gaseous drinks or large meals before lying down or should stop taking agents such as theophylline and mints and other carminatives that cause relaxation of the GE sphincter. In selected patients, more intensive evaluation of GE function is required, and surgical correction of reflux may be deemed necessary; the oropharynx or esophagus may need to be bypassed, or the muscles controlling the laryngeal sphincter may need corrective attention.

SEVERE OR PERSISTENT COUGH

If a cough remains unexplained or is becoming worse after basic evaluation and a trial of appropriate therapy for up to 3 weeks, a chest radiograph is needed. Any suspicious findings require a further diagnostic work-up. A computed tomographic scan and then bronchoscopy may be justified, because an intrabronchial tumor, mass, or other luminal lesion or bronchiectasis may be the cause. Sophisticated pulmonary function tests, exercise studies, inhalation scans, bronchoprovocation challenge tests, and repeated sputum evaluation are not usually required if there is no distinct radiologic abnormality and there are no other respiratory or generalized symptoms besides coughing and its obvious complications. In such frustrating cases, it may be appropriate to treat the patient as a mild case of asthma; a prolonged trial of antitussive and bronchodilator drugs, a steroid, or the use of cromolyn or nedocromil by inhalation is usually required, but patients often become discouraged and seek alternative help. It is possible that some patients with persistent or recurrent, uncontrolled, chronic cough may derive relief from treatments such as chiropractic, homeopathy, common or unusual herbal remedies, acupuncture, or yoga exercises. It is difficult to determine whether the benefit from complementary medical alternatives is a nonspecific placebo effect or is related to the fact that agents and techniques that access the medullary cough center of the brain through its cerebral pathways may have a marked controlling effect on medullary motor output. In some patients, reassuring counseling or the use of sedatives or antidepressants, as well as courses of different antitussives (including newer antihistamines or old, established Chinese herbal cough mixtures), may be worthwhile. However, in all such cases of "idiopathic" cough, the possibility of a serious cause must be periodically reconsidered, or a hidden factor (such as secondhand smoke or exposure to allergens or chemicals) must be repeatedly thought about.

The most severe coughs may be caused by viscous secretions, and their removal may necessitate physical therapy or intubation; bronchoscopy, lavage, or repeated suctioning is required for atelectasis or respiratory failure. Specific infections need to be diagnosed; induction of sputum or bronchoscopy and lavage may be appropriate to provide a culture that will justify subsequent antimicrobial therapy. Pulmonary fibrotic diseases often require biopsy evaluation to direct specific management of conditions such as sarcoidosis.

NONSPECIFIC AGENTS FOR COUGH

Several classes of drugs may be considered for relieving cough, and individual drugs can be selected according to the cause of the cough and the severity of the problem. However, in spite of all the studies of the pharmacologic management of cough, the value of many standard remedies remains uncertain. This is partly because studies of cough management in patients present considerable logistic difficulties, and relatively few laboratories in England, Europe, the United States, and India are carrying out quality evaluations of the mechanisms of and therapies for cough. The findings of competent investigators are all too often not in agreement, and thus not only are many established medications of controversial value, but the introduction of new antitussives is proving to be difficult.

Demulcents

Topical agents based on sugar, honey, or a noncaloric sweetener, flavored with herbal or aromatic agents, are popular as tablets, lozenges, and pastilles. Some incorporate local anesthetics or antitussive agents, but there is no comparative information to suggest that any particular combination is superior.

Herbal Agents

Many practitioners believe that traditional flavorful nonprescription remedies are the best first choice for cough (Table 2). Popular proprietary products with contents such as licorice, menthol, capsaicin (from chili peppers), and caramel are helpful, particularly if pharyngitis or laryngitis is present. Western herbal remedies include coltsfoot, hyssop, mullein, elecampane, and many other plant extracts; these have been used in oral preparations, in topical products, and as cigarettes. Their value is difficult to demonstrate even though coltsfoot (*Tussilago farfara*) contains an inhibitor of the mediator platelet-activating factor, thus suggesting a neurocytokine-directed effect. In China, numerous herbal remedies are used, with products ranging from rhododendron extracts to plants that are unknown in other countries. Lo-Han-Kuo (derived from a gourd), fritillary, and loquat are readily available antitussives that are marketed in the United States. In India, there is excellent evidence to suggest that derivatives of the plant *Adhatoda vasica* (including vasaka) are effective antitussives; their modern derivatives, bromhexine and ambroxol, are used in Europe and other Western countries as mucus-loosening medications. Inhalant mixtures include camphor, eucalyptus, menthol, benzoin, and aloes; these are available in proprietary products such as Vicks VapoRub, Tiger Balm, and Friars' Balsam, which can be used to scent steam. Although such agents are popular, their value is uncertain, but they are unlikely to be harmful unless paraffinaceous products are placed in the nose and aspirated into the lungs.

Mucokinetic Drugs

Numerous expectorants and mucolytics are marketed around the world, but their value in loosening mucus or in alleviating cough remains uncertain. If they loosen mucus and improve expectoration, they may help alleviate ineffective coughing. If they irritate the airway, they may increase the coughing but not benefit the cause of the cough. In the United States, guaifenesin (Robitussin) is popular, and it is often combined with an antitussive. Terpin hydrate is no longer used, and organic iodide (e.g., the preparation Organidin) is not marketed. Although an oral formulation of acetylcysteine is popular in Europe, it is not available in the United States; the inhaled product appears to be less effective in loosening inspissated mucus. Human recombinant dornase alfa (Pulmozyme) is useful for breaking up infected sputum in cystic fibrosis through its topical mucolytic action, but it does not appear to be of value in bronchitis. In general, inhaled mucokinetic drugs, including water or saline, do not have a beneficial effect on cough; indeed, they are liable to induce coughing, and such treatment may not be tolerated in a patient whose cough is caused by an irritable tracheobronchial tree. Hypertonic saline is a protussive agent that can be used to induce production and expectoration of secretions.

Antiallergy Agents

Allergic rhinitis may be accompanied by a cough, and allergic coughs may occur (without rhinitis) as a manifestation of asthma. Such cough-variant asthma may respond to nedocromil or steroid inhalation. Sedating antihistamines may help suppress cough and are particularly useful for nocturnal cough relief. Diphenhydramine and tripelennamine appear to have a specific antitussive effect, and these and other antihistamines are often incorporated into drug mixtures that are used to treat coughs and colds. Their ability to dry nasal secretions in addition to their sedative effects may be beneficial. Nasal ipratropium (Atrovent), which is available for topical therapy to dry the secretions of coryza, may also help relieve coughs that accompany colds. Immunotherapy for asthma desensitization may help relieve chronic cough, but this would occur as part of the total reduction in the asthmatic mediator response.

Bronchodilators

The inflammatory cytokines that mediate the asthmatic response are also responsible for causing activation of the cough reflex. In some asthmatic patients, cough is the primary complaint, even in the absence of regularly expectorated sputum. In bronchitis, the inflammatory mechanisms are based on a neutrophilic response to infection or irritation rather than an eosinophilic response to antigens and other stimuli; expectoration is part of the symptom complex. The use of inhaled beta agonists—whether they are short acting, such as albuterol (Ventolin, Proventil), or long acting, such as salmeterol (Serevent)—reduces bronchospasm and airway congestion and improves mucociliary clearance; the cough of both asthma and bronchitis is thereby improved, because the mucus-induced irritation of cough receptors is diminished. Ipratropium is of major value in bronchitis and emphysema: it can open up the larger airways and thereby enable the patient to generate increased airflow during coughing, thus improving clearance of mucus. Inhaled ipratropium differs from atropine in that it does not cause drying of tracheobronchial secretions, and it generally has a favorable effect on the cough

TABLE 2. **Some Traditional Cough Medications**

Western	Coltsfoot, marshmallow, mullein, slippery elm, horehound, elecampane, eucalyptus, peppermint, echinacea, gentian, primula, sorrel, elder, vervain
Chinese	Ephedra, cinnamon, ginger, loquat, licorice, gingko, mulberry, pinellia, schizandra, fritillary, momordica, coptis, aster, stemona, platycodon, cynanchum, rehmannia, rhododendron
Indian	Vasaka (and ambroxol and bromhexine), peppers, turmeric, amalaki, haritaki, benzoin, tolu, myrrh
Homeopathic	Oscillococcinum, arsenic, bryony, aconite, belladonna, strychnine, phosphorus, tuberculin, sulfur, sepia, burned sponge

of chronic obstructive pulmonary disease (COPD); when used as a bronchodilator, it can be exhaled through the nose to treat any associated rhinitis. Oral bronchodilators, including beta agonists and theophylline, may be better tolerated by some patients whose irritated, hyperactive airways do not permit aerosol therapy because the suspended particles and the deep inhalation can induce a paroxysm of coughing.

Corticosteroids

Inhaled corticosteroids are usually indicated in chronic asthma, especially when persistent symptoms require daily bronchodilator therapy. In asthma, inhaled steroids may be effective in reducing cough, but this is not the case in the majority of patients with bronchitis or COPD. Oral or intramuscular steroids may be needed to control severe asthma, and these drugs may have a benefit in allergic, asthmatic, or postviral cough. However, although clinicians may think that oral steroids benefit the cough of COPD, the evidence suggests that this is an unpredictable outcome that occurs in only 15 to 30% of patients. Oral steroids are sometimes given to patients with incurable lung cancer because they may induce a euphoriant effect, but their use may not result in a direct improvement in the cough.

Analgesics

Reducing chest pain with analgesia allows postthoracotomy patients and those with pleurisy, rib fractures, or chest wall pain to cough out secretions more effectively, thereby reducing the reflex stimulation that is initiated by trapped viscous secretions whose presence induces repetitive, ineffective coughing. Common analgesics, such as aspirin, acetaminophen, and propoxyphene, have little if any antitussive effect. The potent opioid agents heroin,* morphine, and methadone are quite effective; these drugs have a depressive effect on the medullary respiratory center, and they similarly have a depressant effect on the medullary cough center. However, even in COPD, opioids can be given to alleviate pain and cough in effective doses that do not suppress respiration.

SPECIFIC ANTITUSSIVES

Many agents have been reported to be of value in the suppression of cough through direct action on the medullary cough center in the brain or by means of peripheral action on the receptors that mediate cough in the tracheobronchial tree. Not all antitussives can be shown to work as a result of defined actions at either of these sites, and some drugs appear to act at both sites. Current accounts of antitussive agents list more than 40 centrally acting agents and about 20 that act peripherally. Most of these drugs have never been used in the United States, and many are of limited value and have not been favored for use in any country. Thus, only a few antitussives are now available in the proprietary drug formulations listed in standard American drug reference publications (Table 3).

Narcotic Agents

The opiates, which are derived from opium, are the most potent centrally acting antitussives. Heroin* is one of the most effective, and this drug was formerly used with good therapeutic results in terminally ill patients with severe cough and pain caused by lung cancer. Cocaine,† which has useful local anesthetic

---

*Not available in the United States.
†Not FDA approved for this indication.

TABLE 3. **Current Antitussive Drugs**

Drug	Typical Adult Dose	Comments
Narcotics		
Morphine	5–30 mg 3–6 times/d	For severe coughs (e.g., in lung cancer) or cough with pain; larger doses may be needed for intractable condition
Hydromorphone (Dilaudid)	0.75–6 mg 3–8 times/d	Similar to morphine but more potent and therefore rarely needed for cough
Methadone (Dolophine)	5–30 mg 3–6 times/d	Similar to morphine; may be used as a substitute, but not of special value for cough
Hydrocodone (Hycodan)	2.5–10 mg 3–4 times/d	Available only in combination products; extended-release product should have dose limited to 10 mg bid; more addictive than codeine
Codeine	20–30 mg 3–6 times/d	Value of standard dose is uncertain; increased dosage may be needed, but side effects limit value; available alone and in combination products
Non-narcotics		
Dextromethorphan (dormethan)	15–30 mg 3–6 times/d	Best agent for general use; few side effects; available in many combination products
Benzonatate (Tessalon)	100–300 mg 3–4 times/d*	May be needed for chronic intractable cough associated with interstitial lung disease
Carbetapentane (Rynatuss)	30–60 mg 2 times/d	Unusual agent of uncertain effectiveness

* Exceeds dosage recommended by the manufacturer.

properties, may have similar value, but its abuse potential renders it unacceptable as a therapeutic agent. In practice, morphine* is the most valuable agent for severe cough, and its use is particularly indicated when pain, anxiety, and insomnia accompany an intractable cough. Methadone and hydromorphone (Dilaudid) are less effective alternatives, and they have not attained a major role in cough therapeutics.

Codeine is the most interesting of the opiates. This drug has a relatively low addiction potential, but numerous individuals do become habituated to and dependent on codeine if they are given the opportunity. It has long been regarded as an effective antitussive for use in short-lasting coughs or in preterminal fatal conditions in which mild pain control is also required. However, several investigators have been unable to demonstrate a significant antitussive effect in acute URI when codeine is given in generous dosages of 30 to 50 mg four times a day. This surprising finding may be the outcome of the fact that laboratory evaluation of antitussive drugs in patients is difficult, rather than being an indictment of the general impression that codeine is effective. It is clear that many adults who use codeine need to greatly increase the recommended dosage of 20 mg to reach an effective dosing range, and the accompanying psychic effects may present problems. It may be advisable to avoid prescribing codeine-containing cough medications for outpatients and to restrict the use of the drug to inpatient care where its effects can be monitored. Hydrocodone (Hycodan) may be more effective, but it is not clear that this drug offers any advantages over codeine. The other popular narcotic alternatives, oxycodone (Percodan) and meperidine (Demerol), are not recommended for cough suppression. In some countries, pholcodine† is popular but is of dubious value; a variety of additional opiates of uncertain effectiveness are available throughout the world for the treatment of cough. It is unlikely that investigators will agree on a ranking of these agents in terms of antitussive potency and freedom from dangerous side effects, and thus selection of any agent will have to be based on local convention and clinical experience.

Non-narcotic Agents

The most widely used antitussive that has no significant medullary or cerebral effects is dextromethorphan. There is emerging clinical laboratory evidence of the value of this drug, although the common dose of 15 to 30 mg every 4 to 8 hours may need to be increased. Because the drug is usually well tolerated, it should always be used in preference to codeine. Side effects of dextromethorphan may include nausea and dizziness; central depression with respiratory impairment may occur after extremely large doses. This antitussive is usually well tolerated

by children and adults and in patients with respiratory insufficiency.

A valuable peripherally acting, nonsedating antitussive is benzonatate (Tessalon Perles), a local anesthetic drug that is available as capsules. It appears to act on stretch and cough receptors, but it may also have a central effect and may reduce the respiratory reflex response of the carotid body chemoreceptors. The usual dose is 100 mg three times daily, but patients may respond only to higher doses. Toxic effects are mild but include vertigo, headache, and rash. The capsules should not be bitten into because the drug has an unpleasant taste and it will anesthetize the tongue and pharynx for several hours. Benzonatate seems to work best when there is a repetitive, hacking, nonproductive cough or if there are conditions causing hyperreactivity or lung restriction that result in coughing when a deeper breath is taken. Although similar agents are not routinely used as antitussives, several reports have suggested that lidocaine and other local anesthetics relieve cough when they are given by aerosol or, more reliably, intravenously.

Other Cough Remedies

Other agents that had been used for cough in the United States include caramiphen and chlophedianol, but these are no longer marketed. Noscapine and levopropoxyphene may be effective and are usually well tolerated, but they are no longer available. Carbetapentane (pentoxyverine),* which is still available in the United States, is of uncertain value. It is unlikely that any of these agents would ever be considered therapeutically preferable to dextromethorphan or benzonatate.

Antitussive agents are often used in combination mixtures with decongestants, antihistamines, mucokinetic agents, or analgesics. It is sometimes taught that such combinations are undesirable or irrational; thus, it is suggested that sputum loosened up by a mucokinetic drug might move distally if the cough is suppressed. However, antitussives do not suppress cough entirely and they do not interfere with voluntary cough. Therefore, loosened sputum can still be expectorated more readily even if an antitussive is given because the patient can cough productively at will, rather than coughing unproductively at random in the absence of an antitussive. It can be concluded that combination products may be appropriate and effective.

Many agents have been reported to offer some benefit in cough. Inhibitors of prostaglandin synthesis, such as ibuprofen (Motrin),† indomethacin (Indocin),† baclofen (Lioresal),† and sulindac (Clinoril),† have been recommended to treat cough produced by ACE inhibitors, as have calcium channel blockers. Furosemide (Lasix)† and other diuretics, when given by inhalation, have been shown to be effective in

---

*Not FDA approved for this indication.
†Not available in the United States.

---

*Not available in the United States.
†Not FDA approved for this indication.

some forms of asthma, and these agents may improve cough. In the past 5 years, several new agents have received favorable reports, including moguisteine, glaucine, dihydroetorphine, levdropropizine, dextrorphan, and novel antagonists directed at the tachykinin NK2 receptor. Currently, new anticholinergic agents and antihistamines are being evaluated as primary and secondary agents for treatment of idiopathic coughs.

CONCLUSION

Most coughs are self-limited and respond to demulcent or simple over-the-counter cough and cold remedies. Persistent coughs either may signify serious disease that necessitates definitive or radical therapy or can result from unresponsive underlying causes such as airway inflammation or architectural damage that can be managed only by cough suppressive drug therapy. Despite many years of popular use, the value of most antitussive drugs remains uncertain. Morphine is the best agent for severe cough accompanied by pain, and dextromethorphan is currently the most satisfactory agent for nonpainful, nonproductive, aggravating coughs. Most other drugs should be tried only when a trial of dextromethorphan in adequate dosage has shown this drug to be unsatisfactory. It is possible that Chinese or Indian folk medicines will prove to be valuable alternatives for cough relief. There is still a need for more effective, safe, well-tolerated agents for the control of persistent, aggravating coughs that have no underlying treatable disease.

HOARSENESS AND LARYNGITIS

method of
GAYLE E. WOODSON, M.D.
University of Tennessee, Memphis
Memphis, Tennessee

Hoarseness is not a specific disease or symptom but the term for virtually any change in the voice. A rough sound, an increased effort requirement, or a change in pitch is perceived by the patient as hoarseness. There are many different causes, and so hoarseness is commonly encountered in medical practice. Acute hoarseness is most frequently due to laryngitis, inflammation of the voice box. In the majority of patients with laryngitis, expectant conservative management results in recovery within 2 weeks. The specific characteristics of the vocal change and key points in the history serve as clues to the mechanism of the problem and hence guide therapy.

PATHOPHYSIOLOGY

Vocal sound is generated when exhaled air induces passive vibration of the vocal folds (commonly known as the vocal cords). Resonance of the chest, throat, and head modulates sound extensively. Hoarseness can result from impairment of vocal fold vibration or from altered resonance. The requirements for a normal voice are listed in Table 1.

Adequate breath support is required for phonation, but

TABLE 1. **Requirements for a Normal Voice**

Adequate breath support
Appropriate laryngeal closure
Healthy vocal fold mucosa
Control of vocal fold length and tension
Normal resonance

the amount of lung function needed is modest in relation to normal lung capacity. Hence, hoarseness is not a presenting sign of lung disease, but it can be a problem in patients with severely impaired pulmonary function. More often, hoarseness is due to an intrinsic pathologic process in the larynx. If the vocal folds cannot be brought close enough together, there will be a sizeable air leak and the voice will sound breathy. If they are pressed together too tightly, or if the vocal folds are swollen and edematous, more expiratory effort is required, so that speech becomes strained and may sound strangled. Mass lesions, edema, or even alterations in the consistency of mucus can result in irregular vibration and a rough voice. Impaired motor control can lead to tremor or spasms, resulting in a wavery or jerky voice. Inflammation or tumors anywhere in the vocal tract can alter resonance, resulting in abnormalities such as hypernasality or a "hot-potato" voice.

Hoarseness is generally a benign, self-limited problem but can be an emergency. Optimal management requires prompt recognition and treatment of urgent problems, expectant measures for more innocuous conditions, and appropriate evaluation of hoarseness that does not resolve in the expected time course.

VOCAL EMERGENCIES

Hoarseness that is accompanied by stridor, with or without pain or fever, is worrisome. Laryngeal examination is required to look for obstructing disease, such as a tumor or epiglottitis.

A sudden loss or drastic change of voice that occurs during Valsalva's maneuver or extreme vocal effort may be due to a vocal fold hematoma. This most commonly occurs in premenstrual female patients because of hormonal changes in the mucosa and capillaries. However, males can also be affected. Anticoagulant medications and aspirin are risk factors. Vocal fold hematoma can cause significant and permanent hoarseness, particularly if there is a secondary bleed. Outcome is improved by prompt recognition, institution of voice rest, and identification of those large hematomas that require surgical drainage.

Hoarseness that occurs immediately after external trauma, whether blunt, penetrating, or strangulating, may indicate a laryngeal fracture. Sudden airway obstruction is possible, even hours after the injury. Immediate examination is needed, preferably with a flexible endoscope. Endotracheal intubation can create a false passage, with sudden loss of the airway, or it can exacerbate the laryngeal injury. If an airway must be established, a tracheotomy is indicated.

Hoarseness after removal of an endotracheal tube is common and generally benign and self-limited. However, if the patient also has severe pain on swallowing, an arytenoid dislocation must be suspected. Diagnosis is best made by computed tomographic scanning. Immediate treatment is required.

COMMON CAUSES OF LARYNGITIS

Most patients with acute onset of voice impairment have inflammation and swelling of the larynx. In the majority of cases, the cause of the hoarseness can be identified by asking three questions:

1. Have you overused your voice? Attending a football game or a noisy cocktail party, loud singing, and shouting can result in temporary voice loss.

2. Do you have a cold? Direct inflammation of the larynx by a virus is rare, but coughing, throat clearing, drainage of purulent secretions, and mouth breathing due to nasal obstruction can have a significant effect on the larynx.

3. Do you have heartburn? Gastroesophageal reflux is an extremely common cause of hoarseness, both acute and chronic. Many affected patients report no telltale symptoms of heartburn, belching, or ulcers, because inflammation and damage from reflux disease can be isolated to the larynx. Possible cofactors include infection, voice abuse, or trauma as minor as an aspirated potato chip. A typical patient with reflux laryngitis notices hoarseness on awakening in the morning and may also note "morning mouth."

Less common causes of acute hoarseness include allergy, binge smoking, and exposure to chemical irritants. Finally, emotional or psychiatric problems can have myriad vocal effects. Sudden total aphonia, in the absence of any signs of organic disorder, is likely to represent malingering or a conversion disorder.

TREATMENT OF ACUTE HOARSENESS

Most patients with laryngitis eventually recover spontaneously, but appropriate management (Table 2) can hasten the healing process and reduce the chance of permanent voice impairment. The key therapeutic goals are to put the larynx at rest and to control the factors that caused the problem or continue to feed it.

Voice Rest

This is the most important component of treatment for acute laryngitis. The normal fold is uniquely constructed to withstand vibration, but when it is impaired, even a little talking can be traumatic and delay healing. Normal voice use during severe laryngitis is like hiking with blistered feet, wearing ill-fitting shoes. Although healing may eventually occur, calluses or scars may develop. Optimal healing requires elimination of continued trauma. Nevertheless, total voice rest is impractical and can be frustrating to patients. Many are unable to comply and resort to abusive behavior, such as loud whispering or frequent throat clearing in an effort to communicate. In fact, occasional use of easy phonation imparts little or no stress on the vocal folds. Furthermore, total voice rest can lead to atrophy of laryngeal muscles. The optimal program conserves but does not prohibit voice use and is tailored to the severity of the laryngitis.

TABLE 2. **Treatment of Acute Laryngitis**

Voice rest	Antibiotics
Cough suppression	Hydration
Acid suppression	Management of rhinitis

For severe hoarseness, particularly with hematoma or mucosal disruption, the patient should stay home from work or school and avoid the telephone. Whispering is not acceptable. Family members should be conscripted into the plan and instructed to ask yes and no questions, not open-ended ones, and not to yell questions to the patient from the other end of the house.

For less severe hoarseness, restrictions are less stringent. Patients may go to work if their job does not involve much talking and if the work environment is free of atmospheric irritants or particulate matter.

Cough Suppression

Repetitive or vigorous coughing is traumatic to the larynx. If the cough is productive, as in pneumonia or bronchitis, cough suppression is not recommended. However, if a cough is irritative, as in asthma, allergy, or a viral infection, cough suppression can be beneficial. Two to 4 teaspoons of an over-the-counter preparation of guaifenesin and dextromethorphan (Robitussin-DM) is frequently sufficient, but some patients may require codeine or a synthetic narcotic. Cough syrups containing atropine or antihistamine should be avoided, because they tend to dry secretions, resulting in thicker mucus, which leads to more forceful coughing. Furthermore, thick mucus is inadequate lubrication for the vocal folds, so that phonation is traumatic.

Throat clearing should be strongly discouraged. Laryngeal swelling is frequently perceived as "something in the throat" or "postnasal drip." Patients notice a transient feeling of improvement after throat clearing, but the ultimate result is perpetuation of inflammation.

Acid Suppression

For reflux laryngitis, general medical management is indicated, including diet modification, elevation of the head of the bed, voice rest, and stringent acid control. Effective treatment of reflux laryngitis also requires higher doses of acid suppressants than those used in treating peptic ulcers. Even ranitidine (Zantac), 300 mg twice daily, is usually insufficient. The best response is obtained with omeprazole (Prilosec) at 20 mg daily. Medication to facilitate gastric emptying is also recommended, for example, metoclopramide (Reglan), 10 to 15 mg four times a day, before meals and at bedtime.

Reflux laryngitis is a burn and requires time to heal. Reduction or elimination of acidity does not directly promote mucosal healing but merely provides an environment in which healing can occur. Complete resolution may require 6 to 8 weeks. It is important to advise the patients of this before therapy is begun so that they do not become discouraged and discontinue treatment. Acid suppression should continue for a minimum of 2 months and for at least 1 month after resolution of symptoms. Patients who repeatedly develop recurrent reflux laryngitis, despite lifestyle changes, may be candidates for endoscopic fundoplication.

Antibiotics

Purulent secretions can irritate the larynx and superinfect reflux laryngitis. Penicillin is frequently adequate for acute infections, but in the presence of chronic sinusitis, amoxicillin-clavulanate (Augmentin) is preferable. In case of penicillin allergy, appropriate alternative drugs should be used.

Hydration

Adequate liquid intake should be maintained, at least 8 glasses of *water* per day, because even mild degrees of dehydration can result in thick sticky mucus, impairing protective lubrication.

Control of Rhinitis

Nasal congestion can also dehydrate mucus, because mouth breathing bypasses the normal humidification function of the nose. Nasal decongestion should be accomplished by topical or oral sympathomimetic medication. Oral medication, such as pseudoephedrine (Sudafed), has the added benefit of reducing laryngeal swelling. If an antihistamine is necessary to treat allergy, the use of a preparation with little effect on mucus is recommended, such as loratadine (Claritin), 10 mg a day. If excessive watery nasal secretions stimulate coughing, ipratropium bromide (Atrovent) 0.03% nasal spray can dry the nose locally, without affecting laryngeal and bronchial secretions.

WHEN THE SHOW MUST GO ON

Although voice rest is the best recommendation, patients sometimes have a pressing need for continued speech, such as an important presentation or a vocal performance. If laryngeal examination rules out vocal fold hemorrhage or abrasion, it is usually safe to manage vocal fold edema temporarily by oral or parenteral steroids. Prednisone, 40 mg about 4 hours before the event, is usually effective and may be repeated once if necessary. A long-acting topical vasoconstrictor, such as oxymetazoline (Afrin), may also be applied directly to the laryngeal mucosa to further reduce edema. These measures do not promote healing, nor do they protect the vocal folds from sustaining further damage with use.

Cocaine and topical steroids are not recommended in this situation. Although cocaine can achieve impressive decongestion, the accompanying anesthesia eliminates pain feedback, and severe vocal injury may result. Topical administration of steroids is no more effective than systemic administration, and the inhalant preparation can be irritating.

TABLE 3. **Etiology of Chronic Hoarseness**

Vocal abuse	Cancer
Allergy	Laryngeal paralysis
Chronic sinusitis	Systemic illness
Gastroesophageal reflux	Endocrine problems
Nodules	Aging
Polyps	Psychogenic factors
Contact ulcer or granuloma	Habitual misuse
Papilloma	

RECURRENT LARYNGITIS

Patients who have repeated bouts of laryngitis benefit from education in vocal hygiene or actual voice therapy. They should also be screened for contributing conditions, such as allergy, sinusitis, or gastroesophageal reflux.

CHRONIC HOARSENESS

If hoarseness lasts more than a couple of weeks, further evaluation is warranted to determine the cause (Table 3). Laryngeal cancer is primarily a disease of smokers but can affect any adult. In children, the major concern is papilloma, which can lead to airway obstruction if it is not treated. Benign lesions and chronic inflammation are far more common than tumors. The larynx may also be affected by systemic diseases, such as rheumatoid arthritis, or hormonal disorders, such as hypothyroidism or menopause.

Changes in the voice are a natural process of aging. In elderly men, the voice becomes weaker and higher in pitch owing to muscle atrophy and increased stiffness of tissues. The same changes take place in women, but the pitch actually becomes lower because of a second process. During menopause, mucoid edema accumulates in the submucosa of the vocal folds. More severe edema or even polyps occur in women who smoke.

Hoarseness that cannot be attributed to organic diseases may reflect emotional or psychiatric problems. More often, however, the problem is poor vocal habits. Either type of problem can respond well to voice therapy to improve breath support and laryngeal posture.

INSOMNIA

method of
ANDREW WINOKUR, M.D., PH.D.
*Center for Sleep and Respiratory Neurobiology,
University of Pennsylvania School of Medicine
Philadelphia, Pennsylvania*

Insomnia is a commonly encountered clinical problem that is responsible for considerable anguish and anxiety in patients seen in a variety of medical practice settings. Insomnia is associated with and complicates a number of medical and psychiatric disorders and is responsible for a significant cost to society in terms of financial impact in lost work time and productivity and in serious injuries and fatalities related to automobile crashes and industrial accidents caused by impaired functioning secondary to sleepiness. Although complaints of insomnia are common in family practice settings, the majority of patients with significant sleep problems do not report these symptoms to their physician, and recognition of clinically significant insomnia is frequently not achieved during routine office visits. This article begins with a definition of insomnia and a discussion of the public health significance of this problem. The next section reviews the clinical evaluation of insomnia, including consideration of differential diagnostic possibilities and evaluation strategies. Finally, a discussion of treatment options, both pharmacologic and nonpharmacologic, is presented.

OVERVIEW

It should be clearly noted at the outset that the term "insomnia" does not represent a specific diagnosis, but rather a description of a symptom or set of symptoms of unsatisfactory quality of sleep. Typically, complaints of insomnia relate to problems falling asleep (impaired sleep onset), problems waking up frequently during the night (impaired sleep maintenance), waking up too early in the morning (early morning awakening), or a subjective perception of unsatisfactory sleep. The subjective nature of dissatisfaction with sleep represents a significant component of the total insomnia problem. In studies comparing subjective reports by the patient of total sleep time to objective scoring of a laboratory sleep record, many instances have been observed of substantial mismatch between these parameters. Thus, a patient may report having slept only an hour during the previous night, yet be recorded by polysomnographic techniques as having been asleep for 6 hours. This fairly common situation in patients with insomnia is referred to as the "sleep state misperception syndrome." Other clinical complaints associated with poor quality sleep include reports of excessive daytime sleepiness and impaired daytime functioning. When a patient reports any of these complaints in the context of an office visit, it is important to undertake a more detailed investigation to delineate the nature of the sleep problem and to develop an appropriate differential diagnosis, implement a suitable strategy for further diagnostic evaluation, and, finally, tailor a specific treatment plan.

EPIDEMIOLOGIC ASPECTS OF INSOMNIA

A number of epidemiologic studies of insomnia have been carried out, with findings consistently indicating that approximately one third of adults experience some difficulty with sleep during the course of the year. Strikingly, about half of these individuals (i.e., approximately 17%) describe their sleep difficulties as being prominent and persistent. Several studies carried out both in the United States and in Europe have specifically examined complaints of insomnia in patients attending general medical clinics and observed comparable or even higher incidences of insomnia than have been reported in general population surveys. Yet, as reported in a Gallup Poll survey involving 700 patients with insomnia, most patients with sleep difficulties do not discuss these problems with their physicians, and very few patients schedule office visits specifically because of concerns about insomnia. This limited detection of the widespread problem of insomnia is particularly distressing when considered in the context of estimates of the cost to society of untreated insomnia. From strictly eco-

TABLE 1. **Classification of Insomnia on the Basis of Duration of Symptoms**

Transient insomnia: up to several days
Short-term insomnia: up to 3 wk
Chronic insomnia: longer than 3 wk

nomic perspectives, the cost of insomnia has been estimated to be approximately $100 billion per year, with sleepiness-related motor vehicle accidents accounting for a cost of some $50 billion annually. Moreover, such financial estimates do not take into account the cost in terms of human suffering and lost potential in productivity of this treatable yet commonly undiagnosed medical problem.

RECOGNITION AND ASSESSMENT OF INSOMNIA

On the basis of the prevalence and importance of insomnia as a public health problem, it seems appropriate to propose that physicians in primary care settings routinely include specific questions about sleep in all clinical interviews. It is advisable to follow up a general inquiry about a patient's satisfaction with sleep by asking about problems falling asleep, about awakening during the night, about feeling rested and refreshed on arising in the morning, and about level of alertness during the day. If the patient reports problems with any or several of these symptoms, more detailed investigation regarding possible significant sleep-related problems is warranted, as discussed later. For example, it is important to define the chronicity of the sleep symptoms. Convention in the sleep field has involved classifying the duration of insomnia into categories of transient, short term, and chronic (Table 1).

ESTABLISHING THE ETIOLOGY OF INSOMNIA

Once a significant manifestation of insomnia has been established, it is important to attempt to identify the underlying etiology rather than simply prescribing a sedative hypnotic medication to treat the symptoms. In cases of transient or short-term insomnia, acute situational stresses may often be identified that provide adequate explanation for the development of the sleep problem. Moreover, identification of such situational stresses often leads to the formulation of relatively straightforward strategies for effectively coping with the sleep disorder. For patients with chronic insomnia, on the other hand, precipitating stresses may not be readily identifiable, and even in cases in which an initiating stress can be identified, many subsequent physiologic and psychologic factors may have intervened to maintain and even amplify the sleep difficulties.

Many factors may be associated with the initiation or perpetuation of chronic insomnia (Table 2). For example, careful assessment of the patient's daily schedule and cus-

TABLE 2. **Causes of Insomnia**

Stress
Sleep schedule
Indiscretions of sleep hygiene guidelines
Medical disorders
Medications and ingested substances
Lifestyle and circadian rhythm factors
Psychiatric disorders
Primary sleep disorders

TABLE 3. **Sleep Hygiene Guidelines**

Maintain a regular sleep-wake schedule
Avoid naps during the day
Exercise earlier in the day, not in the evening
Avoid alcohol or caffeine consumption in the evening
Avoid heavy or spicy meals too close to bedtime
Have some time for winding down and relaxing before bedtime
Evaluate the conditions of the bedroom to optimize the
    environment for sleep

tomary patterns may shed light on the origin of the sleep problems. Violation of good sleep hygiene guidelines (as reviewed in Table 3) can lead to chronically disrupted sleep patterns. Specific examples of common sleep hygiene deficiencies include irregular sleep schedule, daytime napping, eating a heavy or spicy meal close to bedtime, and exercising vigorously late in the day. In addition, many medical problems may be associated with sleep disruption, including thyroid disorders, gastritis or peptic ulcer disease, and any medical condition associated with chronic pain. Various drugs used to treat other medical problems may produce disrupted sleep patterns, significant examples including sympathomimetic agents, beta blockers, and selective serotonin reuptake inhibitors. It is also important to ask about consumed agents that may alter sleep patterns, including caffeine-containing substances, alcohol, and various recreational drugs. Disturbances in circadian rhythms can underlie complaints of insomnia or nonrestorative sleep. Contemporary lifestyles include numerous situations in which circadian rhythms may be severely strained, such as shift work and jet travel across time zones. Environmental stimuli may also jeopardize well-consolidated sleep patterns. Thus, it is important to inquire about conditions in the bedroom, such as noise, excessive light, or uncomfortable ambient temperature.

An important category to consider in the differential diagnosis of insomnia is psychiatric disorders. Because insomnia is a symptom, not a diagnosis, it must be emphasized that insomnia is a common symptom associated with many psychiatric disorders. In one study involving more than 800 patients with insomnia, 40% were found to have a psychiatric disorder as well, most commonly an anxiety disorder (26%) or depression (14%). From a different perspective, patients with depression usually demonstrate insomnia as a prominent clinical feature. Although early morning awakening has been cited as the most distinctive sleep complaint of depression, initial insomnia (prolonged sleep latency) and middle insomnia (increased number of awakenings during the night) are often observed in depression as well. Moreover, depressed patients often describe sleep as being nonrestorative. In a general practice setting, a vitally important diagnostic challenge is to identify the presence of coexisting depression in the context of insomnia, because some patients focus on their sleep complaints and deny or minimize symptoms of mood disorder per se. In such circumstances, the physician may prescribe a sedative hypnotic drug but may not recommend appropriate treatment for the mood disorder itself. This scenario can lead to a situation in which the insomnia portion of the patient's symptoms is reduced, but effective treatment for the depressive disorder is not initiated. Because clinical depression can be associated with a substantial risk for suicide, potentially tragic consequences can ensue from a treatment approach that is not appropriately broad and well integrated.

A final category that must be considered in the evaluation of insomnia involves a range of primary sleep disorders that are commonly associated with complaints of insomnia, nonrestorative sleep, or excessive daytime sleepiness. Foremost among these primary sleep disorders are obstructive sleep apnea syndrome and periodic leg movement disorder (formerly referred to as nocturnal myoclonus). In the case of both of these disorders, it may be appropriate to have the patient undergo polysomnographic studies to confirm a diagnosis that can be suspected only on the basis of clinical history alone.

TREATMENT OF INSOMNIA

General Comments

As discussed earlier, the foundation of appropriate treatment for insomnia involves making a concerted effort to establish a specific etiologic basis for the sleep problem. In many cases, establishing a causative foundation for the insomnia can then lead to the implementation of a specific and effective treatment strategy. For example, if the sleep problem is found to represent a complication of a medical disorder such as hyperthyroidism, correction of the primary endocrinologic disorder may lead to restoration of normal sleep patterns. When insomnia represents a symptom of underlying major depressive disorder, appropriate antidepressant therapy may lead to improved sleep consolidation in conjunction with elevated mood state. To provide another example, insomnia occurring as a result of sleep hygiene violations or circadian rhythm disruptions (e.g., shift work, jet lag) may respond readily to behavioral modification interventions to remedy these specific circumstances.

It must also be acknowledged that no specific causative factor may be identified in a substantial number of patients with insomnia (perhaps in 50% of cases). In such cases, it is necessary to undertake a treatment plan for a problem that may be viewed as idiopathic insomnia, both to provide some symptomatic relief to the individual suffering with this condition and to break a potentially escalating cycle of sleep disturbance. In general, treatment approaches for idiopathic insomnia are grouped under categories of nonpharmacologic therapy techniques and medication approaches, as discussed in the following sections.

Nonpharmacologic Therapy Techniques

A variety of therapy approaches have been proposed for relief of insomnia (Table 4). Although some of these approaches are probably most appropriately implemented by a specialist in the field of sleep disor-

TABLE 4. **Nonpharmacologic Treatments
for Insomnia**

Sleep hygiene guidelines	Cognitive therapy
Stimulus control	Sleep restriction therapy
Relaxation techniques	Psychotherapy

ders medicine, aspects of several of these techniques can readily be utilized in a family practice setting.

Sleep Hygiene Guidelines. Reviewing with a patient some of the basic elements of proper sleep hygiene can often help to elicit some behavioral changes that may favorably effect sleep patterns. Discussion of sleep hygiene practices can often be carried out in the context of asking a patient with complaints of insomnia to keep a detailed sleep diary for a limited period (e.g., 2 weeks) and then reviewing the information in the diary with the patient. A patient may not be aware of or may have a blind spot about certain behavioral patterns (e.g., irregular bedtime schedule, excess caffeine consumption) that may lead to significant sleep disruption. It often makes sense to attack a complicated sleep disorder by focusing initially on discrete and readily correctable components of the problem.

Stimulus Control. This approach involves some straightforward behavior modification strategies designed both to help reduce the likelihood of experiencing insomnia and to provide the patient with some easily implemented coping methods to help reduce the severity and frustration of episodes of insomnia. Basic elements of the stimulus control method are listed in Table 5. These techniques can effectively be integrated with practical advice about sleep hygiene practices and may be quite useful for some patients. However, for patients with more severe degrees of insomnia, the contributions of sleep hygiene, behavior modification, and stimulus control techniques may be useful components but, by themselves, not sufficiently effective therapeutic modalities.

Relaxation Techniques. A variety of methods, including biofeedback techniques, meditation, and deep muscle relaxation techniques, contain elements in common, including attempting to foster the individual's ability to maintain and enhance a sense of relaxation in the face of potentially increased arousal levels. Although some patients may benefit from working formally with a therapist trained in relaxation techniques, many patients may be able to benefit from a largely self-directed course of relaxation therapy carried out under the general supervision of the primary physician. A variety of self-help materials (e.g., books and tapes) are available to guide an individual in the use of relaxation techniques. Relaxation techniques are generally not effective in directly inducing sleep in patients with insomnia, but these techniques can be quite helpful in allowing the patient to obtain a sense of mastery in inducing a state of heightened relaxation.

Cognitive Therapy. Cognitive therapy was originally developed for application in the treatment of depression, and this modality has been widely accepted as an effective intervention for this indication. Cognitive therapy techniques have been utilized with good results in the treatment of other disorders as well, most notably for various anxiety disorders. The elements of cognitive therapy involve first helping the patient to identify the negatively skewed thought patterns (i.e., cognitions) that typically accompany depression, such as thoughts of helplessness, hopelessness, and low self-esteem. It is believed that the ongoing flood of such negative cognition actually becomes an important component in sustaining and exacerbating the depressive phase. Once the patient has become adept at recognizing the negative cognitions, the next stage in the application of cognitive therapy involves teaching the patient strategies to counter these cognitions, thus neutralizing their pervasive impact.

The use of at least a modified form of cognitive therapy is helpful for virtually all patients suffering with significant insomnia. Most patients with insomnia have some exaggerated and negative cognitions about the meaning of their sleep problem in terms of dire health consequences, the potential for developing even more severe problems (e.g., "I might go crazy"), or other thoughts of catastrophe. Teaching a patient with insomnia to recognize and balance out these distressing negative cognitions often represents a critical step in undoing the potentially vicious circle of insomnia. Frequently, elements of cognitive therapy will be integrated with one or more of the other intervention strategies reviewed in this article. In some cases, referral for a specific, concentrated course of cognitive therapy (often lasting 10 to 12 sessions) is appropriate.

Sleep Restriction Therapy. This technique for insomnia is quite demanding but may be highly effective for some patients. In the application of sleep restriction therapy, the patient and therapist agree on an initial period, set to be deliberately short, that the patient will spend in bed. For example, the starting schedule may require the patient to go to bed at 1 AM and to get up at 6 AM allowing a maximum of 5 hours of sleep. Through the rest of the day, the patient is expected to be up and active, with no napping allowed. This expectation is maintained regardless of how much sleep the patient actually obtains in the 1 AM to 6 AM period. The efficacy of sleep restriction therapy rests on the well-established physiologic need for sleep and the recognition that exposure to sleep deprivation strikingly increases the need for sleep (increases *sleep pressure*). In the context of a sleep restriction therapy paradigm, many of the psychologic barriers that typically prevent sleep from occurring in a tired individual with insomnia are

---

TABLE 5. **Stimulus Control**

Go to bed only when sleepy

Get out of bed and go to a different room and engage in a quiet relaxing activity if unable to fall asleep within a reasonable time interval (e.g., 20 min)

Do not watch television in the bedroom

Get up at a consistent time each morning

Do not nap during the day

Use the bed only for sleep and sexual relations

From Bootzin RR, Perlis MD: Nonpharmacologic treatments of insomnia. The Journal of Clinical Psychiatry *53*(Suppl):37–41, 1992. Copyright 1992, Physicians Postgraduate Press. Reprinted by permission.

removed. Once the individual has developed solid sleep patterns (e.g., sleeping at least 90% of the time) on the initial sleep schedule, the allowed sleep interval is gradually increased. Although this treatment approach requires a high degree of the patient's compliance and persistence and can be rather stressful, it has been found to be quite effective in many individuals with otherwise treatment-refractory insomnia.

Psychotherapy. For some individuals, insomnia occurs in the context of significant psychosocial stressors or personality problems. In such cases, referral for psychotherapy may represent a critical component of the overall treatment strategy. It is quite evident that failing to identify and deal with underlying stresses and psychologic problems is likely to make the patient susceptible to repeated patterns of sleep difficulties.

Pharmacologic Treatment Option

A number of classes of pharmacologic agents have been utilized in the treatment of insomnia, including barbiturates, antipsychotic agents, antihistaminic compounds, chloral hydrate, and the sedating antidepressants (e.g., amitriptyline [Elavil], doxepin [Sinequan], trazodone [Desyrel]). However, many of these drugs have not been demonstrated to have efficacy in the treatment of insomnia, are associated with unacceptable side effects, or both. Much publicity has been directed at the use of melatonin to treat insomnia and some circadian rhythm disorders. Few studies to date have characterized the efficacy of melatonin in the treatment of insomnia, and this compound has not yet been approved for this indication by the Food and Drug Administration. Moreover, the use of at least higher doses of melatonin could be associated with some significant side effect problems, such as suppression of the gonadotropic axis. There does appear to be interesting potential for melatonin or melatonin analogues in the treatment of insomnia or circadian rhythm disorders.

To date, the most widely employed pharmacologic treatments for insomnia have included several of the benzodiazepine compounds and the imidazopyridines. Five benzodiazepines have been evaluated specifically for the treatment of insomnia: triazolam (Halcion), temazepam (Restoril), quazepam (Doral), estazolam (ProSom), and flurazepam (Dalmane). These drugs differ primarily on the basis of half-life (e.g., triazolam is very short acting; flurazepam has a markedly long duration of action) and presence or absence of active metabolites. Familiarity with information about such pharmacokinetic properties of the various benzodiazepine sedative hypnotics may help the physician select one of these options that best suits the needs of a particular patient. To date, only one compound is available in the imidazopyridine category: the short half-life drug zolpidem (Ambien). All of these sedative hypnotic compounds have been demonstrated to be effective in the treatment of insomnia, both by reducing sleep latency (time to fall asleep) and by improving sleep continuity (reduction in nocturnal awakenings).

In general, the sedative hypnotic compounds cited previously all have a relatively benign side effect profile, with the most commonly reported side effects being daytime sedation and ataxia. Caution should be given to the combined use of alcohol and a benzodiazepine sedative hypnotic drug. In addition, because the benzodiazepines have the potential to suppress respiration, these compounds should be avoided in patients with obstructive sleep apnea. Long-term use of benzodiazepine compounds has been reported to be associated with problems with dependence and withdrawal. Thus, it is preferable to limit the duration of treatment with the benzodiazepines. Some suggestions have appeared that zolpidem has lower abuse liability, but further studies are needed to evaluate this possibility.

Conventional guidelines suggest that sedative-hypnotic therapy should be limited to a duration of 4 weeks. It should be noted, however, that some patients with chronic, severe insomnia expect and may require treatment for a considerably longer time. In such cases, the physician must make a considered judgment about the advisability of recommending long-term sedative hypnotic therapy. In a patient who is being treated with a benzodiazepine sedative hypnotic drug for a prolonged period, care must be taken to avoid abrupt discontinuation of the drug regimen.

In summary, the hallmark of effective treatment for insomnia is the identification of symptoms of a sleep problem, careful evaluation of factors underlying the insomnia, development of a specific diagnosis, and then implementation of a treatment program that may involve integration of pharmacologic and other treatment modalities.

PRURITUS
(Itching)

method of
JEFFREY D. BERNHARD, M.D.
University of Massachusetts Medical School
Worcester, Massachusetts

Pruritus (itching) is an unpleasant sensation that evokes the inclination to scratch. Itching is the most common symptom of skin diseases and may also be troublesome in patients without any visible signs of a primary skin problem. The pathophysiologic mechanism of pruritus is incompletely understood. Depending on the disease or trigger factors, different mediators may be involved in the itch sensation. Histamine is an important itch mediator (e.g., in urticaria), but prostaglandins, leukotrienes, vasoactive and neuroactive peptides, kinins, and opioid peptides may contribute to itching in different disease states. This explains why antihistamines (aside from soporific effects) are helpful in urticaria but are ineffective for most other patients with pruritus. Accurate diagnosis is essential for selecting either symptomatic or definitive treatment of itching.

DIAGNOSIS

Before symptomatic therapy for pruritus is initiated, a systematic approach to diagnosis should be undertaken. This can be conducted in a stepwise fashion. If skin disease is present, look for primary lesions that have not been scratched. Are there papules or vesicles? Is there dermatographism (a linear "hive") at the site of scratching? Is the skin dry and scaly? In a patient with acute itching, the most commonly associated skin diseases are urticaria, contact dermatitis, scabies, insect bites, and dry skin. The list of skin disorders that can cause pruritus is extensive and is summarized in Table 1. Many of these disorders have diagnostic clinical appearances, although they may be camouflaged by the effects of rubbing and scratching. Historical points, such as exposure to outside agents (e.g., poison ivy, fiberglass), affected family members (e.g., scabies), drug ingestion, or flea-infested pets, may be helpful in establishing the diagnosis. Overbathing and low ambient humidity (as in heated air in winter) may point to xerosis (dry skin). If a rash is present but is not recognizable, dermatologic consultation should be sought to help establish a specific diagnosis. A skin biopsy may be considered at that point.

When diagnostic primary skin lesions are not present or only nonspecific changes such as secondary eczematization or scratch marks (excoriations) are seen, the possibility that a systemic condition could be causing the pruritus must be considered. This situation can be difficult and perplexing, because skin diseases that have diagnostic primary lesions can sometimes be camouflaged by the effects of rubbing and scratching as well. Chronic renal failure,

TABLE 1. Selected Skin Disorders Associated with Pruritus

Common (Often Acute)

Asteatosis (xerosis, dry skin, "winter itch")
Contact dermatitis (irritant and allergic)
Scabies, pediculosis
Insect bites, flea bites
Urticaria, dermatographism
Varicella
Pityriasis rosea
Sunburn
Miliaria rubra (prickly heat)
Drug hypersensitivity

Common (Often Subacute or Chronic)

Atopic dermatitis (eczema)
Psoriasis
Dermatophytosis (ringworm)
Folliculitis
Lichen planus
Lichen simplex chronicus
Other physical urticarias (e.g., cold, solar, pressure)
Diminutive variants of urticaria (e.g., aquagenic pruritus)

Uncommon or Rare

Dermatitis herpetiformis
Bullous pemphigoid
Polymorphic light eruption
Mycosis fungoides (cutaneous T cell lymphoma)
Mastocytosis
Exfoliative dermatitis
Prurigo nodularis

TABLE 2. Selected Systemic Conditions That May Be Associated with Generalized Pruritus

Condition	Suggested Laboratory Tests
Chronic renal failure	Urinalysis, blood urea nitrogen, creatinine
Cholestatic liver disease	Bilirubin, alkaline phosphatase, aspartate aminotransferase
Hematologic disease	Complete blood count, differential, ferritin
Hyperthyroidism	Thyroid panel
Occult malignant disease (e.g., Hodgkin's disease)	Chest x-ray study (other work-up as indicated by history or physical examination)
Drug reaction	
Infestations, parasitosis	
Pregnancy	
Human immunodeficiency virus (HIV) infection	HIV test
Psychiatric illness	

cholestatic liver disease, hematologic disease, malignant disease (especially Hodgkin's disease), and hyperthyroidism are among the most important and frequent *systemic* causes of generalized pruritus. The history and general physical examination are critically important. Special attention should be paid to constitutional symptoms and to adenopathy and organomegaly. Table 2 lists some of the systemic illnesses that cause itching and an approach to screening laboratory studies. Such a work-up may be indicated in a patient without a diagnosed skin disease who has generalized pruritus occurring daily for more than 2 weeks (pruritus of undetermined origin). Tests should be tailored to the individual patient's presentation. Because human immunodeficiency virus (HIV) infection and acquired immune deficiency syndrome may lead to itching or to exacerbation of pruritic skin diseases, HIV testing may be indicated in some cases.

The possibility of drug-induced itching should not be overlooked. Opiate analgesic agents (e.g., morphine) may cause severe itching without skin lesions. Other drugs that may cause itching include aspirin; quinidine; B-complex vitamins; and drugs that can cause hepatic cholestasis, such as phenothiazines, hormones, and erythromycin estolate (Ilosone). The most common forms of localized pruritus, pruritus ani and pruritus vulvae, are discussed in another article.

SYMPTOMATIC TREATMENT

General Education of the Patient and Topical Therapy

Some environmental factors can make itching worse, no matter what the underlying cause. Skin that is dry is more prone to itching, so that the frequency of bathing should be decreased, deodorant soaps should be discontinued, and milder products such as Dove or Cetaphil cleanser should be substituted. Emollients, moisturizing lotions, and bath oils should be employed whenever dryness may be a trigger factor, even if it is not the only or major cause of itching. The temperature of the bath should not be too hot, because it may temporarily bring relief only to cause the itch to worsen afterward. The addition of baking soda, up to 1 cup per tub bath, or oilated oatmeal bath products (Aveeno) can also be soothing. Older patients should be cautioned about getting into or out of a slippery tub. Towel drying should be done by patting rather than vigorous rubbing. Use of a bath oil or moisturizer applied immediately after bathing to help retain moisture in the skin may also help. Fragrance-free products such as Eucerin cream, DML lotion, fragrance-free Lubriderm, LactiCare, and Vaseline are useful examples. Increasing humidity in the patient's environment through the use of a humidifier or open pans of water may help. Irritating fabrics such as wool and some textured synthetics should be avoided. The use of antistatic fabric softeners that are added to the dryer cycle should be discontinued because these products have been anecdotally associated with itching.

Heat triggers itching, so the patient with pruritus should avoid excessively warm environments by lowering the thermostat, using fewer bed covers, or reducing exercise temporarily. Reduced intake of hot spicy foods, alcohol, and caffeine may be helpful. Emotional stress may also worsen itching of any cause, and patients should be made aware of that fact.

Availability of specific topical treatment of pruritus is limited. Over-the-counter treatments containing anesthetics (such as benzocaine) or antihistamines (diphenhydramine [Benadryl]) should be avoided, because these products can cause contact dermatitis in some individuals. Doxepin (Zonalon) cream can be helpful in localized areas of eczematous dermatitis, but contact dermatitis from this antihistamine can also occur. Preparations containing pramoxine (PrameGel, Prax) or those containing combinations of menthol and camphor (Sarna Anti-Itch), applied several times daily, may give symptomatic relief. When inflammation accompanies xerosis, lotions that also contain hydrocortisone (LactiCare-HC, Sarnol-HC) can be helpful. The addition of a mild or medium-strength corticosteroid cream twice daily for 5 or 6 days is sometimes necessary. The use of more potent topical corticosteroids should be reserved for patients with diagnosed steroid-responsive inflammatory dermatoses, such as psoriasis and acute contact dermatitis. (See specific articles on skin disease.) Topical corticosteroids are not helpful for patients with urticaria. Find out whatever topical products a patient is using, so as not to overlook a subtle contact dermatitis from misguided treatment as a cause of the pruritus.

SYSTEMIC THERAPY

Oral antihistamines are most helpful in histamine-mediated disorders such as urticaria but may also alleviate itching through their sedative effects; for this purpose, traditional agents such as diphenhydramine (Benadryl) and hydroxyzine (Atarax, Vistaril) are often employed. Antihistamines are more helpful if they are taken in adequate dosage at regular intervals, rather than on an as-needed basis. Bed-

time dosing is useful, because itching is often worse at bedtime, and dosages may be increased to tolerance (sedation, dry mouth) under supervision. If no relief is obtained, switching to another type of antihistamine or combining agents of different chemical classes may be helpful. Nonsedating or low-sedating antihistamines such as fexofenadine (Allegra, 60 mg every 12 hours), astemizole (Hismanal, 10 mg at bedtime), and loratadine (Claritin, 10 mg once daily) are useful in chronic urticaria. It takes 6 days for astemizole to reach steady-state plasma concentrations, and thus it is not useful acutely. Loratadine has a rapid onset of action, usually within 2 hours. The nonsedating or low-sedating antihistamines may be suggested for patients in whom there is great concern about sedating side effects of other antihistamines, but they are of limited efficacy for acute itching in my experience. When terfenadine or astemizole is used, possible interactions with other drugs (e.g., erythromycin, ketoconazole) must be avoided. The precise role of some of the newest antihistamines, such as cetirizine (Zyrtec) and fexofenadine remains to be seen, but one advantage is a lower risk for cardiovascular side effects.

Other systemic agents for the treatment of itching should be reserved until a specific diagnosis has been made. Systemic corticosteroids should not be used because they are ineffective, have side effects, and may mask the underlying diagnosis. Tricyclic antidepressant agents, such as doxepin (Sinequan),* have antihistamine properties that may be useful at times and are administered in oral dosages of 10 to 25 mg up to three times daily or in a total dose at bedtime. H_2-histamine antagonists such as cimetidine (Tagamet)* may be useful in treating the itching associated with Hodgkin's disease. Oral cholestyramine (Questran)* may be helpful in controlling itching due to hepatic and sometimes renal disease. At my medical center, ultraviolet B phototherapy is the treatment of choice for itching experienced by some hemodialysis-dependent patients with chronic renal failure and has been helpful in controlling pruritus in some other situations. PUVA (oral methoxsalen photochemotherapy) may be helpful in some patients with severe atopic dermatitis and may be indicated in certain other conditions. It is in the patient's interest to see a dermatologist whenever the diagnosis remains unclear or initial treatment is not effective.†

---

*Not FDA approved for this indication.
†See Bernhard JD: Itch: Mechanisms and Management of Pruritus. New York, McGraw-Hill, 1994.

TINNITUS

method of
JOHN W. HOUSE, M.D.
House Ear Clinic
Los Angeles, California

Tinnitus is a symptom of one or more sounds perceived by the patient in the absence of an external source of the sound. It may be perceived in one ear, in both ears, or in the head. It is important for the physician to know that this is a symptom and not a disease. Tinnitus is usually benign but may represent serious underlying disease. It is most commonly associated with hearing loss, and about 80% of patients with some degree of hearing loss have tinnitus. The tinnitus may be constant, intermittent, steady state, or pulsatile. The frequency of the tinnitus is variable from one patient to another and may vary within the same patient. At times, it may be barely perceptible or may be described as quite loud. There are two types of tinnitus, objective and subjective.

OBJECTIVE TINNITUS

This type of tinnitus can typically be heard by an observer. Objective tinnitus may be of vascular or muscular origin. Vascular tinnitus may arise from either venous or arterial causes or from vascular tumors, such as glomus tympanicum or glomus jugulare tumors. The arterial causes include conditions that produce turbulent flow, such as arterial sclerosis associated with aging, anemia, hyperthyroidism, Paget's disease, aberrant carotid artery, or arteriovenous malformation. The venous causes include a large or exposed jugular bulb on one side and benign intracranial hypertension. The venous-type tinnitus is easily differentiated from arterial if the sound can be stopped or reduced when light pressure is applied over the internal jugular vein on the involved side. Evaluation includes radiographic and ultrasound studies, as indicated. Computed tomography with contrast enhancement and bone program are helpful in identifying erosive lesions or tumors. Magnetic resonance angiography (MRA) and magnetic resonance venography (MRV) are helpful in defining vascular lesions or aberrant vessels. Standard angiography is being performed less often because of the effectiveness of MRA, MRV, and ultrasound studies. This type of tinnitus responds well to treatment aimed at the vascular lesion or correction of the anemia or hyperthyroidism.

Myoclonic activity of the stapedius muscle, the tensor tympani muscle, or the palatal muscle is the cause of muscular tinnitus. This type of tinnitus is characterized by brief periods of clicking, popping, or banging sounds in the ear. Palatal myoclonus can be differentiated from the other types by observing rhythmic contractions of the soft palate that are synchronous with the patient's sounds. While observing the palate, it is important not to have the patient open the mouth widely because this usually stops the myoclonus. It may be possible to observe movement of the tympanic membrane with either the microscope or the tympanometer. Treatment is often successful and is aimed at the offending muscle. By cutting the tendon to the stapedius or tensor tympani muscle, the symptoms are relieved. If the cause is palatal muscle, treatment is more difficult and palliative. Prescribing muscle relaxants or performing myringotomy with tubes may help.

SUBJECTIVE TINNITUS

The majority of tinnitus is subjective, that is, only the patient is able to hear the sound. It is usually associated with some type of hearing loss. In my experience, about 90% of tinnitus patients have a sensorineural hearing loss, about 5% a conductive hearing loss, and about 5% normal hearing.

Because tinnitus is a symptom, the underlying cause must be determined by a history, physical examination, audiogram, and any additional tests that are indicated.

The physical examination includes otoscopy and, at times, auscultation and palpation around the ear and neck. The remainder of the head and neck examination is performed. Tuning fork tests (Rinne and Weber) are routinely performed to determine whether the hearing loss is conductive or sensorineural. The possible causes of a conductive hearing loss with tinnitus are cerumen impaction, otitis externa, otitis media (acute and chronic), chronic otitis media with effusion (serous otitis), and otosclerosis. Some of the causes of sensorineural hearing loss associated with tinnitus include presbycusis (age-related hearing loss); noise-induced hearing loss; ototoxic medications; sudden hearing loss due to either vascular or viral causes; Meniere's disease; and cerebellopontine angle tumors (acoustic neuroma or meningiomas), which are usually associated with unilateral symptoms (hearing loss with or without tinnitus). Patients with unilateral complaints need a neuro-otologic evaluation, such as auditory brain stem audiometry or magnetic resonance imaging with gadolinium enhancement, to rule out a tumor. A blood work-up may be indicated if there is a fluctuating or rapidly progressive hearing loss associated with the tinnitus. This would include a complete blood count with erythrocyte sedimentation rate, a fluorescent treponemal antibody test, and possibly an antinuclear antibody test. These tests are performed to rule out syphilitic or autoimmune hearing loss.

TREATMENT

Because tinnitus is a symptom and not a disease, no single treatment is effective for all. Victor Goodhill, M.D., in 1950 put it very well: "Any management which is based upon a single panacea for the treatment of a symptom and not a disease will result in failure." The important steps in the management of the patient with tinnitus are the evaluation, the examination, and the explanation. The explanation can be of great help when it is accompanied by reassurance that the tinnitus does not represent serious disease and that the patient is not going deaf. About 95% of the patients seen in my office who have tinnitus are not particularly bothered by it. On the other hand, 5% of the patients are driven to distraction by their tinnitus.

If the tinnitus is associated with a hearing loss, amplification with a hearing aid usually helps. The normal environmental sounds mask the tinnitus and at the same time improve the patient's hearing. At night, a noise generator, fan, air conditioner, or radio tuned between stations (to get a static sound) can help mask the tinnitus. Tinnitus maskers are wearable devices that generate sound to help mask the tinnitus. These have limited success in helping reduce the tinnitus. For patients with tinnitus and a hearing loss who find that a masker or hearing aid alone is not helpful, a tinnitus instrument (combination hearing aid and masker) can help to both mask the tinnitus and provide amplification. A promising new tinnitus treatment is auditory habituation as proposed and developed by Pawel Jastreboff, Ph.D., in Baltimore. This involves retraining the auditory system to ignore the tinnitus sounds. Therapeutic noise devices emit stable broadband noise that is softer than the patient's tinnitus. The theory is not to cover the tinnitus but to help the patient learn to ignore it. This training takes time (as long as 1 year), and the technique is in its early stages of development.

I found that for about 80% of a selected group of patients, biofeedback training helps reduce the tinnitus by teaching the patient relaxation techniques. Muscle tension and stress worsen the perceived tinnitus.

Many medications have been tried through the years. There is no single medication that works uniformly in reducing tinnitus. Both my group and Robert Dobie have found that antidepressants are effective in some patients. Most of our severe tinnitus sufferers have sleep problems, are anxious, and are depressed. Small doses of either amitriptyline (Elavil) or nortriptyline (Pamelor) given at bedtime seem to help the patient get through the night and reduce the aggravation of the tinnitus during the day.

Other medications that can help include antianxiety agents such as alprazolam (Xanax), clonazepam (Klonopin), and diazepam (Valium). Because of the potential for abuse and dependence, I rarely prescribe this category of medication.

Additional medications that have been mentioned as possibly helping tinnitus are listed in Table 1. I recently completed a double-blind study using a combination of *Ginkgo biloba* extract, magnesium, and vitamin B_{12} and found that the active treatment group did no better than the placebo group.

In conclusion, there is no sure cure for tinnitus. Many patients have tinnitus, but most learn to ignore it. Most patients find that after an evaluation and explanation with reassurance, they can live with it and learn to ignore it. There is no magic cure, but many avenues of treatment are available to help the patient cope with and overcome the problem of tinnitus.

TABLE 1. Medications That Have Been Proposed to Help Tinnitus*

Anesthetics

Lidocaine (Xylocaine); IV—temporary relief in about 80%
Procaine (Novocain)
Tocainide (Tonocard); oral lidocaine analogue
Flecainide (Tambocor)
Mexiletine (Mexitil); oral lidocaine analogue

Anticonvulsants

Carbamazepine (Tegretol)
Phenytoin (Dilantin)
Primidone (Mysoline)

Diuretics (in Meniere's Disease)

Hydrochlorothiazide with triamterene (Dyazide)

Vitamins and Herbs

Niacin
Misoprostol (synthetic prostaglandin)
Magnesium
Vitamin B_{12}
Ginkgo biloba extract

*Results are inconsistent. None of these drugs is approved by the FDA for this indication.

LOW BACK PAIN

method of
STEPHEN I. ESSES, M.D.
Baylor College of Medicine
Houston, Texas

Musculoskeletal complaints are the most common reason for patients to seek consultation from their primary care physician. Low back pain is the most common musculoskeletal symptom in that group of patients. It is estimated that 80% of adults in North America will have at least one episode of low back pain sufficiently severe that they lose time from work. The cost of low back pain in the United States as a result of time lost from work and permanent disability is estimated to be $75 billion per year.

ACUTE LOW BACK PAIN

In contrast to the situation with patients presenting with other symptoms, it is not usually necessary to make a specific diagnosis for those patients presenting simply with acute low back pain. The Quebec Task Force on Spinal Disorders has classified disorders of the lumbar spine on the basis of symptoms rather than etiology. Class 1 and class 2 disorders are characterized by low back pain without radiation or by low back pain with radiation to the proximal extremity. It is important for the physician to take a detailed history. Specifically, it is necessary to ensure that the patient does not have any systemic symptoms indicative of an infective or neoplastic process. It is important to ensure that there are no unusual symptoms and to confirm that the low back pain is activity related. Class 1 and class 2 disorders are typically mechanical. Patients feel better at rest, and symptoms are exacerbated by bending, twisting, and lifting.

Assuming that the history is compatible with a diagnosis of a class 1 or class 2 disorder, a thorough physical examination is carried out. A note should be made of any unusual finding. A thorough neurologic examination is crucial. Class 1 and class 2 disorders are not associated with nerve root tension signs or with any neurologic deficits. The low back examination is accompanied by evaluation of the hip, sacroiliac, and knee joints.

Many studies have shown that acute low back pain is usually a limited process. Symptoms can be expected to resolve in 80% of patients within 4 to 6 weeks. It is not certain whether any specific modality can accelerate this process. The purpose of initiating treatment is to provide symptomatic relief and to prevent retardation of the healing process.

The triad of treatment is activity modification, physical modalities, and medication. Whereas activity modification often consisted of prolonged bed rest in the past, it is now generally agreed that bed rest should not be instituted for more than 48 hours. Prolonged bed restriction can slow recovery and may lead to debilitation. Patients should be instructed in postural differences. That is, they should understand that sitting may place more stress on the low back than standing or lying. They should understand that forward flexion may increase low back loads. Patients should be encouraged to assume whatever position provides them with maximal comfort. Myriad physical modalities have been advocated for the treatment of acute low back pain. Most are not justified by scientific study. There is good evidence that cryotherapy and heat, in conjunction with exercise, are of some benefit. Therefore, it may be reasonable to recommend a short course of supervised physical therapy to specifically educate the patient how to use heat and cold options at home together with an exercise program. Three groups of medications may be of value in the treatment of acute low back pain: analgesics, nonsteroidal anti-inflammatory agents, and muscle relaxants. For most patients, acetaminophen or aspirin is sufficient in relieving low back symptoms. For those individuals in whom stronger analgesics are necessary, some caution should be exercised. Opioids should be given for only a short time, and patients should be warned about side effects. There are more than 30 nonsteroidal anti-inflammatory agents currently approved by the Food and Drug Administration for use in the United States. This is due, in part, to the fact that response is idiosyncratic. These anti-inflammatories can be subclassified into nine chemical groups. An organized methodical approach to the use of these agents is advised. If a patient does not have significant benefit from an anti-inflammatory within 2 or 3 days, further use of this agent will be of little benefit. Therefore, it is reasonable to switch the patient to a nonsteroidal anti-inflammatory from another chemical class. Some of these agents are categorized in Table 1. Up to 50% of patients taking muscle relaxants have significant complaints of drowsiness and fatigue. Nevertheless, muscle relaxants have been shown to be more effective than placebo in patients with acute low back pain symptoms.

It is important to assure the patient with acute low back pain that this is almost always a self-limited condition. It is not necessary at the time of first evaluation to pursue any imaging studies. After instructing the patient about activity modification and physical modalities and prescribing appropriate medications, it is reasonable to make arrangements for reassessment of the patient in 2 or 3 weeks. At that time, most patients will have demonstrated symptomatic improvement and treatment can be continued as appropriate. For those patients in whom there has been no symptomatic improvement, it is important to repeat the history and physical examination to ensure that there are not constitutional symptoms or abnormal physical findings. Assuming that there are not, treatment should continue with activity modification, physical modalities, and medications. The patient should be reassessed in another 2 or 3 weeks. At that point, most patients will have had significant resolution of symptoms. For those few patients in whom symptoms are still disabling, further investigation should be undertaken. That is, for those patients who continue to have significant low back pain symptoms 6 to 8 weeks after onset, an attempt should be made to provide an etiologic diagnosis. An algorithm for the management of acute low back pain is presented in Figure 1.

CHRONIC LOW BACK PAIN

In contrast to the acute situation, it is advisable for patients with chronic symptoms to be assessed in

TABLE 1. **Nonsteroidal Anti-inflammatory Agents**

Group	Chemical Name	Trade Name
Salicylates	Aspirin	Bayer
	Enteric coated	Ecotrin, Easprin
	Timed release	ZORprin
Substituted salicylates	Diflunisal	Dolobid
	Aspirin with antacid	Ascriptin
Propionic acid derivatives	Ibuprofen	Motrin, Rufen, Advil, Nuprin
	Naproxen	Naprosyn
	Naproxen sodium	Anaprox
	Fenoprofen calcium	Nalfon
	Ketoprofen	Orudis
	Flurbiprofen	Ansaid
	Oxaprozin	Daypro
Pyrrole acetic acid derivatives	Sulindac	Clinoril
	Indomethacin	Indocin
	Tolmetin sodium	Tolectin
	Diclofenac	Voltaren
	Ketorolac tromethamine	Toradol
Oxicam	Piroxicam	Feldene
Fenamate	Meclofenamate sodium	Meclomen
Pyrazolones	Phenylbutazone*	Butazolidin
Pyranocarboxylic acid	Etodolac	Lodine
Naphthylalkanones	Nabumetone	Relafen

* Not available in the United States.
From Esses SI: Textbook of Spinal Disorders. Philadelphia, JB Lippincott Co, 1995, p 144.

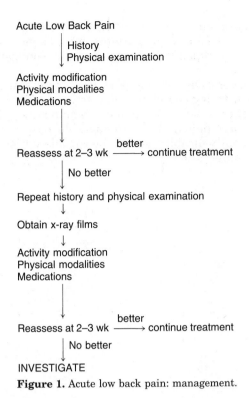

Figure 1. Acute low back pain: management.

an effort to arrive at an anatomic or etiologic diagnosis. Most instances of chronic low back pain in the adult are thought to be due to degenerative disk disease. Other causes include spondylolisthesis, spinal stenosis, herniated nucleus pulposus, and degenerative scoliosis. For the purpose of this discussion, I consider only patients with isolated back pain and exclude patients who have radicular or cauda equina symptoms.

In addition to a thorough history and physical examination, it is worthwhile to consider imaging modalities in the work-up of the chronic low back pain sufferer. However, the identification of an abnormality by radiography, computed tomography, or magnetic resonance imaging does not necessarily mean that it is the source of the symptoms. As the sensitivity of imaging studies increases, so does the number of abnormal findings that can be identified in asymptomatic individuals. The challenge to the clinician is to correlate imaging findings with the history and physical examination findings to accurately identify pain generators.

Most patients can be adequately treated by the triad of lifestyle modification, physical modalities, and medication. In terms of lifestyle modification, there is ample literature that identifies risk factors for the development of chronic low back pain. Activities and work that require prolonged sitting, activities and work that require repetitive bending, and activities and work that involve vibration have been shown to be associated with an increased frequency of chronic low back pain. It is useful, therefore, to educate the patient in an attempt to reduce these activities. In addition, the evidence is clear that smoking increases the risk for chronic low back pain. Therefore, patients need to desist from tobacco and nicotine in any form.

The mainstay of physical modalities for the patient with chronic low back pain is exercise. The frequency and severity of chronic low back pain are decreased in individuals who exhibit good cardiovascular fitness, strong abdominal musculature, and good paravertebral strength. All patients should be made aware of this and instructed to carry out a balanced, organized, and regular exercise program.

The frequency of complications from nonsteroidal anti-inflammatory agents increases with duration of use. Therefore, nonsteroidal agents are best used intermittently. They are relatively contraindicated in patients with renal insufficiency, hypertension, or gastrointestinal intolerance. Regular blood work is advised in those patients taking these medicines for more than 6 weeks.

For those patients whose symptoms are not adequately controlled by the triad of treatment described, other nonoperative options should be considered. These may include pain management techniques such as biofeedback, transcutaneous electrical nerve stimulation, acupuncture, lumbar orthoses, and manipulation.

It is reasonable to consider surgical fusion in those patients with single-level degenerative disk disease, spondylolisthesis, and degenerative scoliosis.

LEG PAIN

A clear distinction should be made between those patients presenting with back pain and those patients presenting with back and leg symptoms. If the leg complaints follow a specific dermatomal pattern, it is most likely radicular. The term radicular refers to symptoms that are of nerve root origin. Pain, numbness, and tingling radiating down the back of the leg to the medial aspect of the foot including the great toe usually indicate an L-5 radicular syndrome. Pain, cramping, or numbness in the calf and lateral aspect of the foot is usually indicative of an S-1 radiculopathy.

History taking of patients with leg symptoms should be directed at ascertaining whether the complaints are unilateral or bilateral. It is important to distinguish between claudicant pain and pain that is not made worse by walking. It is worthwhile to document the effect of postural changes on symptoms and to determine whether one root or multiple roots are involved.

The physical evaluation of the patient should consist of a careful neurologic examination. This, together with the history, can almost always localize the specific roots involved. A peripheral vascular examination is important to rule out a circulatory origin of symptoms. Nerve root tension signs often accompany herniated disk disease.

The three most important considerations in determining treatment are the degree of neurologic deficit, the duration of symptoms, and the cause of the neurologic compression. The first two can be determined by history and physical evaluation, whereas the last often requires magnetic resonance imaging.

Leg pain from a herniated nucleus pulposus can almost always be treated nonoperatively. Physical modalities, epidural steroids, nerve root block, and nonsteroidal anti-inflammatory agents can be useful in this regard. It may be reasonable to consider surgi-cal treatment in those patients with long-standing sciatica, nonsmokers, patients who do not receive workers' compensation, and patients younger than 40 years.

Nonoperative treatment is less successful in patients with leg complaints due to bony spinal stenosis. Patients with this diagnosis who have significant neurologic deficit, have intractable pain, and are functionally disabled should be considered for surgical decompression.

The Infectious Diseases

HUMAN IMMUNODEFICIENCY VIRUS INFECTION AND ITS COMPLICATIONS

method of
BRUCE POLSKY, M.D.

Memorial Sloan-Kettering Cancer Center and
Cornell University Medical College
New York, New York

Infection with the human immunodeficiency virus type 1 (HIV-1), a retrovirus, is characterized by a cellular immunodeficiency primarily affecting the number and function of CD4$^+$ cells, a subclass of T lymphocytes. The result, over a variable time, is a progressive decline in the number of CD4$^+$ cells and increased susceptibility of the infected individual to opportunistic infections and neoplasms.

Full-blown acquired immune deficiency syndrome (AIDS) in HIV-infected persons, which is defined according to criteria established by the Centers for Disease Control and Prevention (CDC), includes a diagnosis of any of a variety of infections and neoplasms, dementia, and progressive weight loss (wasting syndrome). In January 1993, the CDC AIDS surveillance case definition of AIDS for persons 13 years of age or older was expanded to include four additional conditions: (1) a CD4$^+$ cell count of less than 200 per mm^3 or a CD4$^+$ lymphocyte percentage of total lymphocytes of less than 14; (2) pulmonary tuberculosis; (3) recurrent pneumonia; and (4) invasive cervical cancer.

In 1993, HIV infection became the leading cause of death among persons aged 25 to 44 years. Between 1981, when AIDS first became a reportable disease, and 1994, a total of 441,528 cases were reported to the CDC.

Because the AIDS epidemic continues to grow, there is a renewed sense of urgency to develop new treatment strategies, both for HIV infection and for AIDS-related illnesses. Because of advances in our knowledge of the structure and metabolic pathways of HIV, it is possible to pursue a rational approach to therapy with the design of drugs that interfere with specific phases of the viral life cycle. The first antiretroviral drug, zidovudine (AZT), was approved for the treatment of HIV infection in 1987. AZT is a nucleoside analogue that inhibits the enzyme reverse transcriptase.

Since the introduction of AZT, several other nucleoside analogues with a similar mechanism of action have become available, including didanosine (ddI), zalcitabine (ddC), stavudine (d4T), and lamivudine (3TC). More recently, clinical trials of drugs that interfere with other points in the viral life cycle have begun. Among the drugs undergoing investigation are non-nucleoside reverse transcriptase inhibitors, protease inhibitors, and integrase inhibitors.

Progress has been made in the management of patients infected with HIV. It is now possible to successfully prevent and treat several of the more common opportunistic infections associated with HIV infection, and better treatment is available for the two most common neoplasms seen in this population of patients, Kaposi's sarcoma (KS) and non-Hodgkin's lymphoma. Strategies have been devised to prevent or forestall weight loss, including the use of effective drugs based on new insights into the metabolic abnormalities observed in HIV-infected individuals.

PATHOGENESIS OF HUMAN IMMUNODEFICIENCY VIRUS INFECTION

Infection with HIV-1 is characterized by a defined pattern of progression to disease. At primary infection, high titers of virion-associated RNA are detected in blood, and a relatively homogeneous population of viral genotypic variants can be found. With the onset of an HIV-1–specific cellular and then humoral response, plasma HIV-1 RNA titers decline rapidly. During the ensuing period of clinical latency, persistent viral replication can be found in blood and in lymphoid organs. The population of genetic variants diversifies owing to mutation and repetitive cycles of viral replication. In time, the immune surveillance mechanism becomes compromised and HIV-1 disease develops.

Despite this common pattern of development, the rate of progression to AIDS varies among HIV-1–infected individuals. Therefore, the persistent viral replication observed during the period of clinical latency is associated with a rapidly declining, slowly declining, or relatively stable CD4$^+$ cell count. Progression to disease has been related to the extent of viral replication, the pathogenicity of the transmitted or persistent virus, and the host immune response.

A number of hypotheses have been put forth to explain the development of AIDS, including the existence of an antigenic diversity threshold, beyond which the immune system is unable to regulate virus growth. Another hypothesis concerns the destruction of infected cells by a vigorous cell-mediated immune response; a third is based on the interplay between virus replication and the host immune response.

To understand the relationship between the virus and the host during the progression to disease, a survey was performed of virologic and immunologic parameters in serial blood samples obtained from a cohort of HIV-1–infected men and from a cohort of children with perinatal HIV-1 infection. As has been observed previously, the extent of viral replication and plasma virion-associated RNA burden at approximately 9 months after the estimated time of primary infection was directly related to the eventual rate of progression to AIDS.

Analysis of the evolution of viral genotypes during the natural history of HIV-1 infection has revealed a relationship between the extent of genetic diversity and the rate of disease progression. In each of the HIV-1–infected individuals who rapidly progressed to AIDS in the above-mentioned survey, there was a limited distribution of genotypic variants. Therefore, despite the high titers of virion-associated HIV-1 RNA in these individuals, there was little genetic variation observable over time.

A survey of cytotoxic T lymphocyte precursor frequencies elicited against proteins expressed from HIV-1 *gag, pol,* and *env* coding regions has demonstrated a direct association between a vigorous immune response and an indolent disease course. It appears, then, that the limited genetic variability and lack of an effective cytotoxic T lymphocyte–mediated immune response in individuals with a rapid rate of progression to AIDS fail to support the hypotheses that it is either antigenic variation or cytotoxic T lymphocyte–mediated immune destruction that accounts for the development of AIDS. Therefore, although high viral replication, limited genetic variation, and a weak immune response have been demonstrated to correlate with a rapid rate of progression to AIDS, the opposite (i.e., low viral replication, a great extent of genetic variation, and a vigorous immune response) correlates with a more indolent disease course.

The use of potent antiretroviral agents has provided further insights into the dynamics of viral replication during the period of clinical latency. The equilibrium achieved between the rapid destruction and replacement of CD4+ T cells, in concert with the more rapid production and clearance of viruses, characterized the interplay of the virus and the host during this time. Therapeutic interventions during this period modify this interaction by allowing the selection of a less fit variant in the population having a pre-existent mutation that confers antiretroviral resistance. Perturbation by a potent antiretroviral compound may have the ultimate consequence of modifying the rate of progression to AIDS.

In contrast, therapeutic intervention during the primary infection, when there is a relatively homogeneous population of genotypic variants, might have a more favorable impact on the virus-host interaction. Therefore, modifying viral replication at a time when there may be a relative lack of potential mutations that confer antiretroviral resistance could change the equilibrium between T cell loss and production. This has the potential of allowing the immune surveillance mechanisms to become engaged, decrease the virion-associated RNA burden, and ultimately modify disease outcome.

These data offer new insights into disease pathogenesis and the dynamics of viral replication, with potential clinical benefits to be gained by therapeutic trials predicated on these paradigms. Therefore, modification of the host environment, by either an augmented immune response or the introduction of potent antiretroviral compounds, might perturb the virus-host relationship and potentially improve the clinical outcome.

ANTIRETROVIRAL THERAPY

Antiretroviral therapy for HIV infection is based on the theory that pharmacologic interventions can be made at various stages in the life cycle of the virus. The effective agents currently available to clinicians are predominantly in the class of nucleoside analogue reverse transcriptase inhibitors. These include AZT, ddI, ddC, d4T, and 3TC. Saquinavir, a protease inhibitor, has also become available. Although the efficacy and safety of these agents are known, a question remains as to when precisely to initiate therapy. Current National Institutes of Health recommendations based on the AIDS Clinical

Trials Group (ACTG) 019 study indicate that therapy, which most commonly would be AZT, should begin when a patient's CD4+ cell count falls below 500 per mm^3 on two consecutive occasions. In light of what is now known about the pathogenesis of HIV infection, this recommendation may not provide optimal therapy.

In the hypothetical course of HIV infection, the virus load rises rapidly immediately after infection. There is an unexpectedly large reservoir of HIV in the lymph nodes, and about 25% of CD4+ lymphocytes are infected with HIV. Only about 1% of these lymphocytes actively produce virus at any one time; thus, there is a large reservoir of latently infected CD4+ lymphocytes that accounts for persistent infection. Any stimulus (e.g., infection, cytokines) that results in activation of the infected CD4+ lymphocytes will enhance viral production, and the HIV burden will increase. CD4+ lymphocytes are destroyed at twice the rate of replacement by the hematopoietic system, despite the considerable capacity of the immune system to regenerate CD4+ lymphocytes. In time, CD4+ lymphocyte replacement cannot keep pace with the rate of destruction.

In early HIV infection, when germinal follicles are intact, the virus is concentrated on the dendritic cells, which then serve as a reservoir of disease, enabling the infection of surrounding CD4+ lymphocytes. By the late stage of HIV infection, no germinal centers remain and essentially all surrounding CD4+ lymphocytes are infected.

Thus, HIV infection is productive from the time of initial infection, and it may be reasonable to treat patients as soon as a diagnosis is made to suppress viral replication early in the disease process and reduce viral load. In an attempt to accomplish this, Swiss investigators treated 68 patients who had acute HIV infection (seroconverters) with 6 months of therapy with either AZT (250 mg twice daily [bid]) or placebo. There was an indication that the AZT-treated patients experienced a better suppression of viral load, as reflected by higher CD4+ lymphocyte counts at 12 months, as well as fewer clinical events compared with the patients receiving placebo.

In contrast, long-term analysis in the ACTG 019 study (median follow-up, 5 years), in which 1637 patients with CD4+ lymphocyte counts of more than 500 per mm^3 were randomized to either AZT (500 mg or 1500 mg) or placebo, revealed no difference in clinical events between the two groups in terms of either AIDS-defining opportunistic infections or death. However, CD4+ lymphocyte counts were higher among the AZT-treated patients; this difference in CD4+ lymphocyte counts continued throughout the course of the study. The findings of this trial would therefore seem to contradict the hypothesis that early antiretroviral therapy will lower viral burden and will ultimately result in fewer clinical events and, hence, increased survival.

There is an explanation for this apparent contradiction. Although nucleoside analogues are effective drugs, monotherapy remains only modestly beneficial

TABLE 1. **Antiretroviral Drugs: Generic and Trade Names**

Generic Name	Drug Class	Abbreviation	Trade Name	Manufacturer	Status
Zidovudine	Nucleoside RT inhibitor	AZT, ZDV	Retrovir	Glaxo-Wellcome	Approved
Didanosine	Nucleoside RT inhibitor	ddI	Videx	Bristol-Myers Squibb	Approved
Zalcitabine	Nucleoside RT inhibitor	ddC	Hivid	Roche	Approved
Stavudine	Nucleoside RT inhibitor	d4T	Zerit	Bristol-Myers Squibb	Approved
Lamivudine	Nucleoside RT inhibitor	3TC	Epivir	Glaxo-Wellcome	Approved in combination with zidovudine
Saquinavir	Protease inhibitor	Ro 31-8959	Invirase	Roche	Approved
Indinavir	Protease inhibitor	MK-639	Crixivan	Merck	Approved
Ritonavir	Protease inhibitor	ABT-538	Norvir	Abbott	Approved
Nelfinavir	Protease inhibitor	AG-1343	Viracept	Agouron	Approved
Nevirapine	NNRTI	NVP	Viramune	Boehringer-Ingelheim	Approved
Delvaridine	NNRTI	DLV	Rescriptor	Upjohn	Approved
Loviride	NNRTI	LVD	N/A	Janssen	Investigational
Adefovir	Nucleotide analogue	bis-POM PMEA	N/A	Gilead	Investigational

Abbreviations: RT = reverse transcriptase; NNRTI = non-nucleoside reverse transcriptase inhibitor; N/A = not applicable.

and efficacy is of limited duration. Studies to date have shown, at best, incomplete suppression of the HIV. Combination therapy with different nucleoside analogues or with newer agents, such as protease inhibitors, administered early in the disease course may profoundly suppress viral replication, translating into prolonged survival. The challenge is to develop effective agents and to bring them into the clinical arena quickly. The following is a brief review of trials of antiretroviral therapy. Tables 1 and 2 list the available antiretroviral agents, their dosages, and common side effects.

Zidovudine (AZT)

The National Institute of Allergy and Infectious Diseases (NIAID) has published guidelines for the initiation of AZT therapy based on the results of ACTG studies 002, 016, and 019. On the basis of the present understanding of the pathogenesis of HIV infection, the recommendation to start antiretroviral therapy after the patient's CD4$^+$ cell count falls below 500 per mm^3 on two consecutive occasions may become obsolete.

Early analysis of ACTG 019, as well as the European-Australian Collaborative Group 020 study, showed that asymptomatic patients with CD4$^+$ cell counts less than 500 per mm^3 who were randomized to receive AZT were less likely to have clinical progression of their disease. However, the results of the Concorde study challenged this conclusion. This trial randomized 1749 patients to either immediate or deferred AZT (1000 mg per day). CD4$^+$ lymphocyte counts were measured as a surrogate marker, and time to the development of AIDS or to death was the primary end point of the study. Patients were followed up for 36 months.

Analysis showed a significant decrease in disease progression at 18 months as well as an improvement in CD4$^+$ lymphocyte counts in the immediate therapy group. However, there was no difference in survival at 36 months (immediate therapy group, 92%; deferred therapy group, 93%), nor was there a difference in progression to AIDS, AIDS-related complex (ARC), or death.

This led the NIAID to recommend that the initia-

TABLE 2. **Antiretroviral Drugs: Dosage and Side Effects**

Generic Name	Usual Adult Dosage	Common Side Effects (Comments)
Zidovudine	200 mg tid	Bone marrow suppression Gastrointestinal upset Headache Myopathy
Didanosine	200 mg bid	Peripheral neuropathy Pancreatitis Diarrhea Take on empty stomach
Zalcitabine	0.75 mg tid	Peripheral neuropathy Pancreatitis Oral ulcers
Stavudine	40 mg bid	Peripheral neuropathy
Lamivudine	150 mg bid	Anemia Gastrointestinal upset
Saquinavir	600 mg tid	Take with a fatty snack
Indinavir	800 mg tid	Kidney stones Take on empty stomach
Ritonavir	600 mg bid	Gastrointestinal upset Refrigerate medication
Nelfinavir	750 mg tid	Diarrhea
Nevirapine	200 mg qd × 2 wk, then 400 mg qd	Rash
Delavirdine	400 mg tid	Rash
Loviride	100 mg tid	Diarrhea
Adefovir	120 mg qd	Gastrointestinal upset

tion of antiretroviral therapy could wait until the CD4[+] lymphocyte counts declined below 500 per mm[3]; if the patient was asymptomatic, therapy could be delayed until either symptoms developed or the CD4[+] lymphocyte count started to decline.

Didanosine (ddI)

One trial has been conducted to evaluate the efficacy of ddI as initial therapy in patients with advanced disease. In ACTG 116A, 617 patients with AIDS or advanced ARC and less than 300 CD4[+] lymphocytes per mm[3] or with asymptomatic infection and less than 200 CD4[+] lymphocytes per mm[3], who had never received AZT or had been receiving AZT for less than 16 weeks, were randomized to receive AZT (1250 mg, then 600 mg per day) or ddI (500 or 750 mg per day). When stratified by prior AZT use, the results indicated that AZT was superior to ddI in AZT-naive patients, but ddI was superior to continued AZT in patients who had received 8 to 16 weeks of prior AZT treatment.

Zalcitabine (ddC)

There is only one study addressing the role of ddC in initial or early therapy for HIV infection. In ACTG 114, 635 patients with AIDS or advanced ARC who had received less than 3 months of AZT therapy were randomized to receive either ddC (2.25 mg per day) or AZT (1200 mg and then 600 mg per day). This trial was prematurely terminated because of the statistically higher mortality rate observed in the ddC treatment group. AZT appeared to be superior to ddC as initial therapy in AZT-naive patients as well as overall.

Didanosine Monotherapy and Combination Therapy

The theorized advantages conferred by combination antiretroviral therapy are numerous. Yarchoan and colleagues studied 41 HIV-infected patients to evaluate simultaneous versus alternating regimens of AZT and ddI. Patients had either AIDS or symptomatic HIV infection and CD4[+] cell counts of less than 350 per mm[3]. The simultaneous regimen consisted of AZT (300 mg per day) plus ddI (250 mg per day); alternating therapy was AZT (600 mg per day for 3 weeks) and then ddI (500 mg per day for 3 weeks). Initial results suggested that simultaneous therapy was superior to the alternating regimen in achieving elevations in CD4[+] lymphocyte counts that persisted for 6 months.

The efficacy of combining nucleoside analogues for initial therapy has also been studied in ACTG 106. AZT monotherapy was compared with several combinations of AZT and ddC in 56 patients with AIDS or ARC and CD4[+] lymphocyte counts of less than 200 per mm[3] who had received no prior antiretroviral therapy. Combination therapy resulted in higher and more sustained increases in CD4[+] lymphocyte counts

than those in the low-dose AZT arm or in prior studies with AZT and ddC monotherapy.

ACTG 175

ACTG 175 is a large clinical trial of 2467 patients, including 1067 who were previously untreated, with CD4[+] cell counts between 200 and 500 per mm[3] (mean, 350) and who were without clinical AIDS. Patients were randomized to receive AZT, 600 mg; ddI tablets, 400 mg; AZT plus ddI; or AZT plus ddC, 2.25 mg daily. The primary end points were a 50% decline in CD4[+] cell count, an AIDS-related event, or death. Mean follow-up was 143 weeks.

There were 565 end points overall, with two thirds occurring in the previously treated patients. More end points occurred in the AZT monotherapy group than in either of the other treatment groups. Overall, the combination of AZT-ddI and AZT-ddC and ddI monotherapy were significantly more effective than AZT monotherapy in preventing all clinical end points, AIDS-defining events, and death. The same pattern of results was observed when the end points were limited to AIDS-defining events and/or death or mortality alone. When the analysis is limited to the previously untreated patients, the results were similar. However, the benefit for mortality was statistically suggestive but not significant.

In a subset of 348 patients in whom virology analyses were performed, the two combination regimens appeared to perform better than either monotherapy. The combination regimen group experienced a 0.7 log decrease in viral load at 1 year. This result was better than that for the ddI monotherapy group. This group, however, achieved better results than patients receiving AZT monotherapy.

This is the first trial in patients without AIDS that demonstrated a survival advantage for two specific treatment regimens compared with AZT monotherapy. The results of this study will change the way HIV-infected patients are treated. Combination therapy in both previously untreated and treated patients has a clear advantage compared with initiating or continuing AZT monotherapy. One of the biggest surprises of this trial was the benefit seen in patients who received ddI monotherapy. They appeared to do as well clinically as patients who received either combination.

Delta Trials

Delta is actually two European trials totaling 3308 patients having less than 350 CD4[+] cells per mm[3] who were randomized to receive AZT monotherapy, AZT plus ddI, or AZT plus ddC. The 2191 previously untreated patients, who were enrolled into Delta I, had a mean CD4[+] cell count of 212 per mm[3]; the 1117 previously treated patients, who were enrolled into Delta II, had a mean CD4[+] cell count of 189 per mm[3]. Median follow-up in both trials was 26 months.

Results of Delta I demonstrated that survival was better with either combination (log rank $P = .0003$); there was no difference in survival between combination groups; disease progression was delayed with combination therapy (log rank $P = .0001$); and AZT plus ddI was better than AZT plus ddC (log rank $P = .03$).

In Delta II, the group of previously treated patients, the preliminary analysis demonstrated no significant differences among the arms in terms of either survival or disease progression. A final analysis of the results is pending. The combined results from Delta I and Delta II yielded a reduction in mortality of approximately 25% in favor of combination therapy. The survival difference appeared to emerge only after 18 months of follow-up.

The results of the Delta studies clearly suggest that the initiation of combination therapy with AZT plus ddI or ddC confers a substantial and highly significant benefit in terms of survival and progression to AIDS compared with AZT monotherapy. Unfortunately, ddI monotherapy was not considered in this study. Nevertheless, either combination regimen performed far better than did AZT alone.

Previously treated patients did not seem to benefit from combination therapy. In contrast to ACTG 175, these patients had more advanced disease and were not followed up for as long a time. Regardless, the Data Safety Monitoring Board for Delta has recommended that both Delta I and Delta II be discontinued on the basis of available data.

Combination Therapy: Lamivudine (3TC) and Zidovudine (AZT)

NUCA 3001

3TC, another of the nucleoside reverse transcriptase inhibitors recently licensed for use in the United States, has been studied as initial monotherapy and in combination with AZT in patients with no prior treatment history. Two nonclinical end-point trials have been completed. In NUCA 3001, an American study of 336 patients with 200 to 500 CD4$^+$ cells per mm^3, subjects received 3TC, 600 mg; AZT, 600 mg; 3TC, 300 mg, plus AZT, 600 mg; or 3TC, 600 mg, plus AZT, 600 mg daily. During the 24 weeks of the study, CD4$^+$ cell counts in both AZT-3TC combination groups were significantly increased compared with either monotherapy arm ($P < .001$). The combination therapies were also associated with more effective lowering of plasma HIV-1 RNA.

The greatest mean reduction in viral load was approximately 1.55 log for the combination groups versus 0.52 log for AZT monotherapy and 1.19 log in the 3TC monotherapy arm. At 24 weeks, the viral load reduction was still about 1.0 log for the combination groups, and only 0.25 and 0.42 for the AZT and 3TC monotherapy groups, respectively.

NUCB 3001, a similarly designed trial performed in Europe, demonstrated nearly identical results.

Although significant advances have been made in the development of antiretroviral therapy for HIV infection, questions remain not only about which treatment should be initiated and when that treatment should begin but also about how therapy should be managed over time. Alternative therapeutic approaches should be considered, most obviously when the patient no longer responds to initial treatment and immunologically and/or clinically "fails." The optimal time for such a change in treatment is still unknown, although it is probably related to increasing viral burden as well as to known clinical and immunologic signs of deterioration. The following is a brief summary of studies that have addressed the impact of changing the treatment regimen in patients who are already receiving antiretroviral therapy.

Changing Monotherapy: Zidovudine (AZT) to Didanosine (ddI)

ACTG 116B/117

The first large clinical trial that examined the effects of changing from one antiretroviral therapy to another was ACTG 116B/117. The working hypothesis of this study was that the efficacy of AZT might diminish in time because of one or more of the following factors: HIV-1 resistance to AZT monotherapy or intolerance to or toxicity of AZT. This trial was designed to assess whether a change of therapy from AZT to ddI after at least 16 weeks of AZT monotherapy decreased the risk for disease progression and/or death. The trial enrolled 913 patients with CD4$^+$ cell counts of less than 300 per mm^3; they were then randomized to receive either 750 mg or 500 mg of ddI or 600 mg of AZT daily. Progression to a new AIDS-defining event or death was delayed in patients who received 500 mg of ddI daily. The relative benefit of switching to ddI was not related to the duration of prior AZT treatment.

D'Aquila and colleagues performed an analysis of a subgroup of 187 patients from ACTG 116/117 who had baseline follow-up viral isolates. The analysis showed that a high-level resistance of HIV-1 to AZT predicted a more rapid clinical progression and death when adjusted for other factors.

The most important risk factors for death were a high level of AZT resistance, syncytium-inducing phenotype, and AIDS diagnosis at entry into the study. The amount of viral load at the initiation of therapy was significantly related to disease progression. A 50% decrease in HIV-1 RNA translated into a 32% decrease in risk of disease progression.

These results from ACTG 116B/117 were inconsistent with the working hypothesis that patients with baseline AZT resistance would experience a clinical benefit when they were subsequently treated with ddI. However, the number of patients with isolates with high-level AZT resistance was too small to fully explain the observed benefit of ddI. Second, high-level AZT resistance was also associated with an increased risk of death in patients who received either treatment. Third, the adjusted relative hazards of ddI assignment were essentially unchanged when the few patients with highly resistant AZT were excluded.

Several conclusions can be drawn from ACTG 116B/117. In patients without prior AIDS, switching to ddI, 500 mg daily, was associated with fewer AIDS-defining events, although no difference in survival was noted. There was an improvement in CD4$^+$ cell count and p24 antigen in both ddI treatment groups relative to those continuing on AZT. The benefits of ddI therapy were independent of duration of prior AZT therapy. Thus, patients with advanced HIV-1 disease may benefit from a change in therapy from AZT to ddI whether or not high-level HIV-1 resistance is present. Furthermore, laboratory assessment of AZT resistance is not necessary for deciding when to switch therapies.

BMS 010

Another clinical trial, Bristol-Myers Squibb (BMS) 010, attempted to address the same issue of measuring the benefit of changing from AZT to ddI monotherapy. In this study, 312 patients with a CD4$^+$ cell count of less than 300 cells per mm^3 who had received AZT for at least 6 months (median, 18 months) were enrolled. In addition, all patients had to have a clinical or immunologic sign associated with deterioration, such as oral thrush or a 50% decline in CD4$^+$ cell count.

Patients were randomized to receive ddI tablets, 600 mg daily (this was subsequently changed to 400 mg daily), or to continue with AZT, 600 mg daily. Overall median duration of follow-up was 47 weeks. Of the 149 patients who reached a study end point, 97 had a new AIDS-defining event, 23 had two HIV-associated diagnoses plus a decrease in CD4$^+$ cell count, and 29 died. Patients who had continued to receive AZT had a 50% higher risk for developing a primary study end point, compared with those who were switched to ddI (relative risk = 1.5; confidence interval = 1.1, 2.0; P = .02). When death was used as a study end point, there was no difference between the two treatments.

Changing Monotherapy: Zidovudine (AZT) to Stavudine (d4T)

BMS 019

On the basis of favorable results observed in phase II studies of d4T, BMS 019, a large phase III clinical end-point trial, was designed to compare the efficacy and safety of d4T therapy in patients who had received prior AZT therapy. This trial enrolled 822 patients with a median CD4$^+$ cell count of 235 per mm^3 and approximately 20 months of prior AZT use. The protocol-defined end points were an AIDS-defining illness, death, or a 50% drop in CD4$^+$ cell count. The dosage of d4T was 40 mg bid; AZT was given 200 mg thrice daily (tid).

The time to reach a protocol-defined end point was longer for patients treated with d4T (P = .002), as was progression to an AIDS-defining event or death (P = .007). There was a trend toward a survival advantage for the d4T-treated patients (P = .07).

These patients had reduced viral titers and sustained improvement in CD4$^+$ cell counts with 40- to 50-cell increases compared with AZT-treated patients throughout the study.

Peripheral neuropathy occurred in 13% of the d4T-treated patients and in 4% of patients treated with AZT. Approximately 50% of patients who developed neuropathy could tolerate d4T at a 50% dose reduction. Nausea, vomiting, myalgias, anemia, and neutropenia were more common in the AZT-treated group. Elevations in liver function test results occurred more frequently in the d4T-treated group, although no patients experienced drug-associated hepatitis.

In the three studies described, there appears to be a clinical, measurable benefit for patients receiving AZT monotherapy if they have their treatment changed after a minimum of 6 months to either ddI or d4T monotherapy. A delay in the development of clinical AIDS as well as in the time to a 50% fall in CD4$^+$ cell counts was evident in all three trials. A trend toward prolonged survival was observed with d4T treatment. Peripheral neuropathy was the most common problem in the patients receiving d4T; this was highly correlated in patients with a diagnosis of AIDS. It is still uncertain when such a therapeutic switch should be undertaken. The BMS 010 study used a clinical event to trigger the switch in therapy; however, in the two larger trials, therapeutic change was based on prior minimal experience with AZT. The duration of prior AZT therapy was not helpful in predicting who would benefit from changing therapy.

In the ACTG 175 trial, changing to ddI monotherapy in treatment-experienced individuals with less advanced disease was associated with a highly significant decrease in mortality as well as a reduction in clinical events and less severe CD4$^+$ cell count decline.

Combination Therapy: Adding Zalcitabine (ddC) to Zidovudine (AZT)

ACTG 155

The first large nucleoside combination study was ACTG 155. In this trial, 1001 patients with less than 300 CD4$^+$ cells per mm^3 and more than 6 months of prior AZT therapy (mean, 18 months) were randomized to receive either daily AZT, 600 mg, plus ddC, 2.25 mg; ddC monotherapy, 2.25 mg; or AZT monotherapy, 600 mg. Patients were stratified according to the presence or absence of symptoms, type of prophylaxis therapy, and duration of prior AZT treatment.

This study did not fulfill the investigators' expectations. After a follow-up of 18 months, no difference among the three treatment groups with respect to the development of AIDS or death was noted (P = .26). In addition, there was no significant difference in time to an end point in any of the stratified subgroups, and no difference in survival was noted among the treatment groups overall (P = .57) or when patients were grouped by pretreatment CD4+ cell counts.

The results of this trial were certainly disappointing. At least, however, it was learned that adding ddC to AZT in treated patients with advanced disease is not beneficial. Other combinations, fortunately, have proved to be much better.

ACTG 175

As discussed in the preceding section, adding ddC to AZT in patients with less advanced disease was associated with a delay in progression of disease but no survival benefit. On the other hand, adding ddI to AZT in this population of patients was associated with a significant reduction in mortality as well as decrease in the number of AIDS-defining events and rate of CD4+ cell loss.

Delta Trials

In the Delta II trial, there was no benefit observed in patients (all with less than 350 CD4+ cells per mm³) when ddI or ddC was added to the AZT. It must be kept in mind that the results presented for the Delta trials are preliminary at this point and await final confirmation.

Combination Therapy: Lamivudine (3TC) and Zidovudine (AZT)

NUCA 3002

3TC is another reverse transcriptase analogue that has recently been studied both as monotherapy and in combination with AZT. NUCA 3002 was an American study of 254 patients with prior AZT experience and CD4+ cell counts between 100 and 300 per mm³. Patients were randomized to receive either AZT, 600 mg per day, plus 3TC, 150 or 300 mg bid, or AZT, 600 mg, plus ddC, 2.25 mg daily. There was no significant increase in the mean actual change from baseline CD4+ cell count in the AZT plus ddC group, whereas the 3TC plus AZT groups experienced an increase that persisted for 48 weeks. At 24 weeks, there was a decrease in CD4+ cell counts in the AZT plus ddC group. At this point, patients were allowed to cross over to an open-label 3TC regimen, and by week 48, the mean actual change in CD4+ cell counts was the same for all three treatment arms. The plasma HIV RNA levels on polymerase chain reaction (PCR) analysis declined by 0.7 log in all three arms at the end of 24 weeks, although the 3TC-containing regimens had a 1.0 log reduction at week 4 that was not sustained.

NUCB 3002

NUCB 3002 was a European study that evaluated the effect of AZT monotherapy compared with 3TC plus AZT in previously treated patients with CD4+ cell counts between 100 and 300 per mm³. Patients were randomized to receive AZT, 600 mg daily, either alone or in combination with 3TC at either 150 or 300 mg bid.

During the "blinded" phase of the trial, the CD4+ cell count dropped 21 per mm³ in the AZT group compared with a 47-cell increase in the combination arms (P = .0001). There was also a 30% decrease in p24 antigen in the AZT group versus an 80% and a 58% decrease in the 150- and 300-mg 3TC groups, respectively (P = .0009). In addition, RNA levels on PCR decreased by 1.0 log in both combination arms.

These studies were not designed as clinical endpoint trials. However, the greater increase in CD4+ cell counts and improved antiviral effect in both combination arms are encouraging and warrant further study of this potent combination.

Combination Therapy: Protease Inhibitors

ACTG 229

ACTG 229 was the first large trial that involved a protease inhibitor. In this study, saquinavir (a protease inhibitor) plus AZT versus saquinavir, AZT, and ddC was compared with AZT plus ddC in 302 patients with CD4+ cell counts between 50 and 350 per mm³ and at least 4 months of prior nucleoside therapy. The study was originally designed to last 24 weeks, but 244 subjects were allowed to continue blinded therapy for an additional 3 to 6 months.

Although there was inadequate power to detect differences in clinical outcome, the triple combination had a greater and more sustained increase in CD4+ cell count and a greater decrease in viral load as measured by PCR of plasma HIV RNA or quantitative HIV peripheral blood mononuclear cell titer. At 48 weeks, the subjects' HIV plasma RNA on the triple combination was 0.26 $\log_{10}$ below baseline on average versus 0.05 $\log_{10}$ below baseline for the saquinavir-AZT group versus a 0.22 $\log_{10}$ increase above baseline for the AZT-ddC group.

In large part on the basis of these data, saquinavir was the first protease inhibitor licensed for use in the United States.

Other Trials

Ritonavir, another protease inhibitor recently approved for use in the United States, has been shown to have significant antiretroviral activity as well as clinical efficacy in patients with advanced HIV infection. In a pivotal trial, ritonavir was administered as 600 mg bid in a placebo-controlled trial to 1090 patients with less than 100 CD4+ cells per mm³ and more than 9 months of prior nucleoside therapy. Patients were allowed to continue with one or two nucleoside reverse transcriptase inhibitors. After a mean of 6.1 months of follow-up, a survival advantage was observed in the ritonavir group (8.4 versus 4.8%; P = .02).

Ritonavir therapy was associated with an initial 1.3 $\log_{10}$ decrease; at 16 weeks, the viral burden was still 0.6 $\log_{10}$ below baseline. The CD4+ cells were 40 to 50 cells per mm³ above baseline at 16 weeks. Ritonavir was relatively well tolerated in this trial. Significant drug interactions are known to occur with ritonavir because of its effect on the hepatic cyto-chrome P-450 system.

Indinavir, another protease inhibitor, has also been granted accelerated approval in the United States because of impressive antiviral activity demonstrated in several phase II studies. In one study, when indinavir 800 mg tid was administered with standard doses of zidovudine and didanosine, the median virus levels in the blood were reduced by 99.9%, or 2.9 $\log_{10}$. Moreover, the level of virus in the blood was below detectable levels in 59% of patients after 5 months of therapy. These patients also experienced significant increases in CD4$^+$ cell counts. Patients had begun the study with a median CD4$^+$ cell count of 150 per mm^3 and on average had treatment-related increases averaging 90 cells per mm^3.

In another trial, indinavir 800 mg tid, alone or combined with AZT, 200 mg tid, and 3TC, 150 mg bid, versus AZT and 3TC administered together, was given to 97 patients with 50 to 400 CD4$^+$ cells per mm^3 and more than 6 months of prior AZT therapy. This study was not designed as a clinical end-point trial; however, at 16 weeks, the CD4$^+$ cell count response in the indinavir-containing groups was approximately 100 cells per mm^3 above baseline, and the viral load was below detectable limits in 85% of the patients assigned to the indinavir-containing triple combination arm. This dramatic antiviral response has not been observed in any other clinical studies to date. Overall, indinavir was well tolerated except for an approximate 2 to 4% annual rate of developing nephrolithiasis.

Summary

In summary, significant advances in antiretroviral therapy have been made and are summarized in Table 1. Three years ago, it was demonstrated that changing from AZT to ddI monotherapy resulted in a delay to progression to an AIDS-defining condition. More recently, impressive data have emerged regarding the benefits of changing from AZT to d4T monotherapy. Most strikingly, however, has been the report of ACTG 175, the first study in which changing therapy from AZT to ddI, ddI plus AZT, or AZT plus ddC resulted not only in a delay to progression of disease but also in an increase in survival time. As observed in the Delta I study and ACTG 175, patients with up to 500 CD4$^+$ cells per mm^3 may also experience a survival benefit if they are treated with ddI monotherapy or with combinations of AZT plus ddI or ddC. The use of the nucleoside therapies in previously treated patients has now clearly shifted toward ddI and d4T, with or without AZT. Future nucleoside combination regimens with 3TC, d4T, and protease inhibitors look promising at present and are under active investigation.

USE OF PLASMA HIV-1 RNA QUANTITATION IN CLINICAL PRACTICE

The commercial availability of HIV-1 RNA quantitation has greatly enhanced the clinician's ability to monitor and, consequently, adjust antiretroviral treatment regimens in individual patients. In the past, combinations of surrogate markers, such as HIV-1 p24 antigen, β_2-microglobulin, and neopterin, among others, were used in conjunction with CD4$^+$ lymphocyte counts in management of patients. All of these markers suffer from low sensitivity; that is, they were measurable in many but not all patients. In addition, changes in each of these measures were only moderately correlated with clinical progression, particularly in early disease (i.e., patients with greater than 500 CD4$^+$ cells per mm^3). HIV-1 RNA, on the other hand, is measurable in nearly all untreated HIV-1–infected individuals, is highly correlated with clinical progression and survival, and mirrors the CD4$^+$ cell count (i.e., decreases in RNA are typically accompanied by rises in CD4$^+$ cells). Because HIV-1 RNA is a more sensitive measure of drug efficacy, changes in this measure anticipate the reciprocal changes in CD4$^+$ cell count, thus allowing the clinician to intervene on the basis of a viral measure (RNA) before measurable evidence of further immune suppression (CD4$^+$ cells).

Advantages of these assays include their substantial precision, a wide dynamic range that can be measured from a few hundred copies up to millions of copies of RNA (enabling measurement over a large scale compared with the range of the p24 antigen or quantitative cultures), and the potential to be performed by most hospital or commercial laboratories. At present, only the Amplicor HIV-1 Monitor (Roche Molecular Systems, Branchburg, NJ) RNA assay has received approval of the Food and Drug Administration; along with other HIV-1 RNA assays, it has only limited availability and is expensive ($150 to $250 per assay). The willingness of third-party payers to cover the cost of these assays varies widely.

Although plasma HIV-1 RNA quantification is a good indicator of drug efficacy, the clinical utility of the marker is not yet completely understood. This assay has the potential to help individualize management of patients and enhance clinical decision-making through demonstration of therapeutic effects. It may be used for prognosis to indicate any decrease in the viral load, and used serially, the assay could track the degree and duration of viral suppression. In addition, the HIV-1 RNA assay could monitor the effects of a change in treatment protocol. Withdrawal of treatment might be considered if viral load remained high despite administration of a number of antiretroviral agents. However, there are few data concerning the optimal viral threshold for the initiation or withdrawal of therapy. Indeed, data from the Multicenter AIDS Cohort Study suggest that there may not be any threshold for disease progression, because even patients with low viral loads progress in time, albeit at a slower rate than those with higher viral loads. Moreover, the real thresholds for treatment benefits, and the amount of needed decrease in the level of plasma HIV-1 RNA to produce positive effects, are still unknown.

Physicians who incorporate the use of plasma HIV-

1 RNA quantitation into their practices should be aware of several important points:

Blood should be collected in yellow-top acid-citrate-dextrose tubes for reverse transcription–PCR (RNA PCR) or in lavender-top (ethylenediaminetetraacetic acid, EDTA) tubes for branched chain DNA (bDNA) assay. Specimens anticoagulated with heparin are unsuitable for the Amplicor HIV-1 Monitor test because heparin inhibits PCR amplification. Whole blood may be stored at room temperature for up to 6 hours. The specimens should be processed by separating the plasma from the whole blood within 6 hours of collection by centrifugation at $1600 \times g$ for 20 minutes at room temperature. The stability of the processed specimens at room temperature has not been characterized; therefore, processed specimens should be immediately frozen at $-20°C$ or colder ($-70°C$ if storing for more than 1 week). Specimens must be shipped frozen (on dry ice) to the reference laboratory.

Although different assays (bDNA and reverse transcription–PCR) correlate well, there are as yet no commonly accepted reference standards. Values from one assay cannot readily be translated into values from another assay. Thus, it is important to show one assay and maintain consistency.

Given the assay variation of $\pm 0.15 \log_{10}$, only a difference of fivefold ($0.7 \log_{10}$) or greater should be considered significant. A sporadic high value may be the result of immune activation due to an intercurrent clinical event (e.g., vaccination, reactivation of herpesvirus infection).

Although additional studies are needed to fully validate the clinical use of plasma HIV-1 RNA assays, available information suggests that these assays may provide useful prognostic information and may help individualize decisions regarding the use of antiretroviral therapy in selected patients. In a disease as complex as HIV infection, no single test can provide all of the information needed to make informed clinical decisions. The appropriate role of plasma HIV assays will be determined in the coming years on the basis of further studies, clinical experience, and cost. However, given these limitations, most would recommend measurement of HIV-1 RNA and CD4$^+$ cell counts every 3 to 4 months as routine monitoring. They should also be measured in the event of clinical changes and before initiating, or changing, therapy and then more frequently (approximately every 3 weeks) until the desired RNA copy number is achieved and CD4$^+$ cell count has stabilized.

OPPORTUNISTIC INFECTION: NEWER DEVELOPMENTS

Most patients with HIV infection will experience, as their disease progresses, an increasing incidence of opportunistic infections. These include *Pneumocystis carinii* pneumonia (PCP), *Mycobacterium avium* complex (MAC) infection, fungal infections, cytomegalovirus disease, KS, and B cell lymphoma. Investigation continues on defining both therapy for infection and prophylaxis. This section concentrates on the most recent, pertinent advances in prophylaxis and treatment. A summary is provided in Table 3.

Pneumocystis carinii Pneumonia

An open-label study by Bozzette and coworkers (ACTG 081) attempted to analyze which prophylactic therapy would be most efficacious. A total of 843 patients received trimethoprim-sulfamethoxazole, dapsone, or aerosolized pentamidine. All patients had CD4$^+$ cell counts of less than 200 per mm^3. Median follow-up was 39 months.

There was no significant difference among initial assigned therapies in the incidence of PCP; overall risk was 18 to 21%. However, in patients with CD4$^+$ cell counts less than 100 per mm^3, a difference between therapies emerged. Initial therapy with trimethoprim-sulfamethoxazole was shown to be 1.7 times more effective than aerosolized pentamidine. Twenty-eight percent of the trimethoprim-sulfamethoxazole–treated patients and 25% of the dapsone-treated patients, regardless of their initial CD4$^+$ cell counts, remained on their assigned therapy at an effective dose for the study's duration. In contrast, about 90% of patients initially treated with aerosolized pentamidine remained on their therapy.

The average attack rate of PCP was 7% per year, the case-fatality rate was 7%, and PCP-related mortality was 1%. The data from this study suggest that the greatest gains in the prevention of PCP are most likely to derive from identifying persons at risk for PCP rather than optimizing the therapy for those who are already receiving care, although optimizing therapy remains an important goal. For patients with CD4$^+$ cell counts less than 100 per mm^3, trimethoprim-sulfamethoxazole or dapsone (100 mg each day) is superior to aerosolized pentamidine. However, for those who are toxoplasmosis IgG-positive, trimethoprim-sulfamethoxazole may be the optimal prophylactic therapy.

Mycobacterium avium Complex Disease

The prevalence of MAC among AIDS patients has been steadily increasing since 1987, and it now appears that it may eventually infect most HIV-positive patients with CD4$^+$ cell counts of less than 100 per mm^3. Disseminated MAC infection contributes substantially to morbidity, in addition to being associated with decreased survival. One of the agents under study for the prophylactic treatment of MAC infection is rifabutin, a semisynthetic rifamycin. Nightingale and associates conducted two randomized, double-blind, multicenter trials of daily prophylactic treatment with either rifabutin (300 mg daily) or placebo. In the first study, MAC bacteremia developed in 24 of 292 patients (8%) who received rifabutin, compared with 51 of 298 patients (17%) who did not. In the second study, bacteremia was noted

TABLE 3. **Prophylaxis for HIV-Associated Opportunistic Infection**

CD4+ Cell Count	Disorder	Treatment	Alternatives
Any amount	Tuberculosis (if tuberculin-positive)	Isoniazid 300 mg + pyridoxine 50 mg/d for 12 mo	Rifampin 600 mg/d for 12 mo (for isoniazid-intolerant or isoniazid-resistant disease)
<200/mm³	*Pneumocystis carinii* pneumonia	Trimethoprim-sulfamethoxazole 1 double-strength tablet 3–7 times/wk	Dapsone 100 mg/d Aerosolized pentamidine 300 mg/mo (dose and frequency depend on nebulizer used) Atovaquone suspension 1500 mg/d
<100/mm³	Toxoplasmosis (if seropositive for *T. gondii*)	Trimethoprim-sulfamethoxazole 1 double-strength tablet 3–7 times/wk (as for *P. carinii* pneumonia prophylaxis)	Dapsone 50 mg + pyrimethamine 50 mg/wk + leucovorin 25 mg/wk
<75/mm³	*Mycobacterium avium* complex infection	Clarithromycin 500 mg bid Azithromycin 1200 mg/wk	Rifabutin 300 mg
<50/mm³	Cytomegalovirus disease (if seropositive for cytomegalovirus and polymerase chain reaction or culture is positive for cytomegalovirus in blood)	Ganciclovir 1000 mg tid	
	Cryptococcosis (in a few unusual occupational or other circumstances, prophylaxis should be considered; a specialist should be consulted)	Fluconazole 100–200 mg/d	Itraconazole 200 mg/d
	Histoplasmosis (in endemic areas)	Itraconazole 200 mg/d	Fluconazole 200 mg/d
	Coccidioidomycosis (in endemic areas)	Fluconazole 200 mg/d	Itraconazole 200 mg/d

in 24 of the 274 rifabutin patients (9%) compared with 51 of the 282 placebo patients (18%).

Treatment with rifabutin significantly delayed fatigue, fever, hospitalization, and decline in both hemoglobin level (by >10%) and the Karnofsky performance score (by 20%). There was no significant difference in overall survival between the groups, although fewer deaths were associated with rifabutin than with placebo. The relative risk for death in the rifabutin group compared with the placebo group was 0.68 (95% confidence interval, 0.43 to 1.06; $P = .086$). Similarly, there was no significant difference in the incidence of adverse events between the two groups. In these studies, the incidence of MAC resistance to rifabutin was not increased in the treated groups.

Clarithromycin (Biaxin) and azithromycin (Zithromax), both macrolides, alone and in combination with rifabutin (Mycobutin), have been studied as alternative MAC prophylaxis therapies. A preliminary analysis of two large phase III clinical trials suggests that clarithromycin alone, 500 mg bid, was more effective than rifabutin alone in reducing the incidence and delaying the time to development of MAC bacteremia or disease. However, no difference in survival was noted. Clarithromycin-resistant strains were identified in 27% of isolates, whereas no resis-

tance was documented in the rifabutin-treated patients. The combination of rifabutin plus clarithromycin did not appear to significantly reduce the rate of development of clarithromycin resistance, was not more effective than clarithromycin alone, and was not tolerated as well as either monotherapy.

In the other large MAC prophylaxis trial, azithromycin, administered in a single weekly 1200-mg dose, was as effective as rifabutin, 300 mg, given on a daily basis. The combination of azithromycin plus rifabutin was more effective than either agent given alone. Resistant isolates in this study were relatively rare. Only 2 of 18 (11%) of azithromycin breakthrough isolates were resistant to azithromycin. No resistance to rifabutin was observed. One must keep in mind that the results of these two trials are, at this time, considered preliminary. A final and complete analysis should be available in the near future.

Clarithromycin has also been studied as a therapy for MAC bacteremia. Chaisson and colleagues evaluated various doses (500, 1000, and 2000 mg bid) and found that this agent markedly decreased MAC bacteremia at 6 weeks. Survival of patients was best with the 500-mg twice-daily dose ($P = .007$). During the first 12 weeks of the study, significantly fewer patients who received this dose died than did those who received higher doses. However, the emergence of clarithromycin-resistant organisms was an important problem, because 46% of all patients developed resistance to this agent by 16 weeks. Thus, the investigators concluded that combination therapy was essential to optimal care of patients. One possible combination would be clarithromycin and ethambutol with or without ciprofloxacin.

Fungal Infections

Invasive fungal infections, in particular with *Cryptococcus neoformans,* are seen in 5 to 10% of AIDS patients. In addition, mucocutaneous candidiasis is present in almost all patients with advanced HIV disease; recurrent infection, especially candidiasis, causes considerable morbidity.

The NIAID AIDS Clinical Trials Group conducted a prospective, randomized study that compared fluconazole (Diflucan) 200 mg per day with clotrimazole troches (Mycelex) 10 mg taken five times daily in 428 patients with CD4$^+$ cell counts less than 200 per mm^3. At a median follow-up of 35 months, invasive fungal infections were seen in 4.1% of the fluconazole-treated patients (9 of 217) versus 11% of the clotrimazole-treated patients (23 of 211). Two cryptococcosis infections were noted in the former group, whereas there were 15 in the latter group. Patients with CD4$^+$ cell counts of 50 per mm^3 or less derived greater benefit from fluconazole therapy than did those with higher counts. In addition, fluconazole was effective in preventing esophageal candidiasis as well as confirmed and presumed oropharyngeal candidiasis. However, there was no significant difference in survival between the two groups of patients. The cost of therapy required to prevent one episode of invasive fungal infection was significant (11,756 doses of fluconazole per infection prevented). The cost per infection prevented was significantly lower only if patients with CD4$^+$ cell counts less than 50 per mm^3 were targeted for fluconazole prophylaxis. Many investigators are concerned about the emergence of fluconazole-resistant *Candida* and *Torulopsis* with fluconazole therapy. Studies to evaluate the clinical importance of fluconazole resistance are under way.

Kaposi's Sarcoma

KS is the most common malignancy associated with AIDS patients; about 15 to 20% will develop KS at some point during the course of their disease. Although KS usually manifests on the skin, this malignancy often involves other areas, such as the gastrointestinal tract and the lungs.

Chang and colleagues used representational difference analysis to isolate unique DNA sequences in more than 90% of KS tissues obtained from AIDS patients. These sequences were not seen in tissue DNA taken from patients not infected with the AIDS virus but were present in 15% of non-KS tissue DNA samples from AIDS patients. These DNA sequences were homologous to but distinct from capsid and tegument protein genes of the Gammaherpesvirinae *Herpesvirus saimiri* and of Epstein-Barr virus. These KS-associated herpesvirus-like sequences appear to define a new human herpesvirus. The same research group has also identified KS-associated herpesvirus sequences in tissue from elderly non–HIV-infected patients with KS, African children with KS, and non–HIV-infected homosexual men with KS.

These intriguing data await confirmation from other research groups but support epidemiologic evidence that KS results from an infectious agent. In addition, these data raise the possibility that future therapy for KS could target the KS-associated herpesvirus.

Cytomegalovirus Disease

For most patients with AIDS, cytomegalovirus (CMV) is an increasingly common complication of their disease. Indeed, CMV retinitis has long been the most common ocular opportunistic infection in this group of patients; in addition, the proportion of these patients who will develop CMV retinitis during the course of their illness is increasing. Currently, about 25% will experience this particular manifestation of CMV at some point in their disease progression. However, recent evidence suggests that close to 40% of patients who are HIV-positive for long periods will develop CMV retinitis.

The additional diagnosis of CMV retinitis, in patients whose quality of life may already be impaired by AIDS, is viewed by many as devastating, because the condition is associated with loss of vision and shorter survival times. Fortunately, however, present therapies have resulted in improved life expectancy; median survival now exceeds 14 months.

Foremost among treatment goals are the preservation of vision, increase in survival, and enhancement of quality of life. Also of concern is maintaining the patient's independence and minimizing treatment-associated complications. Investigators continue to define the best therapeutic options for these patients. This section presents a brief summary of the latest research findings.

A study by Pertel and coworkers, from Northwestern University, has shown that as the CD4$^+$ cell count declines, the cumulative percentage of individuals with CMV retinitis increases dramatically. In patients with CD4$^+$ cell counts below 50 per mm^3, more than 30% developed this complication at 18 months after diagnosis; this number increased to more than 40% at 27 months. Whereas CMV retinitis may also develop in patients with CD4$^+$ cell counts above 50 per mm^3, the incidence is not as great. Thus, CMV retinitis is an ever present threat for HIV-infected patients, but particularly in those whose CD4$^+$ cell count is below 50 per mm^3.

Therapy

The diagnosis is based on clinical presentation of retinitis and ophthalmoscopic examination. Standard therapy has been divided into two phases: the acute induction phase followed by a lifelong, maintenance phase. Treatment in the acute phase, which may last for 2 to 3 weeks depending on the patient's response, consists of ganciclovir (Cytovene), 5 mg per kg intravenously (IV) every 12 hours for 14 days, or foscarnet (Foscavir), 90 mg per kg IV every 12 hours. Maintenance therapy consists of ganciclovir, 5 to 10 mg per kg IV, or foscarnet, 90 to 120 mg per kg daily.

GANCICLOVIR VERSUS FOSCARNET

A comparison study of the efficacy of these two agents during the acute phase of CMV retinitis has shown that the median time to retinitis progression is approximately 2 months with either drug. However, it also showed that the patients who were initially randomized to receive foscarnet had a median survival of 12.6 months versus 8.5 months for the ganciclovir-treated patients. This suggests that foscarnet may be preferable as initial therapy, although some patients experienced difficulty in tolerating this therapy. More than one third of the patients initially randomized to receive foscarnet had to change to ganciclovir. It has been speculated that this increase in median survival is due to the antiretroviral effect of foscarnet.

ACTG 015/915 also showed this same survival effect. Patients in this study were treated with 60, 90, or 120 mg per kg per day of foscarnet as maintenance therapy. Median survival was approximately 12 months with the highest dose, which was significantly longer than with the lower doses. Although greater toxicity was associated with this high dose, it was manageable.

An additional benefit of the higher, 120-mg per kg per day dose was a decreased rate of retinitis progression, evaluated by retinal photographs, compared with the lower dose of 90 mg per kg per day.

COMBINATION THERAPY

Retrospective case series have shown that in patients who have relapsed at various stages, the median time to recurrence is 80 to 120 days with combination therapy compared with about 60 days for primary single-agent therapy with either ganciclovir or foscarnet. These observations led to a controlled trial that randomized relapsed patients to maintenance therapy with 10 mg per kg per day of ganciclovir, 120 mg per kg per day of foscarnet, or 90 mg per kg per day of foscarnet and 5 mg per kg per day of ganciclovir in combination. Results from this trial showed that the median time to retinitis progression was 4.8 months for the combination therapy versus 1.5 and 1.2 months for the foscarnet and ganciclovir arms, respectively. No difference in survival or visual acuity was noted among the three arms. However, quality-of-life data suggested that patients who received the combination therapy thought that their daily lives were adversely affected by the fact that two drugs needed to be administered.

ORAL GANCICLOVIR

Introduction of oral ganciclovir for maintenance therapy of CMV retinitis has yielded some encouraging results. Patients receive oral ganciclovir after an induction course of IV ganciclovir.

Oral ganciclovir is associated with a risk for a more rapid rate of CMV retinitis progression and should be used only in those patients for whom this risk is balanced by the benefit associated with avoiding daily IV infusions. Oral ganciclovir is not recommended for sight-threatening retinitis in zone 1. Patients who receive this formulation should be examined frequently, at a minimal interval of every 4 weeks.

CIDOFOVIR

Attention has turned to the use of a recently approved drug, cidofovir (HPMPC). One study randomized 48 newly diagnosed patients with CMV retinitis to either immediate or deferred therapy. Therapy consisted of HPMPC, 5 mg per kg per week IV for 2 weeks, followed by maintenance therapy of 5 mg per kg every other week. One of the advantages with this agent is its long half-life, which permits intermittent administration. All patients in this study received oral probenecid, 1.0 gram four times daily (qid) with hydration, to counteract the nephrotoxicity associated with HPMPC administration.

Time to retinitis progression was among the longest yet observed with a systemic agent. However, serious toxicity due either to HPMPC itself or to probenecid was a limiting factor in this study. Further trials will be necessary to determine how best to use this drug.

GANCICLOVIR THERAPY BY INTRAOCULAR DEVICE

Intravitreal ganciclovir has also come under investigation. Patients receive 200 μg per week by a 30-gauge needle. Although this therapy has been shown to be effective, weekly injections are required, potentially increasing the possibility of infection or retinal detachment. To prevent these complications, an intraocular device was developed to deliver ganciclovir.

This intraocular device is a polyvinyl alcohol–coated pellet containing 6 mg of ganciclovir, which is carried in an ethylene vinyl acetate disk. It is available as an 8-month device, which delivers ganciclovir at a rate of 1 μg per hour.

A 1993 pilot study reported the treatment of 30 eyes in 22 patients: 17 had retinitis progression with IV ganciclovir; 5 had newly diagnosed retinitis; and 8 were treated with bilateral implants. Retinitis stabilization was achieved in 27 of 30 eyes (90%). Median time to retinitis progression was 133 days; however, seven patients (32%) developed systemic CMV disease, a major complication of local therapy.

On the basis of the promising results from this pilot study, the National Eye Institute conducted a multicenter trial that studied the use of the ganciclovir intraocular implant in patients with either unilateral or bilateral CMV retinitis and small peripheral lesions. Patients with bilateral disease had one eye treated immediately while therapy for the other eye was deferred. Median time to retinitis progression was 15 days for the deferred therapy arm compared with 225 days for the immediate therapy arm ($P < .00001$). Development of retinitis in the eye that did not receive the implant occurred in 61% of patients at a median time of 203 days. Median survival was 259 days, which is significantly less than that currently achievable with systemic therapy.

Visceral CMV disease occurred in 31% of patients at a median time of 248 days; four other patients were found to have disseminated disease at autopsy.

Retinal detachment occurred in seven eyes (18%), five of these at 30 to 64 days after surgery. However, this is probably a surgical complication rather than a complication of disease.

Primary Prophylaxis

GANCICLOVIR (CYTOVENE)

Standard doses of oral ganciclovir have also been studied for primary prophylaxis against CMV disease. Spector and coworkers randomized patients to receive either oral ganciclovir, 1000 mg per kg every 8 hours (486 patients), or placebo (239 patients). Median CD4$^+$ cell count was 21 per mm^3 for the ganciclovir-treated patients and 23 per mm^3 for the placebo patients. Ganciclovir resulted in about a 50% decrease in the recurrence of all CMV disease (20% of ganciclovir-treated patients versus 39% of placebo patients) as well as CMV retinitis (18% versus 39%). An interim analysis showed a trend toward increased survival in the ganciclovir patients; however, this difference was not apparent in the final analysis. Interestingly, the only patients in the placebo group who developed CMV disease had positive CMV cultures in either blood or urine. This group may benefit from prophylactic treatment with oral ganciclovir.

A similar study sponsored by the NIAID, Community Programs for Clinical Research on AIDS (CPCRA), failed to show a benefit. This study did not mandate ophthalmologic examinations, except for symptoms, and may be tainted by a dropout rate of nearly 80%. Despite the lack of benefit observed in the CPCRA study, oral ganciclovir is approved for the indication of prevention of CMV disease in individuals with advanced HIV infection at risk for developing CMV disease.

VALACYCLOVIR (VALTREX)

ACTG 204 studied the use of valacyclovir (VACV) as prophylactic therapy for CMV disease in patients with advanced HIV disease (CD4$^+$ cell count less than 100 per mm^3). In this trial, 1227 patients were randomized to receive one of the following regimens: VACV 2 grams qid, acyclovir (ACV) 800 mg qid, or ACV 400 mg bid. After a preliminary analysis was performed, VACV was found to be associated with a significantly increased mortality compared with the lowest dose of ACV. However, this association was not apparent when the final analysis was completed. It appears that although patients died of AIDS, they did not die of any specific toxicity due to VACV. On the basis of this observation, the study was halted by the Data and Safety Monitoring Board. Final analysis of confirmed CMV end points showed a trend toward a protective effect of VACV, leaving the role for this drug in CMV prophylaxis uncertain.

Future Investigations

Research continues on further defining the role of primary prophylactic treatment. In addition, ongoing studies regarding optimal treatment of CMV retinitis focus on several strategies: the use of oral ganciclovir, the ganciclovir intraocular device, cidofovir, lobucavir, and anti-CMV monoclonal antibodies.

These strategies can be combined in a number of scenarios, such as induction therapy with IV ganciclovir or foscarnet, followed by maintenance oral ganciclovir with IV reinduction as needed to avoid reactivation. Another possibility would be a ganciclovir intraocular implant plus oral ganciclovir for induction and maintenance therapy, with intermittent pre-emptive IV therapy to prevent reactivation. A third approach is IV induction therapy with or without a ganciclovir intraocular implant, followed by maintenance therapy of oral ganciclovir plus an implant, with intermittent pre-emptive IV therapy to prevent reactivation and visceral CMV disease. The aim of all of these prospective strategies is to decrease the number of reactivations, because each time this occurs, additional retinal tissue is lost, resulting in decreased visual acuity.

CONCLUSION

The rapid accrual of basic information concerning HIV-1 biology and opportunistic pathogens has led to an explosion in our ability to diagnose, prevent, and treat HIV disease and its associated complications. We can expect research in this rapidly evolving field to lead to further advances in the months and years to follow.

ACKNOWLEDGMENTS

The author is grateful to Dr. Robert L. Murphy for helpful discussions and to Ms. Penny Baron and Ms. Patricia Scurvin for invaluable assistance in preparation of this manuscript.

AMEBIASIS
method of
JONATHAN I. RAVDIN, M.D.
University of Minnesota Hospital and Clinics
Minneapolis, Minnesota

Amebiasis is a human disease due to the enteric protozoan *Entamoeba histolytica*. There are two morphologically identical *Entamoeba* species infecting humans, the noninvasive *Entamoeba dispar* and *E. histolytica*. Together they infect 10% of the world's population; approximately 1 in 10 of those infected harbors *E. histolytica*. *E. dispar* has never been associated with invasive colitis or liver abscess; intestinal infection spontaneously clears without treatment in 8 to 12 months. Apparently, all individuals with *E. histolytica* infection mount a serum antibody response, yet only 1 in 10 goes on to develop systemic invasive amebiasis. It is unknown whether clearance of *Entamoeba* infection, spontaneously or by chemotherapy, results in any degree of host immunity to prevent reinfection.

EPIDEMIOLOGY

It is important for clinicians to identify individuals at greater risk for infection and patients who are more likely to suffer severe invasive disease when they are infected. The infective dose can be as little as a single cyst, although a higher inoculum results in a shorter incubation period (1 to 3 days). High-risk groups for acquisition of infection include travelers to or immigrants from highly endemic areas (such as Mexico, India, Bangladesh, South Africa, and South America), sexually promiscuous individuals who engage in oral-anal or anal-genital-oral sex, chronically institutionalized populations (especially the mentally challenged), and Mexican Americans in the southwestern United States. Individuals who become at risk for fulminant amebiasis once they are infected include pregnant women, the malnourished, the very young (<1 year), and patients receiving corticosteroid therapy. Whether infection with human immunodeficiency virus results in increased frequency or severity of invasive amebiasis remains unclear.

CLINICAL SYNDROMES

The main clinical syndromes that result from *E. histolytica* infection include asymptomatic intestinal infection, acute amebic rectocolitis, chronic intestinal amebiasis, and amebic liver abscess. Infections of the peritoneum, lung, and pericardium are unusual manifestations resulting from extension of an amebic liver abscess or colonic perforation. Lung or brain abscesses are rare presentations resulting from hematogenous dissemination. In general, 60 to 90% of individuals with asymptomatic intestinal infection harbor *E. dispar*. Such patients are detected by routine or incidental stool examination. *E. dispar* infection does not elicit a serum antiamebic antibody response. Positive stool microscopy and serologic test results for antiamebic antibodies suggest infection with *E. histolytica*.

Acute amebic rectocolitis is characterized by bloody mucus in stools, tenesmus, and abdominal pain, with the onset of symptoms occurring in 7 to 10 days rather than more acutely. Only one third of patients are febrile; virtually all have stools positive for occult blood. Fulminant colitis is characterized by colonic dilatation, toxemia, and peritonitis (often with associated perforation). Chronic intestinal amebiasis is clinically identical to idiopathic inflammatory bowel disease. The disease can last for years, is intermittent in nature, and is characterized by abdominal pain with bloody diarrhea. The mistaken treatment of such patients with corticosteroids can result in fulminant disease. Ameboma, another form of chronic intestinal amebiasis, presents as a focal colonic mass, usually in the right colon, which is often mistaken clinically for colonic carcinoma. Amebic liver abscess, which presents acutely with right upper quadrant pain and fever, is indistinguishable from infection of the biliary tract. Patients with a more chronic infection have abdominal pain and weight loss. A minority are febrile, and many are initially misdiagnosed as having primary or metastatic liver cancer. Amebic liver abscess can be differentiated from pyogenic infection by its occurrence at any age, its association with specific epidemiologic risk factors, the finding of *E. histolytica* in the stool (20 to 60%), and the presence of serum antigen and antiamebic antibodies.

DIAGNOSIS

Diagnosis of intestinal infection still rests on expert microscopy of fecal samples. However, errors are frequent, and multiple stool samples are required. The finding of hematophagous (presence of ingested erythrocytes) trophozoites by microscopy is highly specific for amebic colitis. Antigen detection tests using enzyme-linked immunosorbent assays demonstrate *E. histolytica* antigen in serum and feces of patients with amebic liver abscess and colitis; a commercial assay for fecal testing is available from Tech-Lab (Blacksburg, Virginia).

Serologic testing is extremely helpful in the diagnosis of invasive amebiasis or asymptomatic pathogenic infection. Ninety percent of patients with invasive amebiasis are seropositive by the seventh day of illness. Asymptomatic patients harboring *E. histolytica* are also seropositive. In nonendemic areas, serologic testing is a cost-effective way to differentiate inflammatory bowel disease from chronic intestinal amebiasis. After the treatment of invasive amebiasis by most methods, patients remain seropositive for years, which is why up to 25% of noninfected control subjects in endemic areas have serum antiamebic antibodies. However, a negative test result does reduce the likelihood of invasive amebiasis.

Colonoscopy with scrapings or biopsy of the ulcer edge is the "gold standard" for diagnosis and is especially helpful in acute colitis or to rule out amebiasis before treatment of presumed inflammatory bowel disease with corticosteroids. A periodic acid–Schiff stain, which highlights trophozoites in tissues, should always be requested. Not only are barium studies not useful in diagnosis, but they also prevent any yield in stool examinations for ova and parasites for 1 to 2 weeks. Because it differentiates biliary tract disease from a primary liver process, abdominal ultrasonography is the most important study in evaluation of patients with right upper quadrant pain and fever. Amebic liver abscesses commonly appear as multiple nonhomogeneous defects by modern imaging techniques, especially in acute disease of less than 10 days' duration. Computed tomography (CT) and magnetic resonance imaging add little in evaluation at increased cost and radiation exposure. Amebic liver abscess cannot be differentiated from necrotic hepatoma or pyogenic abscess by imaging alone. The serologic results and the presence of epidemiologic risk factors are usually sufficient to establish the diagnosis. Well above 90% of patients will be seropositive after 7 days of symptomatic illness. If necessary, fine-needle aspiration under CT guidance can be used to rule out pyogenic disease, but this approach is rarely required for making an accurate diagnosis. Amebic liver abscesses contain proteinaceous fluid (not pus), and trophozoites are usually not found because they are in the tissues at the periphery of the lesion.

TREATMENT

Treatment of amebiasis is complicated by the need to use multiple agents and the lack of familiarity of physicians with an appropriate therapeutic response.

TABLE 1. **Drugs Recommended for Treatment of Amebiasis by Site of Action**

Drug	Advantages and Disadvantages
Luminal amebicides	
Diloxanide furoate (Furamide)	Low toxicity; high efficacy; available only from CDC
Paromomycin (Humatin)	Nonabsorbable; useful in pregnancy
Diiodohydroxyquin (Diiodoquin, Yodoxin)	20-d course required; potential optic toxicity
Useful in intestinal disease only	
Tetracyclines	Must combine with luminal agent against liver abscess
Erythromycin	
Active in all tissues	
Metronidazole (Flagyl)	Effective; in vitro resistance not described; frequent nausea and vomiting
Tinidazole (Simplotan)	Antabuse effect with ethanol Combine with luminal agent

Abbreviation: CDC = Centers for Disease Control and Prevention.

Pharmacology of Antiamebic Agents

The drugs recommended for use in treatment of amebiasis are listed in Table 1. Luminal agents include diloxanide furoate, paromomycin, and diiodohydroxyquin. Diloxanide furoate* is highly efficacious (95% clearance of patients), relatively nontoxic, and clearly the drug of choice to eradicate *E. histolytica* from the intestinal lumen. However, it is not widely available except through the Drug Service at the Centers for Disease Control and Prevention in Atlanta, Georgia (telephone, 404-639-3670 during the daytime and 404-639-2888 in off-hours). Paromomycin, an oral aminoglycoside, is effective in clearing asymptomatic infection and is not absorbed in the setting of little or no inflammation. Therefore, this drug is especially helpful if one elects to treat asymptomatic infection in pregnant women. Paromomycin may cause mild gastrointestinal irritation or fungal overgrowth. Diiodohydroxyquin has been used extensively but requires high compliance to complete a 20-day course. Its accessibility is limited in the United States. This drug can cause optic atrophy, and I prefer to avoid its use for this reason. The tetracyclines and erythromycins have a long history of successful treatment of invasive intestinal disease; however, they are not nearly as active in vitro against trophozoites as metronidazole is and are ineffective in liver abscess. Therefore, these agents are usually used as second-line drugs in combination with a luminal agent to treat mild symptomatic amebic colitis. Given the risks of recurrent or chronic infection, I would reserve them for patients who experience neurotoxicity or otherwise cannot tolerate metronidazole. The nitroimidazoles are the mainstays of therapy for invasive amebiasis. They are directly amebicidal in vitro, penetrate well into all tissues, and have shown no parasite resistance to their amebicidal activity. However, gastrointestinal intolerance is common, and individuals must be cautioned to avoid ethanol owing to a disulfiram (Antabuse) effect. These agents are metabolized in the liver, and high serum levels are associated with neurotoxicity, including seizures. However, most patients tolerate these drugs, and they have been used for years in the treatment of trichomoniasis. Carcinogenic risks suggested by in vitro mutagenesis studies have not been borne out by long-term follow-up (10 to 20 years); nevertheless, caution in use of metronidazoles should be exercised. Teratogenesis is a concern; however, uncontrolled studies suggested reasonable safety during the third trimester. Tinidazole is better tolerated and highly efficacious but is not currently available in the United States.

Emetines were historically used to treat invasive amebiasis. Although directly amebicidal, they are no longer recommended because of significant cardiovascular toxicity (hypotension, precordial chest pain, tachycardia). In addition, parenteral therapy with hospitalization is necessary, and neuromuscular toxicity is common. There are no studies that demonstrate that the addition of emetines to metronidazole improves the outcome in invasive amebiasis or is necessary in instances of initial treatment failure.

Asymptomatic Infection

This is an area of ongoing controversy. There is no evidence that infection with *E. dispar* represents a health risk to the index case or close contacts. However, long-term follow-up studies to assess symptoms and general health status have not been performed. The possibility of asymptomatic *E. histolytica* infection can be addressed by testing for serum antiamebic antibodies. A positive amebic serologic test result or detection of *E. histolytica*–specific antigen in feces is an indication for presumptive therapy, even in an endemic area. Treatment of asymptomatic infected patients who have negative results on Hemoccult and serologic testing should be individualized. In an endemic area, there are no indications for treating such individuals, but treatment is recommended when there is adequate sanitation and the risk for reinfection is low. This recommendation is based on the lack of follow-up studies. For seronegative individuals, treatment with a luminal agent (see Table 2 for regimens) is adequate. In asymptomatic seropositive individuals with no evidence of invasive disease, again a luminal agent is adequate. However, treatment of colitis is indicated if hematophagous trophozoites or occult blood is found in stool, even if the patient is asymptomatic. This may be the only circumstance in which use of a tetracycline with a luminal agent seems a reasonable alternative to metronidazole.

Acute or Chronic Amebic Colitis

Metronidazole (see Table 2) is recommended for all invasive *E. histolytica* infections. Treatment with a

*Not available in the United States.

TABLE 2. **Therapeutic Regimens for Adults with Amebiasis**

Asymptomatic Infection
1. Diloxanide furoate, 500 mg PO tid for 10 d
2. Paromomycin, 10 mg/kg PO tid for 10 d
3. Diiodohydroxyquin, 650 mg PO tid for 20 d

Amebic Colitis
4. Metronidazole, 750 mg PO tid for 7 d followed by 1, 2, or 3
5. Doxycycline, 250 mg PO bid for 14 d followed by 1, 2, or 3

Invasive Liver Abscess
6. Metronidazole, 750 mg PO tid for 7–10 d, followed by 1, 2, or 3
7. Metronidazole, 2.4 gm PO once daily for 2 d, followed by 1, 2, or 3

luminal agent must follow, especially if shorter courses of metronidazole are used. It is unwise to use both agents simultaneously owing to gastrointestinal intolerance, but there is no direct contraindication if compliance is a major issue. Patients respond promptly to metronidazole therapy; there is no benefit from adding additional tissue amebicides. In patients with fulminant amebiasis, intestinal leakage and bacterial peritonitis may necessitate broader antibacterial therapy. Surgery is usually not indicated because it is difficult to handle colonic tissues and conservative management is more likely to be successful. The only (rare) exception is toxic megacolon, often a result of inadvertent corticosteroid therapy, which may require a total colectomy. Localized chronic amebiasis (ameboma) responds well to therapy with metronidazole.

It is imperative that successful clearance of infection be documented because relapses occur. At least two separate stool examinations or follow-up antigen detection tests should be performed after therapy to assess the patient's outcome. As mentioned, serum antiamebic antibody titers remain elevated for years and are not helpful in assessing the resolution of disease. In patients with persistent nonspecific abdominal complaints or underlying inflammatory bowel disease, post-treatment colonoscopy with biopsy is necessary to rule out relapse. In addition, occasional patients may experience the onset of an idiopathic colitis after treatment in which amebae cannot be demonstrated in biopsy samples of tissue. These patients do not respond to metronidazole, and standard therapy for inflammatory bowel disease is also usually not helpful. They are difficult to manage; however, their symptoms often resolve within a year after cure of the amebic infection. This syndrome is presumably an autoimmune phenomenon: circulating amebic antigen-antibody complexes have been identified during colonic amebiasis.

Amebic Liver Abscess

The overwhelming majority of patients with amebic liver abscess respond to therapy with metronidazole (see Table 2) with gradual defervescence, de-

creased pain, and improved appetite during a 3- to 5-day period. There is no need to add potentially toxic agents such as chloroquine or dehydroemetine. A lack of response to metronidazole indicates a need to reconsider the diagnosis and perform a fine-needle aspiration of the abscess under CT guidance. Patients with amebic liver abscess who respond promptly to aspiration should still receive a complete course of metronidazole therapy, and all patients should be treated with a luminal agent after completion of metronidazole therapy. Studies have suggested that intestinal colonization, leading to a recurrence of amebic liver abscess, is more frequent than previously recognized. Regardless of whether the stool examination was initially positive, a complete course of diloxanide furoate or paromomycin is essential.

Whether fine-needle aspiration of the liver abscess should be done immediately on presentation depends on the experience and skill of the physician and the resources of the local medical center. Although such aspiration is unnecessary in 90% of individuals, it is occasionally recommended. Examples include large abscesses with only a thin capsule of liver preventing rupture, a patient in extreme distress requiring rapid relief, and last, a high likelihood that primary or secondary bacterial infection is present. Complications of amebic liver abscess such as peritonitis or lung involvement are best treated conservatively. However, an empyema or pericardial effusion must be drained. Amebic pericarditis is a fulminant disease that is often misdiagnosed; ultrasonography revealing a left lobe liver abscess suggests the diagnosis, and immediate action is necessary.

Once the patient responds, there is no need to monitor the hepatic lesion by expensive imaging studies. This creates undue anxiety and expense, because the lesion usually takes months to resolve. If the patient remains asymptomatic, there is no indication for therapy for a persistent defect, even 6 months after treatment. Only a recurrence of symptoms merits investigation.

GIARDIASIS

method of
MARTIN S. WOLFE, M.D.
Traveler's Medical Service of Washington, D.C., and George Washington University Medical School
Washington, D.C.

Giardia lamblia is the most commonly reported pathogenic intestinal protozoan in the United States. Infection is spread directly from person to person by fecal-oral contamination with cysts or indirectly by transmission in water and occasionally food. Particular situations contributing to infection include foreign travel to highly endemic areas; campers and hikers drinking water contaminated by other humans or by such reservoir animals as beavers and muskrats; community-wide outbreaks resulting from fecally contaminated central water supplies; children infecting each other within nursery schools and other institutions, and then infecting other family members at home; and immunodeficiency.

After cysts are ingested, trophozoites emerge from these cysts in the upper small bowel and attach to the duodenal and jejunal mucosa. A number of factors, both host and parasite, contribute to pathogenic changes, which may include enterocyte damage, villous atrophy, and crypt hyperplasia. These changes lead to malabsorption of sugars and fats and general intestinal irritation.

Symptoms can vary from person to person, depending on inoculum size, duration of infection, and individual host and perhaps parasite factors. The incubation period generally varies from about 9 to 15 days. In the acute stage, there is initially a feeling of intestinal uneasiness, followed by anorexia and nausea. Low-grade fever may be present. Subsequent acute symptoms may include explosive, watery, foul-smelling diarrhea; marked intestinal rumbling; abdominal distention; passage of excessive foul gas and perhaps foul belching; and occurrence of upper or middle epigastric cramps. The acute stage may last only 3 or 4 days, can resemble other causes of traveler's diarrhea, and is often not recognized as being due to giardiasis. Although some acute infections may clear spontaneously, a long-standing subacute or chronic infection may develop. This phase may involve 2 years or more of intermittent diarrhea and other symptoms. In individuals returned from endemic areas, the acute stage may not be recalled, and they can present with persistent or recurrent mild to moderate symptoms. During this chronic state, anorexia, malabsorption, weight loss, and marked fatigue may be present, in addition to characteristic intermittent foul mushy stools and distention and foul gas. As stated by an experienced worker on giardiasis, "the symptomatology of giardiasis is rich and unpredictable; individual variability and the intermittent nature and changing of the symptoms are characteristic." Many infections disappear after variable periods, and about 15% of infected adults and up to 50% of infected young children remain asymptomatic cyst passers. The duration of the asymptomatic cyst-passing state has not been determined.

Diagnosis can be confirmed in the majority of the cases by well-performed stool examinations. A series of three stools, collected in preservative, should be collected on alternate days. Because G. lamblia cysts and less commonly trophozoites are usually shed in the stool on a periodic basis in chronic infections, in some cases examination of even six or more stools may not reveal the organism. Continued negative results of stool examination cannot rule out G. lamblia as the causative agent. A test using enzyme immunoassay is available to detect G. lamblia fecal antigen in either fresh or preserved stool specimens. High specificity and sensitivity have been reported with this method, and it should be carried out in complement with routine stool examinations. In some cryptic cases unable to be confirmed by these techniques, examination of fluid from the area of the duodenal-jejunal junction may reveal G. lamblia trophozoites. Fluid can be obtained from the duodenal string test (Entero-Test) or by endoscopy. A small bowel mucosal biopsy may also be performed. Even after use of all these techniques, some G. lamblia cases may be unable to be parasitologically confirmed. In patients with strong epidemiologic and clinical evidence of giardiasis, marked improvement and apparent cure may follow empirical treatment with specific anti-Giardia drugs to be discussed.

TREATMENT

At present, there are only two commercially available drugs in the United States for treating giardiasis, metronidazole (Flagyl) and furazolidone (Furoxone). Quinacrine (Atabrine) production has been discontinued by the manufacturer, but it may be obtained through some other sources. A number of nitroimidazole compounds, including tinidazole (Fasigyn), ornidazole (Tiberal), and secnidazole (Flagentyl), have been found effective abroad but are not available in the United States. Paromomycin (Humatin), a Food and Drug Administration (FDA)–approved drug, had variable effectiveness in studies abroad and has been used in the United States for treating giardiasis during pregnancy (Table 1). Other FDA-approved drugs evaluated against G. lamblia include mebendazole (Vermox) and albendazole (Albenza).

Metronidazole is a nitroimidazole, available as both a generic and a trade name (Flagyl) product. Although considered the treatment of choice for giardiasis, metronidazole has never been approved by the FDA for this indication. The adult dose is 250 mg three times a day for 7 days. Cure rates are in the 85 to 90% range, but there is evidence of parasite resistance by some clones of G. lamblia. This dose of metronidazole is generally well tolerated. Side effects can include a metallic taste, dark urine, and gastrointestinal symptoms. Alcohol use during treatment is contraindicated because of the disulfiram (Antabuse)–like effect of metronidazole. Questions regarding potential carcinogenic and mutagenic effects of metronidazole have arisen, but careful observation and follow-up of treated patients have shown no increased risk.

Furazolidone is a nitrofuran antibiotic whose major indication for use in the United States is giardiasis. It is the only anti-Giardia drug available in liquid form, making it of particular use in young children. Cure rates have ranged from 75 to 90%. Adverse reactions include gastrointestinal symptoms, fever, rash, and occasionally urticaria, and the urine may become brown. Furazolidone is a monoamine oxidase inhibitor. A disulfiram-like reaction

TABLE 1. **Drugs Used for Giardiasis in the United States**

Drug	Adult Dose	Pediatric Dose	Availability
Metronidazole	250 mg tid × 7 d	5 mg/kg tid × 7 d	Flagyl (Searle) (tablet)
Furazolidone	100 mg (tablet) qid × 7 d	1.25 mg/kg qid × 7 d (liquid)	Furoxone (Roberts) (liquid and tablets)
Quinacrine	100 mg tid × 5 d	2 mg/kg tid × 5 d	See text footnote
Paromomycin	500 mg tid × 7 d	10 mg/kg tid × 7 d	Humatin (Parke-Davis) (capsules)

can occur with concomitant alcohol ingestion, and patients with glucose-6-phosphate dehydrogenase deficiency may develop hemolysis. Furazolidone has caused mammary tumors in rats, and its safety has been questioned; however, it remains an FDA-approved drug for giardiasis. The dosage for adults is 100 mg four times a day for 7 days, and that for children is 1.25 mg per kg four times a day for 7 days.

Quinacrine has a long history of use against *G. lamblia* and is the most effective drug for this condition, with cure rates of 90 to 95%. Unfortunately, for reasons not well explained, the major manufacturer ceased production, and quinacrine has become commercially unavailable worldwide. However, quinacrine in powder form placed in 100-mg gelatin capsules is available from particular sources.* Also tempering enthusiasm for its use as the drug of choice are more frequent side effects. Common side effects include gastrointestinal discomfort, headache, and dizziness. Less frequent but more disturbing untoward reactions include vomiting, fever, and rash. The urine may become bright yellow. In a large personal series of giardiasis patients treated with a 7-day course of quinacrine, toxic psychosis with either depression or excitation occurred in 1.5% of adults. Toxic psychosis and other side effects have been much less common in a more recently used 5-day course, which appears to be equally effective as the standard 7-day course. Some cases of chronic giardiasis persisting after repeated courses of metronidazole and quinacrine alone have been successfully treated with a combined course of metronidazole and quinacrine.

Paromomycin is a poorly absorbed aminoglycoside antibiotic found useful in treating a number of pathogenic intestinal protozoa. Studies abroad using paromomycin for giardiasis showed variable results. Few reports of its use in the United States for giardiasis have been published. Paromomycin does not appear to be nearly as effective as the preceding anti-*Giardia* drugs, but none of these other drugs can be used in pregnancy with completely ensured safety to the fetus. Because paromomycin is poorly absorbed, its use in a few pregnant women with giardiasis requiring treatment has been reported; it has been suggested that paromomycin should be the first treatment of choice in this situation, in a dose of 500 mg three times a day for 7 days. However, a good effect remains to be proved, with only a few pregnant women treated with paromomycin described so far. When treatment of a pregnant woman with severe symptoms from giardiasis that could possibly prove detrimental to the pregnancy is necessary, I have had good success in using quinacrine.

Various nitroimidazole drugs used abroad are not available in the United States, and FDA approval for them is not expected to be attempted. The most widely used of these nitroimidazoles, which are in the same family of drugs as metronidazole, is tinidazole. In a single 2-gram adult dose, comparative studies overseas have shown tinidazole in its short course to be as effective as and better tolerated than metronidazole. Good effect and tolerance are also reported for the related nitroimidazoles ornidazole and secnidazole.

Mebendazole and albendazole are benzimidazole derivatives that have had a few trials against *G. lamblia* in children and adults. Results were better in children than in adults. Further well-controlled studies in a larger number of *Giardia*-positive subjects should be carried out with these drugs, which are both FDA approved and available in the United States.

Asymptomatic cyst passers, particularly young children and food handlers, are potential sources of infection to others and may themselves possibly develop spontaneous symptoms. Although the need to treat asymptomatic carriers is controversial, many physicians prefer to treat all infected individuals living in a nonendemic area.

In some individuals with an exposure history and classic symptoms of giardiasis, it is not possible to confirm infection by repeated stool examinations, by examination of duodenal contents or biopsy, or by finding *G. lamblia* stool antigen. It has been well recognized by many workers that some *G. lamblia* infections are cryptic, perhaps involving the biliary tree. In the absence of other pathogenic intestinal parasites or other recognized causes, and before embarking on an often time-consuming and expensive thorough gastrointestinal work-up, an empirical course of metronidazole or quinacrine should be tried. At times, this can lead to highly gratifying results.

In those with proven *G. lamblia* parasites before treatment, as a check for cure, a series of three stool examinations on alternate days should be performed approximately 4 weeks after completion of treatment. With proven treatment failure (or possible reinfection), re-treatment with a different drug should be carried out. When *Giardia*-like symptoms persist in the absence of proven *G. lamblia* parasites on posttreatment examinations, aftereffects such as lactose intolerance or secondary intestinal yeast infection should be considered.

BACTEREMIA AND SEPTICEMIA

method of
JAMES LEGGETT, M.D.
*Providence Portland Medical Center and Oregon
    Health Sciences University*
Portland, Oregon

Bacteremia, the presence of bacteria in the bloodstream, is a commonplace event; it occurs normally not only after daily tooth-brushing or bowel movements but also after simple procedures such as tooth extraction or manipulation

---

*Quinacrine is available from (1) Priority Pharmacy (telephone, 1-800-487-7113); (2) Medical Center Pharmacy, 800 Howard Avenue, New Haven, CT 06511 (telephone, 1-203-785-6816).

of the gastrointestinal or genitourinary tract. Bacteremia is fortunately most often transient owing to the host's prompt systemic response to infection and the filtering action of the reticuloendothelial system amplified by a cascade of inflammatory mediators, cytokines, and vasoactive agents. Septicemia refers to the physiologic consequences of severe bloodstream infection with bacteria or other pathogens. In the majority of septic patients, the host's defenses prevail and the invaders are destroyed. In the weaker or less fortunate, the host's system is overwhelmed and the immune response becomes chaotic, resulting in a downward spiral of hypotension, impaired organ perfusion, and death. To enhance the septic patient's chance of survival, a careful search for the source of sepsis is imperative both to guide antibiotic therapy and to allow appropriate adjunctive therapy, such as drainage of abscesses. The history and physical examination are the most valuable diagnostic tools. For instance, a history of dysuria and flank pain suggests a urinary source, whereas a mass in the left lower quadrant with pain and fever suggests diverticulitis.

SEPSIS

Clinically detectable bacteremia is usually a result of spillage into the blood from an extravascular site of infection (e.g., abscess, urinary tract infection, necrotizing skin infection) rather than a sustained intravascular infection (e.g., endocarditis). Although localizing symptoms and signs often accompany generalized sepsis, it is still difficult to accurately predict the presence of bacteremia in a septic patient. For example, only one third of patients enrolled in clinical studies of agents to treat gram-negative bacteremia actually had such an infection. Another third had nonbacteremic gram-negative infections, 10% had gram-positive infections, and nearly 20% had no infection.

The 25 to 60% mortality associated with advanced sepsis has prompted efforts at its earlier recognition. The sepsis syndrome defines a constellation of features (Table 1), including hypothermia or hyperthermia; tachycardia; tachypnea; a presumed site of infection; and evidence of inadequate perfusion manifested by either poor or altered cerebral function, arterial hypoxia, elevated plasma lactate level, or urine output less than 30 mL per hour. The sepsis syndrome results from the host response to pathogenic microorganisms, their components (e.g., endotoxin, peptidoglycans), or their toxins (e.g., the toxic shock syndrome toxin) in the blood or tissues. Because this inflammatory reaction may also accompany noninfectious illnesses, such as pancreatitis, trauma, or thermal injury, it is often referred to as the systemic inflammatory response syndrome.

TABLE 1. Definition of Sepsis Syndrome

Clinical evidence of infection
Tachypnea (>20 breaths/min)
Tachycardia (>90 beats/min)
Hyperthermia (>38.3°C, or 101°F) or hypothermia
  (<35.6°C, or 96°F)
Evidence of inadequate organ perfusion including one or more
  of the following:
  Elevated plasma lactate
  Hypoxemia (PaO$_2$ < 75 mm Hg) without other
    pulmonary disease as a cause
  Oliguria (urine output <30 mL/h or 0.5 mL/kg of body
    weight)
  Poor or altered cerebral function

The diagnosis does not require the presence of a positive blood culture; the point is to detect the condition in its early manifestations before blood cultures are positive. Patients with the sepsis syndrome should be admitted for close monitoring (in many cases to the intensive care unit) and should have blood cultures and appropriate tests performed to localize the source of infection (e.g., chest radiograph, Gram's stain and culture of sputum, urinalysis, joint aspiration, lumbar puncture). Antibiotic therapy should be based on the likely source of infection and Gram's stain results when possible (see "Antibiotic Therapy").

Septic shock occurs when sepsis is accompanied by hypotension, a systolic blood pressure less than 90 mm Hg or a decrease of 40 mm Hg from baseline. Shock is a complication of sepsis in almost 50% of patients and is the most common cause of adult respiratory distress syndrome (ARDS) and of death in the intensive care unit. In the United States, 400,000 people develop sepsis and 200,000 develop septic shock each year.

Early in septic shock, the systemic vascular resistance falls and the cardiac output increases. Management at this point consists of rapid fluid administration; fluid requirements may be as high as 6 to 8 liters per day. Placement of a pulmonary artery catheter may be important in determining optimal filling pressures for the left side of the heart in these patients, because central venous pressures frequently fail to correlate with wedge pressures. A wedge pressure of 10 to 15 mm Hg is usually optimal, but each patient must be assessed individually. In patients who remain hypotensive in spite of aggressive fluid resuscitation, dopamine at doses of 5 to 15 µg per kg per minute exerts both beta-adrenergic and alpha-adrenergic effects.

Forty to 60% of patients with septic shock develop ARDS, characterized by refractory hypoxemia, diffuse pulmonary infiltrates, and a normal wedge pressure. Mechanical ventilation with positive end-expiratory pressure may be necessary to maintain adequate oxygenation. Although high-dose steroids and other anti-inflammatory medications have been employed to suppress the inflammatory response in experimental protocols in patients with ARDS, none has been shown to be effective to date. The majority of patients who die of septic shock have multiple organ failure resulting from hypoperfusion, microvascular injury induced by the body's inflammatory response (disseminated intravascular coagulation), and ongoing release of toxic products from invading organisms. The most common pattern is sequential pulmonary, hepatic, and renal failure; mortality ranges from 80 to 100% with failure of three or more organs.

BLOOD CULTURES

Blood cultures are the "gold standard" for diagnosing bacteremia. Their maximal usefulness depends on a number of factors, including the timing, number obtained, volume of blood, sterile technique, culture media, and proper interpretation. Bacteremia may be classified as transient, intermittent, or continuous. Transient bacteremia commonly occurs early in the course of localized infections (such as pyelonephritis or pneumonia), after manipulation of infected or colonized tissue or mucosal surfaces (as with tooth extraction or endoscopy), or in the course of daily events such as tooth-brushing. Intermittent bacteremia is characteristic of undrained abscesses. Continuous bacteremia is the hallmark of endovascular infections such as endocarditis, septic thrombophlebitis, mycotic aneurysms, or intravascular catheter infections. Introduction of bacteria into the bloodstream results in the synthesis of cytokines that cause fever and other systemic responses to sepsis within 30 to 90 minutes. If bacteremia is transient or intermittent, culture of a blood sample drawn after the fever spike may be negative. Because bacteremia in the patient suspected of having intermittent or transient bacteremia is unpredictable, the traditional practice of obtaining blood samples for culture after a fever spike may be no better than obtaining them at random intervals. In patients with continuous bacteremia, the timing of the cultures is of little significance, by definition, and blood samples may be obtained from separate venipuncture sites a few minutes apart before the institution of antibiotics. In patients with *Staphylococcus aureus* bacteremia due to endovascular infections, blood cultures will remain positive for several days; in bacteremias with other organisms, cultures should be negative soon after the first dose of antibiotics.

The requisite number of cultures depends on the clinical setting. In patients with true sepsis, roughly 90% of bacteremic episodes are detected by the first blood culture (10 mL of blood), 99% by the first two cultures (20 mL), and nearly 100% by the first three cultures (30 mL). In nearly all cases, two cultures suffice (see Table 2 for more specific guidelines). The correct interpretation of blood culture results depends on proper interpretation by the physician. The sensitivity (true-positive rate) of blood cultures depends predominantly on the volume of blood obtained; at least 10 mL per culture is recommended. The specificity of blood cultures (true-negative rate) depends on the physician's ability to distinguish false-positive cultures from true-positive cultures. False-positive cultures are those that yield organisms not consistent with a clinical infection. The false-positive rate among all blood cultures, positive and negative, is reported to be 1 to 8.9%. The percentage of positive cultures that are falsely positive is much higher and has been reported to be as high as 47%. The most common false-positive organisms consist of skin and mouth flora, which can either contaminate blood cultures or cause nonsignificant bacteremias (Table 3). Therefore, cultures from normal hosts yielding skin flora such as diphtheroids, *Staphylococcus epidermidis*, or *Bacillus* species are nearly always false-positive due to nonpathogenic strains. Half of *Clostridium* species and of viridans streptococci give false-positive results. (However, in patients who are immunocompromised or who have prosthetic devices, diphtheroids, *S. epidermidis*, and others may be true pathogens.) On the other hand, *Escherichia coli*, *Klebsiella pneumoniae*, *Bacteroides* species, *Streptococcus pyogenes*, and *Streptococcus pneumoniae* are rarely contaminants and should be considered true pathogens

TABLE 2. Guidelines for Number of Blood Cultures

One blood culture is rarely, if ever, sufficient.

Two blood cultures are necessary and sufficient to either rule out or establish a diagnosis of bacteremia when the probability of bacteremia is low to moderate (as in patients with pneumonia or gastrointestinal sepsis).

Three blood cultures should be obtained to rule out continuous bacteremia (such as with endocarditis) or when the probability of bacteremia is high.

Four (or more) blood cultures should be obtained if the probability of bacteremia is high and the anticipated pathogens are also common contaminants (as in prosthetic valve endocarditis) or if the patient has received antibiotics in the last 2 wk.

TABLE 3. Interpretation of Blood Culture Results

Blood culture isolates likely to be contaminants
  Diphtheroids
  Staphylococcus epidermidis
  Bacillus species
Blood culture isolates likely to be true pathogens
  Staphylococcus aureus
  Streptococcus pyogenes
  Streptococcus pneumoniae
  Enterococcus
  Enterobacteriaceae (*Escherichia coli, Klebsiella, Proteus, Serratia, Enterobacter*)
  Pseudomonas
  Gram-negative anaerobes (*Bacteroides*)
Blood culture isolates with intermediate probability of being contaminants (about 50% are true pathogens)
  Clostridia
  Viridans streptococci

when isolated. Contaminants may also be identified by their delayed growth (resulting in positive cultures after 48 to 72 hours of incubation) and rare isolation from simultaneous or subsequent cultures (for instance, the organism grows in only one of four bottles). Multiple skin organisms isolated from a single blood culture also suggest contamination. Polymicrobial bacteremia with nonskin organisms, although rare, suggests significant gastrointestinal disease, especially if *Bacteroides* is present, and should not be discounted.

ANTIBIOTIC THERAPY

The antimicrobial spectrum of an antibiotic is the most important factor in its selection; additional factors can modify the choice, such as mechanism of antimicrobial activity and pharmacologic properties as well as allergies, physiologic conditions of the host, and cost of the drug. A bacteriostatic drug inhibits growth of the pathogen without killing outright, whereas a bactericidal drug kills pathogens directly. Bactericidal agents should be used in bacteremic patients, especially those with endocarditis, as well as in patients with impaired host defenses or meningitis. When possible, avoid nephrotoxic drugs in patients with renal impairment and hepatotoxic drugs in patients with liver disease. The patient's statements about allergic reactions to antibiotics must be given serious consideration. In most cases of genuine allergy to an antibiotic of first choice, chemically unrelated but effective alternative regimens are available. Although many infections can be treated with a single antibiotic, there are specific cases in which antimicrobial combinations should be considered. Intra-abdominal infections are often due to a mixture of bacteria, and the combination of ampicillin, clindamycin, and gentamicin is classic; however, newer broad-spectrum β-lactams alone are also effective. Multiple antibiotics are indicated when the synergistic activity of two or more drugs may bring an infection under control more rapidly or more effectively than a single drug. Such synergistic combinations are most often applied to endocarditis and to infections due to *Pseudomonas aeruginosa*. For instance, in the case of enterococcal endocarditis, ampicillin alters the cell wall, allowing gentamicin to penetrate the bacteria and inhibit protein synthesis at the ribosomal level. Neither ampicillin nor gentamicin is effective alone. For *Pseudomonas*, the combination of an antipseudomonal penicillin with an aminoglycoside provides similar synergistic effects. Antimicrobial combinations may also be employed when a subpopulation of resistant bacterial mutants is likely to emerge during therapy with a single drug, such as occurs during single-drug therapy with *P. aeruginosa* and *Enterobacter* and *Serratia* species. Theoretically, use of combination therapy poses a risk for antimicrobial antagonism, chemical incompatibility, or chemical inactivation; however, such adverse effects have rarely been observed clinically. The optimal length of therapy has not been clearly determined for many bacterial infections. In general, 1 to 2 weeks is sufficient. Unnecessarily prolonging antimicrobial therapy increases the risk for toxic effects of the drug and for superinfection with resistant organisms.

Empirical antibiotics are usually administered before blood culture results are known. The choice of antibiotic depends on the site of infection and epidemiologic considerations (e.g., age, community-acquired versus hospital-acquired infection, use of intravenous drugs). Because it is not possible to distinguish grampositive sepsis from gram-negative sepsis clinically, broad-spectrum coverage is essential until the infecting organism is identified. In general, streptococci, staphylococci, and gram-negative bacilli must be covered if there are no clinical clues to the etiology of bacteremia. The lungs and the abdomen are frequently the source of infection in patients in whom the source of sepsis is not found, even after a thorough evaluation. Table 4 lists guidelines for empirical treatment of sepsis. Empirical treatment of urosepsis should cover gram-negative bacilli and enterococci, with the initial choice of antibiotic based on Gram's stain of the urine, if possible. In addition to these organisms, empirical therapy for intra-abdominal sepsis should cover anaerobes. Empirical therapy for pneumonia should be directed at pneumococci and common gram-negative pathogens. Empirical therapy for presumed cardiovascular infections should include staphylococcal coverage. Empirical coverage of sepsis in immunocompromised patients is difficult because of the wide range of organisms that cause infections; blood cultures and appropriate cultures of other sites are imperative to direct antimicrobial therapy. Neutropenic patients must be treated with antibiotics active against *Pseudomonas*. Once the pathogen is identified, antibiotics should be tailored from broad-spectrum to narrower-spectrum coverage to prevent superinfections with more resistant bacteria or fungi. When the patient becomes afebrile, intravenous antibiotics may be converted to oral formulations if there

TABLE 4. **Empirical Intravenous Antibiotics for Sepsis**

Infection	Organisms	Antibiotics
Community Acquired		
Urinary	Enterobacteriaceae*	Ceftriaxone (Rocephin)†
	Enterococcus	Ampicillin + gentamicin
Pulmonary	*Streptococcus pneumoniae*	Penicillin G; ceftriaxone†
	Klebsiella, Haemophilus influenzae	Ceftriaxone†
	Staphylococcus aureus	Nafcillin (Unipen)‡
Abdominal	Enterobacteriaceae, anaerobes	Ampicillin + gentamicin‡ + clindamycin (Cleocin) or metronidazole (Flagyl)
	Enterococcus	Ampicillin-sulbactam (Unasyn); ticarcillin-clavulanate (Timentin)§; imipenem-cilastatin (Primaxin)
Meningitis (adult)	*S. pneumoniae, Neisseria meningitidis*	Ceftriaxone† (+ vancomycin if ceftriaxone-resistant pneumococci suspected)
Unspecified source	Enterobacteriaceae, *S. aureus, S. pneumoniae,* other streptococci	Ceftriaxone†; ampicillin-sulbactam; cefazolin (Ancef) + gentamicin‖
Endocarditis (native valve) Nonintravenous drug abuser		
Subacute	Viridans streptococci, *Streptococcus bovis, Enterococcus*	Penicillin G or ampicillin + gentamicin
Acute	*S. aureus, Enterococcus, S. pneumoniae*	Nafcillin‡ + gentamicin
Intravenous drug abuser	*S. aureus,* Enterobacteriaceae	Nafcillin‡ + gentamicin
Hospital Acquired		
Intravascular catheter sepsis	*Staphylococcus epidermidis, S. aureus*	Vancomycin
Unspecified site	Enterobacteriaceae, *S. aureus*	Ceftriaxone† + gentamicin‖; ticarcillin-clavulanate§; ampicillin-sulbactam; imipenem
Neutropenic patient	Enterobacteriaceae and *Pseudomonas*	Ticarcillin (Ticar) or ceftazidime (Fortaz)† + tobramycin‖; imipenem; equivalent regimen

* Enterobacteriaceae include *Escherichia coli, Klebsiella, Enterobacter, Salmonella,* and other bacteria commonly isolated from enteric specimens.
† Or equivalent (e.g., cefotaxime, ceftizoxime).
‡ Vancomycin should be used for penicillin-allergic patients or for methicillin-resistant staphylococcus.
§ Or equivalent (piperacillin-tazobactam).
‖ Peak aminoglycoside levels should be at least 6–8 µg/mL.

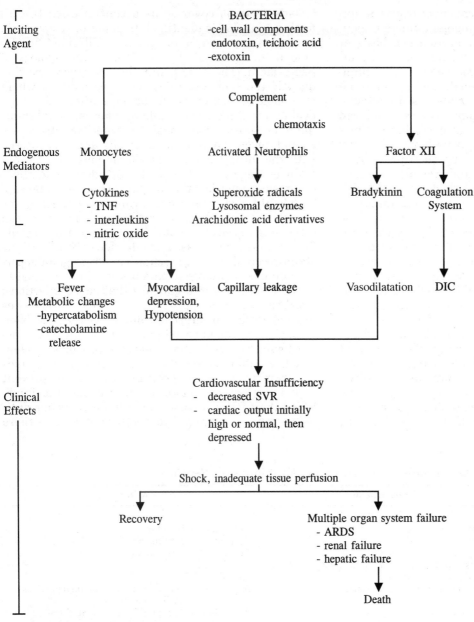

Figure 1. Pathogenesis of sepsis.

ARDS = adult respiratory distress syndrome
TNF = tumor necrosis factor
DIC = disseminated intravascular coagulation
SVR = systemic vascular resistance

is no endovascular focus or undrained abscess. *S. aureus* bacteremia may require a more prolonged intravenous course (often 1 to 4 weeks) than bacteremia caused by other organisms.

In many cases, antibiotic therapy will be ineffective unless the focus of infection is removed. For instance, abscesses must be drained, dead tissue must be débrided, infected joints must be serially aspirated or surgically drained, infected lines must be removed, and empyema must be treated with a chest tube.

EXPERIMENTAL THERAPIES

In spite of the availability of effective antibiotics against most organisms causing sepsis, mortality re-

mains high, 10 to 20%. Researchers have therefore focused on intervening in that part of the *host* response that causes tissue damage.

Figure 1 shows a proposed sequence of pathogenetic steps leading from infection to septic shock. Bacterial cell wall components (endotoxin in gram-negative bacteria, teichoic acid or peptidoglycan in gram-positive bacteria) introduced into the bloodstream lead to complement system activation, which incites a series of inflammatory events, including vasodilatation and increased vascular permeability, platelet aggregation, and activation of neutrophils. Activated neutrophils then release arachidonic acid derivatives, cytotoxic superoxide radicals, and lysosomal enzymes that damage the microvasculature and result in capillary leakage—a process presumed to be important in the pathogenesis of ARDS.

Macrophages play a pivotal role in the pathogenesis of sepsis. Once activated by binding to bacterial endotoxin or other molecules, they release cytokines into the system, producing fever, metabolic changes, and hormonal changes as well as activating coagulation pathways (sometimes resulting in disseminated intravascular coagulation) and causing cardiovascular depression. Cytokines, including tumor necrosis factor and the interleukins, are important mediators of the inflammatory response to sepsis.

Several adjunctive therapies have been investigated in the hope of reducing the morbidity and mortality associated with sepsis. High-dose steroids have shown no benefit in several well-controlled trials in patients with early septic shock or ARDS; in some studies, deleterious consequences were observed. Administration of monoclonal antibodies to endotoxin core glycolipid or to the interleukin-1 receptor has not been shown to significantly reduce mortality in patients with gram-negative bacteremia. Early in the course of sepsis, when the antibody must be given to be effective, it is as yet impossible to determine which patients have gram-negative bacteremia. In the absence of well-defined criteria for the early recognition of gram-negative bacteremia, the optimal use of such antibodies remains a problem.

BRUCELLOSIS

method of
EDWARD J. YOUNG, M.D.
Baylor College of Medicine and VA Medical
    Center
Houston, Texas

Brucellosis is a disease of animals (zoonosis) that is transmittable to humans. The disease exists worldwide but is especially prevalent in the Mediterranean basin, the Arabian peninsula, the Indian subcontinent, and parts of Mexico and Central and South America. Programs designed to control and eradicate bovine brucellosis have dramatically reduced the frequency of human infection in the United States.

Humans contract brucellosis by direct contact with infected animals, their secretions, and carcasses. Other modes of transmission include inhalation of contaminated aerosols and ingestion of unpasteurized milk or dairy products, such as cheese. Whereas brucellosis was once principally an occupational hazard for persons engaged in the livestock industry, such as farmers, ranchers, veterinarians, and abattoir workers, its epidemiology in the United States has changed. The majority of cases currently occur among people of Hispanic descent, with the ingestion of unpasteurized goat milk cheese being the major risk factor. Brucellosis has long been recognized to be a risk for laboratory personnel, and Biohazard Level 3 precautions are recommended when handling clinical specimens.

Although closely related genetically, four species of *Brucella* are differentiated by their preference for natural hosts: *B. abortus* (cattle), *B. melitensis* (goats and sheep),

B. suis (swine), and *B. canis* (dogs). For reasons that are not entirely clear, infection with *B. melitensis* causes the most serious disease. *Brucella* species are small, gram-negative coccobacilli that respire aerobically; some species require additional CO_2 for primary isolation. They lack flagellae, spores, exotoxins, and native plasmids, and the principal virulence factor is cell wall lipopolysaccharide (endotoxin). They are facultative intracellular pathogens that have the ability to survive and multiply within phagocytic cells of the host. Brucellae are phagocytosed by neutrophils, but they resist intracellular killing by mechanisms that are not well understood. Within the infected host, they are rapidly localized within monocytes and macrophages of the reticuloendothelial system (RES). Consequently, many complications of brucellosis involve organs rich in elements of the RES, such as lymph nodes, spleen, liver, kidneys, and bone marrow. Although humoral antibodies play a role in resistance, the primary mechanism of recovery is cell-mediated immunity.

Brucellosis is a systemic infection that can involve any organ or tissue of the body. Symptoms are largely nonspecific and usually begin within 2 to 3 weeks after inoculation. In about half of the cases, the onset of disease is insidious, developing in weeks to months. The disease is characterized by multiple somatic complaints, such as fatigue, malaise, body aches, and depression. In contrast, abnormal physical findings can be few, notably, fever, sweats, lymphadenopathy, and occasionally hepatosplenomegaly. The fever pattern waxes and wanes during several days, giving rise to the term "undulant fever." When symptoms related to a single organ system predominate, the disease is referred to as localized. Osteoarticular localization is the most common complication.

TREATMENT

Antimicrobial therapy relieves symptoms, shortens the duration of illness, and decreases the frequency of complications, some of which (e.g., endocarditis and meningitis) can be life-threatening. A variety of drugs are active against *Brucella* in vitro; however, the results of routine susceptibility tests do not always predict clinical efficacy. Moreover, the intracellular location of *Brucella* appears to provide some protection against the action of certain classes of drugs. Consequently, β-lactam antibiotics, such as penicillin and cephalosporins, are generally ineffective despite in vitro activity.

The tetracyclines remain the most effective class of antibiotics for the treatment of human brucellosis, and most strains of *Brucella* are inhibited by 0.1 μg per mL or less. Because tetracyclines are bacteriostatic, they are usually used in combination with another drug, such as an aminoglycoside, rifampin,* or trimethoprim-sulfamethoxazole (TMP-SMZ).*

The traditional therapy is tetracycline HCl (500 mg four times per day orally for 6 weeks) in combination with streptomycin (1 gram per day intramuscularly for 2 to 3 weeks). Currently, doxycycline (Vibramycin), 200 mg per day orally for 6 weeks, has largely replaced tetracycline HCl because of its longer half-life and fewer adverse side effects. In addition, many authorities have replaced streptomy-

---

*Not FDA approved for this indication.

cin with gentamicin (Garamycin), 5 mg per kg per day intravenously or intramuscularly for 2 to 3 weeks; however, there are no controlled studies comparing the efficacy of the two aminoglycosides.

Rifampin (Rifadin) is active against *Brucella*, penetrates cell membranes, and is bactericidal. In 1986, the World Health Organization recommended the combination of doxycycline (200 mg per day) plus rifampin (600 to 900 mg per day), each administered orally for 45 days, as the treatment of choice. Although some studies have shown this combination to be comparable to doxycycline plus streptomycin, others have reported it to result in higher rates of relapse.

TMP-SMZ (Bactrim, Septra) in a fixed combination of 80 mg of trimethoprim and 400 mg of sulfamethoxazole is also active against *Brucella*. The usual dose is 4 tablets (or 2 tablets of the double-strength dose) daily for 45 days; however, some authorities have reported unacceptably high rates of relapse with this drug.

The fluoroquinolones vary in their activity against *Brucella* in vitro, but ciprofloxacin (Cipro)* and ofloxacin (Floxin),* among others, show favorable minimal inhibitory concentrations. Unfortunately, when they are used alone in cases of brucellosis, the relapse rates are high, and antibiotic-resistant strains of *Brucella* have emerged in rare instances. Consequently, quinolones should be used only in combination with other drugs, and their role in treatment remains to be determined.

SPECIAL SITUATIONS

Childhood Brucellosis

The tetracyclines are contraindicated in children younger than 8 years because of the potential for irreversible staining of deciduous teeth. In this regard, doxycycline appears to bind less well to enamel than tetracycline HCl does, but this does not entirely obviate this concern. Nevertheless, some authorities have treated childhood brucellosis with doxycycline and streptomycin or gentamicin with favorable results. Others prefer to use TMP-SMZ, but the risk for relapse remains high. The combination of TMP-SMZ plus rifampin appears to be a reasonable alternative, but there is little published experience with this regimen.

Pregnancy

Brucellosis during pregnancy can result in spontaneous abortion, although there is little evidence that it occurs more commonly than with other bacteremic infections. The same problems of tetracycline use with childhood brucellosis apply to pregnancy as well. In addition, the drugs commonly used to treat brucellosis are not approved for use in pregnancy. Nevertheless, doxycycline and an aminoglycoside

---

*Not FDA approved for this indication.

have been used successfully during pregnancy. TMP-SMZ has also been used in this setting and, when combined with rifampin, appears to offer a safe alternative.

COMPLICATIONS

Osteoarticular Brucellosis

Complications involving bones and joints occur in 25 to 50% of patients with brucellosis, but rarely do they present special problems in treatment. The majority of patients respond to routine anti-*Brucella* chemotherapy. Surgical intervention is rarely necessary except to drain septic joint effusions or large, symptomatic paraspinal abscesses. The indications for surgery of paraspinal abscesses are neurologic dysfunction, continued fever and pain after adequate antibiotic therapy, and spinal instability.

Neurobrucellosis

A variety of neurologic syndromes have been reported in patients with brucellosis, of which acute or chronic meningitis is the most common. Although central nervous system involvement occurs in less than 5% of cases, it poses special problems owing to the need to achieve bactericidal concentrations of drugs. Most agents commonly used in brucellosis do not penetrate the blood-brain barrier well. Most authorities recommend doxycycline, streptomycin, and rifampin. TMP-SMZ has also been used, but it should not be the sole agent. There is no agreement on the duration of therapy; however, treatment should not be discontinued before 6 weeks and is often required for 6 to 8 months. Although the value of adding corticosteroids has not been proved, some authors give them for complicated cases.

Endocarditis

Another complication of brucellosis requiring bactericidal concentrations of antibiotics is endocarditis. Although rare, endocarditis is reportedly the most common cause of fatal brucellosis. Although some patients have been treated successfully with antibiotics alone, the majority require valve replacement surgery as well. Triple therapy with doxycycline, an aminoglycoside, and rifampin or TMP-SMZ is generally recommended, with treatment continued for periods ranging from 6 weeks to 9 months. After valve replacement, antibiotics are often continued for periods of weeks to months.

RELAPSE

Most patients are cured by a full course of therapy as long as antibiotics are continued for at least 6 weeks. A minority will have a delayed convalescence, despite declining titers of antibodies and absent objective signs of illness. In some cases, relapses occur after the completion of therapy, even when the patient is compliant with treatment. Because relapse is rarely due to the emergence of antibiotic-resistant strains, most patients are cured by repeating the treatment with the same drugs. Chronic localized infection can occur, with relapses of objective signs of disease during long periods. In some cases of chronic brucellosis, surgical drainage of localized disease may be required.

PROPHYLAXIS

Persons in high-risk occupations are advised to use precautions in handling potentially infected animals or their carcasses. The general population should avoid unpasteurized dairy products, especially those originating in brucellosis-endemic areas. Attenuated live *Brucella* vaccines are available for immunizing livestock, but vaccination of humans is not recommended. Accidental self-inoculation with veterinary vaccines (*B. abortus* strain 19 and *B. melitensis* strain Rev-1) can cause brucellosis in humans.

ADVERSE REACTIONS TO THERAPY

On occasion, the initiation of treatment for brucellosis is followed by a transient worsening of symptoms (Herxheimer-like reaction). This reaction is rarely severe and is not a contraindication for continuing therapy.

IMMUNOTHERAPY

Before the advent of effective chemotherapy, immune serum, vaccines, and a variety of antigen preparations were in vogue for treating human brucellosis. There is no evidence of efficacy for these products, and their use is not recommended.

CONJUNCTIVITIS

method of
TERRENCE P. O'BRIEN, M.D.
The Wilmer Eye Institute, Johns Hopkins University School of Medicine
Baltimore, Maryland

Conjunctivitis, the most common ocular inflammation, involves all ages and is worldwide in occurrence. The principal causes of acute conjunctivitis are introduction of a wide spectrum of exogenous microbes, exposure to numerous potential allergens, and irritative toxic stimuli. The strategy for accurate diagnosis and management of conjunctivitis includes distinguishing between an acute and chronic pace of inflammation, identification of any precipitating events, consideration of the role of any antecedent medication, and use of the principal ocular signs with identification of the key distinctive conjunctival signs. The principal ocular signs in external diseases of the eye include skin and mucous membrane involvement, orbital involvement, regional lymphadenopathy, type and amount of conjunctival discharge, morphologic pattern of conjunctival inflammation, and type of corneal epithelial abnormality.

Infectious conjunctivitis may cause significant morbidity, depending in part on the type of invading organism and local ocular defense mechanisms. The normal flora of the conjunctiva, various sources of infection in conjunctivitis, and factors important in the resistance of the conjunctiva to infections have been well described.

ETIOLOGIC AGENTS

The numerous agents that may cause conjunctivitis are listed in Table 1.

CLINICAL MANIFESTATIONS

The clinical findings and course of infection are influenced by the pathogenic features of the exogenous microorganisms. The most obvious clinical manifestation of conjunctivitis is hyperemia of the conjunctiva. The dilata-

TABLE 1. **Etiologic Agents of Conjunctivitis**

Bacteria
  Streptococcus
  Streptococcus aureus
  Haemophilus influenzae
  Neisseria gonorrhoeae
  Haemophilus aegyptius (Koch-Weeks)
  Haemophilus ducreyi
  Neisseria meningitidis
  Streptococci of the viridans group
  Proteus vulgaris
  Morax-Axenfeld bacillus (*Moraxella lacunata*)
  Corynebacterium diphtheriae
  Mycobacterium tuberculosis
  Francisella tularensis
  Treponema pallidum
  Branhamella catarrhalis
  Shigella flexneri
  Yersinia enterocolitica
  Staphylococcus epidermidis
  Acinetobacter calcoaceticus var. *anitratus*
  Aeromonas hydrophila
  Peptostreptococcus
  Propionibacterium
  Cat-scratch bacillus
Viruses
  Adenoviridae
  Poxviruses (variola, vaccinia, molluscum contagiosum viruses)
  Herpesviruses (herpes simplex, varicella-zoster, Epstein-Barr viruses)
  Papillomaviruses
  Influenza virus
  Paramyxoviruses (measles, mumps, Newcastle disease viruses)
  Picornaviruses (echovirus, enterovirus, coxsackievirus, and poliovirus)
Chlamydia trachomatis
Fungi
  Candida species
  Sporothrix schenckii
  Rhinosporidium seeberi
  Cryptococcus
Parasites
  Onchocerca volvulus
  Loa
  Wuchereria bancrofti
  Oestrus ovis (myiasis)
  Microsporidia
    Nosema species
    Encephalitozoon species

tion and congestion of the vessels are greater near the periphery of the bulbar conjunctiva and become less marked as the limbus is approached.

The presence of secretion is almost always a feature of conjunctivitis. This is due to an exudation of inflammatory cells and a fibrin-rich edematous fluid from the blood, and the exudate is combined with denuded epithelial cells and mucus. The secretion may be purulent, mucopurulent, fibrinous, or serosanguineous, depending on the cause and severity of the disease. When the exudate dries, the eyelids may stick together.

Conjunctival edema (chemosis) may be present in parts of the conjunctiva that are freely movable over the globe and lids. The normal transparency of the conjunctiva may be lost, and it may appear thickened owing to the infiltration of the tissues with leukocytes. If there is diffuse leukocytic infiltration of the conjunctival stroma, with hyperplasia of the overlying epithelium, papillae form. A papilla contains a central blood vessel in its core. This vessel branches on the surface of the papilla. Papillae usually occur in the tarsal conjunctiva. The conjunctiva may have a velvety appearance from numerous small papillae. When large, the papillae have the appearance of cobblestone excrescences. This is unusual in acute infectious conjunctivitis but more common in allergic and chronic conjunctivitis. Papillae are nonspecific conjunctival signs but are most commonly observed with bacterial infection and allergy.

The conjunctiva contains lymphatic tissue that may be stimulated by various microbial antigens to form a follicle. Normal conjunctiva has an occasional follicle in its substantia propria, especially in the fornices. In certain forms of conjunctivitis, especially viral, chlamydial, or toxic, a follicular reaction may predominate. Follicles and papillae are differentiated clinically by appearance; follicles resemble smooth, glistening bumps, whereas papillae are smaller (<1 mm) and red with a central vascular core.

Membrane formation is also seen in some cases of conjunctivitis, especially with viral and some bacterial causes. This membrane consists of a superficial fibrinous layer connected to subconjunctival granulation tissue. When this membrane is excised, a raw bleeding surface is exposed.

Corneal involvement may occur in conjunctivitis, especially viral, because of the proximity of the corneal epithelium to the inflamed tarsal and limbal conjunctivae. Symptoms of corneal involvement include a gritty foreign body sensation, photophobia, diminished vision, and pain. The various forms of conjunctivitis have many of the aforementioned signs and symptoms in common. Awareness of the principal ocular signs with selection of the most distinctive conjunctival sign can narrow the differential diagnosis.

Bacterial Conjunctivitis

Bacterial conjunctivitis is among the most common types of ocular infection. Pathogenesis typically involves exogenous routes of infection with airborne fomites, contact with upper respiratory tract infections, hand-to-eye contact, and possible relationship with genital tract infections. Endogenous routes of infection occur less frequently with spread from adjacent structures such as the face and eyelids, lacrimal drainage apparatus, and paranasal sinuses. Hematogenous routes of infection in acute bacterial conjunctivitis are rare.

The principal causes of acute conjunctivitis in the normal host include *Staphylococcus aureus, Streptococcus pneumoniae, Neisseria gonorrhoeae,* and *Haemophilus influen-*

zae. Age-related factors are important determinants of causative organisms. In neonates, there is a notorious invalidity of clinical signs because of the immature immunologic system. There is a frequency of *Neisseria* and *Chlamydia* infections in the newborn. In children, there is an opportunity for severe conjunctivitis caused by *H. influenzae. S. pneumoniae* and occasionally *S. aureus* may also cause acute conjunctivitis in children. In young adults, there may be a frequency of *Neisseria* and *Chlamydia* infections.

In adults, the most common bacterial isolates from an acute conjunctivitis are *S. pneumoniae, S. aureus,* and *Staphylococcus epidermidis.* The role of the last two organisms in causation is, however, disputed.

The bacterial etiology of chronic bacterial conjunctivitis is less well defined.

Anaerobic bacteria have been isolated from conjunctivitis patients in association with aerobic organisms thought to be the cause of the conjunctivitis. The same organisms have been isolated in immunodeficient patients, in whom acute conjunctivitis and chronic conjunctivitis are more common than in normal patients. Table 1 identifies bacteria that probably have been responsible for conjunctivitides.

The clinical significance of certain organisms isolated in studies of bacterial cultures during conjunctivitis remains incompletely determined. However, early in the course of infection, bacterial and viral conjunctivitis may not have distinctive clinical signs to differentiate the conditions.

Investigations into the cause of epidemics of bacterial conjunctivitis have improved to better establish, for example, *S. pneumoniae, Pseudomonas aeruginosa,* and *Moraxella.*

In acute bacterial conjunctivitis, it is helpful to assess the severity of inflammation on the basis of the rate of evolution of signs and certain distinctive signs including corneal involvement.

In nonsevere bacterial conjunctivitis, there is minimal to no lid edema, scant purulent discharge with moderate conjunctival hyperemia, and a normal cornea. In contrast, severe conjunctivitis is characterized often by marked lid edema with copious purulent discharge, marked conjunctival hyperemia, chemosis, membrane formation, and suppurative or nonsuppurative keratitis.

The principal causes of nonsevere bacterial conjunctivitis are *S. aureus, S. pneumoniae, Haemophilus* species (especially after age 5 years), and *Moraxella* species.

Severe bacterial conjunctivitis is most often caused by *Neisseria* species, *H. influenzae* in children, *Streptococcus pyogenes,* and *S. aureus.*

Severe conjunctivitis caused by *N. gonorrhoeae* or *Neisseria meningitidis* deserves special recognition. Infection with *Neisseria* may result in markedly swollen eyelids, extreme hyperemia and chemosis, and a profuse purulent discharge. The massively swollen conjunctiva infiltrated with polymorphonuclear neutrophils may become draped over the peripheral cornea at the limbus. The action of lytic enzymes from the neutrophils may cause serious complications in untreated gonococcal conjunctivitis including corneal ulceration with subsequent perforation. Gonococcal conjunctivitis may occasionally have a prolonged asymptomatic course, in a manner similar to some of the genital infections.

N. meningitidis is an uncommon cause of acute bacterial conjunctivitis. In 84 cases of primary meningococcal conjunctivitis, the male/female ratio was 1.76:1, with 9 neonates, 55 children, and 20 adults. Systemic meningococcal disease developed in 17.8% of the patients, and the overall mortality was 13.3%. Gonococcal conjunctivitis can occur without sexual transmission, although a healthy suspicion for possible sexual abuse should be maintained in prepubertal children. Other *Neisseria* species including *Neisseria cinerea* may cause acute purulent conjunctivitis.

Membrane formation may be seen in any severe infection of the conjunctiva, but it is typically present in infections with streptococci and *Corynebacterium diphtheriae* or with adenovirus. These membranes may lead to a spectrum of changes from fine corneal scarring to obliteration of the fornices and permanent dry eye states. In contrast to most other types of conjunctivitis, pain is a common symptom with *C. diphtheriae* infection. Diphtheritic conjunctivitis does not occur as the sole manifestation of diphtheria, and so other manifestations of the disease should be sought. Widespread immunization programs have made diphtheritic conjunctivitis extremely rare.

Moraxella lacunata produces a localized "angular" conjunctivitis associated with fissuring and dermatitis of the external canthi and a scanty conjunctival discharge. *Moraxella* conjunctival infection may be incorrectly diagnosed as chlamydial, epidemic keratoconjunctivitis, and herpes simplex virus infections. Although *Moraxella* conjunctivitis is associated with adolescent girls, 13 of 27 female patients with culture-proven *Moraxella* infection (48%) were 20 years or older. *Moraxella* conjunctivitis can occur in epidemics from sharing contaminated eye makeup.

Certain nonpyogenic organisms (*Mycobacterium tuberculosis, Francisella tularensis, Treponema pallidum*) produce an atypical clinical picture characterized by unilateral conjunctival nodules that tend to ulcerate. Moderate localized conjunctival injection, minimal discharge, and a palpable preauricular lymph node on the affected side are present. Nonsyphilitic spirochetal infection with *Borrelia burgdorferi* has reportedly caused conjunctivitis in association with Lyme disease.

The pleomorphic gram-negative cat-scratch disease bacillus, first observed in lymph nodes, now conclusively identified as *Bartonella henselae*, produces a unilateral follicular conjunctivitis associated with prominent enlargement of the ipsilateral preauricular lymph node. *Yersinia* infection has been implicated in a syndrome similar to Reiter's syndrome and consisting of a self-limited conjunctivitis, acute myalgia, fever, gastrointestinal symptoms, prolonged anterior uveitis, polyarthritis, sacroiliitis, and HLA-B27 association. Similar syndrome complexes were seen within family groups. *Yersinia enterocolitica* has also been associated with an isolated conjunctivitis.

Haemophilus ducreyi, Pasteurella multocida, F. tularensis, N. meningitidis, streptococci, *Acinetobacter calcoaceticus (Herellea vaginicola),* and *Aeromonas hydrophila* have caused isolated cases of acute conjunctivitis.

Fungal Conjunctivitis

Primary fungal conjunctivitis is infrequently encountered clinically, although *Candida* species and others (see Table 1) may be isolated from the conjunctiva. Blastomycosis involving the eyelid may cause a granulomatous conjunctivitis. Lid or conjunctival nodules are the usual form of ocular involvement with *Sporothrix schenckii. Rhinosporidium seeberi* may cause a characteristic granulomatous inflammatory reaction in the conjunctiva. Other fungi are rarely recovered from cultures in immunocompromised individuals.

Viral Conjunctivitis

Viral conjunctivitis is common, causing 20% of nonepidemic cases of conjunctivitis in one study in children and 14% of cases in adult patients in another study. The morphologic pattern of associated corneal changes, the time course, systemic involvement, and epidemic characteristics will usually permit presumptive clinical diagnosis of viral conjunctivitis. The actual causative virus usually cannot be determined by ocular morphologic characteristics alone, and definitive diagnosis requires cultures and serologic studies. Most viral conjunctivitides are self-limited but highly contagious, with potential for causing considerable morbidity. The discharge is usually serous rather than mucoid or purulent. A generalized conjunctival hyperemia, moderate tearing, and mild itching are present. Follicle formation stimulated by viral antigen may be prominent. Regional lymphadenopathy with preauricular and submandibular node enlargement is common, and the conjunctivitis is occasionally associated with an upper respiratory tract infection. The preauricular node is usually exquisitely tender to palpation.

Adenoviruses are responsible for the most frequent epidemics of viral conjunctivitis in the United States and are a major occupational hazard for eye care professionals.

Serotypes of adenoviruses typically associated with pharyngoconjunctival fever are 3 and 7, with occasional involvement by types 1, 2, 4, 5, 6, 8, and 14. The clinical complex of pharyngitis, fever, and conjunctivitis with inferior forniceal follicles and, rarely, keratitis may help identify this conjunctivitis. Spontaneous resolution within 1 to 2 weeks is the rule. Outbreaks among children may occur after swimming pool inoculation or hand-to-eye contact.

Epidemic keratoconjunctivitis has most commonly resulted from infection with serotype 8, but types 2, 3, 4, 7, 9, 10, 11, 14, 16, 19, and 29 have been reported. The clinical picture includes pharyngitis, preauricular lymphadenopathy, and follicular conjunctivitis, and there is a 7- to 10-day incubation period with a 5- to 12-day interval before characteristic (but inconsistent) corneal subepithelial infiltrates develop. These epidemics are sometimes propagated by eye health care personnel. Despite a wide spectrum of symptoms ranging from severe photophobia to mild irritation only, this disease is usually self-limited and is rarely associated with visual loss from corneal changes. Occasional reports have described raised intraocular pressure and chronic keratitis and Stevens-Johnson syndrome as a result of epidemic keratoconjunctivitis. Chronic adenovirus conjunctivitis has also been reported.

Reports of epidemics in Florida have emphasized the emergence of a picornavirus as a factor in epidemic hemorrhagic conjunctivitis in the United States. Previous reports have been mainly from Africa. Enterovirus type 70, coxsackievirus A24, and adenovirus 11 have all resulted in a similar clinical picture. This consists of bilateral follicular conjunctivitis of sudden onset, with (rarely) corneal changes and systemic symptoms, a short (4- to 5-day) symptomatic course, and bulbar conjunctival hemorrhages. Spontaneous resolution with low morbidity is the usual course, although occasional reports have described Bell's palsy, radiculomyelitis, cranial nerve palsies, and other types of central nervous system involvement.

Ocular infection with vaccinia virus occurs when the virus is accidentally transferred from the site of medical inoculation to the eye. Vesicles appear on the lid margin, and a conjunctivitis may follow. Conjunctivitis without lid lesions has also been reported.

Molluscum contagiosum virus produces small, waxy, elevated lid margin nodules with umbilicated centers that are associated with a chronic follicular conjunctivitis caused by the toxic effect of shed incomplete virions.

Herpes simplex virus types 1 and 2, varicella-zoster virus, and Epstein-Barr virus can cause conjunctivitis. Primary herpes simplex is responsible for the majority of cases of nonepidemic follicular conjunctivitis in young children. Vesicular lid lesions, preauricular lymphadenopathy, and transient keratitis may be noted. The conjunctivitis is self-limited and is rarely associated with significant morbidity.

In patients with chickenpox, papules may develop on the lids and conjunctiva and at the limbus during the infection. These papules may become pustules and ulcerate. Vesicles may be found on the conjunctiva, particularly on the semilunar fold. Four percent of patients with chickenpox have conjunctival and corneal manifestations. In herpes zoster ophthalmicus, a follicular conjunctivitis with regional adenopathy rarely occurs. In less than 5% of patients with infectious mononucleosis, a mild conjunctivitis is present.

Human papillomavirus may produce lesions on the tarsal and bulbar conjunctivae and on the lid margin. A catarrhal conjunctivitis may result, and the cornea may show multiple punctate erosions. The presence of viral antigen and DNA sequences in some dysplastic epithelial lesions of the conjunctiva has raised concern that the virus may have a role in the development of conjunctival epithelial malignant neoplasms, similar to its suspected role in the female genital tract.

Congenital rubella is associated with numerous ocular abnormalities. Epidemic rubella in young children has produced a follicular conjunctivitis associated with occasional corneal epithelial changes.

The influenza viruses often cause catarrhal conjunctivitis and occasionally an acute follicular conjunctivitis. This ocular manifestation of influenza has been reported in both 48% and 60% of patients.

Infections due to the measles (rubeola) virus may be associated with mild paralimbal conjunctival epithelial erosion; the epithelia contain measles antigens that develop during the prodrome before the rash. An epithelial keratitis with photophobia may occur after the rash. Koplik spots may be found on the semilunar fold.

Conjunctivitis occurs rarely with mumps. Newcastle disease virus (which causes a fatal pneumoencephalitis in fowl) may produce a self-limited, unilateral follicular conjunctivitis in humans. Echovirus 11 and poliovirus have occasionally been described as a cause of follicular conjunctivitis.

Parinaud's oculoglandular syndrome is a clinical complex of conjunctivitis, prominent preauricular lymphadenopathy, and a febrile illness with various possible causes, including infectious mononucleosis, cat-scratch fever, syphilis, tuberculosis, and sarcoidosis.

Chlamydial Conjunctivitis

Trachoma, one of the leading causes of blindness in the world, is caused by a chlamydial organism that has a low infectivity. In the United States, the disease is largely confined to certain Native American populations that are characterized by poverty and poor communal hygiene. Repeated infections appear necessary to establish clinical trachoma. The conjunctivitis is characterized by a follicular reaction in the superior tarsal conjunctiva that is often associated with a concurrent papillary response. As follicles resolve, they appear to be replaced with fine subconjunctival scars. The degree of scarring seems to be related to the intensity of the follicular response and also to the presence of secondary bacterial infection. The subconjunctival scarring may in time lead to distortion of the tarsal plate and result in trichiasis.

Also associated with trachoma is the development of a superior limbic pannus with opacification of the corneal stroma and neovascularization. Follicles may occur in the limbus, and when these resolve, a clear depression persists (Herbert's pit).

Inclusion conjunctivitis is a fairly common infection caused by *Chlamydia trachomatis* that is most often sexually transmitted. Because an infant may acquire the organism during passage through the birth canal, it is one of the causes of ophthalmia neonatorum. Because the conjunctiva in the newborn does not form follicles, the injected appearance of this conjunctivitis in newborns is nonspecific. In adults, numerous papillae and follicles form on the tarsal conjunctiva and are more pronounced on the lower. The disease is usually bilateral, and the discharge is often profuse. Inclusion conjunctivitis is differentiated from trachoma by two important features: (1) corneal scarring rarely occurs in inclusion conjunctivitis; and (2) in trachoma, the upper tarsal conjunctiva is more involved than the lower, although inclusion conjunctivitis may occasionally take on the characteristics of trachoma, and various corneal changes have been described in inclusion conjunctivitis. Associated urethritis and cervicitis are common.

Conjunctivitis is a rare manifestation of systemic lymphogranuloma venereum that is caused by certain immunotypes (L1, L2, L3) of *C. trachomatis*. Moderate unilateral conjunctival injection, slight conjunctival discharge, and extreme edema of the upper and lower lids are present. In addition, ipsilateral preauricular, parotid, and submaxillary lymphadenopathy is present. Types A, B, Ba, and C have been most commonly found in hyperendemic areas of trachoma. Lymphogranuloma venereum conjunctivitis has caused marginal keratitis with corneal perforation in a human immunodeficiency virus–positive individual.

Parasitic Conjunctivitis

A number of ocular parasites may cause conjunctivitis. Blepharoconjunctivitis due to *Leishmania donovani* in association with nodules of post–kala azar dermal leishmaniasis can occur as a result of infection of the conjunctiva by spread from contaminated fingers. Parasites are being recovered in increasing frequency from the conjunctiva of individuals with the acquired immune deficiency syndrome (AIDS). Microsporidia are small ubiquitous obligate intracellular parasites that usually cause infections in animals and rarely in humans. *Encephalitozoon* species may cause a mild conjunctivitis with punctate keratopathy in patients with AIDS. The symptoms may mimic those of blepharitis or dry eye, and a high index of suspicion should be maintained to diagnose this parasitic keratoconjunctivitis in immunodeficient individuals. Cryptosporidial enteritis has also been complicated by conjunctivitis. Ophthalmomyiasis, nematode, and trematode infections have been described.

Ophthalmia Neonatorum

The incidence of acute conjunctivitis of the newborn (ophthalmia neonatorum) is reported to be as high as 12% of all newborns. It has been most commonly the result of mild chemical irritation after ocular silver nitrate prophylaxis. This self-limited conjunctivitis appears within the first 24 hours, and it lasts 1 to 2 days. However, chlamydial conjunctivitis is becoming much more common, with an incidence of approximately 2.8% of all births at one clinic and occurring in more than 35% of the infants who are born to mothers with proven chlamydial cervicitis. This has been substantiated by other studies. The onset generally occurs within 5 to 19 days, with no pathologic features except for an association with other systemic chlamydial infections such as pneumonia and otitis media. It has been suggested that the organism in these cases gains entry to the neonate through the conjunctival mucosa. There have been reports of occasional cases of chlamydial conjunctivitis in infants delivered by cesarean section.

Bacterial conjunctivitis is most often the result of *S. aureus* infection, with *S. pneumoniae* and *H. influenzae* the next most common. There are no pathognomonic features of these infections, and they may occur as early as 24 hours after birth. Streptococcal infections may be associated with acute dacryocystitis of the newborn, and *Pseudomonas* species have been reported as an occasional cause. Cases of staphylococcal scalded skin syndrome have been attributed to primary staphylococcal conjunctivitis. *H. influenzae* conjunctivitis has been implicated in neonatal meningitis. *Shigella flexneri* has caused ethmoiditis and conjunctivitis. *Branhamella catarrhalis* infection is being more frequently diagnosed and has been confused with true gonococcal ophthalmia neonatorum.

The prevailing incidence of gonococcal ophthalmia neonatorum is not known, but it is usually seen 1 to 2 days after birth and is characterized by a florid course and the threat of corneal ulceration and perforation. Recent cases of penicillin-resistant strains and occasional cases with a deceptively mild course have made diagnosis and management more difficult.

Infants born to mothers with herpes simplex virus cervicitis may develop a conjunctivitis within a few days of birth. The conjunctivitis is usually self-limited but may be associated with corneal epithelial changes and, rarely, stromal keratitis.

Other Infective and Noninfective Conjunctivitides

Conjunctival inflammation (chemosis and injection and discharge) is seen as a result of many noninfectious conditions but particularly as an allergic mucosal response. The agents responsible include drugs and devices such as hard and soft contact lenses, contact lens–sterilizing solutions (usually the preservative thimerosal), and prostheses that cause giant papillary conjunctivitis. Other agents implicated include topical timolol, atropine, antiviral agents, and other drugs; cosmetics; and external allergens that cause vernal keratoconjunctivitis. Conjunctivitis may occur as a response to toxic agents such as gentian violet, latex, and ultraviolet irradiation. Phlyctenular keratoconjunctivitis has occurred in patients with increased tuberculin sensitivity and staphylococcal hypersensitivity.

The precise mechanisms eliciting conjunctivitis in numerous other conditions with fairly specific clinical features have not been conclusively identified. These include keratoconjunctivitis sicca, superior limbic keratoconjunctivitis, ligneous conjunctivitis, mucocutaneous lymph node syndrome, and Reiter's syndrome. Immune-mediated conjunctivitis has been implicated in mucous membrane pemphigoid and in the conjunctivitis associated with graft-versus-host disease in bone marrow transplant patients.

DIFFERENTIAL DIAGNOSIS

Other serious, sight-threatening conditions that present as "red eye" may superficially resemble a conjunctivitis. The points of difference are highlighted in Table 2. Chronic, unilateral conjunctivitis in which a specific diagnosis is not made should alert the physician to the possibility of a meibomian gland carcinoma.

LABORATORY INVESTIGATIONS

Mild, nonsevere conjunctivitis is not routinely investigated and is often treated empirically without benefit of knowledge from microbial culture. Reports differ on the value of culturing suspected bacterial conjunctivitis. In nonsevere conjunctivitis, a calcium alginate swab dipped in trypticase soy broth may be used to obtain material from the superior and inferior tarsal conjunctivae. Cultures should be obtained from both eyes and plated on chocolate agar. In severe conjunctivitis, scrapings of the superior and inferior tarsal conjunctivae should be taken after the administration of topical proparacaine hydrochloride, 0.5% for diagnostic smears, as well as microbial culture. Cultures are usually taken from both conjunctival sacs and occasionally separately from both lids in suspected conjunctivitis. Chlamydial cultures are usually taken with a dry calcium alginate swab, which is then placed in special *Chlamydia* transport medium before processing for cell culture.

All cases of suspected ophthalmia neonatorum should have cultures and smears performed for bacteria, chlamydiae, and herpes simplex virus. Acute and convalescent serologic tests for adenovirus and picornavirus may help in diagnosing epidemic conjunctivitis, but these are generally not required because of the self-limited nature of the infection, the nonspecific treatment available, and the diagnostic characteristics of the epidemic features. Serodiagnostic testing of tears in serum by using microimmunofluorescent tests has been described for patients with *C. trachomatis* inclusion conjunctivitis. Serologic testing for SS-A and SS-B autoantibodies has assisted in the early diagnosis of keratoconjunctivitis sicca that is a prodrome of Sjögren's syndrome.

In a conjunctival scraping from a normal healthy eye, epithelial cells and occasional goblet cells are present. In

TABLE 2. **Comparison of Conjunctivitis and Other Conditions**

Characteristic	Conjunctivitis	Uveitis	Acute Angle-Closure Glaucoma
Prominent symptoms	Discharge, irritation	Photophobia, visual loss	Pain, visual loss
Vision	Usually normal	Normal and occasionally decreased	Markedly reduced
Ocular injection	Conjunctival injection generalized	Paralimbal injection (ciliary flush)	Paralimbal injection
Cornea	Usually clear	Usually clear	Edematous and cloudy
Pupil	Normal	May be normal or small	Usually mid-dilated, irregular, and immobile
Intraocular pressure	Normal	Normal or slightly elevated	Markedly elevated

acute bacterial infection, the scraping shows large numbers of neutrophils. Bacteria may be present within or outside leukocytes. In chronic bacterial infections, there is a decrease in neutrophils and an increase in lymphocytes and large mononuclear cells. In viral conjunctivitis, lymphocytes and monocytes are predominant. In herpes simplex virus infections, multinucleated epithelial cells may be seen. In chlamydial infections, a mixed inflammatory cell population (polymorphonuclear leukocytes and lymphocytes) is present, and basophilic intracytoplasmic inclusion bodies may be seen in epithelial cells; the latter finding is common in children and less common in adults. Immunofluorescent techniques provide more sensitivity in identification. Topically applied fluorescein does not appear to have an effect on fluorescent monoclonal antibodies in the diagnosis of chlamydial conjunctivitis. In allergic conjunctivitis, scrapings characteristically reveal eosinophils. They are found in greatest abundance in vernal conjunctivitis. Between attacks of vernal conjunctivitis, mast cells and no eosinophils are seen.

Scrapings from patients with keratoconjunctivitis sicca and superior limbic keratoconjunctivitis reveal keratinized epithelial cells or condensed chromatin patterns when the Papanicolaou staining technique is used.

Impression cytology may offer an alternative to the conjunctival scraping method. Immunoelectron microscopy and immunofluorescent techniques may aid in diagnosing viral conjunctivitis.

TREATMENT

Most types of mild bacterial conjunctivitis and most types of viral conjunctivitis are usually self-limited, benign conditions that perhaps require no treatment. Topical gentamicin or tobramycin for gram-negative rod infections and erythromycin, bacitracin, polymyxin B–trimethoprim, or neomycin-polymyxin for gram-positive infections, given every 2 to 4 hours for 7 to 10 days, are usually effective. Often an organism reported to be resistant to a specific antibiotic in the laboratory will respond to that antibiotic clinically because of the high concentrations achievable in the tear film by topical application.

Gonococcal conjunctivitis requires urgent therapy with parenteral penicillin G, topical penicillin, and frequent instillations of normal saline for lavage. Penicillinase-producing *N. gonorrhoeae* strains require systemic ceftriaxone or another third-generation cephalosporin. A single intramuscular dose of 125 mg of ceftriaxone resulted in a 100% cure rate for gonococcal ophthalmia neonatorum without the need for concomitant topical therapy.

Herpes simplex virus conjunctivitis may be treated with topical trifluridine every 2 hours for 7 days, although this condition is usually benign and self-limited.

Adult inclusion conjunctivitis requires a 1-week course of doxycycline 100 mg twice daily; in pregnant or lactating women, erythromycin or sulfamethoxazole may be substituted orally. Adjunctive topical tetracycline ointment or erythromycin drops may be prescribed. A similar therapy is effective in treating trachoma, but prevention of reinfection and bacterial superinfection is equally important. Macrolide antibiotics having long serum half-lives and favorable tissue penetration (e.g., azithromycin, clarithromycin, and roxithromycin) are under investigation for a potential role in therapy for trachoma in developing nations.

Because interferon and interferon inducers have been shown to be largely ineffective in therapy for viral conjunctivitis, the search continues for an effective broad-spectrum antiviral preparation for ocular use.

Allergic and immune-mediated conjunctivitis responds best to topical corticosteroids. The long-term use of topical steroids may be associated with glaucoma and cataracts, whereas short-term use may accelerate herpes simplex epithelial keratitis. Nonsteroidal anti-inflammatory agents such as aspirin and cromolyn sodium, ketorolac tromethamine, and others are useful adjunctive measures.

PROPHYLAXIS OF OPHTHALMIA NEONATORUM

There is considerable debate over the relative efficacy of 1% silver nitrate versus topical antibiotics such as 0.5% erythromycin or 1% tetracyclines. Silver nitrate is still extremely effective, particularly against gonococcal infection, but it has little impact on the increasing incidence of chlamydial infections. Topical erythromycin seems the most effective agent in preventing this infection. In infants born to mothers with known genital chlamydial infection, the routine use of erythromycin ointment will eliminate chlamydial conjunctivitis, but systemic erythromycin estolate is preferred to prevent nasopharyngeal colonization.

Children born to mothers with known gonococcal genital infections should be treated with parenteral penicillin or ceftriaxone, depending on susceptibility testing results.

VARICELLA
(Chickenpox)

method of
THOMAS H. BELHORN, M.D., Ph.D.
University of Texas Health Science Center
Houston, Texas

Varicella (chickenpox) and herpes zoster (shingles) are infections caused by the herpesvirus varicella-zoster virus (VZV). Varicella, the disease associated with the initial infection, is a common, highly communicable illness of childhood characterized by a familiar vesicular rash. Zoster, a typically painful vesicular rash in a dermatome distribution, occurs later in life due to reactivation of latent virus. Although chickenpox is usually viewed as a benign disease, complications certainly occur and may have significant consequences, especially in the immunocompromised host. Immunoprophylaxis and/or antiviral therapy in selected patients may reduce the incidence and morbidity of complications.

VARICELLA IN THE NORMAL HOST

Diagnosis

The characteristic exanthem of chickenpox in the normal host rarely requires the use of laboratory tests for diagnosis. A prodrome of fever, malaise, coryza, and anorexia may precede the onset of the exanthem by 24 to 48 hours but is often not seen in children. The pruritic rash of chickenpox begins with lesions on the trunk, face, and/or scalp (often hidden by hair). These are followed over a period of 3 to 6 days by successive crops of lesions developing in these areas and less densely on the extremities. Lesions on mucosal surfaces are quite common. Most lesions progress from an initial macular or maculopapular stage (present for only a few hours) to the characteristic vesicular lesion (present for 1 to 3 days), and then to a dry, crusted form. Vesicles initially contain clear fluid but later become cloudy and pustular in appearance. Lesions in various stages are often present simultaneously. The total number of lesions varies greatly, but the average is between 200 and 400; subsequent cases in families often involve many more vesicles than the index case, perhaps because of a greater inoculum due to the more intense exposure.

If documentation of VZV infection is necessary, viral culture of vesicle fluid is the "gold standard" but may require several days for confirmation. Results from examination of cells scraped from the base of a vesicle and stained with fluorescent antibody can be available in 1 or 2 hours. Both techniques require the use of experienced personnel in a diagnostic virology laboratory. An alternative technique involves the preparation of scrapings from the lesion base by air-drying, fixing with ethanol or methanol, and staining with Giemsa or Wright's stain (Tzanck's smear). Examination for multinucleated giant cells and intranuclear inclusions can be performed rapidly but does not differentiate VZV-infected from herpes simplex virus–infected cells.

Treatment

Management of varicella in most children is symptomatic and does not require specific antiviral therapy. Daily bathing is recommended to keep lesions clean and to relieve discomfort, especially when vaginitis or urethritis is present. The addition of baking soda or colloidal oatmeal to bath water, as well as the use of cool compresses or calamine lotion, or both, after bathing, may be helpful in alleviating pruritus. Preparations containing steroids should be avoided. Oral antihistamines may also be of benefit in severe pruritus, especially if the child is having difficulty sleeping, but should be used judiciously due to the risk of masking neurologic complications of varicella. Fingernails should be kept trimmed and clean to decrease the risk of superinfection associated with scratching. Fever usually does not require treatment, but, if treatment is necessary, acetaminophen may

be helpful; salicylates (aspirin) should be avoided due to the reported association with Reye's syndrome.

Oral acyclovir (Zovirax) has been shown to be somewhat beneficial in reducing the number and duration of vesicles, pruritus, and time to healing, as well as the duration of systemic symptoms, in the normal host. However, drug therapy must be initiated early after the onset of rash to be effective. Oral acyclovir should be considered only for selected patients at risk of severe varicella; such patients include children older than 11 years and healthy adults, patients with chronic pulmonary or cutaneous disorders, and patients receiving corticosteroids or chronic salicylate therapy. The oral antiviral agents famciclovir (Famvir) and valacyclovir (Valtrex) are approved for the use of herpes zoster; these and other agents may eventually have a role in the treatment of varicella.

Complications

The most common complication seen in varicella is bacterial superinfection of skin lesions, most commonly by *Streptococcus pyogenes* or *Staphylococcus aureus*. The usual presentation is localized impetiginous lesions, but cellulitis, staphylococcal scalded skin syndrome, and scarlet fever also occur. Hallmarks of superinfection include persistent or secondary fever, vesicles of large diameter, and advancing margins of erythema and tenderness. Bacteremia may lead to infection at secondary sites (e.g., septic arthritis, osteomyelitis, pneumonia, meningitis). Cultures of infected lesions need to be obtained before initiation of antibiotic therapy; cultures from additional sites such as blood, cerebrospinal fluid, or joint fluid should be obtained, depending on the clinical presentation. Initial antibiotic therapy would include a β-lactamase–resistant penicillin or cephalosporin or amoxicillin-clavulanate (Augmentin). Antibiotic dosage and route depend on the clinical presentation.

The most common neurologic complication of varicella is ataxia secondary to cerebellitis. Symptoms of ataxia with occasional slurred speech and nystagmus can develop at any time during or soon after the disease onset, but they usually present from 5 to 10 days after onset of skin lesions. The disease is self-limited, and symptoms usually resolve in 1 to 4 weeks. Encephalitis, a more serious complication, usually presents with personality changes, often with rapid progression to seizures and loss of consciousness. Increased intracranial pressure may necessitate intensive care management with attention to fluid restriction and the use of mannitol, steroids, and/or hyperventilation. If cerebrospinal fluid is obtained for analysis, only a moderate lymphocytosis and slight elevation in protein are usually noted. Treatment is mainly supportive, and antiviral therapy is of unproven benefit, although many would employ intravenous acyclovir for encephalitis. If death due to complications of increased intracranial pressure can be averted, full recovery is often obtained. Additional uncommon neurologic complications of varicella include Guillain-Barré syndrome, cranial nerve palsies, and transverse myelitis.

Approximately 20 to 30% of cases of Reye's syndrome occur in association with varicella. Clinically, Reye's syndrome has many similarities to encephalitis; laboratory evaluation of liver enzymes and serum ammonia levels may help to differentiate these two entities. The association of this syndrome with medications containing salicylates has contraindicated the use of these drugs in varicella. Management of Reye's syndrome, as in encephalitis, involves the provision of basic supportive care to manage increased intracranial pressure. Antiviral drugs are not likely to be helpful.

Varicella lesions occasionally occur on or adjacent to the conjunctivae; such lesions usually resolve without complications. However, ocular involvement may include keratoconjunctivitis or uveitis. If ocular involvement is suspected, consultation of an ophthalmologist is recommended for definition of the extent of corneal involvement and treatment with a topical antiviral agent.

Approximately 15% of healthy adults will have evidence of pulmonary involvement with varicella, whereas fewer children have this complication. The spectrum of disease ranges from asymptomatic radiographic abnormalities (manifested as a pattern of multiple nodular hilar and perihilar densities) to severe pulmonary compromise requiring supplemental oxygenation and ventilation. Inasmuch as active viral replication in lung tissue is thought to play a role in the disease process, antiviral therapy may be indicated in symptomatic pulmonary disease. Oral acyclovir is recommended for adolescents and adults with varicella because the illness may be more severe than in children.

A variety of hematologic and hemorrhagic complications may infrequently complicate varicella in the immunologically normal host. Thrombocytopenia with associated hemorrhage at the base of the lesions and purpura fulminans may necessitate transfusion of blood products, a full evaluation to rule out bacterial septicemia, and intensive care management. Transient thrombocytopenic purpura and Henoch-Schönlein purpura have both occurred after varicella. Myocarditis and nephritis are quite rare but important complications. Arthritis of nonbacterial etiology may also be manifest after varicella; the presence of bacterial pathogens must be excluded, but no antiviral treatment is required.

VARICELLA IN HIGH-RISK POPULATIONS

Pregnant Women and Neonates

Varicella is uncommon during pregnancy because most women of childbearing age are immune to VZV. However, pregnant women with varicella may develop pneumonitis, and spontaneous abortion of the fetus can occur with varicella during the first half of pregnancy. In addition, infection during the first half of pregnancy may be associated with approximately a 2% risk of fetal malformations. Common abnormalities of congenital infection include skin lesions in a dermatome distribution, a variety of eye and musculoskeletal malformations, central nervous system effects, and intrauterine growth retardation. Maternal varicella occurring near the time of delivery places the infant at risk for severe, disseminated infection.

Although of unproven efficacy, passive immunoprophylaxis with varicella-zoster immune globulin (VZIG) should be administered to the pregnant varicella-susceptible woman exposed to varicella. Such maternal immunoprophylaxis would be expected to modify maternal disease, although protection of the fetus has not been proved. VZIG should also be administered as soon as possible after birth to the neonate delivered to a woman who has had the onset of varicella from 5 days before to 2 days after delivery. If progression of varicella in the neonate ensues, intravenous acyclovir should be begun. Young infants lacking sufficient varicella antibody due to, for example, delivery before 28 weeks of gestation or lack of immunity in the mother should also be considered candidates for VZIG on significant varicella exposure. Treatment of the pregnant woman with varicella must be considered on a case-by-case basis; intravenous acyclovir should be considered in severe disease, as the potential benefits appear to outweigh the known risks of the drug to the developing fetus.

Immunocompromised Hosts

In the immunocompromised population, VZV infection can lead to progressive varicella, a devastating illness characterized by clinical involvement of multiple organ systems (such as pneumonitis, hepatitis, and encephalitis), severe hemorrhagic varicella, persisting crops of vesicles, and high mortality. The patients at highest risk are those with a deficiency in cellular immune function, whether due to a primary defect or acquired. In addition to specific congenital immunodeficiencies, diseases such as leukemia, lymphoma, and human immunodeficiency virus infection; the use of immunosuppressive or cytotoxic agents or radiation therapy; and severe malnutrition with protein loss are processes predisposing to an increased risk of this potentially lethal complication. Corticosteroids administered in the treatment of asthma or juvenile rheumatoid arthritis may not greatly increase the risk of progressive disease, although 2.0 mg of prednisone per kg per day has been reported to be associated with this complication in children with asthma. To prevent progressive varicella, significantly immunocompromised patients should receive immunoprophylaxis with VZIG if exposed to varicella and should receive intravenous antiviral therapy after the onset of symptoms or signs indicative of VZV infection.

IMMUNOPROPHYLAXIS AND ANTIVIRAL THERAPY

Passive immunoprophylaxis, when necessary, is achieved through the use of VZIG, supplied in vials containing 125 units. The dosage is 1 vial (125 units) for each 10 kg of body weight given intramuscularly, with a maximal dosage of 5 vials (625 units). Children weighing less than 10 kg should receive 1 vial (125 units). VZIG is most effective when given within 48 hours of exposure and may not be effective if administered more than 96 hours after exposure.

Although both intravenous acyclovir and vidarabine (Vira-A)* are considered effective against varicella, acyclovir is the preferred drug because of the greater ease of administration. The recommended dosage of intravenous acyclovir for varicella is 500 mg per m^2 per dose given every 8 hours (10 mg per kg per dose every 8 hours for children younger than 1 year of age). The medication should be infused over at least 1 hour and the patient kept well hydrated to avoid crystallization in the kidney and renal complications. Delay in starting therapy should be avoided because antiviral therapy begun early in varicella is more efficacious.

Oral acyclovir, available in both tablet and suspension forms, has less bioavailability but exhibits a low risk of toxicity. The dosage of oral acyclovir for treatment of uncomplicated varicella is 20 mg per kg per dose to a maximum of 800 mg per dose four times daily for 5 days. As noted previously, antiviral agents such as famciclovir, valacyclovir, and newer agents in development may eventually have a role in the treatment of varicella. Early institution of therapy appears optimal if not necessary for efficacy.

DISEASE PREVENTION

Infection Control in the Hospital Setting

The high rate of complications seen in immunocompromised patients with varicella coupled with the highly communicable nature of the virus necessitates strict enforcement of infection control policies to prevent transmission of the disease in high-risk settings. Risk in a given setting will depend on the proportion of susceptible patients and the number of susceptible patients who are immunocompromised, the risk of nosocomial spread being greatest in a tertiary care pediatric setting (or a newborn nursery) and far less in a nursing home for the elderly. The virus is spread both by direct contact and by the airborne route. A person developing varicella is infectious from 1 to 2 days before the onset of lesions until all lesions are crusted. All exposed varicella-susceptible patients should be placed in isolation from days 8 through 21 postexposure. Because administration of VZIG may lengthen the incubation period, patients who receive VZIG are usually isolated for a longer period until 28 days after exposure.

Varicella Vaccine

A live attenuated varicella vaccine (Varivax) was licensed by the Food and Drug Administration in

---

*Not FDA approved for this indication.

1995. This vaccine is currently recommended as part of the routine immunizations for healthy children as well as adults who are varicella susceptible (refer to the manufacturer's recommendations regarding indications, contraindications, adverse effects, and dosage). Research is under way to develop and evaluate alternative vaccines as well as to address the possible effect of immunization of seropositive elderly adults to reduce the incidence of herpes zoster.

CHOLERA

method of
FREDERIK P. L. VAN LOON, M.D., Ph.D., M.P.H., M.B.A.
Centers for Disease Control and Prevention
Atlanta, Georgia

Cholera is an acute watery diarrhea caused by infection of the small intestine with *Vibrio cholerae*. Although sporadic cases of cholera have been reported in communities along the Gulf Coast of the United States as well as in other industrialized countries, the disease is most common in developing countries where fecal contamination of water supplies is widespread.

PATHOGENESIS

The port of entry for the vibrio is the mouth; spread occurs fecal-orally. Severity of disease depends on the inoculum ingested; 10^6 bacilli are more likely than a low inoculum to cause severe illness. Vibrios are acid sensitive, but once past the gastric barrier and in the small intestine, they colonize the mucosa—a process that is facilitated by specific colonization factors—and release cholera toxin. This toxin is a protein, consisting of an active (A) subunit and five binding (B) subunits, that attaches to the G_{M1} ganglioside receptor at the lining of the mucosal cells. It triggers a cascade of reactions involving the release of neurotransmitters including cyclic adenosine monophosphate, prostaglandins, serotonin, and calmodulin. The ensuing increase in intestinal chloride secretion and decrease in sodium chloride absorption are accompanied by water excretion that leads to diarrhea when the volume of fluid secreted by the small intestine surpasses the absorptive capacity of the colon. The volume typically exceeds 1 liter per hour in adults and 10 mL per kg per hour in children. It is intriguing that cholera results from infection yet is not accompanied by systemic manifestations of a cytokine-induced acute phase reaction. Electron microscopic studies of the small intestinal mucosa show prominent widening of intercellular spaces and alteration of apical junctional complexes in the villus epithelium, whereas blebbing of microvillus border and mitochondrial changes are more prominent in the crypt epithelium. Changes that correlate with clinical severity include degranulation of argentaffin cells, mucosal mast cells, and eosinophils; an increase in neutrophil polymorphs; and changes in the enteric nerve fibers and microvasculature. It is suggested that morphologic change of the gut in the recently emerged non-O1 *V. cholerae* infection is more severe than in infection caused by *V. cholerae* O1.

TABLE 1. **Classification of Dehydration and Fluid Deficit Based on Clinical Signs and Symptoms**

Sign or Symptom	Sign or Symptom for Degree of Dehydration		
	Mild or None	*Moderate*	*Severe*
Approximate absolute fluid deficit (%)	≤50 mL/kg (<5%)	51–90 mL/kg (5–7%)	>90 mL/kg (10%)
Mentation	Alert	Restless or lethargic	Infants or young children may be comatose; older children and adults are apprehensive
Voice	Normal	High pitched	Absent (aphonia)
Thirst	Present	Present	Present
Radial pulse	Normal	Rapid	Rapid and feeble or impalpable
Respiratory pattern	Normal	Tachypneic	Tachypneic, labored (Kussmaul's)
Blood pressure	Normal	Normal	Low or absent (shock)
Mucous membranes	Moist	Dry	Dry
Elasticity of subcutaneous tissue	Pinch retracts immediately	Pinch retracts slowly	Pinch retracts slowly; washerwoman's fingers
Eyes	Normal	Sunken	Sunken
Urine flow	Normal	Scant and dark	Scant or absent

CLINICAL SYMPTOMS

The spectrum of illness varies from mild disease with no or hardly any symptoms to severe disease (cholera gravis) when the voluminous painless watery diarrhea leads to dehydration and even death within a few hours (Table 1). Associated symptoms include nausea, vomiting (especially early in the illness), and muscle cramps followed by signs of hypovolemic shock, such as a weak radial pulse, undetectable blood pressure, depressed mental status, and ultimately coma. As a result of the metabolic acidosis, hyperventilation (Kussmaul's breathing) may occur. The case-fatality rate for untreated cholera gravis is 50%. Cholera is in principle a self-limited disease if the dehydration is sufficiently remedied.

Cholera stool is not malodorous and is often described as rice-water stool because of small flecks of mucus but little fecal matter; bloody stool is not suggestive of cholera. Because the vibrio does not invade the epithelial lining of the intestine, there is little inflammatory response; hence, the stool contains few if any leukocytes, and patients are afebrile. The stool is isotonic with plasma; the sodium concentration is slightly lower and bicarbonate and potassium concentrations are higher than those found in plasma (Table 2).

Suspicion of cholera increases if there are other cases of cholera in the area, if the patient is from an area of poor sanitation, or if the patient has recently traveled to a cholera-endemic area.

Assessment of Dehydration

The degree of dehydration is assessed on the basis of physical signs (see Table 1) and measurement of stool, vomitus, and urine output. Measurement of stool output is facilitated by the use of a "cholera cot." This plastic-lined jute cot contains a hole in the middle through which stool is collected into a calibrated bucket. Monitoring stool losses every 2 to 4 hours may assist in ensuring that fluid replacement proportional to stool losses is given.

Complications

Complications from cholera are largely due to inadequate rehydration. Acute tubular necrosis with renal failure can result if the rate of rehydration is too low or if the rehydration solution does not contain salts.

Metabolic abnormalities can also occur. Hypokalemia is the result of loss of potassium in the stool but may initially

TABLE 2. **Electrolyte Composition of Cholera Stool in Adults and Children and of Rehydration Solutions (Concentration in mmol/L)**

Cholera Stool	Na$^+$	K$^+$	Cl$^-$	HCO$_3^-$	Carbohydrate
Adults	135	15	100	45	—
Children	105	25	90	30	—
Rehydration Fluid	**Na$^+$**	**K$^+$**	**Cl$^-$**	**Citrate**	**Carbohydrate**
Cereal ORS*	90	20	80	10†	20–50
Glucose ORS*	90	20	80	10	111
Lactated Ringer's	131	41	11	29	—
Dhaka solution	133	13	98	48	—
Saline‡	154	—	154		—

*Glucose ORS contains (per liter) NaCl 3.5 gm, KCl 1.5 gm, trisodium citrate 2.9 gm, and glucose 20 gm, with a total osmolality of 311 Osm/L. The electrolytes in cereal ORS are the same, but the glucose is replaced by a cereal (e.g., rice) 40–80 gm/L. Cereal (Ceralyte) ORS has a total osmolality of about 220–250 Osm/L.

†Either sodium bicarbonate 2.5 gm (which provides 30 mmol of bicarbonate) or trisodium citrate 2.9 gm (which provides 10 mmol of citrate) can be used as the base. The World Health Organization prefers citrate.

‡Normal saline only should be used for patients in shock when lactated Ringer's solution or another polyelectrolyte solution is not available. ORS is to be started immediately to replace potassium and base, which are not included in saline.

Abbreviation: ORS = oral rehydration solution.

be masked by the concomitant acidosis. The acidosis results from both bicarbonate loss in the stool and increased lactate production due to anaerobic glycolysis. Restoration of the circulation will diminish lactate production, and the bicarbonate contained in the intravenous solution will replenish plasma bicarbonate concentrations. Excess bicarbonate therapy can lead to tetany as a result of a decrease in the proportion of ionized to bound calcium. Halting the bicarbonate infusion will result in the resolution of the tetany. Pulmonary edema may occur if saline rather than lactated Ringer's is used and the metabolic acidosis is not corrected. Generalized edema can occur if excessive intravenous fluids are given. Ileus, paralytic bladder, and cardiac arrhythmias may occur as a result of hypokalemia when the rehydration fluids do not contain sufficient potassium. Cardiac arrhythmias can also result from hyperkalemia if renal failure is not recognized. Shock from cholera can precipitate abortion in pregnant women, although this is less likely to occur if rehydration is prompt. Severe hypoglycemia due to deficient gluconeogenesis can result in seizures and other neurologic abnormalities. Hypoglycemia is most common in malnourished children who have not eaten for several hours and have depleted their glycogen stores.

Hyperglycemia at admission has been found as a common feature in some settings. Septicemia is rare but has been described in a patient concurrently infected by *V. cholerae* O139 Bengal and *Shigella boydii*; as an extraintestinal manifestation, it is ascribed to the fact that *V. cholerae* O139, in contrast to *V. cholerae* O1, contains a capsulated polysaccharide.

MICROBIOLOGY

V. cholerae is a gram-negative, comma-shaped rod (formerly called *Vibrio comma*) belonging to the family Vibrionaceae. The diagnosis is confirmed by identifying *V. cholerae* from a stool culture on special media (thiosulfate citrate bile salts sucrose agar). For rapid diagnosis, darkfield examination of a fresh, unstained stool specimen is highly sensitive and specific; typical is the "shooting star" phenomenon caused by the motility of the vibrio's single polar flagellum. Cholera SMART is a rapid, colorimetric immunodiagnostic kit suitable for the direct detection of the presence of *V. cholerae* O1 in clinical specimens. A new immunochromatographic strip test (QUIX) is claimed to be the most simple, rapid, sensitive, and specific immunochromatographic test currently available for the detection of *V. cholerae*. In advanced settings, serologic tests are available for diagnosis; toxigenic *V. cholerae* serogroup O1 can be subdivided into El Tor and classical biotypes and Ogawa and Inaba serotypes. Two monoclonal antibody–based rapid immunodiagnostic test kits, BengalScreen, a coagglutination test, and Bengal DFA, a direct fluorescent antibody test, have been developed for direct detection of *V. cholerae* O139. For higher yield, rectal swabs are preferred to stool samples for both culture and rapid diagnosis. Other Vibrionaceae can also cause diarrhea, but only toxigenic *V. cholerae* belonging to serogroup O1 or to serogroup O139 has been associated with epidemic cholera. Other serogroups of *V. cholerae* as well as nontoxigenic *V. cholerae* O1 and O139 do not cause epidemic cholera, although they may cause individual cases of diarrhea. In epidemic settings in developing countries, a bacteriologic diagnosis is not indicated in all suspected cases because the management of dehydrating diarrhea is guided by the extent of fluid loss rather than by the nature of the infecting organism. By contrast, in individual cases of suspected cholera in the developed world, the diagnosis should be confirmed with culture and reported to the national health authorities.

EPIDEMIOLOGY

Since 1817, cholera has raged in seven pandemics, with possibly an eighth one emerging superimposed on the seventh. The first six were caused by the classical biotype and originated in cholera's homeland, Bengal; the seventh and current one is caused by the El Tor strain and began in 1961 in Indonesia to gradually affect most of Asia and Africa. In 1991, this pandemic reached South America, where cholera had not been seen for more than 100 years, and has since spread over the whole of Latin America where it is accompanied by an emerging diversity in the vibrio's electrophoretic types. In its wake, hundreds of importations have been reported in the United States. In Latin America, despite the epidemic's rapid spread, well-established case management has kept fatality rates low (about 1%). In contrast, cholera in Africa has been sporadic, and fatality rates tend to be higher (about 10%). In the Rwandan refugee camps in eastern Zaire in 1994, an estimated 50,000 persons died during the first several weeks of an explosive cholera epidemic, in the absence of adequate health facilities and oral rehydration. In 1992, a novel *V. cholerae* variant O139 (synonym Bengal) emerged in southern Asia where marine ecosystems in the Bay of Bengal were experiencing a pandemic of coastal algal blooms, apparently harboring and amplifying the agent, as a reflection of what ecologists refer to as "environmental distress syndrome." Studies using the random amplified polymorphic DNA fingerprinting method have suggested that this *V. cholerae* O139 strain has emerged from a common origin associated with the El Tor strain. This was the first epidemic caused by a serogroup other than O1 and occurring in populations assumed to be largely immune to *V. cholerae* O1. The Bengal strain has potential for pandemic spread because it has now affected areas throughout the Indian subcontinent, neighboring states, and other parts of Asia, with imported cases as far as the United States and Western Europe. It might be illustrative of the relative virulence of the three strains that the El Tor strain nearly completely replaced the classical strain in cholera-endemic Bangladesh during the late 1980s and that, in turn, the Bengal strain has nearly replaced the El Tor strain during the 1990s.

RISK FACTORS

The following risk factors have relevance for the management of patients.

Breast-feeding

Exclusive breast-feeding provides important protection to infants not because of transmission of maternal antibodies but because of the lesser exposure to contaminated food and water. Mothers should be encouraged to continue breast-feeding their children during episodes of cholera.

ABO Blood Type

Persons with blood group O have a higher risk for El Tor cholera than do persons with blood group A, B, or AB.

Strain Biospecificity

V. cholerae El Tor can survive longer in humans and in the environment and is more infectious than classical strains. An episode of classical cholera protects nearly entirely against recurrent cholera of either biotype; an episode of cholera El Tor does not protect against future attacks. The impact of a *V. cholerae* O139 infection on the risk for a subsequent *V. cholerae* infection, either O1 or non-O1, has not been determined yet.

Gastric Acid Output

Persons with impaired gastric function (e.g., after gastric surgery or while receiving antacid or acid-suppressing medication) have a substantially increased risk because of the loss of the gastric acid barrier. In addition, *Helicobacter pylori* gastritis is associated with a significant increase in the risk for life-threatening cholera but only among persons lacking natural vibriocidal immunity.

Age

Children are more likely to have only subclinical infection or mild diarrhea; adults tend to develop more severe disease and require hospitalization.

TREATMENT

The treatment of cholera patients consists of two components: rehydration, which is critical; and antimicrobial therapy, which is optional and intended to shorten the duration of illness.

Rehydration in the Acute Phase

Depending on the severity of the dehydration (see Table 1), intravenous or oral rehydration is preferred, and the choice of solution and rate of administration are determined. Effective fluid replacement can be expected to reduce mortality to less than 1% of severely affected individuals, compared with 50% or more when no treatment is provided. Return to a status of full hydration must be achieved in 4 hours of the beginning of treatment, with half of the fluid replacement occurring within the first hour. Analysis of the electrolyte loss in cholera stool has provided clues for the composition of rehydration solutions, oral and intravenous (see Table 2). The stool is generally isotonic and has electrolyte concentrations that are similar to those of serum.

Mild and moderately dehydrated patients can be treated with use of oral rehydration solution (ORS), which has three basic components: sugars, salts, and water. The sugar acts physiologically as the vehicle for salts to be absorbed by the mucosal cell, and water follows passively. The World Health Organization (WHO) and the United Nation's Children's Fund promote standard ORS, which comes in packages (see Table 2). Alternative formulations of ORS have also been developed. Solutions in which sugar is substituted by starch decrease the purge rate and the duration of diarrhea significantly. Similarly, studies have suggested that reduced osmolarity ORS may be more effective than standard ORS in reducing stool output. Partial replacement of glucose by the amino acid glutamine has the same effectiveness as standard ORS but has metabolic advantages. Homemade

solutions lack the potassium and bicarbonate salts and are often inaccurately prepared ("a fist of sugar and a pinch of salt in a pint of water").

ORS is intended to replace only the stool losses. Patients are therefore encouraged to drink additional fluids such as water. Infants should continue to be breast-fed or use formula, and all patients should resume eating as soon as possible.

Severely dehydrated patients should be treated intravenously. The optimal intravenous fluid is an isotonic, polyelectrolyte solution containing a base and potassium. Commonly available examples include lactated Ringer's and the Dhaka solution* (see Table 2).

Providing rapid rehydration requires one or sometimes multiple intravenous infusions. When intravenous solutions and equipment are not available, severely dehydrated patients may be treated through a nasogastric tube with use of the intravenous rate of rehydration. Subcutaneous and intraperitoneal parenteral fluids should not be used, because absorption from these sites is not sufficiently rapid to restore circulation.

Maintenance Hydration

Once rehydration is achieved, continuous stool losses have to be replaced. Patients receiving intravenous therapy may begin ORS treatment; patients receiving ORS should continue with ORS until the diarrhea stops.

Antimicrobials

Antibiotic treatment is optional and serves to shorten the illness and save rehydration fluids; incomplete courses have contributed to antibiotic resistance. Options are shown in Table 3 and are guided by local sensitivity patterns. Single-dose treatment has higher compliance of patients. Tetracyclines and quinolones are not recommended during pregnancy; at the recommended doses, tetracycline is not harmful to children. During epidemics, prophylactic antibiotics should be used for the immediate family only and be limited to a single-treatment dose.

Other Drugs

Not recommended in cholera are the following drugs: activated charcoal, kaolin, loperamide (Imodium), diphenoxylate (Lomotil), dopamine, norepinephrine, high-dose steroids, and colloid intravenous fluids.

PREVENTION

The persistence and penetrance of the current cholera pandemic serve as a marker for the inadequate sanitation in most of the world for which future prospects are undermined by the impact of international

---

*Not available in the United States.

TABLE 3. **Antimicrobial Agents Used in the Treatment of Cholera**

Agent	Adult Dose	Dose for Children <12 Years
Doxycycline*	300 mg as a single dose or 100 mg bid × 3 d	Do not use
Tetracycline	500 mg qid × 3 d	12.5 mg/kg qid × 3 d
Furazolidone (Furoxone)†	100 mg qid × 3 d	1.25 mg/kg qid × 3 d
TMP-SMZ (Bactrim, Septra)‡§	TMP 160 mg + SMZ 800 mg bid × 3 d	TMP 5 mg/kg + SMZ 25 mg/kg bid × 3 d
Ciprofloxacin (Cipro)‡‖	500 mg bid × 3 d	Do not use
Erythromycin‡¶	250 mg qid × 3 d	Do not use

* The drug of choice for most situations, because a single dose can be used.
† The drug of choice in pregnant women.
‡ Not FDA approved for this indication.
§ The preferred drug for children.
‖ This fluoroquinolone is the reserve for strains resistant to all other antibiotics.
¶ Next best alternative in case of multiple resistance.
Abbreviation: TMP-SMZ = trimethoprim-sulfamethoxazole.

debt on ailing economies. Because cholera is difficult to eradicate from water, it is likely to remain a serious threat to public health for some time. This holds particularly true for Latin America, where 73% of the population carries the predisposing blood type O. Measures to prevent cholera at the community and household levels include separation of sewage and water systems; disinfection of drinking and cooking water through boiling or addition of alum potash; bucket chlorination at untreated water sources; avoidance of commercial ice used by street vendors; safe food preparation, particularly of seafood (shellfish), using a core temperature of 60°C or 170°F, and of vegetables and fruits; basic sanitation including use of designated defecation areas; hygiene measures such as hand washing with soap; active case finding through community outreach; and effective case management of ill patients with the use of oral rehydration. During epidemics, bodies of persons dying of cholera should be disinfected and rapidly buried, and community leaders should be instructed to discourage the consumption of food served at gatherings including funerals.

Vaccines

The currently licensed, parenteral, killed cholera vaccine is no longer recommended by WHO because of its limited protective effect (50% for about 3 to 6 months) and ensuing false sense of security. To induce mucosal immunity, oral vaccines, both inactivated (WC/BS) and live (CVD103), have been developed and field tested; they show no side effects and have longer lasting protection than the parenteral vaccine. Vaccines that include the toxin's B subunit have been proved to provide cross-protection against traveler's diarrhea due to enterotoxigenic *Escherichia coli*. Before the use of cholera vaccines is recommended for public health purposes, several considerations have to be taken into account. The cost-effectiveness of the vaccine needs to be weighed against the cost-effectiveness of other preventive measures; the safety of live vaccines in populations with human immunodeficiency virus infection is questioned; vaccination may induce a transient state of enhanced susceptibility; and the new oral vaccines still have a delayed onset of protection of a limited level and duration. In light of these considerations, new guidelines need to be developed for the use of cholera vaccines, particularly in emergency settings such as refugee camps established overnight.

DIPHTHERIA

method of
GARY D. OVERTURF, M.D.
University of New Mexico–School of Medicine
Albuquerque, New Mexico

Diphtheria, an acute infection caused by *Corynebacterium diphtheriae*, is characterized by symptoms localized to the respiratory tract and by toxin-induced neurologic, renal, and cardiac injury. Diphtheria toxin is an extracellular phage-mediated protein consisting of an enzymatically active A domain and binding B domain. The infection is acquired by contact with a human carrier (endemic carrier rate, 3 to 5%) or person with active disease. The bacteria may be transmitted by respiratory droplets or contact with infected skin lesions. Although diphtheria occurs worldwide, it is currently epidemic in newly independent states of the former Soviet Union and eastern Europe, with more than 35,000 cases in 1995.

The period of communicability in untreated individuals is 2 to 6 weeks. The incubation period is 2 to 7 days. The usual portal of entry is the nose or mouth or, occasionally, the conjunctivae, skin, or genital mucosa. The organism remains localized to mucosal or cutaneous surfaces. A localized inflammatory response results in tissue necrosis with formation of the characteristic diphtheritic pseudomembrane in the upper respiratory tract. Toxin produced and absorbed at the local site of infection is distributed hematogenously, causing injury to the heart, nervous system, or kidneys. Thus, the severity of disease and resultant symptoms depend on the site and extent of the primary respiratory infection, the immunization status of the infected individual, and the degree of toxin-induced injury. To avoid continuing toxigenic injury, the diagnosis of diphtheria and the decision to administer antitoxin should be made on the basis of clinical history and findings and not await cultural confirmation. Definitive diagnosis requires the isolation of *C. diphtheriae* on selective media and the proof of toxigenicity (Elek agar diffusion test) of the isolated strain.

TREATMENT

Antitoxin Administration

Successful treatment of diphtheria is predicated on (1) neutralization of free toxin and (2) elimination of further toxin production by eradication of the organism. The only specific treatment available is antitoxin of equine origin (diphtheria equine antitoxin). Antitoxin is delivered preferably by the intravenous route in a single dose. A history of prior sensitization or exposure to horses or horse serum should be sought. If the history is positive, testing for horse serum hypersensitivity should first be performed with either a scratch test or intracutaneous injection of dilute antitoxin. The scratch test is performed with application of 1 drop of a 1:100 saline solution to the site of a superficial scratch, prick, or puncture on the volar aspect of the forearm. A positive test response is a wheal with surrounding erythema at least 3 mm larger than a control test response with normal saline (at 15 to 20 minutes after application). For those patients with a history of possible horse serum hypersensitivity, a smaller intracutaneous injection of 0.02 mL of a 1:1000 saline dilution of antitoxin may be administered. Erythema greater than 10 mm or a wheal within 20 minutes is a positive reaction. For those patients with a negative history or for those with an initially negative intradermal test reaction with dilute material, the intracutaneous injection should be performed or repeated, respectively, by injection of 0.02 mL of a 1:100 dilution.

If the patient is hypersensitive to horse serum, desensitization is required. Desensitization regimens require adequate preparation for management of anaphylaxis (e.g., availability of resuscitative and monitoring equipment and aqueous epinephrine 1:1000) and are optimally performed in a monitored setting. A recommended regimen employing increasing intravenous doses administered at 15-minute intervals is shown in Table 1. If no reaction occurs, the remaining dose is given by slow intravenous infusion. Patients may benefit from premedication with antihistamines with or without the addition of corticosteroids. Intravenous administration results in higher levels in saliva, more rapid neutralization of toxin, and subsequent detoxification of horse serum products.

The choice of the therapeutic dosage of equine antitoxin is empirical (Table 2). Administration is based on the site and duration of infection and degree of toxin-induced injury, not the age or size of the patient.

Antitoxin is available in the United States from the Centers for Disease Control and Prevention, Atlanta, Georgia (404–332–4555). An immediate reaction can be seen in up to 16% of patients, including a variety of rashes, fever, and anaphylaxis; a serum

TABLE 1. Suggested Intravenous* Dosage Schedule of Diphtheria Equine Antitoxin for Desensitization

Dose	Amount (mL)	Dilution	Alternative Route
1	0.10	1:1000	Intradermal
2	0.30	1:1000	Intradermal
3	0.60	1:1000	Subcutaneous
4	0.10	1:100	Subcutaneous
5	0.30	1:100	Subcutaneous
6	0.60	1:100	Subcutaneous
7	0.10	1:10	Subcutaneous
8	0.30	1:10	Subcutaneous
9	0.60	1:10	Subcutaneous
10	0.10	Undiluted	Subcutaneous
11	0.20	Undiluted	Subcutaneous
12	0.60	Undiluted	Intramuscular
13	1.0	Undiluted	Intramuscular

*The intravenous route is preferred because of better control.

sickness delayed reaction (rash, urticaria, fever, and arthralgia or arthritis) may occur in 10 to 20% of children or adults. Serum sickness characteristically occurs at 5 to 21 days after infusion and may be treated symptomatically with acetaminophen, aspirin, ibuprofen, or, in severe cases, corticosteroids.

Antibiotic Therapy

Antibiotics are important to eradicate the organism and prevent further toxin production. Erythromycin and penicillin are equally effective. Erythromycin may be given orally or intravenously at a dosage of 40 to 50 mg per kg per day in four divided doses (maximum, 2.0 grams per day). Penicillin may be given as aqueous penicillin, 100,000 to 150,000 units per kg per day divided in four doses (maximum, 10 million units), or as procaine penicillin G, 25,000 to 50,000 units per kg per day intramuscularly in two divided doses (maximum, 1.2 million units per dose). Both penicillin and erythromycin should be given for a total of 14 days. Elimination of the organism should be documented by three consecutive (daily) negative cultures after cessation of therapy. Clindamycin (Cleocin), fluoroquinolines, rifampin (Rifadin), and newer macrolides (clarithromycin [Biaxin], azithromycin [Zithromax]) have good in vitro activity against diphtheria organisms and may be better tolerated than erythromycin, but they have not been critically evaluated in clinical infection or carriage.

TABLE 2. Recommended Dosage of Diphtheria Antitoxin for Treatment

Clinical Indication	Antitoxin Dose
Pharyngeal or laryngeal disease of 48 h duration or less	40,000 units
Nasopharyngeal lesions	40,000–60,000 units
Extensive disease of more than 3 d duration or brawny neck swelling	80,000–120,000 units

In cutaneous diphtheria, lesions should be cleaned vigorously with soap and water. Most authorities recommend the administration of oral erythromycin or penicillin V for 10 days. Antitoxin therapy is of unproven value for this form of diphtheria, but some authorities recommend the administration of 20,000 to 40,000 units. Because of its uncertain value, antitoxin should not be given to patients who are sensitive to horse serum by history or skin testing.

Supportive Therapy

Patients with diphtheria should be hospitalized for horse serum and antibiotic administration as well as for careful monitoring. Isolation is recommended with measures to prevent airborne spread for the duration of hospitalization or until the completion of antibiotic therapy. Isolation should continue until two negative cultures for *C. diphtheriae* are obtained from both the nasopharynx and the throat 24 hours apart after cessation of therapy.

Delays in therapy are associated with an increased risk for myocardiopathy and bulbar and peripheral paralysis. Continuous cardiac monitoring should be employed during acute hospitalization; thereafter, serial electrocardiograms and/or echocardiograms should be obtained two or three times per week to assess for cardiac arrhythmias and myocardial function for up to 4 to 6 weeks. Patients with diphtheria may be successfully digitalized if congestive heart failure develops. In severe cases, prednisone (1 to 2.0 mg per kg per day) for up to 2 weeks has been employed, but its therapeutic efficacy is unproved. Serial urinalysis and renal functional screens should also be employed to detect nephropathy, and serial neurologic examinations should be carefully performed to detect any evidence of neuropathy. Maintenance of adequate hydration and nutrition, including parenteral nutrition if necessary, should be provided because palatal paralysis may complicate oral hydration or alimentation. Patients with laryngeal disease may require diagnostic or therapeutic bronchoscopy and/or intubation to ensure an unobstructed airway (e.g., necrotic nasal or pharyngeal membrane may dislodge and obstruct the airway).

Contacts

A history of symptoms and immunization status should be sought in all contacts. Cultures should be performed in contacts regardless of immunization status. Persons with positive cultures should be treated with either oral erythromycin or penicillin V for 7 days or a single intramuscular dose of benzathine penicillin G (600,000 units for those weighing less than 30 kg and 1.2 million units for those weighing more than 30 kg). Asymptomatic, previously immunized household or other close contacts should receive a booster dose of dT (adults and children older than 7 years) or DTaP, DPT, or DT (children younger than 7 years) (see the section on prevention). Asymptomatic close contacts who are unimmunized or not fully immunized, or whose immunization status is unknown, should have cultures performed and be treated with the antibiotic regimens used in carriers. Cultures should be repeated after treatment. Active immunization with DPT, DTaP, DT, or dT should be initiated or boosted appropriately for the age of the contact. Contacts who cannot be kept under close surveillance should be given benzathine penicillin G as noted earlier and a dose of an appropriate immunizing agent, depending on age and immunization status.

PREVENTION

Universal immunization with the diphtheria toxoid is an effective control measure. Up to the seventh birthday, children should receive DTaP or DPT (or DT for those in whom pertussis immunization is contraindicated) according to the currently approved schedule at 2, 4, 6, and 15 to 18 months of age, repeated at 4 to 6 years. After age 7 years, booster immunization with dT toxoid is recommended at 10-year intervals and/or with administration of tetanus prophylaxis for wounds. Childhood preparations of diphtheria toxin (DT, DTaP, or DPT) contain 6.7 to 12.5 flocculating units (Lf) of diphtheria toxoid per dose, compared with preparations of vaccine for older children and adults (dT) that contain no more than 2 Lf per dose. A primary series of immunization for older children and adults who have not previously been immunized is 2 doses given at 1- to 2-month intervals and a booster dose at 6 to 12 months.

FOOD-BORNE ILLNESS

method of
GARY L. SIMON, M.D., Ph.D.
George Washington University Medical Center
Washington, D.C.

A wide variety of chemicals, microbial toxins, and pathogenic microorganisms have been implicated as etiologic agents of food-borne illness. The clinical manifestations of such illnesses are predominantly gastrointestinal, although neurologic symptoms are frequently noted in patients who have ingested toxins.

The onset of disease is usually heralded by nausea, vomiting, abdominal cramps, and diarrhea. In some individuals, especially the very young and the very old, dehydration may be severe and hypotension may be present. Systemic symptoms such as fever, chills, and rigors may occur, depending on the specific etiologic agent. Paresthesias, weakness, and even paralysis may be present in those patients who have ingested neurologic toxins.

Identification of the specific microbial agent is important from both a therapeutic and a public health standpoint. Criteria that help to establish the etiologic diagnosis include (1) an epidemiologic and dietary history, including the type and preparation of the suspected food, recent travel, season of the year, and similar symptoms in companions or family members. It may be necessary to contact the local health department in some cases. (2) The clinical features of the illness should be defined; including suspected incubation period, type and severity of gastrointestinal symptoms, and presence of extraintestinal manifestations. (3) Appropriate specimens of blood, feces, and gastric aspirate and samples of the suspected food, if available, should be sent for laboratory confirmation of the diagnosis.

TREATMENT

The mainstay of therapy for patients with food-borne illness is supportive care. Most cases are self-limited so that only symptomatic therapy may be necessary. Vital signs are carefully monitored to ensure adequate hydration, and when appropriate, efforts should be made to remove unabsorbed toxin. In some patients, specific antimicrobial therapy may be warranted.

The degree of hydration can be assessed by examination of skin turgor and mucous membranes and by measurement of heart rate and blood pressure in several positions to demonstrate orthostatic changes. The volume of stool output or vomitus as reported by the patient is rarely accurate, whereas reports of decreased urine output can be helpful. Prompt repletion of fluid and electrolytes should be given to restore intravascular volume in the dehydrated patient. Pulse, blood pressure, urine output, and respiratory status should be monitored to ensure the adequacy of fluid replacement and to avoid overhydration.

Rehydration may be accomplished either orally or parenterally, depending on the severity of illness, available facilities, and the patient's ability to tolerate an oral preparation. For most individuals, oral rehydration therapy (ORT) is perfectly acceptable and provides a simple, inexpensive approach to mild dehydration. An oral rehydration solution can be prepared with use of commercially available packets (Jianas Brothers Packaging Co., Kansas City, MO) or by mixing 3.5 grams of NaCl, 1.5 grams of KCl, 2.5 grams of $NaHCO_3$, and 20 grams of glucose in 1 liter of boiled water. Sucrose (table sugar) can be substituted for glucose; a home recipe for an equivalent oral replacement solution is 4 level tablespoons of sugar, ¾ tablespoon of salt, 1 teaspoon of sodium bicarbonate, and 1 cup of orange juice in 1 liter of water. Cereal flour (50 to 60 grams or 200 grams of boiled mashed potato can be substituted for table sugar, which may help to reduce fluid output. Packets of a food-based ORT product using rice can also be purchased (Cera Products, Columbia, MD). Infants who are not severely ill can be treated with commercially available oral rehydration solutions such as Pedialyte or Lytren.

Hospitalization and intravenous rehydration are necessary for individuals who are severely dehydrated, especially infants, young children, and elderly patients. Children with severe hypernatremia must be closely monitored because brisk rehydration can result in a rapid decrease in serum sodium leading to cerebral edema.

In some patients with toxigenic food poisoning, unabsorbed toxin may be present in the gastrointestinal tract. Syrup of ipecac, 30 mg orally, or apomorphine,* 5 mg subcutaneously, is an effective emetic. To avoid aspiration of gastric contents, these agents should not be used in any patient who is neurologically impaired. Gastric lavage and activated charcoal may be administered to aid in removal of toxin. Cathartics such as magnesium citrate or sodium sulfate are effective at speeding transit through the gut.

Persistent nausea and vomiting can be controlled with antiemetics. Promethazine (Phenergan), 25 mg every 4 to 6 hours given intramuscular, orally, or rectally, or prochlorperazine (Compazine), 5 to 10 mg orally, 25 mg by rectal suppository, or 10 mg intramuscularly, may be given to adults. Trimethobenzamide hydrochloride (Tigan), 250 mg orally or 200 mg rectally, can be used as an alternative agent in children. These drugs should be avoided in children younger than 2 years.

The use of antidiarrheal agents is controversial. In many patients with food-borne illness, diarrhea is relatively brief and self-limited, and it may actually aid in removing toxin and pathogenic microorganisms. Antidiarrheal agents, such as loperamide hydrochloride (Imodium), 4 mg followed by 2 mg after each stool to a maximal daily dose of 16 mg; diphenoxylate hydrochloride (Lomotil) with atropine, 5 mg every 6 hours; or paregoric, 4 mL every 2 hours, may be used in selected patients with moderate or severe persistent diarrhea. These agents reduce peristalsis and are contraindicated in patients with fever, fecal leukocytes, or other features that suggest the presence of an invasive pathogen such as *Campylobacter*, *Salmonella*, *Shigella*, or *Entamoeba histolytica*. Bismuth subsalicylate (Pepto-Bismol), 2 tablespoons or 2 tablets every 30 to 60 minutes up to 8 doses, has been used in patients with traveler's diarrhea with relief of diarrheal symptoms. This drug should not be used in patients with aspirin sensitivity, renal failure, or gout or in individuals receiving warfarin (Coumadin) or oral hypoglycemic agents.

MICROBIAL AGENTS OR THEIR TOXINS

Food-borne Viral Infections

Several outbreaks of food-borne viral gastroenteritis have been reported in recent years. Norwalk-like virus has been associated with the ingestion of contaminated water or ice and consumption of oysters in Florida and freshly cut fruit on a cruise ship. The incubation period ranges from 18 to 72 hours. Illness is characterized by nausea and abdominal cramping, followed by vomiting and diarrhea. Low-grade fever is common. Symptoms are self-limited and resolve within 2 to 3 days. Antiperistaltic agents may be prescribed, but their benefit is unknown.

Astroviruses are another group of viral agents that have been transmitted in food or water. Nausea, diarrhea, headache, and malaise are characteristic; vom-

---

*Not yet approved for use in the United States.

iting is less frequently seen. The incubation period is 3 to 4 days, and symptoms usually resolve within 5 days after onset.

Hepatitis, especially hepatitis A and E, may be transmitted through contaminated food or water. These topics are covered elsewhere.

Bacterial Infections: Early Onset (<16 Hours)

Enterotoxigenic strains of *Staphylococcus aureus* are associated with the acute onset of nausea, vomiting, and diarrhea, usually within 1 to 6 hours of ingestion of the preformed toxin. Vomiting and diarrhea are each seen in approximately three fourths of patients with staphylococcal disease, but fever and other systemic symptoms are not commonly found.

Staphylococcal food poisoning is rarely attributable to commercially prepared foods but usually results from contamination of food by an infected or colonized food handler followed by improper storage at room temperature. This allows the bacteria to multiply and produce toxin. High protein concentrations favor the growth of staphylococci. Dairy products, meats and salads (such as ham, poultry, and egg salad), and cream-filled pastries are often implicated as the vehicles of infection. Foods that are contaminated with enterotoxigenic staphylococci taste and smell normal. Culture of stool or vomitus may reveal staphylococci, but this organism can also be present in the normal flora of healthy individuals so that definitive proof requires evidence of enterotoxin production. If cultures are obtained from either the suspected food or food handler, the phage type should be tested to demonstrate that it is the same as that found in the patient. Quantitative cultures that reveal 10^5 CFU or greater of staphylococci per gram of food are strongly suggestive of this syndrome.

Bacillus cereus food poisoning may present in two distinct clinical syndromes. A short-acting emetic form of the illness due to ingestion of preformed toxin mimics staphylococcal food poisoning and is characterized primarily by nausea and vomiting with onset within 1 to 6 hours of ingestion. This syndrome is usually associated with eating reheated fried rice.

There is a second form of illness with a long incubation period attributable to ingestion of *B. cereus* in which diarrhea and abdominal cramps are the prominent clinical features. Vomiting may occur in nearly one third of patients with the diarrheal form of *B. cereus* disease. This illness usually occurs 8 to 16 hours after ingestion and is more frequently associated with proteinaceous foods including vegetables, sauces, and puddings. In the long-acting syndrome, illness occurs as a result of toxin formation in vivo.

Meats, meat products, or poultry may be contaminated by *Clostridium perfringens*, which causes illness characterized by abdominal cramps and diarrhea 8 to 16 hours after ingestion. This longer incubation time is attributable to production of toxin in vivo.

These illnesses are self-limited and usually resolve within 1 to 2 days. Therapy is aimed at maintaining adequate intravascular volume with fluid replacement and providing symptomatic relief with antiemetic or antiperistaltic agents as necessary. Antibiotics have no role in the treatment of these intoxications.

Bacterial Infections: Late Onset (>16 Hours)

Vibrio cholerae, the prototypic diarrheal illness, may occur in individuals who have recently traveled to an endemic area. The organism has been isolated from the bayous of Louisiana, and infection can occur as a result of eating contaminated shellfish. Massive fluid loss results from the effects of the cholera enterotoxin, and rehydration is of paramount importance in the treatment of this illness. Intravenous therapy is usually required with either lactated Ringer's or Dhaka solution (0.5% NaCl, 0.4% $NaHCO_3$, 0.1% KCl). Oral replacement therapy can be used in patients with mild disease (when the volume of stool is less than 100 mL per kg per 24 hours). Antibiotics are of benefit in ameliorating symptoms, reducing stool volume, and shortening the duration of excretion of the organism. Tetracycline, 250 mg every 6 hours or 2 grams once daily for 2 days, is the regimen of choice for adults; children should receive ampicillin, 50 mg per kg per day in divided doses. Trimethoprim-sulfamethoxazole (Bactrim, Septra) or a quinolone may be a useful alternative agent; however, quinolones should not be used in young children because of their effects on cartilage formation.

Another vibrio species, *Vibrio parahaemolyticus*, has an enterotoxin and invasive properties. This organism is halophilic and is frequently found in coastal waters. Infection occurs when contaminated seafood, especially crab or shrimp, is eaten raw or is inadequately cooked and then stored at room temperature for several hours before it is eaten. Clinical illness usually occurs within 48 hours of ingestion of contaminated seafood and is characterized by abdominal cramps and watery, explosive diarrhea. The disease is self-limited, and no treatment other than supportive measures is necessary. Antimicrobial agents have little impact on the severity or duration of symptoms.

Infection with organisms that produce their effects by tissue invasion, such as *Campylobacter*, *Salmonella*, and *Shigella*, is characterized by fever, abdominal cramps, and diarrhea. Hematochezia may be seen in patients with these invasive pathogenic organisms. Vomiting may occur, but less frequently than with staphylococcal or *Bacillus* intoxications. In general, patients with these invasive forms of enteric disease tend to have a longer incubation period, usually more than 16 hours and occasionally several days. The diagnosis of an invasive enteric pathogen may be suspected by the presence of fecal leukocytes.

Confirmation is made by isolation of the pathogen from stool cultures.

Salmonella gastroenteritis is the most frequently identified food-borne enteric infection in the United States. Poultry, eggs, beef, and dairy products are frequently implicated as vehicles of transmission. *Salmonella* gastroenteritis is rarely treated inasmuch as most antimicrobial agents have little impact on the duration of illness and tend to prolong asymptomatic carriage of the organism. All bacteremic patients should be treated, however. In addition, patients who should receive specific antimicrobial therapy include neonates; elderly subjects; individuals with hemoglobinopathies, lymphoproliferative disorders, human immunodeficiency virus infection, and prosthetic joints or valves; transplant recipients; and patients receiving immunosuppressive therapy. Parenteral therapy with a new cephalosporin antibiotic such as ceftriaxone (Rocephin), 1 gram daily, is effective for bacteremic infection. Useful alternative agents include trimethoprim-sulfamethoxazole, 80 mg of trimethoprim and 400 mg of sulfamethoxazole twice daily, or ciprofloxacin (Cipro), 500 mg twice daily. In children, trimethoprim-sulfamethoxazole can be used. The dose is 8 mg per kg of trimethoprim and 40 mg per kg of sulfamethoxazole in 24 hours given in two daily doses.

Like *Salmonella* gastroenteritis, *Campylobacter* infection has been associated with poultry. The treatment of campylobacteriosis is not well defined. Erythromycin, 500 mg every 6 hours, and ciprofloxacin (Cipro), 500 mg twice daily, are active in vitro but may have little impact on the course of the illness, especially when antibiotics are started several days after the onset of symptoms.

Shigella infections are highly contagious and, unlike *Salmonella* or *Campylobacter* infection, may occur as a result of direct person-to-person spread. Identification of *Shigella* in a clinical specimen should be followed by specific antimicrobial therapy, which not only shortens the duration of illness, but also reduces the number of organisms present in fecal specimens, thereby lowering the secondary attack rate. Both trimethoprim-sulfamethoxazole and ciprofloxacin are effective agents, but sensitivity testing should be done because of the frequent occurrence of microbial resistance.

Escherichia coli

E. coli has been implicated as the etiologic agent in a variety of diarrheal syndromes. Enteroinvasive *E. coli* penetrates intestinal cells and produces a clinical illness similar to that seen with *Shigella*. Outbreaks in relation to contaminated food have been described. Enterotoxigenic *E. coli* (ETEC) is the most commonly identified agent of traveler's diarrhea. Enteroadherent isolates, which do not produce enterotoxin but rather adhere closely to the enterocyte surface and cause destruction of the microvilli, have also been associated with diarrhea in travelers. Disease due to enterohemorrhagic *E. coli* (EHEC)

has been recognized since 1982 when hemorrhagic colitis associated with eating undercooked hamburgers from a fast-food restaurant was reported. This outbreak was due to contamination of the meat with *E. coli* serotype O157:H7. Numerous additional cases have been reported, and an association between EHEC and hemolytic-uremic syndrome has been demonstrated.

In general, these *E. coli*–related syndromes benefit from treatment with antibiotics. Trimethoprim-sulfamethoxazole, ampicillin, tetracycline, or one of the quinolones such as ciprofloxacin can be used. However, a report has suggested that hemolytic-uremic syndrome is more common among patients with EHEC who receive antibiotics.

Traveler's Diarrhea

Acute, watery diarrhea may occur in up to 60% of travelers to developing countries. ETEC is the most frequently identified etiologic agent, although other pathogens may also be encountered. The incubation period for traveler's diarrhea due to ETEC is usually less than 48 hours. Untreated, infection may last 5 to 7 days.

Careful attention to diet is the best method for avoiding traveler's diarrhea. Boiled or bottled water, especially carbonated beverages, is safer than untreated tap water. Raw fruits and vegetables, inadequately cooked or cold meats, and dairy products should be avoided.

Most cases are self-limited, and dehydration is usually not a significant problem. Treatment with antibiotics may shorten the duration of illness. Useful agents for travelers with this syndrome are doxycycline (Vibramycin), 100 mg twice daily; trimethoprim-sulfamethoxazole, 1 double-strength tablet twice daily; or a quinolone such as ciprofloxacin, 500 mg twice daily.

Cryptosporidiosis

Cryptosporidiosis is a protozoal infection that has been recognized to cause a profuse watery diarrhea. Outbreaks of cryptosporidiosis have been associated with ingestion of contaminated water. In one outbreak in Wisconsin, it was estimated that 403,000 individuals became ill. Symptoms usually resolve within 10 days in immunocompetent hosts. In patients with the acquired immune deficiency syndrome, diarrhea may be intractable. Therapeutic regimens that may be useful in patients with gastrointestinal cryptosporidiosis include paromomycin (Humatin), bovine colostrum,* and octreotide (Sandostatin), but further study is necessary.

Botulism

Botulism occurs most commonly as a result of eating contaminated home-processed fruits, vegetables, or meats. Ingestion of botulinum toxin is charac-

---

*Not yet approved for use in the United States.

terized by nausea and vomiting followed by symptoms of dry mouth, weakness, diplopia, and dysphagia. The illness may progress rapidly, with respiratory compromise requiring ventilatory support. The incubation period may vary from 6 hours to 8 days, depending on the quantity of toxin ingested.

Infant botulism is caused by ingestion of *Clostridium botulinum* spores that germinate and produce toxin in vivo. It is recommended that infants do not receive honey because it may contain *C. botulinum*.

The mainstay of therapy is intensive monitoring and supportive care. Removal of unabsorbed toxin by cathartics and emetics may be beneficial. A trivalent A, B, and E antiserum is available from the Centers for Disease Control and Prevention.

CHEMICAL INTOXICATIONS

Heavy metals such as copper, zinc, tin, and cadmium directly irritate the gastric mucosa and result in the rapid onset of abdominal cramps, nausea, and vomiting, usually within 5 to 15 minutes of ingestion. The inadvertent ingestion of these substances has been associated with the storage of acidic beverages such as fruit punch or citric juices in galvanized metal cans, from which the metal is leached by the acid in the juice or punch. Corroded tubing in old vending machines that were dispensing soft drinks by the cup has also been implicated. Antiemetics are contraindicated in this condition because the symptoms will resolve within a few hours after emetic activity removes the offending agent.

Monosodium glutamate is the putative agent of the Chinese restaurant syndrome. Headache, flushing, diaphoresis, and a burning sensation of the skin may be evident within 10 to 15 minutes of ingestion. There is no specific therapy, and symptoms resolve within a few hours.

SEAFOOD-RELATED SYNDROMES

Ciguatera Fish Poisoning

Ciguatera fish poisoning is characterized by gastrointestinal and neurologic symptoms after the ingestion of fish contaminated with ciguatoxin, a neurotoxin from the dinoflagellate *Gambierdiscus toxicus*. Ciguatoxin is found only in fish living within 30 degrees of the equator. Most cases have been associated with ingestion of large carnivorous fish such as red snapper, amberjack, grouper, and barracuda. Ciguatoxin is not affected by heating or cooling, and it may persist for several weeks; it is difficult to detect because it does not alter the taste, color, or odor of contaminated fish.

Gastrointestinal symptoms including nausea, vomiting, diarrhea, and abdominal pain are usually first noted within 1 to 6 hours of ingestion. These symptoms are followed by pruritus; paresthesias of the extremities, mouth, tongue, and throat; shooting pains in the legs; and sensation of looseness and pain in the teeth. Other characteristic symptoms include

dry mouth, blurred vision, photophobia, bradycardia, hypotension, and temperature reversal (e.g., ice cream tastes hot). Severe cases may progress to coma and require mechanical ventilation. Ciguatoxin has been transmitted by breast milk and through sexual intercourse.

The duration of illness is variable. Most patients recover within a few weeks; however, some individuals may note persistence of neurologic symptoms for more than 6 months. Intermittent recrudescence of symptoms can occur for a period of months to years. Chronic symptoms tend to occur more frequently in persons who had more severe initial symptoms or a longer duration of symptoms.

Toxin should be removed with emetics or by gastric lavage if the patient is seen within 4 hours of ingestion. Cathartics and enemas may also be used to help remove unabsorbed toxin. Atropine may be used to treat severe bradycardia. In the acute setting, intravenous infusion of mannitol (1 gram per kg of 20% solution, given in 45 minutes) has been noted to have a dramatic effect on neurologic symptoms. In patients with life-threatening weakness and low blood cholinesterase concentrations, pralidoxime chloride (Protopam), 1 to 2 grams in 100 mL of saline, may be given intravenously. Chronic symptoms may be treated with amitriptyline (Elavil), tocainide (Tonocard), imipramine (Tofranil), nifedipine (Procardia), and alprazolam (Xanax), although further studies are needed to define the benefit of these agents.

Scombroid Fish Poisoning

Scombroid fish poisoning is a histamine reaction due to ingestion of fish flesh containing histidine that has undergone decarboxylation by marine bacteria. Scombrotoxicosis occurs most commonly after ingestion of fish from the families Scombridae and Scomberesocidae, which includes tuna, mackerel, skipjack, and bonito. The syndrome is also seen with other nonscombroid species, such as mahi-mahi, bluefish, and salmon.

The incubation period of scombroid fish poisoning varies from 10 minutes to a few hours. Symptoms include the sudden onset of flushing, tingling and burning sensations around the mouth, headache, nausea, vomiting, palpitations, and occasionally swelling of the face and tongue. The illness is self-limited and resolves within 6 to 12 hours. Antihistamines are effective and may reduce the severity and the duration of symptoms. Although overt spoilage of fish is not necessary, toxic fish have been noted to have a peppery taste, which should be used as a warning to stop eating.

Puffer Fish Poisoning

Tetrodotoxin intoxication may occur after the ingestion of improperly prepared puffer fish. The clinical syndrome is characterized by the rapid onset of weakness, paresthesias, and abdominal pain. In severe cases, there is ascending paralysis with respiratory failure and death. A 60% mortality has been reported with this intoxication.

Paralytic Shellfish Poisoning

Paralytic shellfish poisoning (PSP) is caused by eating bivalve mollusks (mussels, clams, oysters, scallops) containing a neurotoxin, saxitoxin, that is produced by toxigenic dinoflagellates. Blooms of the toxic dinoflagellates (red tides) occur in the Northeast and along the West Coast in late spring and summer, after which the shellfish become toxic and remain so for several weeks thereafter. The toxin is heat stable and not affected by cooking.

Symptoms of PSP occur within 1 to 10 hours of ingestion and include nausea, vomiting, circumoral paresthesias, and paresthesias of the extremities. Ataxia, dysphonia, dysphagia, and mental status changes may occur. Severe cases may be accompanied by paralysis and respiratory compromise.

Treatment includes gastric lavage and cathartics to remove unabsorbed toxin. Symptoms usually resolve within hours to a few days.

Neurotoxic Shellfish Poisoning

Neurotoxic shellfish poisoning occurs within a few hours of ingestion of shellfish harvested from the Gulf of Mexico and the Atlantic coast of Florida that have been contaminated by brevetoxin, which is also produced by a dinoflagellate. Symptoms of neurotoxic shellfish poisoning are similar to those of PSP but less severe. Paralysis and respiratory failure do not occur, and symptoms usually resolve within a few hours.

Amnesic Shellfish Poisoning

Ingestion of shellfish harvested from the Atlantic coast of Canada containing domoic acid has been reported to cause a syndrome of abdominal cramps, nausea, vomiting, diarrhea, headache, confusion, and loss of short-term memory. Severe anterograde memory deficits along with preservation of other cognitive functions have been noted in patients who have experienced this intoxication. Coma and cardiovascular instability have been noted in severe cases. There is no specific therapy, but Canadian authorities regularly analyze shellfish for domoic acid and close contaminated beds.

Diarrheic Shellfish Poisoning

Ingestion of mussels, scallops, or clams that produce okadaic acid and dinophysistoxin 1 causes symptoms of nausea, vomiting, diarrhea, and abdominal pain. To date, all cases of this syndrome have been reported in Japan and Europe.

Mushroom Poisoning

Seven established groups of toxic mushrooms elaborate different toxins and produce different clinical syndromes. Many mushroom intoxications produce a self-limited gastrointestinal syndrome of nausea, vomiting, abdominal cramps, and diarrhea that requires only supportive care. However, if there is a suspicion of mushroom poisoning, a local poison control center should be contacted because some ingestions may be fatal and specific therapy may be lifesaving.

Ingestion of the muscarine-containing mushrooms *Clitocybe* species and *Inocybe* species may be associated with the development of an anticholinergic syndrome. Symptoms of parasympathetic hyperactivity such as sweating, salivation, lacrimation, and bradycardia may develop 30 minutes to 2 hours after ingestion. Severe cases may require treatment with atropine, 1 to 2 mg every 2 to 6 hours as warranted.

Psilocybin, psilocin, and other indoles are toxins associated with mushrooms from the *Psilocybe* and *Panaeolus* families. Mood elevation, hallucinations, hyperkinetic activity, and muscle weakness occur within 30 to 90 minutes after ingestion of these substances. Symptomatic therapy with benzodiazepines may be administered to relieve agitation.

Amatoxins and phallotoxins are found in *Amanita phalloides* as well as in several other species. These toxins produce a biphasic illness in which the first phase is characterized by abdominal pain, vomiting, and diarrhea occurring 6 to 12 hours after ingestion. These symptoms resolve within 24 hours. After a brief respite of 1 to 2 days, renal and hepatic failure ensues, which has a mortality of 30 to 50%. Hemolysis and methemoglobinemia may also be seen during the latter stages of illness. Hemoperfusion may be useful in removing toxin.

Amanita species that contain ibotenic acid and isoxazole derivatives may cause a syndrome of confusion, restlessness, dizziness, and visual disturbances. In more severe cases, there may be ataxia, stupor, and convulsions. Barbiturates and benzodiazepines should be avoided because they tend to exacerbate the symptoms. Severely affected individuals may be treated with physostigmine (Antilirium) 0.5 to 1.0 mg intramuscularly or intravenously.

Coprine, a substance produced by *Coprinus* species, causes a disulfiram-like reaction after alcohol ingestion. Headache, nausea and vomiting, and flushing may persist for 5 days after ingestion. Therapy is to simply avoid alcohol.

Mushrooms of the genus *Gyromitra* contain gyromitrin, which is converted in vivo to a competitive inhibitor of pyridoxal phosphate, methylhydrazine. Nausea and vomiting occur within 2 to 12 hours of ingestion, followed by hemolysis with methemoglobinemia and hepatic failure. Neurologic symptoms such as convulsions may be treated with intravenous pyridoxine hydrochloride, 25 mg per kg.

Orellanine is a toxin produced by mushrooms of the genus *Cortinarius* that causes thirst, nausea, headache, abdominal pain, and visual disturbances. The incubation period may be as long as 3 to 5 days.

Other Fungal Poisoning

Claviceps purpurea, a fungus that contaminates wheat and rye, produces ergot, which is an alpha-adrenergic smooth muscle vasoconstrictor. Headache, muscle and abdominal pain, paresthesias, and convulsions may occur after ergot ingestion. In severe cases, there may be ischemic necrosis and gangrene. Treatment consists of anticoagulation and the use of vasodilators such as intravenous nitroprusside titrated against blood pressure.

Aflatoxin, a fungus found in peanut butter, may also contaminate corn and other grains in the tropics. Ingestion of aflatoxin is associated with gastrointestinal bleeding, hepatic injury, and the development of hepatoma.

Tricothecenes are heat-stable mycotoxins that may contaminate grains in colder climates. Symptoms of nausea, vomiting, and bloody diarrhea may follow ingestion.

Plant Poisoning

A number of plants or plant products that may be ingested are capable of causing a wide variety of clinical syndromes. The Italian broad (fava) bean has been associated with acute hemolytic crisis in individuals with glucose-6-phosphate dehydrogenase deficiency. Lathyrism is a spastic paraplegia that follows chronic ingestion of *Lathyrus sativus* (sweet pea). Early symptoms of muscle spasm, cramps, and leg weakness may be followed by signs of degeneration of the posterolateral tracts of the spinal cord. Neostigmine methylsulfate (Prostigmin), 0.5 mg subcutaneously, may be beneficial.

Ingestion of leaves from rhubarb, beets, spinach, or the houseplants philodendron and dieffenbachia can result in oxalic acid poisoning. Intravenous fluids should be given to prevent renal tubular cell damage; calcium gluconate, 10 mL of a 10% solution, can be given if tetany develops. Oral calcium reduces oxalate concentrations by precipitating calcium oxalate in the gastrointestinal tract.

Solanine is present in the leaves and fruit of the Jerusalem cherry; the leaves and stems of tomatoes; tubers, vines, and leaves of potatoes; and jimson weed, which may be ingested by humans who drink milk from cattle that have eaten jimson weed. Intoxication is characterized by headache, abdominal pain, diarrhea, and confusion. Treatment is supportive.

Digitalis intoxication can occur in patients who prepare home-brewed teas that contain foxglove or oleander. These individuals need to be admitted for electrocardiographic monitoring and treatment, which may include potassium, antiarrhythmics, temporary pacemaker insertion, and administration of antidigoxin antibody. The benefit of the last in this situation is unknown, and advice should be obtained from Glaxo-Wellcome before the drug is administered.

Cyanide poisoning may occur after the ingestion of large numbers of seeds from fruits and vegetables.

NECROTIZING SKIN AND SOFT TISSUE INFECTIONS

method of
ROBERT E. CONDON, M.D., M.S.
Medical College of Wisconsin
Milwaukee, Wisconsin

Necrotizing infections are a group of uncommon, rapidly progressive, potentially life-threatening diseases that are best treated initially with high doses of intravenous penicillin G plus meropenem and clindamycin coupled with early and repeated débridement if there is involvement of subcutaneous fat, fascia, or muscle. The sites of primary infection (in descending order of frequency) are the abdominal wall, perineum, and extremities (especially the feet in diabetics). Secondary hematogenous infections occur at sites of recent trauma (may be minimal), at pressure points (iliac crest, ischial tuberosity, heel, elbow, occiput), in joints, or in the lungs.

A high index of suspicion must be maintained regarding any patient exhibiting skin erythema or tissue tenderness, especially if one or more risk factors for necrotizing infection are also present. The risk factors include insulin-dependent diabetes mellitus, alcohol or drug abuse, immunosuppression due to drugs or to other disease, chronic renal failure, peripheral vascular disease, older age, lymphoma, and colitis. The portal of entry may be obvious, such as a surgical or traumatic wound, but these infections may also begin through only a minor break in the skin. In cases of colitis or lymphoma, the portal of entry is through involved bowel. No portal of entry can be identified in one fifth of patients.

Treatment is influenced by the depth of infection and the presence of necrosis more than by the specific bacteria involved. Early, aggressive intervention is needed because these infections may be fulminating in their course; the rate of progression can be astonishingly rapid. Tissue necrosis is due to toxins (enzymes) secreted by the infecting bacteria and to thrombosis of blood vessels in and around the infected area. In addition to causing local death of infected tissues, toxins also enter the circulation and generate profound systemic effects that can culminate in multiple organ failure and death.

CLASSIFICATION

The taxonomy of necrotizing infections is complex and confusing. In simplified terms, there are two broad categories: the cellulitis group and the fasciitis-myonecrosis group. It can be difficult to distinguish clinically among the many syndromes within each of these two disease groups, but an exact diagnosis is not important because it is not needed to initiate treatment. Diagnostic classification can be deferred until more information about the histologic type, the results of culture, and the outcome of treatment is available.

Cellulitis Group

These infections involve the skin (epidermis and dermis; occasionally, immediately adjacent subcutaneous fat) and have a reasonably good prognosis if treatment is not delayed. They are characterized by erythema that typically shows a well-defined advancing margin. Edema, usually pitting in character, often involves a wider area than does the erythema. Fever, leukocytosis, and, later, development of systemic toxicity (confusion, hypotension) occur regularly. Sometimes skin blisters and bullae appear, or there may be central necrosis of skin that subsequently sloughs, leaving an ulcer.

This group of infections includes impetigo, streptococcal cellulitis, the scalded skin (epidermolysis) syndrome, ecthyma gangrenosum, and similar entities. These are typically monomicrobial infections due to staphylococci or streptococci. Nonbacterial lesions such as a brown recluse spider bite and pyoderma gangrenosum need to be differentiated.

Fasciitis-Myonecrosis Group

These infections involve the deeper parts of the subcutaneous fat, fascia, or muscle. They continue to be associated with a mortality risk on the order of 10% if adequate treatment is effected early, but the mortality risk exceeds 40% if treatment is delayed by as little as 24 hours. Fasciitis-myonecrosis group infections are characterized by extreme and constant pain that is disproportionate to the local signs of infection. Early signs of systemic toxicity (confusion, delirium, hypotension, renal failure) are accompanied by fever and leukocytosis. Edema, sometimes producing a woody texture in involved tissues, is always present but may not be prominent. Gas derived from bacterial metabolism is frequently present, and subcutaneous crepitus can be detected in some patients. Spontaneous dissection occurs, lifting the subcutaneous fat free from the underlying fascia, and spreads rapidly centrally along fascial planes. A thin layer of slightly turbid "dishwater" fluid is found here, and it can be detected on computed tomographic examination. Skin changes of dusky erythema, bluish brown discoloration progressing to black necrosis, appear with or after signs of systemic toxicity. These skin changes are due to thrombosis and lymphatic obstruction in the underlying subcutaneous fat. Late signs in this group of necrotizing infections are anemia secondary to hemolysis, coagulopathy, hematuria or myoglobinuria, and cutaneous anesthesia.

Infections in this group can be polymicrobic or monomicrobic. The organisms are typically gram-positive in monomicrobic infections and include staphylococci, streptococci, peptostreptococci, and clostridia. In the polymicrobic infections, a mixed aerobic-anaerobic flora, usually of fecal origin, is recovered in culture. This group of infections includes clostridial cellulitis, anaerobic (peptostreptococcal) cellulitis, necrotizing fecal fasciitis, streptococcal fasciitis, synergistic gangrene, clostridial myonecrosis (gas gangrene), and related entities. Mucormycosis, a fungal necrotizing infection, mimics the clinical signs and symptoms of the bacterial necrotizing infections but has a worse prognosis.

STEPS IN INITIAL MANAGEMENT

1. Call a Surgeon

The advice of a knowledgeable general surgeon is helpful in differentiating the various diagnostic entities. Further, the skills of a surgeon are needed in the management of the more serious forms of these infections.

2. Insert a Central Venous Line

The central line provides secure access for the administration of antibiotics and other drugs in these patients whose condition may become unstable without warning. A subclavian catheter is preferred to one inserted in the jugular vein because it can remain in place for longer periods and causes less difficulty for the patient. The central line can also be used as a simple monitor of central venous pressure.

3. Start Intravenous Antibiotics

Penicillin G, 2.4 million units intravenously (IV) over 15 to 30 minutes, followed by 1.0 million units every hour as a continuous infusion

Meropenem (Merrem), 2.0 grams IV in the next 30 minutes; repeat 1.0 gram every 6 hours

Clindamycin (Cleocin), 900 mg IV in the next 30 minutes; repeat every 8 hours

Because the bacteria causing the infection are not identified at this stage, administration of this three-drug redundant regimen of antibiotics is appropriate as initial therapy. A more specifically targeted antibiotic regimen can be selected when the initial clinical course is known and sensitivity data from initial cultures become available. Clindamycin is preferred to metronidazole because of its activity in reducing the synthesis of toxins by staphylococci and streptococci. If staphylococci are documented in culture, substitute nafcillin or vancomycin, depending on the sensitivity data, for penicillin. If the patient has documented hypersensitivity or major allergy (anaphylaxis, serum sickness, exfoliative dermatitis, urticaria) to β-lactam antibiotics, use high doses of alternatives (in order of preference) such as ciprofloxacin (Cipro), chloramphenicol (Chloromycetin), an aminoglycoside (ineffective in anaerobic infections), or doxycycline (Vibramycin).

4. Start Fluid Resuscitation

Use normal saline initially, shifting to lactated Ringer's solution when reasonably normal renal function is demonstrated. The first liter of fluid should be given as rapidly as possible. The rate of administration is then adjusted according to the response. Intravenous fluid administration should be continued rapidly until there has been a response in the pulse and blood pressure and adequate urine output is recorded. The usual error in fluid resuscitation is to administer too little volume too slowly, especially in older patients.

5. Start Monitoring

Insert a Foley catheter to monitor urine output. If the patient shows hemodynamic instability, insertion of a Swan-Ganz catheter through a second central venous puncture and insertion of a radial artery catheter may be needed.

6. Administer Tetanus Prophylaxis

Give a booster dose (0.5 mL) of adsorbed diphtheria-tetanus toxoid (DT) unless the patient is known to have been immunized and to have received a booster within the last 10 years. If there is any doubt, give a booster dose. If the patient has not previously been immunized, administer 250 units of human tetanus immune globulin (Hyper-Tet) and start immunization with tetanus toxoid (use DTP in infants).

7. Determine the Extent of Disease

Solicit a history of trauma, however trivial. Do a focused physical examination, inspecting carefully for an entry site (do not forget the vagina and rectum as potential entry sites). Record the current state of the apparently infected tissues and plan to make serial recordings of the infection as it progresses and, it is hoped, regresses under treatment. Initial diagnostic studies should include a hematocrit, white blood cell count, differential white blood cell count, and absolute platelet count; prothrombin and partial thromboplastin times; and creatinine, creatine kinase (CK), lactate dehydrogenase (LDH), serum albumin, and calcium determinations. Hemolysis may result in a decreasing hematocrit as the infection progresses. Coagulopathy or disseminated intravascular coagulation may occur, and these baseline studies are helpful in following such events. If there is myositis, the CK and LDH values will be markedly elevated. Low albumin concentration is frequently found; serum calcium levels may be even lower than can be explained by the low albumin concentrations. Plain films are sometimes helpful to detect gas in tissue, but treatment should never be delayed just to get confirming radiographs.

8. Draw Blood Samples for Cultures

Blood samples for two sets of cultures should be drawn from two separate carefully prepared sites, yielding a total of four sets of initial blood cultures.

9. Decide on the Most Likely Diagnosis

On the basis of the clinical findings, make a diagnosis of an infection in the cellulitis group or, alternatively, in the fasciitis-myonecrosis group.

10. Treatment of Cellulitis Group Infections

These infections usually respond to the antibiotic therapy initiated in step 3. If there is a pre-existing wound, that wound should be explored with a blunt instrument to determine whether any deep necrosis

is present or whether the subcutaneous fat is easily separable from the underlying fascia (these findings indicate an infection in the fasciitis-myonecrosis group). Perform a biopsy of the advancing skin margins of infection under local anesthesia using a small dermatologic punch. The biopsy specimen should be sent for aerobic and anaerobic cultures as well as for histologic examination. Advance notice to the laboratory about processing this specimen is often helpful. Radiographs may be obtained to determine whether there is gas in the involved tissue (the presence of gas heightens the suspicion that fasciitis-myonecrosis group infection is present). Observe the patient for the effects of the antibiotic treatment. The expectation is that the patient will stabilize in 2 to 6 hours and begin to improve clinically in 24 to 48 hours. Continued instability, progression of the infection, or failure to respond as expected should lead to exploration (see step 11). Topical mupirocin (Bactroban) may be helpful if there is incipient necrosis or ulceration of the skin.

11. If Unsure, Explore

Because the treatment of deeper infections is markedly different from that of superficial infections, it is important to accurately classify the group of necrotizing infection affecting the patient. If a firm diagnostic decision cannot be made, or if the patient is not responding to initial treatment for cellulitis, then exploration under general anesthesia is appropriate. It is better to have an unnecessary scar and survive than to die because more radical treatment was delayed.

After establishing general anesthesia and the usual preparation of an operative field, incise through the center of the affected area down to the underlying fascia following the lines of skin tension. Inspect the subcutaneous fat for necrosis and probe with a finger along the surface of the fascia. If the fat is still adherent to the fascia and there is no evidence of necrosis in the deeper layers, the patient probably has a cellulitis group infection. On the other hand, findings of necrosis of the subcutaneous fat (dull and slightly discolored), thrombosis of vessels, and necrotic fascia (dull gray with a shaggy stringy surface) that is easily undermined and separated from the subjacent fascia by blunt finger dissection, accompanied by thin brownish or gray turbid fluid or fluid containing gas bubbles, indicate the presence of a fasciitis-myonecrosis group infection. Open the fascia to inspect the muscle if there is any question of myositis.

12. Treatment of Fasciitis-Myonecrosis

Any pre-existing wound is the route for exploration or, as indicated before, a new incision is made across the central portion of the affected area and carried initially down to the underlying fascia. Smears for Gram's stain and aerobic and anaerobic culture are obtained of any fluid and from tissue surfaces. All obviously necrotic tissue needs to be débrided as quickly as possible. Samples of the excised tissue are sent for aerobic and anaerobic culture as well as for histologic examination. The boundary of subcutaneous fat necrosis usually is not clearly demarcated; excision should be continued until fat that bleeds normally has been encountered. The fluid found in these infections may have no odor, may be "mousy" (a sweet, musty smell associated with streptococcal infections), or may be pungent (gases released by fecal anaerobes).

The fascia should be opened to inspect the underlying muscle. If myositis is present (muscles soft and mushy, little or no bleeding, brownish discoloration), bold excision of the entire muscle or muscle group needs to be done. The overall objective of the initial operative débridement is to preserve as much viable tissue as possible but to remove all necrotic tissues. Amputation is necessarily employed under wartime conditions but can sometimes be avoided in civilian practice if prompt excision of all involved muscles is done. Amputation may still be needed, however, especially when treatment has been delayed for several hours after onset of the infection. After débridement, the wound is packed open with wet saline dressings. If full-thickness excision of the abdominal wall is necessary, temporary closure with a device such as the artificial burr and wound coverage with plastic film can be used. The initial débridement is rarely definitive. Daily re-exploration under general anesthesia in the operating room should be conducted until all necrotic tissue has been removed, the wound is clean and granulating, and the patient's clinical state is stable.

13. Start Parenteral or Enteral Nutrition

The energy requirement of patients suffering necrotizing infections is enormous and cannot be brought into immediate balance. However, the administration of parenteral or enteral nutrition regimens sufficient to ensure an intake of about 2000 calories in a typical adult is helpful and should be initiated at the start of the overall therapy program. Anticipate that patients with these terrible infections will need nutritional supplementation for 2 or 3 weeks. My personal preference is to use parenteral nutrition through a central line. Enteral nutrition is a viable alternative, usually administered through a nasal jejunal tube, in patients who do not have advanced paralytic ileus as a complication of their infection.

14. Consider Hyperbaric Oxygen Therapy

Application of hyperbaric oxygen therapy should never delay the initial débridement required in patients with a fasciitis-myonecrosis group infection. Hyperbaric oxygen treatment is the subject of mixed anecdotal reports in the literature; there have been no reports of controlled clinical trials. If a hyperbaric chamber is readily available, it can be used because there is some suggestion that this therapy may decrease the volume of tissue that needs to be débrided. However, because the efficacy of hyperbaric oxygen treatment is not established, it is probably unwarranted to transport patients over long distances simply to secure such treatment.

15. Gather Updated Information

A MEDLINE search, using "fasciitis, necrotizing" as the search string and checking the "reviews" box, can be conducted through GRATEFUL MED or through your hospital librarian to provide access to current information regarding the management of these complicated cases.

INFLUENZA

method of
THOMAS R. CATE, M.D.
Baylor College of Medicine
Houston, Texas

Influenza outbreaks of varying severity occur every year during the fall and winter in areas with temperate climates. The type A and/or B influenza viruses that cause these outbreaks can be transmitted person to person by aerosol or close contact, and the speed of modern travel facilitates spread of the virus between communities and continents. Propagation of influenza within a community commonly involves dissemination of the virus among schoolchildren who then carry it home and to other activities. Increases in school and industrial absenteeism, visits to physicians' offices and emergency centers for respiratory illness, hospitalizations for respiratory illness, and pneumonia-influenza deaths occur during mild to moderate influenza epidemics when 10 to 15% of the population becomes infected. Severe epidemics can have attack rates of 20% or more. The severity of an epidemic depends largely on the degree of immunity to the influenza virus or viruses circulating in the population.

The type A and B designations of influenza viruses are based on antigenically stable internal proteins. Antibodies that develop against these internal proteins after infection are not protective against subsequent infection, although cell-mediated immune responses to them facilitate elimination of the viruses from the body. Protection against infection depends largely on antibodies to the two major glycoproteins that project from the lipid envelop of the virions, hemagglutinin (HA) and neuraminidase (NA). The most protective antibodies are those to the HA, which can prevent infection by blocking attachment of virions to cells. Antibodies to NA also contribute by impairing release of virions from infected cells, thus limiting spread of the infection. The HA and NA glycoproteins of both type A and type B influenza viruses undergo frequent minor antigenic alterations (antigenic drift) because of point mutations in the viral genome. This drift can cause variable reductions in the effectiveness of antibodies induced by prior infections and is a primary factor determining the severity of the yearly influenza outbreaks.

Infections with influenza A viruses also occur in avian and lower animal hosts. The viruses involved can have HA and/or NA glycoproteins similar to those of current or past human strains or ones that are completely distinct antigenically. Exchange of viral gene segments between one of these viruses and a human strain during a dual infection can result in a virus that grows well in humans and has a totally different HA from that of strains currently circulating in humans (antigenic shift); NA may or may not exhibit a concomitant shift. Immunity of humans to infection with such a "new" influenza A virus subtype is greatly reduced or absent. Such new influenza A subtypes have caused severe, worldwide epidemics (pandemics) and displaced the preceding subtype at 1- to 3-decade intervals during the past century, the most recent occasions being the 1958 shift from H1N1 to H2N2 viruses and the 1968 shift from H2N2 to H3N2 viruses. H1N1 viruses reappeared in 1977 and have co-circulated with H3N2 viruses up to the present.

DISEASE

The onset of influenza illness usually occurs 1 to 3 days after exposure. Although influenza viruses primarily infect respiratory epithelial cells, systemic manifestations of the infection are typically prominent. Classic symptoms in adolescents and young adults include the abrupt onset of fever, rasping cough, myalgias, and general malaise; some nasal obstruction and pharyngeal irritation may be present. However, the presentation can differ, particularly at the extremes of life. Young children may present with fever, irritability, cough, and rhinorrhea or sometimes with fever alone; vomiting and loose stools may also occur, although the pathogenesis is uncertain. Among the very old, lethargy, confusion, anorexia, and/or unexplained fever may be the primary manifestations rather than respiratory symptoms. Acute, uncomplicated influenza usually lasts 3 to 5 days, but cough and lethargy can persist for several additional days or weeks. Measurable decreases in pulmonary function occur during uncomplicated influenza, with or without the presence of transient interstitial infiltrates on the chest film, and can also require weeks to resolve.

An uncommon but severe complication of influenza is primary influenza pneumonia. Findings include diffuse pulmonary infiltrates and acute respiratory failure that develop in 1 to 2 days as a progression of the acute illness. Primary influenza pneumonia is most likely to be seen during severe influenza epidemics, usually in patients with conditions causing pulmonary vascular congestion, and it carries a high mortality rate. Much more frequent complications of influenza are secondary bacterial infections including otitis media, sinusitis, bronchitis, and pneumonia. The bacteria involved in these infections are similar to those found during noninfluenza periods; pneumococci are most frequent, but the frequency of *Staphylococcus aureus* infections, which have a relatively high morbidity and mortality, is greater than that in noninfluenza periods. Secondary bacterial infections most often appear 4 to 6 days after the onset of influenza, when the virus infection seems to be clearing, and are manifested by a recurrence of fever and development of localizing symptoms and signs.

Persons at increased risk for severe influenza and secondary complications include children younger than 1 year; persons 65 years old or older; persons of any age who have chronic cardiovascular or pulmonary disorders; and persons who have required hospitalization in the past year for chronic metabolic disease, renal dysfunction, hemoglobinopathy, or immunosuppression. Physiologic changes during pregnancy can also predispose to complications of influenza, particularly during the third trimester and early puerperium. With regard to immunosuppression, persons infected with human immunodeficiency virus have not been particularly prone to severe influenza virus disease, although secondary bacterial infections in such patients can be quite severe.

DIAGNOSIS

A variety of respiratory viruses can cause influenza-like illnesses, but influenza viruses tend to displace the others during a moderate to severe influenza epidemic. Hence, most influenza-like illnesses during such an epidemic are caused by influenza virus infection. Information about the influenza virus strains circulating is available from local health authorities or the Centers for Disease Control and Prevention, and it is not usually necessary to prove the etiologic diagnosis to make decisions about therapy or prophylaxis. However, viral diagnostic tests may be desirable in certain situations, such as at the beginning of an outbreak to identify the circulating strains, during a mild outbreak when other respiratory viruses are not fully displaced, or during a combined influenza A and B epidemic when a decision about whether to use amantadine or rimantadine is needed.

Influenza viruses can usually be isolated from respiratory secretions during the first 2 to 3 days of illness by growth in embryonated eggs or appropriate tissue cultures, but rarely after 5 to 7 days. The secretion specimens are generally collected by gargle, throat swab, or nasal wash (instill 2 to 5 mL of a balanced salt solution into each nostril with the head tilted back, and then catch the effluent in a cup when the head is brought forward and the nose is blown gently). If viral transport medium is not available, addition to the specimens of broth intended for bacterial cultures helps stabilize the virus. Specimens should be transported to the laboratory in wet ice as soon as possible. The laboratory will be able to report isolation of an influenza virus within 3 to 4 days for a majority of those specimens that are ultimately positive. When rapid diagnosis of influenza A virus infection is desirable, enzyme immunoassay kits suitable for use in an office are available.

Retrospective confirmation of influenza virus infection can also be accomplished by demonstration of an increase in the titer of antibody to the virus in convalescent serum (2 to 3 weeks after illness onset) relative to that in acute serum. This is an important tool for epidemiologic studies, but the delays inherent in serodiagnosis make it less useful for routine clinical purposes. Nevertheless, serodiagnosis may be the only means for confirming that an illness was due to influenza virus infection when the patient presents 5 days or more after onset, because cultures are often negative.

PREVENTION AND TREATMENT

Vaccine

The primary means for attempting to reduce the impact of influenza is administration of an inactivated (killed-virus) influenza virus vaccine. The formulation of these vaccines each year is adjusted to contain antigens of influenza viruses judged from worldwide surveillance to be most likely to circulate during the upcoming season. Current vaccines contain antigens of three influenza viruses, A/H1N1, A/H3N2, and type B. Each of the chosen virus strains is grown in embryonated eggs, highly purified, and rendered noninfectious (inactivated). Some manufacturers then lyse (split) the virions by dissolving the lipid coat and partially or fully purify HA and NA from the preparation. Thus, the vaccines available include whole-virus (Fluzone), subvirion (Fluogen, Fluzone), and purified surface antigen (Fluvirin) preparations, respectively. Reactogenicity of the different vaccine preparations in persons older than 12 years is similar, and any one of them may be used in persons of this age range. In children 12 years old or younger, use of one of the split-virus vaccines is recommended because of an increased likelihood of febrile reactions in children given whole-virus vaccine. Children younger than 9 years should receive 2 injections a month apart if they are receiving their first influenza vaccination, but no advantage has been found for a booster vaccination in older individuals.

Influenza vaccine should be administered intramuscularly in the deltoid or, for young children, in the anterolateral aspect of the thigh. A quarter or so of recipients of the vaccine will have soreness or tenderness at the injection site lasting 1 to 2 days. A small number, perhaps 1 in 20, will develop malaise and/or fever; this type of reaction usually begins 6 to 12 hours after vaccination, lasts 1 to 2 days, and can be relieved with acetaminophen. Although some will think they have developed influenza from the vaccination, this is not possible because the vaccine contains no live virus. Immediate allergic-type reactions have occurred rarely after vaccination, most likely due to traces of egg protein remaining in the vaccine, and persons with severe egg allergy should not receive the vaccine. A low (1 per 100,000) but significant association of Guillain-Barré syndrome (GBS) with receipt of swine influenza vaccine was observed in 1976. Although no clear association of GBS with subsequent influenza vaccines has been found, persons who have suffered GBS once are at greater risk than the general population for developing it again and should be offered influenza vaccine only for strong indications.

The aim of current vaccination policy is not to prevent an epidemic but rather to reduce the severe consequences of influenza, such as exacerbation of congestive heart failure or chronic obstructive pulmonary disease, pneumonia, or death. Persons at greatest risk for such complications (see "Disease") are primary targets for annual vaccination. Vaccinations of infants and children are reserved for those with underlying heart or lung disease. A particularly high potential exists for spread of influenza yielding high morbidity and mortality rates in facilities housing elderly and/or other high-risk persons. Influenza vaccine provides about 70% protection against influenza in healthy persons younger than 65 years when the match between vaccine and epidemic strains is good. Vaccine-induced protection against influenza in high-risk populations is often only about half as high (30 to 40%) but is usually higher against severe consequences of influenza such as hospitalization and

death (50 to 60% and 70 to 80% protection, respectively). Moreover, achieving high vaccination rates in facilities such as nursing homes has been shown to be capable of preventing influenza outbreaks in the facility through herd immunity.

Equally important as vaccinating high-risk patients is the vaccination of persons who live and work with them to reduce the possibility that virus will be brought in and transmitted to the patients. Included among these are physicians, nurses, support personnel, and family members who have contact with the high-risk patient.

Other persons for whom influenza vaccine is a strong consideration are those who provide essential services and those who will be traveling in areas where influenza may be active. Children who are receiving aspirin on a regular basis should be offered the vaccine, because Reye's syndrome has occurred in such children in association with influenza. The vaccine may also be offered to anyone who wishes to reduce the likelihood of becoming ill with influenza.

Antibody responses to influenza vaccine may be present as early as a week but generally require 2 to 4 weeks to become maximal. A slow decline in serum antibody titers then occurs during the next several months. It is uncommon for significant influenza activity to occur in the United States before December. Thus, optimal timing for influenza vaccination to provide the highest antibody titers against the viruses during most epidemics is mid-October to mid-November. However, administration of the vaccine to high-risk patients is more important than its precise timing and may be done from September through the onset of the epidemic if necessary to ensure its receipt. When vaccination is delayed until after an epidemic has begun, temporary administration of an antiviral agent may be used for protection until an antibody response has had time to develop (see later).

Many patients who are candidates for influenza vaccine are also candidates for pneumococcal vaccine, although revaccinations with the pneumococcal vaccine are generally at 6-year intervals rather than annually as with influenza vaccine. If a patient is due to receive pneumococcal vaccine, it may be administered at the same time as influenza vaccine, but in a different site.

Antiviral Agents

Two antiviral agents with specific activity against influenza A (but not type B) viruses are available, amantadine (Symmetrel) and rimantadine (Flumadine). The two agents inhibit replication of influenza A viruses through the same mechanism, and each can induce virus resistance that crosses with the other. Both are administered orally as capsules, tablets, or syrup and can cause nausea and/or anorexia in a few patients. Each can provide about 70 to 90% protection against influenza illness when it is taken regularly on a daily basis, and each can reduce the severity and duration of influenza A virus illness if it is begun therapeutically within 48 hours of illness onset.

Despite their similarities, important differences exist between these antiviral agents. Amantadine is excreted unchanged by the kidneys, whereas about 75% of rimantadine is metabolized by the liver before it and its metabolites are excreted by the kidneys. Amantadine has therapeutic activity against Parkinson's disease and drug-induced extrapyramidal reactions whereas rimantadine does not, and amantadine is about twice as likely as rimantadine (10 to 15% versus 5 to 10%, respectively) to cause central nervous system side effects such as nervousness, anxiety, difficulty concentrating, or light-headedness. If high blood levels of either drug accumulate, which is most likely to happen in patients with renal insufficiency, more severe central nervous system side effects including seizures may occur.

Amantadine and rimantadine serve as backup means for prophylaxis against influenza A virus infection, with vaccine being the primary means. Situations in which one of these agents should be considered for prophylaxis include the following: for 2 to 3 weeks after vaccination (i.e., until antibody has had time to develop) when vaccination has been delayed until after the onset of an influenza epidemic; in persons not expected to respond to vaccine because of immunodeficiency; and in persons for whom vaccine is contraindicated because of severe egg allergy or a previous severe vaccine reaction. The agents may also be used for outbreak control within facilities such as nursing homes; administration of amantadine or rimantadine to all residents of the facility, whether or not they had received vaccine, has been shown to be capable of aborting an influenza A outbreak within the facility.

When amantadine or rimantadine is used therapeutically, it is important to begin the therapy as soon as possible after onset of influenza illness, certainly within 48 hours, to obtain a therapeutic effect. Later administration, such as when complications occur, has not been shown to be of benefit. Drug-resistant virus may appear after 5 to 7 days of therapy, and stopping therapy 1 to 2 days after symptoms abate is recommended in an effort to minimize pressure toward development of this resistance. However, because resistance may occur, patients undergoing treatment with amantadine or rimantadine should be separated as much as possible from those who may be dependent on one of these agents for prophylaxis.

For persons 10 to 64 years of age who have normal renal and hepatic function, standard dosing of both amantadine and rimantadine is 100 mg orally twice a day for prophylaxis or therapy. For younger children, the dosing of each drug is 5 mg per kg per day in two divided doses not to exceed 150 mg per day. For persons 65 years of age and older, the daily dose of each drug is reduced to 100 mg once daily because of the natural decline in renal function that occurs with aging. The package insert should be consulted for amantadine dosage reductions in patients with a creatinine clearance of 50 mL per minute or less. For rimantadine, the daily dose should be halved for severe hepatic dysfunction and/or a creatinine clearance of 10 mL per minute or less.

Other Measures

Rest is important in the management of influenza illness and also serves to reduce dissemination of the virus. Increased fluid intake is necessary because of losses due to fever, and fluid is important for maintaining mucociliary clearance. Pseudoephedrine can be useful for reducing congestion and promoting evacuation of secretions. An antihistamine may be indicated if excessive secretions are interfering with rest, but too much reduction in secretions may impair mucociliary clearance. An antipyretic analgesic such as acetaminophen may be given as necessary for comfort and rest. Aspirin should be avoided in children because of its association with Reye's syndrome.

LEISHMANIASIS
method of
ROBERT N. DAVIDSON, M.D.
Imperial College School of Medicine and
Northwick Park Hospital
Harrow, Middlesex, England

BIOLOGY AND ECOLOGY

Leishmania protozoa cause visceral, cutaneous, and mucocutaneous infections. Female phlebotomine sandflies infect humans when injecting promastigotes in their saliva into the skin during feeding. Host phagocytes take up the promastigotes (flagellate stage) of *Leishmania,* which become amastigotes, able to survive and reproduce within the parasitophorous vacuoles of macrophages. The clinical outcome is determined by both the host cellular immune response and the species of *Leishmania:* some are dermatotropic, others viscerotropic. Most species produce more than one syndrome, although there are typical patterns of disease. Host cellular immunity determines whether clinical or subclinical infection occurs; whether the disease is visceral, cutaneous, or mucocutaneous, whether lesions are few or diffuse; and whether response to treatment is complete or partial.

The diagnosis of leishmaniasis is suggested by the clinical features and supported by serologic or skin tests, but wherever possible, it should be confirmed by finding or culturing the parasite. Amastigotes (Leishman-Donovan bodies) measure 2 to 3 μm in length and are found within macrophages in tissue sections. Amastigotes lie free in smears, because infected macrophages burst while being smeared. Nuclei and kinetoplasts of amastigotes stain blue with hematoxylin and eosin, red with Giemsa. *Histoplasma* is the main source of mistaken identification; however, *Histoplasma* lacks these structures.

About 10 million cases of cutaneous leishmaniasis (CL) and 400,000 cases of visceral leishmaniasis (kala-azar; VL) occur worldwide annually. Both VL and CL are increasing because of environmental changes. In Brazil, the increase in VL and CL is due to deforestation, which brings humans into contact with forest reservoirs and vectors of *Leishmania braziliensis* and other species. In North Africa and the Middle East, irrigation projects have increased the numbers of rodents, leading to marked increases in CL caused by *Leishmania major*. Breakdown of the infrastructure in Afghanistan has caused outbreaks of urban CL due to *Leishmania tropica*. Reduction of DDT spraying against malaria mosquitoes in India has been blamed for the current large epidemic of VL caused by *Leishmania donovani*. Since 1988, there has been a major epidemic of *L. donovani* VL in south Sudan brought on by famine, civil war, and ecologic change. In Europe, VL caused by *Leishmania infantum* is increasing, and half the new cases are co-infected with human immunodeficiency virus (HIV). HIV co-infection has also been reported among VL cases from Africa and also among CL, VL, and mucocutaneous leishmaniasis (MCL) cases from South America.

Visceral Leishmaniasis

In VL, the amastigotes disseminate throughout the reticuloendothelial system. After an incubation period of weeks to months (range, 10 days to >2 years), the patient develops pyrexia, wasting, and hepatosplenomegaly that may become massive. Lymphadenopathy is common in the Sudan. Males and females are equally affected, with a predominance of children and infants in Europe and Brazil. Patients report fever, malaise, abdominal discomfort, diarrhea, cough, and epistaxis. Laboratory tests reveal pancytopenia, polyclonal hypergammaglobulinemia, and hypoalbuminemia. The erythrocyte sedimentation rate (ESR) and C-reactive protein levels are elevated. In 95% of cases, serology for *Leishmania* is positive at high titers with use of the direct agglutination test, immunofluorescent antibody test (IFAT), or enzyme-linked immunosorbent assay. The leishmanin skin test result is invariably negative, indicating antigen-specific anergy and an absence of cell-mediated immunity. The diagnosis is made by finding amastigotes by microscopy of aspirates of spleen, bone marrow, or lymph node or a positive *Leishmania* culture from these sites. Although parasites are in greatest number in the spleen, bone marrow aspiration is safer. After weeks to months of illness, most patients with VL die, often with uncontrolled bleeding or secondary pneumonia, tuberculosis, or dysentery. Serologic and leishmanin skin test surveys indicate that subclinical self-healing infection occurs more frequently than do clinical cases. For example, in the Mediterranean countries, approximately 30% of adults living in rural areas typically have a positive leishmanin skin test response, indicating good cellular immunity against *Leishmania,* and presumptive evidence of prior subclinical infection with *L. infantum*. In the same areas, typically about 30% of dogs are actively and chronically infected with *Leishmania*. In epidemics with *L. donovani*, however, most infections are symptomatic, and mortality is high.

VL occurs as an opportunistic infection among immunosuppressed individuals: those co-infected with HIV, those receiving corticosteroids, and patients who have undergone organ transplantation or thymectomy. Travel to an endemic area may have been years previously. Clinical features in HIV-positive patients are often atypical; symptoms may be vague, laboratory abnormalities less severe, and hepatosplenomegaly unimpressive or absent. Amastigotes may be found unexpectedly in bone marrow aspirates of febrile HIV-positive patients or in circulating neutrophils or gut mucosa. *Leishmania* serology is negative in a third of immunosuppressed patients. Such patients may respond well to antileishmanial treatment, only to relapse 2 to 12 months later. Alternatively, response to treatment may be incomplete, or the patient may be totally nonresponsive or suffer exaggerated drug toxicity. Nine U.S. soldiers who served in the Persian Gulf area in 1990 to 1991 developed systemic infection caused by viscerotropic *L. tropica,* the cause of urban CL in the Middle East. They had nonspecific febrile illness with fatigue, arthralgia, and diarrhea. Some soldiers recovered spontaneously; others progressed to a chronic condition with adenopathy or splenomegaly. Most responded to treatment with sodium stibogluconate.

After successful treatment of VL due to *L. donovani,* a minority of patients develop a rash called post–kala-azar dermal leishmaniasis (PKDL). This occurs within a few weeks or months of stopping treatment in Africa or months to years later in India. PKDL may occasionally be acute and severe, with desquamation of skin and mucosae. More commonly, there are hypopigmented patches, nodules, and plaques. Parasites are scanty.

Successful treatment of VL results in defervescence within a week; by 14 days, the clinical and laboratory abnormalities should improve. Parasite clearance should be established before treatment is stopped. Clinical improvement should be sustained after treatment, although slight splenomegaly may persist for more than a year. By 6 to 12 months, there should be a fall in *Leishmania* IFAT titer and a positive leishmanin test response. The patient should be re-examined 1, 3, 6, and 12 months after treatment. The patient's body weight, spleen size, full blood count, serum albumin concentration, and ESR are all sensitive markers of recurrent VL. A relapse rate of less than 5% is expected in VL in immunocompetent patients, but more than 80% of HIV–co-infected patients will relapse. Almost all relapses occur within 6 months.

Cutaneous Leishmaniasis

In CL, amastigotes multiply in macrophages near the site of inoculation, typically on the arms, legs, face, or ears. Lesions may be nodular or ulcerative; they may be single, or there may be multiple satellite nodules or lymphangitic spread. The most typical lesion of CL is a chronic ulcer 2 to 5 cm in diameter with raised, indurated margins. The ulcer may be covered by a dry crust or have a serous or purulent exudate. The ulcers are painful if they are large or secondarily infected. The histologic picture is of intense lymphoid and monocytic infiltrate, with granulomas. The diagnosis of CL is confirmed by finding amastigotes in a biopsy specimen or on touch impression smears made from the biopsy tissue. An alternative is to perform a slit-skin smear. Amastigotes are most abundant in the dermis near the raised ulcer edge and may be scanty in old lesions. The base of the ulcer and secondarily infected lesions are avoided because parasite yield is low. In CL, *Leishmania* serology may be weakly positive, but the leishmanin skin test result is usually positive. A "tissue paper" scar remains after healing.

In the Middle East, zoonotic CL is caused by *L. major* and is linked to living or working near gerbil burrows. In towns in the same areas, person-to-person transmission of CL due to *L. tropica* occurs commonly. *L. infantum* occasionally causes CL in Europe, often in the elderly. *Leishmania aethiopica* causes CL in Ethiopia and parts of Kenya.

CL occurs in South and Central America, the Caribbean, and Mexico and as far north as Texas. CL in the Americas is mainly caused by members of the *L. mexicana* complex (*L. mexicana mexicana, L. mexicana amazonensis, L. mexi-*

cana venezuelensis) and the *L. braziliensis* complex *(L. braziliensis braziliensis, L. braziliensis panamensis, L. braziliensis guyanensis, L. braziliensis peruviana).* Speciation of the parasite in the Americas is important, because MCL can occur after *L. braziliensis* CL.

Two chronic forms of CL occur. Diffuse cutaneous leishmaniasis (DCL) is rare but disfiguring. Widespread dermal plaques containing huge numbers of amastigotes persist for decades. DCL patients are anergic to *Leishmania* antigen but do not have visceral dissemination or systemic symptoms. DCL is caused mainly by *L. aethiopica* in Africa and *L. amazonensis* in South and Central America. Leishmaniasis recidivans is a chronic nonhealing or relapsing cutaneous infection seen mainly with *L. tropica;* patients are hypersensitive to parasite antigens, and organisms are scanty.

The spontaneous healing rate is different for each species. Typically, cutaneous lesions caused by *L. major* heal within 5 months, *L. mexicana* within 8 months, and *L. tropica* and *L. braziliensis* within 1 year. Treatment is necessary only if the lesions are large, multiple, disfiguring, or over a joint. CL due to *L. braziliensis* must be treated systemically to reduce the risk for subsequent MCL. Heat and cold treatments, laser and diathermy, and careful curettage have been advocated to accelerate natural healing. Removing the crusts is of no benefit.

Mucocutaneous Leishmaniasis

MCL (espundia) occurs in approximately 3 to 10% of cases of CL due to *L. braziliensis braziliensis;* it is most common in Peru and Bolivia. The mucosal lesions usually begin months to years after CL has healed, but cases of simultaneous CL and MCL occur, as do those with no history of CL. The tip of the nose, nasal cartilage, or upper lip is usually involved first, with a painless induration or ulceration. MCL may remain static or may gradually extend into the nasopharynx, palate, uvula, larynx, and upper airways. Mutilating destruction of the nose may occur. Biopsies of the lesions show a chronic inflammatory and granulomatous infiltrate with scanty amastigotes. Cultures of biopsy specimens are usually positive for *L. braziliensis,* but this may require repeated attempts. Results of both *Leishmania* serology and the leishmanin skin test are usually positive.

A less severe degree of oral or nasal mucosal involvement rarely occurs with other species causing CL, such as *L. infantum.* This often indicates an underlying defect of host immunity.

Because untreated MCL usually progresses to cause disfiguring lesions, early treatment is important. MCL responds slowly to treatment, and relapses are common. Corticosteroids should be used if the larynx or airways are involved, because edema often occurs at the start of effective therapy. Relapse may occur many months to several years after treatment, and clinical follow-up with repeated biopsies may be necessary. Falling *Leishmania* IFAT titers in 6 to 12 months are encouraging evidence of cure in MCL.

TREATMENT

First-Line Drugs

Antimonials

Since the 1940s, the first-line drugs for all forms of leishmaniasis have been the pentavalent antimonials. In English-speaking countries, sodium stibo-gluconate (Pentostam), containing 100 mg of pentavalent antimony per mL, is used. In India, an identical compound is called sodium antimony gluconate (Albert David Ltd. Calcutta). In other countries, meglumine antimonate (Glucantime, Rhône-Poulenc, Spain, and Specia, France; Glucantim, Farmitalia Carlo Erba, Milan) is used; this contains 85 mg of pentavalent antimony per mL. It is assumed that these drugs are identical in activity and toxicity, but they have never been directly compared in patients. In the United States, virtually all cases of leishmaniasis are treated with sodium stibogluconate. This is available only through the Drug Service of the Centers for Disease Control and Prevention in Atlanta, Georgia (telephone, 404-639-3670). As systemic treatment of VL, CL, and early lesions of MCL, 20 mg of pentavalent antimony per kg is traditionally used as a single daily dose for 28 days. However, the kinetics of pentavalent antimony suggest that twice- or thrice-daily administration is logical, and studies in VL have shown superiority of such regimens over once-daily administration. Intravenous injections are less painful than intramuscular. Indian VL is treated for 40 days or longer, and courses of up to 3 months of pentavalent antimony are used for PKDL. Primary resistance to pentavalent antimony is seen in approximately 1% of cases in Africa and approximately 10% in India. Secondary pentavalent antimony resistance is likely to develop in relapsed patients unless they are re-treated thoroughly. Undertreatment with low doses and interrupted courses often lead to relapse. Children tolerate pentavalent antimony better than adults do and may be given higher doses according to body surface area. Before starting treatment, patients should be evaluated clinically, and baseline full blood count, biochemistry, and electrocardiogram should be obtained. If no significant abnormalities are found, therapy can begin. Patients should be hospitalized during systemic pentavalent antimonial therapy, and blood tests and electrocardiography should be performed twice weekly. Hospital-based pentavalent antimonial treatment is usually impossible in poor countries, where it is administered by a nurse on an outpatient basis without the facilities for monitoring toxicity. Serious adverse events are rare, and deaths due to pentavalent antimony are very rare, even in severely debilitated VL patients. Toxicity is reversible and includes elevation of serum amylase and liver enzymes levels, arthralgia and myalgia, thrombocytopenia, leukopenia, anorexia, and thrombophlebitis. Patients may complain of lethargy, headache, nausea, vomiting, metallic taste, or pruritus. Toxicity can usually be managed by interrupting pentavalent antimonial treatment for 1 to 2 days and reducing dosage slightly. Acute renal failure, thrombocytopenia, arthritis, and exfoliative dermatitis occur occasionally. Pancreatitis has been recognized as a complication of pentavalent antimonial therapy; asymptomatic hyperamylasemia is common, but symptomatic and even fatal pentavalent antimonial–associated pancreatitis has been reported.

When it is used intralesionally in CL, approximately 1 mL of undiluted pentavalent antimonial is infiltrated into the base and edges of a CL lesion; the injections are repeated each 2 to 3 days for up to 2 to 3 weeks. There are no systemic side effects, but the injections are painful.

Amphotericin B

Amphotericin B deoxycholate (Fungizone) is a powerful antileishmanial and is an alternative first-line drug in VL. Amphotericin B is remarkably nontoxic in the regimens used in Indian VL, which range from 14 daily doses of 0.5 mg per kg to 20 doses of 1 mg per kg on alternate days. Amphotericin B is the drug of choice (to total doses of 30 mg per kg) in advanced MCL, in which pentavalent antimonial therapy has a high failure rate. Amphotericin B has not been systematically assessed in CL or PKDL.

Lipid-Associated Amphotericin B*

These compounds are all different, but all are taken up by macrophages and target amphotericin B to the site of infection, achieving high levels in liver and spleen. All have lower toxicity than amphotericin B but are expensive. Liposomal amphotericin B (AmBisome) is rapidly effective and nontoxic in VL in Europe and of value in Sudan. The recommended regimen is a total dose of 20 to 30 mg per kg AmBisome given as 5 or more daily doses of 3 to 4 mg per kg in 10 to 21 days. AmBisome may be considered the drug of first choice in VL in the following situations: when the reduced hospital stay (5 days or less) outweighs the drug costs; when toxicity of pentavalent antimony or amphotericin B is unacceptable; when the patient is moribund (AmBisome leads to rapid clinical improvement); when the patient is unresponsive to or has relapsed after pentavalent antimonial therapy. A few complicated cases of CL and MCL have been successfully treated with longer courses of AmBisome. Amphotericin B cholesterol dispersion (Amphocil) has been used in Brazilian VL as 2 mg per kg per day for 7 or 10 days. Fever, chills, and respiratory distress were common in children younger than 3 years and were partly preventable by pretreatment with nonsteroidal anti-inflammatory drugs. Amphotericin B lipid complex (Abelcet) has been used successfully in Indian VL in a regimen of 3 mg per kg on alternate days for 5 doses.

Second-Line Drugs*

Aminosidine (paromomycin [Humatin]†) may be synergistic with pentavalent antimony. The most widely studied regimen in VL is aminosidine 15 to 17 mg per kg daily plus pentavalent antimony 20 mg per kg daily, given together for 14 to 20 days. Aminosidine alone is probably inadequate in VL or

---

*Note: Abelcet, allopurinol, aminosidine, Amphocil, itraconazole, and ketoconazole are not listed for use in leishmaniasis in the manufacturer's official directives. AmBisome is being considered for a product license for VL at the time of writing.

†Not FDA approved for this indication.

CL. Aminosidine is not currently being manufactured.

Pentamidine (Pentam)* is too weak to be routinely used in VL. In American CL, short courses of pentamidine are effective: 2 mg per kg on alternate days for 7 doses or 3 mg per kg on alternate days for 4 doses.

Immunotherapy

Interferon-γ added to pentavalent antimony improves cure rates in relapsed or pentavalent antimony–unresponsive VL and MCL cases, but toxicity and expense exclude it from routine use. Granulocyte-macrophage colony-stimulating factor combined with pentavalent antimony in VL treatment induces a quicker rise in leukocytes and fewer secondary infections, but it cannot be recommended for routine use.

Oral Agents

Ketoconazole (Nizoral) is effective in CL caused by *L. major* and *L. mexicana* but less so against *L. tropica*, *L. aethiopica*, and *L. braziliensis*. Itraconazole has similar efficacy but is better tolerated. Neither itraconazole (Sporanox) nor ketoconazole can reliably cure VL or PKDL, and there are no studies in MCL. Allopurinol has been assessed in all forms of leishmaniasis, but without consistent benefit.

Topical Treatment

Topical aminosidine 15% in methylbenzethonium chloride applied twice daily for 10 to 30 days is effective in *L. major* CL. Preparations without methylbenzethonium chloride are of little value.

---

*Not FDA approved for this indication.

LEPROSY
(Hansen's Disease)

method of
S. K. NOORDEEN, M.B., B.S., D.P.H., M.P.H.
World Health Organization
Geneva, Switzerland

Leprosy is an age-old disease affecting large populations in Asia, Africa, and Latin America. It is estimated that in 1996, there were about 1.4 million patients with leprosy in the world. A small number of cases occur in the southern United States, mainly in Louisiana, Texas, and California, and also in Hawaii; the large majority of leprosy patients diagnosed in the United States, however, come from immigrant communities.

Leprosy as a chronic disease affects mainly the skin, mucous membranes, and peripheral nerves, although in extremely advanced states, it can affect most systems of the body. The disease is caused by *Mycobacterium leprae*, an intracellular acid-fast organism. The human being is the only significant reservoir of infection, although natural leprosy is known to occur in the nine-banded armadillo, found particularly in Louisiana. The disease is transmitted from human to human by means of inhalation of organisms released through nasal discharges of patients with multibacillary leprosy and also by skin-to-skin contact. Leprosy has a long incubation period, sometimes as long as 20 years.

CLINICAL MANIFESTATIONS

The clinical manifestations of leprosy vary widely, depending on the cellular immunity of the individual, and occur in a spectrum of disease that is classified as lepromatous leprosy, in which the immune response is low; borderline leprosy, in which the immune response is moderate; and tuberculoid leprosy, in which the immune response is high. Further subclassifications of the spectrum, according to Ridley-Jopling classification, are polar lepromatous leprosy (LL), borderline lepromatous (BL) leprosy, midborderline (BB) leprosy, borderline tuberculoid (BT) leprosy, and polar tuberculoid (TT) leprosy. In addition, an early form of leprosy called indeterminate (I) leprosy is recognized. For the purposes of chemotherapy, the disease has been broadly classified into multibacillary (MB) leprosy, consisting of LL, BL, BB leprosy, and a proportion of BT leprosy cases, in which the skin smears show acid-fast bacilli (AFB), and paucibacillary (PB) leprosy, consisting of I, TT, and a proportion of BT leprosy cases in which skin smears do not show any AFB. In general, in MB leprosy, the skin lesions, which consist of macules, papules, and nodules as well as diffuse infiltration, are numerous with varying degrees of sensory loss. In PB leprosy, the skin lesions are anesthetic, consist mostly of well-defined macules and papules, and are limited in number. In both MB and PB leprosy, peripheral nerves such as ulnar, lateral popliteal, and facial nerves are affected, leading to sensory loss over the limbs and paralysis of the small muscles of the hands and feet, which in turn results in classic deformities of leprosy such as clawhand. Involvement of the facial nerve may lead to lagophthalmos, exposure keratitis, and, if unattended, ultimately blindness. Extensive sensory loss over the limbs may lead to such problems as trophic ulcers of the feet and loss of digits.

DIAGNOSIS

The diagnosis of leprosy is relatively easy in a large majority of cases. Examination comprises inspection of the skin lesions, palpation of the nerve trunks, and testing for sensory loss for light touch, pain, and temperature, as well as collection of skin smears for evidence of AFB. Leprosy is diagnosed on the basis of characteristic skin lesions, sensory loss, nerve thickening, and presence of AFB in skin smears. Histopathologic examination of lesions can often be quite useful.

COMPLICATIONS

Leprosy patients suffer from complications during the course of the disease, the most important of which are lepra reactions, which consist of two distinct entities. The first, referred to as reversal reaction (RR), or type I reaction, is seen mostly in BT leprosy and is characterized by the occurrence of erythematous lesions with edema, either afresh or over the existing skin lesions, and often accompanied by severe neuritis. The second, referred to as erythema nodosum leprosum (ENL), or type II reaction, is seen mostly in LL and BL leprosy; is characterized by evanescent, tender, and erythematous skin nodules; and

is often accompanied by systemic features such as fever, malaise, and nerve pain. A third type of reaction, called the Lucio phenomenon, occurs among lepromatous patients mainly in Central America; it is due to occurrence of vasculitis and is characterized by punched-out skin ulcers resulting from hemorrhagic infarcts. Lepra reactions, if not properly treated, may result in deformities. Other complications in MB leprosy include neuritis, iridocyclitis, arthritis, and rhinitis. The major complication in PB leprosy, apart from RR, is neuritis leading to deformities.

TREATMENT OF LEPROSY

The treatment of leprosy itself is primarily through chemotherapy employing a combination of drugs. The treatment of leprosy patients, however, should encompass all the problems faced by the patients, including complications and deformities as well as the psychologic and social effects.

Until the 1940s, the treatment of leprosy was a frustrating experience with no effective drugs available. The advent of sulfone drugs, of which dapsone is the most important, made leprosy treatment effective, although the treatment period had to last for several years and was often lifelong. The subsequent discovery of highly effective antileprosy drugs such as rifampin and clofazimine changed the situation further. The widespread employment of monotherapy with dapsone in the 1950s, 1960s, and 1970s, however, resulted in the emergence of resistance of *M. leprae* to sulfones, making dapsone treatment increasingly ineffective. This challenge has since been met through treatment of leprosy with a combination of drugs referred to as multidrug therapy (MDT), as recommended by the World Health Organization (WHO) in 1981. WHO/MDT has been widely implemented in disease control programs, and about 8 million patients have been cured through this approach so far.

The standard WHO/MDT for MB leprosy consists of a 24-month treatment with the following agents:

Rifampin (Rifadin): 600 mg once a month, supervised
Dapsone: 100 mg daily, self-administered
Clofazimine (Lamprene): 300 mg once a month, supervised, and 50 mg daily, self-administered

The standard WHO/MDT for PB leprosy consists of rifampin, 600 mg once a month, supervised, for 6 months, plus dapsone, 100 mg daily, self-administered, for 6 months.

As mentioned earlier, the WHO/MDT regimens have been found to be quite effective, and in general, there is no need to try other variations. In case of any specific need to try new regimens, however, it is important to ensure that patients receive combinations of effective drugs with three drugs for MB leprosy and two for PB leprosy. The following discussion deals with individual drugs employed in the treatment of leprosy, and others that have potential to be employed in the future.

Dapsone

Dapsone is a synthetase inhibitor in the folate synthesis of *M. leprae*. The dose is 1 to 2 mg per kg of body weight, with a general adult dose of 100 mg per day, in which dose it acts essentially as a bacteriostatic substance, although with weak bactericidal properties. The drug is extremely well absorbed, is generally well tolerated with few side effects, and can be administered even during pregnancy. The side effects attributable to dapsone include hemolytic anemia, leukopenia, fixed drug eruptions, peripheral neuropathy, exfoliative dermatitis, nephritis, hepatitis, and psychosis. The hemolytic anemia is particularly important for patients with complete glucose-6-phosphate dehydrogenase deficiency. The dapsone syndrome reported by some as occurring around the fifth week of treatment is quite rare and consists of exfoliative dermatitis, lymphadenopathy, and hepatitis with potentially fatal consequences. In such instances, dapsone should be immediately stopped, and steroids should be started.

Clofazimine

Clofazimine, a bright red dye and an iminophenazine derivative, is reasonably well absorbed when formulated in a microcrystalline oil-wax base. Clofazimine also has anti-inflammatory properties and is therefore a useful drug for the treatment of ENL or type II reactions. The adult dose of clofazimine is 50 to 100 mg per day for treatment of leprosy itself and up to 300 mg per day for the treatment of type II reactions. In WHO/MDT, the dose is 50 mg daily together with a loading dose of 300 mg once a month. The drug is essentially bacteriostatic with weak bactericidal properties. The antileprosy effect of the drug is almost the same as that of dapsone. Only rare cases of resistance of *M. leprae* to clofazimine have been reported so far. Among the side effects of clofazimine, the most important is the reddish black pigmentation of the skin produced by deposition of the drug in the skin. After therapy is stopped, the discoloration disappears during a period of 6 to 12 months. Other side effects of clofazimine include dryness of the skin, ichthyosis, abdominal pain, and diarrhea. The drug can be administered during pregnancy.

Rifampin

Rifampin is the most potent antileprosy drug to date. It acts by inhibiting the DNA-dependent RNA polymerase of the organisms, thereby interfering with bacterial RNA synthesis. The drug is rapidly absorbed from the gastrointestinal tract. Rifampin has high bactericidal activity against *M. leprae* that is far superior to its activity against *Mycobacterium tuberculosis*. A single dose of 600 to 1200 mg of rifampin is capable of killing 99.9% of the organisms. It is because of this extremely high bactericidal activity that the WHO/MDT regimen uses the drug only once a month at a dose of 600 mg for adults. At the dose and interval used in WHO/MDT, the drug is extremely well tolerated, and the rare side effects include rashes, drowsiness, thrombocytopenia, and hepatitis. Rifampin also causes red coloration of the urine. The "flu syndrome" often reported in the treatment of tuberculosis with rifampin is quite rare in the treatment of leprosy employing WHO/MDT. Rifampin can be safely administered during pregnancy. Although this drug is highly bactericidal, it should not be employed as monotherapy, because bacterial resistance can emerge quite rapidly. It is therefore extremely important to use rifampin only as part of MDT.

Ofloxacin*

Ofloxacin (Floxin) is an orally administered antibacterial drug belonging to the group of fluorinated quinolones. It acts by inhibiting the enzyme DNA gyrase, which controls supercoiling of DNA in bacteria. Among the fluoroquinolones, ofloxacin is the most promising agent in the treatment of leprosy, as demonstrated in animal experiments and short-term clinical trials that show its bactericidal activity as being next only to that of rifampin. It is effective at a dose of 400 mg per day. As with other antileprosy drugs, ofloxacin should not be given as monotherapy. A large-scale, WHO-supported, multicenter trial is currently under way to find out whether or not a combination of rifampin and ofloxacin could reduce the treatment period of MB leprosy to just 1 month. The side effects attributed to ofloxacin include gastrointestinal pain, diarrhea, hypersensitivity reactions, and vertigo.

Minocycline*

Minocycline (Minocin) is a semisynthetic tetracycline that has been found to have significant bacterial activity against *M. leprae* similar to that of ofloxacin. It is effective at a dose of 100 mg per day. Side effects are discoloration of teeth in children, gastrointestinal symptoms, and central nervous system complaints, including dizziness. Clinical trials are under way evaluating minocycline in combination with rifampin and ofloxacin.

Clarithromycin*

Clarithromycin (Biaxin) is a macrolide identified to have both in vitro and in vivo bactericidal activity against *M. leprae*, probably at the same level as those of ofloxacin and minocycline. It is readily absorbed from the gastrointestinal tract. The dose commonly employed is 500 mg per day. Common side effects are nausea, vomiting, and diarrhea.

TREATMENT OF COMPLICATIONS

Complications of leprosy, most of which lead to deformities if unattended, need prompt and effective

*Not FDA approved for this indication.

treatment. Education of patients to identify problems early and seek treatment is crucial to the prevention of sequelae. Apart from specific complications, such as type I and type II reactions, neuritis, and arthritis, which can cause permanent incapacitation, the occurrence of peripheral sensory loss over the extremities, which is considered part of the disease, has lifelong consequences in terms of risk of injury, ulceration, and loss of digits.

Treatment of Type I or Reversal Reaction

The most important aim in the treatment of type I reaction is to prevent nerve damage through treatment of the acute neuritis that is part of most reactions, as well as to control inflammation of the skin lesions. There is no need to interrupt antileprosy treatment during a reaction. In mild reactions, patients should be treated just with analgesics, particularly when there is no evidence of neuritis. In severe reactions, particularly when there is evidence of acute neuritis with pain, tenderness, and loss of nerve function, the patient should be hospitalized whenever possible, and treatment with steroids initiated together with analgesics. The painful nerves should be rested, and the affected limb splinted. Treatment with steroids should preferably start with 40 mg daily, which should be maintained for at least 2 weeks, and depending on the response, the dose can be reduced every 1 to 2 weeks by 5 to 10 mg. Most patients with severe reactions require at least 12 weeks of treatment with steroids before treatment can be completely withdrawn.

Treatment of Type II or ENL Reactions

Although type II reactions are less important from the point of view of nerve damage, the consequences of repeated and severe reactions can be quite grave in view of the associated systemic effects. Mild reactions can be easily managed on an ambulatory basis by use of analgesics and drugs such as chloroquine (Aralen),* 150 mg three times a day, or antimonials (e.g., stibophen,† containing 8.5 mg of antimony per mL given in a dose of 2 to 3 mL intramuscularly on alternate days for a maximal total dose of 30 mL). Thalidomide,‡ in a dose of 400 mg daily, is quite effective in controlling ENL reactions. This drug should never be given to women of childbearing age because of its teratogenic effects.

Patients with severe ENL reactions require hospitalization. The treatment of choice for such patients is thalidomide, which can be administered for prolonged periods. The alternative to this is treatment with either steroids or clofazimine§ in doses of 300 mg per day. Both carry significant risks for patients who are treated for long periods. Patients given ste-

roid therapy may become steroid dependent, making withdrawal of the drug difficult. Long-term use of clofazimine in high doses can cause severe gastrointestinal side effects. Often, a judicious combination of any two of thalidomide, prednisolone, and clofazimine may help in reducing the dosage of the drugs and, ultimately, in their withdrawal.

Neuritis

Inflammation of the peripheral nerve trunk with enlargement, pain, and tenderness can occur by itself in the course of either MB or PB leprosy or may accompany either type I or type II reactions. The treatment of choice in neuritis is prednisolone. If pain is intractable and persistent, surgical intervention through nerve decompression will be of value. Patients with leprosy in general should be closely monitored for sensory and motor changes, because some of these changes can occur insidiously without acute neuritis. This phenomenon, described as "quiet nerve paralysis," also requires steroids in appropriate doses.

Iridocyclitis

Apart from exposure keratitis and other complications arising from lagophthalmos, iridocyclitis is the most important cause of blindness in leprosy and therefore should be treated promptly and vigorously. Acute iridocyclitis should be treated with mydriatics, such as 1% atropine or 0.25% scopolamine, and anti-inflammatory drugs, such as 1% hydrocortisone.* Chronic iridocyclitis should be treated along similar lines but for longer periods.

DEFORMITIES IN LEPROSY

The common paralytic deformities in leprosy are clawhand, footdrop, lagophthalmos, and wristdrop. The common disabilities due to sensory loss over the extremities are trophic ulcers and absorption of digits. In addition, the disease process can cause problems such as depressed nose, loss of eyebrows, gynecomastia, and blindness resulting from lagophthalmos and iridocyclitis.

Once deformities and disabilities set in, their management poses major problems. Every effort should be made, therefore, to prevent deformities through early treatment of complications. Care of anesthetic hands and feet calls for constant education of patients and use of appropriate footwear. Physiotherapy and splinting have important roles to play in preventing and controlling deformities. Reconstructive surgery, through a number of effective surgical procedures, has enabled correction of deformities of hands, feet, nose, and eyes. Re-education, physiotherapy, and occupational therapy are important adjuncts to surgical correction of deformities.

---

*Not FDA approved for this indication.
†Not available in the United States.
‡Not yet approved for use in the United States.
§Exceeds dosage recommended by the manufacturer.

---

*Ophthalmic form not available in the United States.

LEPROSY CONTROL

The strategy of leprosy control today involves essentially secondary prevention through early detection of cases and treatment of patients with effective drugs, so that the reservoirs of infection can be eliminated and the transmission of infection interrupted. So far, there is no primary preventive strategy available for leprosy, although bacille Calmette-Guérin itself is known to have a protective effect against the disease, particularly in certain parts of the world. The widespread application of WHO-recommended MDT in the last 10 years has had a significant impact in reducing the disease burden in the world, raising hopes of eliminating the disease as a public health problem in the not too distant future.

MALARIA

method of
MALCOLM MOLYNEUX, M.D.
Queen Elizabeth Central Hospital
Chichiri, Blantyre, Malawi

THE PARASITE

Four species of *Plasmodium* may cause human malaria: *P. falciparum, P. vivax, P. ovale,* and *P. malariae.* The usual route of infection is through the bite of a female anopheline mosquito carrying sporozoites of the parasite in its salivary glands. Sporozoites rapidly invade the human host's hepatocytes, where they multiply and release large numbers of merozoites into the bloodstream. Merozoites invade erythrocytes, in which they grow through early ring stages to mature trophozoites and then divide (schizogony). The resulting schizont ruptures the erythrocyte, and merozoites are again released into the bloodstream to invade more red blood cells. This asexual cycle is repeated with a periodicity that differs between parasite species. Some parasites develop into gametocytes, undergoing no further replication until ingested by the feeding mosquito, when a sexual cycle is completed and sporozoites accumulate in the salivary glands. In the human host, a proportion of the intrahepatic parasites of two species, *P. vivax* and *P. ovale,* may fail to develop into schizonts; these remain dormant as hypnozoites, which may develop and cause relapses of malaria after intervals of months or years.

The incubation period (from mosquito bite to first symptom) is usually about 10 to 15 days, although it may occasionally be as short as 7 days for falciparum malaria. Much longer incubation periods can occur in partially immune people and in those who have taken prophylactic antimalarial drugs.

Although usually inoculated by mosquito bites, malaria parasites may also be transmitted transplacentally, by blood transfusion, through needle sharing, and occasionally in laboratory accidents.

PATHOGENESIS

Fever in malaria results from the release of cytokines by host macrophages, when macrophages are stimulated by parasite components released during the rupture of schizont-containing erythrocytes. An important difference between *P. falciparum* and other plasmodia is that erythrocytes infected with maturing *P. falciparum* develop altered surface characteristics, resulting in their adherence to the endothelial linings of venules and capillaries in deep organs, including the brain, lungs, liver, gut, and bone marrow. This sequestration protects parasites from destruction by the spleen and may thus account for the higher parasite densities that occur in *P. falciparum* infections than in other malarias. Sequestration may also be responsible for the dysfunction of cerebral and other tissues that is characteristic of severe falciparum malaria. In malaria due to the other three species of *Plasmodium,* sequestration does not occur and organ failure is rare. High plasma concentrations of cytokines (including tumor necrosis factor and interleukin-6) are found in severe malaria, levels being particularly high in fatal cases. Excessive cytokine activity may contribute to the pathogenesis of severe malaria.

EPIDEMIOLOGY

Malaria is transmitted in most tropical areas of the world. *P. falciparum* predominates in Africa and is also common in South America and Southeast Asia. *P. vivax* is the most common species in the Indian subcontinent, but falciparum malaria also occurs there. In endemic areas with intense transmission, most adults are semi-immune; immunity is manifested as reduced susceptibility to infection and also as increased tolerance of parasitemia. Newborn infants are protected by maternal antibody and by the fact that parasites grow less well in fetal than in adult hemoglobin; infants become increasingly susceptible to malaria during later infancy and early childhood, when the most severe illnesses occur. About a million young children are believed to die of *P. falciparum* infections every year in Africa alone. Semi-immune adults who leave an endemic area appear to lose their immunity within a few years.

Travelers from a malaria-free territory to an endemic area are susceptible to malaria and, in the case of *P. falciparum,* to severe and complicated disease.

CLINICAL FEATURES

All species of malaria parasite, including *P. falciparum,* may cause nonspecific fever, chills, malaise, headache, and myalgia. There is sometimes vomiting and diarrhea. Fever is commonly without any pattern, or there may be spikes each day. The classic 2- or 3-day periodicity is seen only in more protracted illness. The liver and spleen may be moderately enlarged, and the patient may be anemic. There is no rash or lymph node enlargement.

In falciparum malaria, severe complications may rapidly develop, and the disease is potentially lethal.

Falciparum Malaria

The uncomplicated illness resembles the other malarias. Severe disease is characterized by the development of any of a number of complications (Table 1). Suspected falciparum malaria in a nonimmune subject therefore requires urgent diagnosis and treatment.

In children in the endemic areas of Africa, two complications of falciparum malaria predominate: cerebral malaria (characterized by convulsions and coma) and severe anemia. Hypoglycemia and acidosis are common features of cerebral malaria. In nonimmune adults, it is more common for severe malaria to consist of several organ complications, each requiring attention in management.

TABLE 1. **Clinical Features of Severe (Complicated) Falciparum Malaria***

Principal Features	Other Manifestations
Cerebral malaria (unrousable coma, convulsions)	Impaired consciousness (but rousable)
Severe anemia	Prostration
Renal failure	Jaundice
Respiratory distress syndrome	Hyperpyrexia
Hypoglycemia	Any seizure
Shock	
Spontaneous bleeding	
Repeated seizures	
Acidemia and acidosis	
Visible hemoglobinuria	

*Malaria is severe by definition if any of the principal features is present. The other manifestations indicate increased risk compared with mild or uncomplicated malaria.

DIAGNOSIS AND INVESTIGATIONS

Malaria must be considered in any patient who develops a fever after travel to an endemic area or after receiving a blood transfusion. A single day or even an airport stop in a malarious territory can be sufficient for inoculation by mosquito to have occurred. Exposure must have been at least 7 days before the illness, but an interval of several months is not uncommon, and illness may be delayed several years in the nonfalciparum malarias.

Uncomplicated malaria must be distinguished from fevers of viral, bacterial, and parasitic origin, of which the most common in returning travelers are gastroenteritis and hepatitis; others include typhoid, rickettsial infections, relapsing fever, and acute schistosomiasis. Complicated falciparum malaria must be distinguished from encephalopathies—meningitis, viral encephalitis, rabies, typhoid psychosis, heat stroke—and from other causes of renal failure, respiratory distress syndrome, hypoglycemia, intravascular hemolysis, hemolytic anemia, or disseminated intravascular coagulation.

Failure to take an adequate travel history and to consider the possibility of malaria may have serious or tragic consequences. Diagnosis depends on the demonstration of parasites in peripheral blood films, although rarely films may be negative in a patient with severe falciparum malaria. Thick and thin blood films should be taken immediately and stained with Romanowsky's stain. An assessment of the density (percentage of erythrocytes parasitized) helps with the planning of treatment. Anemia is common; thrombocytopenia is almost invariable in falciparum and common in vivax malaria; there may be leukopenia, although neutrophil leukocytosis occurs in severe disease. White blood cells commonly contain characteristically refractile hemozoin pigment.

In patients with severe falciparum malaria, investigations should be directed at assessing renal function, glycemic status, and pulmonary function. Lumbar puncture is necessary in the comatose patient to exclude other encephalopathies, and blood should be cultured because bacteremia may complicate severe malaria.

TREATMENT

Therapy must combine specific antiparasitic drugs and supportive measures.

Antimalarial Drugs. The available drugs and the stages of the parasite against which they act are listed in Table 2. Drugs acting against the red blood cell stages of the parasite are commonly called schizonticides, although some drugs in this category probably act on the parasite before it reaches the schizont stage of development. The aim of treatment is to achieve a therapeutic plasma concentration of an effective schizonticide as quickly and as safely as possible and to maintain plasma levels of the drug for long enough to clear asexual parasites from the blood and prevent their subsequent recrudescence. No attempt should be made to eliminate gametocytes, which may persist in the blood for days or weeks after successful treatment. In the case of vivax or ovale malaria, radical cure in addition requires a drug (primaquine) to eliminate hepatic hypnozoites.

Malaria due to *Plasmodium vivax*, *Plasmodium ovale*, or *Plasmodium malariae*

Nonspecific measures include analgesic and antipyretic drugs and fluid replacement if required. Chloroquine is the antimalarial drug of choice for nonfalciparum malarias acquired in most parts of the world. Chloroquine-resistant *P. vivax* has, however, been encountered with increasing frequency in Papua New Guinea, and alternative chemotherapy (mefloquine [Lariam] or oral quinine) may be needed for patients in whom chloroquine proves to be ineffective. Drug dosage schedules are given in Table 3. Chloroquine should be taken by mouth if possible. In patients unable to take oral treatment, chloroquine may be given by slow intravenous infusion (5 mg of chloroquine base per kg of body weight infused in 6 hours, repeated to a total of 25 mg per kg [30 hours]) or in small, repeated doses by subcutaneous or intramuscular injection (3.5 mg of base per kg every 6 hours, to a maximum of 25 mg per kg).

In patients with *P. vivax* or *P. ovale* infections, primaquine should then be given to eliminate hepatic hypnozoites. This may be considered unnecessary in

TABLE 2. **Antimalarial Drugs and Their Chief Site of Action in the Parasite Life Cycle**

Site of Action	Mode of Action	Drugs
Asexual (blood-stage) parasite	Unknown; may inhibit the parasite's enzyme heme polymerase	Chloroquine Quinidine Quinine Amodiaquine* Mefloquine Halofantrine* Artemisinins*
Hepatic-stage parasite	"Tissue schizonticide"— folate antagonists	Proguanil* Pyrimethamine Sulfonamides Sulfones
Hypnozoites	Mechanism unknown	Primaquine
Gametocytes	Mechanism unknown	Primaquine Artemisinins*

*Not available in the United States.

TABLE 3. **Antimalarial Drugs for Treatment of Patients Who Can Take Medication by Mouth***

Drug	Dosage (Given for Base Content of Drug)
Chloroquine	10 mg/kg, then 5 mg/kg after 6, 24, and 48 h (usual adult doses in 150-mg tablets: 4, 2, 2, 2)
Mefloquine (Lariam)	15 mg/kg divided into 2 equal doses given 6 h apart
Pyrimethamine-sulfadoxine (Fansidar)	Pyrimethamine 1.5 mg/kg, sulfadoxine 30 mg/kg, as a single dose (usual adult dose, 3 tablets)
Quinine	10 mg/kg q 8 h for 7 d
Halofantrine†	8 mg/kg q 6 h for 3 doses (usual adult dose, 2 tablets × 3)
Primaquine	0.25 mg/kg daily for: 5 days (Indian subcontinent) 14 days (Mediterranean and South America) 21 days (West Pacific and Southeast Asia)

*See text for recommended schedules.
†Not available in the United States.

patients who will be living in an area where reinfection is almost inevitable. Primaquine may cause severe hemolysis in individuals with glucose-6-phosphate dehydrogenase (G6PD) deficiency; the red blood cell G6PD level should be checked before primaquine is prescribed. In patients with G6PD deficiency, the likelihood of relapses can be reduced by giving chloroquine and proguanil* in prophylactic doses for a period of 3 months.

Malaria due to *Plasmodium falciparum*

Uncomplicated Falciparum Malaria

Correct treatment must be regarded as a matter of urgency because of the possibility that complicated disease may develop. Because chloroquine resistance is now prevalent in most parts of the world, a drug other than chloroquine should be given as the first line of treatment of falciparum malaria, regardless of the geographic origin of the parasite. The drug of choice is mefloquine; alternatives are pyrimethamine-sulfadoxine or quinine (or quinidine). For doses and schedules, see Table 3. If possible, the drug should be taken orally. A patient who cannot take drugs by mouth should be given treatment as for severe and complicated malaria until oral treatment can be resumed.

In areas where *P. falciparum* is resistant or partially resistant to many drugs, artemisinin derivatives* are useful, especially when given in combination with mefloquine. A regimen effective in parts of Thailand is artesunate 4 mg per kg (or artemisinin 10 mg per kg) daily for 3 days plus mefloquine 15 to 25 mg per kg as a single dose on day 2 or 3.

*Not available in the United States.

Severe (Complicated) Falciparum Malaria

For practical purposes, malaria should be regarded as severe if the patient is too weak or sick to take drugs by mouth or if any of the complications listed in Table 1 is present. Patients with falciparum malaria may have several complications at once, and additional complications may develop during treatment.

Management requires a combination of general supportive care, specific antimalarial chemotherapy, and the identification and treatment of complications both before and during treatment.

ANTIMALARIAL DRUGS FOR SEVERE FALCIPARUM MALARIA

The first requirement is for an effective schizonticidal drug, in a dosage and by a route sufficient to achieve therapeutic plasma levels quickly and safely. Quinine is the drug of choice in most countries. Because parenteral quinine is not available in the United States, the recommended drug in the United States is quinidine.

Quinidine gluconate or quinine dihydrochloride is administered by slow intravenous infusion (Table 4). Most patients tolerate the regimen well, but careful attention should be paid to cardiac function and glycemic status. Although quinidine is more cardiotoxic than quinine, this effect rarely proves to be a problem during treatment of malaria. Prolongation of the electrocardiographic QT_C interval beyond 0.6 second, or of the QRS duration beyond 25% of the baseline value, is an indication for slowing the infusion rate of quinidine. Plasma quinidine levels may be monitored if possible and should not exceed 6 mg per liter.

TABLE 4. **Drug Regimens for Treatment of Patients with Severe or Complicated Falciparum Malaria**

Agent	Dosage and Schedule
Quinidine	10 mg of quinidine gluconate salt (= 6.2 mg of base)/kg infused intravenously in 2 h (loading dose*), then 0.02 mg (salt)/kg/min by constant infusion until the patient can take treatment by mouth (quinine sulfate 10 mg/kg q 8 h) to complete a 7-d course of antimalarial drugs
Quinine	20 mg/kg of quinine dihydrochloride salt† (= 16.7 mg/kg of quinine base) infused intravenously in 4 h (loading dose*), then 10 mg/kg of salt infused in 4 h q 12 h until patient can take oral quinine to complete a 7-d course
Tetracycline or pyrimethamine-sulfadoxine or mefloquine	Should be added as oral treatment, in standard dosage (see Table 3), for patients coming from areas where partial quinine resistance is common (e.g., Southeast Asia)

*Use half the initial (loading) dose if the patient has already received quinine or quinidine in the preceding 12 h.
†Not available in the United States.

Oral treatment should be substituted as soon as the patient is well enough to take it.

If intravenous infusion is impossible, quinine dihydrochloride* can be given by intramuscular injection into one or both thighs. For this purpose, quinine dihydrochloride should be diluted in sterile water to a concentration of 50 mg (salt) per mL. Half of the loading dose can be given immediately and half after 4 hours; thereafter, doses of 10 mg (salt) per kg can be given every 12 hours until oral therapy is possible.

Artemisinin drugs are effective against parasites resistant to other antimalarials and can be valuable for the treatment of severe falciparum malaria. Regimens used in parts of Southeast Asia include artemether (by intramuscular injection) and artesunate (by intravenous infusion). These drugs are not yet available in the United States.

SUPPORTIVE MEASURES IN SEVERE FALCIPARUM MALARIA

Fluid Balance. The total volume of fluid infused during and between drug administrations should be adjusted to provide for the fluid requirements of the patient, assessed by clinical observations, precise monitoring of urine output, and, when necessary, central venous pressure recordings. Volumes of other fluids—e.g., transfused blood—given in the course of the management of the patient must be taken into account in calculating fluid input. In a patient given intramuscular quinine, fluid and glucose therapy must be maintained, if necessary by the nasogastric route. Fluid balance is of critical importance in patients who develop acute renal failure, pulmonary edema, or respiratory distress syndrome.

Anticonvulsants. In adults with cerebral malaria, a single intramuscular injection of phenobarbital reduces the likelihood of subsequent seizures. The same effect has not yet been demonstrated in children, but prophylaxis against seizures in the comatose child should be considered (e.g., phenobarbital, 15 mg per kg intramuscularly). If a seizure occurs in a patient with cerebral malaria, possible triggering causes (hyperpyrexia, hypoglycemia, hyponatremia) should be sought and corrected, and an anticonvulsant drug given to prevent further episodes.

Antipyretics. Moderate fever is not harmful, but a core temperature above 39°C should be treated by sponging with tepid water and fanning and with an antipyretic drug. Rectal acetaminophen (12 mg per kg every 4 hours in a child; 0.5 to 1 gram every 4 hours in an adult; maximum of 4 doses in 24 hours) is a useful and safe regimen.

RECOGNITION AND MANAGEMENT OF COMPLICATIONS IN FALCIPARUM MALARIA

Careful clinical assessment is essential to identify complications (1) at the time of presentation and (2) during the course of treatment.

Cerebral Malaria. This syndrome is characterized by altered consciousness, ranging from delirium to profound unrousable coma. The syndrome may develop rapidly, especially in young children. Seizures, which may be focal or generalized, are common. Coma may be accompanied by a variety of physical signs, including abnormalities of conjugate gaze, posturing of limbs, muscle hypertonicity, and opisthotonos. Retinal hemorrhages may be present, and macular and extramacular edema is usual. Papilledema is occasionally seen. Pupillary light reflexes and corneal reflexes may be lost in the most deeply comatose patients. The mechanisms responsible for cerebral dysfunction remain unknown. The intracranial pressure is commonly high, especially in children, but there is no evidence that this is the mechanism of coma or death or that specific therapy directed against raised intracranial pressure is beneficial. All the features of cerebral malaria may be mimicked by hypoglycemia, which is an additional complication in some patients (see later), especially young children and pregnant women. The blood glucose level must be measured initially and at repeated intervals during treatment. Acidosis and acidemia are commonly present in the patient with cerebral malaria (see later).

An individual with cerebral malaria needs meticulous application of the principles of care for the unconscious patient. It is helpful to monitor the depth of coma frequently, using the Glasgow Coma Scale or a suitable modification for children. Other complications of falciparum malaria are common in patients with cerebral complications and must therefore be looked for regularly.

Severe Anemia. All parasitized red blood cells are destroyed either by rupture of the schizont or by splenic removal. The life span of unparasitized cells is also commonly reduced, and erythropoiesis is impaired. Anemia may therefore develop rapidly, especially in patients with hyperparasitemia. The hematocrit or hemoglobin levels should be monitored frequently, and infusions of packed red blood cells should be given if necessary.

Spontaneous Bleeding. This complication is due to disseminated intravascular coagulation and is identified by measurement of platelets, fibrinogen, and fibrin degradation products in the peripheral blood. Appropriate treatment with fresh-frozen plasma, platelet-rich plasma, or fresh whole blood must be given.

Acute Renal Failure. Patients particularly susceptible to this complication are those with hypotension or shock, commonly associated with septicemia. Renal failure is usually the result of acute tubular necrosis. Early recognition allows attempts to restore renal function with intravenous fluids, diuretics, and, if necessary, pressor drugs. Once renal failure is established, management is the same as for acute tubular necrosis of any cause. Dialysis is commonly required. In patients with renal failure, the doses of quinidine or quinine should be reduced to half. If possible, blood levels of antimalarial drugs should be monitored and further dosages adjusted accordingly. Plasma quinidine levels should be kept below 6 mg

*Not available in the United States.

per liter and quinine concentrations below 15 mg per liter.

Acidosis and Acidemia. These commonly accompany other complications of falciparum malaria. In some cases, there is adequate respiratory compensation for metabolic acidosis; in others, compensatory mechanisms are insufficient and acidemia develops, manifested clinically by deep breathing. The cause of acidosis is usually tissue hypoxia through inadequate tissue perfusion and/or anemia. Prompt management of fluid deficit and anemia, together with treatment of the malaria, usually proves sufficient to correct acidosis without the need to administer alkali.

Respiratory Distress Syndrome. This grave complication resembles pulmonary edema, from which it must be distinguished by measurement of central venous and pulmonary wedge pressures. The respiratory distress syndrome is not due to fluid overload (although fluid overload may coexist). There is tachypnea with hypoxemia, with or without audible crackles in the lung fields and with characteristic diffuse bilateral radiographic shadows spreading from the lung hila. Any abnormal fluid balance must be corrected, but intubation and artificial ventilation are likely to be necessary, and the prognosis is poor even with these measures.

Hyperparasitemia. The prognosis in falciparum malaria is worst in patients with high parasite counts in the peripheral blood. Exchange transfusion has been used in a number of centers. This procedure, using 5 to 10 liters of donor blood, reduces parasitemia dramatically. The risks of using multiple blood donations must be recognized, and no properly controlled trial has yet been done to prove that exchange transfusion is beneficial. In a patient with extremely high parasitemia (>15% erythrocytes parasitized), exchange transfusion seems logically appropriate and has been successful in a number of reported cases.

Shock. A small proportion of patients with complicated falciparum malaria develop a shock state, with hypotension and peripheral vasoconstriction. Septicemia is commonly responsible, especially but not only in patients with indwelling catheters or intravascular lines. Blood must be cultured, fluid balance assessed, and a broad-spectrum antibiotic given while bacteriologic results are awaited.

Intravascular Hemolysis and Hemoglobinuria. Red blood cells are destroyed by parasites and also by autoimmune lysis. If cell breakdown is extremely rapid, free hemoglobin accumulates in the blood and appears in the urine. Management requires attention to renal function, fluid balance, and the possible need for blood (red blood cell) transfusion.

Jaundice. In adults with severe malaria, jaundice is not uncommon. It is usually of mild degree, and hepatic failure is almost unknown. The importance of this sign is in differential diagnosis (a diagnosis of hepatitis in a patient whose jaundice is due to malaria can be a tragic error). No treatment specific for this complication is needed or available.

Hypoglycemia. This condition may complicate severe malaria in any patient; children are particularly susceptible. Hypoglycemia may also develop in a patient receiving quinidine or quinine, as a result of hyperinsulinemia induced by the drug. Hypoglycemia must be recognized and treated with intravenous 50% glucose in a dose sufficient to restore and maintain normoglycemia.

Inappropriate Treatment of Severe Malaria

Some therapies still survive in current practice despite evidence that they are ineffective or potentially dangerous. The most common of these are heparin and dexamethasone, which should not be used in the treatment of severe malaria.

Unwanted Effects of Antimalarial Drugs

Quinidine and Quinine. The most important toxic effect is hypoglycemia due to drug-induced pancreatic insulin secretion. Pregnant women are particularly susceptible to this complication. Cardiotoxic effects, which are greater with quinidine than with quinine, are confined to prolongation of the QT interval in most individuals but may become clinically significant in those with ischemic heart disease or in patients taking digoxin. If quinidine or quinine is infused too rapidly in any patient, severe hypotension may result. Thrombocytopenia is a rare toxic effect (moderate thrombocytopenia is also a usual feature of untreated falciparum malaria). Therapeutic doses of either drug invariably cause cinchonism—tinnitus, high-tone deafness, and vertigo. These symptoms are reversible and do not indicate a need to stop treatment. Overdose of either drug may cause blindness and deafness.

Mefloquine (Lariam). Minor gastrointestinal symptoms are common. Some individuals develop altered sleep patterns or minor degrees of incoordination. Disabling encephalopathy is a recognized but rare idiosyncratic complication. The drug is therefore not recommended for persons for whom such toxicity would be disastrous—e.g., airline pilots—and for individuals with a chronic neurologic or psychiatric disorder. Mefloquine should be avoided in patients taking beta blockers. Mefloquine should not be given during the first trimester of pregnancy: this is a policy of caution; because no toxicity to the fetus has been demonstrated, a history of taking mefloquine during the first trimester is not sufficient grounds for recommending abortion. Mefloquine can be prescribed for prophylaxis or treatment in the second and third trimesters of pregnancy.

Chloroquine. Excessively rapid infusion may cause profound hypotension and cardiac arrest. A prophylactic dose of 300 mg of base weekly if continued for about 6 years (total dose, 100 grams) is believed to endanger retinal macular function, and alternative prophylaxis is recommended after this interval. Chloroquine may exacerbate psoriasis. Pruritus is a troublesome side effect in about 40% of black-skinned people.

Primaquine. Primaquine may cause severe hemolysis in individuals with red blood cell G6PD deficiency.

Proguanil. Proguanil* has few toxic effects. Its use is associated with mouth ulcers in some people.

Pyrimethamine-Dapsone (Maloprim).* This combination causes transient methemoglobinemia in persons with red blood cell NADH methemoglobin reductase deficiency. A small number of patients, most of them taking 2 tablets per week for prophylaxis (double the usual dose), have developed agranulocytosis.

Pyrimethamine-Sulfadoxine (Fansidar). When used weekly as a prophylactic, this agent has been associated with potentially fatal Stevens-Johnson syndrome and with toxic epidermal necrolysis.

Halofantrine.* Halofantrine causes gastrointestinal upset in a minority of patients. Transient slight elevation of serum transaminase values has been reported. The drug should not be used in pregnancy and is not validated as suitable for complicated malaria.

ADVICE TO TRAVELERS

Malaria is a risk for any individual traveling to an endemic area, even for a period as short as an airport stopover. The World Health Organization annually publishes a book (*Vaccination Certificate Requirements and Health Advice for International Travellers*) with information about current malaria transmission worldwide.

Intending travelers should be advised (1) to minimize mosquito bites in endemic areas by use of bed nets, house screens, and protective clothing; (2) to take regular prophylactic antimalarial drugs for the specified time (see the next section); and (3) to understand that no prophylaxis is fully protective; a fever could still be due to malaria and should be reported immediately, whether during or after travel.

Chemoprophylaxis

Recommendations in the United States have changed. The use of weekly chloroquine is no longer advised for most parts of the world because of the increased prevalence of chloroquine-resistant *P. falciparum*. Weekly mefloquine (adult dose 250 mg) is now the preferred recommendation for most areas. Mefloquine should not be given to pregnant women or young children, for whom chloroquine, 5 mg per kg weekly, remains the safest available drug. (For other contraindications to use of mefloquine, see earlier discussion under "Unwanted Effects of Antimalarial Drugs.") In Britain, weekly chloroquine (adults 300 mg of base) and daily proguanil* (adults 200 mg) remain the prophylaxis of choice for most areas, with mefloquine as an alternative for areas of intense transmission of chloroquine-resistant *P. falciparum*. Pyrimethamine-dapsone and pyrimethamine-sulfonamide combinations are no longer recommended for

prophylaxis because of the significant risk for toxicity (see earlier).

Prophylactic drugs should be taken for at least a week before travel and continued for at least a month after leaving the transmission area.

BACTERIAL MENINGITIS

method of
W. MICHAEL SCHELD, M.D.
University of Virginia School of Medicine
Charlottesville, Virginia

Despite the introduction of newer antimicrobial agents, the morbidity and mortality associated with bacterial meningitis remain unacceptably high. For example, approximately 60% of infants who survive gram-negative bacillary meningitis have developmental disabilities and/or neurologic sequelae. Similarly, in a review of 493 episodes of bacterial meningitis in adults, the overall case-fatality rate was 25%. This brief discussion highlights epidemiologic trends of therapeutic importance, considers the potential impact of new diagnostic tests, and focuses on the management of bacterial meningitis with antimicrobial agents including the role of adjunctive therapy.

EPIDEMIOLOGIC TRENDS

In 1990, the Centers for Disease Control and Prevention published a multistate surveillance study of bacterial meningitis based on data collected in 1986 (Table 1). Although these data reflect a prospective laboratory-based study performed in five states and Los Angeles County and are the latest published information, more recent trends have rendered the results out of date. In 1986, *Haemophilus influenzae* was the most common cause of bacterial meningitis, accounting for 45% of cases with an overall fatality rate of 3%. *Streptococcus pneumoniae* (18%) and *Neisseria meningitidis* (14%) were isolated less commonly with case-fatality rates in the 15 to 20% range. The incidence rates for specific pathogens were most influenced by age. In 1986, approximately 15,000 cases of bacterial meningitis occurred in the United States, and most cases were documented at the extremes of life (<1 month of age and >60 years of age).

The frequency of meningitis due to *H. influenzae* in children has declined dramatically because of widespread use of *H. influenzae* type b vaccines. For example, in the United

TABLE 1. **Bacterial Meningitis: Five States and Los Angeles County, 1986**

Organism	Total (%)	Case-Fatality Rate (%)
Haemophilus influenzae	45	3
Streptococcus pneumoniae	18	19
Neisseria meningitidis	14	13
Group B streptococci	5.7	12
Listeria monocytogenes	3.2	22
Other	15	28

Adapted from Wenger JD, Hightower AW, Facklam RR, et al: Bacterial meningitis in the United States, 1986: Report of a multistate surveillance study. J Infect Dis *162*:1316–1323, 1990. University of Chicago, publisher.

*Not available in the United States.

TABLE 2. **Changing Epidemiology of Bacterial Meningitis: United States***

Organism	Incidence/100,000 Population	
	1986	1995
Haemophilus influenzae	2.9	0.2
Neisseria meningitidis	0.9	0.6
Streptococcus pneumoniae	1.1	1.1

*Data for 1995 represent race- and age-adjusted estimates and refer to surveillance for all pathogens listed from six counties in Maryland, eight in Georgia, five in Tennessee, and three in San Francisco. For San Francisco, surveillance occurred from October 1994 through September 1995.

Data from Schuchat A, Robinson KA, Wenger JD, et al: Bacterial meningitis in the United States in 1995. N Engl J Med *337*:970–976, 1997; and Wenger JD, Hightower AW, Facklam RR, et al: Bacterial meningitis in the United States, 1986: Report of a multistate surveillance study. J Infect Dis *162*:1316–1323, 1990.

States as stated in one report, there was an 82% reduction in the incidence of *H. influenzae* meningitis in children 5 years of age and younger from 1985 through 1991. The changing epidemiology of meningitis from 1986 through 1995 is displayed in Table 2. These data, yet unpublished, were first presented at an international infectious diseases meeting in September 1996. The incidence per 100,000 population for *H. influenzae* disease has declined more than 95% in the past decade. This is the greatest achievement in pediatric infectious diseases in this generation, and the scientists most responsible for this result received the Lasker Award in 1996. As can be seen, the overall incidence of pneumococcal and meningococcal meningitis has remained relatively stable in the United States during this interval. As shown in Table 3, the mortality for pneumococcal meningitis has remained approximately 20% during the past 10 years, but a dramatic decline in the mortality rate associated with meningococcal meningitis and meningitis due to group B streptococci *(Streptococcus agalactiae)* has been documented. Mortality associated with meningitis due to *Listeria monocytogenes* has remained relatively stable. Despite the overall reduction in *H. influenzae* disease, the overall rate of invasive disease due to *S. pneumoniae* and *S. agalactiae* has increased in the past 10 years (Table 4), whereas the incidence of invasive meningococcal disease has remained relatively stable. These epidemiologic trends have profound implications for the treatment of bacterial meningitis. *H. influenzae* meningitis has almost disappeared from the United States. Meningitis due to pneumococci and meningococci is now found more frequently in children.

TABLE 3. **Mortality for Bacterial Meningitis Caused by Selected Pathogens, 1986–1995**

Organism	Mortality (%)	
	1986	1995
Streptococcus pneumoniae	19	21
Neisseria meningitidis	13	3
Streptococcus agalactiae	12	7
Listeria monocytogenes	23	15

Data from Schuchat A, Robinson KA, Wenger JD, et al: Bacterial meningitis in the United States in 1995. N Engl J Med *337*:970–976, 1997; and Wenger JD, Hightower AW, Facklam RR, et al: Bacterial meningitis in the United States, 1986: Report of a multistate surveillance study. J Infect Dis *162*:1316–1323, 1990.

TABLE 4. **Invasive Disease Caused by Selected Pathogens, 1986–1995***

Organism	Incidence/100,000 Population	
	1986	1995
Streptococcus pneumoniae	15.0	26.1
Streptococcus agalactiae	3.7	8.1
Neisseria meningitidis	1.3	1.3
Listeria monocytogenes	0.7	0.5

*Data for 1995 represent race- and age-adjusted estimates and refer to surveillance for all pathogens listed from six counties in Maryland, eight in Georgia, five in Tennessee, and three in San Francisco. For San Francisco, surveillance occurred from October 1994 through September 1995.

Data from Schuchat A, Robinson KA, Wenger JD, et al: Bacterial meningitis in the United States in 1995. N Engl J Med *337*:970–976, 1997; and Wenger JD, Hightower AW, Facklam RR, et al: Bacterial meningitis in the United States, 1986: Report of a multistate surveillance study. J Infect Dis *162*:1316–1323, 1990.

Although penicillin resistance was first documented in *S. pneumoniae* in the late 1960s, the incidence of infections with *S. pneumoniae* resistant to penicillin, other β-lactam antibiotics, and other agents has increased worldwide in the last decade. This resistance is mediated not by β-lactamase production but by alterations in the penicillin binding proteins involved in bacterial cell wall synthesis. The global spread of penicillin-resistant pneumococci has important implications for the empirical treatment of meningitis (see later).

DIAGNOSTIC EVALUATION

The diagnosis of bacterial meningitis still rests on examination of the cerebrospinal fluid (CSF); the typical CSF abnormalities in patients with bacterial meningitis are shown in Table 5. In patients with typical CSF findings and a negative Gram stain, several other tests are available to assist in making an etiologic diagnosis, including counterimmunoelectrophoresis or latex agglutination tests for the detection of the antigens of common meningeal pathogens. The overall sensitivity of these tests ranges from 50 to 100%, but they are highly specific. Latex agglutination is currently favored. A positive test result establishes the diagnosis of bacterial meningitis caused by a specific pathogen, although a negative test result does not rule out this diagnosis. Examination of petechiae, if present, by scrapings with a touch preparation technique and proper staining will detect meningococci in approximately 70% of cases of meningococcemia. Similarly, in suspected meningococcemia, the organism may be apparent on the peripheral blood smear, especially a buffy coat preparation. The differential diagnosis of fever, altered sensorium, and petechial

TABLE 5. **Typical Cerebrospinal Fluid Findings in Patients with Bacterial Meningitis**

Cerebrospinal Fluid Parameter	Typical Findings
Opening pressure	>180 mm H$_2$O
Leukocyte count	1000–5000/mm^3 (range <100 to >10,000)
Percentage of neutrophils	≥80%
Protein concentration	100–500 mg/dL
Glucose concentration	≤40 mg/dL
Gram's stain	Positive in 60–90%
Culture	Positive in 70–85%

TABLE 6. **Differential Diagnosis of Fever, Altered Sensorium, and Petechial Rash**

Meningococcal disease
Rickettsial infections (Rocky Mountain spotted fever, others)
Staphylococcus aureus endocarditis
Streptococcus pneumoniae or *Haemophilus influenzae* infection
  (especially with splenectomy)
Septic shock
Viral meningitis
Viral hemorrhagic fevers
"Noninfectious": thrombotic thrombocytopenic purpura,
  hemolytic-uremic syndrome, vasculitis, others

rash is shown in Table 6. This condition should be considered a medical emergency and promptly evaluated.

Several newer techniques have been proposed for the diagnosis of bacterial meningitis when the Gram stain of the CSF is negative. Elevation of the concentration of C-reactive protein in CSF is highly sensitive for the diagnosis of bacterial meningitis but is not specific. Nevertheless, a normal CSF C-reactive protein concentration excludes bacterial meningitis with nearly 99% certainty in the acute phase. CSF concentrations of tumor necrosis factor appear to be elevated in bacterial but not viral meningitis. The potential use of this technique in separating partially treated bacterial from viral meningitis remains uncertain but is promising. Similarly, the polymerase chain reaction (PCR) for the diagnosis of bacterial meningitis in the absence of a positive CSF Gram stain, latex agglutination test result, or culture may prove useful in the future. PCR for the diagnosis of tuberculous meningitis is particularly attractive because current diagnostic modalities are suboptimal.

INITIAL APPROACH TO MANAGEMENT

A strategy, in algorithmic form, for the initial management of patients with suspected bacterial meningitis is shown in Figure 1. When a patient presents with clinical features suggestive of bacterial meningitis and displays an acute presentation (i.e., ≤24 hours from first symptom to presentation and/or stupor or coma), blood samples for two sets of cultures should be immediately obtained and the patient pre-

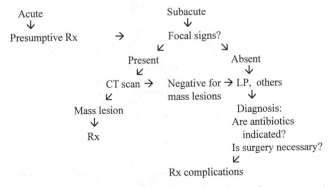

Recognition of Meningitis

Figure 1. An algorithm for the initial strategy of management for patients with suspected bacterial meningitis. *Abbreviations:* CT = computed tomography; LP = lumbar puncture; Rx = therapy.

sumptively treated while lumbar puncture is performed. If the presentation is more subacute (i.e., >24 hours from the onset of symptoms to presentation, minimal alteration in mental status), a rapid neurologic examination should be performed. If focal findings are present (e.g., hemiparesis) or papilledema is documented, the patient should be evaluated first with computed tomography (CT). If bacterial meningitis is a strong consideration, blood samples should be drawn for cultures and the patient presumptively treated while undergoing CT. Appropriate treatment should be administered if a mass lesion is documented. If the CT result is normal or focal signs are absent on neurologic examination, the patient should immediately be subjected to lumbar puncture. On the basis of the results (CSF formula, Gram's stain, or antigen detection tests), empirical and/or specific treatment should be started. The interval from the onset of evaluation to the first dose of antimicrobial agent should not exceed 30 minutes, although a delay in therapy has not been conclusively documented to adversely affect outcome in multiple studies in the medical literature. Nevertheless, in the absence of compelling clinical data and in the best interest of the patient, antimicrobial therapy should be initiated promptly in patients with suspected bacterial meningitis.

EMPIRICAL ANTIMICROBIAL THERAPY

When lumbar puncture is delayed or Gram's stain of the CSF is nondiagnostic, empirical therapy for presumed bacterial meningitis is essential and should be directed to the most likely pathogens based on the patient's age and the underlying host status (Table 7). In neonates, the major pathogens are group B streptococci, *Escherichia coli,* and *L. monocytogenes*; the empirical antimicrobial regimen of choice is ampicillin plus cefotaxime (Claforan), although some neonatologists still prefer ampicillin plus an aminoglycoside. Ceftriaxone is avoided in this age group because of concerns regarding protein binding and displacement of bilirubin. In older infants, the neonatal pathogens are joined by the three major meningeal pathogens, and ampicillin plus a third-generation cephalosporin is preferred. In children and young adults, a third-generation cephalosporin is often administered alone, although the addition of vancomycin must be considered owing to the emergence of penicillin-resistant pneumococci (see later). Ampicillin plus chloramphenicol is probably inadequate. In older adults (i.e., >50 years), the pneumococcus is the most frequently isolated pathogen from CSF, but the organisms listed are more common in this age group than in younger adults; therefore, ampicillin plus a third-generation cephalosporin is the regimen of choice. These recommendations may require modification under special circumstances, most notably when penicillin-resistant pneumococci are prevalent in the community. In immunocompromised patients, such as those with a lymphoreticular

TABLE 7. **Common Pathogens and Empirical Therapeutic Recommendations Based on Age in Patients with Bacterial Meningitis***

Age	Common Bacterial Pathogens	Empirical Antimicrobial Therapy
0–4 wk	*Streptococcus agalactiae, Escherichia coli, Listeria monocytogenes, Klebsiella pneumoniae*	Ampicillin plus cefotaxime, or ampicillin plus an aminoglycoside
4–12 wk	*S. agalactiae, E. coli, L. monocytogenes, Haemophilus influenzae, Streptococcus pneumoniae, Neisseria meningitidis*	Ampicillin plus a third-generation cephalosporin†
3 mo–18 y	*S. pneumoniae, N. meningitidis, H. influenzae*	Third-generation cephalosporin,† or ampicillin plus chloramphenicol
18–50 y	*S. pneumoniae, N. meningitidis*	Third-generation cephalosporin ± ampicillin‡
>50 y	*S. pneumoniae, N. meningitidis, L. monocytogenes,* aerobic gram-negative bacilli	Ampicillin plus a third-generation cephalosporin†

*Vancomycin should be added to empirical therapeutic regimens when pneumococcal meningitis is suspected with strains that are highly resistant to penicillin or cephalosporins.
†Cefotaxime or ceftriaxone.
‡Add ampicillin if meningitis caused by *L. monocytogenes* is suspected.

malignant neoplasm or receiving cytotoxic or high-dose glucocorticoid therapy, *Listeria* is a major consideration and ampicillin should be added to any regimen. In penicillin-allergic patients, the drug of choice for potential *L. monocytogenes* meningitis is high-dose trimethoprim-sulfamethoxazole (Bactrim, Septra). For patients with recent head trauma or neurosurgery or those with indwelling CSF shunts, broad-spectrum antibiotics effective against both gram-positive and gram-negative organisms including staphylococci should be initiated (e.g., vancomycin [Vancocin] plus ceftazidime [Fortaz]). If identifiable bacteria are seen on Gram's stain of the CSF, antibiotic therapy remains empirical but should be directed toward the presumptive pathogen. These regimens are shown in Table 8 and are discussed in more detail in the following.

PATHOGEN-SPECIFIC THERAPY

Streptococcus pneumoniae

The recommendations for antimicrobial therapy for pneumococcal meningitis have been altered on the basis of changes in the pneumococcal susceptibility pattern to penicillin G. The susceptibility to penicillin G is based on the minimal inhibitory concentration (MIC) of this agent. Strains with an MIC less than 0.1 μg per mL are considered susceptible. When the MIC is 0.1 to 1.0 μg per mL, the strains are termed relatively or intermediately resistant; strains with an MIC of 2 μg per mL or greater are considered highly resistant. Strains of pneumococci that are relatively or highly resistant to penicillin are at least as highly invasive as susceptible organisms. The most recent data in the United States document penicillin

TABLE 8. **Specific Antimicrobial Therapy for Bacterial Meningitis**

Bacterial Pathogen	Standard Therapy	Alternative Therapy
Streptococcus pneumoniae		
Penicillin MIC ≤0.1 μg/mL	Penicillin G or ampicillin	Third-generation cephalosporin*; chloramphenicol; vancomycin
Penicillin MIC 0.1–1.0 μg/mL	Third-generation cephalosporin*	Vancomycin
Penicillin MIC ≥2.0 μg/mL	Vancomycin plus a third-generation cephalosporin*	Meropenem†
Neisseria meningitidis	Penicillin G or ampicillin	Third-generation cephalosporin*; chloramphenicol; fluoroquinolone
Haemophilus influenzae		
β-Lactamase–negative	Ampicillin	Third-generation cephalosporin*; chloramphenicol; aztreonam
β-Lactamase–positive	Third-generation cephalosporin*	Chloramphenicol; aztreonam; fluoroquinolone
Enterobacteriaceae	Third-generation cephalosporin*	Aztreonam; fluoroquinolone; trimethoprim-sulfamethoxazole
Pseudomonas aeruginosa	Ceftazidime‡	Aztreonam; fluoroquinolone‡
Listeria monocytogenes	Ampicillin or penicillin G‡	Trimethoprim-sulfamethoxazole
Streptotoccus agalactiae	Ampicillin or penicillin G‡	Third-generation cephalosporin*; vancomycin
Staphylococcus aureus		
Methicillin sensitive	Nafcillin or oxacillin	Vancomycin
Methicillin resistant	Vancomycin	
Staphylococcus epidermidis	Vancomycin§	

*Cefotaxime or ceftriaxone.
†Currently under study in patients with pneumococcal meningitis.
‡Addition of an aminoglycoside should be considered.
§Addition of rifampin should be considered.
Abbreviation: MIC = minimal inhibitory concentration.

TABLE 9. **Proportion of Pneumococcal Isolates Resistant to Selected Antimicrobial Agents, Atlanta, 1994**

Drug	% Resistant*
Penicillin	25 (7)
Cefotaxime	9 (4)
Erythromycin, clarithromycin	15
Trimethoprim-sulfamethoxazole	26
Tetracycline	8

*Numbers in parentheses indicate the percentage of strains with *high level* resistance.

Based on data from Hofmann J, Cetron MS, Farley MM, et al: The prevalence of drug-resistant *Streptococcus pneumoniae* in Atlanta. N Engl J Med 333:481–486, 1995.

resistance rates of approximately 25% overall among pneumococci (Table 9); higher rates have been reported from Spain, eastern Europe, South Africa, Japan, and other areas of the world. Factors that have been shown to predispose to the development of resistance include age younger than 10 or older than 50 years, immunosuppression, prolonged hospital stay, children in day care settings, infection by serotypes 14 and 23, and frequent or prophylactic use of antimicrobial therapy (e.g., for the prevention of otitis media).

Because of these considerations, penicillin, ampicillin, and related agents can no longer be recommended as empirical antimicrobial therapy when *S. pneumoniae* is considered a likely pathogen in patients with bacterial meningitis. Chloramphenicol, despite long-standing worldwide use, has proved disappointing in several areas, especially in South Africa where a poor outcome has been documented in approximately 80% of children with penicillin-resistant pneumococcal meningitis treated with this agent. The third-generation cephalosporins cefotaxime and ceftriaxone (Rocephin) have been effective in the therapy for meningitis caused by relatively penicillin resistant pneumococci. Unfortunately, several reports of pneumococcal strains in patients with meningitis with relatively low MICs for the third-generation cephalosporins (approximately 0.5 to 1 μg per mL) have documented failures with conventional therapy with these agents. The current guidelines by the National Committee for Clinical Laboratory Standards state that CSF isolates of *S. pneumoniae* with MICs for cefotaxime or ceftriaxone of greater than 0.5 μg per mL be considered intermediately resistant to cephalosporins. Some regard this recommendation as too conservative. Nevertheless, third-generation cephalosporins are recommended for meningitis due to intermediately resistant strains (see Table 8). Pneumococcal isolates resistant to vancomycin have not been described, and this agent is commonly employed in the empirical regimens for adults and children when resistant pneumococci are of concern. CSF penetration of vancomycin in adults has been somewhat erratic and is reduced in the presence of dexamethasone therapy. Therefore, van-

comycin should never be used alone in the empirical treatment of meningitis, especially when dexamethasone is administered as an adjunctive treatment. In experimental pneumococcal meningitis, the combination of vancomycin and ceftriaxone was synergistic when the disease was induced with ceftriaxone-resistant strains.

Several other agents have been investigated for the treatment of pneumococcal meningitis. Although imipenem has been used successfully, the proconvulsant activity of this drug precludes its use in patients with central nervous system infection. Meropenem (Merrem) appears to be less epileptogenic and has been evaluated with promising results, although only a few patients with resistant pneumococcal strains have been treated with this agent. Newer fluoroquinolones such as trovafloxacin* appear to penetrate into the CSF in therapeutic concentrations and may be useful in the future. Trovafloxacin has also been used orally in therapy for meningococcal meningitis.

The empirical regimen for pneumococcal meningitis suspected to be caused by strains highly resistant to penicillin or cephalosporins remains controversial. The combination of vancomycin plus a third-generation cephalosporin (cefotaxime or ceftriaxone) is recommended at present. Some authorities have also suggested the addition of rifampin to this empirical regimen, but rifampin may be antagonistic when it is used in combination against some pneumococcal strains and is not preferred currently. Follow-up lumbar puncture to document clearance of the organism is essential in all cases of suspected penicillin-resistant pneumococcal meningitis. Again, once susceptibility studies are available, antimicrobial therapy can be modified (see Table 8).

Neisseria meningitidis

The antimicrobial agents of choice for the treatment of meningococcal meningitis remain penicillin G and ampicillin. Although meningococcal strains are now emerging that are relatively resistant to penicillin G (i.e., MIC range of 0.1 to 1 μg per mL), they remain unusual in the United States, and the clinical significance of these resistant isolates is unclear because patients with meningitis caused by these strains have recovered with standard penicillin therapy. Third-generation cephalosporins are also acceptable as empirical therapy for meningococcal meningitis. Newer quinolones are not recommended as first-line agents pending further clinical experience.

Haemophilus influenzae

Approximately one third of *H. influenzae* type b strains in the United States produce β-lactamase and are therefore resistant to ampicillin and related agents. Resistance to chloramphenicol is unusual. The second-generation cephalosporin cefuroxime (Zinacef) was initially found to be as efficacious as the

---

*Not available in the United States.

combination of ampicillin plus chloramphenicol in childhood bacterial meningitis caused predominantly by *H. influenzae* type b, but subsequent studies have questioned the efficacy of this agent, and ceftriaxone or cefotaxime is now considered the drug of choice. These agents sterilize the CSF more rapidly and are associated with a lower rate of hearing loss compared with older cephalosporins such as cefuroxime.

Enteric Gram-Negative Bacilli

Before the early 1980s, the outcome of therapy for bacterial meningitis caused by gram-negative aerobic bacilli was often poor. Chloramphenicol was ineffective because it was often bacteriostatic against these isolates, and aminoglycosides were not highly effective because of inadequate CSF concentrations. With the advent of the broad-spectrum cephalosporins, clinical outcomes were remarkably improved (85 to 90% success rates) owing to the high activity of these agents against gram-negative pathogens and their high CSF penetration. Ceftazidime (Fortaz) (and perhaps cefepime [Maxipime], pending further data) must be considered the drug of choice for *Pseudomonas aeruginosa* meningitis, often in combination with an aminoglycoside against this nosocomial pathogen.

Several other agents have been employed successfully in patients with enteric gram-negative bacillary meningitis; these include aztreonam (Azactam), imipenem (Primaxin) (to be avoided for the reasons cited before), meropenem, newer cephalosporins such as cefepime, and fluoroquinolones. In patients who fail to respond, intrathecal or intraventricular aminoglycosides or alternative systemic antimicrobial therapy may be necessary and should be based on susceptibility studies.

Listeria monocytogenes

Ampicillin or penicillin remains the agent of choice for a documented *L. monocytogenes* meningitis. However, neither agent is bactericidal against *Listeria,* and mortality rates remain as high as 30%. Therefore, gentamicin should be combined with ampicillin for this disease. In penicillin-allergic patients, trimethoprim-sulfamethoxazole is the agent of choice. Despite susceptibility data to the contrary, chloramphenicol and vancomycin have proved ineffective for patients with systemic *Listeria* infection. Meropenem is active in vitro and in experimental animal models of *Listeria* meningitis, but there are inadequate human data at present to recommend its use as a first-line agent.

Streptococcus agalactiae

For neonates with meningitis due to group B streptococci, the combination of ampicillin and gentamicin is the therapy of choice because of documented in vitro synergy and reports of penicillin-tolerant strains. For adults, the benefit of the combination therapy over penicillin or ampicillin alone is un-

TABLE 10. **Guidelines for Duration of Antibiotic Therapy**

Pathogen	Suggested Duration (d)
Haemophilus influenzae	7
Neisseria meningitidis	5–7
Streptococcus pneumoniae	10–14
Listeria monocytogenes	14–21
Group B streptococci	14–21
Gram-negative bacilli*	21

*Other than *H. influenzae.*

proved, and mortality is chiefly influenced by the presence of underlying disease.

DURATION OF ANTIMICROBIAL THERAPY

The duration of antimicrobial therapy for patients with bacterial meningitis is based largely on tradition rather than rigorous scientific evidence. Nevertheless, the suggested duration of antimicrobial therapy for each of the major meningeal pathogens is shown in Table 10.

ADJUNCTIVE THERAPY

As stated before, the morbidity and mortality from bacterial meningitis remain unacceptably high. Multiple studies in experimental animal models of infection conducted during the past 2 decades have elucidated many aspects of the pathogenesis and pathophysiology of bacterial meningitis. These studies have documented the inflammatory potential of the gram-positive cell wall and gram-negative lipopolysaccharide as mediated through host molecules, such as the proinflammatory cytokines interleukin-1, interleukin-6, and tumor necrosis factor. Similarly, adjunctive corticosteroid therapy has been shown to be effective in attenuating many of the pathophysiologic consequences during experimental meningitis, such as subarachnoid space inflammation, increased intracranial pressure, and cerebral edema.

On the basis of these experimental studies, multiple clinical trials have been undertaken to determine the effects of adjunctive dexamethasone or similar agents on outcome in patients with bacterial meningitis. Several major controversies remain, despite the accumulation of this clinical information. The majority of children enrolled in these trials were infected with *H. influenzae,* a pathogen that is disappearing from the United States as a cause of invasive infection. The benefits of dexamethasone in children infected with other pathogens, especially *S. pneumoniae,* are not as compelling, although trends suggest a reduction in audiologic and neurologic sequelae. Furthermore, the role of adjunctive glucocorticosteroid therapy for adults and neonates is less clear because these populations of patients have not been studied in adequate detail. Adjunctive dexamethasone in a dose of 0.15 mg per kg every 6 hours for 2 to 4 days is recommended in children older than 2 months with suspected bacterial meningitis, particularly those suspected of being infected with *H. influenzae*. On the basis of a meta-analysis (in press), dexamethasone should be initiated intravenously simultaneously with or slightly before the first dose of antimicrobial agent. When the delay in dexamethasone administration exceeds 3 to 4 hours beyond the first dose of antimicrobial agent, most beneficial effects are lost; therefore, the agent is not recommended in this setting. Data on the use of dexamethasone in the neonatal period are lacking. In adults, the benefits are less convincing, and dexamethasone reduces the penetration of several important agents such as vancomycin into the CSF. If dexamethasone is chosen as a component of the empirical regimen administered to adults with suspected bacterial meningitis, a combination regimen that covers penicillin-resistant pneumococci should be selected. Dexamethasone is appropriate when other indications for its use are present in patients with bacterial meningitis, such as a marked increase in intracranial pressure or the presence of cerebral edema at CT. When severe sepsis or septic shock is suspected or documented, corticosteroids should be avoided because the outcome is adversely affected. Plasmapheresis or plasma exchange has been used in small series of patients with meningococcemia and severe sepsis or septic shock (purpura fulminans). The initial results are extremely promising, but the use of these modalities in this desperately ill population of patients must be considered experimental at present.

INFECTIOUS MONONUCLEOSIS

method of
CIRO V. SUMAYA, M.D., M.P.H.T.M.
University of Texas Health Science Center
San Antonio, Texas

Infectious mononucleosis (IM) is the prototypic primary symptomatic infection produced by the Epstein-Barr virus. IM is diagnosed by a triad of characteristic clinical, hematologic, and serologic findings. The typical clinical manifestations include fever, malaise, cervical lymphadenitis, tonsillopharyngitis, and splenic and/or liver enlargement. Children, particularly the very young, may also present with additional findings, including increased occurrence of rashes, respiratory tract infections, and abdominal pain. Hematologic features include a relative lymphocytosis and presence of atypical lymphocytes equal to or greater than 10% of the leukocytes. The serologic findings include a positive typical heterophil antibody test, although this antibody response may not be detected until 1 to 2 weeks into the disease course or it remains undetectable (as is often the case of children younger than 4 years). In these instances, determination of Epstein-Barr virus–specific antibody titers may be required to make a satisfactory diagnosis. Acute IM is self-limiting in almost all cases, with patients recovering in 2 to 4 weeks. Complications of the respiratory system (upper airway obstruction, pneumonia), neurologic system (meningoencephalitis, Bell's palsy, Guillain-Barré syndrome), and hematologic system (thrombocytopenia, granulocytopenia) occur occasionally. Fortunately, these complications are usually short in duration and seldom produce permanent sequelae. Splenic rupture is noted in about 0.2% of patients. Very rarely, the IM episode in some patients with or even without an underlying immunocompromised condition can result in severe, prolonged multiorgan dysfunction that is potentially fatal.

TREATMENT

Routine Infectious Mononucleosis

Uncomplicated IM is managed principally by measures to control or minimize symptoms. Aspirin or acetaminophen can be used to control fever as well as to alleviate discomfort from headache, throat inflammation, or muscle and joint irritation. Gargling with warm saline water also provides some relief from pharyngeal pain. Reduction of activity and bed rest are usually dictated by the tolerance of the patient. Contact sports or activities with a potential for trauma or stress to the abdomen (vigorous exercise, heavy lifting) should be avoided during the period that the spleen is palpable and thus presumably enlarged.

The small percentage of patients with group A beta-hemolytic streptococcal superinfection of the throat should be treated with penicillin (oral penicillin V 250 to 500 mg given four times a day for 10 days) or, alternatively, erythromycin at equivalent doses after documentation of this infection by throat culture or antigen detection. Parenteral benzathine penicillin may be necessary if the patient refuses to or cannot swallow. Ampicillin is not recommended because it may elicit a hypersensitivity-related maculopapular rash.

Corticosteroids are not recommended for routine use in uncomplicated infectious mononucleosis. The few isolated reports of the efficacy of metronidazole, tinidazole, and cimetidine require more critical evaluation before general use of these agents is considered.

Complicated Infectious Mononucleosis

In addition to the above-mentioned considerations for uncomplicated IM, for some patients who are severely symptomatic short-term corticosteroid therapy may provide apparent relief. The corticosteroid therapy can be given orally or intravenously in doses equivalent to 40 mg of prednisone per m^2 per day, with tapering to complete the therapy during 1 to 2 weeks. Patients with stridor caused by massively enlarged tonsils or paratracheal adenopathy or with hematologic or neurologic complications constitute those for whom corticosteroids have been used more commonly.

The insertion of an artificial airway is replacing emergency tonsillectomy as the treatment of choice for complete airway obstruction produced by profound upper respiratory tract inflammation. The rare complication of traumatic or spontaneous splenic rupture is managed by traditional splenectomy or, as more recently introduced, nonoperative means through blood transfusion maintenance.

In the extremely rare instance that a life-threatening, multiorgan dysfunctional state results from the IM episode, high-dose intravenous acyclovir (Zovirax) (e.g., 1500 mg per m^2 per day divided every 8 hours) should be used, although the evidence for benefit is controversial. Preliminary studies of the use of anti–B cell monoclonal antibodies and irradiated transplant donor leukocytes, along with reduction of the patient's immunosuppressive medication (if being administered), have shown variable benefit.

PREVENTION

Patients with a recent history (within about 6 months) of IM should not donate blood. There is no requirement for isolation of hospitalized patients with IM. Investigations are ongoing to produce a suitable vaccine against the causative agent of IM.

CHRONIC FATIGUE SYNDROME

method of
ANTHONY L. KOMAROFF, M.D.
Brigham and Women's Hospital and Harvard
*   Medical School*
Boston, Massachusetts

FATIGUE IN A PRIMARY CARE PRACTICE

Everyone experiences fatigue. Furthermore, nearly everyone occasionally experiences a fatigue that is thought to be "unnatural," not clearly explained by the mental, emotional, and physical stresses of the previous days. Such fatigue is usually transient. The complaint of chronic fatigue accounts for 10 to 15 million office visits per year in the United States. Primary psychiatric disorders, particularly depression and anxiety, along with overwork, are the cause of most cases of chronic fatigue in a general medical practice. Moreover, primary psychiatric disorders presenting with somatic symptoms frequently go undiagnosed and untreated; unrecognized and untreated major depression is an important public health problem.

On occasion, various "organic" conditions can also produce fatigue, for example, occult malignant neoplasms, anemia, and thyroid disorders. However, in an office practice, this accounts for less than 5% of all patients presenting with the complaint of fatigue.

CHRONIC FATIGUE SYNDROME

There has been growing discussion of another illness that many believe may have an organic basis: chronic fatigue syndrome (CFS). Some patients and clinicians have adopted the name "chronic fatigue and immune dysfunction syndrome," but CFS is the preferred name. The illness is also similar to the condition that the British call "myalgic encephalomyelitis."

CFS is controversial because no causal agent and no

TABLE 1. **Definition of Chronic Fatigue Syndrome**

Classify as chronic fatigue syndrome if both of the following criteria are met:
  Unexplained persistent or relapsing fatigue of new or definite onset that is not due to ongoing exertion, is not relieved by rest, and results in a substantial reduction in previous levels of activity
                                 and
  Four or more of the following symptoms are concurrently present for 6 mo or longer:
    Impaired memory or concentration that impairs everyday activities
    Sore throat
    Tender cervical or axillary lymph nodes
    Muscle pain
    Multijoint pain
    New headaches lasting more than 24 h
    Unrefreshing sleep
    Postexertional malaise

From Fukuda K, Straus SE, Hickie I, et al: The chronic fatigue syndrome: A comprehensive approach to its definition and study. Ann Intern Med *121*:953–959, 1994.

diagnostic laboratory test have been identified. A formal case definition of the illness has been developed by the Centers for Disease Control and Prevention (Table 1). The illness is characterized by at least 6 months of exceptional fatigue, with several associated chronic symptoms. Chronic diseases that would exclude the diagnosis of CFS include untreated hypothyroidism, sleep apnea, chronic active hepatitis, any psychotic disorder, dementia, anorexia nervosa or bulimia nervosa, recent substance abuse, and severe obesity. Bipolar affective disorder excludes a diagnosis of CFS, but nonpsychotic unipolar major depression or anxiety disorders do not. As so defined, patients with CFS represent a small fraction (1 to 3%) of all patients seeking medical care for the complaint of chronic fatigue.

Patients with CFS may be of any age, of either sex, and from all walks of life; the typical patient is a 35-year-old white woman. In my experience, the onset is often sudden, frequently after an acute "viral" syndrome. In unusual cases, CFS follows in the wake not of a nondescript "flulike" illness but of a well-defined acute infectious illness, including acute infectious mononucleosis and Lyme disease (despite adequate antibacterial therapy and the resolution of Lyme disease–specific symptoms).

CFS is associated with a wide range of dysfunction. As a group, patients with CFS report functional limitations that are at least as striking as those of patients with congestive heart failure, diabetes mellitus, myocardial infarction, and multiple sclerosis. Some patients appear to be completely disabled by the fatigue, cognitive impairment, muscle weakness, and pain.

Although CFS is currently defined only by a constellation of symptoms, and although no diagnostic test with adequate accuracy has yet been developed, there is growing evidence of objective biologic abnormalities in patients with CFS. Various imaging and functional studies of the central nervous system and immune system have been reported. In my experience, a number of laboratory findings clearly distinguish patients with CFS from healthy control subjects (and, in some cases, from comparison group patients with various fatiguing psychiatric and organic diseases): low levels of circulating immune complexes, elevated total complement (CH_{50}), elevated IgG, atypical lymphocytosis, elevated alkaline phosphatase, low lactate dehydrogenase, elevated total cholesterol, and low levels of antinuclear antibody. No infectious agent has been convincingly shown to be a cause of CFS. Nevertheless, there is evidence from controlled studies of the reactivation of several chronic viral infections in CFS.

A National Institutes of Health panel has recommended that a patient with debilitating and protracted chronic fatigue, as described, should have the following diagnostic tests: complete blood count, manual differential white blood cell count, erythrocyte sedimentation rate, chemistry panel, thyroid-stimulating hormone, antinuclear antibody, rheumatoid factor (if arthralgias), and urinalysis. These tests can help identify well-recognized organic diseases. Moreover, as indicated, some may also provide clues regarding the diagnosis of CFS, although none constitutes a diagnostic test.

MANAGEMENT OF CHRONIC FATIGUE SYNDROME

Nonpharmacologic Management

Management of the patient with CFS requires more than pharmacotherapy. First, the clinician must make a personal judgment as to whether patients are accurately relating their symptoms—both those that they admit to and those that they deny. CFS is an illness defined only by symptoms. Thus, an occasional patient seeking secondary gain may fabricate a "perfect story" for CFS. Somewhat more commonly, patients who have been told that they are suffering from major depression and who find that diagnosis to be stigmatizing read about CFS in the media and come to believe that it explains their fatigue. So, the first task of the clinician is to make an admittedly arbitrary judgment as to the veracity of the symptoms reported. In my experience, with CFS and other illnesses, it is generally wisest to believe what the patient tells you.

It is therapeutic for the clinician to listen to the patient, take seriously the patient's recounting of the illness, and explain honestly what is known and not known about the illness. The growing number of studies finding objective abnormalities in patients with CFS have convinced me that there is an underlying biologically based illness: there is "something wrong," even if the pathogenesis is still unknown. It is antitherapeutic for the clinician to dismiss any patient's symptoms out of hand, even when the clinician is convinced that the patient is suffering from a primary psychiatric disorder with somatizing features. This may be particularly true with CFS, which is a "delegitimizing" illness. This delegitimization probably augments a patient's perception of symptoms and diminishes his or her sense of self-worth. It is an enormously frustrating thing, for both patient and clinician, when there is no definitive explanation for symptoms. The busy clinician can easily become impatient when dealing with any presenting complaint that does not have an obvious diagnosis. However, especially when a definitive therapeutic technology is not at hand, there is no substitute for patient and sympathetic listening and explanation.

In Table 2 are listed some nonpharmacologic treatments of CFS. Perhaps the most important nonpharmacologic treatment is to encourage patients to avoid unusual physical or emotional stress and to pace themselves; each day should have a regular routine. Patients should be encouraged to be as active and involved as they feel is possible, and the clinician may need to spend time explaining to employers why a scaled down, part-time work schedule is necessary. Modest regular exercise, to avoid deconditioning, is important.

One study from the United Kingdom reported encouraging results from the use of cognitive-behavioral therapy; other prior studies, however, had been disappointing, and the efficacy of such therapy is therapist dependent.

Pharmacologic Therapy

No treatment has been proved to benefit patients with CFS in large randomized controlled trials that have been replicated by other investigators in other populations of patients. Moreover, without a better understanding of the pathogenesis of CFS, it is unlikely that definitive treatment will be identified. Indeed, the pharmacologic treatment of CFS primarily involves the treatment of the symptoms associated with CFS. In my experience, patients with CFS are unusually sensitive to any drug or substance (e.g., alcohol) that affects the central nervous system; one should start with a low dose and then gradually escalate it as necessary.

Low-Dose Tricyclic Agents

The most widely used treatment of CFS is sedating tricyclic antidepressant agents in low doses: amitriptyline (Elavil)* or doxepin (Sinequan),* 5 to 20 mg at bedtime. For unusually low doses, the liquid form of the medication may be necessary. Low-dose tricyclic agents have been proved efficacious in randomized trials of a similar illness (fibromyalgia) and in a number of sleep disorders. No such trials have been

---

*Not FDA approved for this indication.

TABLE 2. **Steps in Managing the Patient with Chronic Fatigue Syndrome**

Establish the diagnosis
Symptomatic treatment
   Medications for depression, anxiety, pain, sleep, allergies
   Avoid exotic untested remedies
   Cognitive-behavioral therapy
Provide reassurance and emotional support
   Acceptance of symptoms
   Avoid confrontational approach
   Referral to support groups and counseling
Lifestyle management
   Apply stress reduction
   Restructure activities
   Make realistic goals
Prevent further disability
   Graded exercise program
   Physical therapy
Regular follow-up
Continue to rule out other medical problems

conducted in patients with CFS. In my anecdotal experience, most patients immediately notice that their sleep is less frequently interrupted and that they awaken feeling somewhat more refreshed.

Patients with concomitant depression do not report an improvement in the core symptoms of depression when given these low doses of tricyclic agents. Patients should be warned that during the first week of therapy, even extremely low doses of tricyclics may cause them to feel groggy in the morning; that reaction usually dissipates after about 1 week. When this reaction does not dissipate, patients can be switched to a less sedating tricyclic agent, such as desipramine (Norpramin),* 20 to 50 mg at bedtime, or to the triazolopyridine antidepressant trazodone (Desyrel),* 25 to 50 mg at bedtime.

Antidepressant Agents

Half or more of patients with CFS develop major depression in the months and years after the onset of their illness, although only a minority have experienced an episode of depression in the years before their illness. When patients are suffering from depression, antidepressant therapy is indicated. Again, one should start any antidepressant at an unusually low dose and gradually increase it. In my experience, tricyclic agents can rarely be tolerated in conventional antidepressant doses, but selective serotonin reuptake inhibitors are better tolerated. Sertraline (Zoloft), fluoxetine (Prozac), and paroxetine (Paxil) have been used the most. Some colleagues have reported good results with the combined serotonin and norepinephrine uptake inhibitor venlafaxine (Effexor). Despite this, the only randomized trial of antidepressant therapy in CFS, which used fluoxetine, found no benefit in either the fatigue or depression.

Although I have seen many patients with CFS and depression in whom the depression is successfully treated, I have seen no patient whose entire symptom complex appears to have been cured by antidepressant therapy.

Anxiolytic Agents

Panic disorder and generalized anxiety disorder may be more common in patients with CFS, after the onset of the illness, than in the general population. In such patients, careful use of alprazolam (Xanax), clonazepam (Klonopin), or other benzodiazepines is indicated—with care taken to start at a low dose and to avoid escalating the regimen beyond normal dose levels.

Nonsteroidal Anti-inflammatory Drugs

The majority of patients with CFS experience myalgias, arthralgias, headaches, and migratory paresthesias. For some, the pain is the most debilitating aspect of their illness. In most patients, nonsteroidal anti-inflammatory drugs (NSAIDs) seem to provide a measure of relief. The less expensive NSAIDs, particularly naproxen (Naprosyn) and ibuprofen (Motrin),

appear to be just as efficacious as the more expensive NSAIDs.

Antimicrobial Therapy

Because there is no proven infectious cause of CFS, it is not surprising that antimicrobial agents are rarely used. One randomized controlled study found no benefit from acyclovir (Zovirax); however, that antiviral drug has little or no in vitro efficacy against those viruses that studies have found to be reactivated in patients with CFS.

Immunomodulation Therapy

Several controlled trials of intravenous immune globulin* have been tried, on the premise that some kind of immune dysregulation may explain CFS. However, only one study showed a small benefit, and the same investigators have subsequently published a second study with negative findings. There are no data supporting the use of other immunomodulation treatments such as interferon or transfer factor. A randomized trial did not find low-dose corticosteroid* therapy to be beneficial.

Antiallergy Therapy

Many patients with CFS have experienced atopic symptoms since childhood, and the atopic symptoms often flare in CFS. Nonsedating antihistamines* are useful in such patients. Elimination diets have not been studied.

Antihypotensive Therapy

A substantial fraction of patients with CFS have modest abnormalities of the autonomic nervous system, leading to neurally mediated hypotension. Whereas syncope is relatively uncommon in patients with CFS, dizziness and dysequilibrium—particularly associated with postural change—are common. It has been my anecdotal experience that these symptoms may benefit from therapy that increases the vascular space: adding salt to the diet, or taking fludrocortisone (Florinef),* a salt-retaining steroid. At this writing, a randomized trial of fludrocortisone is under way.

SUMMARY

The chief complaint of chronic fatigue is common in any primary care practice. Most patients seeking medical care for chronic fatigue are suffering from depression or overwork. The illness called CFS is uncommon and is of uncertain etiology. Growing evidence indicates that it has a biologic basis and that the central nervous system and immune system are involved. At the same time, many patients with CFS suffer from depression.

There are no proven therapies for CFS, but substantial anecdotal experience indicates that low doses of tricyclic agents can improve the quality of sleep and thereby improve a patient's level of func-

---

*Not FDA approved for this indication.

*Not FDA approved for this indication.

tion. NSAIDs can help mitigate pain from headaches, myalgias, and arthralgias. Patients who suffer from depression along with CFS should be treated with antidepressant therapy, but one randomized trial indicated that the depression associated with CFS may be resistant to selective serotonin reuptake inhibitor antidepressants.

An important part of the treatment of CFS is non-pharmacologic. The clinician should pay sympathetic attention to the patient's description of the illness. The clinician should also help the patient set realistic goals, to reduce stresses, to develop a regular schedule of work and sleep, and to maintain and gradually increase activity levels.

MUMPS

method of
H. DAVID WILSON, M.D.
University of North Dakota School of Medicine and Health Sciences
Grand Forks, North Dakota

Mumps is a generalized, communicable infection caused by the mumps paramyxovirus with a tropism for glandular and nervous tissues. It is usually diagnosed in children or young adults from the appearance of a painful swelling in one or both parotid glands that lasts 5 to 7 days. The submandibular glands are principally affected in 10 to 15% of cases, and rarely, the sublingual glands alone are involved. Subclinical infection occurs in 30 to 40% of people; thus, many persons who believe they are susceptible are really immune.

The incubation period is usually 16 to 18 days (range, 12 to 25 days). The infected individual is communicable from a day or two (rarely as long as 7 days) before the onset of swelling and for 5 to 7 days after disease is apparent. Full recovery is the rule and results in lifelong immunity. Recurrent bouts of parotitis usually indicate infection with another virus (parainfluenza, coxsackievirus, and others) or another disease, idiopathic recurrent parotitis.

DIAGNOSIS

The swollen parotid glands that obscure the mandibular angle and the glandular pain that occurs when salivation is stimulated are the clinical hallmarks. The area around the openings of Stensen's and/or Wharton's duct may be seen as erythematous and swollen. The virus may be cultured from urine, from saliva, and from cerebrospinal fluid if meningitis is present. A fourfold rise in serum antibody titer between acute and convalescent serum specimens, as measured by complement fixation or hemagglutination inhibition, indicates recent infection. Enzyme-linked immunosorbent assay, neutralization tests, and other tests can indicate immunity. An elevated serum amylase value may also indicate acute infection.

TREATMENT

There is no specific treatment for mumps. Therefore, symptomatic measures are used when needed. Eating soft and bland foods and avoiding sour, spicy, or other foods that cause pain are the rule. Ice packs applied over the affected glands may be soothing in some cases. Treatment for pain and fever with acetaminophen or other analgesics is helpful.

COMPLICATIONS AND THEIR TREATMENT

Meningitis is the most common complication, occurring in about 10% of patients, and can occur in the absence of parotid swelling. Treatment is supportive, with analgesia for headache and fluids, oral or intravenous, as required for dehydration. *Encephalitis* is rare but severe, with 1 to 2% mortality and 25% of survivors having neurologic sequelae. The only treatment measures would be directed toward reducing cerebral edema. *Epididymo-orchitis* is a common complication in postpubertal males (20 to 30%), resulting in some degree of testicular atrophy in about half of those affected. It is characterized by high fever, pain, and rapid swelling of the testis. In more than two thirds of cases, testicular swelling is unilateral, and it usually follows parotitis by 1 to 10 days. Sterility is rare, and impotence is not a consequence of mumps. Treatment is with bed rest, physical support for the testis, ice packs if beneficial, and pain medications (including narcotics) as needed. Severe pain may be alleviated with 1% procaine hydrochloride block of the spermatic cord. There is no convincing evidence for the use of systemic steroids, and the use of interferon alfa-2b requires more study. *Deafness,* seen as transient loss of high-frequency tones, has been reported in approximately 4% of cases in a military population. Unilateral permanent hearing loss occurs in 1 in 20,000 cases. There is no treatment for the acute hearing loss. *Other complications* are oophoritis (in 7% of postpubertal females), pancreatitis, thyroiditis, mastitis, myocarditis, nephritis, and arthritis. Rarely, aqueductal stenosis and hydrocephalus develop after central nervous system infection.

PREVENTION

Live attenuated mumps vaccine (Jeryl Lynn strain) in the United States, given either as monovalent vaccine or combined with measles and rubella (MMR) vaccine, has been quite effective in preventing mumps disease. The number of cases of mumps has been reduced by 98 to 99% since routine vaccination was begun in 1977. The number of cases reported yearly in the United States is now approximately 1500 (1993 and 1994). Most cases occur in persons who have not been immunized, with rare cases due to waning immunity. Mumps occurring in those who have been immunized are the result of failure to respond to mumps vaccine; because the efficacy of the vaccine is approximately 90 to 95%, one would find 1 person in 10 to 20 recipients still susceptible. This should be virtually eliminated with the standard booster dose of MMR now recommended.

All children older than 12 months and other susceptible persons should now be immunized, and the vaccine is recommended at 15 months of age as MMR vaccine. A second dose of MMR is given to children at entry to school (kindergarten) or middle school. All persons should be considered susceptible unless they have documentation of (1) physician-diagnosed mumps, (2) immunization with mumps vaccine after 12 months of age, or (3) laboratory evidence of mumps immunity. One can reasonably assume that almost all people born before 1957 are naturally immune. When there is doubt about susceptibility, immunization may be performed with either monovalent vaccine or MMR, because the vaccine is quite safe, and if the patient is immune, the vaccine will simply boost protective antibody.

Mumps vaccine is produced in chick embryo cell culture. Adverse reactions to the vaccine are uncommon with the strain used in the United States. One should consult authoritative sources for direction regarding immunization of persons who have had anaphylactic reactions to eggs or neomycin. The virus is not present in the secretions of immunized children. Immunization of susceptible persons after exposure may not provide protection but is indicated. Because the vaccine contains live virus, it should not be given to pregnant women, patients receiving immunosuppressive therapy, or those with congenital or acquired immunodeficiencies. Children with mild illness and low-grade fevers may safely be immunized according to standard guidelines. Patients infected with human immunodeficiency virus should be immunized with MMR vaccine unless otherwise indicated.

EXTERNAL OTITIS

method of
CHARLES P. KIMMELMAN, M.D.
Manhattan Eye, Ear and Throat Hospital and
  Cornell Medical College
New York, New York

Otitis externa is an inflammatory condition of the external auditory canal that afflicts almost every human being at some time. The canal is a blind-ending, skin-lined invagination that terminates at the tympanic membrane. Its function is to direct sound waves gathered by the pinna to the tympanic membrane. The lateral half of the canal is supported by cartilage, and the skin contains additional elements, such as hair, sebaceous glands, and modified apocrine sweat glands. The products of the latter two glands combine with desquamated skin to form a protective coat of cerumen. The medial canal skin is thin and devoid of adnexae, with dermis lying directly on the periosteum of the tympanic bone. Because the canal is a cul-de-sac, lateral migration of cerumen and desquamated epithelium is required to keep the canal patent. This process is unique to the external canal, and interference with the migration leads to many of the disorders of the canal. Canal

problems are also the result of automanipulation with excessive removal of cerumen, leading to a breach of the protective barrier to microbial invasion. Loss of cerumen also induces itching of the canal, with resultant scratching and additional inflammation.

INFECTIOUS CAUSES

The most common presentation of external otitis is a painful, itchy ear with hearing loss. It most commonly occurs in the summer, when excessive moisture from sweating and swimming leads to obstruction of the pilosebaceous units in the lateral portion of the external auditory canal. In this setting, there is proliferation of local bacterial flora, evoking a cellulitis of the skin with swelling and occlusion of the canal. The most commonly seen bacteria are *Staphylococcus epidermidis*, *Staphylococcus aureus*, and gram-negative bacilli, such as *Pseudomonas aeruginosa*. Fungi, especially *Aspergillus* and *Candida* species, are especially prevalent in the moist external auditory canal and are common causes of external otitis. When the inflammation is localized to the hair follicles alone, small abscesses may form and require drainage. More commonly, there is a diffuse cellulitis causing a generalized edema of the canal and eventually a purulent exudate containing desquamated skin. When fungal elements are present, they may be distinguished by their characteristic fruiting bodies and dark, matlike appearance. When there is a question of the etiologic agent, a culture is indicated.

Occasionally, otitis externa has a viral causation, most often herpes simplex virus or varicella-zoster virus (herpes zoster). Herpes zoster oticus is characterized by a vesicular eruption of the pinna and external auditory canal, frequently with a facial paralysis. The external canal component of the disorder is usually of lesser importance, but the neuralgic pain associated with this condition and the need to treat the facial paralysis with corticosteroids mandate its immediate identification.

The key to the treatment of an infectious external otitis is suction débridement of infected material in the canal under microscopic guidance. This allows contact of an appropriate antimicrobial topical preparation with the inflamed skin. In cases of bacterial external otitis, a suspension of polymyxin, neomycin, and hydrocortisone (Cortisporin) is preferred. Fungal infections respond to acidification of the ear canal with an acetic acid preparation (VōSol HC Otic) or a more specific antifungal agent, such as nystatin or tolnaftate (Tinactin). Analgesics for severe pain should also be prescribed, and the ear should be kept scrupulously dry for at least 1 week with an occlusive plug during bathing. Swimming should be avoided until the infection has resolved. Débridement may have to be repeated every few days in severe cases.

In immunocompromised individuals, the external canal infection tends to be caused by *P. aeruginosa*, which may become invasive, leading to osteomyelitis of the temporal bone. This condition has been called malignant or necrotizing external otitis. The classic presentation is in a diabetic who has had a prolonged period of ear pain, discharge, and hearing loss. In any diabetic or immunocompromised individual with an external otitis that does not respond within a few days, this diagnosis should be considered. Evaluation in this case would include a culture to determine the organism and its sensitivities, computed tomography of the temporal bone to detect bony erosion, and biopsy of the characteristic granulation tissue at the bony-cartilaginous junction to exclude the possibility of a neoplasm. Treatment should be started with débridement; systemic antibiotics, such as ciprofloxacin, to eradicate the *Pseudomonas* organism; and topical antipseudomonal agents such as ciprofloxacin ophthalmic (Ciloxan).* Once the infection extends deep into the temporal bone, intravenous antibiotics (tobramycin with or without ticarcillin, ceftazidime) are required for at least 6 weeks to control and eradicate the infection. Surgical intervention is limited to repeated débridement of necrotic tissue or drainage of an abscess. Extensive surgery rarely improves the outcome.

Malignant external otitis is life-threatening; the infection can insidiously progress to involve the skull base, cranial nerves, dural venous sinuses, deep cervical fascial spaces, and opposite temporal bone. The end point of therapy for malignant external otitis is determined by the absence of obvious inflammatory changes in the external auditory canal, cessation of pain, and a normal gallium radionuclide scan. The last is sensitive to inflammation and will remain positive when the bony infection is still present. Despite prolonged intensive therapy for many months, a small percentage of patients may still succumb to this disease.

CONTACT DERMATITIS

Rarely, an external otitis seems to worsen during treatment, and the exudate becomes more profuse; the possibility of a contact dermatitis to topical therapy should be considered. Extension of the inflammation onto the pinna and face is not unusual in this case. The antimicrobial drop should be discontinued and substituted with an acidifying preparation (VōSol, Domeboro), and a systemic antibiotic (ciprofloxacin) should be added. Other foreign substances, such as chemical hair treatments and hearing aids, may also initiate contact dermatitis. The treatment is removal of the offending agent, débridement of the canal, and application of a corticosteroid cream or suspension.

TRAUMA

Trauma to the external auditory canal is another cause of inflammation. This is usually the result of the use of cotton-tipped swabs or other objects to remove impacted cerumen or to relieve itching in the

*Not FDA approved for this indication.

external canal. The delicate skin is easily torn, and a secondary bacterial infection can ensue. Trauma can also be caused by the retention of a foreign body (usually in children) or by the entry of an insect. The foreign body must be removed under microscopic control, and antibiotic drops should be administered. Because a struggling insect causes pain, it should be immobilized by several drops of lidocaine applied to the ear canal before removal.

ATOPIC DERMATITIS

Atopic dermatitis is an occasional cause of external canal inflammation. This poorly understood disease may have an allergic basis, but it also seems to be exacerbated by emotional stress or physical factors such as chemicals. It is recurrent and is characterized by severe itching and subsequent thickening of the skin with erythema. Treatment involves corticosteroid drops or creams and, occasionally, surgical excision of the chronically inflamed skin when the canal is irreversibly narrowed or stenotic. Occasionally, autoimmune skin disorders such as pemphigus, lichen planus, and scleroderma may affect the external auditory canal. They are usually seen along with systemic manifestations, but the ear involvement may be severe. Treatment with topical corticosteroid preparations and ear canal débridement is indicated.

IMPAIRED SKIN MIGRATION

As mentioned previously, the normal lateral migration of canal skin is crucial to the maintenance of a normal external auditory canal. This process can be overwhelmed in psoriasis, in which the excessive proliferation of skin rapidly fills the canal with a keratin plug. This plug needs to be removed frequently and the skin treated with topical corticosteroids. Sometimes the canal skin fails to migrate for obscure reasons, and a keratin plug quickly forms; the designation keratosis obturans has been applied to this condition. It may be associated with bronchiectasis and sinusitis. As with other disorders, frequent débridement of the plug is required; often the condition spontaneously resolves. Lateral migration of canal skin is also impaired when the bony canal contains an exostosis, or bony thickening. These proliferative lesions occur in swimmers from the repeated contact of the canal with cold water, which stimulates new periosteal bone growth. The canal stenosis leads to a build-up of migrating keratin debris, which serves as a culture medium for microbes. Removal of larger exostoses is required if infections are frequent.

CHOLESTEATOMA

A cholesteatoma of the external auditory canal is an aggressive change in the skin of the medial canal with bony invasion and destruction. There is eventual erosion of the inferior medial bony canal so that the deeper middle ear structures become exposed.

This condition usually occurs in elderly individuals and can be managed by frequent débridement and corticosteroid drops. Surgical removal of the invasive skin with canal reconstruction may be required.

CONGENITAL MALFORMATIONS

In rare instances, congenital malformations of the first branchial cleft apparatus may lead to canal swelling and infection. The first branchial cleft normally gives rise to the external auditory canal. The remnants or duplications of first cleft structures have an intimate relationship with the parotid gland and facial nerve. After resolution of the acute inflammation, evaluation with computed tomography may reveal a component of the lesion in the parotid or periauricular region. Sometimes, there is a porelike opening leading from the external canal into a sinus tract with or without an attached cyst. Surgical extirpation of the lesion will prevent recurrent infections, and the operating surgeon must be able to follow the tract through the parotid gland with dissection and preservation of the facial nerve.

REFRACTORY OTITIS

Occasionally, a case of external otitis is particularly refractory to treatment. The application of various types of antimicrobial drops, use of corticosteroid drops, and frequent débridement may fail to resolve the inflammation. When the canal is severely swollen, the use of a wick for 24 hours often helps draw the drops into the medial portion of the canal. A culture can be helpful in guiding therapy, because a resistant or unusual organism may be present. The possibility of a fungal etiology should also be considered in these instances. Malignant external otitis, although unlikely in an immunocompetent individual, should also be entertained. Sometimes the canal is extremely sensitive to the various types of topical medications, and all topical preparations may have to be stopped. When the presumed infection appears to be extending beyond the confines of the skin of the external auditory canal, systemic therapy with an appropriate antibiotic or antifungal is indicated. This should be based on culture and sensitivity results. Often, ciprofloxacin is used initially because of its excellent activity against *Pseudomonas*.

TUMOR

If the inflammation continues to fail to respond, the possibility of a neoplasm should also be considered. These tumors usually arise in the setting of prolonged external otitis and may be indistinguishable from a purely inflammatory process. A biopsy and a high index of suspicion are the best means of identifying these lesions. The most common diseases are squamous cell carcinoma in the medial canal and basal cell carcinoma in the region of the external auditory meatus; adenocarcinoma arising from the cerumen glands and melanoma are also seen. Treatment modalities include surgical extirpation with or without radiation therapy.

PLAGUE

method of
WILLIAM P. REED, M.D.
Veterans Affairs Medical Center
Albuquerque, New Mexico

Plague is a worldwide disease that was imported into the United States from Asia around 1900. Initially the disease occurred largely in California, but now most of the cases occur in New Mexico. Plague has also been acquired in California, Colorado, Arizona, Utah, Oregon, and a few other locations. Fewer than 40 cases per year have been diagnosed in this country during the past 50 years. The seriousness of the disease is illustrated by the high mortality in Europe, where the Black Death was estimated to have killed 25 million persons, or about one quarter of the population, in the mid-14th century. At that time, plague occurred as a rat-flea-rat epidemic that was readily transmitted to human beings in an urban setting. The epidemiology is now quite different, because plague largely exists in the United States as a flea-transmitted epizootic involving rodents and other wild animals. Humans and domestic pets only occasionally become infected. When domestic pets in rural or semirural areas come into contact with dead or ill flea-infested animals infected with plague, the fleas may be brought home and subsequently infect humans. Most cases occur in the warmer months, and many are acquired within about 1 mile of home. Other cases are seen in people whose occupation brings them in contact with infected animals, or through hunting and recreational activities. Males and females are about equally infected, and about 60% of the cases occur in persons younger than 20 years. Although plague has been sylvatic in the United States since the 1920s, urban epidemics remain possible, especially in view of the fact that urban rodent populations have occasionally been found to be infected with the organism.

CLINICAL MANIFESTATIONS

A history of possible exposure is usually present and has occurred 2 to 7 days before the patient seeks medical attention. Fever is usually present, and 85 to 90% of the infected people have painful lymphadenopathy, often with an area of surrounding edema and erythema. Inguinal-femoral nodes are most commonly involved, but axillary, cervical, epitrochlear, and other nodes can also be involved. Even mediastinal node enlargement may be demonstrable by radiography. Single-node involvement is quite common, but multiple nodes may be found, a situation that leads to a poorer prognosis. Between 10 and 15% of patients have septicemic plague, in which no lymphadenopathy is detected on initial examination but blood cultures are positive. These patients may present only with fever, malaise, nausea, vomiting, diarrhea, or even shock.

Primary infection of the lung can be acquired from aerosol spread of the organisms, but fortunately, this is uncommon in the United States. Primary pneumonic plague can have an extremely rapid course, with death in 2 to 3 days. Pulmonary infiltrates or mediastinal adenopathy occurs in approximately 10% of patients with bubonic or septicemic plague.

The diagnosis of plague requires a high level of suspicion. A history of having been in a setting where exposure is possible is quite common, but the flea bite itself is usually unrecognized either by history or on physical examination. Fever and the usually characteristic bubo are readily recognizable, but at times, there may be no bubo, or it may simply be missed on examination. This is especially true when the patient has been in a distant area where plague is more likely and has now returned to a place where it is quite rare. An initial rapid diagnosis may be made by aspirating the bubo under strict precautions with personnel wearing protective clothing, including masks. Bacteriologic stains using the Gram or, preferably, the Wayson method may show organisms with characteristic bipolar staining. However, a fluorescent antibody stain is more satisfactory and can usually be arranged through state public health laboratories. Aspirated material should be cultured, and at least two blood cultures should be obtained. The laboratory should be informed that plague is suspected. Blood cultures are positive in about 80% of cases, but growth may require 2 to 3 days of incubation. Occasionally, the level of bacteremia is so high that organisms can be seen microscopically in the blood. Incorrect initial diagnoses include streptococcal or staphylococcal lymphadenitis, tularemia, incarcerated inguinal hernia, acute appendicitis, cat-scratch fever, and sepsis of unknown origin. Serologic diagnostic techniques are readily available and accurate, but the tests do not become positive until the second week of illness.

TREATMENT

When bubonic plague is untreated, the mortality rate is in the range of 50 to 60%. Thus, patients who are at risk and have a characteristic disease must be treated as rapidly as possible even in the absence of a definitive diagnosis. Such a patient should initially be strictly isolated, even one who has no cough or pulmonary infiltrate. The isolation may be relaxed after 48 hours of treatment if there are no signs of pulmonary disease. No treatment has ever been shown to be superior to intramuscular streptomycin, 30 mg per kg per day in two divided doses. Clinical experience suggests that other aminoglycosides are as effective, but clinical studies are lacking. When the patient presents in shock and absorption of intramuscular drugs is questionable, it is probably preferable to use intravenous gentamicin (Garamycin),* at a single daily dose of 5.1 mg per kg. Doxycycline (Vibramycin),* 2 to 4 mg per kg per day in two divided doses, or chloramphenicol,* 25 to 60 mg per kg per day in four divided intravenous or oral doses, is also effective, and these agents are commonly given in addition to the aminoglycoside. When meningitis is suspected or proved or when abscesses or unusual locations are involved, chloramphenicol should be given because of its excellent penetration into all tissue sites and abscesses. Trimethoprim-sulfamethoxazole (Bactrim, Septra)* may also be effective. Superinfection of buboes with other organisms can occur. Antibiotic sensitivity tests are not necessarily a good guide for antibiotic treatment of

*Not FDA approved for this indication.

plague. For instance, the organism is often reported as sensitive to ampicillin, but this drug as well as some other penicillins and cephalosporins are clinically disappointing. In patients with mild disease or rapid improvement, the aminoglycoside may be stopped in 3 to 5 days, and oral therapy with one of the other drugs continued for a total of 10 days of treatment. Public health authorities should be notified about suspected or proven cases so that they can conduct appropriate surveillance.

PREVENTION

The best way to prevent plague is to avoid situations in which it may be acquired. Persons in endemic areas should avoid wild rodents, carnivores, and especially carcasses during summer. Persons who have rural or semirural homes in such areas should take measures to remove potential rodent food and living places from around their homes. Appropriate measures should be taken to control fleas on household pets. A vaccine is available and has been shown to reduce the frequency and severity of plague, and it may be indicated for individuals whose occupation places them at high risk for the disease.

A major problem exists when people have been exposed to a patient with proven plague. Household contacts are considered to have about a 5% chance of developing plague, which is also likely to be flea-borne. Health care and laboratory workers may also be at risk, and others who might be at risk could include people who have been in a waiting room with a patient who has a cough and pulmonary infiltrates due to plague. A common practice is to treat such high-risk contacts with tetracycline* (15 mg per kg per day) or a sulfonamide* such as sulfamethoxazole (Gantanol)* or trimethoprim-sulfamethoxazole* at a daily sulfamethoxazole dose of 20 to 40 mg per kg for 5 to 7 days.

*Not FDA approved for this indication.

PSITTACOSIS

method of
ROBIN McKENZIE, M.D.
Johns Hopkins University School of Medicine
Baltimore, Maryland

Chlamydiae are intracellular bacteria. The genus *Chlamydia* contains three species: *Chlamydia trachomatis*, *Chlamydia pneumoniae*, and *Chlamydia psittaci*. *C. trachomatis*, well recognized as a cause of ocular trachoma and sexually transmitted diseases, is also a common cause of neonatal pneumonia. Neonatal infection is acquired at birth from mothers with genital infection.

A newly discovered, but not new, species, *C. pneumoniae* is a common cause of community-acquired pneumonia. Serologic studies in different countries suggest that infection with *C. pneumoniae* is common after age 5 years, individuals may be reinfected, and almost everyone is eventually infected. Although asymptomatic and mild infections occur frequently, *C. pneumoniae* has been shown in various studies to cause 6 to 12% of community-acquired pneumonia. It is, therefore, a much more common cause of pneumonia than are the other two *Chlamydia* species. Unlike *C. psittaci,* it has no bird or animal reservoir.

C. psittaci causes psittacosis, a systemic zoonosis. This organism, which frequently infects birds, only occasionally spreads to humans and other mammals. The commonly used term psittacosis derives from the Greek word for parrot, *psittakos.* "Ornithosis" more accurately refers to all birds as possible sources of human infection. Rarely, other animals infect humans. Persons at greatest risk are owners of pet birds, those who work with poultry (especially turkeys and ducks), abattoir workers, and veterinarians. Anyone, however, who has contact with a bird, especially a sick bird, is at risk. Infection occurs by inhalation of dried feces or nasal or lacrimal secretions, in which the organism can survive for long periods. Exposure may be indirect. Cases have occurred in persons who merely entered a room where infected birds had been. Occasional cases have been reported after exposure to infected sheep, cows, cats, and other humans. However, some cases without bird contact diagnosed as psittacosis by the genus-specific complement fixation test have been shown by more specific tests to be caused by *C. pneumoniae.*

PRESENTATION AND DIAGNOSIS

Human infection with C. *psittaci* may be aymptomatic or may produce severe, even fatal, systemic illness. The incubation period is generally 7 to 10 days with a range of 4 to 29 days. The most commonly reported illness is pneumonia. Onset is frequently abrupt, with flulike symptoms: fever, chills, headache, and myalgias. Headache may be severe enough to elicit lumbar puncture. Cough is often nonproductive initially and frequently delayed, occurring 4 or more days after the onset of illness. Some patients experience nausea, vomiting, or diarrhea. Rare complications include endocarditis, myocarditis, pericarditis, hepatitis, reactive arthritis, and a variety of neurologic abnormalities, such as cranial nerve palsies, transverse myelitis, and encephalitis.

A relative bradycardia may be present. Severely ill patients may be confused. Auscultation of the chest frequently reveals only a few crackles. Splenomegaly, present in a minority of cases, is a helpful clue. Cutaneous eruptions, including blanching maculopapules (Horder's spots), urticaria, erythema nodosum, and erythema multiforme, are occasionally present.

The white blood cell count is usually normal or only slightly elevated, although a left shift is often present. Hepatic enzyme values are elevated in approximately one half of cases. If examined, cerebrospinal fluid is usually normal; the protein value is elevated in a minority of cases. The chest radiograph often shows an infiltrate confined to a single lower lobe.

A diagnosis of psittacosis should be considered in anyone with pneumonia or a severe systemic illness who has had contact with birds. Culturing the organism from blood, sputum, or pleural fluid is difficult and dangerous to laboratory personnel. The diagnosis, therefore, is usually made serologically. The most commonly used serologic test is the complement fixation test, with a fourfold increase in titer to at least 1:32 being considered positive. Because this test does not distinguish among the three species of chlamydiae, such a rise in titer may also have resulted from infection with *C. pneumoniae,* a more common cause of pneumo-

nia. Microimmunofluorescent IgG and IgM tests are more species specific, but cross-reactivity still causes false-positive results. Because all strains of *C. psittaci* are not represented, false-negative results also occur. Rapid detection of antigen in sputum has been accomplished by using the enzyme-linked immunosorbent assay and polymerase chain reaction techniques.

TREATMENT

The preferred treatment for adults is doxycycline (Vibramycin), 100 mg twice daily, or tetracycline, 500 mg four times daily, for 10 to 21 days. Erythromycin,* 500 mg four times daily, is an alternative treatment but may be less effective. Clarithromycin (Biaxin),* 250 to 500 mg twice daily, or azithromycin (Zithromax),* 500 mg the first day followed by 250 mg daily thereafter for 10 to 21 days, may be efficacious, although there is little experience with these agents. Although patients have been treated with chloramphenicol and rifampin (Rifadin),* relapses have occurred. Penicillins and cephalosporins are ineffective. With appropriate treatment, patients generally improve in 24 to 48 hours, and the mortality of 20% in untreated patients drops to 1%.

Preventive measures should include quarantine and long-term antibiotic prophylaxis for all imported birds. Many birds, however, are imported without adequate antibiotics. All cases of psittacosis should be reported and fully investigated, and all ill birds should be treated with antibiotics.

---

*Not FDA approved for this indication.

Q FEVER

method of
ROBERT C. KIMBROUGH, III, M.D.
Texas Tech University Health Sciences Center
Lubbock, Texas

Q fever is a zoonotic illness of humans that produces pneumonia, granulomatous hepatitis, a flulike syndrome, and meningoencephalitis. The chronic illness may be manifested by blood culture–negative endocarditis, infections of vascular aneurysms and vascular prostheses, and osteomyelitis. The acute illness is a self-limited disease, but the chronic illness is quite prolonged and severe enough to cause mortality exceeding 65%. The etiologic agent of Q fever is a gram-negative bacterium that is an obligant intracellular organism. It is classified in the family Rickettsiaceae and is named *Coxiella burnetii.* The illnesses caused by this *Rickettsia* organism differ from those of other *Rickettsia* species in that no rash is produced.

C. burnetii is highly infectious. It survives for long periods despite drying, heat, sun, and various chemical exposures. The organism is carried by cattle, sheep, and goats, and has been reported to be carried by cats and other animals. It may also be carried in ticks. The organism is found in body fluids, excreta, meat, uterus, and the placenta of carrier animals. Drying of these products and the aerosolization of the blood and postpartum discharges lead

TABLE 1. **Therapy for Acute Q Fever**

Antibiotic	Dose	Route	Duration
Tetracycline	500 mg q 6 h	Oral	2–3 wk
Doxycycline (Vibramycin)	100 mg q 12 h	Oral	2–3 wk
Co-trimoxazole (Bactrim or Septra)	1 double-strength tablet q 12 h	Oral	2–3 wk
Erythromycin	500 mg q 6 h	Oral	2–3 wk

to infection in humans by inhalation of the dust or of aerosolized organisms or by the drinking of unpasteurized milk. Workers in dairies, slaughterhouses, and veterinary practices, as well as farmers and laboratory personnel are at highest risk. The illness may be asymptomatic in animals and is asymptomatic for ticks. In humans, however, it manifests as a self-limited pneumonia or flulike illness or a chronic illness that may lead to endocarditis.

The incubation period is 10 to 40 days with an average of 20 days. The acute illness is that of a gradual onset of various nonspecific or flulike symptoms characterized by fever (temperature as high as 104°F) and severe headache with retrobulbar pain. No rash is apparent. The usual illness is that of a gradual onset of atypical pneumonia or the appearance of granulomatous hepatitis. Chronic Q fever may have few specific signs or symptoms.

The diagnosis of Q fever is usually based on a history of exposure and appropriate serologic testing. The organism lives in two phases, with phase I being the infectious phase and phase II being the organism that has been passed in egg yolk cultures. Antibodies to both phases are present in both the acute and the chronic forms; however, antibodies to phase II are higher in the acute illness, and antibodies to phase I are present in higher levels only in the chronic form of the illness. Antibodies may be detected by complement fixation, indirect immunofluorescence assay (IFA), or enzyme-linked immunosorbent assay (ELISA). The IFA and ELISA are the most accurate.

TREATMENT

The acute illness is self-limited. Unfortunately, there is no way to predict whether the acute illness may progress to one of the chronic illnesses. Thus, it is recommended that the acute illness be treated (Table 1). It is difficult to perform susceptibility testing with *C. burnetii*, because the organism requires strict intracellular growth. However, the use of antibiotics that control other rickettsial illnesses has been successful in controlling the acute illness. More recent methods have enabled susceptibility testing to

be performed, and these tests have confirmed the organisms' sensitivity to various antibiotics that have been proved useful in a clinical setting.

Tetracycline and its analogues have been the treatment of choice, with erythromycin and co-trimoxazole being useful alternatives. The quinolone antibiotics have also been found to be useful. Neither the tetracyclines nor the quinolones should be used for children younger than 10 to 12 years. None of the antibiotics used alone is effective for the chronic illness or endocarditis. All should be used in the acute illness for 2 to 3 weeks.

The treatment of chronic Q fever and endocarditis is quite prolonged and may require prosthesis or valve replacement (Table 2). The combination of tetracycline or one of its analogues plus rifampin, used for approximately 3 years, has been shown to render heart valves sterile. Co-trimoxazole plus rifampin has also been found to be effective, as have the quinolones plus rifampin. None of these drugs is bactericidal when used alone. In susceptibility testing, tetracycline and its analogues, rifampin, and co-trimoxazole were found to be effective against all strains tested. However, there was varying sensitivity to chloramphenicol, azithromycin, and the quinolones.

PREVENTION

There is no vaccine approved for human use in the United States. Vaccine has been successfully used in Australia. However, some animal vaccines are available in the United States. Because most animals are asymptomatic, it is difficult to screen all herds or vaccinate all animals to eradicate the infection. Therefore, attempts at prevention should be directed to persons in high-risk occupational groups. Inhalation of aerosolized body fluids and products of concep-

TABLE 2. **Therapy for Chronic Q Fever***

Antibiotic	Dose	Route	Duration (y)
Doxycycline (Vibramycin)	100 mg q 12 h	Intravenous or oral	3
Quinolone (various)	Varies with drug	Intravenous or oral	3
Co-trimoxazole (Bactrim or Septra)	1 double-strength tablet or intravenous equivalent q 12 h	Intravenous or oral	3
	plus		
Rifampin (Rifadin)	300–600 mg q 12 h	Intravenous or oral	3

*Endocarditis usually requires valve replacement. Infected prosthesis requires removal and replacement of the prosthesis.

tion of the animals should be reduced. Workers in research settings, particularly those using pregnant sheep, should be serologically screened at routine intervals for asymptomatic disease.

RABIES

method of
SUZANNE R. JENKINS, V.M.D., M.P.H.
Virginia Department of Health, Office of
    Epidemiology
Richmond, Virginia

Although only 30 cases of human rabies were diagnosed in the United States from 1980 to 1996, animal bites are quite common; between 1 and 4.5 million occur each year. Thus, the clinician is more likely to be faced with a decision about the management of a potential rabies exposure than with the diagnosis and treatment of the actual disease. Rabies among animals, particularly wild animals, is common in this country. In 1995, only 8% of the 7881 animals reported as rabid were domestic; however, exposures to domestic animals, especially dogs and cats, account for the majority of human postexposure treatments.

Rabies is caused by a rhabdovirus that can infect any warm-blooded animal but tends to predominate in a particular species in a defined geographic area. For example, there is a raccoon rabies outbreak affecting all of the East Coast states; skunk rabies exists in a wide band through the middle part of the country as well as in California; and coyote rabies has been spreading in Texas. Although the predominant species may make up more than 85% of the animal rabies cases in an area, spillover to any other mammal, including humans, is possible. Also, there is always the potential for isolated cases of rabies to occur among bats or in an individual animal that has been bitten by a rabid bat.

Ecotypes and variants of rabies virus are now being defined through the use of panels of monoclonal antibodies and by nucleotide sequencing of polymerase chain reaction–amplified virus. These techniques can help explain the distribution of rabies among various animal species and identify the source of human infections. Of the 30 humans diagnosed with rabies in the United States since 1980, 12 are presumed to have acquired the infection from dogs in another country, 1 was infected with a skunk variant, and 2 were infected with the U.S./Mexico border canine strain; the remaining 15 human rabies cases were associated with various bat variants of virus, most commonly a rabies variant found in the relatively uncommon silver-haired bat.

POSTEXPOSURE DECISION-MAKING

The rabies biologics currently available in the United States are relatively safe, but because of the potential for reactions and the high cost of postexposure prophylaxis, the decision to treat should not be undertaken lightly. Each potential exposure should be evaluated on a case-by-case basis to decide the most appropriate action (Figure 1). Consultation with local or state public health officials who are familiar with the epidemiology of rabies in the spe-cific area and the availability of biologics should be sought.

The first part of the decision-making process is to ascertain whether an exposure actually took place. In rabid animals, rabies virus is present in concentrations that are considered to be infectious in the saliva, salivary glands, brain, and, less often, the spinal cord or large peripheral nerves of animals such as cattle and horses. The virus usually enters the body through broken skin; it rarely enters through intact mucous membranes. Thus, the most likely route of entry is via the bite of a rabid animal or contamination of a fresh open wound by saliva. Petting a rabid animal or coming in contact with its blood, urine, or feces does not constitute an exposure. Aerosol transmission of rabies has occurred only under special circumstances in which there were high concentrations of suspended droplets carrying viral particles, such as in laboratories with concentrated virus used for vaccine production, and bat caves containing unusually high numbers of bats. Infections have also resulted from corneal transplants.

If it is established that a true exposure has taken place, the next step is to ascertain the likelihood that the animal could transmit rabies. In dogs and cats, signs of rabies usually accompany the shedding of virus in saliva. Rarely, the onset of signs can be delayed for up to 5 days. If a dog or cat that bites someone is considered to be normal by a veterinarian, animal control officer, or public health official, it should be placed in confinement and observed for 10 days. As long as no signs of illness or behavioral changes indicative of rabies occur, rabies postexposure treatment of the exposed person is not necessary. A dog or cat that shows signs at the time of the bite or develops them during the period of confinement should be euthanized immediately, and the head should be shipped to an appropriate laboratory for testing. The 10-day confinement applies to both vaccinated and unvaccinated animals. Although the risk of rabies in a vaccinated dog or cat is extremely low, vaccine failures do occur, most commonly in young animals that have received only an initial rabies vaccination.

If the exposure occurred from a dog or cat that is not available for observation or testing (e.g., a stray animal that cannot be located or a pet that disappears), the decision about postexposure prophylaxis should be based on the presence of animal rabies in the area and the circumstances of the biting incident, that is, whether the animal was behaving normally and whether the bite was provoked. The expertise of local or state public health officials should always be sought in these cases.

Although exposures from other domestic animals such as livestock have the potential for transmitting rabies, the risk of acquiring the disease from these species is extremely low, and treatment of the person is not usually indicated unless the animal is symptomatic or its brain is found to be positive when examined for virus. Because the period of rabies virus shedding in wild and exotic animals is unknown,

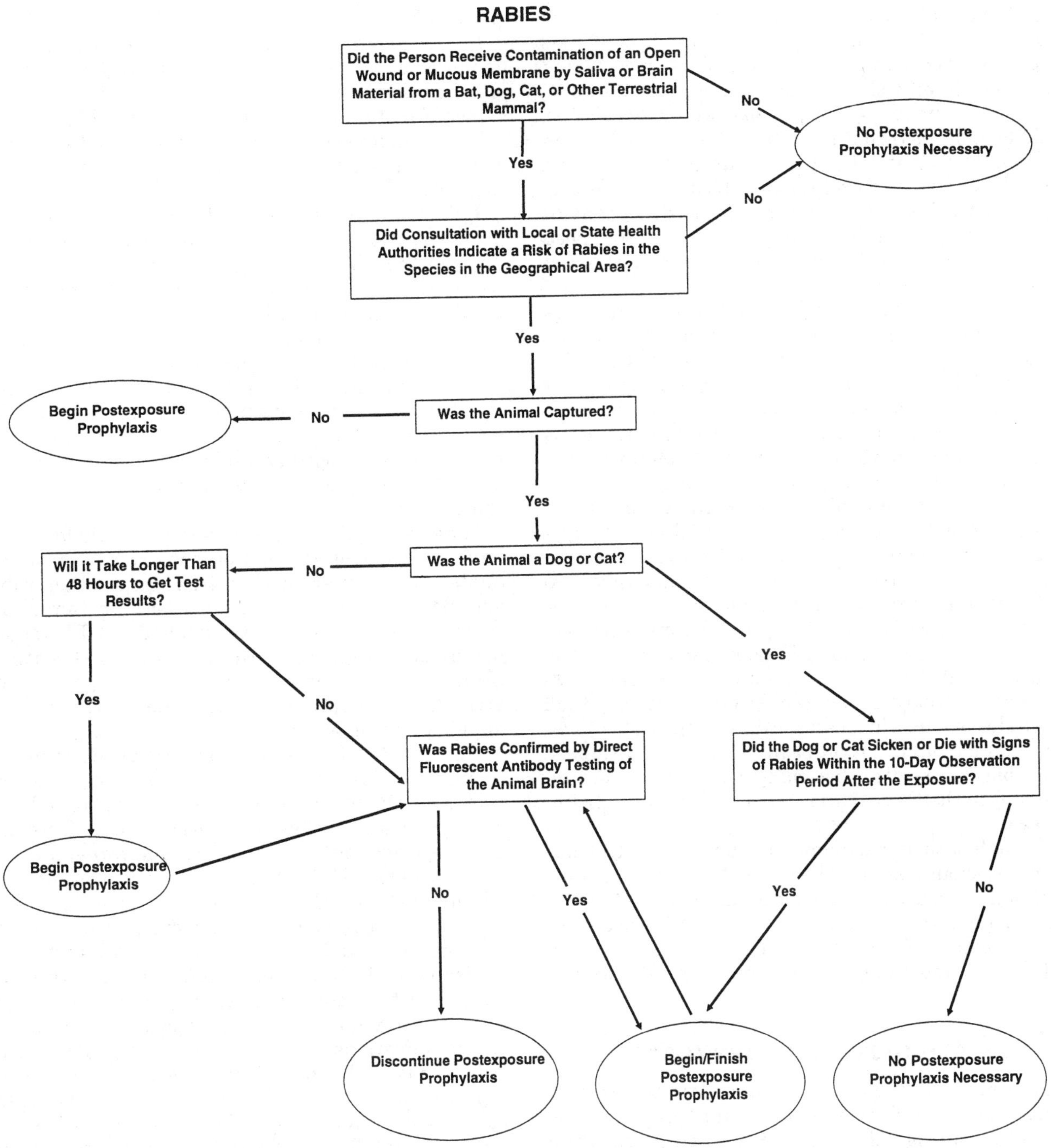

RABIES

Figure 1. *Note:* Consult accompanying text before using this algorithm.

even those that are kept as pets cannot be managed the same way as dogs and cats. Pet skunks, foxes, raccoons, and other wild carnivores that bite humans should, under most circumstances, be euthanized and tested for rabies.

The major wildlife reservoirs of rabies in this country are skunks, raccoons, foxes, coyotes, and bats, and exposure from any of these animals should be considered a high rabies risk. Unless the animal's brain can be submitted for rabies testing, postexposure prophylaxis should always be instituted when a person has been bitten by one of these species. Expo-

sures to bats appear to require an even higher index of suspicion. After reports of rabies in persons who had been in the proximity of bats but were not aware of a bite from the animal, public health officials began recommending that postexposure prophylaxis be considered if a bite or scratch from a bat that tested positive or was not available for testing could not be ruled out. Examples of such situations are (1) a sleeping individual awakes to find a bat in the room and (2) an adult witnesses a bat in a room with a previously unattended child, a mentally challenged person, or an intoxicated individual.

Animals that are unlikely to be rabid and for which exposure rarely requires postexposure prophylaxis include hooved mammals (such as deer, moose, and antelope), small rodents (such as mice, rats, gerbils, hamsters, guinea pigs, squirrels, and chipmunks), and lagomorphs (rabbits and hares). Despite the high number of rodent bites that occur in this country, there has never been a human rabies case resulting from such a bite. Abnormal or aggressive behavior by any of these animals might indicate the need for postexposure prophylaxis if the animal was not available for testing.

Woodchucks (groundhogs) and beavers are large rodents that account for the majority of rabid rodents in the United States, particularly in association with the mid-Atlantic raccoon outbreak. The potential for transmission from these animals is unknown. Bites by these species in areas where wildlife rabies is endemic require postexposure prophylaxis unless the animal is found to be negative on testing.

The testing of animal brains for rabies should be carried out in laboratories that are familiar and experienced with the procedure. In the United States, the exquisitely sensitive direct fluorescent antibody (FA) test has replaced the microscopic examination for Negri bodies, which yielded up to 20% false-positive and false-negative results. In some laboratories, the mouse inoculation test is still done as part of a quality control program, but the 21-day waiting period precludes its use in postexposure prophylaxis decision-making. Inoculation of in vitro cultured mouse neuroblastoma cells is becoming a more common supplement to the FA test and can provide results within 8 days.

Local health department and animal control authorities should be contacted to institute and monitor confinement periods or to capture animals and advise on the preparation and shipment of the heads for rabies testing. A specimen should be refrigerated, not frozen, and the brain should never be placed in a fixative.

POSTEXPOSURE PROPHYLAXIS

Treatment for exposure to rabies has two components, local wound treatment and immunization. The risk of acquiring rabies can be reduced markedly if the wound is immediately and thoroughly washed with soap and water. In animal studies, the use of water or saline alone was not as effective as soap and water.

Two products are used for immunization of persons who have had no prior experience with rabies biologics, human rabies immune globulin (HRIG) and vaccine. HRIG (Hyperab, Imogam) is administered on the first day of treatment (designated day 0) to confer passive immunity until the body responds to the rabies vaccine (approximately 7 to 10 days after the initial vaccination). The dose of HRIG is 20 IU per kg of body weight. If anatomically possible, up to half of the HRIG dose should be infiltrated around the wound; the remainder should be given deep in the gluteal area. Under no circumstances should the HRIG be given in the same site as the vaccine, where it might compromise vaccine activity. HRIG is supplied in 2-mL (300-IU) and 10-mL (1500-IU) vials, which are standardized to contain 150 IU per mL. If HRIG is inadvertently not given on day 0, it can be administered up to the eighth day after the first dose of vaccine.

Rabies vaccine is administered in a series of five 1-mL injections during a 28-day period (days 0, 3, 7, 14, and 28). Two vaccines are currently licensed for use in the United States, human diploid cell vaccine (HDCV; Imovax, distributed by Connaught Laboratories) and rabies vaccine, adsorbed (RVA; distributed by SmithKline Beecham). Administration of either vaccine should be by the intramuscular route in the deltoid region. For small children, the anterolateral upper thigh can be used. Vaccine failures have been associated with administration in gluteal muscles. RVA has not been tested in children younger than 6 years.

Persons requiring postexposure prophylaxis who have a history of vaccination with HDCV or an adequate postvaccination titer from some other rabies vaccine should receive only two 1-mL intramuscular doses of vaccine given on days 0 and 3. HRIG should not be administered in these cases. Post-treatment titers are recommended only to evaluate persons who are immunocompromised and who may not mount an adequate response.

Up to 50% of persons who receive postexposure prophylaxis may report mild symptomatic reactions such as headache, nausea, myalgias, abdominal pain, and dizziness. Rarely, more serious side effects have been reported, but none has been life-threatening. At least one case of Guillain-Barré syndrome after the administration of HDCV has been reported with no permanent sequelae. Immune complex–like illness has been reported in about 6% of persons who have a history of HDCV vaccination and then receive a booster of the same vaccine. Pregnancy, existing illness, and previous allergy to rabies vaccine are not contraindications for postexposure prophylaxis if the person has had a bona fide exposure to rabies. Patients with a history of allergic reactions should be closely monitored during postexposure prophylaxis. If a different brand of vaccine is available, its use may avert a reaction. Otherwise, allergic reactions can be controlled with antihistamines, epinephrine, or corticosteroids. Corticosteroids should be used only as a last resort, because they may interfere with the production of rabies antibodies.

PRE-EXPOSURE PROPHYLAXIS

Rabies vaccines can be used for pre-exposure immunization of persons who are likely to experience an inapparent exposure, such as wildlife workers, veterinarians and their staff members, animal control officers, rabies diagnostic laboratory workers, spelunkers, and others having direct contact with animals at high risk for having rabies. Pre-exposure immunization of such populations may offer some protection for minor, unrecognized exposures and will reduce the postexposure regimen for recognized exposures. Travelers to foreign countries who will be spending more than 30 days in areas with endemic rabies should also receive rabies pre-exposure immunization. This immunization may offer protection if there are delays in receiving postexposure treatment or if HRIG is not available. A history of pre-exposure immunization does not eliminate the need for postexposure treatment after a known exposure. However, the need for HRIG is eliminated, and only 2 doses of vaccine are required, 1 on day 0 and 1 on day 3.

Pre-exposure immunization consists of three 1-mL intramuscular doses of HDCV or RVA given in the deltoid region on days 0, 7, and 28. HDCV (Imovax Rabies ID Vaccine) may also be given in three 0.1-mL intradermal doses in the deltoid region by using the same schedule as that for the 1-mL intramuscular doses. Travelers should either receive the 1-mL intramuscular series or complete the 0.1-mL intradermal series at least 30 days before departure. Postvaccination serologic testing is not recommended unless the vaccinated person is immunocompromised. For persons who have a continuing potential for exposure, a booster dose should be considered every 2 years. Because of the risk of immune complex–like illness from boosters, a titer should be obtained and a booster administered only if the titer is inadequate. Either HDCV (1 mL intramuscularly or 0.1 mL intradermally) or RVA (1 mL intramuscularly) can be administered as a booster.

CLINICAL DISEASE IN HUMANS

Although human rabies is rare in the United States, it should be included in any differential diagnosis of a person with a rapidly progressive encephalitis even if there is no history of an exposure to an infected animal. Of the 30 patients with human rabies diagnosed in the United States since 1980, 23 did not report an animal bite. This probably reflects an inadequate history, instead of nonbite transmission of the disease.

Fortunately, humans do not appear to be very susceptible to rabies. The probability of developing rabies from an animal with confirmed rabies varies from less than 1% for contamination of minor wounds to more than 80% for severe bites by rabid wolves. The risk of developing clinical disease depends on the amount and variant of virus that is inoculated, the anatomic site of the inoculation, the amount of innervation at the site, and other viral and host factors. Once symptoms develop, there is little likelihood of recovery. Only two recoveries have been documented in the United States, one complete and the other with permanent sequelae; both patients had received some form of either pre-exposure or postexposure prophylaxis. Bats may be more capable than other mammals of transmitting rabies. In vitro studies have shown that silver-haired bat rabies virus may cause disease when only a small amount of virus is superficially inoculated.

Although some symptoms of rabies may be considered to be pathognomonic, such as hydrophobia and aerophobia, most symptoms are nonspecific and so varied that the diagnosis of rabies is rarely entertained until late in the disease or is not recognized until after death, when histopathologic slides of the brain may reveal Negri bodies. Clinical rabies in humans is classically divided into five stages: incubation period, prodrome, acute neurologic phase, coma, and recovery or death. The usual incubation period is between 20 and 90 days, although it can be as short as 9 days or as long as many years.

The initial symptoms, experienced during the 2- to 10-day prodrome, are the most nonspecific and may include malaise, fatigue, headache, anorexia, fever, cough, chills, sore throat, abdominal pain, nausea, vomiting, or diarrhea. Approximately 50% of patients report pain or paresthesia at the site of inoculation. Neurologic involvement may be suggested by apprehension, anxiety, agitation, irritability, nervousness, insomnia, or depression. The first objective signs of neurologic involvement include hyperactivity, disorientation, hallucinations, seizures, bizarre behavior, nuchal rigidity, and paralysis. In most cases, hyperactive episodes either occur spontaneously or are precipitated by various stimuli. It is during this time that attempts to drink may produce severe spasms of the pharynx or larynx. Fever (temperature >100°F) occurs in almost all patients. As the disease progresses (unless respiratory or cardiac arrest causes the patient's death), paralysis develops, and mental status deteriorates from confusion to disorientation, stupor, and finally coma. Throughout the acute neurologic period, the mental status alternates between severe obtundation and relative normality. Coma occurs 4 to 10 days after onset of symptoms. In the absence of intensive supportive care, death can occur as early as 7 days after the first appearance of symptoms. With care, most patients survive for another week.

Rabies can be diagnosed by detection of antigen in direct immunofluorescent antibody–stained impressions of corneal epithelium or neck skin biopsies, isolation of virus from saliva, or demonstration of a significant titer to rabies virus in cerebrospinal fluid or serum (in the absence of a history of passive or active immunization). If these tests become positive, they usually do so late in the course of illness.

If rabies is suspected in a patient, state public health authorities should be notified to assist in evaluating the patient, provide information on proper hospital isolation procedures, and facilitate the rapid processing of laboratory tests for rabies.

RAT-BITE FEVER

method of
KAREN A. HOLBROOK, M.D.

Montefiore Medical Center
Bronx, New York

Rat-bite fever is an uncommon, systemic, febrile illness caused by either *Streptobacillus moniliformis* or *Spirillum minus*. It is typically acquired through the bite or scratch of a rat.

EPIDEMIOLOGY AND MICROBIOLOGY

S. moniliformis, a pleomorphic gram-negative bacillus that can form filaments and beadlike chains with fusiform swellings, is the etiologic agent of most of the cases of rat-bite fever in the United States. This organism colonizes the nasopharynx of 50 to 100% of both laboratory and wild rats. Although most infections are contracted from rats, some cases occur after contact with other small rodents or carnivores that prey on the rodents. Haverhill fever, a variant of rat-bite fever, occurs after oral ingestion of *S. moniliformis* (e.g., food or water contaminated with rat feces).

S. minus, a short, tightly coiled gram-negative spiral rod, rarely causes disease in the United States but is responsible for most cases of rat-bite fever in Asia. Transmission requires contact with rodents because oral ingestion of organisms leading to disease has never been documented.

CLINICAL PRESENTATION

Streptobacillary disease presents soon after the rat bite, usually within 10 days, although the incubation period ranges from 1 to 22 days. At the time of presentation, the wound has typically healed, and patients frequently do not recall a bite. Sudden onset of fever, chills, headaches, vomiting, and severe migratory arthralgias and myalgias herald the illness. Two to 4 days later, a nonpruritic, maculopapular, morbilliform, or petechial rash occurs over the palms, soles, and extremities. Approximately half of patients experience either asymmetrical polyarthritis or a true septic arthritis that usually involves the knees, ankles, elbows, wrists, or shoulders. In untreated disease, the fever typically resolves after 3 to 5 days; the other symptoms resolve within 2 weeks. Fever or arthritis occasionally continues to relapse for long periods. In addition to these symptoms, patients with Haverhill fever typically have pharyngitis and more severe vomiting.

Infection due to *S. minus* differs from streptobacillary disease in that 1 to 4 weeks after the rat bite and initial healing, the wound site becomes painful, swollen, purple, and associated with local adenopathy. It progresses to ulceration and eschar formation. Arthritis and myalgias also rarely occur. The rash may be blotchy, violaceous, or sometimes urticarial and typically occurs over the face, scalp, and trunk. In untreated disease, fever regularly recurs for months.

Serious complications of both infections include endocarditis, myocarditis, pericarditis, meningitis, pneumonia, amnionitis, abscesses in most organs, and anemia. Mortality in untreated cases ranges from 6 to 13%.

Leptospirosis represents the leading alternative diagnosis in cases with known rat exposure. Without the rat-bite history and depending on the signs and symptoms displayed, the differential diagnosis includes meningococcemia, enteric fever, drug reaction, viral exanthem, Rocky Mountain spotted fever, secondary syphilis, disseminated gonococcal infection, Lyme disease, brucellosis, septic arthritis, infective endocarditis, collagen-vascular disease, acute rheumatic fever, malaria, and lymphoma.

DIAGNOSIS

Direct visualization of organisms in appropriately stained samples of blood, exudate, or lymph node biopsy specimens assists with the diagnosis of *S. moniliformis* infection and provides the only laboratory evidence available for diagnosing *S. minus* infection. One can see *S. moniliformis* with Giemsa, Wayson, or Gram's stain. *S. moniliformis* infection is confirmed by culturing the organism in enriched media. Alternatively, a diagnosis can be made by identifying specific agglutinins that appear within 10 days of illness and disappear after 1 to 3 months. An initial titer of 1:80 or greater or a fourfold rise in titer is considered positive.

TREATMENT

Treatment of all bite wounds should include good cleaning, irrigation, débridement, and assessment of the need for tetanus prophylaxis. Both *S. moniliformis* and *S. minus* are susceptible to penicillin. Historically, procaine penicillin (600,000 units intramuscularly every 12 hours for 10 to 14 days) was used for treatment. Currently, however, serious infections should probably be treated with intravenous penicillin (600,000 units every 6 hours), and less serious infections could be treated with oral penicillin or ampicillin (500 mg four times daily). Penicillin-allergic patients can be treated with tetracycline (500 mg every 6 hours) or streptomycin (7.5 mg per kg intramuscularly every 12 hours). In vitro data suggest that erythromycin, ciprofloxacin (Cipro), chloramphenicol, or cephalosporins may be effective, but few clinical data exist.

RELAPSING FEVER

method of
MALCOLM T. FOSTER, JR., M.D.

University of Florida Health Science Center
Jacksonville, Florida

Human relapsing fever is a vector-borne systemic spirochetal disease characterized by recurrent episodes of fever and caused by many different strains of *Borrelia recurrentis.* It is transmitted to humans by the body louse, *Pediculus humanus corporis,* or by soft ticks of the Ornithodoros family. Louse-borne relapsing fever (LBRF) is transmitted by the crushing of an infected louse, which thus contaminates the bite wound. Its prevalence depends on conditions favoring heavy infestations of body lice. Epidemics occur in Asia, Africa, and South America.

The endemic tick-borne relapsing fever (TBRF) is transmitted likewise, but by the bite of an argasid (soft) tick. Rodents, chipmunks, and tree squirrels serve as reservoirs through transovarial transmission. TBRF occurs in Central and South America, the Near East and Middle East,

Africa, and the western United States. In the United States, species are vector specific; the most common are *Ornithodoros hermsi*, *Ornithodoros turicata*, and *Ornithodoros parkeri*. Outbreaks have been reported at the north rim of the Grand Canyon in Arizona and in west Texas caves. Individuals at risk are campers using log cabins or seasonally occupied mountain homes.

DIAGNOSIS

Presentation varies, ranging from mild to fulminating disease. Typical features are sudden onset of fever, headache, ocular pain, cough and chest pain, myalgia, and gastrointestinal symptoms, including nausea and vomiting. Conjunctival suffusion, pain in the gastrocnemius muscle, splenomegaly, and liver and heart involvement are all common. After an incubation period of approximately 1 week, the patient is markedly febrile for 3 to 6 days; this is followed by an afebrile period of 5 to 10 days, and then another febrile episode. LBRF has longer incubation periods and febrile episodes. TBRF may have from 3 to 10 relapses. A truncal petechial rash may present during the initial febrile episode.

Laboratory diagnosis is made by demonstrating the spirochete by darkfield microscopy or in Giemsa or Wright's stained thick and thin smears. Because of the antigenic shifts of the *Borrelia* species, serology is unreliable. The organisms may exhibit titers to the *Proteus* OXK antigen. Other laboratory tests used with limited availability are indirect fluorescent microscopy, Western blot, analysis of DNA-DNA hybridization and ribosomal RNA gene restriction patterns, and cultivation on "Kelly" media.

Differential diagnosis includes Colorado tick fever, dengue fever, malaria, typhus, leptospirosis, ehrlichiosis, and other rickettsial infections.

TREATMENT

Management consists of supportive care, antibiotic therapy, therapy of systemic symptoms, and treatment of the Jarisch-Herxheimer reaction and other complications.

Supportive Care

Because most patients are acutely ill, bed rest and proper fluid and electrolyte balance are mandatory. Systemic relief of pain and vomiting will assist in ensuring proper nutrition. Hospitalization is indicated because of possible life-threatening complications that necessitate close observation by nursing and medical staff. These complications are disseminated intravascular coagulation and splenic rupture.

Antimicrobial Therapy

Tetracyclines, erythromycin, chloramphenicol, and penicillin are effective in the treatment of relapsing fever. Tetracyclines are the drugs of choice. Erythromycin is an effective alternative therapy. See Table 1 for antibiotic treatment guidelines for TBRF. LBRF can be treated with a single dose of any of the antibiotics listed in Table 1. Ceftriaxone (Rocephin) has also been shown to work. The fatality rate for treated relapsing fever is less than 5%. Untreated LBRF has a case-fatality rate of greater than 50%. The rapid destruction and clearance of the spirochetes can provoke a severe Jarisch-Herxheimer reaction. During the late febrile stage, when the Jarisch-Herxheimer reaction is more likely to occur, small doses of procaine penicillin G,* such as 50,000 units intramuscularly every 8 hours for 6 doses, has been recommended.

Systemic Symptoms

Control of fever usually is indicated only when the temperature approaches 40°C (104°F) taken orally. Tepid water soaks are the safest form of antipyretic therapy. Hypothermic blankets may also be used if extreme temperature elevations greater than 40°C (104°F) occur. Nausea and vomiting can be managed with antiemetics such as promethazine (Phenergan), 25 mg every 4 to 6 hours rectally or intramuscularly.

Dehydration should be treated with appropriate intravenous electrolyte solutions. Clinical appearance, blood pressure, heart rate, urinary output, and central venous pressure are useful clinical observations for indicating hydration.

Pain may be moderately severe but can be controlled with nonsalicylate analgesics, such as acetaminophen, 650 mg every 4 hours orally. Salicylates should be avoided.

---

*Not FDA approved for this indication.

TABLE 1. **Treatment Guidelines for (Tick-Borne) Relapsing Fever**

Drug	Adult Dose	Pediatric Dose	Duration (d)
Tetracycline*	500 mg q 6 h IV/PO	6.25–12.5 mg kg q 6 h PO 5–7.5 mg/kg q 6 h IV	5–10
Erythromycin†	500 mg q 6 h IV/PO	7.5–12.5 mg/kg q 6 h PO 3.75–12.5 mg/kg q 6 h IV	5–10
Doxycycline*	100 mg q 12 h IV/PO	1.1–2.2 mg/kg q 12 h IV/PO	5–10
Chloramphenicol‡	12.5–25 mg/kg q 6 h IV/PO	Same as adult	5–10
Penicillin G†	0.5–1 gm q 6 h PO 20 million U/d × 10 d IV	100,000–250,000 U/kg/d (given in doses q 4–6 h)	10

*Contraindicated in pregnant women and in children younger than 8 y.
†Not FDA approved for this infection.
‡Incidence of aplastic anemia is reported at 1:24,500–40,800.

Jarisch-Herxheimer Reaction

Typically, patients who exhibit the Jarisch-Herxheimer reaction received tetracycline during the late febrile period or between relapses and displayed no adverse reaction for several hours. The reaction is caused by the rapid destruction of the spirochetes. It is characterized by sudden chill, temperature elevation, and tachycardia. After a short time, profound vasodilatation follows, which may result in shock. Direct measurements have shown the cardiac output to be increased and the total peripheral resistance to be decreased during this state. The phenomenon usually lasts from 8 to 12 hours, and recovery ensues. Hypotension may be controlled with appropriate intravenous fluid therapy. Patients in shock should receive oxygen, and older patients with heart failure may require digitalization. Corticosteroid therapy has not proved effective in treating the Jarisch-Herxheimer reaction.

Other Complications

Disseminated intravascular coagulation (DIC) rarely occurs. However, any hemorrhagic phenomenon occurring in a patient with relapsing fever should suggest DIC. Therapy consists of the following measures: (1) control of the infection with antibiotics, (2) anticoagulation with heparin, 600 to 850 USP units per kg every 24 hours by intravenous infusion, and (3) transfusion (if indicated) with fresh blood, platelet-rich plasma, or platelet concentrates.

Prolonged prothrombin time without DIC is fairly common in this entity. This can be reversed by the administration of 10 to 20 mg of vitamin K_1 oxide intramuscularly. Should intense abdominal pain occur in a patient with splenomegaly, one should consider splenic rupture. Splenectomy should be performed on an emergency basis.

PREVENTION

Controlling tick and louse population with pesticides is the keystone of control of relapsing fever. Personal protection includes using repellents and permethrin (Elimite) on clothing and bedding in endemic areas. Antibiotic chemoprophylaxis with tetracycline may be initiated when there is suspicion of exposure. Health care workers should follow universal precautions with a hospitalized patient. Isolation is not required.

RHEUMATIC FEVER

method of
HARRY R. HILL, M.D.
University of Utah School of Medicine
Salt Lake City, Utah

Acute rheumatic fever (ARF) is one of the leading causes of acquired heart disease in young people in the world. Rheumatic fever is a nonsuppurative sequela of a group A streptococcal pharyngitis that may involve the joints, skin, heart, and central nervous system, resulting in migratory polyarthritis, erythema marginatum, subcutaneous nodules, carditis, and chorea. The incidence of rheumatic fever has declined in developed countries in the past 30 years but remains high in developing countries. Moreover, a resurgence of ARF has occurred in several areas of the United States during the past decade, suggesting that physicians should not become complacent about streptococcal infections and their nonsuppurative complications.

The peak incidence of ARF follows that of streptococcal pharyngitis, residing between 5 and 15 years of age, although rarely, individuals younger than 3 years and older than 15 years do suffer new attacks. There appears to be an inherited susceptibility to develop ARF, in that as many as 30 to 50% of patients have a family history of the disease. The exact mode of inheritance of this susceptibility has not been completely deciphered.

PRIMARY PREVENTION

ARF may follow group A streptococcal pharyngitis but does not come after skin infection due to these organisms. This feature has led to some speculation on the link between the pharynx and the heart. Unfortunately, the signs and symptoms of group A streptococcal pharyngitis may vary widely from the classic onset of sore throat, fever, enlarged tender anterior cervical lymphadenopathy, and palatal petechiae to asymptomatic acquisition of the organisms. In fact, during the resurgence of ARF in the area my colleagues and I serve, a minority of our patients even noted a preceding respiratory infection. Thus, a high index of suspicion of streptococcal respiratory infection must be maintained by deliverers of health care.

Although some studies may claim slightly better results, I suggest that most clinicians have only a 50% chance of correctly diagnosing a group A streptococcal pharyngitis on the basis of clinical findings alone. Thus, it is essential that in all patients suspected of having group A disease, a throat culture be performed. Furthermore, it should be remembered that group A streptococcal antigen detection tests are only 80% to, at best, 90% sensitive, so all negative results must be confirmed by culture on sheep blood agar plates.

Primary prevention of ARF in patients with proven group A streptococcal pharyngitis depends on prompt (less than 10 days after acquisition) and prolonged (at least 10 days) therapy. The drug of choice in treating group A streptococcal pharyngitis remains penicillin, because resistant strains have not been described. The use of broad-spectrum penicillins and cephalosporins offers no advantages over penicillin; their use should be discouraged, in most cases. Penicillin V, in a dose of 250 mg or 400,000 units every 8 hours for 10 full days, is adequate for both children and adults. If twice-a-day dosing is preferred, 500 mg bid can be utilized. If compliance may be a problem, during outbreaks of disease, or if there is a family history of ARF, a better choice may be long-acting benzathine penicillin G, in a dose of 1.2 million units intramuscularly for patients weighing more than 60 pounds and 600,000 units for those weighing less than 60 pounds. In the penicillin-allergic individual, erythromycin, 50 mg per kg per day in three or four divided doses up to 1 gram per day for 10 full days, may be used. Clindamycin (Cleocin) is an alternative. Oral cephalosporins may also be employed, but there is 5 to 10% cross-sensitivity in penicillin-allergic individuals, so caution must be maintained.

Again, a therapeutic concentration of antibiotic must be maintained for 10 full days to eradicate group A streptococci from the pharynx. Such a regimen prevents more than 90% of cases of ARF. In endemic circumstances, 15% to as high as 25% of school-age children may be carrying group A streptococci during late winter or spring. Thus, not uncommonly, children who present to their physicians with pharyngitis due to other causes may be culture-positive for group A streptococci. It is almost impossible to distinguish these "carriers" from patients with acute streptococcal infections without the use of serologic studies, which require blood sampling and are expensive. Thus, a 10-day course of antibiotics is probably indicated in these individuals. These carriers may be much more difficult to treat successfully, because their organisms are more dormant and antibiotics are less effective. It is debatable, therefore, whether those for whom such treatment fails should receive another course of therapy. If one elects to try to eradicate the streptococci remaining after a full course of therapy, the regimen should likely comprise both penicillin and clindamycin or rifampin.

RECOGNITION

One of the most difficult problems involved in the appropriate management of ARF is recognizing and firmly establishing the diagnosis of the disease. The revised Jones criteria of the American Heart Association (Table 1) are useful in establishing a firm diagnosis of ARF in most cases. The presence of two major or one major and two minor criteria along with

TABLE 1. **Revised Jones' Criteria for the Diagnosis of the Initial Attack of Rheumatic Fever**

Major Manifestations	Minor Manifestations
Carditis	Fever
Polyarthritis	Arthralgia
Chorea	Elevated erythrocyte sedimentation rate or C-reactive protein value
Subcutaneous nodules	Prolonged PR interval

plus

Supporting evidence of preceding streptococcal infection: positive throat culture for group A streptococcus or elevated or rising antistreptococcal antibody serum titer

Adapted from the Special Writing Group of the Committee on Rheumatic Fever, Endocarditis, and Kawasaki Disease of the Council on Cardiovascular Disease in the Young of the American Heart Association: Guidelines for the diagnosis of rheumatic fever. Jones criteria, 1992 update. JAMA *268*:2069–2073, 1992. Copyright 1992, American Medical Association.

culture or serologic evidence of a preceding streptococcal infection indicates a strong probability of the disease.

The average time between the acute streptococcal infection and the onset of ARF is 18 days; when chorea is the major manifestation, the time may be as long as 3 to even 12 months. Thus, seldom does one obtain a positive group A streptococcal throat culture at the time of diagnosis of ARF. In fact, if one is really trying to isolate the strain that caused the rheumatic fever in a particular patient, performing cultures in the patient's siblings may be more rewarding than performing them in the patient.

Still, throat culture should be performed in all new suspected cases of ARF, and serum should be obtained for streptococcal antibody studies. The classic antistreptolysin O test and the newer, and probably better, anti–DNase B assay should both be employed. The latter test value remains elevated for 2 to 3 months or longer and so is the one of choice in patients with chorea. If both tests are employed, well over 95% of patients with ARF have a positive antibody test confirming the presence of a preceding streptococcal infection.

Carditis, which occurs in approximately 50% of patients, is clearly the most important manifestation of ARF, because it alone leads to permanent abnormalities, including rheumatic heart disease. Although pancarditis may occur, carditis in children and young adults is almost always manifested by mitral regurgitation. This disorder is indicated by a new, high-frequency, systolic murmur at the apex with transmission to the left axilla. Regurgitant flow across the mitral valve can be confirmed by Doppler echocardiography, which may also be of value in cases of silent mitral regurgitation. In patients older than 30 years, the predominant manifestation of cardiac disease is mitral stenosis due to low-grade inflammation associated with fusion and deformity of the mitral leaflets. Thus, a new murmur or a change in a previous murmur is required to make the diagnosis in the adult.

Arthritis occurs in as many as 70% of patients with ARF but is nonspecific, because many other disorders have similar manifestations. In general, the arthritis in ARF is asymmetrical, involves the large joints, and is fleeting or migratory in nature. The joints are painful, red, and warm, but permanent damage does not occur. The arthritis of ARF is exquisitely sensitive to salicylate therapy, so aspirin should not be administered before a firm diagnosis of ARF is made. Later, after the arthritis is well documented, a trial of salicylates usually results in disappearance of the arthritis within 24 to 48 hours.

Sydenham's chorea occurs in 15 to 30% of ARF patients and probably results from inflammatory changes in the caudate nucleus and basal ganglia. Patients suffer from choreiform, involuntary, purposeless movements and emotional lability lasting from 2 to 4 weeks or longer.

The skin manifestations of ARF, which include subcutaneous nodules and erythema marginatum, occur in 3% and 5% of patients, respectively. In the large series of cases seen by us in Utah, skin manifestations, although specific for the disease, seldom were of value in establishing the diagnosis, because they most often occur along with other major manifestations.

TREATMENT

After throat cultures and blood samples for serology have been obtained, the patient with suspected ARF should be treated for the preceding streptococcal infection whether or not the culture is positive, to eradicate any remaining group A streptococci from the upper respiratory tract or lymph nodes. This is best accomplished with 1.2 million units of long-acting benzathine penicillin, which not only treats the acute infection but also provides the first month's prophylaxis. Alternatively, penicillin G or, preferably, penicillin V, in a dose of 250 mg (400,000 units) three or four times per day for 10 full days, or, in the penicillin-allergic individual, erythromycin, 50 mg per kg per day in three or four divided doses for 10 days (maximum, 1 gram per day), will suffice. The patient will then need prophylaxis as described later.

Treatment of the patient with ARF then depends upon the nature and severity of the manifestations. In general, during acute carditis or arthritis, bed rest is recommended. Return to normal activity should be encouraged once the acute manifestations of disease have resolved. Although vigorous physical activity is contraindicated initially, prolonged confinement should be discouraged.

Suppression of the inflammatory response in ARF is carried out by using salicylates or glucocorticoids. Both are capable of suppressing acute manifestations of the disease and, thus, if utilized too early can obscure the diagnosis. Therefore, the patient should be seen by individuals experienced in making the diagnosis of ARF, such as rheumatologists, cardiologists, or infectious disease or immunology specialists, before initiation of immunosuppressive therapy. An inappropriate diagnosis of ARF results in unnecessary prophylaxis against streptococcal infection for the patient well into adulthood as well as continuing concern about the development of rheumatic heart disease. In contrast, failure to diagnose ARF in the patient suffering from the disease may result in failure to administer prophylaxis, a recurrence of disease, and an increased chance for significant cardiac damage. Thus, the patient with suspected ARF should be examined thoroughly so that the correct diagnosis is established firmly.

Carditis

With the possible exception of obsessive-compulsive disorders, which may follow rheumatic chorea, carditis is the single long-term sequela of ARF. Salicylates (aspirin, Bufferin, Ecotrin) or corticosteroids (prednisone) are employed in treating carditis, depending on the severity of the illness. The efficacy of nonsteroidal anti-inflammatory agents such as ibu-

profen has not been well studied in ARF. In general, salicylates are employed when there is no cardiomegaly and no evidence of congestive heart failure.

Aspirin is administered initially in a dose of 100 mg per kg per day in four divided doses for the first 2 to 3 days. The dose may then be tapered to 70 to 80 mg per kg per day, which should be sufficient to maintain a salicylate concentration of 20 to 25 mg per dL. The salicylate concentration should be assessed 4 to 5 days after initiation of therapy, because absorption may vary, and some patients may require more or less of the drug to maintain appropriate concentrations. Therapy should be maintained for 2 to 4 weeks, depending on the response, or until the acute phase reactants, erythrocyte sedimentation rate and C-reactive protein value, return to normal. The dose should then be tapered during 4 weeks to prevent rebound. Should disease activity or acute phase reactant values increase, the salicylate dose should be returned to the maximal level as previously described.

Moderate to severe carditis, in which there is evidence of cardiomegaly or congestive heart failure, is most often treated with oral steroids. Although many cardiologists believe that such therapy may be life-saving, there is no documentation that steroids alter the incidence of residual cardiac disease from ARF. Oral prednisone is given at a dose of 2 mg per kg per day in 1 to 4 doses. The drug is continued until disease activity has disappeared and acute phase reactants such as the erythrocyte sedimentation rate and C-reactive protein value have returned to normal. This usually requires at least 2 weeks, after which one gradually tapers the steroid during 2 to 3 weeks. Aspirin therapy should be instituted at 70 to 80 mg per kg per day at the start of the steroid taper and continued for 2 to 3 weeks after steroids are discontinued to prevent rebound. The doses of prednisone utilized are always associated with significant side effects, including moon facies, hirsutism, and even hypertension, which should be watched for and treated. Antacids may be used to prevent ulcer disease from the steroids.

Congestive heart failure is managed with digoxin, diuretics, and oxygen therapy. Because the inflamed myocardium may be more sensitive, digitalization is carried out using a maintenance dose in an attempt to avoid arrhythmias. The total digitalizing dose is in the range of 0.02 to 0.03 mg per kg, with a maximal total dose of 1.5 mg. Maintenance is usually one fourth of the digitalizing dose and is given in two equally divided doses.

Usually, patients with active carditis are initially confined to bed. As evidence of disease activity declines, gradual ambulation is indicated. Prolonged bed rest is not necessary, although activity should remain light to moderate.

Arthritis

The arthritis of ARF is usually exquisitely sensitive to salicylates. In patients who do not have evidence of serious carditis, the arthritis usually responds to 70 to 80 mg of aspirin per kg per day. The response is often dramatic and rapid. If the arthritis does not improve in the first 2 to 3 days of salicylate therapy, the diagnosis of ARF should be reviewed closely for evidence of some other collagen-vascular or infectious disorder. Full-dose aspirin therapy should be continued for 2 to 3 weeks and then gradually tapered during the next month; the patient should be closely followed up for evidence of an increase in disease activity or acute phase reactants, such as the erythrocyte sedimentation rate or C-reactive protein concentration. If relapse occurs, full-dose (70 to 80 mg per kg per day) aspirin therapy is reinstituted. Glucocorticoids are not indicated in patients with arthritis who do not have accompanying moderate to severe carditis. Bed rest is indicated only during the active phase of the arthritis.

Sydenham's Chorea

Sydenham's chorea is a usually self-limited manifestation of ARF occurring in 20 to 30% of cases. It usually lasts several months but may persist for as long as a year. In mild cases, treatment may not be necessary, or the patient may be kept home from school in a more tranquil, nonstressful environment. More severe cases may require sedative or anticonvulsant therapy. Phenobarbital or haloperidol is most often employed, but the doses necessary for control of symptoms vary significantly from patient to patient. Haloperidol has significant toxic effects, including extrapyramidal reactions and dyskinesia, so it should likely be used only when the patient is under close observation in the hospital. More recently, valproate and carbamazepine have also been employed. Although steroids have generally not been recommended for isolated chorea, we have observed beneficial results, on occasion, with doses of prednisone like those employed for carditis.

SECONDARY PREVENTION

Recurrent ARF occurs in from 5% to as high as 50% of cases. Furthermore, the incidence of cardiac damage resulting in rheumatic heart disease increases with each episode of ARF. Thus, it is critical that subsequent infections with group A streptococci be prevented. Because there is still no safe and efficacious vaccine for group A streptococci (in fact, some of the early vaccine trials against group A streptococci resulted in higher attack rates for rheumatic fever after subsequent streptococcal infections), we physicians must rely on antibiotic prophylaxis, with its attendant problems of drug reactions and the development of microbial resistance.

Optimal prophylaxis results from the use of 1.2 million units of intramuscular long-acting benzathine penicillin every 4 weeks. Some even recommend this dose on an every-3-week basis* if exposure

*Exceeds dosage recommended by the manufacturer.

is likely to be high in crowded situations or developing countries. Oral penicillin G or V, or erythromycin in penicillin-allergic individuals, in doses of 250 mg twice a day may also be sufficient. Oral administration of the penicillin may result in increased resistance of oral viridans streptococci, which must be considered when prophylaxis for oral procedures is given to patients with cardiac valve disease. Compliance is also a major problem for oral compared with intramuscular penicillin therapy. Group A streptococcal resistance to erythromycin is also a problem, which makes this form of prophylaxis less than optimal. Sulfisoxazole (1 gram daily) is actually the second best choice after intramuscular benzathine penicillin prophylaxis, even though sulfonamides should not be used to treat an acute streptococcal infection.

Allergic rashes and even anaphylactic reactions may occur with use of the antibiotics. Because the recurrence rate is much higher during the first 5 years after the initial attack of ARF, it is recommended that intramuscular benzathine penicillin prophylaxis be used for at least 5 years in patients with a history of carditis. When the patient reaches young adulthood, some physicians switch to oral prophylaxis or even discontinue prophylaxis. Although there has been a great deal of discussion about when one can discontinue prophylactic therapy, I believe that it should be continued indefinitely, especially in the patient with any evidence of cardiac involvement. Compliance in maintaining the prophylactic regimen depends on thorough education of the patient and/or the parents. This is especially true in high-risk situations in which there is crowding, such as in military camps, schools, inner cities, and developing countries.

FOLLOW-UP AND SPECIAL HAZARDS

The patient with ARF should be thoroughly educated as to the seriousness of the disease and the need for close follow-up, continuing antibiotic prophylaxis, and periodic examination for evidence of valvular disease. Initially, patients should be seen at least briefly every 3 to 4 weeks when they receive their intramuscular prophylaxis. A more thorough examination for residual cardiac effects should also be carried out at least on a yearly basis, which may even include echocardiography if indicated.

Patients with evidence of valve involvement should be cautioned to maintain good dental and oral hygiene and to have prophylaxis for endocarditis when undergoing dental manipulations or gastrointestinal or genitourinary procedures. Recommendations for antibiotic prophylaxis to prevent bacterial endocarditis are discussed elsewhere.

Thus, appropriate primary prevention of ARF requires a high index of suspicion of group A streptococcal respiratory infection, liberal use of throat cultures, and prompt appropriate antibiotic therapy of adequate duration.

Management also depends on a high index of suspicion of ARF along with a definitive diagnosis of the disease based on Jones' modified criteria published by the American Heart Association (see Table 1). Therapy is then aimed at suppression of inflammation with salicylates or, in more serious cases with moderate to severe carditis, steroids. Thereafter, secondary prophylaxis is essential to prevent recurrences of disease, which increase the incidence and severity of valvular damage. In spite of all of our efforts, sophisticated diagnostic tests, and potent antibiotics, infection with the group A streptococcus and its most serious sequelae, ARF and rheumatic heart disease, continue to be a major problem throughout the world.

LYME DISEASE

method of
ALLEN C. STEERE, M.D.
Tufts University School of Medicine, New England Medical Center
Boston, Massachusetts

Lyme disease is a tick-transmitted spirochetal infection that occurs in North America, Europe, and Asia. It is now the most common vector-borne disease in the United States, with approximately 10,000 new cases reported each year. Although sporadic cases occur in many states, most are clustered in endemic coastal areas in the northeastern United States from Massachusetts to Maryland and in areas of Wisconsin and Minnesota. The infection usually begins in summer with a characteristic expanding skin lesion, erythema migrans (EM). After several days to weeks, the spirochete may spread hematogenously to many different sites, particularly to other skin sites, the nervous system, heart, or joints. Serologic testing is the most practical laboratory aid in diagnosis. The infection can usually be treated successfully with appropriate oral antibiotic therapy, except for neurologic abnormalities, which seem to require intravenous therapy.

ETIOLOGIC AGENT

Borrelia burgdorferi, the causative agent of Lyme disease, is a fastidious, micro-aerophilic spirochetal bacterium that may be cultured in a complex, liquid medium called Barbour-Stoenner-Kelly (BSK) medium. *B. burgdorferi* has been cultured readily from skin biopsy samples of EM early in the infection, but culture from other sites has been difficult later in the illness. Three genomic groups of *B. burgdorferi sensu lato* have now been identified, and more may exist. To date, all North American strains have belonged to the first group, *B. burgdorferi sensu stricto*. Although all three groups have been found in Europe, most isolates there have been group 2, *Borrelia garinii,* or group 3, *Borrelia afzelii,* strains. These differences may well account for regional variations in the clinical picture of Lyme borreliosis.

DISEASE VECTOR

The vectors of Lyme borreliosis are several closely related ixodid ticks that are part of the *Ixodes ricinus* complex. In the northeastern and midwestern United States,

Ixodes dammini (also called *Ixodes scapularis*) is the vector, and *Ixodes pacificus* is the vector in the West. In Europe, *I. ricinus* is the primary vector, as *Ixodes persulcatus* is in Asia. Immature *I. dammini* larvae and nymphs feed primarily on white-footed mice, and adults usually feed on larger mammals, especially white-tailed deer. However, the tick may also feed on other animals and on humans.

During the last several decades, Lyme disease has spread and has caused focal outbreaks, particularly in the northeastern United States. The marked increase in deer populations is thought to be the major reason for the emergence of Lyme disease in epidemic form in the late 20th century. *I. dammini* continues to invade new areas, and the ultimate limit of this spread is not known.

CLINICAL MANIFESTATIONS

Early Infection: Stage 1 (Localized Infection)

After an incubation period of 3 to 32 days, EM, which occurs at the site of the tick bite, usually begins as a red macule or papule that expands to form a large annular lesion, most often with a bright red outer border and partial central clearing. Because of the small size of ixodid ticks, most patients do not remember the preceding tick bite. The center of the lesion sometimes becomes intensely erythematous and indurated, vesicular, or necrotic. In other instances, the expanding lesion remains an even, intense red; several red rings are found within the outside one; or the central area turns blue before it clears. Although the lesion can be located anywhere, the thigh, groin, and axilla are particularly common sites. The lesion is warm but not often painful. Perhaps as many as 25% of patients lack this characteristic skin manifestation of the disorder.

Early Infection: Stage 2 (Disseminated Infection)

Within days to weeks after the onset of EM, the organism often spreads hematogenously to many different sites. Affected patients may develop secondary annular skin lesions, which are similar in appearance to the initial lesion. Skin involvement is commonly accompanied by severe headache, mild neck stiffness, fever, chills, migratory musculoskeletal pain, arthralgias, and profound malaise and fatigue. Less common manifestations are generalized lymphadenopathy or splenomegaly, hepatitis, sore throat, nonproductive cough, conjunctivitis, iritis, and testicular swelling. Except for fatigue and lethargy, which are often constant, the early signs and symptoms of Lyme disease are typically intermittent and changing. Even in untreated patients, the early symptoms usually improve or disappear within weeks.

Symptoms suggestive of meningeal irritation may occur early in Lyme disease when EM is present, but they are usually not associated with a cerebrospinal fluid (CSF) pleocytosis or objective neurologic deficit. After several weeks to months, about 15% of untreated patients develop frank neurologic abnormalities, including meningitis, subtle encephalitic signs, cranial neuritis (including bilateral facial palsy), motor or sensory radiculoneuropathy, mononeuritis multiplex, or myelitis, alone or in various combinations. The usual pattern consists of fluctuating symptoms of meningitis accompanied by facial palsy and peripheral radiculoneuropathy. CSF shows a lymphocytic pleocytosis, often with elevated protein and normal or slightly low glucose values. These early neurologic abnormalities usually resolve completely within months, but chronic neurologic disease may occur later.

Within several weeks after the onset of illness, about 8% of patients develop cardiac involvement. The most common abnormality is fluctuating degrees of atrioventricular block (first-degree, Wenckebach's, or complete heart block). Some patients have more diffuse cardiac involvement, such as electrocardiographic changes of acute myopericarditis, left ventricular dysfunction on radionuclide scans, or, rarely, cardiomegaly or pancarditis. Cardiac involvement usually lasts only a few weeks but may recur.

Late Infection: Stage 3 (Persistent Infection)

Months after the onset of infection, about 60% of patients in the United States who have not received antibiotic treatment develop frank arthritis. The typical pattern is intermittent attacks of oligoarticular arthritis in large joints, especially the knees, lasting weeks to months in a given joint. Small joints and periarticular sites also may be affected, primarily during early attacks. The number of patients who continue to have recurrent attacks decreases each year. However, in a small percentage of patients, involvement in large joints, usually one or both knees, becomes chronic and may lead to erosion of cartilage and bone. These patients have an increased frequency of the class II major histocompatibility complex allele HLA-DR4.

Although less common, chronic neurologic involvement may also occur months to years after the onset of infection, sometimes after long periods of latent infection. The most common form of chronic central nervous system involvement is a subtle encephalopathy affecting memory, mood, or sleep, often accompanied by an axonal polyneuropathy manifested as either distal paresthesias or spinal radicular pain. Patients with encephalopathy often have evidence of memory impairment on neuropsychologic tests and abnormal CSF analyses. In those with polyneuropathy, electromyography generally shows extensive abnormalities of proximal and distal nerve segments. The prolonged disease course of chronic neuroborreliosis, following periods of latent infection, is reminiscent of tertiary neurosyphilis.

DIAGNOSIS

Serodiagnosis

The diagnosis of Lyme disease is usually based on the presence of a characteristic clinical picture, exposure in an endemic area, and a positive antibody response to *B. burgdorferi*. The specific immune response in Lyme disease develops slowly, and only about 40% of patients with EM have a positive IgM response to *B. burgdorferi* in acute phase serum samples. However, a higher percentage of patients (approximately 60 to 70%) have IgM reactivity to the spirochete in convalescent serum samples 2 to 4 weeks later, even after antibiotic treatment. The best serologic evidence for early infection is a significant change in response between acute and convalescent serum samples tested together on the same plate. After 4 weeks of active infection, almost all patients have IgG reactivity with the spirochete; a positive IgM response alone should not be used to support the diagnosis after that time.

Because serologic testing for Lyme disease has a marked risk of false-positive results, the Centers for Disease Control and Prevention now recommends that all equivocal or positive results by enzyme-linked immunosorbent assay also be tested by Western blotting. For a positive IgM blot result, patients are required to have at least 2 of 3 bands (23 [OspC], 39, or 41 kilodaltons). A positive IgG blot is defined by the presence of at least 5 of the 10 most common IgG bands (18, 23 [OspC], 28, 30, 39, 41 [fla], 45, 58 [not GroEL], 66, and 93 kilodaltons).

The limitation of serologic testing is that it does not distinguish active from inactive disease. Because patients with Lyme disease often remain seropositive for years after antibiotic treatment, a positive test result for Lyme disease may cause diagnostic confusion if the patient subsequently develops another illness, particularly another illness with joint or neurologic symptoms.

Polymerase Chain Reaction

Because of the limitations of serologic testing, a test is needed that identifies the spirochete itself. In most bacterial infections, culture serves this purpose. However, *B. burgdorferi* has been cultured regularly only from skin biopsy samples of EM obtained early in the infection. Detection of *B. burgdorferi* DNA from joint fluid by polymerase chain reaction (PCR) has shown promise as a substitute for culture in patients with Lyme arthritis, but the test is not as sensitive in detecting spirochetal DNA in CSF samples in patients with neuroborreliosis. PCR is still being researched for the testing of blood or urine samples. The great problem with PCR is the risk of exogenous contamination causing false-positive results. For this reason, PCR results must be interpreted with caution. The test is not yet routinely available.

DIFFERENTIAL DIAGNOSIS

A common problem in diagnosis is mistaking fibromyalgia or chronic fatigue syndrome for Lyme disease. This problem is compounded by the fact that a small percentage of patients develop fibromyalgia in association with or soon after EM or Lyme arthritis, suggesting that *B. burgdorferi* infection is one of the stressful events that may trigger this chronic pain syndrome. Lyme arthritis and fibromylagia are quite different clinically. Lyme arthritis typically causes marked joint swelling in one or a few joints at a time with little in the way of systemic symptoms. This clinical picture is most like Reiter's syndrome or reactive arthritis in adults or pauciarticular juvenile rheumatoid arthritis in children. In comparison, patients with fibromyalgia often have marked fatigue, severe headache, diffuse musculoskeletal pain, stiffness and pain in many joints, diffuse dysesthesias, difficulty with concentration, and sleep disturbance. On physical examination, such patients have multiple symmetrical tender points in characteristic locations, but they lack evidence of joint inflammation.

TREATMENT RECOMMENDATIONS

Early Lyme Disease

The various manifestations of Lyme disease can usually be treated successfully with oral antibiotic therapy, except for objective neurologic abnormalities, which seem to require intravenous therapy (Table 1). For early Lyme disease, doxycycline, 100 mg twice a day, is recommended for patients older than 8 years and for nonpregnant women. Amoxicillin, 500 mg three times a day; cefuroxime axetil, 500 mg twice a day; and erythromycin, 250 mg four times a day, are second, third, and fourth choices as alternatives, respectively. In children, amoxicillin is effective (50 mg per kg per day, but not more than 2 grams

TABLE 1. **Treatment Regimens for Lyme Disease***

Early Infection (Local or Disseminated)

Adults	Doxycycline (Vibramycin), 100 mg orally 2 times/d for 10–30 d†
	Amoxicillin,‡ 500 mg orally 3 times/d for 10–30 d†
	Alternatives in case of doxycycline or amoxicillin allergy:
	Cefuroxime acetil (Ceftin),‡ 500 mg orally twice daily for 10–30 d†
	Erythromycin,‡ 150 mg orally 4 times a day for 10–30 d†
Children (age 8 y or less)	Amoxicillin, 250 mg orally 3 times a day or 20 mg/kg/d in divided doses for 10–30 d†
	Alternative in case of penicillin allergy:
	Cefuroxime acetil, 125 mg orally twice daily for 10–30 d†
	Erythromycin, 250 mg orally 3 times a day or 30 mg/kg/d in divided doses for 10–30 d†

Arthritis (Intermittent or Chronic)

	Doxycycline, 100 mg orally 2 times/d for 30–60 d
	Amoxicillin, 500 mg orally 4 times/d for 30–60 d
	or
	Ceftriaxone (Rocephin),‡ 2 gm IV once a day for 30 d
	Penicillin G, 20 million U IV in 4 divided doses daily for 30 d

Neurologic Abnormalities (Early or Late)

	Ceftriaxone, 2 gm IV once a day for 30 d
	Penicillin G, 20 million U IV in 4 divided doses daily for 30 d
	Alternative in case of ceftriaxone or penicillin allergy:
	Doxycycline, 100 mg orally 3 times a day for 30 d§
Facial palsy alone	Oral regimens may be adequate

Cardiac Abnormalities

First-degree AV block (PR interval >0.3 s)	Oral regimens, as for early infection
High-degree AV block	Ceftriaxone, 2 gm IV once a day for 30 d‖
	Penicillin G, 20 million U IV in 4 divided doses daily for 30 d‖

*Treatment failures have occurred with any of the regimens given, and a second course of therapy may be necessary.
†For localized infection of the skin, 10 d of therapy is generally adequate, but for disseminated infection, 20–30 d of treatment is recommended.
‡Not FDA approved for this indication.
§In my experience, this regimen is ineffective for the treatment of late neurologic abnormalities of Lyme disease.
‖Once the cardiac abnormalities have stabilized, the course may be completed with oral therapy.

per day) in divided doses; in patients with penicillin allergy, cefuroxime axetil or erythromycin may be used. For patients with infection localized to the skin, 10 days of therapy is generally sufficient, but for patients with disseminated infection, 20 to 30 days of therapy is recommended. Approximately 15% of patients experience a Jarisch-Herxheimer–like reaction during the first 24 hours of therapy.

Co-infection

The Lyme disease tick *I. scapularis* may also transmit at least two other pathogens, *Babesia microti* and a newly recognized *Ehrlichia* agent. The principal clinical clue that the patient may have co-infection is the presence of more severe flulike symptoms. In that case, a blood count should be done. *Ehrlichia* often causes leukopenia and thrombocytopenia, and *B. microti* may cause thrombocytopenia and, in severe cases, hemolytic anemia. An advantage of the doxycycline regimen for the treatment of Lyme disease is that it is also the drug of choice for the treatment of *Ehrlichia*. *B. microti* may be treated with clindamycin and quinine.

Lyme Arthritis

Oral doxycycline or amoxicillin, given for 30 days, is usually effective for the treatment of Lyme arthritis (see Table 1). However, this therapy is not ade-

quate if the patient has concomitant neuroborreliosis. In that case, intravenous ceftriaxone or penicillin should be used. If the arthritis fails to respond to a 1-month course of oral antibiotic therapy, a second course should be given, or intravenous therapy should be tried. However, a small percentage of patients with arthritis, particularly those with the HLA-DR4 allele and an immune response to the outer surface proteins OspA or OspB of the spirochete, may not respond to either oral or intravenous antimicrobial therapy. If the patient still has a swollen joint, usually the knee, after two courses of oral therapy or one course each of oral and intravenous therapies and if the PCR test for joint fluid is negative, I prescribe anti-inflammatory agents. Synovectomy may also be successful in these patients.

Neuroborreliosis

For objective neurologic abnormalities, with the possible exception of facial palsy alone, parenteral antibiotic therapy seems to be necessary (see Table 1). Intravenous ceftriaxone, 2 grams per day for 4 weeks, is most commonly used for this purpose, but intravenous cefotaxime, 2 grams three times a day, or intravenous penicillin G, 20 million units per day in four divided doses, for the same duration may also be effective. The advantages of ceftriaxone are its high level of activity against *B. burgdorferi*, excellent penetration of the brain parenchyma, and long serum half-life, which permits once-a-day dosing. The disadvantages are its expense and the potential side effects of granulocytopenia, antibiotic-associated colitis, and biliary sludging. An additional risk of intravenous therapy is catheter sepsis, which may be life-threatening.

Cardiac Abnormalities

In patients with high-degree atrioventricular block or a PR interval of greater than 0.3 second, intravenous therapy for at least part of the course and cardiac monitoring are recommended (see Table 1). In patients with complete heart block or congestive heart failure, glucocorticoids may be of benefit if the patient does not improve with antimicrobial therapy alone within 24 hours.

Asymptomatic Infection

It is unclear how and whether asymptomatic infection should be treated, but asymptomatic patients are often given a course of oral antibiotics.

Pregnancy

The appropriate treatment for Lyme disease during pregnancy is also unclear. Because the risk of maternal-fetal transmission seems to be quite low, standard therapy for the stage and manifestation of the illness may be sufficient.

Relapse

Relapse may occur with any of the antibiotic regimens for Lyme disease, and a second course of therapy may be necessary. However, there is no evidence that many courses of antibiotics are necessary in the treatment of Lyme disease. In addition, in patients who develop chronic fatigue syndrome or fibromyalgia after Lyme disease, further antibiotic therapy does not seem to be of benefit.

Tick Bites

The risk of infection with *B. burgdorferi* after a recognized tick bite is so low that prophylactic antibiotics are not routinely indicated. However, if the tick is engorged, if follow-up is difficult, or if the patient is quite anxious about developing Lyme disease, amoxicillin or doxycycline therapy for 10 days is likely to prevent the occurrence of this infection.

Vaccine Development

A vaccine for Lyme disease is currently being tested. In experimental animal models, vaccination with recombinant OspA has been shown to protect the host from infection with *B. burgdorferi*. In phase I and II trials, this vaccine has been shown to be immunogenic and safe in human subjects. Two manufacturers are currently completing phase III trials to assess the efficacy and safety of the vaccine in large numbers of human subjects.

ROCKY MOUNTAIN SPOTTED FEVER

method of
LISA G. KAPLOWITZ, M.D.
Division of Infectious Diseases, Medical College of Virginia
Richmond, Virginia

Rocky Mountain spotted fever is the most prevalent and severe rickettsial disease in the United States. Although the disease was initially described and studied in the Rocky Mountain states of Idaho and Montana, most cases in the past 50 years have occurred in the Piedmont plateau region of the southeastern United States. The etiologic agent is *Rickettsia rickettsii*, an obligate intracellular parasite transmitted to humans by the bite of an adult tick. The ticks that usually transmit the infection are the dog tick *Dermacentor variabilis*, in the eastern United States, and the wood tick *Dermacentor andersoni*, in the western United States, though other tick species have been implicated in transmission of this infection.

The risk of acquiring disease from any single tick bite is small. Even in endemic areas, only a small percentage of ticks carry the rickettsial organism; each infected tick must feed for a prolonged period, usually 2 hours or more, before rickettsiae are activated and inoculated into the bloodstream. The organisms invade and proliferate within vascular endothelial cells, with the development of a diffuse necrotizing vasculitis. Vasculitis and thrombosis can occur in any organ system, accounting for the systemic nature of the infection.

The peak occurrence of Rocky Mountain spotted fever is in the summer months, with most cases appearing between April and October, the time of peak tick activity. All age groups can be affected, although most cases occur in children and adolescents, probably because of increased tick exposure for those younger than 20 years. The incidence of this infection increased in the 1960s and 1970s, peaked about 1980, and has shown a steady decrease since then.

CLINICAL MANIFESTATIONS

The incubation period between the tick bite and onset of clinical symptoms ranges from 3 to 14 days. Clinical severity of disease can range from mild to quite severe with a fatal outcome. The initial symptoms of Rocky Mountain spotted fever are relatively nonspecific and include malaise, diffuse myalgias, headache that is frequently severe, and fever (temperature that often is as high as 102 to 104°F). Gastrointestinal symptoms are common, with approximately 75% of patients having symptoms of nausea, vomiting, diarrhea, or abdominal pain. Neurologic symptoms, including lethargy and mental status changes, are not infrequent and can progress to seizures and coma in patients with advanced disease. Hypotension caused by hypovolemia can occur and may result in renal insufficiency due to acute tubular necrosis. Multiorgan involvement is common with advanced disease and is due to the vasculitis that results from rickettsial infection of the vascular endothelium in multiple organ systems. This vasculitis can result in pneumonitis, myositis, skin necrosis, and coagulopathy as well as the gastrointestinal and central nervous system complications mentioned previously.

The presence of a rash is considered a hallmark of the infection, through a rash usually does not appear until 3 to 6 days into the illness and as many as 10% of patients are never affected with a rash. The rash usually begins on the extremities, initially presenting as macular lesions that progress to petechiae or purpura in patients with more advanced disease.

DIAGNOSIS

Serologic tests remain the major means of definitively diagnosing Rocky Mountain spotted fever. Currently, the standard serologic test is the indirect fluorescent antibody test; the latex agglutination technique is also accurate. Antibodies to Weil-Felix antigens, such as OX19, are nonspecific, and complement-fixing antibodies are insensitive; neither test is clinically useful at present. Serologic tests do not become positive until 7 to 10 days after the onset of clinical disease and are not useful in making a diagnosis of Rocky Mountain spotted fever early in the course of the illness. Biopsy of the rash with immunofluorescent rickettsial antibody staining can give a rapid diagnosis when the test is positive, with an overall sensitivity of about 70%; this test is limited in availability and can be done only when a rash is present. In more advanced disease, thrombocytopenia, hyponatremia, and a significant increase in immature white blood cells may be seen, though none of these findings is specific for Rocky Mountain spotted fever. Other laboratory techniques to diagnose rickettsial disease have been developed but are not readily available, including polymerase chain reaction detection of rickettsial DNA in blood and biopsy specimens, immunocytologic identification of rickettsial organisms in endothelial cells, and isolation of rickettsiae. In most cases, specific therapy must be initiated on the basis of clinical presentation plus a history of possible tick exposure in an endemic area in the spring or summer months.

In the preantibiotic era, mortality from Rocky Mountain spotted fever was estimated to be 20%. With the advent of effective antibiotic therapy, the mortality has been between 3 and 5%. Mortality is higher for patients older than 40 years and for black men; higher mortality rates and more fulminant disease noted in some black men may be related to glucose-6-phosphate dehydrogenase deficiency and related hemolysis. Successful outcome of infection correlates with early diagnosis and early institution of appropriate therapy.

TREATMENT

Specific Antirickettsial Therapy

The only antibiotics that have been proved effective for the therapy of Rocky Mountain spotted fever are chloramphenicol and the tetracyclines. Both are rickettsiostatic, and they are equally effective in the treatment of this infection. Antibiotic therapy should be instituted as early as possible in the course of the illness. Administration of appropriate antibiotic therapy before the seventh day of symptoms usually results in complete recovery. Most deaths from Rocky Mountain spotted fever occur in the second week of illness, because the diagnosis is not considered early in the course and institution of specific therapy is delayed.

Doxycycline (Vibramycin), a long-acting tetracycline, is considered the drug of choice in the treatment of Rocky Mountain spotted fever for older children (more than 8 years of age) and for adults with mild or moderately severe illness who can tolerate oral medication. Doxycycline and other tetracyclines should not be used during pregnancy or in patients with tetracycline allergy. Doxycycline offers some advantages over generic tetracycline, which is also effective therapy. Doxycycline is administered twice a day and can be given to patients with renal insufficiency because excretion is predominantly nonrenal. Both the oral and the intravenous doses are 100 mg twice a day after an initial loading dose of 200 mg. Oral doxycycline may cause less gastrointestinal irritation than tetracycline. The cost of doxycycline is higher than that of generic tetracycline but doxycycline is generally better tolerated.

All tetracyclines can cause varying degrees of gastrointestinal irritation. They should not be administered with milk products, vitamin and mineral preparations, or antacids containing metallic salts because of decreased absorption. Tetracyclines can affect fetal bone and tooth development and are contraindicated in pregnancy. They can also cause tooth defects and staining when given to children younger than 8 years, although the risk is greatest for very young children. The risk of tooth staining appears to be directly related to the total amount of tetracycline medication ingested. If the diagnosis of Rocky Mountain spotted fever is relatively certain, a course of tetracycline can be given to a young child if one wishes to avoid chloramphenicol toxicity. Other side effects of tetracycline therapy are photosensitivity and, less commonly, hypersensitivity reactions and hepatic damage. Most reports of hepatotoxicity have been after high-dose intravenous tetracycline therapy given to pregnant women.

Chloramphenicol, the other antibiotic effective in treating this infection, is administered at a dose of 50 to 100 mg per kg per day in four divided doses, orally or intravenously. The major toxicity of chloramphenicol is hematologic. In an extremely small number of patients, aplastic anemia develops weeks to months after chloramphenicol therapy as an idiosyncratic reaction to the drug; this may occur after intravenous or oral therapy. More common is a dose-related suppression of the bone marrow that can be manifested by anemia, leukopenia, or, less commonly, thrombocytopenia and that is reversible on cessation of therapy. Chloramphenicol is the treatment of choice for pregnant women with Rocky Mountain spotted fever. It is also commonly used to treat young children because of concern about tooth staining after tetracycline therapy.

Patients with Rocky Mountain spotted fever usually begin to show clinical improvement within 24 to 48 hours of initiating treatment, although fever may persist for many days after therapy is begun. Treatment is usually prescribed for 7 to 10 days; antibiotic therapy should be continued until the patient is afebrile for at least 48 hours. Relapses are unusual but may occur if antibiotic therapy is discontinued too soon.

Because Rocky Mountain spotted fever is a systemic disease, the differential diagnosis for patients with this infection is frequently extensive. Early in the illness, the differential diagnosis often includes systemic viral infections because of gastrointestinal symptoms, fever, myalgias, and headache. With more advanced disease, meningococcemia, bacterial sepsis, meningitis, and other vasculitides must be considered because of multiorgan involvement and the common presence of a macular or petechial-purpuric rash. It is important to recognize that standard therapies for bacterial sepsis, including penicillins, cephalosporins, and aminoglycoside antibiotics, have no antirickettsial activity. Sulfonamides also have no antirickettsial activity and are actually thought to exacerbate rickettsial infections. Fluoroquinolones have shown some activity against rickettsiae in cell culture and have been used to treat other rickettsial infections, but no data exist regarding their use in the treatment of Rocky Mountain spotted fever.

Ehrlichiosis, caused by another tick-borne rickettsial organism of the genus *Ehrichia,* is being recognized increasingly in the United States as an illness that is clinically similar to Rocky Mountain spotted fever. Ehrlichiosis has many of the same systemic symptoms as Rocky Mountain spotted fever, although the incidence of rash is much less, occurring in 8% and 36% of cases of granulocytic ehrlichiosis and monocytic ehrlichiosis, respectively. Treatment of ehrlichiosis is the same as treatment of Rocky Mountain spotted fever.

Supportive Care

Because Rocky Mountain spotted fever is a systemic vasculitis, it can cause hypotension, hypoproteinemia, vascular collapse, and renal failure through intravascular volume depletion. It is essential to maintain adequate blood volume, and patients may require large amounts of intravenous fluids. Renal failure, when it occurs, is virtually always due to hypotension and hypovolemia and can be prevented by maintaining good renal perfusion. Hyponatremia may also occur from hypotension and hypovolemia and resolves with prompt intravascular volume repletion in most cases. Peripheral edema as well as noncardiogenic pulmonary edema can result from leakage of isotonic fluid into the extravascular space. Edema resolves gradually with adequate therapy of the rickettsial infection.

Thrombocytopenia and coagulopathy can occur as a result of the disseminated vasculitis. Heparin and dextran therapies have been used to manage the coagulopathy associated with Rocky Mountain spotted fever, but no controlled studies of these approaches are available, and their use is controversial. Optimal management of the coagulation defects is therapy of the underlying infection.

Corticosteroids have been employed for patients with severe disease. No controlled studies of corticosteroid use in Rocky Mountain spotted fever are available, and it is not clear whether these agents have any effect on survival.

PREVENTION

The only effective prophylaxis against Rocky Mountain spotted fever is the prevention of tick attachment to the skin or prompt removal of a tick once it becomes attached. Effective measures include (1) use of tick repellents on clothing and exposed parts of the body, (2) covering as much of the body as possible to prevent tick attachment, and (3) daily inspection of the entire body, especially scalp, hairline, and areas where gaps in clothing occur, to remove attached ticks promptly. Twice-daily inspection with prompt tick removal can be especially important for young children living in endemic areas. Ticks should be removed not with bare fingers but with a tissue, gauze, or forceps, if necessary. The tick should not be crushed in direct contact with the skin, because tick secretions may be inoculated into small breaks in the skin and transmit rickettsial organisms.

There is no role for antibiotic administration immediately after a tick bite. Few ticks are actually infected, and even if organisms have been inoculated, administration of antibiotics before any symptoms have occurred will only prolong the incubation period, not prevent disease. Once symptoms appear, it is appropriate to initiate therapy as soon as possible.

At present, there is no commercially available vaccine for this infection. Acquisition of Rocky Mountain spotted fever probably confers lifelong immunity.

RUBELLA AND CONGENITAL RUBELLA

method of
PETER MORGAN-CAPNER, B.Sc., M.B., B.S.
Royal Preston Hospital
Preston, United Kingdom

Rubella (German measles) is now an uncommon infection in countries that have achieved a high rate of measles, mumps, and rubella (MMR) vaccination in infants. It must still be considered, however, on all occasions when rashes or contact with rubelliform illness occurs during pregnancy, as clusters of congenital rubella in the United States demonstrate.

CLINICAL MANIFESTATIONS

Up to 50% of cases of rubella in children are subclinical, but with increasing age, the proportion of subclinical infection falls, and in a majority of adults, infection is symptomatic. Rubella usually presents as a maculopapular, pinkish red rash with an incubation period of 14 to 21 days (usually 15 to 17 days). The rash starts on the face and neck but rapidly spreads to involve the body and limbs. The individual spots may coalesce, but the rash usually clears within 3 to 4 days. Itching is uncommon. The rash is often preceded by a few days of nonspecific illness with fever and upper respiratory tract symptoms. Conjunctivitis can occur but is seldom as severe as that seen in measles. Lymphadenopathy is common, with the suboccipital nodes most often involved. It frequently precedes the rash and may persist for some days. Fever is usually mild and, particularly in children, may be absent. Children usually have only mild disease with little or no systemic upset and only a fleeting rash.

COMPLICATIONS

The major complication of rubella is the potential for adverse effects on the fetus when infection occurs early in pregnancy (see later). Although arthralgia is rare in children, it occurs in up to 30% of adults. The small joints are most commonly involved, particularly the hands and wrists. Although the joint symptoms usually resolve within a month, they can persist for much longer. Thrombocytopenia and postinfectious encephalitis are rare complications, the latter occurring in about 1 in 10,000 cases. Infection in the immunocompromised patient is not unduly severe, nor does it have an unusual presentation.

DIFFERENTIAL DIAGNOSIS

The clinical diagnosis of rubella is notoriously unreliable, even during epidemics. Infection with other viruses, such as enteroviruses, particularly echoviruses, parvovirus B19, and even measles virus, can be easily confused with rubella. Differentiating the rash of parvovirus B19 infection from that of rubella is particularly problematic in adults, with arthralgia of small joints a common complication of both, and the characteristic malar erythema of parvovirus B19 infection in children a rare manifestation in adults. Nonspecific pinkish red macular rashes are not uncommon, particularly in children, and may also be due to noninfective causes such as allergy. As rubella becomes increasingly rare, further difficulties arise, because the infection may not even be considered in the differential diagnosis by medical practitioners unfamiliar with its manifestations.

CONGENITAL RUBELLA

Primary rubella in the first 16 weeks of pregnancy presents a major risk to the fetus. Although transplacental infection can occur throughout pregnancy, the risk of fetal damage varies with gestation. Infection in the first 8 weeks causes intrauterine death or major malformations in up to 85% of fetuses. The risk falls progressively with gestational age, so that at 12 to 16 weeks, the risk is 20%, and the only damage likely is sensorineural deafness. Beyond 16 weeks, although occasional cases of deafness may be attributable to intrauterine infection, the risk to the fetus is remote and is probably close to zero for infections after 24 weeks of gestation. Rubella before conception carries minimal, if any, risk to the fetus.

Infection in the first 12 weeks is associated with a wide range of congenital abnormalities. The classic triad of the congenital rubella syndrome consists of deformities of the eye (cataract, micro-ophthalmia, chorioretinitis), heart (patent ductus arteriosus, pulmonary artery stenosis), and ear (sensorineural deafness). Neurologic complications such as microencephaly and mental retardation also occur, and a wide range of other manifestations may be present (intrauterine growth retardation, purpura, hepatosplenomegaly). Further problems that may develop after birth include immune-mediated pneumonitis, progressive rubella panencephalitis, and diabetes mellitus.

EPIDEMIOLOGY

Patients are infectious for 7 days before and after onset of rash. Transmission is by direct nasopharyngeal droplet spread, with no evidence for survival of infectious virus in the environment or spread by fomite. There is no animal reservoir. Infants with congenital rubella can remain infected for many years, although infectivity for susceptible contacts is negligible after 1 year of age, and failure to isolate virus may be demonstrated in even younger patients. Before widespread infant immunization, epidemics of rubella were seen every 7 to 10 years, but the current pattern is one of low-level endemic infection with localized outbreaks, infection being most common in the spring.

DIAGNOSIS

Primary Rubella

Because clinical diagnosis is so unreliable, laboratory investigation must be performed to make the specific diagnosis. As has been demonstrated in recent clusters, a history of past vaccination or positive antibody screening, even if documented, does not necessarily exclude recent rubella. Hence, it is essential to investigate all rubelliform rashes in pregnancy. Because subclinical primary rubella can occur and damage the fetus, it is wise to also investigate all pregnant contacts of patients with rubelliform illness. If possible, the source patient should also be tested to ascertain the validity of the diagnosis of rubella.

Virus isolation has no place in the diagnosis of postnatal primary rubella, because it is unreliable and may take some weeks. Diagnosis is serologic, and serum should be obtained as soon as possible after contact or onset of illness. Procedures and tests vary by laboratory, but it is essential for correct testing and interpretation of results that full clinical details are given, including any past testing and immunization. Most laboratories test either for total antibody by hemagglutination inhibition (HI) or for specific IgG by a wide variety of tests and, if the titer is high enough, for specific IgM. The detection of specific IgM is usually considered indicative of recent primary rubella, but all specific IgM assays may occasionally give false-positive results, and care is needed in their interpretation. False-positive specific IgM results can occur in infectious mononucleosis and parvovirus B19 infection, both of which may be clinically confused with rubella. Depending on the results obtained with the first serum, it is often necessary to repeat tests 1 to 4 weeks later. The final interpretation depends on the serologic results taken in conjunction with the clinical details and history of antibody and vaccination.

Reinfection

Reinfection is usually diagnosed in the laboratory by demonstrating a rise in antibody titer after recent contact with rubella by someone who has had natural rubella or successful immunization. The risk to the fetus posed by reinfection in early pregnancy is ill defined but likely to be less than 10%, substantially less than the risk with primary rubella. Reinfection is rarely symptomatic, but the differentiation of primary rubella from reinfection in the asymptomatic patient is critical in determining proper treatment. Routine rubella antibody tests may not be able to distinguish these conditions, however, because rubella-specific IgM can often be detected in reinfections, albeit usually at a lower concentration than in primary rubella.

If primary rubella or reinfection is diagnosed in pregnancy, further management depends on counseling of the patient, including assessment of the degree and type of risk to the fetus and the possible prognosis for the infant.

Congenital Rubella

Isolation of virus from urine, throat swab, or tissue is of value in diagnosing congenital rubella, but sufficient virologic expertise for reliable isolation and identification is often not readily available. The detection of specific IgM in neonatal or infant serum is highly reliable, because almost all infants with congenital rubella are seropositive for the first 3 months of life, and most remain so for 6 months. At older ages, but before administration of MMR, persistence of specific IgG or total antibody is diagnostic, because maternal antibody declines to negativity during the first year of life.

Rubella Antibody Screening

To determine whether a patient is susceptible to rubella, and hence should be immunized, testing for rubella-specific IgG or total antibody is required. There are many reliable assays, including HI, latex agglutination, radial hemolysis, and enzyme-linked immunosorbent assay. Sensitivity of the assays varies, and debate continues about the protective efficacy of low concentrations of antibody. Although immunization may be advised for those with low concentrations of antibody (less than 15 IU), it may not boost their antibody levels. Protection against primary rubella can be assumed if two or more doses of vaccine have been given, even if the antibody concentration does not increase.

TREATMENT

There is no justification for the routine administration of gamma globulin to susceptible women after contact with rubella. Although there may be some attenuation of illness, no prophylactic effect on or reduced transmission to the fetus has been demonstrated.

Antiviral drugs have not been used for the treatment of postnatal or congenital rubella.

RUBELLA VACCINE

Rubella virus vaccine (RA 27/3 strain) (Meruvax) is available either as a component of MMR or as a single vaccine. It induces protection in more than 95% of recipients. Widespread administration of MMR vaccine to infants at age 12 to 15 months has had a major impact on the incidence of rubella. To ensure a continued low incidence, it is necessary to maintain high immunization levels by enforcing school entry laws and targeting socioeconomically deprived groups. Continued efforts must also be made to identify susceptible adolescent and adult women who would benefit from immunization. Screening in occupational health departments, prenatal clinics, family planning services, and college health services should continue.

Rubella vaccine is a live attenuated virus, and

rarely, a mild rubelliform illness is seen 2 to 3 weeks after immunization. Arthralgia may occur, but an association with long-term arthritis is disputed and seems unlikely. Administration during pregnancy is contraindicated, and an immunized woman should avoid pregnancy for 1 month afterward. If inadvertent immunization in pregnancy does occur, the risk to the fetus is remote; no congenital abnormalities have been found in term infants (maximal risk is 2%, similar to that for nonexposed infants), although in occasional cases, the fetus may have been infected.

Vaccination in immunocompromised individuals, including those infected with human immunodeficiency virus, has not been associated with significant side effects, but further guidance should be sought if immunization of such individuals is considered.

Immunization should be postponed for 3 months after administration of intramuscular gamma globulin or blood transfusion. Anti-D antibody does not interfere with development of immunity, although follow-up serologic testing is advisable. Vaccine virus cannot be transmitted between the immunized individual and susceptible contacts.

MEASLES
method of
JAMES BARRY HANSHAW, M.D.
Memorial Hospital
Worcester, Massachusetts

Measles is an acute disease caused by an RNA virus with one antigenic type. It is classified as a morbillivirus of the Paramyxoviridae family. The illness is characterized by a course of approximately 7 days with high fever, coryza, conjunctivitis, and cough. There is a characteristic enanthema (Koplik spots) and exanthem (maculopapular rash). Death from measles in the United States declined before the use of the measles vaccine, presumably because of antibiotics and improved nutrition. In developing countries, measles is still a life-threatening disease with a case-fatality rate of 3 to 5% in countries with high infant mortality rates. Major factors in this mortality rate are thought to be poor nutritional status with a relatively high prevalence of vitamin A deficiency, a heavy disease burden from other infectious diseases, crowding and intensity of exposure, and lack of access to appropriate care.

EPIDEMIOLOGY

The wide use of measles vaccine in the United States since 1963 resulted in a 99% decrease in the incidence of the disease by 1981. Before the introduction of the vaccine, approximately 500,000 cases were reported annually. In 1989 and 1990, outbreaks of measles occurred among poor, inner-city preschool children. These outbreaks represented a public health failure rather than a failure of the vaccine to protect. Most cases reported in recent years have not received 1 dose of vaccine.

Measles remains one of the most contagious of infectious diseases. More than 90% of susceptible household contacts will contract the disease. Exposure in a school, on a bus, or in a hospital results in disease in 25% of susceptible contacts. An infected person is contagious 3 to 5 days before the onset of the rash and for 5 days thereafter. The incubation period is 8 to 12 days after exposure; the rash usually appears an average of 14 days after exposure.

Measles is endemic in most of the world. Epidemics occur every 2 to 3 years in developing countries with peak incidence in the winter and spring months.

PASSIVE IMMUNIZATION

Immune globulin (IG) (Gamastan, Gammar), if given within 6 days of exposure to measles, will prevent or modify the disease. Passive immunization with IG is indicated for susceptible household contacts of measles patients, immunocompromised contacts, and pregnant women in whom the risk for complications is high. The usual dose is 0.25 mL per kg of body weight given intramuscularly. Immunocompromised persons should receive 0.5 mL per kg. (The maximal amount of either dose is 15 mL.) Once the child is older than 12 months, measles vaccination can begin 5 to 6 months after IG is administered.

Patients receiving intravenous IG (Gamimune N, Polygam, Sandoglobulin) at the usual dose of 100 to 400 mL per kg are protected from measles for 3 weeks or more. If 300 to 400 mL per kg is used, active immunization with measles vaccine should not be undertaken for 8 weeks. Larger intravenous IG doses of 1000 mL per kg or more require an interval of 10 to 11 weeks before vaccination should be attempted.

Passive immunization should not be used to control measles outbreaks in schools or communities. Available data suggest that live-virus measles vaccine should be the intervention of choice for control of school or community measles outbreaks. If given within 72 hours after exposure, the vaccine will provide protection in some susceptible individuals exposed to the virus. Subsequent measles infection will be prevented in almost all cases.

ACTIVE IMMUNIZATION

Measles vaccine is prepared from a live, further attenuated measles virus prepared in chick embryo cell culture. It is available as a monovalent vaccine (Attenuvax) or in combination with rubella (MR) and mumps (MMR) vaccines. The MMR is the vaccine of choice for routine vaccination of children. When one dose is administered at 15 months or older, approximately 95% develop serum measles antibody after a mild or inapparent noncommunicable infection. Waning immunity after vaccination does occur but only in a small percentage of individuals.

At present, it is recommended that measles vaccine be given at 15 months (12 months in high-risk areas) and at entry to middle or junior high school unless 2 doses were given after the first birthday. College students should have either serologic evidence of immunity or receipt of 2 doses of measles-containing vaccine given after 12 months of age and at least 1

month apart. Physician-diagnosed disease is no longer accepted in some states, presumably because there is now a generation of physicians with little or no experience with measles.

CONTRAINDICATIONS AND PRECAUTIONS

Pregnancy, compromised immunity, and a history of anaphylactic reaction to neomycin are contraindications to the administration of measles vaccine. Women who are given the vaccine should not become pregnant for at least 30 days. There is a theoretical risk that the live virus from the vaccine could be transmitted to the fetus.

The Committee on Infectious Diseases of the American Academy of Pediatrics recommends testing the child with egg anaphylaxis with a scratch test followed by an intradermal skin test with measles vaccine before immunization. The committee recommends that children with positive skin test reactions undergo desensitization under careful supervision. Studies have indicated that such children can be safely vaccinated without prior skin testing or desensitization. The vaccine should be given, however, in a setting where a rare serious reaction can be treated.

Live measles vaccine can be administered to individuals who received a killed measles vaccine between 1963 and 1967. Such individuals may develop atypical measles, which ranges from a mild illness to an uncommon severe form characterized by fever, pulmonary infiltrates, polyserositis, and a vesicular and/or hemorrhagic rash. Because natural measles is more likely than measles vaccine to result in a more severe type of atypical measles, most authorities advise giving the live-virus vaccine to such patients with adequate warning.

IMMUNOCOMPROMISED PATIENTS

Fatal measles virus infection has occurred after live measles vaccination of children with acquired or congenital disorders of immune function. The former include children with leukemia or lymphoma and those receiving high-dose steroid, radiation, and antimetabolite therapy. Immunocompromised children may not be able to respond to live vaccines, and some may be receiving regular doses of Ig that tend to inactivate the vaccine virus. Because person-to-person transmission of measles vaccine virus does not occur, the siblings and household contacts of immunocompromised children can be vaccinated with MMR. Measles vaccine is recommended for patients with human immunodeficiency virus (HIV) infection at the recommended ages. HIV-infected patients tolerate the vaccine well and may have severe or fatal infections from natural measles.

Mild acute illness with low-grade fever, mild diarrheal illness, a family history of convulsions, breastfeeding, and pregnancy in the mother are *not* contraindications to measles vaccination.

MANAGEMENT OF MEASLES

Although no specific antiviral therapy is available, measles virus is susceptible to ribavirin (Virazole)* in vitro. The drug has been given intravenously and by aerosol to severely affected or immunocompromised patients. Because controlled studies have not yet been done, ribavirin has not been approved by the Food and Drug Administration for the treatment of measles.

In many countries of the world where vitamin A deficiency is present, the administration of this vitamin has reduced the mortality and morbidity from measles. In the United States, the American Academy of Pediatrics Committee on Infectious Diseases recommends that vitamin A supplementation be considered for

1. Infants 6 to 24 months of age hospitalized with measles and its complications (e.g., croup, pneumonia, diarrhea)
2. Patients 6 months of age or older with
   a. Immunodeficiency
   b. Ophthalmologic evidence of vitamin A deficiency
   c. Impaired intestinal absorption
   d. Malnutrition
   e. A history of recent immigration from a country with a high measles mortality rate (1% or greater)

The evidence for the efficacy of 1 dose of vitamin A in oil to prevent measles complications is not as strong as that previously shown for two 200,000-IU doses of water-miscible vitamin A.

Acetaminophen 5 mg per kg should be given every 4 hours for symptomatic relief of fever, headache, and general discomfort.

COMPLICATIONS

If fever continues after the full development of a rash, complications such as bacterial otitis media or pneumonia should be suspected and appropriate antibiotics employed.

Acute measles encephalitis occurs in about 1 per 1000 cases and usually appears in the early convalescent phase of the disease. Neurologic consultation is advisable when this complication is suspected.

Patients requiring intensive care have a guarded prognosis associated with adult respiratory distress syndrome, pneumothorax, and sepsis. Mechanical ventilation should employ the lowest possible inspiratory pressure and fraction of inspired oxygen while accepting an arterial oxygen pressure below 60 mm Hg. Intravenous cefuroxime (Kefurox) should be instituted early in patients requiring intensive care with doses of 750 mg to 1.5 grams every 8 hours for adults and 50 to 100 mg per kg per day in equally divided doses every 6 to 8 hours in children.

---

*Not FDA approved for this indication.

FUTURE CONTROL OF MEASLES

Whereas it may be feasible to eliminate measles with current vaccines, a panel of the world's measles experts have recommended a new strategy for global control of measles. This would involve the development of a safe and effective oral vaccine that is heat stable and able to bypass maternal antibody.

TETANUS

method of
JAMES P. RICHARDSON, M.D., M.P.H.
University of Maryland School of Medicine
Baltimore, Maryland

Tetanus, one of the oldest afflictions of humankind, results from infection with the anaerobic gram-positive organism *Clostridium tetani*. The manifestations of the disease are caused by the neurotoxin elaborated by the organism, not by the infection itself. Tetanus usually presents as increased tone of the masseter muscles, or trismus, hence the former name of lockjaw.

ETIOLOGY

The causative organism of tetanus, *C. tetani,* exists as spores that are resistant to heating and disinfectants and thus are nearly ubiquitous. Spores have been found in animal and human feces, and in soil, dust, human dwellings, and hospitals.

EPIDEMIOLOGY

Tetanus is a rare disease in the United States, with an annual incidence of about 0.02 per 100,000 population. About 50 cases are reported to the Centers for Disease Control and Prevention each year; two thirds of these patients are age 50 years and older. Probably many cases of tetanus go unreported, however. There is a slightly higher incidence of tetanus in men. Today the overall case-fatality rate is about 20 to 30%, but this increases with increasing age, reaching 52% in those older than 60 years.

Worldwide, the disease is much more common due to lower levels of immunization. More than 0.5 million infants succumb to neonatal tetanus every year.

PATHOGENESIS

Tetanus spores gain entrance to the body through injuries to the skin. These injuries are often so minor that they do not result in any medical attention (e.g., a prick from a thorn bush, a minor puncture wound). Because *C. tetani* is an obligate anaerobe, the spores will grow only in areas of low oxygen tension, such as occurs with pressure sores, puncture wounds, or gangrene. Growing, or vegetative, *C. tetani* organisms elaborate tetanospasmin, one of the most potent neurotoxins known, which then spreads via axons to the central nervous system.

Tetanospasmin becomes bound to gangliosides within the central nervous system, suppressing inhibitory influences on the motor neurons and inhibiting acetylcholine release at the motor end plate. This results in reflex irritability, rigidity, and disinhibition of spinal cord reflex arcs.

Autonomic hyperactivity is common, resulting from direct stimulation by tetanospasmin. Hypertension and tachycardia, alternating with periods of hypotension and bradycardia, may occur.

CLINICAL PRESENTATION

The incubation period of tetanus is usually from 3 days to 3 weeks, but tetanus can occur several months after an injury. Cases with shorter incubation periods tend to be the most severe.

Generalized disease is the most common presentation of tetanus (Table 1). Common presenting complaints include trismus, neck rigidity, stiffness, dysphagia, restlessness, and reflex spasms. Risus sardonicus is the characteristic grimace that patients with tetanus may display. These patients show raised eyebrows and a wrinkled forehead with the corners of the mouth pulled up. Muscle rigidity usually starts with the jaw and facial muscles and then spreads to the extensor muscles of the limbs. Neonatal tetanus presents as an inability to suck 3 to 10 days after birth. Tetanic seizures, manifested by tonic muscle contractions, may occur in generalized tetanus. Tetanic seizures differ from major motor seizures in that patients with tetanic seizures remain conscious. This activity may be provoked by noise, light, or examination of the patient. These seizures are extremely painful and portend a poor prognosis if frequent.

As the disease progresses, hypoxia may result from involvement of the respiratory muscles. Airway control is extremely important because laryngospasm may cause further compromise (see later).

Two much less common types of tetanus are localized tetanus and cephalic tetanus. Localized tetanus is characterized by painful spasms of muscles close to the site of injury. This disorder is usually self-limiting and lasts less than 2 weeks, but progression to generalized disease can occur if untreated. Cephalic tetanus is a frequently severe form of localized tetanus. Minor head trauma or chronic otitis media may be the mode of entry of the organism. Cephalic tetanus may present as single or multiple cranial nerve palsies or trismus and often progresses to generalized tetanus if not treated.

DIAGNOSIS

Tetanus is determined by clinical diagnosis; there are no laboratory tests specific for the disease. A history of a

TABLE 1. **Presentations of Tetanus**

Generalized Disease
Trismus
Risus sardonicus
Dysphagia
Opisthotonos
Isolated cranial nerve palsies
Rigidity or stiffness in an extremity
Neck stiffness
Restlessness
Tetanic seizures
Poor sucking (newborns)

Localized Disease
Rigidity or stiffness in an extremity

Cephalic Disease
Single or multiple cranial nerve palsies

predisposing injury and the development of the usual clinical features make the diagnosis clear in most cases. However, as noted earlier, a history of injury is not always present. Laboratory tests such as complete blood counts and routine blood chemistry tests are not helpful. Cultures are positive in only 32 to 50% of patients, and in any event treatment cannot wait for their completion. Absence of any sensory deficits and a clear sensorium support the diagnosis of tetanus. A well-documented history of primary immunization and a booster immunization within the last 10 years makes the diagnosis of tetanus much less likely.

Whereas established generalized tetanus is easily recognized, the diagnosis of early tetanus can present some difficulty. Cranial nerve involvement is common and may confuse the physician. Trismus may result from intraoral disease or an acute reaction to a phenothiazine drug such as chlorpromazine (Thorazine). Muscular stiffness can also be a manifestation of strychnine poisoning, meningitis, hepatic encephalopathy, rabies, and conversion reaction. A delay in the diagnosis of tetanus has occurred in patients presenting with dysphagia. Rigid abdominal muscles may stimulate an acute abdomen.

TREATMENT

Whenever possible, patients with suspected tetanus should be transferred to a facility with experience with this disease. Patients should be kept in a quiet, dark environment. Treatment has the following goals: (1) neutralization of circulating toxin, (2) elimination of the source of toxin by careful surgical excision, (3) prevention of respiratory and metabolic complications, and (4) prevention of muscle spasms.

Tetanus antitoxin should be given to prevent further fixation of the toxin to the central nervous system, although it will not reduce manifestations already present. Three thousand to 6000 units of human tetanus immune globulin (TIG) (Hyper-Tet) should be given intramuscularly as soon as possible. Some authorities recommend giving some of this near the site of the wound. Immunization with tetanus-diphtheria toxoid (Td) or diphtheria-pertussis-tetanus (DPT), as appropriate, should also be given, at a site different from that for TIG (Table 2).

Débridement is important for several reasons. Débridement removes existing organisms, creates an aerobic environment unfavorable for further growth, and secures specimens for culture. Débridement should be delayed until several hours after the administration of antitoxin because tetanospasmin may be released into the bloodstream. Antibiotic therapy is essential to sterilize the wound and reduce bacteremia. The antibiotic of choice is now metronidazole (Flagyl), given at a dose of 7.5 mg per kg every 6 hours after a loading dose of 15 mg per kg has been given. Acceptable alternatives are doxycycline (Vibramycin) and imipenem-cilastatin (Primaxin). Penicillin, once the drug of choice, should not be used because it may worsen γ-aminobutyric acid–induced hypertonia.

Oxygenation is assured by protecting the airway. In all but the mildest of cases, prophylactic intubation should be initiated early. Intubation will usually require sedation with a benzodiazepine (e.g., lora-

TABLE 2. Guide to Tetanus Prophylaxis in Routine Wound Management

History of Adsorbed Tetanus Toxoid (Doses)	Clean, Minor Wounds		All Other Wounds*	
	Td†	TIG	Td†	TIG
Unknown or less than 3 doses	Yes	No	Yes	Yes
More than 3 doses‡	No§	No	No‖	No

*Such as, but not limited to, wounds contaminated from dirt, feces, soil, saliva; puncture wounds, avulsions; and wounds resulting from missiles, crushing, burns, and frostbite.

†For children younger than 7 y; DPT (DT, if pertussis vaccine is contraindicated) is preferred to tetanus toxoid alone. For persons 7 y and older, Td is preferred to tetanus toxoid alone.

‡If only 3 doses of fluid toxoid have been received, a fourth dose of toxoid, preferably an adsorbed toxoid, should be given.

§Yes, if more than 10 y since last dose.

‖Yes, if more than 5 y since last dose. (More frequent boosters are not needed and can accentuate side effects.)

From Diphtheria, tetanus, and pertussis: Recommendations for vaccine use and other preventive measures. Recommendations of the Immunization Practices Advisory Committee (ACIP). MMWR Morb Mortal Wkly Rep 40:1–28, 1991.

zepam [Ativan], 2 mg intravenously) and neuromuscular blockade (e.g., vecuronium [Norcuron], 0.08 to 0.1 mg per kg). Patients requiring more than 10 days of intubation or who have generalized seizures should undergo elective tracheostomy. An oropharyngeal airway will allow removal of secretions and prevent biting in mild cases that do not require intubation.

Control of tonic spasms and tetanic seizures is best achieved with the benzodiazepines. Additional benefits are that these drugs produce sedation and amnesia. Diazepam (Valium) can be given at a dose of 0.5 mg per kg to 15 mg per kg per day intravenously. Alternatively, continuous infusions of lorazepam at a dose of 0.1 to 2.0 mg per hour or midazolam (Versed) at a dose of 0.01 to 1.0 mg per kg per hour can be given. The goal is to control muscle rigidity and inhibition of spasm as well as produce the desired level of sedation.

In patients whose muscle spasms do not respond to sedation, neuromuscular blocking agents, such as vecuronium, are often necessary. These patients will require assisted ventilation, often for several days or weeks. Because neuromuscular blocking agents prevent skeletal muscle movements only and do not reduce pain or provide sedation, it is essential that these patients be monitored closely for adequate pain relief.

Later in the course of the disease, cardiovascular instability may develop through effects on the autonomic nervous system. Both alpha-adrenergic blockade and beta-adrenergic blockade may be necessary with phentolamine (Regitine) and propranolol (Inderal) for treatment of hypertension and tachycardia. Bradycardia may develop as well, requiring placement of a pacemaker. Hypotension may require monitoring of cardiac output and intravenous fluids or pressor agents.

COMPLICATIONS

Supportive care is critical to the prevention of complications. Most of these complications are those common to immobile patients. Attention to nutritional status and frequent turning of the patient will prevent pressure sores. Low-dose heparin should be administered to prevent deep venous thromboses and pulmonary emboli. Physical therapy should be begun as soon as possible to prevent contractures. Fractures and dislocations may result from tetanic seizures, requiring orthopedic management.

Most patients will eventually make a full recovery, but some patients remain hypertonic. It is important that recovering patients complete a primary series of immunizations because having had the disease does not confer immunity (Table 3).

PREVENTION

Prevention of tetanus through immunization is the key to the elimination of tetanus. It is important to distinguish between primary and booster immunization, however. A never-immunized patient requires two additional doses of Td beyond the dose given when the wound is treated (see Table 3). Wounded patients who have never been immunized may require TIG (see Table 2). The elderly population is particularly susceptible, because so many have never been immunized or because their immunity has lapsed.

Physicians should use a case-finding approach to increase tetanus immunization rates. Reminders placed at physicians' desks or computer-generated reminders attached to charts or patients' bills have improved immunization rates. Td should be given whenever tetanus immunization is necessary, to ensure immunity to diphtheria as well as tetanus.

Td is a safe vaccine. Adverse reactions consist primarily of local edema, tenderness, and fever. Anaphylactoid reactions are rare. Most adverse reactions occur in persons with evidence of hyperimmunization. The only contraindications to Td are a history of a neurologic sequela or a severe hypersensitivity reaction after a previous dose.

To reduce neonatal tetanus and protect the mother, pregnant women who are due for a booster should

TABLE 3. Routine Immunization Schedule with Tetanus-Diptheria Toxoid for Persons 7 Years and Older

Dose	Age or Interval
Primary 1	First dose
Primary 2	4–8 wk after first dose*
Primary 3	6–12 mo after second dose*
Boosters	Every 10 y after last dose

*Prolonging the interval does not require restarting series.

Adapted from Diphtheria, tetanus, and pertussis: Recommendations for vaccine use and other preventive measures. Recommendations of the Immunization Practices Advisory Committee (ACIP). MMWR Morb Mortal Wkly Rep 40:1–28, 1991.

receive Td, preferably during the last two trimesters. TIG should be given to pregnant women only when clearly indicated.

PERTUSSIS*
(Whooping Cough)

method of
JAMES W. BASS, M.D., M.P.H.
Tripler Army Medical Center
Honolulu, Hawaii

Pertussis (whooping cough) is a communicable infection of the respiratory tract characterized by severe paroxysms of cough terminating in a gasping stridulous inspiratory effort. This characteristic musical, whooping-like sound is responsible for the term "whooping cough." The term "pertussis" is usually reserved for the clinical illness produced by infection with *Bordetella pertussis;* however, pertussis-like syndromes are also noted in association with infection due to *Bordetella parapertussis, Bordetella bronchiseptica, Chlamydia trachomatis,* adenovirus, respiratory syncytial virus, and combinations of these organisms. When pertussis-like illnesses are associated with agents other than *B. pertussis,* the disease is usually milder and of shorter duration.

Pertussis is spread by the airborne route directly from droplet and droplet nuclei from aerosols generated by the intense cough of infected individuals. It is one of the most highly communicable human diseases. Attack rates in families and in some community outbreaks approach 100% of susceptible contacts. Infection begins when aerosol particles containing viable pertussis organisms settle onto the mucous film overlying the respiratory passages of susceptible individuals. Here they adhere to the cilia of the epithelial cells that line the mucosal surface of the respiratory passages from the nasopharynx to the respiratory bronchioles in the lung. Only here do they replicate. Their presence in large numbers on these surfaces is associated with elaboration of profuse tenacious mucus and ciliostasis, resulting in stagnation of mucus flow and inspissation of air passages. Patchy atelectasis and bronchitis are constant, and secondary bronchopneumonia is common.

Bordetella pertussis organisms are not found beyond the cilia of the respiratory epithelium. Here, several biologically active surface components that play a role in the pathogenesis of the disease are elaborated and absorbed. Several of these components have been studied extensively. The characteristic lymphocytosis associated with pertussis is stimulated by lymphocytosis-promoting factor, now called pertussis toxin (PT); filamentous hemagglutinin (FHA) and a 69-kilodalton nonfimbrial surface protein called pertactin are involved in the attachment of *B. pertussis* organisms to ciliated respiratory epithelial cells; agglutinogens are thought to be associated with type-specific immunity, and tracheal cytotoxin causes ciliostasis and epithelial cell death. PT and FHA are the primary antigens that have been incorporated into effective acellular vaccines. Tracheal cytotoxin appears to be the cause of most

of the destruction of the respiratory tract and respiratory symptoms associated with the disease. As both secretory and humoral antibodies are produced in increasing quantity, pertussis organisms are gradually eliminated from the respiratory passages, ciliary movement is restored, tenacious mucous secretions are diminished, mucous inspissation is resolved, and the airway heals, usually without residua.

CLINICAL MANIFESTATIONS

After an incubation period of 7 to 10 days (range, 5 to 20 days), clinical illness progresses in three stages: (1) the catarrhal, prodromal, or preparoyxsmal stage, (2) the acute paroxysmal or spasmodic cough stage, and (3) the convalescent stage.

The Catarrhal Stage. The catarrhal stage is characterized by a period of 1 day to several days of clear, serous, or mucoid rhinorrhea, nasal congestion, and sneezing followed by cough. During this time, the disease is often indistinguishable from the common cold, and pertussis is seldom suspected unless classic clinical whooping cough has been observed in other members of the family or local community. Later in this stage, the cough grows more severe and persistent, particularly at night, and profuse nasopharyngeal secretions grow thick and tenacious. There is heavy shedding of pertussis organisms in these secretions, and it is at this stage that the patient is most contagious and that the organism is most easily cultured. The catarrhal stage may persist for up to 2 weeks, or it may be so mild that it even goes unrecognized.

The Paroxysmal Stage. The second stage of pertussis rarely begins abruptly without a preceding catarrhal stage. Violent, protracted bouts of coughing occur in distinct paroxysms lasting up to several minutes. There may be only 2 to 5 or up to 40 to 50 episodes a day. Toward the end of these paroxysms, patients often vomit previously swallowed thick, ropy secretions. Severe cough may produce a marked florid venous engorgement of the head and neck. In younger, weaker infants, severe cough paroxysms may not be associated with the characteristic whoop but are more often terminated in exhaustion, vomiting, aspiration, apnea, cyanosis, and loss of consciousness. Without resuscitation, these episodes may result in anoxic brain damage or death. In older children and adults, who have relatively larger upper airways, the characteristic whoop is also often absent. The paroxysmal stage of pertussis may last from only a few days to 3 to 4 weeks.

The Convalescent State. Convalescence begins when chronic cough replaces paroxysms. It usually lasts for 3 to 4 weeks with a decrease in frequency and severity of cough. Rarely, the convalescent stage may persist for months.

COMPLICATIONS

Nonsuppurative Complications. Increased intrathoracic pressure resulting form severe cough paroxysms, hypoxia, and persistent vomiting causes venous engorgement and hypoxemia with petechial hemorrhages, epistaxis, subconjunctival and scleral hemorrhages, and cerebral hemorrhages. Rarely, subarachnoid and subdural hemorrhages with convulsions, transient hemiplegia (Todd's paralysis), encephalopathy, and coma occur.

Marked and prolonged increases in intrathoracic and intra-abdominal pressure with cough paroxysms have been associated with rupture of the diaphragm; interstitial, subcutaneous, or mediastinal emphysema; pneumothorax; umbilical and inguinal hernia; and rectal prolapse. Intractable

---

*The opinions or assertions contained herein are the private views of the authors and are not to be construed as official or as reflecting the views of the Department of the Army or the Department of Defense.

vomiting may produce severe metabolic alkalosis with tetany, aspiration pneumonia, and inanition.

Encephalopathy occurs in about 1% of patients with pertussis. The cause has not been determined. The fact that it is often seen in patients with hyperlymphocytosis suggests that PT may be causally related to this complication of pertussis. Whether the organism elaborates a neurotoxin, which to date has not been identified, or whether encephalopathy is due to intracranial hemorrhage or anoxia secondary to severe cough spasms is debatable. Edema, congestion, and scattered petechial hemorrhages are commonly found in brain tissue of patients who die of pertussis and are consistent with hypoxic brain damage.

Suppurative Complications. Secondary infections of the respiratory tract should be suspected in the patient who develops fever and an elevated erythrocyte sedimentation rate, because uncomplicated pertussis is not associated with fever and the erythrocyte sedimentation rate is either normal or, more commonly, low.

Acute otitis media is common, as is sinusitis. Clinical and radiographic evidence of pneumonia develops in approximately 10% of infants with pertussis. This may be difficult to differentiate from atelectasis, which is usually present in varying degrees. Segmental or lobar atelectasis primarily affects the lower lobes, the right middle lobe, and the lingular segment of the left upper lobe. Serial radiographs may show frequent changes, as some segments re-aerate and others collapse. If soft, fluffy infiltrates develop around these areas of atelectasis and the patient becomes toxic and febrile, secondary bronchopneumonia should be suspected. Treatment should be initiated against bacterial pathogens commonly implicated in the cause of pneumonia.

DIAGNOSIS

The diagnosis of pertussis should be suspected in any person with severe cough and should be considered foremost if the cough occurs in severe paroxysms. It is helpful if there is a history of contact with a person known to have pertussis or if the disease is known to be prevalent in the community. Lack of prior immunization or only partial immunization against pertussis should further increase the likelihood of the diagnosis. In older children and adults, the diagnosis of pertussis should be considered in a person who has had a cough longer than 2 weeks.

An absolute lymphocytosis involving small, mature lymphocytes with counts ranging from 20,000 to greater than 100,000 cells per mm³ is usually seen in the late catarrhal stage and throughout most of the paroxysmal stage. This characteristic lymphocytosis may not be present in infants younger than 6 months old, in partially immunized individuals, and in adults.

Culture

Culture of pertussis organisms from respiratory tract secretions remains the standard for laboratory diagnosis of pertussis. Although this test is highly specific, it is not very sensitive. Culture of *B. pertussis* organisms is best achieved from nasopharyngeal secretions obtained by aspiration during irrigation with phosphate-buffered saline. Culture of calcium alginate swabs inserted through the nose deep enough to reach the posterior pharynx also yields excellent results; Dacron and cotton swabs are not as effective, however, and should not be used. Cough plate specimens and swabs taken from the oropharynx yield less reliable results; these techniques should not be used.

Nasopharyngeal swabs should be smeared directly onto Regan-Lowe medium with and without cephalexin. Fresh Bordet-Gengou medium with and without penicillin may also be used, but it is less effective for isolation of *B. pertussis* and requires special preparation. Culture plates should be streaked and then sealed with masking tape to prevent desiccation during the prolonged incubation required for growth of *B. pertussis* organisms. Characteristic small, pinpoint, metallic-like colonies are first noted after incubation of 72 hours or more at 37°C. Most positive cultures are evident after 5 to 7 days; however, significant additional positive readings have been observed on plates held and read at 12 days. Organisms are most often cultured during the catarrhal stage of illness, when almost pure cultures are obtained. The incidence of positive cultures remains equally high throughout the first week of the paroxysmal stage but decreases thereafter. It is seldom possible to recover the organism more than 3 weeks after the onset of the paroxysmal stage of illness.

Direct Fluorescein-Labeled Antibody Test

Most large medical centers and state laboratories can quickly confirm the presence of *B. pertussis* organisms in nasal secretions by the use of direct fluorescein-conjugated antibody (DFA) staining. This method is compromised by interobserver variability. Both false-positive and false-negative results can occur; however, DFA tests may be more sensitive than culture, and they often remain positive even after effective antibiotic treatment has cleared the patient of viable organisms. DFA staining is probably the best test currently used for immediate presumptive diagnosis of pertussis and permits early management decisions regarding isolation of the patient, administration of pertussis vaccine, and institution of antibiotic treatment and prophylaxis.

Serology

Tests for serologic diagnosis of pertussis infection are now becoming commercially available. Enzyme-linked immunosorbent assay (ELISA) tests for IgG antibodies to PT and FHA may reflect past infection of vaccine administration when a single serum shows levels of antibody significantly above the reference range. A significant elevation of IgM antibody above the reference range indicates concurrent or recent infection or vaccine adminstration. IgA antibodies are not produced as a result of vaccine administration, but only with infection. Because they are short-lived, the finding of IgA antibodies indicates recent infection; however, only about half of patients with pertussis infection develop IgA antibodies. A significant rise in any of these antibodies noted in paired acute and convalescent sera confirms recent infection with *B. pertussis*.

Commercial laboratories in the United States that offer tests for the diagnosis of pertussis infection are as follows: Associated Regional University Pathologists (Salt Lake City, Utah), DFA; Specialty Laboratories (Santa Monica, California), DFA, ELISA—IgG, IgM, and IgA; Microbiology Reference Laboratory (Cypress, California), DFA, ELISA panel including IgA (PT), IgG (PT), IgG (FHA), and IgA (FHA). Antigen preparations and criteria for positivity may vary among commercial laboratories. Some have not published their methods in detail, or the sensitivity and specificity of their tests, in refereed medical journals.

Other tests that have been developed for identification of the organism or its components in nasopharyngeal secretions are DNA hybridization and polymerase chain reaction. Results of these tests are seldom available early enough to guide management decisions, although they are often useful in epidemiologic studies. These tests are both highly sensitive and specific, but they are not currently available for general use.

TREATMENT

Supportive Care

Severe disease and a high incidence of complications occur most often in young infants. Most infants who die are only 2, 3, or 4 months old, so it is wise to hospitalize very young infants with pertussis, particularly those who have severe cough paroxysms with cyanotic and apneic episodes. Gentle suctioning and supplemental oxygen administration are indicated during severe bouts of paroxysmal cough. Fluid depletion from suctioning of secretions, vomiting, and inadequate oral fluid intake may necessitate administration of parenteral fluids and electrolytes. Parenteral hyperalimentation may be necessary to prevent malnutrition in patients with protracted disease. Management of these patients in intensive care settings with experienced and efficient nursing staff is probably the most important factor in survival.

Cough suppressants, expectorants, antispasmodics, sedatives, and mucolytic agents have not been shown to be of benefit. Mist therapy is not helpful, but continuous well-humidified oxygen is indicated for patients who show sustained evidence of hypoxemia. Blood gas determinations should be performed in patients with labored respirations, unstable vital signs, or alterations in mental status. Such patients usually have significant complications, such as atelectasis, bronchopneumonia, and encephalopathy.

Specific Treatment

Pertussis hyperimmune globulin was marketed from the 1940s through the 1970s for treatment of pertussis and for prevention of pertussis in exposed susceptible contacts. More recent, well-controlled clinical trials evaluating the effectiveness of this product for these purposes have failed to show any benefit. The product is no longer recommended, and it is no longer available in the United States. A 1993 report on the use of human hyperimmune serum for treatment of pertussis did show significant benefit, but this product is not available for general use.

Antimicrobial agents that are active against *B. pertussis* organisms in vitro and diffuse in significant concentrations into respiratory tract secretions have been shown to be beneficial in the management of persons with pertussis. Erythromycin, the tetracyclines,* and chloramphenicol have been shown to be effective in achieving early bacteriologic cures; however, no antimicrobial agent alters the subsequent course of the illness if given in the paroxysmal stage of the disease, when the diagnosis is most often first suspected. There is evidence that these drugs may be effective in preventing the disease when ad-

ministered in the incubation period (culture-positive asymptomatic susceptible persons) and in attenuating the disease when given in the catarrhal or preparoxysmal stage of the disease. Their administration to a patient at any stage of pertussis may render the patient noninfectious.

The preceding reasons constitute the rationale for the use of antimicrobials in pertussis, and for these purposes, erythromycin appears to be the most effective and least toxic drug studied to date. There is also evidence that erythromycin may be of value in prophylaxis against pertussis in exposed susceptible individuals. In all of these circumstances, the recommended dose of erythromycin is 40 to 50 mg per kg per day (maximum, 2 grams) orally in four divided doses for 14 days; the drug may be given in two or three divided doses daily if tolerated. Treatment for less than 14 days may be complicated by bacteriologic and clinical relapse.

Activity of clarithromycin (Biaxin)* against pertussis organisms and its concentration in serum and respiratory tract secretions are equal to or greater than those of erythromycin. Limited clinical trials to date also indicate that this drug may be equal to or better than erythromycin for treatment of pertussis. It has a significantly longer half-life, the recommended dosage is 15 mg per kg per day in two divided doses, and it is better tolerated than erythromycin. With these advantages, clarithromycin may become the preferred drug for treatment of pertussis.

Trimethoprim-sulfamethoxazole (TMP-SMZ) (Bactrim, Septra),* given as 8 mg of TMP and 40 mg of SMZ per kg per day in two oral doses for 14 days, is a possible alternative for patients who do not tolerate erythromycin or clarithromycin, but the efficacy of this treatment regimen is unproved. Other antibiotics, such as the penicillins, including ampicillin, and the first-generation cephalosporins, have some activity against *B. pertussis* in vitro but are clinically ineffective (probably owing to poor penetration into respiratory secretions) and should not be used.

Corticosteroids were shown to significantly alter the severity and duration of pertussis in two controlled clinical trials even when treatment was not begun until after the paroxysmal stage of the disease had developed. In one study, betamethasone (Celestone) was given orally at a dose of 0.075 mg per kg per day. In the second study, hydrocortisone sodium succinate (Solu-Cortef) was given intramuscularly at a dose of 30 mg per kg per day for 2 days; the dose was gradually reduced thereafter and discontinued after several days. In both studies, significant reduction in the number and duration of paroxysms was noted in the corticosteroid-treated groups compared with untreated control subjects. Other anecdotal observations attesting to the effectiveness of corticosteroids in the treatment of pertussis have been reported. Additional controlled studies are needed, but it appears that corticosteroids may be beneficial in the treatment of pertussis, particularly in extremely young infants with life-threatening paroxysms. One

---

*Not FDA approved for this indication.

*Not FDA approved for this indication.

of these regimens may be used, or other corticosteroid preparations at comparable dosages should be equally effective.

Albuterol (Ventolin, Proventil) has been shown to be effective in the treatment of pertussis in a number of studies. In one controlled study, albuterol-treated children (1 mg four times daily for children younger than 2 years, and 2 mg four times daily for children older than 2 years) had significantly fewer paroxysms than in non–albuterol-treated controls. In another study, albuterol, 0.5 mg per kg per day in three divided doses, was associated with a better rate of recovery with respect to frequency of paroxysms of coughing and whooping compared with placebo-treated control subjects. A single study that was randomized, double-blind, and cross-over in design failed to show a benefit of albuterol treatment. This study involved nine study patients, only six of whom had culture-positive pertussis and none of whom was critically ill. Failure to show a benefit for albuterol treatment under these circumstances cannot be considered conclusive. A reported study of a patient with pertussis who had severe paroxysmal coughing with cyanosis requiring ventilatory support showed a dramatic effect due to the administration of albuterol, 0.5 mg per kg per day in 3 doses. Additional controlled studies are needed, but it appears that albuterol, in a dosage of 0.3 to 0.5 mg per kg per day in three divided doses, is effective and well tolerated.

PROGNOSIS

The prognosis in uncomplicated pertussis is good. In the United States, the mortality has been less than 1% for the past 3 decades. Except for rare brain damage associated with pertussis encephalopathy or severe hypoxic episodes, there is no other serious permanent residual morbidity. Pulmonary function values return to normal, and there does not appear to be any subsequent predisposition to chronic or recurrent pulmonary infections.

PREVENTION

Pertussis vaccination confers 80 to 90% protection against the disease for 3 years; the protection level decreases thereafter for 12 years, after which no protection is evident. Attempts at active immunization after exposure afford no benefit. Pending the development of a better pertussis vaccine, the only means available for control of pertussis outbreaks are as follows: early identification and isolation of infected individuals; booster pertussis vaccine administration for selected partially immunized individuals younger than 7 years, and attempts at antimicrobial prophylaxis.

Individuals suspected of having pertussis should be placed in respiratory isolation pending laboratory confirmation of the diagnosis. Children younger than 7 years who have had at least four doses of pertussis vaccine should receive a booster dose, usually as diphtheria-tetanus-pertussis (DTP) vaccine, unless the fourth dose has been given within the past 3 years or after the fourth birthday. Children younger than 7 years who have received their third dose 6 months or more before exposure should be given their fourth dose at this time. Children who have had culture-proven pertussis need not receive further pertussis immunization. Anyone older than 7 years should not receive pertussis vaccine.

Attempts at antimicrobial prophylaxis should be initiated in the patient and all significant susceptible contacts using erythromycin in the dosage given and for the duration described previously for treatment. Isolation should be continued for at least 5 days after the start of erythromycin (3 weeks after onset of paroxysms if antimicrobials are not given) in those individuals whose nasopharyngeal smears are shown to be positive for *B. pertussis* organisms by fluorescent microscopy or culture. In populations in which effective pertussis vaccines have decreased the incidence of the disease in preschool and school-age children, young adults with waning vaccine-induced immunity and extremely young infants who have no passive immunity from their mothers are evolving as two major groups with susceptibility to pertussis. Young mothers usually have atypical pertussis, which often goes undiagnosed, and the disease is transmitted to their susceptible newborn infants.

One reported study has shown that administration of erythromycin to mothers with laboratory-confirmed pertussis and to their newborn infants prevented the infants from contracting the disease, an otherwise almost certain probability. The mothers received erythromycin stearate or base in a dose of 250 to 500 mg three times daily, and the infants received 40 mg per kg per day of erythromycin ethylsuccinate in three divided doses, both for 10 days. The medications were well tolerated, and effective antibiotic prophylaxis was provided for the infants, who were at high risk for severe or life-threatening disease.

IMMUNIZATION PRACTICES

method of
JAN EDWIN DRUTZ, M.D.
Baylor College of Medicine
Houston, Texas

Preventive care is considered essential to maintaining patient health and controlling medical costs. Most representative of a successful preventive health care measure has been the national vaccine immunization program. With rapid advances in virology, immunology, cell biology, and genetics, newer and more effective vaccines have been licensed and produced. To stay abreast of ongoing breakthroughs, immunization guidelines from the Advisory Committee on Immunization Practices (ACIP) and the Committee on Infectious Diseases of the American Academy of Pediatrics (AAP) have had to be revised and updated continuously.

A dramatic example of the effect that appropriate immunization has had in preventing disease is the marked de-

TABLE 1. **Recommended Childhood Immunization Schedule,* United States, 1997†**

Vaccine	Birth	1 Month	2 Months	4 Months	6 Months	12 Months	15 Months	18 Months	4-6 Years	11-12 Years	14-16 Years
Hepatitis B‡§	Hep B-1	Hep B-2			Hep B-3					Hep B§	
Diphtheria and tetanus toxoids, and acellular pertussis‖			DTaP or DTP	DTaP or DTP	DTaP or DTP		DTaP or DTP	DTaP or DTP	DTaP or DTP	Td	
Haemophilus influenzae type b¶			Hib	Hib	Hib⁴	Hib					
Poliovirus**			Polio**	Polio		Polio			OPV		
Measles-mumps-rubella††						MMR			MMR	or MMR	
Varicella virus‡‡						Var				Var	

Approved by the Advisory Committee on Immunization Practices (ACIP), the American Academy of Pediatrics (AAP), and the American Academy of Family Physicians (AAFP)

*This schedule indicates the recommended age for routine administration of currently licensed childhood vaccines. Some combination vaccines are available and may be used whenever administration of all components of the vaccine is indicated. Providers should consult the manufacturers' package inserts for detailed recommendations. Vaccines are listed under the routinely recommended ages. Open bars indicate range of acceptable ages for vaccination. Shaded bars indicate catch-up vaccination: at 11–12 y, hepatitis B vaccine should be administered to children who lack a reliable history of chickenpox.

†Use of trade names and commercial sources is for identification only and does not imply endorsement by the Public Health Service or the U.S. Department of Health and Human Services.

‡Infants born to hepatitis B surface antigen (HBsAg)–negative mothers should receive 2.5 µg of Merck vaccine (Recombivax HB) or 10 µg of SmithKline Beecham (SB) vaccine (Engerix-B). The second dose should be administered >1 mo after the first dose. Infants born to HBsAg-positive mothers should receive 0.5 mL of hepatitis B immune globulin (HBIG) within 12 h of birth, and either 5 µg of Merck vaccine (Recombivax HB) or 10 µg of SB vaccine (Energix-B) at a separate site. The second dose is recommended at age 1–2 mo and the third dose at age 6 mo. Infants born to mothers whose HBsAg status is unknown should receive either 5 µg of Merck vaccine (Recombivax HB) or 10 µg of SB vaccine (Energix-B) within 12 h of birth. The second dose of vaccine is recommended at age 1 mo and the third dose at age 6 mo. Blood should be drawn at the time of delivery to determine the mother's HBsAg status; if it is positive, the infant should receive HBIG as soon as possible (no later than age 1 wk). The dosage and timing of subsequent vaccine doses should be based on the mother's HBsAg status.

§Children and adolescents who have not been vaccinated against hepatitis B during infancy may begin the series during any childhood visit. Those who have not previously received 3 doses of hepatitis B vaccine should initiate or complete the series at age 11–12 y. The second dose should be administered at least 1 mo after the first dose, and the third dose should be administered at least 4 mo after the first dose and at least 2 mo after the second dose.

‖Diphtheria and tetanus toxoids and acellular pertussis vaccine (DTaP) is the preferred vaccine for all doses in the vaccination series, including completion of the series in children who have received one or more doses of whole-cell diphtheria and tetanus toxoids and pertussis vaccine (DTP). Whole-cell DTP is an acceptable alternative to DTaP. The fourth dose of DTaP may be administered as early as 12 mo of age provided 6 mo has elapsed since the third dose and if the child is considered unlikely to return at age 15–18 mo. Tetanus and diphtheria toxoid (Td), absorbed, for adult use, is recommended at age 11–12 y if at least 5 y has elapsed since the last dose of DTP, DTaP, or diphtheria and tetanus toxoids. Subsequent routine Td boosters are recommended every 10 y.

¶Three *H. influenzae* type b (Hib) conjugate vaccines are licensed for infant use. If PRP-OMP (PedvaxHIB [Merck]) is administered at ages 2 and 4 mo, a dose at age 6 mo is not required. After completing the primary series, any Hib conjugate vaccine may be used as a booster.

**Two poliovirus vaccines are currently licensed in the United States: inactivated poliovirus vaccine (IPV) and oral poliovirus vaccine (OPV). The following schedules are all acceptable by ACIP, AAP, and AAFP, and parents and providers may choose among them: (1) IPV at ages 2 and 4 mo and OPV at age 4–6 y; (2) IPV at ages 2, 4, and 12–18 mo and at age 4–6 y; and (3) OPV at ages 2, 4, and 6–18 mo and at age 4–6 y. ACIP routinely recommends schedule 1. IPV is the only poliovirus vaccine recommended for immunocompromised persons and their household contacts.

††The second dose of measles-mumps-rubella vaccine is routinely recommended at age 4–6 y or at age 11–12 y but may be administered during any visit provided at least 1 mo has elapsed since receipt of the first dose and that both doses are administered at or after age 12 mo.

‡‡Susceptible children may receive varicella vaccine (Var) during any visit after the first birthday, and unvaccinated persons who lack a reliable history of chickenpox should be vaccinated at age 11–12 y. Susceptible persons aged ≥13 y should receive 2 doses at least 1 mo apart.

crease in the number of invasive *Haemophilus influenzae* type b (Hib) infections since December 1987. The first of a series of Hib conjugate vaccines (HbCVs) was introduced at that time, and since then, the number of cases in children younger than 5 years of age has declined 95%.

Unfortunately, failure on the part of many physicians, health care providers, parents, and guardians to comply with immunization guideline recommendations has contributed to the development of preventable disease in susceptible individuals. A poignant example of the result of failure to immunize or of inadequate immunization was made evident during the 1989 to 1990 U.S. measles epidemic. A change in measles vaccine guidelines since that time and a major effort by health care providers to appropriately immunize patients have resulted in a dramatic decrease in the number of indigenous cases.

In comments to follow, vaccines included in the 1997 childhood immunization recommended schedule (Table 1)—their administration, contraindications, and adverse reactions—are discussed. Specific conditions for which administration of live attenuated vaccines should be avoided are addressed. Attention also is devoted to vaccines other than those included in the standard schedule (influenza, pneumococcal, and meningococcal). Brief mention is made regarding some of the newly approved vaccine combinations, combinations under study, future vaccines being contemplated, and innovative technologies being considered.

STANDARD CHILDHOOD IMMUNIZATIONS

Hepatitis B Vaccine

Nearly a quarter of a million people in the United States contract acute hepatitis B virus (HBV) infection each year. More than 1 million individuals in this country have chronic HBV infection, and more than 4000 die from hepatitis B–induced chronic liver disease and hepatocellular carcinoma. Acute HBV infection can occur at any age, although an increased number of cases occur during adolescence. Chronic HBV infection tends to occur in inverse ratio to the age at which an individual acquires acute infection. The younger a child at the time of the acute infection, the more likely that individual will become a carrier

and die years later from hepatocellular carcinoma or cirrhosis of the liver.

Transmission of HBV occurs primarily through exposure to blood and blood products, through sexual contact, and through vertical transfer from mother to infant at the time of birth. In close contact with other individuals, particularly family members, patients can transmit HBV through contact with open skin lesions and perhaps through mucous membranes by contact with other body fluids, such as saliva.

Two recombinant hepatitis B vaccines, Engerix-B and Recombivax HB, are available for use in the United States. Although these vaccine preparations are supplied in several different concentrations and vial sizes, they can be used interchangeably. Doses vary for each product and between products according to the presence or absence of maternal surface antigen, the age of the patient, and whether the individual is receiving dialysis or is immunocompromised (Table 2). The Food and Drug Administration (FDA) has given approval to the marketing of a combination vaccine containing both Recombivax HB and PedvaxHIB (HbCV).

Standard immunization guideline recommendations include universal childhood HBV immunization. Routine serologic screening of all pregnant women for hepatitis B surface antigen (HBsAg) is now mandatory, because the dose and schedule of the HBV vaccine as well as the need for hepatitis B immune globulin (HBIG) for infants depend on whether the mother is HBsAg-positive or -negative.

The HBV vaccine should be administered in 3 doses: to infants within 48 hours of birth; at 1 to 2 months of age; and at 6 to 18 months of age (Table 3). For infants born to HBsAg-negative mothers, an alternative schedule for vaccine administration is at the time of normal well child examinations, at 2, 4, and 6 to 18 months of age. Ideally, vaccine-induced protection should result in antibody levels of 10 mIU per mL or higher. Adults and children of normal immune status do not need booster doses or routine serologic testing.

TABLE 2. **Recommended Doses of Currently Licensed Hepatitis B Vaccines**

Group	Recombivax HB Dose*		Engerix-B Dose*	
	μg	mL	μg	mL
Infants of HBsAg†-negative mothers and children aged <11 y	2.5	0.5‡	10.0	0.5
Infants of HBsAg-positive mothers; prevention of perinatal infection	5.0	0.5§	10.0	0.5
Children and adolescents aged 11–19 y	5.0	0.5§	20.0	1.0
Adults aged ≥20 y	10.0	1.0§	20.0	1.0
Dialysis patients and other immunocompromised persons	40.0	1.0‖	40.0	2.0¶

*Both vaccines are routinely administered in a 3-dose series. Engerix-B also has been licensed for a 4-dose series administered at 0, 1, 2, and 12 mo.
†Hepatitis B surface antigen.
‡New pediatric formulation.
§Previously licensed formulation; can be used to deliver the appropriate age-specific dose to infants of HBsAg-negative mothers and children aged <11 y.
‖Special formulation.
¶Two 1.0-mL doses administered at one site in a 4-dose schedule at 0, 1, 2, and 6 mo.
Modified from New pediatric formulation of Recombivax HB. MMWR Morb Mortal Wkly Rep *42*:686–687, 1993.

TABLE 3. **Recommended Routine Hepatitis B Immunization Schedules**

Maternal Hepatitis B Surface Antigen Status	Dose	Age
Negative*	1	0–2 d
	2	1–2 mo
	3	6–18 mo
Positive	1†	0 d
	2	1 mo
	3	6 mo

*Alternative schedule: dose one at 1 to 2 months of age, dose two at 4 months, and dose three at 6 to 18 months.

†Hepatitis B immune globulin should also be administered.

Used with permission of the American Academy of Pediatrics from American Academy of Pediatrics Committee on Infectious Diseases: Universal hepatitis B immunization. Pediatrics *89*:795–800, 1992. (Refer to corrected statement regarding the appropriate administration of HBIG to infants whose mothers have unknown HBsAg status [Pediatrics *90*:715, 1992] and Table 1 in Pediatrics *89*:795–799, 1992 regarding recommended dosage of hepatitis B vaccine.)

Infants of HBsAg-positive mothers should receive HBIG shortly after birth and should be immunized with HBV vaccine, preferably within 12 hours but certainly before 7 days of age (see Table 3). At 1 month and 6 months of age, these infants should be given their second and third doses of HBV vaccine, respectively, and at 9 months of age or at least 1 month after the third dose, testing for HBsAg and an anti-HBs antibody level should be obtained. If the HBsAg test is negative and anti-HBs antibody level is lower than 10 mIU per mL, a fourth dose should be administered. If on subsequent testing, the level remains low, up to 2 more doses of HBV vaccine may be given.

An infant born to a mother with unknown HBsAg status should receive the same dose of HBV vaccine as an infant born to an HBsAg-positive mother. Doses and appropriate dates for the next two injections of HBV vaccine depend on subsequent HBsAg testing of the mother. If she is found to be HBsAg-positive, the infant will have to be given HBIG as soon as possible.

In addition to infants, all children, adolescents, and adults who are at significant risk of exposure to HBV infection should be immunized. After the first injection, subsequent doses of HBV should be given at 1 and 6 months. Those at increased risk include heterosexuals with more than one sexual partner in the previous 6 months and those with a recent sexually transmitted disease, homosexual and bisexual males, hemophiliac patients, intravenous drug abusers, and health care workers as well as others with occupational risk.

Diphtheria-Tetanus-Pertussis Vaccine

Combined diphtheria, tetanus, and pertussis (DTP/DTaP) immunization is recommended for all children at 2, 4, and 6 months of age. Booster doses should be given at 15 to 18 months and 4 to 6 years of age. If the fourth dose is given after the patient is 4 years of age, the fifth dose is unnecessary. Should a patient have one of the absolute contraindications to receiving pertussis, diphtheria and tetanus toxoid (DT) is the acceptable alternative. No patient beyond the age of 7 years should receive the pertussis component, owing to an increased possibility of adverse reaction. Such a patient should receive tetanus and the reduced diphtheria toxoid in the form of dT, and subsequent dT doses should be given at 10-year intervals throughout life.

The first combination diphtheria, tetanus, and acellular pertussis (DTaP) vaccine approved for use in the United States was licensed by the FDA in late 1991. Its approved use was only for the fourth and fifth doses in children between the ages of 15 months and 7 years and only in those previously immunized with at least 3 doses of DTP vaccine. Acellular vaccines contain only certain antigens of the whole pertussis bacterium and produce fewer local reactions (erythema and induration at the injection site), fever, and systemic symptoms (drowsiness, irritability, and anorexia). There are now three licensed combined acellular pertussis vaccines in the United States (Acel-Imune, Tripedia, Infanrix). As of April 1997, two of them are approved for the first 4 doses only. One of them (Acel-Imune) is approved for all 5 doses.

In areas of endemicity or during outbreaks of diphtheria or pertussis, DTP may be given as early as 4 weeks of age. Normally, the minimal age is 6 weeks for administration of either DTP or DTaP vaccines or one of the combination vaccines, DTP-HbCV. Minimal intervals for subsequent second, third, and fourth doses are 1 month, 1 month, and 6 months, respectively.

Certain precautions for and specific contraindications to giving DTP or DTaP vaccine should be kept in mind. Mild acute illness with or without fever is not one of them. An anaphylactic reaction to the vaccine or vaccine constituent and encephalopathy (not due to another identifiable cause) within 7 days of administration of a previous DTP or DTaP vaccine are considered true contraindications. Moderate or severe illness with or without fever is considered a temporary contraindication, with immunization given on recovery. Certain conditions are not contraindications but require caution before administration of subsequent doses of either vaccine. Caution should be exercised if a child, within 48 hours of having received a previous dose of DTP or DTaP, developed one of the following: temperature 105°F or higher not attributable to another identifiable cause; collapse or shocklike state; and persistent, inconsolable crying lasting 3 hours or longer. Caution also is warranted if a child had a seizure within 3 days of having received a prior dose of either preparation.

The decision to administer DTP, DTaP, or DT to an infant or child with a recognized, possible, or potential underlying neurologic condition calls for special consideration. Within 2 to 3 days after immunization, some patients appear to be at some increased risk for the appearance of manifestations of the underlying neurologic disorder.

To minimize a febrile response, consideration should be given to administering acetaminophen to patients before they receive the vaccine and every 4 hours for 24 hours thereafter. This applies, in particular, to children with a personal history or family history (siblings or parents) of convulsions.

Polio Vaccine

Indigenous wild polio, at one time a commonly encountered and devastating viral infection, is now virtually nonexistent in the United States. During the last 30 years, standard childhood immunization with oral polio vaccine (OPV) (Orimune) has resulted in significant protective intestinal immunity, and the excretion of virus by vaccinees (for 6 to 7 weeks after OPV administration) has occasionally provided inadvertent benefit by immunizing previously unimmunized contacts.

The 8 to 10 cases of paralytic polio that do occur in the United States each year are all vaccine-associated and due to OPV. Some cases involve the vaccinee, and others involve susceptible contacts. To reduce the incidence of vaccine-associated paralytic polio, the ACIP, in the fall of 1996, recommended that inactivated poliovirus vaccine (IPV) (IPOL) become the vaccine of choice. Accordingly, polio vaccine should be given in 4 doses, with the first 2 doses at 2 and 4 months of age, and the third and fourth doses given at 12 to 18 months and 4 to 6 years of age, respectively. The latter 2 doses can be given as either OPV or IPV. Significant areas of concern regarding the change to injectable polio vaccine involve cost/benefit ratio, compliance by the patient or parent, and increased disease risk among minorities and the economically disadvantaged.

Should the physician, the patient, or the family prefer OPV, it should be given at 2, 4, and 6 months of age with a booster dose at 4 to 6 years. The fourth dose given before school is not needed if the third dose of either IPV or OPV is given after the patient's fourth birthday.

Contraindications to giving OPV include being human immunodeficiency virus (HIV)–positive, having a congenital immunodeficiency, being immunosuppressed by cancer or long-term immunosuppressive therapy, and having an HIV-positive or otherwise immunodeficient household contact. Patients who have previously had an anaphylactoid reaction to OPV or to streptomycin, bacitracin, or neomycin (trace amounts of which are contained in OPV) should not be given the vaccine. The only contraindication to the use of IPV is in a patient with a history of anaphylactoid reaction to neomycin or streptomycin, both of which are contained in trace amounts.

Although high concentrations of passively acquired serum antibodies have blunted serum antibody response to OPV and IPV, parenterally administered immune globulin has had little or no effect on OPV in the intestine. Breast-feeding does not interfere with OPV immunization, and although there is no documented evidence that either OPV or IPV has produced adverse effects in pregnant women or their fetuses, immunization with these vaccines should be avoided. In an epidemic, if a pregnant woman needs protection, OPV is preferred.

Haemophilus influenzae Type B Conjugate Vaccine

Currently, four licensed HbCVs are available in the United States. Variability among them includes the kind of carrier protein used, the polysaccharide molecular size, and the method of saccharide-protein conjugation. To complete the primary series before the age of 7 months, two of these vaccines (HbOC [HibTITER] and PRP-T [ActHIB and OmniHib]) require 3 doses given at 2-month intervals, and one (PRP-OMP [PedVaxHIB]) requires 2 doses with a 2-month interval. If feasible, the same HbCV should be used to complete the primary series. A booster dose at 12 to 15 months of age (or as soon thereafter as possible) is required for each of these vaccines. The fourth HbCV (PRP-D [ProHIBIT]) is licensed for use only in patients 12 months or older. Any one of the four HbCVs can be used for the booster dose regardless of the type of HbCV used previously. The ACIP has identified no contraindications or precautions regarding administration of HbCV.

If the first dose of the primary series is initiated at 7 to 11 months of age, HbOC, PRP-T, and PRP-OMP all require 2 doses at 2-month intervals. A booster dose should be given at 12 to 15 months of age, preferably 2 months after the second dose. For patients who have received only a single dose of HbCV or no vaccine before 1 year of age and who are now 12 to 14 months of age, 2 doses of any of the HbCVs are recommended. Patients who are 15 months up to 60 months old require only a single dose.

For patients with immunologic impairment associated with increased risk of invasive Hib disease, specific guidelines should be followed. Patients who have HIV infection, IgG2 subclass deficiency, bone marrow transplant, sickle cell disease, or splenectomy, or are receiving chemotherapy for malignancies, who are 12 to 59 months of age, and who have received either one or no previous HbCV injection should be given 2 doses of any of the preparations 2 months apart. For patients with sickle cell disease or asplenia who are older than 59 months and have had no previous HbCV, a single dose should be given, and for those with HIV infection, IgG2 subclass deficiency, bone marrow transplant, or malignancy, 2 doses separated by 1 to 2 months are suggested.

Patients with invasive Hib disease who are younger than 2 years of age, regardless of previous history for having received HbCV, should be given HbCV during convalescence according to the age-appropriate schedule for unvaccinated children. Those whose disease occurred at age 24 months or later do not need immunization.

To reduce the number of injections, two combination vaccines containing HbCV and DTP and one containing HbCV and DTaP are available. HbCV-DTP can be used routinely in children 6 weeks to 59 months of age. HbCV-DTaP has been approved for use only as the fourth dose of DTP or DTaP in children 15 months or older.

Measles-Mumps-Rubella Vaccine

Measles, mumps, and rubella live-virus vaccines, although available for separate single-antigen administration, are preferably administered subcutaneously as a combination MMR vaccine. Current guidelines recommend that the vaccine be given as a first dose at 12 to 15 months of age and as a second dose at either 4 to 6 or 11 to 12 years of age. To rapidly complete a 2-dose MMR series, a minimal interval of 1 month is required.

For patients who are older than 12 years, who were born after 1956, or who do not have adequate history or documentation of having received either dose of MMR, 1 or 2 doses should be given. This is particularly true for health care workers, for people in post–high school educational settings, and during epidemics. Special attention should be made to avoid administration to women who are pregnant or are contemplating pregnancy in the next 3 months. The theoretical risks to the fetus should be explained to women of childbearing age for whom MMR vaccination is being considered, but accumulated data from the Centers for Disease Control and Prevention have revealed no case of adverse fetal response.

Parenterally administered immune globulin can blunt or block the host response to certain live-virus vaccines. Suggested guidelines from the Committee on Infectious Diseases of the AAP regarding interval length between administration of various immune globulin preparations and MMR or monovalent measles vaccine should be consulted.

True contraindications to administration of MMR vaccine include pregnancy, known altered immunodeficiency states such as congenital immunodeficiencies, long-term immunosuppressive therapy, and hematologic or solid tumors. Immunization should be temporarily withheld from patients with moderate or severe febrile illnesses until the acute phase has subsided. Patients experiencing thrombocytopenia within 6 weeks of having had MMR vaccine should probably not receive a subsequent dose.

MMR should be administered to all asymptomatic HIV-infected persons and to HIV-infected persons who are not severely immunocompromised and who have no evidence of measles immunity. Routine immunization of the severely immunocompromised HIV-infected individual remains controversial. Should a person in this latter group be at risk for measles exposure during an outbreak, the choice between measles vaccination and immune globulin prophylaxis should be considered.

Reports suggest that anaphylactic reactions to measles-containing vaccines are associated not with hypersensitivity to egg antigens but with some other component of the vaccines. Because MMR and its component vaccines contain hydrolyzed gelatin as a stabilizer and trace amounts of neomycin, extreme caution should be used before the vaccine is given to individuals with a history of anaphylaxis to these additives.

Varicella Vaccine

Varicella-zoster virus (VZV) vaccine (Varivax) was added to the list of standard childhood vaccines in 1995. Before its recommended use, an estimated 3.7 million cases of chickenpox occurred in the United States annually, resulting in nearly 9000 hospitalizations and approximately 100 deaths. A cost-effectiveness study in 1994 employing use of the vaccine estimated a savings to society, in terms of the costs of medical care and time lost from work, at almost $400 million.

VZV vaccine is recommended to be given on a routine basis to all immunocompetent children at 12 to 18 months of age. However, anyone 1 year or older without a history of having had chickenpox can be immunized. Between ages 1 and 13 years, a single subcutaneous injection is required; after age 13, two injections given 4 to 8 weeks apart are needed.

VZV vaccine appears to confer a high rate of protection against severe disease. Seroconversion rates for children 1 to 12 years of age are greater than 95%, and for those older than 12 years, 94%. Ongoing studies from the United States and Japan indicate that antibodies to VZV are present 10 years after immunization in more than 95% of recipients.

Contraindications to giving VZV vaccine include primary or acquired immunocompromised states, pregnancy, moderate or severe illnesses, and a previous anaphylactoid reaction to neomycin. As a precaution, salicylates should not be administered for at least 6 weeks after the vaccine has been given, owing to potential development of Reye's syndrome.

Approximately 7 to 8% of all patients develop a few maculopapular or varicelliform skin lesions within 1 month of immunization. About one fifth of children and up to one third of adolescents and adults express complaints of pain, tenderness, or redness at the injection site. Temperature higher than 102°F, occurring up to 1.5 months after varicella immunization, has been noted in 15% of patients, but because of similar febrile response in placebo recipients, the reaction is not considered significant.

VZV has been recovered from skin lesions of healthy vaccine recipients, yet no clinical case of varicella has occurred in contacts of those vaccinees. Subclinical or extremely mild cases of varicella have been reported in contacts of vaccinees with leukemia. Children with acute lymphocytic leukemia in remission for at least 1 year and with platelet counts higher than 100,000 per mm^3 and lymphocyte counts higher than 700 per mm^3 24 hours before immunization should be considered potential recipients.

OTHER IMMUNIZATIONS

Influenza Vaccine

The trivalent influenza whole-virus (Fluzone) or split-virus (Fluogen) vaccine has two type A and one type B inactivated components. Influenza A virus is classified into subtypes on the basis of two surface antigens, hemagglutinin (H) and neuraminidase (N). Hemagglutinin has three subtypes (H1, H2, H3), and neuraminidase has two subtypes (N1, N2). New variants of influenza virus, particularly type A, emerge each year, necessitating vaccine modification.

Elderly patients and children considered at high risk for severe complications of influenza infection should be immunized yearly. Patients at risk are those with chronic pulmonary diseases or hemodynamically significant cardiac disease, those undergoing immunosuppressive therapy, and those with a hemoglobinopathy. Other persons considered to be at increased risk are patients with chronic metabolic disease, chronic kidney disease, or diabetes mellitus; recipients of long-term aspirin therapy; and HIV-infected patients. The close contacts of high-risk patients also should be immunized.

Influenza vaccine should not be given to children younger than 6 months. For children older than 6 months but younger than 9 years who are being immunized against influenza virus for the first time, 2 doses of the split-virus vaccine should be given intramuscularly 1 month apart. For patients older than 9 years, a single dose of the split-virus vaccine is required. Patients 12 years or older may be given either the whole-virus or split-virus vaccine.

Influenza vaccine does not cause an infection in recipients. Local reaction consists of tenderness at the site of injection lasting approximately 2 days. Delayed hypersensitivity reaction, consisting of rash, tenderness, swelling, and/or redness, due to one of the vaccine components may occur infrequently. Fever, malaise, and myalgia, particularly in recipients not previously exposed to influenza virus antigens, may last for 1 to 2 days. Patients with history of anaphylaxis to eggs or other vaccine components should not be given influenza vaccine. Alternatively, these patients should receive chemoprophylaxis with either amantadine or rimantadine to protect against influenza A.

Pneumococcal Vaccine

Streptococcus pneumoniae is the leading cause of bacterial pneumonia worldwide and among the principal causes of sepsis and meningitis. The current 23-valent pneumococcal polysaccharide vaccine (Pneumovax 23) is considered to be 55 to 60% effective in preventing invasive pneumococcal disease in immunocompetent hosts. It is recommended to be given intramuscularly or subcutaneously to patients 65 years and older and to patients with sickle cell disease, asplenia or splenic dysfunction, chronic renal disease or nephrotic syndrome, immunosuppressed conditions, cerebrospinal fluid leaks, or HIV infection. When elective splenectomy or scheduled chemotherapy or immunotherapy is contemplated, pneumococcal vaccine should be given at least 2 weeks beforehand.

This vaccine is not recommended for children younger than 2 years or for routine reimmunization of patients previously immunized with the 14-valent vaccine. Patients at high risk of fatal pneumococcal infection, however, who have previously received the 14-valent vaccine should be considered candidates for the 23-valent vaccine. Children 10 years or younger who are at high risk of pneumococcal infection and who previously received the 23-valent vaccine should be considered for reimmunization after 3 to 5 years. Similarly, adults, older children, and adolescents at high risk should be considered for reimmunization after 6 years.

Meningococcal Vaccine

Neisseria meningitidis is the leading cause of childhood bacterial meningitis and a major cause of septicemia in North America. The majority of cases of invasive meningococcal disease are equally distributed between serogroups B and C. No vaccine is currently available to prevent group B disease. The only available vaccine in the United States to prevent invasive meningococcal disease is Menomune, containing four purified capsular polysaccharides (A, C, Y, and W-135).

Routine meningococcal immunization is recommended for individuals older than 2 years and at significant risk, including those with terminal complement or properdin deficiencies and anatomic or functional asplenia. If there is an outbreak or cluster of cases of meningococcal disease due to one of the serogroups contained in the vaccine, local or state health authorities will select the target group for vaccination. The vaccine may also be recommended for individuals older than 3 months who are traveling or residing in a country with hyperendemic or epidemic meningococcal disease caused by a vaccine-preventable serogroup.

Meningococcal vaccine should be given subcutaneously. Parents and older patients should be told that vaccine protection may not develop until 2 weeks after immunization. Mild local side effects, such as pain, redness, swelling, and tenderness, may appear at the injection site. Persons allergic to thimerosol (a preservative) should not receive the vaccine.

Antimicrobial prophylaxis is recommended for close contacts of any person with invasive meningococcal disease, including household members, other individuals in the patient's child care centers or nursery school, and persons who were directly exposed to oropharyngeal secretions during the 7 days before onset of disease in the index case. Unless treated with ceftriaxone, the index patient also should receive chemoprophylactic antibiotics before discharge.

Few data are available to determine the need or timing for revaccination when new or continued risks exist. Even if new risk of exposure occurs, adults may not have to be revaccinated for 5 years. Children younger than 4 years and at risk of new or continuous group C exposure should be considered for revaccination after 1 year, whereas those initially immunized at 4 years or older should be revaccinated after 5 years.

SIMULTANEOUS ADMINISTRATION OF VACCINES

Simultaneous administration of any of the vaccines mentioned does not interfere with overall immune response. When injectable vaccines have to be given in the same muscle area, the distance between them should be at least 1 inch. HBV vaccine should be injected intramuscularly in either the anterolateral thigh or the upper arm, not the buttocks. VZV vaccine should not be given at the same injection site as MMR vaccine.

Fever and other local reactions may occur after either DTP or influenza immunization. Because of the difficulty of determining which of the two could be responsible for an adverse reaction, some health care providers prefer administering them 3 days apart. Giving DTaP instead of DTP might avoid the problem.

FUTURE PROSPECTS

Efforts toward the development of conjugate pneumococcal and meningococcal vaccines are under way. Vaccines being investigated or being considered for development include those for rotavirus, respiratory syncytial virus, herpes simplex virus, group B *Streptococcus, Shigella* species, *Escherichia coli, Vibrio cholerae, Borrelia burgdorferi, Mycobacterium tuberculosis*, and malaria. The potential production of multiple combination vaccines, such as VZV-MMR and DTaP-Hib-HBV-IPV, is being evaluated. New vaccine formulation strategies, including the use of polymers, novel adjuvants, and vector systems to enhance the effectiveness of vaccines, are being researched. Such efforts should prove enormously beneficial in helping to eradicate some of the more devastating infections currently plaguing humankind.

TOXOPLASMOSIS

method of
LOUIS M. WEISS, M.D., M.P.H.
*Albert Einstein College of Medicine
Bronx, New York*

Infection with *Toxoplasma gondii,* an apicomplexan protozoan, is highly prevalent throughout the world. In fact, subclinical toxoplasmosis is probably one of the most common parasitic infections of humans. In the United States, the prevalence of infection in adults as determined by seropositivity epidemiologic studies varies from 20 to 70%, depending on the geographic area. In France, the seropositivity rate in women older than 35 years is 95%. This parasitic infection is not limited to humans but is also present in most animal and bird species.

T. gondii was first discovered in the gondi, a North African rodent, by Nicolle in 1908. In the 1930s, the association between congenital toxoplasmosis and retinitis was described, and later, severe disseminated toxoplasmosis was described. Shortly thereafter, a mononucleosis-like adenopathy syndrome and seropositive asymptomatic acute infection were recognized. Iatrogenic immunosuppression with transplantation resulted in the emergence of reactivation toxoplasmosis as a disease entity. Fifteen to 20% of patients with acquired immune deficiency syndrome (AIDS) have developed encephalitis owing to secondary reactivation of latent toxoplasmosis. Data suggests that one third of AIDS patients who are seropositive for *T. gondii* will ultimately develop toxoplasmic encephalitis. Latent *T. gondii* infection in humans is common. In the United States, it has been shown that the yearly antibody acquisition rate is 0.5 to 1%. Of human immunodeficiency virus–positive adults in major urban areas of the United States, 16% are seropositive for *T. gondii.*

The parasite has three morphologic forms: tachyzoite (endozoite), bradyzoite (tissue cyst), and oocyst. In humans, tachyzoites (the rapidly proliferating stage) and bradyzoites (latent stage) are seen. In felines, the definitive host, an enteroepithelial sexual life cycle takes place with the production of infectious oocysts. Oocysts become infectious, i.e., sporulate, in 1 to 21 days after passage, depending on temperature and availability of oxygen. Humans or animals become infected by ingestion of oocyst-contaminated (i.e., cat feces–contaminated) food or water, by ingestion of bradyzoites in inadequately cooked meat, or by transplacental transmission. Transplacental transmission in humans results when a seronegative woman acquires toxoplasmosis during pregnancy. Seropositive women who become pregnant usually do not transmit toxoplasmosis to their children unless they are severely immunosuppressed (e.g., have AIDS). Transmission has also occurred by organ transplantation and laboratory accident. Infection can be prevented by eating only meat that has been well cooked (to more than 60°C) or has been frozen (to less than 20°C) for at least 24 hours. Because sporulation of oocysts takes several days, regular cleaning of cat litter boxes also decreases transmission. Cats kept indoors and fed commercial cat food have a low risk of acquiring and shedding *T. gondii* oocysts.

The early stage of infection is characterized by replication of tachyzoites with subsequent hematogenous dissemination to every organ. Tachyzoites parasitize virtually any cell type. Interferon-γ (IFN-γ) appears to be a critical factor in host defense against this organism. Replication of the tachyzoites is contained by the immune system, and tissue cysts accumulate in the brain, heart, and skeletal muscle cells. Cysts, which may persist for years or for the life of the host, are surrounded by a tough, argyrophilic, cyst wall with a positive periodic acid–Schiff reaction. When a host with chronic toxoplasmosis (seropositive host) becomes immunosuppressed, reactivation of these latent foci (i.e., tissue cysts) occurs, with the transformation of bradyzoites to tachyzoites and the development of reactivation disease, manifesting as either disseminated disease or focal abscesses.

TREATMENT

Most people infected with *T. gondii* are asymptomatic, but a wide spectrum of clinical diseases can result from infection. For purposes of therapy, it is helpful to separate the disease into several categories (Table 1). The decision to treat is based on the location of infection, the immune status of the patient, and whether or not a woman with acute toxoplasmosis is pregnant. The recommended therapies are based on extrapolations from in vitro and animal models (mostly murine), a few large well-controlled clinical studies, and the clinical experience and practice at medical centers experienced in the treatment of *Toxoplasma* infection. The ideal dosage, combination of drugs (Table 2), and length of therapy are not known. In general, the drugs used to treat toxoplasmosis are active against the rapidly replicating tachyzoite stage but have limited efficacy against tissue cysts. Thus, patients treated for toxoplasmosis have latent infection (tissue cysts) at the conclusion of treatment.

Asymptomatic Infection or Latent Infection

Immunocompetent individuals with latent toxoplasmosis as evidenced by positive serology do not require treatment. *Toxoplasma* encephalitis developed in 12% of patients with CD4+ cell counts of 100 per mm^3, 25% of those with counts of 50 to 99 per mm^3, and 45% of those with counts less than 50 per

TABLE 1. *Toxoplasma* Infections and Treatment Indications

Syndrome	Treatment*
Asymptomatic infection (latent infection detected by positive serologic test)	
Immunocompetent host	Not required
AIDS patient (CD4+ cell count < 100/mm^3)	TMP-SMZ
Cardiac transplantation	PYR
Adenopathy, fever, or malaise in the immunocompetent host	Not required†
Disseminated disease (i.e., CNS, heart, or liver) in an immunocompetent host or a laboratory infection with tachyzoites	PYR/SULFA
Infection during pregnancy	SPR-PYR/SULFA‡
Congenital toxoplasmosis	PYR/SULFA§
Ocular toxoplasmosis	PYR/SULFA and steroids
Infection in immunocompromised hosts	
AIDS	PYR/SULFA (see Table 3)
Transplantation	PYR/SULFA
Acute disease	PYR/SULFA

*Recommended primary treatments as described in the text.
†Painful adenopathy may respond to indomethacin; prolonged adenopathy may respond to PYR/SULFA.
‡Infection during pregnancy as determined by seroconversion of the mother is treated with spiramycin. If the fetus is confirmed to have toxoplasmosis by ultrasonography, amniocentesis, or cordocentesis, PYR/SULFA is given alternating with SPR.
§Congenital toxoplasmosis is treated until the infant is 6 to 12 mo old.
Abbreviations: AIDS = acquired immune deficiency syndrome; CNS = central nervous system; PYR = pyrimethamine; SPR = spiramycin; SULFA = sulfonamides; steroids = corticosteroids; TMP-SMZ = trimethoprim-sulfamethoxazole.

mm^3, who were followed up for 18 months. Primary prophylaxis is appropriate for AIDS patients with positive serology for *T. gondii* and CD4+ cell counts of 100 per mm^3 or less. Numerous studies have reported the efficacy of daily trimethoprim-sulfamethoxazole (Bactrim, Septra)* one double-strength tablet daily, for prophylaxis. An alternative is pyrimethamine (Daraprim) (25 mg per week) and dapsone* (100 mg twice a week). In heart transplantation, seronegative recipients of a heart from a seropositive donor have been given pyrimethamine 25 mg per day for 6 weeks after transplantation to prevent reactivation of disease.

Acquired Toxoplasmosis

In immunocompetent individuals, *T. gondii* infection is usually asymptomatic or presents as a mild, self-limited febrile illness characterized by adenopathy, fever, and malaise. Treatment is rarely needed. In the uncommon patient whose symptoms are persistent, however, treatment should be as described for disseminated disease. In an occasional patient, acute toxoplasmosis may manifest as severe disseminated disease with organ dysfunction. Myocarditis, encephalitis, and a sepsis syndrome with shock and hepatitis have been described. In patients with these manifestations, treatment should be given with pyrimethamine, 100 mg as a loading dose and 25 to 50 mg per day, and sulfadiazine or trisulfapyrimidines, 4 to 6 grams per day, for 4 to 6 weeks. Folinic acid, 5 to 10 mg per day, should also be given. Infections acquired through a laboratory accident or blood transfusion should also be treated as just described.

Acquired Toxoplasmosis During Pregnancy

Toxoplasmosis is transmitted to the fetus when a woman acquires the infection after the date of conception. The risk of transmission of toxoplasmosis increases with the trimester in which a woman acquires the infection; therefore, in the first trimester, the risk of fetal infection is 14%, in the second trimester, 29%, and in the third trimester, 59%. The severity of the manifestations of infection falls with each trimester, so the majority of fetal infections in the first trimester result in mental retardation and the TORCH (toxoplasmosis, other agents, rubella, cytomegalovirus, herpes simplex) syndrome, but fetuses infected in the third trimester are asymptomatic at birth. However, follow-up of congenitally infected children who are asymptomatic at birth does show that the majority develop clinical toxoplasmosis with retinitis and/or subtle central nervous system (CNS) effects later in life. Treatment of women who become infected with *T. gondii* during pregnancy decreases the incidence of fetal infection.

Diagnosis of infection acquired during pregnancy requires documentation of (1) seroconversion, (2) a

*Not FDA approved for this indication.

TABLE 2. **Drugs Used in the Treatment of Toxoplasmosis**

Drug	Mode of Action	Metabolism	Adverse Effects
Pyrimethamine (Daraprim)	Inhibits folic acid synthesis via dihydrofolate reductase	Readily absorbed via the gastrointestinal tract; hepatic metabolism, lipid soluble, concentrated in brain parenchyma Serum half-life of 35–175 h, cerebrospinal fluid levels 10–25% of serum levels Serum levels with 25–75 mg/d = 1–4.5 mg/L	Cytopenias (neutropenia, leukopenia, thrombocytopenia) that are dose related and may be ameliorated by folinic acid (leucovorin) administration Headache, nausea, a funny taste in the mouth, rash, and gastrointestinal intolerance Histamine *N*-methyltransferase possibly inhibited by high doses, causing increased histamine levels
Sulfadiazine or trisulfapyrimidine (other sulfonamides are less active in vitro against *Toxoplasma gondii*)	Inhibits folic acid synthesis via dihydrofolic acid synthetase; acts synergistically with pyrimethamine	Readily absorbed via the gastrointestinal tract; penetrates blood-brain barrier	Gastrointestinal tract intolerance, cytopenias, nephrolithiasis, crystalluria (2–4% of patients), interstitial nephritis, rash, Stevens-Johnson syndrome, hypersensitivity reactions Adverse reactions more common in patients with acquired immune deficiency syndrome
Clindamycin (Cleocin)	Unknown; may interact with apicoplast (an organelle) to cause cell death	Readily absorbed via the gastrointestinal tract; excellent tissue penetration	Gastrointestinal tract intolerance, pseudomembranous colitis, rash
Macrolides Spiramycin Clarithromycin (Biaxin) Azithromycin (Zithromax)	Unknown; may interact with apicoplast (an organelle) to cause cell death	Readily absorbed via the gastrointestinal tract; high intracellular and tissue levels Spiramycin placental levels 6.2 mg/L and cord blood levels 0.78 mg/L with a 3 gm/d maternal dose	Gastrointestinal tract intolerance common (nausea, vomiting, diarrhea, abdominal pain) High levels of clarithromycin and azithromycin associated with hearing loss and liver function test abnormalities
Atovaquone (Mepron)	Uncoupling of electron biosynthesis; inhibition of de novo pyrimidine biosynthesis	Poorly absorbed via the gastrointestinal tract; suspension has better bioavailability than tablets; absorption improved by fatty foods	Rash, elevated liver function parameters

rise in *Toxoplasma*-specific IgG titer, or (3) the presence of significant amounts of *Toxoplasma*-specific IgM.*

Studies in France suggest that acutely infected women should be given spiramycin, 3 grams per day divided three times a day, once maternal infection is suspected or diagnosed. Spiramycin should be continued throughout pregnancy. In the United States, spiramycin is available by request from the Food and Drug Administration (phone number: 301-443-9553).

Amniocentesis, fetal blood monitoring, and fetal ultrasonography should be used to assess infection in the fetus. Ultrasonography should be done every 2 to 4 weeks, because ventricular dilatation may develop in as little as 10 days. If fetal toxoplasmosis is diagnosed by (1) demonstration of fetal *Toxoplasma*-specific IgM, (2) culture of *T. gondii* from amniotic fluid or fetal blood, (3) polymerase chain reaction of amniotic fluid or fetal blood, or (4) ultrasonographic evidence of ventricular dilatation, then

specific therapy with pyrimethamine, 50 mg per day, sulfadiazine, 3 grams per day, and folinic acid, 5 to 15 mg per day, should be administered to the mother for 3 weeks, alternating with spiramycin,* 3 grams per day for 3 weeks, until delivery. This regimen significantly reduces the severity of disease seen at birth. The majority of infants born to women treated with this regimen had subclinical disease at birth. Of note, however, is that the majority of women whose ultrasound scans demonstrated fetal hydrocephalus with ventricular dilatation in the second trimester elected to have abortions, and the aborted infants were shown to have severe toxoplasmosis on autopsy examination. An alternative regimen, consisting of spiramycin* 3 grams per day, Fansidar (sulfadoxine 1500 mg and pyrimethamine 75 mg) 3 tablets every 10 days, and folinic acid until delivery, has also been used in France with success. Pyrimethamine should not be used in the first 14 to 16 weeks of pregnancy because of concerns about teratogenicity. Even if the mother receives pyrimethamine and sulfadiazine, a neonate with congenital toxoplasmosis should receive further drug therapy.

*A good review of the diagnostic tests and their utility and interpretation can be found in Remington JS, Klein JO (eds): *Infectious Diseases of the Fetus and Newborn Infant,* 4th ed. Philadelphia, WB Saunders Co, 1995.

*Not available in the United States.

Congenital Toxoplasmosis

It is estimated that 1 per 1000 children born each year in the United States has congenital toxoplasmosis. The cost of caring for all of the cases of congenital toxoplasmosis has been estimated to be $200 to $400 million per year. Even neonates who appear normal at birth (subclinical disease) may later demonstrate serious sequelae (primarily retinitis). The Chicago Collaborative Treatment Trial has demonstrated that treatment of an infant with congenital toxoplasmosis during the first year of life mitigates tissue destruction and ameliorates sequelae.*

In all healthy-appearing infants born to mothers known to have active toxoplasmosis in pregnancy, therapy with pyrimethamine and sulfadiazine for 3 weeks followed by spiramycin or sulfadiazine alone is given until laboratory confirmation or denial of congenital infection can be obtained. Documented congenital toxoplasmosis is treated with pyrimethamine in a loading dose of 2 mg per kg per day for 2 days, followed by 1 mg per kg day or 15 mg per m^2 for 2 months, and then by 15 mg per m^2 or 1 mg per kg three times a week for the next 10 months. In addition, sulfadiazine or trisulfapyrimidine, at 100 mg per kg per day in two divided doses, and folinic acid, 5 mg every other day, are administered. Blood counts should be obtained twice weekly. In severely affected children, a different schedule of pyrimethamine, for 6 months of 1 mg per kg per day, followed by 6 months of 1 mg per kg per day three times a week, is often used. Corticosteroids, 1 mg per kg per day, should be added for patients with active macular disease or active cerebrospinal fluid profiles (protein level of 1 gram per dL or higher).

Ocular Toxoplasmosis

It is believed that local reactivation of toxoplasma cysts in the eye is responsible for ocular toxoplasmosis. Ocular disease can occur, however, with acute infection. Diagnosis is made by observation of classic retinochoroiditis on ophthalmologic examination combined with serologic evidence of toxoplasmosis. Serologic titers may be low in this disease, and occasionally, aqueous humor serology is useful for diagnosis. The retinochoroiditis is self-limited. At present, it is clear that therapy with pyrimethamine, 25 mg per day, sulfadiazine, 4 grams per day (in four divided doses), and folinic acid, 5 to 10 mg per day for 4 weeks, is effective in decreasing the inflammation but does not appear to shorten the time course of the retinitis. Corticosteroids (prednisone, 1 to 2 mg per kg per day) are also indicated if the macula, optic nerve head, or papillomacular bundle is involved. If prednisone is given, the dosage is tapered once pigmentation (healing) begins. Clindamycin (Cleo-

cin),* 1200 mg per day, has been used in place of pyrimethamine, but in a comparative trial, it was inferior to pyrimethamine with sulfadiazine. For ocular disease, tetracycline and spiramycin are not effective.

Toxoplasma Infection in Immunocompromised Hosts

In AIDS patients, *Toxoplasma* encephalitis is a common disease, manifesting as mental status changes and radiographic evidence (computed tomography or magnetic resonance imaging) of ring enhancing lesions in the brain (multiple or single). The clinical presentation of *Toxoplasma* encephalitis often reflects the multifocal involvement of the CNS seen in this disease. These clinical findings include alteration of mental status, seizures, sensory abnormalities, neuropsychiatric disease, cerebellar dysfunction, motor weakness, movement disorders, and transverse myelitis. Usually, the presentation is subacute, with focal neurologic disease reported in 60 to 90% of patients and altered mental status in 60%. In about 30% of patients, seizures are present as an initial manifestation. Most AIDS patients are seropositive for *T. gondii*, and this disease is believed to be due to reactivation of tissue cysts in the brain. No specific serologic test can confirm this diagnosis. In areas where the seroprevalence of *T. gondii* infection is high, *Toxoplasma* encephalitis is often the initial manifestation of AIDS. Most AIDS patients with toxoplasmosis have CD4+ T lymphocyte counts of less than 100 per mm^3. Primary prophylaxis with trimethoprim-sulfamethoxazole* is appropriate for AIDS patients with positive *T. gondii* serology and CD4+ counts of 100 per mm^3 or less.

Therapy is often started empirically with pyrimethamine and sulfadiazine (Table 3), and the diagnosis is confirmed by an improvement with specific antitoxoplasmal therapy. Once specific antitoxoplasmal therapy is started, radiographic improvement should be evident in 7 to 14 days. Treatment is with pyrimethamine, 25 to 100 mg per day, and sulfadiazine, 4 to 6 grams per day. Folinic acid, 10 to 20 mg per day, is also given. Folic acid should not be used, because it could inhibit the action of pyrimethamine on *T. gondii*. When pyrimethamine, 25 mg per day, is used, a loading dose of 100 to 200 mg per day (divided into two daily doses) should be given, owing to the long half-life of this agent. Corticosteroids are often used to control intracranial hypertension due to mass effect. Prophylactic anticonvulsants are not recommended. Because of the wide variation in absorption and half-life of pyrimethamine, many authorities recommend using 75 to 100 mg per day of pyrimethamine combined with sulfadiazine in the setting of *T. gondii* encephalitis in AIDS.

In AIDS patients intolerant to sulfadiazine, there is no standard therapy. Pyrimethamine alone, at dosages of 75 to 100 mg per day, has been utilized with

---

*See McAuley J, Boyer KM, Patel D, et al: Early and longitudinal evaluations of treated infants and children and untreated historical patients with congenital toxoplasmosis: The Chicago Collaborative Treatment Trial. Clin Infect Dis *18*:38–72, 1994; phone Dr. Rima McLeod at the University of Chicago.

---

*Not FDA approved for this indication.

TABLE 3. **Treatment of *Toxoplasma* Encephalitis in Patients with AIDS**

Drug	Dose	
	Acute Treatment (3 to 6 Weeks)	*Maintenance Treatment*
Pyrimethamine	Loading dose of 100–200 mg, then 50–75 mg/d with folinic acid, 10–20 mg/d	25–50 mg/d with folinic acid, 10–20 mg/d
plus		
Sulfadiazine	1–1.5 gm q 6 h	0.5–1.0 gm q 6 h
or		
Clindamycin	600 mg q 6 h	300–600 mg q 6 h
Alternatives		
Pyrimethamine	As above	As above
plus		
Atovaquone	1500 mg twice/d*	750–1500 mg twice/d
or		
Clarithromycin	500 mg twice/d	500 mg twice/d
or		
Azithromycin	1250–1500 mg/d*	1000–1500 mg/d

*Exceeds dosage recommended by the manufacturer.

good results. A prospective randomized study has demonstrated that there was no significant difference in clinical outcome when pyrimethamine plus clindamycin was compared with pyrimethamine plus sulfadiazine. A panel of experts has recommended that pyrimethamine, 50 to 75 mg per day, with clindamycin, 600 mg every 6 hours, be considered the alternative regimen in patients with sulfadiazine intolerance. Desensitization to sulfadiazine has also been reported to be successful in some sulfadiazine-intolerant patients. There are patients in whom *Toxoplasma* encephalitis has progressed when sulfadiazine was stopped despite the use of high-dose pyrimethamine and clindamycin; these patients have generally had a decrease in encephalitis once they restarted sulfadiazine after undergoing desensitization.

A number of other agents have been used in animal models and in case reports for the treatment of toxoplasmosis. Experience suggests that two agents in combination are more effective than monotherapy. The new macrolide-azalide antibiotics azithromycin (Zithromax) and clarithromycin (Biaxin) were effective in a murine model, and the combination of clarithromycin plus pyrimethamine was effective in a small clinical trial. Atovaquone (Mepron),* a hydroxynaphthoquinone, has remarkable activity against *T. gondii* in animal models, and a response rate of 66% was demonstrated in a monotherapy clinical trial of 24 patients with *Toxoplasma* encephalitis. Relapse, however, occurred in 50% of patients who continued to take atovaquone for maintenance therapy. Other drugs with reported efficacy include rifabutin (Mycobutin)*, minocycline (Minocin),* trimetrexate (NeuTrexin), and dapsone.* In addition, recombinant IFN-γ demonstrated efficacy in animal models, especially when combined with anti-*Toxoplasma* drugs. The folic acid antagonists piritrexim and trimetrexate have demonstrated efficacy in in

vitro and in vivo models of toxoplasmosis. Arprinocid, a purine analogue, is an anticoccidial agent that has shown efficacy in mice. 5-Fluorouracil (5-FU)* has efficacy in vitro and was shown to have some effect on *Toxoplasma* encephalitis in a limited trial in France.

After initial therapy, the relapse rate of *Toxoplasma* encephalitis in patients who do not receive maintenance therapy is 50 to 80% at 12 months. Thus, after successful primary therapy, drug dosages are generally decreased for lifelong maintenance therapy. The regimen of pyrimethamine, 25 mg per day, sulfadiazine, 1 gram every 6 hours, and folinic acid, 10 mg per day, is the standard therapy used. In the setting of sulfadiazine intolerance, pyrimethamine and clindamycin, 600 mg every 6 hours, are often used. Alternatives include pyrimethamine-sulfadoxine (Fansidar), 1 tablet three times weekly, pyrimethamine alone, 50 mg per day, pyrimethamine plus atovaquone, 1500 mg every 12 hours, pyrimethamine plus azithromycin, 1200 mg per day, and pyrimethamine plus clarithromycin, 500 mg every 12 hours.

In acute disease in other immunocompromised hosts, pyrimethamine and sulfadiazine are given as described previously for 6 weeks. It is not clear that patients other than AIDS patients are at a high risk for relapse. In heart transplantation, acute disease occurs only when a seronegative recipient receives a heart from a seropositive donor. Therapy for 6 weeks has been effective in these cases. In one transplant center, pyrimethamine alone, at 25 mg per day for 6 weeks after transplantation, has prevented acute toxoplasmosis in seronegative recipients receiving seropositive hearts.

Clearly, less toxic drugs for toxoplasmosis therapy in AIDS patients are needed. In addition, a drug active against the tissue cyst (bradyzoite) would make the radical cure of toxoplasmosis feasible and could be used as prophylaxis in seropositive immunocompromised patients.

*Not FDA approved for this indication.

*Not FDA approved for this indication.

TRICHINOSIS

method of
JAY S. KEYSTONE, M.D.
University of Toronto
Toronto, Ontario, Canada

Trichinosis is an infection with an intestinal nematode acquired by the ingestion of meat containing encysted larvae of *Trichinella spiralis*. The usual source of trichinosis is pigs, but other sources include bears, walruses, boars, horses, and carnivorous wild animals such as hyenas and lions. The severity of infection is proportional to the numbers of ingested larvae. Two phases of infection follow the ingestion of infected meat.

INTESTINAL PHASE

Meat that has undergone acid-pepsin digestion in the stomach liberates previously encysted larvae, which develop into adult worms within the villi of the small intestine. Toward the end of the first week of infection, the enteric phase of trichinosis begins, at about the time that worms release newly formed larvae into the circulation. Patients may experience nausea, vomiting, diarrhea, and abdominal cramps, or no symptoms at all. Larval production continues for several weeks, until the adult females are expelled into the feces. Intestinal symptoms usually last 1 to 2 weeks, although studies suggest that previously infected patients may experience prolonged diarrhea. Intestinal symptoms, if present, usually precede or overlap with the systemic symptoms characteristic of the muscle phase.

MUSCLE PHASE

Symptoms associated with systemic invasion of larvae usually begin to appear during the second week of infection. Clinical manifestations are mainly due to the inflammatory reaction, largely mediated by eosinophils, that is provoked by larval forms. Typically, patients present with periorbital and facial edema, chemosis, and subconjunctival and splinter hemorrhages. In the third week of infection, when larvae encyst in skeletal muscle, patients experience myalgia, muscle swelling, weakness, and fever. Cough, dyspnea, headache, dysphagia, and urticarial skin lesions also occur. Marked eosinophilia usually accompanies the systemic phase. In heavy infections, myocarditis, encephalitis, or pneumonitis may occur. During the convalescent phase, malaise and weakness are not uncommon; symptoms often subside over many weeks or months.

DIAGNOSIS

Trichinosis should be suspected in a patient who has periorbital edema, myalgia, and eosinophilia. Often the patient gives a history of consuming poorly cooked meat; in common-source outbreaks, many people who ate the same food complain of typical symptoms. Although *Trichinella* serology is available, a diagnostic rise in titer does not usually develop for 1 to 2 weeks after the onset of the muscle phase. Encysted larvae in a muscle biopsy may not be demonstrable until 2 to 3 weeks after the onset of symptoms. The optimal method for examining a muscle biopsy specimen is to compress a portion of the unpreserved specimen between two glass slides and examine it under low power for encysted larvae.

TREATMENT

Treatment of trichinosis is unsatisfactory. Because the infection is self-limited in most patients, symptomatic therapy with analgesics, antipyretics, and bed rest is sufficient. For serious infections, especially those with myocarditis or central nervous system manifestations, prednisone, in a dose of 40 to 60 mg per day, is administered with mebendazole (Vermox), in a dose of 200 to 400 mg three times* daily for 3 days, followed by 400 to 500 mg three times daily for 10 days. Albendazole, another benzimidazole derivative that is better absorbed than mebendazole, may be used in a dose of 400 mg twice daily for 14 days. Mebendazole and albendazole appear to reduce further larval release from the intestine but may have little effect on the killing of muscle-dwelling larvae. Thiabendazole should be avoided because of its adverse effects. Controlled trials have not been carried out to determine optimal anthelmintic therapy or even whether such therapy is required at all; in fact, the curative efficacy of antiparasitic drugs has never been convincingly demonstrated. At present, it would be fair to conclude that anthelmintic therapy has little effect on the outcome of trichinosis unless it is begun soon after the infected meat is ingested.

Pork larvae can be killed by heating meat to 55°C (no trace of pink or flesh color) or by freezing meat at −15°C for 3 weeks. Arctic strains may require lower temperatures or more prolonged freezing to eradicate larval cysts. Smoking, salting, and drying are unreliable.

---

*Exceeds dosage recommended by the manufacturer.

TULAREMIA

method of
CHARLES S. BERENSON, M.D.
State University of New York at Buffalo and
Department of Veterans Affairs Western New
York Healthcare System
Buffalo, New York

Tularemia is an acute infectious zoonotic illness caused by a small gram-negative coccobacillus, *Francisella tularensis*. This pathogen was first isolated from wild rodents in Tulare County, California, and reported in 1912. Onset of illness is relatively sudden, including nonspecific findings of fever, chills, headache, myalgias, and fatigue. The incubation period after exposure is 3 to 5 days (range, 1 to 21 days). Classic syndromes of the disease are highly varied and often depend on the route of inoculation, the virulence of the strain, and the immune status of the victim. Division into clinical syndromes is somewhat arbitrary, and considerable overlap often occurs. Ulceroglandular disease, the most common presentation (21 to 87% of cases), is characterized by a painful ulcer at the site of inoculation and painful regional lymphadenopathy. Glandular disease (3 to 20% in the United States) manifests as regional lymphadenopathy, but without a skin ulcer. Typhoidal disease (5 to 30%) may be difficult to diagnose, as patients lack classic lymphadenopathy and skin ulcers and present with systemic symptoms only. Tularemia pneumonia may occur in any form of the disease. Pleural effusions of this syndrome may be confused with those of tuberculous pleurisy. Other syndromes are oculoglandular disease (less than 5%), oropharyngeal disease, and, less commonly, meningitis, osteomyelitis, and pericarditis. Mortality is 1 to 3% with antibiotic treatment of uncomplicated disease but higher with typhoidal tularemia and tularemia complicated by secondary pneumonia. Severity of disease ranges from a mild, self-limited illness to fulminant septic shock or adult respiratory distress syndrome.

F. tularensis is primarily an animal pathogen, particularly of wild animals but also of domestic animals. Lagomorphs (rabbits and hares) and rodents, particularly squirrels, muskrats, and beavers, are the most important reservoirs. Transmission of disease from infected animals to humans may occur via several routes. Arthropod-borne transmission (ticks, deer flies, and mosquitoes) is particularly important in North America, where tick bites account for more than 50% of cases, particularly west of the Mississippi River. Major tick vectors in the United States include the Lone Star tick (*Amblyomma americanum*), the wood tick (*Dermacentor andersoni*), and the dog tick (*Dermacentor variabilis*). Infection may also occur by direct contact with infected animal tissues, inhalation of aerosolized organisms, ingestion of infected meat or water, and bites from infected animals. Disease may begin with the introduction of as few as 10 organisms intradermally or by aerosol.

In the United States, tularemia has been reported in all 50 states but is most concentrated in Arkansas, Missouri, and Oklahoma. Approximately 150 to 300 cases are reported in this country annually. Occupations that pose risk for contracting tularemia include hunting, trapping, farming, veterinary practice, cooking, meat handling, and laboratory work.

Murine models have classically demonstrated a strong role for T lymphocytes and macrophages in clearance of *F. tularensis* and survival after an infection. However, other studies collectively indicate important T lymphocyte–independent host responses that may play a greater role in the early phases of infection. Bacterial lipopolysaccharide and membrane lipoproteins may be involved in eliciting protective host responses.

DIAGNOSIS

Because immediate laboratory diagnosis is often not possible, the diagnosis often rests on strong clinical suspicion, with appropriate history and presentation. In these instances, empirical antibiotic therapy is given before the laboratory diagnosis is made. Definitive laboratory diagnosis may be made by isolation of *F. tularensis* from cultures of blood, lymph node aspirates, pleural fluid, sputum, or ulcers. Media must include special supplements, such as cysteine, to support growth. Because isolation of *F. tularensis* poses a danger to laboratory personnel, the clinical laboratory should be warned of the clinical suspicion to implement precautions to prevent transmission. Serologic diagnosis, demonstrating a single positive agglutinating antibody titer of 1:160 or greater, or a fourfold rise in titer during the ensuing 2 to 6 weeks, has also been used. Agglutination tests may be positive by the end of the second week of illness and peak by 4 to 5 weeks. Antibodies may have low-titer cross-reactivity with antigens of *Brucella, Proteus,* and *Yersinia* species. Reports of persistent immune responses, present years after exposure, indicate that caution is warranted in interpretation of single, intermediate-titer serologic measurements. Direct immunofluorescence of organisms from infected tissues may be available from state public health laboratories. Identification by polymerase chain reaction and by immunoelectron microscopy has also been described and may facilitate rapid diagnosis in the future.

TREATMENT

The drug of first choice for all forms of tularemia, with the possible exception of meningitis, is streptomycin. One study indicated a 97% cure rate and no relapses among individuals treated with streptomycin. The effective dosage in adults is 7.5 to 10 mg per kg intramuscularly every 12 hours for 7 to 14 days. Shorter treatment regimens have been associated with more frequent relapses. Children should receive 20 to 40 mg per kg per day in two divided doses. Severely ill patients may be treated with higher doses (up to 30 mg per kg per day). However, doses greater than 2 grams per day do not improve clinical efficacy and are associated with increased ototoxicity and nephrotoxicity. Dosages must be adjusted for patients with renal insufficiency to minimize toxicities. In rare instances, initiation of streptomycin therapy may induce a Jarisch-Herxheimer reaction.

Tetracycline and chloramphenicol have also been used to treat tularemia. Both are bacteriostatic, possibly accounting for the higher relapse rates associated with their use. Cure rates of 88% and 77%, respectively, have been reported, with tetracycline having a 12% relapse rate. Tetracycline is given at 2 grams per day but should not be used in children younger than 9 years of age, or in pregnant or lactating women. Chloramphenicol, 50 to 100 mg per kg per day intravenously, may be added to streptomycin for the treatment of meningitis.

Studies of the efficacy of alternative agents were in part prompted by lack of availability of streptomycin in the United States for a period before 1993. Gentamicin, 3 to 5 mg per kg per day intravenously in divided doses, is an effective alternative. Reports indicate an 86% cure rate and a 6% relapse rate. By contrast, the cure rate with tobramycin was reported as only 50%.

Third-generation cephalosporins have also been used as alternative agents. One report documented eight cases of treatment failure with outpatient ceftriaxone (Rocephin) therapy despite prior acceptable in vitro susceptibilities. The latter point has prompted caution regarding the clinical usefulness of in vitro susceptibility data in selection of antibiotics to treat tularemia infections.

Case reports have also suggested a role for quinolone antibiotics in treatment of tularemia. Isolated reports of successful treatment offer limited experience but provide encouragement for broader study of quinolones in the treatment of this disease.

Erythromycin has been used with variable success. In vitro susceptibilities have been highly variable. Therefore, use of macrolide antibiotics should not be relied on in seriously ill patients. Poor in vitro susceptibilities and clinical failures have also been documented with penicillins, ceftazidime (Fortaz), and carbapenems (imipenem [Primaxin] and meropenem [Merrem]).

PREVENTION

The best means of preventing tularemia is minimizing direct contact with infected animals. Individuals at risk may avoid exposure by wearing gloves, masks, and protective eye coverings while skinning or processing wild animals. Similarly, avoidance of contaminated wells is essential. Antibiotic prophylaxis for exposed individuals is not recommended. However, because streptomycin given in the incubation period after experimental inoculation is effective, accidental laboratory inoculations may be preventively treated with intramuscular streptomycin. Person-to-person transmission does not occur, so special isolation is not needed for hospitalized patients. Use of insect repellent and tight-fitting clothing around wrists and ankles provides protection against arthropod-borne infection.

A live attenuated vaccine is available through the Centers for Disease Control and Prevention. It has provided partial protection in laboratory workers who work frequently with *F. tularensis*. Its use is not practical for protection against tick-borne tularemia. Murine model data indicate that immune response to the vaccine is relatively specific for *F. tularensis*. Previous infection generally results in lifelong immunity.

SALMONELLOSIS (EXCLUDING TYPHOID FEVER)

method of
DAVID R. HILL, M.D.
*The International Traveler's Medical Service,
University of Connecticut School of Medicine
Farmington, Connecticut*

Salmonellosis refers to a group of infections caused by bacteria of the genus *Salmonella*. Four clinical syndromes are recognized that may overlap one another. The first syndrome is enterocolitis caused by nontyphoid *Salmonella*. The second syndrome is bacteremia with or without focal, extraintestinal infection. Bacteremia can be a complication of enterocolitis. Enteric fever is the third syndrome and is caused primarily by *Salmonella typhi*, although some nontyphi *Salmonella* may also cause this. The final syndrome is a chronic carrier state that can develop after enteric fever and less commonly after enterocolitis.

Salmonellae are members of the family Enterobacteriaceae. They are now considered to be members of one species that contains several subgroups. Within these subgroups are more than 2000 serogroups de-

fined by biochemical determinations and serologic reactivity of the H (flagellar) and O (lipopolysaccharide) antigens. Salmonellae, except *S. typhi*, which is a pathogen only of humans, are widely distributed throughout the animal kingdom, which contributes to many food-borne infections.

Human infection with *Salmonella* usually requires ingestion of a large number of organisms (10^6 to 10^9) in contaminated food and, less frequently, water. Smaller numbers may be sufficient to cause infection in some cases, especially when gastrointestinal mechanisms are compromised secondary to achlorhydria or previous gastroduodenal surgery. Most cases of salmonellosis occur sporadically and are attributed to inappropriate food preparation in the home or in restaurants. Alternatively, other cases occur in outbreak settings. Children younger than 5 years, and particularly younger than 1 year, have the highest incidence of salmonellosis (62 cases per 100,000). Infection is usually secondary to a contaminated food source, which is frequently a poultry product such as chicken or eggs; pork, beef, and unpasteurized dairy products may also transmit *Salmonella*. Contaminated shell eggs have accounted for an increasing number of outbreaks; one outbreak associated with commercial ice cream affected nearly 225,000 persons throughout the United States. *Salmonella enteritidis* is the most common serotype involved in these egg-associated infections. From 1988 to 1992, *Salmonella* accounted for 69% of all bacterial food-borne outbreaks in the United States. Person-to-person spread may occur in groups with poor fecal hygiene.

To prevent infection, foods should be prepared by thorough cooking. They should then be properly stored because organisms may readily multiply in contaminated foods held at room temperature. Liquids should be heated or pasteurized, and all egg dishes should be thoroughly cooked. Pasteurized egg products should be used for recipes that call for uncooked or partially cooked eggs, particularly if they are being prepared in commercial establishments.

Resistance to antibiotics occurs primarily through the transfer of resistance plasmids and has been an increasing problem with *Salmonella*. Much of the resistance has been facilitated by the use of subtherapeutic doses of antibiotics in animal feeds. In the last decade in the United States, 30% or more of human isolates have been resistant to ampicillin, sulfonamides, or tetracyclines. Therefore, susceptibility testing needs to be performed on all isolates, and empirical therapy of severe disease should be initiated after resistance patterns are taken into account.

ENTEROCOLITIS

Clinical Features

Salmonella enterocolitis is the most common clinical syndrome and ranges from mild, self-limited diarrhea to dysentery. Six to 48 hours after ingestion of contaminated food or liquid, gastrointestinal symptoms begin with nausea, abdominal cramps, and diarrhea. Vomiting, headache, myalgias, malaise, chills, and fever (temperature of approximately 38°C) are also common. Diarrhea may be profuse, watery, and dehydrating or, less commonly, may be dysenteric with tenesmus, abdominal tenderness, and the passage of gross blood and mucus. The variation in the clinical picture is probably secondary to the multiple potential mechanisms by which *Salmonella* may cause diarrhea: from elaboration of an enterotoxin with fluid and electrolyte secretion to entry into intestinal epithelial cells with inflammation and tissue damage. Diagnosis is by stool culture. Stools may or may not contain polymorphonuclear leukocytes and occult or gross blood.

Most healthy adults have an uncomplicated course, and symptoms improve without treatment within 48 to 96 hours. However, there are several groups for whom *Salmonella* can cause severe disease or disease complicated by bacteremia and localization to extraintestinal sites. These groups include persons at the extremes of age; children younger than 1 year are particularly susceptible. Elderly, debilitated persons in nursing homes may have a poor outcome; 85% of the deaths in the United States from 1988 to 1992 associated with *S. enteritidis* food-borne outbreaks occurred in nursing home residents. Also at increased risk for severe infection are persons with abnormal cellular and humoral immunity, such as those with cancer, lymphoreticular malignant neoplasm, or human immunodeficiency virus infection; those treated with immunosuppressive drugs; and persons with hemolytic syndromes, especially sickle cell disease.

Treatment

Fluid and Electrolytes

The most important therapeutic modality in diarrhea is the replacement of fluids and electrolytes lost in the diarrheal stools. If possible, this should be done orally with use of a balanced solution of sugar, salt, and water in commercially prepared oral rehydration solutions or packets or in homemade recipes. The World Health Organization oral rehydration solution contains sodium chloride (3.5 grams per liter), potassium chloride (1.5 grams per liter), glucose (20.0 grams per liter), and trisodium citrate (2.9 grams per liter). In cases of enterocolitis in adults, hydration may be the only treatment necessary. As illness improves, the diet can be advanced with caffeine-free liquids, salted crackers, and lactose-free bland foods (bananas, chicken, potatoes, and pasta) given in frequent small meals. If parenteral hydration is necessary, frequent measurement of blood pressure, weight, and urine output and specific gravity should be carried out, particularly with infants.

Antimotility and Antinausea Agents

Antimotility agents such as atropine plus diphenoxylate (Lomotil) or loperamide (Imodium) may slow the diarrhea, relieve severe cramping, and decrease nausea, which can be helpful for some patients. However, they may theoretically prolong or worsen an inflammatory enteritis. Therefore, if there is gross blood or mucus in the stool or temperature above 38.5°C, they should not be used. Bismuth subsalicylate (Pepto-Bismol) has been studied extensively in the treatment of traveler's diarrhea caused by multiple agents and works to decrease the number of diarrheal stools by about 50% in a dose of 30 mL or 2 tablets (262 mg per 15 mL or tablet) orally every half-hour for 8 doses.

Antinausea medications are usually not required. Prochlorperazine (Compazine) may be administered orally (5 to 10 mg three or four times daily), by rectal suppository (25 mg twice daily), or by intramuscular injection (5 to 10 mg every 4 hours as needed). Promethazine hydrochloride (Phenergan) may also be used orally, by suppository, or intramuscularly (25 mg initially, then 12.5 to 25 mg every 4 to 6 hours). Dosages should be adjusted for children.

Antibiotics

Most experts agree that the use of antibiotics in uncomplicated enterocolitis in a healthy person is not necessary. This opinion has been based on clinical experience demonstrating that antibiotics neither shorten nor improve symptoms and may contribute to the development of antimicrobial resistance and increase the risk for symptomatic and bacteriologic relapse. Many of these studies were done with older classes of antibiotics, and it was expected that the quinolone antibiotics would not be associated with these problems because they have excellent in vitro activity against *Salmonella*, including multidrug-resistant isolates, and attain high levels in tissues and macrophages. However, whereas they do have superior clinical efficacy with a tendency toward more rapid cure and return to normal stool patterns, they still may prolong convalescent carriage of organisms. Immunosuppressed patients, neonates, the chronically ill, the elderly, and those with bone and joint prostheses should be treated to avoid potential complications.

Depending on antimicrobial sensitivity patterns, trimethoprim-sulfamethoxazole (TMP-SMZ) (Bactrim, Septra) (4 mg of TMP per kg two times daily for children; 2 single-strength tablets [80 mg of TMP plus 400 mg of SMZ] two times daily for adults), ampicillin (50 to 100 mg per kg per day in 4 doses for children; 500 mg four times daily for adults), or amoxicillin may be taken for 3 to 7 days. The fluoroquinolones norfloxacin (Noroxin, 400 mg), ciprofloxacin (Cipro, 500 mg), and ofloxacin (Floxin, 300 mg) twice daily for 3 to 7 days are also effective and may be the drugs of choice in cases of resistant *Salmonella*. They should not be used in pregnant women. Although they are not approved for use in children younger than 18 years because of concerns about cartilage dysplasia, they may be considered for short-term use in cases that are difficult to treat.

BACTEREMIA AND FOCAL SUPPURATIVE INFECTION

Clinical Features

Bacteremia in acute, uncomplicated enterocolitis occurs in 5 to 10% of infections. It may be more frequent in the pediatric age groups and immunocompromised hosts. Unless the patient falls into high-risk groups, complications are unusual. Therefore, blood cultures are not routinely necessary. Patients who have symptomatic bacteremia complicating enterocolitis present with fever and shaking chills in addition to diarrhea. Certain serogroups, such as *Salmonella dublin* and *Salmonella choleraesuis,* more frequently cause bacteremic infection.

Localization of infection may occur at any site but is uncommon. *Salmonella* can cause pneumonia, empyema, infected aortic aneurysms, septic arthritis, and splenic and hepatic abscesses. When bacteremia occurs in persons older than 50 years, an infected vascular aneurysm, particularly of the abdominal aorta, should be suspected. Osteomyelitis usually occurs in areas of bone infarct, such as may occur in sickle cell disease. Meningitis occurs primarily in infants younger than 5 months. Patients with acquired immune deficiency syndrome (AIDS) may suffer from prolonged gastrointestinal infection with recurrent bacteremia. This syndrome is an AIDS-defining illness.

Treatment

Both bacteremia and localized infection require active intervention to prevent potentially life-threatening sequelae. Parenteral ampicillin (100 to 200 mg per kg per day, divided into 4 to 6 doses) or TMP-SMZ (10 mg of TMP per kg per day in three or four divided doses) is effective if the organism is sensitive. However, cephalosporin and quinolone antibiotics should be used empirically if resistance is suspected. The minimal inhibitory concentration (MIC) against *Salmonella* of the extended-spectrum cephalosporins is often manyfold lower than the MIC of ampicillin or TMP-SMZ. This makes the use of these agents attractive for empirical use and for infections that are difficult to treat, such as meningitis. Ceftriaxone (Rocephin, 1 to 2 grams every 24 hours for adults), cefotaxime (Claforan, 1 to 2 grams every 8 hours for adults), and other third-generation cephalosporins are effective. Parenteral quinolones, ciprofloxacin (400 mg every 12 hours) or ofloxacin (400 mg every 12 hours), can also be used. Because of the potential for bone marrow toxicity, and the availability of excellent alternatives, chloramphenicol is used less frequently for bacteremia and localized infections.

Surgical drainage and débridement are often necessary for some localized infections; vascular reconstruction is required for infected aneurysms. Uncomplicated bacteremia may be treated for 10 to 14 days, meningitis for 2 to 3 weeks, and osteomyelitis and endovascular infection for 4 to 6 weeks or longer. In osteomyelitis and cardiovascular infections, one can initiate therapy parenterally and then, when defervescence has occurred, switch to prolonged oral treatment. AIDS patients may require chronic suppression to prevent relapses.

CARRIER STATE

Asymptomatic excretion of *Salmonella* after nontyphoid enterocolitis (convalescent carriage) occurs for up to 2 months in 5 to 10% of persons. The chronic carrier state (persistence of asymptomatic fecal or urinary carriage of *Salmonella* for longer than 1 year) occurs in less than 1% of adults and in about 5% of children younger than 5 years. Chronic carriage occurs most often with *S. typhi* after typhoid fever (about 3% of cases). Carriers of nontyphoid *Salmonella* are managed in the same fashion as carriers of *S. typhi*.

Convalescent carriers need only maintain strict personal hygiene so that they will not transmit the agent to others. When treatment is necessary for chronic carriers with normal gallbladder function and no evidence of cholelithiasis, ampicillin or TMP-SMZ has traditionally been used. Ampicillin is given in a dose of 100 mg per kg per day in four divided doses with probenecid, 25 mg per kg per day in four divided doses, for up to 4 to 6 weeks. TMP-SMZ is given in doses used to treat enterocolitis; some have combined this with rifampin (600 mg per day in adults) if cholelithiasis is present. High-dose ciprofloxacin (750 mg twice daily) for a month may be effective, even in some cases with gallstones.

If medical attempts at eradication fail in the presence of gallbladder disease, cholecystectomy may be necessary. Even with all of the measures, permanent eradication may be difficult. Patients with *Schistosoma haematobium* may require treatment of their schistosomiasis before one can eradicate urinary *Salmonella*.

TYPHOID FEVER

method of
RICHARD B. HORNICK, M.D.
Orlando Regional Healthcare System
Orlando, Florida

Typhoid fever is a rare disease in the United States but remains a public health problem in those areas of the world where there is the potential for water and food supplies to become contaminated with *Salmonella typhi*. The World Health Organization has estimated the annual number of cases worldwide to be about 33 million. The increasing number of multidrug-resistant strains in the past 10 years has created therapeutic problems. In this article, current recommendations are presented for the immediate choice of antibiotics when a clinical diagnosis has been made.

Typhoid fever is the most common form of enteric fever and is caused by *S. typhi*. Other species, *Salmonella paratyphi A, Salmonella schottmuelleri,* and *Salmonella hirschfeldii* (formerly known as paratyphoid A, B, and C), cause about 10% of the cases. These organisms are ingested, pass through the stomach, and invade epithelial cells in the small and large intestine and especially cells in Peyer's patches. Multiplication occurs in the mononuclear cells, which phagocytose the *S. typhi* organisms and then transport them to the liver, spleen, bone marrow, and lymph nodes. Once the organisms reach these areas of the reticuloendothelial system, they maintain an intracellular locus. Bacteremia ensues from these cells, and the febrile disease evolves.

EPIDEMIOLOGY

Typhoid fever is acquired by consumption of food or water contaminated with *S. typhi*. These organisms come from carriers (a fecal-oral route is operative) who either are convalescing from the disease or are asymptomatic chronic carriers. Many persons who are asymptomatic chronic carriers may not be aware of having had typhoid fever in the past. In the industrialized countries, safe drinking water and control of known carriers (e.g., cannot be food handlers) have markedly reduced the incidence of the disease. Each year for the past 15 years, there have been about 450 cases in the United States. Most of these are imported by non–U.S. citizen immigrants and to a lesser degree by U.S. citizens who travel to countries where the disease is prevalent. In 1994 to 1996, the Indian subcontinent and Mexico have been the most common countries from which these cases arise.

DIAGNOSIS

Typhoid fever is confirmed by isolating the organism from blood cultures, stool specimens, and/or bone marrow. Few *S. typhi* organisms circulate in the blood so that small-volume single specimens may fail to yield the organisms. Patients with severe forms of the disease, septic shock, have the highest yield of positive blood cultures, 90%; those with milder forms range from 60 to 70% positive. Two or three separate specimens of blood for culture are recommended. Higher yields are obtained from bone marrow aspirates because of the localization of these intracellular bacteria in this part of the reticuloendothelial system. Bone marrow specimens obtained 1 year after successful treatment have been culture-positive for latent *S. typhi*. Stool cultures are intermittently positive during the acute disease and in the convalescent phase. At least three specimens need to be negative after completion of therapy to be confident that a carrier state has not developed. String cultures of duodenal secretions produce a yield of 80%. These secretions are mixed with biliary tract drainage; the liver and gallbladder will be shedding organisms into the duodenum. The string culture is also useful for detecting carriers.

For more than 100 years, the Widal test has been used to measure antibodies to the typhoid bacillus. It measures antibodies to both the O (surface) and H (flagellar antigens). This test is not specific because it cross-reacts with many nontyphoid salmonellae O and H antigens. A single serum specimen is considered positive for typhoid fever if the O antibody titer is equal to or greater than 1:320 and/or the H antibody titer is equal to or greater than 1:640. A fourfold or greater titer rise demonstrated in paired serum specimens obtained 2 to 3 weeks apart is diagnostic. The polymerase chain reaction has been shown to detect *S.typhi* DNA in serum specimens in 16 hours. This test is sensitive and specific but not readily available.

PREVENTION

Typhoid fever, like other enteric infections, can be prevented by avoiding high-risk food and drinks. In endemic areas, travelers need to be educated about these potential sources of infection. Eating in hotels catering to tourists is sensible and logical. Buying ice cream or various foods from street vendors is risky. Drinking water (or ice cubes) from sources not certified as potable is very risky. Using bottled water or boiling or chlorinating water eliminates a big risk.

The use of vaccines to prevent typhoid fever has been enhanced by the development of new and effective vaccines (Table 1). However, none has been 100% protective. Their use is recommended for travel to endemic areas and for military and Peace Corps workers and others who will be living in these areas for a prolonged period. The old standard vaccine is not as effective as the two new vaccines. They are preferred.

MANAGEMENT

Antibiotic Therapy

S. typhi, because of its intracellular habitat, is best treated by antibiotics that are able to readily enter various types of cells. Therefore, in vitro, antibiotic sensitivity testing may not provide appropriate therapeutic choices for the clinician. When such tests demonstrate resistance, the antibiotic will obviously not be effective. However, those that demonstrate sensitivity to the strain may also fail to help cure the patient. For example, the aminoglycosides inhibit growth in the in vitro test situation but fail to produce a therapeutic response.

Like all gram-negative bacteria, *S. typhi* has been able to develop resistance to many antibiotics. In 1948, chloramphenicol was shown to successfully treat patients with typhoid fever. An occasional resistant strain was detected in endemic areas in the late 1950s and in the 1960s. In 1972, a large outbreak occurred in Mexico caused by a strain resistant to chloramphenicol. Other outbreaks were documented in other areas, but chloramphenicol was still a valuable drug because it was inexpensive and readily tolerated when given by mouth. Ampicillin or amoxicillin and trimethoprim-sulfamethoxazole (TMP-SMZ) (Bactrim, Septra) were comparable in effecting a cure and widely used. By 1990, increasing numbers of strains, especially from India, Pakistan, Egypt, and the Philippines, were found to be resistant to chloramphenicol, ampicillin, and/or TMP-SMZ. Since 1994, about 35% of such strains tested in England have this resistance pattern. Therefore, none of these antibiotics is recommended for initial treatment of patients with typhoid fever (Table 2).

The recommended choice, especially when there is concern that the *S. typhi* is a multidrug-resistant strain, is a fluoroquinolone. These drugs can achieve high concentrations inside phagocytic cells and in the bile. Relapses are rare. Use of ciprofloxacin or ofloxacin in children is not approved because of concern about damage to cartilage. Reports of tendinitis with an Achilles tendon rupture after the use of

TABLE 1. **Vaccines for Prevention of Typhoid Fever**

Vaccine Type	Dosage	Remarks
Killed—old vaccine (less effective than the newer vaccines)	Two 0.5-mL doses administered 4 wk apart in adults with a booster at 3 y if needed	Provides significant protection to persons living in endemic areas; local pain and fever common
Attenuated (Vivotif)	Four capsules, one administered every other day to be completed 1 wk before departure	Suitable for children; simultaneous use of mefloquine or chloroquine for malaria prophylaxis decreases efficacy
Vi antigen (Typlum Vi)	One injection of 0.5 mL intramuscularly in the deltoid for adults and children; second dose of 0.5 mL after 2 y may be needed if the risk for exposure remains high	Approved for general use; not recommended for children younger than 2 y

fluoroquinolones are increasing and will result in the Food and Drug Administration's requiring a warning in the labeling. In Vietnam, ciprofloxacin and ofloxacin were tested in children. Two-year follow-up studies revealed no joint problems or decrease in height or weight compared with an untreated matched control group. In children with severe disease with multidrug-resistant strains, ciprofloxacin or ofloxacin should be used. As ciprofloxacin is increasingly used for many infections, resistant *S. typhi* strains will evolve; at least five have been identified in India, Pakistan, and Vietnam.

The effectiveness of ampicillin prompted the evaluation of the cephalosporin antibiotics, especially the third-generation group. The efficacy of these antimicrobial agents has been tested in several endemic areas. Various doses and duration of therapy preclude a definitive recommendation. Those trials that were successful in the treatment of children and adults were used for these guidelines. Resistance to cefixime and ceftriaxone has not been reported as yet.

Monobactam Antibiotics

Several studies have shown aztreonam (Azactam) to be therapeutically comparable to chloramphenicol.

For patients infected with sensitive strains of *S. typhi*, the above-mentioned drugs can be used; however, reliable and less expensive are chloramphenicol, ampicillin, and TMP-SMZ. Relapses occur in about 10 to 15% of patients treated with these drugs. Fever reappears in 2 to 3 weeks, but the patient is not as ill as with the primary disease. For therapy, repeat the previous antibiotic for 3 to 5 days. Mild relapses may not need to be treated.

COMPLICATIONS

Intestinal Perforation

The mortality rate is about 20% in countries with endemic disease. The process takes about 2 to 3 weeks to occur mainly in adults and especially if inappropriate or inadequate therapy is used. Prompt surgical treatment is required. Additional antibiotic therapy to cover the anaerobic and aerobic bacterial contamination is needed (metronidazole or clindamycin for the anaerobes, ceftriaxone or ciprofloxacin for the aerobes).

Hemorrhage from sites in the gastrointestinal tract is a rare complication. Management of blood

TABLE 2. **Antibiotic Therapy for Typhoid Fever**

Medication	Dosage	Daily Frequency	Number of Days	Remarks
Multidrug-Resistant S. typhi *Strains*				
Ciprofloxacin (Cipro)	500–750 mg orally	2 times/d	3–7 d	Excellent results expected*
Ofloxacin (Floxacin)	7.5–15 mg/kg orally	3 times/d	3–7 d	Excellent results expected*
Ceftriaxone (Rocephin)	1–3 gm intravenously	1 time/d	3–5 d	Useful for inpatient therapy
Cefixime (Suprax)	10–20 mg/kg orally	2 times/d	8–14 d	For outpatient treatment of uncomplicated cases
Aztreonam (Azactam)	50–70 mg/kg intramuscularly	3 times/d	7–10 d	Effective—slower response than others in this group
Sensitive Strains				
Chloramphenicol (Chloromycetin)	50 mg/kg—oral route preferred	4 times/d	14 d	
Ampicillin	4–6 gm intravenously	1–1.5 gm 4 times/d	10–14 d	
Trimethoprim-sulfamethoxazole (Bactrim, Septra)	1 double-strength tablet orally	2 times/d	14 d	Avoid use in pregnancy

*Check sensitivity with nalidixic acid 10-mg disk. Resistant strains present in India, Pakistan, and Vietnam.

loss is key. Antibiotic therapy will help heal the source.

Chronic Carriers

Patients recovering from the acute disease who have persistently positive stool cultures for 1 year are carriers. Women are more likely than men because of the increased frequency of gallbladder disease in women. Surgical removal, under intravenous ampicillin treatment, of a gallbladder with stones will cure the carrier state in some patients. The *S. typhi* organisms reside in the stones; eradication from those sites by antibiotics is difficult. Chloramphenicol is not effective. A 4- to 6-week course of intravenous ampicillin is effective (60%) if no stones are present. However, even some of those apparent cures had positive stool cultures 2 to 4 years later. Ciprofloxacin and norfloxacin (Noroxin)* have been successfully tested in small numbers of patients who are carriers (ciprofloxacin 750 mg twice daily orally for 28 days, and norfloxacin 400 mg twice daily orally for 28 days). One-year "cure" rates of 80 to 90% were obtained. These results suggest either of the two as the antimicrobial of choice to treat chronic carriers. Additional confirmatory data are needed.

---

*Not FDA approved for this indication.

TYPHUS FEVER

method of
BRUCE H. HAMORY, M.D.
Hershey Medical Center
Hershey, Pennsylvania

Organisms responsible for the clinical syndromes of typhus fever include *Rickettsia prowazekii* (epidemic or louse-borne typhus), *Rickettsia typhi* (endemic, murine, or flea-borne typhus), and *Rickettsia tsutsugamushi* (scrub or mite-borne typhus). These agents have distinct clinical manifestations, geographic distributions, and ecologies. They account for the great majority of typhus group infections. Recrudescence of epidemic typhus (*R. prowazekii*) is called Brill-Zinsser disease. *Rickettsia canada,* an organism related serologically to *R. prowazekii* and *R. typhi,* may cause a spotted fever–like disease in humans.

All these organisms produce diffuse inflammation of the small blood vessels, which probably accounts for most of the physiologic derangements occurring in these illnesses. Rickettsiae are intracellular parasites, and current evidence suggests that available antibiotics suppress their growth but do not kill them. Therefore, general principles of management of patients include (1) prompt and appropriate antimicrobial therapy to control the infection until immunity develops; (2) general supportive measures to correct the physiologic derangements that may occur; and (3) prevention or treatment of complications.

THERAPY

Louse-borne typhus is used as the therapeutic model for all these diseases because it is the most severe, it tends to occur in isolated parts of the world, and it is the classic infection of this group. The other typhus fevers are managed using the same principles, unless otherwise stated.

Clinical Classification of Severity

Particular attention should be paid to the patient's neurologic state, as evidenced by level of consciousness, ability to cooperate, and ability to swallow. Physiologic abnormalities (hypotension or shock, diminished renal or hepatic function, clotting abnormalities), nutritional state, degree of hydration, and evidence of any complications are also evaluated. Duration of illness is important because the duration of antibiotic therapy is influenced by this (see below), and complications tend to occur during the second week of clinical disease.

Cooperative patients with mild, uncomplicated disease can be given oral antimicrobials and fluids. Even patients with severe disease usually can be managed with oral therapy, as long as they are alert and able to swallow. Patients who are uncooperative, are unable to swallow, or have severe complications require additional methods of treatment.

Antirickettsial Therapy

Prompt administration of adequate doses of antirickettsial drugs is the most important factor in successful treatment. It shortens the course of the clinical disease and reduces mortality.

The drugs of choice are the tetracyclines and chloramphenicol. Tetracyclines are the preferred drugs because they do not cause the marrow depression or aplastic anemia reported with chloramphenicol. All other antibiotics, with the possible exception of rifampin, are ineffective against rickettsia. Penicillin, streptomycin, and sulfonamides have been shown to be clinically ineffective. In vitro susceptibility testing of several aminoglycosides, semisynthetic penicillins (including ampicillin), and cephalosporins disclosed no growth inhibition of *R. prowazekii* with clinically achievable concentrations. Except for chloramphenicol, none of the drugs used for the treatment of typhoid fever gives either clinical or in vitro evidence of activity in typhus fever. This is important to consider in those parts of the world where both typhus and typhoid fevers occur with some frequency.

Clinical response to either tetracycline or chloramphenicol is rapid, with defervescence occurring by 36 to 72 hours in epidemic or murine typhus and sooner in scrub typhus. Reports of presumed *R. canada* infections also indicate rapid response to both tetracycline and chloramphenicol. Failure of the patient to respond to therapy indicates (1) mistaken diagnosis, (2) a complication, or (3) a concomitant infection.

Treatment regimens include the following:

1. Doxycycline, a tetracycline derivative available for oral and intravenous use, is the treatment of choice for louse-borne typhus. A single 100-mg oral

dose routinely cures epidemic typhus fever infections at all stages of disease in adults. A single 50-mg oral dose for children up to age 10 years is also curative. There is no reported experience with the use of this drug for infants with typhus.

Limited evidence suggests that a single 200-mg oral dose of doxycycline cures scrub typhus with occasional relapses. However, murine typhus tends to relapse if only one dose is given, so daily doses should be given as discussed later. Note that Rocky Mountain spotted fever is not cured by single-dose therapy and requires daily therapy with doxycycline or another drug.

2. Tetracycline is given orally in four to six divided doses for a daily dose of 25 to 50 mg per kg of body weight. Two grams per day given in divided doses (every 4 to 6 hours) suffices for adults. This drug is poorly absorbed if taken with oral medications that contain divalent cations (such as aluminum or magnesium). Decreased dosage in patients with renal or hepatic dysfunction (not necessary in single-dose doxycycline therapy) is necessary. Superinfections may occur due to changes in microbial flora; long-term therapy of children younger than 8 years should be avoided to prevent staining of developing teeth.

3. Chloramphenicol is given in divided oral doses every 4 to 6 hours for a total daily dose of 50 to 75 mg per kg of body weight. Two grams per day in divided doses suffices for adults. *Caution*: Doses over 25 mg per kg of body weight may be toxic for infants younger than 2 weeks. Dosages may have to be lowered in the presence of hepatic impairment to prevent the accumulation of toxic drug levels.

Patients unable to take oral medications (those who are comatose, delirious, unable to swallow, or vomiting) require special management. Intravenous therapy with tetracycline, 0.5 gram every 12 hours, diluted in 100 mL of 5% dextrose in water or isotonic saline solution and administered over one half hour; or chloramphenicol sodium succinate, 1.0 gram every 8 to 12 hours (diluted to a 10% solution) may be given until the patient is alert and able to swallow. At that time, a single 100-mg oral dose of doxycycline usually suffices to complete therapy. If intravenous medications or fluids are not available, the oral drugs may be given via nasogastric tube.

Duration of Chemotherapy

As noted, drugs used for the treatment of rickettsial infections are rickettsiostatic, providing suppression of the infection until host immune responses can control it. Therefore, optimal duration of chemotherapy is related to (1) the point in the course of the illness at which therapy is started, and (2) the length of drug effect on the particular organism. If therapy is started early in the course of the disease, it must be continued longer than treatment begun late in the course. A reasonable rule of thumb for administering either chloramphenicol or tetracycline therapy is to administer the drug for at least 48 hours after the patient becomes afebrile. The drug should then be continued until the total time from onset of clinical disease is 12 to 14 days, which is roughly the time required for an adequate immune response. This is not the minimal necessary regimen but is used to provide automatic compensation for treatment begun at any stage during the disease.

If drugs are discontinued too soon, the patient may experience a febrile "relapse." This may occur within 12 hours in murine typhus or as long as 6 days after the last dose of therapy in scrub typhus. Relapses respond to retreatment with the same drug and should be treated for at least 48 hours after defervescence. Drug resistance, which is inducible in the laboratory, has not been noted in patients.

Steroids

Use of steroids should be reserved for those instances of neurologic impairment that affect patients' ability to feed themselves or otherwise endanger their health. Examples of this include inability to swallow, coma, and delirium or agitation. Uncontrolled studies indicate that in outpatient settings, corticosteroids in conjunction with appropriate antibiotic therapy may cause rapid reversal of neurologic impairment, enabling faster institution of oral therapy as well as improvement in the state of well-being and more rapid defervescence. There is no evidence that such therapy adversely affects the course of the infection when antibiotics are also used. The regimen is hydrocortisone, 100 mg intravenously, followed by an intramuscular injection of 200 to 300 mg of cortisone acetate, in addition to 500 mg of tetracycline intramuscularly. This is given to comatose or severely ill "uncooperative" patients on admission. Within 24 to 36 hours, the patient is usually able to take oral fluids and food, swallow the last antibiotic dose (100 mg of doxycycline), and regain bowel and bladder control as well as spontaneous movement. Falciparum malaria must be excluded by blood smear before steroid treatment in areas where patients are at risk for both diseases.

Supportive Therapy

In hospital settings in which intravenous fluids and constant nursing supervision are available, the patient can be supported until there is neurologic improvement. The need for hospitalization is determined by the patient's requirements for supportive therapy and nursing care or the presence of any complications. Mild to moderately severe infections, such as murine typhus and Brill-Zinsser disease, can usually be managed at home if the patient is able to take oral fluids. Mild to moderately severe cases of epidemic typhus and scrub typhus also respond well to oral chemotherapy and simple supportive measures such as bed rest, adequate protein and caloric intake, rehydration, and analgesia for myalgias and headache. These patients may be deloused, given chemotherapy, and followed up as outpatients. Patients with altered consciousness or who are unable to take and retain oral medications and those who are so debilitated as to be unable to control their bowel and bladder functions need to be hospitalized. They should be deloused on admission (to be discussed) to prevent spread of disease to other patients and the staff. In the absence of serious underlying disease or concomitant infections, mortality in patients treated early should be essentially zero. When therapy is begun late in the course, deaths still occur despite the most sophisticated supportive therapy.

Nursing Care

Close observation of patients for changes in mental status is warranted to prevent self-inflicted injury. Some patients may be irrational or agitated to the point of attempting self-destruction, and physical restraint may be required. Patients may become irrational after antibiotic therapy has been instituted and even a day or two after defervescence. Comatose patients should be turned frequently to prevent the development of pressure sores and aspiration pneumonitis. The legs should be elevated or placed in support hose to prevent venous stasis and thrombosis. Good oral hygiene is essential.

The patient should be given a diet high in protein and calories. This is important to prevent negative nitrogen balance with attendant muscle loss and hypoproteinemia. In the presence of diminished renal function with azotemia, excessive protein intake should be avoided until renal function improves. Oral fluids sufficient to ensure a urine flow of 1500 mL per day should be given. If the patient cannot take oral liquids within a day or two of instituting therapy, fluids should be given via nasogastric tube or by vein. Comatose or uncooperative patients require intravenous fluids to maintain adequate renal output. These intravenous fluids should be given slowly, and the proper concentrations of electrolytes will be based on urinary output and laboratory determinations. Frequent examinations for signs of congestive heart failure are warranted to avoid overtaxing the cardiovascular system.

Hepatic and Renal Systems

Abnormalities of liver and renal functions are usually transient, responding to antibiotic therapy of the infection. Acute renal failure resulting from massive intravascular hemolysis has been reported in glucose-6-phosphate dehydrogenase–deficient individuals infected with murine or scrub typhus and can be managed with peritoneal dialysis or hemodialysis.

Blood and Cardiovascular System

Typhus group rickettsia cause widespread focal lesions in the small blood vessels. These lesions are presumed to account for the increased vascular permeability, vascular collapse, and clotting abnormalities (from disseminated intravascular coagulation, thrombocytopenia, and diminished hepatic synthesis of clotting factors), which are recognized in several of these infections. Appropriate laboratory tests that pinpoint the specific abnormalities present may allow more rational prevention and management of the

reported complications of hemorrhage, arterial occlusion (gangrene), or thrombophlebitis.

Specific blood component therapy in the form of packed red blood cells for significant anemia and albumin for severe hypoproteinemia is preferred over whole blood or plasma. Heparin has been reported as a treatment for intravascular clotting in a single rickettsial infection.

The management of peripheral vascular collapse, usually in the second week of untreated clinical disease, is empirical. It includes (1) nasal oxygen; (2) plasma expanders such as salt-poor albumin; (3) vasopressor drugs such as norepinephrine bitartrate (Levophed); and (4) corticosteroids.

Pulmonary edema and congestive heart failure are attributed to hypoproteinemia, increased vascular permeability, and myocarditis. After correction of the hypoproteinemia, they can be managed with digitalis. Use of diuretics must be based on the presence of adequate renal function.

Other Complications

Secondary bacterial pneumonias and other bacterial infections are treated with appropriate antibiotics, based on isolation and antibiotic sensitivity testing of the causative organism. Gangrene, decubitus ulcers, and thrombophlebitis are treated by the usual surgical and medical methods. As noted, neurologic deficits usually resolve during convalescence, although personality changes and deafness have been reported to persist in certain patients for months. Those deficits caused by large-vessel disease (hemorrhage or thrombosis) may not resolve.

Prevention and Control Measures

General control measures for epidemic typhus rest on louse control with residual insecticides, isolation and chemotherapy of patients, and attempts to improve personal hygiene, such as bathing and washing clothes.

All patients with epidemic typhus should be deloused with a residual insecticide when first seen. Body lice in different parts of the world are developing resistance to various insecticides, so a knowledge of local resistance patterns is important in making the proper selection. Widely used insecticides include 10% DDT powder, malathion, 1% lindane (γ-hexachlorocyclohexane), and a carbamate (Mobam).

Clothing should be removed from hospitalized patients and autoclaved—heat sterilization will kill the lice, their eggs, and the rickettsia in the louse feces. The patient should be bathed (some hospitals also shave patients' hair if infestation is heavy), deloused, and re-treated at the appropriate intervals with insecticides. If proper delousing and decontamination are performed before admission to the ward and the ward is kept louse free, physicians and nurses need not take special precautions with epidemic typhus patients. During the delousing, however, gowns, gloves, and masks should be worn to protect the operator from the infected lice and their feces. All these articles should be subjected to heat sterilization after use. Isolation of the patient is not necessary if lice are killed and not present on the ward.

Murine (endemic) typhus is controlled by first eliminating rat fleas with insecticides and then controlling rats. If rats are killed before fleas are eliminated, the infected fleas will seek a new host, such as human beings. Personal preventive measures often must suffice for control of scrub and tick typhus. These include avoidance of known habitats of the insect, if possible, or application of repellents to the clothing (benzyl benzoate) and skin (diethyltoluamide, M-1960) if these areas must be entered.

Reports have documented the effectiveness of doxycycline given as a 200-mg oral dose once a week as prophylaxis for scrub typhus (*R. tsutsugamushi*). This is of benefit only for individuals working in areas known to be endemic foci for scrub typhus. No studies of doxycycline prophylaxis have been conducted for other rickettsial diseases.

Currently available commercial killed vaccines for epidemic typhus are variable in potency but do reduce the severity of clinical disease. An experimental live attenuated vaccine (Madrid E) shows promise in epidemic situations but is not yet commercially available. No vaccines are commercially available for preventing murine typhus, scrub typhus, or *R. canada* infections.

The Respiratory System

ACUTE RESPIRATORY FAILURE

method of
MICHAEL C. BOYARS, M.D.
University of Texas Medical Branch
Galveston, Texas

Acute respiratory failure (ARF) is a sudden decompensation of the oxygenation and/or ventilation functions of the respiratory system. This leads to inadequate oxygen delivery and/or carbon dioxide removal, resulting in altered cellular function. Signs may include hypoxia, hypercapnia, and sometimes systemic acidosis. Dyspnea is the most common symptom of ARF but is too nonspecific to be helpful clinically. ARF is a clinical syndrome of acute respiratory decompensation, and as such its diagnosis is made from its clinical presentation more than from laboratory data such as arterial blood gas (ABG) analysis. The patient's chronic baseline pulmonary function, and hence pulmonary reserve, is most important in determining the course of ARF. Whereas an ABG determination on room air showing a PO_2 of 52 mm Hg, PCO_2 of 46 mm Hg, and pH of 7.35 may signify ARF in a 15-year-old asthmatic, it may represent a stable baseline for a 66-year-old patient with moderately advanced emphysema. Despite its limitation, ABG analysis plays an essential role in the diagnosis and follow-up of therapy for ARF. I find it useful clinically to divide causes of ARF into those with normal lungs and those with abnormal lungs (Table 1).

VENTILATORY SUPPORT

Adequate oxygenation and ventilation are the cornerstones of therapy for ARF. What defines adequate oxygenation is a more complex subject. Oxygenation is dependent on several factors, including (1) the partial pressure of arterial oxygen (PaO_2), because this determines oxygen saturation of hemoglobin; (2) the hemoglobin concentration; (3) the cardiac output (CO); (4) the blood pressure; and (5) the distribution of blood flow through the multiple vascular beds. Because tissue oxygenation is dependent on so many variables, it is difficult to determine when we are optimally oxygenating the patient. Calculation of total arterial transport seems to be the best single parameter to accurately assess adequacy of tissue oxygenation in a patient with ARF:

$$O_2 \text{ transport} = CO \times (\text{hemoglobin concentration} \times 1.34 \text{ mL } O_2 \times O_2 \text{ saturation \%}) + 0.003 \times PaO_2$$

Adequacy of alveolar ventilation is generally assessed by the level of $PaCO_2$. With alveolar hyperventilation, there is relative hypocapnia; with alveolar hypoventilation, there is relative hypercapnia.

Treatment of ARF frequently requires intubation and mechanical ventilation. Regardless of the cause, when the patient's clinical parameters fall below those shown in Table 2, intubation and mechanical ventilation should be strongly considered. There are several modes of mechanical ventilation, as shown in Table 3. No one mode has been shown to be superior with respect to morbidity or mortality in clinical trials. They all have relative advantages and disadvantages that may make them more desirable in certain clinical situations. If you are inexperienced with a certain mode of ventilation, it is best to use one with which you are familiar rather than worry about which mode is best in a given clinical situation. Modes of ventilation can be divided into volume or pressure modes. With volume modes (assist/control [A/C] and synchronized intermittent mandatory ventilation [SIMV]), the patient is given a preset tidal volume (V_T) and the pressure rises to whatever is needed to deliver that volume. Pressure-mode ventilation (pressure-control ventilation [PCV] and pres-

TABLE 1. **Causes of Acute Respiratory Failure**

With Normal Lungs	With Abnormal Lungs
Central nervous system causes	Obstructive airways disease
Sedative drug overdose	Asthma
Cerebrovascular disease	Chronic bronchitis
Infection	Emphysema
Tumor	Restrictive airways disease
Neuromuscular causes	Chronic pulmonary fibrosis
Guillain-Barré syndrome	Acute diffuse edema or inflammation
Myasthenia gravis	
Amyotrophic lateral sclerosis	Space-occupying lesions
	Pneumothorax
Drug induced	Pleural effusion
Aminoglycosides	Pneumonia—any cause
Organophosphates	Atelectasis
Muscular causes	Airway obstruction
Myositis	Pleural effusion
Hypophosphatemia	Pulmonary edema
Other causes	Hydrostatic (congestive heart failure)
Upper airway obstruction	Increased microvascular permeability (adult respiratory distress syndrome)
Sleep apnea syndrome	
Enlarged tonsils (children)	
	Pulmonary embolism

TABLE 2. **Guidelines for Initiation of Mechanical Ventilation**

Spontaneous respiratory rate	>30/min
Spontaneous tidal volume	<300 mL
Vital capacity	<20 mL/kg
Negative inspiratory pressure	< -30 cm H_2O
PaO_2	<60 mm Hg on supplemental oxygen
$PaCO_2$	>55 mm Hg or 10 mm Hg above baseline stable value
Poor clearance of secretions or ineffective cough	

sure-support ventilation [PSV]) delivers a predetermined oxygen mixture until a specified peak airway pressure is reached, and the volume delivered varies directly with the stiffness or compliance of the lungs. Bilevel positive airway pressure (Bi-PAP) is a noninvasive mode of ventilation. General guidelines concerning each mode follow.

Bi-PAP is a noninvasive mode of ventilation that may be used to support a patient with ARF and thus prevent the need for intubation and mechanical ventilation. Bi-PAP is delivered by a tight-fitting nasal mask. The patient's respiratory efforts are "sensed" by the Bi-PAP machine, which delivers a higher pressure during inspiration and a lower pressure during expiration. This provides for a measure of end-expiratory pressure that helps keep small airways open and improves gas exchange as well as drives a gas mixture into and out of the lungs. In this way, it works as a pressure respirator. This can decrease the patient's work of breathing and augment ventilation, and it has been reported to decrease the need for intubation and mechanical ventilation in some patients with ARF. The exact indication for this mode of therapy in ARF is not yet determined.

The goal of mechanical ventilation is to return the pH and PCO_2 to their previous stable values while maintaining adequate oxygenation. For volume-mode ventilation, initial settings are as follows. V_T should be set at 7 to 10 mL per kg of ideal body weight. Use lower volumes in patients with obstructive airways disease because the reduced lung compliance gener-

TABLE 3. **Modes of Mechanical Ventilation**

Noninvasive
Bilevel positive airway pressure
Invasive
Volume cycled
  Assist/control
  Synchronized intermittent mandatory ventilation
Pressure cycled
  Pressure-control ventilation
    Inverse ratio ventilation
  Pressure-support ventilation

ates higher airway pressures, which results in a higher frequency of barotrauma. The initial rate should be 8 to 12 breaths per minute. The larger the V_T, the lower the rate. The initial fraction of inspired oxygen (FIO_2) is set at 0.50, and this should be adjusted to maintain a PaO_2 in the range of 60 to 80 mm Hg. Blood samples for initial ABG analysis should be drawn in 30 to 45 minutes and adjustment made as necessary to keep PaO_2 and pH values optimal. Marked respiratory alkalosis should be avoided because this can lead to seizures and cardiac arrhythmias as well as be a negative stimulus to respiration.

A/C is the oldest mode of ventilation. The physician selects a V_T, minimal respiratory rate, and FIO_2. Each time an inspiratory effort is made, the patient gets a machine-delivered breath of predetermined V_T and FIO_2. If the patient's spontaneous rate falls below that set on the ventilator, the patient gets the preset rate. The greatest potential benefit of A/C is that unless the patient cannot make appropriate inspiratory efforts, the patient will not be "underventilated" and run the risk of worsening respiratory failure because of too low a preset rate. On the other hand, some believe that it is more difficult to wean patients from this mode because they tend to be "overventilated."

In the SIMV mode, the physician selects a V_T, respiratory rate, and FIO_2. Unlike in A/C ventilation the rate cannot be increased by the patient's effort. The ventilator senses the patient's effort and delivers the preset V_T when an inspiratory effort is made. If an inspiratory effort is made in between the ventilator breath, the patient gets a V_T proportional to the inspiratory effort. The greater the effort, the greater the V_T. SIMV allows the patient to "actively participate" in respiration, and some think that this makes weaning easier. The most serious concern with SIMV is setting the spontaneous rate too low. If this is done, the patient will have increased work of breathing, which may eventually worsen the respiratory failure and prolong ventilator dependency.

PCV is similar to A/C, but rather than selecting a V_T, the physician chooses a peak inspiratory pressure. Each time the ventilator senses a patient's effort, the oxygen mixture is delivered to a preset peak airway pressure limit. The delivered V_T varies directly with the lung compliance. The more compliant the lungs, the greater the V_T; the stiffer the lungs, the less the V_T. This mode of ventilation guarantees that maximal peak airway pressure will not exceed the preset limit, thus minimizing the risk for barotrauma with resultant pneumothorax, subcutaneous emphysema, decreased venous return, and hemodynamic instability. Because of this, it is most useful in ventilating patients with obstructive airways disease. Initially, set the pressure at 30 cm H_2O, the respiratory rate at 8 to 10, and the FIO_2 at 0.50. Check the ABG values in 30 minutes and make appropriate adjustments to keep the PaO_2 in the 60 to 80 mm Hg range.

PSV delivers a preset pressure in the ventilator

circuit when a patient's inspiratory effort is sensed by the ventilator. This is thought to decrease the patient's work of breathing. PSV can be used alone or combined with SIMV. When it is used in this way, combine a fixed rate volume-mode ventilator with a pressure-mode ventilator to assist the patient's spontaneous breaths. This mode of ventilation has its greatest utility in weaning. The amount of pressure to use initially is in the range of 15 to 25 cm H_2O. This can be increased or decreased on the basis of the patient's clinical status.

Permissive hypercapnia is an acceptable ventilatory strategy in which you ventilate with lower volumes and airway pressures and thus allow hypoventilation, and consequent $PaCO_2$ elevation, to occur. This is done in an effort to lower the mean and peak airway pressures, which decreases the frequency of complications secondary to barotrauma. Critically ill patients can tolerate pH values in the range of 7.10 without significant consequences. Patients with significant heart disease do not tolerate a serum pH of less that 7.25, however. The level of pH, *not* the $PaCO_2$, is the limiting factor.

Inverse ratio ventilation (IRV) is a ventilatory mode that is usually used with PCV. The normal inspiratory and expiratory time ratio (I/E ratio) is reversed, allowing a greater inspiratory than expiratory time. A normal I/E ratio is 1:2 to 1:3. The clinical indications for and exact place of IRV in supporting patients with ARF are controversial, and it should not be used unless one has extensive experience with it.

Intubation causes atelectasis and a fall in functional residual capacity (FRC) by unclear mechanisms. A small amount of positive end-expiratory pressure (PEEP) (2.5 to 5 cm H_2O) has been shown to prevent this and is routinely applied to most patients on ventilators. The use of PEEP may be harmful in some groups of patients. Patients with asthma or chronic obstructive pulmonary disease (COPD) usually have elevated baseline FRCs, and PEEP can worsen the hyperinflation and cause significant barotrauma. In patients with hypovolemia, relatively small increases in intrathoracic pressure may additionally reduce venous return significantly and cause hypotension.

Intubation and mechanical ventilation are uncomfortable and frightening for the patient. Because of this the patient should be sedated and have anxiety relieved. If the patient "fights" the ventilator, this will increase airway pressures, interfere with oxygenation and ventilation, and increase the rate of complications. Experience, personal preference, and the clinical situation dictate the agents used. It is best to use neuromuscular paralysis as a last choice because of the short- and long-term neuropathy and myopathy associated with these agents.

WEANING FROM MECHANICAL VENTILATION

Weaning is as much art as science. When the initial pathologic process that led to the ARF is treated or resolves, the patient is ready for weaning. If there is no objective improvement in this process, the patient will fail weaning attempts. Whereas no one or combination of clinical parameters can accurately predict weaning, I have found some to be clinically helpful (see Table 2). The patient has a greater chance at successful weaning if the spontaneous respiratory rate is 30 per minute or less, the spontaneous V_T is 300 mL or more, the vital capacity (VC) is 20 mL per kg or more, and the negative inspiratory pressure (NIP) is -30 cm H_2O or less. Patients who do not fulfill these criteria may be weaned; however, the better their "weaning parameters," the more likely weaning will be successful.

No one method of weaning has been shown to be uniformly superior in all clinical situations. If the patient is in the SIMV mode, one can simply reduce the SIMV rate progressively as the patient's clinical state allows until the patient is successfully weaned. This same strategy can be used with PSV. When the patient is ventilated with A/C or PCV, it is best to use a T tube trial. The patient is removed from the ventilator and given a T tube for a short time, 5 to 10 minutes initially, before being returned to ventilatory support. If this is tolerated, progressively longer periods of T tube support are used until the patient can breathe with the T tube without respiratory fatigue. The patient is then extubated and prescribed a Venturi or aerosol mask.

ACUTE RESPIRATORY FAILURE WITH NORMAL LUNGS

ARF with normal lungs usually results in a reduction in alveolar ventilation. The ventilatory function of the respiratory system serves to move gas into and out of the lungs during the respiratory cycle. Impulses originating in the "respiratory center" are transmitted down spinal tracts through peripheral nerves to the neuromuscular junction of the muscles of inspiration, causing them to contract. Expiration is a more passive process, effected largely by relaxation of the muscles of inspiration. Regardless of the cause, ventilatory failure leads to inadequate bellows function of the respiratory system, causing alveolar hypoventilation. This reduced ventilation causes inadequate removal of carbon dioxide from the alveoli, resulting in an increase in the alveolar PCO_2 ($PaCO_2$). Because the total barometric pressure is unchanged, this increase in $PaCO_2$ causes a decrease in alveolar PO_2 (PaO_2), which results in a reduction in the PaO_2. The difference or gradient between the alveolar and arterial PO_2 ($PaO_2 - PaO_2$) remains normal in ARF caused by ventilatory failure with normal lungs, whereas it is always widened in ARF caused by ventilatory failure with abnormal lungs. The relationship between PaO_2 and $PaCO_2$ is described in the alveolar air equation (Table 4). Using it, we can calculate the PaO_2 from the ABG values and then determine the alveolar-arterial PO_2 difference. When the alveolar-arterial PO_2 difference is widened (normal = 5 to 15 mm Hg), the ARF is secondary to ventila-

TABLE 4. **Alveolar Air Equation**

P_{AO_2} = alveolar P_{O_2}	F_{IO_2} = fraction of O_2 in inspired air
Pa_{O_2} = arterial P_{O_2}	R = respiratory quotient
Pa_{CO_2} = arterial P_{CO_2}	$P_{AO_2} - Pa_{O_2}$ = alveolar-arterial P_{O_2} difference
P_{IO_2} = partial pressure of inspired O_2	

$$P_{AO_2} = P_{IO_2} - Pa_{CO_2}/R$$

$$P_{AO_2} = (\text{barometric pressure} - \text{water vapor pressure})(F_{IO_2}) - Pa_{CO_2}/R$$

At sea level on room air assuming R = 0.8

$$P_{AO_2} = (760 - 47)(0.21) - Pa_{CO_2}/0.8$$

$$P_{AO_2} = 150 - (Pa_{CO_2})(1.2)$$

Normal $P_{AO_2} - Pa_{O_2}$ = 5 to 15 mm Hg

tory failure with abnormal lungs or oxygenation failure. When the alveolar-arterial P_{O_2} difference is normal, the ARF is secondary to ventilatory failure with normal lungs. Because the alveolar-arterial P_{O_2} difference widens with increasing concentrations of inspired oxygen, it is only clinically useful when the patient is breathing room air.

The rise in Pa_{CO_2} that occurs with ventilatory failure causes a respiratory acidosis. The more severe the ventilatory failure, the greater the rise in Pa_{CO_2} and the more severe the respiratory acidosis. Acutely, every rise in Pa_{CO_2} of 10 mm Hg results in a decrease in pH of approximately 0.08 unit. If the ventilatory insufficiency is more chronic (days, weeks, or longer), the kidneys partially compensate by retaining bicarbonate, and so the fall in pH is not as great. In this situation, for every rise of Pa_{CO_2} of 10 mm Hg, there is a fall in pH of approximately 0.03 unit. Making this kind of calculation helps determine whether the ventilatory failure is acute or chronic.

Spirometry is the optimal way to monitor the day-to-day progression of ARF with normal lungs. VC, forced expiratory volume in 1 second (FEV_1), NIP, and maximal expiratory pressure can be easily and reliably measured at the bedside even in critically ill patients (see Table 2). In addition, they are relatively early indicators of change in the patient's clinical state. These parameters will improve as the ventilatory failure resolves. If they worsen, intubation and mechanical ventilation may be necessary.

The treatment of ARF with normal lungs is mainly supportive. The etiologic process can be treated or addressed in some cases, but frequently one has to support respiration while the primary process resolves. If there is only mild respiratory depression with minimal hypoxemia, and hypercapnia, supplemental oxygen by face mask or nasal cannula will suffice. With more profound degrees of respiratory depression, intubation and mechanical ventilation are required. The decision for intubation is predominantly a clinical one. Guidelines on when to intubate and mechanically ventilate a patient are given in Table 2. Measurement of FEV_1, VC, spontaneous res-

piratory rate and V_T, and NIP made at the bedside can be an invaluable aid. If these parameters deteriorate progressively during hours, this is a strong indication of progressive ventilatory failure and an urgent need for intubation and ventilation before complete respiratory collapse occurs. If the patient's bedside measurements are far outside the limits given in Table 2 and/or there is significant risk for aspiration, then intubation and mechanical ventilation should be considered immediately.

Sedative drug overdose is a frequent cause of ARF with normal lungs. The degree of respiratory depression generally correlates with the stage of coma. The greater the degree of coma and risk for vomiting and aspiration, the stronger the indication for intubation and mechanical ventilation. Naloxone (Narcan) 0.4 to 0.8 mg intravenously (IV) can be administered as a diagnostic test, because it will cause rapid improvement of narcotic sedation.

Central nervous system (CNS) infections are treated with appropriate antimicrobial agents coupled with ventilatory support. CNS tumors, cerebrovascular disease, and central apneas generally do not have a favorable response to specific therapy, and supportive care for the ARF is the mainstay of the treatment. Myasthenia gravis is treated with pyridostigmine (Mestinon), 60 mg three times daily initially. Plasmapheresis is effective in removing circulating antibody and has been found helpful in severely weak myasthenia patients in addition to supportive ventilatory care. Patients with the Guillain-Barré syndrome who develop severe weakness may be helped with plasmapheresis or intravenous immune globulin (0.4 gram per kg per day for 5 days).

Hypophosphatemia and hypokalemia are treated with the appropriate IV electrolyte solutions. Cholinergic crisis secondary to organophosphate poisoning should be managed with atropine, 2 to 5 mg IV. It is repeated every 15 minutes until atropinization occurs. To combat the muscle weakness, pralidoxime (Protopam), 1 gram IV given slowly, is used. It can be repeated three times in 8 to 12 hours if the muscle weakness is not relieved.

ACUTE RESPIRATORY FAILURE WITH ABNORMAL LUNGS

Asthma

Patients with ARF secondary to obstructive airways disease have special needs. The bronchial narrowing causes significant increases in airways resistance and hence work of breathing. Patients with asthma generally have more reversible obstruction than do those with COPD. They are generally younger in age and in better overall baseline health. Findings that indicate increased severity of an asthmatic attack are listed in Table 5.

Rapid IV hydration is always part of initial therapy in severe asthma. These patients are usually moderately dehydrated, which not only contracts their vascular volume but increases the viscosity of their secretions and exacerbates mucous plugging of the airways. In the first hour, 0.9% saline, 500 to 1000 mL, should be given unless it is contraindicated. This is followed by 100 to 200 mL per hour of 0.9% or 0.45% saline as indicated by the patient's cardiovascular and renal status.

Oxygen is administered to keep the minimum PaO_2 in the 60 to 70 mm Hg range, which gives an oxygen saturation of greater than 90%. Unlike for patients with COPD, there is minimal risk for carbon dioxide narcosis with oxygen delivery to patients with asthma. Supplemental oxygen is most conveniently administered by nasal cannula at 1 to 2 liters per minute. The flow rate can be adjusted the basis of

TABLE 6. Initial Drug Therapy in Asthma

IV hydration

Inhaled beta₂ agonists delivered by aerosol mist
  Albuterol (Ventolin), 0.5 mL of a 0.5% solution in 2.5 mL of 0.9% saline
  Metaproterenol (Alupent), 0.3 mL of a 5% solution in 2.5 mL of 0.9% saline
This can be administered q 20 min the first hour and q 2–4 h thereafter.
If the patient cannot use a nebulizer:
  Epinephrine in water 1:1000, 0.3–0.5 mL SC q 20 min for up to 3 doses
  or
  Terbutaline (Brethine), 0.25–0.50 mg SC as above

Intravenous theophylline (aminophylline)
  Loading dose 5–6 mg/kg in 0.9% saline in 20 min
  Initial maintenance dose 0.3–0.6 mg/kg/h
    Lower doses for older patients (>45 y) and those with active liver disease
    Higher doses in younger patients (<30 y); in cigarette smokers; and with certain drugs, e.g., cimetidine (Tagamet), barbiturates
  Obtain theophylline level at 12–24 h and maintain at 15–20 mg/L

Corticosteroids
  Initially 250–1000 mg of hydrocortisone or 50–200 mg of methylprednisolone IV
  Maintenance of 100–400 mg hydrocortisone IV q 4–6 h or 20–80 mg of methylprednisolone q 4–6 h

Inhaled parasympatholytic delivered by aerosol mist
  Ipratropium bromide (Atrovent), 2.5 mL of a 0.02% solution by nebulizer initially and q 2–4 h as indicated by clinical response

TABLE 5. Indications of a Severe Asthmatic Attack

History

Previous recent severe attack
Prolonged attack (>24 h)
Previous steroid treatment within the last 6 mo
Previous hospitalization for asthma within the last 2 y

Physical Examination Findings

Pulsus paradoxus >15 mm Hg
Use of accessory muscles of respiration
Respiratory rate >30/min
Pulse >130/min
*Central cyanosis
*Disturbance of consciousness
*Subcutaneous emphysema
*Pneumothorax
*Silent chest in a tachypneic patient

Laboratory Data

*$PaCO_2$ ≥40 mm Hg
*PaO_2 <60 mm Hg on supplemental oxygen
*FEV_1 <30% predicted and no improvement with bronchodilators
*Vital capacity <1 L
*Electrocardiogram showing P pulmonale and right ventricular strain

*Strongly consider intubation and mechanical ventilation.

the ABG results. Venturi or aerosol masks are also acceptable, although some asthmatic patients tolerate them poorly.

Initial drug therapy for ARF due to asthma is outlined in Table 6. Beta-adrenergic agents are first-line therapy and can be given by nebulizer or subcutaneously if the patient cannot tolerate use of a nebulizer. The nebulized route is preferred in older patients and those with known or suspected cardiac disease. IV theophylline therapy is usually started at the same time. In a patient who is already taking theophylline, a loading dose of 2 mg per kg can be given if there are no obvious signs of xanthine intoxication, such as nausea, vomiting, tremors, or seizures. This raises the serum level 5 to 8 mg per liter. Because of its narrow toxic/therapeutic ratio and variable rate of clearance, one must monitor serum theophylline levels and clinical effect closely.

Parenteral glucocorticoids should be used in all patients with asthma and ARF. Although there is no consensus on the precise dosage or which preparation is optimal, there is agreement that they should be given early, because a beneficial effect will not occur before 4 to 8 hours. Once stabilized, the patient should be switched to oral agents and then tapered slowly in 3 to 4 weeks to prevent rebound bronchospasm. There is little clinical evidence to support a beneficial effect of inhaled ipratroprium bromide (Atrovent) solution in ARF due to asthma; however, because of its negligible side effects, it may be worth a therapeutic trial.

Factors that lead one to consider intubation and mechanical ventilation are marked with an asterisk in Table 5. Special care must be taken because of the high rate of complications due to elevated airways resistance and pressures in asthmatics. The goal of mechanical ventilation is to ventilate the patient at relatively low tidal volumes and respiratory rates. This prevents high airway pressures and excessive work of breathing. A good rule of thumb is to keep the respiratory rate less than 25 per minute and the airway plateau pressure less than 35 cm H_2O. The mode of ventilation used to achieve this is not important, because no one mode has been proved to be superior to any other. ARF due to asthma is a relatively reversible process, and if you support the patient with ventilation while aggressively treating the bronchospasm, your patient is likely to have a favorable outcome.

Chronic Obstructive Pulmonary Disease

ARF in patients with COPD usually results from an acute decompensation complicating their significant chronic underlying disease. Unlike asthmatics, these patients have little capacity to compensate for this insult. Therefore, a seemingly trivial event such as an upper respiratory tract infection may put them in ARF. In many patients, no obvious predisposing event can be found.

Patients with COPD may have chronic hypoxia, hypercapnia, and compensated respiratory acidosis. An ABG analysis at a time when the patient is clinically stable is invaluable. Indwelling arterial lines are useful to continuously monitor blood pressure and provide access for the frequent blood samples that must be drawn. Erythrocytosis (hematocrit greater than 50) is a clue to chronic hypoxia; a bicarbonate level of greater than 30 mEq per liter is a clue to chronic hypercapnia with renal compensation.

Unlike for patients with asthma, carbon dioxide may not be the main respiratory stimulus in patients with COPD, and one must be concerned about the development of carbon dioxide narcosis when administering oxygen. The lowest amount of oxygen needed to keep the Pa_{CO_2} around 60 mm Hg is used. This results in an oxygen saturation of more than 90%. Further increases in oxygen are not necessary because they will result only in increased risk for carbon dioxide narcosis with negligible increase in oxygen delivery.

Venturi and aerosol masks provide oxygen at a fixed concentration and so are the initial treatments of choice. Begin with 24% or 28% oxygen and adjust as indicated by ABG values and clinical response. Be more concerned by the level of pH than P_{CO_2}, because it is the degree of acidosis that causes complications and not the level of P_{CO_2}. Oxygen therapy frequently causes some carbon dioxide retention, which then re-equilibrates at a higher level. If the P_{CO_2} continues

to rise and the pH falls, you should reduce the oxygen concentration or consider mechanical ventilation.

Oxygen delivery by nasal cannula or prongs at a rate of 1 to 3 liters per minute is another option. This may be more comfortable for the patient, but the concentration of oxygen varies with the patient's minute ventilation. As the minute ventilation decreases, the oxygen concentration increases and so does the risk for carbon dioxide narcosis. Because of this, Venturi and aerosol masks are preferred.

Hypercapnia is tolerated well by patients with COPD. Hypoxia and acidosis are stronger indications for intubation and mechanical ventilation. Persistent severe acidosis, hypoxia, confusion, coma, decreased cough effectiveness, respiratory muscle fatigue, and use of accessory muscles of respiration are all indications for intubation and ventilation. The use of the largest possible endotracheal tube is recommended because this will allow more adequate suctioning, decrease resistive forces, and allow decreased work of breathing.

As in asthma, the choice of ventilator mode is not as important as keeping the respiratory rate below 25 per minute and the airway plateau pressure below 35 cm H_2O. The goal is to keep the Pa_{O_2} around 60 mm Hg while avoiding marked respiratory acidosis or alkalosis. The use of bronchodilator therapy as outlined for ARF due to asthma is indicated but generally not as effective.

Adult Respiratory Distress Syndrome

The adult respiratory distress syndrome (ARDS) is the result of increased microvascular permeability secondary to another primary process that results in diffuse lung injury. The pulmonary capillaries are flooded with fluid, which causes impaired oxygenation and decreased lung compliance in the face of normal left-sided cardiac function. The primary process is frequently a systemic infection, but ARDS is the final common pathway of lung injury secondary to a myriad of conditions. The same principles described before guide ventilator management in ARDS. In addition, because of the increased capillary microvascular permeability, one must be careful not to overhydrate these patients because the fluid will end up in the pulmonary capillaries, worsening the pulmonary edema.

Other Causes

For the other causes of ARF with abnormal lungs (see Table 1), the general principles of clinical management of the oxygenation and ventilation defects are the same as outlined earlier. In addition, the primary process needs to be addressed. For example, the patient with pneumonia needs appropriate antibiotics, the patient with significant pneumothorax or pleural effusion needs chest tube drainage, and the patient with pulmonary embolism needs heparin and/or fibrinolytic therapy. The indications for and management of ventilatory support are the same as previously outlined.

A Swan-Ganz catheter can be indispensable in distinguishing cardiogenic from noncardiogenic pulmonary edema as well as being a guide to respiratory and cardiovascular status. Hemodynamic parameters that should be obtained include CO, mixed venous Po_2, pulmonary capillary wedge pressure, central venous pressure, and pulmonary artery pressure. Systemic vascular resistance can be calculated by subtracting central venous pressure from the mean aortic pressure and dividing by the CO.

The treatment of the nonpulmonary factors is essential. Alimentation should be instituted from the onset. Enteral alimentation with a soft feeding tube is best if possible; if not, IV alimentation should be used. Low-dose heparin therapy should be instituted unless it is contraindicated. Last, the use of H_2 blockers to maintain the gastric pH above 4 for prophylaxis against stress ulceration is warranted.

ATELECTASIS

method of
LOREN F. HIRATZKA, M.D.
The Jewish Hospital and The Christ Hospital
Cincinnati, Ohio

Atelectasis is collapse of lung tissue due to absence of air within the alveoli. Atelectasis may involve anatomic segments, lobes, or the whole lung but may also be a miliary process, as in the adult respiratory distress syndrome. Atelectasis may occur in surgical patients as a result of pain and splinting with altered respiratory mechanics, retained airway secretions, and decreased mucociliary clearance. Atelectasis may also result from either intrinsic or extrinsic airway obstruction, so that diagnostic procedures including bronchoscopy should be performed when the cause of atelectasis is in question. Potential problems of hypoxemia and pneumonitis may follow the development of atelectasis and can further prolong and complicate a patient's hospital course.

PREVENTION AND TREATMENT OF ATELECTASIS

The keys to treatment of atelectasis are

1. Prevention in clinical situations in which atelectasis might be anticipated, such as patients undergoing surgical procedures with general endotracheal anesthesia
2. Treatment of underlying conditions causing atelectasis
3. Vigorous treatment once atelectasis is diagnosed

Prevention of atelectasis in surgical patients can be facilitated by systematic preoperative, intraoperative, and postoperative strategies.

Preoperative teaching in techniques of incentive spirometry and coughing as well as in the expectations regarding early postoperative mobilization can be useful. Modification of preoperative risk factors, such as smoking (cessation for 1 to 2 weeks) or chronic sputum production (preoperative antibiotics, if sputum is purulent; pulmonary physiotherapy for symptomatic patients), may also reduce the impact of these factors on postoperative care.

Intraoperative preventive measures include protection of the airway to avoid aspiration, periodic "sighs" to hyperinflate the lung, and removal of retained secretions.

Postoperative preventive measures are directed toward maintenance of clear airways and restoration of ventilatory mechanics to as nearly normal as possible. These measures are also applicable to nonsurgical patients. Early mobilization and ambulation, periodic coughing and deep breathing exercises (including incentive spirometry), and adequate analgesia to facilitate these measures are important and effective in awake, cooperative patients. In unconscious, sedated, or uncooperative patients, avoidance of aspiration by proper positioning and protection of the airway are of paramount importance.

Treatment of atelectasis requires more vigorous and invasive therapy. Methods that increase functional residual capacity include intermittent or continuous positive airway pressure or positive expiratory pressure. Clearing of endobronchial secretions may require frequent suctioning even by endotracheal tube or bronchoscope. Chest percussion and postural drainage may help mobilize secretions and expand dependent lung segments.

Bronchoscopy should be used early when refractory lobar or significant segmental atelectasis is present, particularly when an endobronchial mass or foreign body could be the inciting cause. Insufflation of atelectatic lung by balloon catheters placed in lobar or segmental bronchi has been useful in some cases.

Bronchospasm can be reversed with inhaled beta-adrenergic agonists (e.g., albuterol [Ventolin, Proventil], isoproterenol, terbutaline) and/or intravenous bronchodilators (e.g., theophylline). Tenacious secretions may be liquefied by mucolytic agents (e.g., acetylcysteine [Mucomyst]). The routine and prophylactic use of these measures has not been shown to be cost-effective.

The use of cricothyroid membrane catheters or injections to induce cough may be effective in uncooperative patients but may cause significant laryngospasm. For severe and prolonged respiratory failure, tracheostomy may be required and can facilitate direct tracheobronchial suctioning.

CHRONIC OBSTRUCTIVE PULMONARY DISEASE

method of
RONALD B. GEORGE, M.D.
Louisiana State University School of Medicine
Shreveport, Louisiana

Chronic obstructive pulmonary disease (COPD) is a term used to describe a combination of chronic obstructive bronchitis, emphysema, and bronchospasm usually resulting from years of contact with cigarette smoke and other inhaled irritants. More than 14 million Americans suffer from COPD, and it is now the fourth leading cause of death in the United States. COPD accounted for 4.2% of all deaths in 1991 (more than 90,000 people). Of even greater importance is the chronic, progressive nature of the disorder, leading to severe, prolonged disability, which costs the American economy more than $10 billion per year.

The American Thoracic Society (ATS) has chosen an objective measure of airflow limitation, the 1-second forced expiratory volume (FEV_1) as a percentage of the predicted value, to estimate the degree of disability caused by COPD in a given patient. In the ATS guidelines for management, to which the interested reader is referred,* the recommended treatment is related to the severity of disease.

A STEPPED-CARE APPROACH TO THE MANAGEMENT OF CHRONIC OBSTRUCTIVE PULMONARY DISEASE

This discussion centers on a stepped-care approach to management of patients with COPD based on the severity of disease, symptoms, and response to therapy. This should yield a cost-effective management strategy and prevent the use of ineffective treatment measures while maximizing the lifestyle of the patient. A summary of this recommended approach is shown in Table 1. The following discussion relates the recommended treatment measures to the individual patient's needs.

Step 1: Assessment and Prevention of Further Damage

As with any chronic, progressive disease process, it is important for the clinician to assess the degree of dysfunction and correlate this with the symptoms. Processes that are ongoing and can be corrected should be addressed, and preventive measures should be instituted. The most cost-effective method of assessing the stage of disease in COPD, in addition to the general evaluation of the patient, is spirometry. This consists of a maximal expiratory flow curve, with a flow-volume loop, available in most hospitals and clinics for a reasonable fee. The degree of airflow obstruction is assessed by the FEV_1, the forced vital capacity (FVC), and the FEV_1/FVC ratio. With use of the ATS grading system, stage 1 disease is present if the FEV_1 is more than 50% of the predicted value, and therapy required is usually primarily preventive. Moderate disease, requiring ongoing symptomatic therapy, is present if the FEV_1 is 35 to 50% of the predicted value. If the FEV_1 is below 35% of predicted, complications including exercise hypoxemia and cor pulmonale are likely, and aggressive therapy is indicated.

In assessing the severity of obstruction, it is important to determine the variability of obstruction,

*See Celli BR, Snider GL, Heffner J, et al: Standards for the diagnosis and care of patients with chronic obstructive pulmonary disease. Am J Respir Crit Care Med *152*:S77–S120, 1995.

TABLE 1. A Stepped-Care Approach to the Management of Chronic Obstructive Pulmonary Disease

Step 1: Assessment and Prevention of Further Damage

Baseline assessment
Screen for risk factors
Smoking cessation
Vaccination
Fitness program

Step 2: Symptomatic Therapy for Airflow Obstruction

Anticholinergic agents
Beta-adrenergic agonists
Methylxanthines

Step 3: Corticosteroid Therapy

Systemic corticosteroids
Inhaled corticosteroids

Step 4: Pulmonary Rehabilitation and Oxygen Therapy

Education of the patient
Nutrition
General exercise conditioning
Chest physical therapy
Breathing retraining
Psychosocial support
Long-term oxygen therapy

Step 5: Management of Acute Exacerbations

Oxygenation
Bronchodilator therapy
Corticosteroids
Antibiotics
Mechanical ventilation
Advance directives

and this is usually done by administering a standard bronchodilator and repeating the test. About 10% of patients with COPD have significant reversibility of airflow, and this has major implications for therapy and prognosis. Patients with 20% or more improvement after beta-adrenergic aerosol administration have significant airflow reversibility; if marked responsiveness is present, they are often classified as having "asthmatic bronchitis." Reversibility of airflow can also be determined by reviewing serial spirograms; variation of 20% or more in FEV_1 in time indicates reversibility. In all patients with COPD requiring clinic care, I urge that the clinician obtain a spirogram annually and that a flow-chart be maintained, so that the rate of decline in FEV_1 in time as well as response to various treatment maneuvers can be determined objectively.

Among patients with emphysema, about 1 to 2% have an inherited deficiency of the antiproteinase system, called alpha$_1$-antitrypsin (AAT) deficiency. It is not useful to screen for the presence of AAT deficiency, unless the onset of emphysema is at an early age, especially in women, or unless there is a family history of AAT deficiency. If a homozygous deficiency of AAT is found, replacement therapy is available as a preventive measure, but it is expensive, and long-term results are not yet known.

Because cigarette smoking is the most important cause of COPD, it follows that a major part of management should involve cessation of smoking. In the

Lung Health Study conducted by the National Institutes of Health, cessation of smoking was the single factor associated with improvement in the rate of decline of airflow in time. A recommended protocol for smoking cessation that is applicable to an office practice is shown in Table 2.

The physician should make a clear, unequivocal recommendation to the smoker that he or she *must* quit smoking for health's sake. If significant airflow obstruction is shown on the spirogram, it may be useful to indicate this to the patient. Help the patient choose a quit date, at a time he or she is not expecting any major stress, such as a holiday or weekend. Also useful is a simple pledge written on the patient's record, "I, John Doe, agree to stop smoking completely as of the following date," signed by the patient and witnessed by the physician. At this point, the patient should choose between a self-help program with a physician's support and a group program. Many group programs are available, some at minimal expense, and they are useful if they are available and the patient has the time. Alternatively, a number of self-help booklets, telephone hot lines, and other assistance sources are available from the ATS (call the local lung association), the National Cancer Institute and various other government and volunteer agencies. Follow-up support and evaluation are critical, and the patient should return within a month for repeated counseling. The patient should be encouraged to telephone the office if any unusual stresses or temptations are encountered.

Most smokers are addicted to nicotine, and withdrawal symptoms are common. Nicotine replacement therapy has been shown to be helpful in improving quit rates. Nicotine patches (Nicoderm, Habitrol, Nicotrol, ProStep) are now available in various doses without prescription and are provided with accompanying literature to assist the patient in quitting. The nicotine replacement is designed as a short-term assist and should not be continued past 2 months; patients are often able to do without replacement after as little as 2 weeks. Additional increased quit rates have been reported with other agents such as clonidine, an alpha$_2$-adrenergic agonist, and the anxiolytic drug buspirone, but neither of these is approved by the Food and Drug Administration for use in smoking cessation.

Additional preventive measures for routine use in COPD include a pneumovax injection every 5 or 6 years to prevent pneumococcal infections and annual administration of influenza vaccine. The patient should be encouraged to maintain an active and healthy lifestyle, to avoid household or work place irritants such as passive cigarette smoke or polluted environments, and to partake in a general exercise and fitness program. These can be designed to fit the symptoms and abilities of the patient. Progressive toning exercise (e.g., walking, biking) is useful even for patients whose exercise capacity is limited.

Step 2: Symptomatic Therapy for Airflow Obstruction

Anticholinergic agents cause a lowering of guanosine 3′,5′-cyclic monophosphate in bronchial smooth muscle cells, causing a decrease in muscle tone. When given systemically, they cause several unwanted side effects; however, when given by aerosol as quaternary ammonium derivatives of atropine, their systemic effects are minimal. Ipratropium bromide (Atrovent) is the only such agent currently available in the United States. It is available in a metered-dose inhaler (MDI) and as a nebulizer solution. Its onset of action is slower than that of beta-adrenergic agents (60 to 90 minutes), but its duration of action is longer (6 to 8 hours); its longer duration of effects, wide therapeutic range, low incidence of side effects, and absence of tachyphylaxis make it suitable for use on a regular basis with chronic airflow obstruction. An algorithm for use of bronchodilator therapy in patients with COPD is shown in Figure 1. When given according to the manufacturer's recommendation (2 puffs four times daily), it is an effective bronchodilator in COPD, but many clinicians prescribe it in a higher dosage, such as 4 puffs three times daily, or even more during acute exacerbations.

Whereas the MDI form of ipratropium is as effective as the nebulizer solution, some patients prefer to use the nebulizer solution at least once a day. The administration of nebulized saline may help with

---

TABLE 2. **Protocol for Smoking Cessation**

Initiation

Physician or health care worker should initiate quitting, explaining risks of cigarette smoking for the individual and including a strong admonition. Encourage establishment of a definite quit date. Offer referral for a group program or recommend self-help materials. Nicotine replacement may be offered to control withdrawal symptoms; infrequently, other pharmacologic therapy, such as clonidine or buspirone, may be discussed. Hypnosis may be considered but is of little value as a single-session recourse.

Early Follow-up

Telephone the patient on or within 3–5 d after the quit date. Review progress and counsel regarding recruitment of a support person. Call again 1–2 wk after the quit date. Repeat as needed.

Continuing Reinforcement

Further follow-up should be arranged by the physician or health care worker. The next regular visit should be less than 2 mo after initiating the cessation program. If the patient is abstinent, review and reward success and reinforce prior warnings. May monitor by phone monthly until next visit; continue follow-up at increasing intervals for 12 mo after the quit date.

Failure or Recidivism

If the patient fails to achieve abstinence or does so but relapses, the physician or health care worker should review the program with the patient, emphasizing elements of success and identifying circumstances of failure; explore alternatives (e.g., referral for group therapy).

Adapted from Celli BR, Snider GL, Heffner J, et al: Standards for the diagnosis and care of patients with chronic obstructive pulmonary disease. Am J Respir Crit Care Med 152:S77–S120, 1995.

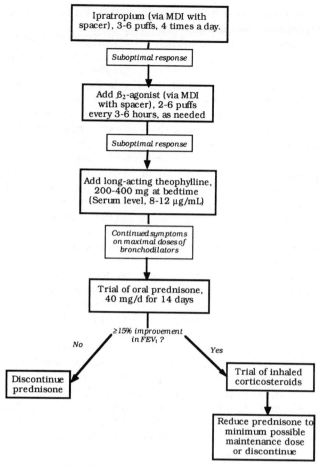

```
┌─────────────────────────────┐
│ Ipratropium (via MDI with   │
│ spacer), 3-6 puffs, 4 times a day. │
└─────────────────────────────┘
         │
   ┌──────────────────┐
   │ Suboptimal response │
   └──────────────────┘
         │
┌─────────────────────────────┐
│ Add β₂-agonist (via MDI     │
│ with spacer), 2-6 puffs     │
│ every 3-6 hours, as needed  │
└─────────────────────────────┘
         │
   ┌──────────────────┐
   │ Suboptimal response │
   └──────────────────┘
         │
┌─────────────────────────────┐
│ Add long-acting theophylline, │
│ 200-400 mg at bedtime        │
│ (Serum level, 8-12 μg/mL)    │
└─────────────────────────────┘
         │
   ┌─────────────────────┐
   │ Continued symptoms   │
   │ on maximal doses of  │
   │ bronchodilators      │
   └─────────────────────┘
         │
┌─────────────────────────────┐
│ Trial of oral prednisone,    │
│ 40 mg/d for 14 days          │
└─────────────────────────────┘
```

Figure 1. Proposed algorithm for the pharmacologic management of stable chronic obstructive pulmonary disease. *Abbreviation:* MDI = metered-dose inhaler. (Adapted with permission from Ferguson GT, Cherniack RM: Management of chronic obstructive pulmonary disease. N Engl J Med *328*:1017–1022, 1993. Copyright 1993 Massachusetts Medical Society. All rights reserved.)

expectoration of sputum and allows administration of larger doses of the drug. Some clinicians prescribe the nebulizer for home use along with the MDI for use away from home.

Beta-adrenergic agonists increase adenosine monophosphate in bronchial smooth muscle cells, resulting in a reduction of bronchomotor tone. When given by inhalation, their onset of action is faster than that of ipratropium bromide, but their duration of action is somewhat shorter (except for salmeterol, which is discussed later), and there is evidence of tachyphylaxis to bronchodilator effects when they are used on a regular basis. For this reason, they are usually recommended for use on an as-needed basis to supplement the effects of ipratropium. Patients should be instructed to carry their beta-adrenergic MDI with them and to use it when symptoms are increased, such as before exercise or physical activity (see Figure 1).

There are several beta₂-specific agents available in MDI form, and in general they provide similar bronchodilation in equivalent dosage. These include metaproterenol (Alupent, Metaprel), albuterol (Ven-

tolin, Proventil), terbutaline (Brethaire, Bricanyl), bitolterol (Tornalate), and pirbuterol (Maxair). Choice of an agent is based on the patient's preference, physician's experience, dosage forms available, and cost. The recommended dose of these agents is 2 puffs by MDI every 4 to 6 hours as needed. Several other dosage forms besides MDI are marketed, including nebulizer solution, dry powder inhaler, and oral and subcutaneous forms.

There is currently a single, extra-long-acting inhaled beta-adrenergic agent on the U.S. market, salmeterol (Serevent). It is available as an MDI, and after 2 inhalations, its bronchodilator effects last up to 12 hours or longer. Its usefulness is somewhat hindered by fears of side effects and tachyphylaxis, but in some cases, such as nocturnal attacks of wheezing in patients with reversible disease, the drug may allow restful sleep and a decrease in symptoms.

Methylxanthines provide an additive effect to the bronchodilator medications. After many decades of use, the exact method of action of theophylline on the bronchi is unclear, but it does relax bronchial smooth muscle to a moderate degree. Additional beneficial effects in COPD patients include an increase in cardiac output, improved contraction and delayed fatigue of the diaphragm, stimulation of the respiratory center, and diuresis. Theophylline is available from a wide variety of manufacturers in an oral sustained-release form, and it is relatively inexpensive for long-term use. Theophylline is generally prescribed in sustained-release form, given once a day at bedtime or twice daily. The usual adult dose is 200 to 300 mg (see later).

Theophylline has a narrow therapeutic window, with significant toxic effects at serum levels above 20 mg per liter. Side effects include nausea, vomiting, insomnia and sleep disturbance, agitation, tremor, seizures, and cardiac dysrhythmias; serum levels must be monitored carefully, especially in patients with associated medical conditions, including elderly patients and those with hepatic dysfunction, congestive heart failure, or febrile illnesses. In addition, a large number of widely prescribed medications, including macrolide and quinolone antibiotics, H₂ blockers, and propranolol, may prolong the serum half-life of theophylline, resulting in toxic side effects. Current recommendations are for maintaining peak serum levels in the range of 8 to 12 μg per mL. Serum should be obtained 4 to 6 hours after an oral dose to determine peak levels, and serum levels should be checked frequently until a stable level is maintained. Even then, any change in the patient's status, or addition of new therapy, is an indication for determining the serum level, as is the onset of any symptoms associated with theophylline toxicity.

Step 3: Corticosteroid Therapy

Ongoing inflammatory changes in the bronchial walls appear to correlate with an increased decline in airflow in at least some patients with obstructive chronic bronchitis. The dominant inflammatory cell in chronic bronchitis appears to be the neutrophil, and increased numbers of activated neutrophils are present during exacerbations of chronic bronchitis. Clinical correlates of an active inflammatory process in patients with chronic bronchitis include the presence of increased neutrophils and/or eosinophils in the sputum, reversibility of airflow obstruction, and a rapid decline in FEV_1 over time.

Studies of clinical response to systemic corticosteroid therapy in patients with stable COPD have yielded varying results; a meta-analysis of reported trials showed that 10% of patients had a 20% or greater improvement in baseline FEV_1 with oral corticosteroid therapy. Patients more likely to respond were those with significant response to inhaled bronchodilator. For a therapeutic trial of oral corticosteroids, a baseline FEV_1 should be recorded and a 2-week course of prednisone 40 mg per day prescribed, with the other baseline therapy continued (see Figure 1). If the FEV_1 improves significantly during this trial period (at least 15% above baseline), the patient is a candidate for long-term inhaled corticosteroid therapy. The inhaled corticosteroids should be given initially in high doses (800 µg of beclomethasone or equivalent per day or more) and later tapered as symptoms permit. Alternate-day oral corticosteroids are sometimes necessary but are associated with a variety of serious side effects, including osteoporosis, hypertension, and glucose intolerance. Repeated attempts at weaning from alternate-day oral corticosteroids should be made, with substitution of high-dose inhaled corticosteroids.

The effects of long-term administration of inhaled corticosteroids in patients with COPD are currently being evaluated in two multicenter studies, one by the European Respiratory Society and the other as an extension of the U.S. Lung Health Study. The use of inhaled corticosteroids as a preventive measure in patients with COPD holds some promise, especially if they are started before the airflow obstruction becomes severe, but improvement has not yet been demonstrated conclusively. It is likely that some patients may benefit (those with clinical signs of ongoing inflammation, including chronic bronchitic patients and asthmatic bronchitic patients), whereas others will not (those with predominant emphysema). Nonsteroidal anti-inflammatory agents such as cromolyn and nedocromil have not been shown to be useful in patients with severe COPD, nor have the new leukotriene antagonists.

Step 4: Pulmonary Rehabilitation and Oxygen Therapy

Patients with severe COPD continue to have dyspnea even with bronchodilator therapy. They are subject to repeated exacerbations requiring antibiotic and systemic corticosteroid therapy. In these patients, a comprehensive rehabilitation program may offer significant benefits. Individual components of such a program may vary and should be tailored to the needs of each patient; the basic elements include education of the patient, nutritional assessment, exercise training, and psychosocial support.

Education is aimed at assisting patients to understand the pathophysiologic process of their disease, to modify risk factors, and to use medications properly. Patients learn to develop practical ways of coping with disabling symptoms and demonstrate improved adherence to the prescribed therapeutic regimen. To be effective, the education program must be a part of a comprehensive rehabilitation program as outlined in the following discussion. Nurses, respiratory therapists, physical therapists, and other allied health personnel are usually better trained to assist patients than are most physicians and often spend more time with the patients. Printed materials, videos, and other teaching materials are available for office and home use. Group discussions are an important part of the program, and "emphysema clubs" are available in many communities to allow patients to share their problems and solutions. The patient is encouraged to live a healthy and active life as symptoms permit, get annual vaccinations, recognize exacerbations early, and avoid smoke and other irritants. During this time, advance directives can be discussed with the patient.

Nutrition is a problem in about 25% of COPD patients, usually those with the most advanced disease, and weight loss has been correlated with early mortality in patients with emphysema. Patients may complain that eating is an effort, and dyspnea may interfere with adequate caloric intake. An early assessment of the nutritional status is indicated; if malnutrition is noted, a dietitian should be consulted to assist the patient in choosing the proper foods. Adequate fluid intake is important, especially during hot weather in elderly patients and in those taking diuretic medications. Timing of food intake may affect absorption of some oral medications, and use of a nebulizer may involve swallowing air, which in turn interferes with adequate food intake. Thus, eating habits should be correlated with therapeutic maneuvers, including exercise.

General exercise conditioning has been shown to increase exercise tolerance, prolong endurance, and improve quality of life, even in patients with advanced COPD. The optimal methods of training and the mechanisms of response to exercise are still being defined, and a variety of methods are used. Reports indicate that a strenuous training program that pushes the patient toward his or her dyspnea-related maximal exercise tolerance is beneficial. With general exercise conditioning, less oxygen is required for a given amount of work, less carbon dioxide and lactate are produced, and a lower ventilatory demand is generated. Exercise training is largely muscle group specific, and lower extremity bicycle or treadmill training will not improve arm-related activities such as dressing, grooming, and bathing.

Chest physical therapy is often included in a general exercise program and involves training the patient, and often family members, in the techniques of postural drainage, deep breathing, coughing, and chest percussion designed to improve expectoration of secretions. Chest physical therapy should follow nebulizer treatments and should be timed so that it does not interfere with other activities. Treatments are often performed at home, on arising in the morning and at bedtime.

Breathing retraining includes instruction in diaphragmatic breathing and pursed-lip breathing, in an attempt to optimize airflow during expiration. Studies have indicated mixed results, and one study found no change in tidal volume or respiratory frequency, a loss of mechanical efficiency, and an increase in dyspnea. Most patients return to their usual method of breathing as soon as the training session is over.

Psychosocial support is an important part of an organized rehabilitation program, because patients with advanced COPD have a variety of symptoms including hopelessness, inability to cope with their disease, and chronic depression. One advantage of a successful exercise program is a decrease in symptoms such as depression, fear, and anxiety. Family members and friends should participate in program activities so that they can help the patient cope with her or his disease. Patients with severe depression may benefit from individual counseling and psychotherapy. Psychotropic drugs should be reserved for those with severe psychologic dysfunction.

Long-term oxygen therapy has been shown to be beneficial in patients with chronic hypoxemia, a common finding during the later stages of COPD. Insurance companies and government guidelines allow reimbursement for home oxygen if the resting PaO_2 is 55 mm Hg or less or if there is evidence of tissue hypoxia (cor pulmonale, secondary polycythemia, impaired mental status). The use of home oxygen must be prescribed by a physician and the rate of flow adjusted to maintain the PaO_2 at 60 mm Hg or greater. Higher flow rates may be required during sleep or with exercise. With an organized exercise program and careful medical therapy, the need for oxygen may decrease over time, and resting PaO_2 should be reassessed after 1 or 2 months. Oxygen may be administered during exercise in a rehabilitation program.

The presence of carbon dioxide retention is a warning sign to most clinicians, who fear respiratory center depression and decreased ventilation when oxygen is given. In general, carbon dioxide retention in severe COPD is the result of ventilation/perfusion imbalance rather than respiratory depression, and hypoxemic patients tolerate home oxygen well. During oxygen administration, there may be a mild rise in carbon dioxide, which is a normal adjustment mechanism to improve the efficiency of ventilation. This is acceptable, and a new, higher level of carbon dioxide is usually maintained. Sedatives should be avoided in patients requiring home oxygen, and the patient and family must be warned never to smoke where oxygen is used because it supports combustion.

Home oxygen can be supplied by an oxygen concentrator, compressed oxygen cylinders, or liquid oxygen. The most cost-effective and reliable method is the oxygen concentrator; it is usually prescribed with backup compressed or liquid oxygen to provide mobility for the patient and for use during mechanical or power failure. Oxygen is usually given by nasal cannula at flow rates of 0.5 to 4 liters per minute.

Transtracheal oxygen (TTO) by small-bore catheter has several advantages over nasal oxygen for home use, including a 50% reduction in oxygen requirement, decreased dyspnea, better exercise tolerance, and improved cosmetic appearance. TTO works by flushing carbon dioxide from the lower trachea and large bronchi, so that the large airways act as an oxygen reservoir, reducing the respiratory dead space. TTO may also work with sleep hypoxemia by bypassing the nose and glottis. Careful management by a health care team is required for optimal insertion and placement of the catheter, and humidification decreases the incidence of mucus ball formation, a common problem with TTO.

Step 5: Management of Acute Exacerbations

Increased dyspnea and cough, often with purulent sputum, fever, and new chest film infiltrates, are characteristic of acute exacerbations of COPD. These are usually the result of intercurrent respiratory infections but may also be due to left-sided heart failure, pneumothorax or rib fracture associated with mild chest trauma, or administration of sedatives. Mortality rates associated with acute exacerbations of COPD are related to age, severity of hypoxemia, presence of cardiac arrhythmias, and need for mechanical ventilation; reports indicate a mortality rate of about 15%. Indications for hospitalization during acute exacerbations and for treatment in an intensive care unit are shown in Tables 3 and 4, which are adapted from the ATS guidelines.

Initial therapy for acute exacerbations includes optimal bronchodilatation, mobilization of secretions, oxygenation, and monitoring of ventilatory status while the causative problem is addressed. Beta agonists have long been the major bronchodilator agents used for acute exacerbations, and these are ideally given by nebulizer aerosol. Because beta agonists have an additive effect when they are combined with ipratropium bromide, both agents should be given and can be combined in the nebulizer. Oxygen should be administered to maintain PaO_2 above 55 mm Hg, with careful monitoring of $PaCO_2$ and acid-base status. Progressively rising $PaCO_2$ or persistent hypoxemia is an indication for mechanical ventilation, unless the patient has indicated that he or she does not want it used.

Intravenous corticosteroids are generally used to optimize the effects of bronchodilator therapy, and several studies indicate that they hasten recovery from acute respiratory failure. Methylprednisolone (Solu-Medrol) in doses of 100 to 125 mg initially and

TABLE 3. **Indications for Hospitalization of Patients with Chronic Obstructive Pulmonary Disease**

Acute exacerbation (increased dyspnea, cough, or sputum production), plus one or more of the following:
 Inadequate response to outpatient management
 In a patient previously mobile, inability to ambulate because of dyspnea
 Inability to eat or sleep because of dyspnea
 Inadequate home care resources
 Serious co-morbid condition
 Prolonged progressive symptoms before emergency visit
 Altered mentation
 Worsening hypoxemia
 New or worsening hypercapnia
New or worsening cor pulmonale unresponsive to outpatient management
Planned invasive surgical or diagnostic procedure requiring analgesics or sedatives that may worsen pulmonary function
Co-morbid condition, e.g., severe steroid myopathy or acute vertebral compression fractures, that has worsened pulmonary function

Adapted from Celli BR, Snider GL, Heffner J, et al: Standards for the diagnosis and care of patients with chronic obstructive pulmonary disease. Am J Respir Crit Care Med 152:S77–S120, 1995.

at 6- to 8-hour intervals is recommended. The role of intravenous theophylline during acute episodes of COPD is debated, but theophylline is added to the bronchodilator regimen in most reported series. Loading doses are contraindicated until baseline serum theophylline levels are available, because the patient may have been receiving oral theophylline at home. As noted before, the optimal serum level is in the range of 8 to 12 μg/mL, and the clinician should be aware that hepatic congestion and a variety of medications may delay excretion of theophylline. Patients commonly fail to eat and drink properly during acute exacerbations of COPD, and this may lead to drying and increased tenaciousness of sputum. Adequate fluid balance should be maintained either orally or parenterally.

Antibiotics are given as part of the therapy for acute exacerbations because respiratory infection is so frequently present, even if signs of infection are minimal. In one large, double-blind study of outpatients with COPD, the addition of antibiotics was

TABLE 4. **Indications for Intensive Care Unit Admission of Patients with Acute Exacerbation of Chronic Obstructive Pulmonary Disease**

Severe dyspnea that responds inadequately to initial emergency therapy
Confusion or lethargy
Respiratory muscle fatigue (especially paradoxical diaphragmatic motion)
Persistent worsening hypoxemia despite supplemental oxygen or severe or worsening respiratory acidosis (pH < 7.30)
Need for noninvasive or invasive assisted mechanical ventilation

Adapted from Celli BR, Snider GL, Heffner J, et al: Standards for the diagnosis and care of patients with chronic obstructive pulmonary disease. Am J Respir Crit Care Med 152:S77–S120, 1995.

associated with more rapid resolution of symptoms and a more rapid improvement of airflow rates. A meta-analysis of randomized trials of antibiotics during COPD exacerbations indicated a small but statistically and clinically significant improvement associated with antibiotic therapy. Many if not most respiratory infections in patients with COPD are viral, but bacteria are often present in the lower airways of these patients, and bacterial infection may follow an initial viral episode. The common pathogenic bacteria isolated from sputum of patients during acute exacerbation are *Streptococcus pneumoniae, Haemophilus influenzae,* and *Moraxella catarrhalis.* A variety of antibiotics are effective for these infections, including tetracyclines, macrolides, β-lactamase–resistant penicillins, cephalosporins, fluoroquinolones, and trimethoprim-sulfamethoxazole (Bactrim, Septra). Antibiotics are often administered parenterally during the early, acute illness in hospitalized patients to guarantee optimal absorption. When recovery begins, an oral form can be substituted.

SURGERY FOR EMPHYSEMA

Thoracotomy for removal of giant bullous disease has long been an option in selected patients who are otherwise well. In these cases, improvement after surgery is rapid and dramatic, although the giant bullae may later recur. Medical and surgical advances have led to the use of thoracic surgical techniques in patients with generalized, severe emphysema. These techniques include lung transplantation and volume reduction surgery of the lungs.

Lung transplantation for severe emphysema has been made possible by improvement in methods of immunosuppression. The realization that single-lung transplantation for emphysema is possible has led to an increase in its use, so that emphysema associated with COPD and AAT deficiency now accounts for about 60% of all single-lung transplants in the United States. Selection criteria include age younger than 60 years, life expectancy without transplantation of 2 years or less, progressive deterioration of clinical status despite optimal medical therapy, emotional stability, and adequate psychosocial support. With increasing experience, some of these restrictions (e.g., the age limit) are becoming less rigid. Survival after transplantation has been reported as 77% at 2 years and 75% at 3 years. Thereafter, survival rates fall, partly owing to rejection problems or infection and partly because of associated nonrespiratory conditions in elderly patients. With time, the incidence of bronchiolitis obliterans, a manifestation of graft rejection, increases, and survival beyond 8 years is rare. At present, the major limitations of lung transplantation for emphysema are the cost of the procedure and the lack of an adequate supply of donor lungs.

Volume reduction surgery has been employed at several large transplant centers because of a lack of donor organs and the fact that many patients died while awaiting a transplant. One commonly used procedure, which the originators call bilateral pneumectomy, involves removing 20 to 30% of the most severely involved areas of each lung through a median sternotomy. Other centers use a thoracostomy technique for tissue resection. Most centers no longer use the laser technique because of its high rate of postoperative complications. After surgical removal, the remaining lung is stapled with a device fitted with bovine pericardium or other materials designed to decrease postoperative air leaks. Several small series of patients have been reported with good short-term results, including a reduction of lung volumes, improvement in flow rates, increase in lung elastic recoil, relief of dyspnea, and improved quality of life.

In centers with successful volume reduction results, selection criteria are rigid, and only about a third of referred patients undergo the procedure. The cost is considerable, and Medicare is not at present reimbursing for volume reduction surgery except as part of an approved research protocol. For these poor surgical candidates with far-advanced disease, preoperative and postoperative care must be extensive. A significant part of the improvement in symptoms is associated with a vigorous preoperative and postoperative rehabilitation program, with careful attention to bronchial hygiene and conditioning exercises. Among the patients reported so far, improvement appears to peak at 6 months to 1 year after surgery, then remain stable, after which deterioration occurs as a result of the underlying lung disease. An ongoing controlled study is examining the long-term benefits of volume reduction surgery versus a vigorous, organized rehabilitation program. Until the results are known, volume reduction surgery should be considered an experimental procedure and should be restricted to a few large centers where lung transplantation programs are under way.

SLEEP APNEA AND HYPOPNEA*

method of
MARK H. SANDERS, M.D.
*University of Pittsburgh School of Medicine and
 Veterans Affairs Medical Center
Pittsburgh, Pennsylvania*

The primary, immediate consequences of total and partial upper airway obstruction during sleep (obstructive apnea and hypopnea, respectively) include sympathetic nervous system activation and sleep disruption associated with the arousal that terminates the event and, often, oxyhemoglobin desaturation. It is generally accepted that these physiologic outcomes lead to the clinical impact of sleep apnea and hypopnea. There is compelling epidemiologic evidence that sleep apnea and hypopnea are prevalent in the general population. Between 1 and 10% of middle-aged individuals have a frequency of apnea plus hypopnea events equal to or in excess of 5 per hour of

*Supported by the Veterans Affairs Medical Research Service and NIH Training Grant NHLBI2T32HL0756311A2.

sleep, and 2 to 4% of the middle-aged working population have sleep apnea and hypopnea with excessive daytime sleepiness. A substantial body of literature strongly suggests that untreated sleep apnea and hypopnea may have serious medical and nonmedical morbidity and mortality. Several studies have concluded that there is a relationship between sleep apnea and hypopnea and systemic hypertension as well as increased cardiovascular and cerebrovascular morbidity and mortality. The morbidity and mortality associated with sleep apnea and hypopnea extend into the nonmedical realm with the recognition that these patients are predisposed to having motor vehicle accidents, presumably owing to sleepiness, decreased vigilance and other manifestations of cognitive dysfunction. Although large prospective trials have not been done, nor may they ever be justified on ethical grounds, smaller studies have suggested that these adverse medical and nonmedical outcomes associated with sleep apnea and hypopnea may be avoided with adequate treatment. Thus, by identifying and successfully treating sleep apnea/hypopnea patients, the clinician will be serving the interests of both the patient and society.

A successful treatment plan is one that prevents the physiologic and clinical sequelae of apnea and hypopnea, including oxyhemoglobin desaturation and arousals, and entails acceptable risks or inconveniences to the patient. In the late 1990s, therapeutic options are varied and diverse in nature, but unfortunately, no single treatment modality is successful in all patients. However, with rare exception, an acceptable if not total alleviation of the consequences of sleep apnea and hypopnea can be achieved in all patients by use of one or a combination of therapies (Table 1). These treatments are discussed in the following sections.

LIFESTYLE AND BEHAVIORAL MODIFICATIONS
Establishing Good Sleep Hygiene

Sleep deprivation has a negative impact on upper airway stability and the arousal response to upper

TABLE 1. **Treatment Options for Obstructive Sleep Apnea and Hypopnea**

Lifestyle and Behavioral Modifications

Weight reduction (dietary modification)
Avoidance of sleep deprivation
Treatment of rhinitis and nasal congestion
Smoking cessation
Avoidance of alcohol, benzodiazepines, ventilatory depressants
When it is shown to be therapeutically efficacious, enforcement of sleeping in the lateral recumbent or head-elevated body position

Medical Therapy

Diagnosis and treatment of hypothyroidism
Positive airway pressure
Oral appliances

Surgical Therapy

Tracheotomy
Weight reduction surgery
Uvulopalatopharyngoplasty
Genioglossal advancement with hyoid myotomy and suspension
Maxillomandibular osteotomy and advancement

Education of the Patient and Follow-up

airway obstruction when an individual eventually does to go to sleep. This leads to more frequent and longer apneas and hypopneas. Although there are no studies to suggest that establishing good "sleep hygiene" may be sufficient therapy for a sleep apnea/hypopnea patient, counseling in this regard is warranted.

Weight Loss

The association between obesity (especially as reflected by body mass index or neck circumference) and sleep apnea and hypopnea has long been recognized. Obesity is associated with increased upper airway resistance, which may decrease after weight reduction. Even modest weight reduction may have a favorable impact on upper airway stability during sleep, and patients should be strongly encouraged to achieve their ideal body weight or body mass index. Dietary counseling should be offered to all overweight patients as part of a general education program regarding the nature and treatment of sleep apnea and hypopnea. Although weight reduction is optimally achieved by dietary and lifestyle modifications, failures are common (considering both commercial weight loss programs and even inhospital-based, medically supervised programs), especially when maintenance of weight loss is considered. Bariatric surgery leading to weight loss has a salutary effect on sleep apnea and hypopnea, awake pulmonary function, and arterial blood gases. If bariatric surgery is considered, it is essential to have an experienced surgical team, including anesthesiologists with expertise in difficult intubations and emergency airway management. Perioperative and postoperative complications may be minimized by administering continuous positive airway pressure (CPAP, see later) before as well as after surgery. As is the case with any sleep apnea and hypopnea patient undergoing surgery, these patients require careful postoperative monitoring and minimization of agents that promote upper airway collapsibility. In addition, studies including results of long-term follow-up and selection criteria of patients based on outcomes for each of the operative procedures employed in bariatric surgery would enhance the utility of this approach.

At present, there are no published trials describing the safety and effectiveness of pharmacologic weight loss agents in sleep apnea/hypopnea patients. Any consideration of using these agents must incorporate the possible development of pulmonary hypertension into the benefit/risk equation, and patients must be provided with all the necessary information to make an informed decision regarding this avenue of treatment.

Avoidance of Agents That Promote Upper Airway Instability During Sleep: Alcohol, Benzodiazepines, and Intravenous Narcotics

Many studies indicate that alcohol consumption increases the frequency and duration of apneas/hypopneas. Thus, until adequate treatment is established, patients should be counseled to abstain from alcohol. Limited data suggest that the requisite level of CPAP to maintain adequate upper airway patency during sleep is unchanged or slightly greater after alcohol consumption. The impact of alcohol consumption on upper airway stability after upper airway surgery for sleep apnea and hypopnea (see later) is even less clear. Thus, even after effective medical or surgical therapy is established, it would seem prudent to advise abstinence. Recognizing that this may be an unrealistic expectation of many patients and although abstinence may be advised, it would be reasonable to counsel that if the patient chooses to consume alcohol, it should be in minimal quantities and appropriately remote from sleep time to permit a return to a zero blood alcohol level before sleep.

Although not all benzodiazepines have been studied with respect to their impact on upper airway stability during sleep, diazepam reduces the neural activation of the upper airway dilator muscles, and flurazepam has been shown to increase apnea frequency in some studies. Like alcohol, this class of agents is best avoided in patients with sleep apnea and hypopnea. Narcotics (particularly intravenously administered) and other ventilatory depressants should be provided to sleep apnea/hypopnea patients only after weighing the risks and benefits and in a monitored environment. If conscious sedation is to be given to a sleep apnea/hypopnea patient (e.g., during colonoscopy, fiberoptic bronchoscopy), the amount should be reduced to the minimal level that is consistent with good, humane medical practice, and the facility should be capable of providing close monitoring in the postprocedure period with immediate availability of an airway management team. If the patient is on CPAP, the device should be brought to the facility and used after if not during the procedure as is practical. If the patient has not been on CPAP, a machine should be available in the recovery area and, if needed, empirically titrated.

Tobacco smoking may also predispose to upper airway instability during sleep. This adds but one more justification for stressing smoking cessation to all patients.

Body Position Therapy

A subset of patients have apneas and hypopneas, episodic oxyhemoglobin desaturation, and sleep fragmentation primarily during sleep in the supine position. Some of these patients will either not accept or not tolerate noninvasive therapies (see later) and either do not wish to have or are not candidates for operative procedures. These individuals may be candidates for body position therapy employing the "sleep ball" technique or one of its many variants. With this technique, one or more tennis balls (or similar objects) are placed in a pocket sewn in the back of the sleeping garment or placed in a sock that is pinned to the back of the garment. If the patient inadvertently rolls onto the back during sleep, he or she will be prompted to resume sleeping on the side. In time, it is hoped that the patient will be "trained" to maintain sleep in the lateral recumbent position and therefore no longer need the ball or sock.

A population of patients may also experience an improvement in sleep apnea and hypopnea while sleeping with the head of the bed elevated at a 30- to 60-degree angle. Even patients who do not exhibit improvement in apnea and hypopnea while asleep in the lateral recumbent position may derive benefit from the "head-up" position. It has been speculated that the occasional patient who does not experience satisfactory upper airway stabilization despite delivery of maximal levels of positive-pressure therapy (e.g., CPAP, see later) may derive improvement at the same or lower pressure during sleep in the head-up or lateral recumbent position.

If the clinician wishes to include body position therapy in the clinical armamentarium for sleep apnea and hypopnea, it is necessary to employ a diagnostic method that permits distinction of body position–dependent sleep apnea and hypopnea.

MEDICAL THERAPIES

Positive Airway Pressure Therapy

Administering air (supplemented with oxygen, if necessary) under pressures that vary from 4 to 20 cm H_2O provides a "pneumatic splint" that maintains acceptable upper airway patency during sleep in almost all sleep apnea/hypopnea patients. The pressure is most commonly provided as a constant pressure, or CPAP, that maintains the same pressure during both inspiration and expiration. In some patients who are not able to tolerate CPAP, bilevel devices are available that permit independent adjustment of inspiratory and expiratory pressure in an effort to deliver the minimal level of expiratory pressure that provides adequate therapy. During sleep, the patient wears a nasal mask, a nasal cannula device, or an oronasal mask through which the positive pressure is delivered. Since the early 1980s, CPAP has been the first-line medical therapy for sleep apnea and hypopnea.

In sleep apnea/hypopnea patients with chronic ventilatory failure as reflected by hypercapnia during wakefulness, CPAP may not provide acceptable oxyhemoglobin saturation during sleep despite maintaining upper airway patency. This is presumably due to alveolar hypoventilation. Modalities that assist or augment ventilation including bilevel positive-pressure devices and portable volume-cycled ventilators may provide successful treatment in these patients. In some individuals, it remains necessary to add supplemental oxygen to the CPAP, bilevel, or portable volume-cycled ventilator system to maintain acceptable oxyhemoglobin saturation during sleep.

The major limitation of positive-pressure treatment is the requirement for the patient's active participation in his or her care. The factors that distinguish compliant from noncompliant patients are not well defined. It appears that the magnitude of the patient's perception of his or her daytime sleepiness and functional impairment as well as of the benefits from CPAP is an important determinant of compliance. Some studies have shown that centers providing more intensive education of patients with respect to the nature of sleep apnea and hypopnea and the consequences of being untreated plus ongoing support after initiation of therapy have populations of patients with greater compliance.

The side effects associated with CPAP therapy include skin abrasions from the mask, leakage at the skin-mask interface (or, when a nasal interface is used, through the mouth), nasal congestion or rhinorrhea, nasal-oral dryness, and discomfort associated with the delivered pressure and the encumbrance of the machine. Most of the adverse effects can be eliminated or mitigated by adjusting the interface, providing humidification, using nasal corticosteroids, or using a bilevel positive-pressure device, alone or in combination. Patients who cannot keep the mouth sufficiently closed to maintain therapeutic pressure or avoid mouth dryness or who cannot breathe exclusively through the nasal route may consider using an oronasal mask. Patients using an oronasal mask should be counseled to avoid oral ingestion for several hours before use of the mask and to contact the physician before the oronasal mask is used in the event of illness associated with repetitive vomiting. This should minimize the likelihood of aspiration of gastric contents. Incorporation of an unobtrusive safety valve into the circuit should be considered in prescribing an oronasal interface to provide for entrainment of fresh air in the event of machine failure. In certain patients with motor deficits that may preclude rapid removal of the mask, a low-pressure alarm should be considered.

"Autotitrating" CPAP devices have been developed. Using various algorithms, these devices automatically adjust the delivered pressure according to what the device detects and identifies as abnormal upper airway function. After a period of upper airway stability, the device adjusts the pressure downward. The objective of autotitrating CPAP is to provide the patient with the minimal amount of pressure that maintains acceptable upper airway patency at any given time. Thus, the pressure fluctuates during the night, and the patient is not subjected to a single high pressure. It is speculated but not yet proved that compliance will be improved on this basis. There have been no published results of large, prospective and controlled trials assessing the value of home use of autotitrating devices. Thus, although autotitrating CPAP is not ready for clinical application in the home setting, clinicians can expect to learn much more about its utility in the near future.

Individual modifications of positive-pressure therapy make this form of treatment tolerable and therefore effective in a number of patients who would otherwise be unable to benefit from it.

Oral Appliance Therapy

There has been interest in and application of oral appliance (OA) therapy for sleep apnea and hypopnea. There is a wide variety in the design of these appliances. Some exclusively maintain the tongue in an anterior position, others advance the mandible and open the bite in an effort to augment pharyngeal cross-sectional area and minimize the likelihood of obstruction during sleep. Approximately 50% of patients experience reasonable therapeutic success with OA therapy. OA therapy is generally not as uniformly successful in maintaining upper airway patency during sleep as CPAP is, particularly in patients with more than moderate sleep apnea and hypopnea. Although OA therapy may not be tolerated by all patients, it may be tolerated by patients who are intolerant of or noncompliant with positive pressure.

Potential side effects of OA therapy include soreness of the teeth and jaw, hypersalivation, temporomandibular joint dysfunction, and alteration of dental occlusion. The absence of suitable dentition, which is necessary for retaining many types of OAs in place during sleep, imposes a limitation on applicability of this form of treatment. Although there are several available off-the-shelf types of OAs, it is important to engage the participation of a knowledgeable dental practitioner in developing a treatment plan including OA therapy. The dental practitioner can assess the baseline status of the patient's temporomandibular joint and dentition to provide insight into the level of risk of OA therapy in this regard as well as to contribute to selecting the optimal type of OA for the individual patient. Objective follow-up evaluation of breathing during sleep should always be done to assess the effectiveness of OA therapy in patients with sleep apnea and hypopnea and to ensure that the frequency of abnormal breathing events has not actually increased.

Pharmacologic Therapy

Unfortunately, with the exception of thyroid replacement therapy in hypothyroid patients, no pharmacologic therapy enhances upper airway stability during sleep to a therapeutically useful degree. The physician should, however, be cognizant of those agents that have been demonstrated to be of little or no therapeutic efficacy in the clinical setting. Such agents include tricyclic antidepressants* (most notably protriptyline [Vivactil]) and ventilatory stimulants such as medroxyprogesterone,* acetazolamide (Diamox),* theophylline, and doxapram (Dopram). The clinical utility of sustained serotonin reuptake inhibitors such as fluoxetine (Prozac) has not yet been convincingly demonstrated. The serotonin precursor L-tryptophan should be avoided in view of its association with the eosinophilia-myalgia syndrome and eosinophilic lung disease.

Hypothyroidism confers a risk for sleep apnea and hypopnea. Several studies have demonstrated improved upper airway patency during sleep after initiation of thyroid replacement therapy. The clinician should be aware that replacement therapy may augment metabolic rate and oxygen demands before there is optimal improvement in upper airway function during sleep. Alternatively, the degree to which replacement therapy restores upper airway patency during sleep is variable across patients, and it is possible that a given patient may have persistent sleep apnea and hypopnea despite reversal of the hypothyroid state. The combination of augmented oxygen demands during sleep in the context of persistent sleep apnea and hypopnea with reduced oxyhemoglobin saturation may set the stage for a variety of problems including myocardial ischemia, dysrhythmias, and arrhythmias. It is therefore necessary to ensure maintenance of upper airway patency during sleep during thyroid replacement therapy (by providing CPAP or OA therapy, for instance) until objective reassessment of the patient's therapeutic requirements is performed.

SURGICAL THERAPIES

Tracheotomy

Because of its invasive nature, the attendant substantial medical and psychosocial morbidity, and the development of medical (see earlier) and other surgical alternatives (see later), this procedure is rarely performed. It is reserved for patients with immediately life-threatening sleep apnea and hypopnea (e.g., life-threatening dysrhythmias) who cannot be treated by alternative means or on whom upper airway surgery (see later) is being performed with the need for immediate guarantee of a patent upper airway in the perioperative period as well as during sleep until assessment of the long-term impact of the surgery.

Uvulopalatopharyngoplasty

In general, uvulopalatopharyngoplasty (UPPP) consists of resection of the uvula and excision of redundant oropharyngeal tissue with trimming of the tonsillar pillars and posterior margin of the soft palate. Hypertrophic tonsillar tissue is also resected. This surgical procedure is designed to enlarge the retropalatal air space. By use of an appropriate definition of successful surgery (reduction of the apnea plus hypopnea frequency to less than 20 or an apnea frequency below 10 and a 50% reduction in apnea plus hypopnea frequency), UPPP is successful in only about 41% of all patients. Patients who appear to have preoperative upper airway obstruction exclusively at the retropalatal level (the region that is specifically addressed by UPPP) have a generally greater likelihood of successful outcome, 52%. Patients with a greater apnea plus hypopnea frequency have a reduced likelihood of successful UPPP. In addition, there is evidence that some patients experi-

---

*Not FDA approved for this indication.

ence a recurrence of sleep apnea and hypopnea in time after UPPP, especially if there is coincident weight gain.

UPPP usually reduces snoring intensity in both nonapneic snorers and sleep apnea/hypopnea patients. Patients may report substantial subjective improvement in daytime alertness after UPPP even when there is no objective evidence of improved breathing during sleep. These factors mean that the physician is deprived of two clinical markers for assessing postoperative success. Thus, patients who undergo UPPP for treatment of sleep apnea and hypopnea should have an objective evaluation of sleep and breathing defining the impact of surgery.

Intraoperative, perioperative, and postoperative complication rates are measurable although relatively low. Potential postoperative complications of UPPP include bleeding, variable degrees of velopharyngeal insufficiency or nasal reflux, voice alterations, stenosis of the nasopharynx, the sensation of a foreign body in the back of the throat, dry throat, and difficulty swallowing. Extreme care should be taken inasmuch as serious postoperative difficulties including death associated with airway obstruction have been reported.

Laser-Assisted Uvulopalatoplasty

This procedure, performed in the office setting with local anesthesia and conscious sedation, involves trimming of soft palate and uvula by use of a laser apparatus. Patients often return at 4- to 6-week intervals for additional sessions. Unfortunately, there are limited data from prospective, controlled studies to provide insight into the effectiveness and safety of this procedure. Many of the published studies do not uniformly identify and distinguish nonapneic snorers from sleep apnea/hypopnea patients in an objective manner, thereby limiting the ability to make conclusions regarding the likelihood of therapeutic success in individual patients. The existing literature suggests that snoring is diminished in more than half of nonapneic snorers and sleep apnea/hypopnea patients and that there is probably a measurable proportion of patients with at least mild sleep apnea and hypopnea who obtain a satisfactory response to laser-assisted uvulopalatoplasty (LAUP). There may also be a measurable number of patients who are worse after LAUP. Complications of LAUP include hemorrhage, velopharyngeal insufficiency, and altered taste. The last two problems are reported to be transient. There are also the potential hazards of sedating a sleep apnea/hypopnea patient in the outpatient environment. At present, the American Sleep Disorders Association, in its standards of practice statement, does not recommend LAUP for treatment of sleep-related breathing disorders.

Genioglossal Advancement with Hyoid Myotomy and Suspension

This procedure repositions the genial tubercle of the mandible to a more anterior location, moving the tongue anteriorly and opening the retrolingual air space. The hyoid bone is stabilized anteriorly by suspending it from the mandible or thyroid cartilage. Most patients described in the literature who underwent genioglossal advancement with hyoid myotomy and suspension (GAHM) had either previous or concomitant UPPP. By use of reasonable criteria for therapeutic success (a postoperative apnea plus hypopnea frequency of 20 or less in conjunction with at least a 50% reduction of apnea plus hypopnea frequency compared with preoperative values and minimal postoperative desaturation), the literature suggests that 60 to 70% of patients have a favorable response. The likelihood of successful surgery is probably negatively influenced by greater body mass index and increasing degrees of craniofacial skeletal deformity. The potential complications of surgery include the airway complications described before as well as temporary anesthesia of the lower teeth, mandibular fracture, and dental injury.

Maxillomandibular Osteotomy and Advancement

Although maxillomandibular osteotomy and advancement (MMO) is performed by some surgeons as an isolated procedure, much of the published literature reports the results of MMO as part of a staged surgical protocol, generally after UPPP with GAHM (see earlier). MMO advances the maxilla as well as the mandible, thereby advancing the mandible and tongue to a greater extent than can be achieved by GAHM. There is some increase in the retropalatal as well as the retrolingual air space. Advancement of the maxilla in conjunction with mandibular advancement maintains dental occlusion. Experienced surgical teams have reported success in more than 90% of patients with relatively short follow-up evaluation after MMO in patients who have failed previous upper airway surgery. It is possible that nonobese patients with more severe mandibular deficiency may be satisfactorily treated by MMO alone, without adjunctive airway surgery. The optimal way to identify these patients remains to be defined, however. The reported complications of MMO include temporary numbness of the cheek and chin.

The literature contains reports from centers with specific experience and expertise in these procedures, and the excellent results and limited frequency and severity of complications may not be extrapolated to general community practice. In addition, data from long-term follow-up are not yet available.

Successful surgical management of sleep apnea and hypopnea depends on not only surgical expertise but also a team of dedicated anesthesia, critical care–pulmonary, and sleep medicine specialists. Success is probably heavily dependent on selection of patients and matching of the individual patient with the optimal surgical procedure. Unfortunately, much remains to be learned in this regard, and patients need to be counseled regarding the risk of therapeutic failure as well as the various potential complications during discussions of surgical options.

EDUCATION OF THE PATIENT AND LEGAL ISSUES

The clinician must be aware of the importance of education of the patient. As noted early in this discussion, sleep apnea/hypopnea patients should be made aware of the nature of their problem and the potential consequences if it is left untreated. This effort may promote willingness to accept and be compliant with treatment. Of course, the relevant lifestyle modifications as well as the wide range of treatment options, including potential risks, benefits, and relative likelihood of success, should be discussed with patients. The physician's legal obligations with respect to issues of impaired motor vehicle operation vary from state to state. The clinician has an obligation to diagnose and treat in the most expeditious fashion those individuals in whom safe motor vehicle operation is in question. The same is true for patients who are engaged in occupations or activities that require vigilance for safety. In addition to compliance with legal obligations, health care providers should counsel those individuals whose alertness is in question not to operate a motor vehicle or other dangerous equipment until appropriate alertness is restored. Patients should also be counseled to notify all current and future providers of their health care that they have sleep apnea and hypopnea to avoid inadvertent prescription of inappropriate pharmacologic agents and to ensure proper monitoring and precautions in the event that surgical procedures are indicated.

PRIMARY LUNG CANCER

method of
JACOB D. BITRAN, M.D.
Lutheran General Hospital, Cancer Care Center
Park Ridge, Illinois

EPIDEMIOLOGY

Lung cancer is a health care problem of global proportions. Trillions of dollars are spent globally in providing care to victims of lung cancer and in lost wages that would be better spent in preventive medicine, prenatal care, and nourishing the world's youth.

Lung cancer is lethal. Within the United States, we are witnessing an epidemic of lung cancer. In 1996, it was estimated that 177,000 individuals (98,900 men and 78,100 women) would be diagnosed with lung cancer and that 154,000 would die of it. Among U.S. women, lung cancer is the leading cause of cancer-related deaths and accounted for an estimated 68,000 deaths in 1996. Although the incidence of lung cancer has decreased in U.S. men, it is increasing at an alarming rate among U.S. women, 78,100 cases in 1996 versus 73,000 in 1995. The increased incidence among women is clearly related to the fact that more women are smoking. In addition, given the popularity of smoking among teenage girls, it is likely that the epidemic of lung cancer will continue into the 21st century. Lung cancer is in the majority of instances preventable, and preventive efforts need to be redoubled to curb the rising tide of smoking among women and teenage girls.

Cigarette smoking accounts for 85% of all lung cancer; the remaining 15% is thought to be linked to either environmental exposure or genetic factors. Environmental exposure to arsenic, asbestos, bis(chloromethyl)ether, chromium, nickel, radon, and vinyl chloride and passive exposure to smoke (secondhand smoke) have been implicated in the increased risk for lung cancer. Most recently, an increased risk for primary lung cancer has been described in patients treated with external beam radiation therapy for Hodgkin's disease and breast cancer. Genetic factors that may contribute to an increased lung cancer risk include individuals who have high levels of 4-debrisoquin hydroxylase and individuals who have a relative deficiency of the MU phenotype of glutathione transferase. Adults who survive childhood retinoblastoma have a 15-fold increased incidence of small cell lung cancer (SCLC) compared with the general population. It is believed that polycyclic aromatic hydrocarbons and *N*-nitrosamines in cigarette smoke lead to DNA damage by adduct formation. In turn, the DNA damage leads to the activation of proto-oncogenes and the inactivation of tumor suppressor genes.

SYMPTOMS AND SIGNS

The symptoms and signs of lung cancer can vary from the complete absence of any symptoms or signs (an incidental lesion found on a chest radiograph that has been obtained for another reason) to the presence of a new or changed cough, dyspnea, hemoptysis, chest pain, shoulder pain, superior vena cava syndrome, Horner's syndrome, Pancoast's syndrome, supraclavicular or cervical lymphadenopathy, unresolving pneumonia or pneumonitis, bone pain, headache, paresis or paralysis, confusion, ataxia, or abdominal pain. Systemic symptoms can include fatigue, weight loss, or cachexia. Paraneoplastic syndromes that are often associated with primary lung cancer include ectopic adrenocorticotropic hormone (ACTH) syndrome, Eaton-Lambert syndrome, dermatomyositis, and acanthosis nigricans.

HISTOLOGIC CLASSIFICATION

It is likely that all lung cancers arise from a common pluripotent cell. Furthermore, it is likely that the phenotypic (histologic) appearance is a function of the various cytogenetic abnormalities that are present and associated proto-oncogenes that are "activated" (see later). The pathologic appearance of a primary lung cancer is of particular importance both for diagnostic purposes and in developing the therapeutic approach. Lung cancers are basically composed of four different subtypes: small cell carcinoma and squamous cell carcinoma, adenocarcinoma, and large cell lung cancer, all of which are referred to as non–small cell lung cancer (NSCLC). Most pathologists employ the World Health Organization classification of lung cancer (Table 1). Many lung cancers, if examined closely, have mixed histologic features.

SCLC accounts for 25% of the lung cancer diagnosed in the United States. The presence of neurosecretory granules on electron microscopy is characteristic of SCLC. Most often, SCLC presents as a central (hilar) lesion. Adenocarcinoma accounts for 40% of all lung cancer diagnosed in the United States, and it is the most frequent lung cancer

TABLE 1. **World Health Organization Histologic Classification of Epithelial Bronchogenic Carcinoma**

Malignant

Squamous cell (epidermal) and spindle cell carcinoma
Small cell
   Oat cell carcinoma (lymphocytic-like)
   Intermediate cell type
   Combined oat cell carcinoma (mixed histologic types, small with squamous or adenocarcinoma)
Adenocarcinoma
   Acinar
   Papillary
   Bronchoalveolar
   Mucinous secreting
Large cell
   Giant cell
   Clear cell
Adenosquamous carcinoma
   Carcinoid
   Bronchial gland carcinoma
   Adenoid cystic
   Mucoepidermoid
Others

Adapted from World Health Organization: Histological Typing of Lung Tumors, 2nd ed. Geneva, WHO, 1981.

that occurs in women. It is associated with cigarette smoking and pulmonary injury. It can arise in a central or peripheral location. Squamous cell lung cancer accounts for 25% of all lung cancer and has been declining in the past 2 decades. Squamous cell lung cancer stains positively for keratin and presents most often as a central lesion. Large cell lung cancer accounts for about 3% of all lung cancers and has an anaplastic appearance. The use of immunohistochemical stains (carcinoembryonic antigen and keratin) permits the accurate identification of poorly differentiated adenocarcinoma or an anaplastic squamous cell lung cancer from large cell lung cancer. Bronchoalveolar carcinoma of the lung is classified as a subtype of adenocarcinoma. The neoplastic cells in bronchoalveolar carcinoma are type II pneumonocytes. Patients with bronchoalveolar carcinoma usually present with alveolar infiltrates or lobar consolidation that is often initially diagnosed as pneumonia. Unresolved pneumonia infiltrates in an adult may be a manifestation of bronchoalveolar carcinoma.

BIOLOGY OF PRIMARY LUNG CANCER

Lung cancers arise from mutational events in the bronchial epithelium during a person's life. Lung cancer represents the culmination of 10 to 20 of such mutational events. In the past decade, scientists have begun to define these events and have begun to construct a hypothesis of how lung cancer develops. It appears that one of the earliest events that leads to bronchial epithelial hyperplasia is allelic loss on the short arm of chromosome 3 (3p) where at least three tumor suppressor genes are present. Allelic loss of 3p coupled with allelic loss on the short arm of chromosome 9 (9p) leads to dysplasia. Mutational events that convert epithelial dysplasia into carcinoma in situ include mutation of the gene for p53 encoding (chromosome 17) and mutational activation of the K-ras oncogene (chromosome 12). At this point, further mutational events and the loss of antecedent cytogenetic events will determine the progression of carcinoma in situ and ultimate phenotypic

appearance (histologic type) of the lung cancer. Deletion of 3p coupled with myc oncogene (N-, c-, and L-myc, chromosome 8q24) activation, mutation of the gene encoding retinoblastoma (chromosome 13), and loss of K-ras activation will lead to the SCLC phenotype. In contrast, persistence of K-ras activation, allelic loss of chromosome 1, and overexpression of c-erb-2 and/or bcl-2 will lead to the NSCLC phenotype.

Growth factors that serve as paracrine (autocrine) promoters of cellular growth include gastrin-releasing peptide (SCLC), epidermal growth factor (SCLC and NSCLC), insulin-like growth factor-1 (SCLC and NSCLC), transforming growth factor-β1 (NSCLC), bombesin, and cholecystokinin (SCLC).

DIAGNOSTIC METHODS AND STAGING OF LUNG CANCER

Patients with lung cancer usually have an abnormal chest radiograph. Stage 0 lung cancer (carcinoma in situ) is exceedingly rare and represents an incidental finding in a patient undergoing bronchoscopy for another indication. If a suspicious lesion is found on chest radiography, obtaining old chest radiographs for comparative purposes is essential. If a lesion has been stable on the chest radiograph for 2 years, further work-up is not necessary. New lesions need to be investigated. A thorough history and physical examination are key to the investigation of a pulmonary nodule or hilar mass. Particular attention should be paid to the lymph node examination (cervical and supraclavicular), the lung examination (localized rales or rhonchi, absent breath sounds), the abdomen (organomegaly), and the neurologic examination. The presence of lymphadenopathy or organomegaly will provide staging information and locate a potential area for biopsy in determining the histologic diagnosis. In the event that the physical examination findings are entirely normal, computized tomography (CT) of the chest to the level of the adrenals should be performed while the physician attempts to arrive at a histologic diagnosis. CT confirms the presence and extent of the pulmonary mass, evaluates the mediastinum for the presence or absence of any lymphadenopathy, and confirms or excludes the presence of other pulmonary nodules. Positron emission tomography (PET) using 2-fluorodeoxyglucose (2-FDG) is helpful in the evaluation of a solitary pulmonary nodule. The absence of any uptake of 2-FDG on a PET scan excludes a malignant neoplastic process with a 99% level of confidence. PET will play an increasingly important role in the staging of lung cancer.

After a histologic diagnosis of lung cancer has been established, further work-up is based on symptoms and signs. Complaints of back pain should prompt a technetium Tc 99m bone scan. A complaint of headache should prompt CT or magnetic resonance imaging (MRI) of the brain. At completion of clinical staging, patients are placed into a clinical stage as described in Table 2. Patients with NSCLC clinical stage I and stage II require further pathologic staging; patients with NSCLC clinical stages IIIA, IIIB, and IV require no further pathologic staging, and treatment decisions can be made on the basis of clinical stage. Patients with SCLC of any stage (with the exception of stage I) are treated with chemotherapy.

PATHOLOGIC STAGING

Fiberoptic bronchoscopy is an accurate and safe technique for rendering a diagnosis of lung cancer in patients with central (hilar) lesions. The bronchoscope can directly

TABLE 2. **International Staging System for Lung Cancer**

Primary Tumor (T)

T0	No evidence of primary tumor
TX	Cancer cell in bronchopulmonary secretions; no tumor seen on chest radiography or bronchoscopy
Tis	Carcinoma in situ
T1	Tumor ≤3 cm in greatest dimension, surrounded by lung tissue; no bronchoscopic evidence of tumor proximal to lobar bronchus
T2	Tumor >3 cm in greatest diameter, or tumor of any size that involves visceral pleura or is associated with atelectasis extending to the hilum (but not involving entire lung); must be ≥2 cm from the carina
T3	Tumor involves chest wall, diaphragm, mediastinal pleura, or pericardium, or is <2 cm from the carina (but does not involve it)
T4	Tumor involves the carina or trachea or invades the mediastinum, heart, great vessels, esophagus, or vertebrae; or there is a malignant pleural effusion

Nodal Involvement (N)

N0	No demonstrable lymph node involvement
N1	Ipsilateral peribronchial or hilar nodes involved
N2	Metastases to ipsilateral mediastinal nodes or subcarinal nodes
N3	Metastases to contralateral hilar, mediastinal, or scalene or supraclavicular nodes

Distant Metastasis (M)

M0	No (known) distant metastasis
M1	Distant metastasis present—specify site(s)

Stages

Stage 0	Tis
Stage I	T1 or T2, N0, M0
Stage II	T1 or T2, N1, M0
Stage IIIA	T3, N0 or N1, M0; or T1–3, N2, M0
Stage IIIB	Any T, N3, M0; or T4, any N1, M0
Stage IV	Any T, any N, M1

Adapted from Mountain CF: A new international staging system for lung cancer. Chest 89:225S–233S, 1986.

visualize the tracheobronchial tree, and hilar masses can be sampled by directed biopsy and/or brush biopsy. Location of the mass relative to the carina is noted, and the carina can be inspected and sampled. Clinical staging of the mediastinum is provided by CT of the chest. The presence of enlarged mediastinal lymph nodes (2 cm or more) is considered pathologic, and histologic confirmation is not always necessary. Mediastinal lymph nodes that are 1 cm or less in size are considered normal, and mediastinoscopy is a low-yield procedure. Mediastinal nodes that are 1.1 to 1.9 cm are considered intermediate in size and represent a "gray area." Such nodes may be reactive or harbor metastases. PET of the mediastinum in patients with nodes of normal or intermediate size will play an increasingly important role in the future.

At present, patients with clinical stage I or stage II lung cancer and mediastinal nodes of indeterminate size require a mediastinoscopy (for right-sided lesions) or mediastinotomy (for left hilar regions) for pathologic confirmation. Mediastinoscopy is a surgical procedure performed under a general anesthetic in which a hollow, rigid instrument is introduced through a small incision in the suprasternal notch and advanced along the pretracheal plane to the level of the carina. Enlarged lymph nodes can be visualized and sampled for biopsy. On the right side, the upper margin of the hilum may be reached, whereas the aortic arch precludes access to the left hilum. Contraindications to mediastinoscopy include superior vena caval obstruction, mediastinal surgery, and previous radiotherapy. A limited parasternal mediastinoscopy can be performed for pathologic or diagnostic staging of left hilar or aortopulmonary window lesions.

Once pathologic staging has been completed and patients have been segregated into clinical-pathologic stage I to IV, the physician is now ready to decide which patients are candidates for surgical treatment and which patients are better suited for alternative therapies.

PREOPERATIVE ASSESSMENT

It is obvious that in planning treatment, one needs to consider the overall health of a patient, the patient's age, and other co-morbid conditions that preclude lung resection. In patients who are identified as potential surgical candidates, preoperative assessment of pulmonary function and estimation of postoperative pulmonary function are necessary. All surgical candidates should have initial pulmonary function tests. Patients who have a preoperative forced expiratory volume in 1 second (FEV_1) of greater than 1.2 liters and a diffusing capacity for carbon monoxide ($DLCO$) of greater than 80% and who do not have hypercapnia or cor pulmonale are clearly surgical candidates independent of the extent of lung resection (lobectomy versus pneumonectomy). Patients who have an FEV_1 of 0.5 liter or less are inoperable, and no further assessment is required. Patients who have an FEV_1 of 0.8 to 1.2 liters or a $DLCO$ of less than 60% are considered borderline operative candidates in whom thoracotomy is considered high risk. Such patients should undergo quantitative ventilation/perfusion lung scans to estimate postoperative pulmonary function. In general, patients who are estimated to have a postoperative FEV_1 of less than 0.5 liter are not operative candidates.

NON–SMALL CELL LUNG CANCER

Treatment of Stages I and II

Patients with stage I or stage II NSCLC account for only 20 to 25% of all patients with newly diagnosed NSCLC. The preferred treatment of such patients who are medically fit is surgical resection. The preferred surgical resection is lobectomy and a sampling of mediastinal lymph nodes. A segmental pulmonary resection is an appropriate alternative if patients do not have the pulmonary reserve to undergo a lobectomy; however, several series have reported a higher local recurrence rate for segmental resections. Pneumonectomies do not confer any advantage to a lobectomy and are indicated only if a lobectomy results in an incomplete resection. The operative mortality (which includes the 30-day postoperative period) from pneumonectomy, lobectomy, and segmental resection is 6.2%, 2.9%, and 1%, respectively. The causes of death include pneumonia, respiratory failure, myocardial infarction, pulmonary embolism, bronchopleural fistula, and empyema. Video-assisted thoracoscopic lobectomy is undergoing evaluation; however, at present, its role in the treatment of stage I and stage II NSCLC is unclear.

Surgical resection for patients with stage I and stage II NSCLC leads to an excellent disease-free survival rate of 60 to 80% for stage I NSCLC and 35 to 50% for stage II NSCLC. There is a better disease-free survival for patients with stage I or stage II squamous cell carcinoma compared with stage I or stage II adenocarcinoma. Additional prognostic factors that may predict recurrence and survival are the presence of K-ras mutations at codon 12 (adenocarcinoma, factor indicating poor prognosis) and overexpression of bcl-2 (positive prognostic factor). Patients with stage I or stage II NSCLC who either are medically unfit or for whatever reason are not surgical candidates should be treated with radiotherapy, at least 60 Gy in 30 fractions (2-Gy fractions). The disease-free survival for patients with stage I or stage II NSCLC treated with radiotherapy is 17 to 32% at 5 years.

To date, there is no role for adjuvant chemotherapy or postoperative radiotherapy in patients with stage I or stage II NSCLC. Patients who have been successfully treated for stage I or stage II NSCLC have a 2 to 3% risk per year of developing a second primary lung cancer. In 10 years, the risk is 20 to 30%. There are ongoing studies to determine the role of cis-retinoic acid and other types of "chemopreventive agents" in stage I or stage II NSCLC. Because such patients represent a high-risk group, they should be followed up at a minimum of every 3 to 4 months for the first 24 months and then every 6 months thereafter.

Treatment of Stages IIIA and IIIB

Stage IIIA T3, N0–1, M0

Patients with stage IIIA NSCLC present a subset of different cohorts, that is, T3, N0, M0; T3, N1, M0; T1–3, N2, M0; T1–3, N3, M0. According a uniform treatment approach to all patients with stage IIIA cannot be recommended. Rather, the treatment approach will vary with the subset of patients. For patients with NSCLC who have tumor directly extending into the chest wall (T3, N0–1, M0), there is consensus that surgical resection of the primary lung cancer and the involved chest wall is indicated. The 5-year survival of such patients is approximately 50%. To date, there is no role for adjuvant postoperative radiotherapy to the chest wall or the resected tumor bed. For patients with Pancoast's tumors (superior sulcus tumors) (T3, N0–1, M0), the treatment consists of preoperative radiotherapy of 30 to 45 Gy followed, if possible, by lung resection with resection usually of the first two ribs. The 5-year survival of patients with Pancoast's tumors is 35 to 45%. Whereas some reports advocate the use of radiotherapy and chemotherapy in the treatment of Pancoast's tumors, no randomized trials have compared the potential additive effect of chemotherapy, and its use cannot be recommended at this time.

Stage IIIA T1–3, N2, M0 and Stage IIIB

Patients with mediastinal nodal (N2) involvement are discovered in two ways. The most common is the detection of mediastinal nodal involvement at chest radiography, chest CT, or mediastinoscopy. Such patients *are not candidates for surgery;* they have inoperable lung cancer and should be treated as described in the following. The other smaller group of N2 patients are those who present as clinical-pathologic stage I or stage II NSCLC and at the time of lung resection and on mediastinal nodal sampling are found to have involved mediastinal lymph nodes. The 5-year survival of this subset of patients is poor, 9 to 12%. No compelling data indicate that this subset of patients has had its natural history altered with the use of postoperative adjuvant chemotherapy, radiotherapy, or both. The recommendation for such patients is close follow-up, and treatment decisions can be made at the time of relapse.

As already stated, the majority of stage IIIA patients, T1–3, N2, M0, and stage IIIB patients are discovered at the time of clinical staging. At present, there have been four prospective randomized trials that have examined the role of chemotherapy followed by radiotherapy or concurrent radiotherapy and chemotherapy in patients with stage IIIA/IIIB NSCLC. These studies are shown in Table 3. The Dillman trial compared two courses of initial chemotherapy with vinblastine (Velban)* and cisplatin (Platinol)* followed by radiotherapy of 60 Gy in 2-Gy daily fractions with radiotherapy alone. This trial was the first to report a statistically significant prolongation of life in patients receiving initial chemotherapy followed by radiotherapy. The trial published by Sause confirmed Dillman's observations. A large multicenter French trial by LeChevalier employing an alternative chemotherapy regimen of cyclophosphamide (Cytoxan),* cisplatin, CCNU (lomustine [CeeNu]),* and vindesine (Eldisine)† showed similar results. Thus, patients with unresectable stage IIIA or stage IIIB NSCLC who have a good overall physical status should be encouraged to participate in the current generation of clinical trials, which are designed to determine the optimal initial chemotherapy and optimal radiotherapy regimens. For patients who choose not to enroll in such studies, initial chemotherapy with cisplatin at 75 to 100 mg per m² every 4 weeks and vinblastine followed by radiotherapy represents the standard of care in 1997. Patients who are debilitated from stage IIIA/IIIB NSCLC are best treated with palliative radiotherapy alone.

The concept of neoadjuvant chemotherapy (preoperative) is not new, and a number of feasibility studies have addressed this concept in stage IIIA patients with NSCLC. After neoadjuvant chemotherapy in most of these feasibility studies, there has been an attempt at surgical resection. In 1994, two small prospective randomized studies showed a survival

---

*Not FDA approved for this indication.
†Investigational drug in the United States.

TABLE 3. **Combined Modality Therapy for Stage IIIA/IIIB Non–Small Cell Lung Cancer: Results of Randomized Trials**

Author	Year	Number of Patients	Comparative Arms	Median Survival (mo)	3-Year Survival (%)	Conclusions
Dillman	1990	155	RT 60 Gy (2-Gy fractions), 77 patients	9.7	11	PV/RT better than RT alone
			PV/RT 60 Gy (2-Gy fractions), 78 patients	13.8	23	
Shacke-Konning	1992	331	RT 30 Gy/10 fractions, 25 Gy/10 fractions, 114 patients	12.0	4	RT + cisplatin better than RT alone
			RT same as above + weekly cisplatin, 110 patients	12.0	15	
			RT same as above + daily cisplatin, 107 patients	14.0	15	
LeChevalier	1991	353	RT 40 Gy/16 fractions, 177 patients	10.0	4	CCVP/RT better than RT alone
			CCVP/RT same as above, 176 patients	12.0	12	
Sause	1995	452	RT 60 Gy (2-Gy fractions), 149 patients	11.4	19	PV/RT better than RT alone and CHART
			PV/RT 60 Gy (2-Gy fractions), 151 patients	13.8	32	
			CHART 1.2 Gy bid to 69.6 Gy, 152 patients	12.3	24	

Abbreviations: CCVP = cyclophosphamide, CCNU, vindesine, and cisplatin; CHART = continuous hyperfractionated accelerated radiation therapy; PV = vinblastine and cisplatin; RT = radiotherapy.

benefit to the use of neoadjuvant chemotherapy followed by surgical resection in a selected group of patients with stage IIIA NSCLC. Subsequently, two larger multi-institutional trials have confirmed the benefit of neoadjuvant chemotherapy followed by surgical resection compared with surgery alone. Patients who received neoadjuvant chemotherapy had a median survival in the range of 26 to 64 months, and the 3- to 5-year survival was 25 to 30%. These results were better than those of the surgery control arm. Patients treated with surgery alone had a median survival of 8 to 12 months and a 3-year survival of 0 to 15%. However, this approach carries with it significant morbidity and a treatment-related mortality of 10 to 15%. Furthermore, it is unknown whether this treatment approach is better or worse than the sequence of chemotherapy followed by radiotherapy in patients with stage IIIA NSCLC. A large multi-institutional phase III trial is currently addressing this question. Therefore, at present, the standard approach in patients with stage IIIA/IIIB NSCLC is initial chemotherapy followed by radiotherapy.

Treatment of Stage IV

After sequential staging, about 40 to 50% of patients with NSCLC will be found to have stage IV disease. For such patients, there is no curative therapy, and the goals should be palliation and an improved quality of life. Seven randomized clinical trials have attempted to answer the question of the value of multiagent chemotherapy compared with best supportive care in NSCLC. These seven trials employed a variety of chemotherapy regimens. During the past 5 years, three meta-analyses of these randomized trials have been performed and reached the following conclusions:

1. In patients without debility from NSCLC (good performance status), there is a 35% and 27% reduction in mortality from NSCLC at 3 and 6 months,

respectively, which is statistically significant; however, the risk reduction diminishes in time.

2. There is an increase in the median survival from 3.9 to 6.7 months, a net gain of 12 weeks.

Because none of the studies performed a quality of life analysis, conclusions cannot be drawn. However, a trial carried out by the National Cancer Institute of Canada and reported by Rapp and colleagues analyzed cost of care and concluded that best supportive care was *more* expensive than one of the chemotherapy arms (cyclophosphamide,* doxorubicin,* and cisplatin* [CAP]). Patients in the supportive care group required more radiotherapy and days in hospital than did patients receiving CAP. The net saving of CAP chemotherapy was $6172 per year of life gained compared with the best supportive care. These data suggest that patients receiving chemotherapy experience a palliation of symptoms and spend less time in the hospital. Thus, in patients who have a good performance status, the current recommendation is that they receive chemotherapy, which is preferably done on an ambulatory basis. Such patients should be encouraged to enroll in clinical trials so that we can advance the state of the art. If patients choose not to enroll in such studies, vinorelbine (Navelbine) is the only drug approved by the Food and Drug Administration for stage IV NSCLC patients. There are a variety of drugs a medical oncologist can choose to attempt to provide palliation. During the past few years, many new chemotherapeutic agents have been developed and released. Many of these new drugs are active drugs in NSCLC (>15% response rate) and include paclitaxel (Taxol),* docetaxel (Taxotere),* gemcitabine,* irinotecan (CPT-11 [Camptosar]),* and topotecan (Hycamtin).* There is the expectation that better treatments will be forthcoming in stage IV NSCLC.

SMALL CELL LUNG CANCER

SCLC represents 20 to 25% of all lung cancers within the United States; the incidence of SCLC in

*Not FDA approved for this indication.

1996 was estimated between 35,000 and 44,000 men and women. SCLC is a distinct clinical-pathologic entity and is almost always associated with cigarette smoking. It has a distinctive histologic appearance with the presence of neuroendocrine granules (electron dense) at electron microscopy and a distinctive cytogenetic alteration that is the deletion of the short arm of chromosome 3 (3p14-21), which in turn leads to overexpression of the c-*myc* oncogene. SCLC is associated with peptide secretion, such as gastrin-releasing peptide (bombesin), and stains positively for neuron-specific enolase and chromogranin A. It is characterized clinically by rapid tumor growth and progression. It is responsive to both chemotherapy and radiotherapy; a large percentage of patients attain a complete response, which represents complete disappearance of all clinical disease. Other clinical features include ectopic hormone production, such as antidiuretic hormone and corticotropin (ACTH). As previously stated, patients with SCLC are staged as limited disease (stages I, II, IIIA, IIIB) and extensive disease (stage IV).

Staging in SCLC consists of a thorough history and physical examination, chest radiography, CT of the chest to the level of the adrenals, bone marrow aspiration and biopsy (to detect occult bone marrow involvement), MRI or CT of the brain, and bone scan. Most recently, the two newer modes of imaging have become available. SCLC expresses receptors for somatostatin. Accordingly, on the basis of this observation, imaging with indium. In 111–radiolabeled octreotide (D-Phe-Cys-Phe-D-Trp-Lys-Thr-Cys-Thr-ol), a somatostatin analogue, has been evaluated in patients with SCLC. The sensitivity of ^{111}In-octreotide is 86%, and specificity is 92%. Radiolabeled octreotide fails in detecting central nervous system (CNS) metastases, and its role in SCLC is still undergoing evaluation. Another imaging agent that has been evaluated in patients with SCLC is ^{99m}Tc-radiolabeled NR-LU-10 (Verluma). Verluma is a monoclonal antibody fragment that recognizes a 40-kilodalton glycoprotein expressed on the cell membrane of SCLC. This imaging agent has a sensitivity of 77% and a specificity of 94%. Whereas comparative studies between ^{111}In-octreotide and Verluma have not been conducted, these imaging techniques may replace conventional CT in the staging of SCLC.

Treatment

The treatment of patients with SCLC is determined on the basis of whether patients have limited or extensive disease. Patients with extensive disease represent about 67% of all patients with SCLC. The treatment of patients with extensive SCLC is chemotherapy with the intent of providing palliation. The chemotherapy regimens in clinical use include cisplatin* plus etoposide (PE); carboplatin* plus etoposide; and cyclophosphamide,* doxorubicin,* and vincristine* (CAV). These regimens induce complete and

partial responses in 60 to 80% of patients (20 to 30% complete response). The median duration of response is 6 to 9 months, and the median survival is 9 to 11 months. The 2-year survival rate is 10%, and the 5-year survival rate is 0 to 2%. For elderly patients or those debilitated by SCLC (poor performance status), a British trial conducted by the Medical Research Council Lung Cancer Working Party showed that oral etoposide resulted in greater toxic effects and an inferior survival compared with CAV. Thus, even in the elderly or in patients with poor performance status, multidrug chemotherapy remains the treatment of choice. The dismal survival of patients with SCLC underscores the importance of finding new and active agents. In the past 5 years, investigators have initiated phase II studies in previously untreated patients with extensive SCLC with the aim of identifying new agents. The design of these studies has been to use the single agent for three or four courses and obviously to continue its use if patients enter a complete or partial response; however, if patients have either stable or progressive disease during the time that the phase II agent is administered, they rapidly cross over to a conventional chemotherapy program such as PE or CAV. It is clear from the analyses of such trials that the use of a phase II agent in previously untreated patients with extensive SCLC does not jeopardize their ability to respond to a more conventional program, nor does it decrease the median survival of 9 to 11 months. As a result of such studies, newer and active chemotherapeutic agents in SCLC include paclitaxel,* docetaxel,* topotecan,* JM-216† (an oral carboplatin analogue), and gemcitabine. Currently, phase II studies are addressing the role of such agents in extensive SCLC.

Patients with SCLC who are found to have limited disease (approximately one third of patients with SCLC) are treated with concurrent chemotherapy and radiotherapy. In the past 9 years, a number of important trials have established the beneficial role of administering concurrent radiotherapy and chemotherapy in patients with limited SCLC. On the basis of a meta-analysis of 13 randomized trials that included more than 2100 patients, the use of radiotherapy decreased mortality from SCLC by 14% and increased survival at 3 years by 5.4%. A randomized trial conducted in Canada addressed the issue of the timing of thoracic irradiation in limited SCLC and concluded that patients who received chemotherapy and radiotherapy beginning on the first day of treatment had a better survival than when the thoracic radiotherapy was delayed. On the basis of the aforementioned meta-analysis and the Canadian trial, the current recommendation is to begin cisplatin* and etoposide (PE) with concurrent thoracic irradiation (to a portal that includes the chest primary, the mediastinum, and both supraclavicular fossae to a total dose of 55 Gy). The PE regimen is continued every 3

---

*Not FDA approved for this indication.

*Not FDA approved for this indication.
†Investigational drug in the United States.

to 4 weeks for a total of six courses. Continuation of PE beyond six courses does not lead to a survival benefit as demonstrated by several randomized trials. Prophylactic cranial irradiation (PCI), 25 Gy in 10 fractions, is administered to these patients because the brain represents a pharmacologic sanctuary and numerous randomized studies have shown that PCI decreases the frequency and morbidity of CNS relapse. Concurrent radiotherapy and PE lead to a 70 to 90% rate of complete response (complete clinical disappearance of all disease). The median survival for all patients with limited SCLC undergoing such treatment is 17 to 20 months; the 2-year and 4-year disease-free survival rates are 40% and 15 to 30%, respectively. This approach is not without toxic effects, which include myelosuppression, esophagitis, and pulmonary fibrosis, which is usually radiographically apparent but usually asymptomatic. The use of PCI can lead to cognitive defects and a slight decrease in IQ. The 5-year disease-free survival for patients with limited SCLC is 12% ± 2%. There is a stepwise decrease in the disease-free survival rate between years 2 and 5 as a result of patients' developing a second non–small cell primary lung cancer. Late relapse (>3 years) of SCLC is distinctly unusual. Patients with limited SCLC who do relapse usually do so within the first 24 to 36 months. Such patients may be candidates for phase II clinical trials or CAV if they have received prior PE. Survival after relapse is usually limited, 4 to 6 months.

The Role of Surgery

Ever since the publication of the British Medical Research Council randomized trial that compared surgical resection with radiotherapy for SCLC, surgery has been abandoned as a mode of treatment for the majority of patients with SCLC. To date, no study has demonstrated that the use of surgery in addition to chemoradiotherapy in patients with limited SCLC has conferred a survival advantage. The only subset of patients with SCLC who should be approached surgically are patients who present with small peripheral lesions (solitary pulmonary nodule). Such patients should undergo pulmonary resection even if a preoperative biopsy shows SCLC. After resection, patients should receive postoperative adjuvant chemotherapy with either cisplatin and etoposide or cyclophosphamide, doxorubicin, and vincristine. The 5-year survival in this small subset of patients with SCLC is 50 to 60%.

CONCLUSION

The advances made in the past decade in the treatment of lung cancer have been small but incremental. The most fundamental advances have been in understanding the molecular events that lead to the malignant lung cancer phenotype. With a better understanding of the stepwise intracellular molecular events that lead to a malignant phenotype, there is no doubt that novel compounds and treatments will be developed to delay and reverse the progression to malignant transformation. It is clinical trials that have brought about small but significant incremental survival in stages IIIA and IIIB NSCLC. Clinical trials require the support of the entire medical community, physicians, nurses, patients, insurers, and managed health care organizations. The sad comment is that only 1.4% of Americans diagnosed with lung cancer participate in a clinical trial. Finally, the identification of new drugs and novel antineoplastic compounds can only happen by supporting and enrolling patients in phase I and phase II studies. Progress in the treatment of lung cancer cannot occur without clinical research.

COCCIDIOIDOMYCOSIS

method of
ROYCE H. JOHNSON, M.D.
University of California, Los Angeles
Los Angeles, California
Kern Medical Center
Bakersfield, California

Coccidioidomycosis was originally described in 1892 and is caused by *Coccidioides immitis*. This dimorphic fungal pathogen causes one of the endemic mycoses. It exists in the soil in the mycelial phase. Mycelia produce specialized structures, arthroconidia, that easily become airborne. These structures may travel as far as 75 miles or more from their origin. Arthroconidia may infect a new hospitable soil site or, if inhaled by a susceptible host, produce a primary pulmonary infection. In tissue, arthroconidia transform to spherules that reproduce by endosporulation. *C. immitis* may be recovered on simple bacteriologic or mycologic media and will grow in the mycelial phase. It is extraordinarily dangerous to work with these cultures unless special precautions are taken because arthroconidia are produced after a few days of in vitro cultivation.

C. immitis has a specific geographic distribution in South, Central, and North America. Most cases seen in the United States are related to exposure in the Southwest. Occasional fomite acquisition occurs at sites distant to the endemic focus. There is no human-to-human or enzootic transmission of the disease.

The predominant pathologic finding is granulomatous inflammation. Spherules with endosporulation are diagnostic pathologically, although these structures are not always easily found in human infection.

Sixty percent of individuals with primary infection have no or trivial symptoms. The remainder develop pulmonary or systemic symptoms within 1 to 3 weeks of exposure. Cough and chest pain are usually the dominant pulmonary features. Alternatively, pulmonary symptoms may be absent or relatively modest, and fever with night sweats and headache may be the more dominant symptoms. Erythema nodosum and less commonly erythema multiforme with arthralgia and arthritis may occur with or without concomitant respiratory symptoms. The chest radiograph in mild cases may show little or no change. In more severe cases, especially those with respiratory symptoms, focal infiltrates often with significant perihilar and even peritracheal lymphadenopathy are demonstrated. Diminishing

TABLE 1. **Chemotherapy for Coccidioidomycosis**

Drug	Route	Dosing		
		Initial	*Maximal*	*Total*
Amphotericin B (Fungizone)	IV	1-mg test dose, then 5–10 mg	1 mg/kg/d, usually not >50 mg	1–3 gm, occasionally more
Ketoconazole 200 mg (Nizoral)	PO	400 mg qd	400 mg	3 mo to years
Fluconazole 200 mg (Diflucan)	PO	400 mg qd	800–1200 mg	3 mo to years
Itraconazole 100 mg (Sporanox)	PO	200 mg bid	200 mg tid	3 mo to years

acute infiltration with persistent or increasing hilar adenopathy defines progressive pulmonary coccidioidomycosis. The disease may also present as an exudative pleural effusion with or without concomitant infiltrate.

Chronic pulmonary involvement also occurs. A residual fibrosis may occur after acute infection. Pulmonary nodules also represent a resolution of acute infection but are often confused with carcinoma both in and at some distance from the endemic area. Pulmonary cavities are frequently seen, and although these may be asymptomatic, they often cause persistent inflammatory symptoms and are occasionally superinfected. They may also develop or present with hemoptysis, which on rare occasion may be severe. These cavities may also rupture and produce pyopneumothorax.

Approximately 5% of all diagnosed cases of symptomatic coccidioidomycosis will disseminate. Fifty percent of disseminated cases will not have a history of diagnosed respiratory infection. Extrapulmonary foci include virtually every structure in the body. Infections of skin, subcutaneous tissue, lymph node, bone, joint, and meninges are the most prevalent.

Meningitis is the most serious manifestation of coccidioidomycosis. Untreated, death is uniform, usually within 1 year. Presentation and cerebrospinal fluid analysis are compatible with a chronic meningitis. Headache is the most common presenting symptom. Alteration in consciousness, psychologic disturbance, fever, stiff neck, and focal neurologic deficits are also common. Cerebrospinal fluid analysis usually reveals a dominant lymphocytic pleocytosis. Early in the course of illness, neutrophils may predominate. Cerebrospinal fluid eosinophilia may also be encountered. Hypoglycorrhachia and an increased protein level complete the typical analysis. Cerebrospinal fluid coccidioidal antibody titer is usually but not invariably elevated. Serum IgG as detected by complement fixation or immunodiffusion antibodies is almost always present in disseminated coccidioidomycosis except in severely immunocompromised patients, especially those with human immunodeficiency virus infection.

TREATMENT

Treatment of coccidioidomycosis is currently less than optimal. The ideal antifungal therapy for this disease would be one that penetrates all body compartments well. It would be desirable to have both an oral and a parenteral dosage form with low toxicity and good bioavailability. Fungicidal agents would be preferred. Unfortunately, currently available therapy includes amphotericin B (Fungizone) and its lipid solubilized congeners, and the azoles, of which ketoconazole (Nizoral), fluconazole (Diflucan),* and itraconazole (Sporanox)* are the most relevant (Table 1).

Primary Disease

It is clear that many cases of primary pulmonary coccidioidomycosis and even cutaneous disease and other disseminated disease of limited extent recover spontaneously. In previous editions of this text, many authors have indicated that primary disease in low-risk individuals perhaps need not be treated. More recent analysis, however, has suggested that therapy may be beneficial for virtually all symptomatic cases of coccidioidomycosis. It has long been agreed that pneumonia of substantial severity or extent or of a duration greater than several weeks is an indication for therapy. The second indication is to diminish the risk for extrapulmonary dissemination. The risk factors for extrapulmonary dissemination are indicated in Table 2. No controlled trials of azoles for primary pulmonary disease have been undertaken. Clinicians have used ketoconazole or fluconazole at doses of 400 mg orally per day for disease of moderate extent or in individuals with significant risk for dissemination. Amphotericin B has been reserved for more severe clinical presentations in individuals with compromised gas exchange, those who have an exceptionally high risk for dissemination, or those in whom azole therapy has failed.

Persistence of a pulmonary cavity for an extended period such as 6 to 24 months, cavity size greater than 3 to 4 cm, or recurrent or severe hemoptysis suggests the need for surgical extirpation with or

---

*Not FDA approved for this indication.

TABLE 2. **Factors That Increase Risk for Dissemination of Coccidioidomyocosis**

Age	Very young and very old
Sex	Male > female
Race	Nonwhite
Skin test response (Spherulin)	Negative > positive
Serum complement fixation titer	≥1:32
Pregnancy	Third trimester and post partum

without concomitant medical therapy. Diabetic patients seem to fare poorly with surgical therapy for cavities, and every attempt is made to avoid surgery in this group of patients.

Nonmeningeal Disseminated Coccidioidomycosis

Virtually all disseminated coccidioidomycosis mandates systemic chemotherapy. Disease with limited severity and extent may be managed by initial azole therapy with ketoconazole 400 mg per day, fluconazole 400 mg per day, or itraconazole 200 mg twice daily. Clinical experience is greater with ketoconazole and fluconazole. There is currently a clinical trial comparing fluconazole and itraconazole in such patients. More extensive and severe disease should be treated with amphotericin B. Failure of either azole or amphotericin B could suggest a trial with the other. Amphotericin B given by local injection or irrigation, particularly in a joint space or surgical site such as osteomyelitis, may prove a beneficial adjunct to primary therapy with intravenous amphotericin; on occasion, it has been used as primary therapy. Since the advent of azoles, the frequency and desirability of local amphotericin as primary therapy have diminished substantially.

Surgical drainage with removal of involucrum and sequestrum is an important part of the treatment of soft tissue infection and osteomyelitis.

Coccidioidal Meningitis

Meningitis is the most difficult treatment problem in coccidioidal disease. The "gold standard" of therapy has historically been the intrathecal administration of amphotericin B. The drug can be administered by lumbar or cisternal puncture or by ventricular or cisternal Ommaya reservoirs. Each route of administration has advantages and disadvantages. Therapy is usually initiated with alternating lumbar and cisternal punctures done on a daily basis with initial doses of 0.1 mg of amphotericin B in 4 mL of D5W. A glucocorticoid such as methylprednisolone (Solu-Medrol) in doses of 5 to 10 mg is often administered as an intrathecal preinjection or concomitant with the amphotericin B. Subsequent amphotericin B doses are increased by 0.1 mg after each cycle of lumbar and cisternal injections as tolerated by the patient. Complications of therapy and problems of the individual patient may necessitate the use of cisternal or ventricular reservoirs as either primary or secondary therapy. More recently published and unpublished reports have found that there is efficacy in the use of fluconazole in treatment of coccidioidal meningitis. There is some limited experience with ketoconazole in the past and more recent limited experience with itraconazole in the treatment of meningitis. However, by far the largest number of patients have been treated with fluconazole because of its superior cerebrospinal fluid penetration; it achieves virtually the same level in cerebrospinal

fluid as in serum. Early attempts at the treatment of meningitis with oral fluconazole were predicated on using the maximal dose approved by the Food and Drug Administration (FDA) of 400 mg. Subsequent experience has suggested that doses of 800 to 1200 mg* per day or even higher are well tolerated and more likely to achieve success.

Antifungal Agents

As noted earlier, three azoles are used in the treatment of coccidioidomycosis. Ketoconazole has been used the longest, is the only azole with FDA approval for coccidioidomycosis, and has the lowest cost. The dose is 400 mg per day for both pulmonary and nonmeningeal disseminated disease of mild and moderate extent. This is administered as two 200-mg tablets. Higher doses have been used in the past, but this is done less commonly today with the advent of the newer azoles. The daily dose of ketoconazole is taken at one time to decrease the suppressive effects of the drug on steroidogenesis, particularly of androgenic steroids. The drug is best absorbed in an acid milieu, and antacid therapy or H_2 blockers preclude absorption. An acidic drink such as cola may promote absorption. Variability in drug absorption may be a factor in the variability of the patient's response to this agent. Gastrointestinal intolerance, gynecomastia, and drug-induced hepatitis (rarely fatal) are major side effects. Monitoring of the patient with routine laboratory studies, particularly liver function tests and determination of serum drug levels, is desirable.

Fluconazole is usually administered as a single daily dose of 400 mg (two 200-mg tablets). Fluconazole is much less affected by the presence of food and pH than are other azoles. The absorption of the drug is substantially more predictable although somewhat variable from patient to patient. The fungal inhibitory concentration of fluconazole is higher than that of itraconazole. As noted before, substantially higher doses of fluconazole have been used in disseminated disease. It is not clear whether doses above 800 to 1200 mg have any additional efficacy, but it is clear that there does seem to be an advantage of these high doses over the usual 400 mg per day dose, and this has been demonstrated in meningitis. Patients taking fluconazole should be monitored with routine laboratory parameters, particularly liver function tests, because hepatotoxic effects have been reported with this drug. This is usually a modest problem, but at least one fatality has been reported.

Itraconazole is the most recent addition to the coccidioidal azole armamentarium. It is usually dosed as two 100-mg capsules taken twice daily. Itraconazole actually has the longest half-life of the azoles discussed here but it is not well absorbed, particularly when it is taken in large doses; hence, its absorption is promoted by splitting the dose. Absorption of itraconazole is improved by acid pH and the presence of

---

*Exceeds dosage recommended by the manufacturer.

food, particularly lipid. Like ketoconazole, the absorption of itraconazole is severely hindered by the use of antacids or H_2 blockers. Itraconazole should be monitored with routine laboratory studies including liver function studies as well as drug level determinations.

Amphotericin B is initiated with a test dose and slowly escalated. This is done because of rare problems with hypotension, hypertension, and possible cardiac injury. A test dose of 1 mg has often been used. After the test dose, if there is no adverse effect, a 5-mg dose is administered and increased at 8 to 12-hour intervals in 10-mg increments until a dose of 1 mg per kg or 50 mg is reached, whichever is least. The drug is then administered at that level on a daily basis until clinical stability is attained. Subsequently, ambulatory therapy three times a week may be undertaken until the total course of therapy is completed. Home amphotericin B therapy has been administered in selected cases with direct nursing supervision.

For relatively mild disease such as a skin lesion, a total dose of 1 gram of amphotericin B may suffice. For more severe lesions and soft tissue infections, 2 grams may be needed. Three grams is most often used for significant osteomyelitis and other severe disseminated disease. Repeated courses of up to 9 grams or more are rarely needed.

The immediate signs of amphotericin B toxicity are fever, chills, nausea, vomiting, and headache. Acetaminophen (Tylenol) 650 mg and diphenhydramine (Benadryl) 50 mg orally are routinely used as premedication. Prochlorperazine (Compazine) 10 mg or metoclopramide (Reglan)* 10 mg orally is added as needed for gastrointestinal symptoms. Severe chills are specifically treated by parenteral meperidine (Demerol) in small doses of 25 to 50 mg intramuscularly administered as premedication or during acute episodes.

One problem with amphotericin B therapy is nephrotoxicity. Creatinine monitoring is crucial. A creatinine level greater than 3.0 mg/dL would indicate a need to discontinue the drug until the level has decreased to below 3.0 mg/dL. Monitoring the blood urea nitrogen is not helpful. The other major toxic effect of the drug is bone marrow suppression, particularly anemia. Evaluation of renal tubular damage, particularly by monitoring of potassium and magnesium levels, and correction of abnormalities are necessary.

Amphotericin B complexed with lipids and liposomes has been under evaluation. Only liposomal amphotericin B (Abelcet)* and amphotericin B cholesteryl (Amphotec) are currently available. The likely role of these products is in patients with significant renal toxicity from standard amphotericin B. These agents might also be used at higher doses when other therapies have failed.

---

*Not FDA approved for this indication.

Discontinuation of Therapy

Typical duration of azole therapy for primary disease is 3 to 6 months, although courses longer than this are certainly not unusual. Amphotericin B for primary disease is usually dosed at the level of 1 gram. It is occasionally continued to higher doses, and in many cases in the recent past, initial amphotericin B has been followed by a continuation course of azole therapy in patients who appear to be only partial responders, particularly those who have persistent elevation of the complement fixation titer. In nonmeningeal disseminated disease, amphotericin B is usually given to a total dose as described before. If a salutary response is not obtained at the conclusion of this therapy, more protracted courses of amphotericin B to very high gram doses have been used in particularly severe disease. More commonly, in mild or moderate cases, follow-up azole therapy has been used. Azole therapy in disseminated disease is usually at least a year, commonly 2 years, and occasionally substantially longer.

In meningeal disease, intrathecal amphotericin B is often used on a declining schedule for a period of years. At this juncture, fluconazole therapy for meningitis is thought to be lifelong.

It is with some hope that we look forward to the availability of newer antifungal agents that are more efficacious than the currently available drugs to ameliorate the morbidity and mortality of this illness.

HISTOPLASMOSIS

method of
LISA A. HAGLUND, M.D.
University of Cincinnati College of Medicine
Cincinnati, Ohio

Infection with the dimorphic fungus *Histoplasma capsulatum* is acquired by inhalation of mycelial fragments or microconidia that are deposited within terminal bronchioles and alveoli. Within days, the mycelial phase elements transform into yeast cells. These forms spread by the lymphohematogenous route within phagocytes to invade the reticuloendothelial system. Thus, most if not all cases of primary infection are disseminated. In tissues, yeast cells commonly evoke an inflammatory response that consists of caseating or noncaseating granulomas. Virtually all the clinical manifestations of histoplasmosis are caused by yeast cells.

Cases of histoplasmosis have been reported from every continent except Antarctica. In the United States, this fungal infection is endemic to the mideastern and south central regions. Variations in the prevalence of infection in these areas are most likely caused by the presence of hyperendemic foci. Point sources for infection include caves, chicken houses, bird roosts, attics, and old buildings. Epidemics have been associated with mechanical disruption of infested areas by bulldozers, with clearing of accumulated bird or bat guano, or with renovation of old buildings.

Infection with *H. capsulatum* produces three distinct

illnesses: acute pulmonary histoplasmosis (APH), chronic pulmonary histoplasmosis (CPH), and progressive disseminated histoplasmosis (PDH). APH often produces an influenza-like illness with cough, but it may be clinically inapparent. Severity of illness can be correlated directly with inoculum size. Each inhaled particle induces a small patch of bronchopneumonia. The primary lesions encapsulate, become necrotic in the center, and subsequently calcify.

CPH develops predominantly in older individuals with structural lung damage such as obstructive lung disease. This form of histoplasmosis is characterized by weight loss, cough with abundant sputum production, and occasionally fever and hemoptysis. It is believed that the yeast phase organisms proliferate in bullae and slowly induce additional destruction of the lung parenchyma. In some cases, *H. capsulatum* may spread through bronchi to the opposite lung.

In PDH, there is widespread involvement of the mononuclear phagocyte system by yeast cells. Two forms of PDH exist. One is an acute form that is associated with high fever, weight loss, hepatosplenomegaly, pancytopenia, and coagulation disturbances. The other form is chronic PDH, which is characterized by low-grade fever, hepatosplenomegaly, and mucocutaneous ulcers. Human immunodeficiency virus (HIV)–infected patients may present with either form and can also manifest skin lesions, pneumonia, and prostatic abscess. Bone marrow and biopsy materials may be misdiagnosed as acute leukemia, lymphoma, or lymphomatoid granulomatosis if silver stains for fungus and fungal cultures are not performed. The mucocutaneous ulcers of histoplasmosis may mimic head and neck cancers, colon cancers, and Crohn's disease and may cause small bowel obstruction and malabsorption.

Serologic tests and fungal cultures are useful in establishing the diagnosis of histoplasmosis. A complement-fixation (CF) titer of 1:8 is considered positive, and a titer of 1:32 strongly suggests active disease. A fourfold rise in CF titers in 4 to 6 weeks is indicative of active histoplasmosis. The immunodiffusion test is less sensitive than the CF test. The presence of an H precipitin band indicates active disease, whereas an M band signifies past or recent infection. Both may be present in acute disease.

In immunosuppressed patients, serology may be of limited value. Histopathologic examination of tissues, particularly bone marrow or liver, is a useful adjunct. Tissues should be silver stained to visualize yeasts. Culture of sputum and any tissue should be performed. The lysis-centrifugation blood culture system (Isolator) can detect *H. capsulatum* in patients with PDH in 1 to 2 weeks. Other blood culture systems (Septi-Chek, BACTEC, and BacT/Alert) will not grow *H. capsulatum* unless the bottles are held 3 to 6 weeks (for example, with use of BACTEC TB media). The polysaccharide antigen detection system (most sensitive when it is performed on urine) is especially useful in identification of those with PDH and can be used to observe the response to therapy. This assay is available commercially only in the Histoplasma Reference Laboratory (Indianapolis, Indiana).

TREATMENT

Acute Pulmonary Histoplasmosis

Because most patients with APH improve spontaneously by 2 weeks, antifungal therapy is not required in most individuals. Bed rest, antipyretics, and cough suppressants are effective for the influenza-like symptoms. Nevertheless, in a few individuals, there is a prolonged illness (>3 weeks) that consists of fever, weight loss, chest pain, and cough. In these patients, antifungal therapy can hasten resolution of disease. Amphotericin B (Fungizone) should be given intravenously in a dose of 50 mg per day or every other day to a total dose of 500 mg, until the patient is asymptomatic for 7 to 10 days. In children, 0.25 mg per kg of body weight of amphotericin B is given on the first day followed by 0.5 mg per kg on day 2 and 1 mg per kg thereafter. Resolution of illness is much more rapid with amphotericin B than with ketoconazole (Nizoral) administered at a dose of 400 mg per day. Itraconazole (Sporanox) 400 mg daily does not markedly shorten the course of APH and may have a higher occurrence of side effects than expected. A brief tapering course of corticosteroids decreases acute high fevers and chest pain dramatically but does not shorten the overall duration of fever.

Certain sequelae may follow acute histoplasmosis. Examples include pericarditis, fibrosing mediastinitis, lymphadenitis, and arthritis. Pericarditis may be manifested approximately 6 weeks after acute exposure to *H. capsulatum*. Yeast cells are rarely detected in pericardium or pericardial fluid. This illness is treated with anti-inflammatory agents such as salicylates or nonsteroidal drugs. Uncommonly, the severity of illness may necessitate the use of corticosteroids. There is no role for antifungal treatment. If cardiac tamponade develops, pericardiocentesis is necessary. Pericardiectomy is indicated for constrictive pericarditis.

Fibrosing mediastinitis is a progressive illness that probably arises from an exuberant host response to the fungus. Proliferation of fibrous tissue leads to constriction of vital structures including bronchi, superior vena cava, and pulmonary arteries. Optimal therapy for this disorder has not been determined. Amphotericin B, surgery, corticosteroids, ketoconazole or itraconazole, or combinations thereof have been used, with inconsistent results. No controlled trials of medical therapy have been done.

Chronic Pulmonary Histoplasmosis

Treatment of patients with cavitary lung disease or CPH should be instituted when there are thick-walled cavities, enlarging pneumonic lesions, progressive declines in pulmonary function, or persistent fever and weight loss. Ketoconazole 400 mg once daily, or itraconazole 200 mg once daily, is curative in high proportions (two thirds to three fourths) of patients when it is given for at least 6 months. Fluconazole therapy is only moderately effective for CPH. If disease progresses during oral therapy or if the patient is immunocompromised, amphotericin B should be substituted. The total amount of amphotericin B given should be 30 to 35 mg per kg of body weight. Surgical resection of involved lung tissue should be considered in those with massive hemoptysis or in those who fail to respond to medical therapy.

Progressive Disseminated Histoplasmosis

If untreated, PDH is fatal in more than 80% of cases. Risk factors for the development of PDH are immunosuppressive drug treatment, lymphoreticular malignant neoplasm, infection with HIV, and age. Less frequently, individuals without known pre-existing immune defects develop PDH. Interestingly, PDH may cause CD4+ lymphocyte depletion in non–HIV-infected individuals that is reversible with therapy. Reactivation is the most frequent cause of PDH; less commonly, overwhelming primary infection produces symptoms of PDH. Most HIV-infected patients have acquired immune deficiency syndrome (AIDS) with CD4+ lymphocyte counts less than 200 per mm³ at the time of diagnosis of PDH. In endemic areas, 5% of AIDS patients are diagnosed with PDH, probably a result of reactivation. However, PDH has been reported in AIDS patients from nonendemic areas such as New York City and San Francisco.

Treatment of choice for PDH depends on severity of presenting illness. In immunocompromised patients as well as in AIDS patients who present ill enough to require hospitalization, amphotericin B remains the initial treatment of choice. However, after response to initial amphotericin B therapy of 1 gram intravenously in 4 to 6 weeks, itraconazole 200 mg twice daily (bid) can be substituted. If the patient cannot tolerate itraconazole or ketoconazole or there is progression of disease while the patient is receiving these drugs, amphotericin B should be given to a total dose of 30 to 35 mg per kg of body weight. In AIDS patients with PDH, itraconazole therapy should be continued indefinitely. In patients with PDH who are less ill or not otherwise immunocompromised, administration of itraconazole 200 mg bid for at least 6 months is generally as efficacious as amphotericin B. AIDS patients with less severe illness at the time of diagnosis of PDH may be given itraconazole 300 mg bid for 3 days followed by 200 mg bid indefinitely. Ketoconazole and fluconazole (Diflucan)* both have unacceptably high failure rates for either initial therapy or chronic suppressive therapy given to patients with AIDS and PDH. PDH may be successfully controlled in 85% of AIDS patients and cured in more than 90% of other patients with use of available drug therapy.

ANTIFUNGAL THERAPY

Amphotericin B

Amphotericin B is a polyene antibiotic for which intravenous administration is required. This drug binds to membrane sterols, especially ergosterol, and increases permeability of fungal membranes, thus leading to loss of cell constituents and lysis of cells. The drug is insoluble in many solutions including saline and should be diluted in 5% dextrose and water at a concentration not to exceed 0.1 mg per mL. There is no loss of bioactivity if it is exposed to light. Although some clinicians begin with a test dose of 1 mg, I prefer to initiate therapy with 10 mg,* which is infused in 2 to 4 hours. If the test dose is tolerated, the dosage is increased by 15 to 20 mg per day until a maximal dose of 0.7 mg per kg is achieved. In adults, a dose of 50 mg given three times per week is generally a well-tolerated regimen. Electrolytes, renal function, and hemoglobin level should be checked two or three times weekly during the first 3 weeks of therapy and then once weekly until completion.

Adverse side effects to amphotericin B that may be encountered include fever, chills, headache, hypotension or hypertension, anorexia, and vomiting. These symptoms are observed frequently during the first few days of therapy and tend to subside thereafter. Fever, chills, and headache may be mitigated by premedication with acetaminophen (Tylenol), 650 mg orally in adults, and diphenhydramine hydrochloride (Benadryl), 25 to 50 mg orally or parenterally, 0.5 to 1 hour before amphotericin B administration. If symptoms persist despite these measures, slowing the rate of infusion may help. Parenteral meperidine (Demerol) or dantrolene (Dantrium) may also abort symptoms, but these drugs should be reserved for difficult cases. In addition, premedication with 400 to 800 mg of ibuprofen (Motrin) or 10 to 25 mg of hydrocortisone (Solu-Cortef) may be added to alleviate side effects. Amphotericin B often causes phlebitis, especially if it is infused through peripheral veins. Addition of 1000 to 2000 units of heparin to the infusion is helpful in reducing phlebitis.

Renal dysfunction is the most serious toxic effect. The glomerular filtration rate is depressed in almost everyone who receives amphotericin B. Adequate hydration and salt intake help to limit nephrotoxic effects. Treatment should not be stopped until the creatinine or serum urea nitrogen concentration exceeds 3.0 mg per dL or 50 mg per dL, respectively. When the creatinine concentration falls to 2.5 mg per dL, the drug may be restarted. Moreover, because only a small fraction of amphotericin B is excreted by the kidneys, the dosage regimen does not need to be modified in renal failure. A high percentage of patients experience hypokalemia secondary to renal tubular damage, and thus potassium and magnesium supplementation is often necessary. This is especially true in patients receiving concomitant treatment with semisynthetic penicillins such as carbenicillin (Geopen) or ticarcillin (Ticar). Amphotericin B also adds to the nephrotoxicity of cyclosporine. Anemia, probably caused by temporary inhibition of renal erythropoietin production, is another side effect of long-term amphotericin B therapy.

One liposomal preparation (Abelcet) and one cholesteryl sulfate complex (Amphotec) of amphotericin B have become available. Because these lipid-based drugs have a lower occurrence of nephrotoxic effects, they are indicated when a patient undergoes a marked elevation of serum creatinine while receiv-

---

*Not FDA approved for this indication.

*Test dose exceeds dosage recommended by the manufacturer.

ing amphotericin B (despite saline prehydration) or when pre-existing renal insufficiency is present (serum creatinine concentration at least 2.5 mg per dL). Efficacy of the lipid-based preparations is no better than that of amphotericin B and is probably similar. The recommended dosage is 5 mg per kg per day, although the optimal dosage is not known.

Ketoconazole

Ketoconazole is an imidazole that inhibits ergosterol synthesis. It offers advantages because it is less toxic than amphotericin B and is administered orally. It is efficacious in the treatment of pulmonary, localized (e.g., infection of oropharynx, bone, lymph nodes), and disseminated histoplasmosis in immunocompetent individuals. Resolution of infection appears to be slower than with amphotericin B. The combination of amphotericin B and ketoconazole does not offer any advantage over therapy with a single agent.

Twenty percent of individuals complain of nausea, vomiting, or anorexia. These symptoms can be reduced by giving the drug in two divided doses rather than in a single dose or by taking the drug with meals or at bedtime. The drug is well absorbed from the gastrointestinal tract, but absorption is diminished by achlorhydria or by drugs that raise gastric pH because the compound must be converted to the hydrochloride salt before it can be absorbed. Administration of ketoconazole with food enhances absorption. Ketoconazole blocks synthesis of testosterone, and high doses of the drug can produce oligospermia, gynecomastia, loss of libido, and loss of sexual potency. In addition, this agent inhibits cortisol secretion. To date, however, permanent hypoadrenalism has been reported in only one patient. Liver enzyme values are elevated transiently in approximately 10% of patients, but there is symptomatic hepatic dysfunction in less than 0.1%. If jaundice or marked elevation of liver enzymes develops, ketoconazole must be discontinued. Otherwise, fatal hepatic necrosis may result. Other drug interactions are discussed later.

Itraconazole

Itraconazole is the newest of the azole antifungal compounds and is approved for use in histoplasmosis, including chronic cavitary pulmonary disease and disseminated, nonmeningeal histoplasmosis. Like amphotericin B, it is a highly lipophilic agent with little plasma protein binding. It is entirely metabolized by the liver. It is available in 100-mg capsules for oral administration only; no intravenous form is available. Because it may take 1 to 2 weeks to reach steady-state concentration, a loading dose of itraconazole 200 mg three times daily for the first 3 days is recommended.

Absorption of itraconazole is a problem. Itraconazole absorption is impaired in the presence of a high gastric pH. Thus, itraconazole serum levels may have to be monitored to demonstrate adequate absorption in the elderly, HIV-infected patients with hypochlorhydria, or patients who have had ulcer operations. Absorption may improve with coadministration of a cola beverage to lower gastric pH. Patients should not be given concurrent antacids, H_2 blockers, or omeprazole (Prilosec). Itraconazole capsules must be taken along with a meal to facilitate absorption; when they are taken on an empty stomach, serum levels are only one third of those achieved after the same dose is taken immediately after a meal. There is no experience yet with tube feedings, but it is not well absorbed through a nasogastic tube. Diarrhea has also been observed to interfere with absorption in some patients. If more than 200 mg per day of itraconazole is given, divided doses are advised. A newly available oral solution containing 10 mg of itraconazole per mL may be better absorbed but it is not approved by the Food and Drug Administration for treatment of histoplasmosis.

Transaminase elevations and cholestatic hepatitis that are reversible on discontinuation of itraconazole have been described. The most common adverse reactions are nausea, vomiting, and rash with dosages up to 400 mg per day. These symptoms occur less frequently with itraconazole than with ketoconazole. Itraconazole-associated impotence and decreased libido have been reported. Reversible edema has also been observed. One case of reversible adrenal insufficiency has occurred with high doses (600 mg per day). No dosage adjustment is necessary in the presence of renal insufficiency, and it is not removed by either peritoneal dialysis or hemodialysis.

Drug interactions in this class of antifungal agents are summarized later, but two important drug interactions are mentioned here. Coadministration of terfenadine (Seldane) or astemizole (Hismanal) with itraconazole or ketoconazole is contraindicated, because it may result in increased levels of the antihistamines, inducing cardiac arrhythmias that may be fatal. Coadministration of rifampin (Rifadin) or phenytoin (Dilantin) has been observed to profoundly decrease serum itraconazole levels by increasing itraconazole metabolism, thus resulting in loss of antifungal efficacy. This effect has also been observed with coadministration of phenytoin and H_2 antagonists. However, a small study of HIV-infected persons found that the pharmacokinetics of zidovudine (Retrovir) were not affected during concomitant administration of itraconazole.

Itraconazole is more efficacious in PDH than in CPH (also the case with amphotericin B), probably because of local factors in the cavitary pulmonary disease that interfere with antifungal therapy. For PDH in AIDS patients, itraconazole has been shown to be useful for both suppressive therapy after induction with amphotericin B and for treatment of patients who are mildly to moderately ill with PDH. Treatment should be given at a dose of 400 mg per day (200 mg bid). There are no studies in pregnant women, and itraconazole should be used in pregnancy only if the potential benefit outweighs the risks because a teratogenic effect has been observed in rats experimentally.

Itraconazole should not be used in the critically ill patient because absorption may be impaired. In the absence of food, absorption of the drug is drastically reduced. In addition, critically ill patients may receive agents that reduce gastric acidity, and this intervention may further impair absorption of the drug. Thus, for several reasons, amphotericin B remains the drug of choice in patients who are extremely ill with histoplasmosis.

Fluconazole

Fluconazole (Diflucan) is a triazole antifungal agent with the same mechanism of activity as ketoconazole and itraconazole. Unlike these agents, however, it has low protein binding, it distributes in the total body water, and 80% of the administered drug is excreted unchanged in the urine. It is available in 50-, 100-, 150-, and 200-mg tablets for oral administration and in a 2 mg per mL intravenous solution. Adverse effects associated with fluconazole include gastrointestinal irritation (anorexia, nausea, and vomiting), hepatitis (usually clinically inapparent transaminase elevations), pruritic rashes, and one possible case of Stevens-Johnson syndrome. Reversible alopecia and chapped lips have been observed with prolonged courses. To date, the interference with human steroidogenesis seen with ketoconazole

has not been reported with either fluconazole or itraconazole.

For maintenance therapy for PDH, fluconazole at doses of 100 to 400 mg per day is less effective than either itraconazole or amphotericin B. Its use should be restricted to patients with mild to moderate disease who have poor tolerance or poor absorption of itraconazole or to those receiving drugs that may potentially interact with itraconazole. In these cases, it seems reasonable to administer a minimal daily dose of 400 mg. With prolonged therapy using high doses of fluconazole, reversible alopecia may be observed.

DRUG INTERACTIONS WITH AZOLE ANTIFUNGAL AGENTS

The principal mechanism of action of the azole compounds is to preferentially inhibit cytochrome P-450 enzymes in fungal organisms. Because these enzymes are also present in mammalian cells, in which they play a key role in metabolic and detoxifying reactions, this class of drugs is well known to interfere with metabolism of other compounds (Table 1).

Severe hypoglycemia has been reported in patients concomitantly receiving azole antifungal agents and oral hypoglycemic agents. Fluconazole, even at low doses (100 mg per day), markedly potentiates the anticoagulant activity of warfarin (Coumadin); itra-

TABLE 1. **Antifungal Azole Pharmacokinetics and Drug Interactions**

Measure	Ketoconazole	Itraconazole	Fluconazole
Dose, route	200-mg tablet PO	100-mg capsule PO	Various PO, IV
Peak serum concentration (µg/mL)	1.7–3.6	0.1	2.5–6.7
Half-life (h)	8	15–40	20–30
Protein bound (%)	99	84–99	11
Requires hydrochloric acid for absorption	Yes	Yes	No
Metabolism	Hepatic	Hepatic	80% renal
Adverse effects	Gastrointestinal upset, hepatitis, oligospermia, decreased steroid levels	Gastrointestinal upset, hypokalemia, impotence, liver function test increases	Gastrointestinal upset, rashes, liver function test increases
Phenytoin (Dilantin)	Increased phenytoin level, decreased ketoconazole level	Increased phenytoin level, decreased itraconazole level	Increased phenytoin level
Warfarin (Coumadin)	Increased anticoagulation	Increased anticoagulation	Increased anticoagulation
Cyclosporine	Increased cyclosporine level	Increased cyclosporine level	Increased cyclosporine level
Carbamazepine (Tegretol)		Decreased itraconazole level	Increased carbamazepine level
Oral hypoglycemics	Increased hypoglycemic effect	Increased hypoglycemic effect	Increased hypoglycemic effect
Digoxin		Increased digoxin level	
Terfenadine (Seldane), astemizole (Hismanal)	Increased antihistamine level with possible result of fatal arrhythmias	Increased antihistamine level with possible result of fatal arrhythmias	Increased antihistamine level
Rifampin, isoniazid	Decreased ketoconazole level	Decreased itraconazole level	Decreased fluconazole level
Cisapride (Propulsid)	Increased cisapride level, with possible result of fatal arrhythmias	Increased cisapride level, with possible result of fatal arrhythmias	Increased cisapride level
Midazolam (Versed), triazolam (Halcion)	Increased sedative effect	Increased sedative effect	
Lovastatin (Mevacor), simvastatin (Zocor)		Possible rhabdomyolysis	
100-mg oral dose cost (average wholesale price)		$6.88	$4.92
200-mg oral dose cost (average wholesale price)	$2.32	$11.25	

conazole may have the same effect. Potentially fatal arrhythmias from elevated levels of the newer antihistamines have been described with itraconazole. Drug interactions with the addition of itraconazole include decreased metabolism and therefore toxic levels of digoxin, phenytoin, and cyclosporine (Sandimmune). Ketoconazole also increases levels of cisapride (Propulsid). Plasma concentrations of azole antifungal agents are reduced when they are given concurrently with isoniazid. Induction of hepatic microsomal enzymes by rifampin produces decreased serum concentrations of ketoconazole. Ketoconazole increases serum concentrations of cyclosporine. Although no studies have been conducted, case reports suggest that the dose of cyclosporine should be reduced by 50% when itraconazole is given. There is no information regarding cross-hypersensitivity among the azole antifungal agents.

BLASTOMYCOSIS

method of
G. DOUGLAS CAMPBELL, JR., M.D.
Louisiana State University Medical Center
Shreveport, Louisiana

Blastomyces dermatitidis, the agent that causes blastomycosis, is a thermally dimorphic fungus widely distributed throughout the eastern half of North America, especially around the Great Lakes and the great river valleys of the Saint Lawrence and the central United States. Blastomycosis has also been documented in South America, Africa, and Asia. Although no reliable skin test exists, sensitive antibody tests suggest that a significant portion of the population in endemic areas has been exposed to *B. dermatitidis* and apparently did not develop clinical disease.

The mycelial form of *B. dermatitidis* exists in moist soil rich in decaying organic material, and aerosolization of spores occurs when the soil is disturbed and conidia are released. Inhalation of an infective aerosol is by far the most common portal of entry in humans. At 37°C, the fungus converts to the yeast form in the lungs, and hematogenous dissemination may occur; the most frequent sites of infection are the skin, bones, genitourinary tract, and reticuloendothelial system. Human-to-human spread is not reported except for rare cases of genitourinary or intrauterine transmission.

Blastomycosis may present as either an acute or a chronic infection. The host response, unlike in most other fungal infections, is pyogranulomatous. The clinical presentation of acute blastomycosis may range from a mild lower respiratory tract infection, to acute pneumonia (indistinguishable from a bacterial infection with alveolar or lobar involvement and the production of purulent, even blood-streaked sputum), to adult respiratory distress syndrome. Chronic pulmonary disease is often more insidious although progressive, with the patient complaining of productive cough, chest pain, low-grade fever, night sweats, and weight loss. Chest radiographs often reveal either lobar or segmental infiltrates, occasionally with cavitation or a mass lesion that mimics tuberculosis or cancer. Extrapulmonary infections, especially of the skin, bones, genito-

urinary tract, and reticuloendothelial system, are reported to occur in about a fourth of cases and are probably more likely if the patient is immunocompromised.

DIAGNOSIS

Patients with blastomycosis not infrequently present after having failed to respond to antimicrobial therapy for presumed bacterial pneumonia and are often suspected of having cancer or tuberculosis. In these settings, in endemic areas, blastomycosis should be considered; pulmonary secretions or pus from draining sinuses and skin lesions should be obtained, mixed with potassium hydroxide, and examined for the characteristic yeast with a refractile cell wall and wide-based mother-daughter junctions. If available, cytologic specimens should be stained with Papanicolaou or Giemsa stains, and pathologic specimens should be stained with periodic acid–Schiff and silver stains. In addition, all material should be cultured at 30°C on enriched media (i.e., Sabhi). Central nervous system (CNS) fluid cultures have a low yield, but biopsies of involved skin, bone, and genitourinary tract are often rewarding.

INDICATIONS FOR TREATMENT

Any patient with evidence of active blastomycosis of more than several weeks' duration, extrathoracic disease, immunosuppression, or severe disease should be treated. Recommendations for therapy are displayed in Table 1.

Azole Antifungal Agents

In the past 20 years, several oral azole agents have been introduced for the treatment of systemic fungal infections. Whereas the azoles are effective agents, they are not as potent as amphotericin B and in severe infections should not be used as first-line drugs or single therapy. The azoles work by suppressing the cytochrome P-450–dependent biosynthesis of a crucial fungal cell wall component, the sterol ergosterol. Since its introduction in 1992, itraconazole (Sporanox) has become the standard therapy for mild to moderate forms of blastomycosis. Itraconazole is available in 100-mg capsules, and standard therapy consists of 200 mg given either once or twice daily with meals for 6 to 12 months depending on the extent of disease and response to therapy. Absorption requires gastric acidity; thus, achlorhydria or the administration of agents that raise gastric pH (antacids, H_2-receptor antagonists, proton pump inhibitors) dramatically reduces absorption. Penetration into the CNS is poor. Itraconazole is reported to be less toxic than previous azoles, such as ketoconazole; the most frequently reported side effects are nausea, vomiting, edema, and hypokalemia. Rare cases of hepatitis have been reported; therefore, monitoring of hepatic enzyme levels should be considered. Hepatitis usually resolves with discontinuation of therapy. Suppression of testosterone or corticosteroid secretion is not reported except when the daily dosage of itraconazole exceeds the standard dose approved by the Food and Drug Administration of 400 mg per day. The dose is not affected by renal failure.

TABLE 1. **Recommended Therapeutic Regimens for Various Forms of Blastomycosis**

Type of Infection	Therapy	Dosages*
Pulmonary Blastomycosis		
Acute pneumonia: progressing or not resolving in several weeks	Itraconazole (Sporanox)	200–400 mg daily for 6 mo
Chronic cavitary, nodular or mass lesion	Itraconazole	200–400 mg daily for 6 mo
Life-threatening pneumonia or immunosuppressed patient	Amphotericin B (Fungizone)	Total dose 2 gm
Extrapulmonary Blastomycosis		
Cutaneous, bone joint, or other organ involvement	Itraconazole	200–400 mg daily for 6 mo
Life-threatening disseminated infection or immunosuppressed patients	Amphotericin B	Total dose 2 gm
All patients with central nervous system infection	Amphotericin B	Total dose 2 gm

*See text for complete discussion. It is necessary to monitor the patient's response to therapy. If the patient does not respond, consider noncompliance or switch from itraconazole to amphotericin B.

Azoles are associated with important drug interactions. Terfenadine (Seldane) and astemizole (Hismanal) should not be used in patients receiving itraconazole because of the risk for serious arrhythmias. Cyclosporine and digoxin levels are increased with itraconazole therapy, and careful monitoring of serum levels of these agents is important. Itraconazole levels may be decreased with the concomitant use of phenytoin, carbamazepine, and rifampin, which can result in treatment failure.

Compliance is important in treating patients with blastomycosis. The azoles are not associated with immediate improvement, and the side effects, especially nausea and anorexia, and the relative expense of the drug may result in the patient's prematurely discontinuing the agent. In patients who do not respond adequately to an azole after the first 1 or 2 months, consider noncompliance. Careful questioning and obtaining a blood level 2 hours after a dose of itraconazole can identify patients who are noncompliant; patients who have unrecognized achlorhydria; or patients who are taking antacids, H_2-receptor antagonists, or proton pump inhibitors.

Amphotericin B

Amphotericin B (Fungizone) is a polyene macrolide antibiotic with broad activity against many fungi. It acts by combining with cytoplasmic sterols, particularly ergosterol, to form channels in fungal cell walls resulting in intracellular leakage and cell death. It remains the most potent antifungal agent available but is associated with a number of side effects. Immediate reactions include nausea, vomiting, headaches, chills, and fever. These reactions tend to decrease with continued therapy or may be reduced by using a more rapid infusion time (2 hours) and premedication with diphenhydramine (Benadryl), 50 mg orally, and aspirin or acetaminophen, 650 mg orally. If no benefit is achieved, then codeine, 30 to 60 mg, or meperidine (Demerol), 15 to 20 mg, intravenously before therapy may decrease symptoms. Phlebitis may be lessened by adding glucocorticoid preparations (hydrocortisone, 50 to 100 mg) to the infusion and alternating peripheral vein administration sites. Dose-related side effects include renal failure, hypo-

kalemia (especially with sodium depletion), hypomagnesemia, and anemia. Replacement of fluid volume (to ensure that the urine output is greater than 30 mL per kg per day) and salts (especially potassium, bicarbonate, and magnesium) reduces the risk for and severity of nephrotoxicity. Anemia is not uncommon and rarely requires treatment or interruption of therapy. Serum blood urea nitrogen (BUN), creatinine, potassium, and magnesium concentrations and hematocrit should be obtained twice weekly for the first month and then weekly throughout the rest of therapy. Because therapy will continue for weeks, I suggest placing a flow sheet on the chart to record the daily dose, cumulative dose, and important laboratory values. Despite the side effects associated with amphotericin B, one clear advantage to amphotericin B therapy is that compliance can be easily documented.

In my experience, the use of an initial test dose followed by gradually increasing doses of amphotericin B (<10 mg) has been of little benefit and delays reaching effective doses. In adult patients, I usually begin amphotericin B therapy at 10 mg, increasing the dose at 10-mg increments until a 50-mg daily dose is achieved. If an effective dose is needed rapidly, I give an initial dose of 0.25 mg per kg of body weight, double the dose on the second day, and give 50 mg on the third day. In general, 50 mg is administered on alternating days or thrice weekly until the total dose is given, but daily and even higher doses may be necessary in the severely ill. Except in severe life-threatening situations, therapy may need to be modified if renal dysfunction is noted. If the BUN concentration is greater than 40 mg per dL or the creatinine concentration is greater than 3 mg per dL, I decrease the dose by 10 mg until renal function has stabilized. A rise in BUN to greater than 50 mg per dL prompts me to stop therapy until renal function improves.

Once amphotericin B is started, it is continued until a total cumulative dose of 1.5 to 2 grams is reached. Initial treatment with 500 mg of amphotericin B followed by a full course of itraconazole has been suggested, but there are currently no clinical studies available to support this approach. I have used this approach in occasional patients, but only after they had experienced an excellent early response to amphotericin B therapy. These patients received itraconazole for an additional 6 months; close observation is necessary during the follow-up period.

Liposomal amphotericin B is now available, but it is expensive. The side effect profile is better, and this drug formulation may be considered in patients with severe disease when higher doses are needed or when side effects limit therapy.

There is little information on treating immunosuppressed patients. Amphotericin B is generally the preferred agent because of its superior activity against *B. dermatitidis*. In patients with the acquired immune deficiency syndrome, blastomycosis is often disseminated and initial therapy should begin with amphotericin B, unless infection is mild. Switching to itraconazole can be considered if early improvement is noted, but thereafter, the patient requires suppressive therapy with itraconazole for life. Renal transplant recipients present a different problem owing to the potential for combined nephrotoxicity of amphotericin B and cyclosporine. In selected patients with mild to moderate disease, itraconazole at 400 mg per day can be instituted, but relapse rates almost certainly will be higher than with amphotericin B, so careful follow-up is necessary. Itraconazole is not effective in patients with involvement of the CNS, and treatment with amphotericin B is required.

PLEURAL EFFUSION AND EMPYEMA THORACIS

method of
DON R. MILLER, M.D.
*University of California, Irvine, College of
   Medicine*
Irvine, California

Pleural effusion, a collection of fluid in the pleural space, is a common clinical feature of many local and systemic diseases including congestive heart failure, bacterial pneumonia, malignant neoplasm, pulmonary embolism, and viral infections. Less frequent causes are cirrhosis, tuberculosis, pancreatitis, and others. Pleural effusion results when the delicate balance between hydrostatic and oncotic pressures in pleural vessels is altered.

A complete history and physical examination may indicate the precise cause of the effusion or provide a rational differential diagnosis for the selection of appropriate studies. Posteroanterior and lateral chest films show obliteration of sulci, and the lateral decubitus view defines the layered fluid. The accuracy of ultrasonography and computed tomography is increasingly helpful in the diagnosis of pulmonary and pleural diseases and in needle or catheter drainage of small loculated collections. Any significant effusion should be promptly sampled by needle aspiration for study.

Effusions may be classified as transudates or exudates on the basis of the protein or lactate dehydrogenase (LDH) concentration in the fluid and serum. Reportedly highly accurate, these criteria (Light) are

1. The ratio of the pleural fluid protein concentration to the serum protein concentration is greater than 0.5.
2. The ratio of the pleural fluid LDH concentration to the serum LDH concentration is greater than 0.6.
3. The pleural fluid LDH concentration is greater than two thirds of the upper limit of normal of the serum LDH concentration.

Exudates have at least one of these criteria, whereas transudates have none. Transudates usually arise from congestive heart failure, cirrhosis, or the nephrotic syndrome, and further tests of the fluid are not needed, the treatment being directed to the underlying cause. Exudates result from a large number of causes and require selected additional tests, depending on the differential diagnosis and the gross and microscopic characteristics of the fluid, which may be diagnostic. These include specific gravity; pH; glucose concentration; white cell count and differential; red cell count; aerobic, anaerobic, and acid-fast bacterial and fungal cultures; Gram's stain; cytologic examination; and lipid and amylase determinations.

The pH may be less than 7.20 in tuberculous, parapneumonic, malignant, and rheumatoid effusions. The glucose level may be below 60 mg per dL in tuberculosis and rheumatoid arthritis. Amylase points to pancreatitis or esophageal perforation. The culture for tubercle bacilli is positive in only 30% of patients with tuberculous pleurisy, which increases to 75% with pleural biopsy. Lymphocytes predominate in cell counts of tuberculosis and rheumatoid arthritis, whereas red cells are prominent in malignant neoplasm, pulmonary embolism, and trauma. Chylothorax has a grossly milky appearance and lipid content greater than that of the plasma. Although the fluid analysis is diagnostic in a large percentage of patients, in others the cause for effusion cannot be established. Test results may be variable with similar diagnoses.

The diagnostic tap should be referenced to the posteroanterior and lateral chest films, avoiding the diaphragm, the heart shadow, and the internal mammary, axillary, and intercostal vessels. If selective studies of the exudative fluid are not diagnostic, closed pleural biopsy, video-assisted thoracoscopy (VAT), or open pleural biopsy may be indicated.

TREATMENT

Empyema

Empyema is a purulent infection of the pleural space that accompanies or follows pneumonia, lung abscess, trauma, thoracic surgery, or chest tube insertion. Its bacterial source may be hematogenous. The mortality rate is reportedly as high as 20%, and it is particularly lethal to the immunocompromised patient (i.e., the elderly, acquired immune deficiency syndrome victims, the debilitated). The organisms involved most frequently are *Streptococcus pneumoniae*, *Staphylococcus aureus*, multiple organisms including anaerobes, and, in children, *Haemophilus influenzae*. Gram-negative bacteria often originate from infections below the diaphragm that extend into the thorax.

Empyema is often the result of delay in the antibiotic treatment of pneumonia. Pleural effusion is common in association with pneumonia (parapneumonic effusion); if small, it may resolve with antibiotics alone. Early and, if necessary, repeated thoracentesis, identification of the organism, and prompt, appropriate antibiotic therapy are necessary to halt the natural progression from thin, serous fluid to thick, fibrinopurulent, and then loculated pus.

"Complicated" parapneumonic effusion refers to that which requires prompt chest tube drainage in addition to parenteral antibiotics. The effusion is recognized on thoracentesis by the purulent appearance or a positive Gram stain. A glucose level below 40 mg per dL and a pH below 7.0 may be seen. After tube drainage, a prompt clinical response is expected, and if it is not forthcoming, the remaining loculations of thick pus must be found and drained by additional tubes, VAT débridement, or open surgical procedure. The pleural instillation of fibrinolytic agents (streptokinase, urokinase) has been reported to aid in coalescing loculations in conjunction with tube drainage, thus avoiding surgical intervention. Complete pulmonary expansion must be maintained to ensure adequate respiratory function and prevention of trapped lung. A persistent space or unexpanded lung sets the stage for fluid collection leading to chronic empyema, thickened pleura, and consideration of the more formidable decortication procedure. Early operation is advocated for immunocompromised patients who respond poorly to tube drainage only. Reports of VAT débridement applied early in the course of complicated effusion and empyema relate its effectiveness in improved results, hastened recovery, and less morbidity than with open surgical drainage. Open surgical drainage remains the "gold standard" against which newer approaches are judged.

Pleural Effusion Caused by Neoplasm

The most frequent causes of malignant pleural effusion are metastatic adenocarcinoma of the lung, breast carcinoma, and the lymphomas. The primary site of origin may be unknown and remain so in 10% of patients. The effusion may be clear or bloody, unilateral or bilateral. Cytologic study of pleural fluid is usually diagnostic, and a positive result for malignant neoplasm is a contraindication to curative definitive therapy for the primary lesion. If the primary tumor has not been located, a search for it should be made. Closed pleural biopsy by use of a special needle, VAT, or open thoracotomy may be indicated when the results of initial and repeated fluid cytologic study are negative.

Systemic chemotherapy and/or radiation will usually be the initial treatment. When systemic therapy does not control the effusion, and rapid symptomatic reaccumulation of the fluid requires repeated thoracentesis, local palliative treatment to block fluid formation by pleurodesis may be indicated. Many substances and procedures have been used to induce pleurodesis, tetracycline* probably the most often. But it is no longer available for parenteral use. Bleomycin (Blenoxane)* is less effective and is expensive.

Talc, either insufflated at the time of VAT or thoracotomy or as a slurry through chest tube, is reported to be 90% effective and is the current agent of choice. Respiratory complications, believed to be dose related, have been reported but have not occurred if the dose is limited to 5 grams. Little long-term follow-up is known.

Pleuroperitoneal shunts (Denver shunt) have selected application, particularly in effusion with trapped lung.

Tuberculosis and Other Effusions

The incidence of tuberculosis and its complications varies with the geographic region. An effusion of acute onset in younger patients without apparent cause may be tuberculous in origin. It is thin and nonpurulent and may fail to show tubercle bacilli on smear or culture. Pleural needle biopsy may be diagnostic of chronic pleural disease of tuberculosis when other measures have failed. With only a positive purified protein derivative skin test response and no other cause for the effusion, multidrug treatment for tuberculosis is indicated. Resolution of the effusion may be supplemented by thoracentesis if required, but chest tube drainage is avoided. Some patients may later be candidates for decortication for residual pleural disease. Epstein's review of 24 patients with tuberculous effusion showed an older population with mean age of 56 years.

Pulmonary embolism is commonly overlooked as a cause of pleural effusion. Although the fluid is classically bloody and has a predominance of polymorphonuclear leukocytes, either or both of these characteristics may be absent. One fourth of the effusions are transudates. The effusion resolves with anticoagulants as given for emboli without effusion.

Intra-abdominal subdiaphragmatic conditions such as hepatic, pancreatic, and subphrenic abscess may communicate with the pleural space and result in pleural effusion. CT and endoscopic retrograde cholangiopancreatography are valuable in the diagnosis and selection of the surgical approach to correct these problems.

Chylothorax has a milky appearance and a lipid content greater than that of the plasma. Various approaches to chylothorax include surgery, VAT, pleuroperitoneal shunting, pleurodesis, and observation. Selection of the appropriate treatment must be based on several factors including the underlying cause.

PRIMARY LUNG ABSCESS

method of
JOHN G. BARTLETT, M.D.
Johns Hopkins University School of Medicine
Baltimore, Maryland

Lung abscess refers to pulmonary necrosis caused by bacteria other than mycobacteria. The usual mechanism of

---

*Not FDA approved for this indication.

detection is by chest radiography or computed tomography (CT) showing a parenchymal infiltrate accompanied by a thick-walled cavity, often with an air-fluid level. The usual clinical features are cough, fever, and sputum production, sometimes accompanied by hemoptysis, pleurisy, weight loss, and leukocytosis. The distinction between primary and secondary lung abscess is determined by associated conditions. Primary lung abscess is most common in patients who are prone to aspiration as a result of compromised consciousness or dysphagia. Secondary lung abscesses represent complications of bronchial obstruction, such as a malignant neoplasm or foreign body, or a systemic disease associated with compromised defense mechanisms, as with organ transplantation, acquired immune deficiency syndrome (AIDS), cancer chemotherapy, or steroid administration.

The bacteriology of lung abscess is variable and often not determined with precision. Most primary lung abscesses are caused by anaerobic bacteria, primarily *Prevotella melaninogenica*; fusobacteria; *Bacteroides* species; and streptococci including aerobic, anaerobic, and microaerophilic streptococci. The bacterial etiology is usually not determined, but putrid sputum, pleural fluid, or breath is considered diagnostic of anaerobic infection; this is found in 60 to 70% of patients with lung abscesses involving anaerobes. Gram-negative bacteria, especially *Klebsiella* and *Pseudomonas aeruginosa*, are relatively common causes in patients with neutropenia, advanced AIDS, and nosocomial pneumonia. Injection drug users commonly have multiple lung abscesses involving *Staphylococcus aureus* representing emboli with tricuspid valve endocarditis.

The diagnostic evaluation depends to a large extent on the clinical setting. Patients with typical clinical features accompanied by putrid sputum have presumed anaerobic infections and are treated empirically for that diagnosis. Symptoms often shared with tuberculosis include chronic cough, fever, and weight loss, and chest films often show upper lobe cavities with or without a pleural effusion. It is often important to exclude *Mycobacterium tuberculosis* with three morning stains and culture for acid-fast bacteria. Common causes of lung abscess, especially in compromised hosts, include *Nocardia, Cryptococcus, Aspergillus,* and gram-negative bacteria. In these cases, more rigorous diagnostic testing is usually advocated, including bronchoscopy with appropriate stains and cultures if results of expectorated sputum studies are negative. Detection of anaerobic bacteria requires appropriate culture of an uncontaminated specimen such as transtracheal aspirate or pleural fluid. Quantitative cultures of bronchoscopic specimens (protected brush or bronchoalveolar lavage fluid specimens) may be adequate, although experience is limited. Expectorated sputum is of no value for detecting anaerobes, but it may be useful because the failure to grow *S. aureus* or gram-negative aerobic bacteria is strong evidence that these organisms are not involved.

TREATMENT

Most patients with primary lung abscess are treated empirically on the basis of the assumption that anaerobic bacteria are responsible. The standard drug for more than 3 decades was penicillin G in doses of 750 mg four times daily by mouth or 10 to 20 million units per day intravenously. More recently, clindamycin has largely supplanted penicillin as the preferred drug on the basis of two comparative therapeutic trials demonstrating a statistically significant advantage for clindamycin in terms of response rates, time to defervescence, and time for elimination of putrid discharge. The standard initial dose of clindamycin (Cleocin) for hospitalized patients is 600 mg intravenously three times daily; when patients are clinically improved, this may be changed to oral clindamycin, 300 mg four times daily. The duration of treatment is arbitrary, but I have witnessed several relapses when patients were treated for arbitrarily defined periods such as 4 to 6 weeks. Consequently, I recommend continuation of treatment until the chest radiograph is clear or there is only a small, stable residual scar. This often requires 2 to 4 months of treatment, most of which is by oral treatment on an outpatient basis. If penicillin is used, the usual dose is 10 to 20 million units of aqueous penicillin G per day until the patient is clinically improved; the long-term outpatient treatment is with penicillin V, 750 mg per day, or amoxicillin, 500 mg three times daily. A disadvantage of penicillin is the inferior results compared with clindamycin in the two clinical trials noted before. In addition, there is a theoretical concern based on in vitro susceptibility of anaerobic bacteria that are commonly involved; about 20 to 25% produce β-lactamase, indicating penicillin resistance.

Alternative drugs that may be used for infections involving anaerobic bacteria include the following: imipenem-cilastatin (Primaxin); meropenem (Merrem), a β-lactam–β-lactamase inhibitor; or chloramphenicol. All of these drugs are active in vitro against virtually all clinically significant anaerobic bacteria, although there is limited clinical experience with these drugs for primary lung abscess. The potential utility of these drugs is important to recognize because they may be attractive as initial treatment in cases in which the role of enteric gram-negative bacteria is unclear. Metronidazole (Flagyl) is active against virtually all anaerobic bacteria, but approximately 50% of patients with primary lung abscess show an inadequate response. This is ascribed to the lack of activity against aerobic and microaerophilic streptococci that are commonly involved in these polymicrobial infections. Thus, if metronidazole is to be used, it should be combined with penicillin. The usual dose of metronidazole is 500 mg two or three times daily by mouth. One drug that has had favorable experience in lung abscess patients for outpatient management is amoxicillin-clavulanate (Augmentin) in a dose of 500 mg three times daily.

Side effects of the drugs that are important to recognize include *Clostridium difficile*–associated diarrhea or colitis with clindamycin, diarrhea that is dose related or associated with *C. difficile* with amoxicillin-clavulanate, and the disulfiram (Antabuse)–like reaction with metronidazole in alcoholic patients.

Drainage

Many patients with lung abscess have empyema that requires drainage. Drainage of the lung abscess is controversial. Bronchoscopy or physical therapy with appropriate positioning of the patient will sometimes yield copious respiratory secretions, and sometimes this may be therapeutically important. However, on rare occasions there may be spillage to other bronchial segments with extension of the pulmonary infection. Thus, postural drainage is encouraged, but with due caution.

Bronchoscopy

A previous recommendation was for routine bronchoscopy in all patients with lung abscess to detect associated lesions such as neoplasms or foreign bodies. At present, bronchoscopy is generally reserved for patients who fail to respond to treatment, for patients with atypical presentations or suspected neoplasms, and for detection of selected microbial pathogens, especially in patients who do not produce expectorated sputum.

Failure to Respond

Patients with primary lung abscess should show subjective improvement within 3 to 5 days and defervescence within 7 to 10 days. Improvement on the chest film is delayed; in fact, there may be extension of the infiltrate with new cavity formation during the first 1 to 2 weeks. The major poor prognostic features are large cavity size (>6 cm in diameter), a debilitated host, and patients with secondary lung abscess. Diagnostic studies in patients who fail to respond include bronchoscopy to detect underlying lesions or an unusual etiologic agent (fungi, *Nocardia*, mycobacteria) and chest CT to define the anatomy. The most common cause of failure to respond is simply a delay in response according to the sequential observations noted before or a host who is unable to respond owing to advanced disease or poor defenses. Reversible causes for failure to respond include the need for drainage, the need for resectional surgery, or a need to change antibiotic treatment. Changes in antibiotic treatment are optimal if they are based on microbiologic studies to define the bacterial agent. Unfortunately, common bacteria involved in lung abscess are difficult to cultivate after antibiotic treatment, and respiratory secretions often contain antibiotic-resistant organisms that simply colonize the airways. It is a mistake to change antibiotic treatment on the basis of each new bacterium recovered from respiratory secretions. Detection of unusual agents is critical, and these include *Legionella, S. aureus*, fungi, *Nocardia*, and mycobacteria. Some patients fail to respond because they have nonbacterial lesions that appear as lung abscesses, such as Wegener's granulomatosis, fluid-containing cysts, pulmonary sequestration, or cavitating neoplasm. Surgery is rarely required in primary lung abscess but should be considered in patients who are unresponsive to antibiotics or have severe hemoptysis.

OTITIS MEDIA

method of
ELLEN R. WALD, M.D.
*University of Pittsburgh School of Medicine and
Children's Hospital of Pittsburgh*
Pittsburgh, Pennsylvania

Otitis media is the second (to the simple upper respiratory infection) most common organic disease presenting to the practitioner who cares for children. More than two thirds of all children will experience a single episode of acute otitis media by the age of 2 years, and one third of these will experience at least three episodes before their second birthday. Children who experience their first episode of acute otitis media early in the first year of life identify themselves as "otitis prone" and are subject to frequent recurrences of acute otitis media, persistent middle ear effusion, and subsequently chronic otitis media.

ACUTE OTITIS MEDIA

Pathogenesis

The current understanding of the pathogenesis of acute otitis media revolves around the concept of eustachian tube dysfunction. The three functions of the eustachian tube include ventilation, protection, and drainage. Under normal circumstances, the middle ear cleft is ventilated during yawning and swallowing. This allows the equilibration of air pressure between the middle ear and nasopharynx. Obstruction of the nasopharyngeal aspect of the eustachian tube impairs ventilation and fosters the development of negative pressure within the middle ear cavity (owing to absorption of oxygen by the respiratory mucosa lining the middle ear). The major risk factor for the development of acute otitis media is a simple upper respiratory infection. Eustachian tube obstruction may result from adenoidal hypertrophy (uncommon), mucosal edema, or impairment of the muscular function of the tensor veli palatini. When negative pressure is present in the middle ear cavity and the eustachian tube opens, nasopharyngeal mucus and bacteria may be aspirated into the middle ear and may initiate an episode of acute otitis media.

Diagnosis

Diagnosis is usually made by otoscopy, but certain symptoms may suggest more careful attention to the examination of the ears. Specific symptoms of ear infection include ear pain, otorrhea, diminished hearing, and vertigo. Nonspecific signs include fever and irritability. However, fever is frequently absent (one third to one half) in children with acute otitis media, and of course, irritability may be difficult to interpret. During the ear evaluation with a pneumatic otoscope, the examiner should systematically consider contour, color, translucence, and mobility. The normal drum is pearly gray, concave, translucent, and freely mobile.

Microbiology

Many studies have been performed to determine the bacteriology of acute otitis media. Table 1 shows the bacterial etiology of acute otitis media for children between 1 month and 6 years of age. *Streptococcus pneumoniae* is most common, followed by *Haemophilus influenzae* and *Moraxella catarrhalis*. The *S. pneumoniae* causing middle ear disease generally belongs to one of six common serotypes that are usually responsible for invasive diseases such as occult bacteremia, pneumonia, and meningitis. Although previously uniformly susceptible to penicillin and other β-lactams, *S. pneumoniae* has been noted to demonstrate increasing resistance to penicillin in many geographic areas both within and outside the United States. In certain areas of the United States, the prevalence of penicillin-resistant pneumococci is 50%. Pneumococci are considered susceptible to penicillin when their minimal inhibitory concentration (MIC) is less than 0.1 μg per mL. Resistance is categorized as intermediate when the MIC is between 0.1 and 1.0 μg per mL and as high-level when the MIC is 2.0 μg per mL or greater. Many strains of pneumococci that are resistant to penicillin are also resistant to cephalosporins, erythromycin, and trimethoprim-sulfamethoxazole.

The *Haemophilus* species that cause acute otitis media are usually nontypeable (rather than *H. influenzae* type b), reflecting the relative prevalence of these bacterial species as colonizers of the nasopharynx. These organisms may be β-lactamase producing and, accordingly, amoxicillin resistant. The prevalence of β-lactamase–producing *H. influenzae* varies geographically (between 10 and 65%) and even from year to year within geographic areas. *M. catarrhalis* is now recognized as an important cause of both acute sinusitis and acute otitis media. *M. catarrhalis* may also be found to produce β-lactamase in 80 to 95% of isolates. *Streptococcus pyogenes* (group A streptococcus) causes acute otitis media in 4 to 8% of cases. Staphylococci (both *Staphylococcus aureus* and *Staphylococcus epidermidis*) are uncommon causes of acute otitis media; when they are implicated as a cause of middle ear effusion, it is imperative to be sure that they are not contaminating flora from the skin of the external canal.

In nearly every series of cases of acute otitis media, approximately 20% of middle ear aspirates are sterile. These cases are clinically and otoscopically indistinguishable from the remainder with positive bacterial cultures. Studies have shown that anaerobes account for approximately 5% of these sterile effusions. Investigations into the viral etiology of otitis, with the use of new viral antigen detection techniques, show viruses to account for nearly 20% of cases of otitis media. In about half of these cases, virus alone is the cause; in the remainder, virus and bacterial agents are demonstrated. *Chlamydia trachomatis* may occasionally cause otitis media in young infants.

The list of bacterial agents causing acute otitis in the age group older than 6 years is shown in Table 2. *H. influenzae* continues to be an important cause of otitis media in older children, adolescents, and adults. Antimicrobial selection should be undertaken with this in mind.

The list of bacterial agents causing acute otitis media in neonates is shown in Table 3. Even in this age group, *S. pneumoniae* and *H. influenzae* are most common. *S. aureus* and gram-negative coliforms may cause infection approximately 20% of the time; the infants at risk for these agents are high-risk neonates who have spent extended periods in the intensive care unit and have required prolonged nasotracheal or nasogastric intubation. Infants who have been discharged from the hospital at 3 or 4 days and have been in the community before acquiring the respiratory infection that leads to otitis media are most likely to have the usual respiratory bacteria causing their ear infection.

Treatment and Follow-up

Antibiotic selection for patients with acute otitis media can be made from those listed in Table 4. Amoxicillin is still a reasonable choice for patients with uncomplicated infection. It works most of the

TABLE 2. Bacterial Isolates in Acute Otitis Media (Ages 6 Years to Adult)

Bacterial Isolates	Percentage
Streptococcus pneumoniae	35
Haemophilus influenzae	35
Streptococcus pyogenes	5
Other	5
Sterile	20

TABLE 1. Bacterial Isolates in Acute Otitis Media (Ages 1 Month to 6 Years)

Bacterial Isolates	Percentage
Streptococcus pneumoniae	30–40
Haemophilus influenzae	20–30
Moraxella catarrhalis	8–18
Streptococcus pyogenes	4–8
Staphylococcus aureus	1–2
Staphylococcus epidermidis	1–2
Sterile	25–35

TABLE 3. Bacterial Isolates in Neonatal Otitis Media

Bacterial Isolates	Percentage
Streptococcus pneumoniae	20
Haemophilus influenzae	15
Moraxella catarrhalis	5
Streptococci (A, B)	3
Staphylococci	8
Enterics	12

TABLE 4. **Antimicrobials and Dosage Schedules for the Treatment of Otitis Media in Children**

Antimicrobial	Dosage
Amoxicillin (Amoxil)	40 mg/kg in 3 divided doses
Amoxicillin–potassium clavulanate (Augmentin)*	Amoxicillin 45 mg/kg + potassium clavulanate 7.5 mg/kg/d in 2 divided doses
Erythromycin-sulfisoxazole (Pediazole)	Erythromycin 50 mg/kg + sulfisoxazole 150 mg/kg/d in 4 divided doses
Trimethoprim-sulfamethoxazole (Bactrim, Septra)	Trimethoprim 8 mg/kg + sulfamethoxazole 40 mg/kg/d in 2 divided doses
Cefuroxime axetil (Ceftin)*	30 mg/kg/d in 2 divided doses
Cefprozil (Cefzil)	30 mg/kg/d in 2 divided doses
Cefixime (Suprax)	8 mg/kg/d in 1 daily dose
Cefpodoxime proxetil (Vantin)*	8 mg/kg/d in 2 divided doses
Ceftibuten (Cedax)	9 mg/kg/d in 1 daily dose
Loracarbef (Lorabid)	30 mg/kg/d in 2 divided doses
Clindamycin (Cleocin)†	30 mg/kg/d in 4 divided doses

*These drugs are preferred in areas where the prevalence of β-lactamase–producing organisms or penicillin-resistant pneumococci is high.

†Clindamycin is preferred when the middle ear isolate is known to be a penicillin-resistant pneumococcus.

time and is inexpensive and extremely safe. For patients who fail to show response to amoxicillin, who live in an area with a high prevalence of β-lactamase–producing bacteria, or who have more complicated infections, alternative choices must be made. The most potent oral antimicrobials with the broadest spectra include amoxicillin–potassium clavulanate, cefuroxime axetil, and cefpodoxime proxetil. In areas with a high prevalence of penicillin-resistant pneumococci, these same antibiotics are preferred. Newer macrolides such as clarithromycin (Biaxin) and azithromycin (Zithromax) should be reserved for children with drug intolerance to the β-lactams. Clindamycin is recommended when the middle ear isolate is known to be a penicillin-resistant *S. pneumoniae*.

Antibiotics have traditionally been prescribed for 10 to 14 days. There has been recent interest in shorter durations of treatment (5 days) for children who are likely to recover quickly, including older children, those without a previous history of ear disease, those presenting in the summer, and those with mild illness. In most cases, a clinical response, that is, relief of otalgia and/or defervescence, is effected within 24 to 72 hours. When tympanocentesis is performed in cases in which clinical response has not occurred, approximately 20% of patients will have a resistant pathogen recovered. The results of tympanocentesis may guide antimicrobial choice in selected cases. Alternatively, if amoxicillin was the initial therapy, a change to an antimicrobial capable of eradicating β-lactamase–producing bacterial species would be advised.

Routine re-evaluation of the patient after 10 days is recommended. If the tympanic membrane appears normal or improved, antimicrobials may be terminated. The persistence of fluid alone, in an asymptomatic child with an improved or normal-appearing tympanic membrane, is not an indication for contin-

ued antimicrobials. Persistent effusion is commonly found at the end of a 10-day course of antimicrobials (50 to 70%) and will last for 3 months in approximately 10% of patients. If the tympanic membrane appears unchanged or worse at the 10-day mark despite clinical improvement, the same antimicrobial should be extended for another week or an alternative antimicrobial selected. Re-evaluation at the end of 7 to 10 days is again indicated.

For children with persistent middle ear effusion, there is concern about sustained hearing loss in time. If a significant hearing loss (>20 decibels bilaterally) is noted for more than 3 months, an intervention is recommended. One alternative is another course of antimicrobials with the thought that bacterial persistence may be causing some cases of persistent effusion. If antimicrobials fail to clear the effusion, myringotomy with or without tympanostomy tube placement is recommended. The tube placement is recommended when myringotomy can be done only under general anesthesia. If myringotomy can be done in the office setting, myringotomy alone should be tried for fluid removal, and tympanostomy tube placement should be reserved for cases in which fluid reaccumulates and persists in the next few months.

RECURRENT ACUTE OTITIS MEDIA

Some infants experience recurrent episodes of acute otitis media with nearly every new upper respiratory infection. When these episodes respond promptly to antimicrobials and middle ear effusion does not persist, each episode can be managed separately. However, if the number of episodes becomes excessive, e.g., more than three episodes in 6 months or more than four episodes in a year, antimicrobial prophylaxis may be undertaken to prevent new symptomatic episodes.

The drugs that have been used for antimicrobial prophylaxis include either sulfisoxazole (Gantrisin), 75 mg per kg per day in two divided doses, or amoxicillin, 20 mg per kg per day as a single nightly dose. Children receiving antimicrobial prophylaxis to prevent acute otitis media should be examined once per month to evaluate the problem of persistent effusion. Although symptomatic episodes of acute otalgia are avoided with antimicrobial prophylaxis, persistent effusion may complicate management and warrant an alternative strategy. If prophylaxis is prescribed, it is worth warning parents that the antimicrobial will not prevent the child from acquiring new viral upper respiratory infections, but it is hoped that these infections will not lead to secondary bacterial complications.

Tympanostomy tube placement is occasionally used to manage recurrent acute otitis media. The provision of sustained middle ear ventilation may allow the middle ear cavity to be restored to a more normal state. The tubes may also prevent structural damage and cholesteatoma from developing in cases of deep retraction pockets in the posterosuperior quadrant of the tympanic membrane.

Complications

The most common complication of otitis media is hearing loss. Some degree of hearing loss probably accompanies each episode of acute otitis media for a variable time. The impact of fluctuating mild hearing loss on language and intellectual development or ultimate cognitive function is unknown. When fluid accumulation persists for months, concern regarding hearing loss increases. Most episodes of acute otitis media lead to temporary and reversible episodes of conductive hearing loss. Rarely, the hearing loss may be sensorineural as well. Permanent conductive or sensorineural hearing loss occasionally results.

Perforation of the tympanic membrane may occur spontaneously in the course of acute otitis media or result after dislodgment of a tympanostomy tube. Small central perforations are associated with minimal hearing loss and usually go on to heal. Peripheral or marginal perforations may result in cholesteatoma formation.

Severe retraction pockets result from high negative pressure in the middle ear cavity and a flaccid tympanic membrane. These pockets may predispose to cholesteatoma formation. Cholesteatomas may cause ossicular damage and may also predispose to chronic suppurative otitis media.

Chronic suppurative otitis media is defined as chronic inflammation of the middle ear and mastoid characterized by persistent otorrhea through a perforated eardrum (>6 weeks) and failure to respond to the usual antibiotics prescribed for acute otitis media. In these cases, the bacterial species isolated from the middle ear cleft may be *Pseudomonas aeruginosa*, *Proteus mirabilis*, or *S. aureus* alone or in some combination. Many patients will respond to topical therapy with an aminoglycoside. If drainage does not cease within a few days, appropriate parenteral antimicrobials (ticarcillin-clavulanate [Timentin]) may be necessary. It is essential to evaluate the ear daily with appropriate aural toileting to determine when the drainage ceases. Parenteral antibiotics should be maintained for 1 week after cessation of the otorrhea.

Subclinical mastoiditis complicates many cases of acute otitis media. Treatment of the primary otitis media is usually effective in managing the mastoid problem. However, mastoiditis may progress to a clinical presentation with characteristic local pain or the formation of a subperiosteal abscess. In the former case, myringotomy plus parenteral antimicrobials may suffice. In the more complicated cases, incision and drainage or mastoidectomy is required in addition to parenteral antimicrobials.

ACUTE BRONCHITIS

method of
RICHARD GLECKMAN, M.D.
Boston University School of Medicine
Boston, Massachusetts

Acute bronchitis, an inflammatory condition of the bronchi, refers to a clinical syndrome whose most distinctive hallmark is the recent onset of cough. This disorder, which has a predilection for occurrence in the winter, is often preceded by headache, sore throat, and coryza; on occasion, it is accompanied by fever and chest discomfort. Bronchitis is usually but not exclusively caused by a respiratory pathogen, predominantly a virus (rhinovirus, coronavirus, adenovirus, influenza virus) and less frequently *Mycoplasma pneumoniae*, *Chlamydia pneumoniae*, *Bordetella pertussis*, *Legionella* species, *Streptococcus pneumoniae*, and *Haemophilus influenzae*. Neither the appearance of the sputum (purulence) nor the measurement of the white cell count is a reliable indicator of the cause of the acute bronchitis (viral versus bacterial).

When wheezing, shortness of breath, and tightness of the chest occur, the disease can resemble an acute attack of asthma. In fact, when these bronchospastic symptoms develop, patients often display spirometric evidence of reversible airway obstruction, which is referred to as "adult acute asthmatic bronchitis." The symptoms of acute infectious bronchitis, consisting of fever, chest discomfort, cough, and shortness of breath, imitate infectious pneumonia, and a chest radiograph is required to precisely distinguish acute bronchitis from pneumonia.

The preponderance of evidence indicates that most healthy individuals experience spontaneous resolution of the bronchitis and do not sustain any sequelae. These patients, with rare exception (such as disease caused by influenza virus), do not have their disease progress into a pneumonia or develop irreversible anatomic abnormalities of the respiratory tract. In contrast, patients with human immunodeficiency virus (HIV) infection are at risk for having their disease evolve into bronchiectasis.

I elect to perform neither blood nor sputum analyses for immunocompetent patients, and I do *not* prescribe an antibiotic. For the nonpregnant patient with "presumed" influenza A bronchitis and symptoms for less than 48 hours, either amantadine (Symmetrel) or rimantadine (Flumadine) should be prescribed. Patients who experience insomnia from "bouts" of coughing can obtain symptomatic improvement from an antitussive codeine-containing medication, and patients who have symptoms consistent with adult acute asthmatic bronchitis are candidates for inhaled bronchodilator therapy.

Most physicians feel pressure to prescribe an antibiotic, however, because the public has the expectation of receiving a "magic bullet" to hasten the resolution of the infection. Patients should be reassured that most infections are viral and will not respond to an antibiotic. In addition, physicians are concerned that some of these episodes of acute bronchitis are precipitated by *potentially* treatable organisms (*M. pneumoniae, C. pneumoniae, B. pertussis*). Although there are no rapid, readily available ways, either clinical or laboratory, to distinguish these etiologic agents, and although there are no convincing data that antibiotic treatment accelerates the resolution of the symptoms of acute bronchitis caused by *M. pneumoniae* or *C. pneumoniae*, clinicians often elect to administer a course of an antimicrobial (e.g., erythromycin, clarithromycin, azithromycin, doxycycline, cefaclor, cefuroxime, loracarbef, trimethoprim-sulfamethoxazole). I believe that this approach has no scientific foundation, adds to medical costs, fosters the emergence of resistant organisms, and contributes to toxic effects of the drug, such as skin eruptions and gastrointestinal adverse events.

Many patients, with or without antimicrobial therapy, will cough for weeks. If a patient fails to improve within 4 to 5 days, efforts should be made to confirm the diagnosis, exclude alternative disorders (including pneumonia), and identify specific offending pathogens, such as *B. pertussis*, because patients infected with this bacterium merit antibiotic treatment (erythromycin or trimethoprim-sulfamethoxazole) and serve as a reservoir of infection for nonimmune children and adults.

Acute bronchitis is the most frequent lower respiratory tract illness in HIV-infected patients. These patients typically present with cough, purulent sputum, and low-grade fever. Their sputum culture often grows *S. pneumoniae, H. influenzae*, or *Pseudomonas aeruginosa*. They should receive an antibiotic. Unfortunately, however, they are prone to recurrences. When HIV-infected patients with acute bronchitis manifest cough and shortness of breath *unaccompanied* by purulent sputum, an effort needs to be made to distinguish this disease from *Pneumocystis carinii* pneumonia in which the chest radiograph is normal.

ACUTE EXACERBATION OF CHRONIC BRONCHITIS

When a patient with known chronic bronchitis experiences a syndrome consisting of the abrupt development of fatigue, chest tightness, worsening cough, and dyspnea accompanied by an increased volume and/or purulence of sputum, an "exacerbation" has been defined. The syndrome does not require all these elements, and although infections precipitate some of these exacerbations, most exacerbations are unassociated with fever. The exacerbation not only produces uncomfortable and disabling symptoms, but can result in lost work time, significant financial costs, and hospitalization. The 7.5 million Americans with chronic bronchitis are not a homogeneous group. Some of these individuals escape exacerbations, some have one or two winter exacerbations, and others have numerous episodes per year.

Certainly not all exacerbations are precipitated by an infectious event. Those organisms most frequently associated with the exacerbation of chronic bronchitis include viruses, *M. pneumoniae, H. influenzae, S. pneumoniae*, and *Branhamella (Moraxella) catarrhalis*. Limited data suggest a role for *Haemophilus parainfluenzae* and, rarely, *C. pneumoniae*.

As a general rule, there is no compelling need to analyze the blood or sputum or to obtain a chest x-ray study during the first encounter with a patient who does not appear seriously ill. A blood gas determination would be appropriate for patients experiencing insomnia, agitation, or increasing dyspnea.

For more than 50 years, physicians have prescribed antimicrobial agents to patients with chronic bronchitis who were experiencing an exacerbation, but the efficacy of this treatment has remained a subject of controversy. It has been difficult to assess the value of administering an antimicrobial to these patients because there is no precise definition of an exacerbation, not all exacerbations are caused by a bacterial infection, patients' symptoms are often relieved by comedications, and meaningful end points of treatment are difficult to identify. In addition, there are few published clinical trials, and the available investigations have some design defects. My interpretation of the published randomized trials is that antibiotic treatment exerts a modest but statistically significant clinical improvement. Antimicrobials appear to have their greatest impact on therapy for the patient experiencing a more severe exacerbation, not simply increased sputum production or a change in the appearance of the sputum but both of these features plus increased shortness of breath. Antimicrobials have accelerated the rate of clinical resolution and reduced the need for additional medication, return visits, and hospitalization.

Table 1 lists the macrolides, aminopenicillins, cephalosporins, carbacephem, fluoroquinolones, trimethoprim-sulfamethoxazole combination, and tetracyclines that clinicians prescribe for patients experiencing an exacerbation of chronic bronchitis. There are no convincing scientific data to indicate that any one of these oral agents produces enhanced clinical resolution compared with the others. Features of the host and antimicrobial that influence drug selection include the following: the patient's history of drug allergy; the drug's track record; the drug's potential to initiate untoward events or undesirable drug-drug interactions; the drug's spectrum of activity; the ease of compliance; and the drug's costs.

Trimethoprim-sulfamethoxazole and doxycycline appear to be appealing drugs. They inhibit the growth of the majority of bacteria incriminated in the exacerbation of chronic bronchitis, are an appropriate selection for the penicillin-allergic patient, are prescribed as a twice-daily regimen, are relatively safe compounds, have an established track record, and are inexpensive antimicrobials. With regard to trimethoprim-sulfamethoxazole, however, some patients develop hypersensitivity reactions (fever, rash) or gastrointestinal untoward events, and there is a risk for interaction when there is coadministration with warfarin (Coumadin), cyclosporine (Sandim-

TABLE 1. **Antimicrobial Agents for Exacerbation of Chronic Bronchitis**

Generic Name	Trade Name
Macrolides	
Erythromycin	E-Mycin, Ery-Tab, E-Base, Ilotycin, PCE, Robimycin
Clarithromycin	Biaxin
Azithromycin	Zithromax
Dirithromycin	Dynabac
Cephalosporins	
Cefaclor	Ceclor
Cefuroxime	Ceftin
Cefixime	Suprax
Cefprozil	Cefzil
Cefpodoxime	Vantin
Ceftibuten	Cedax
Carbacephem	
Loracarbef	Lorabid
Aminopenicillins	
Ampicillin	Omnipen, Polycillin, Principen, Totacillin
Amoxicillin	Amoxil, Polymox, Trimox, Wymox
Amoxicillin-clavulanate	Augmentin
Bacampicillin	Spectrobid
Fluoroquinolones	
Ciprofloxacin	Cipro
Ofloxacin	Floxin
Lomefloxacin	Maxaquin
Levofloxacin	Levaquin
Sparfloxacin	Zagam
Trimethoprim-sulfamethoxazole	Bactrim, Septra, Cotrim
Tetracyclines	
Doxycycline	Vibramycin
Minocycline	Minocin
Tetracycline	

mune), phenytoin (Dilantin), methotrexate, and oral hypoglycemic agents. In addition, older patients are at greater risk of experiencing trimethoprim-sulfamethoxazole–induced blood dyscrasias and hyperkalemia. Doxycycline has a potential to cause gastrointestinal toxic effects. Treatment with either of these compounds can be restricted to approximately 1 week.

Ancillary treatment consists of encouraging smoking cessation. The use of a bronchodilator, such as ipratropium (Atrovent) or a beta-adrenergic sympathomimetic agent, may confer some additional benefit. The value of drinking copious fluids or taking an expectorant is undocumented. Patients usually improve clinically within 4 days and achieve complete resolution of the exacerbation within 2 weeks.

When a patient fails to demonstrate any improvement within 5 days, the clinician should consider the following: incorrect diagnosis (perhaps pneumonia, neoplasm, or congestive heart failure); an issue with compliance; inappropriate antimicrobial selection (organism resistant to the medication prescribed); diminished antimicrobial bioavailability (the coadministration of iron, antacids, didanosine [ddI, Vi-

dex], and multivitamins with zinc decreases the absorption of tetracyclines and fluoroquinolones); and excessive bronchospasm and bronchial secretions.

Patients with chronic bronchitis are candidates for an annual influenza immunization as well as a pneumococcal vaccine, although the value of pneumococcal vaccine for these patients is controversial. Another potential preventive measure is to offer the patient antibiotic prophylaxis, with an agent such as tetracycline, ampicillin, amoxicillin, or trimethoprim-sulfamethoxazole prescribed once daily either four times a week or daily during the winter. The published scientific data are "soft" here, however. Antibiotic prophylaxis should be restricted to the patient who experiences four or more exacerbations per year.

BACTERIAL PNEUMONIA

method of
STEPHEN B. GREENBERG, M.D.
Baylor College of Medicine
Houston, Texas

Acute pneumonia occurs in approximately 3 million persons in the United States each year. Of those affected, 20% are hospitalized. As the sixth leading cause of death in this country, it remains a major public health problem. Certain groups are particularly prone to acquiring pneumonia: the elderly, the immunosuppressed, and those with underlying diseases such as diabetes mellitus and chronic obstructive pulmonary disease (COPD). Patients with these underlying conditions or those on mechanical ventilation have an increased risk for nosocomial pneumonia. Bacterial pneumonia is the third most common hospital-acquired infection.

ETIOLOGY

Adherent bacteria that colonize the upper airway are aspirated into the lower airway and alveoli, where they multiply. Some bacteria such as *Pseudomonas aeruginosa* can colonize the trachea directly. *Mycobacterium tuberculosis* and *Legionella* species reach the lung through inhalation of airborne droplets. Outbreaks of pneumococcal pneumonia in closed populations, such as in prisons, suggest the possibility of aerosolization of pneumococci into the lower airways.

Community-acquired pneumonias differ from nosocomial pneumonias in the organisms isolated (Table 1). Although the frequency varies widely in published series, *Streptococcus pneumoniae* probably accounts for well above half of community-acquired pneumonias. Of the remaining bacterial isolates, *Haemophilus influenzae*, *Staphylococcus aureus*, enteric gram-negative rods, and anaerobes are most frequently cultured. Viruses probably account for 8 to 10% of community-acquired pneumonias. *Chlamydia pneumoniae*, *Mycoplasma pneumoniae*, *Coxiella burnetii* (Q fever), and *Legionella* species are responsible for approximately 30% of cases. In many published series, no identifiable pathogen is found in 25% of cases.

Although bacterial pneumonia affects the young and old disproportionately, all age groups are candidates for this infection. Specific etiologic agents can be suggested on the basis of a knowledge of the patient's age, season, geo-

TABLE 1. **Etiology of Community-Acquired and Nosocomial Pneumonias**

Agent	Community Acquired (%)	Nosocomial (%)
Streptococcus pneumoniae	33–67	6
Mycoplasma pneumoniae	9	—
Haemophilus influenzae	7	5
Virus	7	—
Legionella species	6	—
Chlamydia species	6	—
Staphylococcus aureus	3	8
Aerobic gram-negative bacteria	5	80

graphic location, and underlying conditions. Predisposition to community-acquired pneumonia is increased by alcoholism, malnutrition, and recent hospitalization. Smoking and recent respiratory viral infections are thought to be important factors contributing to decreased pulmonary clearance of bacteria. Diminished neutrophil function and phagocytic capacity have been reported with diabetes mellitus, chronic steroid use, cirrhosis, and renal failure. Production of specific immunoglobulins may be diminished in human immunodeficiency virus (HIV)–infected patients, in lymphoma or myeloma patients, and with common variable immunodeficiency syndrome.

Patients with COPD or a smoking history are prone to *H. influenzae*, *Branhamella (Moraxella) catarrhalis*, and *Legionella* infections. Gram-negative bacilli are found more commonly in debilitated and alcoholic patients. *S. aureus* is more common after influenza virus infection and in intravenous drug users. *Legionella* species, *M. pneumoniae*, and *C. pneumoniae* are identified more commonly in summer and fall. A history of exposure to birds should suggest psittacosis; to rabbits, tularemia; to cattle, Q fever; and to water-heating units, *Legionella* infection. HIV infection changes the spectrum of organisms causing community-acquired pneumonia to *Pneumocystis carinii*, *M. tuberculosis*, pneumococci, and endemic fungi.

Most nosocomial pneumonias are caused by aerobic gram-negative bacilli. More than one bacterium is isolated from the lower respiratory tract in 40% of nosocomial pneumonias. The mortality rate has not changed for the past 2 decades and remains approximately 50%.

DIAGNOSIS

Clinical signs and symptoms of acute bacterial pneumonia include fever, chills, productive cough, and pleuritic chest pain. Physical examination reveals an acutely ill, febrile patient with tachypnea. A new pulmonary infiltrate on chest radiographs is common.

Several studies have attempted to define indications for hospitalization in patients with community-acquired pneumonia. Severe vital sign abnormalities such as tachycardia (>140 beats per minute), decreased systolic blood pressure (<90 mm Hg), and tachypnea (>30 breaths per minute) are indications for admission. Altered mental status and arterial hypoxemia (Po_2 < 60 mm Hg) are also indications for admission. Acute electrolyte, hematologic, or metabolic laboratory abnormalities are also reasons for hospitalization. Any acute coexisting medical condition or related suppurative infection, i.e., empyema, septic arthritis, meningitis, or endocarditis, should also be a criterion for hospitalizing a patient with acute pneumonia. Increased mortal-

ity has been noted in patients with bacterial pneumonia who are 60 years old or have multiple lobes involved.

There are no differentiating clinical characteristics among the common bacterial pneumonias. Sputum and blood cultures should be obtained. Peripheral leukocytosis is common, but leukopenia can occur. Debate concerning the utility of Gram's stain in the diagnosis of bacterial pneumonia continues. Proponents for the use of Gram's stain for diagnostic purposes give the following arguments: (1) a specimen that is diagnostic can be obtained in more than 50% of cases; (2) patients are better off with a known diagnosis; and (3) there are problems with empirical treatment. Those who do not use Gram's stain for diagnosis of bacterial pneumonia state the following: (1) 50% of patients with community-acquired pneumonia cannot produce sputum; (2) the Gram stain is reliable in only 50 to 67% of cases; (3) few physicians are currently competent to interpret the Gram stain; and (4) newer antimicrobials are not too toxic. Most authorities agree that an adequate sputum sample should have fewer than 10 squamous epithelial cells and more than 25 polymorphonuclear leukocytes per low-power field. In ventilated patients, quantitative bacteriology from bronchoalveolar lavage fluid or protected brush specimens can help in determining the cause of nosocomial pneumonias.

No one chest x-ray finding is specific or unique to any one bacterial species. Lobar infiltrates are common, but diffuse bronchoalveolar infiltrates can occur. Cavitation is described with *S. aureus*, *S. pneumoniae*, anaerobes, and *M. tuberculosis*. Parapneumonic effusions are common, especially with *S. pneumoniae* and *S. aureus*.

TREATMENT

Community-Acquired Pneumonia

In 1993, the American Thoracic Society published guidelines for empirical antimicrobial therapy for adults with community-acquired pneumonia (Table 2). Initial therapy is to be guided by the likely pathogen in a specific epidemiologic setting. Patients without a co-morbid condition and younger than 60 years are to receive a macrolide or tetracycline if they are allergic to or intolerant of macrolides. The newer macrolides, clarithromycin or azithromycin, should be used if there is intolerance of erythromycin and in smokers. Patients with a co-morbid condition such as COPD or bronchiectasis and/or older than 60 years should receive a second-generation cephalosporin or trimethoprim-sulfamethoxazole or a β-lactam–β-lactamase inhibitor with or without a macrolide. Patients with lung conditions are prone to infection with *H. influenzae*, *S. aureus*, *M. catarrhalis*, and *Klebsiella pneumoniae* in addition to *S. pneumoniae*. These pathogens should respond to second-generation cephalosporins.

Penicillin-resistant pneumococci are increasing in frequency throughout the United States. Macrolides are still effective for 98% of penicillin-sensitive pneumococci and 50% of penicillin-resistant pneumococci. Newer fluoroquinolones are effective against penicillin-resistant pneumococci, as are the third-generation cephalosporins cefotaxime (Claforan) and ceftriaxone (Rocephin).

Patients requiring hospitalization usually have se-

TABLE 2. **Recommendations for Empirical Treatment of Community-Acquired Pneumonia**

Outpatient pneumonia without comorbidity* and age ≤60 years
  Preferred: macrolide: erythromycin; alternative (clarithromycin or azithromycin) with erythromycin intolerance and smokers (to treat *H. influenzae*)
  Alternative: tetracycline

Outpatient pneumonia with comorbidity† and/or age ≥60 years
  Second-generation cephalosporin or trimethoprim-sulfamethoxazole, or β-lactam–β-lactamase inhibitor with or without erythromycin or other macrolide if *Legionella* is a concern

Hospitalized patients
  Second- or third-generation cephalosporin or β-lactam–β-lactamase inhibitor with or without erythromycin if legionellosis is a concern; rifampin may be added if *Legionella* is documented

Severe community-acquired pneumonia‡
  Macrolide (with rifampin if legionellosis) plus third-generation cephalosporin with anti-*Pseudomonas* activity or other antipseudomonal agent such as imipenem or ciprofloxacin plus an aminoglycoside

*Excludes patients with risk for human immunodeficiency virus infection.
†Comorbid illness includes chronic obstructive lung disease, diabetes mellitus, renal insufficiency, congestive heart failure, hospitalization within past year, postsplenectomy state, chronic alcohol abuse, malnutrition, altered mental status, and suspected aspiration.
‡Respiratory rate > 30/min, PaO_2/FiO_2 ratio < 250 mm Hg, requirement for mechanical ventilation, radiograph showing bilateral or multiple lobe involvement, systolic blood pressure < 90 mm Hg or diastolic < 60 mm Hg, requirement for vasopressors > 4 hours, or renal failure.
From Niederman MS, Bass JB Jr, Campbell GD, et al: Guidelines for the initial management of adults with community-acquired pneumonia: Diagnosis, assessment of severity, and initial antimicrobial therapy. American Thoracic Society. Medical Section of the American Lung Association. Am Rev Respir Dis 148:1418–1426, 1993.

vere community-acquired pneumonia. Severe community-acquired pneumonia often presents with tachypnea, hypoxemia, shock, and oliguria. Multilobar radiographic involvement is more common. If mechanical ventilation or close monitoring is needed, the patient will require intensive care unit (ICU) care. Although *S. pneumoniae* is still a common cause of severe community-acquired pneumonia, *H. influenzae*, gram-negative bacilli, and *S. aureus* are isolated in increasing numbers.

If severe community-acquired pneumonia occurs in patients younger than 60 years and without co-morbid conditions, initial treatment could be a macrolide plus a third-generation cephalosporin (ceftriaxone or cefotaxime) or high-dose penicillin plus a quinolone. If *Legionella* is documented, rifampin should be added. If *Pseudomonas* is possible, a third-generation cephalosporin (ceftazidime [Fortaz]) or carbapenem (imipenem-cilastatin [Primaxin] or meropenem [Merrem]) or quinolones (ciprofloxacin [Cipro] or ofloxacin [Floxin]) should be added to a macrolide. Patients in the ICU with co-morbid conditions and older than 60 years should have an aminoglycoside added to one of the regimens for better anti-*Pseudomonas* coverage.

Duration of treatment for most patients with community-acquired pneumonia should be 5 to 7 days. Parenteral antibiotics can be switched to oral agents when the patient has improved clinically and the

fever has abated. With clinical improvement and no complications, the patient can complete the course of antibiotics at home. Home intravenous antibiotic therapy can be used in patients well enough to be discharged but in whom parenteral antibiotics are indicated. A cephalosporin with a long half-life (e.g., ceftriaxone) may be useful.

Nosocomial Pneumonia

The mortality rate for nosocomial pneumonia has not changed significantly in recent years. Host factors and the use of appropriate antibiotics are important for recovery. Certain gram-negative bacteria such as *Pseudomonas, Enterobacter,* and *Acinetobacter* species are associated with a high mortality rate and a poorer response to antibiotics. Presumptive therapy should include a cephalosporin such as ceftazidime (Fortaz) or cefuroxime (Zinacef) plus an aminoglycoside. Other broad-spectrum antibiotics could be used: imipenem, ticarcillin-clavulanate (Timentin), or aztreonam (Azactam). After confirmation of a specific pathogen, the antibiotic regimen can be adjusted to the least expensive, least toxic, and most effective combination.

Nonresponse to Treatment

There are several possible reasons for patients not to respond to antibiotic therapy. The disease may be too far advanced at the time of treatment. It is uncommon for the wrong antibiotic selection or microbial diagnosis to be the reason for a poor response. A patient who is debilitated, is immunosuppressed, or has severe associated disease may not respond. Complicated pneumonia with parapneumonic effusion or bronchial obstruction may not respond to antibiotics alone. Noninfectious diseases can occasionally mimic pneumonia, and the diagnosis can be delayed. These noninfectious diseases include pulmonary infarction, congestive heart failure, Wegener's granulomatosis, sarcoidosis, and atelectasis. The mortality rate for hospitalized patients with community-acquired or nosocomial pneumonia remains high despite excellent antibiotics. Newer, innovative preventive measures and treatment options are being tested to improve the outcome in this serious infection.

VIRAL RESPIRATORY INFECTIONS

method of
ROBERT B. COUCH, M.D.
Baylor College of Medicine
Houston, Texas

Viral infection is the most common cause of acute respiratory illness. Such illnesses are more common in children than in adults and during the winter than during the summer in temperate climates. The viruses causing most viral respiratory illnesses are the rhinoviruses, coronaviruses, influenza viruses, parainfluenza viruses, respiratory syncytial virus, and a number of adenoviruses and enteroviruses. Infection may be asymptomatic or exhibit one of a variety of syndromes or combinations of syndromes. Typical viral infection syndromes are the common cold, pharyngitis, upper respiratory illness, laryngitis, laryngotracheobronchitis (croup), tracheobronchitis, bronchiolitis, and influenza. Pneumonia may also be caused by a virus infection. Certain viruses exhibit a tendency to produce similar illnesses, and this may aid in guiding diagnosis and therapy. At present, specific antiviral therapy is available for severe bronchiolitis and pneumonia in infants caused by respiratory syncytial virus and acute influenza caused by an influenza A virus. Rapid diagnostic tests that have high sensitivity for virus detection in young children with more severe illness are available for both of these.

GENERAL PRINCIPLES OF TREATMENT

Severe viral pneumonia leading to death can occur, but most respiratory viral infections are self-limited and followed by complete recovery. Because specific antivirals are not available for most causative viruses and most of these self-limited illnesses are mild, the guiding principle of treatment is to ameliorate symptoms until recovery occurs. Thus, an important consideration is to do no harm. In keeping with these principles, it is my practice to employ as few medications as possible and to attempt to alleviate only the distressing symptoms. Because most "cold remedies" include a variety of medications in combination, many of uncertain benefit, it is preferable to avoid them.

Antimicrobial agents should not be used during the acute phase of viral respiratory disease. These agents have no antiviral effect and in all probability do not prevent the uncommon case of secondary bacterial infection. Moreover, if secondary bacterial disease develops during their use, it is usually with a resistant organism. In addition, the use of antimicrobials may result in toxic effects or sensitize the patient to a valuable therapeutic agent. Demanding patients will usually accept the judgment of a thoughtful physician in this regard.

Isolation of persons with viral respiratory disease is impractical because of the omnipresence of these infectious agents, but a reduction in activities, frequent hand washing, and efforts to prevent secretion spread by ill persons may impair transmission to others.

TREATMENT OF SPECIFIC SYMPTOMS
Malaise and Fatigue

Activity should be curtailed in keeping with the extent of the symptoms. Bed rest is indicated in those patients with fever. Adequate diet should be maintained and oral fluids encouraged.

Fever

Acetaminophen is preferred for therapy because of the association of acetylsalicylic acid (aspirin) with Reye's syndrome after influenza in children and sometimes adults. For persons with body temperature greater than 101.5°F, acetaminophen is given in doses of 0.6 gram every 4 to 6 hours to adults. For infants and children, dosages are 40 mg for those 0 to 3 months, 80 mg for those 4 to 11 months, 120 mg for those 12 to 23 months, 160 mg for those 2 to 3 years, 240 mg for those 4 to 5 years, 320 mg for those 6 to 8 years, 400 mg for those 9 to 10 years, and 480 mg for those 11 to 12 years. If preferred, aspirin in doses of 0.6 gram every 4 to 6 hours may be used for adults. In individuals with nausea and vomiting, acetaminophen suppositories may be used at 4- to 6-hour intervals; dosages are 80 mg every 6 hours for infants 3 to 11 months, 80 mg every 4 hours for those 1 to 3 years, 120 mg every 4 to 6 hours for those 3 to 6 years, 325 mg every 4 to 6 hours for those 6 to 12 years, and 325 to 650 mg every 4 to 6 hours for adults. Nonsteroidal anti-inflammatory drugs are an alternative for control of fever. Ibuprofen in dosages of 200 to 400 mg every 4 to 6 hours may be used by adults and 5 to 10 mg per kg every 6 to 8 hours by children. Reduction of high fever may additionally require sponging with tepid water or alcohol; these methods should be employed vigorously to reduce high fever in infants and small children to avoid febrile convulsions.

Headache

Acetaminophen or ibuprofen in the dosages listed for fever are effective for control of headache in most persons. Aspirin in the doses listed is an alternative for adults. On occasion, codeine, 32 or 64 mg every 4 to 6 hours orally or by injection, will be necessary to control pain; when it is combined with 25 mg of promethazine (Phenergan), severe headache in adults is usually relieved.

Nasal Obstruction

Humidification of room air with a portable humidifier should be provided. Cool mist humidifiers are preferable so that the mist may be directed toward the resting or sleeping patient. Phenylephrine nose drops in a 0.25% solution should be used in patients with sufficient nasal obstruction to necessitate mouth breathing. In infants, 2 drops should be instilled into each nostril, with the head extended, 15 minutes before feeding and at bedtime. After instillation, the head should be rotated from side to side for a few seconds. Four or 5 drops of 0.25% phenylephrine, 0.1% xylometazoline (Otrivin), or 0.05% oxymetazoline (Afrin) is satisfactory for adults. Phenylephrine may be used three or four times daily, but the other two topical medications are used every 12 hours. Nose drops should be used for no more than 4 or 5 days because overuse will result in lack of effectiveness and rebound nasal congestion.

Rhinorrhea

Rhinorrhea uncommonly requires medication. The irritating effect of secretions on the face and upper lip may be reduced by using bland creams. If treatment is thought necessary, oral antihistamine therapy is frequently beneficial. Chlorpheniramine, 4 mg every 6 hours, is recommended for adults with use of 8-mg enteric-coated tablets at bedtime. Children younger than 12 years should be given 2 mg and infants 1 mg as fractions of a tablet or as a syrup (2 mg per 5 mL). The selective histamine H_1-receptor antagonist loratadine (Claritin), 10 mg once a day, may be used in persons older than 12 years if somnolence must be avoided.

Sore Throat

Warm saltwater gargles (½ teaspoonful of salt to ½ glass of warm water) and humidification of air are frequently sufficient to relieve sore throat. Analgesics such as ibuprofen, acetaminophen, or aspirin (adults only), in doses already given, may sometimes be helpful.

Hoarseness

Persons with hoarseness should avoid speaking and are more comfortable in humidified air.

Cough

Troublesome cough should be treated with an expectorant and humidified air. Guaifenesin (Robitussin) is recommended as an expectorant. For severe cough requiring a suppressant, guaifenesin with dextromethorphan (Robitussin-DM) is recommended. Dosage of each for adults is 2 teaspoonfuls every 4 to 6 hours. Dosages are halved for children 6 to 12 years and quartered for those 2 to 6 years. Guaifenesin only is recommended for infants.

Respiratory Distress

Respiratory distress due to viral respiratory infection is rarely encountered except in infants and young children. If it is encountered in an adult, it is because of mucous plugs in the trachea or major bronchi, pneumothorax induced by coughing, or an unrelated complication. If mucous plugs are not removed by humidification, postural drainage, and vigorous coughing, aspiration for removal via bronchoscopy or intubation is indicated. Respiratory distress attributable to viral bronchiolitis or pneumonia is common in infants and small children and frequently requires hospitalization. Supplementary oxygen is usually required to correct hypoxemia. Heavy mist should be provided, and the patients should be given 0.45% saline solution intravenously. A trial of nebulized *l*-epinephrine should be employed for persistent distress (see "Croup" for dosage). Corticosteroids are not beneficial. Gentle suctioning may be used as the child begins to raise secretions.

Croup

In children with croup, humidified air is helpful, and on occasion heavy mist in the shower stall or bathroom is necessary to facilitate air exchange. If humidification is inadequate, relief of the spasm of croup may be provided by inhalation of nebulized epinephrine. Because this is not easily done in the home, hospitalization is recommended so that oxygen and steroids may also be given if needed. Three to 5 mL of 1:1000 *l*-epinephrine in saline is given by nebulizer and repeated at 2-hour intervals as needed. Observation for possible rebound obstruction is required. At admission, 0.6 mg per kg of dexamethasone (Decadron) should also be given intramuscularly for severe illness.

Complications

Secondary bacterial infections sometimes follow a viral respiratory illness and result in otitis media, sinusitis, or pneumonia. They usually occur 5 to 10 days after onset of the acute viral infection and frequently follow a period of improvement. Appropriate antimicrobial agents are indicated for these conditions.

Persistent nasal discharge and productive cough often occur after proven acute viral respiratory illness without evidence of one of the clinical entities given before. When the nasal discharge and sputum are purulent, a common practice is to administer antimicrobial agents for 2 to 4 days; prompt relief from the symptoms frequently results. In such circumstances, amoxicillin is recommended because it is economical and usually effective.

SPECIFIC ANTIVIRAL THERAPY

Respiratory Syncytial Virus Infection

Ribavirin by small-particle aerosol is effective for treatment of acute bronchiolitis and pneumonia in infants caused by respiratory syncytial virus infection. Treatment is recommended for hospitalized patients and is administered into a tent, oxygen hood, mask, or ventilator for 12 to 20 hours a day until clinical improvement occurs, usually 2 to 5 days. A small-particle aerosol generator with recommended reservoir drug concentrations is available from ICN Pharmaceuticals (Costa Mesa, CA). Treatment is well tolerated.

Influenza A

Amantadine (Symmetrel) and rimantadine (Flumadine) are effective for prophylaxis and treatment of influenza A. Each is recommended as a 200-mg dose initially and 100 mg twice daily thereafter for 3 to 5 days for treatment and 100 mg twice daily for prophylaxis of healthy persons 10 to 65 years. Those older than 65 years should be given 100 mg daily; 5 mg per kg twice daily is recommended for prophylaxis with either drug for those 1 to 10 years, but only amantadine at that same dosage is approved for treatment of young children. Neither drug is approved for those younger than 1 year. Reductions in dosage of amantadine are required for persons with underlying renal disease (consult the package insert for dosing).

Administration of influenza vaccine is preferred for prevention of influenza. However, amantadine and rimantadine are alternatives for prevention of influenza A, but they must be used throughout the exposure period. This is generally 4 to 8 weeks for community exposure, 2 to 4 weeks for population exposure such as in a nursing home, and 10 days for exposure to an active case such as in the home. Rimantadine is preferred for prophylaxis because of equal effectiveness and fewer adverse reactions. Amantadine causes mild and sometimes severe central nervous system symptoms at recommended doses; rimantadine induces few reactions. Treatment hastens clearance of symptoms if it is started within 48 hours of illness onset. Although not proven to be beneficial, a 3- to 5-day course of treatment is recommended for acutely ill elderly persons and those with significant underlying disease, even if it is started after 48 hours of symptoms. Because of risk for emergence of resistant virus, treatment of young children to whom persons with underlying disease may be exposed is not recommended.

VIRAL AND MYCOPLASMAL PNEUMONIAS

method of
ROBERT C. WELLIVER, M.D.
State University of New York at Buffalo School of Medicine and Biomedical Sciences and Children's Hospital of Buffalo
Buffalo, New York

VIRAL PNEUMONIAS

Etiologic Agents

Viruses are the most common causes of community-acquired pneumonia and are probably still the most frequent cause of hospital-acquired pneumonia. Although essentially any respiratory virus may infrequently cause pneumonia, the agents responsible for the majority of cases of pneumonia in various age groups are indicated in Table 1.

Clinical and Laboratory Diagnosis

Respiratory syncytial virus (RSV) infection occurs, in temperate climates, in annual outbreaks essentially from December through April. In the tropics,

TABLE 1. Etiologic Agents in Viral Pneumonia

Age or Condition	Relative Frequency*
Infancy and early childhood	
Respiratory syncytial virus	+ + + +
Parainfluenza viruses	+ +
Influenza virus type A	+ +
Adenovirus	+
Adolescence and early adulthood	
Influenza virus type A	+ +
Adenovirus	+ +
Elderly	
Influenza virus type A	+ + + +
Respiratory syncytial virus	+
Immunocompromised, any age	
Cytomegalovirus	+ + + +
Herpes simplex virus	+ +
Varicella-zoster virus	+ +
Epstein-Barr virus	+
Respiratory syncytial virus	+

*Range is + for relatively uncommon to + + + +, very common.

cases may occur throughout the year. In otherwise normal hosts, the hallmark of RSV infection is the presence of airway obstruction with wheezing on auscultation and hyperinflation (often with patchy atelectasis) on chest radiographs. In infants with cardiac disease, diffuse interstitial infiltrates are more commonly observed. A definitive diagnosis may be made by identification of viral antigen in respiratory secretions with use of enzyme-linked immunosorbent assay techniques or in exfoliated airway epithelial cells by immunofluorescence. Commercially available kits for both of these techniques are at least as accurate as, and far more rapid than, conventional cell culture or serologic techniques.

Influenza virus infections also occur in winter outbreaks, which are often sufficiently extensive to result in school closings or recognizable increases in mortality rates among the elderly. Influenza virus infection is often suggested by the patient's complaints of headache, severe myalgia, and prostration out of proportion to the degree of respiratory symptoms. Chest radiographs reveal diffuse, interstitial infiltrates. Lobar consolidation suggests the presence of bacterial superinfection. As for RSV, a specific diagnosis of influenza virus infection can often be made much earlier by antigen detection techniques than by standard cell culture or serology.

Members of the herpes group of viruses, especially cytomegalovirus (CMV), herpes simplex virus, varicella-zoster virus, and to a somewhat lesser extent Epstein-Barr virus, cause particularly severe, life-threatening pneumonia in subjects with suppressed function of T lymphocytes. The technique of polymerase chain reaction is useful for the rapid diagnosis of CMV infection but is not yet widely available. A diagnosis of infection by each of these agents can be made by application of antigen detection techniques to various clinical specimens. The shell vial technique often accelerates the rate of identification of some of these agents in cell culture.

Hantavirus pneumonia is an uncommon illness

that may occur in association with renal failure and capillary leak syndromes. The other viruses listed in Table 1 cause pneumonia infrequently and rarely cause recognizable clinical syndromes. A specific diagnosis of parainfluenza virus and adenovirus infection can sometimes be made by use of antigen detection techniques or cell culture. However, illness caused by these agents is usually mild in nature, and no specific forms of therapy are available.

Treatment

Respiratory Syncytial Virus Infection

Most infants hospitalized with RSV infection will improve with supplemental oxygen and replacement of fluid deficits, and they will be ready for discharge as soon as oral fluid intake is adequate. Ribavirin (Virazole) is a guanosine analogue with in vitro activity against a wide variety of viruses. It is licensed for treatment of serious RSV infection in infants with underlying heart or lung disease, premature birth (probably those infants born at less than 32 weeks' gestation), and chronic conditions that would lessen their ability to survive severe respiratory tract infections. The drug is administered by aerosol (Table 2) with use of a special generator supplied by the manufacturer.

TABLE 2. **Therapeutic Agents in Viral Pneumonia**

Virus	Drug	Dose
Respiratory syncytial virus	Ribavirin (Virazole)	6 gm/d by aerosol
Influenza virus	Amantadine (Symmetrel)	100 mg PO q 12 h (adults <65 y)
		100 mg/d PO (adults ≥65 y)
		5–8 mg/kg/d PO divided q 12 h (children)
		See package insert if creatinine clearance ≤ 50 mL/min
	Rimantadine (Flumadine)	100 mg PO q 12 h (adults <65 y)
		100–200 mg/d PO (adults ≥65 y)
		No approved dose for children
		See package insert if creatinine clearance ≤ 10 mL/min
Cytomegalovirus	Ganciclovir (Cytovene) plus IV immune globulin or cytomegalovirus immune globulin (CytoGam)	5 mg/kg IV q 12 h
		150 mg/kg/dose
		150 mg/kg/dose
Varicella-zoster virus	Acyclovir (Zovirax)	10 mg/kg IV q 8 h; reduce dosage with renal insufficiency
Herpes simplex virus	Acyclovir (Zovirax)	5 mg/kg IV q 8 h; reduce dosage with renal insufficiency

The usefulness of ribavirin therapy has been subjected to substantial challenge. The apparent improvements in illness are generally small, with most studies failing to demonstrate statistically significant reductions in hospital stays, days receiving intensive care, or days requiring ventilator assistance. More important, it is not clear whether the differences in outcome in controlled studies occurred because the treated groups derived benefit from ribavirin or because the control subjects deteriorated while receiving aerosolized water, which is known to cause temporary bronchospasm in subjects with reactive airway disease. Moreover, the drug is extremely expensive, costing approximately $1500 per day of administration. If ribavirin is to be administered to infants on ventilators, special care must be taken to avoid obstruction of ventilator circuits, because aerosolized ribavirin can precipitate in endotracheal tubes and in ventilators.

Ribavirin is probably not entirely ineffective, but cost/benefit concerns should be taken into account when use of the drug is considered. Most infants with RSV infection, even those requiring intensive care, will recover without ribavirin therapy, and they should probably not be treated. Preliminary studies of immunocompromised children indicate that substantial mortality occurs from RSV infection in this population and that mortality may be improved when ribavirin is administered in conjunction with intravenous immune globulin containing neutralizing antibodies to RSV. This approach to treatment would be extremely expensive, and no statement can be made at this time regarding its effectiveness.

Bacterial superinfection is an uncommon event in RSV infection, and the use of antibiotics in an attempt to prevent this cannot be defended.

Influenza Virus Infection

In otherwise healthy individuals, influenza virus pneumonia is usually mild in nature. Only supportive management, including rest and adequate fluid intake, is required. Control of cough may be attempted with any of the nonprescription cough suppressants, but the efficacy of many of these is in question. The use of acetaminophen (Tylenol and others) may be helpful in reducing fever, myalgia, and malaise. Salicylates should be avoided in children because of the association of influenza virus infection, salicylate use, and the development of Reye's syndrome.

In contrast, influenza pneumonia may be life-threatening in individuals 65 years of age and older and those with underlying cardiac or pulmonary disease, immunodeficiency, hemoglobinopathies, metabolic diseases (including diabetes mellitus), or chronic renal disease. Specific antiviral therapy with amantadine (Symmetrel and others) or rimantadine (Flumadine) should be considered for influenza virus infection in these patients as well as for otherwise healthy persons with relatively debilitating forms of influenza (see Table 2). The effectiveness of these drugs has been demonstrated only when therapy is instituted within 48 hours of the onset of illness. Treatment should be continued for 5 to 7 days. The use of the lower recommended doses listed in Table 2 may avoid the central nervous stimulation and gastrointestinal irritation commonly seen when these drugs are used, particularly in the elderly.

Amantadine and rimantadine are effective only against influenza virus type A. There is limited information on the use of ribavirin in influenza, but it is active in vitro against type B strains.

Secondary bacterial pneumonia occurs more commonly after influenza virus (and measles virus) infection than after any of the other common respiratory viruses.

Viral Infections in Immunocompromised Patients

Viral pneumonia in patients with deficient T lymphocyte function (either as a result of an underlying disease or from chemotherapy) is likely to be severe, and treatment should be undertaken in institutions with appropriate resources for specific diagnosis and management of complications. Useful agents in the management of CMV, varicella-zoster, and herpes simplex pneumonia are listed in Table 2. There are anecdotal reports of recovery from prolonged parainfluenza virus infection in immunocompromised patients after the use of ribavirin.

Other Considerations

Hantavirus pneumonia is frequently fatal and is currently treated with ribavirin in the absence of supporting data. Likewise, measles pneumonia, which is uncommon in vaccinated populations, may also improve after the administration of ribavirin.

MYCOPLASMAL PNEUMONIA

Clinical and Laboratory Diagnosis

Mycoplasma pneumoniae is responsible for approximately 15% of all episodes of pneumonia. Whereas bacterial pneumonias are more common at the extremes of age, mycoplasmal pneumonia occurs most commonly in the 5- to 19-year age group, with progressively fewer cases seen with increasing age. Cases occur year-round, with somewhat of an increase in the autumn months. There are no truly distinctive clinical features, although illness develops slowly, and there is often a discrepancy in the degree of reported symptoms, auscultatory findings, and extent of radiographic infiltrate. Chest radiographs most often reveal patchy lobar infiltrates, which are usually unilateral. The presence of large pleural effusions suggests another diagnosis. Illness may be particularly severe in patients with sickle cell hemoglobinopathy. A specific diagnosis can be made by recovery of the agent in culture or by serologic means, but this usually requires up to 2 weeks and is therefore not of benefit to the clinician.

TABLE 3. **Antibiotics Effective in Mycoplasmal Pneumonia**

Antibiotic	Dose
Tetracycline (Achromycin)	500 mg PO q 6 h for 10–14 d (adults) 25–50 mg/kg/d PO divided q 6 h (children older than 8 y)
Erythromycin (E.E.S.)	400 mg PO q 6 h for 10–14 d (adults) 10 mg/kg PO q 6 h (children)
Azithromycin (Zithromax)	500 mg PO on day 1, then 250 mg on d 2–5 (adults)
Clarithromycin (Biaxin)	250 mg PO q 12 h for 7–14 d (adults) 7.5 mg/kg PO q 12 h (children)

Treatment

Although mycoplasmal pneumonia will almost always resolve without specific therapy, the cough and malaise are nevertheless often prolonged. The use of the antibiotics listed in Table 3 will reduce the duration of clinical findings by half. However, tetracyclines (Achromycin and others) cannot be used in children younger than 9 years, and erythromycin (E.E.S. and others) is often not tolerated by individuals of any age. Newer macrolide antibiotics such as azithromycin (Zithromax) and clarithromycin (Biaxin) have antimycoplasmal activity similar to that of erythromycin but are better tolerated and require fewer doses. Ciprofloxacin (Cipro) and other early quinolone antibiotics have been demonstrated to have reasonable effectiveness in small studies of mycoplasmal pneumonia, but newer derivatives may have better activity.

LEGIONELLOSIS
(Legionnaires' Disease and Pontiac Fever)
method of
ROBERT R. MUDER, M.D.
Pittsburgh VA Medical Center and University of Pittsburgh School of Medicine
Pittsburgh, Pennsylvania

Bacteria of the genus *Legionella* are fastidious aerobic gram-negative rods that are widely distributed in natural and artificial aquatic environments. Human disease primarily involves the respiratory tract, with two distinct clinical syndromes. Legionnaires' disease refers to bacterial pneumonia caused by members of the genus. Pontiac fever is a self-limited febrile illness resembling influenza. Although there are 40 species within the genus *Legionella* and multiple serogroups within some species, 90% of human infections are caused by *Legionella pneumophila*, with 80% of these caused by serogroup 1. The majority of the remaining cases are caused by *Legionella micdadei*, *Legionella longbeachae*, *Legionella bozemanii*, and *Legionella dumoffii*.

EPIDEMIOLOGY

Legionella species occur naturally in water and soil. Artificial aquatic habitats include water distribution systems (hot-water tanks, pipes and faucets), cooling towers, evaporative condensers, and whirlpool baths. Humans acquire infection from environmental sources; human-to-human transmission has not been demonstrated. Possible modes of transmission include aspiration and inhalation of contaminated aerosols. *Legionella* species account for approximately 7% of adult community-acquired pneumonias; the estimated incidence of infection is 6.1 per 100,000 population per year. Although the majority of cases are sporadic, point-source epidemics occur. Endemic nosocomial disease often occurs in hospitals in which there is colonization of the water system by *Legionella*. Risk factors for *Legionella* pneumonia include advanced age, male sex, cigarette smoking, chronic pulmonary disease, use of immunosuppressive medication, malignant disease, chronic renal failure, and acquired immune deficiency syndrome.

Pontiac fever is most frequently recognized as an epidemic illness affecting multiple persons exposed to an aerosol contaminated with *Legionella*. Although sporadic cases have been documented, recognition is difficult because of the nonspecific and self-limited nature of the clinical illness.

CLINICAL MANIFESTATIONS

The incubation period of legionnaires' disease is 2 to 10 days after exposure. Nearly all patients are febrile at presentation. Cough is typically nonproductive initially, but 50% or more of patients produce sputum within several days of presentation. Chest pain and dyspnea occur in about half of patients. The presentation may mimic pulmonary embolism, particularly in immunocompromised patients. Diarrhea and abdominal pain are common; myalgias may be prominent. A variety of other extrapulmonary syndromes have been reported during the course of pneumonia, including acute renal failure, obtundation, cerebellar ataxia, peripheral neuropathy, rhabdomyolysis, hemolytic anemia, and thrombotic thrombocytopenic purpura. However, there is no distinctive clinical syndrome that permits differentiation of legionnaires' disease from other causes of bacterial pneumonia. Microbiologically documented extrapulmonary infection is rare. Reported cases include endocarditis, pericarditis, soft tissue infection, and hemodialysis shunt infection.

Pontiac fever occurs 1 to 2 days after exposure to a *Legionella*-contaminated aerosol. Patients abruptly develop fever, chills, myalgia, headache, and malaise. Although patients often complain of nonproductive cough and chest pain, radiographic evidence of pneumonia is absent. The disease is self-limited; symptoms resolve in 2 to 5 days.

DIAGNOSIS

Legionnaires' disease is not readily distinguishable from other pneumonias on the basis of clinical presentation. *Legionella* species are fastidious and will not grow on most artificial media routinely used in the diagnosis of pneumonia. The organisms take up Gram's stain poorly and are rarely visualized in clinical specimens. Thus, specialized diagnostic tests are needed to confirm the diagnosis. Buffered charcoal–yeast extract agar with added antibiotics to inhibit commensal floral permits growth from expectorated sputum in 70% of cases. Pretreatment of the specimen with acid improves sensitivity. Growth occurs in 3 to 5 days; the isolate is confirmed as a *Legionella* species by direct fluorescent antibody staining or slide agglutination.

Direct fluorescent antibody staining of respiratory secretions permits visualization of the organisms in 30 to 70% of cases. Rapid diagnosis of infection due to *L. pneumophila* serogroup 1 can be accomplished by detection of *Legionella* antigen in urine. Sensitivity is 80% and specificity is 99%. The urinary antigen test is not useful for diagnosis of infection due to other serogroups or species. Serologic diagnosis is obtained by the finding of a fourfold rise in anti-*Legionella* titers in acute and convalescent samples of serum obtained 4 to 6 weeks apart.

Pontiac fever is diagnosed by documentation of seroconversion in the appropriate clinical and epidemiologic setting.

TREATMENT

The most frequently used antibiotic is erythromycin. The initial dose is 1 gram intravenously every 6 hours until clinical response is apparent. Therapy can then be continued with oral erythromycin, 500 mg every 6 hours. Patients who are immunocompromised, have multilobar pulmonary involvement, or require mechanical ventilation should also receive rifampin (Rifadin),* 600 mg orally twice daily.† Minimal duration of therapy is 2 weeks in immunologically normal patients and 3 weeks in those who are immunocompromised. Shorter courses may be associated with relapse. Erythromycin therapy may be associated with thrombophlebitis and gastrointestinal upset. Patients with renal or hepatic failure may develop reversible hearing loss. In addition, erythromycin may interfere with the metabolism of antirejection drugs, such as cyclosporine, used in transplantation.

Fluoroquinolone antimicrobials have excellent in vitro and in vivo activity that is superior to that of erythromycin; in addition, fluoroquinolones do not interact with most antirejection medications. Transplant recipients, patients intolerant of erythromycin, and patients failing to respond to erythromycin therapy should receive ciprofloxacin (Cipro), 400 mg intravenously or 750 mg orally twice daily. Although there are no randomized comparative trials of therapy for *Legionella* infection, ciprofloxacin may also be preferable to erythromycin in other groups of immunocompromised patients and in patients with multilobar pulmonary involvement. Critically ill patients may benefit from the addition of rifampin to ciprofloxacin. Rifampin affects the metabolism of a large number of other drugs, including cyclosporine.

Other agents potentially useful in the treatment of *Legionella* infection include tetracycline and trimethoprim-sulfamethoxazole (Bactrim, Septra). The newer macrolide agents azithromycin (Zithromax) and clarithromycin (Biaxin) show promise as therapeutic agents on the basis of in vitro susceptibility studies and reports of clinical efficacy.

---

*Not FDA approved for this indication.
†Exceeds dosage recommended by the manufacturer.

Pontiac fever resolves spontaneously; antimicrobial therapy is not indicated.

PREVENTION

Prevention of legionnaires' disease is best accomplished by preventing exposure of susceptible patients to environmental sources of the organism. Routine treatment of cooling towers with biocides for the purpose of *Legionella* control is of uncertain efficacy as a public health measure. Colonization of a hospital water system with *L. pneumophila* predicts the occurrence of nosocomial legionellosis. Periodic culture surveillance of hospital water supplies for *Legionella* is advisable. Isolation of *Legionella* from hospital water makes surveillance for cases of nosocomial legionellosis mandatory. Identification of cases indicates the need for decontamination of the water system. Decontamination methods include periodic elevation of hot-water temperature to 70°C and flushing of distal sites or treatment with a silver-copper ion generator.

Although animal studies indicate that development of an anti-*Legionella* vaccine is feasible, no vaccine is currently available.

PULMONARY EMBOLISM

method of
WILLIAM H. GEERTS, M.D.
*Sunnybrook Health Science Centre, University of
   Toronto*
Toronto, Ontario, Canada

Deep venous thrombosis (DVT) and pulmonary embolism (PE) are common and potentially lethal components of the same disease process, venous thromboembolism (VTE). PE is the third leading cause of hospital death and the most common preventable cause.

The risk factors for VTE have generally been well characterized (Table 1). Previous VTE predisposes to recurrence, although the majority of patients with previous DVT who have new or worsening leg symptoms have postphlebitic syndrome rather than recurrent thrombosis. Malignant disease is a well-known risk factor for VTE, but chemotherapy itself is also thrombogenic, as is radiotherapy if the radiation field includes a large vein. Heart failure and respiratory failure as well as exacerbations of chronic lung disease also predispose to thrombosis. Although the risk for thromboembolism is slightly increased in pregnancy, the risk in the postpartum period is far greater. Whether there is a true association between currently used doses of estrogen-containing contraceptives and thromboembolism is unknown for women who do not have a molecular hypercoagulable state. There are no data supporting such an association with postmenopausal hormone replacement therapy, and this treatment need not be avoided in patients with a current or past history of thromboembolism.

A coagulation system disorder should be considered in the presence of a positive family history, recurrent episodes of thromboembolism, thrombosis at unusual sites, or unexplained VTE especially in patients younger than 50 years.

TABLE 1. **Risk Factors for Venous Thromboembolism**

Clinical Factors

Previous thromboembolism
Surgery
Trauma
Immobility: bed rest, stroke, paralysis
Malignant disease and its treatment
Increased age
Heart and respiratory failure
Pregnancy and postpartum period
High-dose estrogens
Inflammatory bowel disease
Varicose veins
Central venous lines or injury

Coagulation System Factors

Resistance to activated protein C (factor V Leiden)
Antiphospholipid antibody syndrome
Deficiencies of
   Antithrombin III
   Protein C
   Protein S
   Heparin cofactor II
   Factor XII
Dysfibrinogenemia
Fibrinolytic dysfunction
   Decreased or abnormal plasminogen
   Decreased plasminogen activator
   Increased plasminogen activator inhibitor
Myeloproliferative disorders
   Polycythemia vera
   Primary thrombocytosis
Homocyst(e)inemia
Heparin-induced thrombocytopenia

By far the most common molecular hypercoagulable state is activated protein C resistance (factor V Leiden), an inherited abnormality resulting from a single amino acid substitution in the coagulation cofactor, factor V. The mutation does not allow factor V to be inhibited by the endogenous anticoagulant, activated protein C. This abnormality is found in at least half of the cases in which hypercoagulability is suspected, in 20% of patients with their first episode of thrombosis, and in 5 to 7% of the normal white population. The risk for thrombosis in heterozygotes with the factor V allele is increased 5- to 10-fold; the risk in homozygotes is even higher.

The other relatively common coagulation disorder is the antiphospholipid antibody syndrome (which includes lupus anticoagulants and anticardiolipin antibody). The presence of these antibodies may result in venous or arterial thrombosis, stroke, recurrent fetal loss, thrombocytopenia, and prolongation of the partial thromboplastin time (PTT).

The relationships between thromboembolic risk factors, DVT, and PE have been defined (Figure 1). For PE, the causative DVT originates in the deep veins of the legs in more than 90% of cases; a small proportion of emboli arise in the veins of the arms or pelvis, in the inferior vena cava, or in the right side of the heart. Proximal DVT plays an essential role in the development of PE, fatal PE, and chronic venous insufficiency and is therefore the condition most critical to diagnose, to treat, and to prevent.

PROPHYLAXIS

Because PE is common, usually occurs without warning, may lead to disastrous consequences, and is associated with significant resource expenditure, the routine use of

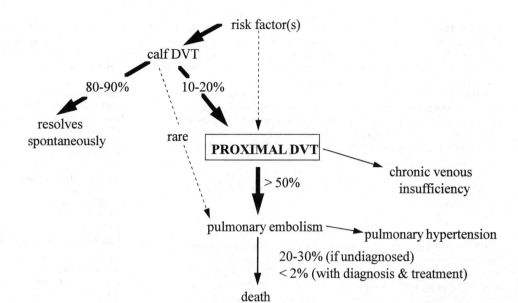

Figure 1. Venous thromboembolism. DVT = deep venous thrombosis.

effective, safe, and cost-effective methods of prophylaxis is essential for patients at risk (Table 2).

Low-dose subcutaneous heparin (5000 units every 12 hours) remains the prophylactic method of choice for most medical and general surgical patients who are immobilized for longer than 24 hours. For higher risk general surgery patients, including those having prolonged surgery (especially for malignant neoplasm) and those with prior VTE, low-dose heparin is associated with a significant failure rate. Other options to consider in this situation include

TABLE 2. **Thromboprophylaxis**

Risk Setting	Recommended Prophylaxis Approaches
Medical Patients (bed rest, heart or respiratory failure)	*Heparin 5000 U SC bid
Acute Myocardial Infarction	*Heparin 5000 U SC bid *or* *Full anticoagulation (heparin → warfarin)
Stroke	
Hemorrhagic	*Graduated compression stockings Intermittent pneumatic compression device
Nonhemorrhagic	*LMWH, enoxaparin (Lovenox), dalteparin (Fragmin) Heparin 5000 U SC bid
Major General, Gynecologic, or Urologic Surgery	
Usual risk	*Heparin 5000 U SC bid
High risk	*Heparin 7500 U SC bid Heparin 5000 U SC tid LMWH, enoxaparin (Lovenox), dalteparin (Fragmin) Heparin 5000 U SC bid or tid + stockings
Neurosurgery	*Graduated compression stockings Intermittent pneumatic compression device Heparin 5000 U SC bid
Orthopedic Surgery	
Hip arthroplasty or fracture	*LMWH, enoxaparin (Lovenox), dalteparin (Fragmin) *Warfarin (INR 2–3) Adjusted-dose heparin (PTT 35–40 s)
Knee arthroplasty	*LMWH, enoxaparin (Lovenox), dalteparin (Fragmin) Intermittent pneumatic compression device Warfarin (INR 2–3)
Major Trauma	
Central nervous system bleeding	*Graduated compression stockings → LMWH Intermittent compression device → LMWH
Others	*LMWH, enoxaparin (Lovenox), dalteparin (Fragmin) → warfarin

*Best option or, where there are inadequate data, my preference.
Abbreviations: LMWH = low-molecular-weight heparin; INR = International Normalized Ratio; PTT = partial thromboplastin time.

heparin three times daily, low-molecular-weight heparin (LMWH), or the combination of low-dose heparin with either graduated compression stockings or intermittent pneumatic compression, although my preference is to use heparin at 7500 units subcutaneously twice daily.

Patients with hip fracture, arthroplasty of the hip or knee, or major trauma are poorly protected by low-dose heparin, graduated compression stockings, and aspirin. Hip surgery patients should receive prophylaxis with either warfarin (aiming for an International Normalized Ratio [INR] between 2.0 and 3.0) or LMWH. Although the optimal duration of prophylaxis for these patients is still controversial, I usually continue prophylaxis for 3 to 4 weeks after surgery.

DIAGNOSIS

PE is one of the most commonly misdiagnosed conditions in medicine, especially in patients with concomitant cardiac, pulmonary, or malignant disease. The diagnosis is not even considered before death in 70 to 95% of cases of fatal PE. At the same time, the majority of patients with clinically suspected PE have this condition ruled out by objective diagnostic testing.

The clinical features of PE are nonspecific (Table 3), and the differential diagnostic possibilities are numerous (Table 4). The first step in approaching this problem is to consider the diagnosis in every patient with unexplained cardiorespiratory symptoms. The second step is to strive to never miss large pulmonary emboli or proximal DVT, the precursor for hemodynamically important PE.

Once a suspicion of PE is raised, an examination especially directed toward the chest (pleural rub, right ventricular dysfunction) and the legs (swelling, tenderness) is performed. The chest radiograph and electrocardiogram are rarely diagnostic, although they occasionally detect alternative conditions, and the chest film may be useful in the interpretation of the lung scan. It has definitively been shown that arterial blood gas analysis should not be used to confirm or exclude PE once this diagnosis has been considered. Patients with large emboli may have normal results on blood gas analysis, whereas the findings of hypoxemia and a wide alveolar-arterial oxygen gradient are also seen in many of the conditions in the differential diagnosis.

TABLE 3. **Presentations of Pulmonary Embolism**

Asymptomatic
"Minor" pulmonary embolism
Transient dyspnea
Pleuritic chest pain
Cough
Hemoptysis
"Major" pulmonary embolism
Apprehension
Severe dyspnea
Ischemic chest pain
Syncope
Sudden death
Other
Arrhythmia
Fever
Right-sided heart failure
Mental confusion
Bronchospasm
Shock
Disseminated intravascular coagulation
Paradoxical arterial embolism

TABLE 4. **Differential Diagnoses of Pulmonary Embolism**

"Minor" Pulmonary Embolism

Pneumonia
Acute bronchitis
Left-sided heart failure
Postoperative atelectasis
Pleural effusion
Hyperventilation
Esophageal spasm
Musculoskeletal chest wall pain
Viral or immune pleuritis
Pericarditis
Acute asthma
Bronchiectasis
Lung cancer

"Major" Pulmonary Embolism

Acute myocardial infarction
Arrhythmias
Pulmonary edema
Exacerbation of chronic obstructive lung disease
Pneumothorax
Sepsis
Pericardial effusion or tamponade
Aortic dissection

Ventilation/Perfusion Lung Scanning

Lung scanning has high sensitivity (95%) but low specificity (10%) for PE. The interpretation of lung scans can be simplified into three patterns: normal perfusion (PE ruled out); high probability, defined as one or more segmental or greater perfusion defects with relatively normal ventilation (associated with a probability of PE exceeding 85%); and nondiagnostic (Figure 2). The nondiagnostic category includes such labels as "nonhigh," "intermediate," "indeterminate," and "low probability" and is associated with a frequency of PE of 10 to 40%. A normal or high-probability lung scan result is useful, but at least half of all scans fit into the nondiagnostic category. Although the physician's assessment of the likelihood of PE has some predictive value, combining all of the clinical data with the lung scan result still does not clarify the diagnosis in 60% of patients with suspected PE.

Venous Imaging and Pulmonary Angiography

The next step for most patients with nondiagnostic lung scans is to assess for the presence of lower extremity DVT by use of venous ultrasonography. If this test discovers DVT, treatment should be initiated. The majority of patients with nondiagnostic scans, however, will have normal findings on lower extremity ultrasonography. One option to consider at this point is pulmonary angiography (if it is essential to be certain that PE is present or not). Although this option may seem to be the most sensible approach, we do not often need to be absolutely certain that PE is present. I consider angiography in patients with continuing risk factors for thrombosis coupled with a high risk for bleeding, those who cannot be observed with serial leg ultrasonography, and those who present with unexplained recurrent cardiorespiratory symptoms. Although pulmonary angiography is generally safe (mortality 0.25% and serious morbidity 2%), it has major limitations: there is a requirement for considerable technical expertise, it is nondiagnostic in a significant percentage of cases, and its routine use in all patients with nondiagnostic scans is not

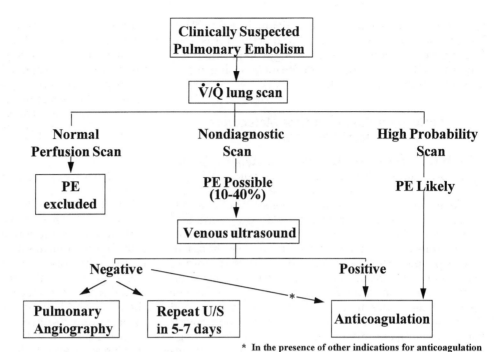

Figure 2. Diagnosis of pulmonary embolism (PE). U/S = ultrasonography; V̇/Q̇ = ventilation/perfusion.

unacceptable to most clinicians. Transesophageal echocardiography and spiral computed tomography may occasionally assist in the diagnosis of large pulmonary emboli but are much less useful in the diagnosis of smaller emboli.

An alternative that I commonly use for patients with nondiagnostic scans involves reassessment in 5 to 7 days with a repeated venous ultrasound examination. The rationale for using serial leg ultrasonography in the management of patients with suspected PE is based on the knowledge that the overwhelming majority of pulmonary emboli arise in the proximal deep veins of the legs; that as long as proximal DVT is not present, the risk for a subsequent pulmonary embolus will be low; and that the treatment of patients with PE is primarily treatment of the causative DVT rather than the PE itself. If repeated venous imaging findings remain normal, anticoagulation can be safely withheld. Patients at high risk for other potential sources of emboli such as the right side of the heart, around central venous lines, or the pelvic veins require further testing.

Many patients with suspected PE have underlying conditions that are themselves indications for anticoagulation (e.g., after orthopedic surgery or major trauma, recent myocardial infarction, atrial fibrillation, or cardiomyopathy). If such patients present with possible PE and there is no contraindication, I usually recommend full anticoagulation for at least the period of risk rather than proceed to further investigations. Finally, blood testing for D dimer, a degradation product of the effect of plasmin on fibrin, has high sensitivity for acute VTE although specificity is low. In patients with nondiagnostic lung scans, a normal plasma D-dimer level excludes clinically important VTE; a positive test result indicates the need for further investigation.

TREATMENT

General Supportive Measures

Hypoxemic patients with PE should have supplemental oxygen, and those with pleuritic chest pain often require parenteral narcotic analgesics. Enforced bed rest has not been shown to be beneficial, and my practice is to aggressively mobilize patients the day after admission. Resuscitation of the hemodynamically compromised patient should initially involve administration of a vasopressor agent such as norepinephrine or epinephrine with or without the inotrope dobutamine. Volume expansion may worsen right ventricular function and therefore must be done cautiously.

Traditional Anticoagulation

The primary management objective in patients with acute PE is the prevention of recurrent emboli by inhibiting further clot formation. Anticoagulation should commence as soon as the diagnosis of DVT or PE is seriously considered, especially if there will be a delay in obtaining the objective diagnostic test. The traditional approach involves an intravenous heparin bolus of 5000 units followed by a continuous infusion starting at 18 units per kg per hour. The target PTT range is two to three times the control value. Starting with 1000 units per hour will render two thirds of patients subtherapeutic, a situation associated with a 14-fold increased risk for recurrent VTE. On the other hand, a supratherapeutic PTT has not been associated with an increased risk for bleeding. The first PTT is obtained 4 to 6 hours after the start of treatment and then every 6 hours until the target range is reached. Use of a heparin nomogram most efficiently guides dosage adjustment.

Patients treated with heparin require a daily platelet count to look for heparin-induced thrombocytopenia (suggested by a greater than 30% fall in platelet count from the pretreatment baseline). If this life- and limb-threatening condition is suspected, heparin should be discontinued and acute anticoagulation using the low-molecular-weight heparinoid danaparoid (Orgaran)* or the defibrinogenating agent ancrod (Arvin)* instituted.

Anticoagulation with Low-Molecular-Weight Heparin

LMWHs (enoxaparin [Lovenox], dalteparin [Fragmin]) provide effective treatment for both DVT and PE with a number of advantages over standard heparin. When it is injected subcutaneously, the bioavailability of LMWH exceeds 90% (30% for heparin), and these agents have a longer half-life and a much more predictable dose-response effect than does heparin. These properties have resulted in LMWHs' being given as treatment for VTE in a fixed dose based on body weight (generally 200 anti–factor Xa units per kg every 24 hours in a single dose or two divided doses) without the need for either laboratory monitoring or subsequent dosage adjustment. A large number of clinical trials have confirmed that fixed-dose, body weight–adjusted, subcutaneous LMWH is superior therapy to intravenous heparin and is more cost-effective in the initial treatment of VTE. When the data from comparative studies are reviewed, LMWH, given for the 5 to 7 days it takes to achieve therapeutic oral anticoagulation, is associated with a reduced risk for recurrent thromboembolism, lower risk for bleeding, and decreased all-cause mortality.

Large randomized trials have demonstrated that patient-administered subcutaneous LMWH on an outpatient basis is as effective and safe as traditional hospital therapy with intravenous heparin but with enormous cost savings. Therefore, LMWH is now the preferred initial treatment of DVT and PE. No laboratory monitoring is required when LMWH is used, and the risk for heparin-induced thrombocytopenia is so low that I do not obtain platelet counts. Approximately 60 to 80% of outpatients with these conditions can now have anticoagulation without hospital admission. Even if patients require admission for other reasons, significant cost savings accrue with the replacement of intravenous heparin by LMWH. How-

*Not FDA approved for this indication.

ever, each hospital embarking on outpatient therapy with LMWH must have the infrastructure in place to carry this out safely and efficiently. An "expert" team with the responsibility for this program must be in place to screen potentially eligible patients, to educate the patients in the self-injection of LMWH, and to supervise them at least by telephone on a daily basis during the first week of therapy.

Thrombolytic and Mechanical Therapy

The use of intravenous thrombolytic therapy results in accelerated early resolution of pulmonary emboli and reduction in right ventricular dysfunction. In the treatment of DVT or PE, however, thrombolytic therapy is infrequently used because the short-term benefits are generally small, long-term benefits are uncertain, bleeding risks are increased, the costs and logistical problems associated with this intervention are great, and the majority of patients with PE do well with anticoagulant therapy alone. I therefore reserve lytic therapy for patients who have extensive PE with hypotension or right ventricular failure and no absolute contraindications. The optimal regimens for administering thrombolytic therapy have not been established (Table 5). My preference is to use a brief intravenous infusion of either streptokinase (1.5 million units during 60 minutes) or recombinant tissue plasminogen activator (1 mg per kg during 15 minutes) for patients with massive PE or to use intraembolus, catheter-directed lysis (urokinase 100,000 units per hour for 12 to 48 hours) for major emboli when the patient is stable enough to tolerate transport to the vascular radiology suite. Other endovascular procedures with promise include percutaneous embolus extraction, mechanical clot lysis, and catheter fragmentation coupled with thrombolysis for significant residual disease.

The only indication for surgical embolectomy is massive PE in a patient for whom thrombolytic therapy is contraindicated or has been unsuccessful. Vena caval filter insertion is indicated in patients with proximal DVT and an absolute contraindication to anticoagulation or with major bleeding while receiving anticoagulants. Once the risk for bleeding decreases, the addition of anticoagulation is neces-

TABLE 5. **Thrombolytic Therapy Regimens for Pulmonary Embolism**

Drug	Intravenous Infusions	Bolus Regimens	Local Catheter Infusions
Streptokinase (Kabikinase, Streptase)	250,000 U in 30 min followed by 100,000 U/h for 12–36 h*	1.5 million U in 60 min	10,000–50,000 U/h
Urokinase (Abbokinase)	4400 U/kg in 10 min followed by 4400 U/kg/h for 12–36 h*	3 million U in 2 h	50,000–150,000 U/h
Tissue plasminogen activator (Activase)	100 mg in 2 h*	0.6–1 mg/kg in 15 min	3 mg/h

*FDA approved.

TABLE 6. **Practical Oral Anticoagulation**

Initiate warfarin the same day as heparin.

Start with 5–10 mg, approximately twice the expected maintenance dose.

Check INR the next day.

Repeat loading dose if INR is unchanged.

Check INR daily until value is in target range.

Reduce the dose when INR starts to rise.

Try to predict maintenance dose rather than reacting to each day's INR.

Overlap LMWH or heparin with warfarin until at least 2 consecutive INR values are 2.0–3.0.

Prescribe single-strength warfarin tablets.

Recommend a laboratory that uses a sensitive thromboplastin (ISI 1.0–1.5) as the prothrombin time reagent.

Explain rationale for anticoagulation, need for compliance, and blood testing.

Provide the patient with written information and an anticoagulant calendar to record number of tablets daily, results of INR values, and the date of the next blood test.

Avoid overreacting to INR values that are just outside target range.

Attempt to monitor stable patients once every 4–6 wk.

Abbreviation: ISI = International Sensitivity Index.
Modified from Geerts WH, Jay RM: Oral anticoagulants in the prevention and treatment of venous thromboembolism. *In* Poller L, Hirsh J (eds): Oral Anticoagulants. London, Edward Arnold, 1996, pp 97–122.

sary to prevent recurrence or progression of the underlying DVT.

Oral Anticoagulation

Warfarin (Coumadin) is generally commenced on the day the diagnosis of PE is made with a dose approximately twice the expected maintenance dose (Table 6). As soon as the prothrombin time starts to increase, the dose of warfarin is reduced toward the expected maintenance dose. The heparin or LMWH and warfarin are overlapped for at least 5 days and until the INR has been greater than 2.0 for at least 2 days.

Patients must have a detailed discussion about the indications for anticoagulation, the potential risks and warning signs for bleeding, and the importance of regular INR testing and compliance with the prescribed dose of warfarin. I do not advise any restriction in diet or activity level (apart from contact sports), and I do not discourage alcohol use in moderation.

Duration of Anticoagulation

Although the optimal duration of oral anticoagulation for DVT and PE has not been clearly established, clinical trials have demonstrated that anticoagulation for 3 to 6 months is associated with fewer recurrent thromboembolic events than 4 to 6 weeks of therapy; that patients with reversible risk factors for the original episode (surgery, trauma, bed rest) require a shorter course of treatment than do those with an ongoing risk factor (including uncontrolled

malignant disease) or with unexplained thromboembolism; and that patients with poor resolution of the thrombosis may benefit from more prolonged duration of anticoagulation. There is no evidence that patients with PE require longer therapy than do those with DVT. I individualize the duration of therapy and base it on the number of previous thromboembolic events, reversal of thromboembolic risk factors, resolution of the DVT or PE, and risk for bleeding. The first time I reassess the duration of therapy is generally 3 months after the acute event. If, at this point, the risk factor has resolved and the findings on perfusion lung scan (or venous ultrasound scan) have essentially normalized, I discontinue the warfarin. Patients with ongoing risk factors and those with more than two episodes of VTE remain anticoagulated, and it is also my practice to continue warfarin as long as significant residual embolism or DVT is still present.

Two clinical situations warrant consideration of alternative methods of anticoagulation. Oral anticoagulants are contraindicated during pregnancy because they produce a skeletal embryopathy and fetal central nervous system bleeding. Full-dose subcutaneous heparin or preferably LMWH is used in this setting. Patients with uncontrolled malignant disease commonly have recurrent thrombosis despite anticoagulation with warfarin. I also use full-dose subcutaneous LMWH or heparin when warfarin has failed in these patients.

SARCOIDOSIS

method of
OM P. SHARMA, M.D.
University of Southern California School of Medicine
Los Angeles, California

Sarcoidosis is a systemic granulomatous disease. Its cause is not known. It most commonly affects young adults and manifests with bilateral hilar lymphadenopathy, pulmonary infiltration, reticuloendothelial involvement, and eye and skin lesions. Myocardial and central nervous system lesions are less frequent. About 10 to 20% of patients have hypercalcemia. Immunologic alterations include peripheral depression of delayed-type hypersensitivity, imbalance of OKT4/OKT8 subsets, influx of T4 helper cells to the sites of inflammation, hyperactivity of B cells, and presence of serum immune complexes.

The course and prognosis of sarcoidosis correlate well with the mode of onset and clinical involvement. An acute onset with hilar adenopathy and erythema nodosum and uveitis usually portends a self-limited course and spontaneous resolution; an insidious onset may be followed by progressive fibrosis with diffuse pulmonary infiltration, hepatosplenomegaly, skin lesions, and bone cysts.

DIAGNOSIS

Any consideration for treating sarcoidosis should be preceded by establishing the accurate diagnosis based on the following criteria: (1) compatible clinical or radiologic picture, or both; (2) histologic evidence of noncaseating granulomas by either an appropriate biopsy or a Kveim-Siltzbach test; and (3) negative special stains and cultures (acid-fast bacilli, fungi, bacteria, protozoa) of tissue specimens. If all three steps are not performed, the diagnosis of sarcoidosis remains in doubt because clinical or radiologic features suggest too wide a differential diagnosis, and noncaseating granulomas may be induced by many bacteria, fungi, viruses, chemicals, and organic dust particles. Once the diagnosis is established, an attempt should be made to assess the activity, severity, and extent of the granulomatous process.

EVALUATION OF DISEASE ACTIVITY AND SEVERITY

The four techniques that are useful in assessing the extent and severity of granulomatous inflammation include determination of serum angiotensin-converting enzyme (SACE), gallium Ga 67 scans, bronchoalveolar lavage (BAL), and high-resolution computed tomography (HRCT). SACE, BAL analysis, and ^{67}Ga scans reflect different aspects of sarcoid activity. There is considerable uncertainty about how the three methods correlate with each other. SACE does not accurately reflect activity of the disease as assessed by the BAL lymphocyte count. There is an approximate correlation between the results of ^{67}Ga scanning and SACE activity but not between ^{67}Ga lung scans and BAL lymphocyte counts. These results are not surprising in view of the distinctive tissue sources of these markers, namely, the blood, the lung tissue, and the lavage fluid. HRCT is the most modern imaging technique, providing outstanding resolution of the lung's morphologic features. These tests are of little help in establishing the specific diagnosis of sarcoidosis. The technique of positron emission tomography with fluorine 18–labeled fluoro-2-deoxy-D-glucose has not yet found a place in the management of sarcoidosis.

NATURAL HISTORY

For evaluation of the natural course of pulmonary sarcoidosis, patients must be selected and monitored while they are still in the early stages of the disease, without any type of treatment, for a long time. In a British study, 125 patients with sarcoidosis were followed up for more than 2 years. Spontaneous radiographic improvement in a mean time of 1 year occurred in 71% of patients with hilar nodes and in 50% of those with pulmonary infiltration. The outlook was much better in those patients who presented with erythema nodosum. None of the patients who had spontaneous remission experienced relapse. Pulmonary infiltration, if it persists for more than 2 years, is unlikely to remit without therapy. The prognosis is poor in American black persons, particularly women, especially in those who at the time of the initial discovery have pulmonary infiltration and disease involving more than three organ systems.

TREATMENT

Pulmonary Involvement

Lungs are the most frequently involved organs; 9 of every 10 patients with sarcoidosis have intrathoracic involvement. Conventionally, chest radiographic appearances are classified into the following four stages: stage 0, normal findings on chest radiographs; stage I, bilateral hilar adenopathy; stage II, bilateral hilar adenopathy and parenchymal involvement; stage III, parenchymal involvement only; and stage IV, extensive fibrosis, bullae formation, and cystic changes.

Stage I. Asymptomatic patients with bilateral hilar lymphadenopathy with or without erythema nodosum but without extrapulmonary involvement should be left untreated. Patients with fever and joint pains respond to nonsteroidal anti-inflammatory agents. On occasion, prednisone, 15 to 20 mg per day, may be needed to control symptoms that do not respond to anti-inflammatory drugs. Symptoms of cough and dyspnea may be associated with airway obstruction—even in this early stage—and should be treated with corticosteroids. In a few of these cases, inhalational corticosteroids are found to be effective.

Stage II. Patients with bilateral hilar adenopathy and infiltration and symptoms (cough, dyspnea, chest pain, exercise intolerance) should be treated with corticosteroids. Patients who are asymptomatic and have only mild impairment of lung function need only to be observed. However, if deterioration of lung function occurs in a 3-month period, the treatment should be instituted.

Patients who are asymptomatic but have severe impairment of lung function need treatment. Serial chest radiographs and lung function measurement should be performed to establish the maximal response before the drug dosage is tapered to the maintenance level.

Stage III. Patients with diffuse pulmonary infiltration usually have symptoms along with lung function abnormalities and almost always need treatment. A few of these patients recover, but most of them require long-term therapy.

Stage IV. Patients with extensive fibrosis and bullae formation respond either poorly or not at all to corticosteroids and immunosuppressive therapy. However, the treatment should be given at least once to improve symptoms if possible. Some of these patients need lung transplantation. Bronchiectasis, hemoptysis, and aspergilloma are treated conservatively with appropriate antibacterial and antifungal agents. If antifungal agents fail, hemoptysis should be managed with bronchial artery embolization. If the lung function is adequate, massive hemoptysis will require resectional surgery.

Lung Transplantation

Single- or double-lung transplantation should be considered as early as possible in patients with stage III and stage IV sarcoidosis with cor pulmonale and inexorable progression. Although there have been many reports of recurrent sarcoidosis in lung allografts, the exact frequency is not known. Furthermore, these recurrences of sarcoidosis respond well to therapy.

Extrapulmonary Involvement

Indications for the treatment of extrapulmonary involvement are relatively clear. Ocular, neurologic, cardiac, and upper airway involvement almost always necessitates treatment with corticosteroids, often in higher doses (see "Corticosteroid Therapy") and for a long time. Glandular involvement, splenic enlargement, parotid swelling, and cutaneous lesions respond to modest doses (see "Corticosteroid Therapy"). Asymptomatic hepatic involvement requires no therapy, but regular follow-up evaluation must be provided.

Corticosteroid Therapy

Sarcoidosis is sensitive to corticosteroids. I give 30 to 40 mg of prednisone daily in a single dose, gradually reducing to a maintenance level of 10 to 15 mg during a period of 6 months. Higher doses (60 to 80 mg daily) are needed to control severe ocular, neurologic, and myocardial lesions and malignant hypercalcemia. Relapse is common and is evidenced by reappearance of clinical signs, chest radiograph abnormality, impairment in lung function, or elevated levels of angiotensin-converting enzyme. If a relapse occurs, prednisone is increased to the previously high level sufficient to control the recurrence. Although an alternate-day regimen is effective in producing considerable reduction of side effects, daily treatment is recommended to ensure increased compliance by the patient. In selected cases with no extrapulmonary involvement and mildly impaired lung function, inhalational corticosteroids improve lung functions and suppress cough.

Drugs Other Than Corticosteroids

Chloroquine (Aralen),* hydroxychloroquine (Plaquenil),* and methotrexate* are given to patients who either do not respond to prednisone or experience severe corticosteroid-induced side effects. I have used all three drugs in those two situations mentioned and also as an initial treatment of chronic skin lesions. Chloroquine administration rarely leads to retinopathy; hydroxychloroquine almost never causes ocular involvement. However, frequent eye examinations (every 3 months) are mandatory if either of the drugs is used. Hydroxychloroquine or chloroquine should not be given to patients with retinitis. Hydroxychloroquine is particularly useful in patients with sarcoidosis and non–insulin-dependent diabetes mellitus because the drug, by increasing peripheral glucose use and suppressing hepatic gluconeogenesis, makes hyperglycemia manageable. In patients receiving methotrexate, close monitoring of the white blood cell count and liver function is required. The drug should be discontinued if the white blood cell count goes below 3000 to 3500 per mm³. In patients who cannot tolerate any of the aforementioned drugs or when contraindications to use exist, I use azathioprine (Imuran),* 100 to 150 mg daily by mouth. More information is needed about indications and precautions before these drugs can be recommended as the routine initial therapy for sarcoidosis.

---

*Not FDA approved for this indication.

SPECIAL SITUATIONS

Children

Sarcoidosis is not rare among children younger than 15 years. The younger children tend to have extensive, systemic disease, with a less favorable prognosis. Corticosteroids are useful in suppressing the inflammation. Chloroquine, hydroxychloroquine, methotrexate, and azathioprine are not indicated.

The Elderly

Sarcoidosis carries a low mortality rate, and many patients live with it into the later years. A malignant disease of the lung, stomach, intestine, and even uterus may give rise to a granulomatous reaction in draining lymph nodes.

Pregnancy

Pregnancy has a favorable effect on the disease. Many patients improve and are able to discontinue or curtail corticosteroid therapy. The disease does not have any damaging effect on gestation or on the fetus. In a few patients, the disease worsens after parturition but responds well to corticosteroids.

Infection

The frequency of tuberculosis and other bacterial and viral infections in persons with sarcoidosis is not higher than that in the general population. Prophylactic isoniazid therapy is indicated for patients with sarcoidosis who have positive tuberculin test responses and are prescribed corticosteroids. Aspergilloma is the common fungal colonization in chronic fibrotic sarcoidosis.

Myocardial Sarcoidosis

Granulomatous infiltration of the myocardium may remain clinically silent or it may cause heart block, fatal arrhythmias, and sudden death. Endomyocardial biopsy, thallium (rest and exercise) imaging, ⁶⁷Ga scanning, and magnetic resonance imaging have all been used to assess cardiac sarcoidosis. Prednisone at a dose of 80 to 100 mg daily should be the initial dose. After 6 to 8 weeks, the dosage is gradually reduced on the basis of the results of repeated thallium scans. If the patient's disease is steroid resistant or severe side effects appear, hydroxychloroquine 200 mg twice a day may be added to the regimen. A pacemaker defibrillator should be inserted and be continued after the drug therapy is discontinued.

Neurosarcoidosis

This unpredictable complication of sarcoidosis also requires high dosage of prednisone. The disease, however, does not always respond to any therapy. Irradiation of the brain and the spinal cord has been used with some success.

SILICOSIS

method of
JOHN E. PARKER, M.D.

*National Institute for Occupational Safety and
 Health and West Virginia University School of
 Medicine*
Morgantown, West Virginia

Silicosis is a fibrotic disease of the lungs caused by the inhalation of, retention of, and pulmonary reaction to crystalline silica. Despite extensive knowledge about the cause of this pneumoconiosis (respiratory exposures to silica-containing dusts), this serious and potentially fatal occupational lung disease is tragically still seen even today, in the last part of this century in the United States and throughout the world. Silica, or silicon dioxide, is the predominant component of the earth's crust. The three important crystalline forms of silica are quartz, tridymite, and cristobalite. These forms are also called free silica to distinguish them from the silicates. The silica content in different rock formations, such as sandstone, granite, and slate, varies from 20% to nearly 100%. Occupational exposure to silica particles of respirable size (0.5 to 5 μm) is associated with mining, quarrying, drilling, and tunneling operations. Silica exposure is also a potential hazard to sandblasters, stonecutters, and pottery, foundry, ground silica, and refractory workers. The national or worldwide prevalence of silicosis is unknown, but more than 2 million workers in the United States alone are employed in trades at risk for the development of silicosis; in the developing world, cumulative estimates exceed 1 million cases of the disease.

The precise pathogenic mechanism for the development of silicosis remains uncertain. Abundant evidence implicates the interaction between pulmonary alveolar macrophages and silica particles deposited in the lung. It is proposed that surface properties of the silica particle activate macrophages. These cells then release chemotactic factors and inflammatory mediators that result in a further cellular response by polymorphonuclear leukocytes, lymphocytes, and additional macrophages. Fibroblast-stimulating factors are released that promote hyalinization and collagen deposition. The resulting pathologic silicotic lesion is the hyaline nodule, which contains a central acellular zone with extracellular silica surrounded by whorls of collagen and fibroblasts and an active peripheral zone composed of macrophages, fibroblasts, plasma cells, and additional extracellular silica. Impaired macrophage function also plays a role in susceptibility to infectious organisms such as *Mycobacterium tuberculosis* and *Nocardia asteroides*.

There is mounting evidence that freshly fractured silica may be more toxic than aged silica, perhaps related to reactive radical groups on the cleavage planes of freshly fractured silica. This may offer a pathogenic explanation for the observation of cases of advanced disease in both sandblasters and rock drillers where exposures to recently fractured silica are particularly intense.

FORMS OF DISEASE: CLINICAL PICTURE

Chronic silicosis is often asymptomatic and presents as a radiographic abnormality with small (<10 mm), rounded opacities predominantly in the upper lobes. A history of 15 years or more since onset of exposure is common. Results of pulmonary function testing may be normal or may show mild restriction. Less commonly, mild obstruction to airflow or reduced diffusing capacity may be present. Chronic nodular silicosis not infrequently progresses to more advanced disease or progressive massive fibrosis.

Complicated silicosis, also called progressive massive fibrosis, is more likely to present with exertional dyspnea. Progressive massive fibrosis is characterized by nodular opacities greater than 1 cm on the chest radiograph and commonly involves reduced carbon monoxide diffusing capacity, reduced arterial oxygen tension at rest or with exercise, and marked combined obstruction and restriction on spirometry or lung volume measurement. Distortion of the bronchial tree may also lead to airways obstruction and productive cough. Recurrent bacterial infection not unlike that seen in bronchiectasis may occur. Weight loss and cavitation of the large opacities should prompt concern for tuberculosis or other mycobacterial infection. Pneumothorax may be a life-threatening complication, because the fibrotic lung may be difficult to re-expand. Hypoxemic respiratory failure with cor pulmonale is a common terminal event.

Accelerated silicosis may appear after more intense exposures of shorter (5 to 10 years) duration. Symptoms, radiographic findings, and physiologic measurements are similar to those seen in the complicated form. Deterioration in lung function is more rapid, and in some countries, as many as 25% of patients with accelerated disease may develop mycobacterial infection. Autoimmune diseases, including scleroderma and rheumatoid arthritis, are seen with silicosis, often of the accelerated type. The progression of radiographic abnormalities and functional impairment can be rapid when autoimmune disease is associated with silicosis.

Acute silicosis may develop within 6 months to 2 years of massive silica exposure. Dramatic dyspnea, weakness, and weight loss are often presenting symptoms. The radiographic findings of diffuse alveolar filling differ from those in the more chronic forms of silicosis. Histologic findings similar to pulmonary alveolar proteinosis have been described, and extrapulmonary (renal and hepatic) abnormalities are reported. Rapid progression to severe hypoxemic ventilatory failure is the usual course. The potential for mycobacterial infection in acute silicosis requires constant vigilance.

PREVENTION

There is no specific therapy for silicosis. Prevention remains the cornerstone of eliminating this occupational lung disease. The education of workers and employers regarding the hazards of silica dust exposure and measures to control exposure is important. Improved ventilation and local exhaust, process enclosure, wet techniques, personal protection including the proper selection of respirators, and, where possible, industrial substitution of agents less hazardous than silica reduce exposure.

Silicosis is a reportable disease in many states. Even in the absence of legal reporting requirements, cases of silicosis should be viewed as sentinel health events and should initiate work site evaluations to reduce exposures that may be surprisingly excessive even for current workers. Medical examinations of coworkers may also identify additional cases of early or, at times, advanced disease. If silicosis is recognized in a worker, limiting future significant exposure is advisable. Unfortunately, the disease may progress even

---

All material in this chapter is in the public domain, with the exception of any borrowed figures or tables.

without further silica exposure. In the United States, finding a case of silicosis, especially the acute or accelerated form, should prompt notification of state or federal agencies, such as the Occupational Safety and Health Administration, the Mine Safety and Health Administration, or the National Institute for Occupational Safety and Health (NIOSH) to obtain work place evaluations to protect other workers also at risk. NIOSH maintains a toll-free number, 1-800-35-NIOSH, for occupational safety and health information and assistance with work place "health hazard evaluations." In other nations, cases should also be reported by physicians to relevant public health authorities to address primary prevention efforts.

TREATMENT

When prevention has been unsuccessful and silicosis has developed, therapy is directed largely at complications of the disease. Therapeutic measures are similar to those commonly used in the management of airway obstruction, infection, pneumothorax, hypoxemia, and respiratory failure complicating other pulmonary disease. Historically, the inhalation of aerosolized aluminum has been unsuccessful as a specific therapy for silicosis. Polyvinyl pyridine N-oxide, a polymer that has protected laboratory animals, is not available for use in humans. Laboratory work with tetrandrine has shown in vivo reduction in fibrosis and collagen synthesis in silica-exposed animals treated with this drug. However, strong evidence of human efficacy is currently lacking, and this drug is not available in the United States. The search for a specific therapy for silicosis to date has been unrewarding.

If obstructive airway disease with bronchospasm develops, bronchodilator therapy is indicated. Inhaled selective beta$_2$-adrenergic agents, such as albuterol (Ventolin, Proventil), 2 inhalations every 4 to 6 hours, may be helpful. Oral long-acting theophylline preparations, given twice daily, to achieve a blood level of 10 to 20 µg per mL may be beneficial in some patients in combination with inhaled beta agonists.

Episodes of acute bronchitis, commonly caused by *Streptococcus pneumoniae* or *Haemophilus influenzae*, can be treated with ampicillin 250 to 500 mg every 6 hours for a 10-day course. Erythromycin, trimethoprim-sulfamethoxazole (Bactrim, Septra), ciprofloxacin (Cipro), and other antibiotics are also useful for treatment of initial or recurrent episodes of infectious bronchitis. If infection does not improve on empirical therapy, re-evaluation of sputum with Gram's stain, culture, and sensitivity tests should be performed. Pneumococcal and influenza vaccinations are recommended.

Airway secretions causing copious, tenacious sputum production and occasionally disabling cough should be managed with time-honored methods of adequate hydration, humidification, and postural drainage. Cessation of smoking is clearly important and must be strongly encouraged.

Tuberculosis is a common and serious complication, especially in complicated, accelerated, and acute silicosis. Patients with silicosis who have a significant tuberculin skin reaction but no clinical, bacteriologic, or radiographic evidence of active disease should be treated with isoniazid (INH) or rifampin (Rimactane, Rifadin) preventive therapy. These antimicrobials should be given for a minimum of 6 months to 1 year. Some physicians recommend lifelong preventive therapy for tuberculin skin test–positive patients with silicosis. Silicotic patients receiving glucocorticoids should also be considered for INH or rifampin preventive therapy.

The diagnosis of active tuberculosis infection in patients with silicosis can be difficult. Clinical symptoms of weight loss, fever, sweats, and malaise should prompt radiographic evaluation and sputum acid-fast bacilli stains and cultures. Radiographic changes, including enlargement or cavitation of progressive massive fibrosis lesions or nodular opacities, are of particular concern. Bacteriologic studies on expectorated sputum may not always be reliable in silicotuberculosis. Fiberoptic bronchoscopy to obtain additional specimens for culture and study may often be helpful in establishing a diagnosis of active disease.

Proven active tuberculosis and clinically suspected disease should be treated with appropriate antimicrobials (see the article on tuberculosis), now commonly including three or four drugs such as INH, rifampin, pyrazinamide, and ethambutol for a minimum of 6 to 9 months. Because of the difficulties in treating tuberculosis in the setting of silicosis, many authorities have recommended more prolonged courses. Antituberculous therapy, of course, should always be guided by laboratory studies of sensitivity, especially with the increasing recognition of multidrug-resistant organisms. Initiation of therapy before bacteriologic confirmation is prudent in silicotic patients with clinical signs compatible with active tuberculosis. Careful long-term follow-up with chest radiographs, bacteriologic cultures, and monitoring of clinical symptoms is imperative in view of numerous reports of recurrent pulmonary tuberculosis in silicotic patients after the completion of conventional therapeutic courses of antimicrobials.

Hypoxemia should be treated with supplemental oxygen to prevent the development of polycythemia, to delay or prevent development of pulmonary hypertension and cor pulmonale, and to improve exercise tolerance. The goal of oxygen therapy should be to elevate the Po$_2$ above 60 mm Hg. Two to 4 liters per minute of oxygen by nasal cannula often achieves this level of arterial oxygenation. Measurement of arterial blood gases should guide the selection of inspired oxygen concentrations. Portable and home oxygen systems are widely available for managing these patients.

Ventilatory support for respiratory failure is indicated when it is precipitated by a treatable complication. Pneumothorax, spontaneous and ventilator related, is usually treated by chest tube insertion. Bronchopleural fistula may develop, and surgical consultation and management should be considered.

Acute silicosis may rapidly progress to respiratory failure. When this disease resembles pulmonary alveolar proteinosis and severe hypoxemia is present, aggressive therapy has included selective whole-lung lavage with the patient under general anesthesia in an attempt to improve gas exchange and remove alveolar debris. Although it is appealing in concept, the efficacy of whole-lung lavage remains to be established. Glucocorticoid therapy has also been used for acute silicosis; however, it is still of unproven benefit. Prednisone has been used at dosages of 40 to 60 mg per day for 1 to 2 months and, if accompanied by evidence of clinical improvement, has been tapered to 15 to 20 mg per day and continued for 6 months to 1 year. Early, rigorous initial evaluation for tuberculosis and other mycobacterial infection cannot be overemphasized. INH or rifampin should be given while steroids are administered. Empirical therapy with three or four antituberculous drugs pending results of cultures for 6 weeks may be appropriate in the life-threatening acute form of disease.

Some young patients with end-stage silicosis may be considered candidates for lung or heart-lung transplantation by centers experienced with this procedure. Early referral and evaluation for this intervention may be offered to selected patients.

The discussion of an aggressive and high-technology therapeutic intervention such as whole-lung lavage and transplantation serves to dramatically underscore the serious and potentially fatal nature of silicosis as well as emphasize the crucial role for primary prevention.

HYPERSENSITIVITY PNEUMONITIS
(Allergic Alveolitis)

method of
H. BENFER KALTREIDER, M.D.
VA Medical Center San Francisco and School of Medicine, University of California, San Francisco
San Francisco, California

DEFINITION AND ETIOLOGY

Hypersensitivity pneumonitis, or allergic alveolitis, constitutes a group of inflammatory interstitial lung diseases that result from allergic or hypersensitivity immune reactions to the repeated inhalation or ingestion of a variety of antigens derived from fungal, bacterial, animal protein, or reactive chemical sources. A selected listing of examples of hypersensitivity pneumonitis and the major etiologic agents responsible for their pathogenesis are shown in Table 1. The most important etiologic agents are (1) thermophilic actinomycetes, which are responsible for farmer's lung, bagassosis, and humidifier lung; (2) avian serum proteins, which induce bird fancier's lung; (3) fungi such as *Aspergillus* and *Penicillium* species, which cause malt worker's and cheese worker's lung; and (4) reactive chemical compounds such as toluene diisocyanate and certain drugs. A large number of additional environmental agents have been associated on occasion with the development

TABLE 1. **Representative Syndromes of Hypersensitivity Pneumonitis**

Clinical Syndromes by Etiologic Category	Major Causative Agents	Environmental Source
Thermophilic Actinomycetes		
Farmer's lung	*Faeni rectivirgula* Thermoactinomyces vulgaris*	Moldy hay
Bagassosis	*Thermoactinomyces sacchari, T. vulgaris*	Moldy pressed sugar cane
Humidifier lung	*T. vulgaris, Thermoactinomyces candidus*	Contaminated humidifiers, air conditioners
Avian Proteins		
Bird fancier's lung	Avian proteins	Bird droppings, feathers
Fungi		
Malt worker's lung	*Aspergillus clavatus*	Moldy malt
Cheese worker's lung	*Penicillium casei*	Cheese mold
Suberosis	*Penicillium frequentans*	Moldy cork
Reactive Chemicals and Drugs		
Hypersensitivity pneumonitis	Toluene diisocyanate Trimellitic anhydride	Plastics industry
	Amiodarone, gold, minocycline	Medications

*Formerly *Micropolyspora faeni.*

of hypersensitivity pneumonitis. Regardless of the precise etiologic agent or the environmental setting in which it is encountered, the pathogenesis and clinical manifestations of the resultant hypersensitivity pneumonitis are identical.

PATHOGENESIS

Hypersensitivity pneumonitis is an allergic inflammatory and granulomatous interstitial lung disease for which the inciting antigen is often identifiable. The pathogenicity of an environmental antigen is dictated by its chemical composition (usually an organic particle or a reactive chemical), particle size, and the dose and duration of exposure. The susceptibility of the host to allergic lung injury is also of critical importance, because only a minority of equally exposed individuals develop pneumonitis. The pathogenesis of hypersensitivity pneumonitis requires ongoing or repeated exposure to the offending antigen. During the initial sensitizing exposures, the host generates appropriate immune responses to the antigen, which consist of specific antibody and sensitized T lymphocytes. Subsequent antigen exposure of sensitized individuals can produce lung injury in those who are predisposed to develop hypersensitivity immune reactions.

DIAGNOSIS
Clinical

Two distinct clinical syndromes, with different presentations and manifestations, are recognizable: acute and subacute-chronic hypersensitivity pneumonitis. The different manifestations are primarily determined by the intensity and frequency of antigen exposure. Episodes of acute hypersensitivity pneumonitis result from intermittent intense exposure and are reversible. Acutely, symptoms consist of a flulike illness characterized by dyspnea, chest tightness, and a nonproductive cough accompanied by fever, chills, malaise, and myalgias that occur 4 to 6 hours after inhalation of antigen. There are signs of fever, tachypnea, cyanosis, and bibasilar crackles in the lungs. The diagnosis is readily apparent when the characteristic illness occurs 4 to 6 hours after exposure to a suspect environmental antigen and the symptoms resolve with cessation of exposure. Otherwise, the clinical syndrome is nonspecific and indistinguishable from an acute respiratory infection.

Subacute-chronic hypersensitivity pneumonitis results from chronic, low-level exposure to antigen. The onset is insidious, with few if any symptoms during the early stages of the disease process. In the later stages, after interstitial inflammation and fibrosis have been established, symptoms of increasing dyspnea on exertion, fatigue, anorexia, cough, and weight loss appear. Physical signs include restriction of ventilation, bibasilar crackles, and eventually signs of right-sided heart failure. The clinical findings usually do not bear an obvious temporal relationship to antigen exposure and are nonspecific in that they are characteristic of interstitial lung diseases of a variety of causes. Only a detailed occupational, environmental, and drug ingestion history coupled with a high index of suspicion will lead to the correct identification of the cause of the lung disease.

Radiographic

The chest radiograph in acute disease may be normal or reveal ill-defined air-space nodularity or consolidation diffusely at the lung bases. In subacute disease, it shows a diffuse, fine nodular or reticulonodular pattern. In chronic hypersensitivity pneumonitis, there are reduced lung volumes, diffuse or patchy interstitial fibrosis, and, at advanced stages, honeycombing. These radiographic findings, although characteristic, are nonspecific.

If the chest radiograph is normal in acute disease, high-resolution computed tomography (HRCT) of the chest offers a remarkably sensitive tool for detecting early interstitial and air-space changes. In subacute hypersensitivity pneumonitis, HRCT often reveals characteristic patchy ground-glass and nodular opacities in a centrilobular distribution throughout the lungs. In chronic disease, there are findings of fibrosis with superimposed ground-glass nodular opacities. HRCT is useful for determining the activity, extent, and progression of the lung disease.

Physiologic

Pulmonary physiologic abnormalities are those of a restrictive ventilatory defect characterized by reductions in the vital capacity, the total lung capacity, and the diffusing capacity for carbon monoxide. Airways obstruction is absent or mild. Moderate hypoxemia and mild hypocapnia are often present. In acute disease, physiologic changes revert to normal between episodes. In chronic disease, physiologic abnormalities are progressive and largely irreversible.

Laboratory

Routine laboratory studies are nonspecific. Acutely, there is a neutrophilic leukocytosis; the white blood cell count is normal in subacute-chronic disease. Eosinophilia is distinctly unusual at any stage of the disease. There may be a polyclonal increase in immunoglobulins, but the serum concentration of IgE is normal. Immunologic studies reveal serum precipitating antibodies against the suspect antigen in more than 90% of cases. Commercial precipitin batteries for thermophilic organisms, avian antigens, and molds are available, but their sensitivity depends on the quality and quantity of antigens used for testing. The presence of precipitins indicates intense exposure to antigen and provides an important clue to etiology but does not establish a causal relationship between antigen exposure and lung disease. Bronchoalveolar lavage reveals a marked increase in the percentages of lymphocytes (up to 80% total cells), the majority of which are T cells. In the absence of a characteristic clinical syndrome, such as frequently occurs in subacute-chronic disease, a lung biopsy showing characteristic alveolar and peribronchiolar lymphocytic infiltrations may be necessary to suggest the diagnosis of hypersensitivity pneumonitis. Inhalation provocation with highly purified antigen preparations under controlled laboratory conditions elicits the reproduction of the acute clinical syndrome and, although investigational, can definitively establish the causal etiologic role of an environmental antigen.

TREATMENT

Antigen Avoidance

The mainstays of treatment are early and accurate diagnosis, avoidance of continued exposure to the offending antigen, and corticosteroid therapy. The maneuvers used to establish an accurate diagnosis will suggest the appropriate therapeutic program. An accurate diagnosis of acute hypersensitivity pneumonitis may be suspected clinically on the basis of a high index of suspicion, a thorough environmental and drug history, and the onset of the typical clinical syndrome several hours after exposure to the suspect antigen. A presumptive diagnosis will be established by observing amelioration of symptoms after removal of the patient from the suspect environment, followed by exacerbation of symptoms after reentry into the environment. Strong supporting evidence for the correct etiologic agent can be obtained from serum precipitin analysis. A positive test result indicates intense exposure to the antigen and, in the proper clinical setting, suggests a causal relation between exposure and disease. Inhalation provocation is definitive but investigational, and it should be reserved for selected cases in which the causal relationship between antigen and lung disease must be established.

An accurate diagnosis having been established and the offending agent and environment having been identified, measures to avoid exposure should be designed and instituted. Avoidance of antigen exposure is most important and may be accomplished by eliminating the offending antigen or its source from the work place or domestic environment, discontinuing suspect drugs, removing the individual from the environment, using a respiratory protective device, changing the nature of employment in the work place, or when all else fails, changing the patient's occupation or residence on a trial basis or permanently. When avoidance is successful, the syndrome of acute hypersensitivity pneumonitis will resolve completely and spontaneously. Subacute disease will relentlessly progress unless exposure to the offending antigen is completely eliminated. Subacute-chronic disease may not resolve spontaneously and will usually require additional therapy with corticosteroids.

Drug Therapy

Mild episodes of acute pneumonitis will resolve spontaneously on removal of the patient from the offending environment. Resolution of severe episodes of acute hypersensitivity pneumonitis can be hastened by a brief course of oral or parenteral corticosteroid therapy, in addition to oxygen and other supportive measures. Such patients can be treated safely with a brief, rapidly tapering course of prednisone, 0.5 mg per kg per day for 7 to 14 days, depending on the severity of illness. Subacute-chronic hypersensitivity pneumonitis, like other inflammatory interstitial lung diseases, requires moderate doses of prednisone, 1.0 mg per kg per day for 4 to 6 weeks, followed by gradual reduction to a maintenance dose of 10 to 20 mg per day. An objective response should be evident after 4 to 6 weeks, in which case maintenance therapy should be continued until no further improvement occurs. If lung disease flares during tapering or after discontinuation of steroid therapy, the patient should be maintained with the lowest effective dose of prednisone indefinitely. The effectiveness of therapy is monitored by measuring clinical, radiographic, and physiologic parameters. Current practice dictates prompt and aggressive treatment of both the acute and subacute-chronic forms of hypersensitivity pneumonitis to prevent progression to fibrosis. The long-term beneficial effects of corticosteroids on arresting disease progression are encouraging; however, they remain to be definitively established.

SINUSITIS

method of
ALAN H. SHIKANI, M.D.
The Johns Hopkins Medical Institutions
Baltimore, Maryland

Sinusitis is defined as an inflammation of the lining of the membranes of any of the paranasal sinuses. The sinuses are lined with ciliated stratified columnar epithelium and are continuous with the upper respiratory tract through the sinus ostia. Inflammation causes mucosal edema and increased sinonasal secretion. Whereas the most common cause is an upper respiratory tract infection, other etiologies include an acute exacerbation of allergic rhinitis, dental infection or manipulation, and trauma to the sinuses. If sinus obstruction occurs, the retained secretion results in a milieu that is well suited for bacterial growth, and bacterial sinusitis occurs.

Underlying host factors are significant in the genesis of sinusitis. General predisposing causes include immunodeficiency, acetylsalicylic acid–asthma–polyposis triad, abnormal mucociliary clearance secondary to ciliary structural abnormalities as in Kartagener's syndrome, and secretory disturbances such as those in cystic fibrosis. Local anatomic factors are also significant. The importance of severe septal deviation has been recognized for some time, but localized abnormalities in the anterior ethmoid–middle meatal area appear to be even more important.

The anterior ethmoid–middle meatal complex (ostiomeatal complex) is a key area in the pathogenesis of sinusitis. The ostiomeatal complex contains the narrow channels that provide for mucociliary clearance and ventilation of the anterior ethmoid, maxillary, and frontal sinuses. Relatively minor swelling of the mucosa in this area, such as that associated with viral upper respiratory tract infections or allergic rhinitis, may lead to frontal or maxillary sinus obstruction and secondary disease within these sinuses. Nasal foreign bodies, including nasogastric tubes, nasotracheal tubes, and nasal packing, also risk blocking the ostiomeatal complex and causing nosocomial sinusitis. When the sinus drainage is obstructed, mucus, inflammatory cells, and bacteria accumulate and oxygen tension in the sinuses is reduced. Opsonization, phagocytosis of bacteria, and immunoglobulin-dependent activities are impaired. Drainage and ventilation of the major paranasal sinuses depend on the patency of the ostiomeatal complex. It is therefore imperative that this area be carefully evaluated by diagnostic endoscopy and computed tomography (CT) before surgical intervention is contemplated on the sinuses. If such an evaluation reveals an underlying ostiomeatal cause for chronic or recurrent disease, intranasal removal of the cause typically allows the secondary mucosal disease to resolve.

Sinusitis can be classified as acute or chronic on the basis of the duration of the infection. Even though multiple organisms have been isolated from infected sinuses, a "normal flora" has been cultured from healthy uninfected sinuses (including *Streptococcus pneumoniae; Haemophilus influenzae; Staphylococcus aureus*; and anaerobes such as *Bacteroides*, anaerobic gram-positive cocci, and *Fusobacterium*), but the bacterial titer of resident flora is usually low. When bacterial titers exceed 1000 cfu per mL, they are truly pathogenic. The bacteria implicated as primary pathogens in acute sinusitis are *S. pneumoniae, H. influenzae,* and *Branhamella (Moraxella) catarrhalis. Bacteroides* species and *S. aureus* are found in 8 to 10% of acute sinusitis cases. In contrast, chronic sinusitis is usually associated with anaerobes, most commonly *Bacteroides* species, anaerobic gram-positive cocci, *Fusobacterium* species, *Streptococcus, Veillonella,* and *Corynebacterium* species. Gram-negative bacteria predominate in nosocomial sinusitis, including *Pseudomonas aeruginosa, Klebsiella pneumoniae,* and *Enterobacter* species. The bacterial growth on cultures of specimens obtained from the nose or nasopharynx and growth on those obtained with sinus aspiration or open antrostomy frequently do not correlate, unless gross purulent discharge is visible through the sinus ostium and is available for culture. Hence, the decision about initial management is often a clinical one, based on the history and physical examination findings. Other organisms can infect the sinuses rarely, including *Actinomyces* species and *Nocardia* species. There should be a high index of suspicion for fungal sinusitis (e.g., sinusitis caused by *Aspergillus, Bipolaris, Candida, Mucor, Penicillium*) for nonresponders to antibiotic therapy and for immunocompromised patients.

DIAGNOSIS

The symptoms of acute sinusitis are usually localized to the region of the sinus involved and may include discomfort, pain, headache, and tenderness. In infection of deeper structures such as the posterior ethmoids and sphenoid, symptoms are deep in the head or referred to the occiput. Acute sinusitis is also typically accompanied by systemic signs such as fever, leukocytosis, and lassitude along with purulent nasal discharge. In addition, the patient may complain of smell disorder, pain with mastication, toothache, and fever. The symptoms of chronic sinusitis, on the other hand, tend to be more vague and poorly localized. In both types of sinusitis, one may have suppurative rhinorrhea, nasal obstruction, postnasal drainage, and pharyngitis. When a sinus is acutely infected, physical examination may reveal sinus tenderness, erythema and swelling of overlying skin, and purulent nasal exudate. Transillumination sometimes provides information about the condition of the maxillary and frontal sinuses. Endoscopic examination of the nose and the sinuses with the telescope is the most reliable method to differentiate purulence, mucus, serous fluid, and thickened mucosa. Nasal endoscopy is also critical in the evaluation of the key ostiomeatal area and in identification and biopsy of suspicious lesions.

Complementary to the physical examination are radiologic studies including conventional sinus radiographs and CT scans. The conventional (or plain film) examination usually consists of Waters', Caldwell's, lateral, and basal views of the sinuses. These views give excellent visualization of the frontal and maxillary sinuses and moderately good visualization of the sphenoid. However, plain film radiographs provide poor visualization of the ethmoid sinus as a result of density averaging. Plain films are therefore useful for diagnosing frontal and maxillary sinus disease but are of limited use in the diagnosis of disease in the important area of the ostiomeatal complex.

The most appropriate method for the diagnosis of ostiomeatal complex disease is CT, and this radiologic study is necessary to diagnose local underlying causes of recurrent or chronic sinusitis. CT is usually best performed after acute changes have been treated. The scan is performed in the coronal plane without intravenous contrast enhancement and is viewed with magnification of the sinus area; window settings are similar to those used to visualize the lung. These parameters optimize demonstration of the fine anatomy of the area and allow not only visualization of gross disease but, more important, identification of minor disease and anatomic obstruction in key areas.

Magnetic resonance imaging is not currently the study of choice for the evaluation of sinus disease. Although magnetic resonance imaging is useful in the differentiation of soft tissue disease, it does not demonstrate the bone, whereas CT allows excellent visualization of the fine bony anatomy and its important anatomic variants. Bony changes may also occur as a result of disease. Inflammatory disease typically expands bone and causes a reactive osteitis, whereas bone destruction is more suggestive of a malignant lesion, although such a lesion may also occur with severe infections and with mucoceles. The use of intravenous contrast enhancement during sinus CT is indicated if there may be an intracranial complication.

TREATMENT

Nonsurgical Treatment

Early treatment is medical and consists of the use of antibiotics and decongestants and the avoidance of any exacerbating environmental factors. Oral decongestants such as pseudoephedrine or phenylpropanolamine are helpful but should be used with care in hypertensive patients. In older male patients, these drugs may cause urinary retention. A nasal spray (e.g., oxymetazoline [Afrin]) may be added but should be used for no more than 3 to 5 days. A broad-spectrum antibiotic is typically chosen to cover the usual sinus pathogens (H. influenzae, S. pneumoniae, and B. catarrhalis). Amoxicillin 500 mg orally three times daily may be used as an initial treatment, but I am noticing an increasing incidence of resistance to penicillins. Cephalosporins provide more powerful alternatives for nonresponders. I favor cefuroxime (Ceftin) 250 to 500 mg twice daily, cefpodoxime (Vantin) 200 to 400 mg twice daily, loracarbef (Lorabid) 200 to 400 mg twice daily, or cefaclor (Ceclor) 500 mg three times daily. Another good alternative is amoxicillin–clavulanate potassium (Augmentin) 500 mg three times daily. Clarithromycin (Biaxin) 250 to 500 mg twice daily or an azithromycin (Zithromax) pack (Z-PAK) may be given to patients who are allergic to penicillins. Time-honored remedies such as inhalation of steam or mist are often not prescribed but may aid both comfort and drainage. Patients with signs and symptoms suggestive of allergic sinusitis and patients with present chronic sinusitis are also treated with a nasal steroid spray, such as fluticasone (Flonase), beclomethasone (Beconase, Vancenase), triamcinolone (Nasacort), budesonide (Rhinocort), or flunisolide (Nasarel).

If medical treatment fails to relieve the symptoms of maxillary sinusitis or pansinusitis, a repeated course with a stronger antibiotic is initiated. Irrigation of the maxillary sinus is performed when a patient is immunosuppressed or has an underlying immunodeficiency to allow accurate culture in acute sinusitis. This method washes out the inspissated material and allows accurate culture.

Acute ethmoid sinusitis, particularly in children, may lead to periorbital or infraorbital abscess, but such a complication is rare outside the pediatric age group. However, acute frontal and sphenoid sinusitis should be considered a medical emergency at any age because of the potential for disease in these sinuses to spread intracranially. Patients with acute symptomatic frontal and sphenoid sinusitis are usually hospitalized and given intravenous rather than oral antibiotic therapy. Failure to improve with medical therapy requires surgical drainage. In the case of acute, poorly responding frontal sinusitis, frontal sinus trephine and irrigation are performed. The irrigation catheter may be left in place for several days. In persistent sphenoid sinusitis, sphenoidotomy is performed.

Whereas acute sinusitis frequently demonstrates a heavy bacterial growth of a predominant pathogen, chronic sinusitis is typically a polymicrobial infection in which anaerobes are often present. Antibiotic therapy is therefore adjusted accordingly, and prolonged therapy (2 to 6 weeks or more) may be required. The prolonged use of topical steroids and short bursts of oral steroid therapy may also help to reduce swelling and relieve ostiomeatal obstruction. Allergic patients also benefit from use of antihistamines and desensitization. Smoke and other environmental pollutants may be exacerbating factors and are to be avoided. Because the most frequent local cause of chronic sinusitis is ostiomeatal disease and the extent of the underlying ostiomeatal disease may be limited, nasal endoscopy and CT are of particular value in these patients. Endoscopy provides the ability to visualize the middle meatus and adjacent ethmoid structure and to identify areas of persistent infection and edema. It allows the response to medical therapy to be accurately monitored and permits culture to be performed with precision. This anatomic area also varies widely, and anatomic abnormalities that narrow the ostiomeatal channels and predispose to infection can be identified. CT provides complementary information about the deeper sinuses and ostiomeatal structures. However, in interpreting CT findings, it must be remembered that asymptomatic mucosal thickening may be evident on a CT scan and is not predictive of clinically significant sinus disease.

Endoscopy also provides the ability to accurately visualize disease within the maxillary or sphenoid sinus for an accurate diagnosis of unusual radiographic findings. Maxillary sinuscopy is performed by a cannula inserted sublabially under local anesthesia. Biopsies can be performed and cysts removed. Sphenoid sinuscopy may be performed via a trocar introduced intranasally or after intranasal sphenoidotomy.

Surgical Treatment

The importance of managing the underlying problems, whether these are irritation, allergic factors, or structural nasal deformities, cannot be overemphasized. The goal of treatment is restoration of normal ventilation and mucociliary clearance and ultimately reversal of mucosal disease. Although the predominant symptoms and disease are often in the maxillary or frontal sinus, careful endoscopic evaluation and CT frequently reveal underlying disease in the ostiomeatal area. This improved diagnostic accuracy has reduced the need for surgical procedures aimed at the major sinuses. Even when the disease within these sinuses appears to be extensive, the initial approach is often intranasal removal of the underlying ostiomeatal problem. This approach has been termed "functional endonasal surgery" or, when it is performed under endoscopic visualization, "functional endoscopic surgery."

The channels for sinus ventilation and mucociliary clearance within the ostiomeatal complex are narrow and tortuous. Minor underlying disease in this area may therefore cause extensive secondary changes. Thus, localized obstruction in the narrow opening of the frontal recess may give rise to an extensive frontal sinus mucocele. In identifying the relative importance of ostiomeatal disease in chronic or recurrent acute sinusitis, the site of disease is thus more relevant than the extent.

Indications for functional surgery include sinusitis that persists despite adequate medical therapy and documented recurrent acute sinusitis with related structural or inflammatory abnormalities in the ostiomeatal unit. The functional approach can usually be performed with local anesthesia without external incision and dramatically reduces morbidity compared with standard open surgical techniques. Damage to normal anatomy is minimized, and packing is usually not required. This type of surgery, however, is complicated and requires special skills if the risks to adjacent critical structures are to be minimized. After surgery, the secondarily involved mucosa usually recovers slowly. The extent of surgery performed with this approach varies from a limited procedure to complete sphenoethmoidectomy with opening of both maxillary and frontal sinuses.

Indications for external sinus surgery include osteomyelitis, orbital complications, intracranial complications, and failure of the functional approach. Numerous techniques for cleaning the different sinuses have been described. The frontal sinus may be approached by an external frontoethmoidectomy by using a curvilinear incision in the area of the medial canthus. It can also be approached more completely by an incision across the eyebrows or behind the hairline. In the latter case, the anterior bony wall of the sinus is incised and reflected anteriorly to provide access. The maxillary sinus is typically approached by a sublabial incision (Caldwell-Luc), and the ethmoid by an incision on the side of the nose (external ethmoidectomy). Unfortunately, these procedures, particularly the frontal sinus osteoplasty, may create permanent changes in the sinuses that can be difficult to differentiate radiologically from disease recurrence.

COMPLICATIONS OF SINUSITIS

One of the more common complications of sinusitis, primarily in children, is the spread of ethmoid infection into the orbit. The first indication of orbital involvement is inflammatory edema of the eyelids. Progression of the infection may be rapid with chemosis, ophthalmoplegia, and even visual loss. In the early cellulitic stage of the disease, intravenous antibiotic therapy is appropriate. However, careful evaluation and an orbital CT scan are required to rule out a subperiosteal abscess or intraorbital abscess, both of which require prompt surgical drainage.

Purulent frontal sinusitis may result in extension of the infection through the anterior wall and presentation as Pott's puffy tumor. Inflammatory sinus disease may also spread intracranially and result in meningitis or epidural, subdural, or brain abscess. The precise frequency of intracranial complications is not known. However, sinusitis is reported to be the source of 35 to 65% of subdural abscesses. Such complications, although uncommon, are not rare. Intracranial complications are most likely to occur from acute frontal sinus disease, but they also occur from the sphenoid or, less frequently, the ethmoid sinus. These complications are most common in adolescent patients, and there is male predominance. If there is a clinical suggestion of intracranial spread, lumbar puncture and intravenous contrast–enhanced CT or magnetic resonance imaging should be performed. Magnetic resonance imaging is more sensitive for identifying early intracranial disease and epidural abscess. If intracranial infection occurs, early surgical drainage of the sinuses is usually performed; when indicated, it can be combined with surgical drainage of the intracranial collection.

STREPTOCOCCAL PHARYNGITIS

method of
MICHAEL A. GERBER, M.D.
*University of Connecticut School of Medicine
and Connecticut Children's Medical Center
Hartford, Connecticut*

Pharyngitis is one of the most common reasons for patients to visit primary health care providers. Although most cases are caused by viruses, group A beta-hemolytic streptococci (GABHS) are the most common agents of bacterial pharyngitis, the only commonly occurring form of acute pharyngitis for which antimicrobial therapy is definitely indicated. Therefore, when the physician is confronted with a patient with acute pharyngitis, the clinical decision that usually needs to be made is whether the pharyngitis is attributable to GABHS. GABHS pharyngitis is important not only because of the acute morbidity associated with it but also because it may be followed by nonsuppurative sequelae—acute rheumatic fever or acute glomerulonephritis. GABHS pharyngitis is spread by person-to-person contact with infectious nasal or oral secretions and is more common in situations of crowding, such as in schools, and during the colder months of the year.

DIAGNOSIS

It is extremely difficult to distinguish GABHS pharyngitis from other forms of acute pharyngitis on the basis of clinical findings alone. Therefore, an accurate diagnosis depends on the performance of a throat culture or antigen detection test. However, the throat culture or antigen detection test cannot distinguish between patients with bona fide streptococcal infections and those who are streptococcal carriers. Patients who are streptococcal carriers pose no danger to themselves or to others. They do not develop acute rheumatic fever, and they rarely spread the organism to contacts. Consequently, they usually do not need to be identified or treated. To minimize the number of streptococcal carriers who have cultures and are subsequently treated unnecessarily with antimicrobials, throat cultures or antigen detection tests should be performed selectively.

In attempting to decide whether to perform a laboratory test on a patient presenting with acute pharyngitis, the epidemiologic and clinical findings should be considered before the test is performed. GABHS pharyngitis is primarily a disease of children between 5 and 15 years of age; in temperate climates, it usually occurs in the winter and early spring. A history of close contact with a patient with well-documented GABHS pharyngitis is helpful, as is an awareness of a high prevalence of GABHS infections in the community. Patients with GABHS pharyngitis commonly present with sore throat (generally of sudden onset), pain on swallowing, and fever. Headache, nausea, vomiting, and abdominal pain may also be present, especially in children. On examination, patients have tonsillopharyngeal erythema, with or without exudate, and tender, enlarged anterior cervical lymph nodes. Other findings may include a beefy red swollen uvula, petechiae on the palate, excoriated nares (especially in infants), and a scarlatiniform rash. However, none of these findings is specific for GABHS pharyngitis, and they may occur with other upper respiratory infections as well. Conversely, clinical features such as conjunctivitis, cough, hoarseness, coryza, anterior stomatitis, discrete ulcerative lesions, viral exanthem, and diarrhea strongly suggest a virus rather than GABHS as the etiologic agent. Testing usually need not be performed on patients with acute pharyngitis whose clinical and epidemiologic features do not suggest GABHS as the cause.

It is usually not necessary to perform a throat culture (or rapid antigen test) on or to treat household contacts of a patient with GABHS pharyngitis who are asymptomatic. Laboratory testing of asymptomatic family contacts with treatment of those whose test results are positive is advisable only when there is someone in the family with a history of rheumatic fever, during outbreaks of either acute rheumatic fever or poststreptococcal acute glomerulonephritis, during outbreaks of GABHS pharyngitis in closed or semiclosed communities, and when "Ping-Pong" spread of GABHS has been occurring within a family. Only symptomatic household contacts of a patient with GABHS pharyngitis should have a culture (or rapid antigen test) performed and be treated if results are positive.

THERAPY

Objectives

There are several reasons for attempting to diagnose and treat GABHS pharyngitis. (1) It has been established that eradication of the GABHS from the upper respiratory tract of a patient with acute pharyngitis will prevent that patient from developing acute rheumatic fever. However, antimicrobial therapy has not been shown to be effective in preventing the other nonsuppurative sequela of pharyngitis—poststreptococcal glomerulonephritis. (2) Antimicrobial therapy helps to prevent the suppurative sequelae of GABHS pharyngitis, such as peritonsillar abscess, retropharyngeal abscess, and cervical lymphadenitis. These complications were relatively common in the preantibiotic era, but their frequency has declined markedly with the use of antimicrobial therapy. (3) Eradication of the infecting GABHS from the patient's upper respiratory tract with antimicrobial therapy prevents spread of that organism to other individuals. (4) Antimicrobial therapy, particularly if it is begun early in the disease, can shorten the clinical course of the illness.

Specific Agents

The oral antimicrobial of choice is penicillin V (phenoxymethylpenicillin) (Table 1). All patients should

TABLE 1. **Treatment of Group A Beta-Hemolytic Streptococcal Pharyngitis**

Category	Dose	Mode	Duration
Benzathine penicillin G	600,000 U for patients ≤27 kg (60 lb) 1,200,000 U for patients >27 kg (60 lb) *or*	Intramuscular	Once
Penicillin V (phenoxy-methylpenicillin)	Children: 250 mg 2–3 times/d Adolescents and adults: 500 mg 2–3 times/d	Oral	10 d
For Individuals Allergic to Penicillin			
Erythromycin Estolate (Ilosone)	20–40 mg/kg/d 2–4 times/d (maximum, 1 gm/d) *or*	Oral	10 d
Ethylsuccinate (E.E.S.)	40 mg/kg/d 2–4 times/d (maximum, 1 gm/d)	Oral	10 d

From Dajani A, Taubert K, Ferrieri P, et al: Treatment of acute streptococcal pharyngitis and prevention of rheumatic fever: A statement for health professionals. Reproduced by permission of Pediatrics 96:758–764, copyright 1995.

continue to take the penicillin regularly for an entire 10-day period, even though they will likely be asymptomatic after the first few days. Although the broader spectrum penicillins, ampicillin and amoxicillin, are often used for the treatment of GABHS pharyngitis because they taste much better than penicillin V, they offer no microbiologic advantage over penicillin V. Because of problems with compliance with a 10-day oral regimen, the most effective treatment of GABHS pharyngitis is a single intramuscular injection of benzathine penicillin G (see Table 1). Preparations containing procaine penicillin in addition to benzathine penicillin G are associated with decreased pain at the injection site. If such mixtures are used, care must be taken to provide the required amount of benzathine penicillin G. The combination of 900,000 units of benzathine penicillin G and 300,000 units of procaine penicillin is satisfactory for most children, but the efficacy of this combination in adolescents and adults requires further study. Orally administered erythromycin is indicated for patients allergic to penicillin (see Table 1). Other agents shown to be effective in the treatment of GABHS pharyngitis include the new macrolides azithromycin (Zithromax) administered as a once-daily regimen and clarithromycin (Biaxin) administered as a twice-daily regimen.

A 10-day course of a narrow-spectrum oral cephalosporin is an acceptable alternative, particularly for individuals allergic to penicillin. However, as many as 15% of penicillin-allergic persons are also allergic to cephalosporins. Therefore, a cephalosporin should not be administered to patients with immediate, anaphylactic-type hypersensitivity to penicillin.

Reports have suggested that a 5-day course of azithromycin or of selected oral cephalosporins is comparable to a 10-day course of oral penicillin in eradicating GABHS from the pharynx. However, further studies are warranted to expand and confirm these observations before these regimens can be recommended for routine use. The new macrolides and most oral cephalosporins are considerably more expensive than penicillin and have a wider range of antibacterial activity, both of which preclude recommending them for routine use in persons with GABHS who are not allergic to penicillin.

Certain antimicrobials are not recommended for the treatment of GABHS pharyngitis. Tetracyclines and trimethoprim-sulfamethoxazole (Bactrim, Septra) have been shown to be ineffective in the treatment of this disease. The sulfonamides, although effective as a continuous prophylaxis for prevention of recurrent attacks of rheumatic fever, will not eradicate the streptococci from the upper respiratory tract and should not be used for the treatment of GABHS pharyngitis. Penicillinase-resistant penicillins are considerably more expensive and offer no advantage over penicillin V, even in patients who harbor penicillinase-producing staphylococci in their upper respiratory tract; therefore, they should not be used.

Scarlet fever is simply GABHS pharyngitis with a rash, and the antimicrobial therapy should be identical to that for routine GABHS pharyngitis.

Treatment Failures

Routine throat culturing (or rapid antigen testing) of asymptomatic individuals after completion of antimicrobial therapy for GABHS pharyngitis is not necessary. Only those patients who have a return of signs and symptoms of acute pharyngitis within the succeeding few weeks should return for reassessment. Should such a symptomatic patient again have a positive culture or antigen detection test result for GABHS, there are several possible explanations: persistence of the streptococcal carrier state with an intercurrent viral pharyngitis; noncompliance with the prescribed antimicrobial regimen; or a new infection with GABHS acquired from family, classroom, or community contacts. A second episode of acute pharyngitis with the original infecting GABHS strain (i.e., treatment failure) cannot be ruled out, but this occurs only rarely. For a single episode of symptomatic culture or rapid test–confirmed GABHS pharyngitis occurring shortly after completion of a course of appropriate antimicrobial therapy, any of the agents listed in Table 2 is appropriate. Because the patient's compliance with oral antimicrobials is often an issue, a regimen employing intramuscular benzathine penicillin G should be considered. For a single repeated episode, it is usually not necessary to reculture the throat (or repeat the antigen detection test) after the

TABLE 2. **Eradication of Group A Beta-Hemolytic Streptococcal Carrier State**

Agent	Dose	Mode	Duration
Clindamycin (Cleocin)	20 mg/kg/d in 3 doses	Oral	10 d
Rifampin (Rifadin) *plus*	20 mg/kg/d in 2 doses	Oral	4 d
Benzathine penicillin G	600,000 U for patients ≤27 kg (60 lb) 1,200,000 U for patients >27 kg (60 lb)	Intramuscular	Once
Penicillin V (phenoxy-methylpenicillin)	Children: 250 mg 2–3 times/d Adolescents and adults: 500 mg 2–3 times/d	Oral	10 d
plus Rifampin	20 mg/kg/d in a single dose	Oral	4 d (last 4 d of penicillin regimen)

second course of therapy unless the patient remains or again becomes symptomatic.

Streptococcal Carriers

During the winter and spring in temperate climates, as many as 20% of asymptomatic school-age children may be streptococcal carriers. These individuals have GABHS present in their pharynx but have no evidence of an immunologic reaction to this organism. They may be colonized by GABHS for several months and during that period may experience episodes of intercurrent viral pharyngitis. When tested, these patients have GABHS in their pharynx and would appear to be suffering from acute GABHS pharyngitis. Streptococcal carriers are unlikely to spread the organism to their close contacts and are at low risk, if any, for developing suppurative or nonsuppurative (e.g., acute rheumatic fever) complications. Streptococcal carriers do not ordinarily require antimicrobial therapy. In addition, it is more difficult to eradicate GABHS from the upper respiratory tracts of streptococcal carriers than from those with acute GABHS pharyngitis. This has been shown to be true for penicillin therapy and may also be true for some other antimicrobials.

Eradication of the streptococcal carrier state may be desirable when the family has a history of rheumatic fever, when Ping-Pong spread of GABHS has taken place within a family, when a family has an inordinate amount of anxiety about GABHS, when outbreaks of GABHS occur in closed or semiclosed communities, or when tonsillectomy is being considered only because of chronic carriage of GABHS. A short course of rifampin in conjunction with penicillin has been shown to be effective in eradicating the streptococcal carrier state. A 10-day course of oral clindamycin has also been shown to be effective (see Table 2).

Recurrent Pharyngitis

An often challenging situation is the individual who experiences multiple episodes of laboratory-confirmed GABHS pharyngitis within a period of months to years. It is likely that most of these patients are chronic GABHS carriers experiencing intercurrent viral infections. Information regarding the clinical and epidemiologic findings with each of these episodes, the serologic response to GABHS extracellular antigens, the clinical response to antibiotic therapy, and the presence or absence of GABHS in throat cultures taken during asymptomatic intervals is helpful in distinguishing persistent GABHS carriage from repeated episodes of GABHS pharyngitis. Serotyping of repeated streptococcal isolates from an individual patient may also assist in making this distinction, but such studies are available only from specialized research laboratories.

When a physician suspects that Ping-Pong spread is causing multiple repeated episodes of GABHS pharyngitis within a family, simultaneously obtaining cultures from all family contacts and treating those whose cultures are positive may be helpful. There is no credible evidence that family pets are reservoirs for GABHS or that they contribute to spread of GABHS within the family.

Continuous antimicrobial prophylaxis is not recommended for patients experiencing repeated episodes of GABHS pharyngitis because there is insufficient evidence to show that it is effective. Surgical removal of the tonsils may be considered in the rare patient whose symptomatic episodes do not diminish in frequency in time and in whom no alternative explanation for the recurrent pharyngitis is evident. Tonsillectomy may decrease recurrences of symptomatic pharyngitis in selected patients, but only for a limited time.

TUBERCULOSIS AND OTHER MYCOBACTERIAL DISEASES

method of
JOHN G. WEG, M.D.
University of Michigan Medical Center
Ann Arbor, Michigan

TUBERCULOSIS

Tuberculosis (TB) has ably demonstrated that it is the phoenix of infectious diseases. After a decline from 84,000 to 22,255 reported cases of TB in the United States from 1953 to 1984, the number of cases increased 18%, approximately 4400, from 1985 to 1991 and peaked at 26,673 (10.46 per 100,000) in 1992. Concomitant with this increase was a reported increase in drug resistance: 14.2% of cases to one or more drugs; 9.5% to isoniazid (INH) or rifampin (RIF); and 3.5% to both INH and RIF, multidrug-resistant tuberculosis (MDR TB).

TB is also a disease of paradox. The increased incidence was generally limited to large metropolitan areas and our southern border while other areas showed a continued decline in cases. New York City (NYC) accounted for 14% of the increase through 1993. In contrast, 15 states had case rates of 3.5 per 100,000 or less, and 14 states had rates of 3.6 to 5.9 per 100,000. From 1958 to 1969, 5.8% of U.S. naval recruits were tuberculin reactors compared with 2.5% in 1990. In men, it was 5.2% among blacks, 5.4% among Hispanics, 26.4% among Asian–Pacific Islanders, and 0.8% among whites. It was greater in foreign-born recruits, 19.2%, than in U.S.-born recruits, 1.6%.

Resistance to INH or RIF was found in 107 counties in 33 states, and MDR TB was found in 35 counties in 13 states; NYC accounted for 61.4% of the nation's MDR TB in 1991. A report, however, has documented the spread of MDR TB from NYC by a patient in Denver, Colorado; by patients in Florida and Nevada; and by health care workers in Atlanta, Georgia, and Miami, Florida. This raises the specter of widespread MDR TB in the United States.

The increased incidence of TB and MDR TB can be traced to

1. The increase in human immunodeficiency virus (HIV) disease, particularly in injection drug users
2. The high incidence in racial and ethnic minorities: non-Hispanic blacks, Hispanics, Asian–Pacific Islanders, Native Americans, and Alaskan natives, especially among those younger than 35 years
3. The foreign-born (their proportion of U.S. TB cases increased from 21.6% in 1986 to 29.6% in 1993)—about two thirds from Mexico, the Philippines, Vietnam, People's Republic of China, South Korea, and Haiti, the majority identified in their first 5 years in the United States
4. Our population 65 years of age or older, particularly those in nursing homes
5. The homeless and those in jails
6. The abandonment of well-documented means of preventing the transmission of TB in health care facilities—the spread of the majority of MDR TB in NYC has been traced to just four hospitals
7. Errors in medical decision-making by physicians—addition of a single drug to a failing regimen, inadequate primary regimen, failure to recognize initial or acquired resistance, failure to recognize and respond to nonadherence (noncompliance), failure to provide indicated INH prophylaxis or inappropriate prophylaxis (one drug with disease, or INH when the index case has INH drug resistance)
8. The most critical, the radical decline of the essential infrastructure for the prevention and elimination of TB—the public health services provided by federal, state, county, and city governments—at one NYC hospital in 1988, 89% of patients discharged

on TB treatment were lost to follow-up and did not complete therapy; in contrast, Baltimore, which maintained its public health services, preserved a continuing decline in incidence

The incidence of TB has been decreasing since 1993 because of the reallocation of governmental resources; the reinstitution of procedures to prevent TB transmission in health care facilities; and the dramatic growth of directly observed therapy (DOT), particularly in high-incidence areas, in high-risk populations, and for those likely to be nonadherent to therapy. The total number of reported cases in the United States in 1995 was 22,813 (8.7 per 100,000); the estimate for 1996 is approximately 20,155. The incidence of resistance to INH has decreased to 7.6%, and the incidence of MDR TB to 1.4%. From 1992 to 1994, there has been a 21% decrease in NYC cases and a remarkable 44% decrease in MDR TB. This decrease has been attributed primarily to the interruption in the transmission of TB and to DOT.

Practicing Physician

The practicing physician plays the preeminent role in (1) identifying patients with TB, (2) reporting them to the health department, (3) ensuring successful completion of therapy, and (4) initiating plans for contact investigation. This physician must ensure initial susceptibility testing; prescribe appropriate drug therapy to prevent the emergence of resistance; compare susceptibility test results with the initial regimen; monitor carefully to identify failing regimens or nonadherence; and seek consultation with a physician expert in the care of complicated cases, such as patients with drug-resistant TB or MDR TB (Table 1).

Mycobacteriology Laboratory

The mycobacteriology laboratory plays an essential secondary role in providing high-quality smear and

TABLE 1. **Principles of Tuberculosis Therapy**

Think tuberculosis with compatible presentation, especially in high-risk groups.
Report every case of tuberculosis to the health department.
Partner with the health department
  Free drugs
  Contact investigation
  Directly observed therapy
  Prevalence of drug resistance in the community
  Mycobacteriology services
Test for all new isolates for drug susceptibility.
Initiate therapy with isoniazid, rifampin, pyrazinamide, and ethambutol (or streptomycin in children too young to monitor for visual acuity) for 2 mo, followed by 4 mo of isoniazid and rifampin. Ethambutol may be withheld if certain conditions are met (see text).
Consult an expert in the treatment of tuberculosis if drug resistance, especially multidrug-resistant tuberculosis, is identified (five or more drugs may be needed) or a regimen is failing (two or three drugs to which the organism is susceptible should be added).
Isolate pulmonary and laryngeal tuberculosis suspects immediately.

culture techniques. This requires rapid laboratory methods: fluorescent acid-fast staining, liquid medium for primary culture, radiometric or similar systems (e.g., BACTEC), and susceptibility testing for first-line drugs.

The Food and Drug Administration (FDA) has approved a nucleic acid amplification test, the amplified *Mycobacterium tuberculosis* direct (MTD) test (Gen-Probe, San Diego, CA), for use along with cultures on respiratory specimens that are positive on smear from untreated patients. This test has had a 95.5% sensitivity and 100% specificity in clinical trials. However, this includes some MTD test–positive specimens that were culture-negative with other specimens being positive. Other reports have indicated low positivity with non-TB mycobacteria. Another test, Amplicor (Roche Diagnostic Systems, Basel, Switzerland), is in the process of being approved. Limited data suggest that these tests are less sensitive for smear-negative specimens, nonrespiratory specimens, or specimens from treated patients. A polymerase chain reaction assay of peripheral blood specimens (not commercially available) correctly identified 39 of 41 patients with proven pulmonary TB, 63% of whom were smear-negative; 43% of these patients were HIV infected. The sensitivity and specificity were 95% and 89%, respectively. The appropriate role of nucleic acid amplification testing awaits further study.

The laboratory should be able by law to report positive cultures to the health department. In addition, I recommend that a clinician expert at each hospital or health care facility be notified of each positive culture and act in an oversight role to be sure that the patient's physician is aware of the culture and has initiated appropriate action. This is especially valuable for cultures reported after patients have been discharged.

Health Department

Although the practicing physician has the preeminent role in treating TB, the state and local health departments have the primary responsibility for the prevention and control of TB. Their highest priority is the identification and treatment (ensuring completion of therapy) of persons with TB. They are responsible for contact investigation, screening of high-risk individuals, and provision of appropriate preventive therapy. They must also develop overall TB policy and collect data to monitor outcomes. Whereas these responsibilities are public health mandates, TB control programs must respect the individual patient-physician relationship. If patients indicate that they wish to be under the care of their physician, the TB control program should partner with them to achieve mutual goals. The principles of TB therapy are provided in Table 1. Because the incidence of TB is low in many parts of the country, it may escape consideration. This also occurs in large metropolitan areas in hospitals not primarily responsible for TB.

Drug Therapy for Disease

Daily Self-administered Therapy

The best regimen is a 6-month course of INH, RIF, pyrazinamide (PZA), and ethambutol (EMB) or streptomycin (SM) in children too young to test for visual acuity for 2 months followed by INH and RIF for 4 months. This regimen is successful even with INH resistance. EMB (or SM) can be discontinued if the organisms are susceptible. An alternative is to withhold EMB if the likelihood of drug-resistant TB is low. This is defined as (1) less than 4% primary resistance (organisms from patients never treated for TB) and (2) the patient had no previous TB drug treatment, is not from a country with a high prevalence of drug resistance, and had no known exposure to a drug-resistant case. The local or state health department is the source of information on drug resistance and may be able to assist in determining the patient-related elements just described. Prescribing a four-drug initial course until drug susceptibility studies are available generally offers a higher likelihood of avoiding drug resistance with a low risk for drug toxicity and increases the efficiency of members of the health care team. Patients should have baseline measurements of hepatic enzyme activities and bilirubin level, a complete blood count, and a platelet estimate or platelet count. A serum creatinine concentration should be obtained if SM or other aminoglycosides are used; a uric acid level determination if PZA is used; and visual acuity testing and red-green color discrimination if EMB is used (formal ophthalmologic evaluation is not necessary). If the findings on baseline assessment are normal, laboratory studies need not be done again unless the clinical findings at monthly evaluations for toxic drug effects warrant a repeat. These monthly visits should include detailed review of medication ingestion to ensure adherence. Daily self-administration of medications is appropriate for patients in whom concerns about adherence do not arise after careful inquiry. Such individuals will generally have a stable home, family unit, and work or school environment. A combination form of INH-RIF is recommended to improve adherence and avoid resistance that might develop if only one of these agents is used.

An alternative acceptable 9-month regimen is INH and RIF. EMB (SM in children too young to test for visual acuity) should be given until drug susceptibilities are available. This alternative regimen should be reserved for people who cannot or should not take PZA. If the organisms are INH resistant, RIF and EMB should be given for 12 months. Patients with silicotuberculosis should have therapy extended at least 2 months.

Directly Observed Therapy

Adherence is of concern in patients with the following problems: homelessness, drug addiction, alcoholism, psychiatric or psychosocial dysfunction, communication difficulty, history of poor adherence, migrant status, unemployment, low income, low socioeconomic status, members of a minority, and cultural characteristics (Hispanic and other cultures believing in folk illness and/or faith healers). There is extremely convincing evidence that DOT achieves well in excess of 90% completion of the prescribed drug regimen. Not only has it been shown to avoid increasing the number of patients with drug resistance or MDR TB, but it has also dramatically reduced its prevalence in areas with high rates of MDR TB. DOT is also appropriate for patients in whom initial treatment has failed and for those with drug-resistant TB and MDR TB.

Two effective regimens are available. INH, RIF, PZA, and EMB (or SM) are given daily for 2 weeks, followed by the four drugs given twice a week for 6 weeks, followed by INH and RIF twice a week for 16 weeks. All the drugs must be given by DOT. The second effective DOT intermittent regimen uses INH, RIF, PZA, and EMB (or SM) three times a week for 6 months.

Intermittent therapy must be directly observed. It is best handled through the department of health. The observer is usually a health care provider, although any reliable individual may be designated to serve this function. The usual site for DOT is a clinic, but the use of other sites can be effective, such as schools, drug treatment facilities, prisons, places of employment, nursing homes, physicians' offices, or patients' homes (place of residence).

Whereas the success of DOT is without question, it ought not be a requirement for all patients. Such a position infringes on the individual's rights. Its effectiveness has been demonstrated in "worst case" scenarios such as NYC. In Baltimore, DOT has resulted in the greatest decline (50%) in TB incidence in large U.S. cities and rare (0.57%) MDR TB. In the late 1960s in Houston, 95% 2-year drug completion was achieved with self-administered therapy and adaptable outreach programs. In Massachusetts, a public health nurse case management approach with the majority of patients receiving self-administered therapy—incorporating selective use of DOT and providing a multiservice, highly structured, long-term care facility when necessary—has also been highly successful. Hospitalization has been voluntary, but court-ordered hospitalization is also available. A spectrum of care options would seem to serve most communities with highly effective therapy for TB in a cooperative partnership between the patient, his or her social unit (if available), the practicing physician, and the health department.

Smear- and Culture-Negative Pulmonary Tuberculosis

In the past a person with a pulmonary parenchymal infiltrate compatible with TB and a "positive" purified protein derivative (PPD) intermediate skin test response was given INH for 12 months as secondary prevention. Such patients have more recently been categorized as having smear- and culture-negative "active" tuberculosis because a substantial number (7 to 41%) become smear- and/or culture-positive

with clinical disease. Data are also available to solidly support the efficacy of a 4-month course of treatment with INH and RIF, adding EMB (or SM) until results of susceptibility studies return. This approach is more likely to be completed because it is shorter and avoids the anomalous position of treating disease with a lesser number of organisms for a longer period than regular treatment.

Evaluating Treatment Response

Sputum smears and cultures should be obtained at least monthly until sputum cultures are negative for 2 months. Sputum cultures from patients receiving INH- and RIF-containing regimens become negative at 2 months in more than 85% of cases. If cultures are negative after 2 months, at least one further culture should be obtained at completion of therapy along with a chest radiograph to serve as a baseline for potential future evaluations. Further scheduled follow-up is not necessary for those with a prompt satisfactory response who do not have risk factors for reactivation. If the patient is immunosuppressed (e.g., HIV disease, lymphoma), has a large residual on a chest radiograph, or was slow to respond, a 6-month follow-up chest radiograph and sputum smear and culture (if there is sputum) should be obtained. All patients, after successful completion of therapy, should be advised to seek medical attention if prolonged cough, fever, weight loss, or even prolonged malaise or fatigue develops and to inform their physician of their history of TB and its treatment.

If cultures are positive after 2 months, a thorough re-evaluation is necessary. It should include repeated drug susceptibility studies, chest radiography, and re-evaluation of the adherence to therapy. If drug resistance is not identified, it is strongly recommended that therapy be given under DOT. If drug resistance is identified, the patient should receive at least two drugs to which the organisms are susceptible after consultation with an expert in the treatment of TB. Subsequent treatment should be by DOT, and the expert consultant should continue to advise on management.

Extrapulmonary Tuberculosis

Extrapulmonary TB is effectively treated with the same 6-month or alternative 9-month regimen used for pulmonary TB. In children, a 12-month course of therapy is recommended for miliary, bone and joint, and meningeal TB.

Corticosteroids

The use of corticosteroids reduces the likelihood of constrictive TB pericarditis and the neurologic sequelae of TB meningitis. Corticosteroids have also been shown to be of benefit in patients with TB who are in an acutely toxic condition by reducing fevers, enhancing weight gain, and decreasing generalized toxic effects. These patients generally have extensive cavitary disease and/or hematogenous dissemination. Reported doses have ranged from 20 to 60 mg per day for a period of about 3 weeks. Corticosteroids have not altered outcome when they were given to patients with TB pleural effusions.

Pregnancy

Although INH, RIF, and EMB cross the placenta, there is no evidence that they have teratogenic effects. PZA is recommended internationally, but this drug is given a C category by the FDA ("use only if clearly necessary") because animal reproduction studies have not been performed. SM is the only antituberculous drug documented to harm the fetus; it interferes with ear development and may cause deafness. The other aminoglycosides are likely to have the same effect. At present, other antituberculous drugs such as ethionamide and cycloserine cannot be recommended because of inadequate information. Nursing need not be discontinued because of TB therapy.

Patients with HIV Infection and AIDS

Patients with HIV infection and those with acquired immune deficiency syndrome (AIDS) with susceptible organisms should receive a 6-month regimen of therapy. The majority of these patients should receive DOT because of concomitant problems such as injection drug use. They require careful monitoring of response to therapy. Extension of therapy is recommended if response is slow, e.g., cultures are positive at 2 months and beyond. TB and AIDS frequently coexist, but there is wide geographic variation. Nationally, approximately 1 in 10 patients with TB has AIDS, but in NYC it is about 1 in 4. Nationally, 1 in 20 patients with AIDS has TB, but in NYC it is about 1 in 10. In about 90% of cases, TB is identified in the 2 years before or first year after the diagnosis of AIDS. Five states account for more than 75% of the matched cases—New York including NYC, New Jersey, Florida, Texas, and California. TB therapy is effective in patients with HIV infection or AIDS, especially those receiving DOT and those who have completed at least 8 weeks of therapy. Time to conversion of sputum to negative and relapse rates are the same as in patients without HIV infection or AIDS. However, mortality due to the HIV infection and AIDS is appreciable, and TB contributes to the mortality if it is not treated or receives only brief treatment. In patients with HIV infection or AIDS, TB may be rapidly fatal.

Protease Inhibitors and Rifamycins

Protease inhibitors (PIs), e.g., saquinavir, ritonavir, indinavir, and nelfinavir,* retard the metabolism of rifamycins. Rifamycins induce the hepatic cytochrome P-450 oxidases that accelerate the metabolism of the PIs, resulting in subtherapeutic PI levels that may reduce their effectiveness or increase the risk for PI resistance. PIs conversely retard the metabolism of rifamycin, resulting in high serum rifamycin levels, which may cause uveitis. Recommendations to resolve this serious concern are in

flux. If a patient has not started a PI, one should consider delaying its use until a minimal 6-month RIF-containing regimen has been successfully completed. For the patient already receiving a PI, various alternatives are being suggested, although sufficient data to support them are not available, e.g., (1) discontinue the PI, which could result in deterioration of the patient and the development of PI resistance; (2) use a four-drug RIF-containing regimen for at least 2 months or until cultures are negative, then continue INH and EMB for an additional 16 months; or (3) continue the PI using only indinavir 800 mg every 8 hours and treat with a four-drug regimen using rifabutin 150 mg per day instead of RIF (rifabutin is not FDA approved for TB), with measurement of serum rifabutin levels if possible. An expert Public Health Service–Infectious Disease Society working group has met (November 1996). Additional information is available from the Centers for Disease Control and Prevention (404-639-8123). Clearly, the complexities of these interactions warrant direction of therapy with both PIs and anti-tuberculous drugs by an expert.

Drug Resistance or Failure

Patients who have drug-resistant TB or MDR TB should be under the care of or have care guided by an expert in TB. These patients should have DOT, and as previously noted, this is best accomplished by or with the assistance of the health department. The drug selection process must be on an individual basis. The current reports on MDR TB are generally confounded by a large proportion of patients with concomitant HIV infection and AIDS. However, one report of a small number of patients with MDR TB but without HIV infection or AIDS showed 96% clinical response with negative cultures when they were done. Other studies reported overall response rates of 50 to 65% with many of the patients having HIV infection or AIDS. However, if effective drugs are used, up to 100% sputum conversion has been reported with 88% survival at 4 months or later.

Treatment failure is defined as continuing positive cultures after 5 to 6 months of what is believed to be effective therapy on the basis of initial susceptibility studies. Patients with treatment failure require repeated susceptibility studies. Some physicians add three new drugs while waiting for these (a reasonable practice when results took months), whereas others continue with the initial regimen if the patient is stable.

Relapse

Relapse is defined as recurrence of TB on smear or culture in a person who had previously been successfully tested, i.e., negative smears and cultures at the end of treatment. Radiographic progression should also be considered a relapse even with negative cultures if other diseases are excluded by a thorough evaluation usually including fiberoptic bronchoscopy with bronchoalveolar lavage and transbronchial biopsy. These patients should be started on a standard

---

*Not available in the United States.

6-month or alternative 9-month regimen while awaiting results of susceptibility studies. Organisms from patients who have relapsed usually do not develop resistance.

The Drugs

Table 2 lists the commonly used drugs with daily dose, side effects, and drug interactions. RIF impairs the effectiveness of oral contraceptives, warfarin, imidazole, antifungals, azathioprine, cyclosporine, digoxin, propranolol, quinidine, theophylline, diazepam, glucocorticoids, haloperidol, opioids, and tolbutamide and may increase the levels of trimethoprim-sulfamethoxazole. The recommended adult doses for the two-times-a-week regimen are INH 900 mg maximum (15 mg per kg); RIF 600 mg maximum (10 mg per kg); PZA 4 grams* maximum (50 to 70 mg per kg); EMB 2.5 grams* maximum (50 mg per kg); or SM 1.5 grams maximum (25 to 30 mg per kg). The recommended doses for the three-times-a-week regimen in adults are the same for INH, RIF, and PZA; for EMB 2.5 grams maximum (25 to 30 mg per kg) or SM 1 gram maximum (25 to 30 mg per kg).

Other drugs have been shown to be effective against *M. tuberculosis* but have not yet been evaluated with the same rigor as the standard drugs. Amikacin is bactericidal; 15 mg per kg for 5 of 7 days is the recommended dose. Its side effects are similar to those of the other aminoglycosides, with nephrotoxicity the major concern. Ofloxacin (Floxin), ciprofloxacin (Cipro), rifabutin (Mycobutin), and amoxicillin-clavulanate (Augmentin) have also been shown to be effective in vitro. Clofazimine (Lamprene), which is slowly bactericidal for *Mycobacterium leprae*, also inhibits *M. tuberculosis*. The newer macrolides clarithromycin and azithromycin also have in vitro effectiveness (see section on treatment of *Mycobacterium avium-intracellulare* [MAI] disease).

Preventive Therapy

The recommendations for the use of INH 300 mg per day for 6 months (9 months in children according to the American Academy of Pediatrics) are based on clinical risk factors and the measured diameter of induration resulting from a PPD intermediate skin test (Table 3). A significant (positive) PPD skin test response is an indicator of infection with mycobacteria (mycobacteria other than *M. tuberculosis* may cross-react with the PPD tuberculin used in the skin test). The interpretation of the PPD skin test result has evolved in the last 2 decades by incorporating (1) the likelihood that a given diameter of induration represents infection with *M. tuberculosis*; (2) the clinical information concerning an individual's risk for infection, e.g., close exposure to a patient with smear-positive TB, HIV infection, AIDS, or other immunocompromised conditions; and (3) the goals of providing preventive therapy to those at greatest risk and avoiding such therapy in those at low risk to achieve the best cost/benefit ratio in terms of both money and potential morbidity. The following patients should not receive INH preventive therapy: (1) patients who had previous adequate therapy or preventive therapy with INH; (2) patients with previous INH hepatitis; associated drug fever, rash, or arthritis; or unstable active hepatitis; and (3) patients whose contacts have INH-resistant TB or MDR TB.

INH 300 mg daily should be provided for only a month at a time. At monthly visits, patients should be asked if they have had anorexia, nausea, or vomiting; dark urine; jaundice; rash; numbness and tingling of hands or feet; fatigue or weakness; abdominal discomfort, pain, or tenderness (especially in the right upper quadrant); or fever. Laboratory monitoring is unnecessary unless there is increased concern for hepatotoxicity, i.e., daily alcohol consumption, chronic liver disease, or age 35 years or older. INH can also be given by DOT at a dose of 15 mg per kg twice a week.

The use of RIF 600 mg per day is recommended for close contacts of patients with INH-resistant organisms; some physicians also give EMB. The most appropriate therapy for close contacts of patients with MDR TB is less clear. Some would just observe because a proven treatment is not available. Others would give 6 months of PZA and EMB. Perhaps the most prudent approach is to select a 6-month, two-drug regimen with one drug that is bactericidal, if possible, on the basis of susceptibility studies of the index case's organisms.

The role of bacille Calmette-Guérin (BCG) continues to create differences of opinion. There is current agreement, however, to recommend BCG for infants and children younger than 5 years (1) with negative PPD skin test results who have a high risk for intimate or prolonged exposure to patients who are not treated or who are receiving ineffective treatment and (2) when the rate of new infections is more than 1% per year and in whom the standard programs do not work. Others would consider individuals frequently exposed to untreated infectious TB, e.g., hospital personnel including house staff, workers in homeless shelters, and others.

Prevention of Transmission

The most effective means of preventing transmission of TB is the early diagnosis and effective treatment of every person with TB disease; this is *chemical isolation*. The most likely disseminator of TB is the person with laryngeal or pulmonary TB that is not promptly recognized. Any patient in whom infectious TB (pulmonary and laryngeal) is suspected should be promptly isolated and maintained in isolation until infectious TB is reasonably excluded, e.g., three adequate sputum samples or a bronchoalveolar lavage specimen negative for mycobacteria with use of the rhodamine-auramine staining technique or a transbronchial biopsy specimen that has no granu-

---

*Exceeds dosage recommended by the manufacturer.

TABLE 2. **Antituberculosis Drugs, Their Side Effects, and Drug Interactions**

Drug	Dosage (Adult Daily)*	Side Effects (Usual)	Drug Interactions	Remarks
Isoniazid†	5–10 mg/kg (300–600 mg)	Hepatitis, peripheral neuritis, hypersensitivity, convulsions (with overdose)	Isoniazid and phenytoin ↑ concentrations of both; isoniazid ↑ concentration of carbamazepine	Add pyridoxine 25 mg/d in pregnancy, alcoholism, uremia, malnutrition, diabetes; 50–100 mg to treat neuropathy
Rifampin (Rifadin)	600 mg once/d (in children, 10–20 mg/kg to a maximum of 600 mg)	Hepatitis, gastrointestinal upset, rash; rarely thrombocytopenia, cholestatic jaundice	Multiple (see text)	Extremely effective; drug interactions: birth control pills, warfarin, tolbutamide, corticosteroids, methadone, digitoxin
Pyrazinamide†	20–35 mg/kg (not to exceed 3 gm)	Hyperuricemia, hepatotoxicity, arthralgia, rash, gastrointestinal upset		Salicylates for arthralgia
Ethambutol (Myambutol)‡	15 mg/kg	Optic neuritis (reversible with discontinuation of drug; rare at dose of 15 mg/kg), rash		Ocular history and ophthalmoscopic examination before use; visual acuity, red-green color discrimination (Snellen chart); ↓ dose if renal insufficiency
Streptomycin†	0.75–1.0 gm (usually given for initial 60 d); cumulative dose ≤120 gm	Otic and vestibular toxicity, vertigo, tinnitus, decreased hearing (nephrotoxicity—rare)	Ototoxicity ↑ with ethacrynic acid, furosemide, and mannitol; additive toxicity with other aminoglycosides	Side effects more common in older patients (>60 y); decrease dose or avoid drug if renal insufficiency is present
p-Aminosalicylic acid (aminosalicylic acid)§	12–16 gm (150 mg/kg)	Gastrointestinal upset, sensitivity (rash), hepatotoxicity, sodium load	↓ Vitamin B₁₂ absorption	For gastrointestinal upset, temporarily reduce dose; orphan drug (manufactured by Jacobus Pharmaceutical Co., Princeton, NJ)
Ethionamide (Trecator-SC)§	750–1000 mg (15–20 mg/kg)	Gastrointestinal symptoms, hepatotoxicity, hypersensitivity (rash), arthralgias, impotence, gynecomastia, photosensitivity, metallic taste		May ↓ gastrointestinal symptoms by ↑ dose slowly, give at bedtime with antiemetic 0.5 h before; temporarily stop or reduce dose with gastrointestinal upset; monitor alanine and aspartate aminotransferases monthly
Cycloserine (Seromycin)§	750–1000 mg (15–20 mg/kg)	Personality changes, psychosis, convulsions, peripheral neuropathy, rash	Decreases phenytoin metabolism	Pyridoxine, 150 mg/d to ↓ neuropathy; mental problems are more common with predisposition; monitor blood levels if poor renal function
Capreomycin (Capastat)†	1 gm (15–30 mg/kg) for 60 to 120 d, followed by 1 gm 2 to 3 times/wk (750 mg if >60 y)	Ototoxicity, nephrotoxicity, vestibulotoxicity, and hepatotoxicity, hypersensitivity, hypokalemia	As for streptomycin	Effective; frequent cross-resistance with viomycin, also kanamycin; not for pediatric use; see also remarks for streptomycin; audiogram baseline and q 2 mo
Viomycin†	1 gm q 12 h twice/wk	Similar to those of streptomycin, but nephrotoxicity is more common; hypokalemia, hypocalcemia	As for streptomycin	As for streptomycin; not currently available in the United States
Kanamycin (Kantrex)†	0.5–1 gm (15–30 mg/kg) as for streptomycin	Similar to those of streptomycin	As for streptomycin	Rarely used; avoid concomitant ethacrynic acid, furosemide, or mercurial diuretics and mannitol

*See also manufacturers' official directives.
†Bactericidal.
‡May be bactericidal at high dose.
§Bacteriostatic.

TABLE 3. **Indications for Preventive Therapy**

≤5 mm of Induration (primary prophylaxis–prevention of infection)

Children and adolescents in close contact with a newly diagnosed infectious TB patient; if repeated PPD skin test response is <5 mm at 12 wk, stop INH.

HIV-infected and AIDS patients with close contact with a newly diagnosed infectious TB patient: INH × 12 mo*

5–9 mm of Induration (secondary prophylaxis–prevention of disease)

HIV infection and AIDS*

Risk factors for HIV infection and AIDS

Other close contacts of a newly diagnosed infectious TB patient†

Fibrotic lesions on chest radiographs (see text for smear-negative and culture-negative active TB)

≥10 mm of Induration

Infants and children <4 y

PPD converters with an increase in induration of ≥10 mm within 2 y, <35 y; increase of 15 mm >35 y

Diabetes mellitus—especially brittle diabetes

Prolonged adrenal steroids >15 mg of prednisone or equivalent >2–3 wk

Other immunosuppressive therapy

Some hematologic and reticuloendothelial diseases, e.g., leukemia, lymphoma

Injection drug users who are HIV-negative

End-stage renal disease

Rapid weight loss of chronic malnutrition, e.g., after gastrectomy, malabsorption, intestinal bypass for weight loss

Foreign-born persons from high-prevalence countries

Medically underserved low-income populations

Residents of long-term care facilities

Some suggest preventive therapy for staff of long-term care facilities who have induration of ≥10 mm and for those ≤35 y (I suggest <20 y) with induration of ≥15 mm.

---

*AIDS patients frequently (>60%) have skin test anergy including negative PPD skin test results in the majority of those with TB.

†With pregnancy, delay prophylaxis to after delivery unless recently infected or with HIV infection or AIDS.

Abbreviations: AIDS = acquired immune deficiency syndrome; HIV = human immunodeficiency virus; INH = isoniazid; PPD = purified protein derivative; TB = tuberculosis.

---

loma or negative TB tissue stains; one need not wait for cultures to return to discontinue isolation.

Institutional responsibilities for preventing transmission include

1. Administrative planning to reduce exposure of the largest number of health care workers through written policies, implementing effective isolation techniques for health care workers (e.g., proper wearing of individual respiratory protection devices), keeping isolation room doors closed, and educating and screening health care workers about TB

2. Use of appropriate engineering controls for isolation and treatment rooms: local exhaust ventilation (minimum of 6 changes per hour; new construction, 12 or more per hour); negative pressure in room to control direction of airflow; diluting or decontaminating air by general ventilation; and cleaning air by high-efficiency particulate air filtration or upper room ultraviolet germicidal eradication

Personal respiratory protection is a responsibility shared by the institution (making available respira-

tory protection devices that meet federal guidelines) and the individual (wearing the mask correctly, i.e., fitted tightly over nose, chin, and cheeks, not pulled down below the nose; wearing the mask whenever in an infectious TB patient's room or when such a patient is in a treatment room, not putting the mask on during bronchoscopy and taking it off when the bronchoscope is withdrawn while the unmasked patient is still in the room). Alternatively, the patient should wear a mask in his or her room, in the treatment room (when possible), and when being transported through the facility for necessary procedures. Cleaning, disinfecting, and sterilizing of equipment used in care of the patient should follow standard practices.

OTHER MYCOBACTERIAL INFECTIONS

A diagnosis of disease due to mycobacteria other than *M. tuberculosis* requires (1) the presence of disease not attributable to another cause, (2) more than one isolation of the same species in adequate numbers, or (3) isolation from diseased tissue.

Mycobacterium kansasii disease is usually seen in association with underlying lung disease, such as chronic obstructive lung disease. It has been recognized as a complication of HIV infection and AIDS. *M. kansasii* generally responds well to antituberculous chemotherapy. RIF and EMB in standard doses with or without INH for 12 months results in negative sputum cultures in 3 to 5 months with a relapse rate of 3 to 10%. Relapse rates are higher if RIF is not in the regimen and for 9 months of treatment versus 12 months. Continuing treatment for 18 months does not improve the results. In patients with AIDS, *M. kansasii* is more likely if CD4+ lymphocyte counts are low, about 50 per mm³. This is similar to MAI disease and contrasts with TB, which is usually found close to the time of diagnosis of HIV infection with CD4+ cell counts near normal.

Mycobacterium avium-intracellulare Disease

MAI disease also occurs most commonly in patients with underlying lung disease and is a common complication of late-stage AIDS when CD4+ counts are about 50 to 100 per mm³; it occurs in about 22% of AIDS patients. The following regimen has been recommended: clarithromycin 500 mg twice daily or 750 mg daily, EMB 25 mg per kg daily, clofazimine* 100 to 200 mg daily, and SM 10 to 12 mg per kg daily or amikacin* 12 to 15 mg per kg three times a week for 2 months followed by clarithromycin 750 mg daily, EMB 15 mg per kg daily, and clofazimine 50 to 100 mg daily for 18 to 24 months. More recently, HIV-infected patients with MAI bacteremia treated with rifabutin 300 mg daily, EMB 15 mg per kg daily,

---

*Exceeds dosage recommended by the manufacturer; not approved for this use by the FDA.

and clarithromycin 1000 mg twice daily developed negative blood cultures in 69% overall and in 78% of those who received the drugs for 3 weeks, with a median survival of 8.6 months. The dose of rifabutin (Mycobutin) was reduced from 600 to 300 mg because of the development of uveitis in about 37% of those at the high dose versus 4% at 300 mg. The uveitis resolved with discontinuation of the rifabutin and corticosteroid eye drops. Currently, a modification of this regimen is being considered: rifabutin 600 mg daily for 2 to 4 weeks to shorten the time to blood sterilization and reduction of the dose of clarithromycin to 500 mg twice daily (the approved dose in the United States). Rifabutin reduces serum clarithromycin levels by about half, whereas clarithromycin increases the serum concentration of rifabutin 2 to 3 times. Although this three-drug regimen has not been studied in patients without HIV infection, it would be expected to be at least as effective and to avoid the need for an intramuscular drug; the duration of such a regimen is not known.

Rifabutin, azithromycin, and clarithromycin have been shown to be effective in preventing MAI bacteremia (disseminated MAI disease) in patients with HIV infection and should be given when the CD4$^+$ count is 75 per mm^3 or less. The last two result in drug resistance. Some recommend combinations of one of these macrolides with rifabutin, especially when the CD4$^+$ cell count is extremely low, about 10 per mm^3.

Section 4

The Cardiovascular System

ACQUIRED DISEASES OF THE AORTA

method of
MICHAEL E. DeBAKEY, M.D., and
CHARLES H. McCOLLUM, M.D.

Baylor College of Medicine
Houston, Texas

Acquired diseases of the aorta, which may affect a significant number of people, may be classified into two major categories: aneurysmal and occlusive disease. Atherosclerosis is the major cause of this disease. It may be associated with a degenerative process that increases with age. Other causes include infection, inflammation, trauma, cystic medial necrosis, and previous aortic surgery. Abnormal genetic factors, which produce molecular changes that in turn cause alterations in elastin and collagen of the aorta, have also been identified in some families. Among the risk factors that have been associated with this disease are hypertension, tobacco use, and hyperlipidemia. In addition, patients with aortic diseases often have concomitant peripheral arterial occlusive or aneurysmal disease, as well as coronary artery disease.

Aortic aneurysms may be asymptomatic or may cause symptoms by expansion of the aneurysm or compression of adjacent structures. Ultimately, if the patient is not treated, rupture and death may occur. Manifestations of occlusive disease of the aorta are claudication or tissue loss in the legs with or without renal or visceral arterial ischemia. Such manifestations may produce hypertension, renal failure, or ischemia with or without necrosis of the intestines.

Surgical treatment for acquired aortic disease is well standardized, with a low operative risk and excellent results. Depending on the nature and extent of the disease, resection with graft replacement is indicated primarily for aneurysmal disease, whereas bypass grafting is usually used for occlusive disease. Several types of prosthetic grafts are available. Our preference is the Dacron graft, which is available in various sizes and in two types of fabric. The knitted Dacron velour graft is preferable under normal conditions of blood coagulation. The nonporous, woven graft is used in aneurysmal disease when systemic heparinization is necessary. Albumin-, gelatin-, and collagen-impregnated grafts cause less bleeding at implantation and provide better porosity for healing.

Preoperative evaluation of patients with acquired aortic disease is important. Many of these patients are elderly and have pre-existing or associated diseases. Cardiac, pulmonary, and renal artery problems are common, and hypertension, diabetes, and a history of stroke may also be present. The principal cause of death after major aortic surgery is cardiac arrest. Therefore, thorough preoperative examination, including cardiac function with stress or dipyridamole thallium echocardiography and possibly coronary arteriography, is important. Correction of cardiac risk factors will improve the survival rate in patients undergoing major aortic surgery. Complete evaluation of the pulmonary and renal status is critical. Patients who have had a stroke or symptoms of cerebrovascular insufficiency should be similarly evaluated. Identification of coagulation abnormalities will reduce perioperative hemorrhage or thrombosis. Maximal preoperative medical treatment of these associated medical problems can vastly improve surgical results.

Close cooperation between the surgeon and anesthesiologist is mandatory for successful treatment. Appropriate monitoring of the arterial blood pressure, central venous pressure, and pulmonary artery and capillary wedge pressures provides better management of intraoperative cardiac function. Monitoring of the arterial blood gas levels, electrolyte levels, body core temperature, and urinary output is also important. A modern blood bank provides appropriate use of component blood replacement to correct intraoperative coagulopathy. Pharmacologic support is valuable in reducing the cardiac afterload when the aorta is cross-clamped. Postoperative care of these patients in the intensive care unit is extremely important.

ANEURYSMS

Specific patterns of aneurysmal disease depending on the site have been observed. Aneurysms develop in order of decreasing frequency in the following sites: abdominal aorta, descending thoracic aorta, ascending aorta, thoracoabdominal aorta, and aortic arch, as well as in dissecting aortic aneurysms. Morphologically, aneurysms are classified into three types: (1) fusiform (spindle shaped), which involve the entire circumference of the aorta; (2) sacciform, which are characterized by a pouchlike protrusion from a narrow opening in the aortic wall; and (3) dissecting aortic, which are characterized by intramural separation, usually within the medial layer.

Abdominal Aortic Aneurysms

Most published reports about abdominal aortic aneurysms have indicated an increase in their incidence. These aneurysms tend to be fusiform, and most are located in the infrarenal abdominal aorta. They may extend distally to involve the iliac arteries. Aneurysms may cause pain in the abdomen or back, or pain may be referred to the thigh or scrotum. Complete thrombosis of an infrarenal abdominal aorta may produce symptoms of ischemia in the legs, and distal embolization of the atheromatous plaque, with or without intraluminal thrombus material, may produce signs of distal ischemia. An infrarenal abdominal aortic aneurysm may be detected on physical examination as a pulsatile abdominal aortic mass. Most abdominal aortic aneurysms are asymptomatic and are diagnosed incidentally during other diagnostic studies, such as plain radiography of the abdomen, abdominal ultrasonography, computed tomography (CT), or magnetic resonance imaging (MRI). Usually, abdominal aortography is performed to define the exact location and extent of the aneurysm and to evaluate possible occlusive disease of the renal artery, mesenteric artery, or iliac arteries of the legs. Occasionally, the clinical manifestations of infrarenal abdominal aortic aneurysms are those of inflammatory aneurysms, or those of a fistula in the intestine or inferior vena cava. The most common complication of an infrarenal aortic aneurysm is rupture, which may be manifested as a classic triad of pulsatile abdominal mass, abdominal or back pain, and hypotension. The mortality rate for ruptured abdominal aortic aneurysms is often in excess of 50%.

Because most aneurysms are asymptomatic at the time of diagnosis, there is some controversy regarding the timing for elective resection. Many authors agree that a localized enlargement of the aorta more than twice the normal diameter of 2 cm represents an infrarenal abdominal aortic aneurysm. The risk of rupture of abdominal aortic aneurysms is directly related to the size of the aneurysm. A 6-cm aneurysm is considered large and is an indication for operation unless extenuating medical risks exist. Because a small abdominal aortic aneurysm (less than 5 cm) can rupture, most authorities agree that it should be surgically resected if it becomes symptomatic or if it enlarges by more than 0.5 cm a year. Age alone is not a contraindication to surgical resection of infrarenal abdominal aortic aneurysms if the patient's general condition is satisfactory. Contraindications to elective surgical resection include severe cardiac, cerebral, pulmonary, or renal disease; uncontrolled malignant disease; and other severe or disabling diseases. The mortality rate for elective nonruptured aneurysm of the abdominal aorta is less than 2 to 3%.

Treatment

Treatment is essentially surgical and consists of resection of the aneurysm and graft replacement. A Dacron tube graft is used if the common iliac arteries are not affected; otherwise, a bifurcation graft is used.

Endovascular techniques were recently introduced to repair the aneurysm endoprosthetically. The prosthesis, which is introduced through the common femoral artery, is secured to the normal aortic wall above the aneurysm and distally beyond the aneurysmal disease. Both straight (tube) and bifurcation grafts have been employed. The completion of prospective randomized multicenter trial studies is required before the efficacy of these endovascular grafts can be recommended with confidence.

Descending Thoracic Aortic Aneurysm

Aneurysms of the descending thoracic aorta are second in frequency only to infrarenal abdominal aortic aneurysms. The former develop distal to the left subclavian artery and extend distally for varying lengths to the diaphragm. Most aneurysms in this area are due to atherosclerosis or medial degenerative disease. Other causes may be trauma, infection, and aortitis. The most common morphologic type is fusiform, although sacciform and dissecting aneurysms may also occur at this site. These aneurysms are seen most often in men in the sixth to eighth decades of life. About 25% of patients with an aneurysm of the descending thoracic aorta also have aneurysms of the infrarenal abdominal aorta. Approximately one third of the patients with an aneurysm of the descending thoracic aorta are asymptomatic, the disease being diagnosed by plain radiography of the chest. Pain, which is due to compression or erosion of surrounding structures, is the most common symptom. Patients may complain of cough, hemoptysis, dysphagia, or hematemesis. CT or MRI is exceedingly useful in identifying the characteristics of the aneurysm of the descending thoracic aorta, but contrast aortography remains an essential diagnostic tool in providing information regarding the precise site and extent of the disease.

Treatment

Surgical repair of these aneurysms should be considered if the patient is symptomatic or if the transverse diameter of the aneurysm is more than two times that of the medial descending thoracic aorta. Treatment consists of excision of the diseased segment of the aorta and replacement with the proper size of woven or albumin-coated Dacron graft. The use of atrial femoral bypass, which provides distal profusion, minimizes the risk of ischemia to the spinal cord and renal failure. Paraplegia or paralysis occurs in about 3 to 5% of the patients. The long-term results of surgical resection are excellent.

Ascending Aortic Aneurysms

Acquired aneurysms of the ascending aorta may be due to medial degeneration, atherosclerosis, or aortic dissection. Although syphilis used to be a major cause of aortic aneurysms, this cause is seldom seen today. These aneurysms may be asymptomatic, or symptoms may develop as a result of compression of the tracheobronchial tree, the esophagus, or the superior vena cava. Patients with associated aortic valvular insufficiency may have heart failure. Any aneurysm larger than 5 cm in diameter should be considered for surgical resection.

A plain radiograph of the chest often suggests aneurysm of the ascending aorta, and CT or MRI is extremely useful in identifying the extent of the aneurysm. Contrast aortography–ascending coronary arteriography is usually performed.

Treatment

Treatment is surgical, consisting of resection of the aneurysm and replacement with a woven or albumin-coated Dacron graft. If the patient also has aortic insufficiency or a sinus of Valsalva aneurysm, a composite valve graft, requiring reattachment of the coronary arteries, is used. Cardiopulmonary bypass, cardioplegia, and hypothermia are used. The long-term results of this operation have been gratifying.

Thoracoabdominal Aneurysms

Thoracoabdominal aneurysms, which are usually fusiform, involve different portions of the descending thoracic and abdominal aorta. Crawford's classification provides a better understanding of the surgical risks and the dreaded complications of paraplegia, parapesis, or both. Type I involves most of the descending thoracic and upper abdominal aorta above the renal arteries. Type II involves most of the descending thoracic aorta and most or all of the abdominal aorta; this type has the highest incidence of neurologic complications. Type III involves the distal descending aorta and most of the abdominal aorta. Type IV involves most or all of the abdominal aorta, including the visceral vessel segment.

The causes of these aneurysms are usually degeneration, atherosclerosis, and aortic dissection. Occasional causes are trauma, infection, and aortitis. Most of these aneurysms are fusiform. Without surgical resection, the 2-year survival rate is about 24%, with half of these deaths due to rupture of the aneurysm.

Thoracoabdominal aneurysms may be asymptomatic. Most, however, produce symptoms before rupture. The patient may complain of pain in the chest, abdomen, flank, or back, or symptoms may be related to compression of adjacent structures, such as the tracheobronchial tree, esophagus, or recurrent laryngeal nerve, the last causing hoarseness. Rarely, the diagnosis is made by palpation of the abdominal aortic component. A plain radiograph of the chest showing widening of the descending thoracic aorta is most common. MRI or CT provides a more exact diagnosis, including the location and extent of the aneurysm. Total contrast aortography in multiple views is necessary for complete evaluation of associated disease of the renal, visceral, or iliac arteries.

Treatment

Treatment is surgical, consisting primarily of graft replacement. A combined thoracoabdominal incision is usually used. A Carlens (double-lumen endotracheal) tube provides deflation of the left lung and selective ventilation of the right lung.

Paraplegia, paresis, or both are the most dreaded complications of operation for thoracoabdominal aneurysms. A number of factors are involved, including the aortic clamp time and the extent of the aorta replaced. Among the methods that have been advocated to minimize neurologic complications are atrial-femoral bypass, femoral-to-femoral bypass, cerebrospinal fluid drainage, and somatosensory evoked potential monitoring. Distal aortic perfusion, reimplantation of critical spinal arteries, and drainage of cerebrospinal fluid are particularly valuable. The incidence of paraplegia or paresis is 31% in type II aneurysms but significantly less in other types of thoracoabdominal aneurysms when the simple cross-clamp technique is used. Woven Dacron grafts are employed. An island of aortic tissue containing the renal and visceral vessels, as well as spinal arteries, can often be incorporated onto the main graft. This difficult major surgical procedure can now be performed with an expected survival rate of more than 90%.

Transverse Aortic Arch Aneurysms

Aneurysms of the transverse aortic arch are usually fusiform, but occasionally a sacciform aneurysm may occur along the lesser curvature of the aorta. The cause of these aneurysms is related to medial degeneration, atherosclerosis, or aortic dissection. An abnormal mediastinal mass on routine radiography may initiate a diagnostic work-up. Ultimately, CT, MRI, or contrast aortography is required to completely evaluate the aorta and the brachiocephalic arteries.

Treatment

Surgical treatment consists of resection of the involved aorta and reattachment with an island of aorta to the brachiocephalic arteries. Cardiopulmonary bypass, profound hypothermia, retrograde cerebral perfusion, and circulatory arrest are mandatory in the surgical treatment of these difficult surgical cases. If the descending thoracic aorta is concomitantly involved, the "elephant trunk" technique is used to facilitate the subsequent staged repair of the descending thoracic aorta. Close cooperation between the anesthesiologist and perfusionist is imperative in maintaining the body temperature, blood volume, and coagulation factors. This operation can be done with astonishingly good results and long-term survival.

Aortic Transection

Traumatic injuries of the aorta are increasing in frequency and recognition. Most patients with this injury die immediately. Only a small number tamponade sufficiently to reach medical facilities. Transection usually occurs just distal to the left subclavian artery after deceleration injuries from high-speed motor vehicle accidents or falls from heights. The diagnosis may be suspected if the radiograph shows widening of the mediastinum or deviation of the esophagus, trachea, or superior vena cava. Contrast aortography confirms the diagnosis. CT, MRI, or transesophagram ultrasonography may also provide information. Immediate surgical repair is mandatory. The operation consists of primary repair of a localized tear or limited segmental resection of the injured aorta and replacement with a woven or albumin-coated Dacron graft. In the care of the patient with acute aortic transection, the method for minimizing spinal cord ischemia is controversial. The use of an atrial-femoral bypass is recommended. In patients with acute aortic transection who survive, a chronic false aneurysm may develop many years later manifested as a posterior mediastinal mass.

Treatment

Treatment of these chronic post-traumatic thoracic aneurysms is the same as that for descending thoracic aortic aneurysms.

Dissecting Aortic Aneurysms

Dissecting aneurysms of the aorta are characterized by an intimal tear with hemorrhagic intramural separation of the medial layer of the aortic wall. The intimal tear originates, with decreasing frequency, in the ascending aorta, the descending aorta, and the aortic arch. The dissection usually extends distally but may extend proximally and creates a false lumen. Initial dissection may result in rupture and fatal hemorrhage. The dissection may also rupture into the pericardium to involve the aortic valve or coronary arteries and produce cardiac tamponade, acute aortic valvular insufficiency, heart failure, or occlusion of the coronary arteries. Distal dissection may cause obstruction of the major brachiocephalic arteries and cause a stroke or occlusion of the renal or mesenteric arteries followed by renal failure, mesenteric infarction, or occlusion of the iliac arteries with resulting ischemia in the limbs. The predominant underlying pathologic condition is medial degeneration in Marfan's syndrome. Most patients have associated uncontrolled hypertension. Additional risk factors include pregnancy, coarctation, and idiopathic kyphoscoliosis. The initial course of the disease has an extremely grave prognosis, with death in 50% of patients within the first 2 days of onset. A small percentage of patients survive a few years without treatment. Aortic dissection occurs twice as often in men as in women, and most patients are in the fourth to seventh decades of life.

The DeBakey classification of aortic dissection is as follows: type I, the dissecting process involves the entire aorta, usually originating in the ascending aorta, but it may begin anywhere in the aorta and extend both proximally and distally; type II, the dissecting process is limited to the ascending aorta (aortic valvular insufficiency can occur with both types); type III, the intimal tear usually arises in the descending thoracic aorta at or just distal to the left subclavian artery and may extend distally to the diaphragm or the aortic bifurcation.

Treatment

Medical treatment is indicated initially in patients with uncomplicated aortic dissection, particularly in those with aneurysms of the descending thoracic aorta, evidence of imminent rupture, or occlusion of a major aortic branch. Medical treatment includes controlling the blood pressure and reducing cardiac contractility with nitroprusside and propranolol. The goal is to stabilize the patient's condition so that elective surgical resection can be performed if surgical intervention is necessary. If there is evidence of imminent rupture with pain indicating continued dissection or occlusion of a major branch of the aorta, emergency surgery is imperative.

If the diagnosis of aortic dissection is suspected, contrast aortography usually gives the surgeon the necessary information to treat the patient. In addition, CT, MRI, or transesophageal ultrasonography is useful for defining the location and extent of the aortic dissection.

Treatment of types I and II aortic dissection is surgical after initial stabilization. There is a high incidence of rupture into the mediastinum or pericardium with tamponade or involvement of the aortic valve and heart failure. Operation consists of resection of the proximal segment of the ascending aorta and replacement with a woven Dacron graft, including obliteration of the false lumen by approximation of the inner and outer walls with the use of cardiopulmonary bypass and cardioplegia. Some patients require concomitant aortic valve replacement and reattachment of the coronary arteries.

In type III dissection, patients are initially treated medically to control hypertension and cardiac contractility. Surgical treatment is required in patients who have complications with continued pain, suggesting further dissection; evidence of compromise of perfusion to the mesenteric/renal arteries or legs; or continued enlargement of the false lumen. Resection of the descending thoracic aorta, with obliteration of the distal false lumen and replacement with a woven or albumin-coated Dacron graft, is the procedure of choice.

All patients with a history of dissection of the aorta should be examined annually with serial CT scans to evaluate the aorta and false lumen for evidence of further aortic disease. Most of these patients require control of hypertension. Surgical results of treatment of aortic dissection have been extremely gratifying with minimal perioperative morbidity and good long-term results.

OCCLUSIVE DISEASE OF THE ABDOMINAL AORTA

Occlusive disease of the abdominal aorta is usually caused by atherosclerosis and is generally associated with occlusive disease of the iliac arteries. For more than 50% of patients, the superficial femoral artery or more distal arteries are also diseased. Abdominal aortic occlusion is much more common in men than in women. Many of these patients have associated carotid or coronary occlusive disease, as well as hypertension and diabetes, and most patients smoke. The clinical manifestations depend on the extent, location, and duration of the disease. Claudication (muscle pain in the legs) is precipitated by exercise and relieved by short periods of rest. It is the first and most common symptom and may involve muscles of the hip, buttocks, thigh, or calf. Sexual impotence is a complaint in men. Physical findings invariably include the reduction or absence of femoral or pedal pulses and perhaps a bruit over the lower part of the abdomen or femoral arteries. Atrophy of the subcutaneous tissue and muscles of the legs, loss of hair, and changes in toenails are common. Pallor on elevation of the legs and rubor on dependency are usually noted as the occlusive disease progresses and generally is accompanied by distal superficial, femoral, popliteal, or tibial arterial disease. The patients may have evidence of limb-threatening ischemia with rest pain, ulceration, and gangrene. Isolated aortofemoral occlusive disease without distal arterial occlusive disease seldom produces limb-threatening ischemia.

The differential diagnosis includes neurogenic claudication (which is caused by spinal stenosis or other neuropathy), chronic compartment syndromes, and other back problems. A few patients with atherosclerotic occlusive disease of the aorta may have minimal stenosis but consult a physician because of distal microemboli secondary to atheroembolism, the blue toe syndrome.

The diagnosis can generally be suspected from an appropriate history and physical examination. Currently, noninvasive studies are not only used as screening tests for occlusive disease of the legs but aid in diagnostic accuracy and provide physiologic evaluation of the severity of the disease. Ankle or brachial indices, segmental limb pressures, and pulse volume recordings provide useful information. Ultrasonic imaging is available in some vascular laboratories. Abdominal aortography and bilateral femoral arteriography, however, remain essential for the vascular surgeon to plan the appropriate operation. As for other patients with vascular diseases, the general evaluation of the patient's cardiac, pulmonary, renal, and hepatic function is essential. Extracranial occlusive vascular disease or coagulation defects must be identified.

Treatment

Nonoperative treatment includes a regular exercise program and especially an attempt to get patients to stop smoking. A number of studies have shown the importance of cessation of the use of tobacco in improving symptoms in patients with arterial occlusive disease of the legs and to improve results after surgical intervention. There are no effective drugs for pharmacologic treatment of claudication at this time, but most patients are urged to take one 5-grain tablet of acetylsalicylic acid (aspirin) daily because of its antiplatelet effect on the cause of atherosclerosis.

Fortunately, occlusive disease tends to be segmental and localized. This permits effective surgical treatment with restoration of circulation by the bypass technique. A DeBakey knitted Dacron velour bifurcation graft is anastomosed to the infrarenal abdominal aorta. The two limbs of the bifurcation graft are attached distally to the external iliac or common femoral arteries by end-to-end anastomosis. Associated renal artery disease or superficial femoral artery disease can be treated by additional bypass grafts. Endovascular techniques, which are increasing in popularity, consist of percutaneous transluminal angioplasty, particularly of the iliac arteries. The use of an intraluminal stent seems to improve the long-term patency.

Eighty-five to 90% graft patency can be expected at 5 years for aortic bifurcation grafts. The leading cause of death after operation is the result of coronary artery disease. Five-year patency rates for aortofemoral bypass grafts of 60 to 90% can be expected, as in most other patients with vascular disease.

ANGINA PECTORIS

method of
CHARLES R. LAMBERT, M.D., PH.D.
University of Florida and Health First Heart
*   Institute*
Melbourne, Florida

Angina pectoris is a symptom complex associated with myocardial ischemia. Classically, it consists of a pressure-type discomfort that is usually substernal, although it may originate from or radiate to the epigastrium, jaw, neck, back, or arm. Anginal "equivalents" may include dyspnea, palpitations, dizziness, or other cardiac symptoms. The differential diagnosis of angina pectoris includes pulmonary, pericardial, musculoskeletal, pleural, gastrointestinal, and great vessel pathology. Angina pectoris is generally classified into stable and unstable categories. Stable angina is usually exertional with a relatively constant threshold for precipitation. Patients with stable angina have a relatively predictable symptom complex and are generally able to adjust their day-to-day activities and medication regimens to avoid its onset. Unstable angina represents a change in this stable pattern or the new onset of angina pectoris in a previously asymptomatic individual. Changes may include an increase in frequency or intensity of angina, the occurrence of symptoms at rest, a lower exercise threshold for provocation, or the onset of nocturnal symptoms. Most authorities consider angina occurring after myocardial infarction as unstable. Angina may occur in a similar pattern in patients with Prinzmetal's or variant angina. Stable angina, unstable angina, and Prinzmetal's angina all result from myocardial ischemia; however, pathophysiologic mechanisms differ and the approach to treatment of these clinical syndromes may differ as well.

PATHOPHYSIOLOGY OF STABLE ANGINA PECTORIS

Large coronary angiographic studies of patients presenting for evaluation of chronic stable angina consistently reveal severe epicardial coronary atherosclerosis as the major finding. In the Emory University database of 1586 patients catheterized for the first time for evaluation of stable angina pectoris, 9% had no disease, 3% had mild disease, 4% had moderate disease, and 84% had significant disease (>75% area reduction) in at least one major epicardial coronary artery. Furthermore, several investigators have shown that the morphology of coronary artery stenoses can be linked to the clinical syndrome present for a given patient. These findings suggest that stable angina pectoris is more often associated with a "stable" coronary stenosis characterized angiographically by smooth, usually concentric borders, not usually associated with plaque rupture, intramural hemorrhage, or thrombus. Thus, stable angina pectoris is most likely to be associated with severe epicardial coronary atherosclerotic obstruction; however, plaque morphology tends to be "stable" and not associated with marked eccentricity, thrombus, or ulceration.

In the normal heart, the epicardial coronary arteries offer little resistance to blood flow and serve largely as conductance vessels. In most patients with stable angina pectoris, as noted earlier, major atherosclerotic lesions are present within these vessels and a major limitation to coronary blood flow may occur, especially during periods of increased metabolic demand. If an increasingly severe stenosis is imposed on an epicardial coronary artery, resting blood flow is affected little until the luminal diameter has been severely reduced by about 90%. Peak hyperemic blood flow is limited much earlier at a diameter reduction of approximately 50%. Vasomotor tone and hydrodynamic factors may also affect the importance of a given coronary artery stenosis. With appreciation of the dynamic nature of coronary stenoses, many pathophysiologic mediators have been proposed as instigators of ischemia in patients with coronary artery disease. Such potential mediators include the sympathetic nervous system, histamine, serotonin, thromboxane, leukotrienes, and basic alteration of smooth muscle activational processes. Some vasodilators require intact endothelium to exert their effects on vascular smooth muscle. These substances are thought to cause the release of an endothelium-derived relaxing factor (EDRF). In the absence of endothelium, a substance that usually causes vasodilatation when introduced via the luminal surface of a vessel may cause vasoconstriction because of the lack of EDRF. Such observations have been made in atherosclerotic human coronary arteries studied in vitro as well as in patients studied in the cardiac catheterization laboratory. These observations suggest that an important pathophysiologic mechanism for the production of ischemia in coronary artery disease may be the loss of normal endothelial vasodilator function as a result of atherosclerotic injury.

Besides the obvious link between coronary atherosclerotic lesions and flow-related myocardial ischemia in patients with angina pectoris, several other pathophysiologic mechanisms may be important. One factor is the transmural distribution of resting myocardial blood flow from the epicardium to the endocardium. Because of greater systolic compressive forces and resultant wall stress, the distribution of blood flow to the subendocardium is about 1.25 times greater than to the epicardium. This preferential subendocardial flow is dependent on vasodilatation of vessels in this region, and thus the subendocardium has less coronary flow reserve to respond to further stress. Because of this, factors such as lowering of coronary perfusion pressure, elevation of left ventricular end-diastolic pressure, and tachycardia all tend to make the subendocardium ischemic before affecting the epicardial layers. In the presence of coronary artery obstruction, the effective subendocardial perfusion pressure is determined by the gradient distal to the stenosis and the left ventricular end-diastolic pressure. If ischemia occurs and left ventricular end-diastolic pressure begins to rise, a vicious circle may be set up whereby the effective subendocardial perfusion pressure is reduced, further intensifying ischemia, which further raises end-diastolic pressure and so forth. Subendocardial ischemia also plays an important role in the genesis of certain forms of nonatheromatous angina, such as that seen with severe left ventricular hypertrophy.

In patients with stable angina pectoris, most significant pharmacologic interventions are targeted at the determinants of myocardial oxygen demand. At the bedside or in the office these determinants are approximated by heart rate, blood pressure, and volume status. With exercise, heart rate and blood pressure increase with a fall in peripheral vascular resistance and increase in cardiac output. Precipitation of ischemia in this circumstance is usually a function of increased metabolic demand by the myocardium, although dynamic coronary mechanisms may also contribute as noted in the preceding section. Ischemia resulting from increased myocardial oxygen demand may also be a function of inadequate collateral development. A primary mediator of demand-side ischemia in many patients with stable angina is the sympathetic nervous system through direct influence on heart rate, contractility, and afterload. Many investigations have established that the majority of ischemic episodes in patients with stable angina pectoris are not accompanied by angina but are asymptomatic or silent. Thus, clinical inquiries regarding symptoms may be inadquate in assessing the true ischemic burden in a given patient.

A discussion of the pathophysiology of myocardial ischemia would not be complete without mention of circadian patterns of ischemic events. Definite circadian variation has been described for myocardial infarction, sudden cardiac death, thrombotic stroke, Prinzmetal's angina, and transient myocardial ischemia in patients with stable angina. The majority of such events appear to cluster in the morning hours after awakening. Although ischemia tends to track the circadian variation in heart rate and blood pressure, patients are more likely to become ischemic in the morning than in the afternoon with the same heart rate and blood pressure. If the circadian variation in heart rate is abolished by beta-adrenergic blockade, most ischemia is abolished; however, that which remains has frequency characteristics different from those of the previously dominant circadian pattern. This observation suggests a heterogeneous etiology for the total ischemic burden in such patients. Although platelet activation may play a role in the circadian variation of ischemia in some patients, pharmacologic trials designed to alter this mechanism have had variable results. Detailed examination of ambulatory recordings shows episodes of ischemia that are followed by and not preceded by an increase in heart rate, suggesting a possible supply-side mechanism. Time-related variation in coronary artery tone may also play a role in modulating circadian variation of myocardial ischemia. Overall, currently available data suggest that such variation is mediated by a combination of factors, which may include heart rate, blood pressure, platelet activation, coronary blood flow, mental activity, and dynamic alterations in coronary artery stenoses.

PATHOPHYSIOLOGY OF UNSTABLE ANGINA PECTORIS

Coronary angiography in patients with unstable angina reveals lesions with eccentric geometry, irregular or scal-

TABLE 1. **Commonly Used Nitrates**

Medication	Recommended Dosage (mg)	Onset of Action (min)	Peak Action (min)	Duration of Action
Sublingual NTG	0.3–0.8	2–5	4–8	10–30 min
Sublingual ISDN	2.5–10	5–20	15–60	45–120 min
Sublingual PTN	10–40	5–30	15–60	45 min
Sublingual ET	5–10	5	15–30	30–180 min
Oral NTG spray	0.4	2–5	4–8	10–30 min
Buccal NTG	1–3	2–5	4–10	30–300 min
Oral ISDN	10–60	15–45	45–120	2–6 h
Oral ISMN	20	60	60–240	7–12 h
Oral NTG	6.5–19.5	20–45	45–120	2–6 h
NTG ointment (2%)	0.5–2 in	15–60	30–120	3–8 h
NTG disks (transdermal)	10–20 mg	30–60	60–180	Up to 24 h

Abbreviations: NTG = nitroglycerin; ISDN = isosorbide dinitrate; PTN = pentaerythritol tetranitrate; ET = erythrityl tetranitrate; ISMN = isosorbide mononitrate.

loped borders, unstable plaque geometry, and a high incidence of thrombus. The mechanisms by which stable plaques become unstable are the object of intense investigation and appear to be multifactorial. In any event, these coronary angiographic findings are associated clinically with worsening ischemia either at rest or with minimal exertion. Although all of the pathophysiologic mechanisms described for stable angina also apply, limitation of blood flow caused by the coronary lesions just described appears to be of particular importance in unstable angina.

PATHOPHYSIOLOGY OF VARIANT ANGINA

Variant or Prinzmetal's angina is associated with coronary vasoconstriction or spasm, which is usually focal and manifested by rest pain with associated transient electrocardiographic alterations. Although this syndrome may occur with angiographically normal coronary arteries, it is most often seen in conjunction with some degree of underlying coronary atherosclerosis. Variant angina may progress to an unstable ischemic syndrome such as unstable angina or myocardial infarction by mechanisms discussed earlier.

ANTIANGINAL MEDICAL THERAPY

Nitrates

Nitrates are among the oldest and most widely used antianginals and are available in a variety of preparations (Tables 1 and 2). Nitrates act principally as vasodilators affecting venous capacitance vessels. Some effect may be demonstrated on the peripheral and coronary arterial systems, although the latter probably plays a minor role in antianginal clinical efficacy. When given acutely, nitrates reduce venous return, lower cardiac output, reduce systemic arterial pressure, and may have a variable effect on heart rate. Care must be taken during administration of nitrates to patients with diminished cardiac reserve and/or hypovolemia.

Acute nitrate administration is most commonly done by the sublingual route, although spray or intravenous administration may also be utilized, if available. The clinical effects of nitroglycerin and its metabolites are similar with these three routes of administration from a practical standpoint. Continu-

ous nitroglycerin administration is usually done in the acute setting with intravenous infusion. Careful blood pressure monitoring must accompany this practice, and this therapy is most commonly used for unstable ischemic syndromes in the intensive care setting. Topical or percutaneous administration of nitroglycerin in a paste may also be useful in this setting. Patch or transdermal administration is not generally of use in the acute or subacute setting because of slow onset of action and difficulty in adjusting dosage. In addition, tolerance commonly

TABLE 2. **Commonly Used Commercial Nitrate Preparations**

Product	Manufacturer	Dosage Forms
Transdermal		
Nitro-Dur	Key	5 cm² (0.1 mg/h)
		10 cm² (0.2 mg/h)
		15 cm² (0.3 mg/h)
		20 cm² (0.4 mg/h)
		30 cm² (0.6 mg/h)
		40 cm² (0.8 mg/h)
Deponit (NTG)	Schwarz	16 cm² (0.2 mg/h)
		32 cm² (0.4 mg/h)
Transderm-Nitro	Ciba Geneva	0.1 mg/h
		0.2 mg/h
		0.4 mg/h
		0.6 mg/h
Nitro-Bid ointment	Hoechst Marion Roussel	2%
Isosorbide dinitrate		
Dilatrate-SR	Schwarz	40-mg capsules
Isosorbide SL tablets	Wyeth-Ayerst	2.5- and 5-mg
Isordil Tembids	Wyeth-Ayerst	40-mg capsules and tablets
Isordil Titradose	Wyeth-Ayerst	5-, 10-, 20-, and 40-mg tablets
Sorbitrate chewable	Zeneca	5- and 10-mg tablets
Sorbitrate sublingual	Zeneca	2.5- and 5-mg tablets
Sorbitrate oral	Zeneca	5-, 10-, 20-, 30-, and 40-mg tablets
Isosorbide mononitrate		
Imdur	Key	30-, 60-, and 120-mg tablets
Ismo	Wyeth-Ayerst	20-mg tablets

develops with continuous transdermal systems unless care is taken to provide a nitrate-free interval. Tolerance is best avoided with these systems by removal of the patch at bedtime. Oral nitrate preparations such as isosorbide dinitrate (Isordil), pentaerythritol tetranitrate, erythrityl tetranitrate, and isosorbide mononitrate (Ismo) offer convenient dosing intervals and are associated, in general, with fewer tolerance problems, although a nitrate-free interval is still needed. This interval should be 12 to 14 hours regardless of the preparation. These agents are most often used for chronic therapy. Sublingual isosorbide dinitrate tablets are best used for prevention of angina when activity is anticipated. Nitrates have side effects that include reflex tachycardia, headache, and flushing. Tolerance develops to most of these effects in most patients, and careful dose titration can be used to minimize them.

Beta Blockers

Beta blockers are widely used in patients with ischemic heart disease because of their clinical efficacy with regard to symptomatic and objective control of ischemia as well as documented value in secondary prevention. Beta blockers differ primarily with respect to beta$_1$-receptor (cardiac) selectivity, alpha-blocker activity, solubility, intrinsic sympathomimetic activity, and membrane-stabilizing activity. Beta blockers are available in different formulations and vary widely in pharmacologic properties, as outlined in Table 3.

Beta blockers reduce the resting heart rate, depending on the degree of resting adrenergic tone present and the dose administered. They also produce a marked reduction in heart rate at any level of exercise and in the peak heart rate attainable. Drugs with and without beta$_1$ specificity appear to reduce heart rate equally during rest and exercise, whereas agents with intrinsic sympathomimetic activity may have less effect on heart rate during periods of low adrenergic tone (e.g., sleep). Beta blockers generally produce a small reduction in resting cardiac output and a large reduction in exercise cardiac output. Similar changes are seen in blood pressure and are probably secondary to cardiac output, because systemic vascular resistance is usually unchanged or slightly increased with beta blockade during exercise. Beta blockers have little direct effect on left ventricular diastolic function but do reduce contractile state and must be used with caution in patients with significant left ventricular dysfunction. Beta blockers may increase the ventricular fibrillation threshold, decrease automatic arrhythmias by reducing phase 4 depolarization, reduce afterdepolarizations, and alter refractoriness. Sotalol has unique class III antiarrhythmic properties, which result in efficacy for certain atrial and ventricular arrhythmias. Side effects and related problems with beta-blocker therapy are common and are listed in Table 4. Many of these may be avoided or minimized by trying alternative dosing or drugs with different solubilities or selectivities.

Calcium Blockers

Calcium blockers all inhibit entry of calcium into the cell; however, the receptors and subcellular mechanisms involved may differ between compounds. From a clinical standpoint, a classification scheme including verapamil, diltiazem, and the dihydropyridines as three separate groups is useful. Calcium blockers all act as vasodilators, as negative inotropic agents, and to depress conduction. The in vivo dose-response relationships for these various effects are markedly different between the classes, and thus the effect seen clinically may be different. In clinical

TABLE 3. **Commonly Used Beta-Adrenergic Blockers**

Drug	Beta Receptor Blocked (Cardiac Selectivity)	Membrane-Stabilizing Activity*	Intrinsic Sympathomimetic Activity*	Lipid Solubility†	Serum Half-Life (h)	Duration of Action (h)	Protein Binding (%)	Usual Oral Dosage Range (mg/d)
Acebutolol (Sectral)	1‡	+	+	Low	7–10	24	26	400–1800
Atenolol (Tenormin)	1‡	−	−	Low	5–9	24	6–16	100–200
Betaxolol (Kerlone)	1‡	−	−	Mod	12–22	23–25	50–60	10–40
Carteolol (Cartrol)	1 and 2	−	+	Low	5–7	72	23–30	2.5–10
Esmolol (Brevibloc)	1‡	−	−	Low	9 (min)	10–20 (min)	55	None
Labetalol§ (Normodyne, Trandate)	1 and 2	+	−	Mod	3–4	8–12	50	150–1200
Metoprolol (Lopressor, Toprol)	1‡	±	−	Mod	2–6	10–12	13	150–400
Nadolol (Corgard)	1 and 2	−	−	Low	14–24	39	20	80–240
Penbutolol (Levatol)	1 and 2	+	+	High	12–20	>24	99	40–60
Pindolol (Visken)	1 and 2	±	+ + +	Mod	3–4	8	57	10–20
Sotalol (Betapace)	1 and 2	−	−	Low	5–13	24	5	240–480
Timolol (Blocadren)	1 and 2	−	−	Mod	3–4	15	10	15–45
Bisoprolol (Zebeta)	1‡	±	−	Mod	9–12	24	30	2.5–20

*+ = present; − = absent; ± = weak to variable response.
†Mod indicates moderate.
‡Blocks beta$_2$ receptors at higher doses of therapeutic range.
§Has postsynaptic alpha$_1$-adrenergic blocking ability.

TABLE 4. **Side Effects and Adverse Reactions with Beta-Blocker Therapy**

Cardiovascular manifestations (beta$_1$ effects)	Sexual dysfunction
Bradycardia	Impotence
Hypotension	Neuromuscular effects
Ventricular dysfunction	Myasthenic syndrome
Peripheral vascular manifestations (beta$_2$ effects)	Worsening of myasthenia gravis or myotonia
Increased total peripheral resistance	Practolol syndrome
Decreased blood supply to extremities	Psoriasis-like lesions
Muscle fatigue	Ocular disorders
Respiratory dysfunction (beta$_2$ effects)	Sclerosing peritonitis
Bronchospasm	Overdosage
Dyspnea	Bradycardia
Carbohydrate homeostasis (beta$_2$ effects)	Hypotension
Inhibition of insulin release	Low-output cardiac failure
Inhibition of metabolic response to hypoglycemia	Cardiogenic shock
Inhibition of hemodynamic response to hypoglycemia	Bronchospasm
Central nervous system effects	Grand mal seizures
Vivid or disturbing dreams	Beta-blocker withdrawal
Lethargy	Rebound hypertension
Depression	Rebound angina
Acute confusion	Use in pregnancy
Hallucinations	Low birth weight
Gastrointestinal effects	Neonatal bradycardia
Mild indigestion	Neonatal hypoglycemia
Nausea	Use in elderly persons
Constipation	May require dosage reduction
Skin reactions (uncommon)	

doses, verapamil is the most depressant from the myocardial (negative inotropic) and conduction standpoints. The dihydropyridines offer little myocardial or conduction depression but are much more potent arterial vasodilators. Diltiazem is intermediate with respect to these effects. It follows, therefore, that verapamil must be avoided in patients with bradycardia and compromised left ventricular function. On the other hand, if myocardial depression is a desired characteristic, as in a patient with severe hypertension, left ventricular hypertrophy, and diastolic dysfunction, verapamil might be preferred. If a predominant arterial vasodilator effect is desired, the dihydropyridines might be the agents of choice.

Calcium blockers are effective for hypertension as well as ischemic heart disease. During exercise they tend to prolong the time to ischemia by increasing the time taken to reach a given workload as defined by heart rate and blood pressure. Calcium blockers may or may not increase coronary blood flow, although the second-generation dihydropyridines display some coronary vascular selectivity. The dihidropyridines may provoke a reflex increase in heart rate because of their potent vasodilator effects. This is generally not seen with chronic administration and may differ between agents, but it may be a problem acutely. Care should be taken with administration of dihydropyridines to non–beta-blocked patients with severe coronary artery disease to avoid worsening or precipitating ischemia. Dosing and pharmacokinetic information is outlined in Table 5. Diltiazem, nicardipine, and verapamil are available in intravenous preparations. Dosing adjustments may be needed when calcium blockers are used in conjunction with digoxin, cimetidine, or quinidine. Side effects include headache, edema, bradycardia, worsening of ventric-

ular function, flushing, palpitations, and hypotension. Severe cardiovascular side effects can be reversed with intravenous calcium administration. Nimodipine is a dihydropyridine calcium blocker approved for use in subarachnoid hemmorhage.

APPROACH TO TREATMENT

General Principles

All patients with angina pectoris of any variety should be evaluated with respect to underlying factors that may precipitate or exacerbate ischemia. These include hypertension, tachycardia, hyperthyroidism, anemia, smoking, hypoxia, drug use (sympathomimetics, cocaine), and hypotension. An initial evaluation generally includes stress testing of some variety unless the patient is acutely ill. The heart rate and blood pressure response to exercise may be helpful in choosing therapeutic agents.

Stable Angina

Initial monotherapy for stable angina may include agents of the nitrate, beta-blocker, or calcium-blocker class. The most innocuous side effect profile may be associated with calcium-blocker therapy, and many physicians use these agents as first-line therapy. Objective testing usually shows beta blockers to be more effective as monotherapy. Patients are also instructed on the use of nitroglycerin and generally given aspirin unless a contraindication exists. If symptoms persist, pending other indicated testing, a second agent may be added to an adequate dose of the primary compound. Nitrates or a dihydropyridine calcium blocker is generally added to beta blockers,

TABLE 5. **Commonly Used Calcium Blockers**

Parameter	Diltiazem	Nifedipine	Verapamil	Isradapine	Nicardipine	Amlodipine
T max (h)	1–4 6–11 (SR)	0.5–4 6 (SR)	0.5–1 7–9 (SR) 11 (Covera)	1–3	0.5–2 1–4 (SR)	6–12
Bioavailability (%)	24–74	43–65 29–85 (SR)	13–35	16–18	35	64–90
Protein binding (%)	77–93	92–98	83–92	97	>98	93
Half-life (h)	2–7	2–3 6 (SR)	2–7	5–11	0.75–2 8.6 (SR)	30–50
Excretion						
Renal	40	90	70	65	60	60
Fecal	60	10	16	30	35	40
Usual daily dose (mg)	180–360	30–90	120–360	5–10	60–120	5–10
Usual starting dose	Cardizem 30 mg qid Cardizem SR 60 mg bid Cardizem CD 120 mg qd Dilacor XR 120 mg qd	Adalat 10 mg tid Adalat CC 30 mg qd Procardia 10 mg tid Procardia XL 30 mg qd	Calan 40 mg tid Calan SR 180 qd Covera-HS 180 mg qd Isoptin 40 mg tid Isoptin SR 180 mg qd Verelan 120 mg qd	DynaCirc 2.5 mg bid	Cardene 20 mg tid Cardene SR 30 mg bid	Norvasc 5 mg qd

Abbreviations: T max = time to maximal concentration; SR = sustained release.

and nitrates are generally added to calcium blockers. Care must be used in adding calcium antagonists with negative effects on conduction and ventricular function (verapamil > diltiazem) to beta blockers. Triple therapy with nitrates, beta blockers, and calcium blockers may be needed for some patients. The principles of pathophysiology outlined earlier are of primary importance when titrating such therapy. One can alter preload, afterload, and heart rate to a desired effect with careful alterations in compound therapy.

Unstable Angina

Patients with unstable angina require rigorous control of the determinants of myocardial oxygen demand as noted earlier. Beta-blocker therapy is a mainstay in this setting, and rapid-acting agents such as esmolol may be of use. Calcium blockers may also be useful, especially for patients who may develop a non–Q wave myocardial infarction without congestive heart failure. Intravenous nitroglycerin is considered standard therapy; however, attention must be paid to volume status because such patients are often dehydrated and may respond to small doses of nitroglycerin with profound falls in systemic blood pressure. Intravenous heparin and aspirin are also considered standard therapy in the unstable ischemic syndromes. This makes sense in view of the pathophysiology, and multiple clinical studies have supported use of these agents in unstable angina. With initial control of symptoms, oral therapy can generally be instituted early for such patients and must be individualized on the basis of clinical presentation, pathophysiology, and coronary anatomy, if known.

Cardiac Catheterization and Revascularization

Patients with stable angina are generally evaluated with stress testing, and the advisability of cardiac catheterization depends on those findings and the clinical scenario. Published guidelines are available for selecting patients for invasive evaluation. Patients with high-risk anatomy as determined by cardiac catheterization may require revascularization with catheter technology (angioplasty, atherectomy) or with coronary artery bypass surgery. The indications for these procedures are in constant evolution; however, they generally include severe ischemia during stress with or without normal left ventricular function.

Unstable patients commonly undergo angiography in the United States, although noninvasive evaluation has been shown to be effective and safe if medical therapy is successful in converting an unstable to a stable patient. Revascularization may be indicated for patients with unstable angina, depending on clinical factors and coronary anatomy. Both angioplasty and bypass surgery have been shown to be effective in selected groups of patients with unstable angina; however, the decision to proceed with revascularization must be individualized.

CARDIAC ARREST: SUDDEN CARDIAC DEATH

method of
ROGER D. WHITE, M.D.
Mayo Medical School and Mayo Clinic
Rochester, Minnesota

Sudden cardiac death (SCD) is the term used to denote unexpected cardiovascular collapse culminating in cardiorespiratory arrest. According to the American Heart Association (AHA), SCD claims approximately 250,000 lives each year. Although it may follow the onset of ischemic signs and/or symptoms, it may occur without preceding warning signs of impending collapse and without a prior history of ischemic cardiac disease. The majority of these events occur outside the hospital and therefore are out-of-hospital cardiac arrests. Whereas there are many possible causes of out-of-hospital cardiac arrest, coronary artery disease, usually without acute myocardial infarction, is the most frequent cause. At onset, ventricular tachyarrhythmias are the presenting electrical derangement in more than 80% of these episodes, most commonly monomorphic ventricular tachycardia (VT) that then degenerates into ventricular fibrillation (VF) (Figure 1). Bradyarrhythmias initiate cardiac arrest in 18% of patients. The most frequent presenting SCD arrhythmia, VF, is fortunately also the most treatable, and therefore an aggressive effort is warranted in treating patients experiencing SCD. In well-organized emergency medical services (EMS) systems, 40% or more of patients in out-of-hospital cardiac arrest with VF as the presenting rhythm can be resuscitated and discharged without neurologic impairment. The likelihood of survival is directly dependent on rapid and sequential implementation of the AHA chain of survival; its critical links are rapid EMS access by calling for help (911 phone call), prompt bystander cardiopulmonary resuscitation (CPR), early defibrillation, and follow-up advanced cardiac life support (ACLS) care (Figure 2). Early defibrillation has emerged as the most critical lifesaving intervention that has the potential for substantially increasing survival from SCD caused by VF. A major national initiative is needed to implement this intervention on a widespread scale to improve survival from cardiac arrest. The thrust of this presentation is to describe an approach to cardiac arrest that will maximize the likelihood of survival by emphasis on the strategic employment of early defibrillation. However, because the benefit of rapid defibrillation frequently depends on the integration of the other components of the chain of survival, these components need to be understood as well.

The victim who is most likely to survive cardiac arrest is one whose arrest is witnessed and caused by VF, for whom EMS is called immediately (early access), who receives prompt CPR by bystanders (early CPR), who is defibrillated within 6 to 8 minutes of collapse (early defibrillation), and finally who receives follow-up stabilizing ACLS treatment (early advanced care) as needed. The last might include administration of antiarrhythmic drugs, endotracheal intubation, or other definitive interventions. Each of these components is now discussed to develop an action plan that will enable as many patients as possible to be among those most likely to survive a cardiac arrest.

EARLY ACCESS

As soon as a victim is observed to be unresponsive, the EMS system should be called, ideally by the universal emergency number 911. If this number is not yet established in one's community, then all citizens should have posted by their telephones the number to call to access the EMS system.

EARLY CARDIOPULMONARY RESUSCITATION

Preservation of cerebral viability during the arrested state is totally dependent on delivery of oxygenated blood to the brain by ventilation and external chest compression. Surely it is reasonable to assume that all physicians are knowledgeable and skillful in the performance of CPR (basic life support). It is a regrettable experience for an arrested patient to have a spontaneous circulation restored by

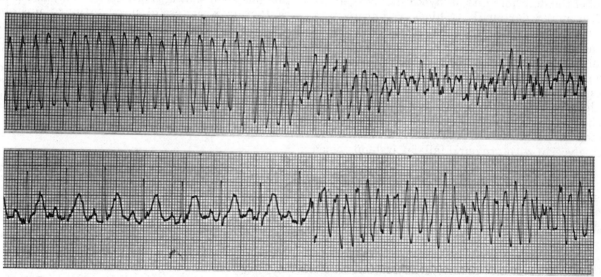

Figure 1. Degeneration of monomorphic ventricular tachycardia into ventricular fibrillation (*top*). Onset of ventricular fibrillation from normal sinus rhythm without preceding ventricular tachycardia (*bottom*).

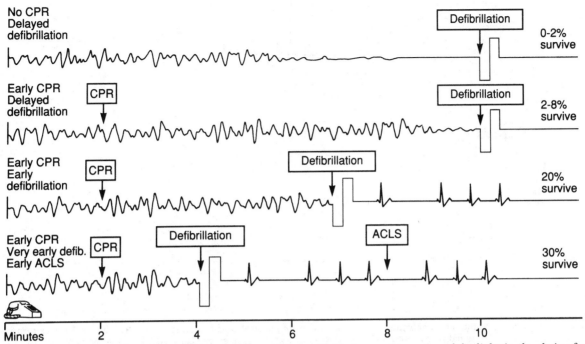

Figure 2. Dependency of survival from cardiac arrest in ventricular fibrillation on integration of the links in the chain of survival: early access to care, early cardiopulmonary resuscitation (CPR), early defibrillation, and early definitive (advanced cardiac life support [ACLS]) care. (Reproduced with permission. © Textbook of Basic Life Support for Healthcare Providers, 1994. Copyright American Heart Association.)

defibrillation only to die or vegetate from irreversible ischemic brain injury. Whereas it is acknowledged that CPR is only a "holding" function, awaiting more definitive interventions, it can be the major determinant of whether a patient awakens without neurologic deficit after cardiac arrest. It behooves all physicians to avail themselves of the opportunity to learn this skill and to periodically (every 1 or 2 years) be updated in the performance of CPR. New CPR techniques are being investigated clinically. They include circumferential thoracic compression (vest CPR) and active compression-decompression CPR. The active compression-decompression CPR procedure held initial promise in preliminary clinical studies, but large-scale investigations have failed to confirm any benefit compared with standard CPR. At this time, no alterative to standard (AHA) CPR has been shown to be advantageous.

EARLY DEFIBRILLATION

The most significant advance in improving the chances for survival from VF cardiac arrest has been the implementation of early defibrillation programs in out-of-hospital settings. Automated external defibrillators (AEDs) make possible the delivery of defibrillatory shocks rapidly, effectively, and safely. AEDs are attached to the chest wall by means of cables connected to adhesive conductive electrode pads that are used to both monitor the rhythm and deliver shocks. The rhythm is automatically analyzed by a microprocessor-based algorithm program. If a treatable rhythm (VF or pulseless VT with a rate beyond

the cutoff) is detected, the AED capacitor is automatically charged, and the operator is requested visually (screen display) and audibly (voice synthesizer) to deliver a shock. After the shock, most devices are programmed to automatically reanalyze the rhythm to determine whether a shockable rhythm is still present. If so, the cycle is repeated, and again a third time if needed. Thus, a total of three shocks can be delivered rapidly and without interruption if needed. After a third shock, or after any shock that terminates VF, the device calls for a pulse check. If none is present, CPR is performed for 1 minute, then the analyze-shock cycle can be repeated. The microprocessor-based algorithms that analyze the rhythm have a high degree of both specificity (98%) and sensitivity (>90%). AEDs are battery powered and therefore portable, lightweight, and easy to operate. New versions require minimal maintenance. AEDs are available with event documentation systems such as dual-channel (voice and electrocardiographic) cassette tape recorders and memory modules or event cards (PCMCIA cards) that store times and electrocardiographic data for a subsequent printout and review (Figure 3).

Improved survival from VF cardiac arrest depends on early defibrillation. All areas for care of patients should be equipped with AEDs, including physicians' offices. In out-of-hospital settings, AEDs are carried in basic life support ambulances and by many first-responder EMS personnel, such as firefighters and police officers. It is evident that physicians seeing patients in their offices or in outpatient clinics would be well advised to consider placement of AEDs in

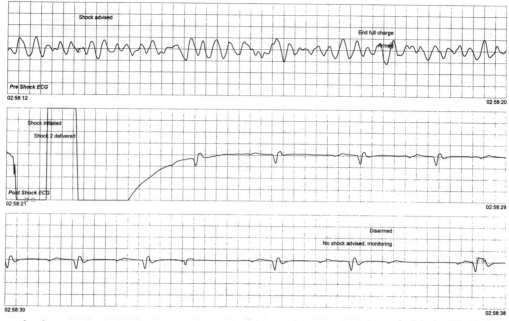

Figure 3. Example of a printout of a defibrillation event in an out-of-hospital cardiac arrest caused by VF. The VF was terminated by the second biphasic shock. These data were obtained from the device's PCMCIA memory card. *Abbreviation:* ECG = electrocardiogram.

those settings and to have office or clinic staff, as well as themselves, trained in their proper operation and maintenance. AEDs can be purchased for $3000 to $4000, including accessories such as spare batteries and extra sets of electrodes.

There is a form of VT that can lead to cardiac arrest that necessitates an awareness of modes of presentation, etiology, and intervention. This is torsades de pointes, a form of polymorphic ventricular tachycardia (PVT) caused by prolonged repolarization, manifest electrocardiographically as QT-interval prolongation. It is characterized by typical "twisting of the points" QRS complexes on the electrocardiogram. The patient may have paroxysms of this tachycardia, between which the QT-interval prolongation is evident. When the disorder is suspected, a search should be made for a cause (Table 1 and Figure 4). Sustained episodes of torsades can cause cardiac arrest and should be treated with defibrillation using the same doses of energy as specified for VF and pulseless VT. Magnesium sulfate (1 to 2 grams intravenously) can be injected to control the episodes of torsades, or if it

is available, overdrive atrial or ventricular pacing can suppress the tachycardia. PVT can occur without QT prolongation, e.g., after acute myocardial infarction, in which case standard antiarrhythmic therapy with lidocaine, procainamide, or bretylium is used. The primary care physician must therefore be alert not only to the electrocardiographic appearance of PVT but also to the etiologic mechanisms that define the PVT as torsades and thus lead to treatment with magnesium sulfate and/or overdrive pacing.

EARLY ADVANCED CARDIAC LIFE SUPPORT CARE

In many patients experiencing VF cardiac arrest, prompt defibrillation is all that is required to restore a spontaneous circulation. After this, an intravenous line can be initiated and lidocaine injected to reduce the risk for recurrent VF. In some patients, more definitive and aggressive interventions will be required, such as additional drugs and airway control and ventilation. Whereas endotracheal intubation is

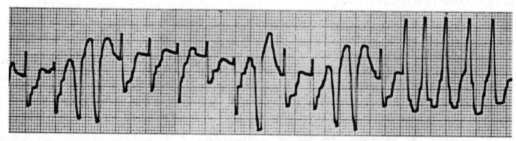

Figure 4. Polymorphic ventricular tachycardia (torsades) accompanying a massive subarachnoid hemorrhage. The electrocardiogram revealed a prolonged QT interval and U waves (K^+ 2.7 mEq/L), along with frequent nonsustained eruptions of torsades. (From Asplin BR, White RD: Subarachnoid hemorrhage: Atypical presentation associated with rapidly changing cardiac arrhythmias. Am J Emerg Med 12:370–373, 1994.)

TABLE 1. **Causes of Torsades de Pointes**

Congenital Prolonged QT Syndromes
Romano-Ward
Jervell and Lange-Nielson

Acquired Prolonged QT Interval
Drug induced
  Quinidine
  Procainamide (Pronestyl)
  Disopyramide (Norpace)
  Sotalol (Betapace)
  Bepridil (Vascor)
  Amiodarone (Cordarone)
  Phenothiazines
    Thioridazine (Mellaril)
    Chlorpromazine (Thorazine)
  Tricyclic antidepressants
    Amitriptyline
    Imipramine
  Cisapride (Propulsid)
  Lithium
  Terfenadine (Seldane) and astemizole
    (Hismanal) in combination with
    ketoconazole (Nizoral), itraconazole
    (Sporanox), erythromycin, or hepatic disease
Electrolyte derangements
  Hypokalemia
  Hypomagnesemia
  Hypocalcemia
Neurologic
  Subarachnoid hemorrhage
  Cerebrovascular accident
Bradycardia of any cause
  Sinus or junctional
  Atrioventricular block
Any combination of the above, e.g., subarachnoid
  hemorrhage with bradycardia and
  hypokalemia

the intervention of choice for airway protection and for both oxygenation and ventilation, it should not be attempted by persons who are not trained in this skill. Instead, a mask with a one-way valve can be used to ventilate the patient with a mouth-to-mask technique. Bag-valve mask devices are difficult to use effectively by one person, and their use in this manner is discouraged. Flow-restricted (peak flow rate, 40 liters per minute), oxygen-powered, manually cycled ventilation devices can be used by one person more effectively than bag-valve masks. These devices also have the advantage of delivering 100% oxygen. They are an alternative to masks with one-way valves if persons are trained in their use. Also, a multilumen airway such as the esophageal-tracheal tube (Combitube) can be inserted by trained persons to protect the airway if endotracheal intubation cannot be accomplished. All of these skills are incorporated in the AHA ACLS training program. Primary care physicians are strongly encouraged to avail themselves of this training opportunity to become thoroughly acquainted with all of these ACLS procedures and devices.

OTHER FORMS OF CARDIAC ARREST (PULSELESS ELECTRICAL ACTIVITY AND ASYSTOLE)

As discussed, VF is the most common and treatable presenting rhythm in SCD and cardiac arrest. However, other presentations include bradyarrhythmias with pulselessness (pulseless electrical activity) and asystole. These, of course, are not treatable with defibrillation. In pulseless electrical activity, which by definition is some form of electrical activity on the electrocardiogram without palpable pulses, a concerted effort must be made to identify a potentially correctable cause, such as hypovolemia (e.g., exsanguination from concealed or evident hemorrhage), tension pneumothorax after trauma or attempted subclavian venous puncture, acute pulmonary thromboembolism, or cardiac tamponade from trauma or secondary to ventricular rupture with acute myocardial infarction. Survival after left ventricular rupture and tamponade is dependent on suspicion, diagnosis, and immediate intervention.

Asystole is most commonly an irreversible derangement secondary to long-standing hypoxia. However, even here, a rapid search should be initiated for a treatable cause. For example, successful resuscitation has been described after prolonged asystolic cardiac arrest associated with hyperkalemia. External pacing can be tried, but it has not been shown to alter outcome from this form of arrest.

SUMMARY

SCD and cardiac arrest are most commonly the consequence of coronary artery disease. VF is the most frequent presenting rhythm, and VF is often correctable with rapid interventions centered on early defibrillation. AEDs provide a means for rapid delivery of defibrillatory shocks to persons in VF cardiac arrest and constitute the single most important means for improving survival from VF arrest. All areas for care of patients, including physicians' offices and outpatient clinics, should be equipped with AEDs. In pulseless electrical activity or asystolic arrest, a rapid assessment should be made to determine whether a potentially correctable cause of arrest is present.

ATRIAL FIBRILLATION

method of
MARSHALL S. STANTON, M.D.
Mayo Clinic
Rochester, Minnesota

Many causes exist for atrial fibrillation (Table 1), but the important causes to exclude in most patients presenting with their first episode are thyrotoxicosis and structural heart disease. The history and physical examination usually point to the underlying etiology, if one is to be found. Important ancillary tests are thyroid function tests (i.e., sensitive thyroid-stimulating hormone [TSH]) and an echocardiogram. Unless otherwise suspected, coronary artery disease need not be excluded in the patient presenting with new-onset atrial fibrillation, as it is quite unusual for coronary artery disease by itself, without concomitant left

TABLE 1. **Common Causes of Atrial Fibrillation**

Cardiac	Systemic Diseases
Hypertension	Thyrotoxicosis
Ischemic heart disease	Alcohol (holiday heart
Cardiomyopathy	syndrome)
Valvular disease	Chronic lung disease
Wolff-Parkinson-White syndrome	Electrolyte abnormality
Atrial septal defect	Idiopathic
Tachycardia-bradycardia syndrome	
(sick sinus syndrome)	

ventricular dysfunction or acute infarction, to be responsible for this arrhythmia.

Beyond diagnosing the cause of atrial fibrillation, the physician must decide (1) how to control the rapid ventricular response that usually accompanies the untreated arrhythmia, (2) whether and how to try to prevent recurrence, and (3) how to minimize the risk of stroke or systemic embolism that exists in these patients.

CONTROL OF VENTRICULAR RESPONSE

Why Control the Ventricular Response in Atrial Fibrillation

Maintaining a well-controlled ventricular response has two goals: (1) improving the patient's symptoms and/or exercise tolerance and (2) preventing ventricular dysfunction.

During rapid ventricular rates, systolic and diastolic functions are impaired. Further, ischemia may occur in patients with coronary artery disease or those with ventricular hypertrophy. Blunting the ventricular response helps optimize cardiac performance. Although many patients with atrial fibrillation and a rapid ventricular response complain of palpitations, fatigue, or dyspnea, a substantial number report no symptoms. The clinician must be wary that although patients claim to be asymptomatic, they may still have reduced exercise tolerance. Studies have shown an increase of about 50% in treadmill exercise time when the ventricular rate is brought under control.

Ventricular dysfunction can arise from a prolonged rapid ventricular rate, a so-called tachycardia-induced cardiomyopathy. This is a well-studied phenomenon in experimental models in which rapid pacing is used to create a cardiomyopathy. Whenever a patient presents with rapid atrial fibrillation and a dilated cardiomyopathy, the fast rate must be considered as a possible cause, as this is a potentially reversible form of ventricular dysfunction. Of course, it is also possible that the atrial fibrillation is the result rather than the cause of the cardiomyopathy. In either case, controlling the ventricular response is an essential part of the patient's management.

Pharmacologic Control

Three main categories of drugs are used to block the atrioventricular (AV) node in an attempt to slow the ventricular response in atrial fibrillation: digitalis glycosides (predominantly digoxin [Lanoxin]), beta-adrenergic blockers, and calcium channel blockers (Table 2). When these drugs are used, it should be remembered that none of them has been shown to be effective in preventing recurrence of atrial fibrillation. The only exception is that meta-analysis has shown that prophylactic use of beta-adrenergic blocking drugs prevents atrial tachyarrhythmias after cardiac surgery. Further, it is probably a misconception that these drugs will convert an acute episode back to sinus rhythm.

Beta-adrenergic blocking drugs are effective in slowing the ventricular response. Acutely, the only ones that are available for intravenous administration are propranolol (Inderal), metoprolol (Lopressor, Toprol), atenolol (Tenormin), and esmolol (Brevibloc). These agents may be particularly useful when atrial fibrillation complicates hyperthyroidism or other hyperadrenergic states (e.g., acute myocardial infarction, after operation, sepsis). Intrinsic sympathomimetic activity is a characteristic of some beta blockers (e.g., acebutolol [Sectral]) whereby the drug blocks the beta-adrenergic receptor but at the same time provides mild tonic stimulation. This results in a lesser reduction in resting heart rate but still adequately blunts sympathetic effects during exertion or other stress. Beta blockers with intrinsic sympathomimetic activity may be useful in patients with relative bradycardia at rest in whom beta-adrenoceptor blockade is desired.

The calcium channel blocking drugs that can control the ventricular rate are verapamil and diltiazem, and they are equally effective. Verapamil and diltiazem are available in intravenous as well as oral preparations. Both have negative inotropic effects, with that of verapamil probably being somewhat more potent than that of diltiazem. The dihydropyridines (e.g., nifedipine [Procardia]) are not effective in atrial fibrillation.

Digoxin has two effects on the AV node. The first action, occurring at lower doses, is the indirect effect

TABLE 2. **Treatment of Atrial Fibrillation**

Control of Ventricular Rate
Atrioventricular (AV) nodal blocking drugs
  Beta-adrenergic blocking drugs (e.g., propranolol [Inderal],
    metoprolol [Lopressor])
  Calcium channel blocking drugs (verapamil [Isoptin, Calan,
    Verelan], diltiazem [Cardizem, Dilacor])
  Digoxin [Lanoxin]
Catheter ablation or modification of the AV node

Maintenance or Restoration of Sinus Rhythm
Antiarrhythmic drugs
  Class IA: quinidine (Quinaglute, Quinidex), disopyramide
    (Norpace), procainamide (Procan, Pronestyl)
  Class IC: flecainide (Tambocor), propafenone (Rythmol)
  Class III: amiodarone (Cordarone), sotalol (Betapace),
    ibutilide (Corvert)
Maze surgical procedure
Catheter maze procedure ?
Implantable atrial defibrillator

of increased vagal tone. With higher doses, the more direct action of digoxin on slowing AV nodal conduction occurs. This fact is of more than just academic interest. When a patient is being monitored at rest, it may appear that an adequate blocking effect on the AV node is present. However, when that patient walks, the ventricular rate may increase dramatically if only the vagal effects of digoxin are present. Thus, it is important to note the ventricular response during exercise before concluding that the patient's heart rate is "well controlled."

Digoxin, by itself, is probably not effective in restoring sinus rhythm. In new-onset atrial fibrillation, about 50% of patients spontaneously revert to sinus rhythm within 24 hours without treatment, and a randomized study has shown no difference in reversion rates between digoxin and placebo. Further, the entire idea of whether digoxin controls the ventricular response at all during recurrences has been called into question. As digoxin shortens action potential duration and refractoriness in the atria, it is conceivable that it may cause atrial proarrhythmia and worsen the frequency and duration of a patient's paroxysms of atrial fibrillation.

Most comparative studies between the different types of AV nodal blocking drugs have shown no difference between beta-adrenergic blocking drugs and calcium channel blockers. Digoxin typically does not control the ventricular response as well as the other drugs, particularly during exercise. The best role for digoxin in atrial fibrillation may be in the patient with left ventricular dysfunction or as adjunctive therapy with a beta-blocking drug or calcium channel blocking drug.

Adenosine (Adenocard) is a potent AV nodal blocker, but its effects dissipate quite rapidly (less than 30 seconds) and thus it has no therapeutic use in atrial fibrillation. Clonidine (Catapres),* a central alpha$_2$-receptor agonist that reduces sympathetic nervous outflow, has been shown in one small study to slow the ventricular response, but its more routine use in this situation should await further studies.

Atrial fibrillation in patients with the Wolff-Parkinson-White syndrome presents a special case, and acute management and chronic management differ from those of atrial fibrillation in other settings. The aforementioned drugs should not be used to control the ventricular response, as they all may precipitate an increase in the ventricular rate and possible degeneration to ventricular fibrillation. Digoxin enhances conduction over accessory pathways in about one third of patients, slows conduction in about one third, and has no effect in the other third. The specific effect of digoxin in any given patient cannot be predicted a priori. The calcium channel blockers can increase the ventricular response by causing hypotension with resultant reflex sympathetic activation. Beta-adrenergic blockers, as well as digoxin and calcium channel blockers, by blocking conduction over the AV node can decrease retrograde concealed con-

duction into the accessory pathway that may have been helping blunt conduction over the accessory pathway.

Nonpharmacologic Approaches

When the ventricular response during atrial fibrillation cannot be controlled pharmacologically, a procedure can be performed in the electrophysiology laboratory that permanently interrupts conduction from the atria to the ventricles. This procedure, *catheter ablation of the AV junction,* is relatively easy to accomplish with use of local anesthesia by the delivery of radiofrequency energy through a catheter placed near the AV node. Because this results in complete AV block, permanent pacemaker implantation is required afterward. Typically, a rate-responsive ventricular pacemaker is placed. If the patient has paroxysmal atrial fibrillation, a dual-chamber pacemaker with mode-switching capability should be used so that AV synchrony can be maintained when the patient has sinus rhythm. Mode switching is a function available in most newer pacemakers by which atrial fibrillation can be detected and results in the pacemaker automatically changing its pacing mode from dual chamber (atrial and ventricular) to single chamber (ventricular). When sinus rhythm returns, the pacemaker senses this and reverts back to the dual-chamber mode, allowing tracking of the patient's native sinus rate. As atrial fibrillation persists after catheter ablation of the AV junction, the risk of thromboembolism is unchanged, and thus aspirin or warfarin therapy still needs to be considered (see later).

Newer approaches using catheter ablation to modify the AV junction so as to slow the ventricular response without creating complete AV block are being attempted. The goal is to attain rate control but avoid a pacemaker. Some investigators have reported success with this technique, but late occurrence of AV block has been reported, and this approach does not have universal acceptance. The irregular ventricular rhythm that remains after AV node modification (as opposed to the regular paced rhythm after AV node ablation) may cause persistent symptoms in some patients.

PREVENTION OF RECURRENCE

A noble goal in the treatment of patients with atrial fibrillation is to prevent recurrence of the arrhythmia. Two important points need to be kept in mind in this regard: (1) treatment of such patients has never been shown to prolong survival or decrease the incidence of stroke or peripheral embolism; (2) the drugs used to prevent recurrence may actually cause new arrhythmias (proarrhythmia).

A meta-analysis of six randomized, controlled trials of quinidine has shown that 1 year after cardioversion 50% of quinidine-treated patients remained in sinus rhythm compared with only 25% of control patients ($P < .001$). However, it was noted that death

---

*Not FDA approved for this indication.

rates were higher in the quinidine group: total mortality 2.9% versus 0.8%; sudden death, 0.8% versus 0.0%. Although this study does point out the potential problem of proarrhythmia seen with antiarrhythmic drug therapy, caution must be used so as not to overinterpret the problem, as the total number of patients suffering sudden death was small (3 of 413 patients).

The decision to treat atrial fibrillation is thus made with the intent of reducing symptoms. As with controlling the ventricular response in asymptomatic patients, exercise tolerance also increases once sinus rhythm is restored. Although preventing any recurrence is the best outcome, it is sometimes necessary to settle for a reduction in the frequency of recurrence. It is useful for the patient to be aware of this possible secondary goal of therapy so that any recurrence is not necessarily viewed as a complete failure. Aside from amiodarone, no one antiarrhythmic drug has been shown to be more effective than another in preventing recurrent atrial fibrillation, and 1-year recurrence rates are in the range of 50 to 70%. Thus, choice of an antiarrhythmic drug is made based on characteristics of the patient and side effects of the drugs. Generally, in patients without coronary artery disease and with normal ventricular function, I will choose a class IC agent (e.g., propafenone [Rythmol]), flecainide [Tambocor]) as first-line therapy. In those patients with coronary artery disease and/or ventricular dysfunction, I begin with a class IA drug (e.g., quinidine) or sotalol (Betapace), although sotalol should not be used in the setting of severe left ventricular dysfunction. Because of the proarrhythmic potential of all antiarrhythmic drugs, therapy is begun in the hospital while the patient's cardiac rhythm is monitored. Consideration can be given to initiation of class IC agents as outpatient therapy in those who have no coronary artery disease and normal cardiac anatomy and function. This is because the incidence of serious proarrhythmia in that specific setting is extremely low. However, it is important to involve the patient in this decision. If a class IC drug is begun as an outpatient therapy, it is best to have the patient return after 3 days of therapy to obtain an electrocardiogram to assess the extent of QRS prolongation (up to 20% beyond baseline is acceptable) and a treadmill exercise test to screen for proarrhythmia. Some arrhythmologists argue that amiodarone can be started on an outpatient basis in individuals without structural heart disease; however, this point is debated.

If neither a class IA nor a class IC drug provides the desired control, amiodarone (Cordarone) often prevents recurrent arrhythmia. In addition, amiodarone is effective at blocking the AV node and slowing the ventricular response. Although the success of amiodarone is greater than for any other drug, side effects are more prevalent. Some of the most prevalent and/or troublesome are pulmonary fibrosis, hepatitis, and hypo- or hyperthyroidism. During follow-up of patients using amiodarone, it is best to assess them every 3 months during the first year of therapy and every 6 months thereafter. At each visit, in addition to a brief history and physical examination aimed at uncovering side effects, a chest radiograph, liver functions tests, and sensitive TSH should be obtained. I initiate amiodarone therapy in the hospital under continuous electrocardiographic monitoring with a loading dose of 800 mg twice a day for 4 days. The patient is then dismissed and receives 400 mg daily with the plan to reduce the maintenance dose to 300 or 200 mg daily within 6 months. Alternatively, some clinicians begin with 200 mg daily without a loading dose. This latter approach takes longer for the patient to attain a maximal antiarrhythmic effect. Ibutilide (Corvert) has been approved for acute conversion of atrial fibrillation. It is available only as an intravenous preparation.

Nonpharmacologic Approaches

The maze procedure has been developed to prevent recurrences of atrial fibrillation. This operation involves incisions, resuturing, and the placement of cryolesions at different anatomic locations throughout the atria. The strategic placement of these lesions prevents the occurrence of the reentrant wavefronts needed to support atrial fibrillation. Sinus rhythm is maintained, and AV conduction is intact in most patients. Long-term prophylaxis against thromboembolism does not appear necessary. Some patients may have early recurrence of atrial fibrillation, but this is likely related to the surgery and due to a different mechanism than the patient's original arrhythmia. This postoperative atrial fibrillation typically resolves within a couple of months. Initial reports are promising, with cure rates greater than 95%. Experience is growing rapidly at some centers, but long-term follow-up is lacking.

Catheter ablation within the atrium to cure atrial fibrillation is being investigated. Analogous to the surgical maze procedure, this technique aims to create multiple lines of block within the atria that prevent atrial fibrillation from occurring. The lines are strategically placed so that the sinus impulse can still traverse the right atrium to the AV node, and AV synchrony is maintained. At present, the catheter maze is early in its investigation. Many more patients and longer follow-up times are needed to determine where this therapy will fit into the treatment of atrial fibrillation. It has the potential to become a major therapeutic advance in the therapy of atrial fibrillation in the next few years.

Implantable defibrillators to treat atrial fibrillation are under investigation. Whether patients will accept the discomfort of the defibrillation shocks remains to be seen.

STROKE PREVENTION

Acute Conversion to Sinus Rhythm

Electrical cardioversion of atrial fibrillation can be associated with embolic events. Whether the same risk exists for medical cardioversion using antiarrhythmic drugs is unknown but should be assumed until data prove otherwise. Exactly how long a person can be in atrial fibrillation before developing a risk of embolism during cardioversion is unclear. If the arrhythmia has been present for more than 24 hours or for an unknown duration, it is safest to proceed as though the risk is increased. In such a situation, oral anticoagulation with warfarin should be accomplished with the International Normalized Ratio (INR) in the 2.0 to 3.5 range for 3 to 4 weeks before attempting reversion to sinus rhythm. Embolic events after cardioversion can occur a week or more after the procedure; thus, anticoagulation should be maintained for an additional 4 weeks and perhaps longer based on the assessment of whether chronic prophylaxis is necessary.

In some instances, there may be a more urgent need to restore sinus rhythm, or there may be a contraindication to long-term anticoagulation. When cardioversion is contemplated in such situations, transesophageal echocardiography (TEE) may be useful in its ability to identify atrial thrombi that would almost always lead to deferral of cardioversion. The ability to detect atrial thrombi is enhanced by using a multiplane system and by the experience of the operator. A negative TEE result reduces but does not exclude the possibility of an embolic event with cardioversion. When a patient has not had adequate anticoagulation with warfarin, heparin should be used during the cardioversion, as there is suggestive evidence that electrical shocks may be thrombogenic.

Chronic Prophylaxis

Patients with nonrheumatic atrial fibrillation have a risk of stroke or peripheral embolism of 3 to 6% per year, which is about five times that of people in sinus rhythm. Those who have lone atrial fibrillation, defined as age younger than 60 years and no clinical heart disease or hypertension, appear to be at extremely low risk and probably do not need prophylaxis. Because of the increased incidence of embolism in all other patients, anticoagulant or antiplatelet therapy is strongly encouraged.

Numerous studies have shown that warfarin reduces the incidence of embolism by 64 to 86%. Most of these studies aimed to keep the prothrombin time ratio at 1.2 to 1.5 times control (INR 1.5 to 3.0). A meta-analysis of the major anticoagulation trials suggests that an INR of 2.0 to 3.5 provides the greatest protection against embolism with the lowest risk of hemorrhage. The incidence of major bleeding episodes with warfarin was 1.3 to 1.5% per year, and that of intracranial hemorrhage was 0.5% per year. The results concerning aspirin's efficacy are conflicting. One large study (Stroke Prevention in Atrial Fibrillation I [SPAF I]) showed a benefit to aspirin, 325 mg per day, compared with placebo; another study (AFASAK) reported no improvement with aspirin, 75 mg per day. SPAF II compared warfarin (pro-

thrombin time 1.3 to 1.8 times control) with aspirin, 325 mg per day, and found that in patients 75 years old or younger, warfarin tended to have a lower rate of stroke or peripheral embolism (1.3% per year versus 1.9% per year) but not significantly so ($P = .24$). Likewise, in patients older than 75 years, the primary event rate was nonsignificantly lower in the warfarin group (3.6% per year versus 4.8% per year, $P = .41$). Thus, the results of SPAF II imply that the event rate for patients aged 75 years or younger is low enough with aspirin, 325 mg per day, that warfarin does not appear to add any benefit. This is particularly so when these patients have no clinical predictors of thromboembolism: history of hypertension, recent heart failure, or prior thromboembolism (0.5% per year event rate in the absence of those predictors). Diabetes mellitus is a predictor of thromboembolism in some studies. It is noteworthy that the presence of paroxysmal as opposed to chronic atrial fibrillation does not appear to affect the thromboembolic potential. Results of SPAF III show that the combination of low-dose warfarin and aspirin is not as effective as standard-dose warfarin.

The results of echocardiography can help stratify for thromboembolic risk. Global left ventricular dysfunction or an enlarged left atrium (more than 2.5 cm per m²) identifies people at increased risk. Reports have also shown that spontaneous echo contrast ("smoke") seen in the left atrium is an independent predictor of thromboembolism in atrial fibrillation, increasing the risk fourfold. This finding can be detected by TEE in 25 to 60% of cases.

Although the use of warfarin versus aspirin must be individualized and the patient should be part of the decision-making process, the following general approach is reasonable. Patients younger than 75 years with none of the risk factors just discussed are at low risk for embolism and can be treated with aspirin. Those younger than 75 years, with any of the risks, should receive warfarin. Patients older than 75 years are at increased risk of major hemorrhage from warfarin and, although they may be at some increased risk of stroke due to their age, in the absence of other risks may best be treated with aspirin. The elderly patient with risk factors presents a particularly difficult therapeutic problem, and the decision of warfarin versus aspirin must take into consideration the patient's long-term outlook, concomitant medical problems, gait, and overall balance.

PREMATURE BEATS

method of
JOHN A. YEUNG-LAI-WAH, M.B., Ch.B.
University of British Columbia and St. Paul's Hospital
Vancouver, British Columbia, Canada

Premature beats are beats that occur early in the cardiac cycle and originate from a site other than the sinus node.

They are termed "supraventricular" if they arise anywhere from the atrium (premature atrial contractions [PACs]) to the His bundle. Premature beats that originate from below the His bundle are termed "premature ventricular contractions" (PVCs).

PREMATURE SUPRAVENTRICULAR COMPLEXES

Diagnosis

Premature supraventricular complexes are recognized on the electrocardiogram (ECG) by the presence of an early P wave, morphologically different from the sinus P wave. They may precede, coincide with, or shortly follow the QRS complexes. Premature supraventricular impulses usually conduct just like the sinus impulse down the His bundle and Purkinje fibers to activate the ventricle. Thus, they give rise to a normal QRS complex. When a premature beat occurs early in diastole, it may reach the atrioventricular node when it is still refractory; it is blocked, and the P wave has no subsequent QRS complex. Or the premature atrial impulse may reach the Purkinje system when one of the bundle branches is still refractory; the QRS complex becomes wide as in bundle branch block. This is termed a "PAC with aberrant conduction."

Clinical Features

Premature supraventricular beats of various origins have similar clinical features and management. They occur commonly in otherwise normal hearts. At times, they can be associated with structural heart disease, for example, cardiomyopathy, myocardial ischemia and infarction, and mitral valve disease. They may be caused by increased left atrial pressure secondary to increased left ventricular end-diastolic pressure. Thus, they may herald left ventricular failure in unstable settings such as acute myocardial infarction (MI). PACs occur commonly in chronic pulmonary disease and renal failure. They are sometimes more frequent during emotional upset or in the presence of medications, in particular, sympathomimetic drugs, alcohol, or caffeine. PACs have been recorded in up to 60% of young adults without heart disease, but only about 2% had more than 100 PACs in 24 hours. The prevalence increased with age. More than 80% of patients older than 90 years had more than 100 PACs per 24 hours.

PACs are mostly asymptomatic. The most common symptoms are palpitations, usually described as skipped beats. At times, PACs can induce paroxysmal supraventricular tachycardia, atrial flutter, or atrial fibrillation. Rarely, frequent PACs can give rise to dizziness. Anxiety and hyperventilation may sometimes be the cause for the symptoms.

Management

In patients with supraventricular premature beats and otherwise normal hearts, removal of obvious precipitating factors such as caffeine or alcohol and reassurance are the mainstays of management. Class I and III antiarrhythmic agents are best avoided because risk for death from proarrhythmia may far outweigh the benefits (Tables 1 and 2).

If the patient remains symptomatic, a beta blocker such as atenolol (Tenormin) 25 to 50 mg once daily or verapamil SR (Isoptin SR) 120 to 240 mg once daily orally may be tried. An anxiolytic agent such as clonazepam (Klonopin) 0.5 to 1 mg twice daily orally may be required. When PACs are still symptomatic, sotalol (Betapace) with a dose ranging from 80 to 160 mg three times daily or propafenone (Rythmol) at 150 to 300 mg three times daily may be used. Close monitoring for proarrhythmic effect and heart failure is mandatory. It is advisable to use the minimal dose possible. These drugs are best avoided in patients with left ventricular ejection fractions (LVEFs) below 30%.

If the patient's symptoms are mainly due to supra-

TABLE 1. **Oral Antiarrhythmic Agents**

Vaughan-Williams Class	Generic Name (Trade Name)	Usual Starting Dose (mg)	Usual Maximal Dose (mg)
IA	Quinidine sulfate (Quinora)	200 q 6 h	400 q 6 h
	Quinidine gluconate (Quinaglute)	324 q 8 h	648 q 8 h
	Quinidine sulfate, long-acting (Quinidex)	300 q 8 h	1200 q 12 h
	Procainamide (Pronestyl)	250 q 4–6 h	750 q 4–6 h
	Procainamide, sustained release (Procan SR, Pronestyl-SR)	500 q 8 h	1000 q 6 h
	Disopyramide (Norpace)*	100 q 6 h	200 q 6 h
IB	Mexiletine (Mexitil)	100 q 6 h	200 q 6 h
	Tocainide (Tonocard)	400 q 8 h	600 q 8 h
IC	Flecainide (Tambocor)†	50 q 12 h	100 q 12 h
	Encainide (Enkaid)†	25 q 8 h	50 q 6 h
	Propafenone (Rythmol)	150 tid	300 tid
II	Propranolol (Inderal)	40 bid	120 bid
	Atenolol (Tenormin)*	25 qd	100 qd
III	Sotalol (Betapace)	80 bid	160 tid

*Dosage reductions are necessary with renal impairment.
†Currently indicated only for severe, life-threatening arrhythmias that cannot be controlled with alternative drugs.

TABLE 2. **Common Adverse Effects of Antiarrhythmic Agents**

	Adverse Effects	Effect on Electrocardiogram
Quinidine	Diarrhea, nausea, headache, visual and auditory symptoms, fever, rash, thrombocytopenia, torsades de pointes	Prolongs QRS complex, QT interval
Procainamide	Gastrointestinal symptoms, fever, hypotension, arthralgia, rash, lupus-like syndrome, abdominal cramps, torsades de pointes, agranulocytosis	Prolongs QRS complex, QT interval
Disopyramide	Anticholinergic symptoms, torsades de pointes, heart failure	Prolongs QRS complex, QT interval
Class IB agents (mexiletine, tocainide)	Gastrointestinal upset, nervousness, tremor, dizziness, loss of balance, sleep disturbance, hepatotoxicity, fever, blood dyscrasias	No change in QRS complex. May shorten QT interval
Class IC agents (propafenone, flecainide, encainide)	Heart failure, aggravation of arrhythmia, sustained ventricular tachycardia, dizziness, blurred vision	Prolong PR interval, QRS complex at low plasma levels
Beta blockers	Bradycardia, atrioventricular block, bronchospasm, heart failure, fatigue, worsening of intermittent claudication, impotence, vivid dreams	Prolong PR interval, atrioventricular block
Sotalol	Same as beta blockers (fatigue common) plus torsades de pointes and sudden death	Prolongs PR, QT interval

ventricular tachycardias induced by the PACs, the therapy should be directed specifically to the tachycardias. Blocked PACs may cause bradycardia and are sometimes misdiagnosed as sinus node dysfunction. Pacing therapy should be considered only if the patient is symptomatic.

PREMATURE VENTRICULAR COMPLEXES OR CONTRACTIONS

Diagnosis

PVCs are recognized on the ECG by the presence of QRS complexes different from those in sinus rhythm. They are not consistently preceded by premature P waves. The timing of the sinus P wave remains undisturbed, unless the PVC is conducted retrogradely to the atrium and sinus node. If all PVCs are of the same form they are termed "monomorphic" or "unifocal." When the PVC forms vary, they are described as polymorphic, multimorphic, or multifocal.

Clinical Features

PVCs are often asymptomatic and are found when patients are examined for other purposes. Symptomatic patients complain of palpitations described as feeling their hearts "stop or skip" followed by "strong beats" or "thumps." PVCs may cause "pulsations in the neck" because of cannon waves. They may produce "difficulty breathing" or give the patient "the urge to take deep sighs." PVCs can occur frequently as in bigeminy or in nonsustained ventricular tachycardia (VT). They may then cause more severe symptoms including lightheadedness and syncope.

PVCs may be worsened by medications such as aminophylline; sympathomimetic drugs; electrolyte disturbances (hypokalemia); emotional upset; stress; and excess of caffeine, alcohol, and tobacco.

The main concern with PVCs is their potential for initiating life-threatening VT or ventricular fibrillation (VF). It is important to determine whether they are likely to be benign or malignant. This evaluation is usually influenced by the presence or absence of structural heart disease. PVCs that occur near the peak of the T wave of the previous complex (R-on-T phenomenon) were originally described to carry a high risk for inducing VF. This is probably relevant only in patients with acute ischemic events and is of no particular predictive value in situations unrelated to acute ischemia.

PREMATURE VENTRICULAR CONTRACTIONS WITHOUT HEART DISEASE

PVCs have been shown to occur in up to 60% of healthy individuals with no structural heart disease, and their prevalence increases with age. Exercise often decreases the number of PVCs or the patient's awareness of their presence or both.

Some patients have a specific type of PVC. These are of left bundle branch block and right axis morphology, indicating that they originate from the right ventricular outflow tract. They are usually sensitive to catecholamines. If a treadmill test is performed, these PVCs can become more frequent during exercise or even develop into sustained monomorphic VT. The PVCs or VT may resolve with rest or with a beta blocker. They are often well tolerated, and the VTs are unlikely to cause a cardiac arrest. Sometimes these PVCs are suppressed by the sinus rate on exercise and become more frequent as the sinus node slows down during the recovery phase.

Similarly, sleep can be associated with a decrease or increase in the frequency of PVCs. A quiet environment or lying in the left lateral position can make the patient more aware of postextrasystolic "pounding of the heart."

Management

The management is based on avoidance of obvious aggravating factors such as *excess* caffeine, alcohol, and stress. It is important to reassure the patients that PVCs are associated with little or no increased risk for cardiac sudden death. Therapy is instituted mainly for symptomatic purposes and has not been shown to prolong life. In fact, drugs have proarrhythmic effects that can be life-threatening. An ECG recording of the PVCs would help determine treatment of the PVCs in symptomatic patients. If they arise from the right ventricular outflow tract, the treatment of choice for these PVCs is electrophysiologic mapping and catheter ablation, which is safe and has a success rate above 85%.

The drug of choice for PVCs is a beta blocker such as atenolol (Tenormin) 25 to 50 mg orally once daily. If this is ineffective, I usually use sotalol (Betapace) 80 to 160 mg three times daily. The next drug of choice is mexiletine (Mexitil) at 100 mg three times daily to 200 mg four times daily. Class IA drugs such as quinidine may be used but can cause torsades de pointes. Class IC drugs such as flecainide (Tambocor) and propafenone are also effective. Initiation of class IC drugs is best left to specialists in the field (see Tables 1 and 2).

PREMATURE VENTRICULAR CONTRACTIONS WITH HEART DISEASE

Coronary Artery Disease

During exercise testing, PVCs occur in approximately 50% of patients who have coronary artery disease compared with about 30% of patients with normal hearts. The prognostic significance of these PVCs is still undetermined.

Post-MI studies showed that the presence of frequent and complex PVCs (ventricular bigeminy, couplets, multiform or early PVCs) is associated with higher mortality. There is some controversy as to whether this association results from a direct causal relationship to the PVCs or whether the complex PVCs are just a marker of more severe left ventricular dysfunction and more severe coronary artery disease. More recently, PVCs with frequency as low as 3 to 10 per hour were associated with increased sudden death and total mortality.

Management

Class I antiarrhythmic drugs are best avoided. Many studies using different class I antiarrhythmic drugs failed to demonstrate any benefit in patients after MI. In the Cardiac Arrhythmia Suppression Trial, patients were enrolled 6 days to 2 years after an MI if they had at least six PVCs per hour and no VT longer than 15 beats on a Holter recording.

Although the PVCs were effectively suppressed by antiarrhythmic agents including flecainide, the study had to be terminated because of greater than twofold mortality in the actively treated group compared with the group receiving placebo.

Beta blockers have been shown to reduce PVCs during the first year after an acute MI. They are the only antiarrhythmic drug class that have consistently decreased mortality. Such benefit has been shown with a variety of beta blockers including timolol (Blocadren), propranolol (Inderal), metoprolol (Lopressor), sotalol (Betapace), and acebutolol (Sectral). Interestingly, patients who have had heart failure had a greater reduction of mortality than did those without. Protection from sudden death was significant even 2 years after MI. Anterior MIs benefit more than inferior MIs. I initiate atenolol 50 mg once daily orally or metoprolol 50 mg twice daily orally as soon as possible after the onset of an MI. If the patient has had a large MI but no overt heart failure, I would start with metoprolol 25 mg twice daily orally. If heart failure is present, I would wait for it to resolve before trying a beta blocker. In some patients treated with a beta blocker, the sinus rate at rest would not decrease below 70 per minute despite higher doses, for example, more than 100 mg of atenolol per day. This does not necessarily mean that they are not beta blocked. Their sinus rate would not increase on exercise.

Two studies reported data regarding the role of amiodarone (Cordarone) in the treatment of PVCs after MI. In the Canadian Amiodarone Myocardial Infarction Arrhythmia Trial, 1202 patients were enrolled within 6 to 45 days after MI and if they had at least 10 PVCs per hour or one episode of nonsustained VT of 3 to 10 beats on a Holter monitor. After loading with amiodarone, the dose was 300 to 400 mg per day at 4 months and about 200 mg per day at 12 months after MI. Amiodarone reduced arrhythmic death by 48% compared with placebo (3.3% in the amiodarone group and 6% in the placebo group). The overall mortality was reduced by 21% but did not reach statistical significance. In the European Myocardial Infarction Amiodarone Trial, which enrolled patients 15 to 21 days after MI with LVEF of 40% or less, the amiodarone dosage was similar. Amiodarone reduced arrhythmic deaths significantly over placebo but made no difference to total mortality. Because amiodarone did not affect total mortality, it should not be used routinely in patients with PVCs after MI. Further electrophysiologic evaluation is recommended in patients with frequent PVCs or nonsustained VT.

During an acute MI, the term "warning arrhythmias" has been used to describe PVCs that are multiform, are R-on-T, or occur more than five per minute or in salvos of two or more beats. However, they are absent in half of the patients who develop VF. Antiarrhythmic drugs are used for PVCs mainly within the first 6 hours of onset of an MI. I start with lidocaine at a loading dose of 1 to 2 mg per kg at a rate of 25 to 50 mg per minute, followed by a maintenance infusion of 2 to 4 mg per minute. If the initial bolus is ineffective, up to two more boluses of 25 mg may be given at 5- to 10-minute intervals. Maintenance doses should be reduced by about half in patients with low cardiac output, with hepatic disease, or receiving drugs that decrease metabolism of lidocaine such as cimetidine (Tagamet) and propranolol.

If lidocaine fails to suppress PVCs or if the patients have VT, I use a loading dose of procainamide (Pronestyl) up to 10 mg per kg at a rate of 25 to 50 mg per minute. The maintenance rate of infusion is 2 to 4 mg per minute.

Non–Coronary Artery–Related Premature Ventricular Contractions

Patients who have frequent PVCs should be screened for conditions such as arrhythmogenic right ventricular dysplasia or cardiomyopathy, which can lead to life-threatening ventricular arrhythmias. This applies even if the patients are young and have no other cardiac symptoms. Further electrophysiologic evaluation is required in these patients.

GENERAL APPROACH TO PREMATURE VENTRICULAR CONTRACTIONS

It is initially important to determine frequency, severity of symptoms, and presence of a family history of sudden death and to establish the presence or absence of structural heart disease. An echocardiogram, 24-hour Holter monitoring, and exercise stress test are often useful in assessment of frequent PVCs. In the absence of structural heart disease, drugs are used for symptomatic purposes only. There can be marked day-to-day variation in the frequency of PVCs in an individual.

Serial ECGs are required to monitor electrophysiologic effects of drugs, for example, QT interval for class IA and III antiarrhythmic agents and QRS width for class IC drugs.

HEART BLOCK

method of
GERALD V. NACCARELLI, M.D.
*Pennsylvania State University College of
    Medicine*
Hershey, Pennsylvania

Bradyarrhythmias secondary to atrioventricular (AV) block at the level of the AV node or distal to the bundle of His account for a large number of patients who have bradyarrhythmias. In this chapter, I review basic and anatomic concepts, clinical profiles, and therapeutic strategies relevant to the recognition and treatment of patients with heart block.

ATRIOVENTRICULAR NODAL DYSFUNCTION

Anatomic Considerations

The AV node lies beneath the right atrial endocardium at the apex of the triangle of Koch, which is formed by the tendon of Todaro and the septal leaflet of the tricuspid valve. This positions the AV node directly above the insertion of the septal leaflet of the tricuspid valve and anterior to the ostium of the coronary sinus. The blood supply to the AV node is by the AV nodal artery, a branch of the right coronary artery in 90% of hearts, with the remaining 10% arising from the circumflex artery. Like the sinus node, the AV node is richly innervated by sympathetic and parasympathetic fibers. The sinus node and AV node are both influenced by the right and left vagus nerves and stellate ganglia. However, stimulation of the nerves on the right has less effect on AV nodal conduction than on sinus nodal rate. Conversely, left-sided autonomic stimulation exerts stronger influence on AV nodal conduction than on sinus rate.

The His bundle is contained within the connective tissue of the central fibrous body and membranous septum. It courses in the base of the membranous septum or along the left side of the crest of the interventricular septum in most cases. The anatomy of the left bundle branch is subject to much variability. The fibers generally travel as a broad band onto the left septum below the noncoronary aortic cusp. The right bundle branch extends unbranched from the His bundle, traveling down the right side of the interventricular septum to the apex of the right ventricle and base of the anterior papillary muscle. Discrete bifascicular subdivisions with anterosuperior and posteroinferior branches of the left bundle branch are not the norm. Anatomically, there may be no clear divisions. Despite this anatomic variability, the concept of the left anterior and posterior fascicular blocks remains clinically useful. The bundle branches end in Purkinje fibers, forming a network over the surface of the endocardium of the ventricles. The His bundle has a dual blood supply from branches of the anterior and posterior descending coronary arteries. Dual blood supply from the left and right coronary arteries is the usual case for the bundle branches.

Electrocardiographic and Electrophysiologic Findings

Normal AV Conduction

On the surface electrocardiogram, the PR interval is normally between 120 and 200 milliseconds in duration. This interval reflects the conduction time from the high right atrium to the point of ventricular activation. To measure the different components of the conduction system that the PR interval includes, intracardiac tracings from the high right atrium and His bundle region are needed. The PA interval, measured from the high right atrial electrogram to the low right atrial deflection in the His bundle electrogram, gives an indirect approximation of the right atrial conduction time. The AH interval (50 to 130 milliseconds) reflects conduction time through the AV node, and the HV interval (35 to 55 milliseconds) represents conduction time from the proximal His bundle to the ventricular myocardium.

First-Degree AV Block

First-degree AV block on the surface electrocardiogram is characterized as a PR interval longer than 0.2 second in adults or longer than 0.18 second in children. Each P wave is followed by a QRS complex with a constant, prolonged interval. PR prolongation is usually due to delay within the AV node. On the His bundle electrogram, this would be seen as an AH interval longer than 130 milliseconds with a normal HV interval. In cases in which first-degree AV block is seen in the presence of a bundle branch block, a His bundle electrogram is necessary to localize the site of block. Infranodal conduction delay is present in 45% of these cases. In addition, intra-hisian conduction delay can cause first-degree AV block.

Second-Degree AV Block

TYPE I SECOND-DEGREE AV BLOCK

Type I second-degree or Wenckebach's AV block features progressive prolongation of the PR interval before failure of an atrial impulse to be conducted to the ventricles. The PR interval immediately after the block returns to its baseline interval, and the sequence begins again. This block is almost always within the AV node when a narrow QRS complex is present. Intra-hisian block is the rare exception. When type I block is seen with a bundle branch block, the block is still more likely to be in the AV, node, but it could also be localized below the His bundle. A His bundle electrogram would be needed to accurately identify the level of block. Type I second-degree block in the AV node is characterized by progressive prolongation of the AH interval until an atrial deflection is not followed by a His bundle or ventricular deflection. In type I block secondary to block below the His bundle, progressive prolongation of the HV interval is followed by an H deflection without an associated ventricular depolarization.

TYPE II SECOND-DEGREE AV BLOCK

Type II, or Mobitz II, second-degree AV block is characterized on the surface electrocardiogram by a constant PR interval followed by sudden failure of a P wave to be conducted to the ventricles. The P-P interval remains constant, and the pause including the blocked P wave equals two P-P intervals. Mobitz II block is usually associated with bundle branch block or bifascicular block. In a majority of these cases, the site of block is within or below the His bundle.

2:1 AV BLOCK

Fixed 2:1 AV block poses a diagnostic dilemma because it is usually impossible to classify as type I or II block by a surface electrogram alone. A narrow QRS complex and accompanying type I second-degree block are highly suggestive of block at the AV nodal level. A 2:1 block associated with a wide QRS complex is likely to be infranodal. A definitive diagnosis can be made only with an intracardiac recording at the His bundle region.

High-Degree AV Block

Nonconduction of two or more consecutive P waves when AV synchrony is otherwise maintained is termed high-degree AV block. The level of block can be at the AV node or His-Purkinje system. When high-degree AV block is due to block in the AV node, QRS complexes of the conducted beats are usually narrow, a Wenckebach periodicity is also seen, and atropine administration produces 1:1 conduction. Features pointing toward block in the His-Purkinje system are conducted beats with bundle branch block and no improvement in block with atropine. His bundle recordings are sometimes needed to confirm the site of block.

Third-Degree AV Block

Third-degree, or complete, AV block is seen on the surface electrogram as completely dissociated P waves and QRS complexes, each firing at their own pacemaker rate. The atrial impulse is never conducted to the ventricles. Congenital complete heart block is characterized by a narrow QRS complex with an escape rate between 40 and 60 beats per minute, which tends to increase with exercise or atropine. This is consistent with block within the AV node. Acquired complete heart block is usually associated with block in the His-Purkinje system, resulting in a wide QRS complex with an escape rate between 20 and 40 beats per minute. The intracardiac electrogram will show His bundle deflections consistently following the atrial electrograms, but with the ventricular depolarization completely dissociated from these (block below the His bundle). In contrast, His bundle potentials consistently precede each ventricular depolarization in complete heart block at the AV nodal level, with the atrial electrograms dissociated from the HV complexes. The sinus rate is faster than the ventricular rate in patients with complete heart block.

Pathophysiology

Table 1 lists the majority of causes of AV block that have been identified. In each case, the abnormality may vary from a delay in conduction to intermittent or complete conduction failure.

Clinical Profile

Incidence

PR prolongation, or first-degree AV block, is rarely found in young healthy adults, but the incidence

TABLE 1. Causes of Atrioventricular Block

Drug effects: digoxin, beta blockers, certain calcium channel blockers, membrane-active antiarrhythmic drugs

Ischemic heart disease: acute myocardial infarction and chronic coronary artery disease

Idiopathic fibrosis of the conduction system—Lenègre's and Lev's diseases

Congenital heart disease: congenital complete heart block, ostium primum atrial septal defect, transposition of the great vessels, maternal systemic lupus erythematosus

Calcific valvular disease

Cardiomyopathy

Infiltrative disease: amyloidosis, sarcoidosis, hemochromatosis

Infectious and inflammatory diseases: endocarditis, myocarditis (Chagas' disease, Lyme disease, rheumatic fever, tuberculosis, measles, mumps)

Collagen-vascular diseases: scleroderma, rheumatoid arthritis, Reiter's syndrome, systemic lupus erythematosus, ankylosing spondylitis, polymyositis

Metabolic: hyperkalemia, hypermagnesemia

Endocrine: Addison's disease

Trauma: cardiac surgery, radiation, catheter trauma, catheter ablation

Tumors: mesothelioma, Hodgkin's disease, malignant melanoma, rhabdomyosarcoma

Neurally mediated: carotid sinus syndrome, vasovagal syncope

Neuromyopathic disorders: myotonic muscular dystrophy, slowly progressive X-linked muscular dystrophy

---

increases with age and in those with heart disease. An epidemiologic study involving a large population of asymptomatic male pilots revealed PR intervals longer than 0.2 second in only 0.52%. In the Tecumsah study, 2% of adults older than 20 years were found to have a PR interval of 0.22 second or longer. Other studies have shown a 5% incidence of first-degree AV block in men older than 60 years and as high as 10% in older patients with cardiac disease.

In a study of healthy pilots, type II second-degree block was found to be extremely rare. In contrast, type I second-degree block can be seen in young athletes at rest and has been documented by ambulatory Holter monitoring in healthy patients during rest or sleep. The Wenckebach periodicity in these settings disappears with exercise and should be considered a normal variant. In a population of patients with heart disease, the incidence of second-degree AV block (types I and II) was 2.7%.

Congenital complete heart block is estimated to occur in 1 of 15,000 to 25,000 live births, with a 60% female predominance. Acquired complete heart block is rarely seen in young individuals without heart disease. The highest incidence occurs in the seventh decade, and there is a 60% male predominance.

Symptoms

Individuals with first-degree AV block are asymptomatic. Symptoms of dizziness or syncope usually occur with acquired high-grade or complete AV block. With time, the majority of these patients will experience a Stokes-Adams attack. Other symptoms can occur as a result of low cardiac output, including fatigue, congestive heart failure, dyspnea on exertion, angina, or even mental status changes.

Diagnostic Techniques

Because the prognosis and treatment differ in AV block depending on whether block is within the AV node or infranodal, determining the site of block is important. In many cases, this can be done by long-term electrocardiographic monitoring techniques.

Exercise testing is a useful tool to help confirm the level of block that is already suspected in second- or third-degree block due to a narrow or wide QRS complex. Patients with presumed type I block or congenital complete heart block and a normal QRS complex usually enjoy an increased ventricular rate with exercise. On the other hand, patients with acquired complete heart block and a wide QRS complex usually show minimal or no increase in ventricular rate. Exercise and atropine worsen infranodal block owing to the change in the rate of the impulses being conducted through the AV node.

An electrophysiologic study is indicated in a patient with suspected high-grade AV block as the cause of syncope or presyncope when documentation cannot be obtained noninvasively. In patients with coronary artery disease, it may be unclear whether symptoms are secondary to AV block or ventricular tachycardia, and an electrophysiology study can be useful in establishing the diagnosis. Some patients with known second- or third-degree block may benefit from an invasive study to localize the site of AV block to help determine therapy or assess prognosis. Once symptoms and AV block are correlated by electrocardiography, further documentation by invasive studies is not required, unless additional information, as discussed before, is needed. Others who should not undergo electrophysiologic studies are asymptomatic patients with a transient Wenckebach block associated with increased vagal tone.

Natural History of Atrioventricular Blocks

The prognosis of any AV block is primarily dependent on the extent of the associated heart disease. First-degree AV block is usually benign. However, first-degree AV block can be found in conjunction with bifascicular block or infranodal disease, therefore increasing the risk for progression to complete heart block.

Type I second-degree AV block is generally benign, usually being transiently observed in the setting of acute inferior myocardial infarction or associated with increased vagal tone in healthy, athletic individuals. However, as with first-degree AV block, when type I AV block occurs in association with bifascicular or trifascicular block, the risk for progression to complete heart block is significantly increased because of probable infranodal disease. Type II second-degree AV block, usually seen with bundle branch block and associated with acute anterior myocardial infarction, carries a high risk for progression to advanced or complete AV block. Congenital complete heart block carries a much more favorable prognosis than the acquired form.

Principles of Management

Pacing is the mainstay of treatment for symptomatic heart block. Medical therapy is effective only as a short-term emergency measure until pacing can be accomplished. Before permanent pacing is instituted, the possibility of a reversible cause of the heart block should be investigated (see Table 1).

The key point in the decision to provide permanent pacing in AV block is the presence of symptoms (Table 2). Patients with complete heart block and syncope have clearly been shown to have improved survival with permanent pacing. The decision to pace is not always clear-cut in dealing with the asymptomatic patient. The American College of Cardiology–American Hospital Association Task Force report is helpful in providing some general guidelines for pacing patients with AV block (see Table 2). Table 3 lists indications for pacing after myocardial infarction.

BUNDLE BRANCH BLOCKS

Although the trifascicular concept is not consistent with pathologic findings, it remains useful clinically. "Block" is more accurately described as slowed conduction in one or more portions of the fascicles, or partial blocks. Electrocardiographic criteria have been established for recognition of right and left bundle branch blocks and hemiblocks. Bifascicular block is defined as conduction delay in two of the fascicles: right bundle branch block with left anterior fascicular block, right bundle branch block with left poste-

TABLE 2. Indications for Permanent Pacing in Acquired Atrioventricular Block

Class I

Symptomatic complete heart block (including associated congestive heart failure, angina, or confusional states)
Asystole ≥3 s or escape rhythm <40 bpm in asymptomatic patients with complete heart block
Symptomatic second-degree AV block (regardless of site of block)
Atrial tachycardia with associated symptomatic high-degree AV block

Class II

Asymptomatic complete heart block with ventricular rate >40 bpm
Asymptomatic type II second-degree AV block
Asymptomatic type I second-degree AV block at intra–His bundle or infra–His bundle levels

Class III

First-degree AV block
Asymptomatic type I second-degree AV block at the level of the AV node

Class I indications are conditions for which it is generally agreed that pacing is needed. Class II indications are conditions associated with varying opinions as to the necessity of pacing. Class III indications are conditions for which pacing is thought not to be indicated.

TABLE 3. Indications for Permanent Pacing After Myocardial Infarction

Class I

Persistent high-grade or complete AV block with bilateral bundle branch block (infranodal)
Transient high-grade AV block associated with bundle branch block

Class II

Persistent high-grade block at the AV nodal level

Class III

Transient AV block without intraventricular conduction defect
Transient AV block with isolated left anterior (or posterior) fascicular block
New left anterior (or posterior) fascicular block without AV block
First-degree AV block with new bundle branch block

rior fascicular block, or left bundle branch block. Trifascicular block is recognized with slowed conduction in three fascicles, namely, PR prolongation in addition to bifascicular block. In some cases, progressive slowing of multiple areas of conduction can result in complete heart block. Acquired intraventricular conduction delay is most commonly a product of idiopathic degenerative conduction disease. The incidence is 0.6% in the total population and increases with age (up to 2% in those older than 60 years). There is a high association with structural heart disease, especially coronary artery disease.

Right bundle branch block is more common than left bundle branch block. It rarely progresses to AV block or produces symptoms. Left bundle branch block is less common than right bundle branch block but is commonly associated with heart disease and an increased mortality rate that rises significantly when the abnormality is newly acquired. Left anterior fascicular block is more frequently found than right bundle branch block. Left posterior fascicular block is seen less frequently than left bundle branch block and is almost always associated with right bundle branch block.

Right bundle branch block in association with left anterior fascicular block is the most common type of bifascicular block; however, only 6% of these cases go on to complete heart block. Right bundle branch block with left posterior fascicular block is rare, but progression to complete heart block is higher presumably owing to more widespread conduction disease. Patients with left bundle branch block and left axis deviation have a 6% incidence of progressing to complete heart block. Those with left bundle branch block alone have a much lower rate of progression.

The prognosis of patients with bifascicular block depends on the extent of underlying heart disease. There is no group in which a high incidence of progression to AV block can be predicted by surface electrocardiography alone. However, the His bundle electrogram is useful in identifying a group at higher risk for developing complete AV block. If the HV interval is found to be markedly prolonged (>100

TABLE 4. **Indications for Permanent Pacing in Bifascicular and Trifascicular Block**

Class I

Bifascicular block with intermittent, symptomatic complete heart block

Bifascicular or trifascicular block with asymptomatic, intermittent type II second-degree AV block

Class II

Bifascicular or trifascicular block in syncope patient in which complete heart block is the presumed (but not proven) etiology

HV interval >100 ms

Pacing-induced block below the His bundle

Class III

Asymptomatic fascicular block with first-degree AV block

---

milliseconds), or if block below the His is seen during atrial pacing, prophylactic pacing is indicated because of a high progression of complete heart block. Indications for pacing in patients with bundle branch block are listed in Table 4.

TACHYARRHYTHMIAS

method of
JOHN H. McANULTY, M.D.
The Oregon Health Sciences University
Portland, Oregon

APPROACH TO THE ARRHYTHMIA PATIENTS
(Table 1)

Immediate Concerns

Some arrhythmias have immediate, potentially severe consequences. Hemodynamic stability has to be the first concern. In trying to think of some way to remind myself of what to do, I start with the question Is there time to think? The irony, of course, is that if there is *no* time to think, immediate action must be taken. A patient in severe hemodynamic distress requires emergency resuscitation measures. If stability of the patient allows, the next approach is to document the rhythm. A rhythm strip should

TABLE 1. **Arrhythmia Management**

Immediate	Chronic
Ask One Question:	*Ask Two Questions:*
Is there time to think?	1. What is the rhythm trying to tell us? That is, what is the cause?
No Take immediate lifesaving action (cardioversion, CPR)	*Outside the body causes* Drugs, drugs, drugs *Inside the body causes* Metabolic abnormalities Endocrine abnormalities *Cardiac causes*
Yes Record and interpret rhythm Apply specific therapy	2. Is treatment needed? For symptoms? For safety?

Abbreviation: CPR = cardiopulmonary resuscitation.

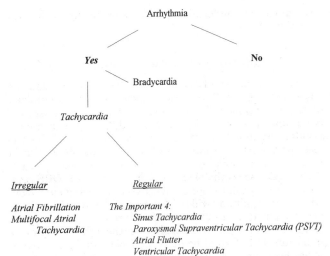

Figure 1. Analysis of arrhythmia on the electrocardiogram (ECG).

be recorded, and if at all possible, more than one lead (preferably 12 leads) should be recorded. The rules for diagnosis of the tachycardias follow, but as shown in Figure 1, there are some important first questions. First, even with the electrocardiogram (ECG) in hand, it is worth determining whether there is, or is not, an arrhythmia. Many patients have been treated for arrhythmias when none occurred; artifact was misinterpreted as an arrhythmia. If it is convincing that an arrhythmia did occur, it is next appropriate to classify it as slow or fast and then to attempt to classify it as to the specific type of arrhythmia (Figure 1).

Chronic Concerns

Once an arrhythmia is terminated, or if the patient is stabilized, the "chronic" phase of management ensues and two additional questions are appropriate.

1. What is the rhythm trying to tell us? That is, what is the cause? Whereas the rhythm itself may be important, it may simply be a marker for something else that should be addressed. This is a concern whether the rhythm is or was atrial premature beats or ventricular fibrillation. In an approach that seems too simple-minded to put into an article like this (but does happen to be that used by me), causes can originate from *outside* the body, from *inside* the body, and finally as the result of a *cardiac* abnormality. The point of this approach is that to treat rhythms when they are only secondary to other problems may not be appropriate. In considering outside of the body causes, drugs are the overwhelming explanation, and when drugs do not explain the problems, drugs should be considered again. Arrhythmias are commonly caused by prescription drugs, over-the-counter drugs, caffeine, tobacco, or illicit or recreational drugs. Causes inside the body that are potentially correctable include metabolic and endocrine abnormalities, particularly thyroid problems. And finally, an arrhythmia may be a marker for a cardiac abnormality that requires treatment. Although not totally satisfying, if a cause cannot be found, a patient can at times be comforted by knowing there is no dangerous underlying cause.

2. Is treatment required? Many arrhythmias do not require treatment. Treatment should be considered if the

rhythm causes intolerable symptoms or increases the risk of sudden death.

DIAGNOSIS OF TACHYCARDIAS

Treatment is usually safer and more effective when the rhythm is defined. Start with assessment of the regularity of the tachycardia. Is the rhythm regular or irregular? Sometimes determination of this is difficult because even regular rhythms have minor rate variation, but if there is less than a 10% variability of R-R intervals, for the most part, a rhythm can be classified within the regular category. Next, assess the QRS duration. A "narrow" QRS complex (≤0.10 second) defines the rhythm as being supraventricular in origin; a "wide" QRS complex may occur with a ventricular or a supraventricular rhythm. Identification of P waves and their relationship to the QRS complex is important but often difficult; on occasion, an esophageal or atrial lead can help. The response to a vagal maneuver (5 to 10 seconds of firm brisk massage of a carotid vessel without a bruit) will help in diagnosis and sometimes in treatment of the regular tachyarrhythmias. A drug challenge can also safely achieve diagnosis and treatment (Table 2). Short-acting drugs are preferable when feasible ("if you're wrong, you're not wrong for long"). Adenosine (Adenocard 12 mg by rapid intravenous [IV] bolus) is almost always the most appropriate. Esmolol (Brevibloc 0.5 mg per kg bolus followed by drip of 0.05 to 0.2 mg per kg per minute) is a short-acting alternative. Although not short acting, verapamil (Isoptin or Calan 2.5- to 5-mg bolus, repeat with 5 to 10 mg at 10 minutes) can be used for *narrow* QRS complex rhythms.

Irregular Tachycardias

Chaotically irregular rhythms are usually atrial fibrillation. The R-R interval patterns are unpredictable, and there are no recognizable consistent P waves. Atrial flutter with extremely variable ventricular conduction can occasionally appear to be atrial fibrillation (the diagnosis is made by looking for a regular P wave pattern). Multifocal atrial tachycardia can also present as a chaotically irregular rhythm. It is not atrial fibrillation because P waves are distinct (usually three or more P wave morphologies). For the most part, however, whether the QRS is narrow or wide, if the ventricular response rate is chaotically irregular, assuming the rhythm to be atrial fibrillation is appropriate.

Regular Tachycardias

These are the most difficult to define, are common, and are the most interesting! Although they are intimidating, there is good news. For all practical purposes, it is necessary to remember the rules for only four—they compose 95% of the regular clinical tachycardias (Table 3).

Sinus Tachycardia. In the nonexercising patient, sinus tachycardia is usually 150 beats per minute or less. In the young, or in those receiving large amounts of sympathomimetic agents, it may be as fast as 160 or 170 beats per minute, but for every increment greater than 150 beats per minute, the diagnosis of sinus tachycardia becomes less secure. When identified, the P waves (upright or "positive" in leads I and II) have a 1:1 relationship to the QRS. On occasion, a vagal maneuver or adenosine will result in transient, gradual slowing of the sinus node (and thus the P and QRS complexes). On rare occasions, the adenosine may cause transient atrioventricular (AV) block defining the P wave and its rate.

Paroxysmal Supraventricular Tachycardia (PSVT). This rhythm, also known as paroxysmal atrial tachycardia (PAT), is due almost exclusively to the mechanisms of reentry within the AV node ("AV node reentry" based on "dual" AV node pathways) or reentry using an accessory pathway ("AV reentry" using an accessory pathway connecting the atrium to the ventricle; this accessory pathway, also called a Kent bundle, occasionally results in pre-excitation on the sinus rhythm ECG, leading to the diagnosis of the Wolff-Parkinson-White syndrome). In either case, the rules for paroxysmal supraventricular tachycardia are about the same. There is a 1:1 P to QRS relationship (again when P waves can be seen), and the rate of each ranges from 150 to 250 beats per minute (occasionally 130 to 260 beats per minute). When the P waves are seen, they immediately follow the QRS (generally by less than 150 milliseconds; thus, these are "short RP" tachycardias). The QRS may be narrow or wide. An excellent vagal maneuver may not affect the rhythm, but the expected response is an abrupt termination of the rhythm with return to sinus rhythm. Adenosine defines and stops PSVT almost 95% of the time. There can be clues in the QRS and the ST-T segments to suggest the rhythm mechanism (AV node reentry versus AV reentry), but management approaches are not greatly affected by this differentiation.

Atrial Flutter. A red-light rule: a QRS or pulse of 150 beats per minute is atrial flutter until proved otherwise. This rule is applicable because atrial flutter is common, the atrial rate often approximates 300 beats per minute (it is "allowed" to be between 250 and 350 beats per minute), and the AV node generally allows 2:1 conduction; thus, the ventricular response rate of around 150 beats per minute. When the rule is ignored, a search for two P waves may not occur, and the diagnosis is often missed (the reason for the rule). The QRS complex may be narrow or wide. A vagal maneuver or adenosine may have no effect, but a transient slowing of the ventricular response with no effect of the P (or flutter) waves is diagnostic. There are different types of atrial flutter, but a common ("typical") form results in the "sawtooth" pattern of the baseline (the flutter waves) best seen in the inferior leads.

Ventricular Tachycardia. The QRS complex is always wide (exceptions are quite rare). The ventricular rate can be as slow as 100 beats per minute and as fast as 300 beats per minute. (Some call a rate faster than 250 beats per minute ventricular flutter.) If P waves can be seen and they are clearly slower than the ventricular rate, the diagnosis is reasonably secure. P waves, however, are often difficult to recognize; even if they are found, there can be a 1:1 P to QRS relationship owing to the retrograde ventricular to atrial conduction observed in 10 to 30% of ventricular tachycardias. Ventricular tachycardia usually (95% of the time) does not respond to a vagal maneuver or adenosine.

Unexplained Wide QRS Complex Tachycardia. Although there are only four important common clinical regular tachycardias, it is this rhythm that is the most difficult to explain and treat because it can be any of the others. The ECG rules (see Table 3) may make the diagnosis obvious. When this rhythm is encountered, it is most important to consider the clinical status. If the patient has known coronary artery disease, and especially if the patient has had a previous myocardial infarction, the rhythm should be diagnosed and treated as ventricular tachycardia. There are many rules for determining whether a wide QRS complex tachycardia is supraventricular or ventricular in ori-

TABLE 2. **Drugs Used to Treat Tachyarrhythmias**

Drug	Dose	Comment
AV-Node–Blocking Drugs		
INTRAVENOUS		
Adenosine (Adenocard)	12 mg rapid "push"	The rapid push (followed immediately by rapid flush if a peripheral vein is used) improves the chance of response. If no response to 12 mg in a large person (arbitrarily >75 kg), 18 mg can be given.
Calcium channel blockers		
Verapamil (Calan, Isoptin)	5-mg bolus; repeat with 5 or 10 mg if no response	Avoid in undiagnosed regular wide QRS tachycardia.
Diltiazem (Cardizem)	10- to 20-mg bolus followed by infusion of 10–15 mg/h	
Beta blockers		
Metoprolol (Lopressor)	5 mg IV q 5 min × 3	Avoid when reactive airway disease is a concern. CHF is not an absolute contraindication but should be monitored and treated. If there is concern about either (airway disease or CHF), esmolol is the appropriate choice because of its 10-min half-life.
Propranolol (Inderal)	0.15 mg/kg bolus	
Esmolol (Brevibloc)	0.5 mg/kg bolus followed by infusion of 0.5–2.0 mg/kg/min	
ORAL		
Beta blockers		If there is concern about toxicity, start with short-acting agents and, if tolerated, switch to once-daily preparations.
Atenolol (Tenormin)*	50–100 mg once daily	There are 14 beta-blocking preparations; I use these almost exclusively because on the basis of efficacy, side effect profile, and expense, there are no advantages to the others. If intrinsic sympathomimetic activity is desired, acebutalol (200–400 mg qd) is effective.
Metoprolol (Lopressor)	25–50 mg tid of the short-acting preparation or 50–200 mg of the once-daily preparations	
Calcium blockers		
Verapamil, sustained-release (Calan SR)*	180–360 mg qd	Verapamil is generally more effective.
Diltiazem, sustained-release (Cardizem SR)*		
Digoxin	0.25 mg qd	Load with 1–1.5 mg in first 24 h. Daily dose lower with renal failure.
Antiarrhythmia Drugs		
INTRAVENOUS		
Lidocaine (Xylocaine)	1.5 mg/kg bolus, repeat ½ in 15 min and infuse at 0.05 mg/kg/min	Whereas mg/kg dosing is optimal, an initial dose of 50 mg (small person), 75 mg (medium-sized person), or 100 mg (large person) is more practical with administration of one half to two thirds of that dose at 15 min.
Procainamide (Pronestyl)	15 mg/kg IV in 30 min and then infuse at 0.08 mg/kg/min	May contribute to hypertension.
Bretylium (Bretylol)	5 mg/kg bolus followed by infusion of 1–2 mg/min	
Amiodarone (Cordarone)	150-mg IV bolus followed by infusion of 1 mg/min for 6 h, then 0.75 mg/min	
ORAL		
Flecainide (Tambocor)	100–150 mg bid	
Mexiletine (Mexitil)	250 mg tid	Important to take with meals to prevent gastric instability.
Sotalol (Betapace)	80 mg bid × 3 d; increase to 160 mg bid if needed for desired effect	The beta-blocker effect is approximately two thirds of that of propranolol.
Amiodarone (Cordarone)	400 mg tid × 2 wk, then 400 mg bid × 2 wk, then 400 mg qd (for VT or VF) or 200–400 mg qd for supraventricular rhythm	

*Not FDA approved for this indication.
Abbreviations: CHF = congestive heart failure; VT = ventricular tachycardia; VF = ventricular fibrillation.

TABLE 3. **The "Important" Four Regular Tachycardias**

| Tachycardia | Onset and Termination | Rate (bpm)* | | QRS Width | Response to Vagal Maneuver or to Adenosine |
		P Wave	QRS Complex		
Sinus tachycardia	Gradual	100–150	100–150	Narrow or wide	None or transient gradual slowing
Paroxysmal supraventricular tachycardia (PSVT)	Abrupt	150–250	150–250	Narrow or wide	None or abrupt termination
Atrial flutter	Abrupt	250–350	<P wave rate: often one half the P wave rate	Narrow or wide	None or transient ventricular slowing
Ventricular tachycardia	Abrupt	≤ QRS rate	100–300	Wide	None

*These values apply about 95% of the time. Sinus tachycardia will occasionally be greater than 150, but the farther it strays above this value, the stronger other rhythms should be considered. Likewise, PSVT may be less than 150, but the same thought process applies. Wide QRS ≥0.12 s.

gin. A ventricular origin is more likely if the QRS width is greater than 0.14 second (recognizing that it is often difficult to assess a QRS width during a tachycardia), if there is a left axis deviation in the limb leads, or if there is a concordance of appearance of the QRS morphologies (either all positive or all negative) in the precordial leads. Other rules are both difficult to remember and apply infrequently enough that they are less useful. Diagnostic procedures can again include transesophageal or atrial recordings of the atrial complex. A drug challenge with adenosine (12 mg IV) can be helpful but—a warning—verapamil should *not* routinely be used as a diagnostic maneuver because of potential hypotension and negative inotropic effects from the drug.

MANAGEMENT OF TACHYARRHYTHMIAS
(See Table 2 for Drug Doses)

Sinus Tachycardia

Do not treat it. Look for and correct the cause (see Figure 1). If a patient is having angina, the first recommendation can be ignored and beta-blocker therapy is appropriate. Rare patients have chronic symptomatic sinus tachycardia unexplained despite an exhaustive search for a cause. Again, beta-blocker therapy may decrease associated symptoms. If not, or if the drug is poorly tolerated or ineffective, catheter ablation techniques can be applied to stop the rhythm or to cause AV block (a pacemaker is required if AV block is created).

Paroxysmal Supraventricular Tachycardia

Patients, of course, learn that they can often stop PSVT with their own vagal maneuver (in particular, a Valsalva maneuver). If a patient presents for medical care with this arrhythmia, a Valsalva maneuver or carotid massage (5 to 10 seconds of firm, almost painful massage) may provide the diagnosis and treatment. IV adenosine or verapamil is effective more than 90% (almost 95%) of the time. IV beta blockers (esmolol, metoprolol,* propranolol) may also

convert the rhythm. Digoxin is less effective and takes 2 to 3 hours to have any effect. A refractory rhythm with deteriorating hemodynamics should be treated with synchronized, direct-current (DC) cardioversion (100 joules, after deep sedation using anterior-posterior paddles).

After an episode of PSVT, a decision about chronic management is required. Daily antiarrhythmic therapy is not appropriate for a first or rare episode. If an individual tolerated the rhythm well, an argument can be made for giving no therapy other than instruction about a vagal maneuver. An alternative is to provide an individual with medication on an as-needed basis—a beta blocker (propranolol 160 mg or metoprolol 100 mg). The patient should be advised to try a vagal maneuver if the rhythm occurs. If the rhythm does not stop, the patient should take the medication and then relax for 1.5 hours. Vagal maneuvers should be tried again. The combination of the drug, the time, the relaxation, and the maneuvers may be enough to convert the rhythm back to normal and avoid a hospital visit. Individuals bothered by recurrent episodes should be treated with a daily AV-node–blocking agent (beta blockers or verapamil). If an accessory AV pathway is potentially a part of the rhythm mechanism, it is optimal to avoid digoxin or verapamil because they can speed conduction through this pathway—a problem if the individual should develop atrial fibrillation.

Radiofrequency catheter ablation is an increasingly used alternative for chronic management. When the mechanism of the rhythm is accessory pathway or dual AV nodal conduction, success again hovers around 95%. Currently, indications for its use include drug failure for control of the rhythms, drug side effects, or an unwillingness to take long-term medications. It is also indicated in the person who is limiting his or her life because of constant concern that an arrhythmia will occur. Although expensive (often $10,000 to $12,000 per procedure), this approach is low risk (rare valve damage, extremely rare death, and rare need for permanent pacemaker); may decrease expense in the long term; and has freed many patients from rhythms, limitations, and apprehension.

*Not FDA approved for this indication.

Atrial Fibrillation

Although treatment of the rhythm for hemodynamic stability is often a pressing concern, it still seems important to first emphasize the need for *stroke prevention* with this rhythm. This issue should be addressed each time a patient with atrial fibrillation is seen. A concept: *Once an atrial fibrillation patient, always an atrial fibrillation patient.* In considering stroke prevention, this concept is particularly important because there is no evidence that the 3 to 8% per year chance of a stroke is any less when a patient is in sinus rhythm. Fortunately, antithrombotic therapy can reduce the risk of this complication by 70% with reasonable bleeding complication rates (1 to 2% per year).

A large amount of recently accumulated information influences treatment recommendations. I use the following approaches as general rules. In patients with chronic atrial fibrillation, whether persistent or intermittent (paroxysmal), antithrombotic therapy is addressed with each interaction. If an atrial fibrillation patient has one of the risk factors that increase the risk of thromboemboli (has left ventricular dysfunction, uncontrolled systolic hypertension [blood pressure above 160 mm Hg], or a previous thromboembolic episode, or is a woman older than 75 years) and is a reasonable warfarin (Coumadin) candidate, use of that drug maintaining an International Normalized Ratio of 2 to 3 is recommended. A previous thromboembolism is the factor of greatest concern and the most important reason to attempt to use warfarin. If an atrial fibrillation patient does not have one of these risk factors, aspirin 325 mg per day offers stroke prevention. If an individual has one of the risk factors but is a poor warfarin candidate, again, aspirin 325 mg per day is appropriate treatment. A patient with "lone" atrial fibrillation (atrial fibrillation occurring in individuals younger than 60 years with no recognizable heart disease) is at such low risk of an embolus that an argument can be made for no treatment. Still, it is recommended that the patient be treated with aspirin 325 mg per day. If a patient goes for some prolonged time with no recognized atrial fibrillation (for example, longer than 6 months to a year), it could again be argued that antithrombotic therapy could be stopped, but until more is known (some large prospective studies are addressing this issue), antithrombotic therapy is recommended for life.

There is less information available on which to base the decision about antithrombotic therapy requirements at the time of a cardioversion. If it can be certain that the atrial fibrillation has existed for a short time (somewhat arbitrarily chosen as less than 48 hours), cardioversion can be performed without initiating antithrombotic therapy (although the therapy should be initiated for the long term). If the duration of atrial fibrillation is uncertain or known to be greater than 48 hours, when possible, rate control should be achieved, warfarin therapy started, and the patient returned in 4 to 6 weeks for an elective cardioversion. If the logistics of this delay are difficult, transesophageal echocardiography can be performed, and if there is no intra-atrial thrombus, the cardioversion can be performed without anticoagulation. This approach is expensive and, in most situations, not required.

Acute Atrial Fibrillation

Most individuals presenting with this rhythm have a ventricular response rate between 100 and 200 beats per minute with some associated symptoms. If there is severe hemodynamic compromise, urgent cardioversion is required (synchronized 200 joules, DC energy using anterior-posterior paddles in a sedated patient). Rate control is preferable in most patients with verapamil (5 mg IV followed in 10 minutes by 5 to 10 mg IV) or diltiazem (10 to 20 mg IV followed by an IV drip at 1 to 2 mg per minute). If an individual is hypotensive, vasodilator drugs must be used with caution, but in almost all cases, the hypotension is related to the rate, and the pressure will improve as the rate is controlled. At this point, the patient is either in sinus rhythm or in atrial fibrillation with a controlled ventricular response (depending on the approach used). In either case, this is still an atrial fibrillation patient.

If the patient remains in atrial fibrillation, cardioversion can be considered if the rhythm is thought to have been present less than 48 hours. If the rhythm duration is longer or uncertain, the rate should be controlled with an oral regimen (verapamil, beta blocker, or digoxin; see Table 2), and warfarin therapy should be started. If an individual is asymptomatic while in atrial fibrillation, an argument can be made for simply maintaining rate control and continuing treatment for prevention of stroke. There are also arguments for cardioversion (currently large ongoing prospective studies are evaluating which approach is optimal). Until the answers are known, at least one attempt to achieve normal sinus rhythm seems appropriate. After 4 to 6 weeks of warfarin therapy, cardioversion can be performed (generally requiring only a few hours under hospital observation). If sinus rhythm is achieved, warfarin should be continued for 2 weeks (to allow time for recovery of atrial contractile function), and then the appropriate long-term antithrombotic program should be initiated (see earlier). If sinus rhythm is maintained for 3 months, the rate control medication can be stopped (unless the patient tolerated the initial atrial fibrillation with a fast response poorly, in which case long-term continuation of medication is appropriate). If the patient is not successfully cardioverted and remains asymptomatic, atrial fibrillation can be accepted with reasonable rate control and attention to stroke prevention. If a patient is symptomatic despite rate control, initiation of an oral antiarrhythmic drug is appropriate. Because all antiarrhythmic drugs have the potential 1 to 2% risk of creating ventricular arrhythmias, the issue of hospitalization for initiation of the drug should be considered. This is not practical in most cases, and hospitalization should be reserved for the individual who has associated severe heart failure or perhaps a recent severe ischemia when the chance of the proarrhythmic effect of the drug may be enhanced.

Flecainide (Tambocor) is usually an appropriate first drug. It has the advantage of being effective with a twice-daily regimen and with a low side effect profile. It should be avoided in those with *severe* heart failure (it has a negative inotropic effect) and in those with recent significant ischemia. When evaluated in recently ischemic patients in the Cardiac Arrhythmia Suppression Trial, it was shown to be proarrhythmic. Other available drugs were not assessed in that trial, so it is not clear that they are any safer for use. Once flecainide is started, the patient can be brought back in a few days for an attempt at repeated cardioversion. If sinus rhythm is achieved, long-term antiarrhythmic drug therapy is warranted. If flecainide fails, sotalol or amiodarone is a reasonable next choice. The list of complications associated with amiodarone is long, and some are severe (potentially severe lung disease, liver disease, or possibly optic neuritis). The risks of using either drug would have to be balanced against the hope for benefit of making an individual feel better.

Many patients have reasonable freedom from symptoms with rate control alone. If drugs are not effective, AV node ablation has a high success rate, although it does obligate the patient to a permanent pacemaker; rate modification with AV node ablation techniques is of uncertain benefit. In a rare individual unwilling to accept atrial fibrillation, a surgical atrial dissection procedure (the maze procedure) has been applied with success in eliminating this rhythm.

Atrial Flutter

Atrial flutter is atrial fibrillation. Of course that is not true, but the statement is made because management should be nearly identical. The differences are worth discussion. First, there is less known about the thromboembolic risk with this rhythm. Because emboli have occurred when the rhythm is chronic and at the time of cardioversion, and because many people with atrial flutter frequently have episodes of atrial fibrillation, the antithrombotic regimen just presented for atrial fibrillation is also recommended for patients with atrial flutter. A second difference with atrial flutter is that it is often more difficult to control the ventricular response rate with the AV-node–blocking drugs—a reason to consider cardioversion earlier. A third difference is that some atrial flutters, particularly those with the typical form with the appearance of negative flutter waves in the inferior leads (sawtooth pattern), with the atrial rate being approximately 300 beats per minute, lend themselves to the possibility of elimination with atrial catheter ablation techniques. The ablation can eliminate the rhythm mechanism but allow maintenance of AV conduction. If that does not work, as

with atrial fibrillation, an AV node ablation can be performed, although this results in the need for permanent ventricular pacing.

Ventricular Tachycardia

When ventricular tachycardia is associated with significant hemodynamic embarrassment, immediate sedation followed by cardioversion (synchronized DC 100 to 200 joules) is the treatment of choice. In the patient with sufficiently stable hemodynamics, drug therapy using IV lidocaine (Xylocaine), procainamide (Pronestyl), or amiodarone (Cordarone), in that order, is appropriate. In the refractory patient or in a patient with recurrent rhythms, IV beta blockers can also be helpful.

Chronic Therapy

Ventricular tachycardia resulting from coronary artery disease or cardiomyopathies has a 20 to 40% chance of recurrence in the first year. Treatment can reduce the mortality to 5 to 15% in that year. Therapeutic options include drug therapy—amiodarone or sotalol (Betapace)—or an implantable cardioverter defibrillator (ICD). The just completed AVID trial (antiarrhythmics vs. implantable defibrillator trial) demonstrated improved survival with the device, compared with drug therapy. Quality of life and financial impact are still being assessed, but, on the basis of this study, an ICD is the preferred treatment in suitable candidates.

An individual will occasionally present with exercise-induced ventricular tachycardia. Particularly when it has an appearance of coming from the right ventricular outflow track (usually a left bundle branch block morphology with an inferiorly directed axis), beta-blocker therapy can be highly effective. If these rhythms are recurrent, they can often be eliminated with radiofrequency catheter ablation.

Another somewhat unusual tachycardia is that arising from the inferior aspect of the left side of the ventricular septum (generally a right bundle branch block morphology with a superior axis). These rhythms respond to treatment with verapamil and can also be treated with catheter ablation.

Ventricular Fibrillation

Complete life support and emergency treatment are of course required. Early defibrillation offers the best chance of survival. Cardiopulmonary resuscitative measures should be undertaken until conversion of the rhythm to normal can be achieved. A sudden death rate of 20 to 40% in the next year can be reduced to 5 to 15% with drug therapy—again sotalol or amiodarone—or with insertion of the ICD. The previously mentioned AVID trial also demonstrated improved survival when the ICD was used to treat survivors of ventricular fibrillation.

Nonsustained Ventricular Tachycardia

The role and optimal treatment of this rhythm are not yet fully understood. In the patient with recurrent unacceptable symptoms, drug therapy may be beneficial, and sotalol or amiodarone is most likely to be effective. Alternatives (quinidine, procainamide, mexiletine, or propranolol) are less likely to be effective and have their own set of potential side effects. In the patient with this rhythm with associated coronary artery disease and a reduced ejection fraction (below 0.35), electrophysiologic testing may determine those whose life would be better protected with an implantable defibrillator (i.e., those in whom sustained ventricular tachycardia can be induced and not suppressed by procainamide in the rhythm laboratory).

THE OTHER FIVE PERCENT

These uncommon rhythms still occur often enough that a comment in regard to each seems appropriate. They are often dangerous and even more difficult to treat than the more common rhythms and thus fortunately *are* rare.

The Rapid Irregular Wide QRS Tachycardia (Often with a Rate Above 250 Beats per Minute)

Irregularity makes ventricular tachycardia an unlikely diagnosis, so atrial fibrillation, as noted before, should be considered. The rapid rate suggests that conduction may be not through the AV node but rather through an accessory pathway. AV-node–blocking drugs will not work and may actually exacerbate the rhythms by increasing accessory pathway conduction or by decreasing blood pressure and ventricular function. The treatment of choice for this rhythm is DC cardioversion. IV procainamide or lidocaine can block accessory pathway conduction in some patients.

Torsades de Pointes

This is perhaps the most confusing of all rhythms; different causes of this rhythm require opposite treatments. The rhythm is recognized by a rapid wide QRS complex tachycardia with a gradually changing morphology. It usually recurs as repetitive nonsustained episodes, so cardioversion should be avoided (and frequently is ineffective). It is difficult to differentiate from a "polymorphic" ventricular tachycardia; the presence of a prolonged QT interval on the sinus rhythm electrocardiogram (a Qt_e >500 milliseconds) is the major reason to consider the rhythm as torsades de pointes. This prolonged QT interval syndrome can be "acquired" and due to drugs (quinidine, class IA antiarrhythmic agents, tricyclic antidepressants, phenothiazine drugs, and the antihistamines astemizole [Hismanal] and terfenadine [Seldane] particularly when used in combination with a macrolide antibiotic) or to metabolic abnormalities (hypokalemia, hypomagnesemia). Treatment consists of identification of and stopping the offending agent, use of magnesium sulfate (2 to 4 grams IV), and potassium repletion. Until the effect of the drug dissipates, the torsades de pointes may be suppressed by initiation of isoproterenol or atrial pacing (to a heart rate of 120 beats per minute).

Torsades de pointes can also occur as the result of a congenital abnormal prolonged QT interval. This should be suspected if these rhythms are documented in the young, in those with a history of recurrent unexplained syncope, and in those with a family history of syncope or early sudden death. In patients with a congenital prolonged QT syndrome, the rhythm is often induced by sudden increase in adrenergic tone, e.g., when an affected person is startled by an alarm. IV beta-blocking agents will suppress the rhythm acutely. Chronic beta-blocker therapy should be initiated. In patients with the chronic syndrome and recurrent rhythms, if beta-blocker therapy does not work, an implantable defibrillator is an occasional consideration.

Abnormal Sinus Node and Atrial Rhythms

Sinus tachycardia, PSVT, atrial flutter, and atrial fibrillation have been discussed. There are other supraventricular rhythms. Sinoatrial reentry tachycardia can appear to be sinus tachycardia but is distinguished by its abrupt onset and termination. Beta-blocking agents or an antiarrhythmia agent can on occasion correct the rhythm. Atrial tachycardia may appear to be PSVT, but it behaves more like atrial flutter. The P waves may be more apparent than they are with PSVT and often are midway between QRS complexes (a "long RP" tachycardia). AV-node–blocking agents do not stop the rhythm (as they may with PSVT) but rather cause an increase in AV block. These rhythms can occur as the result of drug toxicity (e.g., digitalis). In general, treatment should consist of AV nodal blockade (with verapamil or beta blockers) and antiarrhythmia drugs; catheter ablation techniques can eliminate some of these rhythms.

CONGENITAL HEART DISEASE

method of
JEFFREY A. TOWBIN, M.D.
Baylor College of Medicine
Houston, Texas

GENETICS

Congenital heart disease (CHD) was previously considered to be due to multifactorial inheritance (i.e., multiple genetic and environmental effects combined to cause the underlying disease), with greater than 90% of affected patients having this type of inheritance. During the past decade, however, it has become increasingly clear that many of these cardiac abnormalities are single-gene disorders. In many cases, the disease-causing genes have been identified. Furthermore, a significant percentage of children with CHD have associated dysmorphic features that should be identified by the examiner.

The prevalence of CHD is approximately five cases per 1000 live births (excluding bicuspid aortic valve and mitral valve prolapse), with higher prevalences rates seen in aborted fetuses. The most common form of CHD is ventricular septal defect (VSD) (which is discussed later), an abnormality that causes increased pulmonary blood flow but patients retain normal color (i.e., are acyanotic); approximately one third of newborns with CHD, however, present with cyanosis.

CLINICAL EVALUATION

The initial evaluation of any infant or child with suspected CHD should include a comprehensive history, family history, physical examination (including four-extremity blood pressure measurement), posteroanterior and lateral chest radiography, 15-lead electrocardiogram, and pulse oximetry. The physical examination should be performed in a quiet environment, and particular attention should be given to the child's vital signs and growth curve, general appearance (cyanotic vs. acyanotic; well-nourished vs. wasted; dysmorphic vs. nondysmorphic), and state of well-being (comfortable vs. distressed), and also to the cardiac (see later) and pulmonary examination (depth and rate of breathing, use of accessory respiratory muscles, presence of rales or stridor), abdominal examination (location and size of liver; location of stomach), femoral pulses (intensity and presence of radiofemoral delay), and distal extremities (cyanosis, clubbing, edema).

The cardiac examination should proceed in an orderly manner of evaluation as follows: (1) inspection of the chest for detection of precordial bulging, visualization of the cardiac impulses, signs of previous surgery, and recognition of abnormalities such as pectus excavatum and widely spaced nipples; (2) palpation for thrills, apical impulse (noting the location and intensity), and the presence or absence of a left parasternal impulse (also called a right ventricular impulse or tap); and (3) auscultation, proceeding from apex to base or vice versa. When auscultating the heart of a child, the examiner should pay close attention to the quality of the first (S_1) and second (S_2) heart sounds and the presence of third (S_3) or fourth (S_4), heart sounds, the so-called gallop rhythms. The S_2 should be evaluated for its intensity, whether it is single or split, and its variation with respiration. In addition, the presence of clicks must be appreciated when present. Systolic murmurs are quantified on a scale of 1 to 6 based on intensity, with murmurs of grade 4 or above associated with the presence of a thrill. Regurgitant (holosystolic) murmurs begin with S_1 and, therefore, obscure S_1. On the other hand, ejection murmurs begin after S_1. Diastolic murmurs (which occur after S_2) are quantified on a scale of 1 to 4, with grade 4 murmurs associated with the presence of a thrill. Continuous murmurs extend through both systole and diastole. Localization of the murmurs to the classic mitral (apex), tricuspid (mid–left sternal border), pulmonic (upper left sternal border), and aortic (upper right sternal border) areas is helpful, along with a description of the pitch (high frequency, midfrequency, low frequency), harshness, and shape (plateau, crescendo-decrescendo) of the murmur. Auscultation over the posterior thorax, supraclavicular regions, suprasternal notch, carotids, and, in infants, the head, is also important.

Cyanosis is detected clinically when at least 3 grams per

dL of desaturated hemoglobin is present. Central cyanosis, best seen in the buccal mucosa or tongue, must be differentiated from peripheral cyanosis (acrocyanosis), which is usually a normal finding in infants and children. Noninvasive pulse oximetry is easily performed and diagnostic of the level of cyanosis. Typically, oxygen saturations should be greater than 90% in neonates and 95% in infants and children. If cyanosis is present in infants, the hyperoxia test should be performed to help differentiate cardiac from pulmonary disease. This test is performed by obtaining preductal (right radial) arterial blood gas measurements both before and after the neonate is placed in 100% oxygen. Infants with lung disease usually increase their partial oxygen pressures in arterial blood to greater than 150 mm Hg, whereas infants with cardiac disease cannot. The diagnosis of cyanosis in an infant with CHD differentiates those children with likely underlying cyanotic cardiac disease from those children without cyanosis (i.e., cyanotic CHD vs. acyanotic CHD). These patients can be further subdivided into those with increased and those with decreased pulmonary vascularity.

ACYANOTIC CONGENITAL HEART DISEASE WITH INCREASED PULMONARY VASCULARITY

Several CHDs present without cyanosis and increased pulmonary vascularity. The most common defects in this category are (1) VSD, (2) atrial septal defect (ASD), (3) patent ductus arteriosus (PDA), and (4) atrioventricular septal defect (AVSD). These four lesions account for the majority of CHD cases.

Ventricular Septal Defect

VSD is the most common form of CHD, occurring in 32% in children with heart disease. The ventricular septum is a complex structure that can be described embryologically as having four major regions: (1) the inlet septum, located posteriorly and superiorly between the tricuspid and mitral valves; (2) the outlet septum, located anteriorly beneath the aortic and pulmonary valves; (3) the trabecular septum, located inferiorly; and (4) the membranous septum, located in the subaortic region and beneath the septal leaflet of the tricuspid valve. The largest part of the ventricular septum is the trabecular region, and fusion of the inlet, outlet, and trabecular septa occurs in the membranous region.

Patients with a VSD have a dependent left-to-right shunt, meaning that the relative pressures and resistances of both the systemic and the pulmonary circulations determine the amount and direction of ventricular level shunting. At birth, when the pulmonary vascular pressures and resistances are high, little left-to-right ventricular shunting occurs. During the first 2 to 6 weeks of life, pulmonary pressure and vascular resistances drop, creating a pressure difference between the left and right ventricles and, therefore, allowing shunting from left to right. The amount of ventricular shunting also depends on the size of the VSD, with larger defects allowing more blood to shunt. Lastly, other associated cardiac lesions may alter the amount and direction of shunting.

The clinical signs and symptoms of children with VSD are the result of the amount of left-to-right ventricular shunting (i.e., the amount of pulmonary blood flow). Neonates are often without symptoms (due to the high pulmonary vascular resistance), and only as pulmonary pressures and vascular resistances drop do clinical symptoms develop. Beyond the neonatal period, children with a VSD can be categorized into four physiologic groups: (1) small VSD, (2) moderate VSD, (3) large VSD, and (4) VSD with pulmonary vascular obstructive disease (Eisenmenger's syndrome).

Children with a small VSD are asymptomatic. On physical examination, they are found to be normal with the exception of a loud (grade 3 or higher) holosystolic murmur. The vast majority of these defects close completely with time, most within the first few months of life. The only risk is the development of subacute bacterial endocarditis (SBE), for which these children require prophylaxis.

Children with a moderate VSD are often symptomatic. Infants often take longer to feed, and they may have inadequate weight gain in relation to their linear growth. These children also have a higher frequency of pulmonary infections. On physical examination, mild tachypnea may be found. A hyperdynamic impulse is usually present in the midaxillary line. A loud (grade 3 to 4/6) holosystolic murmur is present, and a diastolic rumble may also be audible. Mild hepatomegaly is commonly found. Most of these defects diminish in size, and some close completely as late as young adulthood. As these defects become smaller, the patient's symptoms often disappear. A small percentage of children require surgical closure. For symptomatic children, the use of digoxin and diuretics is helpful. Caloric intake must be recorded frequently along with weight gain, and in children with poor growth, hypercaloric formula (24 to 30 calories per ounce) should be given with a goal of approximately 130 to 150 calories per kg per day. These children are at risk for SBE and require prophylaxis.

Children with a large VSD are all symptomatic. These infants typically fail to thrive, and pulmonary infections are common. On physical examination, a hyperdynamic impulse is found laterally displaced. A loud (grade 3 to 4/6) holosystolic murmur is present with a prominent (grade 2 to 4/4) diastolic rumble at the apex. These children are tachypneic with retractions; rales may be present on auscultation in children (less common in infants). Marked hepatomegaly is typically found. These defects often diminish in size, but surgical closure is often required to prevent pulmonary vascular obstructive disease. Medical therapy should be initiated early and maximized. This includes using digoxin, diuretics, and hypercaloric formula (30 calories per ounce) with a goal of approximately 140 to 150 calories per kg per day. These children are at risk for SBE and require prophylaxis.

Eisenmenger's syndrome develops when a large VSD is left unrepaired and pulmonary hypertension and irreversible pulmonary vascular obstructive disease develop with resultant right-to-left ventricular shunting and cyanosis. Death follows as a result of pulmonary hemorrhage, infections, and/or paradoxical emboli. Fortunately, only rarely do children younger than 3 years develop this disease. In those who do, large defects may be identified by echocardiography; few symptoms exist, however, due to pulmonary hypertension (and, hence, less left-to-right shunting). This entity is most often seen in previously undiagnosed adolescents and adults with large VSDs.

The diagnosis of VSD is often made clinically. An electrocardiogram (ECG) often reveals left atrial and left ventricular volume overload. Chest radiography reveals cardiomegaly with increased pulmonary vascularity if the left-to-right shunt is significant. Confirmation of the diagnosis is made using echocardiography. Technologic advances in equipment and image processing have allowed excellent visualization of the entire ventricular septum. Color Doppler ultrasonography has improved the detection of even tiny VSDs, and pulsed Doppler ultrasonography allows the estimation of right ventricular and pulmonary artery systolic pressures. Cardiac catheterization is usually not required in the management of children with VSD. This procedure is reserved for those patients with multiple VSDs or in those in whom the question of pulmonary vascular obstructive disease exists and the measurement of pulmonary artery pressures, resistances, and flow is desired. In some centers, VSD closure using a device placed by catheter into the defect may be a consideration.

With advances in the medical and surgical care of children with CHD, cardiothoracic surgery is now being performed safely, even in small infants. Indications for surgical closure of a VSD include (1) uncontrolled congestive heart failure, (2) increased pulmonary vascular resistance with a risk for the development of pulmonary vascular obstructive disease, (3) failure to thrive despite maximal medical therapy, (4) recurrent pulmonary infections, (5) endocarditis, and (6) paradoxical emboli. Follow-up with a pediatric cardiologist is required. Right ventricular infundibular stenosis (including double-chambered right ventricle) develops in approximately 20% of patients, even after spontaneous or surgical closure of the VSD. In addition, a subaortic membrane can develop in association with a VSD. SBE prophylaxis can be discontinued 6 months after surgical closure of a VSD assuming no residual defects are present. Typically, no restriction to the child's activity is necessary in the asymptomatic child or in children after VSD closure (spontaneous or surgical).

Atrial Septal Defect

ASD is the third most common form of CHD, occurring in 8% of children with heart disease. ASDs are found more frequently in girls than in boys (2:1) and may occur as an isolated lesion or in association with other cardiac anomalies.

ASDs occur in three separate locations in the atrial septum. Ostium primum defects are located in the lower third of the atrial septum near the atrioventricular valves. Ostium secundum defects are found in the midportion of the septum. Sinus venosus defects occur in the posterior portion of the septum adjacent to the venae cavae. Ostium secundum defects are the most common type found.

The direction and amount of atrial level shunting are determined by the relative compliances of the right and left ventricles and the size of the defect. Typically, the right ventricle is more compliant, and therefore predominantly left-to-right shunting occurs.

Most children with an ASD are asymptomatic. They typically present to the primary care physician with a heart murmur. Atrial arrhythmias are present more frequently in older children and adults. In about 6% of patients with large, unrepaired ASDs, irreversible pulmonary vascular obstructive disease develops, typically in adulthood.

On physical examination, these children are found to have a hyperdynamic subxiphoid impulse. There is a normal S_1, but a fixed and widely split S_2 is present. Often a grade 2 to 3 systolic ejection murmur is heard in the pulmonic region as the result of the increased flow of blood that must traverse the normal pulmonary valve, creating a "relative pulmonary stenosis." An ECG usually reveals right atrial and right ventricular enlargement (rSR' pattern in lead V_1). A chest radiograph often reveals cardiomegaly with increased pulmonary vascularity and a prominent main pulmonary artery segment. Confirmation of the diagnosis is made by using echocardiography, during which the location and size of the defect and the degree of right ventricular volume overload are assessed. Color-flow Doppler echocardiography is a useful adjunct to the two-dimensional echocardiogram.

In children with signs of pulmonary overcirculation, medical therapy is indicated and usually includes digoxin and diuretics. Closure of ASDs is most commonly performed in early childhood, usually after the age of 5 years.

Indications for closure of an ASD are (1) right ventricular volume overload, (2) arrhythmias, (3) paradoxical emboli, and (4) elevated pulmonary vascular resistance. Closure is typically performed surgically with little morbidity or mortality. ASD closure in the cardiac catheterization laboratory using closure devices is performed in some centers. SBE prophylaxis is not recommended by the American Heart Association for an isolated ASD. No restriction to the child's activity is necessary. In children who have had repairs, atrial arrhythmias may occur, and monitoring for this should be performed periodically.

Patent Ductus Arteriosus

Approximately 2% of children with CHD have an isolated PDA. Premature infants have a high incidence of PDA that is inversely proportional to their gestational age. The ductus arteriosus is a normal embryologic structure connecting the main pulmonary artery to the descending aorta. In normal term infants this structure closes within the first few days of life. Patients with a PDA have left-to-right shunting dependent on the size of the PDA and pressures in the descending aorta and pulmonary artery.

Most infants with a large PDA are symptomatic with signs of congestive heart failure. Many infants and children with smaller PDAs are asymptomatic and present to the physician with only a heart murmur. Patients with large PDAs left untreated develop irreversible pulmonary vascular obstructive disease in young adulthood.

On physical examination, children with a PDA are found to have a hyperdynamic apical impulse. The heart sounds are normal. Often a grade 3 to 4/6 continuous murmur is heard best in the pulmonic region. The pulses are bounding. In patients with congestive heart failure, tachypnea, pulmonary edema, and hepatomegaly are present along with the murmur and a gallop rhythm.

An ECG often reveals left atrial and left ventricular enlargement, and chest radiography demonstrates cardiomegaly with increased pulmonary blood flow. Confirmation of the diagnosis is made by using echocardiography. All patients with a PDA require closure with medications, surgery, or interventional cardiac catheterization. Indomethacin (Indocin) is successful in closing most PDAs in premature infants, and surgical closure is only occasionally necessary. Surgical ligation is extremely effective with essentially no morbidity or mortality. Newer interventional catheterization techniques using either PDA closure devices or coils are being used at select centers with reasonable success. The risk for SBE is high in patients with a PDA and is the rationale for recommending closure of all PDAs. Until closure is accomplished, these patients require SBE prophylaxis. Asymptomatic children require no restriction to activity.

Atrioventricular Septal Defect

AVSD occurs in 7% of children with CHD and is commonly found in children with Down syndrome. The defect, which is also known as endomyocardial cushion defect or atrioventricular canal, consists of a large defect in the atrioventricular septum along with a common atrioventricular valve. The clinical presentation, physical examination, and medical treatment are similar to those of children with a large VSD. The ECG demonstrates a superior axis, and chest radiography may demonstrate cardiomegaly and pulmonary vascular overcirculation. Echocardiography is used to confirm the diagnosis and assess the surgical anatomy of the defect. Cardiac catheterization is rarely necessary but may be needed to measure the pulmonary artery pressure and resistance or to calculate the amount of systemic-to-pulmonary shunting. Surgical repair is required in infancy, ideally at 3 to 6 months of age. In children with Down syndrome, pulmonary hypertension may develop after 6 months of age. SBE prophylaxis is necessary preoperatively but may be discontinued if no residual lesions exist 6 months postoperatively.

ACYANOTIC CONGENITAL HEART DISEASE WITH VENTRICULAR OUTFLOW TRACT OBSTRUCTION

Ventricular outflow tract obstruction occurs in both the left and the right ventricles. Obstruction to either ventricle can occur in isolation or in combination with other defects at the (1) subvalvular, (2) valvular, or (3) supravalvular levels.

Aortic Stenosis

Aortic stenosis (AS) occurs in 3% of children with CHD. The commissures of the aortic valve are fused, resulting in a thickened, domed, stenotic orifice. The presenting symptoms and the findings on physical examination are variable and related roughly to the degree of narrowing of the valve. In infants with mild AS, an ejection click and a harsh systolic ejection murmur are present at the right upper sternal border. The intensity of the murmur increases with the severity of the disease, and thrills can be felt in the suprasternal notch in patients with moderate or severe AS. Infants with critical AS present in shock at birth. Often, a murmur is difficult to appreciate because of little forward flow across the valve. Patients with severe AS may complain of substernal chest pain, typically with exercise, and are at risk for sudden death. An ECG often reveals left ventricular hypertrophy with ST-T wave changes. Echocardiography is used to confirm the diagnosis, assess the severity of the lesion and the size of the aortic annulus, and calculate pressure gradients from the left ventricle to the aorta using Doppler techniques. In infants with critical AS, endocardial fibroelastosis and poor ventricular function are common. In some patients, left ventricular outflow tract obstruction occurs at the subvalvular or supravalvular region, with a normal aortic valve. Cardiac catheterization in patients with valvular AS is usually reserved for intervention rather than diagnosis because the treatment of choice for these patients is balloon valvuloplasty. This procedure is quite effective with good initial and long-term results. Surgery is recommended for those in whom the annulus and valve are extremely small and require valve replacement or in whom interventional catheterization was unsuccessful. Exercise is restricted in patients with moderate or severe disease, and SBE prophylaxis is required.

Coarctation of the Aorta

Coarctation of the aorta (CoA) occurs in 5% of children with CHD. CoA is a constriction of the descending aorta that usually occurs opposite the site of the ductus arteriosus–ligamentum arteriosum. The symptoms in these patients are variable. Typically, children with mild disease have no symptoms, whereas infants with critical CoA present with shock in the first week of life after spontaneous closure of the ductus arteriosus. The classic physical findings are right upper extremity hypertension, discrepant upper extremity–to–lower extremity blood pressure (with the upper extremity blood pressure significantly higher), and diminished or absent femoral pulses. The heart sounds are normal. In the left supraclavicular region, a variable grade 2 to 4/6 systolic ejection murmur that spills into diastole is usually present. An ECG reveals left ventricular hypertrophy. A chest radiograph in older patients may reveal cardiac enlargement, rib notching, and the posterior indention of the descending aorta (so-called 3 sign). The diagnosis is confirmed by echocardiography or magnetic resonance imaging techniques. Pressure gradients across the CoA are calculated using Doppler techniques. Cardiac catheterization is usually reserved for patients undergoing intervention (i.e., balloon angioplasty). Prostaglandin E_1 infusion is lifesaving for neonates with critical CoA who are in shock, because of its ability to open and maintain the patency of the ductus arteriosus and, therefore, allow blood flow into the descending aorta. Treatment of hypertension is frequently necessary and usually responsive to beta-receptor blockade. Hypertension may persist even after successful repair. Therapy for CoA includes surgical repair or balloon angioplasty. Increasingly, interventional cardiologists have been successful in treating this lesion with balloon dilatation. Early and long-term results for balloon angioplasty are good except in neonates and young infants (younger than 6 months). Long term, a significant number of repaired patients develop restenosis requiring balloon angioplasty and/or surgery. Isometric exercises and contact sports are prohibited for these patients. SBE prophylaxis is required lifelong.

Pulmonary Stenosis

Pulmonary stenosis (PS) is the second most common form of CHD, occurring in 9% of children with heart disease. The pulmonary valve is abnormal, with fusion of the commissures resulting in a thickened, domed, stenotic orifice. Except for newborns with critical PS, most children with PS are asymptomatic. A prominent subxiphoid impulse and right ventricular tap may be palpated. On auscultation, an ejection click and a grade 3 to 5/6 systolic ejection murmur are found to be present at the left upper sternal border with radiation to the back. The intensity and duration of the murmur increase with the severity of the disease. Neonates with critical PS present with cyanosis due to right-to-left atrial shunting through the patent foramen ovale at birth. A murmur is often difficult to appreciate because of the lack of blood flow across the severely obstructed valve. An ECG reveals right atrial and right ventricular hypertrophy. The diagnosis of PS is made by using echocardiography, and Doppler techniques can be used to assess the severity of the lesion by calculating pressure gradients across the valve. Balloon valvuloplasty is the treatment of choice for these patients. This procedure is usually curative with excellent long-term results. SBE prophylaxis is required for all except those with mild PS.

CYANOTIC CONGENITAL HEART DISEASE WITH DECREASED PULMONARY VASCULARITY

Patients with cyanotic CHD and decreased pulmonary vascularity have obstructed pulmonary blood flow and right-to-left shunting of blood at either the atrial or the ventricular level. In the neonatal period, children with this category of defects are usually intensely cyanotic with hyperpnea but not dyspnea. This presentation is due to the decrease in pulmonary blood flow and the absence of congestive heart failure.

Tetralogy of Fallot

Tetralogy of Fallot (TOF) is the most common form of cyanotic CHD, occurring in 7% of children with CHD. This anomaly consists of (1) pulmonary stenosis (subvalvular, valvular, supravalvular); (2) VSD; (3) overriding of the ventricular septum by the aorta; and (4) right ventricular hypertrophy. Patients present with different degrees of cyanosis depending on the severity of the pulmonary stenosis. A hypercyanotic spell, or "tetralogy spell," is a characteristic sequence of clinical events that begins with irritability and hyperpnea followed by a prolonged period of intense cyanosis leading to syncope.

On physical examination, the patient may appear cyanotic if the degree of pulmonary stenosis is more than mild. A prominent subxiphoid impulse is palpated. S_1 is normal, but S_2 is single. A systolic ejection click (if the obstruction is valvular) and a grade 2 to 4/6 (depending on the degree of pulmonary stenosis) systolic ejection murmur are heard at the left upper sternal border. Clubbing of the distal extremities is present in older children with long-standing cyanosis.

Pulse oximetry documents the degree of cyanosis, whereas the chest radiograph often reveals a boot-shaped heart with an absent main pulmonary artery shadow and decreased pulmonary vascularity. A right aortic arch is found in 25% of children with TOF. An ECG demonstrates right atrial and right ventricular enlargement. Echocardiography is used to diagnose the defect and to assess the severity of the individual components of the lesion. Cardiac catheterization and angiography are still performed frequently in these children to assess and/or confirm the severity of the individual components of the defect.

Medical treatment is lifesaving in a child with a hypercyanotic spell. Initially, the child should be calmed and comforted and placed in a knee-to-chest position. Maximal supplemental oxygen by face mask is then given. If the spell continues, morphine is given intramuscularly at a dose of 0.1 mg per kg. If the spell persists, then more aggressive therapy is initiated. This includes rapid placement of an intravenous catheter by the most experienced personnel followed by intravenous fluid administration (10 to 20 mL per kg of 0.9% saline) and sodium bicarbonate administration (1 mEq per kg). Anemia (hemoglobin less than 10 grams per dL), when present, often precipitates a hypercyanotic spell, and blood transfusion may be required.

Surgical repair of this defect is indicated for any child with hypercyanotic spells or increasing cyanosis (typically oxygen saturations less than 75%). In the past, the approach to these patients had been a palliative operation involving placement of a modified Blalock-Taussig shunt (Gore-Tex tube connection between the innominate artery and the pulmonary artery) in infancy followed by definitive repair (pulmonary valvotomy with resection of right ventricular infundibular muscle bundles and VSD closure) in older childhood (3 to 4 years of age). With advancements in the combined medical and surgical management of younger infants, definitive repair is now commonly being performed in infancy as the only surgical procedure. Immediate and long-term results for these children are excellent. SBE prophylaxis is required lifelong, and these children are prohibited from participating in strenuous sports.

Tricuspid Atresia

Tricuspid atresia is a rare form of cyanotic CHD in which the tricuspid valve orifice is not patent. A patent foramen ovale or ASD is present to allow systemic venous blood to shunt from right to left. The right ventricle and pulmonary outflow tract are typically hypoplastic unless a large VSD is present. These patients present in the immediate neonatal period with marked cyanosis. The cardiac examination is variable and nonspecific. An ECG reveals leftward axis deviation and left ventricular hypertrophy. The diagnosis is made by echocardiography. Catheterization is required infrequently and is reserved for infants who require balloon atrial septostomy because of restriction of blood flow across the atrial septum. Initial medical therapy includes the initiation of prostaglandin E_1 (alprostadil [Prostin VR Pediatric]) infusion (0.05 µg per kg per minute) to maintain the patency of the ductus arteriosus. Palliative surgery is performed in the first week of life and consists of placement of a modified Blalock-Taussig shunt. A modified Fontan operation is performed in children at approximately 2 years of age. The modified Fontan operation allows complete bypass of the right side of the heart by directing inferior and superior venae cavae flow into the pulmonary arteries. These children require lifelong SBE prophylaxis and are restricted from strenuous activities.

CYANOTIC CONGENITAL HEART DISEASE WITH INCREASED PULMONARY VASCULARITY

Cardiac lesions with cyanosis and increased pulmonary vascularity can be divided further into those with increased (1) pulmonary arterial vascularity (transposition of the great arteries and truncus arteriosus [TA]) or (2) pulmonary venous vascularity (total anomalous pulmonary venous connection [TAPVC] and hypoplastic left heart syndrome). Along with cyanosis, children in this category are usually dyspneic because of congestive heart failure associated with pulmonary congestion.

Transposition of the Great Arteries

In transposition of the great arteries, the aorta arises from the right ventricle, whereas the pulmonary artery arises from the left ventricle. Under these circumstances, the pulmonary and systemic circulations are configured in parallel rather than in series, resulting in cyanotic blood's being recirculated back to the systemic circulation rather than passing through the pulmonary circulation and becoming oxygenated. These neonates present immediately after birth with deep cyanosis. The cardiac examination and ECG are often nonspecific. The classic chest radiography reveals an "egg on a string" appearance consisting of a globular heart with a narrow mediastinum. The diagnosis is made with echocardiography. Medical management involves stabilization of the neonate and the initiation of prostaglandin E_1 infusion (0.05 µg per kg per minute) while balloon septostomy is awaited. Catheterization is usually undertaken to perform a balloon atrial septostomy. The infants are typically stabilized after balloon septostomy and undergo surgical repair of the defect in the first week of life. The arterial switch operation in which the aorta is connected to the left ventricle and the pulmonary artery to the right ventricle is currently the surgical procedure of choice. Immediate and intermediate-term outcomes are good. These children require lifelong SBE prophylaxis and are restricted from strenuous activities.

Truncus Arteriosus

TA is a rare form of CHD in which a single-valved vessel is located above both right and left ventricles via a VSD, allowing common egress of blood from both ventricles. This common vessel, the TA, gives rise to the aorta, coronary arteries, and pulmonary arteries. A significant percentage of these patients have DiGeorge's syndrome (thymic hypoplasia, third and fourth pharyngeal pouch defects) or other similar syndromes lumped under the term "CATCH-22" (cardiac, abnormal facies, thymic hypoplasia, cleft palate, hypocalcemia, 22q11 deletions) and should be evaluated immediately for hypocalcemia secondary to hypoparathyroidism and T cell immune deficiency. These children should receive only irradiated blood cell transfusions so as to prevent the development of graft-versus-host disease. Cyanosis in these patients is often mild, and most infants present with symptoms of congestive heart failure and a heart murmur. A prominent right ventricular impulse is palpable, and S_1 and S_2 are single. An ejection click and continuous grade 3/6 murmur are often heard. The murmur is also appreciated well over the back bilaterally. An ECG shows biventricular hypertrophy, and the chest radiograph demonstrates a right aortic arch in one third of patients. Echocardiography is diagnostic, and cardiac catheterization is frequently not required. Initial medical management involves control of the congestive heart failure with digoxin and diuretics. Definitive surgical repair can usually be performed soon after diagnosis and involves placement of a valved homograft conduit from the right ventricle to the main pulmonary artery, which has been separated from the TA. The VSD is closed so as to direct the left ventricular blood into the TA. The long-term outcome is good in patients without immune deficiency. Subsequent surgical procedures are necessary to change the size of the conduit as the children grow. These patients require SBE prophylaxis for a lifetime and are restricted from strenuous activity.

Total Anomalous Pulmonary Venous Connection

Patients with TAPVC, a rare form of CHD, have their entire supply of oxygenated pulmonary venous blood returning to the systemic venous circulation. This admixture of oxygenated and desaturated blood produces cyanosis. The severity of the cyanosis increases if there is obstruction to the return of the pulmonary venous blood (above or below the diaphragm), as commonly occurs. Neonates with TAPVC frequently present in extremis with severe cyanosis. Physical examination results are variable. The ECG is nonspecific, often showing right atrial and right ventricular enlargement. The chest radiograph in patients with obstruction of the pulmonary veins reveals a small heart with diffuse bilateral pulmonary edema. When performed meticulously, echocardiography is diagnostic. Cardiac catheterization is performed only when the pulmonary venous drainage cannot be determined with certainty. Surgical repair is done immediately on presentation with good long-term results. After complete recovery, no SBE prophylaxis or restriction of activity is required.

Hypoplastic Left Heart Syndrome

Hypoplastic left heart syndrome occurs in 4% of children with CHD and comprises stenosis or atresia of the mitral and/or aortic valves, CoA, and hypoplasia of the left ventricle. Neonates present within the first few days of life, typically with mild cyanosis and a shocklike state after the PDA begins to close. Physical examination reveals a prominent right ventricular impulse, single S_1 and S_2, a gallop rhythm, and a systolic ejection murmur in the pulmonic region. All pulses are diminished, and hepatomegaly is frequent. The ECG reveals right ventricular hypertrophy with a paucity of left ventricular forces and occasionally ischemic changes. The chest radiograph usually shows signs of pulmonary venous congestion. Echocardiography is diagnostic and is used to evaluate the severity of the individual components of the syndrome. Cardiac catheterization is rarely required. Initial medical management is lifesaving. Control of the airway and mechanical ventilation are commonly needed. Prostaglandin E_1 infusion (0.05 μg per kg per minute) is begun and the state of shock treated with fluid administration (bolus of 10 to 20 mL per kg of 0.9% saline) and inotropic support (dopamine infusion of 3 to 10 μg per kg per minute). Surgical treatment for this disease is variable and controversial. In some centers, no therapy is offered and the neonates die after intensive support is withdrawn. Cardiac transplantation at a few centers has had some success, but the limited number of donor organs and lifelong immunosuppression are of major concern. In other select centers, a staged surgical approach similar to that for children with tricuspid atresia has been undertaken. With this approach, neonates undergo the palliative Norwood operation (anastomosis of the divided main pulmonary artery of the aorta, aortic arch reconstruction, atrial septectomy, modified Blalock-Taussig shunt). This procedure transforms the right ventricle into the single pumping chamber for both the systemic circulation and, via the shunt, the pulmonary circulation. At 3 to 6 months of life, the infant proceeds to the bidirectional Glenn operation (anastomosis of the superior vena cava to the pulmonary arteries) with takedown of the Blalock-Taussig shunt followed by the modified Fontan operation at 2 years of age. In some centers the results have been promising. SBE prophylaxis and restriction of strenuous exercising are lifelong.

HYPERTROPHIC CARDIOMYOPATHY

method of
LAWRENCE S. COHEN, M.D.
Yale University School of Medicine
New Haven, Connecticut

Isolated descriptions of patients with probable hypertrophic cardiomyopathy appeared in the European medical literature in the mid-19th century. But it was in 1907 that Schmincke definitively described severe diffuse hypertrophy in the hearts of two women: he considered the disorder to be congenital in origin and responsible for left ventricular outflow tract obstruction. As is often the case with scientific discoveries, interest in this syndrome did not ignite until almost 50 years later when the ability to define the hemodynamics in patients with this entity in the cardiac catheterization laboratory became a reality. These latter investigations initiated a series of studies into the nature of the disease, its patterns of inheritance, the presence or absence of true obstruction, its medical and surgical treatments, and its natural history. Controversies surrounding the nature of the syndrome spawned a variety of terms to describe hypertrophic cardiomyopathy—idiopathic hypertrophic subaortic stenosis, hypertrophic obstructive cardiomyopathy, muscular subaortic stenosis, and asymmetric septal hypertrophy, to name a few. Most early investigators stressed the dual concepts of left ventricular hypertrophy and dynamic subaortic stenosis. Careful analysis of left ventricular angiograms identified that the basis for the subaortic obstruction was systolic apposition of the anterior leaflet of the mitral valve against the hypertrophied interventricular septum.

As further understanding of the disease developed, it became clear that some symptomatic patients with hypertrophied ventricles might not evidence any features of left ventricular outflow tract obstruction. These observations led to the thesis that abnormalities in left ventricular compliance might also contribute to the abnormal pathophysiology of these patients. The concept of diastolic dysfunction contributing to left-sided heart failure became an increasingly attractive explanation in certain patients. The introduction of M-mode echocardiography opened a new era in the diagnosis and understanding of hypertrophic cardiomyopathy. Asymmetrical septal hypertrophy was a consistent feature of the disease whether or not patients were symptomatic and whether or not outflow tract obstruction was present. Systolic anterior motion of the mitral valve was seen most frequently in the subset of patients who had outflow tract obstruction. The echocardiogram allowed for extensive screening of family members and helped demonstrate that the disease is transmitted as an autosomal dominant trait with a high degree of penetrance. The preceding introduction to this disease entity can be summarized as follows: Hypertrophic cardiomyopathy should be thought of as a primary myocardial disease resulting in a nondilated, hypertrophied ventricle (usually asymmetrical), with or without dynamic outflow tract obstruction, and usually of a familial nature, manifesting typical clinical signs and symptoms with a characteristic clinical course and response to treatment modalities.

Patients with hypertrophic cardiomyopathy most often present with dyspnea, angina, or dizziness (presyncope). Other symptoms such as edema or palpitations are less frequent. In greater than two thirds of patients, dyspnea is the predominant symptom, and in the majority of patients it is the presenting symptom. Dyspnea and paroxysmal nocturnal dyspnea are a consequence of decreased compliance of the left ventricle with consequent increase in left ventricular filling pressure. This leads to elevation of left atrial and pulmonary venous pressures. Chest pain is a frequent symptom and is likely due to a mismatch between coronary artery supply and the excessive demands of a hypertrophied myocardium. The chest pain may be more prolonged than the usual angina caused by ischemic heart disease. It may worsen after administration of sublingual nitroglycerin. The pain may not be associated with physical or emotional stress but may begin after the cessation of physical activity. It may be made worse by standing and be improved by lying down. Syncope or presyncope is the third most common symptom. This symptom may have a variety of pathophysiologic determinants. It may be secondary to cardiac arrhythmias or to low cardiac output caused by a sudden increase in subvalvular gradient or by decreased cardiac compliance.

In patients with left ventricular outflow tract obstruction, the use of either physiologic maneuvers or pharmacologic agents at the bedside can be quite useful. Any intervention that decreases left ventricular volume (preload) or decreases systemic arterial pressure (afterload) or increases left ventricular ejection velocity (contractility) will augment the resting outflow tract gradient. Conversely, any intervention that increases left ventricular volume, increases systemic arterial pressure, or diminishes left ventricular contractility will decrease the resting outflow tract gradient. An understanding of the foregoing makes interpretation of the physical examination more rational.

At physical examination, the heart is generally enlarged. The precordial impulse is often displaced laterally. A presystolic impulse is often present, corresponding to atrial systole with an augmentation of blood flow into a poorly compliant ventricle. In some patients, there is a late systolic impulse leading to a triple apical impulse. A systolic thrill is present frequently and is felt most regularly at the cardiac apex. A thrill is present in many patients with obstruction but is not present in patients without an obstructive component to their disease.

Examination of the jugular venous pulse may reveal a prominent "a" wave that augments with inspiration. This reflects the diminished compliance of the right ventricle. The arterial pulses are brisk, and the carotid pulse may have a double impulse in patients with obstruction. An atrial gallop (fourth heart sound) is extremely common in patients with and without obstruction. A diastolic filling gallop (third heart sound) is appreciated somewhat less frequently. The second heart sound is at times paradoxically split.

A systolic murmur is present in all patients with obstruction and may vary in intensity, depending on the magnitude of the subvalvular gradient. The murmur is most prominent at either the lower sternal border or at the cardiac apex. For reasons stated earlier related to the pathophysiology of the disease, the murmur often increases with standing, the Valsalva maneuver, tachycardia, and a postextrasystolic beat. Conversely, squatting, isometric handgrip, and bradycardia decrease the intensity of the murmur. In a minority of patients, a diastolic rumble may be present, probably related to abnormalities in flow across the mitral valve secondary to a poorly compliant left ventricle.

Most patients have an abnormal resting 12-lead electrocardiogram, even if they are asymptomatic. The most common electrocardiographic abnormalities are left ventricular hypertrophy and ST and T wave abnormalities. Because of asymmetrical hypertrophy of the left ventricle, patients may have large Q waves in the anterior, lateral, or inferior leads. This finding, especially in young patients, is a distinct clue to the diagnosis of the disease. Other frequent electrocardiographic abnormalities are left atrial or right atrial enlargement, left axis deviation, or PR prolongation. Sudden death is uncommon in patients with ventricular arrhythmias other than sustained ventricular tachycardia. The presence of sustained ventricular tachycardia on a Holter monitor identifies a subgroup of patients with as high as an 8% annual mortality rate. There are no specific radiologic findings, but the chest radiograph may mimic mitral stenosis, mitral regurgitation, or congestive cardiomyopathy. Most patients have an enlarged left ventricle and left atrium, and about half have evidence of right ventricular enlargement as well. At left ventricular cineangiography, the shape of the left ventricle may be quite variable but is always abnormal. In end-diastole, there is frequently the typical banana-shaped ventricle (ballerina shape), with end-systolic cavity obliteration. Systolic anterior motion of the mitral valve may be seen in the left anterior oblique projection. Mitral regurgitation is seen in between half and all patients in reported series.

The hemodynamic findings in this disease are unique.

Systolic pressure gradients in the right ventricular outflow tract may be present in approximately 15% of patients with hypertrophic cardiomyopathy. The degree of right-sided obstruction is usually less than 30 mm Hg and does not contribute to clinical symptoms.

Considerable controversy surrounded the question of whether left ventricular pressure gradients were real or spurious, caused by catheter entrapment in the left ventricle. The result of numerous investigations clarified the issue. It is now clear that there are patients with hypertrophic cardiomyopathy who have true obstruction caused by apposition of the anterior leaflet of the mitral valve and the hypertrophied interventricular septum. Other patients have generalized cardiac hypertrophy but do not develop obstruction. Further understanding of the natural history of this disease has demonstrated that some patients who have normal or supranormal systolic function early in their disease may develop impaired systolic function late in their disease. The impaired systolic function may be due to myocardial fibrosis and/or myocardial ischemia. The clinical picture in these patients mimics that of patients with a dilated cardiomyopathy. There is left ventricular dilatation, cardiac output is low, and filling pressures are elevated.

Mitral regurgitation is commonly present in obstructive cardiomyopathy and less commonly present in the nonobstructive variety. There is a direct relationship between the severity of the outflow tract gradient and the degree of mitral regurgitation. The gradient is initiated by the anterior mitral leaflet–septal coaptation. This anterior movement leads to faulty midsystolic coaptation of the two mitral leaflets and consequent mitral regurgitation.

Abnormalities in diastolic function are often present in this disease and at times may dominate the hemodynamic picture. The thickened left ventricle has decreased compliance, and myocardial fibrosis leads to an increase in muscle stiffness.

In patients with a subvalvular gradient, there is a marked variability of outflow tract obstruction that can be demonstrated during cardiac catheterization and after physiologic or pharmacologic interventions. Interventions that (1) increase cardiac contractility, (2) decrease preload (smaller diastolic chamber size), or (3) decrease afterload (lower aortic diastolic pressure) will augment the left ventricular–aortic gradient. Conversely, interventions that (1) decrease contractility, (2) increase left ventricular size, or (3) increase aortic diastolic pressures will lessen the gradient. Therefore, digitalis, sympathomimetic amines, nitroglycerin, the Valsalva maneuver, and standing will augment the gradient. Conversely, beta-adrenergic receptor blockade, calcium channel blockers (verapamil), phenylephrine, squatting, and isometric handgrip will lessen obstruction.

Echocardiography has been the most useful laboratory examination in the detection and tracking of patients with this entity. The finding of anterior motion of the anterior mitral leaflet, beginning with the onset of ejection and reaching its peak on contacting the interventricular septum in midsystole, was one of the first echo abnormalities described. The finding of asymmetrical septal hypertrophy became synonymous with hypertrophic cardiomyopathy. The ratio of the thickness of the interventricular septum to the thickness of the posterior free wall is greater than or equal to 1:3. Furthermore, most patients have a septal thickness of 15 mm or more. In addition to its thickness, the interventricular septum has decreased systolic excursion. In patients with systolic obstruction, there is premature closure of the aortic valve. Further, there is a prolonged relaxation time index, the time from end-systolic dimension to mitral valve opening. Transesophageal studies are valuable in defining further abnormalities of the mitral valve and in guiding intraoperative procedures.

The natural history of patients with this entity is quite variable. The rate of progression of the disease may be more rapid in children and young adults. The discovery of a heart murmur usually antedates the onset of symptoms by years. The natural history at any stage may be punctuated by the occurrence of sudden death. The risk factors for sudden death are considered to be a "malignant" family history, young age, syncope, evidence of myocardial ischemia, increased septal thickness, sustained ventricular tachycardia on electrophysiologic testing, and ventricular tachycardia on ambulatory monitoring if associated with altered consciousness. The appearance of atrial fibrillation will often initiate symptoms in a previously asymptomatic individual. Infective endocarditis may occur, especially on the mitral valve. Transmural myocardial infarction or pulmonary or systemic embolization may have a negative impact on the clinical course. Sudden death may be due to atrial or ventricular tachyarrhythmias, bradyarrhythmias, heart block, obstruction to left ventricular outflow, diastolic dysfunction, and myocardial ischemia. This last factor is achieving greater significance in most studies. Early studies placed the annual mortality at 3 to 4%, but with wider use of echocardiography to establish the diagnosis, the annual mortality is probably somewhat lower at 1 to 2%.

Studies have identified a genetic abnormality in this disease. There is strong evidence that mutations in the β major histocompatibility complex (β-MHC) gene are responsible for many of the familial forms of the entity. Multiple families have been shown to be genetically linked to the β-MHC locus on chromosome 14. Affected members of a family have the same mutation and unaffected members do not. This β-MHC mutation is not present in the general population. Hypertrophic cardiomyopathy is an autosomal dominant disease, so that half of the offspring of an affected individual inherit the disease. The other half are normal.

TREATMENT

Treatment of patients with hypertrophic cardiomyopathy is aimed at alleviation of cardiac symptoms and prevention of sudden death. For the past 30 years, the mainstay of therapy has been the use of beta-adrenergic blocking agents. These drugs decrease cardiac contractility, slow the heart rate, and therefore allow for increased ventricular filling and end-diastolic size. Although strictly controlled randomized trials have not been carried out, it is generally acknowledged that beta-blocking drugs are the mainstay of therapy for patients with this disorder. Calcium channel blocking agents, particularly verapamil (Isoptin, Calan), have been used to good advantage in patients with this disorder. Drugs in this class inhibit the inward transmembrane flow of calcium ions in cardiac muscle, in smooth muscle of the coronary and systemic arteries, and in cells of the intracardiac conduction system. There is some enthusiasm for the use of verapamil because of its negative inotropic, chronotropic, and muscular relaxant qualities. In patients with diastolic dysfunction, verapamil may have unique qualities. The negative inotropic

effect of disopyramide (Norpace), a class IA antiarrhythmic agent, has led to its use in patients with systolic obstruction.

Dual-chamber pacing has been extensively studied and used in patients with hypertrophic cardiomyopathy. The exact mechanics by which the obstructive gradient is decreased is unknown but may be related to decreased or paradoxical septal motion. The long-term efficacy of this therapy is still unknown. A cornerstone of its success is complete ventricular capture. Therefore, in patients with normal or prolonged PR intervals, it is more successful. In patients with short PR intervals, the hemodynamic benefits are more difficult to achieve.

For the past 30 years, surgical intervention has offered help to symptomatic patients. It is now generally agreed that the operation of choice is transaortic ventriculomyotomy and myectomy. The operation reduces resting and provoked peak systolic gradients. Relief of obstruction is associated with improvement in mitral regurgitation and in all the echocardiographic indices of obstruction. Although prolongation of life has not been proved, most clinicians believe that in the symptomatic patient, the operation has improved the prognosis.

MITRAL VALVE PROLAPSE

method of
CHARLES F. WOOLEY, M.D.
The Ohio State University College of Medicine
Columbus, Ohio

THE FLOPPY MITRAL VALVE, MITRAL VALVE PROLAPSE, AND MITRAL VALVULAR REGURGITATION

Three major themes in our understanding of mitral valvular disease have been identified during the past 50 years (Figure 1):

1. The floppy mitral valve (FMV) was recognized as a discrete pathologic entity producing mitral valve dysfunction.
2. This form of mitral valve dysfunction resulted in mitral valve prolapse (MVP) into the left atrium.
3. The FMV with MVP resulted in a specific form of mitral valvular regurgitation (MVR).

Each cardiac valvular lesion has its own story, its own lineage. Murmur identification was correlated with anatomic pathology in the 19th century, and diagnostic profiles were developed in patients with valvular heart disease. This reliance on autopsy confirmation was effective in patients with inflammatory valvular lesions of rheumatic or syphilitic origin who died at relatively young ages. The FMV was the exception to the rule, because identifying the FMV as a discrete pathologic entity distinct from rheumatic mitral valvular disease was a gradual process, and the long natural history of this lesion was not apparent when the life span was short. Similarly, although the hypothesis that the mitral valve prolapsed into the left atrium was advanced in the 19th century, the proof

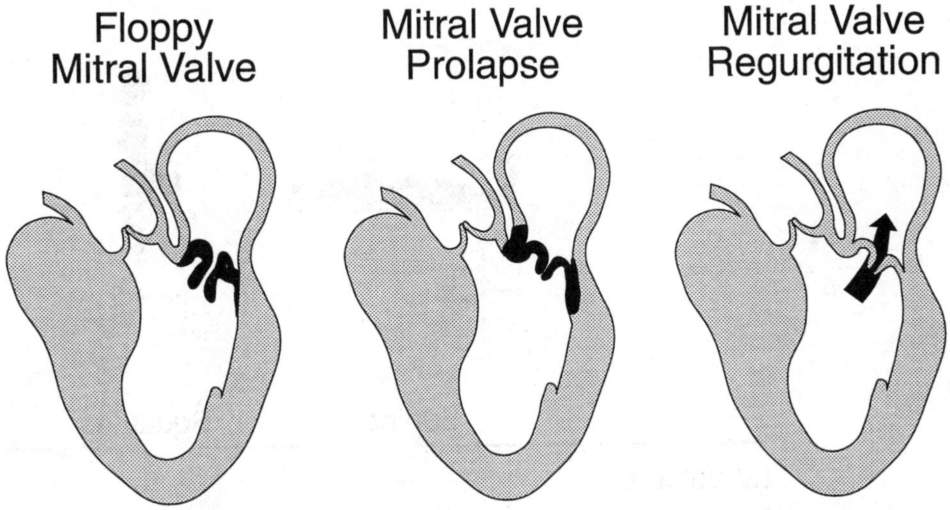

Floppy Mitral Valve

Mitral Valve Prolapse

Mitral Valve Regurgitation

Figure 1. Floppy mitral valve, mitral valve prolapse, mitral valve regurgitation triad. Emphasis is on the central role of the floppy mitral valve.

awaited 20th century surgical observations and imaging techniques.

The impact of newer diagnostic technology during the early 20th century—the clinical use of the x-ray, the electrocardiogram, and the phonocardiogram—was followed at midcentury by clinical use of cardiac catheterization, angiography, and cardiac surgery. The process accelerated with the introduction of increasingly sophisticated imaging techniques.

The Floppy Mitral Valve

Description and definition of the FMV began with the pathologists and morphologists who had the advantage of seeing and handling the FMV at autopsy. They pointed out the discrete nature of FMV in the 1940s and emphasized that these valves were not the result of rheumatic fever. They recognized the clinical correlates, which included the long natural history of the disorder, the susceptibility of the FMV to infectious endocarditis, and the late onset of rapidly progressive congestive heart failure associated with progressive MVR. The idea that there were multiple causes of MVR was slow to develop, however, and although FMV morphology and the clinical implications were well described in the 1940s, the clinicians' preoccupation with rheumatic fever as the predominant cause of valvular heart disease obscured the FMV etiologic and pathodynamic significance for another 2 decades.

The early cardiovascular surgeons were the first to visualize the mitral valve in the beating heart, and they used the term "floppy valve syndrome" in 1965 to describe patients with significant mitral and aortic valvular regurgitation due to myxomatous transformation of the mitral and aortic valves. The mechanism for valvular regurgitation noted at surgery was considered to be "valve prolapse." Visualization of the redundant FMV prolapsing into the left atrium resulted in the introduction of descriptive terminology, including "floppy valve" as a term for myxomatous changes in mitral valve tissue and mitral valve "prolapse" as the mechanism for MVR. Emphasis was placed on the etiologic significance of the connective tissue changes in the FMV rather than on the traditional rheumatic or inflammatory etiology.

The Clinicians

The clinicians' approach to the FMV arose from an auscultatory dilemma. Apical systolic sounds, described dur-

ing the 19th century, were called systolic clicks or systolic gallop sounds. However, their significance was uncertain, and they were considered extracardiac in origin. Whereas the loud, apical holosystolic murmur of advanced MVR that was transmitted to the axilla and the back was well recognized by 19th century auscultators, the fact that apical midsystolic or late systolic murmurs were not transmitted puzzled auscultators for 150 years. As a result, apical systolic clicks and nontransmitted apical midsystolic and late systolic murmurs were long considered to be "extracardiac," "innocent," or "functional." During the 1960s, systematic study of patients with apical midsystolic or late systolic clicks and apical midsystolic and late systolic murmurs showed that these auscultatory phenomena were of intracardiac origin, associated with the FMV prolapsing into the left atrium (MVP). These early auscultatory tenets were established by use of phonocardiographic recordings correlated with left ventricular angiography, i.e., the diagnoses were based on coherence among auscultation, phonocardiography, and angiography—an important distinction in diagnostic specificity and sensitivity.

The systolic clicks correlated with the abrupt termination of the motion of the FMV apparatus into the left atrium; the midsystolic or late systolic murmurs were due to mitral regurgitation occurring during middle or late systole (Figure 2). Thus, clinicians had important physical diagnostic criteria for a clinical approach to patients with FMV producing MVP with or without MVR.

Postural Auscultatory Dynamics and Correlates

Dynamic auscultatory changes occur in patients with FMV-MVP-MVR. The timing and intensity of the systolic click or clicks and the duration and intensity of the apical midsystolic or late systolic murmurs change with changes in body posture (see Figure 2). These changes are often dramatic, reflecting changes in the timing of the MVP and changes in the timing and extent of the MVR. In general, these auscultatory and hemodynamic changes parallel the expected changes in left ventricular volume and left ventricular dynamics with changes in body posture. As a result, dynamic cardiac auscultation expands the role of cardiac physical diagnosis in patients with MVP.

Cardiac Imaging

Prolapse of the FMV into the left atrium, first visualized under direct observation at surgery, was confirmed with

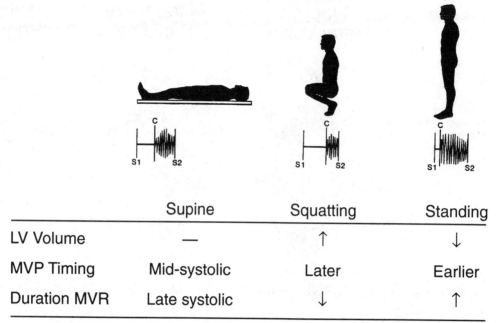

	Supine	Squatting	Standing
LV Volume	—	↑	↓
MVP Timing	Mid-systolic	Later	Earlier
Duration MVR	Late systolic	↓	↑

*c = systolic click; S₁ = first heart sound; S₂ = second heart sound

Figure 2. FMV-MVP: a postural auscultatory complex. *Abbreviation:* LV = left ventricular.

left ventricular cineangiography during the 1960s. These observations were based on small numbers of patients, all of whom had clear-cut auscultatory findings verified by phonocardiography. With time, the angiographic criteria for normal mitral valve morphology and function were established, and a reasonable degree of consensus was reached about FMV-MVP angiographic criteria. These criteria were based on the clinical auscultatory, phonocardiographic, and angiographic correlates.

The advent of ultrasonography provided new imaging modalities for definition of mitral valve function and dysfunction. Major problems in diagnostic specificity and sensitivity were introduced with the early M-mode imaging modalities when the imaging studies were dissociated from the established pathologic criteria for the FMV and from the clinical auscultatory-phonocardiographic-angiographic criteria. A period of diagnostic confusion followed during which the prevalence of "MVP" by use of M-mode criteria was grossly exaggerated.

Currently, Doppler echocardiographic studies using the transthoracic or transesophageal approach and incorporating FMV pathologic criteria with strict FMV-MVP criteria and color-flow imaging with analysis of MVR jet phenomena provide valuable additions to diagnostic precision. Three-dimensional echo imaging of the mitral valve provides even greater definition of individual valve leaflet scallops. FMV patients without MVR at rest may develop MVP with exercise, extending the value of such diagnostic testing. The net effect of informed imaging studies has been a refocusing of attention of the central role of the FMV in the pathogenesis of MVP, enhancing the diagnosis of the FMV-MVP-MVR triad.

Awareness of the evolution in these diagnostic steps is requisite to understanding the inter-relationships within the FMV-MVP-MVR triad, because diagnostic criteria change as technology advances. Clinicians who follow rigid criteria for the clinical, auscultatory, phonocardiographic, angiographic, or Doppler echocardiographic definition of patients with FMV producing MVP with or without MVR

are enhancing diagnostic sensitivity and specificity. As a result, much of the controversy surrounding the FMV-MVP-MVR triad is diminishing.

The Floppy Mitral Valve Characteristics: Clinical Implications

What are the characteristics of the FMV that form the bases for mitral valve dysfunction, specifically MVP and MVR? FMV pathology includes myxomatous degeneration, collagen disruption and dissolution, proteoglycan accumulation, and changes in the extracellular matrix. These intrinsic structural and organizational tissue abnormalities result in a spectrum of pathologic change involving the entire mitral valve complex (Figure 3). As a result, the FMV surface area is greater than normal, and the FMV is thicker than the normal mitral valve.

Abnormal stress-strain relationships of the mitral valve leaflets and support structures provide the setting for valve stretching or redundancy, chordal elongation, and chordal rupture. Redundancy of the enlarged anterior, posterior, or both mitral leaflets, or one or more of the posterior leaflet scallops, or elongated mitral chordae results in MVP. FMV enlargement and redundancy may occur with or without mitral annular enlargement. Valve surface changes that occur as the result of the intrinsic valve pathologic process alter valve surface endothelium and provide the environment for the complications of infectious endocarditis and thromboemboli.

The Clinical Setting

The FMV may occur as an isolated phenomenon; as a familial disorder; associated with congenital cardiac abnormalities; as the cardiac manifestation of a well-defined heritable disorder of connective tissue, such as the Marfan syndrome; as the cardiac manifestation of incompletely defined connective tissue disorders; within the setting that we refer to as a congenital cardiac defect; or in association

Floppy Mitral Valve
Content – Comprehension – Implications

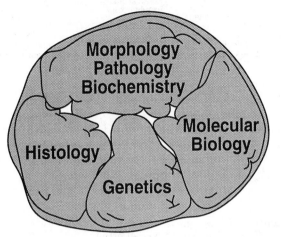

Figure 3. FMV: tissue characteristics reflect basic morphology, pathology, and biochemistry regulated by molecular biologic and genetic factors.

with autonomic nervous system disorders and vasomotor instability. These clinical settings require the clinician to perform careful history taking, pedigree analysis where appropriate, and comprehensive physical examination.

The occurrence of the FMV-MVP in families, frequently as an autosomal dominant trait, is well recognized and has important diagnostic implications. As yet, FMV genetic diagnostic testing has not entered clinical practice, but such approaches open up diagnostic pathways that will be part of the 21st century cardiologist's armamentarium. Separating the click-murmur auscultatory findings of the FMV-MVP-MVR triad from the so-called innocent murmurs in young children and adolescents continues to be a diagnostic challenge and a source of incorrect or missed diagnoses. This becomes apparent in long-term studies when adults with the triad recall being told of an "innocent" murmur in childhood and adolescence.

FMV-MVP-MVR: The Natural History

The FMV-MVP association may lead to progressive mitral valvular dysfunction and progressive MVR in time;

however, it may take seven or eight decades before the individual patient's natural history is defined. FMVs have been documented as one of the leading causes of MVR requiring mitral valve surgery in the United States.

Surface phenomena occur as complications in patients with FMVs. The FMV is particularly vulnerable to infection, is a common site for infectious endocarditis, and has emerged as a universal etiologic factor for infectious endocarditis. Surface thrombi and thromboembolic phenomena are also valve surface complications of FMV.

Progressive MVR, left atrial and left ventricular failure, atrial and ventricular arrhythmias, and FMV chordal rupture occur as late complications in certain patients with FMV. Identification of the FMV-MVP-MVR patients at high risk for these complications is obviously a high-priority issue in the care and management of these patients.

FMV-MVP-MVR: Classification

The classification of cardiovascular disease is in constant evolution, and our textbooks and literature do not always reflect the dynamics of this process. At present, we classify patients with the FMV-MVP-MVR triad in two general categories.

The first category includes those patients whose symptoms, physical findings, laboratory abnormalities, and clinical course are directly related to the mitral valve dysfunction and complications associated with the FMV-MVP-MVR triad (Table 1).

The second category includes those patients with FMV-MVP whose symptoms cannot be explained on the basis of valvular abnormality alone but result from the occurrence of, or coexistence of, various forms of neuroendocrine or autonomic nervous system dysfunction.

The demonstration of MVP with imaging studies without any clinical correlates and without FMV characteristics may occur in individuals with decreased intravascular volumes, small left ventricular chamber size, or hyperdynamic circulatory states. These situations are not considered to fall within the FMV-MVP-MVR triad and are not discussed further.

This classification scheme is clinically useful, with important therapeutic implications.

THERAPEUTIC IMPLICATIONS

For all of the reasons noted in the preceding discussion, the FMV may be dangerous to one's health.

TABLE 1. **Classification of Floppy Mitral Valve, Mitral Valve Prolapse, Mitral Valvular Regurgitation (FMV-MVP-MVR)**

FMV-MVP-MVR	FMV-MVR-MVP Syndrome
Common mitral valve abnormality with a spectrum of structural and functional changes, mild to severe	Patients with MVP
The basis for	Symptom complex: chest pain, palpitations, arrhythmias, fatigue, exercise intolerance, dyspnea, postural phenomena, syncope-presyncope, neuropsychiatric symptoms
Systolic click; midsystolic to late systolic murmur	Neuroendocrine or autonomic dysfunction (high catecholamine levels, catecholamine regulation abnormality, hyper-response to adrenergic stimulation, parasympathetic abnormality, baroreflex modulation abnormality, renin-aldosterone regulation abnormality, decreased intravascular volume, decreased ventricular diastolic volume in the upright posture, atrial natriuretic factor secretion abnormality) may provide explanation for symptoms
Mild or progressive mitral valve dysfunction	
Progressive mitral regurgitation, atrial fibrillation, congestive heart failure	
Infectious endocarditis	
Embolic phenomena	
Characterized by long natural history	
Possibly heritable, or associated with heritable disorders of connective tissue	
Conduction system involvement possibly leading to arrhythmias and conduction defects	MVP—a possible marker for autonomic dysfunction

To understand the long-term significance of the FMV, both the patient and the physician must live a long time—thus the need for long-term periodic follow-up, which will frequently clarify matters that are unclear in an initial evaluation.

The primary concern is the certainty of the diagnosis (Figure 4). Does this individual have an FMV? Does the FMV prolapse into the left atrium? Does the mitral valve leak because of FMV dysfunction? If so, how severe is the leak? Is the individual symptomatic? Are the symptoms related to valvular dysfunction, or are the symptoms more likely related to autonomic dysfunction or neuroendocrine abnormalities? Answering these questions may require assessment of left atrial and left ventricular function. Each question and each answer call forth a different therapeutic response.

From the clinical viewpoint, if the individual has a mitral systolic click or clicks with a midsystolic or late systolic apical murmur, this person should have further evaluation including postural auscultation and a contemporary imaging study. If you are uncertain about the auscultatory findings, do not confuse the issue with an inappropriate diagnosis. Either defer a diagnosis and re-examine the individual on a follow-up basis or refer the person to someone with more experience in this area.

If the individual is shown to have an FMV, and there is auscultatory-imaging coherence, then the primary emphasis is on explanation and prevention (Figure 5). This individual should receive appropriate infectious endocarditis prophylaxis according to the most recent antibiotic usage format established by the American Heart Association.

If the FMV results in MVP with MVR, then the explanation and prevention approach is supplemented by management. Infectious endocarditis prophylaxis is indicated, along with documentation of the extent of the valvular dysfunction. These individuals, whether symptomatic or not, may require more sophisticated imaging studies, exercise testing, or hemodynamic and angiographic assessment.

Floppy Mitral Valve / Mitral Valve Prolapse /
Mitral Valvular Regurgitation (FMV/MVP/MVR):
Diagnosis

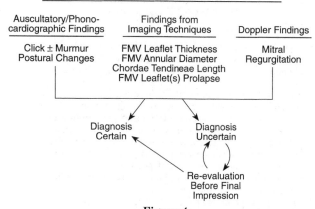

Figure 4.

Floppy Mitral Valve / Mitral Valve Prolapse /
Mitral Valvular Regurgitation (FMV/MVP/MVR):
Management

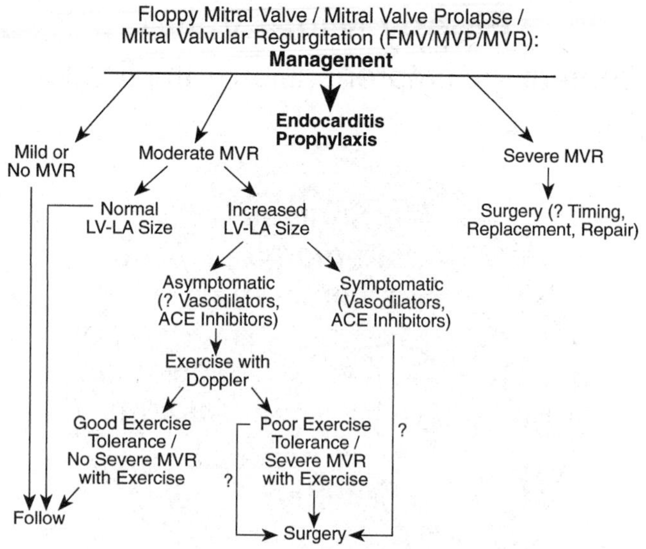

Figure 5. *Abbreviations:* ACE = angiotensin-converting enzyme; LV-LA = left ventricular–left atrial.

Individuals with a history of atrial or ventricular arrhythmias should be evaluated with contemporary electrophysiologic monitoring or testing. Patients with a history of syncope, lightheadedness, or unexplained collapse or who are post resuscitation require extensive postural or tilt-table testing.

As is always the case, evaluation of the individual patient and diagnostic certainty precede rational therapy.

CONGESTIVE HEART FAILURE

method of
GARY S. FRANCIS, M.D.
University of Minnesota Medical School
Minneapolis, Minnesota

Congestive heart failure is a clinical syndrome characterized by cardiac dysfunction, breathlessness, and fatigue. It is one of the most common diagnoses, affecting 1% of the general population in the United States and 10% of the population aged 65 years and older. Virtually any form of heart disease can lead to heart failure. In the advanced stages it is characterized by a large dilated heart, increased left ventricular filling pressures, a reduced cardiac output, and edema. However, there is no physical finding or single laboratory test that is diagnostic of heart failure. The syndrome is being increasingly recognized in patients with normal systolic function who demonstrate features of diastolic dysfunction. It is therefore necessary during the initial evaluation of patients with breathlessness and fatigue to perform echocardiography. This test not only characterizes the size and performance of the heart but can usually distinguish between classic heart failure due to left ventricular systolic dysfunction and heart failure due to diastolic dysfunction. Diastolic dysfunction and systolic dysfunction often coexist. Nevertheless, the demographics, presenting symptoms, prognosis, and therapy may be quite different for patients with heart failure who have normal systolic function compared with those with heart failure and reduced left ventricular function.

HEART FAILURE WITH NORMAL SYSTOLIC FUNCTION (DIASTOLIC DYSFUNCTION OR DIASTOLIC HEART FAILURE)

Typically, patients with pure diastolic dysfunction or diastolic heart failure are older and have associated hypertension. They are more often women. Left ventricular hypertrophy is usually present, and the left ventricular ejection fraction is normal or even increased. Mitral regurgitation is often present and may be responsible for preserving left ventricular systolic function. Other causes of diastolic heart failure include hypertrophic cardiomyopathy and infiltrative cardiomyopathies such as amyloid or sarcoidosis. Patients with diastolic heart failure can usually be identified by echocardiography. In addition to preservation of left ventricular systolic function, left ventricular hypertrophy with impairment of diastolic relaxation and left ventricular filling is generally apparent by echocardiography. Although there are no uniformly agreed on echocardiographic criteria for diastolic heart failure, a constellation of echocardiographic findings including abnormal filling patterns and left ventricular hypertrophy supports the diagnosis of diastolic heart failure.

The prognosis of patients with diastolic heart failure is seemingly better than that of patients who have heart failure due to left ventricular systolic dysfunction. The management of diastolic heart failure is more controversial, however, because there are fewer data available on this topic. When hypertension is present, it should be treated. Angiotensin-converting enzyme (ACE) inhibitors, calcium channel blockers, diuretics, and beta-adrenergic blockers may all find a niche for individual patients with diastolic heart failure. Beta-adrenergic blockers tend to improve diastolic function in part by improving left ventricular filling as a consequence of reduced heart rate. In some cases, e.g., hypertrophic cardiomyopathy or idiopathic hypertrophic subaortic stenosis, beta-adrenergic blockers are the treatment of choice. Sometimes vasodilators and diuretics may adversely affect patients with diastolic heart failure by reducing filling pressure excessively. A careful echocardiographic examination is therefore critical to the proper diagnosis and management of patients with diastolic dysfunction or heart failure.

ASYMPTOMATIC LEFT VENTRICULAR SYSTOLIC DYSFUNCTION

Many patients go through an asymptomatic or a minimally symptomatic period before the development of overt heart failure. For example, patients may sustain acute myocardial infarction and have a long latent period of left ventricular remodeling lasting several years. Ultimately, the full-blown syndrome of heart failure becomes characterized by breathlessness, fatigue, cardiomegaly, and circulatory congestion. However, it is now clear that many patients are asymptomatic or minimally symptomatic during the evolution of left ventricular remodeling. We now know, based on the Studies of Left Ventricular Dysfunction (SOLVD), that such patients may benefit from the use of ACE inhibitors. Data from the large SOLVD trial indicate that treatment with ACE inhibitors delays the onset of heart failure and reduces the need for hospitalization. It is also possible that ACE inhibitor therapy may retard the progressive development of left ventricular dilatation and dysfunction, thus allowing the patient to be free from heart

failure exacerbation. Such patients should be monitored carefully and should be counseled about the nature of the syndrome and what to expect in the way of symptoms, should they occur. The treatment of asymptomatic or minimally symptomatic left ventricular dysfunction with ACE inhibitors is a new concept of emerging importance. In general, the lower the ejection fraction, the more benefit one can expect from ACE inhibitors. A left ventricular ejection fraction of less than 35 to 40% is an indication to institute ACE inhibitor therapy even in the absence of symptoms. Virtually all patients with left ventricular dysfunction should be considered for ACE inhibitor therapy, unless contraindicated because of hyperkalemia or shock.

HEART FAILURE DUE TO IMPAIRED LEFT VENTRICULAR SYSTOLIC FUNCTION

The majority of patients with heart failure develop progressive cardiomegaly, increased left ventricular filling pressures, a low cardiac output, and circulatory congestion. It is important to recognize that a number of factors can precipitate decompensation in patients who have been previously stable (Table 1). These factors include dietary indiscretion, particularly increased salt intake; infectious diseases such as influenza and pneumonia; arrhythmias such as atrial fibrillation; the injudicious use of agents that are known to have negative inotropic effects such as calcium channel blockers; and the imprudent use of sodium-retaining agents such as nonsteroidal anti-inflammatory agents. Acute myocardial ischemia can also cause decompensation in a previously stable patient. All these factors must be considered and corrected (if possible) when evaluating the patient with worsening heart failure.

Despite current efforts to reduce hospitalization rates, heart failure is a potentially lethal disorder that invariably leads to hospitalization for many patients (Table 2). Hospitalization should be considered in patients with tachypnea due to pulmonary congestion or hypoxemia, patients with acute co-morbid conditions such as pneumonia or decompensated lung disease, patients with acute myocardial ischemia, and patients with symptomatic hypotension and/or syncope. In many cases, patients with mild to moderate decompensation can be improved by adjusting the diuretic dosage or adding nonloop diuretics such as metolazone (Zaroxolyn). The most common cause for diuretic resistance is excessive dietary sodium. Hospitalization can frequently be avoided if time is taken to counsel the patient on the importance of dietary discretion. Patients should be advised to weigh themselves daily and in many cases may be able to alter their diuretic dose based on their daily

TABLE 1. **Causes of Acute Decompensation of Heart Failure**

Drug and sodium noncompliance; lack of information given to patient about diet, medications, and so forth
Concurrent infections (e.g., pneumonia, influenza) and other co-morbid conditions
Atrial fibrillation and other arrhythmias
Acute myocardial ischemia and/or infarction
Nonsteroidal anti-inflammatory drugs
Endocrine abnormalities (e.g., uncontrolled diabetes mellitus, hyperthyroidism, hypothyroidism)
Excessive alcohol use
Uncorrected high blood pressure
Obesity
Negative inotropic drugs (e.g., verapamil, nifedipine, diltiazem, beta-adrenergic blockers)

TABLE 2. **Indications for Hospitalization for Heart Failure**

Clinical or electrocardiographic evidence of acute myocardial ischemia
Pulmonary edema or severe respiratory distress
Oxygen saturation below 90% (not due to pulmonary disease)
Severe complicating medical illnesses (e.g., pneumonia)
Anasarca
Symptomatic hypotension or syncope
Heart failure refractory to outpatient therapy
Inadequate social support for safe outpatient management

fluctuations in weight and symptoms. This is analogous to diabetic patients who participate in the management of their insulin therapy.

THERAPY

General Measures

Patients with heart failure tend to retain sodium. With sodium retention comes fluid retention. First and foremost, nearly all patients at some point during the natural course of heart failure require sodium restriction. A 2-gram low-sodium diet is usually sufficient, but sometimes even more stringent sodium restriction is necessary. Fluid restriction is rarely necessary unless the patient is hyponatremic with a serum sodium level of less than 130 mEq per liter. Patients who are overweight should be encouraged to lose weight. Despite symptoms of heart failure, patients should be encouraged to remain active with isotonic exercises but should avoid isometric exercises. For example, any work against gravity such as lifting or working with the arms above the head should be avoided. Patients with heart failure are also at risk of developing hypovolemia due to overvigorous diuretic therapy. They should be warned regarding the signs and symptoms of hypovolemia, and an attempt should be made to determine and maintain an optimal "dry weight."

Angiotensin-Converting Enzyme Inhibitors

Virtually every patient with heart failure should be treated with an ACE inhibitor unless it is contraindicated. These agents are relatively well tolerated, and they are now considered the cornerstone therapy for patients with heart failure (Table 3). In some cases, when there is no obvious salt or water retention, ACE inhibitors can be used without diuretics. However, most patients require a combination of an ACE inhibitor and a diuretic as standard therapy for heart failure.

There has been a tendency for physicians to under-

TABLE 3. **Medications Commonly Used for Heart Failure**

Drug	Initial Dose (mg)	Target Dose (mg)	Recommended Maximal Dose (mg)	Major Adverse Reactions
Thiazide diuretics				
Hydrochlorothiazide (Oretic)	25 qd	As needed	50 qd	Postural hypotension, hypokalemia, hyperglycemia, hyperuricemia, rash
Chlorthalidone (Hygroton)	25 qd	As needed	50 qd	Rare severe reaction with pancreatitis, bone marrow suppression, and anaphylaxis
Loop diuretics				
Furosemide (Lasix)	10–40 qd	As needed	240 bid	Same as thiazide diuretics
Bumetanide (Bumex)	0.5–1.0 qd	As needed	10 qd	
Ethacrynic acid (Edecrin)	50 qd	As needed	200 bid	
Torsemide (Demadex)	20 qd	As needed	40 bid	
Thiazide-related diuretic				
Metolazone (Zaroxolyn)	2.5	As needed	10 qd	Same as thiazide diuretics
Potassium-sparing diuretics				
Spironolactone (Aldactone)	25 qd	As needed	100 bid	Hyperkalemia, especially if administered with ACE inhibitor; rash; gynecomastia (spironolactone only)
Triamterene (Dyrenium)	50 qd	As needed	100 bid	
Amiloride (Midamor)	5 qd	As needed	40 qd	
ACE inhibitors				
Enalapril (Vasotec)	2.5 bid	10 bid	20 bid	Hypotension, hyperkalemia, renal insufficiency, cough, rash, angioedema, neutropenia
Captopril (Capoten)	6.25–12.5 tid	50 tid	100 tid	
Lisinopril (Zestril, Prinivil)	5 qd	20 qd	40 qd	
Quinapril (Accupril)	5 bid	20 bid	20 bid	
Ramipril (Altace)	2.5 qd	10–20 qd	10–20 qd	
Fosinopril (Monopril)	10 qd	10–20 qd	40 qd	
Benazepril (Lotensin)	10 qd	10–20 qd	10–20 bid	
Digoxin	0.125 qd	As needed	As needed	Cardiotoxicity, confusion, nausea, anorexia, visual disturbances
Hydralazine	10–25 tid	75 tid or qid	100 tid or qid	Headache, nausea, dizziness, tachycardia, lupus-like syndrome
Isosorbide dinitrate (Isordil)	10 tid	40 tid	80 tid	Headache, hypotension, flushing
Isosorbide mononitrate (Imdur)	30 qd	60 qd	120 qd	Headache, hypotension, flushing
Isosorbide mononitrate (Ismo)	10 bid	20–40 bid	40 bid	Headache, hypotension, flushing

Abbreviation: ACE = angiotensin-converting enzyme.

dose ACE inhibitors for the treatment of heart failure. The doses recommended in Table 3 have been derived through experience with clinical trials. Although it is possible that smaller doses are safe and effective, there simply are no data to support using such a strategy. On the other hand, it is clear that some patients will not tolerate a full-dose ACE inhibitor because of symptomatic hypotension, azotemia, cough, rash, or other untoward side effects. In every case, however, an attempt should be made to gradually titrate the ACE inhibitor up to a dose that has been demonstrated to be safe and effective. It is expected that some patients will develop small incremental changes in blood urea nitrogen (BUN) and serum creatinine levels. Usually these changes are mild and do not require any adjustment of the ACE inhibitor dose. In some cases, it will be necessary to reduce the diuretic dose if progressive azotemia ensues. Like a small increase in BUN and serum creatinine levels, mild hypotension is an expected consequence of ACE inhibitor therapy. In the absence of symptoms, hypotension per se is not considered a reason to withdraw ACE inhibitors.

Diuretics

Diuretics remain a mainstay of treatment for heart failure, although there are occasional patients who do not demonstrate fluid retention and therefore do not require them. For very mild heart failure, a thiazide diuretic may be satisfactory, but in most cases a loop diuretic such as furosemide, bumetanide, or torsemide is necessary. Patients with advanced heart failure often need twice-daily dosing with a loop diuretic. The dose of diuretic may have to be periodically adjusted based on the patient's perceived needs. Daily weights and careful examination of the neck veins can serve as useful guides for modification of diuretic therapy.

As heart failure worsens, it is often necessary to add a nonloop diuretic such as metolazone 2.5 to 10 mg per day. Metolazone should be taken 0.5 hour before the loop diuretic to allow maximal synergy between the two drugs. Often this results in substantial diuresis, in which case metolazone can be discontinued once the patient's condition stabilizes. Potassium-sparing diuretics such as spironolactone (Aldactone), triamterene (Dyrenium), and amiloride (Midamor) may be useful adjunctive treatment, particularly in patients who are prone to hypokalemia. If potassium-sparing agents are not employed, it is usually necessary to add supplemental potassium chloride, often in a dose of 20 mEq twice a day. I find it useful to keep the serum potassium level near 4.5 mEq per liter, where it seemingly may have some antiarrhythmic property.

Digitalis

Although digitalis has been available for more than 200 years, controversy persists regarding its use in heart failure. Today there is no question that digitalis has important positive inotropic effects and is useful in the treatment of patients with heart failure. However, despite the results of the recent Digitalis Investigators Group (DIG) study (i.e., no overall effect on mortality), there is still some uncertainty about the role of digitalis and the management of patients with heart failure. Digoxin has the potential to reduce death from pump dysfunction and reduce the need for hospitalization (from the DIG study). However, patients with excessive digoxin blood levels are clearly at risk for heightened mortality. At this time it is not certain whether this is a direct consequence of excessive digoxin or is related to the inability to clear digoxin by patients with advanced heart failure who are simply more likely to die because they are nearer the terminal stages of their disease. Despite these uncertainties about the use of digitalis, it is generally recommended as a routine therapy for patients with symptomatic heart failure due to left ventricular dysfunction. Digoxin levels in excess of 2 ng per mL should probably be avoided.

Direct-Acting Vasodilators

There is continued interest in using direct-acting vasodilators as adjunctive therapy for the management of symptomatic heart failure. Long-acting nitrate preparations such as isosorbide dinitrate (Isordil) or isosorbide 5-mononitrate (Ismo) continue to be widely used in the management of patients with advanced heart failure. Occasionally, hydralazine (Apresoline) is also added in small doses of 10 mg every 6 hours. Hydralazine should be gradually titrated to a dose of 50 to 100 mg four times a day if tolerated. Calcium channel blockers continue to be a subject of study as potential therapy for heart failure, but no firm recommendation can be forthcoming at this time for their use as primary therapy for heart failure. Results of one trial suggest that amlodipine (Norvasc) at 10 mg a day may benefit selected patients with nonischemic cardiomyopathy. This hypothesis is being further tested in clinical trials.

Beta-Adrenergic Blockers

Clinical trials have suggested that beta-adrenergic blocking drugs may improve the survival of patients with heart failure. Beta blockers should be started in extremely small doses and gradually titrated up to the maximal dose over several weeks to months. Clinical trials with various beta-adrenergic blockers are currently ongoing, and until the result of these studies are made available, these drugs should be considered investigational. Nevertheless, beta-adrenergic blocking drugs appear quite promising for the treatment of heart failure. They must be used cautiously, as some patients develop worsening heart failure during the initiation of therapy and during the up-titration phase.

Nitroprusside, Dobutamine, and Milrinone

Patients hospitalized with severe heart failure may require treatment with nitroprusside (Nipride), dobutamine (Dobutrex), or milrinone (Primacor) administered intravenously for 48 to 72 hours. These drugs have highly varying pharmacologic profiles and are generally used only in the intensive care unit where patients can be invasively monitored. However, some physicians give positive inotropic agents such as dobutamine and milrinone to outpatients, either as intermittent infusions or as a continuous infusion in low doses. To date, there are no data assessing either the efficacy or the safety of this treatment strategy. In general, dobutamine and milrinone are used in an outpatient setting in those patients who are awaiting heart transplantation and are under the supervision of an experienced heart failure team.

Summary

In summary, the treatment of heart failure has changed radically in the past 10 to 15 years. ACE inhibitors have now emerged as the cornerstone of therapy. Clinical trials continue to explore additional new therapies, and diuretics, digitalis, and vasodilators still have an important role. Routine anticoagulation for heart failure is not recommended, but this is because we have no data to either support or refute such use. Selected patients with atrial fibrillation, mitral stenosis, or a history of previous systemic emboli should be considered for systemic anticoagulation with warfarin (Coumadin). Moreover, there appears to be benefit from warfarin in patients with extremely low left ventricular ejection fractions. On balance, however, there are not sufficient data to make a firm recommendation regarding anticoagulation. Antiarrhythmic therapy is not recommended for patients with ventricular arrhythmias unless the arrhythmias are symptomatic. Such patients usually need referral to an arrhythmia specialist. In my experience, frequent and close follow-up of patients with heart failure, with much assistance from nurses, can reduce the need for hospitalization and can improve the quality of life of these patients.

INFECTIVE ENDOCARDITIS

method of
HENRY F. CHAMBERS, M.D.
*University of California, San Francisco, and
San Francisco General Hospital
San Francisco, California*

PATHOGENESIS AND ETIOLOGY

Infective endocarditis is an infection of the cardiac valves or endocardium. Endocarditis usually occurs on damaged or abnormal valves or endocardial surfaces. Aortic and mitral valves tend to be involved, because they are most often affected by congenital or acquired valvular abnormalities.

TABLE 1. **Predisposing Conditions Associated with High and Moderate Risk for Infective Endocarditis**

More Common	Less Common
Mitral valve prolapse	Rheumatic heart disease
Degenerative valvular disease	Idiopathic hypertrophic subaortic stenosis
Intravenous drug abuse	Pulmonary-to-systemic shunts*
Prosthetic valve*	Coarctation of aorta
Congenital abnormalities† (valvular or septal defect)	Previous endocarditis*
	Complex congenital cyanotic heart disease*

*Indicates lesions at high risk for endocarditis.
†Not atrial septal defect.

Rheumatic valvular heart disease used to be the condition most frequently associated with endocarditis. Now that rheumatic heart disease is relatively uncommon, mitral valve prolapse, congenital and degenerative valvular disease, and valve prosthesis are more important (Table 1).

Endothelial damage resulting from one or more predisposing conditions promotes local deposition of platelets and fibrin to form a sterile vegetation. Bacteria transiently in the blood can attach and adhere to this vegetation. In the absence of cellular host defenses, bacteria multiply and achieve a density of approximately a billion cells per gram of vegetation.

Endocarditis in 90% or more of cases is caused by staphylococci, streptococci, and enterococci (Table 2). This relatively narrow spectrum is probably because these organisms express specific receptors for attachment and adherence to damaged valve surfaces.

Viridans streptococci usually cause subacute endocarditis, characterized by low-grade fevers, generalized weakness, and malaise progressing for a period of weeks. *Staphylococcus aureus* more commonly causes acute endocarditis with high fevers and other signs and symptoms of systemic infection progressing for a few days. Enterococci and nonviridans streptococci may produce either acute or subacute infection.

Intravenous drug abuse strongly predisposes to endocarditis caused by *S. aureus*, which is isolated in 60% or more of cases. If the tricuspid valve is infected, *S. aureus* is almost always the cause.

The etiology of prosthetic valve endocarditis differs from that of native valve endocarditis. Coagulase-negative

TABLE 2. **Approximate Percentages for Organisms Causing Endocarditis**

Organisms	Native Valve	Prosthetic Valve* <2 Months	Prosthetic Valve* >2 Months
Viridans and other streptococci	60	10	30
Staphylococcus aureus	25	20	15
Enterococci	10	5	10
Coagulase-negative staphylococci	<1	30	20
Gram-negative organisms†	5	15	10
Candida species	<1	10	5
Other	<1	10	10

*Time after valve implantation.
†HACEK organisms (*Haemophilus, Actinobacillus, Cardiobacterium, Eikenella,* and *Kingella* species) for native valve endocarditis and other gram-negative aerobic bacilli for prosthetic valve endocarditis.

staphylococci, aerobic gram-negative rods, and fungi, which rarely infect native valves, are relatively frequent in prosthetic valve endocarditis, particularly in cases occurring within the first 2 months of valve implantation.

CLINICAL FEATURES

The clinical presentation of endocarditis depends on the valve that is infected and on the bacterial etiology. In aortic or mitral valve endocarditis, a diastolic or pathologic systolic murmur is heard most of the time. Systemic embolization of vegetation occurs in approximately 20% of cases. Peripheral stigmas of endocarditis (Roth's spots, Janeway's lesions, Osler's nodes, cutaneous and subconjunctival petechiae) occur in 25 to 50% of cases.

Signs and symptoms of pulmonary embolism and pneumonia predominate in tricuspid valve endocarditis. A murmur typical of tricuspid regurgitation will be heard in only 50% of cases. The chest film will usually show infiltrates, pleural effusion, or cavitation. Peripheral stigmas of endocarditis are rarely present unless the patient also has concomitant mitral or aortic valve involvement or a right-to-left shunt.

An acute presentation suggests *S. aureus* infection. Extracardiac foci of infection (e.g., osteomyelitis, septic arthritis, skin or soft tissue infection) are also more common with *S. aureus*.

The presentation may be atypical. A murmur may sound innocent or may even be absent. Fever can be minimal. Symptoms often resemble other nonspecific febrile illnesses. Heart failure, stroke, or aseptic meningitis may be prominent features.

Endocarditis should be included in the differential diagnosis of bacteremia caused by viridans streptococci, enterococci, or *S. aureus*. If a predisposing condition is present or if no source for bacteremia is identified, the patient should be treated presumptively for probable endocarditis.

DIAGNOSIS

Short of histopathologic examination, blood culture is the definitive test for diagnosis of endocarditis. Three blood cultures are sufficient to isolate the causative organism in 95 to 99% of untreated cases. Negative blood cultures will occur in 1 to 5% of cases, usually because of recent antibiotic therapy (Table 3).

TABLE 3. **Causes of Culture-Negative Endocarditis**

Antimicrobial therapy before obtaining cultures
Fastidious organisms
  Anaerobic bacteria
  Nutritionally variant streptococci
  HACEK and other fastidious organisms
  Brucella species
  Bartonella henselae and *Bartonella quintana*
Chlamydiae, rickettsiae, or fungi
  Chlamydia psittaci (psittacosis)
  Coxiella burnetii (Q fever)
  Fungi (e.g., *Aspergillus* species)
Chronic endocarditis
Other disorders
  Marantic endocarditis
  Atrial myxoma
  Libman-Sacks endocarditis
  Incorrect diagnosis

Abbreviation: HACEK = *Haemophilus, Actinobacillus, Cardiobacterium, Eikenella,* and *Kingella* species.

Echocardiography can be useful in managing the patient with suspected endocarditis. The valve or valves that are infected may be determined by echocardiography when physical findings are nonlocalizing. Surface (i.e., M-mode and two-dimensional) echocardiography (30 to 75%) is too insensitive to exclude the diagnosis of endocarditis but can provide evidence to support it. Transesophageal echocardiography is more sensitive (sensitivity up to 90 to 95%) than surface echocardiography in detecting valvular vegetations and is the only reliable noninvasive means for diagnosing complications such as fistula, valve ring abscess, or myocardial abscess and for evaluating prosthetic valves. Echocardiographic measurements of cardiac function and, to a lesser extent, vegetation size may help in assessing need for surgical intervention.

Other laboratory tests are too insensitive and nonspecific to be of much use. An elevated erythrocyte sedimentation rate, mild anemia, mildly elevated white blood cell count, hematuria, and evidence of renal dysfunction are common in endocarditis and numerous other diseases.

APPROACH TO THE PATIENT

The patient suspected of having endocarditis should have at least three separate samples of blood cultured before antibiotics are begun. In acute cases or if risk of death or complication from untreated endocarditis is a significant possibility, empirical therapy should be started as soon as cultures have been obtained. Even in subacute cases, little is gained by delaying therapy. However, if a stable patient has recently been treated with antibiotics, it is reasonable to obtain several additional cultures in an effort to isolate the causative organism and to await results before beginning therapy.

For acute native valve endocarditis, empirical therapy should include antibiotics that are bactericidal against streptococci, staphylococci, and enterococci. The three-drug combination of nafcillin (or oxacillin) plus penicillin plus gentamicin can be used (see Table 4 for doses). Penicillin and gentamicin are needed for enterococci because they are resistant to β-lactamase–stable penicillins and are not killed by penicillin alone. Nafcillin can be omitted for subacute endocarditis in which *S. aureus* is unlikely. For the penicillin-allergic patient, vancomycin will substitute for both nafcillin and penicillin.

Empirical therapy for endocarditis in the intravenous drug abuser must be active against *S. aureus*. For tricuspid valve endocarditis, which is almost always caused by *S. aureus*, nafcillin in combination with gentamicin is adequate, unless there is a high prevalence of methicillin-resistant *S. aureus* in the community, in which case vancomycin should be used.

If the patient has a prosthetic valve, agents should be active against staphylococci, both *S. aureus* and coagulase-negative staphylococci, which may be methicillin resistant, and gram-negative organisms. Vancomycin, gentamicin, and rifampin are recommended as initial therapy.

Optimal management of patients with endocarditis requires a team approach. Consultation with cardiologists, cardiovascular surgeons, and infectious dis-

TABLE 4. **Definitive Therapy for Bacterial Endocarditis***

Organism and Regimen	Comments
Penicillin-Susceptible Viridans Streptococci *(MIC of ≤0.1 μg/mL)*	
Penicillin 2 million units IV q 4 h for 4 wk	Time-honored regimen for native valve endocarditis; also effective for other penicillin-susceptible non-viridans streptococci
Ceftriaxone 2 gm IV once daily for 4 wk	Uncomplicated infection with viridans streptococci, candidate for outpatient therapy; penicillin allergy
Penicillin 2 million units IV q 4 h for 2 wk *plus* Gentamicin 1 mg/kg IV q 8 h for 2 wk	Uncomplicated patient with no renal insufficiency, eighth cranial nerve deficit, prosthetic valve infection, CNS complications, severe heart failure; age <65 y; strain not nutritionally variant; viridans streptococci and *Streptococcus bovis* only
Penicillin 2 million units IV q 4 h for 4 wk *plus* Gentamicin 1 mg/kg IV q 8 h for 4 wk	Nutritionally variant strain or prosthetic valve
Vancomycin 1 gm IV q 12 h for 4 wk	Penicillin allergy
Relatively Penicillin Resistant Streptococci *(0.1 μg/mL < MIC ≤ 0.5 μg/mL)*	
Penicillin 2 million units IV q 4 h for 4 wk *plus* Gentamicin 1 mg/kg IV q 8 h for 2 wk	For MIC of >0.5 μg/mL, gentamicin for 4 wk
Vancomycin 1 gm IV q 12 h for 4 wk	Penicillin allergy; to avoid gentamicin
Enterococci, Penicillin-Resistant Streptococci *(MIC of >0.5 μg/mL)*	
Penicillin† 2 million units IV q 4 h for 4 wk *plus* Gentamicin 1 mg/kg IV q 8 h for 4 wk	Increase duration to 6 wk for symptoms lasting longer than 3 mo in enterococcal endocarditis; 6 wk for prosthetic valve infection
Vancomycin 1 gm IV q 12 h for 4 wk *plus* Gentamicin 1 mg/kg IV q 8 h for 4 wk‡	Penicillin allergy; desensitization to penicillin also an option
Staphylococcus aureus	
Nafcillin 1.5 gm IV q 4 h for 4 wk *plus* Gentamicin 1 mg/kg IV q 8 h for 5–7 d	Methicillin-susceptible strain; omit gentamicin for significant renal insufficiency
Vancomycin 1 gm IV q 12 h for 4 wk	Penicillin allergy or methicillin-resistant strain
Nafcillin 1.5 gm IV q 4 h for 2 wk *plus* Gentamicin 1 mg/kg IV q 8 h for 2 wk	Methicillin-susceptible strain; intravenous drug abuser, no renal insufficiency, tricuspid valve infection only, no extrapulmonary infection
Nafcillin 1.5 gm IV q 4 h for 6 wk *plus* Gentamicin 1 mg/kg IV q 8 h for 2 wk *plus* Rifampin 300 mg PO or IV q 12 h for 6 wk	Prosthetic valve for methicillin-susceptible strain; use vancomycin instead of nafcillin for methicillin-resistant strain
Coagulase-Negative Staphylococci, Prosthetic Valve Infection	
Nafcillin 1.5 gm IV q 4 h for 6 wk *plus* Gentamicin 1 mg/kg IV q 8 h for 2 wk *plus* Rifampin 300 mg orally or IV q 12 h for 6 wk	Only if isolate is susceptible to methicillin; vancomycin regimen recommended in cases of uncertain methicillin susceptibility
Vancomycin 1 gm IV q 12 h for 6 wk *plus* Gentamicin 1 mg/kg IV q 8 h for 2 wk *plus* Rifampin 300 mg PO or IV q 12 h for 6 wk	Methicillin-resistant isolate
HACEK Strains	
Ampicillin 2 gm IV q 4 h for 4 wk	Some authorities' recommendation: add gentamicin 1 mg/kg q 8 h IV
Ceftriaxone 2 gm IV once daily for 4 wk	Penicillin allergy; recommendation based on in vitro susceptibility data

*Dosages are for patients with normal renal function. Lower adjusted doses are needed for renal insufficiency for all drugs except nafcillin, rifampin, and ceftriaxone. Gentamicin doses should be adjusted to achieve a serum concentration of 3 μg per mL 30 min after dosing.

†Ampicillin 12 gm/d may be used instead of penicillin.

‡Need for the addition of an aminoglycoside has not been demonstrated for penicillin-resistant streptococci.

Abbreviations: CNS = central nervous system; MIC = minimal inhibitory concentration; HACEK = *Haemophilus, Actinobacillus, Cardiobacterium, Eikenella,* and *Kingella* species.

ease specialists should be sought for advice concerning proper therapy, need for further diagnostic studies, or indications for surgery.

MEDICAL THERAPY

Endocarditis should be treated with an established regimen whenever possible. Clinical experience with most of the regimens discussed in this article has shown them to be effective. Special tests (e.g., serum bactericidal titers) to document serum bactericidal activity are unnecessary.

Streptococci

For penicillin-susceptible strains of viridans streptococci and *Streptococcus bovis*, the main therapeutic consideration is whether to use penicillin alone or in combination with low-dose aminoglycoside, either streptomycin or gentamicin. For most patients, penicillin plus aminoglycoside for 2 weeks is as effective as penicillin alone for 4 weeks, with relapse rates of 1 to 2% with either regimen. Gentamicin is preferred by many authorities because its nephrotoxicity is reversible and more easily managed than the irreversible vestibular toxicity of streptomycin. Penicillin alone for 2 weeks has a relapse rate as high as 20 to 50% and should not be used.

Two-week penicillin plus aminoglycoside therapy is not appropriate for all patients. To avoid aminoglycoside toxicity, penicillin alone for 4 weeks may be more suitable for patients 65 years of age and older and for those with either pre-existing renal insufficiency or eighth cranial nerve damage. A 2-gram once-daily dose of ceftriaxone for 4 weeks for patients with uncomplicated, penicillin-susceptible viridans group streptococcal endocarditis is also effective. Two-week therapy has not been studied in patients with severe heart failure, brain abscess, stroke, or mycotic aneurysm. Penicillin for 4 weeks, plus aminoglycoside for the first 2 weeks according to some sources, is recommended if these complications are present. Penicillin for 4 weeks plus gentamicin for 2 weeks or vancomycin for 4 weeks is recommended for endocarditis caused by streptococci that are relatively resistant to penicillin (minimal inhibitory concentration [MIC] of >0.1 μg per mL).

Prosthetic valve endocarditis and endocarditis caused by nutritionally variant streptococci should not be treated with 2-week regimens because the relapse rate is unacceptably high. A 4-week penicillin-gentamicin combination regimen is recommended. Infection caused by penicillin-resistant strains of viridans streptococci with an MIC of 1 μg per mL or higher should also be treated with the penicillin-gentamicin combination for 4 weeks.

Vancomycin can be used for penicillin-allergic patients, for patients at risk for significant aminoglycoside toxicity, and for infections caused by penicillin-resistant strains. Two-week vancomycin-aminoglycoside combination regimens have not been studied and cannot be recommended.

Pneumococci and non-viridans streptococci occasionally cause endocarditis. Two-week combination regimens have not been studied for these organisms and should not be used. A 4-week regimen of penicillin will be effective in most cases. Addition of low-dose gentamicin has been recommended for group B streptococcal infections.

Staphylococcus aureus

For methicillin-susceptible strains, nafcillin or oxacillin administered for 4 weeks is usually effective. For penicillin-allergic patients, vancomycin can be used. Vancomycin is the only proven effective drug for methicillin-resistant strains.

The role of combination regimens in *S. aureus* endocarditis remains unclear. Several studies have now shown that nafcillin or oxacillin plus tobramycin or gentamicin given for 2 weeks has a cure rate similar to 4-week courses of single-drug regimens in selected cases of tricuspid valve endocarditis in drug abusers (i.e., susceptible organism, no evidence of mitral or aortic valve involvement, no osteomyelitis or other significant nonpulmonary infection). Whether the aminoglycoside is even necessary is not established, but too few data documenting the efficacy of a penicillinase-resistant penicillin alone for 2 weeks preclude recommending such a regimen at this time.

Enterococci

For enterococcal endocarditis, the relapse rate is unacceptably high if penicillin alone is used. Penicillin plus streptomycin or low-dose gentamicin (higher doses are more toxic but not more effective) for at least 4 weeks is recommended. Patients with symptoms of endocarditis for 3 months or longer or with prosthetic valves may be more likely to relapse, and 6 weeks of therapy may be necessary.

Limited clinical data indicate that vancomycin may be an effective alternative to penicillin for the penicillin-allergic patient. Alternatively, desensitizing the patient to penicillin is also reasonable because of the much greater clinical experience with penicillin.

Enterococci can be resistant to multiple antibiotics. Streptomycin resistance is most common, but gentamicin resistance also occurs. Whichever aminoglycoside is used, susceptibility should be documented. Endocarditis caused by enterococci resistant to both gentamicin (MIC of >500 μg per mL) and streptomycin (MIC of >1000 μg per mL) may be almost impossible to cure medically. It is not clear how these infections should be treated. High-dose ampicillin (e.g., 20 to 30 grams per day administered by continuous infusion) plus surgery has been successful anecdotally.

Almost all strains of enterococci exhibit some level of resistance to penicillin. Synergism between penicillin and an aminoglycoside produces bactericidal activity that is effective for treatment of endocarditis. The penicillin (and ampicillin) MIC at which this synergism is lost and the combination is no longer bactericidal is not well defined. Enterococcal strains with penicillin or ampicillin MICs of 64 μg per mL or higher are encountered with increasing frequency. Efficacy of the traditional penicillin-aminoglycoside regimen for endocarditis caused by such strains and whether vancomycin should be used instead of penicillin are unknown. Patients receiving a penicillin-aminoglycoside combination for treatment of endocarditis caused by a highly penicillin resistant strain should be closely monitored for treatment failure by blood culture during and after therapy to document sterilization of infection.

β-Lactamase–producing penicillin-resistant enterococci and vancomycin-resistant enterococci in particular are a growing problem. A penicillin–β-lactamase inhibitor (e.g., ampicillin-sulbactam [Unasyn]) in combination with gentamicin is active in vitro against β-lactamase–producing penicillin-resistant strains and should also be clinically effective. Alternatively, vancomycin can be used.

Unfortunately, the majority of vancomycin-resistant enterococci are also resistant to penicillin and aminoglycosides and virtually every other drug. Endocarditis caused by vancomycin-resistant strains is probably incurable with conventional agents, and early surgical intervention is probably necessary for cure. An investigational agent, Synercid, which is a combination of two streptogramins, quinupristin and dalfopristin,* is active in vitro against vancomycin-resistant strains of *Enterococcus faecium*, but not *Enterococcus faecalis*. It is available on a compassionate use basis for treatment of infection caused by vancomycin-resistant *E. faecium*. Efficacy of Synercid for treatment of endocarditis is unknown, but because there are no other alternatives, use of Synercid should be considered.

Gram-Negative Organisms

Fastidious gram-negative coccobacilli, the so-called HACEK group (*Haemophilus, Actinobacillus, Cardiobacterium, Eikenella*, and *Kingella* species), occasionally cause native valve endocarditis. In vitro, they are susceptible to ampicillin, cephalosporins, aminoglycosides, and penicillin-aminoglycoside combinations. Ampicillin plus gentamicin for 4 weeks is sometimes recommended, but ampicillin alone is also effective. An ampicillin regimen should not be used if the strain produces β-lactamase. Ceftriaxone is highly active in vitro and is a suitable alternative for both β-lactamase–negative and β-lactamase–positive strains.

Gonococcal and nongonococcal strains of *Neisseria* are rare causes of endocarditis. Penicillin 20 million units a day in six divided doses for 4 weeks will be effective for non–β-lactamase–producing strains. Data on treatment of endocarditis caused by β-lactamase–producing strains of gonococci are not available, but on the basis of in vitro susceptibility, ceftri-

---

*Not yet approved for use in the United States.

axone 2 grams intravenously once a day should be effective.

Gram-negative aerobes are an uncommon cause of native valve endocarditis. Endocarditis due to these organisms is difficult to cure medically, and early surgery may be indicated. With few clinical data as a guide, the choice of antimicrobial agents is usually based on results of susceptibility tests. Third-generation cephalosporins and aminoglycosides are among the most active drugs in vitro, and cephalosporin-aminoglycoside combinations are generally used.

Prosthetic Valve Endocarditis

Coagulase-negative staphylococci, a common cause of prosthetic valve endocarditis, are routinely resistant to methicillin. β-Lactam antibiotics should not be used unless the isolate has been proved to be susceptible. Susceptibility testing may not always be reliable, and if there is doubt, vancomycin should be used. A combination of vancomycin and rifampin for 6 weeks and gentamicin for the first 2 weeks is the regimen of choice.

Culture-Negative Endocarditis

In approximately 5% of cases of endocarditis, no organism will be isolated from blood cultures. Failure to culture an organism from blood should lead to consideration of other diseases, but if a patient has otherwise compatible physical and laboratory findings, a diagnosis of endocarditis can be made.

The differential diagnosis of culture-negative endocarditis is extensive (see Table 3). If endocarditis seems likely and blood cultures have not grown an organism after 3 days, cultures should be supplemented with thiol (if this has not been done) and incubated for 3 weeks before they are determined to be negative. Fastidious and slow-growing organisms may require prolonged incubation before growth can be detected.

A careful history and a more extensive evaluation for unusual causes of culture-negative endocarditis should be initiated. In the absence of a specific diagnosis, empirical therapy is directed against both enterococci and viridans streptococci. A 4-week course of penicillin (or vancomycin for the penicillin-allergic patient) plus gentamicin would be given. If *S. aureus* is a possibility (e.g., right-sided endocarditis, acute clinical course, history of intravenous drug abuse, lack of clinical response to penicillin plus aminoglycoside), then nafcillin should be added or vancomycin substituted for penicillin. For culture-negative prosthetic valve endocarditis, a three-drug regimen of vancomycin, gentamicin, and rifampin should be given for coverage of coagulase-negative staphylococci.

SURGICAL MANAGEMENT

Death from infective endocarditis is usually due to heart failure. Heart failure that is not readily corrected by medical therapy is unlikely to be controlled except by surgical intervention.

Delaying surgery with the intention of sterilizing the valve site before prosthetic valve implantation is a flawed strategy. Chances are that myocardial function will continue to deteriorate and that the patient either will die before the operation or will be unable to survive it. The risk of recurrence of endocarditis after valve implantation during active endocarditis is approximately 10%, much less than the risk of death from uncontrolled heart failure.

Complications of endocarditis associated with significant risk of serious heart failure or persistent infection unresponsive to medical therapy are also indications for early surgical intervention. These include sinus of Valsalva aneurysm, perivalvular abscess, atrioventricular block, and prosthetic valve instability or dehiscence.

Other indications for surgery are more controversial. Endocarditis caused by gram-negative aerobes, fungi, and multidrug-resistant organisms such as aminoglycoside- or vancomycin-resistant enterococci can be difficult to cure with medical therapy alone. Surgical removal of the infected valve should be strongly considered in these cases. Occasionally, antibiotics will not control infection with other organisms (e.g., *S. aureus*), and surgery may be necessary.

Other predictors of increased morbidity and mortality have been proposed as surgical indications. These are aortic valve infection, nonstreptococcal etiology, presence of large vegetations on an echocardiogram, and prosthetic valve infection. Unless heart failure, persistent infection unresponsive to antibiotics, or recurrent embolization is also present, these other indications on their own probably do not warrant surgical intervention.

Surgery solely to prevent embolization of vegetations is probably inadvisable. Prosthetic valve implantation substitutes one risk for others. Risk of embolism must be weighed against the risks of dying from surgery, of endocarditis occurring on the prosthetic valve, of systemic anticoagulation, and of the need for reoperation should the prosthesis fail or if a bioprosthesis is used.

Some patients do poorly with valve implantation and may not be suitable candidates for valve replacement. Relative contraindications to valve replacement are active intravenous drug abuse, because reinfection is likely; bleeding aneurysm or massive stroke, because of the risk of bleeding with systemic anticoagulation during and after surgery; and multiple prior implantations, because of technical limitations of sewing yet another valve into tissue already weakened from prior surgeries.

In some cases, a procedure other than valve replacement can be successful. Excision of the tricuspid valve without replacement to eradicate persistent infection may be an option if the patient does not have right-sided heart failure. Vegetectomy, with or without valvuloplasty, may be feasible. These procedures should be undertaken, however, only with recognition that prosthetic valve replacement may be necessary depending on findings at operation.

Antibiotic therapy after valve replacement for active endocarditis has not been well studied. If a full course of therapy has been administered and there is no evidence of ongoing infection, then additional antimicrobial therapy after surgery is probably unnecessary. If the patient has received less than a week of antibiotics before surgery, then a 4- to 6-week course of antibiotics after operation would be advisable. If the patient has received 2 weeks or more of therapy, culture of the operative site is sterile, and the Gram stain shows no organisms, then therapy for 2 weeks after valve implantation is probably sufficient. If either the culture or the Gram stain is positive, a full 4- to 6-week course of therapy after valve replacement would be recommended.

COMPLICATIONS OF ENDOCARDITIS

Stroke, systemic embolism, mycotic aneurysm, myocardial infarction, congestive heart failure, renal insufficiency, metastatic infection, and persistent or recurrent fever are relatively common complications of endocarditis. Many complications can be managed as they would be for patients without endocarditis. Those for which management may differ are discussed here.

Embolization to kidneys and spleen is common. Although usually clinically silent, this can cause abdominal pain. Other than antibiotics, no specific therapy is required unless there is obstruction causing vascular insufficiency, which is an indication for surgery. Management of embolization to other peripheral arteries is similar.

Embolic strokes will occur in approximately 25% of cases of endocarditis. Like other embolic events, strokes tend to occur early in the course of infection but have also been reported weeks to months after successful antimicrobial therapy. Appropriate studies (e.g., computed tomography, magnetic resonance imaging, arteriography, or lumbar puncture) should be obtained to exclude a brain abscess or mycotic aneurysm. Valve surgery may be indicated for patients with two or more embolic events. Because of the risk of hemorrhagic stroke, anticoagulants are absolutely contraindicated for prevention or treatment of embolic stroke.

Brain abscess is an uncommon complication of endocarditis. These abscesses tend to be multiple and small and usually respond to antibiotics. Large abscesses producing a mass effect should be surgically drained.

Surgical resection is indicated for peripheral mycotic aneurysms. Aneurysms of cerebral vessels that have bled or are causing a mass effect should be resected if possible. Relative contraindications to resection of a cerebral aneurysm are if the patient is moribund, if the aneurysm is asymptomatic, or if the aneurysm cannot be resected without producing major neurologic deficit.

Persistent or recurrent fever during treatment of

TABLE 5. **Regimens for Prophylaxis of Endocarditis**

Amoxicillin 2 gm PO 1 h before procedure	Well-tolerated oral regimen for most patients undergoing dental, oral, or respiratory tract procedures or moderate-risk patients undergoing GI or GU procedures
Ampicillin 2 gm IV 1 h before procedure	For patients unable to take oral medications and undergoing dental, oral, or respiratory tract procedures or moderate-risk patients undergoing GI or GU procedures
Clindamycin 600 mg PO 1 h before procedure	Oral regimen for most penicillin-allergic patients undergoing dental, oral, or respiratory tract procedures May also be given IV for patients unable to take oral medications
Vancomycin 1 gm IV 1 h before procedure	Parenteral regimen for penicillin-allergic moderate-risk patients undergoing GI or GU procedures
Ampicillin 2 gm IV or IM *plus* Gentamicin 1.5 mg/kg IV or IM 0.5 h before procedure Repeat ampicillin 1 gm IV or amoxicillin 1 gm PO in 6 h	Parenteral regimen for high-risk patients undergoing GI or GU procedures
Vancomycin 1 gm IV *plus* Gentamicin 1.5 mg/kg IV or IM 1 h before procedure	Parenteral regimen for penicillin-allergic high-risk patients undergoing GI or GU procedures

Abbreviations: GI = gastrointestinal; GU = genitourinary.

endocarditis occurs in up to half of patients. Clinical signs and symptoms pointing to a potential extracardiac source should be pursued with appropriate imaging studies. Blood cultures should be obtained to rule out persistent bacteremia. Perivalvular abscess, myocardial abscess, and persistently infected vegetation are potential cardiac sources that would be indications for surgery. If no source of fever is found, which is often the case, and the patient is otherwise responding to therapy, then no specific intervention other than to complete the prescribed course of treatment is needed.

PREVENTION OF ENDOCARDITIS

It is the standard of practice to administer antibiotics to prevent endocarditis in patients with predisposing abnormalities who are undergoing procedures that can cause bacteremia. No clinical data prove that this practice is effective except for patients with prosthetic valves. Nevertheless, antimicrobial prophylaxis is recommended in a variety of circumstances.

Dental, oral, respiratory tract, and esophageal procedures and genitourinary and gastrointestinal tract procedures that are likely to cause bacteremia are the two general categories for which prophylaxis is recommended. Surgical procedures involving contaminated or infected tissues also warrant prophylaxis. Antibiotics are selected for activity against the organisms that commonly cause endocarditis: viridans streptococci, enterococci, and staphylococci.

An oral or a parenteral regimen may be used. Parenteral regimens are preferable for the highest risk patients (e.g., prosthetic valve, previous episode of endocarditis, complex cyanotic congenital heart disease, systemic-to-pulmonary shunts). Oral and single-agent regimens are appropriate for patients with moderate risk. The American Heart Association and the *Medical Letter* regularly publish recommendations for prophylaxis. These resources should be consulted for details, particularly concerning the specific procedures for which prophylaxis is indicated. Typical regimens are shown in Table 5.

Prophylaxis before dental procedures has received the most attention. Poor dental hygiene probably poses a more constant and greater risk than does the occasional dental procedure. Therefore, patients who have conditions predisposing to endocarditis should have regular examinations to detect and treat early dental or gingival disease that may be a source of bacteremia.

HYPERTENSION

method of
NORMAN M. KAPLAN, M.D.
The University of Texas Southwestern Medical Center at Dallas
Dallas, Texas

Most people develop hypertension before they die, and we now know for certain that reduction of their elevated blood pressure (BP) will protect against the cardiovascular complications of the disease. Therefore, the treatment of hypertension, already the most common cause of visits to physicians in the United States, will assume an even greater role in clinical practice. There are three major reasons for this greater role for the treatment of hypertension:

Less than 25% of U.S. hypertensive persons now have their condition under adequate control. In a survey of a representative sample of the U.S. adult population, of those identified as hypertensive, only 67% had been aware of the diagnosis, only 50% were being treated, and only 21% had a BP of below 140/90 mm Hg.

There has been a large increase in the numbers of elderly persons, the most rapidly expanding part of the population, more than half of whom have hypertension. In most the high pressure is predominantly or purely systolic, but such elevations are known to lead quickly to cardiovascular trouble, and the results of large controlled trials published in the early 1990s have proved the protective value of antihypertensive treatment in elderly hypertensive patients.

As attempts are made to reduce the high costs of treating end-stage diseases with ever more expensive but usually only transiently effective procedures, the attraction of low-cost and more permanently effective preventive care will surely grow. For those who have hypertension, preventive care will usually involve drug therapy. Such preventive care cannot now or likely never will involve the use of drug therapy for the larger population at risk for developing hypertension. Fortunately, the evidence for the ability of lifestyle changes to prevent the usual rise in pressure with age is becoming strong enough to make these worthwhile for the entire population. This chapter covers only the treatment of those who have hypertension, but the same lifestyle modifications used for them are appropriate for those at risk of developing the condition.

For those who develop hypertension, treatment is usually effective in lowering the BP, even though long-term control of the condition remains difficult because of the inherent problem of keeping asymptomatic people on a lifelong and often expensive regimen that does not provide immediate benefits. Only a small number, perhaps 5%, of patients are resistant to appropriate therapy, and almost all of them can eventually overcome the cause of their resistance.

I describe 10 guidelines that will make it possible to effectively treat almost all hypertensive patients (Table 1). Treatment must start with a careful ascertainment of the usual level of BP as part of a much broader assessment of overall cardiovascular risk. Only then can an appropriate therapeutic regimen be formulated and applied. That regimen almost always should start with lifestyle modifications. If they are not sufficient, active antihypertensive drug therapy is needed, with the ability now as never before to control hypertension with once-a-day, easy to take medications that should not impose bothersome side effects.

ADEQUATE MEASUREMENT OF BLOOD PRESSURE

Obviously, the decision to treat must be based, at least in part if not entirely, on the BP. Unfortunately that is often the weakest link in the process, with too few BPs measured, all of them in the physician's office. This leads to overdiagnosis of hypertension, because initial readings are usually higher, with as many as 80% of readings taken in the office being higher than those taken out of the office—the white coat effect. Fully 20 to 40% of patients

TABLE 1. Ten Guidelines for Managing Hypertension

1. Take enough out-of-office readings to ensure diagnosis.
2. Assess overall cardiovascular risk to determine need for therapy.
3. Have the patient start with and continue lifestyle modifications.
4. Choose the initial drug that best fits each patient's needs.
5. Start with a low dose and titrate slowly—particularly with elderly patients.
6. Use a low dose of a long-acting diuretic as the second drug if not the first.
7. Always use 24-h lasting formulations to cover AM surge.
8. Monitor therapy by home-recorded blood pressures.
9. Aim for a goal of 130–140/80–85 mm Hg, except in patients who need even lower blood pressure.
10. Ascertain and overcome causes for resistance to therapy.

with repeatedly high office readings are normotensive out of the office, i.e., they have white coat hypertension.

White coat hypertensive patients have a higher likelihood of developing persistent hypertension, but they should not now be labeled as hypertensive or begun on drug therapy. They should be strongly advised to use appropriate lifestyle modifications and to remain under surveillance.

To identify those with white coat hypertension, readings out of the office are needed. Automatically recorded readings with an ambulatory monitor can accurately ascertain the BP status in 1 day, but the cost of the procedure continues to preclude its widespread use. Readily available, inexpensive ($30 to $40), semiautomatic devices do almost as well but require 3 to 4 weeks of readings, taken at various times of day during usual activities, including stressful ones. The average of such readings can be fairly easily ascertained, and, if it is above 140/90 mm Hg, the diagnosis is established. Some patients have only occasional high readings: if more than one third are above 140/90 mm Hg, the diagnosis is probable.

If only office readings are used, careful attention must be given to technique (Table 2). These guidelines also apply to home readings, and the patient's readings should be checked against an office manometer.

ASSESSMENT OF OVERALL RISK

For the past 50 years, since it became possible to lower BP, the decision to begin treatment has almost always been based simply on the level of BP, usually measured by a few readings taken in the physician's office. The pressure indicating a need for therapy has gradually fallen as evidence for the value of lowering progressively lower degrees of hypertension has been reported from clinical trials and as easier to take and more effective therapies have become available. In the 1940s and 1950s, only near-malignant hypertension could be treated with the potent but disruptive agents then available. In the late 1950s, diuretics and reserpine were marketed and it became practical to treat less severe hypertension. As beta blockers and then alpha blockers, calcium channel blockers (CCBs), and angiotensin-converting enzyme (ACE) inhibitors became available in the 1970s and 1980s, even milder degrees of hypertension became amenable to active therapy.

However, a dark side to the increasing treatment of milder degrees of hypertension has become obvious as drug therapy has been given in placebo-controlled trials to patients with milder degrees of hypertension. In such patients with less inherent risk for developing cardiovascular complications even if their hypertension were left untreated, less and less protection has been provided, so that the incidence of coronary disease may actually have been *increased* in those low-risk patients given drug therapy. Therefore, the need to consider more than just the level of BP has become obvious in the desire to provide drug therapy to only those who will derive benefit rather than harm.

Such a targeted approach, based on overall risk status, goes against an epidemiologic approach based on the known eventual increase in risk with every increment of BP, starting at levels as low as 110/70 compared with 120/80 mm Hg. On purely epidemiologic grounds, pressures as low as 130/85 mm Hg ought to be lowered. This argument, however, fails to account for the obvious side effects and biochemical mischief induced by even the mildest antihypertensive drugs, which make their wholesale application unwise and likely to increase risks.

Current therapy, in particular the use of much lower

TABLE 2. **Guidelines for Measurement of Blood Pressure**

Patient-Related Conditions
Posture
Initially, particularly in patients older than 65 y, diabetic, or receiving antihypertensive therapy, check for postural changes by taking readings after 5 min supine, then immediately and 2 min after they stand.
For routine follow-up, sitting pressure measurements are recommended. The patient should sit quietly with the back supported for 5 min and the arm supported at the level of the heart.
Circumstances
No caffeine during the hour preceding the reading.
No smoking during the 15 min preceding the reading.
No exogenous adrenergic stimulants (e.g., phenylephrine in nasal decongestants or eye drops for pupillary dilatation).
A quiet, warm setting.
Home readings taken under varied circumstances and 24-h ambulatory recordings may be preferable and more accurate in predicting subsequent cardiovascular disease.
Equipment
Cuff size
Bladder should encircle and cover two thirds of the length of the arm; if it does not, place the bladder over the brachial artery. If the bladder is too small, high readings may result.
Manometer
Aneroid gauges should be calibrated every 6 mo against a mercury manometer.
For infants, use ultrasound equipment (e.g., Doppler method).
Technique
Number of readings
On each occasion, take at least two readings, separated by as much time as is practical. If readings vary by more than 5 mm Hg, take additional readings until two are close.
For diagnosis, obtain three sets of readings at least 1 wk apart.
Initially, take pressure in both arms; if pressures differ, use the arm with the higher pressure.
If the arm pressure is elevated, take pressure in one leg, particularly in patients younger than 30.
Performance
Inflate the bladder quickly to a pressure 20 mm Hg above the systolic pressure, as recognized by disappearance of the radial pulse.
Deflate the bladder 3 mm Hg every second.
Record the Korotkoff phase V (disappearance), except in children, in whom use of phase IV (muffling) may be preferable.
If the Korotkoff sounds are weak, have the patient raise the arm and open and close the hand 5–10 times; then inflate the bladder quickly.
Recordings
Note the pressure, patient's position, which arm, cuff size, e.g., 140/90, seated, right arm, large adult cuff.

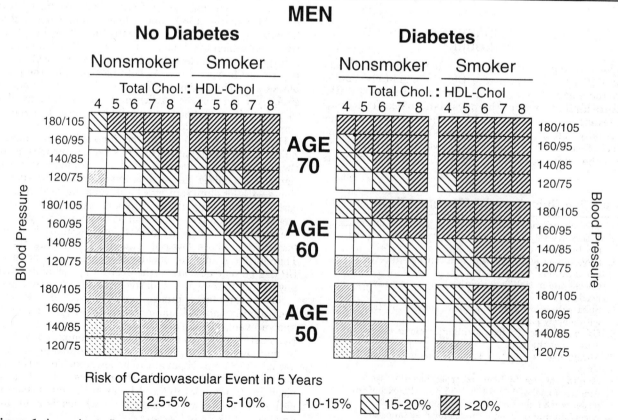

Figure 1. Approximate 5-year risk of a major cardiovascular event in men based on blood pressure level, age, and risk factor status as to diabetes, smoking and ratio of total cholesterol to high-density lipoprotein (HDL) cholesterol. *Abbreviation:* Chol = cholesterol. (From New Zealand Core Services Committee, Ministry of Health, Wellington, NZ.)

TABLE 3. **Overall Guide to Work-up for Secondary Causes of Hypertension**

| | Diagnostic Procedure | |
Diagnosis	*Initial*	*Additional*
Chronic renal disease	Urinalysis, serum, creatinine level, renal sonography	Isotopic renogram, renal biopsy
Renovascular disease	Isotopic renogram and plasma renin level before and 1 h after captopril	Aortogram
Coarctation	Blood pressure in legs	Aortogram
Primary aldosteronism	Levels of plasma potassium, plasma renin and aldosterone (ratio)	Levels of urinary potassium, plasma or urinary aldosterone after saline load; adrenal computed tomography (CT) and scintiscans
Cushing's syndrome	AM plasma cortisol level after 1 mg of dexamethasone at bedtime	Urinary cortisol level after variable doses of dexamethasone; adrenal CT and scintiscans
Pheochromocytoma	Spot urine test for metanephrine	Levels of urinary catechols; levels of plasma catechols, basal and after 0.3 mg of clonidine; adrenal CT and scintiscans

doses of diuretics than were used in the trials from 1965 to 1990, will likely be less hazardous. In the Framingham cohort, progressively greater protection against cardiovascular mortality has been observed in each decade from 1950 to 1990 among those given antihypertensive therapy compared with those not given such therapy.

Nonetheless, until benefit can be shown for those with minimally elevated pressures and low overall cardiovascular risk, a targeted approach seems correct. Perhaps the best constructed such approach has been provided by the New Zealand Core Services Committee. They have used the Framingham risk data to construct a nomogram of overall absolute risk during a 5-year interval with various levels of BP from 120/75 to 180/105 mm Hg in either men or women at ages from 30 up to 70 years, based on the presence or absence of diabetes, cigarette smoking, and an abnormal ratio of total cholesterol to high-density lipoprotein cholesterol (Figure 1).

On the basis of data from clinical trials of the therapy of hypertension, they proposed active drug therapy for only those whose overall absolute risk status is predictive of a 10% or greater likelihood of a major cardiovascular event in the next 5 years. Valid arguments have been made against the implications of withholding needed therapy from younger patients who would eventually derive protection and providing unneeded therapy to many older patients who likely would not be helped by treatment. Although the New Zealand Committee's recommendations may not be perfect, they are certainly better than using BP levels alone in making the decision to start active drug therapy. In clinical practice, such a targeted approach would translate into starting active drug therapy for many elderly patients who are at relatively great immediate risk for hypertension-related cardiovascular catastrophes, even if they have few other risk factors and not extremely high levels of BP. As seen in Figure 1, some younger patients with higher pressures but few other risk factors might not be given drug therapy. On the other hand, a younger diabetic patient with an abnormal lipid profile would be a candidate for antihypertensive therapy even with minimal hypertension.

RULING OUT SECONDARY CAUSES

As part of the initial history, physical examination, and laboratory work used in the ascertainment of overall risk, hints of the presence of various secondary forms of hypertension are also obtained. If they are present, additional

evaluation is needed (Table 3). For most, no more laboratory work than hematocrit, urinalysis, an electrocardiogram, and measurements of levels of blood electrolytes, glucose, creatinine, and total and high-density lipoprotein cholesterol are needed.

LIFESTYLE MODIFICATIONS

All hypertensive patients should be given adequate instructions and constant encouragement to make appropriate modifications in their lifestyle (Table 4). Whether these modifications, in themselves, protect against cardiovascular damage has not been proved in controlled trials (except for smoking cessation), but they clearly reduce the degree of overall risk and lower the BP in enough patients to warrant their enthusiastic use.

Smoking Cessation

Cigarettes kill more often through cardiovascular causes than through cancer. The contribution of the pressor effect of smoking to the increase in heart attacks and strokes has not been appreciated for a simple reason: no one is allowed to smoke in places where BPs are measured, so the relatively short pressor effect of smoking is unrecognized (Figure 2). The time shown in Figure 2 is 15 minutes; by 30 minutes the pressor effect of that cigarette is over. However, a persistent rise in pressure occurs throughout the day when smokers continue to smoke their average of 20 cigarettes or more.

TABLE 4. **Lifestyle Modifications for Treatment of Hypertension**

Stop smoking
Lose weight, particularly for upper body obesity
Reduce sodium intake to 110 mmol/d (2.4 gm of sodium or 6 gm of NaCl)
Moderate alcohol intake to no more than two usual portions per day
Exercise (isotonic) regularly
Increase potassium intake from fresh fruits and vegetables
Maintain adequate calcium and magnesium intake

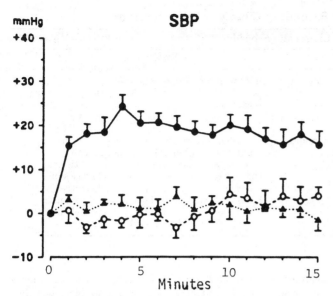

Figure 2. The effect on systolic blood pressure (SBP) of smoking a cigarette for the first 2 minutes (●) compared with no activity (○) or sham smoking (▲) in 10 normotensive smokers. (From Groppelli A, Giorgi DM, Omboni S, et al: Persistent blood pressure increase induced by heavy smoking. J Hypertens *10*:495–499, 1992. © Rapid Science Publishers Ltd.)

Therefore, smokers should be told of this effect and asked to observe the rise in pressure while they smoke, hopefully as an additional motivation to quit. If they will not quit smoking, their "smoking BP" should be used as the level for diagnosis and treatment, not the artificially lower level taken in the absence of smoking for 30 minutes or longer during the office visit.

Weight Reduction

Even small amounts of excess weight may raise BP, and the loss of even a few pounds may lower BP. Caution is needed with diet pills, although no systemic pressor effect has been noted with dexfenfluramine (Redux).

Moderate Sodium Restriction

Cutting out highly salted foods (easier to do today than in the past because all processed foods are labeled) and leaving out salt in cooking and at the table usually lower sodium intake enough to accomplish the major benefits of moderate sodium restriction: lowering of the BP by itself, enhancing the efficacy of other agents, reducing potassium wastage from diuretics, and reducing renal calcium excretion. No harm has ever been shown from a daily sodium intake at the recommended level of 2400 mg (6000 mg of sodium chloride), not so low as to set off the renin-angiotensin mechanism but low enough to return the daily intake closer to the natural level ingested before food processing began a few hundred years ago.

Regular Aerobic Exercise

Exercise lowers BP by itself and aids in weight reduction, which further lowers BP. If starting from a sedentary status, patients should be told to gradually increase to a strenuous level maintained for at least 30 minutes three times a week to achieve cardiovascular fitness. The more the better for weight loss.

Moderation of Alcohol Intake

Too much alcohol—more than three usual portions a day of whiskey, wine, or beer—raises BP and leads to all sorts of alcohol-induced trouble. Just enough alcohol—up to one drink a day for women, up to two a day for men—will not raise BP or cause alcohol-related disease but will protect against coronary disease. Therefore, those who drink in moderation should be encouraged to do so; those who drink too much should be strongly advised to reduce or eliminate their intake. Men younger than 30 years and women with a strong family history of breast cancer are best advised not to drink at all, the former because young men often are binge-drinkers, the latter because in epidemiologic surveys even small amounts of alcohol have been associated with a small increase in breast cancer.

Maintenance of Adequate Intakes of Potassium, Calcium, and Magnesium

Supplemental potassium will likely lower BP, but it is too expensive. Fresh foods, high in potassium, low in sodium, should be substituted for processed foods, mostly low in potassium, high in sodium.

Supplemental calcium does not lower BP, but those who consume too little calcium may develop more hypertension and osteoporosis.

Supplemental magnesium probably does not lower BP, but magnesium deficiency may be deleterious in multiple ways.

INITIAL CHOICE OF DRUG

Only a few of the many choices available (Table 5) are *not* recommended for initial therapy. Those include the centrally acting alpha₂ agonists, which have too many intrinsic side effects, and direct vasodilators, which set off too many reactive side effects including tachycardia and volume retention.

Individualized Therapy

Moderate doses of any of the drugs approved for the treatment of hypertension, listed in Table 5, provide about a 10% reduction in BP for about 60% of the overall hypertensive population. This equal potency is guaranteed by the Food and Drug Administration's approval process and the pharmaceutical marketers' need to provide drugs that demonstrate a clear effect, so physicians will use them,

TABLE 5. **Oral Antihypertensive Drugs**

Drug	Trade Name	Dose Range (mg/d)	Frequency (per Day)	Side Effects
Diuretics (Partial List)				Biochemical abnormalities:
Hydrochlorothiazide	HydroDIURIL, Esidrix	12.5–50	1	↓ potassium, ↑ cholesterol, ↑ glucose
Chlorthalidone*	Hygroton	12.5–50	1	Rare: blood dyscrasias, photosensitivity,
Metolazone*	Mykrox, Diulo	0.5–10	1	pancreatitis
Indapamide	Lozol	2.5	1	(Less if any hypercholesterolemia)
Furosemide	Lasix	40–240	2–3	(Short duration of action)
Torsemide	Demadex	5–40	1–2	(Longer duration of action)
Potassium-Sparing Agents (Plus Thiazide)				
Spironolactone	Aldactazide	25–100	1	Hyperkalemia, gynecomastia
Triamterine	Dyrenium, Dyazide, Maxzide	25–100	1	Hyperkalemia
Amiloride	Moduretic	5–10	1	Hyperkalemia
Adrenergic Inhibitors				
Peripheral				
Reserpine	Serpasil	0.05–0.25	1	Sedation, depression
Guanethidine	Ismelin	10–150	1	Orthostatic hypotension, diarrhea
Guanadrel	Hylorel	10–75	2	Orthostatic hypotension, diarrhea
Central alpha agonists				
Methyldopa	Aldomet	500–3000	2	Hepatic and "autoimmune" disorders
Clonidine	Catapres	0.2–1.2	2–3	Sedation, dry mouth, withdrawal
Guanabenz	Wytensin	8–32	2	Sedation, dry mouth, withdrawal
Guanfacine*	Tenex	1–3	1	Sedation, dry mouth, withdrawal
Alpha blockers				
Doxazosin*	Cardura	1–20	1	Postural hypotension (mainly with first dose), lassitude
Prazosin	Minipress	2–20	2–3	Postural hypotension (mainly with first dose), lassitude
Terazosin	Hytrin	1–20	1	Postural hypotension (mainly with first dose), lassitude
Beta blockers				
Acebutolol*	Sectral	200–800	1	Serious (all beta blockers):
Atenolol	Tenormin	25–100	2	bronchospasm, congestive heart
Betaxolol*	Kerlone	5–20	1	failure, masking of insulin-induced
Bisiprolol*	Zebeta	2.5–10	1	hypokalemia, depression
Carteolol	Cartrol	2.5–10	1	Less serious (all beta blockers): poor
Metoprolol*	Lopressor, Toprol XL	50–300	2;1	peripheral circulation, insomnia,
Nadolol*	Corgard	40–320	1	fatigue, decreased exercise tolerance,
Penbutolol	Levatol	10–20	1	hypertriglyceridemia, decreased HDL
Pindolol	Visken	10–60	1	(except with ISA agents)
Propranolol	Inderal	40–480	2	
Timolol	Blocadren	20–60	2	
Combined alpha and beta blockers				
Labetalol	Normodyne, Trandate	200–1200	2	Postural hypotension, beta-blocking side effects
Carvedilol	Coreg	12.5–50	2	Postural hypotension, beta-blocking side effects
Direct Vasodilators				
Hydralazine	Apresoline	50–400	2	Headaches, tachycardia, lupus syndrome
Minoxidil	Loniten	5–100	1	Headaches, fluid retention, hirsutism
Calcium Channel Blockers				
Verapamil (SR)	Isoptin, Calan; Verelan	90–480	2;1	Constipation, conduction defects
Diltiazem (SR and CD)	Cardizem; Dilacor, Tiazac	120–240	2;1	Nausea, headache, conduction defects
Dihydropyridines				
Amlodipine*	Norvasc	2.5–10	1	Flush, headache, local ankle edema
Felodipine	Plendil	5–20	1	Flush, headache, local ankle edema
Isradipine	DynaCirc	5–20	2	Flush, headache, local ankle edema
Nicardipine (SR)	Cardene	60–90	2	Flush, headache, local ankle edema
Nifedipine (XL)	Procardia XL, Adalat CC	30–120	1	Flush, headache, local ankle edema
Nisoldipine	Sular	20–60	1	Flush, headache, local ankle edema
Angiotensin-Converting Enzyme Inhibitors				
Benazepril	Lotensin	5–40	1	Cough, rash, loss of taste
Captopril	Capoten	25–150	3	Rare: leucopenia, proteinuria
Enalapril	Vasotec	5–40	2	Rare: leucopenia, proteinuria
Fosinopril	Monopril	10–40	1	Rare: leucopenia, proteinuria

Table continued on following page

TABLE 5. **Oral Antihypertensive Drugs** *Continued*

Drug	Trade Name	Dose Range (mg/d)	Frequency (per Day)	Side Effects
Angiotensin-Converting Enzyme Inhibitors Continued				
Lisinopril	Prinivil, Zestril	5–40	1	Rare: leukopenia, proteinuria
Moexipril	Univasc	2.5–10	2	Rare: leukopenia, proteinuria
Quinapril	Accupril	5–80	1–2	Rare: leukopenia, proteinuria
Ramipril	Altace	1.25–20	1	Rare: leukopenia, proteinuria
Trandolapril*	Mavik	1–4	1	Rare: leukopenia, proteinuria
Angiotensin-Receptor Blockers				
Losartan	Cozaar	50–100	1–2	No cough, but angioedema occurs
Valsartan	Diovan	80–320	1	No cough, but angioedema occurs

*Inherently long acting.

Abbreviations: SR = slow release; CD = controlled delivery; XL = extended duration; HDL = high-density lipoprotein; ISA = intrinsic sympathomimetic activity.

but not too great an effect, so patients will tolerate them.

The choice of drug should be made on the basis of the individual patient's need, in turn based on the presence of certain demographic features or one or more coexisting conditions (Table 6). Older and black hypertensive patients have been found to respond particularly well to diuretics and CCBs and somewhat less to beta blockers and ACE inhibitors. This lesser response can be augmented by the addition of even a small dose of diuretic, in keeping with the increasing use of low-dose combinations, as described later.

The partial list of coexisting conditions in Table 6 includes a few that may be aggravated by certain drugs, which should usually be avoided in these patients: diuretics or beta blockers may worsen diabetic control and dyslipidemia. Many of the coexisting conditions can be helped by certain drugs, which should therefore be used in these patients: ACE inhibitors improve congestive heart failure, diabetic nephropathy, and the post–myocardial infarction state; alpha blockers improve dyslipidemia and prostatism; beta blockers are indicated for angina and after myocar-

dial infarction; CCBs are useful for angina, cyclosporine-induced hypertension, and patients who need nonsteroidal anti-inflammatory drugs (NSAIDs), which may interfere with the effectiveness of all other classes but CCBs.

On the other hand, for the third to half of hypertensive patients who have no specific indication for or against a certain choice, a diuretic or beta blocker is preferred (Figure 3). This preference is based on the richly documented ability of diuretic- and, to a lesser degree, beta-blocker–based therapy to reduce cardiovascular morbidity and mortality. All of the 19 completed randomized clinical trials involved a diuretic, about half a beta blocker. The marked reduction in cardiovascular events achieved with low doses of diuretic, 12.5 to 15 mg of hydrochlorothiazide or its equivalent, in the most recently completed three trials in elderly patients is particularly impressive and is the basis for the preference given them in Table 6.

Proper, large-scale, controlled studies are now in process examining the new classes of drugs, including angiotensin II–receptor blockers. As the results of these trials become available, likely beginning in late 1997 or early 1998, the current preference for

TABLE 6. **Recommendations for Selection of Initial Antihypertensive Drug for Patients with Various Coexisting Conditions**

Coexisting Condition	Diuretic	Beta Blocker	Alpha Blocker	ACEI	Calcium Channel Blockers	
					Verapamil, Diltiazem	*Dihydropyridine*
Older age	+ +	±	+	+	+	+
Black race	+ +	±	+	±	+ +	+ +
Angina	+	+ +	+	+	+ +	+ +
Post-MI	+	+ +	+	+	+	−
CHF	+ +	±	+	+ +	−	±
Cerebrovascular disease	+	+	±	+	+	+
Renal disease	+ +	±	+	+ +*	+	+
Diabetes	±	−	+ +	+ +	+	+
Dyslipidemia	−	−	+ +	+	+	+
Prostatism			+ +			

*Caution if renovascular disease has not been excluded.

Abbreviations: ACEI = angiotensin-converting enzyme inhibitor; MI = myocardial infarction; CHF = congestive heart failure; + + = preferred; + = suitable; ± = caution needed; − = usually not advised.

JNC V Treatment Algorithm

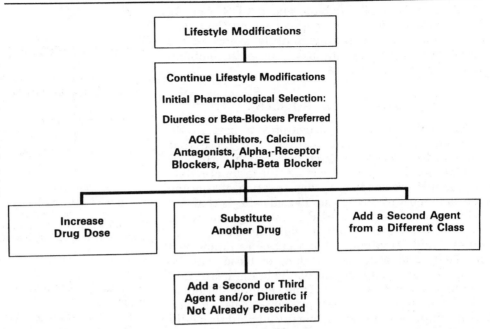

Figure 3. Joint National Committee treatment algorithm. *Abbreviation:* ACE = angiotensin-converting enzyme. (From The fifth report of the Joint National Committee on Detection, Evaluation, and Treatment of High Blood Pressure [JNC V]. Arch Intern Med *153*:154–183, 1993.)

diuretics and beta blockers may be altered if any of the newer drugs are found to be superior. For now, however, I agree with the statement in the fifth report of the Joint National Committee on Detection, Evaluation, and Treatment of High Blood Pressure: "Because diuretics and β-blockers are the only classes of drugs that have been used in long-term controlled clinical trials and shown to reduce morbidity and mortality, they are recommended as first choice agents unless they are contraindicated or unacceptable, or unless there are special indications for other agents."

Individual patients may or may not be among the 60% who respond to any given drug. Therefore, if a reasonable response is not observed with a moderate dose of the first choice, the logical action is to stop the first drug and substitute another from a different class (see Figure 3). Such substitution makes better sense than simply adding another drug, in the old-fashioned stepped-care approach.

On the other hand, if the response to a moderate dose of the first choice is only partial and no significant side effects have been noted, a second agent of another class should be added. More about this is covered under "Resistant Hypertension."

Low-Dose Combination

Rather than starting with a moderate dose of the first choice, two drugs may be given in combination to increase the efficacy of each while keeping side effects to a minimum (Figure 4). As shown in this idealized diagram, a small dose (A) of a drug provides only about 40% of the desired reduction in BP, but

dose-dependent side effects are minimal (A'). If the dose of the same drug is doubled (up to level B), an additional antihypertensive effect is obtained but at the price of significant side effects (B').

A more logical move would be to add a low dose of a second agent, with another set of dose-dependent side effects. Thereby, the total efficacy of the two drugs, each in low dose, is considerable while the side effects are minimized. This goal has been achieved, first with low doses of a diuretic and a beta

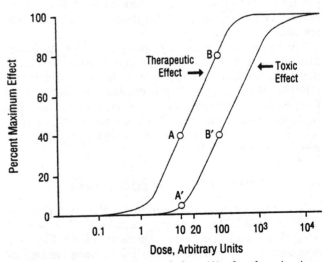

Figure 4. When a suboptimal dose (A) of a drug is given, minimal side effects (A') are seen. If a larger dose is given to achieve a larger effect (B), the side effects also increase (B'). If low doses of two different types of drugs that provide additive effects are given, the full therapeutic goal is obtained but side effects reflect the low dose of each agent. (From Fagan TC: Remembering the lessons of basic pharmacology. Arch Intern Med *154*:1430–1431, 1994. Copyright 1994, American Medical Association.)

blocker in the preparation Ziac, later with combinations of a diuretic and an ACE inhibitor (Lotensin HCT), and an ACE inhibitor and a CCB (Lotrel). More such low-dose combinations are on their way to the market, and they will likely overcome the resistance that many physicians have to combinations of antihypertensives.

START LOW, GO SLOW

As noted, low doses of drugs provide partial efficacy but fewer side effects (except for those that are not dose dependent such as a cough with ACE inhibitors). Even more important, the gradual reduction in BP provided by a slow titration of therapy prevents most of the nonspecific side effects that are related to lowering of the BP by all drugs too much, too fast. These include fatigue, light-headedness, dizziness, and impotence. When pressure is lowered markedly and abruptly, the flow of blood may be reduced to such vital organs as the brain, heart, and genitals. Over a period of time, autoregulation of blood flow often allows lower pressures to be achieved while maintaining organ perfusion, but initially symptoms may appear when the BP is lowered markedly even if the BP remains above "hypertensive" levels. If a patient with a BP of 180/120 mm Hg has a rapid reduction to 140/90 mm Hg, tissue hypoperfusion that produces ischemic symptoms may occur.

The problem is even more likely to occur in elderly patients whose autoregulatory ability has been blunted by atherosclerosis and a loss of reflex sensitivity. Therefore, even smaller doses of drugs should be given to elderly patients, perhaps one half of the usual low starting dose. Slow titration of the dose, for most patients with uncomplicated disease at a monthly interval, should bring the pressure down gradually, thereby achieving control with fewer side effects. A 3- to 6-month total titration period is reasonable.

Those patients with extremely high BP and significant target organ damage may present a therapeutic two-edged sword: if the BP is not reduced quickly, the already ischemic organs may suffer from further hypoperfusion. Such patients need close attention, often an increase in their medication every few days with monitoring of cerebral, cardiac, and renal function.

DIURETIC AS SECOND DRUG

If a diuretic was not chosen as the first drug, a diuretic should be strongly considered if a second drug is needed. The most common reason for poor response to multiple drugs is inadequate control of intravascular volume from too little or no diuretic. Many hypertensive patients start off with an expanded vascular volume, a consequence of multiple factors:

Reduced renal excretory capacity that may be the underlying cause of "essential" hypertension and that

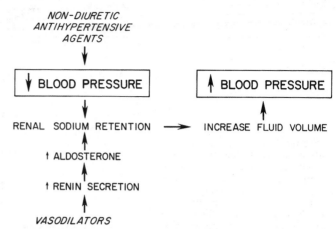

Figure 5. The manner by which nondiuretic antihypertensive agents may lose their effectiveness by renal sodium retention. (From Kaplan NM: Clinical Hypertension, 6th ed. Baltimore, Williams & Wilkins, 1994, p 201.)

is usually aggravated by hypertensive nephrosclerosis.

Excessive dietary sodium intake.

Reactive sodium retention. This reflects the inherent response of the hypertensive kidneys to a fall in BP—an increase in sodium reabsorption in a misguided attempt to restore the lower BP (Figure 5).

As a result of these forces, what starts off in the untreated state as a tightly filled, constricted vascular bed with a high pressure ends up as a dilated vascular bed (from the antihypertensives that work by vasodilatation, including ACE inhibitors, alpha blockers, and CCBs) that is just as tightly filled, and therefore with just as high a pressure. Some patients can get along without a diuretic—if renal function is intact, if sodium intake is not excessive, and if they take antihypertensive agents that either blunt the renin-aldosterone mechanism that accentuates sodium retention (beta blockers, ACE inhibitors, or angiotensin II–receptor blockers) or have a modest natriuretic effect of their own (CCBs).

Most patients, however, will need a diuretic, maybe as little as 6.25 or 12.5 mg of hydrochlorothiazide if renal function is good but a lot more if renal function is impaired. In those with renal impairment, a stronger, loop diuretic may be needed. Often a single, once-a-day dose of furosemide (Lasix) is used. Because that provides only a few hours of diuretic action, the patient thereafter retains all the sodium and water excreted while the diuretic was working. At the end of the 24 hours, the vascular volume and BP are unchanged.

Therefore, long-acting diuretics are needed: hydrochlorothiazide or indapamide (Lozol) work well for those with good renal function; torsemide (Demadex) or, even better, metolazone (Zaroxolyn, Diulo) work well for those with renal impairment, reflected by a serum creatinine level above 1.5 mg/DL. Obviously, diuretics should be given in the morning to reduce nocturia and with potassium-sparing agents unless renal function is impaired.

LONG-ACTING FORMULATIONS

As with diuretics, long-acting agents of all classes should be used for the following reasons:

Adherence to therapy is enhanced. Patients will more likely take a drug once a day than three times a day.

The cost of therapy is often cheaper. Once-a-day trandolapril (Mavik) costs one third as much as 2 doses of enalapril (Vasotec).

The control of hypertension is persistent and smooth, rather than intermittent and erratic.

The abrupt rise in BP on awakening from sleep in the early morning is blunted, thereby hopefully reducing the excess in major cardiovascular catastrophes (sudden death, strokes, and myocardial infarction) that occurs during these hours.

Long-acting, once-a-day formulations are available in every category of antihypertensive drugs (see Table 5). There is a special advantage in using drugs with inherently long durations of action, beyond 24 hours. These include chlorthalidone (Hygroton), betaxolol (Kerlone), amlodipine (Norvasc), trandolapril, and doxazosin (Cardura). The reason is that if patients skip a dose—as they often do—the antihypertensive effect of these drugs will last for the next 24 hours, avoiding any rebound from the loss of drug effect or precipitous fall in BP when the dose is restarted.

Some inherently short-acting drugs have been formulated into longer acting preparations, e.g., verapamil SODAS (Verelan), and nifedipine GITS (Procardia XL). If a dose of these agents is missed, the antihypertensive effect will not persist much beyond 24 hours, so there is reason to use inherently long-acting drugs.

Such long-acting agents can be taken anytime, but I prefer early in the morning so patients can more easily remember to take their medications. If they are prescribed once-daily agents that have a fairly quick and abrupt onset of action, such as felodipine XL (Plendil), they should not take them at bedtime because the effect of the medication will add to the fall in BP that usually occurs spontaneously during sleep, lowering the BP so much as to induce nocturnal ischemia.

A new formulation of verapamil (Covera-HS) that releases its content after 5 to 6 hours has been marketed for bedtime dosing to ensure control of BP in the early morning. The idea is attractive, but the same effect can be achieved by an agent such as Verelan that works throughout the 24 hours.

If more than one drug is needed, all should be long-acting and all should be taken in the early morning. Almost every hypertensive patient should have controlled BP with one dose of medications a day.

HOME RECORDINGS

Once therapy has been started, the response should be monitored, if at all possible, by home BP readings, taken with one of the readily available inexpensive, semiautomatic devices, e.g., AND UA-702, the model that was top-rated in the October 1996 *Consumer Reports*, is sold for less than $40. Patients should bring the home device to the office and measure BP in one arm while the nurse measures it with a mercury manometer in the other arm. Thereby, both the accuracy of the devices and the patient's technique can be ensured.

After a week on any new regimen, a number of seated readings should be taken throughout one day and early the next morning to ensure that the BP is being kept down but not lowered too much.

Once the adequacy of the regimen is established, only an occasional seated reading, perhaps once a week, need be taken unless symptoms are noted. An early morning reading, taken after arising and ambulating a bit but before intake of the day's antihypertensive drugs, is the most useful one because it will ensure the adequacy of control at the end of the dosing interval, at the most critical time for cardiovascular events related to the rise in BP after sleep.

If symptoms of postural or postprandial hypotension—dizziness, weakness, unsteadiness—are noted, the BP should be taken while the patient is supine or seated and again after a few minutes of quiet standing, holding onto a chair if necessary for support. If the standing BP falls by more than 20/10 mm Hg, therapy should be manipulated to avoid such decreases. Obviously, elderly and diabetic patients should be checked for such hypotension before therapy is started and, if it is present, corrective measures taken before antihypertensive therapy is begun. These corrective measures, in addition to arising slowly, may need to include sleeping with the head of the bed elevated, eating only small meals, performing isometric exercise before standing, and wearing support hose. If hypotension persists, additional diagnostic testing and therapeutic maneuvers may be needed.

Most home readings, perhaps 80%, are lower than office readings. Home readings are quite comparable to automatically recorded ambulatory readings, both techniques used out of the office to avoid the white coat effect of office readings. As noted earlier, the white coat effect can lead to overdiagnosis of hypertension. It can also lead to overtreatment, causing some patients to be deemed unresponsive or resistant when, in fact, their BP is well controlled. Therefore, I increasingly use the patient's home readings, faxed or mailed to the office every month, to monitor the response to therapy. Changes in the regimen can safely be made, reducing the frequency and costs of office visits.

If home readings are not feasible, as in many teaching hospitals where patients cannot afford to buy devices, the patient should come to the office as early in the morning as possible, without that day's medication, to check for the adequacy of coverage for the full 24 hours. The occasional recording of a late morning or afternoon BP may give either false security if the regimen is only providing 12 to 18 hours of coverage or false insecurity if the white coat effect results in higher readings than are present away from the office.

GOAL OF THERAPY

The final issue for most patients is how low to bring the BP for maximal protection against hypertension-induced cardiovascular damage. Some would say, "As low as the patient will tolerate," with the assumption that the epidemiologic evidence for less cardiovascular disease the lower the BP in the untreated state translates to the treated state as well. As noted at the beginning of this chapter, treatment may invoke trouble, either from medication side effects or from tissue hypoperfusion from a lower BP.

With newer medications and generally lower doses, side effects should be less and less of a problem. However, tissue hypoperfusion may not go away, regardless of how the BP is lowered. The problem in relation to coronary disease has been described as a "J curve," with progressively fewer coronary events as the diastolic BP (DBP) is lowered to a level about 85 mm Hg and then an increase in events as the pressure falls below 85 mm Hg. Some argue that the increase in coronary mortality below a DBP of 85 mm Hg may reflect a weakened, damaged myocardium, unable to maintain cardiac output, and therefore a premonitor of mortality unrelated to the effects of therapy. A study, the Hypertension Optimal Treatment (HOT) trial, designed to document the J curve in a prospective controlled manner is near completion and perhaps will soon settle the issue.

In the meantime, I believe that a J curve exists for coronary disease. No J curve has been seen for cerebrovascular or renal disease and, for maximal protection against stroke and nephrosclerosis, the lower the pressure perhaps the better. However, the heart is uniquely susceptible to ischemia when perfusion pressure is lowered. Unlike the brain or kidneys, the heart hypertrophies with hypertension and therefore requires more blood flow; the heart cannot extract more oxygen when flow is lowered because the normal heart already extracts as much as possible; the heart, particularly with atherosclerosis of coronary arteries, cannot autoregulate its blood flow efficiently, so that when perfusion pressure falls, blood flow may fall as well. These features make the heart uniquely susceptible to a J curve and, until definitive proof against its presence is shown, the prudent course is to keep the DBP no lower than 85 mm Hg in the majority of hypertensive patients, whose major threat is from coronary disease.

On the other hand, patients whose major threat is from advancing renal damage, e.g., diabetic patients with nephropathy or black patients with nephrosclerosis, may be better protected from progressive glomerulosclerosis by a lowering of systemic BP to much lower levels, perhaps as low as 110/70 mm Hg. Certainly, the BP should be brought down to near 120/80 mm Hg. Therapy in these patients should include an ACE inhibitor, which, although it lowers

TABLE 7. **Causes of Inadequate Responsiveness to Therapy**

Pseudoresistance
  White coat or office elevations
  Pseudohypertension in elderly patients
Nonadherence to therapy
  Side effects of medication
  Cost of medication
  Lack of consistent and continuous primary care
  Inconvenient and chaotic dosing schedules
  Instructions not understood
  Inadequate patient education
  Organic brain syndrome (e.g., memory deficit)
Drug-related causes
  Doses too low
  Inappropriate combinations (e.g., two centrally acting adrenergic inhibitors)
  Rapid inactivation (e.g., hydralazine)
  Drug interactions

Nonsteroidal anti-inflammatory drugs	Oral contraceptives
Sympathomimetics	Adrenal steroids
Nasal decongestants	Licorice (e.g., chewing tobacco)
Appetite suppressants	Cyclosporine
Cocaine	Erythropoietin
Caffeine	Cholestyramine
Antidepressants (MAO inhibitors, tricyclics)	

  Excessive volume contraction with stimulation of renin-aldosterone
  Hypokalemia (usually diuretic induced)
  Rebound after clonidine withdrawal
Associated conditions
  Smoking
  Increasing obesity
  Sleep apnea
  Insulin resistance with hyperinsulinemia
  Ethanol intake more than 1 oz/d (>3 portions)
  Anxiety-induced hyperventilation or panic attacks
  Chronic pain
  Intense vasconstriction (Raynaud's, arteritis)
Secondary hypertension
  Renal insufficiency
  Renovascular hypertension
  Pheochromocytoma
  Primary aldosteronism
Volume overload
  Excess sodium intake
  Progressive renal damage (nephrosclerosis)
  Fluid retention from reduction of blood pressure
  Inadequate diuretic therapy

Abbreviation: MAO = monoamine oxidase.

systemic pressure, also has a greater effect on reducing the pressure in the efferent vessels leaving the glomerulus, thereby protecting even better against progressive glomerulosclerosis. Preliminary evidence suggests that combining an ACE inhibitor with a CCB may be even better because the CCB will have a greater vasodilating effect on the afferent vessels and thereby preserve renal blood flow while the ACE inhibitor lowers intraglomerular pressure.

In the elderly patient with isolated systolic hypertension, data from clinical trials suggest a goal of 140 to 145 mm Hg for the systolic pressure with little regard needed for the diastolic level. Obviously, hypotensive symptoms should be looked for and avoided.

RESISTANT HYPERTENSION

For a small but important group of patients, hypertension does not respond well to presumably adequate therapy. Resistance, defined as a DBP above 90 mm Hg despite three or more drugs in reasonable doses, can arise from multiple causes (Table 7). The first is "pseudoresistance" from the exclusive use of office readings that are higher because of the white coat effect. Therefore, if at all possible, the presence of true resistance should be documented by readings out of the office before additional studies or more aggressive treatment is pursued.

Patients may not adhere to therapy for reasons related to the physician's behavior (a confusing regimen of multiple drugs taken at multiple times throughout the day), medication characteristics (intolerable side effects), or patients' negligence (missed appointments, failure to refill prescriptions).

Resistance may arise from inadequacies of the medications. Some are inherent to the drug, in particular a short duration of action. Others are imposed by drug interactions, most commonly from NSAIDs or sympathomimetics.

The BP may not respond because of interference from other conditions. Hypertensive patients who smoke, gain weight, or drink too much alcohol may overwhelm the effects of their antihypertensive therapy. Obesity is often associated with sleep apnea and is always accompanied by insulin resistance, both of which may worsen hypertension.

Secondary forms of hypertension may arise and make primary (essential) hypertension resistant to previously effective therapy. The most common of these is renal insufficiency from hypertensive nephrosclerosis or diabetic nephropathy. The most difficult to recognize is renovascular hypertension, which must always be looked for when hypertension is severe and resistant, particularly if accompanied by unexplained renal insufficiency.

As noted previously, the most common cause of resistance is inadequate diuretic to overcome the multiple forces that cause volume overload. Most often, resistance can be overcome if volume is controlled.

THE CALCIUM CHANNEL BLOCKER CONTROVERSY

An additional cause of loss of control of hypertension has appeared: concerns about the safety of CCBs that have caused some practitioners to discontinue their use and thereby lose control of their patients' hypertension. These concerns have arisen in part from well-grounded evidence of the adverse effects of large doses of short-acting nifedipine when given to hemodynamically vulnerable patients after an acute myocardial infarction. Even more concerns have been engendered by case-control and cohort studies that have suggested an increase in the frequency of heart attacks and cancer with short-acting CCBs. These uncontrolled studies cannot prove causality, and I

TABLE 8. **Potential Harmful Effects of Calcium Channel Blockers**

Effect	Short-Acting Nifedipine	Long-Acting Agents
Proischemic effect	Unlikely	No
Negative inotropic effect	Yes	Minimal
Effects on rhythm	Unproven	No
Prohemorrhagic effects	Unproven	No
Marked hypotension	Yes	No
Reflex increase in sympathetic activity	Yes	No

strongly believe they are biased by the presence of more pre-existing coronary disease in those patients who received CCBs compared with those who received other drugs.

All these putative claims have been made against short-acting CCBs, which were never approved for the treatment of hypertension. The currently widely used (and approved) long-acting formulations act quite differently (Table 8) and therefore should not be blamed for the largely unproven sins of the short-acting agents. Prospective controlled studies have now shown no increases but rather decreases in coronary and other mortality in patients given long-acting CCBs for either heart failure (the PRAISE [prospective randomized amlodipine survival evaluation] study) or hypertension (the STONE [Shanghai trial of nifedipine in the elderly] study). Therefore, I believe long-acting CCBs can be used without concern about their safety, when they are indicated (see Table 6).

CONCLUSION

On paper, the treatment of hypertension should be fairly easy. In practice, most hypertension is not being successfully treated, in part because of the asymptomatic nature of the condition and the need for lifelong therapy. If the commonsense guidelines described in this chapter are followed, we should be able to do a better job, thereby protecting more patients from premature cardiovascular disease.

ACUTE EVOLVING MYOCARDIAL INFARCTION

method of
PREDIMAN K. SHAH, M.D.
Cedars-Sinai Medical Center and UCLA School of Medicine
Los Angeles, California

Acute myocardial infarction (AMI) is a common complication of atherosclerotic coronary artery disease and often the first clinical expression of coronary artery disease. In the past 3 decades, there have been several advances in the management of patients with an AMI that have contributed to a steady decline in the short-term and long-term mortality. These advances began with the introduction of coronary care units in the late 1960s, which along with the nearly contemporaneous introduction of cardiopulmonary resuscitation, defibrillators, and antiarrhythmic drugs reduced mortality from about 30 to 40% in the pre–coronary care unit era to about 15 to 20%. The last 15 years have witnessed yet another major reduction in postinfarction mortality and morbidity as the importance of restoration of blood flow to the ischemic myocardium early in the evolution of myocardial infarction was recognized. In this article, the management of patients in the early hours of evolution of AMI with an emphasis on reperfusion therapy is discussed.

PATHOPHYSIOLOGY OF ACUTE MYOCARDIAL INFARCTION

Despite the early descriptions of coronary artery thrombosis in AMI, dating back to the turn of the century, the primary role of coronary thrombosis in the pathophysiology of AMI was doubted by several leading cardiac pathologists. The landmark study of DeWood and colleagues, wherein the high prevalence of total or subtotal thrombotic coronary artery occlusion was documented by early coronary angiography and from the findings at coronary artery bypass surgery, largely helped revive the concept that coronary artery thrombus plays a major role in the abrupt occlusion of atherosclerotic coronary arteries, thereby initiating AMI. It is now generally recognized that fissure or rupture of the fibrous cap of an atherosclerotic plaque is a critical event that leads to activation of local hemostatic mechanisms with the formation of intramural and intraluminal platelet-fibrin thrombus, which contributes to an abrupt total or near-total coronary artery occlusion. Plaque disruption may occur in severely or only mildly stenotic plaques; the lipid-rich soft plaques with macrophage infiltration are particularly vulnerable. The magnitude of thrombotic response appears to be, at least in part, determined by the depth of plaque fissure, the thrombogenicity of the plaque constituents (tissue factor–containing lipid core and collagen are highly thrombogenic), the severity of local atherosclerotic stenosis, and the shear rate as well as the circulating state of coagulability and fibrinolytic activity. The precise mechanisms of plaque disruption are incompletely understood but may include hemodynamic stresses, abnormal matrix regulation with increased matrix breakdown by matrix-degrading metalloproteinases (collagenases, gelatinases, stromelysin) produced by inflammatory cells such as macrophages, and reduced matrix synthesis resulting from reduced function or number of smooth muscle cells through mechanisms such as apoptosis (programmed cell death). The consequences of coronary artery occlusion, in turn, may be influenced by the adequacy of collaterals as well as by the duration and completeness of luminal occlusion.

After an abrupt cessation of nutrient flow, the myocardium supplied by the culprit coronary artery becomes ischemic, with subendocardial to subepicardial spread of necrosis occurring in a time-dependent wave front phenomenon. The precise time course of transmural spread of necrosis will depend on residual flow (through collaterals or antegrade), and the eventual size of myocardial infarction is thus determined by the duration of coronary artery occlusion, residual flow, and the area at risk. Several studies have shown that infarct size and its correlates (such as ventricular function, size, and shape) are the

major determinants of short- and long-term prognosis in AMI.

REPERFUSION THERAPY FOR EVOLVING ACUTE MYOCARDIAL INFARCTION

The rationale of reperfusion therapy for AMI derives from the following facts: abrupt thrombotic coronary occlusion initiates AMI; myocardial infarction evolves in a finite time after the onset of coronary artery occlusion; and timely restoration of nutrient flow to the ischemic myocardium can abort the transmural spread of the necrotic wave front, leading to a reduction in infarct size, preservation of ventricular function, attenuation of adverse changes in ventricular shape and size (remodeling), and reduced electrical vulnerability to lethal arrhythmias, which reduces mortality and morbidity (Table 1). The available methods of accomplishing reperfusion in AMI include thrombolytic therapy, percutaneous transluminal coronary angioplasty (PTCA), and surgical revascularization. Intravenous thrombolytic therapy is the most convenient, least expensive, and most widely applicable form of reperfusion therapy for patients with AMI, although prompt PTCA can achieve similar or better outcomes, especially in selected subsets of patients.

Thrombolytic Therapy

Thrombolytic therapy had been tried for the treatment of AMI in the early 1950s and 1960s, but the results were generally inconclusive, perhaps because of varying inclusion criteria and inclusion of patients hours to days after the initial AMI. Interest in coronary thrombolysis was, however, rejuvenated by the clinical and experimental observations of Chazov, Ganz, and Rentrop, who demonstrated the feasibility and success of intracoronary thrombolysis. In the last nearly 15 years, intravenous thrombolytic therapy has been a subject of intense investigation, and sev-

TABLE 1. **Mechanisms of Mortality Reduction with Thrombolytic Therapy in Acute Myocardial Infarction**

Myocardial salvage and preservation of ventricular function
Attenuation of infarct remodeling, expansion, ventricular dilatation
Reduced electrical instability
    Lower frequency of spontaneous ventricular tachycardia or ventricular fibrillation
    Lower frequency of late potentials
    Lower frequency of inducible ventricular tachycardia
Others
    Reduced frequency of rupture except with late therapy (>12 h)
    Reduced frequency of mural thrombus and embolic complications
    Improved infarct healing
    Open artery may serve as a source of collaterals in future

TABLE 2. **Selected Controlled Trials of Thrombolytic Therapy in Acute Myocardial Infarction**

Trial	Number	Short-term Mortality		Follow-up Interval (d)	Reduction (%)	Reduction (%) of Subgroup by Time to Therapy
		Treatment (%)	Control (%)			
GISSI (SK)	11,712	10.7	13.0	21	18	<1 h = 47 0–3 h = 23 3–6 h = 17 6–12 h = −3
ISIS-2 (SK ± aspirin)	17,187	9.1	11.8	35	23	<1 h = 42 <4 h = 32 4–12 h = 13 12–24 h = 19
ASSET (t-PA)	5,011	7.2	9.8	30	26	<3 h = 26 3–5 h = 24
ECSG (t-PA + aspirin)	721	2.8	5.7	14	51	<3 h = 82 3–5 h = 8
AIMS (APSAC)	1,004	6.4	12.2	30	47	<4 h = 41 4–6 h = 52

Abbreviations: GISSI = Gruppo Italiano per lo Studio della Streptochinasi nell' Infarto Miocardico; ISIS-2 = Second International Study of Infarct Survival; ASSET = Anglo Scandinavian Study of Early Thrombolysis; ECSG = European Cooperative Study Group; AIMS = APSAC Intervention Mortality Study; SK = streptokinase; t-PA = tissue plasminogen activator; APSAC = anisoylated plasminogen streptokinase activator complex.

eral controlled clinical trials have provided unequivocal evidence that such therapy significantly reduces short- and long-term mortality and morbidity after AMI.

The beneficial effects of thrombolytic therapy are largely due to restoration of culprit artery patency with brisk flow (Thrombolysis in Myocardial Infarction [TIMI] grade 3 flow). Mortality reduction has been documented in groups of patients with AMI who receive thrombolysis within the first 12 hours after the onset of symptoms of AMI (Table 2). The greatest relative reduction in mortality has been shown to occur in patients who receive therapy within the first 60 to 90 minutes after the onset of symptoms of AMI. With the exception of the second International Study of Infarct Survival (ISIS-2), most other studies have failed to demonstrate a significant mortality reduction in patients with AMI who receive thrombolytic therapy after 12 hours of onset of symptoms. In fact, a meta-analysis of several trials has suggested that the risk for cardiac rupture may be increased when the time from onset of symptoms to treatment exceeds 10 to 12 hours, although this has since been challenged by the results of other trials. The reduction in mortality has been shown to occur in those with an anterior as well as an inferior location of myocardial infarction, in young as well as in older patients (older than 70 to 75 years), in patients with or without a prior additional infarction, and in patients with an AMI who present with a left bundle branch block. Comparative trials of the two most commonly used thrombolytic agents (streptokinase and tissue plasminogen activator [t-PA]) have shown that in general, both agents are effective; t-PA is modestly more effective in terms of an overall effect on mortality (Table 3). The salient characteristics of the streptokinase and t-PA are compared in Table 4.

In the United States, APSAC (anisoylated plasminogen streptokinase activator complex) has been essentially discontinued because it offered few advantages over streptokinase and was considerably more expensive than streptokinase. Overall, the substantially lower cost of streptokinase and slightly lower risk for cerebral hemorrhage justify its use as the first-line thrombolytic agent in all but a few circumstances.

Mechanisms of Mortality Reduction by Reperfusion

Several studies have suggested that restoration of arterial patency results in improved clinical outcome, especially when the flow through the culprit vessel is of TIMI grade 3 quality (flow similar to that of normal vessels). Salvage of ischemic myocardium with a reduction in the infarct size and preservation or improvement in regional and global ventricular function is generally believed to be an important mechanism by which timely reperfusion reduces mortality in AMI (see Table 1). However, reduction in ventricular remodeling and dilatation, reduced vulnerability to spontaneous as well as inducible ventricular arrhythmias, improved infarct healing and reduced risk for cardiac rupture (except perhaps with late therapy), and reduction in mural thrombosis and embolic complications may also contribute in this regard, particularly when mortality reduction appears to occur in the absence of a demonstrable significant improvement in ventricular function. In addition, an open infarct artery may serve as a source of collaterals in the future.

Conjunctive Therapy with Thrombolysis

It has been demonstrated that during thrombolytic therapy, while the lytic effects of the thrombolytic

TABLE 3. **Direct Comparative Trials of Commonly Used Thrombolytic Agents**

ISIS-3 Study	SK	t-PA (deuteplase)*	APSAC
Numbers randomized	13,295	13,290	13,328
5-wk mortality (%)	10.5	10.3	10.6
Adverse drug effects			
Any allergy (%)	3.7	0.8	5.2†
Any hypotension (%)	12	7.1	12.6†
Any CVA (%)	1.1	1.5	1.5†
Probable cerebral bleeds (%)	0.3	0.7	0.6†
Reinfarction (%)	3.6	3.1	3.8†
GISSI-2 Study	**SK**	**t-PA (alteplase)**	
Numbers randomized	6199	6182	
Hospital mortality (%)	9	8.6	
Stroke (%)	1.1	0.9	
Major bleeds (%)	0.5	1	
GUSTO-I Study	**t-PA + IV Heparin**	**SK + IV Heparin**	**SK + SC Heparin**
Numbers	10,396	10,410	9841
Mortality at 30 d (%)	6.3	7.3	7.3
With stroke (%)	1.6	1.4	1.2
With hemorrhagic CVA (%)	0.7	0.6	0.5
With death or nonfatal CVA (%)	7.2	8.2	8.0

*Not available in the United States.
†Statistically significant.
Abbreviations: GUSTO-I = Global Utilization of Streptokinase and Tissue Plasminogen Activator for Occluded Coronary Arteries; alteplase (Activase) = Genentech single-chain recombinant t-PA; deuteplase = Burroughs Wellcome double-chain recombinant t-PA; SK = streptokinase (Kabikinase); APSAC (Eminase) = anisoylated plasminogen streptokinase activator complex; CVA = cerebrovascular accident.

agents are trying to lyse the coronary thrombus, there is ongoing platelet activation and fibrin deposition that can lead to rethrombosis. The net outcome after the administration of thrombolytic agents is thus dependent on the competing effects of lysis and ongoing rethrombosis. Rethrombosis contributes to slow lysis, failure of lysis, and lysis followed by reocclusion (Table 5). Therefore, conjunctive use of antithrombotic agents such as aspirin and heparin is generally considered important for optimizing the results of thrombolytic therapy. The ISIS-2 study clearly demonstrated that use of aspirin by itself reduced mortality in AMI by about 20%, and addition of aspirin to streptokinase was additive in terms of mortality reduction (Table 6). The Antiplatelet Trialists Collaborative Group has examined data from a large number of trials and concluded that the relative risk for death is reduced by approximately 24% (from 17% in placebo to 13% with aspirin) when aspirin is used in patients with a history of myocar-

TABLE 4. **Comparative Features of Commonly Used Thrombolytic Drugs**

	SK	APSAC	t-PA
Coronary patency rate (%)			
90 min	55	65	75
2–3 h	80	?	80
24 h	85	90	85
Mean time to lysis	70 min	70 min	45 min
Hypotensive effect	+ + +	+ +	−
Antigenicity	+ + +	+ + +	−
Circulating half-life	20 min	100 min	6 min
Fibrinogen depletion and systemic lytic state	+ + + +	+ + + +	+ +
Need for conjunctive heparin	±	−	+ +
Reocclusion	+ +	+	+ + +
Ease of administration	+	+ + +	+
Bleeding (except intracranial)	+ +	+ +	+ +
Intracranial bleeding	+ *	+	+ +
Mortality reduction	+ + +	+ + +	+ + +
Cost	$200	$1700	$2200

*The large ISIS-3 study has suggested that streptokinase may carry the lowest relative risk for intracranial bleeding rate.
Abbreviations: SK = streptokinase; APSAC = anisoylated plasminogen streptokinase activator complex; t-PA = tissue plasminogen activator.

TABLE 5. **Current Limitations of Thrombolytic Therapy in Acute Myocardial Infarction**

Underuse because
  Contraindicated in many
  AMI diagnosis not always made on initial presentation
  Late presentation
  Misconceptions regarding age and risks
Slow thrombolysis with limited myocardial salvage
  Average time from treatment to reperfusion with t-PA = 45 min
  Average time from treatment to reperfusion with SK and APSAC = 70 min
Failure of lysis in 15–40% of patients, including incomplete reperfusion (TIMI grade 2 flow) with a high associated mortality
Reocclusion in 5–15% of patients with a high associated mortality and morbidity
Bleeding, especially intracranial
Reperfusion injury (controversial)

TABLE 6. **Beneficial Effects of Aspirin with and Without Thrombolysis in Acute Myocardial Infarction**

Drug	5-Week Vascular Mortality (%)
Placebo (n = 4300)	13.2
Aspirin only (n = 4295)	10.7
Streptokinase only (n = 4300)	10.4
Aspirin + streptokinase (n = 4292)	8

*Second International Study of Infarct Survival (ISIS-2 trial).

dial infarction. The optimal dose of aspirin to achieve a rapid antiplatelet effect appears to be 160 to 320 mg, given with or immediately before administration of the thrombolytic agent. After that, a lower dose of aspirin, such as 80 mg daily, may be sufficient to maintain the antiplatelet effects. Every patient with myocardial infarction should receive aspirin therapy indefinitely.

Several studies have suggested that the conjunctive use of intravenous heparin with thrombolytic therapy improves coronary patency rate, but its impact on survival and reinfarction (particularly when patients are also receiving adequate doses of aspirin) has been somewhat controversial. The ISIS-3 and the Gruppo Italiano per lo Studio della Streptochinasi nell' Infarto-2 (GISSI-2) studies tested the value of subcutaneous heparin (initiated 4 hours after thrombolytic therapy was begun in the case of ISIS-3 and 12 hours after thrombolysis was begun in the case of GISSI-2), and the pooled data suggest a modest additive benefit and a slight increase in the incidence of bleeding. In a subset of patients included in the ISIS-3 trial, patients did receive intravenous heparin, and the results did not appear to be substantively different from subcutaneous heparin. Notwithstanding these uncertainties regarding heparin, it is the current practice in the United States to use intravenous heparin with t-PA and subcutaneous or intravenous heparin with streptokinase.

Given the many limitations of intravenous heparin (inconsistent dose response, inability to inhibit clot-bound thrombin, risk for heparin-induced thrombocytopenia and neutralization of heparin effect by platelet-derived mediators, need for antithrombin III to mediate antithrombin effects), more potent direct inhibitors of thrombin capable of inhibiting free as well as clot-bound thrombin, such as Hirudin and Hirulog, have been tested as conjunctive agents with thrombolytic therapy. The results, in general, have shown either marginal or no clear-cut superiority of recombinant Hirudin over intravenous heparin in terms of clinical outcomes when used with t-PA for AMI; in fact, concern over an increased risk for bleeding with these potent agents has considerably dampened enthusiasm.

Prehospital Initiation of Thrombolysis

After the first report by Koren and Weiss, prehospital (at home or in the ambulance) initiation of throm-

bolytic therapy in an attempt to reduce delay between the time at onset of symptoms and initiation of thrombolytic therapy has been studied by several investigators with variable results. The results of a randomized trial conducted by the Myocardial Infarction Triage and Intervention investigators demonstrated that using t-PA along with aspirin and intravenous heparin, mortality was only 1% when therapy was initiated within 70 minutes of onset of symptoms compared with 10% when therapy was initiated later than 70 minutes after the onset of symptoms regardless of whether the therapy was begun in the ambulance or the emergency department. These data confirm previous findings of the Gruppo Italiano per lo Studio della Streptochinasi nell' Infarto Miocardico (GISSI-1) and ISIS-2 studies, in which the largest reduction in mortality was observed in patients receiving thrombolytic therapy within 1 hour of onset of symptoms, emphasizing the need for early initiation of therapy. Because prehospital initiation of thrombolytic therapy requires considerable logistic organization, it has not been implemented on a wide scale.

ADJUNCTIVE AGENTS (Table 7)

Nitroglycerin

Nitrates reduce ventricular loading conditions as well as reduce coronary artery tone and may thus produce a beneficial effect in AMI by reducing ventricular dysfunction and remodeling as well as by favorably influencing the myocardial oxygen demand and supply relationship. In addition, nitrates may exert an antiplatelet effect, which could contribute to their overall beneficial effect in AMI. Pooled data from six small randomized trials of intravenous nitroglycerin in AMI had suggested an overall 35% reduction in mortality; however, these studies were done without thrombolytic therapy, and the additive benefits of intravenous nitroglycerin in patients receiving thrombolytic therapy remained largely unknown, although some studies have suggested a beneficial additive effect in terms of preventing intermittent occlusion and better preservation of left ventricular function. Two large clinical trials have examined the benefits of either oral sustained-release isosorbide mononitrate (ISIS-4, n = 58,050) or intravenous nitrogycerin followed by transdermal nitroglycerin (GISSI-3, n = 19,394) in patients with AMI. There was no overall significant effect on mortality, although there was a modest reduction in the frequency of angina. However, in both studies, 50 to 60% of patients who were not randomized to receive nitrates in fact received nitrates that could have obscured a true effect on mortality. In view of these findings, routine use of intravenous or long-acting nitrates may not be cost-effective, whereas limiting their use to patients with hypertension, congestive heart failure, or recurrent ischemia would seem to be more appropriate. When nitrates are used in AMI, hypotension should be meticulously avoided because

TABLE 7. **A Meta-analysis of Randomized Trials of Drug Therapy Administered During and After Acute Myocardial Infarction**

Drug Class and Time Administered	Number of Trials	Number of Patients	Relative Risk of Death (95% CI)	P Value	Strength of Evidence*
Beta blockers					
During MI	29	28,970	0.87 (0.77–0.98)	.02	A
After MI	26	24,298	0.77 (0.70–0.84)	<.001	A
ACE inhibitors					
During MI	15	100,963	0.94 (0.89–0.98)	.006	A
After MI (patients with left ventricular dysfunction)	3	5,986	0.78 (0.70–0.86)	<.001	A
Nitrates (during MI)	22	81,908	0.94 (0.90–0.99)	.03	B
Calcium channel blockers (during and after MI)	24	20,342	1.04 (0.95–1.14)	.41	A
Antiarrhythmic drugs					
Lidocaine (during MI)	14	9,155	1.38 (0.98–1.95)	>.05	C
Class I drugs (after MI)	18	6,300	1.21 (1.01–1.44)	.04	A
Amiodarone (after MI)	9	1,557	0.71 (0.51–0.97)	.03	C
Magnesium (during MI)	11	61,860	1.02 (0.96–1.08)	>.05	A

*The strength of the evidence in each meta-analysis was graded as follows: a score of A indicates that a randomized trial of adequate size supports the meta-analysis; B that data from one or more randomized trials of adequate size do not support the meta-analysis; and C that no large randomized trial was conducted.

Abbreviations: ACE = angiotensin-converting enzyme; CI = confidence interval; MI = myocardial infarction.

Adapted with permission from Hennekens CH, Albert CM, Godfried SL, et al: Adjunctive drug therapy of acute myocardial infarction—evidence from clinical trials. N Engl J Med *335:*1660–1667, 1996. Copyright 1996 Massachusetts Medical Society. All rights reserved.

such an effect could also produce a deleterious effect on coronary perfusion to the ischemic zone, especially when the perfusion is collateral dependent or when arterial pressure is particularly preload dependent, as in patients with a right ventricular infarction complicating inferior myocardial infarction.

Beta Blockers

Beta blockers may have a beneficial effect in patients with AMI by reducing myocardial oxygen demand, reducing myocardial wall stress, and antagonizing the arrhythmogenic effects of catecholamines. A meta-analysis of 29 trials of beta blockers (28 of which were conducted before widespread use of aspirin and thrombolytic therapy) in AMI showed a 13% ($P = .02$) reduction in overall mortality in patients assigned to early treatment with beta blockers. Several studies have suggested that beta blockers may reduce early postinfarct adverse events (death, nonfatal cardiac arrest, ad nonfatal reinfarction) by about 16%. At least one of the trials (ISIS-1) has suggested that early intravenous beta blockade may reduce post–myocardial infarction mortality by reducing the occurrence of cardiac rupture and ventricular fibrillation. The results of the TIMI study, which investigated the effects of early versus delayed administration of beta blockers in patients with AMI receiving t-PA as a thrombolytic agent, suggested a modest beneficial effect in favor of early intravenous beta blockade in terms of reduction of reinfarction, although mortality was not significantly different.

Beta-blocker therapy begun 1 to 4 weeks after an AMI has been shown to reduce mortality by about 23% ($P < .001$), with effects maintained for several years and particularly evident in high-risk patients.

In view of these findings, predischarge initiation and long-term use of beta blockers should be considered in all AMI patients—provided that there are no contraindications such as bradycardia, atrioventricular block, significant hypotension, or congestive heart failure or other noncardiac contraindications such as bronchospastic lung disease—and continued for several years after discharge.

Calcium Channel Blockers

Calcium channel blockers could be expected to be beneficial in patients with an AMI because of their favorable effects on the myocardial oxygen supply and demand relationship as well as their effects in preventing cellular calcium overload; however, pooled data from all trials, both short-term and long-term trials, involving the prophylactic use of calcium channel blockers in AMI have in general indicated no benefit. In fact, the use of nifedipine (Procardia, Adalat), in AMI and the use of diltiazem (Cardizem) in patients with evidence of left ventricular dysfunction may increase mortality. Results of one trial and a subgroup analysis of another trial have, however, suggested that patients with non–Q wave AMI and those without a depressed left ventricular function may experience a reduction in reinfarction rate and mortality rate, respectively, with the use of diltiazem. Furthermore, the additive benefit of calcium blockers in patients with AMI receiving thrombolytic and/or antithrombotic therapy has not been convincingly demonstrated. In balance, therefore, the case for a routine and prophylactic use of calcium blockers in evolving AMI is less convincing, and potential for harm does exist.

Angiotensin-Converting Enzyme Inhibitors

Angiotensin-converting enzyme (ACE) inhibitors reduce progressive ventricular dilatation and remodeling after myocardial infarction and in some studies have also been shown to reduce myocardial reinfarction by a mechanism that is not well understood. Several clinical trials have shown that ACE inhibitors reduce progressive ventricular dilatation, incidence of congestive heart failure, and short- and long-term mortality, especially in patients with large myocardial infarcts and in those with overt or subclinical left ventricular dysfunction. Therefore, ACE inhibitor therapy should be considered for patients with AMI, especially when there is evidence of overt or subclinical left ventricular dysfunction. Contraindications include hypotension, renal dysfunction, bilateral renal artery stenosis, and known allergy or idiosyncrasy. Therapy may be begun within the first 24 hours and continued indefinitely if it is well tolerated. Because symptomatic hypotension and reversible azotemia may occur with ACE inhibitor therapy, blood pressure and renal function should be carefully monitored during therapy.

Intravenous Lidocaine

Prophylactic use of intravenous or intramuscular lidocaine to prevent ventricular tachycardia or ventricular fibrillation in AMI has been shown to be effective in reducing the incidence of such arrhythmic events. However, the overall mortality appears to have been unaffected or possibly adversely affected, perhaps owing to increased risk for asystolic events with lidocaine. Therefore, in general, prophylactic use of lidocaine in patients with AMI, even in the presence of complex ventricular ectopy, cannot be safely recommended except perhaps in patients who have already suffered a cardiac arrest or sustained ventricular tachycardia.

Oral Antiarrhythmic Drugs

Despite the well-known adverse prognostic implications of frequent premature ventricular beats (> 10 per hour) in postinfarct patients, suppression of premature ventricular beats with class I antiarrhythmic drugs has actually resulted in 21% increase in mortality based on a meta-analysis of trials involving 6300 postinfarct patients. Results of treatment with sotalol (Betapace) and class III drugs with beta-blocking effects have been similarly disappointing. On the other hand, a meta-analysis of trials involving the use of amiodarone (Cordarone), another class III drug, in more than 1500 postinfarct patients observed a 21% overall reduction in mortality. Two large postinfarct trials of amiodarone, the European Myocardial Infarction Amiodarone Trial (EMIAT) and the Canadian Amiodarone Myocardial Infarction Trial (CAMIAT), have been completed, and the results have been presented in a preliminary form at the annual scientific sessions of the American College of Cardiology in 1996. In the CAMIAT trial, amiodarone resulted in a significant reduction in the combined incidence of arrhythmic deaths plus resuscitated ventricular fibrillation at 2 years, whereas the EMIAT trial showed no reduction in total mortality with amiodarone despite a significant reduction in the secondary end-point of arrhythmic deaths plus resuscitated cardiac arrest. Therefore, uncertainty continues regarding the overall benefits of prophylactic amiodarone in high-risk postinfarct patients.

Intravenous Magnesium

Magnesium has several effects that could produce a favorable impact in patients with AMI. These include vasodilator, antiplatelet, antiarrhythmic, and membrane-stabilizing effects. Several small studies provided conflicting data until the second Leicester Intravenous Magnesium Intervention Trial (LIMIT-2) was completed. The results of this medium-sized randomized trial showed that intravenous magnesium given during AMI reduces mortality. However, these results have not been confirmed in the much larger ISIS-4 trial in which magnesium therapy, if anything, led to a statistically insignificant 6% increase in mortality. The conflicting effects have been attributed to varying intervals between the onset of symptoms, thrombolytic therapy, and magnesium therapy. Pending completion of additional ongoing trials of magnesium therapy in which some of the potential limitations of the ISIS-4 trial may have been overcome, routine prophylactic administration of magnesium to patients with AMI does not appear warranted.

Oral Anticoagulants

Results of several early small trials and the more recently completed trials of warfarin in postinfarct patients that did not involve the use of aspirin have shown about a 20% overall reduction in mortality rate and about 45% reduction in reinfarction rate with oral anticoagulation; however, the relative benefits compared with aspirin or incremental benefits over aspirin are not clear. In view of the established safety, efficacy, low cost, and ease of use of aspirin, routine use of warfarin therapy is not recommended in the postinfarct patient. However, patients at high risk for thromboembolic complications after myocardial infarction (large anterior infarcts; infarcts with serious left ventricular dysfunction, with or without mural thrombus; and infarcts complicated by sustained or prolonged atrial fibrillation) may benefit from oral anticoagulation titrated to an International Normalized Ratio of 2.5 to 3.5.

"Reperfusion Injury" and Interventions to Reduce It

It has been suggested that reperfusion may damage reversibly injured myocytes, contributing to necrosis possibly by the release of toxic oxygen radicals,

TABLE 8. **Indications for Percutaneous Transluminal Coronary Angioplasty in Acute Myocardial Infarction**

Primary PTCA

Contraindications to thrombolysis
When AMI occurs during catheterization
Cardiogenic shock
Routinely especially in high-risk patients

After Thrombolysis

Failed thrombolysis (salvage PTCA)
For recurrent ischemia or reocclusion
Routinely for residual stenosis regardless of whether spontaneous or provocable ischemia is present (controversial)

intracellular calcium overload, microvascular injury, and leukocyte plugging leading to the no-reflow phenomenon and through other ill-defined mechanisms. However, the very existence of reperfusion injury has been questioned by others, and drugs aimed at reducing damaging effects of toxic oxygen radicals (free radical scavengers such as superoxide dismutase) or reducing calcium overload or reducing leukocyte function (leukocyte plugging may contribute to the no-reflow phenomenon) have yielded either negative or conflicting results. The concept of reperfusion injury remains a subject of continued investigation. However, it is clear that the benefits of timely reperfusion in AMI clearly exceed those of no reperfusion.

ROLE OF PERCUTANEOUS TRANSLUMINAL CORONARY ANGIOPLASTY IN ACUTE MYOCARDIAL INFARCTION (Table 8)

There are several clinical circumstances in which PTCA is indicated in a patient with AMI.

Primary PTCA

Primary PTCA without preceding thrombolytic therapy has been applied to patients with evolving AMI instead of thrombolytic therapy and has been successful in restoring infarct artery patency with TIMI grade 3 flow in well above 80 to 90% of patients with a reasonably low mortality. Nonrandomized studies of primary PTCA alone or in combination with thrombolytic therapy have suggested a substantially reduced mortality in patients with AMI presenting in cardiogenic shock. The potential drawback for primary PTCA includes the inherent delay involved in the implementation of such an approach. Several randomized clinical trials comparing thrombolytic therapy with direct or primary PTCA have been completed (Tables 9 and 10). In general, these randomized trials conducted at experienced centers by skilled interventional cardiologists have shown that compared with thrombolytic therapy, primary PTCA applied to patients with AMI results in a high rate of culprit artery patency (>90%), with the majority (about 90%) achieving TIMI grade 3 flow; reduced mortality, particularly in high-risk patients (age >70 years, sinus tachycardia, large anterior infarction); reduced risk for reinfarction; reduced incidence of intracranial hemorrhage; reduced length of hospital stay; and reduced overall cost of care. Large-scale registry cohort studies and the large Global Use of Strategies to Open Occluded Coronary Arteries (GUSTO-IIb) trial comparing thrombolysis and primary PTCA in a real-world setting using front-loaded t-PA, however, have revealed a much more modest and less impressive superiority of primary PTCA versus thrombolytic therapy. Thus, primary PTCA should be strongly considered for patients with AMI who have an indication for reperfusion but have a contraindication for thrombolysis, patients in whom acute coronary occlusion occurs during cardiac catheterization, and patients with cardiogenic shock. Notwithstanding these recommendations, in institutions where primary PTCA can be performed expeditiously (within 40 to 60 minutes of presentation), with a high success and a low complication rate, it is a reasonable (preferable in high-risk patients) alternative to thrombolytic therapy.

Salvage or Rescue PTCA

When thrombolytic therapy fails to accomplish reperfusion in a timely fashion, urgent PTCA is often used as the next therapeutic strategy. Such a strategy of rescue PTCA is successful in 80 to 90% of

TABLE 9. **Randomized Trials of Primary Percutaneous Transluminal Coronary Angioplasty Versus Thrombolytic Therapy in Acute Myocardial Infarction**

Variable	Grines	Zijlstra	Gibbons	Ribeiro
Number of patients	395	301	108	100
Exclusion criteria	Shock, LBBB	age >75 y	Shock	Prior CABG age >75 y
Lytic agent	t-PA	SK	t-PA	SK
Time from symptom onset to randomization	PTCA: 60 min	PTCA: 61 min	?	PTCA: 238 min
	t-PA: 30 min	SK: 30 min		SK: 179 min
Hospital mortality (%)	PTCA: 2.6	PTCA: 2.0	PTCA: 2.0	PTCA: 6.0
	t-PA: 6.5	SK: 7.0	t-PA: 0.0	SK: 2.0
Reinfarction (%)	PTCA: 2.6	PTCA: 1.0	PTCA: 0.0	PTCA: ?
	t-PA: 6.5	SK: 10.0	t-PA: 4.0	SK: ?

Abbreviations: LBBB = left bundle branch block; CABG = coronary artery bypass surgery.

TABLE 10. Randomized Comparison of Front-Loaded t-PA and Primary PTCA in Acute Myocardial Infarction in GUSTO-IIb Trial

Event	PTCA (n = 565)	t-PA (n = 573)	Reduction (%)
Death	5.7%	7%	18.6
Death or disabling CVA	5.9%	7.9%	25.3
Death or CVA or recurrent MI	9.6%	13.1%	26.7

Abbreviations: GUSTO-IIb = Global Use of Strategies to Open Occluded Coronary Arteries; CVA = cerebrovascular accident; MI = myocardial infarction.

TABLE 12. Trials Comparing Immediate Post-Thrombolysis (t-PA) PTCA with Deferred PTCA

Variable	TAMI	ECSG	TIMI-IIA
Number of patients	386	367	389
Immediate PTCA			
Hospital mortality (%)	4	7	8
Reocclusion (%)	11	12.5	Not reported
LVEF (%)	53	51	50
Deferred PTCA			
Hospital mortality (%)	1	3	5
Reocclusion (%)	13	11	Not reported
LVEF (%)	56	51	49

Abbreviations: TAMI = Thrombolysis and Angioplasty in Myocardial Infarction; ECSG = European Cooperative Study Group; TIMI = Thrombolysis in Myocardial Infarction; LVEF = left ventricular ejection fraction.

cases, but mortality remains high, especially when it fails (Table 11). Furthermore, patients undergoing rescue PTCA face a relatively high risk for early reocclusion, and left ventricular function rarely improves. Some investigators have suggested that if a combination of thrombolytic agents such as t-PA plus urokinase is used, the safety and efficacy of rescue PTCA may be enhanced with a much reduced risk for early reocclusion. Precisely how long one should wait before considering thrombolysis a failure is also not entirely clear. My observations would suggest that most patients who reperfuse after administration of t-PA do so within about 1.5 hours, whereas patients receiving streptokinase reperfuse within 3 hours. Thus, one could argue that patients should be observed for 1.5 to 3 hours, depending on the thrombolytic agent used. However, this is an area of controversy. In my institution, the patients who are clinically and hemodynamically stable are observed for about 1.5 hours before rescue PTCA is considered for a failure of thrombolysis. However, patients in shock or severe pump failure receive thrombolytic therapy en route to the cardiac catheterization laboratory.

PTCA After Successful Thrombolysis

Immediately after successful thrombolytic therapy, the site of original coronary artery occlusion generally demonstrates a critical underlying stenosis that is composed of the residual unlysed thrombus and the underlying fissured coronary plaque. PTCA of this residual stenosis immediately after thrombolysis does not reduce the risk for reocclusion and in fact is associated with an increased mortality and morbidity; hence, in patients who have undergone successful thrombolysis, immediate cardiac catheterization and PTCA is neither necessary nor advisable (Table 12). However, with improvements in interventional techniques, increasing use of intracoronary stents, and increasing use of potent antiplatelet therapy such as an antibody against the platelet glycoprotein IIb-IIIa receptor (ReoPro or abciximab or 7E3), PTCA soon after thrombolytic therapy may be safer and more effective than in the past.

Conservative Versus Aggressive Therapy After Successful Thrombolysis

After successful thrombolytic therapy, patients with uncomplicated disease may be managed in a conservative fashion or with aggressive invasive intervention. The conservative approach consists of noninvasive risk stratification using stress testing on day 5 to 7 with cardiac catheterization in patients with evidence of significant residual provocable ischemia. After cardiac catheterization and depending on coronary anatomy, one may choose PTCA or coronary artery bypass surgery. In the more aggressive strategy, all postinfarct patients undergo coronary

TABLE 11. Review of Trials of Salvage Percutaneous Transluminal Coronary Angioplasty for Thrombolysis Failure in Acute Myocardial Infarction

Lytic Agent	Number of Patients	Success	Reocclusion	Change in LVEF	Mortality (%)
SK or UK or combination	308	260/308 (84%)	31/223 (14%)	−1	11.2
t-PA only	252	191/252 (76%)	38/157 (24%)	−1	9.5
Total	560	451/560 (80%)	69/380 (18%)	−1	10.6

Abbreviations: UK = urokinase; LVEF = left ventricular ejection fraction.
Adapted from Ellis SG, Van de Werf F, Ribeiro-daSilva E, Topol EJ: Present status of rescue coronary angioplasty: Current polarization of opinion and randomized trials. Reprinted with permission from the American College of Cardiology (Journal of the American College of Cardiology, 1992, Vol 19, Pages 681–686).

angiography routinely on day 3 to 5 without prior provocative testing. The results of a comparative randomized trial, the TIMI-IIB study, have shown that the outcome of patients is similar whether a conservative approach or an aggressive approach is used. Thus, it appears that patients could be managed conservatively without need for aggressive intervention except in patients with spontaneous or provocable postinfarction ischemia.

NEW DIRECTIONS IN REPERFUSION THERAPY

Several new strategies for achieving infarct artery patency are currently under investigation. These include the use of high-dose intravenous heparin without lytic agents, use of more potent antithrombotic agents such IIb-IIIa platelet receptor–blocking drugs such as ReoPro (a monoclonal chimeric antibody) alone or with lytic therapy, and use of direct thrombin inhibitors such as Hirudin, new lytic agents such as staphylokinase, mutants of t-PA (r-PA, TNK t-PA, nt-PA), and intracoronary stents. The precise role of these strategies will be defined by currently ongoing studies.

OTHER INTERVENTIONS IN ACUTE MYOCARDIAL INFARCTION

Intra-aortic Balloon Counterpulsation

Intra-aortic balloon counterpulsation is a useful circulatory assist device that maintains or augments coronary artery perfusion pressure by augmenting aortic pressure during cardiac diastole and reduces ventricular afterload during systole. The net result of these effects is to stabilize the acutely ischemic patient, which then allows subsequent definitive diagnostic and therapeutic interventions to be carried out with considerably more safety. Intra-aortic balloon counterpulsation is indicated in patients with AMI with severe recurrent and ongoing ischemia associated with severe hemodynamic compromise (hypotension, severe congestive heart failure), acute severe mitral regurgitation, or ventricular septal rupture and as an adjunct to high-risk PTCA (Table 13).

Other Circulatory Assist Devices

Devices such as the percutaneous cardiopulmonary bypass system, the left- and right-sided heart assist

TABLE 13. Indications for Intra-aortic Balloon Pumping in Acute Myocardial Infarction

AMI complicated by
  Severe pump failure and shock
  Severe recurrent or ongoing peri-infarction ischemia
  Acute severe mitral regurgitation
  Acute septal rupture
AMI patient undergoing high-risk angioplasty
AMI patient with threatening coronary anatomy
  undergoing cardiac surgery

TABLE 14. Indications for Urgent Surgery in Acute Myocardial Infarction

AMI complicated by
  Mechanical lesions (papillary muscle rupture, septal rupture, free wall rupture)
  Recurrent or ongoing peri-infarction ischemia
  Severe pump failure related to mechanical lesions and/or peri-infarction ischemia
Evolving AMI (as a routine intervention for reperfusion)*

*Controversial and practiced only at a limited number of centers.

device, and the Hemochron pump are other techniques for providing temporary circulatory assist to patients with acute ischemic syndromes during periods of severe hemodynamic compromise and often as a bridge to subsequent surgery.

Surgery in Acute Myocardial Infarction

Although a limited number of medical centers continue to perform urgent coronary artery bypass surgery during evolving AMI with good short-term and long-term results, urgent surgery in AMI is generally reserved in most medical centers for patients with serious complications of myocardial infarction, such as the development of acute severe mitral regurgitation with or without papillary muscle rupture, acute septal rupture, free wall rupture especially when it is subacute or associated with a pseudoaneurysm, refractory cardiogenic shock in a relatively young patient, and postinfarction recurrent severe ischemia when such ischemia cannot be managed with nonsurgical means such as drugs and PTCA. Surgery may also be performed in the subacute phase in patients with an AMI in whom severe multivessel disease or left main-stem disease has been demonstrated during in-hospital angiography (Table 14).

ROLE OF RISK FACTOR MODIFICATION AFTER ACUTE MYOCARDIAL INFARCTION

Active and aggressive risk factor modification after myocardial infarction must be considered for all patients to reduce the incidence of recurrent events and improve long-term outcome and reduce resource use. In this regard, smoking cessation, use of a Mediterranean-style diet and diet low in animal fat and enriched with fruits and vegetables, and drug-induced lipid modification have been proved to be particularly beneficial. The Scandinavian Simvastatin Survival Study (4S) trial and the Cholesterol and Recurrent Events (CARE) trial have clearly established the substantive (24 to 40%) reduction in overall mortality and cardiovascular mortality and non-fatal myocardial infarction events in post–myocardial infarction patients with normal or average levels of cholesterol (CARE) or mild to moderate elevations in cholesterol (4S) using hydroxymethylglutaryl–coenzyme A reductase inhibitors (simvastatin [Zocor] in the 4S study and pravastatin [Pravachol] in the CARE study) to reduce low-density lipoprotein cholesterol levels. These beneficial effects were observed in both sexes, in diabetic as well as in nondiabetic patients, and in younger (<60 years) as well as in older (60 to 75 years) patients. A reduction in the incidence of stroke and heart failure as well as in the need for PTCA and coronary bypass surgery with the use of lipid-lowering therapy was also demonstrated. On the basis of these data, lipid lowering should be seriously considered for all patients with AMI.

Although several experimental and epidemiologic studies have suggested potential benefits of antioxidant therapy, unambiguous proof of efficacy and safety of such interventions is still unavailable. A small trial of vitamin E in postinfarct patients demonstrated a significant reduction in nonfatal reinfarction rate, although overall mortality was not reduced. Currently ongoing prospective trials should be better able to clarify the role of antioxidant vitamins in patients with known coronary artery disease. Similarly, experimental and epidemiologic studies have suggested that estrogen replacement therapy is likely to reduce cardiovascular events by 40 to 50% in the postmenopausal state with only a slight risk for breast or uterine cancer. Currently ongoing prospective randomized trials should provide more definitive answers within the next few years. Other interventions that are likely to be beneficial include control of diabetes and hypertension, regular exercise, weight loss, and stress reduction.

APPENDIX

Practical Guidelines for the Use of Reperfusion Therapy in Acute Myocardial Infarction

Indications

AMI with onset of symptoms within the preceding 12 hours

Patients may be considered beyond the 12-hour window if (1) ischemic symptoms are recurrent, intermittent, or ongoing (suggestive of intermittent coronary occlusion and a stuttering pattern of infarct evolution) or (2) the patient presents with severe pump failure, i.e., pulmonary edema or shock.

Diagnosis of AMI should be reasonably secure (compatible symptoms and electrocardiographic changes); when in doubt, consider doing two-dimensional echocardiography or taking the patient to the cardiac catheterization laboratory.

Acute pericarditis, aortic dissection or acute pulmonary embolism, Prinzmetal's angina, and at times acute myocarditis and cholecystitis may mimic the diagnosis of AMI.

Contraindications

ABSOLUTE

Any history of cerebrovascular accident, intracranial arteriovenous malformation or aneurysm, intra-

cranial tumor (some investigators include patients with cerbrovascular accidents that occurred more than 6 to 12 months before)

Head or spinal injury or surgery within the preceding 3 to 6 months

Hypertension with blood pressure exceeding 200/110 mm Hg

Severe bleeding diathesis

Serious internal bleeding within preceding 3 months

Advanced liver or renal disease

Pregnancy

Known thoracic or abdominal aortic aneurysm

RELATIVE

Each such case should be judged on its own merits, weighing potential risks and benefits.

Prolonged and traumatic cardiopulmonary resuscitation

Severe diabetic retinopathy

Recent major surgery or organ biopsy (within preceding 3 months)

Small elderly women with an uncomplicated myocardial infarction (controversial)

DRUG SPECIFIC

Because of their antigenicity (which may increase the risk for allergic reactions and decrease efficacy of lytic effect), streptokinase or APSAC (Eminase) should not be reused from 2 days to until after at least 1 year from prior use. This does not apply to t-PA or urokinase, which are nonantigenic and hence can be used repeatedly.

Because rapid infusion of streptokinase as well as APSAC can produce serious hypotension, t-PA should be preferred in hypotensive patients.

Protocol Steps

1. Establish the diagnosis and rule out contraindications.
2. Obtain baseline laboratory blood samples and an electrocardiogram.
3. Start two intravenous lines in one arm (avoid femoral, subclavian, or jugular punctures).
4. Monitor blood pressure at frequent intervals (every 2 to 5 minutes, preferably with an automatic instrument such as a Dynamap) using the other arm. Cardiac rate and rhythm should be monitored continuously.
5. Administer 160 to 320 mg of aspirin orally (chewable may be preferred for rapid absorption). Aspirin should be continued thereafter at 80 to 160 mg daily.
6. An intravenous bolus of heparin 5000 units should be administered, especially if t-PA is used. Use of intravenous heparin with streptokinase is less certain.
7. Initiate thrombolytic therapy
   a. Streptokinase: 1.5 to 3 million units by intravenous infusion in 30 to 60 minutes; slow

infusion rate or temporarily stop infusion if blood pressure falls significantly. Trendelenburg's position or temporary pressor support may also be necessary in some cases.

   b. t-PA: 10 mg bolus and 90 mg infusion in 60 to 90 minutes.

8. Other adjunctive therapy

   a. Intravenous herapin infusion (beginning after the lytic agent has been infused) at 1000 units per hour for 8 to 10 hours and thereafter adjust infusion rate to maintain a partial thromboplastin time of 60 to 80 seconds (use of intravenous heparin with streptokinase may not produce a clear-cut benefit); the infusion may be continued for 48 to 72 hours. The role of subcutaneous heparin relative to intravenous heparin is unclear.

   b. Intravenous nitroglycerin should be considered if the patient is hypertensive, is evolving a large anterior infarction, or has manifestations of heart failure; however, hypotension must be avoided by careful monitoring of blood pressure and adjustment of infusion rate. The infusion may be continued for 48 to 72 hours.

   c. Intravenous beta blockade may be initiated (in the absence of contraindications, such as bradycardia below 50 beats per minute, atrioventricular block, congestive heart failure, systolic blood pressure below 100 mm Hg, history of asthma, or severe obstructive lung disease) with metoprolol given as 5 mg every 5 minutes to a total of 15 mg if tolerated. Oral metoprolol may then be continued at 50 to 100 mg per day indefinitely.

   d. Consider oral ACE inhibitor therapy, starting with low doses, in patients with depressed left ventricular ejection fraction or overt heart failure. Therapy may be started within 24 hours in the absence of contraindications. Blood pressure and renal function should be monitored during treatment.

9. Monitor the patient's symptoms, electrocardiogram, and cardiac rate and rhythm at 5 to 10 minute intervals for evidence of reperfusion, which is indicated by (1) a rapid decrease in symptoms along with (2) a rapid decrease in ST elevation (>50% decrease compared with maximal ST elevation within 60 minutes of onset of decrease). Because ST segments frequently fluctuate before and during lytic therapy, ST segments must be monitored frequently for a reliable detection of reperfusion.

   a. Other bedside markers of reperfusion that may be observed in some patients are (1) sudden sinus bradycardia with hypotension (Bezold-Jarisch reflex) with reperfusion of the right coronary artery; (2) accelerated idioventricular rhythm (consecutive ventricular ectopic beats beginning with a late coupling interval and occurring at a regular rate of 100 per minute or less)

10. Consider salvage PTCA if no evidence of reperfusion occurs within 90 minutes or sooner if the patient is hemodynamically compromised. Patients presenting in severe pulmonary edema or shock with their AMI should be immediately taken for acute PTCA whether or not thrombolytic therapy has been administered. Supportive therapy (e.g., inotropes, intra-aortic balloon pumping, oxygen intubation) should be initiated in patients with severe hemodynamic compromise when necessary.

11. Consider primary PTCA if the patient has a contraindication for thrombolysis or is in cardiogenic shock or if it can be performed within 60 minutes of presentation by an experienced operator, especially when high-risk features (i.e., anterior location, sinus tachycardia, age older than 70 years) are present.

CARE AFTER MYOCARDIAL INFARCTION

method of
BERNARD R. CHAITMAN, M.D.
Saint Louis University School of Medicine
St. Louis, Missouri

In the United States, 13.5 million Americans have coronary heart disease, the leading cause of death in the United States. Nearly 1.5 million Americans sustain myocardial infarction (MI) each year, of which almost 500,000 episodes are fatal. MI can occur at a young age: 5% occur in people younger than 40 years, and 45% in people younger than 65 years. Acute management of patients with MI has evolved rapidly, with aggressive use of thrombolytic therapy, or direct coronary angioplasty in the acute setting. The early use of coronary revascularization for patients with spontaneous or noninvasive test–induced myocardial ischemia of at least moderate severity has significantly reduced morbidity and mortality after MI. One of the primary roles of the physician evaluating an early postinfarct survivor is to determine the extent of left ventricular dysfunction, functional capacity, extent of residual ischemic myocardium, and eligibility for cardiac rehabilitation, particularly multifactorial programs that modify adverse atherosclerotic risk profiles. Pharmacologic therapy should be reviewed and compounds known to prolong life and reduce morbidity chosen.

DRUG THERAPY AFTER ACUTE MYOCARDIAL INFARCTION

Antiplatelet and Anticoagulant Therapy

Mortality rates in the 2 to 3 years after acute MI are reduced by 20 to 25% with the use of aspirin therapy regardless of whether initial thrombolytic therapy is used. The recommended dose is 160 to 325 mg of aspirin on admission and 81 to 325 mg orally indefinitely. In aspirin-intolerant patients, ticlopidine (Ticlid)* 250 mg twice daily, or warfarin may be used. Ticlopidine should not be first-line therapy because of its cost and side effect profile. Other antiplatelet compounds such as sulfinpyrazone (Anturane) and dipyridamole (Persantine) have not been shown to reduce myocardial ischemic events after infarction. Although coronary thrombosis is a critical factor in the development of acute MI, oral anticoagulants have not been shown to be more beneficial than antiplatelet drugs in preventing reinfarction. In the postinfarct setting, oral anticoagulants are indicated for patients with large anterior wall infarcts, severe left ventricular dysfunction, congestive heart failure, history of prior systemic or pulmonary embolism, or two-dimensional echocardiographic evidence of mural thrombi. The International Normalized Ratio should be maintained at 2.5 to 3.0.

Beta-Adrenergic Blocking Drugs

The Beta Blocker Pooling Project, which combined the results of nine randomized clinical trials of beta-adrenergic blocking drugs after acute MI, demonstrated a 24% reduction in total mortality. The greatest benefit of beta-adrenergic blocking drugs is observed in higher-risk patients with electrical or mechanical complications after infarction, patients with prior MI, and patients with compensated heart failure. Although low-risk postinfarction patients also benefit from beta-adrenergic blocking drugs, the absolute benefit in terms of mortality risk reduction is considerably smaller. Major contraindications to beta-adrenergic blocking drugs include insulin-dependent diabetes, severe bronchospasm or uncompensated heart failure, and clinically significant bradyarrhythmias or hypotension. Recommended dosing regimens shown to be effective are metoprolol (Lopressor) 100 mg twice daily, timolol (Blocadren) 10 mg twice daily, propranolol (Inderal) 40 to 80 mg three times daily, and atenolol (Tenormin), 50 mg twice daily. Drugs should be titrated up to maximal effective dosage if tolerated. Beta-adrenergic blocking drugs with intrinsic sympathomimetic activities should be avoided in the postinfarct setting. Nonselective beta-adrenergic blockers such as propranolol and nadolol (Corgard)* produce systemic side effects such as fatigue and depression more frequently than do cardioselective beta-adrenergic blocking drugs.

Angiotensin-Converting Enzyme Inhibitors

Angiotensin-converting enzyme (ACE) inhibitors reduce mortality rates after acute MI, particularly in patients with anterior MI, those with an ejection fraction less than 40%, and those with a prior history of heart failure symptoms. Overall mortality is reduced by 20 to 25%, heart failure symptoms are reduced by approximately 20%, and hospital readmissions are reduced by a similar extent. The routine use of ACE inhibitor therapy in postinfarct survivors with relatively minor degrees of left ventricular dysfunction to reduce mortality risk is not clear at present and is the subject of a large multicenter clinical trial. Recommended dosing regimens include captopril (Capoten)* 12.5 to 50 mg three times daily, enalapril (Vasotec)* 5 to 10 mg twice daily, ramipril (Altace)* 2.5 to 5 mg twice daily, lisinopril (Prinivil, Zestril) 2.5 to 10 mg daily, trandolapril (Mavik)* 1 to 4 mg daily, and zofenopril† 7.5 to 30 mg twice daily. ACE inhibitors should be started at small doses and titrated up to the effective dose.

Mortality benefits of ACE inhibitors are additive to those achieved with aspirin and beta blockers. Adverse reactions such as hypotension or chronic cough are a class effect, and a reduction in dose is recommended. If symptoms persist the ACE inhibitor should be stopped and either an angiotensin II blocker, such as losartan (Cozaar)* 25 to 50 mg twice daily, or a vasodilator such as hydralazine 25 to 50 mg four times daily should be considered. The combination of the vasodilator hydralazine and nitrate therapy appears to improve symptoms of congestive heart failure without increasing mortality.

Calcium Channel Blockers

Current guidelines for postinfarct management do not recommend the routine use of calcium channel blockers. Specifically, short-acting nifedipine is contraindicated and may be associated with a significant increased mortality risk. In postinfarct survivors with a left ventricular ejection fraction less than 30%, nifedipine (Procardia), diltiazem (Cardizem), and verapamil (Isoptin) have not been shown to improve survival and may be detrimental in some patients. Amlodipine (Norvasc), 5 to 10 mg daily, has been used in patients with severe chronic heart failure and an ejection fraction less than 30% and has not been shown to have an adverse impact on survival.

Nitrates

Sublingual nitroglycerin should be routinely prescribed at the time of hospital discharge in all postinfarct survivors. In patients with residual myocardial ischemia or significant left ventricular dysfunction, long-acting nitrate therapy (e.g., isosorbide dinitrate [Isordil], isosorbide mononitrate [Ismo]) should be considered.

Antiarrhythmic Drug Therapy

Chronic antiarrhythmic drug therapy after acute MI for asymptomatic nonsustained ventricular tachycardia or isolated premature ventricular beats is not recommended with the exception of beta-adrenergic blocking drugs. In patients with symptomatic

---

*Not FDA approved for this indication.

---

*Not FDA approved for this indication.
†Not available in the United States.

TABLE 1. **Minimal Guidelines for Risk Stratification**

Risk	Characteristics
Low	No significant left ventricular dysfunction (i.e., ejection fraction ≥50%)
	No resting or exercise-induced myocardial ischemia manifestations such as angina and/or ST segment displacement
	No resting or exercise-induced complex arrhythmias
	Uncomplicated myocardial infarction, coronary artery bypass surgery, angioplasty, or atherectomy
	Functional capacity >6 METs on graded exercise test 3 wk or more after clinical event
Intermediate	Mild to moderately depressed left ventricular function (ejection fraction 31–49%)
	Functional capacity <5–6 METs on graded exercise test 3 wk or more after clinical event
	Failure to comply with exercise intensity prescription
	Exercise-induced myocardial ischemia (1–2 mm ST segment depression) or reversible ischemic defects (echocardiographic or nuclear radiography)
High	Severely depressed left ventricular function (ejection fraction ≤30%)
	Complex ventricular arrhythmias at rest or appearing or increasing with exercise
	Decrease in systolic blood pressure of >15 mm Hg during exercise or failure to rise with increasing exercise workloads
	Survivor of sudden cardiac death
	Myocardial infarction complicated by congestive heart failure, cardiogenic shock, and/or complex ventricular arrhythmias
	Severe coronary artery disease and marked exercise-induced myocardial ischemia (>2-mm ST segment depression)

Abbreviation: MET = metabolic equivalent unit.
From McNeer JF, Margolis JR, Lee KL, et al: The role of the exercise test in the evaluation of patients for ischemic heart disease. Circulation 57:64–70, 1978. Reproduced with permission from Circulation. Copyright 1978 American Heart Association.

nonsustained ventricular tachycardia, or ventricular tachycardia, amiodarone (Cordarone) or possibly sotalol (Betapace) may be used. In many patients, however, an automatic implantable cardiodefibrillator is recommended.

CARDIAC REHABILITATION

The beneficial effects of exercise training include an increase in the arterial oxygen saturation and improved oxygen uptake by peripheral tissues. The improved efficiency of oxygen transport and utilization by peripheral tissues results in a decrease in the cardiac output required to perform a certain level of exercise. Cardiac rehabilitation in postinfarct survivors improves exercise tolerance, cardiac symptoms, blood lipid levels, and psychosocial well-being. A multifactorial program that reduces stress and cigarette smoking is associated with a 20% reduction in mortality. Although the benefits of a multifactorial cardiac rehabilitation program are well established, only 30 to 35% of postinfarct patients are currently enrolled.

Phase I rehabilitation begins in the early in-hospital postinfarct phase with range-of-motion exercises and a progressive increase in activities designed to prevent physical deconditioning and the decreases in plasma volume that occur with bed rest. Early mobilization reduces the risk of thromboembolic complications and autonomic dysfunction.

Phase II structured outpatient multifactorial programs of exercise training and risk factor counseling and education are typically initiated 1 to 3 weeks after hospital discharge with a duration ranging from a minimum of 4 to 6 weeks to 6 months or more. The most consistent benefit of exercise training occurs when it is done three times weekly for 12 or more weeks' duration with aerobic exercise training sessions of 20 to 40 minutes at an intensity approximating 70 to 85% of the baseline exercise test heart rate. Exercise training intensities in the 50 to 70% target heart rate range rather than 70 to 85% have been shown to effect comparable improvements in functional capacity and endurance, may provide greater safety during unsupervised exercise, and are likely to promote longer term adherence to exercise programs. Medically supervised programs are recommended for moderate- to high-risk patients (Table 1). Electrocardiographic monitoring is recommended in higher risk patients (Table 2). Strength training improves skeletal muscle strength and endurance in clinically stable coronary patients, and training measures designed to increase musculoskeletal strength can safely be included in the exercise-based rehabilitation of stable coronary patients when appropriate instruction and surveillance are provided. The American College of Sports Training recommends that 8 to 10 resistive exercises of the major muscle groups be included in the rehabilitation program 2 days per week. Strength training is of particular importance to patients whose occupation involves physical labor.

In phase III cardiac rehabilitation, the goal is to develop a lifelong pattern of regular aerobic exercise and further modify risk factors. Phase III rehabilitation may be undertaken in a community program or at home.

TABLE 2. **Criteria for Electrocardiographic Monitoring**

1. Severely depressed left ventricular function (ejection fraction <30%)
2. Resting complex ventricular arrhythmia
3. Ventricular arrhythmias appearing or increasing with exercise
4. Decrease in systolic blood pressure with exercise
5. Survivors of sudden cardiac death
6. Survivors of myocardial infarction complicated by congestive heart failure, cardiogenic shock, serious ventricular arrhythmias, or some combination of the three
7. Severe coronary artery disease and marked exercise-induced ischemia (ST segment depression ≥2 mm)
8. Inability to self-monitor heart rate because of physical or intellectual impairment

From Parmley WW: Position report on cardiac rehabilitation: Recommendations of the American College of Cardiology on cardiovascular rehabilitation. Reprinted with permission from the American College of Cardiology (Journal of the American College of Cardiology, 1986, Vol 7, pages 451–453).

Components of cardiac rehabilitation services include exercise training, education, counseling, and behavioral interventions designed to optimize risk factor status, including improvements in blood lipid and lipoprotein profiles; dietary modification and physical activity in obese patients over 120% of their ideal body weight for height; blood glucose and blood pressure levels; and cessation of smoking. The program should be designed to reduce stress and anxiety and lessen depressive symptoms, seen in approximately 33 to 50% of postinfarct survivors. Depression is associated with increased mortality and morbidity after MI.

SMOKING CESSATION

Smoking doubles total mortality and the risk of recurrent infarction and sudden death in postinfarct patients. The risk of recurrent MI decreases immediately on smoking cessation and within 3 years reaches that of survivors of MI who have never smoked. Smoking cessation rates are highest among patients who receive strong and repeated advice to quit smoking from health care professionals. Complete cessation of smoking is strongly encouraged for patients and their families, and counseling, nicotine replacement, and behavioral modification programs should be used to achieve this goal. However, only 16 to 26% of patients stop smoking after an MI.

LIPID MANAGEMENT

In postinfarct survivors, the lipid profile may take 4 to 6 weeks to stabilize. Once a lipid profile is established, the primary goal is to reduce low-density lipoprotein (LDL) cholesterol less than 100 mg per dL, increase high-density lipoprotein (HDL) cholesterol to greater than 35 mg per dL, and reduce triglyceride levels to less than 200 mg per dL. Secondary coronary prevention trials have shown significant reductions in fatal cardiac events, nonfatal MI, the need for coronary revascularization, and stroke with achievement of LDL cholesterol levels less than 100 to 125 mg per dL, with the greatest reduction in patients with the highest LDL cholesterol values pretreatment. The American Heart Association stepped dietary approach should be used with drug therapy (a statin [HMG-CoA reductase inhibitor], a resin [bile acid sequestrant], or niacin) for elevated LDL cholesterol with normal or mildly elevated triglyceride levels, and combined drug therapy with a fibrate in patients with elevated triglyceride levels (400 mg per dL). Weight reduction and physical activity are important components of lipid management.

DIABETES MELLITUS

Diabetes results in endothelial dysfunction and accelerated platelet deposition, with advanced glycosylation proteins promoting inflammatory cell recruitment and smooth muscle proliferation. Intensive treatment of elevated blood glucose levels delays the onset and slows the progression of diabetic retinopathy, nephropathy, and neuropathy in patients with insulin-dependent diabetes. These complications can be reduced by dietary management, combined with the use of either oral hypoglycemics or insulin therapy when appropriate to target hemoglobin A_{1c} levels less than 8.5%. Hemoglobin A_{1c} levels to monitor long-term diabetes control are more stable than random blood glucose levels, which may be influenced by physical activity levels, carbohydrate intake, or the timing of blood sampling.

HYPERTENSION

In hypertensive patients, weight control, physical activity, alcohol moderation, and moderate sodium restriction are indicated in all patients with blood pressures greater than 140/90 mm Hg. Target therapy should be individualized according to age, race, and choice of initial therapy or combination therapy to achieve the target blood pressure. The choice of blood pressure medication in postinfarct survivors should take into consideration the fact that beta-adrenergic blocking drugs and ACE inhibitors have been shown to prolong life in the postinfarct setting.

HORMONE REPLACEMENT THERAPY

Hormone replacement therapy should be considered in all postmenopausal women with individualized recommendations titrated against other health risks. Estrogen therapy has potential benefits on the lipid profile, with elevation of HDL levels, antioxidant effects, inhibition of smooth muscle hyperplasia, and reversal of impaired vasodilatory responses in the endothelium. In type IV hyperlipidemia, estrogen may aggravate hypertriglyceridemia. Large-scale randomized clinical trials are necessary to firmly establish the routine use of estrogen supplementation for postmenopausal women in secondary prevention after infarction.

ANTIOXIDANTS

Vitamin E (α-tocopherol) may have a role in the prevention of atherosclerosis through inhibition of oxidation of LDL. In the Cambridge Heart Antioxidant Study, 400 to 800 IU daily significantly reduced the risk of cardiovascular death and nonfatal MI in patients with angiographically proven coronary disease. The beneficial effect was primarily due to reduction of nonfatal MI. The effect of α-tocopherol treatment in the postinfarct setting requires further study.

PERICARDITIS

method of
DAVID H. SPODICK, M.D., D.Sc.
University of Massachusetts Medical School
Worcester, Massachusetts

Treatment of pericarditis is aimed at (1) suppressing symptoms, (2) relieving cardiac compression by pericardial effusion or constriction, and (3) controlling or destroying the etiologic agents and processes.

SUPPRESSION OF SYMPTOMS
Pain, Fever, and Discomfort

Pain is managed by using the lowest effective doses of individual or combined analgesic agents. Except in some patients with surgically induced pericarditis, escalation to maximal dosages and combined therapy with simpler medications should be attempted before resorting to corticosteroid treatment. Careful attention to contraindications and monitoring for side effects are mandatory, particularly for anti-inflammatory agents and especially for nonsteroidal agents. In any case, management of symptoms should be commensurate with the patient's distress. Frequently, in mild cases no symptomatic treatment is necessary.

Nonsteroidal anti-inflammatory drugs (NSAIDs) are the mainstay of treatment of both pain and inflammation (in patients with fever, aspirin should be considered first—325 to 650 mg every 4 to 6 hours). The principal NSAID of value, ibuprofen, has the best side effect profile and the largest dose range among patients who can tolerate it, beginning with 800 mg every 8 hours and increasing to every 6 hours with the option of raising the dose to 1000 mg.* Otherwise, any NSAID may be tried with the exception of indomethacin (Indocin) in adults, a drug that often works but that reduces coronary flow and increases the size of experimental myocardial infarcts. If pain is refractory or severe before the effects of these agents become manifest (usually a matter of a few hours), an icebag on the precordium occasionally suffices (not to be used in patients with ischemic heart disease). Otherwise, codeine, 60 mg every 4 hours, is particularly useful if there is a distressing cough, or morphine sulfate, 10 to 15 mg intramuscularly every 4 to 6 hours, or pentazocine (Talwin), 50 mg every 2 hours for up to 10 doses† a day may be tried. Tranquilizers may be needed for anxious patients who are not taking an opiate, notably those with heart disease, related or unrelated, who are often worried by any chest discomfort.

Occasional marked nausea or vomiting may require a 5- to 25-mg suppository of prochlorperazine (Compazine). Palpitations are uncommon and usually subside after suppression of pain. Important rhythm disturbances occur only in patients with underlying valvular or myocardial disease (including myocarditis); these patients require specific antiarrhythmic agents if the arrhythmia causes hemodynamic impairment or is unusually distressing.

Large nontamponading effusions may cause thoracic or abdominal distress requiring a palliative pericardiocentesis.

---

*Exceeds dosage recommended by the manufacturer. Rarely needed except in corticosteroid-dependent cases (see later).
†Exceeds dosage recommended by the manufacturer.

Corticosteroid agents should be a last resort (unless pericarditis is produced by a syndrome for which such treatment is necessary) because of the growing number of individuals with chronic recurrent or incessant pericarditis who are "hooked" on an agent, usually prednisone, and cannot discontinue it without experiencing disabling discomfort.

RELIEF OF CARDIAC COMPRESSION
Acute Cardiac Tamponade

Acute cardiac tamponade is a major emergency requiring removal of pericardial fluid by paracentesis or surgical drainage. The technique of pericardiocentesis should be learned from an experienced mentor. In any case, needle drainage should always include a pericardial catheter to remain in situ for continuous drainage until the effusion ceases. The echocardiogram can demonstrate the optimal site for needle-catheter drainage, which is at the subxiphoid location in approximately 50% of patients. However, *surgical drainage is safest.* Until recently, most experience has been with a subxyphoid incision, which is extrapleural and extraperitoneal and permits a resection of a large specimen of pericardium and inspection manually or by scope of the pericardial cavity and both layers of the pericardium. In any case, except in an emergency, needle paracentesis should be avoided if there is less than a 5-mm depth of anterior effusion fluid. Another option is thoracoscopic drainage, which also permits both resection of large amounts of pericardium and creation of a window into the adjacent pleural cavity, usually the left. Pericardial windows can also be made with a double-balloon technique via a pericardial catheter.

Medical therapy supporting the heart and circulation during cardiac tamponade remains controversial and has not been conclusively demonstrated to be effective except in patients who are dehydrated. In any case, the administration of oxygen, blood volume expansion, and the use of inotropic agents have increased the ejection fraction, especially when this treatment is combined with afterload reduction. Theoretically, dobutamine (Dobutrex) is the best agent; however, *there is no substitute for drainage.*

Under certain conditions, open thoracotomy with pericardial resection is necessary; these conditions are (1) recurrence of tamponade after partial (subxiphoid) pericardial resection, (2) recurrence of malignant pericardial effusion, (3) tamponade in dialyzed uremic patients who are unresponsive to increased dialysis and intrapericardial instillation of a corticosteroid, and (4) *almost every patient with severe suppurative pericarditis (particularly children).* If cardiac compression can be even partially relieved by needle drainage, this procedure is optimal before general anesthesia is induced. Anti-inotropic and anticoagulant treatments must be discontinued.

Chronic or Recurrent Acute Cardiac Tamponade

Although pericardiocentesis may be a temporary expedient, recurrent tamponade or epicardial constriction often makes pericardiectomy mandatory. Although extremely ill patients may undergo a window operation with fenestration of the pericardium into the adjacent pleural cavity, *all pericardial windows eventually close.* Therefore, the widest excision is best, preferably through a thoracoscope unless other conditions make thoracotomy necessary.

Constrictive Pericarditis (Chronic, Subacute, or Acute)

All patients recovering from any kind of acute pericarditis (excepting rheumatic) should be followed indefinitely because of the possibility of eventual constriction. Naturally, some causes, for example, tuberculosis, require a more intense follow-up. Patients with only asymptomatic pericardial thickening and calcification do not require treatment even if the calcification is extensive. However, they should be followed up especially closely.

The definitive treatment is extensive (complete or quasi-complete) pericardiectomy. In occasional patients with mild acute constriction (and there is some evidence that this occurs frequently, although subclinically, after many instances of acute pericarditis), the syndrome resolves spontaneously or with anti-inflammatory management. In patients with definite constriction, the usual measures to relieve heart failure and systemic congestion may be tried, paying careful attention to avoidance of overdosing and side effects. In truly chronic cases (now quite rare in developed countries) ascites may require abdominal paracentesis. The patient's clinical response is the best guide to optimal control. However, the presence of advanced liver involvement and atrial fibrillation, as seen in chronic cases, reduces the chances of surgery's being successful in the long term.

Chronic Pericardial Effusion

Chronic, apparently nontamponading, effusion may be present for very long periods, even many years, with no effect on the patient's quality of life, although in some cases reduction of lung volume induces a restrictive pulmonary defect. A number of cases have been observed in which progressive, rapid, or even sudden decompensation occurs, causing cardiac compression, so that there is a tendency to favor early surgery. Naturally, etiologic sources should be sought, particularly hypothyroidism, although most cases are idiopathic.* A few cases are due to cholesterol pericarditis or chylopericardium and are for some reason asymptomatic or minimally symptomatic.

CONTROL OR DESTRUCTION OF ETIOLOGIC AGENTS AND PROCESSES

Table 1 shows the broad etiologic range of pericardial disease, which falls into 10 major categories,

---

TABLE 1. Etiologic Categories of Acute Pericarditis

Idiopathic (syndrome; resembles viral pericarditis)*
Infectious
Parasitic
Vasculitis–connective tissue disease group
Immunopathies; hypersensitivity (including drug-related) states
Diseases of contiguous structures
Metabolic
Neoplastic
Traumatic (direct and indirect)
Of uncertain origin or associated with syndromes of uncertain pathogenesis

---

*Ultimately, nothing is truly idiopathic.

indicating the *involvement of the pericardium in every kind of medical and surgical disorder.* This list should be learned as a catechism because every new case of pericardial disease will fall into one of these categories, which may not be immediately apparent. Fortunately, the great majority of acute cases are idiopathic; when pericarditis is part of a generalized disorder, appropriate specific treatment, if available, is indicated. For example, drug-related "hypersensitivity" pericarditis calls for discontinuance of the drug. For infectious forms of pericarditis, most antibiotics tested produce effective levels in pericardial fluid when given orally or intravenously.

Idiopathic Pericarditis*

In idiopathic pericarditis the exact cause is never determined, although viral pericarditis probably accounts for most cases. The main therapeutic problems are pain, recurrences (sometimes for years), occasional tamponade, and constriction. Corticosteroid dependency occurs mainly in this group. All female patients with this syndrome should undergo screening tests and follow-up for systemic lupus erythematosus.

Pericarditis Caused by Living Agents

Viral Pericarditis. Viral pericarditis, usually diagnosed by inference from the epidemiologic and serologic findings, usually has no specific therapy. When a specific agent, such as Epstein-Barr virus, is identified, acyclovir (Zovirax) may be effective. Most cases are self-limiting, although occasionally pericarditis is combined with significant myocarditis (myopericarditis).

Nontuberculous Bacterial, Fungal, and Parasitic Pericarditis. Mortality in patients with purulent pericarditis has been reduced from almost 100% to well under 50% by surgical drainage alone. Antibiotics have further cut the remainder drastically. Because this condition remains dangerous, particularly in children and in immunocompromised hosts, rapid control is essential. Pus must be removed from the pericardium, preferably by surgery. Antimicrobial

---

*Ultimately, nothing is truly idiopathic.

treatment should be matched to organisms found in the pericardial drainage or the bloodstream. While proof is awaited, treatment with oxacillin (Bactocill), 1 gram every 3 hours,* plus gentamicin (Garamycin), beginning with 6 mg per kg per day,* may be attempted with subsequent dosages adjusted according to serum assay or creatinine level. For penicillin-sensitive patients, cephalothin sodium (Keflin) may be substituted for oxacillin. However, specific treatment should be instituted as soon as possible.

Fungal pericarditis and parasitic pericarditis require specific therapeutic agents plus surgical excision and drainage.

Tuberculous Pericarditis. Tuberculous pericarditis, whether seriously suspected or actually demonstrated, requires vigorous antituberculous therapy, usually with multiple drug regimens. Pericarditis in patients with acquired immune deficiency syndrome (AIDS) is becoming more common and is often produced by mycobacteria, particularly "atypical" organisms requiring special therapeutic protocols (bacterial and viral infections of the usual kinds also occur in AIDS patients).

Because of the tendency of tuberculous pericarditis to provoke constriction, early surgery is necessary if the symptomatic constitutional response is poor or if fluid reaccumulates despite multiple drainage procedures (painless cases seem to follow a more insidious chronic course). In any case, patients who are known to have had tuberculous pericarditis must be followed up indefinitely for late complications.

Pericarditis in the Vasculitis–Connective Tissue Disease Group

Here the treatment is sometimes disease specific, although anti-inflammatory treatment, notably with corticosteroid therapy in the most severe cases, is usually successful. In patients with rheumatic pericarditis, antistreptococcal therapy is added.

Drug-Related Pericarditis

An increasing number of drugs have been associated with acute pericarditis. The major ones are procainamide, hydralazine, certain antineoplastic agents, phenytoin, and some antibiotics. Some of these can also cause constriction. The offending agent must be discontinued.

Diseases of Contiguous Structures

Pericarditis in the course of pleural and pulmonary disease requires attacks on the originating process. The course of acute pericarditis is followed with frequent electrocardiograms and enzyme studies, which should be examined for evidence of myocardial infarction. (Computer reports on electrocardiograms

should always be overread by an experienced electrocardiographer because the computer frequently either misses the diagnosis or identifies acute pericarditis as "anterolateral infarct," and antithrombotic and anticoagulant therapies have been given, sometimes provoking a life-threatening hemopericardium with tamponade.)

Metabolic Pericarditis

Classic uremic pericarditis is usually well controlled by chronic dialysis, but tamponade requires aspiration, and the occasional constriction requires pericardiectomy. A pericardial effusion may be decompensated to frank tamponade by rapid hemorrhage or by dialysis if fluid is removed too rapidly from the intravascular compartment. The success with this form of treatment contrasts with *dialysis pericarditis,* in which continued dialysis does not suffice, and the patient may have to undergo drainage with instillation of a nonabsorbable corticosteroid or eventual pericardial resection. Occasionally switching from hemodialysis to peritoneal dialysis solves the problem (the latter for unknown reasons is associated much less often with induction of pericarditis). *Myxedema,* a rare cause of pericardial effusion, is usually without detectable inflammation. Treatment is thyroid hormone replacement.

Traumatic Pericarditis

Direct trauma, wounds of the heart and pericardium, requires emergency pericardiocentesis, treatment of shock, and early surgical drainage and repair. The surgical approach with careful inspection of the pericardium, heart, and adjacent structures is nearly always the safest and most successful because cardiac wounds can be temporarily stopped by clotting and later insidiously or suddenly result in hemopericardium. *Indirect trauma* caused by blunt blows to the chest should be observed and managed like idiopathic pericarditis. *Iatrogenic indirect trauma* is due to radiation therapy of lesions in the vicinity and produces all forms of pericarditis, the most insidious being delayed tamponade and constriction, which should be treated as outlined previously.

Pericarditis of Uncertain Origin

There is a great variety of patients in this category, for example, cholesterol pericarditis, which occurs in association with rheumatoid arthritis, myxedema, or tuberculosis but is usually idiopathic. This is treated by drainage of effusions and resection of the pericardium. Another example is pericarditis associated with thalassemia major (relatively frequent in younger patients), which is treated like idiopathic pericarditis. Most patients in this group mainly require specific therapy of the associated condition.

---

*Exceeds dosage recommended by the manufacturer.

PERIPHERAL ARTERIAL DISEASE

method of
JAMES C. STANLEY, M.D.
University of Michigan
Ann Arbor, Michigan

CHRONIC ARTERIOSCLEROTIC OCCLUSIVE DISEASE OF LOWER EXTREMITY ARTERIES (Table 1)

Arteriosclerotic macrovascular occlusive disease commonly affects the extremity arteries in elderly persons. Nearly 10% of individuals older than 70 years exhibit symptomatic lower extremity occlusive disease. This disease, like that affecting the coronary and carotid circulations, is most likely to develop in people who smoke and those with diabetes, lipid disorders, or hypertension. Blood flow alterations are also important, in that arteriosclerotic disease is usually first evident, and later most severe, at origins and branchings of arteries, with lesser degrees of disease affecting the intervening segments. Fortunately, such focal disease is more easily treated by operation or catheter angioplasty than is diffuse disease.

Men are affected with lower extremity arteriosclerotic occlusive disease twice as often as women. Clinical symptoms evolve when the tissue's metabolic needs exceed the oxygen delivery capacity of the blood flow. Claudication is the usual first manifestation, representing reproducible pain in a muscle group precipitated by a fixed degree of walking, with relief after a brief period of rest. Rest pain, a more advanced form of ischemia, occurs when the occlusive process develops more rapidly or is more extensive and collateral vessels are insufficient to supply the tissue's basal needs. This is classically manifest by pain in the distal foot (metatarsalgia) occurring at nighttime. In this setting, reduced cardiac output during sleep causes mean perfusion pressures to fall below critical capillary closing pressures and results in severe tissue ischemia of such a degree that the foot pain awakens the patient. Many patients with rest pain, in an attempt to lessen their discomfort, sleep with their foot hanging over the edge of the bed, or sleep in a chair with their foot in a dependent position. Actual tissue loss and gangrene are the most serious manifestations of this disease. However, only 5% of individuals with claudication not subjected to therapeutic interventions develop extremity gangrene during a 5-year time period. The incidence of limb-threatening gangrene in diabetic patients is approximately twice that of nondiabetic persons.

Pallor, cool skin, decreased muscle mass, and loss of secondary skin appendages, including hair, reflect chronically reduced extremity blood flow, but these are often inconsistent findings among such patients. Although diminished peripheral pulses are usually evident, a more objective means of quantitating impaired blood flow is to compare the posterior tibial or dorsalis pedis arterial blood pressure with that of the brachial artery. In normal individuals, the ratio established by this comparison, the so-called ankle/brachial index, is usually 1.0 or slightly greater. Pressures are established by the use of a Doppler stethoscope. A decrease in the index to the 0.6 range is typical of claudication. Rest pain ensues with indices in the 0.25 range. Impending tissue loss or actual gangrene is a frequent accompaniment once the index is 0.1 or less. In addition, the typical triphasic Doppler waveform associated with normal blood flow is lost as the occlusive state progresses, first to a biphasic waveform and then to a monophasic waveform. Arteriography facilitates planning of operative or percutaneous catheter-based treatment but in general should not be used as a primary diagnostic test. In fact, simple Doppler ankle/brachial pressure measurements and waveform assessments usually define the extent and location of clinically relevant disease.

Nonoperative therapy should be offered to the majority of patients with lower extremity arteriosclerotic occlusive disease that has not progressed to rest pain or tissue loss. Cessation of smoking, control of hypertension, treatment of severe hyperlipoproteinemias, and maintenance of euglycemia in diabetic patients are important in managing these patients. Pentoxifylline (Trental), a drug that increases red blood cell deformability, has been advocated as a means of increasing a patient's exercise tolerance to impaired extremity blood flow. Although a few studies exist with statistical evidence that this may be the case, this drug has not proved to be useful clinically. Similarly, vasodilators have no value in treating symptomatic lower extremity occlusive disease.

The most efficacious nonoperative treatment for lower extremity arteriosclerosis associated with claudication is an active exercise program, in the form of relatively vigorous walking for as little as 20 minutes twice a day. Patients should be encouraged to walk fast enough to develop pain after 5 minutes or so, with cessation of walking at that point for a few minutes until the pain disappears. They should then resume walking and repeat this pattern of walking and resting until 20 minutes of actual walking has been achieved. Slow walking without the development of pain will not be beneficial to the patient. The pace of walking varies from patient to patient, and in a given patient the pace or distance walked in-

TABLE 1. **Chronic Lower Extremity Arteriosclerotic Occlusive Disease**

1. Male/female ratio 2:1
2. Clinical manifestations
   Claudication (calf discomfort most common; ankle/brachial index 0.6; 5% of patients progress to gangrene)
   Rest pain (nocturnal metatarsalgia; ankle/brachial index 0.25; impending tissue loss)
   Gangrene (ankle/brachial index 0.1; amputation inevitable)
3. Nonoperative treatment for nondisabling claudication: walking exercise program beneficial in 80%
4. Treatment for disabling claudication or rest pain: percutaneous catheter angioplasty or bypass grafting (most often aortobifemoral, femoropopliteal, or femorotibial reconstructions)

creases as the collateral circulation improves. This physical activity facilitates the development of collateral vessels and reduces the severity of claudication in 80% of patients.

Percutaneous transluminal balloon angioplasty is an important means of treating select patients with lower extremity arteriosclerotic occlusive disease. This involves fracture of the arteriosclerotic plaque and is most successful in treating focal lesions, especially those affecting the iliac artery. It is less valuable for treating femoral, popliteal, or tibial artery occlusive disease. Complications attending balloon angioplasty occur in less than 10% of cases, with initial successes generally occurring in more than 75% of these patients. Unfortunately, percutaneous balloon angioplasty of smaller vessels is durable treatment in only half the cases because of later restenosis.

Surgical therapy for peripheral vascular occlusive disease affecting the lower extremities is justified only among patients manifesting disabling claudication, rest pain, or tissue loss. Various operations including bypasses or endarterectomy are possible, depending on the site and extent of disease. Arteriosclerosis of the lower extremities may be categorized as to the anatomic location of the most severe obstructive lesions, being divided into patients exhibiting (1) Leriche's syndrome, (2) generalized aortoiliac occlusive disease, and (3) femoropopliteal or tibioperoneal occlusive disease.

Leriche's syndrome is associated with occlusion of the terminal infrarenal aorta, occurring as a result of severe arteriosclerotic disease. Men with Leriche's syndrome most often have lower extremity fatigue (not claudication), lower extremity muscular atrophy, trophic skin changes with pallor of their legs and feet, and an inability to sustain an erection. A similar clinical pattern is seen in women without the erectile dysfunction component. Most patients are in the 35- to 60-year age range. Treatment consists of an aortoiliac endarterectomy or an aortobifemoral bypass with a synthetic vascular graft. These procedures can be undertaken with a mortality less than 2% and a 5-year graft patency rate of 95%.

Generalized aortoiliac arteriosclerotic occlusive disease, so-called inflow disease because it affects inflow of blood into the lower extremities, usually involves patients in the 60- to 70-year age group. Lower extremity claudication is more common than tissue loss, with the latter often occurring as a consequence of additional tandem occlusive lesions in the more distal extremity arteries. If the disease is limited to the common iliac arteries, balloon angioplasty, often with a stent, is successful in 80% of cases. In patients with more extensive disease, treatment usually encompasses an aortobifemoral bypass with a synthetic graft. This procedure can be undertaken with a 2 to 3% operative mortality rate and a 5-year graft patency rate approaching 90%. Aortoiliac endarterectomy provides a similar outcome but in patients with diffuse disease is more technically difficult to perform than an aortobifemoral bypass. In high-risk patients

with other serious medical illnesses such as cardiac disease that render them poor anesthetic and operative candidates, alternative therapies should be considered, including extra-anatomic revascularizations in the form of axillobifemoral or femorofemoral bypasses. The surgical risks are reduced with these extra-anatomic reconstructions. However, in the case of axillofemoral bypasses the long-term patency rates are slightly less than with direct aortic reconstructions.

Femoropopliteal and tibioperoneal arteriosclerotic occlusive disease is called outflow disease because it affects the vascular outflow within the lower extremity. It is most often manifest by calf or foot claudication due to superficial femoral or infrapopliteal arterial disease, respectively. Rest pain and tissue loss are more likely to accompany diseases of outflow vessels than with aortoiliac disease. Treatment usually entails a bypass procedure using a saphenous vein or synthetic graft for above-knee procedures, or an autologous saphenous vein bypass either as a reversed conduit or in the in situ position for below-knee reconstructions. Although these procedures involve dissections only within the subcutaneous tissues, operative mortality is in the 3 to 5% level. Cardiac events are the most serious complications attending these operations. In this regard, patients with both occlusive and aneurysmal lesions of the aorta or distal arteries should undergo careful preoperative cardiac evaluation, often including assessments of myocardial ischemia by noninvasive means, to ensure the absence of precarious coronary artery disease that if untreated might compromise the patient's subsequent care. This is particularly true in patients with diabetes and all individuals with symptoms suggesting coronary artery disease.

ACUTE EMBOLIC OCCLUSIVE DISEASE OF LOWER EXTREMITY ARTERIES
(Table 2)

Acute embolic occlusions of the aorta and distal arteries must be differentiated from acute thromboses of pre-existent atherosclerotic occlusive lesions. The latter usually occur in patients who have a pre-existing history of claudication or rest pain suggesting antecedent chronic extremity ischemia. Patients with extremity embolism often present as emergencies with the "five p's." These are pain, pallor, paresthesias, paralysis, and pulseless extremi-

TABLE 2. **Acute Lower Extremity Embolic Occlusive Disease**

1. Source of macroemboli: atrial fibrillation 90%
2. Site of obstruction: femoral artery 40%, popliteal artery 20%, aortic bifurcation 10%
3. Prophylactic early (heparin) and long-term (warfarin) anticoagulation
4. Mortality from underlying cardiac disease: 10–15%
5. Treatment: balloon catheter embolectomy with 85–90% limb salvage

ties. The discomfort and the color and temperature changes invariably occur distal to the site of actual arterial occlusion, with collateral vessels usually affording adequate circulation in the region of the obstruction itself.

Macroembolism is due to arteriosclerotic heart disease and associated atrial fibrillation in 90% of cases. In this situation, stagnant atrial blood may clot and subsequently become dislodged into the systemic circulation. Ventricular aneurysm thrombus and endocardial clot accompanying transmural myocardial infarctions are less common sources of emboli. The site of embolic obstruction is the aorta in 10% of patients, the femoral artery in 40%, and the popliteal artery in 20%. Mortality associated with peripheral arterial embolism ranges from 10 to 15%, usually due directly to the coexisting cardiac disease, not limb ischemia.

Treatment of macroembolism usually involves advancing a Fogarty balloon catheter beyond the embolic occlusion, inflating the balloon, and subsequently extracting the obstructing material and associated thrombus. This usually can be accomplished with local anesthesia. Limb salvage occurs in 85 to 90% of these patients. The in-hospital rate of further embolic episodes in patients not having immediate anticoagulation approaches 30%. To lessen the likelihood of recurrent embolism, all patients presenting with acute embolic disease should have immediate anticoagulation with heparin and subsequently be maintained with long-term anticoagulant therapy with warfarin.

Atheroembolism is a second form of extremity embolism. In these individuals, dislodged debris from aneurysms or extensive occlusive lesions become entrapped in small distal arteries having diameters of 50 to 200 μm. Atheroembolism may occur spontaneously or follow arterial manipulations during vascular operations or during catheterization procedures. These emboli frequently cause severe pain and may result in focal cutaneous infarctions. Occasionally a reddish blue appearance of a digit occurs due to sluggish capillary blood flow. The latter is referred to as the blue toe syndrome when affecting digits of the foot.

Treatment of atheroembolism is somewhat ill defined. Most physicians prescribe antiplatelet agents, such as aspirin, as a means of lessening recurrent embolism. This therapy may impair the stability of the fibrous cap over soft heterogenous atheromatous plaques and increase the susceptibility of subsequent embolism. Nevertheless, the thrombotic extension of the embolic occlusion is likely to be much less in patients taking antiplatelet drugs. If multiple episodes of atheroembolism are associated with tissue loss, elimination of the embolic source by aneurysmectomy or bypass and exclusion of the vessel that is the source of the emboli is justified.

ANEURYSMS OF THE AORTA AND FEMORAL AND POPLITEAL ARTERIES
(Table 3)

Aortic aneurysms are thought to be related to genetic and acquired defects in elastin and collagen

TABLE 3. Aneurysmal Disease

Aortic Aneurysms

1. Male/female ratio 4 : 1
2. Location: ascending aorta 5%, descending aorta 12%, thoracoabdominal aorta 2.5%, infrarenal abdominal aorta 80%
3. Associated femoropopliteal artery aneurysms 2%, associated lower extremity occlusive disease 20%
4. Most aneurysms are asymptomatic
5. Rupture rate of 20–30% in 2–3 y with diameter 5 cm (emergent operative mortality for ruptured aneurysm: 45–55%)
6. Treatment: elective aneurysmectomy: 95–98% survival

Femoral Artery Aneurysms

1. Male patients, bilateral 70%
2. Associated aortic aneurysms 85%, associated popliteal artery aneurysms 45%
3. Thrombotic occlusion or distal embolization 15%
4. Treatment: elective aneurysmectomy and interposition grafting

Popliteal Artery Aneurysms

1. Male patients, bilateral 45%
2. Associated aortic aneurysms 60%, associated popliteal artery aneurysms 40%
3. Thromboembolism resulting in amputation 33%, thrombosis and claudication 33%
4. Treatment: elective aneurysmectomy or aneurysm exclusion and bypass

metabolism, with 15 to 20% of affected patients having a family member who was similarly afflicted. Nevertheless, most of these aneurysms exhibit arteriosclerosis. Arteriosclerosis is probably a secondary event in aortic aneurysms, but once present it clearly contributes to further vessel wall weakening. Among these aneurysms, the ascending aorta is involved in 5% of cases, the descending thoracic aorta in 12%, the thoracoabdominal aorta in 2.5%, and the infrarenal aorta in 80%. The iliac arteries are also involved in 20% of the latter lesions. Men appear to be affected four times as often as women. In general, women with aortic aneurysms are likely to be a decade older than men with these aneurysms.

The diagnosis of an aortic aneurysm should be considered when the lateral aortic pulsations on abdominal examination or radiographic evidence of calcifications of the aortic walls suggests such a lesion. In regard to the latter, a lateral abdominal radiograph is more useful than an anteroposterior abdominal radiograph. Certain imaging studies should be pursued to objectively document the presence and size of a suspected aortic aneurysm. Ultrasonography is presently the most cost-effective manner to identify these lesions. Computed tomography and magnetic resonance angiography are more costly but provide additional anatomic information regarding the extent of an aneurysm and involvement of its branches. Arteriography, because of intramural thrombus, may give the appearance of a relatively normal aortic lumen. Arteriography should be restricted to preoperative planning of surgical therapy in these patients and not used as a diagnostic test for aortic aneurysmal disease.

Most aortic aneurysms are asymptomatic, often recognized as incidental findings during imaging studies for other diseases, or as painless pulsatile masses during routine physical examinations. With expansion, they may be associated with back and abdominal or flank pain. Lower extremity pain is not a manifestation of an uncomplicated aortic aneurysm. However, in 20% of these cases, coexistent peripheral arterial occlusive disease may produce extremity discomfort. Coincidental femoral and popliteal artery aneurysms affect approximately 2% of patients with aortic aneurysms. Multiple aneurysmal disease, such as the latter, is usually observed in men.

Rupture of aortic aneurysms appears related in part to size. In general, aneurysms 5 cm or greater in diameter carry a 20 to 30% risk of rupture during a 2- to 3-year period. Aneurysms larger than 6 cm diameter have a slightly greater than 40% risk of rupture. Aneurysms 4 cm in diameter may rupture but have a less clearly defined natural history. Many 3- to 4-cm aneurysms can be followed annually with serial ultrasonography or some other form of imaging without undue risk to the patient. The presence of diastolic hypertension or chronic obstructive pulmonary emphysema is associated with an increased risk of aneurysmal rupture.

Operation is recommended for all aortic aneurysms 5 cm or larger and those whose diameter increases more than 4 mm during a 12-month period. Operative treatment usually entails aneurysmectomy and interposition aortoaortic or aortoiliac reconstruction using a synthetic vascular graft. Surgical mortality for elective treatment of aortic aneurysms is in the 2 to 5% range. Percutaneous insertion of grafts by endovascular means awaits further technologic advances and follow-up evaluation before being considered applicable to conventional practice. Once patients have symptomatic aneurysms, the operative mortality increases to 7 to 15%. The mortality accompanying operative treatment after rupture ranges from 45 to 55%. In addition, approximately 30% of patients experiencing rupture do not survive long enough to reach the operating room. Abdominal aortic aneurysmectomy is lifesaving. Those individuals undergoing elective resection have 1-, 3-, and 5-year survival rates of 77, 64, and 48%, respectively. Individuals not subjected to operative intervention have survival rates at these same time periods of 55, 30, and 18%, respectively. Approximately 35% of patients with abdominal aortic aneurysms not subjected to surgical treatment succumb from later aneurysmal rupture.

Femoral artery aneurysms occur almost exclusively in men. The cause of these aneurysms is poorly defined but is likely related to abnormalities in elastin and collagen metabolism. Most femoral artery aneurysms exhibit arteriosclerotic changes, but these are though to represent a secondary process rather than a cause of these lesions. Femoral artery aneurysms usually present as a discrete pulsatile groin mass. Most importantly, 85% of patients with a femoral artery aneurysm have an associated life-threatening aortic aneurysm. Femoral artery aneurysms are bilateral approximately 70% of the time, and associated popliteal aneurysms occur in 45% of patients. Femoral artery aneurysms rarely rupture but often contain large quantities of mural thrombus that in approximately 15% of cases progresses to femoral artery occlusion or is the source of distal arterial emboli. All femoral artery aneurysms greater than 3 cm in diameter are appropriately treated by excision and arterial reconstruction with interposition synthetic or autologous vein grafts. Smaller asymptomatic aneurysms may be followed up without a need for operative intervention.

Popliteal artery aneurysms are associated with aortic aneurysms in nearly 60% of patients and exhibit concomitant femoral artery aneurysms nearly 40% of the time. Popliteal artery aneurysms are bilateral in 45% of cases. These lesions invariably occur in men. Like the cause of other aneurysms, their cause may be linked to a defect in elastin and collagen metabolism, although arteriosclerosis is a common histologic finding. Popliteal artery aneurysms are limb threatening. Both local thrombosis and distal embolism lead to irreparable tissue injury and subsequent extremity amputation in one third of these patients. Another third of these patients develop symptomatic leg and foot claudication. The remaining third are asymptomatic at the time their aneurysms are recognized. Rupture is an exceedingly rare complication of a popliteal artery aneurysm. Most all popliteal artery aneurysms greater than 2 cm in diameter should be treated operatively. Surgical therapy includes an interposition or bypass graft procedure with exclusion of the aneurysm. The latter eliminates subsequent embolic dislodgment of thrombus from the aneurysm. Although femoral and popliteal artery aneurysms are limb threatening and not life-threatening, it is important to remember that they are frequently associated with life-threatening abdominal aortic aneurysms.

DEEP VENOUS THROMBOSIS OF THE LOWER EXTREMITIES

method of
G. PATRICK CLAGETT, M.D.
*University of Texas Southwestern Medical Center
Dallas, Texas*

Venous thromboembolism is a major cause of death and morbidity in the United States. Pulmonary embolism (PE) causes death in more than 100,000 patients each year in the United States and contributes to the death of another 100,000. However, these estimates may be low because the disease is most often clinically silent, with PE unsuspected in 70 to 80% of patients whose conditions are diagnosed at autopsy. Fatal PE may be the most common, preventable cause of hospital death. PE and deep venous thrombosis (DVT) are particularly common in the elderly population;

TABLE 1. **Risk Factors for Development of Deep Venous Thrombosis**

Clinical Risk Factors

Age >40 y	Malignancy
Immobility or paralysis	Operations on the pelvis or leg
Congestive heart failure	Oral contraceptive use
Surgery and other trauma	Obesity
Advanced age (>70 y)	Varicose veins
Prior venous thromboembolism	

both increase with age with no special predilection for sex or race. In addition to causing acute morbidity and mortality, venous thromboembolism can result in long-term disability. Recurrent venous thromboembolism occurs in 20 to 30% of patients 5 to 8 years after the initial episode, and chronic venous insufficiency occurs in 10 to 30%.

ETIOLOGIC FACTORS

Stasis of blood, venous endothelial damage and dysfunction, and blood changes are major causes of DVT. These elements are apparent in considering clinical risk factors in individual patients who have been shown to be predisposed to DVT (Table 1).

Stasis of venous blood flow and pooling of blood in the lower extremities are common among hospitalized patients. Immobility, bed rest, paralysis, and congestive heart failure engender this condition. In patients undergoing operation, general anesthesia and muscle paralysis lead to pooling of blood in the lower extremities, an effect exacerbated by pronounced increases in intra-abdominal pressure during insufflation for laparoscopic procedures. The increased risk of DVT in patients with a history of venous thromboembolism and in those with varicose veins can be related to endothelial dysfunction, as well as to stasis of blood flow from chronic obstruction and to venous valvular insufficiency. A number of congenital and acquired alterations in hemostasis mechanisms have been identified that also predispose patients to DVT (Table 2). Prothrombotic or hypercoagulable states occur when deficiencies in coagulation inhibitors exist, when imbalances occur in the fibrinolytic system, when substances are present that accelerate coagulation or platelet reactions, and when diffuse endothelial dysfunction exists. Hypercoagulable states can be classified into two broad categories, hereditary and acquired. Genetic abnormalities underlie the hereditary conditions, and the biochemical abnormalities are generally fixed and persistent, and yet the clinical thrombotic events

TABLE 2. **Hypercoagulable States**

Hereditary Disorders	Acquired Disorders or Secondary Hypercoagulable States
Antithrombin III deficiency	Myeloproliferative disorders
Protein C deficiency	Malignancy
Activated protein C resistance (factor V Leiden)	Lupus anticoagulant
	Antiphospholipid antibodies
Protein S deficiency	Heparin-induced thrombocytopenia with thrombosis
Congenital fibrinolytic disorders	Nephrotic syndrome
Dysfibrinogenemia	
Homocystinuria	

are episodic. Many of these patients have a family history of venous thromboembolism, and they may present with unusual clinical scenarios such as DVT at a young age, recurrent DVT, or venous thrombosis in unusual locations such as the mesenteric veins. Patients with hereditary conditions have a greater risk for DVT when placed in circumstances, such as the postoperative state and immobility, that ordinarily predispose to DVT. The most common hereditary condition predisposing to DVT is the factor V gene mutation (factor V Leiden) that underlies activated protein C resistance and has been found in 3 to 7% of large populations. In addition to accounting for a large number of cases of spontaneous venous thrombosis, it probably contributes to postoperative venous thrombosis in large numbers of patients. An example of the additive effects of circumstantial and genetic risk factors causing DVT is found in pregnancy. It has been estimated that 60% of women who have DVT during pregnancy have activated protein C resistance and the factor V Leiden abnormality.

Acquired hypercoagulable states accompany other clinical conditions such as malignancy, myeloproliferative disorders, pregnancy, and the nephrotic syndrome. These disorders are considered to have multiple causes related to hyperviscosity, elaboration of procoagulants, and inactivation of elements that lead to alterations in the balance between coagulation and fibrinolysis. In some cases, the development of DVT may precede the appearance of the associated medical condition. For example, there is an important association between recurrent, idiopathic DVT and the subsequent development of clinically overt cancer.

Clinical risk factors are highly prevalent in hospitalized patients, and they are additive. For example, an elderly patient with a history of congestive heart failure has a higher risk of developing DVT after elective surgery than does a 30-year-old patient with varicose veins. Older patients with hip fractures and those undergoing major orthopedic procedures have the highest risk of venous thromboembolism. This risk is attributable in part to additive risk factors of trauma, advanced age, and immobility. Extraskeletal trauma is also associated with high DVT risk. DVT has been shown to be a common complication after major trauma of all types, with up to 60% of patients having venographically proven leg thrombi and 18% having proximal DVT. DVT risk is highest among trauma patients with injuries of the spinal cord, head, and lower extremities.

Venous thrombi arise most often in the soleal veins of the calf or behind valve cusps in the tibial veins. Although the risk of embolization in patients with isolated calf vein DVT is small, up to 20 to 30% of these patients have propagation of thrombi into the popliteal or more proximal veins, where embolic potential becomes a significant risk. Not all DVT originates in calf veins. In orthopedic patients, thrombi most often originate in veins contiguous with the area of orthopedic trauma. In patients with pelvic and hip fractures, as well as those undergoing hip replacement procedures, proximal DVT is present in 20 to 40% of patients who are unprotected with prophylactic measures. Fatal PE occurs in 3 to 13% of such patients. In general surgery patients, the overall incidence of DVT among patients who do not receive antithrombotic prophylaxis is 25 to 30%, and this is most often confined to leg veins. Seven percent develop above-knee DVT and 2% have PE, of which approximately one half are fatal.

DIAGNOSIS

The clinical diagnosis of DVT is nonspecific, and objective tests are required to confirm the diagnosis before therapy is instituted. The classic symptoms of pain, swelling, and increased warmth are unreliable. More than half of the patients who are suspected of having DVT on clinical grounds do not have a confirmed diagnosis on objective testing. However, a careful history and physical examination are mandatory to exclude other causes of leg symptoms, such as infection, hematoma, leg trauma, and congestive heart failure.

The standard for diagnosis of DVT is ascending phlebography, which is highly accurate in detecting calf vein thrombi as well as thrombi involving the more proximal venous segments. Phlebography is invasive, uncomfortable, and associated with contrast allergies in a small percentage of patients. Occasionally, it can cause DVT because of vein wall damage. Phlebography cannot be used on a repeated basis, and it is not appropriate, therefore, for monitoring patients with serial studies.

Duplex scanning, with and without color-flow contrast, is highly accurate in the diagnosis of DVT and has replaced contrast venography in many circumstances. The duplex scan combines B-mode ultrasonography with a real-time, Doppler color-flow image to achieve a color-coded image of the tissue being examined. The overall sensitivity for detecting proximal DVT in symptomatic patients is greater than 95%, and the overall specificity is nearly 100%. It is much less sensitive in asymptomatic patients, probably because of partially occlusive thrombus, and is unreliable for screening patients after orthopedic surgery. Sensitivity of the test in such circumstances is approximately 60%. Duplex scanning is also less accurate in detecting calf vein thrombi. It is also problematic in imaging thrombi in iliac veins or the vena cava, because bowel gas interferes with direct visualization of these structures. However, abnormal Doppler flow patterns in the femoral veins may indirectly aid in the diagnosis of thrombi at more proximal levels. Most authorities consider duplex ultrasonography to be sufficiently sensitive and specific to confirm or rule out proximal DVT in symptomatic patients. This test is an excellent choice for following up patients with calf vein DVT to detect proximal extension of the thrombus.

Other objective tests for the diagnosis of DVT include iodine 125 fibrinogen scanning, impedance plethysmography, computed tomography (CT), and magnetic resonance imaging (MRI). ^{125}I-radiolabled fibrinogen scanning has been widely used in the past but has been withdrawn from the market because of the potential transmission of infectious agents from fibrinogen donor pools. Fibrinogen scanning is most sensitive in detecting distal thrombi; it is less sensitive in detecting DVT above the midthigh. Impedance plethysmography has been recommended for detecting proximal DVT. However, it has been found to lack sensitivity when used as a screening test for patients at high risk for DVT because the test misses large thrombi that are not completely occlusive. Impedance plethysmography may still be used for serial monitoring of patients with distal DVT to detect proximal extension. CT and MRI are not cost-effective for routine DVT screening or serially monitoring patients with calf vein DVT. However, both may be useful in special cases. For example, CT is useful for detection of thrombi in iliac veins and the vena cava. MRI has been found to have a nearly 100% sensitivity and specificity for proximal DVT and has been useful in patients with pelvic fractures who may have thrombi in internal iliac veins that would not be detected by venography or indirectly by duplex ultrasonography.

PREVENTION

The rationale for prophylaxis of venous thromboembolism is based on the clinically silent nature of the disease. Both DVT and PE manifest few specific symptoms, and the clinical diagnosis is insensitive and unreliable. To rely on the diagnosis and treatment of established venous thromboembolism may expose susceptible patients to unacceptable risks. The first manifestation of the disease may be fatal PE. Although anticoagulant therapy is highly effective in treating venous thromboembolism, most patients who die of PE do so within 30 minutes of the acute event, too soon for anticoagulation to be effective. An alternative to prophylaxis would be to use surveillance tests such as impedance plethysmography or duplex ultrasonography in high-risk patients. Although attractive, this approach is expensive and can be applied to only limited numbers of patients at risk. In addition, impedance plethysmography and duplex ultrasonography have been shown to have only moderate sensitivity and positive predictive value when used in asymptomatic, high-risk patients such as those undergoing major orthopedic surgery. Most experts believe that broad application of effective methods of prevention is more cost-effective than selective, intensive surveillance.

Appropriate DVT prophylaxis is based on stratification of patients according to the presence of risk factors (Table 3). In low-risk patients who are undergoing minor operations, are younger than 40 years, and have no clinical risk factors, no specific prophylaxis other than early ambulation is necessary. Moderate-risk patients include those undergoing major surgery who are older than 40 years but have no additional clinical risk factors or medical patients hospitalized at bed rest for more than 2 to 3 days who also do not have additional risk factors. Graduated elastic compression stockings, low-dose subcutaneous unfractionated heparin (5000 units every 12 hours), and intermittent pneumatic compression are appropriate choices in such patients. High-risk patients would include those undergoing major surgery who are older than 40 years who have additional risk factors, or patients with myocardial infarction or other acute medical conditions necessitating bed rest. These patients would be appropriately treated with low-dose unfractionated heparin (5000 units every 8 hours), low-molecular-weight heparin (LMWH) administered once daily, and intermittent pneumatic compression. The most critical category of patients is those at extremely high risk of venous thromboembolism. This group would include patients older than 40 years who have the specific risk factors of previous venous thromboembolic or malignant disease; those undergoing major orthopedic surgery (particularly those undergoing hip or knee replacement); patients with hip fracture, stroke, or spinal cord injury; and patients with multiple trauma. These patients need intensive prophylaxis; appropriate choices are LMWH (given twice daily); warfarin (Coumadin) anticoagulation; intermittent pneumatic compression combined with low-dose heparin or LMWH prophylaxis; and adjusted-dose heparin. Antithrombotic regimens are presented in Table 4, and recommended

TABLE 3. **Classification of Level of Risk of Thromboembolic Event Based on Published Data**

Thromboembolic Event	Low Risk (%)	Moderate Risk (%)	High Risk (%)	Very High Risk (%)
	Uncomplicated surgery in patients <40 y old with no other risk factors	Major surgery in patients >40 y old with no other risk factors	Major surgery in patients >40 y old with additional risk factors or myocardial infarction	Major surgery in patients >40 y old plus previous thromboembolism, malignant disease, orthopedic surgery, hip fracture, stroke, or spinal cord injury
Calf vein thrombosis	2	10–20	20–40	40–80
Proximal vein thrombosis	0.4	2–4	4–8	10–20
Clinical pulmonary embolus	0.2	1–2	2–4	4–10
Fatal pulmonary embolus	0.002	0.1–0.4	0.4–1.0	1–5

From Clagett GP, Anderson Jr FA, Heit J, et al: Prevention of venous thromboembolism. Chest *108*:312S–334S, 1995.

prophylaxis for specific conditions is outlined in Table 5.

TREATMENT

The goals of treatment in patients with DVT are to prevent PE and to restore venous function. Maintenance of venous patency and valvular competence are necessary to reduce postphlebitic sequelae. All patients with DVT should be placed at bed rest with the legs elevated until symptoms subside. Anticoagulation is the mainstay of treatment in proximal DVT

TABLE 4. **Antithrombotic Regimens to Prevent Venous Thromboembolism**

Method	Description
Low-dose heparin	5000 U heparin given SC q 8–12 h, starting 1–2 h before operation
Adjusted-dose subcutaneous heparin	3500 U heparin given SC q 8 h with postoperative dose adjustments by ±500 U to maintain APTT at high-normal values
Low-molecular-weight heparin and heparinoids	Various doses, depending on preparation given SC once or twice daily
Moderate-dose perioperative warfarin	Start moderate daily dose (5 mg) the day of or the day after operation; adjust dose for prothrombin time ratio of 1.3–1.5 (INR 2–3) by day 5
Pre- and postoperative two-step warfarin	Start 1–2.5 mg/d 5–14 d before operation, aiming for 2–3 s increase in prothrombin time at time of operation; give 2.5–5 mg/d, aiming for prothrombin time ratio of 1.3–1.5 (INR 2–3) in postoperative period
Minidose warfarin	Start 1 mg/d 10–14 d before operation, aiming for INR = 1.5 after operation
Intermittent pneumatic compression and/or elastic stocking	Start immediately before operation, and continue until fully ambulatory

Abbreviations: APTT = activated partial thromboplastin time; INR = International Normalized Ratio.

(DVT involving the popliteal and more cephalad veins). Isolated calf vein DVT that remains confined to the calf is associated with a low risk of clinically evident PE (<1%) or recurrent DVT (2%). However, most authorities believe that patients with symptomatic calf vein thrombosis should be treated with full anticoagulant therapy. Most patients with asymptomatic calf vein DVT can be managed with leg elevation alone if serial noninvasive testing is used to detect proximal extension of the thrombus. This occurs in approximately 20% of patients, and anticoagulation is begun in this circumstance. Anticoagulation should also be used in patients with isolated calf vein DVT in whom serial noninvasive testing cannot be performed.

A combination of continuous intravenous heparin and oral warfarin is the standard anticoagulant therapy for DVT. Heparin and warfarin begun simultaneously is appropriate in patients who are medically stable. This allows shortening the hospital stay to 5 to 7 days, during which the warfarin dosage is adjusted. Exceptions to simultaneous administration of warfarin and heparin include patients who require immediate medical or surgical intervention (such as thrombolysis or insertion of a vena cava filter), patients in the intensive care unit who have multiple invasive lines, and patients with conditions that predispose them to major bleeding.

Immediate, aggressive heparin therapy is necessary to halt the thrombotic process and to prevent embolization. The critical therapeutic level of heparin as measured by the activated partial thromboplastin time (APTT) is 1.5 times the control value, and it is important to establish this level within the first 24 hours of treatment. There is considerable variability in the APTT response to different heparin blood levels in individual patients, and dosages to achieve therapeutic levels are generally higher within the first 24 to 48 hours after presentation. Aggressive therapy based on monitoring the APTT is important. Failure to achieve an APTT ratio of 1.5 is associated with an unacceptably high risk of recur-

TABLE 5. **Recommended Prophylaxis for Venous Thromboembolism**

Classification	Description	Prophylaxis Options*
Low risk	Uncomplicated surgery in patients <40 y (no other risk factors)	No specific prophylaxis Early ambulation
Moderate risk	Major surgery in patients >40 y old and medical patients at bed rest for 2–3 d (no other risk factors)	Elastic stockings or heparin 5000 U SC bid or IPC
High risk	Major surgery in patients >40 y old and/or one or more of the following: MI, CHF Immobility (>3 d) Elective neurosurgery	Heparin 5000 U SC tid *or* IPC *or* LMWH
Very high risk	Major surgery in patients >40 y old and/or one or more of the following: History of DVT and/or PE Fx: pelvis, femur, tibia Malignancy (not skin) Major trauma Spinal cord injury Paralytic stroke Orthopedic Total hip arthroplasty Total knee arthroplasty	LMWH *or* Warfarin *and* IPC or elastic stockings LMWH or warfarin or adjusted-dose heparin, LMWH or IPC LMWH or IPC

*Prophylaxis until patient is fully ambulatory.
Abbreviations: LMWH = low-molecular-weight heparin; IPC = intermittent pneumatic compression; MI = myocardial infarction; CHF = congestive heart failure; Fx = fracture; DVT = deep venous thrombosis; PE = pulmonary embolism.

rent venous thromboembolism; in contrast, there is little or no association between supratherapeutic APTT responses (an APTT ratio of 2.5 or more) and the risk of bleeding. Bleeding during treatment with heparin depends more on underlying clinical risk factors such as recent surgery or active lesions predisposing to gastrointestinal or genital urinary bleeding than on the level of the APTT.

An excellent protocol for the initiation of continuous heparin therapy is outlined in Table 6, and a heparin dose titration scheme based on the APTT is displayed in Table 7. The use of a heparin nomogram, as opposed to standardized dosing of heparin, guarantees that virtually all patients will achieve a therapeutic heparin level as measured by the APTT within the first 24 hours.

Warfarin is usually begun as an oral dose of 10 mg per day for 2 days. There is a delay in the anticoagulant effect because of the half-life of the coagulation factors whose hepatic synthesis is reduced by warfarin administration. To shorten the duration of hospitalization, one can start warfarin simultaneously with continuous heparin administration; the warfarin dose is then adjusted according to the one-stage prothrombin time, which is adjusted to a level according to the International Normalized Ratio (INR) of 2 to 3. It is possible to predict dose requirements based on observations of the prothrombin time response after a fixed dose of warfarin over an interval of a few days. A simple guideline for estimating maintenance dose requirements is as follows. An individual who rapidly achieves a high therapeutic prothrombin time (INR > 2.5) after 2 doses of 10 mg is likely to be a slow metabolizer of warfarin and requires a low maintenance dose (<5 mg daily). The opposite holds for those who show little elevation of

the prothrombin time (INR < 1.5) after 2 doses. These patients usually require 5 mg or more daily. Once stabilized, the prothrombin time should be checked every 2 weeks.

Oral anticoagulation should be maintained for at least 3 months to reduce the risk of recurrent venous thromboembolism. Some patients require continued

TABLE 6. **Intravenous Heparin Protocol for Patients with Venous Thromboembolism**

1. Initial IV heparin bolus: 5000 U
2. Continuous IV heparin infusion: begin at 42 mL/h of 20,000 U (1680 U/h) in 500 mL of diluent (24-h heparin dose of 40,320 U), except in the following patients in whom the heparin infusion is begun at a rate of 31 mL/h (1240 U/h) (i.e., a 12-h dose of 29,760 U)
   a. Patients who have undergone surgery within the previous 2 wk
   b. Patients with a previous history of peptic ulcer disease, gastrointestinal bleeding, or genitourinary bleeding
   c. Patients with recent stroke (i.e., thrombotic stroke within the previous 2 wk)
   d. Patients with a platelet count <150,000 mm³
   e. Patients with miscellaneous reasons for a high risk of bleeding (e.g., invasive line, hepatic failure)
3. The APTT is obtained in all patients as follows:
   a. At 4 h after beginning heparin; the heparin dose is then adjusted according to the scheme shown in Table 7
   b. From 4 to 6 h after implementing the first dosage adjustment
   c. The APTT is then obtained as indicated by the scheme (Table 7) for the first 24 h of therapy
   d. Thereafter, the APTT is obtained once daily, unless the patient is subtherapeutic, in which case the APTT should be repeated 4 h after increasing the heparin dose

Abbreviation: APTT = activated partial thromboplastin time.
From Hull R, Raskob G, Rosenbloom D, et al: Optimal therapeutic level of heparin therapy in patients with venous thrombosis. Arch Intern Med 152:1589–1595, 1992. Copyright 1992, American Medical Association.

TABLE 7. Intravenous Heparin Dose-Titration Scheme Using Activated Partial Thromboplastin Time for Patients with Venous Thromboembolism

| APTT (s) | IV Infusion* | | Additional Action |
	Rate Change (mL/h)	Dose Change (U/24 h)	
≤45	+6	+5760	Repeat APTT in 4–6 h
46–54	+3	+2880	Repeat APTT in 4–6 h
55–85	0	0	None†
86–110	−3	−2880	Stop heparin for 1 h
			Repeat APTT 4–6 h after restarting heparin
>110	−6	−5760	Stop heparin for 1 h
			Repeat APTT 4–6 h after restarting heparin

* Heparin concentration of 20,000 U in 500 mL = 40 U/mL.
† During the first 24 h, repeat APTT in 4–6 h. Thereafter, the APTT is done once daily, unless below therapeutic levels.
Abbreviation: APTT = activated partial thromboplastin time.
From Hull R, Raskob G, Rosenbloom D, et al: Optimal therapeutic level of heparin therapy in patients with venous thrombosis. Arch Intern Med 152:1589–1595, 1992. Copyright 1992, American Medical Association.

anticoagulation for 6 months or longer, depending on the degree of venous thrombosis and the presence of continued risk factors. A single DVT recurrence should probably warrant anticoagulation for 1 year. Patients with recurrence should also be aggressively studied for hypercoagulable conditions, and those with defined hypercoagulable states or multiple DVT recurrences may require lifelong anticoagulation. The risk of bleeding is related more to the intensity of anticoagulation than the duration of warfarin therapy.

LMWHs* may supplant continuous intravenous unfractionated heparin therapy for the initial treatment of DVT. The LMWHs are given subcutaneously and have a predictably high absorption rate and a prolonged duration of action. They can be administered by injection once or twice daily for the treatment of DVT and do not require laboratory monitoring. Eliminating the need for continuous intravenous infusion and for laboratory monitoring will allow patients to be discharged earlier and eventually lead to the outpatient treatment of DVT. Because the findings associated with any individual LMWH preparation cannot be extrapolated to all LMWHs, each preparation must be evaluated in separate clinical trials. These are appearing with greater frequency, and it is anticipated that LMWHs will be approved for use in the treatment of DVT in the near future. Dosage will depend on the individual preparation approved for use.

All patients receiving heparin therapy should be carefully followed up with platelet counts obtained daily. Heparin-induced thrombocytopenia and thrombosis are infrequent, but disastrous, complications with high morbidity and mortality. The diagnosis is made on the basis of a significant decline in platelet count in the absence of other etiologic factors, usually to a platelet count of less than 100,000 per mm³. However, there is no specific cutoff for the platelet count that establishes the diagnosis. Heparin-associated thrombocytopenia with thrombosis may be preceded by a large, rapid decline in platelet count without overt thrombocytopenia (for example, a decline in platelet count from 400,000 to 150,000 per mm³). A significant decline in platelet count in 2 to 3 days should raise the suspicion of heparin-associated thrombocytopenia. The complication can also occur with LMWH.

The indications for use of thrombolytic agents in the initial treatment of venous thromboembolism remain undefined. Thrombolytic agents have been associated with a more rapid restoration of vein patency compared with anticoagulants alone. However, a number of clinical trials have shown no significant improvement in venous function and no reduction in postphlebitic sequelae in patients treated with thrombolytic agents compared with those treated with heparin alone. Thrombolytic agents do not offer more protection than heparin against PE. The higher incidence of bleeding complications in patients receiving thrombolytic agents makes this option less attractive in most cases. At present thrombolytic therapy should be restricted to patients with extensive DVT such as those with phlegmasia cerulea dolens who have minimal bleeding risk.

Deep Venous Thrombosis During Pregnancy

Standard heparin therapy remains the initial treatment of choice in pregnant patients with documented venous thromboembolism. Heparin has the advantage in that it is unable to cross the placenta. In contrast, warfarin crosses the placental barrier and causes fetal complications. In the first trimester, warfarin exposure is associated with embryopathies such as stippled epiphyses and nasal and limb hypoplasia. Exposure during the second trimester is associated with central nervous system abnormalities. In the third trimester, rates of spontaneous abortion and stillbirths are elevated, probably as a result of hemorrhage.

Because warfarin therapy is contraindicated throughout pregnancy, therapeutic adjusted-dose heparin therapy has become the standard long-term therapy. Patients suffering venous thromboembo-

---

*Not FDA approved for this indication.

lism during pregnancy are treated with initial heparin therapy (see Tables 6 and 7) for 6 days followed by adjusted-dose subcutaneous heparin every 12 hours. Subcutaneous therapeutic heparin (initial dose, 12,500 to 20,000 units every 12 hours) is monitored by the APTT, the midinterval APTT being adjusted to the therapeutic range. The duration of long-term therapy is determined by the need to protect the patient during the remainder of pregnancy, and for 4 to 6 weeks post partum. Subcutaneous heparin prophylaxis (5000 units every 8 to 12 hours) is recommended during pregnancy and 4 to 6 weeks post partum in patients with a history of venous thromboembolism.

Inferior Vena Caval Interruption

In patients who cannot receive anticoagulation or who experience recurrent DVT or PE while receiving adequate anticoagulant therapy, interruption or sieving of the inferior vena cava offers protection against PE. A number of options are available, including surgical plication or interruption, placement of partially occluding external clip devices, transluminal balloon occlusion, and placement of intraluminal filter devices. Interruption of the inferior vena cava is associated with significant morbidity, and surgical plication and placement of partially occluding external devices have a substantial risk of subsequent caval occlusion.

Because filter devices offer a high degree of protection against PE while maintaining a caval patency, they have achieved an overwhelming popularity in PE prophylaxis. Current indications for insertion of a vena cava filter are listed in Table 8. Although there are a large number of approved filter devices, the greatest experience has been reported with the original stainless steel device developed by Greenfield. The Greenfield filter is associated with long-term caval patency of 98% and a recurrent PE incidence of 4%. The filter is placed transvenously, by either venous cutdown or percutaneous introduction. The newer titanium Greenfield filter was developed for percutaneous insertion using a No. 12 French catheter introduced through a No. 14 French sheath. A modification of the hook design has improved filter stabilization, reducing the incidence of filter migration and caval wall penetration.

The filter is usually deployed below the level of the renal veins, but it has also been placed without problems in the suprarenal vena cava and in the superior vena cava. Because the filter does nothing to treat leg vein DVT, it is desirable to maintain patients with long-term anticoagulation after filter

TABLE 8. **Indications for Insertion of a Vena Cava Filter**

Absolute Indications

DVT or documented thromboembolism in a patient who has a contraindication to anticoagulation

Recurrent thromboembolism despite adequate anticoagulation

Complications of anticoagulation requiring therapy to be discontinued

Failure of another form of caval interruption

Patient who has had a pulmonary embolectomy

Relative Indications

High-risk patients with a free-floating iliofemoral and/or vena caval thrombus demonstrated by venography

Patients with a propagating iliofemoral thrombus despite adequate anticoagulation

Chronic pulmonary embolism in a patient with pulmonary hypertension and cor pulmonale

Patients with occlusion of more than 50% of the pulmonary vascular bed who would not tolerate any additional thrombus

Presence of recurrent septic embolism

Abbreviation: DVT = deep venous thrombosis.
Modified from Greenfield LJ, Whitehall TA: New developments in caval interruption: Current indications and new techniques for filter placement. *In* Veith FJ (ed): Current Critical Problems in Vascular Surgery, Vol 4. St Louis, Quality Medical Publishing, 1992, pp 113–121.

placement to reduce the risk of developing the postthrombotic syndrome and caval occlusion.

Late Treatment of Deep Venous Thrombosis

During the late phases of DVT treatment, education of the patient and long-term avoidance of venous stasis are important to prevent recurrent DVT and minimize the risk of postphlebitic symptoms. Approximately one third of patients have some degree of edema, pigmentation, varicosities, and abnormal venous hemodynamics 5 to 10 years after a single episode of DVT. Five to 10% develop ankle ulcerations. Avoidance of stasis is important to reduce venous hypertension and to control leg edema. Patients should be instructed to elevate the involved extremity whenever possible and to avoid extended periods of sitting with the legs dependent, such as on long car or airplane trips. The use of graduated compression stockings may be beneficial in controlling edema, which if untreated can lead to skin fibrosis and eventual ulceration. Because a history of venous thromboembolism is a lifelong risk factor for DVT, patients should be instructed to seek medical advice immediately should they develop recurrent symptoms. In addition, when they are placed in high-risk situations such as hospitalization for surgery or other problems, they should be counseled to inform their treating physicians of their predisposition to DVT so that they can receive aggressive prophylaxis.

The Blood and Spleen

APLASTIC ANEMIA

method of
LYLE L. SENSENBRENNER, M.D.
University of Maryland School of Medicine
Baltimore, Maryland

Aplastic anemia is a clinical syndrome characterized by pancytopenia of varying degree and a demonstrated hypoplastic marrow with no evidence of infiltrating disease. What hematopoietic cells remain must show no evidence of dysplasia. Macrocytosis may be seen in the erythroid lines, but no dyserythropoiesis or dysplastic changes of the granulocytic or megakaryocytic lines should be present. Chromosomal analysis of those hematopoietic cells present in the marrow must show no clonal abnormalities (e.g., deletions, translocations).

Aplastic anemia is classified in several ways (Table 1). The two most commonly used classifications are by severity of the pancytopenia (severe, super severe, and not severe or moderate) and etiologic, that is, whether there is an inherited condition predisposing to the disorder or the disease is acquired in the absence of a recognized underlying predisposition (inherited versus acquired aplastic anemia).

The end result of the pathogenic process is the failure of the marrow to produce an adequate number of precursors and mature cells. Toxins and other marrow-damaging agents act either by directly destroying the earliest stem cells in the marrow or by causing nonlethal damage to progenitor cells, exposing antigens that induce an autoimmune destruction of early marrow cells. Whatever the pathogenesis or etiology, replacement of stem cells from a normal donor appears able to correct the defect, because allogeneic marrow transplantation has been reported to be successful in restoring normal hematopoiesis in all forms of aplastic anemia.

CLINICAL PRESENTATION

A complication of one of the cytopenias usually results in the symptoms that compel the patient to seek medical attention. The most common presenting feature is bleeding secondary to thrombocytopenia. This is first manifested by either petechiae, especially of the dependent portions of the body, or minor bleeding from other sources, such as the gums during tooth-brushing. The petechiae frequently progress to ecchymoses, and the patient has no history of trauma to explain their presence.

The second most common presenting symptom is frequent or severe infections with no clear explanation. These infections are commonly at the sites of minor trauma, such as a small cut or a skin or mucosal abrasion. They frequently occur in the mouth, throat, nasal passages, and sinuses.

Anemia along with its symptoms of fatigue, shortness of breath on exertion, and weakness is occasionally the factor initiating the patient's visit to the physician's office.

DIAGNOSIS

The diagnosis of aplastic anemia is made by a complete blood count to determine the severity of pancytopenia. In addition, a careful inspection of the peripheral blood smear and marrow aspirate is essential to rule out any dysplastic changes. A bone marrow biopsy is essential to accurately assess cellularity and to detect the presence of any infiltrating diseases, such as metastatic cancer, leukemia, or lymphoma. Chromosomal analysis of the marrow aspirate cells should also be done to rule out clonal dysplastic disorders. Careful attention should be paid to the physical examination to rule out Fanconi's anemia. If the patient is younger than 30 years or there is any suspicion that Fanconi's anemia might be the underlying cause (short stature, history of or presence of extra or missing digits on the hands, numerous café au lait spots, or congenital renal abnormalities), a clastogen-induced chromosomal breakage study of peripheral blood lymphocytes should be done to exclude the disorder. A careful history, elucidating an underlying etiology or familial incidence, is of value for determining the type of aplastic anemia, because the approach to therapy in some cases varies with the etiology of the disorder.

TABLE 1. **Classification of Aplastic Anemia**

Severity

Super severe	Neutrophils <200/mm^3
	Platelets <20,000/mm^3
	Reticulocytes <40,000/mm^3
Severe (2 of 3)	Neutrophils <500/mm^3
	Platelets <20,000/mm^3
	Reticulocytes <40,000/mm^3
Moderate	Pancytopenia less than severe

Etiologic Classification

Acquired aplastic anemia
  Idiopathic
  Secondary to a recognized etiologic agent
    Toxins and chemicals—benzene, trinitrotoluene, chlorophenol pesticides
    Drugs—chloramphenicol, hydantoins, gold, carbamazepine, phenylbutazone, sulfonamides, penicillamine, cancer chemotherapeutics
    Viruses—Epstein-Barr virus, hepatitis (not hepatitis A, B, C, or G)
    Autoimmune disorders
    Radiation
    Pregnancy
Inherited aplastic anemia
  Fanconi's anemia
  Dyskeratosis congenita
  Shwachman-Diamond syndrome
  Amegakaryocytic thrombocytopenia
  Familial aplastic anemia

THERAPY

Supportive Care

Blood Product Support (Table 2)

Because pancytopenia is the major manifestation of aplastic anemia, supportive measures are directed primarily at correcting bleeding, infections, and anemia. Thrombocytopenic bleeding can be a serious and even lethal complication of aplastic anemia, and it is corrected primarily by the use of platelet transfusions. Major bleeding almost never occurs in patients with aplastic anemia in whom the platelet count is higher than 20,000 per mm³. Significant bleeding usually occurs only when the platelet count has fallen to 5000 per mm³ or less.

Platelet transfusions can and often do lead to severe alloimmunization, resulting in refractoriness to further platelet infusions. The fewer transfusions given the patient, the less likely that alloimmunization will result. Therefore, my colleagues and I give platelet transfusions only if one of the following conditions is present: (1) the platelet count is 5000 per mm³ or less, (2) the patient is bleeding, (3) the patient is febrile with a platelet count of 10,000 per mm³ or less, (4) the patient has demonstrated bleeding at a platelet count greater than 5000 per mm³ and the count is now that low, or (5) the patient is to undergo a procedure that could cause bleeding, such as surgery, a diagnostic "scoping" procedure, or tooth extraction.

To prevent alloimmunization, the use of leukocyte-depleted platelet products should be standard practice for any transfusion for aplastic anemia patients. If platelet support is required, 10-minute post-transfusion platelet counts are obtained to determine whether an adequate incremental rise in platelet count is obtained with each transfusion. If a poor response to the transfused platelets is detected, studies of lymphocytotoxic antibody should be carried out. If evidence of severe alloimmunization is detected, the use of either crossmatched platelets or of platelets matched for the class I HLA antigens may be required to obtain an adequate increment in the platelet count with transfusion.

Alloimmunization becomes a severe problem for patients who might be candidates for allogeneic bone marrow transplantation. Many of the antigens that are important for rejection of transfused platelets are also responsible for the rejection of an allogeneic marrow graft. Thus, it has been shown that the fewer the number of platelet transfusions a patient with aplastic anemia has received, the more likely that patient is to accept an allograft. It is important that patients who might be candidates for a transplant receive as few platelet transfusions as possible and that all such transfusions be leukocyte depleted.

As the disease progresses, red blood cell transfusions are required. Most patients can tolerate a slowly developing anemia as long as the hemoglobin level remains above 7 grams per dL. If the patient is symptomatic from the anemia at a level greater than 7 grams per dL and is unable to carry out normal activities of daily living, transfusions of red blood cells are indicated. In patients in whom bleeding is a problem, or who are to undergo a procedure that could result in bleeding, the hemoglobin level should be kept at least 2 grams per dL higher, that is, above 9 grams per dL or 2 grams per dL above the symptomatic level if that level is higher than 7 grams per dL.

All red blood cell products should be leukocyte depleted to prevent alloimmunization. Each unit of red blood cells contains about 250 mg of iron, an element the body has no mechanism for removing. If iron stores develop to a high level, damage to pancreas, liver, and heart can result, with lethal consequences. To prevent such complications, chelation therapy should be instituted early in the course of the disease. At present, the only chelating agent available is deferoxamine (Desferal), which must be administered either quite slowly intravenously or by subcutaneous infusion. The usual dose of deferoxamine is 1.5 to 2.5 grams per day given subcutaneously and using a portable pump to administer the drug. Chelation therapy should begin after 20 to 50 units of red blood cells has been administered or when the serum ferritin level is greater than 600 ng per mL.

For the severely neutropenic patient, meticulous care should be taken to prevent infections, including careful cleansing and prevention of breaks in the skin if at all possible. Finger or earlobe sticks to obtain blood should be avoided. Careful hand washing is essential, as are good oral hygiene and dental care to prevent infectious sites from developing. The use of prophylactic antibiotics is to be avoided except for coverage during an invasive procedure such as

TABLE 2. **Therapeutic Approaches to Aplastic Anemia**

Immunosuppressive Regimens

ATG, 40 mg/kg/d IV × 4 d, plus cyclosporine, 2–5 mg/kg/d IV, or 2.5–7.5 mg/kg q 12 h PO for 3–4 mo
or
Cyclophosphamide, 45 mg/kg/d × 4 d IV over 1–2 h

Supportive Care

Transfusions	Use leukocyte-depleted products. For potential transplant patients, use only CMV-negative products unless patient and/or donor are CMV-positive.
Platelets	Only if patient is bleeding or count < 5000/mm³, or if count < 10,000/mm³ and patient is febrile, or if count < 50,000/mm³ and patient is to undergo a surgical procedure.
Red blood cells	When hemoglobin < 7.0 gm/dL or patient is symptomatic from anemia (9.0 gm/dL if patient is having bleeding problems).
Neutropenic fever	Imipenem, 500–1000 mg q 6 h IV
	or
	Ceftazidime, 1–2 gm q 8 h IV
	If fever persists, add vancomycin, 1 gm q 12 h IV
	If fever persists, add amphotericin, 0.75 mg/kg/d IV

Abbreviations: ATG = antithymocyte globulin; CMV = cytomegalovirus.

tooth extraction or colonoscopy. The use of antifungal prophylaxis with an agent such as fluconazole (Diflucan) can and often does lead to overgrowth of resistant fungi. Infections that do occur in neutropenic patients must be treated promptly with empirically chosen broad-spectrum antibiotics while awaiting the results of cultures of blood, urine, throat, sputum, and any potentially infected site. Imipenem (Primaxin), 500 to 1000 mg intravenously every 6 hours, or ceftazidime (Fortaz, Tazicef, or Tazidime), 1.0 to 2.0 grams every 8 hours intravenously, is an effective empirical antibiotic regimen that can be used while awaiting culture results. If after 48 to 72 hours the patient remains febrile with little in the way of signs of improvement, vancomycin (Vancocin, Vancoled), 1 gram every 12 hours intravenously, is added to cover possible gram-positive organisms. If fever continues more than 72 hours longer with the double-antibiotic regimen and a source and organism have not been determined, or if the patient's condition appears to be deteriorating, antifungal coverage with amphotericin B (Fungizone), 0.25 to 0.75 mg per kg per day intravenously, should be added. If the patient demonstrates a serious infection with an organism shown to be resistant to antibiotics, granulocyte transfusions may be considered, but they are associated with severe reactions in addition to alloimmunization. In patients with no defined period of neutropenia, granulocytes are frequently ineffective in the long run.

Blood products can jeopardize a later marrow transplant by transmitting cytomegalovirus (CMV) as well as other viruses with the transfusions. Marrow recipients who are serologically negative for CMV and who have a donor who is negative have the best chance of not having problems with the virus during the transplantation. Therefore, all blood products given to a patient with aplastic anemia should be from a CMV-negative donor until the CMV serologic status of the patient has been established. If the patient is CMV-negative or of indeterminate status, all blood products should be CMV-negative. If CMV-negative products are not available and transfusion is necessary, a filter to remove any white blood cells should be used in the administration of the product. If the patient or the donor is serologically CMV-positive, the status of the blood product is not important. Because family members could share minor antigens with the donor, antigens that the patient may not have, family members should not be used as blood product donors for potential transplant candidates.

Hematopoietic Growth Factors

If the granulocyte count is less than 500 per mm³, granulocyte colony-stimulating factor (Neupogen) or granulocyte-macrophage colony-stimulating factor (Leukine) may be used to temporally raise the granulocyte counts. The usual dosage is 250 µg per m² per day given subcutaneously. However, this dosage rarely causes a rise in the hemoglobin level or the platelet count, and the granulocyte count drops back to the pretreatment level shortly after the drug is stopped.

Specific Therapy (Table 3)

Bone Marrow Transplantation

For patients younger than 55 years who have severe acquired aplastic anemia and for whom an HLA-identical donor is available, the therapy of choice is marrow transplantation. A sibling donor is preferred. If none is available, one can occasionally find a perfectly matched donor in the unrelated donor registry. Because the earlier in the course of the disease one attempts transplantation, the more successful the procedure is, one should refer all potential transplant patients to a transplant center immediately after making the diagnosis of severe aplastic anemia. With allogeneic marrow transplantation utilizing an HLA-matched sibling donor, one expects a long-term disease-free survival of greater than 75%. If radiation is not utilized in the regimen to prepare the patient for transplantation, the rate of post-transplantation neoplastic complications is low (<5%).

Patients with inherited forms of aplastic anemia are also candidates for marrow transplantation if a suitable donor can be found. However, it is essential to determine the underlying disease process, such as Fanconi's anemia, because patients with such processes are exceedingly sensitive to agents such as cyclophosphamide and radiation, and they must be prepared for transplantation with a much milder regimen.

TABLE 3. **Approach for Treating Patients with Aplastic Anemia**

I. Severe aplastic anemia.
  A. If patient is younger than 55 years, perform HLA typing of siblings and other potential family member matches.
    1. If a match, proceed to marrow (stem cell) transplantation.
    2. If no match in family, proceed to immunosuppressive therapy and begin searching the unrelated donor registries for a marrow donor.
      a. If anemia responds to immunosuppressive therapy, follow patient with no further therapy.
      b. If anemia fails to respond to immunosuppressive therapy, give supportive therapy while pursuing an unrelated marrow donor. Consider androgens, cytokines, or experimental therapies.
  B. If patient is 55 years or older, give immunosuppressive therapy along with supportive care.
    1. If anemia responds to immunosuppressive therapy, follow patient with no further therapy.
    2. If anemia fails to respond to immunosuppressive therapy, give supportive therapy and consider androgens, cytokines, or experimental therapies.
II. Moderate aplastic anemia.
  A. Transfusion independent: observe patient.
  B. Transfusion dependent: immunosuppressive therapy.
    1. If anemia responds, observe patient.
    2. If no response and the transfusion requirements are more frequent than once a month, consider androgens, cytokines, or experimental therapies. If patient is younger than 55 years, consider for transplantation.

Immunosuppressive Therapy

If the patient with acquired severe aplastic anemia is older than 55 years, or no donor for a younger patient can be readily identified, immunosuppressive therapy should first be attempted. The most commonly used regimen for immunosuppression is antithymocyte globulin (ATG) (Atgam), 40 mg per kg per day intravenously for 4 consecutive days, followed by 3 to 4 months of cyclosporine (Sandimmune),* starting at 5 mg per kg per day as a continuous infusion, and after 5 days gradually tapering the dose to maintain a blood level of between 150 and 450 ng per mL of whole blood. If the patient can tolerate the drug orally, it may be given in doses of 5 to 10 mg per kg every 12 hours. Careful attention to blood levels of cyclosporine and creatinine is necessary, with adjustments in the cyclosporine dose if toxicity occurs. Serum sickness, manifested as arthralgias, arthritis, fever, proteinuria, and rash, is a common complication of ATG therapy and is treated with a steroid such as prednisone or methylprednisolone (Solu-Medrol) at a dose of 0.5 to 1.0 mg per kg per day. This dose should be tapered and the steroid discontinued as soon as the process subsides.

If a patient has not shown response to the therapy by 4 months after starting the cyclosporine, it should be stopped. If, however, the patient has shown a response, the cyclosporine is tapered slowly, being reduced by no more than 5% a week, while the blood counts are carefully monitored and higher doses are instituted if the counts begin to fall. Another immunosuppressive regimen reported to be quite effective in a small series of patients with severe acquired aplastic anemia is the use of cyclophosphamide (Cytoxan),* 45 mg per kg per day for 4 days given as an intravenous infusion over 1 to 2 hours. The patients in the small series who showed a response to cyclophosphamide had no episodes of relapse of disease and no late clonal disorders.

Immunosuppressive therapy has been tried in patients with aplastic anemia secondary to Fanconi's anemia, with little success.

Androgens

Androgens either alone or in combination with immunosuppressive therapy have had some degree of efficacy, but the results have been extremely variable. Reported results vary from no response to more than 30% of patients showing response. The most commonly used agents are oxymethalone (Anadrol-50), at a dose of 3 to 5 mg per kg per day orally. At present, however, this compound is no longer available in the United States. Nandrolone deconate (Deca-Durabolin), a compound that is as effective as oxymethalone, is available and possibly has less hepatotoxicity. It is given intramuscularly (deep in the buttocks), a potential problem in patients with pancytopenia. The dosage is 3 to 5 mg per kg weekly for up to 12 weeks. We have also used danazol (Dano-

crine),* 400 to 800 mg per day orally, with some success.

Androgens have been shown to be effective in Fanconi's anemia as well and have resulted in remissions of the pancytopenia for months to even years in some patients.

---

*Not yet approved for use in the United States.

IRON DEFICIENCY ANEMIA

method of
JAMES D. COOK, M.D.
University of Kansas Medical Center
Kansas City, Kansas

Iron deficiency remains the most common cause of anemia throughout the world, both in the population as a whole and in patients receiving medical care. In most patients, iron deficiency anemia is easy to diagnose and simple to treat. Severe long-standing iron deficiency anemia can occasionally be suspected clinically in patients who present with pica, dysphagia, glossitis, cheilosis, or koilonychia, but the diagnosis is almost always made in the clinical laboratory. One of the cardinal rules of clinical medicine is that it is as important to determine the cause of iron deficiency anemia than it is to correct it.

IRON BALANCE

The content of total body iron in adults averages 50 mg per kg in men and roughly 20% less in women. More than three quarters of body iron is contained in functional iron complexes, the most important being hemoglobin in circulating red blood cells. The remaining body iron is contained in a storage compartment located in the reticuloendothelial cells of the liver, spleen, and bone marrow. The size of iron stores can be estimated reliably in healthy individuals from the serum ferritin concentration; 1 µg of serum ferritin per liter corresponds to 8 to 10 mg of storage iron. Iron stores in women of the childbearing age average about 300 mg, with 20 to 30% of women having no reserves. Men accumulate an average of 1000 mg of storage iron by their early twenties, after which there is a slow continuing rise with advancing age. After menopause, iron stores in women increase rapidly, approaching the levels in men within 5 to 10 years. There is no mechanism for excreting an unwanted excess of body iron. Consequently, the amount of storage iron is controlled entirely by the intestinal absorption of iron, which is tightly regulated to maintain body iron within narrow limits.

Basal iron loss, which occurs primarily from the gastrointestinal tract, averages 1 mg daily in both sexes, added to which is a loss of 0.5 mg daily in women through menstruation. Nutritional iron deficiency refers to the inability of dietary iron absorption to supply the iron required to replace physiologic losses. Because the latter are greatly increased during periods of rapid body growth or gestation, iron deficiency is more common in infants and toddlers and during pregnancy, when iron is needed for the expansion of the maternal blood volume and growth of the placenta and fetus.

Whether or not iron deficiency develops in the presence of increased iron requirements depends on the extent to which increased absorption of dietary iron can compensate.

---

*Not yet approved for use in the United States.

The iron content of the American diet averages 6 mg per 1000 calories and is largely independent of socioeconomic status. In men, only 5% of this iron must be retained to offset normal daily losses, whereas more than 10% must be absorbed in women of childbearing age. Ceiling absorption of dietary iron in patients with severe iron deficiency is 3 to 4 mg daily. Between 10 and 20% of dietary iron is in the form of heme, which is absorbed as an intact porphyrin complex and is therefore highly bioavailable. The larger nonheme fraction of dietary iron is much less available for assimilation and is greatly influenced by dietary ligands, which either enhance (ascorbic acid, meat, poultry, fish) or reduce (bran, tea, coffee) the solubility and therefore absorption of food iron.

CAUSES OF IRON DEFICIENCY

The main challenge for the physician who encounters iron deficiency anemia is to distinguish between the physiologic form, in which iron requirements exceed the absorptive capacity for iron by the intestinal tract, and the pathologic form, in which an underlying disease process is responsible for excessive iron loss. The key risk factors for physiologic iron deficiency are accelerated growth rate, pregnancy, and excessive menstrual loss. An exhaustive search for an underlying gastrointestinal lesion is seldom justified when iron deficiency anemia first occurs in infants or young adolescents or in pregnant or premenopausal women. Other factors that can contribute to the development of iron deficiency in these settings are chronic aspirin use, intense and prolonged aerobic training, frequent blood donations, reduced caloric intake, and consumption of a diet of low iron bioavailability. However, it should be noted that even strict vegetarians seldom develop iron deficiency anemia solely on a dietary basis.

With the preceding exceptions, the detection of iron deficiency anemia requires a careful search for an underlying pathologic cause. When an explanation for iron deficiency anemia is not readily apparent, fecal occult blood tests and upper and lower gastrointestinal endoscopy are indicated to search for a bleeding gastrointestinal lesion, which accounts for roughly one third of cases of pathologic iron deficiency anemia. Most of the remaining cases are due to vaginal blood loss or remain undiagnosed despite extensive investigation.

DIAGNOSIS

Because the demands of the erythroid marrow must be fully satisfied before iron stores can accumulate, the absence of storage iron, as defined as a serum ferritin level below 20 µg per liter in an anemic patient, is conclusive evidence of iron deficiency anemia. Several other laboratory indices reflect the iron-deficient state: hypochromia and microcytosis on the peripheral blood smear, reduced mean corpuscular volume, low serum iron, elevated total iron-binding capacity, low transferrin saturation, elevated red blood cell distribution width, increased serum transferrin receptors, and increased free erythrocyte protoporphyrin level. However, because none of these measurements is entirely specific for iron deficiency anemia, they are useful only for gauging the severity and duration of the iron lack. The only laboratory test required to diagnose iron deficiency anemia in addition to the hemoglobin concentration or hematocrit is the serum ferritin measurement, which should always be performed not only to diagnose iron deficiency anemia but also to avoid the risk of prescribing iron for patients with an iron-loading hypochromic anemia such as thalassemia or sideroblastic anemia.

The most common problem in recognizing iron deficiency in an anemic patient is when the serum ferritin level is increased to within the normal range because of inflammatory, neoplastic, or hepatic disease. Serum ferritin values above 150 µg per liter exclude iron deficiency, but lower values, between 20 and 150 µg per liter, may or may not be due to iron deficiency. In this situation, hematologists usually perform a bone marrow examination to diagnose iron deficiency on the basis of the absence of stainable iron. Studies indicate that the serum transferrin receptor level and/or the receptor/ferritin ratio can be used to detect iron deficiency even in the presence of chronic disease. The wider availability of this new test will be helpful in avoiding the need for a costly and unpleasant bone marrow examination of the patient in whom iron deficiency is suspected.

ORAL IRON THERAPY

Oral iron treatment promptly alleviates iron deficiency in the vast majority of cases. Ferrous rather than ferric salts are preferred because of their greater solubility and hence better absorption. Ferrous sulfate is preferred by most physicians because of its low cost and high assimilation. The greatest obstacle with oral iron therapy is the gastrointestinal side effects of iron. The most troublesome symptoms are nausea and epigastric discomfort, which occur within 30 to 60 minutes of taking iron. The frequency and severity of these symptoms are proportional to the dose of iron and are believed to reflect the concentration of ionized iron in the stomach or duodenum. The symptoms can be reduced by taking iron with food that complexes iron and thereby reduces its absorption by 60 to 80% compared with the fasting state. Symptoms referable to the lower gastrointestinal tract, such as constipation or diarrhea, are not related to dose and should not be used as a reason for discontinuing oral iron therapy.

It is important to tailor the regimen of oral iron to the severity of the anemia. Maximal absorption occurs when 300 mg of ferrous sulfate (60 mg of elemental iron) is taken three times daily between meals and at bedtime. Severely deficient patients can retain as much as 30 to 40 mg of iron daily on this regimen, although absorption declines progressively as the deficiency is corrected. The disadvantage of using maximal doses of iron is that at least one third of patients experience significant side effects that reduce compliance and may lead the patients to refuse further oral iron treatment. Consequently, if the anemia is not severe and the patient is not symptomatic, it is preferable to start with a preparation such as ferrous gluconate, which contains one third less elemental iron. If patients agree to take iron initially between meals and at bedtime to achieve a more rapid hematologic response, they should be advised to take iron with their meals if side effects persist after 3 to 4 days of therapy. Because there is seldom any urgency about correcting iron deficiency, a single iron tablet at bedtime usually eliminates side effects and still provides enough iron to increase the hemoglobin concentration by 10 grams per liter every 2 to 3 weeks.

Because of the high prevalence of iron deficiency and the large potential pharmaceutical market for iron, there have been continuing efforts to develop preparations that are more effective or have fewer side effects. In general, these efforts have not been successful. Absorption is increased when ascorbic acid is added to the iron preparation, but so are the side effects. Slow-release preparations often have fewer side effects, because the release of iron in the gut is delayed until it is beyond the area of maximal mucosal iron uptake in the duodenum; consequently, absorption is significantly lower. This is commonly the case with enteric-coated iron preparations, from which the absorption of iron is invariably low. A gastric delivery system of delayed-release iron that largely eliminates upper gastrointestinal symptoms and is better absorbed than ferrous sulfate when given with food has been developed but is not yet available in the United States.

ASSESSING THERAPEUTIC RESPONSE

The rate of hematologic response to oral iron therapy depends on the severity of the deficiency, the intensity of the therapeutic regimen, and the extent to which the factors responsible for the deficiency have been corrected. In patients with severe anemia, the hemoglobin concentration should increase by 10 grams per liter each week with full therapeutic doses of iron, and the anemia should be fully corrected within 6 to 8 weeks. Unlike the brisk reticulocyte response to the treatment of folic acid or vitamin B_{12} deficiency, the modest increase after treatment of iron deficiency anemia is not reliable in gauging the therapeutic response. When the hemoglobin concentration has returned to within the normal range, serum ferritin measurements are helpful in determining the end point of treatment; ferritin should be monitored so the iron therapy can be stopped rather than simply being continued indefinitely. A reasonable end point of treatment is to restock iron reserves to 500 mg in an average-sized adult, which is equivalent to a serum ferritin concentration of 50 to 60 µg per liter.

True therapeutic failures of oral iron therapy are relatively uncommon. The usual cause is poor compliance with treatment, which may not be easy to determine. Compliance can be improved by taking the time to instruct the patient initially about the importance of taking the iron regularly and discussing ways that side effects can be reduced. It is preferable to write a prescription for iron and to give only sufficient medication to last until the next visit. This provides a guide to compliance, because patients seldom request a refill if they have an unused supply of iron.

The possibility of a defect in iron absorption is often considered in those who show no response to oral therapy, but such defects occur only rarely. Pa-

tients with a prior total gastrectomy have a severe defect in iron absorption, but those with a partial gastrectomy or achlorhydria can absorb iron normally if it is given separately from food. If there is a strong reason to suspect malabsorption, an iron absorption test should be performed by giving 100 mg of elemental iron the morning after an overnight fast and obtaining a serum iron determination 1 and 2 hours later. If the baseline value is less than 50 µg per dL, and the serum iron level fails to increase by at least 100 µg per dL, malabsorption is likely to be present. A biopsy of the small intestine should then be performed, because intestinal disorders such as celiac disease can manifest as iron deficiency anemia.

PARENTERAL IRON THERAPY

Parenteral iron treatment is occasionally required in patients who either refuse to take oral iron because of gastrointestinal side effects or who continue to have uncontrollable blood loss. There is no evidence that parenteral iron produces a faster hematologic response in patients who absorb iron normally and who tolerate full therapeutic doses. Parenteral iron is far more expensive than oral therapy, because it must be given under careful medical supervision to manage the serious and sometimes fatal anaphylactic reactions. Parenteral iron should be used in preference to repeated blood transfusions but should never be given as a matter of convenience for the patient or physician.

The only available preparation in the United States at present is iron dextran (InFeD), a colloidal iron complex containing 50 mg of iron per mL. The manufacturer currently recommends that no more than 100 mg of iron be given intramuscularly each day, which is highly impractical in patients who often need more than 2 grams of iron to replenish body iron. Most physicians therefore resort to total dose infusion by the intravenous route by diluting 500 to 2000 mg* of iron dextran in 500 mL of normal saline. The most serious potential complication is anaphylaxis, which typically occurs within a few minutes of beginning the infusion. Consequently, 20 to 30 mL of the diluted solution should be given slowly over 3 to 5 minutes, the infusion stopped for 15 to 30 minutes, and the remainder then given over 2 to 3 hours. Resuscitation capability must be immediately available. Parenteral iron should not be given to patients with rheumatoid arthritis, because it can produce a severe exacerbation of the disease. Approximately one third of patients receiving total dose infusion develop mild delayed reactions such as myalgia, arthralgia, and fever within 24 to 48 hours, but these symptoms usually respond promptly to simple measures such as use of a nonsteroidal anti-inflammatory agent. In patients with recurrent iron deficiency anemia, the timing of subsequent infusions is best determined by monitoring the rate of decline in the serum ferritin concentration after each treatment.

---

*Exceeds dosage recommended by the manufacturer.

AUTOIMMUNE HEMOLYTIC ANEMIA

method of
CHARLES H. PACKMAN, M.D.

*University of Rochester School of Medicine and
Dentistry and Strong Memorial Hospital
Rochester, New York*

Autoimmune hemolytic anemia (AIHA) is a collection of diseases in which shortened red blood cell (RBC) survival is mediated by autoantibodies. The entities that constitute AIHA are classified primarily by the temperature at which the autoantibodies bind most efficiently to the patient's RBCs. In adults, most cases (80 to 90%) are mediated by antibodies that react optimally with RBCs at 37°C (warm-reactive autoantibodies). Patients with cryopathic hemolytic syndromes exhibit autoantibodies that bind more avidly to RBCs at temperatures below 37°C (cold-reactive autoantibodies). The warm- and cold-antibody distinctions are further classified by the presence or absence of underlying diseases. When no recognizable underlying disease is evident, the AIHA is designated "primary" or "idiopathic." The term "secondary" is used when the AIHA is a manifestation or complication of an underlying disorder. Primary (idiopathic) AIHA and secondary AIHA occur with approximately equal frequency. Finally, certain drugs may also cause immune destruction of RBCs by three different mechanisms. True autoantibodies are involved in only one of these mechanisms. The hapten–drug adsorption mechanism and the ternary (immune) complex mechanism involve antibodies directed primarily against drugs or their metabolites rather than RBC antigens. The classification of the immune hemolytic anemias is shown in Table 1.

CLINICAL FEATURES AND DIAGNOSIS

The annual incidence of AIHA is approximately one or two cases per 100,000 population. It occurs in people of all ages, with a peak incidence in the seventh decade. No racial predisposition is known, and familial occurrence is rare.

In warm-antibody AIHA, the presenting complaints are usually referable to the anemia itself. The onset of symptoms is typically insidious over months, but occasional patients may experience sudden symptoms of severe anemia and jaundice over a few days. In secondary cases, the symptoms and signs of the underlying disease may overshadow the hemolytic anemia. The physical examination is often normal. Modest splenomegaly may be noted in patients with relatively severe hemolytic anemia. Patients with acute hemolysis may exhibit fever, pallor, hyperpnea, angina, tachycardia, hepatosplenomegaly, heart failure, and jaundice. In secondary cases, other physical findings may be contributed by the associated disorder.

Patients with cold agglutinin disease usually exhibit chronic hemolytic anemia with or without jaundice, but some patients experience episodic, acute hemolysis with hemoglobinuria induced by chilling. Acrocyanosis is sometimes seen, owing to sludging of RBCs in the cutaneous circulation. Hemolysis in patients with *Mycoplasma pneumoniae* infections is acute in onset, often appearing as the patient is recovering from pneumonia and lasting 1 to 3 weeks. Hemolytic anemia in infectious mononucleosis can occur at any time within the first 3 weeks of illness. Splenomegaly, which is most characteristic of lymphoma and infectious mononucleosis, may also occur in idiopathic cold agglutinin disease.

Paroxysmal cold hemoglobinuria (PCH) is a chronic illness characterized by periodic episodes of massive hemolysis after cold exposure. It occurs in an idiopathic form and in patients with congenital or tertiary syphilis. Donath-Landsteiner hemolytic anemia is a related disorder that occurs more commonly in children or young adults; it manifests as an acute, self-limited hemolytic anemia usually after a viral syndrome. In both diseases, paroxysms are characterized by prominent constitutional symptoms, including aching pains in the back or legs, abdominal cramps, headaches, and chills and fever occurring a few minutes to several hours after cold exposure. The urine typically contains hemoglobin. The constitutional symptoms and hemoglobinuria generally last a few hours.

Drug-induced immune hemolytic anemias are usually slow in onset. However, those caused by the ternary (immune) complex mechanism are characterized by a rapid onset after only a few days of drug exposure, or after a single dose in patients who have taken the drug previously. Some common drugs implicated in immune RBC injury are shown in Table 2.

LABORATORY FEATURES

General

In both warm-antibody and cold-antibody AIHA, the anemia can be mild or severe, with hemoglobin levels occasionally as low as 3 to 4 grams per dL. Patients with drug-induced immune hemolysis mediated by the hapten–drug adsorption mechanism or by true autoantibodies usually exhibit mildly depressed hemoglobin levels, whereas those with hemolysis mediated by the ternary (immune) complex mechanism may have severe, life-threatening anemia. Polychromasia on the blood smear indicates reticulocytosis, reflecting an increased rate of RBC production. Spherocytes are usually seen as well. Most patients exhibit mild leukocytosis and neutrophilia; occasionally, leukopenia and neutropenia are noted. Platelet counts are usually normal.

TABLE 1. **Diseases Characterized by Immune-Mediated Red Blood Cell Destruction**

I. Autoimmune hemolytic anemia due to warm-reactive autoantibodies
  A. Primary (idiopathic)
  B. Secondary
    1. Lymphoproliferative disorders
    2. Connective tissue disorders (especially systemic lupus erythematosus)
    3. Nonlymphoid neoplasms (e.g., ovarian tumors)
    4. Chronic inflammatory diseases (e.g., ulcerative colitis)
II. Autoimmune hemolytic anemia due to cold-reactive autoantibodies (cryopathic hemolytic syndromes)
  A. Primary (idiopathic) cold agglutinin disease
  B. Secondary cold agglutinin disease
    1. Lymphoproliferative disorders
    2. Infections (*Mycoplasma pneumoniae* infection, infectious mononucleosis)
  C. Paroxysmal cold hemoglobulinuria (primary or associated with syphilis)
  D. Donath-Landsteiner hemolytic anemia (associated with viral syndromes)
III. Drug-induced immune hemolytic anemia
  A. Hapten–drug adsorption
  B. Ternary (immune) complex
  C. True autoantibody induction

TABLE 2. **Drug-Induced Immune Hematologic Anemia**

Mechanism	Examples of Causative Drugs*
Hapten–drug adsorption	Penicillins
	Cephalosporins
	Tolbutamide
Ternary (immune complex)	Quinine
	Quinidine
	Cephalosporins
	Chlorpropamide
True autoantibody induction	Methyldopa
	Levodopa
	Cephalosporins
	Procainamide
Uncertain	Acetaminophen
	Thiazides
	Ibuprofen
	Erythromycin
	Omeprazole

*Listed are examples of commonly used drugs that are well documented to cause immune hemolysis. The list is incomplete; many other drugs have been implicated. In general, in patients with immune hemolytic anemia, any recently ingested drug should be considered etiologically suspect until proved otherwise.

Although not usually indicated, marrow examination may reveal an underlying lymphoproliferative disorder.

The reticulocyte count is usually elevated, but transient reticulocytopenia may be seen early in approximately one third of patients with AIHA for unknown reasons. Usually, reticulocytes appear in the circulation of such patients in a few days. Reticulocytopenia may also be seen in patients with marrow function compromise related to infection, toxic chemicals, or nutritional deficiency. These patients must be monitored carefully and transfused promptly (see later), because life-threatening anemia may develop quickly in patients with hemolysis and decreased RBC production.

The total bilirubin value is often mildly increased, up to 5 mg per dL, and is chiefly unconjugated (indirect). Bile is not detected in the urine unless serum conjugated (direct) bilirubin is increased. Serum haptoglobin levels are typically low, and lactate dehydrogenase levels are usually elevated. In warm-antibody AIHA and in cold agglutinin disease, hemoglobinuria is encountered only in those uncommon patients who develop hyperacute hemolysis. In patients with PCH or Donath-Landsteiner hemolytic anemia, hemoglobinuria is characteristic, starting shortly after chilling. Hemoglobinuria may be a prominent feature of drug-induced hemolysis due to the ternary (immune) complex mechanism and may cause renal failure.

Serologic Features

The diagnosis of AIHA depends on the demonstration of an immune response directed against autologous RBCs. The evidence for this usually comes in the form of a direct antiglobulin reaction (Coombs' test) or demonstration of direct agglutinins or hemolysins in the patient's serum.

Warm-Antibody AIHA and the Direct Antiglobulin Test. Most patients with warm-antibody AIHA exhibit neither direct agglutinins nor hemolysins. Rather, their RBCs are coated with nonagglutinating antibodies, almost always of the IgG class, and/or complement components. Antibodies and complement components on patients' RBCs are detected by antiglobulin serum (Coombs' reagent), which cross-links the RBCs to produce visible agglutina-

tion. This procedure is called the direct antiglobulin (Coombs') test. The "broad-spectrum" antiglobulin (Coombs') reagent detects both immunoglobulin and complement components (principally C3). More specific reagents that detect *only* IgG or complement may be used to refine the pattern of RBC coating. Three *major* patterns of direct antiglobulin reaction have been noted in warm-antibody AIHA: RBCs coated with IgG alone; RBCs coated with IgG plus complement components; and RBCs coated with complement components alone.

In patients with warm-antibody AIHA, the autoantibody exists in a reversible, dynamic equilibrium between RBCs and plasma. If sufficient "free" autoantibody is present in the plasma or serum of these patients, it may be detected by the indirect antiglobulin test. In general, the presence of plasma autoantibody may be viewed as "overflow" or excess above that bound to RBCs. Thus, patients with a positive indirect antiglobulin test due to a warm-reactive autoantibody must also have a positive direct antiglobulin test. A patient who exhibits a serum anti-RBC antibody (positive indirect antiglobulin reaction) in the presence of a negative direct antiglobulin reaction probably does not have an autoimmune process but rather an alloantibody stimulated by prior transfusion or pregnancy.

Cryopathic Hemolytic Syndromes: Direct Agglutinins and Hemolysins. Direct agglutinins, as the name implies, directly agglutinate normal or autologous human RBCs. These antibodies, largely of the IgM class, are present in patients with cold agglutinin disease. Cold agglutinins cause RBCs to agglutinate maximally at 0 to 5°C. In patients with chronic cold agglutinin disease, the serum cold agglutinin titers are commonly 1:10,000 or higher and may reach 1:1,000,000 or more. The direct antiglobulin test is positive only with anticomplement reagents. The antibody itself (i.e., the cold agglutinin) is not detected by the antiglobulin test, because the antibody molecules readily dissociate from the RBCs during the washing steps of the standard antiglobulin test procedure. In contrast, complement components are covalently bound to target RBCs and cannot be washed off.

In PCH and Donath-Landsteiner hemolytic anemia, the patient's serum contains hemolysins, antibodies that lyse RBCs in the presence of complement. The direct antiglobulin reaction may be positive during or briefly after an acute attack, because of the coating of surviving RBCs with complement. The antibody is a nonagglutinating IgG that binds only in the cold. It is detected by the biphasic Donath-Landsteiner test, in which the patient's fresh serum is incubated with RBCs initially at 4°C and then warmed to 37°C. Intense hemolysis follows.

Drug-Induced Immune Hemolytic Anemia. The serologic findings in drug-induced immune hemolytic anemia vary according to the mechanism. When hemolysis is mediated through the hapten–drug adsorption mechanism, the direct antiglobulin test is positive for IgG alone. The indirect antiglobulin test is positive only when the test RBCs have been previously coated with the drug. In hemolysis mediated by the ternary (immune) complex mechanism, the direct antiglobulin test is positive only for complement components. The drug does not bind in measurable quantity to the RBC membrane, but if the drug is included in the mixture with test RBCs and fresh serum as a source of complement, the cells become coated with complement components, which can then be detected by an antiglobulin reagent. The term "ternary complex" is derived from the observation that in certain of these cases, a trimolecular complex of antibody, drug, or metabolite and a specific RBC membrane antigen must be present for complement deposition and hemolysis to occur. In patients with drug-induced immune hemolysis mediated by autoantibody induction, the direct antiglobulin reaction is generally positive for IgG alone. The direct antiglobulin test may be positive in as many as 25 to 30% of patients receiving methyldopa (Aldomet), the most common drug to induce autoantibodies, but less than 1% of these patients actually have hemolysis. The indirect antiglobulin reaction is almost always positive in those who do have hemolysis.

TREATMENT

Warm-Antibody Autoimmune Hemolytic Anemia

Transfusion

The clinical consequences of anemia are related to both the severity of the anemia and the rapidity with which it develops. Most patients with AIHA are in little danger of circulatory failure, because the anemia usually develops over a sufficient time to allow cardiovascular compensation to occur. It is not usually necessary to transfuse these patients. The best guide to the need for blood transfusion is the patient's clinical condition rather than a predetermined hematocrit or hemoglobin level. In patients with significant co-morbid disease such as coronary artery disease with angina, or in patients who suddenly develop severe anemia and exhibit signs and symptoms of circulatory failure, transfusion is often required and may prove lifesaving. As noted previously, transfusion should be considered early in a patient with AIHA and reticulocytopenia, because the anemia may become severe quite rapidly.

Transfusion of RBCs in AIHA presents two problems: the issue of crossmatching and the likelihood of rapid hemolysis of transfused cells. It is usually impossible to find truly serocompatible donor blood. The autoantibody in the patient's serum usually reacts with all potential donor RBCs except in those unusual cases in which the autoantibody exhibits specificity for a defined blood group antigen and binds only to cells exhibiting that antigen. Without such specificity, candidate units of blood should be chosen on the basis of least incompatibility with the patient's serum in crossmatch testing. Furthermore, before such an incompatible unit is transfused, it is also essential to assay the patient's serum for an alloantibody that could cause a severe hemolytic transfusion reaction directed toward the donor RBCs. Alloantibodies are more likely found in patients with a history of pregnancy or prior transfusion. Once selected, packed RBCs should be infused very slowly while the patient is monitored for evidence of a hemolytic transfusion reaction. The transfused cells are often destroyed as rapidly as the patient's own cells. Nonetheless, the temporarily increased hemoglobin level may maintain the patient's oxygen-carrying capacity during the time required for more definitive therapy to become effective.

Corticosteroids

Corticosteroids cause cessation or slowing of hemolysis in about two thirds of patients. About 20% of patients with warm-antibody AIHA achieve a complete remission with corticosteroids. About 10% show minimal or no response. Treatment is initiated with oral prednisone, 1 to 2 mg per kg daily. Critically ill patients with severe hemolysis should receive intravenous methylprednisolone, 2 to 4 mg per kg in divided doses in the first 24 to 48 hours. High doses of prednisone may be required for 10 to 14 days. When the hemoglobin level begins to increase, the prednisone dose may be decreased in fairly large steps to approximately 30 mg per day. With continued response, the prednisone dose is further decreased by 5 mg per day each week, to a dose of 15 to 20 mg daily. This dose should be continued for 8 to 12 weeks after the acute hemolytic episode has subsided. The patient may then be weaned from the drug during 4 to 8 weeks. If continued corticosteroid therapy is needed, treatment on an alternate-day schedule may be helpful, for example, 20 to 40 mg of prednisone every other day. Alternate-day therapy causes fewer corticosteroid side effects but should be attempted only after the patient maintains a stable hemoglobin level with daily prednisone in a dose range of 15 to 20 mg per day. Many patients achieve complete remission of hemolysis, but relapses often occur after discontinuation of corticosteroids. Patients should be followed up for several years after treatment. If relapse occurs, the patient may require further corticosteroid therapy and eventually splenectomy, or immunosuppression.

Splenectomy

About one third of patients with warm-antibody AIHA require prednisone in doses greater than 15 mg daily to maintain an acceptable hemoglobin concentration. Such patients are candidates for splenectomy. It is usually reasonable to continue corticosteroids for 4 to 8 weeks and wait for a response. If the patient's clinical condition deteriorates, the anemia is extremely severe, or there is no response to prednisone, splenectomy should be done sooner. Approximately two thirds of splenectomized patients have a partial or complete remission, but relapses are disappointingly common. After splenectomy, some patients maintain acceptable hemoglobin levels only with further prednisone treatment, albeit at lower dosage than required before splenectomy.

After splenectomy, there is a slightly increased risk of pneumococcal sepsis, more likely in children than in adults. Pneumococcal vaccine is generally given before surgery. Prophylactic penicillin (250 to 500 mg daily) is also of value in children.

Cytotoxic Immunosuppressive Drugs

Cytotoxic immunosuppressive therapy is not universally accepted, but responses to immunosuppressive drugs have been observed in some patients who do not to respond to corticosteroids. It is important to note that most cases of warm-antibody AIHA respond to corticosteroids and/or splenectomy. Cytotoxic immunosuppressive therapy is usually considered only for those patients who have no response to glucocorticoids and splenectomy, or for those patients who are poor surgical risks. The most commonly used drugs are cyclophosphamide (Cytoxan),* 1.5 to 2 mg per kg, or azathioprine (Imuran),* 1.5 to 2 mg per kg, given daily. If the patient tolerates the drug, treatment may be continued for up to 6 months in hopes of a response. When response occurs, the drug dose may be slowly decreased during 2 to 3 months. If there is no response, the alternative drug may be similarly tried. Cyclophosphamide and azathioprine cause marrow suppression, so the patient's blood counts must be monitored closely during therapy. Both agents increase the risk of subsequent neoplasia, and cyclophosphamide may also cause severe hemorrhagic cystitis. Women of childbearing age should avoid pregnancy while taking cytotoxic immunosuppressive agents.

Other Therapies

Plasma exchange (plasmapheresis) has been used in warm-antibody AIHA. Improvement has been noted in a few cases, but its use remains controversial. The literature contains anecdotal reports of short-term successful treatment with high-dose intravenous gamma globulin, as well as reports of treatment failures. Danazol (Danocrine),* a nonvirilizing androgen, is also reported as useful in uncontrolled studies and in case reports. Intravenous gamma globulin and danazol may be used in cases unresponsive to other therapies.

Cryopathic Hemolytic Syndromes

Keeping the patient warm, particularly the extremities, provides symptomatic relief. This may be the only measure required in patients with mild chronic hemolysis, who generally have a benign course and survive for many years. When a cold agglutinin is associated with a lymphoproliferative disorder, treatment of the underlying neoplasm often corrects the hemolysis. Interferon alfa-2b (Intron A)* was remarkably successful in one patient with idiopathic cold agglutinin disease, and this approach deserves further trials. Successful therapy with cyclophosphamide* or chlorambucil (Leukeran) has been reported in a few instances. Splenectomy and corticosteroids are generally disappointing, although exceptions have been reported. RBC transfusions, as in warm-antibody AIHA, are generally reserved for patients who have severe anemia and are in danger of cardiorespiratory complications. The use of washed RBCs may avoid replenishing depleted complement components, which could reactivate the hemolytic process. Plasma exchange (with replacement by albumin-containing saline) has been tried in refractory cases. The procedure may temporarily slow the rate of hemolysis but does not provide long-term benefit. The postinfectious forms of cold agglutinin disease are usually self-limited, with recovery expected in a few weeks. When massive hemoglobinuria is compli-

cated by acute renal failure, a period of hemodialysis may be required.

Acute attacks in both chronic and transient forms of PCH may be prevented by avoidance of cold. Corticosteroids and splenectomy have not been useful. PCH associated with syphilis often responds to effective treatment of the syphilis. Patients with chronic idiopathic PCH may survive for many years in spite of occasional paroxysms of hemolysis. Donath-Landsteiner hemolytic anemia is usually self-limited.

Drug-Induced Immune Hemolytic Anemia

Discontinuation of the offending drug is usually all that is required. This measure is particularly important and potentially lifesaving in patients with severe hemolysis mediated by the ternary (immune) complex mechanism. In such patients, hemoglobinuria may lead to renal failure requiring a period of dialysis. Corticosteroids are generally unnecessary and of questionable efficacy. Transfusions should be reserved for the unusual circumstance of severe, life-threatening anemia. Crossmatching may present a problem, as with warm-antibody AIHA, in patients with a strongly positive indirect antiglobulin test. Patients with hemolytic anemia due to the hapten–drug adsorption mechanism should have a compatible crossmatch, because the serum antibody reacts only with drug-coated cells. In hemolysis due to ternary complex or hapten–drug adsorption mechanisms, the direct antiglobulin test becomes negative once the drug is cleared from the circulation, usually a few days after it is discontinued. Hemolysis due to autoantibodies induced by methyldopa ceases promptly after the drug is discontinued. However, the autoantibodies may remain in the patient, as evidenced by a positive direct antiglobulin test, for weeks or months.

NONIMMUNE HEMOLYTIC ANEMIA

method of
KOUICHI R. TANAKA, M.D.
Harbor–UCLA Medical Center
Torrance, California

Given a patient with anemia in whom there is reticulocytosis and a negative direct Coombs antiglobulin test result, the diagnosis of nonimmune hemolytic anemia (NIHA) is often applied. This is akin to the use of the term nonspherocytic hemolytic anemia when only hereditary spherocytosis (HS) was recognized as an entity and all others were considered to be nonspherocytic. So it is with NIHA—a heterogeneous group of hemolytic disorders other than immune-mediated hemolysis. For appropriate therapy to be instituted, specific diagnosis is paramount.

Recent blood loss and response to a hematinic unbeknown to the patient need to be excluded. Hemorrhage into deep tissues or ruptured ectopic pregnancy with elevated indirect bilirubin levels and reticulocytosis may mimic non-

---

*Not FDA approved for this indication.

immune hemolysis until careful study is done. In hemolytic disorders, anemia is not always present because the normal bone marrow can compensate for premature destruction of erythrocytes by increasing the production of erythrocytes about eight times.

Examination of a well-prepared, well-stained peripheral blood smear often provides valuable clues to direct a cost-effective approach to determine the specific cause. The mean corpuscular volume (MCV) viewed in the light of reticulocytosis (1% chronic reticulocytosis increases the MCV 1 fL) is helpful in suspecting concomitant iron or folate deficiency or incidental presence of α-thalassemia. An elevated mean corpuscular hemoglobin concentration (MCHC) level is suggestive of HS.

Table 1 lists the major categories and clinically important disorders constituting the NIHAs. The list is not meant to be exhaustive.

HEREDITARY MEMBRANE DISORDERS

The erythrocyte membrane is a mixture of phospholipids, unesterified cholesterol, and glycolipids ar-

TABLE 1. **Nonimmune Hemolytic Anemias**

Hereditary Disorders

Membrane Disorders

Hereditary spherocytosis
Hereditary elliptocytosis
Hereditary ovalocytosis
Abetalipoproteinemia

Enzyme Disorders

Glucose-6-phosphate dehydrogenase deficiency
Pyruvate kinase deficiency
Other enzymopathies

Hemoglobin Disorders

Sickle cell disease (see separate article)
Hemoglobin CC disease
Hemoglobin EE syndrome
Unstable hemoglobins
Hemoglobin M disorders

Acquired Disorders

Paroxysmal Nocturnal Hemoglobinuria

Fragmentation Syndromes

Big-vessel disease or trauma
Mechanical heart valve or other prostheses
Severe aortic or mitral valvular disease
Bongo drumming, karate
Small-vessel disorders or microangiopathy
Thrombotic thrombocytopenic purpura–hemolytic-uremic syndrome
Disseminated intravascular coagulation
Malignant hypertension
Malignant neoplasm
Eclampsia

Infections

Malaria
Babesiosis
Bartonellosis
Clostridial disease

Miscellaneous

Copper
Arsine poisoning
Lead intoxication
Hypophosphatemia
Brown recluse spider bites

ranged in a bilayer and contains 10 to 15 major proteins and many minor ones. Examination of the peripheral blood smear is the most useful test for detecting membrane defects. Almost all membrane disorders alter cell shape, such as spherocytes, elliptocytes, and acanthocytes.

HS is clinically the most important disorder. It may present at any age. In neonates, excessive jaundice sometimes requires an exchange transfusion. After the neonatal period, most patients develop partially compensated hemolysis with mild to moderate anemia. The disease occurs in all races but is particularly common in northern Europeans. About 75% of the affected families demonstrate a classic autosomal dominant pattern. The primary molecular defects in HS involve the "vertical" connections between spectrin, ankyrin, protein 4.2, and band 3 that link the lipid bilayer and the membrane skeleton. Abnormalities in each of these proteins have been observed in HS, and increasing numbers of mutations are being described. Clinical severity varies widely, reflecting the great variety of causative mutations and variable compensation by the normal allele in the usual dominant disorders.

Complications include aplastic crises often severe enough to threaten heart failure and require transfusion. They are usually caused by parvovirus B19, which invades erythropoietic stem cells. Megaloblastic crises due to inadequate dietary intake of folic acid occur rarely in HS or other hemolytic anemias. Gallstones are common at a young age; ultrasonography is the most reliable method for detecting bilirubin stones. Only 50% are radiopaque.

Diagnosis is not difficult in the patient with anemia, jaundice, splenomegaly, and spherocytes present on the blood smear. However, many patients with HS are not anemic or are borderline anemic, and hyperbilirubinemia is present in only 50 to 60%. An elevated reticulocyte count is a more dependable sign of hemolysis. If spherocytes are noted, the osmotic fragility test is only confirmatory and not essential. If HS is suspected by history or MCHC level of 36 g/dL or greater and the unincubated osmotic fragility test result is normal or only slightly increased, then the incubated osmotic fragility is almost always abnormal and is the most reliable available diagnostic test.

HS of the classic type is the only hereditary hemolytic anemia in which splenectomy produces a clinical cure in all patients. If anemia is not eliminated or the reticulocyte count does not decrease to near-normal levels (1 to 3%), then the diagnosis of HS was in error or there is a complicating factor. A relapse several or more years later suggests an accessory spleen that has grown to 20 grams or more to cause clinically significant hemolysis.

The important practical issue is when and in whom splenectomy should be recommended. The risk for postsplenectomy sepsis is greater in infancy and early childhood; splenectomy should thus be delayed until the age of 5 years or more if possible, even if repeated transfusions are required. I recommend splenectomy for all patients with severe HS (hemoglobin level <8 grams per dL). Splenectomy is also recommended for patients with moderate HS (hemoglobin level 8 to 11 grams per dL) between the ages of 10 and 60 years unless there are medical contraindications to surgery. Whether patients with moderate, asymptomatic anemia should have a splenectomy remains controversial. In my experience, however, I have recommended splenectomy for children older than 8 years or so with even minimal anemia but with reticulocytosis of 4% or greater. In every instance, the anemia has been clinically cured as expected, but more important, the children have improved their school performance or behavior, they have greater stamina comparable to their peers, and the risk for traumatic rupture of the spleen has been eliminated. In my experience in adults with mild anemia, splenectomy has resulted in a state of well-being not previously experienced by the patient. In the older adult, I discuss the pros and cons and leave the final decision to the patient.

Partial splenectomy may eventually be an effective compromise, but more experience and longer follow-up are needed. Laparoscopic splenectomy is being performed in increasing numbers and is the preferred method in some centers. The benefits, which include shortened hospitalization and improved cosmetic appearance, must be balanced against the risks of longer surgery and anesthesia and problems with control of bleeding.

All patients recommended for splenectomy should receive polyvalent pneumococcal polysaccharide vaccine (Pnu-Imune 23 or equivalent, 0.5 mL intramuscularly or subcutaneously) about 1 month before operation. The vaccine, however, is not effective in patients younger than 2 years. Immunization with meningococcal vaccine (Menomune-A/C/Y/W-135 or equivalent, 0.5 mL intramuscularly) is also recommended, especially in children.

Long-term prophylaxis against pneumococcal infection after splenectomy is recommended with penicillin VK (125 mg orally twice daily for children younger than 5 years and 250 mg orally twice daily for children older than 5 years and young adults), even in individuals who have been vaccinated. I do not prescribe oral penicillin prophylaxis in adults, but the duration of prophylactic therapy in children and usage in adults are controversial issues. In HS patients with ongoing hemolysis, I recommend folic acid (1 mg orally per day) prophylactically.

Hereditary elliptocytosis (HE) is more common than HS but is less important clinically. Only about 10 to 15% of patients have significant hemolysis. Four clinical forms of HE have been recognized: mild HE, hereditary pyropoikilocytosis (HPP), spherocytic HE, and Southeast Asian ovalocytosis. Common HE is clearly the most prevalent form of HE. In most heterozygous carriers, prominent elliptocytosis is noted by the clinical laboratory as an incidental finding when a blood count is performed; there is no anemia or splenomegaly and only mild hemolysis is present. In general, common HE and HPP are caused by defects in the "horizontal" interactions that hold the membrane skeleton together. Many specific defects have been identified in α spectrin and in protein 4.1. The rare recessive hemolytic syndrome of HPP demonstrates striking erythrocyte fragmentation (MCV 45 to 75 fL), bizarre poikilocytosis, a marked defect in spectrin self-association, and heat-sensitive erythrocytes. The hemolysis is decreased but not completely cured by splenectomy. Spherocytic elliptocytosis is a relatively rare autosomal dominant disorder with features of both HS and HE. Splenectomy is curative as in HS. Southeast Asian ovalocytosis is an autosomal dominant disorder that is asymptomatic and is quite common (approximately 30%) in some Asian populations such as those in Melanesia and Malaysia. The rigid ovalocytes resist invasion by malarial parasites. Splenectomy is indicated only in severe cases of HE or HPP and should be delayed preferably to the fifth year or later, because spontaneous regression occurs in some infants with HPP.

Acanthocytosis in abetalipoproteinemia, a rare autosomal recessive disorder, is secondary to a primary molecular defect involving absence of apolipoprotein B in plasma. Progressive neurologic abnormalities lead to death in the second or third decade.

HEREDITARY ENZYME DISORDERS

Glucose-6-phosphate dehydrogenase (G6PD) deficiency is by far the most common enzymopathy in the world. In the United States, G6PD deficiency is prevalent in African-Americans, people of Mediterranean ancestry, and individuals from Southeast Asia. G6PD catalyzes the first step in the hexose monophosphate pathway, producing NADPH, which is required for the maintenance of reduced glutathione. Reduced glutathione is essential for protecting erythrocytes against oxidative insults. On the basis of gene analysis, about 100 variants have been identified, most of them demonstrating one or two missense mutations. The gene is X linked; thus, males are more often affected. G6PD deficiency can be diagnosed by a simple screening test. The test may not be reliable after an acute hemolytic event because the residual younger erythrocytes have greater activity. Three classes of G6PD are important clinically: class 1, severe deficiency associated with chronic hemolytic anemia (CHA); class 2, moderate deficiency, Mediterranean type associated with favism; class 3, mild deficiency, prototype being G6PD A− among African-Americans. Although CHA due to G6PD deficiency is rare, class 1 G6PD and pyruvate kinase (PK) deficiencies in about equal numbers account for 90% of CHA due to erythroenzymopathies.

Major clinical manifestations for the common class 2 and class 3 types of G6PD deficiency are neonatal jaundice and an acute hemolytic anemia developing after infection or after ingestion of fava beans or certain drugs. Some of the more important drugs and chemicals that can or do not induce hemolytic anemia are listed in Table 2. Spontaneous recovery is the rule after elimination of the triggering event, but

TABLE 2. **Important Drugs and Chemicals That Can Induce Hemolytic Anemia or Be Given Safely to Individuals with Glucose-6-Phosphate Dehydrogenase Deficiency**

Can Induce Hemolytic Anemia

Dapsone
Doxorubicin hydrochloride (Adriamycin)
Furazolidone (Furoxone)
Methylene blue
Nalidixic acid (NegGram)
Nitrofurantoin (Furadantin)
Phenazopyridine hydrochloride (Pyridium)
Primaquine
Sulfamethoxazole

Can Be Given Safely*

Acetaminophen
Aspirin
Chloroquine
Sulfisoxazole (Gantrisin)
Trimethoprim
Vitamin K

*In therapeutic doses to those individuals without chronic hemolytic anemia.

erythrocyte transfusions may be necessary in severe cases. Splenectomy is not curative but is of partial benefit in some patients with CHA.

PK deficiency is the most common enzymopathy of the Embden-Meyerhof pathway causing CHA. The disorder occurs worldwide. Lifelong chronic hemolysis of variable severity is the rule; a particularly severe form occurs among the Amish in the United States. PK deficiency is inherited as an autosomal recessive disorder. Increasing numbers of gene mutations (mostly missense) are being described. In the absence of consanguinity, clinically affected PK individuals are usually compound heterozygotes for two mutant alleles. Defective PK catalysis in affected erythrocytes results in elevated concentrations of 2,3-diphosphoglycerate and decreased ATP. Quantitative in vitro assays of erythrocyte PK are necessary for diagnosis.

Therapy in affected PK subjects is directed at the patient and not at the hemoglobin or hematocrit level, because the elevated 2,3-diphosphoglycerate level enhances oxygen delivery to tissues. Erythrocyte transfusions should be kept to the minimum while maintaining a reasonable quality of life. Splenectomy provides only modest benefit; hemolysis continues, and reticulocytosis may even increase. Nonetheless, there is slight to moderate improvement in the anemia, which may be lifesaving in the most severely affected patients or may diminish or even eliminate transfusion requirements. Splenectomy should be considered only in patients with significant chronic transfusion requirements. Vaccination and folate supplementation are as discussed for HS.

Many other erythroenzymopathies involving the glycolytic pathway, pentose phosphate shunt, glutathione, and nucleotide metabolism have been documented but are all rare. The only CHA due to enzymopathy that may be suspected strongly from initial examination of the peripheral blood smear is pyrimidine nucleotidase deficiency, which is characterized by marked basophilic stippling of erythrocytes as in acute lead poisoning. In fact, lead readily inhibits pyrimidine nucleotidase, thus producing similar basophilic stippling.

HEMOGLOBIN DISORDERS

Sickle cell disease is discussed elsewhere. Hemoglobin CC disease occurs in 1 of 6000 African-Americans; it is characterized by marked targeting of microcytic erythrocytes, mild anemia, and splenomegaly. Hemoglobin E is common in Southeast Asia. Individuals with hemoglobin EE also demonstrate marked targeting of microcytic erythrocytes but are not anemic or have only borderline anemia. The unstable hemoglobin mutants that result in congenital Heinz's body hemolytic anemias are one of the largest groups of mutants (although each is rare). Hemoglobin Köln is perhaps the most prevalent. The isopropanol test is a simple screening test. Therapy depends on severity. Oxidative stresses should be avoided as in G6PD deficiency. When splenectomy is indicated, most patients experience significant improvement after the surgery. Hemoglobin mutations with a propensity to form methemoglobin (e.g., hemoglobin M Boston) have been known for many years because of their phenotypic manifestations (cyanotic skin and blood). However, these syndromes are usually without other clinical effect.

ACQUIRED DISORDERS
Paroxysmal Nocturnal Hemoglobinuria

Paroxysmal nocturnal hemoglobinuria (PNH) is an acquired clonal disorder characterized by an intrinsic erythrocyte membrane defect resulting in intravascular hemolysis and complicated by venous thromboses. Although uncommon, PNH should be considered whenever NIHA is associated with cytopenias, a hypoplastic state is associated with hemolysis, or a hypercoagulable state is accompanied by pancytopenia.

The primary lesion in PNH is a somatic mutation of the *PIGA* gene, which codes an enzyme necessary for the synthesis of the glycophosphatidylinositol (GPI) anchor. All GPI-linked proteins are deficient on the membrane of affected hematopoietic cells. One of these proteins, the membrane inhibitor of reactive lysis (MIRL, or CD59) is of major importance in preventing attack to the membrane by the C5b,6,7,8,9 complement complex. Thus, CD59 deficiency explains the increase in complement-mediated lysis of PNH erythrocytes and resultant intravascular hemolysis, hemoglobinuria, and hemosiderinuria characteristic of the disorder.

PNH is usually a disease of young adults, but I have seen patients ranging from age 9 to 68 years. In most cases, the patient presents as a problem in the differential diagnosis of NIHA. In many instances, the passing of dark urine may have been unnoticed by the patient or its presence not specifically elicited by the physician. Once PNH is suspected, the sucrose hemolysis test and acid hemolysis (Ham's) test usually establish the diagnosis. More recently, flow cytometry has been used to demonstrate the deficiency in PNH erythrocytes of GPI-linked proteins such as CD59, CD48, and CD55. This technique is quantitative, is sensitive, and can detect affected peripheral blood granulocytes (best with anti-CD14) and lymphocytes. The leukocyte alkaline phosphatase score is low and erythrocyte acetylcholinesterase activity is decreased, because both are GPI-anchored proteins. The most common causes of death are thrombosis or hemorrhage associated with severe thrombocytopenia. PNH patients may gradually develop an aplastic bone marrow, whereas about 30% of aplastic anemia patients eventually develop PNH. Appropriate therapy depends on the symptoms. The only curative treatment is bone marrow transplantation, which is a valid option for patients who have a donor available and who are willing to accept the attendant risks. However, about 15% have a spontaneous recovery; thus, the decision for transplantation is often difficult and an individual matter. For those not slated for transplantation, treatment is supportive. Erythrocyte transfusion is indicated only when the hemoglobin level falls below the tolerated level of the individual patient. On-line white cell filters should be used for all transfusions. Patients should receive iron supplements unless they are being transfused. Prednisone at a dose of 20 to 40 mg every other day should be tried for anemic patients with evidence of hemolysis, but the use of prednisone is controversial. Some patients respond to androgens; danazol (Danocrine)* 400 mg per day is best tolerated. Thrombolytic agents (tissue plasminogen activator, streptokinase, or urokinase) should be used as soon as possible for patients with acute thrombosis. Therapy with heparin and warfarin (Coumadin) should be instituted and heparin discontinued after 7 days. The optimal duration of warfarin therapy is not known; 6 months for the initial episode of documented thrombosis is reasonable. PNH patients with an aplastic presentation should receive antithymocyte globulin* (15 mg per kg per day for 8 days or 40 mg per kg† per day for 4 days).

Fragmentation Syndromes

Fragmentation syndromes may be divided into big-vessel disorders or traumatic hemolysis and small-vessel disease or microangiopathy (see Table 1). Patients present with varying degrees of NIHA with evidence of erythrocyte fragmentation on blood smears. The differential diagnosis of fragmentation hemolysis can usually be deduced from the clinical setting. A prosthetic heart valve or occasionally severe aortic stenosis or even mitral valvular disease

---

*Not FDA approved for this indication.
†Exceeds dosage recommended by the manufacturer.

may cause the fragmentation syndrome. Prolonged physical activity of various kinds, e.g., bongo drumming or karate, may be the cause. Among small-vessel disorders, patients with malignant hypertension, eclampsia, thrombotic thrombocytopenic purpura, and disseminated intravascular coagulation may develop the fragmentation syndrome because of slicing of erythrocytes by fibrin strands in small vessels. Therapy is mainly directed at the underlying disease or event.

Infections, Toxins, and Other Causes

Malaria is by far the most common infectious cause of hemolytic anemia worldwide. Direct parasitization by *Plasmodium falciparum, Plasmodium vivax,* or *Plasmodium malariae* causes erythrocyte lysis both intravascularly and extravascularly. Babesiosis occurs along the coast of New England and is caused by *Babesia microti,* which invades the erythrocyte and induces hemolysis. *B. microti* is transmitted from deer mice to people by hard ticks and occasionally by transfusion of blood or components. Infection in splenectomized patients can lead to catastrophic intravascular hemolysis and acute renal failure. In bartonellosis, the organism attaches to the surface of the erythrocyte and produces lysis. *Clostridium perfringens* septicemia invariably produces cataclysmic, often fatal, intravascular hemolysis. Suspicion of the complication is raised after septic abortion, biliary tract disease, perforated viscus, and any situation that engenders anaerobic tissue necrosis. Sudden massive release of unbound copper from the liver in Wilson's disease results in hemolytic episodes. Drinking of ritual waters containing copper sulfate has caused severe hemolytic anemia. Exposure to arsine vapor (garlicky odor) during processing of certain metals or manufacturing of fertilizers may cause acute intravascular hemolysis. Heavy lead exposure may be associated with significant hemolysis, but the primary cause of the anemia is impaired heme production. Severe hypophosphatemia typically occurs after initiation of therapy without phosphate supplementation in an alcoholic patient. Erythrocyte ATP levels decrease, resulting in hemolysis. The brown recluse spider in southwestern sections of the United States injects a venom that often causes severe spherocytic anemia. Management in all the disorders described rests on establishing the diagnosis followed by appropriate therapy.

PERNICIOUS ANEMIA AND OTHER MEGALOBLASTIC ANEMIAS

method of
EUGENE P. FRENKEL, M.D.
The University of Texas Southwestern Medical Center
Dallas, Texas

Classically, pernicious anemia and related anemias involve macrocytic megaloblastic hematopoiesis, wherein

DNA synthesis is defective (delayed) and RNA synthesis continues producing dissociation between cytoplasmic and nuclear maturation. The etiologic mechanisms producing megaloblastosis involve pathophysiologic changes beyond the bone marrow, and these may occur in the absence of anemia. In essence, the molecular and biochemical mechanisms of megaloblastosis involve all organs and can be especially evident in the central nervous system.

ETIOLOGIC MECHANISMS OF MEGALOBLASTIC STATES

Although a detailed list of the etiologic basis of megaloblastosis is shown in Table 1, virtually all of the cases relate to vitamin B_{12} (cobalamin) or folate deficiency or defects in their transport or metabolism. In general, transport defects are rare and relate to cobalamin (primarily, congenital absence of transcobalamin II, the physiologic transport protein for vitamin B_{12}). Transport and receptor binding are known for folate; to date, however, no clinical sequelae have been defined, although the neural tube defect may be one. By contrast, many drugs interfere with the cobalamin-folate–dependent metabolic pathway (especially chemotherapeutic agents such as methotrexate and fluorouracil).

CLINICAL FEATURES OF COBALAMIN OR FOLATE DEFICIENCY

Deficiency of either cobalamin or folate produces a megaloblastic anemia. Other clinical features are shown in Table 2. The noteworthy difference between cobalamin and folate deficiencies is the occurrence of acquired neurologic injury. It is now evident that a significant presentation in cobalamin deficiency is with clinical neurologic features, and these may be seen when no hematologic changes are present. This is particularly true in the aged. Similarly, congenital neural tube defects are now known to result from folate deficiency during pregnancy in the absence of a megaloblastic anemia in the mother.

LABORATORY DIAGNOSIS IN MEGALOBLASTIC STATES

Megaloblastic anemia is characterized by macro-ovalocytosis and anisocytosis (elevated red blood cell distribution width) of circulating red blood cells. Because the defective DNA synthesis is expressed in all cells, hypersegmentation of polymorphonuclear leukocytes is common, and as the anemia progresses, leukopenia and thrombocytopenia often develop. The biochemical defect from either cobalamin or folate deficiency produces ineffective hemato-

TABLE 1. **Etiologic Mechanisms of Megaloblastic States**

Common Mechanisms

Deficiency or defects in transport or metabolism of vitamin B_{12} (cobalamin)
Deficiency or alteration of folate metabolism

Rare Mechanisms

Alteration of reductive conversion of ribotide to deoxyribotide
Erythroleukemia (Di Guglielmo's syndrome)
Arsenic intoxication
Alterations of orotic aid metabolism
Idiopathic (refractory) megaloblastosis

TABLE 2. **Clinical Features of Cobalamin and Folate Deficiencies**

Cobalamin (Vitamin B_{12}) Deficiency	Folate Deficiency
Megaloblastic anemia	Megaloblastic anemia
Neurologic lesions	Neurologic lesions
Posterolateral spinal column dysmyelinization (paresthesia, loss of vibratory and positional sense, deep tendon reflexes and ataxia)	Congenital neural tube defects
Peripheral neuropathy	Other clinical events
Cerebral defects (depression, irritability, and memory loss)	Increased spontaneous abortions and abruptio placentae
Other clinical events	Decreased weight and body length of infant
Glossitis and papillary atrophy	
Hyperpigmentation of skin	
Pseudotumor cerebri (headaches)	

poiesis, resulting in increased serum iron, ferritin, lactate dehydrogenase, muramidase, and indirect bilirubin values, and reduced haptoglobin and alkaline phosphatase values. The nuclear-cytoplasmic dissociation produces a large cell with a fibrillar nucleus and abundant cytoplasm; this characterizes all cells with a high turnover rate. Thus, mucosa appears "macrocytic," and uterine cervical smears from affected patients have sometimes been considered malignant.

The primary differential diagnostic approach is the identification of deficiency of cobalamin or folate. Serum assays of each have served as important initial laboratory tests. This statement presumes that the clinical history has eliminated exposure to recent chemotherapeutic and metabolic inhibitor drugs. The serum cobalamin assay has been the clinical diagnostic test to identify the deficient state, although animal models have long shown significant tissue depletion before a major reduction in serum levels occur. Problems of assay sensitivity and, to a lesser degree, specificity have been recognized. Although at least 90% of cobalamin-deficient patients have serum levels less than 200 pg per mL, truly deficient patients have been recognized with values in the range of 200 to 300 pg per mL, and 1% of deficient patients have normal levels. Although specificity is less of a problem, folate deficiency, pregnancy, and dysproteinemias often cause reduced cobalamin values in the absence of true deficiency.

Even more problematic is the serum folate measurement. Dietary deprivation for even a few days, significant alcohol ingestion, and chronic hemolytic states reduce the serum level in the absence of a tissue deficiency state. Therefore, the red blood cell folate level has been used as a measure of tissue deficiency; unfortunately, it is also insensitive, especially with alcoholism and during pregnancy.

As a result of these problems of sensitivity and specificity, assays of metabolic products of the biochemical pathways relevant to cobalamin and folate have been shown to be a more reliable measure of deficiency. Serum methylmalonic acid (MMA), the product of propionate catabolism mediated by adenosylcobalamin, increases with tissue deficiency of cobalamin. Serum total homocysteine (HCYS), the metabolism of which requires both methylcobalamin and folate, is increased in both vitamin B_{12} and folate deficiencies, with a sensitivity of greater than 99%. The assays do have technical problems and are inaccurate in renal insufficiency. However, in circumstances of atypical or subtle clinical presentation, particularly when anemia is not present, assays of MMA and HCYS provide the most reliable clinical evaluation of tissue deficiency of cobalamin or folate. Therefore, these assays become quite important in neuropsychiatric syndromes, advanced age, and pregnancy, in which clinical features consistent with cobalamin or folate deficiency or borderline serum vitamin assays are found.

Once the deficiency state is identified, the pathophysiologic mechanism whereby it has occurred must be defined, because this will determine the duration of therapy required. Most of the altered metabolic states are therapy induced, so the clinical history can eliminate those; for the others, tests of function are helpful (Table 3).

GENERAL PRINCIPLES OF THERAPY

The first and most critical therapeutic concern is the clinical stability of the patient who presents with severe anemia or rapidly progressive neurologic deficit, especially one in whom an impending or "pseudo" spinal cord transection appears to be developing. Because megaloblastic anemias develop slowly, compensatory cardiopulmonary responses are often associated with only modest symptoms, even when patients present with hemoglobin levels below 3 or 4 grams per dL. Often the impulse is to "quickly treat with multiple hematemics" while awaiting diagnostic data from the laboratory. The appropriate approach is to recognize that even with a specific diagnosis and therapy, the red blood cell values will not improve for at least 7 to 14 days. The red blood cell needs must be judged solely on the cardiopulmo-

nary and cerebral functional status of the patient; if required, cautious transfusion is the urgent treatment of choice. Commonly, only a single unit of packed red blood cells is needed. Transfusions should be given slowly (during 3 to 4 hours), because rapid volume shifts may precipitate functional problems related to the precarious hemodynamic status of such patients.

Rarely, the neurologic deterioration of the patient poses urgency of therapy. Such rapid progression virtually defines the etiology to be due to cobalamin. Fulminating neurologic progression can be seen with nitrous oxide anesthesia (which produces inhibition of cobalamin-dependent enzymes) or with folate therapy inappropriately given when cobalamin was the cause of the megaloblastic anemia. Although rare, if progression appears rapid, serum should be collected and treatment with cobalamin instituted.

The second important principle is the requirement for a specific etiologic diagnosis. The pathophysiologic mechanism that produced the defect must be defined. Such delineation is necessary to determine reversibility of the cause and duration of therapy (e.g., short term, lifetime). Thus, (genetic) pernicious anemia demands a lifetime of cobalamin replacement therapy, whereas cobalamin deficiency due to jejunal diverticula can be approached with short-term vitamin B_{12} therapy, antibiotics, and the consideration of surgical repair.

The third issue relates to an understanding of the rate and pattern of repair of the clinical abnormalities. If the anemia fails to respond in the expected time frame, the question of an incorrect diagnosis or an unrecognized associated lesion must be considered. Thus, iron deficiency goes unrecognized when associated with megaloblastosis; it will, however, result in suboptimal therapeutic response to the iden-

TABLE 3. **Pathophysiologic Mechanisms of Cobalamin and Folate Deficiencies**

Deficiency	Mechanism	Laboratory Evaluation*
Cobalamin		
Deficient intake	Dietary deficiency (vegans: absence of all animal protein)	History
Deficient absorption	Intrinsic factor (IF) deficiency (e.g., pernicious anemia, gastric atrophy, long use of H_2 blockers)	Serum IF antibodies
		Gastric IF after pentagastrin, Schilling's I, II
	Defective food proteolysis and vitamin B_{12} liberation (e.g., the "aged" stomach)	Schilling's test with protein-bound vitamin B_{12}
	Cleavage of vitamin B_{12}–IF complex (e.g., stasis states: small bowel diverticula, fish tapeworm)	Schilling's III
	Defect of ileal absorption site (e.g., resection, enteritis)	Schilling's I, II
Defective transport	Transcobalamin (TC) deficiency	TCII assay
Enzymatic defects	Congenital defects of cobalamin enzymes	Assays of adenosylcobalamin and methylcobalamin enzymes
	Acquired defects (e.g., nitrous oxide anesthesia)	History
Folate		
Deficient intake	Dietary deficiency	History
Deficient absorption	Malabsorption states	Small bowel biopsy
	Drug interference	History
Increased folate loss	Renal dialysis	History
Increased folate requirement	Pregnancy	History
	Alcoholism	History

*Schilling's I measures urinary radiocobalamin excretion after an oral dose of radiolabeled vitamin B_{12}. Schilling's II is the same assay but in which oral radiolabeled vitamin B_{12} is given with intrinsic factor. Schilling's III is the test done after 2 wk of antibiotics.

tified cause. This can be particularly noteworthy in cobalamin deficiency, in which patients with pernicious anemia have an increased risk of gastric cancer, and the finding of iron deficiency may provide the clue to its diagnostic pursuit.

Fourth, the serial follow-up of patients after therapeutic restitution requires an understanding of the natural history of the underlying disease status. Education of patients to the need for therapy and follow-up can be done only when the physician understands the cause and mechanism. Such education is important, because the ease with which repair can be achieved sometimes belies the significance of the problem. For instance, patients with pernicious anemia have an increased incidence of gastric cancer and have the potential to develop endocrinopathies (especially hypothyroidism and hypoadrenalism) secondary to organ-related autoantibodies. Thus, they will need a lifetime of therapy and serial clinical evaluations.

Finally, the concept of a therapeutic trial in patients with megaloblastic states has evolved from the era of "shotgun" multihematemic therapy to our present view of the need to define the physiologic significance of a possible deficiency state. Subtle or atypical presentation of cobalamin deficiency, particularly in the elderly, in whom anemia may be absent and neurologic change prominent, as well as the absence of true tissue deficiency in some patients with low serum vitamin B_{12} values has expanded the need for a clear diagnosis. Metabolite assays are of particular value in such suspected circumstances. An elevated MMA or HCYS value can be used as a parameter for a trial of therapy; correction of the defect should similarly correct the metabolic abnormality in 10 to 14 days. This allows affirmation of the diagnosis and confirms the presence of tissue deficiency. I do not favor therapeutic trials with *both* vitamin B_{12} and folate, because such approaches still leave unanswered the clinical question of specificity. A sequential trial (first with vitamin B_{12} and then, if needed, with folate) allows reasonable characterization under these circumstances.

TREATMENT OF COBALAMIN (VITAMIN B_{12}) DEFICIENCY

Normal total body cobalamin stores (primarily in liver and bone marrow) range between 7 and 15 mg. Clinically significant deficiency is expressed when tissue stores are reduced to 30 to 50% of normal. The goal of therapy is to replete tissue stores. With each dose of cobalamin, however, the percentage of the given dose retained by tissues declines. Therefore, significantly greater amounts of cobalamin must be administered than one would calculate from the amount known to exist in total body tissues. In essence, fractional urinary excretion of an administered dose increases as the stores are progressively repleted. The fractional retention is better when temporal gaps (i.e., daily or every few days) exist between doses. These physiologic issues help explain

the variable repletion schedules found in the literature and further allow the clinician to adopt a sequence most appropriate to the patient and the related clinical issues.

Because virtually all mechanisms of cobalamin deficiency relate to decreased absorption, the initial therapy should begin with cyanocobalamin (or hydroxycobalamin), 1 mg (1000 μg) given subcutaneously or intramuscularly. This is rapidly absorbed from either site, with peak serum levels approximately 1 hour after injection; after this initial dose, approximately 65% will be retained. Intravenous injection produces a much greater urinary loss and should not be used. A simple repletion schedule from that point is 1 mg given daily or every other day during the first 2 weeks and then weekly for the next month, by which time normal peripheral hematologic values are expected.

Thereafter, the pathophysiologic mechanism of the deficiency determines the approach to future therapy. For most patients, if gastric intrinsic factor secretion is defective (e.g., in pernicious anemia), cobalamin must be given for life. Monthly or bimonthly injections (subcutaneous or intramuscular) of 1 mg provide simple, inexpensive, and effective therapy that requires no special monitoring. In patients with neurologic deficit, more frequent administration of cobalamin has been used in the first 6 months, when neurologic repair is at the maximum. It must be emphasized that such an increased frequency is empirical, with no supportive data. Similarly, shortening the interval between injections, often requested by elderly patients who express having an "improved sense of well-being" with the treatment, has no special support. The elderly often have cobalamin deficiency due to ineffective liberation of cobalamin bound to protein in food. In these patients, the absorption of crystalline vitamin B_{12} is normal. In such patients, as well as for the strict vegan (i.e., no animal product ingestion), oral cobalamin can be utilized after tissue stores have been repleted with parenteral therapy. Oral 1-mg (1000-μg) tablets are available for such use and should be given daily.

Increased daily cobalamin requirements occur in pregnancy and lactation, thyrotoxicosis, and liver or renal disease (especially if protein loss is extensive). Because tissue concentrations of cobalamin are in the milligram range and daily requirements are in the microgram range, the normal stores are adequate for 1 to 3 years in the absence of supplementation. Deficiency is therefore uncommonly associated with such an increased need, except in pregnancy in a vegan, because cobalamin deficiency can occur in the infant of a clinically asymptomatic mother.

Side effects of cobalamin therapy are incredibly rare. Patients with the extremely rare early Leber disease (hereditary optic nerve atrophy) have been reported in the past to have increased atrophy with institution of high-dose therapy. Rarely, pruritus and rash have occurred. Anaphylactic shock has been reported.

Short-term sequelae of repletion therapy in megaloblastic states occur regardless of the etiology of the deficiency. These include hypokalemia and hyperuricemia, especially in the first 48 to 72 hours of therapy. Therefore, potassium supplementation is wise when therapy is started.

TREATMENT OF FOLATE DEFICIENCY

Normal total tissue stores of folate are approximately 5000 µg (5 mg) with a projected daily requirement of 100 to 200 µg. Folate deficiency therefore develops more quickly with dietary deprivation than does cobalamin deficiency. Because most clinical circumstances of folate deficiency are due to inadequate intake or drug interference, oral repletion is the usual mode, with 1-mg (or 5-mg) folic acid pills (the commonly available form) per day. In general, 1 mg per day provides a significant excess, and allows repletion of tissue stores. In known malabsorption syndromes, the 5-mg daily folic acid oral dose is preferable. An intravenous formulation is available in a 15-mg dose form. In general, tissue stores can be repleted easily in a few weeks with daily oral therapy; therefore, the duration of therapy is then determined by the continued presence of cause.

Folate prophylaxis is recommended throughout pregnancy, in which at least 600 µg of folic acid per day is desirable because of the potential to eliminate neural tube defects. For a patient in whom a previous pregnancy has been associated with a neural tube defect, it is recommended that 4 mg per day be used, beginning 4 weeks before the pregnancy and continuing at least through the first 3 months. High doses of folate (greater than 500 µg per day) have allegedly reduced zinc absorption; thus, mineral supplementation during pregnancy is appropriate. Another circumstance that merits folate prophylaxis is in patients undergoing long-standing anticonvulsant therapy. Folate deficiency has been associated with an increased frequency of convulsions. This can be circumvented by giving 1 mg per day of folic acid.

It again merits emphasis that empirical folate therapy in megaloblastic anemia will repair the anemia, but if the correct diagnosis is cobalamin deficiency, a fulminant neurologic deficit may ensue.

SEQUENCE OF REPAIR AFTER THERAPY AND FOLLOW-UP CARE

Table 4 delineates the sequence of repair immediately after institution of therapy in megaloblastic anemia. Because increased incidences of gastric polyps (up to 5%) and gastric cancer (2 to 3%) occur in patients with pernicious anemia, long-term surveillance is needed. Less common is the development of endocrinopathy (especially thyroid or adrenal) secondary to the organ-related autoantibodies. Such surveillance provides for continued education of patients, compliance with treatment, and confirmation that a reversible pathophysiologic mechanism has been corrected.

TABLE 4. Pattern of Repair of Megaloblastic Anemia with Therapy

Time	Response
8–12 h	Decrease in serum iron and ferritin
12–36 h	Hypokalemia; hyperuricemia
24–48 h	Normalization of bone marrow
	Normalization of deoxyuridine suppression
D 2–3	Increased sense of well-being and appetite
	Increased reticulocytes
	Decrease in indirect hyperbilirubenemia
D 5–9	Reticulocyte peak
D 7–10	Decrease in serum lactate dehydrogenase
D 7–14	Decrease in serum methylmalonic acid and total homocysteine
	Increasing red blood cell values
Wk 2–4	Normalization of mean corpuscular volume
	Disappearance of hypersegmented polymorphonuclear leukocytes

THALASSEMIA

method of
EDWARD J. BENZ, JR., M.D.
Johns Hopkins University School of Medicine
Baltimore, Maryland

PATHOPHYSIOLOGY: BASIC MECHANISMS OF HEMOGLOBIN SYNTHESIS

The sequential expression of the different globin genes is responsible for the production of specific types of hemoglobins at different stages of development. At about 12 weeks of gestation, there is a transition from embryonic to fetal hemoglobin, followed at 38 weeks by the switch to adult hemoglobin. Hemoglobin production occurs in bone marrow erythroblasts. The stable accumulation exclusively of fully formed hemoglobin tetramers (e.g., hemoglobin A = $\alpha_2\beta_2$) requires that the production of alpha-like globins equal that of beta-like globins by the globin gene clusters (alpha-like genes on chromosome 16; beta-like genes on chromosome 11) at all times.

Thalassemia syndromes result from deficiencies in the production of either alpha-globin (α-thalassemia) or beta-globin (β-thalassemia) chains. The disease becomes apparent when production of the affected globin is first required during development. α-Thalassemia is thus symptomatic during gestation. Because beta globin is not required before birth, β-thalassemia is asymptomatic until 6 to 12 months after birth.

An obvious consequence of the biosynthetic defect in thalassemia is the microcytosis and hypochromia due to reduced amounts of hemoglobin tetramer in each red blood cell. However, the major pathologic process in the thalassemias is caused by the imbalance of alpha and non-alpha chain accumulation. Aggregation of the *unaffected chains* produced in normal amount occurs because the surplus chains are unable to find a heterologous counterpart to which to bind; these precipitate during erythropoiesis because free globin is far less soluble than intact tetramers. In β-thalassemia, the precipitated alpha globin forms inclusion bodies that damage the red blood cell membrane and cause cell death (ineffective intramedullary erythropoiesis); decreased red blood cell survival also occurs because of uptake in the splenic reticuloendothelial system (splenomegaly). A dramatic expansion of the bone marrow compartment then results from erythropoietin stimulation of further ineffective erythropoiesis. The marrow overgrowth leads to cortical thinning, pathologic fractures, and deformities of bones. Hypersplenism worsens the anemia by causing increased trapping of the formed elements of the blood. An increase in plasma volume, a consequence of the marrow and splenic expansion, also lowers the effective level of hemoglobin.

In α-thalassemic fetuses, excessive gamma globin forms tetramers (γ_4 = hemoglobin Bart's) during the fetal and neonatal period; excess beta globin (β_4 = hemoglobin H) accumulates after birth. Hemoglobin Bart's and hemoglobin H are somewhat more soluble and result in a milder ineffective erythropoiesis than is seen in β-thalassemia. These tetramers, however, exhibit abnormal oxygen binding and sensitivity to oxidant stress (see later).

The alpha-globin gene is duplicated. There is a good correlation between the number of abnormal alpha-globin loci inherited and the clinical presentation. Loss of all four globin genes results in a lethal intrauterine condition, hydrops fetalis. Only hemoglobin Bart's can form; this hemoglobin has a massively left-shifted oxygen dissociation curve that supports almost no oxygen delivery to tissues. Deletion of three alpha loci produces a chronic hemolytic anemia, hemoglobin H disease. Hemoglobin A production is sufficient for survival, but hemoglobin H is moderately unstable and oxidant sensitive, causing hemolysis. Deletion of only one (α-thalassemia-2) or two (α-thalassemia-1) loci is asymptomatic, although the latter condition produces hypochromia and microcytosis.

Severe forms of α-thalassemia are common in Asians and in Mediterranean populations. In black (African) populations, severe disease is almost never seen, even though the α-thalassemia-2 deletion is extremely common (5 to 15% gene frequency). The virtual absence of mutations that inactivate both loci on the same chromosome in black persons explains this discrepancy.

In β-thalassemia, clinically significant disease is seen only when both beta-globin alleles are impaired by mutation. Direct globin gene analysis in affected patients and their families indicates whether the expression of each of the two affected genes is completely absent (β^0-thalassemia) or partially reduced (β^+-thalassemia). A large number of different molecular lesions of the gene, mostly point mutations, cause these defects.

Thalassemia syndromes are commonly graded according to the severity of the anemia. Severe anemia presenting in the first 6 to 9 months after birth (thalassemia major) is usually caused by the inheritance of two seriously impaired beta-globin alleles. The heterozygous state (inheritance of a single defective allele) is characterized by a mild hypochromic and microcytic anemia (thalassemia minor). Under certain circumstances, the "homozygous" state has a milder than usual presentation, for example, when there is a relatively mild reduction in globin synthesis attributable to one or both thalassemic alleles, when there is a higher than usual compensatory increase in gamma chain production, or when the coinheritance of α-thalassemia decreases the net imbalance and alpha- and beta-globin synthesis. This condition, termed "thalassemia intermedia," exhibits stigmas of anemia, hemolysis, and marrow expansion but no requirement for chronic transfusions for survival.

DIAGNOSIS

The diagnosis of severe thalassemia is usually straightforward. The family history, especially in ethnic groups at high risk (Italian, Greek, black, Asian, North African), is often a solid lead. Thalassemia major or thalassemia intermedia is marked by microcytic anemia associated with jaundice, bone deformities, and splenomegaly appearing during gestation (α-thalassemia) or in the first 2 years of life. Hydrops fetalis typically presents as polyhydramnios and fetal distress during the second trimester.

Peripheral blood films show characteristic features that distinguish thalassemia from iron deficiency. For the same level of anemia, thalassemic smears exhibit more pronounced microcytosis with anisocytosis and *relative* hypochromia, punctate basophilic stippling, and a high percentage of target cells (up to 30%). The last two phenomena are less dramatically expressed in iron deficiency. The reticulocyte count is deceptively low for the degree of anemia (2 to 8%) because of the ineffective erythropoiesis. In hemoglobin H disease, the diagnosis can be suspected by in vitro precipitation of hemoglobin H with brilliant cresyl blue.

β-Thalassemia trait (β-thalassemia minor) is recognized by mild anemia (hematocrit of >30) with dramatically low mean corpuscular volume (<75 fL) and erythrocytosis (red blood cell count of $>5 \times 10^6$ per mm^3), near-normal "red blood cell distribution width" and mean corpuscular hemoglobin concentration values, a normal serum iron concentration and total iron-binding capacity, and normal ferritin level. A microcytic blood picture is also seen in cases of congenital sideroblastic anemia, but the classic dimorphic picture and the higher degree of transferrin saturation in this disorder usually permit discrimination.

Hemoglobin electrophoresis, including a quantitative search for the elevation of hemoglobin A and F levels characteristic of β-thalassemia or for hemoglobin H or Bart's, is a useful adjunct, but normal results do not rule out the diagnosis of heterozygous thalassemia. In most heterozygotes, elevations of hemoglobin A_2 and/or hemoglobin F confirm the diagnosis of β-thalassemia. Rare forms of β-thalassemia (e.g., δ β-thalassemia) do not cause elevated hemoglobin A_2 levels. α-Thalassemia trait can be completely silent or similar to β-thalassemia trait, except for an absence of changes in hemoglobin A_2 or F levels. Iron deficiency can mask β-thalassemia trait by decreasing the hemoglobin A_2 level. Coexisting thalassemia trait may thus be overlooked in an iron-deficient individual. If microcytic anemia does not respond completely to iron therapy, hemoglobin electrophoresis should be reconsidered.

The prenatal diagnosis of thalassemia can now be accomplished with a high degree of safety and reliability by direct polymerase chain reaction analysis of fetal DNA obtained by amniocentesis or chorionic villus biopsy. Fetal cell DNA is obtained by amniocentesis after 14 weeks of gestation or by chorionic villus biopsy any time in the first trimester. Direct isolation of fetal cells from maternal blood for DNA analysis by ultrasensitive polymerase chain reaction methods has been shown to be technically feasible but remains clinically unproven as a noninvasive method of antenatal diagnosis.

The large variety of DNA sequence defects that can cause thalassemia require that these analyses be done by experts. Many mutations must be screened to achieve useful predictability. One solid improvement has been the tailoring of these searches within each ethnic group on the basis of molecular epidemiologic surveys. These have shown that a few mutations account for the majority of serious cases within virtually every ethnic group. This greatly simplifies the analyses. The small size of the globin genes also permits rapid and direct DNA sequencing of the inherited alleles in cases in which clear diagnosis is not apparent from the standardized assays. Widespread application of molecular epidemiology, genetic counseling, and antenatal diagnosis has virtually eliminated the appearance of new cases of thalassemias in some areas of the Mediterranean basin.

THERAPY

β-Thalassemia

In heterozygous α- or β-thalassemias, close monitoring of the hematocrit is necessary during pregnancy to avoid a harmful drop, but patients are otherwise asymptomatic. Genetic counseling is mandatory.

Transfusion Therapy

In β-thalassemia major, red blood cell transfusion is the mainstay of supportive therapy. Transfusions should be administered in sufficient quantity and frequency to achieve a hemoglobin level of *at least* 9.3 grams per dL; this level partly suppresses the erythropoietic drive. A regimen that maintains the mean hemoglobin level above 10.5 to 11 grams per dL reduces marrow expansion, leading to a reduction in plasma volume and thus in the amount of blood required to achieve the same level of hemoglobin, especially in splenectomized patients. Bone changes are arrested or even regress, splenomegaly is retarded or recedes, growth improves, and improved physical activity can be expected. The increased transfusional iron load is partially compensated for by decreased gastrointestinal iron absorption. *Most experts maintain patients in the range of 9.5 to 11 grams per dL.*

With regard to initiation of chronic transfusions, one can safely follow the recommendations of the guide of the Cooley's Anemia Foundation: transfusion should be started for a persistent and otherwise unexplained fall in hemoglobin below 7 grams per dL. Patients with higher hemoglobin levels may require chronic transfusions to address significant growth impairment, serious bone changes, or progressive splenomegaly. A maintenance hemoglobin level above 10.5 to 11 grams per dL in nonhypersplenic patients is recommended. Frequent (one or two per week) infusions of small quantities of red blood cells provide the most "physiologic" support, but the psychologic burden, especially for children, and logistical issues render this strategy impractical. In general, transfusion of about 15 mL of red blood cells per kg at 3- to 5-week intervals is feasible for most patients and families. Transfusion records should be kept to measure the annual mean hemoglobin level and the annual blood consumption.

A complete genotype of the patient's red blood cells should be established before any transfusion treatment occurs; this information simplifies later identification of the involved antigens should isoimmunization occur. Only fresh ABO- and Rh₀D-compatible crossmatched blood should be given. I advocate continuous monitoring for isoantibodies to critical red blood cell antigens, using indirect antiglobulin testing. When patients develop febrile reactions during transfusions, filters retaining the leukocytes should be installed or red blood cells frozen in glycerol used instead. If this is unsuccessful, washing the red blood cells is the next option. Aspirin taken before the transfusion often reduces the reaction. Increased transfusion requirements should alert the physician to possible hypersplenism, alloimmunization, or the presence of an accessory spleen. In addition to the rigorous screening of donor blood for hepatitis antigens, patients should be immunized early for hepatitis B. When titers drop to low levels, booster immunizations are suggested. The danger of human immunodeficiency virus (HIV) infection acquired from blood transfusion depends on the incidence of the disease in the donor pool but is favorably influenced by the intensity of the donor blood screening program, which has considerably diminished the risk for HIV infection in the United States. The possible use of irradiated and cytomegalovirus-free preparations is relevant in potential bone marrow transplant candidates and should be approached in that fashion, in consultation with transfusion medicine experts who are conversant with this rapidly evolving area.

Splenectomy

Massive splenomegaly is usually avoided or delayed by a proper hypertransfusion regimen. However, splenic sequestration of donor cells can eventually cause an excessive transfusion requirement. A 50% or greater increase in the transfusion requirements during a 1-year period is the major indication for surgical removal of the spleen. A transfusion requirement of more than 200 mL per kg per year of packed red blood cells is also an indication for splenectomy if there is no serologic evidence of isoimmunization. Significant leukopenia and thrombocytopenia by splenic trapping are other indications, but these rarely occur without the aforementioned increase in the red blood cell requirement.

Splenectomy significantly increases the risk of overwhelming sepsis, especially in young children. Encapsulated pneumococci are responsible in two thirds of the cases. The other two most frequent pathogens are *Haemophilus influenzae* and *Neisseria meningitidis* (meningococcus). *Yersinia enterocolitica* or *Yersinia pseudotuberculosis* is also found, especially in patients undergoing deferoxamine mesylate (Desferal) treatment (these organisms use the iron bound to the chelator). Because the risk of infections is greatest if patients undergo splenectomy during infancy, one should attempt to defer the operation until the age of 6 years.

Polyvalent pneumococcal vaccine should be administered 1 month before splenectomy. Many experts advocate the administration of oral penicillin V (250 mg per day) as prophylaxis after the procedure for at least 2 years in children younger than 10 years. Trimethoprim-sulfamethoxazole is an alternative in case of allergy. Parents should be instructed to seek immediate medical attention when significant fever develops (>101°F). Such patients are at risk for a fulminant course leading to death within 6 hours. Broad-spectrum antibiotics should be given immediately, even before the results of any laboratory investigations are obtained. Splenectomized patients undergoing invasive procedures (e.g., dental work, endoscopy) should be given prophylactic penicillin (or alternative drugs in allergic patients, as stated earlier) for 24 hours before and after the procedure.

Treatment of Iron Overload

Each unit of blood contains approximately 250 mg of iron. A typical hypertransfusion regimen encumbers each patient *each year* with an average of four times the normal total body iron burden. There is no compensatory mechanism of sufficient magnitude to eliminate this iron; the decrease in intestinal absorption typical of the iron overloaded state is inadequate. Indeed, many transfused thalassemic patients continue to absorb dietary iron at high rates, probably because of signals from the expanded erythropoietic drive. By the time most of these patients reach adolescence, their iron stores have risen to toxic levels (transfusional hemosiderosis).

Before effective iron chelation therapy was developed, the dramatic multiorgan toxicity of iron was the major determinant in the fatal progression of the disease. The complications have a more subtle presentation in patients maintained with chelation therapy. Hemosiderosis causes the most striking clinical dysfunction in the endocrine organs, liver, and heart.

One common endocrinologic complication is glucose intolerance. Insulin-dependent diabetes mellitus occurs in a smaller group. Laboratory evidence of primary hypothyroidism, hypoparathyroidism, and other endocrinopathies can often be detected in the absence of symptoms; digoxin refractoriness in such patients should lead one to suspect hypocalcemia on this basis. One should be alert to diminished adrenal reserves during periods of metabolic stress in these patients. Delayed puberty is common and is probably the result of iron deposition in the hypothalamus. Retarded growth in the hypertransfused patients is less striking in the early years but becomes pronounced at puberty. The exact mechanism is unclear.

Hepatic toxicity can lead to cirrhosis, but progression to symptomatic liver disease before the era of sustained chelation therapy was unusual because of the superseding onset of lethal cardiac complications. Subclinical cardiac dysfunction usually begins in the early teens; it is detectable by the reduced ejection fractions in exercising patients or by wall motion anomalies. Onset of clinical symptoms usually begins with arrhythmias or pericarditis, followed by congestive failure in the late teens and death at about the age of 20 years.

The iron chelator deferoxamine mesylate is an effective agent when it is administered as a continuous subcutaneous or intravenous infusion. This maneuver markedly improves urinary iron excretion in comparison with intramuscular injections. When given as a continuous infusion in high enough doses in *most* patients, the drug maintains a negative iron balance despite continuing blood transfusions. When started before 5 to 8 years of age, these regimens are proving to be effective in delaying cardiac disease in some patients, potentially prolonging survival.

In the presence of a significant iron burden before the onset of therapy, complete reversibility of the lesions by deferoxamine cannot be reliably predicted. If therapy is started after 10 years of age, progressive cardiac dysfunction may not be completely prevented. Early initiation of therapy is thus advocated.

Iron overload should be documented first in candidates for iron chelation by a deferoxamine test. The 24-hour urinary excretion after injection of 500 mg of deferoxamine should exceed 1 mg to consider chelation therapy (or the serum ferritin level should be above 1000 ng per mL). Another option, gaining increasing favor and preferred by me, is to start the deferoxamine therapy at the same time as the transfusions.

A small infusion pump is used to administer a dose of about 40 mg per kg per day during a period of 10 hours into the abdominal subcutaneous fat, with rotation of the sites. Hypertonicity of the solution can be prevented by increasing the volume of water for the delivery of a given dose. Local allergic reactions (pruritus, hyperemia) can be suppressed by adding hydrocortisone (up to 2 mg per mL) to the solution or by using topical diphenhydramine. A number of cases of severe arrhythmias and severe congestive heart failure have been temporarily reversed with high-dose (15 mg per kg per hour for 10 hours) deferoxamine through a central venous catheter.

The drug is generally well tolerated. Anaphylactic reactions are rare and can be treated with desensitization. A number of patients treated with high-dose intravenous deferoxamine developed optic and acoustic neuritis, with only partial reversibility. Periodic vision and hearing tests are advocated. If the abnormalities disappear after discontinuation of the drug, the treatment can be cautiously reinitiated, beginning with lower doses.

Iron overload causes depletion of vitamin C. This deficiency inhibits iron release from the reticuloendothelial cells. Sudden availability of vitamin C can lead to a massive, abrupt release of iron, a situation that can cause serious cardiotoxicity. It is therefore advisable to start exogenous vitamin C administration only *after* the first cycle of treatment with deferoxamine. The dose should be about 5 mg per kg, should not exceed 100 mg per day when deferoxamine is given, and should be given only while the deferoxamine infusion is actually in progress. Ascorbate can be replaced by oranges (75 mg per orange) or orange juice (50 mg per 100 mL).

The major problem with deferoxamine therapy is noncompliance because of the inconvenience using the pump. Regular monitoring and psychologic support are important for the success of the treatment. In addition to specialized assistance from social workers and child psychologists, patients' advocacy associations can help the patient cope with the emotional burden of the disease. There is reason to hope that the inconvenience of the present chelation therapy will disappear in the near future. Clinical trials with a promising oral chelator (L1) suggest possible clinical efficacy, although further testing for long-term effectiveness and safety is still in progress.

Thalassemia Intermedia

A number of patients with symptomatic β-thalassemia do not develop a debilitating anemia. These patients should not be committed to a lifelong transfusion regimen. In general, when the hemoglobin level remains above 8 grams per dL, patients lead a relatively normal life. However, regardless of the steady-state hemoglobin level, the patient should be watched closely for signs of bone marrow expansion, increasing spleen size, or growth retardation. These are all indications to initiate transfusion, usually the same regimen used to treat thalassemia major. If the fall of the mean hemoglobin level to unsuitable values parallels an increase in spleen size, splenectomy should be considered. Hypertransfusion can be delayed or avoided by splenectomy in some cases.

The hyperplastic marrow in thalassemia intermedia stimulates intestinal iron absorption, resulting in iron overload. Deferoxamine therapy should probably be started when the ferritin level rises above normal; one or two subcutaneous infusions a week generally suffice. Deferoxamine therapy is stopped during pregnancy, and a regular transfusion regimen during this period should be considered. The avoidance of iron-rich meats (liver and spleen), the ingestion of cereals, and the regular drinking of a cup of tea are advocated by some as dietary measures.

Other complications of chronic hemolysis are relative folate deficiency, gallstones, leg ulcers, and, rarely, compression syndromes. Vitamin deficiency can be avoided by a daily supplement of 1 mg of folic acid. Patients should be evaluated promptly for symptoms suggestive of cholecystitis. In addition to local treatment of leg ulcers, leg elevation and per-oral zinc sulfate are useful; ulcers in a nontransfused patient may require at least temporary hypertransfusion. Radiotherapy may be needed to treat spinal cord compression from marrow expansion in vertebrae.

α-Thalassemia

Often no treatment is indicated with this disorder. The homozygous form is usually lethal in utero. Cases have been described of neonates who were kept alive with exchange transfusions. Patients with hemoglobin H disease usually present with moderate anemia. They should be monitored for worsening of the anemia during infections. If it is persistent and is associated with increasing splenomegaly, splenectomy should be considered; as in other forms of unstable hemoglobin disease, a substantial increase in red blood cell survival and in hemoglobin level often follows removal of the spleen. Another characteristic in common with unstable hemoglobin variants is the sensitivity of hemoglobin H to oxidant stress; drugs such as sulfonamides exacerbate the effect of the infection in worsening the anemia. Oxidant drugs should thus be avoided in this disease. Folic acid supplements are indicated, as in other cases of chronic hemolysis. Iron overload is a real issue in these patients, by analogy to patients with β-thalassemia intermedia, and becomes a major issue in late adolescence and adult life; iron status should thus be monitored even in the absence of transfusions.

EXPERIMENTAL THERAPY

Bone Marrow Transplantation

Allogeneic bone marrow transplantation can be curative by replacing stem cells harboring defective globin genes with normal cells. Transplantation is associated with significant mortality and morbidity resulting from the toxicity of the conditioning regimen and from the pancytopenia and acute and chronic graft-versus-host disease after the procedure. Because of the immediate risks, only a few centers have systematically used this therapeutic option in the last decade. Data emerging from these centers suggest short-term mortality rates of 10 to 15%, with good long-term results in survivors; risk of dying is greatest in patients with the greatest degree of iron overload at the time of transplantation. Organ hemosiderosis is considered the age-related risk factor. Relapse occurred in 13% of the younger patients and 5% of the older ones. Moderate to severe graft-versus-host disease was present in 5% of patients younger than 7 years and in 13% of the older group.

I believe that if a patient has an HLA-matched sibling, marrow transplantation should be considered in the earlier years. The risks of this curative therapeutic modality must be weighed against the lifelong burden of hypertransfusion regimens and iron-chelating therapy. This balance may be shifted in the near future by the introduction of oral chelating agents and by improvement in the transplantation regimens.

Activation of Fetal Globin Synthesis

In a limited number of patients studied for a short period of observation, gamma-globin chain expression was stimulated by the use of the chemotherapeutic agent 5-azacytidine. The increased gamma chain synthesis resulted in a significant decrease in the transfusion requirement that lasted for several days after discontinuation of the drug. Initially, the effect of the drug was thought to be mediated by the DNA hypomethylating activity of this agent, because gamma-globin gene expression was inversely correlated with the methylation status of gamma-globin gene DNA. (DNA *hypermethylation* often correlates with inactivation of a gene.) Other cytotoxic agents (hydroxyurea and cytosine arabinoside) with no direct demethylating activity have subsequently been shown to be efficacious, suggesting strongly that the clinical effect arises from cell selection and reprogramming of globin gene regulation by mechanisms not dependent on demethylating activity. The uncertainty about the carcinogenic side effects resulting from long-term use of these drugs has, until recently, limited this therapy to adult patients with advanced disease in the controlled setting of experimental trials in a few centers. However, significant favorable clinical experiences have been reported with the use of hydroxyurea in sickle cell anemia. These findings suggest that this drug might be useful for wider application to thalassemic patients. Until more information about long-term toxicity and efficacy is available from these studies, this therapy should still be considered experimental and used in major centers in the context of longitudinal studies. Butyric acid derivatives also appear to promote gamma globin synthesis; they are also under active investigation.

Gene Transfer

Many are investigating the biologic mechanisms necessary to achieve the long-term goal of correcting the defective genes in the stem cells of a thalassemic patient. At present, the most efficient system for transferring globin genes in hematopoietic stem cells is the retroviral vector, but many alternative systems are being studied because of disappointing results with this vector. Recent research has defined the major DNA control elements ("locus control region" sequences) that must be introduced with the structural globin sequences in retroviral vectors for controlled, abundant expression in erythroid progenitors. Several important problems must be solved before gene transfer systems can be applied in a curative mode to human thalassemic, hematopoietic stem cells. No definite time frame for the introduction of gene therapy in thalassemia can be anticipated at this moment.

SICKLE CELL DISEASE

method of
GRAHAM R. SERJEANT, M.D.
MRC Laboratories (Jamaica), University of the West Indies
Kingston, Jamaica, West Indies

The experience presented here draws heavily, but not entirely, on Jamaican practice evolved from the management of more than 5000 patients with sickle cell disease. These groups of patients include the Jamaican Cohort Study (approximately 550 children with sickle cell disease followed up from birth) and a large group of patients acquired predominantly by symptomatic referral. With the limited resources available for care, this treatment approach has had to be confined to methods for which there is good scientific and experimental evidence. Costly and often arbitrary therapies such as blood transfusion

have been used only if there was clear evidence of a benefit. It is suggested that the rigorous discipline imposed by limited resources has rarely compromised the quality of medical care. This, then, is a Jamaican perspective of the therapy for sickle cell disease.

PATHOPHYSIOLOGY

The single nucleotide mutation determining the insertion of valine for glutamic acid at the sixth position from the amino terminus of the beta chain significantly changes the behavior of the hemoglobin (Hb) molecule. When deoxygenated, molecules of sickle hemoglobin (HbS) polymerize, raising the internal cellular viscosity, reducing membrane pliability, and distorting the red blood cell (RBC). Such cells have difficulty negotiating capillary beds, resulting in the two independent but closely interrelated pathophysiologic features of the disease, hemolysis and vaso-occlusion.

Hemolysis reduces RBC survival from a normal mean of 120 days to an average of 8 to 12 days, resulting in anemia (average Hb value, 6–9 grams per dL in homozygous sickle cell [SS] disease), jaundice, increased prevalence of pigment gallstones, and expansion of the bone marrow spaces. The expanded bone marrow can change the configuration of some bones, and its metabolic and nutritional demands may compromise growth and development. Generally, the hemolytic features are well tolerated and, with the exception of a superimposed aplastic crisis, rarely lead to mortality. The tendency to compromise blood flow damages the tissue supplied, the features depending on the site of nonperfusion. This ischemia most commonly affects the bone marrow (painful crisis), skin (leg ulceration), spleen (acute and chronic sequestration, impaired function), brain (stroke), and lungs (acute chest syndrome).

GENOTYPES OF SICKLE CELL DISEASE

Among communities in which sickle cell disease is predominantly of African origin, there are four principal genotypes (Table 1). SS disease and sickle cell–β^0-thalassemia manifest the greatest anemia and generally more severe clinical courses, although both show extreme variability in clinical features. Patients with sickle cell–hemoglobin C (SC) disease

TABLE 1. **Major Genotypes of Sickle Cell Disease and Their Frequency in Jamaica**

Genotype	Abbreviated Form	Frequency
Homozygous sickle cell disease	SS disease	1 in 300 births
Sickle cell–hemoglobin C disease	SC disease	1 in 500 births
Sickle cell–β^+-thalassemia	Sβ^+-thalassemia	1 in 3000 births
Sickle cell–β^0-thalassemia	Sβ^0-thalassemia	1 in 7000 births

and sickle cell–β⁺-thalassemia are less anemic, with hemoglobin levels reaching into the normal range, and generally have mild manifestations. Most complications of sickle cell disease occur in all genotypes, although the frequency and severity are greater in the severe forms. The following discussion relates primarily to SS disease, and the complications believed to be related to hemolytic rate are discussed first.

ANEMIA

Steady State

Most patients with SS disease have steady-state hemoglobin levels of 6 to 9 grams per dL. At steady-state levels, symptoms of anemia are unusual, and oxygen carriage appears to be close to normal. This is because HbS within the RBC manifests a low oxygen affinity, becoming almost fully saturated in the lungs but releasing more oxygen per gram of hemoglobin in the periphery compared with normal hemoglobin A (HbA). Furthermore, the severity of anemia correlates with the extent of shift in the oxygen dissociation curve, patients with the largest shifts (lowest affinity) manifesting the lowest hemoglobin levels. These observations imply that erythropoiesis is switched off at submaximal levels (average reticulocyte counts 10 to 12%), not because the bone marrow cannot sustain greater erythropoietic activity, but because higher levels are not necessary to maintain adequate oxygen carriage. Transfusion of patients with hemoglobin at their steady-state levels is therefore not justified on the basis of improving oxygen carriage.

Lowered Hemoglobin Levels

A variety of complications are associated with acute and chronic lowering of hemoglobin below steady-state values. In each case, the physician should seek and treat the cause rather than resorting to the blanket therapy of transfusion. Reticulocyte counts, as indicators of bone marrow activity, are essential to diagnosis, and mean cell volume (MCV) is helpful in distinguishing iron deficiency or megalo-

blastic change from folate deficiency (Table 2). Megaloblastic change should be treated with folic acid. Regular folate supplementation is not practiced in Jamaica, because dietary folate levels appear adequate, but folate supplementation may be given at times of additional requirements, such as rapid growth periods or pregnancy. Unnecessary supplementation should be avoided, and patients encouraged to eat fresh fruit and vegetables.

Iron deficiency may occur without obvious cause and is presumed to be dietary in origin, although causes of iron loss may need investigating. There is usually a rapid response to oral iron therapy. Occasionally, combined iron and folic acid deficiencies may cause diagnostic confusion, because there may be no change in RBC characteristics, but both serum folate and iron levels are low. Supplementation with folate reveals iron-limited erythropoiesis, and the MCV falls; supplementation with iron reveals folate-limited erythropoiesis, and the MCV rises. Aplastic crisis and acute splenic sequestration generally require urgent transfusion and are discussed later. A variety of hypoplastic situations manifest low hemoglobin levels, and low levels but not absence of reticulocytes and can occur with infections and chronic renal failure.

APLASTIC CRISIS

Aplastic crisis affected 30% of patients with SS disease in the Jamaican Cohort Study by the age of 15 years. Defined clinically by marked lowering of hemoglobin level and absence of reticulocytes from the peripheral blood, aplastic crises are most common before 15 years of age, occur in epidemics, and cluster in families. The cause is human parvovirus infection. Bone marrow aplasia lasts 7 to 10 days, and the bone marrow always recovers provided that oxygen carriage is maintained by transfusion. A single unit of blood (1 pint for age 15 years and older; 10 mL/kg for younger than this age) achieves this goal, and the clinical course is so predictable and benign that the transfusion is usually performed as an outpatient procedure; the patient is seen after 3 to 4 days to ensure that the reticulocytosis of spontaneous marrow

TABLE 2. **Features Associated with Lowered Hemoglobin Levels in SS Disease**

Complication	Hb Range (gm/dL)	Reticulocytes (%)	MCV (fL)	Other Features
Normal average	6–9	10–12	75–95	
Acute lowering				
Acute splenic sequestration	1–4	20–30	Unchanged	Splenomegaly, 3–5 cm
Aplastic crisis	2–5	0	Unchanged	
Chronic lowering				
Iron deficiency	4–6	1–8	67–75	Iron stores low
Folate deficiency	3–4	1–10	100–120*	
Chronic hypersplenism	3–5	20–40	Unchanged	Splenomegaly, 5–15 cm
Infection	4–6	1–8	Unchanged	
Chronic renal failure	3–5	1–8	Unchanged	Renal impairment

*Degree of change in MCV is important; some patients with genetically determined microcytosis, such as those with SS and α-thalassemia, with a steady-state MCV of 65 fL may manifest megaloblastic change with a rise in MCV to 85 fL (i.e., increase of 20 fL).

Abbreviations: Hb = hemoglobin; MCV = mean cell volume.

recovery has occurred. The strong family history (50% chance of susceptible siblings being affected within 3 weeks) implies that the patient's siblings with SS should be closely monitored. A human parvovirus vaccine has been developed and is currently undergoing early trials. Recurrence of human parvovirus–induced aplastic crisis has never been described, and immunity appears to be lifelong.

ACUTE SPLENIC SEQUESTRATION

Acute enlargement of the spleen with pooling of a significant proportion of the RBC mass may lead to a life-threatening anemia in young children. In the Jamaican Cohort Study, this complication had affected 25% of children by 2 years and 30% by 5 years of age. If the patient survives the first episode, there is a 50% chance of recurrence, with repeated episodes occurring at shorter intervals. Transfusion of a single unit of blood is the treatment of the acute attack, and splenectomy is recommended after two attacks. Parental education in the detection and significance of acute splenic sequestration (ASS) has reduced mortality from this complication by 90%.

CHRONIC HYPERSPLENISM

Chronic splenic sequestration or hypersplenism differs from ASS in its gradual development, greater degree of splenomegaly, and markedly expanded bone marrow activity, which allows a new hematologic equilibrium but at a greatly increased hemolytic rate (mean RBC life, 1 to 3 days). The metabolic demands of the expanded bone marrow compete with those of growth, which frequently slows or ceases, and rapid increase in growth follows splenectomy. The very low hemoglobin level (3 to 5 grams per dL) is associated with high cardiac output and increased cardiac work. Death may occur from superimposed acute sequestration, incidental aplastic crisis, or hemorrhage consequent to the low platelet counts. Hypersplenism may resolve spontaneously, so the condition is usually monitored for 4 to 6 months to assess any resolution before splenectomy is recommended. Patients may be managed by regular transfusion for a limited period, but splenectomy after a period of monitoring is the preferred option.

CHRONIC RENAL FAILURE

Renal tubular damage is common in SS disease, resulting in an inability to concentrate urine and in other functional tubular abnormalities, but the progressive loss of glomeruli results in chronic renal failure. The most likely mechanism is glomerular hyperfiltration leading to glomerulosclerosis and a progressive fall in glomerular filtration rate with eventual elevation of serum creatinine level. Reduced erythropoietin production by the kidney leads to an increased anemia. This is initially well tolerated; indeed, many patients experience a "honeymoon period" free of painful crises. As hemoglobin falls to a level compromising cardiac function, simple "top-up" transfusion may alleviate symptoms. Patients are often the best judges of when transfusion is required, and 1 to 2 units may be given to raise the hemoglobin to 5 to 6 grams per dL. Higher levels are not necessary, and sudden changes in hematocrit may actually further compromise renal function. The anemia of renal failure has been treated with recombinant human erythropoietin, most effectively given by subcutaneous injection at least twice weekly. The most appropriate dose is not known, experience with this expensive drug in sickle cell disease is limited, and poor response is common. Correction of anemia by this method rather than by transfusion increases circulating HbS. Sudden increases in hemoglobin level may induce iatrogenic painful crises, and careful follow-up by clinicians experienced in the use of this agent is recommended. Where renal replacement therapy is an option, early referral to a renal physician is recommended. The severity of renal impairment in SS disease may be underestimated from serum creatinine levels, which are usually lower than those in normal people. Impaired cardiac or respiratory function may necessitate early entry of an SS patient into a dialysis program. Renal transplantation has been successful in SS disease, although sickle-induced damage may occur in the transplanted kidney.

INFECTIONS

Patients with SS disease are more prone to several bacterial infections. Early loss of the splenic filtering capacity for removing blood-borne antigens results in a tendency to overwhelming septicemia, most commonly with *Streptococcus pneumoniae* and *Haemophilus influenzae* type b (Hib).

Prevention

Pneumococcal septicemia may be prevented in a child with SS by regular penicillin, given in Jamaica by monthly intramuscular depot preparations, from 4 months to 4 years of age (penicillin G benzathine, 300,000 units from 4 months to 3 years; 600,000 units from 3 to 4 years), and then administering the 23-valent pneumococcal vaccine (Pneumovax 23) before stopping the penicillin. It is vital that penicillin prophylaxis is not stopped before the vaccine is given, because the child has little naturally acquired immunity and is therefore especially susceptible to infection. The capsular polysaccharide vaccines appear to be poorly antigenic in children younger than 4 years, and there is no convincing evidence that booster vaccines provoke a better response than the age-related increase in maturity of the immune system. Two factors may cause this policy to be modified in the near future, the increasing frequency of penicillin-resistant pneumococci and the advent of a conjugated pneumococcal vaccine that may be effective when given at 2, 4, and 6 months and that is currently undergoing trial in SS disease.

Hib infection is also increased in SS disease and becomes more apparent with the prevention of pneumococcal disease. Prevention is based on a conjugated Hib vaccine (HibTITER), which appears to induce good antibody levels and the clinical efficacy of which is being assessed. This may be given with other immunizations at 2, 4, and 6 months.

Areas of avascular necrosis of bone have long been known to be susceptible to infection by *Salmonella* species, causing salmonella osteomyelitis (see later). Salmonella septicemia may also occur in the absence of bone involvement, and the low index of suspicion for this organism in a "septicemic" patient may result in high mortality.

Treatment

Septic patients with high fever must be assumed to have infections with *S. pneumoniae*, Hib, or *Salmonella* and should be given suitable antibiotics pending the results of blood culture. Most effective, if available, is ceftriaxone (Rocephin), 100 mg per kg per day twice daily intravenously for at least 7 days. Cheaper alternatives are crystalline penicillin, 200,000 units per kg per day, and chloramphenicol, 75 to 100 mg per kg per day, both intravenously every 6 hours for at least 7 days.

Although infections are commonly associated with reduced bone marrow activity and an increasing anemia, primary therapy must be directed against the cause of the infection and only secondarily against the anemia, which may require transfusion.

JAUNDICE, BILIRUBIN EXCRETION, AND GALLSTONES

The increased bilirubin production consequent to hemolysis is associated with both clinical jaundice and pigment gallstones. The severity of clinical jaundice varies among patients and also in the same patient, becoming more obvious during fever, dehydration, or painful crises. This feature causes concern, but patients may be reassured that such jaundice is a harmless side effect of hemolysis and does not have the serious significance of jaundice in otherwise normal people (e.g., indicative of hepatitis). Occasionally, marked increases in bilirubin level may occur consequent to acute cholestasis or obstruction of the common bile duct by a gallstone. The distinction by ultrasonography is vital, because acute cholestasis generally resolves with conservative therapy, whereas an obstructed common bile duct may need removal at surgery or endoscopy.

Gallstones have been observed in children as young as 3 to 4 years and reached an incidence of 40% by age 20 years in the Jamaican Cohort Study. Most gallstones are asymptomatic, and there is no evidence justifying surgical removal of asymptomatic stones. Cholecystectomy should be performed for specific symptoms, including acute and chronic cholecystitis, empyema, and obstruction of the cystic duct or of the common bile duct. Nonspecific abdominal pain

should not be considered an indication for cholecystectomy, because it frequently coincides with gallstones, but studies have shown that both factors reflect an underlying clinical severity and that they are not causally related. Nonspecific abdominal pain may continue after cholecystectomy for gallstones.

BONE PROBLEMS

Dactylitis

A common early manifestation of SS disease, dactylitis affects 50% of Jamaican Cohort Study children by the age of 2 years. Because it may start in children as young as 3 to 4 months and is almost synonymous with sickle cell disease, it is a common cause of the initial diagnosis of sickle cell disease. Painful swelling of the small bones of the hands and feet affects single or multiple bones and results from bone marrow necrosis. Dactylitis frequently recurs, but attacks become rare after age 5 to 6 years. Generally, clinical and radiologic resolution is complete, although sometimes, probably as a result of superimposed infection, there may be premature fusion of the epiphysis and a permanent shortening and deformity of small bones. Treatment consists of pain relief and reassurance that the complication is not serious.

Painful Crisis

With increasing age, erythropoietic activity ceases in the bone marrow of the small bones of the hands and feet, and greatest activity occurs in the juxta-articular areas of the long bones, the spine, and the flat bones of the sternum, ribs, and pelvis. Avascular necrosis of bone marrow at these sites causes the typical painful crisis that may thus be viewed as the adult counterpart of dactylitis in childhood. It is believed that the necrosis is probably painless but that the inflammatory response associated with the repair and healing of dead bone marrow increases intramedullary pressure and may cause extreme pain. There are well-recognized precipitating factors that, in Jamaica, include skin cooling, dehydration, infection, pregnancy, and the immediate postpartum period. Cold is most common, and many painful crises may be prevented by avoiding getting caught in the rain, not taking cold baths, and keeping warm in winter and at night. Risk factors include a high hemoglobin level, most common in adolescent male patients. The natural history is for pains to become less frequent and less severe after age 30 years, and in most patients, they cease entirely after age 40 years. Patients who seem to be exceptions to this pattern should be carefully assessed for social, psychologic, and other possible factors.

Pain relief is a clinical challenge in the painful crisis. Human response to pain and the ability to cope with pain are notably influenced by many social and cultural factors. Examination of the clinical course in some patients manifesting frequent painful crises in Jamaica shows amelioration of symptoms during periods of social stability and recurrence of pains when support systems disappear. Patients in painful crisis often do not understand the cause or mechanism of the pains, and they experience panic and a sense of impending doom. Patients in painful crisis have stated that they have only to reach the doors of the Sickle Cell Clinic in Jamaica and they start to feel better. It is clear that reassurance can do much to alleviate anxiety and increase the ability to cope with pain.

The objectives of management should therefore be reassurance, treatment or alleviation of any underlying cause if identified, hydration (by intravenous fluid if the patient is vomiting or unable to take fluids orally), and pain relief sufficient to allow the patient to rest and sleep. Most patients keep acetaminophen (Tylenol) at home and have used it before reaching the clinic, but if not, this would be the first line of treatment for all but severe bone pain. Codeine, 30 mg orally, may be helpful in children. Patients with severe bone pains may be given pentazocine (Talwin), 1 mg per kg intramuscularly, or meperidine (Demerol), 1.5 mg per kg intramuscularly,* with further assessment and additional doses after 2 to 3 hours. Anti-inflammatory agents such as diclofenac (Voltaren), 1.5 mg per kg intramuscularly, may relieve pain and reduce narcotic requirements. Most patients are treated in a day care center, where after being monitored for 6 to 7 hours, they are offered the option of admission to hospital or discharge home with the same analgesics in oral form. More than 90% of patients with pain of sufficient severity to require narcotic analgesia in the morning elect to go home in the evening with the assurance that they can return to the day care center on the following day.

Avascular Necrosis of the Femoral Head

Avascular necrosis of bone marrow may also occur in the femoral head and, with continued weight bearing, may result in permanent deformity. Treatment depends on early diagnosis and avoidance of weight bearing for approximately 6 months to allow the femoral head to heal without deformity. Traction may be necessary, but many cases, especially in children and adolescents, may be managed with plaster casts and crutches, alternating a hip spica for 6 weeks with a bent-knee cast for 6 weeks, preventing weight bearing on the affected hip, and allowing the patient to continue attending school. In the belief that a high pressure within the femoral head may exacerbate further necrosis, core decompression of the femoral head has been proposed but is untested in controlled trials. Permanent deformity of the femoral head with persistent pain and limitation of movement may be alleviated by a limited remodeling of the head or osteotomy, but extensive damage and severe symptoms often require total hip replacement (THR). There has been reluctance to perform THR in

younger patients because of concern about life of the prosthesis or the need to revise the operation when such patients are older. Experience suggests that many patients have 10 to 15 years of good function with THR before revision and that the operation should be performed on the basis of severity of symptoms rather than concern about future needs for revision.

Avascular Necrosis of Bone

Avascular necrosis forms part of the spectrum of syndromes resulting from bone marrow necrosis, but rather than the commonly symmetrical distribution of sites seen in the painful crisis, the term "avascular necrosis of bone" is usually reserved to describe involvement of one or two sites that is associated with marked, persistent pain and swelling. Commonly affected sites are the humerus, radius and ulna, clavicle, and tibia. Repeated blood cultures are sterile. Treatment consists of pain relief, restriction of movement, rest of the affected area, and, usually, antibiotics to decrease the risk of secondary infection of dead bone marrow. Differentiating this complication from osteomyelitis may be difficult.

Osteomyelitis

Osteomyelitis, usually caused by *Salmonella* organisms, although occasionally by Hib, *Staphylococcus,* or *Escherichia coli,* is a well-recognized complication. It is believed to be secondary to sterile avascular necrosis. The distribution reflects that of underlying avascular necrosis, most commonly affecting the femur, tibia and fibula, humerus, radius and ulna, small bones of the hands and feet secondary to dactylitis, and, occasionally, femoral head, causing a rapid bone destruction. The diagnosis may be obvious, with gross pain and swelling, high fever, marked radiologic change, suppuration, and positive blood cultures, but some cases are difficult to distinguish from sterile avascular necrosis of bone. There is no acceptable standard for diagnosis in this situation. Treatment requires antibiotics for at least 4 to 6 weeks. Choice of antibiotic is usually based (pending the results of culture) on the typical sensitivity of *Salmonella,* i.e., with chloramphenicol or ampicillin. Surgical drainage and removal of a sequestrum, if formed, are also done. Gentamicin-impregnated beads inserted into the site of osteomyelitis release high concentrations of antibiotic locally, but there is no evidence of their efficacy from controlled trials.

ACUTE CHEST SYNDROME

The acute chest syndrome covers a spectrum of lung disease characterized by fever, cough, pleuritic pain, clinical signs, and radiologic evidence of new pulmonary infiltrates. It is one of the major manifestations of SS disease and a principal cause of death at all ages after 2 years. The pathogenesis includes elements of infection, infarction, fat embolism, and

---

*Intramuscular form not available in the United States.

pulmonary sequestration. A patient's condition may deteriorate rapidly, especially with acute pulmonary sequestration, and should be monitored by pulse oximetry. Respiratory distress with a rapid fall in oxygen saturation is an emergency requiring immediate exchange transfusion (performed in Jamaica manually, with 1 unit of blood removed and 2 units of HbA blood given), which may be repeated after 4 to 6 hours. In successful cases, respiratory distress and a pulmonary "whiteout" may be reversed within 24 hours, indicating an acutely reversible vascular phenomenon. Although evidence of infection is uncommon, all cases of acute chest syndrome should be treated with broad-spectrum antibiotics and physiotherapy. Oxygen is usually given on basic principles, but there is no proof of its benefit. Rib and sternal infarction may also cause pleuritic pain, and voluntary splinting of the chest wall may give rise to secondary atelectasis and the acute chest syndrome. In such cases, incentive spirometry significantly reduces the risks of secondary acute chest syndrome.

BRAIN AND EYES

Stroke

Stroke occurred in 8% of patients in the Jamaican Cohort Study by 14 years and at a median age of 8 years. The risk factors for initial stroke are largely unknown, so prevention is not possible. The risk of recurrence is 50 to 70% within 3 years, and treatment at other centers is currently based on preventing recurrent events through long-term transfusion programs aimed at maintaining HbS levels below 30%. There are many problems with such programs, including the development of alloimmunization, iron overload, maintenance of venous access, transfusion-acquired infections, duration of necessary transfusion, and most appropriate methods of monitoring.

Stroke recurrence has been seen with "successful" programs that maintain HbS levels below 25%. Transfusion reactions continue to be a problem despite the use of leukocyte- and platelet-depleted blood, and some patients develop so many antibodies as to be untransfusable. Prevention of iron overload requires subcutaneous chelation with desferrioxamine and the use of syringe driving pumps for at least 5 nights each week. This treatment is expensive and commonly fails because of lack of compliance in adolescence. Many patients lose peripheral veins and require permanent ports such as Port-A-Caths or Hickman's catheters, both of which are subject to infection and thrombosis.

Transfusion-acquired infections have been reduced by screening of transfused blood, but there remains a period during which infection with human immunodeficiency virus may be undetectable. Cessation of transfusion programs after periods up to 10 to 12 years suggests that the recurrence rate for strokes is higher than if transfusion had never been commenced, resulting in a policy of transfusion for life.

The enormous cost and logistic difficulties with such treatment place it beyond the resources in Jamaica, so long-term transfusion programs are not offered. Exchange transfusion is recommended for the acute event, and a limited transfusion program (approximately 1 unit per month) is offered for 1 year only because of the risks of iron accumulation. A final disadvantage of current therapy is that it cannot be commenced until the child develops the initial stroke.

There is a need to understand the risk factors for initial stroke to institute prevention. This is currently being addressed by two initiatives, a trial of transcranial Doppler ultrasonography to detect cerebral vessel stenoses predictive of stroke and an assessment of the predictive role of upper airway obstruction and episodic hypoxemia in stroke. In the meantime, management of stroke represents a major problem and may justify the risks of bone marrow transplantation (see later).

Eyes

Retinal vaso-occlusion, affecting predominantly the peripheral retina, results in the development of fragile new vessel systems in the periphery supplied by feeding arterioles. These proliferative sickle retinopathy (PSR) lesions may bleed, causing vitreous hemorrhage with transient blurring of vision, and large lesions with associated fibrosis may cause retinal detachment and permanent visual loss. Prevention of these symptoms has led to attempts to render PSR lesions avascular by coagulating the feeding arterioles with a xenon arc or argon laser and also by ablating the ischemic retina with an argon laser. Three trials involving much effort, expense, and potential complications confirmed a significant decrease in the risk of vitreous hemorrhage, but it was clear that although PSR was common (occurring in approximately 70% of adult patients with SC disease), visual loss was relatively rare. It is now recognized that spontaneous nonperfusion (autoinfarction) of these lesions is common, and there is a moratorium on such treatment in Jamaica until the risk factors for autoinfarction are better understood. It is hoped that treatment may be focused on patients in whom spontaneous autoinfarction of PSR lesions is unlikely and in whom the risks of visual loss justify the potential complications of treatment.

LEG ULCERS

Chronic leg ulcers around the ankles are particularly common in Jamaica, affecting 75% of adults with SS disease at some time. They are believed to be multifactorial, with components from trauma, skin infarction, and high venous pressure. Prevention depends on avoiding skin trauma and treating early lesions seriously and intensively. All ulcer swabs yield a variety of bacteria, but these are generally colonizers, and antibiotics do not promote healing unless there is evidence of invasion, such as cellulitis. Standard treatment consists of regular dressing at home twice daily with mild antiseptic agents such as half-strength Eusol* or 0.01% potassium permanganate.* Débridement is achieved when necessary by the use of crushed papaya, which has a proteolytic enzyme. Oral zinc sulfate, 200 mg three times daily, significantly improved healing in a controlled trial. Skin grafting (only pinch grafts, and not split-skin or full-thickness grafts) may be used in clean vascular ulcers, but ambulation before complete healing commonly leads to failure of the pinch grafts. This feature requires complete bed rest in hospital for periods of 2 to 4 months, and the recurrence rate after complete healing is 80 to 90% within 2 years. Complete bed rest always improves ulcer healing, and there is no evidence for a beneficial effect of transfusion or hyperbaric oxygen. In Jamaica, ulceration usually commences in patients between 15 and 20 years of age, at a critical time for education, and there is a direct relationship between age at ulceration and educational attainment. In the absence of the ability to reliably heal ulcers quickly, this secondary educational deprivation may be avoided by persuading teachers and parents to allow children to continue attending school and to dress their ulcers at home at the beginning and end of each day.

PRIAPISM

Involuntary painful erection of the penis unassociated with sexual desire affects approximately 30 to 40% of postpubertal Jamaican male patients with SS disease. It is commonly not reported because of embarrassment or lack of realization that it is related to sickle cell disease. There are two clinical patterns: stuttering priapism, which is generally nocturnal, lasts 3 to 4 hours, is relieved by simple physical measures such as exercise, and is associated with normal intervening sexual function; and major attacks lasting longer than 24 hours, with extreme pain, often penile edema, and usually followed by irreversible damage to the vascular erectile system and impotence. Stuttering attacks are commonly a prodrome for a major attack, although some major attacks occur de novo.

The physician should always inquire directly about stuttering priapism and should reassure patients that these attacks are a common complication of sickle cell disease. If they occur more than 2 nights per week, they may be stopped by stilbestrol.† After the attacks have been stopped, the dose should be rapidly decreased to the minimal amount required to prevent stuttering priapism but allow normal erections and avoid gynecomastia. The usual regimen is 5 mg daily for 3 days to stop the attacks, then 5 mg twice weekly for 2 weeks, 2.5 mg twice weekly for 2 weeks, 2.5 mg weekly for 2 weeks, and then 2.5 mg on alternate weeks for 2 weeks. At that point, the drug is stopped to see whether the attacks return. Cases of priapism vary in the dosage required; some

are controlled by almost homeopathic doses of 1 mg every 3 weeks but attacks recur if this dose is stopped or replaced by a placebo. An alternative but more expensive approach is the use of injections of luteinizing hormone–releasing hormone, but these have not been tested in controlled trials. Lack of understanding of the association of stuttering priapism with sickle cell disease and the anxiety involved may result in frequent painful crises, otherwise uncharacteristic of the patient, which resolve with the successful prevention of priapism with stilbestrol.

Major attacks do not respond to stilbestrol and require surgical relief, which should be minimal. Aspiration and irrigation of the corpora by wide-bore needles allow detumescence, and a spongiosocavernosal shunt is a simple procedure giving more permanent relief. In the past, surgical drainage was avoided in the belief that it induced impotence, but this complication is now recognized to result from the permanent damage to the erectile vascular system. Vascular function may recover in patients sustaining major attacks before the age of 15 years, and occasionally, other patients recover some erectile function in 1 to 2 years after a major attack; usually, however, impotence results. Ejaculation is normal, and the mechanical problems of impotence may be treated with penile prostheses. The dense fibrosis of the corpora renders insertion of even simple rigid prostheses, such as the Small-Carrion prosthesis, difficult, and there is no place for the more sophisticated pneumatic penile prostheses.

PREGNANCY AND CONTRACEPTION
Pregnancy

Sexual development is retarded in patients with sickle cell disease, with a mean delay in menarche of 2.5 years. The interval between first unprotected sexual exposure and pregnancy is similar in SS disease and normal control subjects, contrary to the concept of relative infertility in this condition. Pregnancy is associated with a higher risk of painful crises and acute chest syndrome, especially in the third trimester and the immediate postpartum period. The risk of fetal loss is increased at every stage of pregnancy, and the infant is usually of low birth weight. Delivery should be by the normal vaginal route unless there are obstetric contraindications. All mothers should receive regular antenatal care with daily supplementation with iron and folic acid and should be booked for delivery in a hospital. There is no evidence that prophylactic transfusion improves fetal outcome, and this measure is not performed in Jamaican management of pregnancy in sickle cell disease. Many pregnant women with SS disease continue in good health throughout pregnancy and have normal deliveries, but some are seriously ill, and the maternal mortality in Jamaica is 1%.

Contraception

Patients requesting contraception should be given the best methods available. The frequent assumption

---

*Not available in the United States.
†Not FDA approved for this indication.

that there are serious risks to contraception in SS disease is unjustified, and the risks of pregnancy, although small, far outweigh the theoretical risks of contraception. The injectable contraceptive medroxyprogesterone (Depo-Provera), which is not only an effective contraceptive agent but also increases RBC survival and decreases bone pain in SS disease, is the method of choice. Many Jamaican patients prefer to have regular menstruation and choose the low-estrogen pill. Those requiring longer lasting methods are offered the intrauterine device, or tubal ligation if a permanent method is requested.

SURGERY AND ANESTHESIA

Surgery is performed as infrequently as possible in patients with SS disease, conservative management being preferred for asymptomatic gallstones and non-specific abdominal pain. Common causes of surgery are splenectomy, orthopedic procedures, and operations unassociated with sickle cell disease, such as tonsillectomy and adenoidectomy. Elective surgery should be performed only with the patient clinically well and at a steady-state hemoglobin level. Preoperative transfusion is not performed, but blood is cross-matched to replace that lost at surgery. Most patients are preoxygenated before induction, and close monitoring is essential in the immediate postoperative period, when anesthesia-induced respiratory depression is common. Continued oxygenation and physiotherapy are important after upper abdominal surgery to prevent postoperative acute chest syndrome. The randomized study of transfusion in the Cooperative Study of Sickle Cell Disease in the United States found no difference between preoperative simple transfusion and exchange transfusion but did not assess a group without transfusion. Jamaican experience without transfusion shows a morbidity similar to that observed in transfused groups elsewhere, casting doubt on the value of routine preoperative transfusion.

DIAGNOSIS AND COUNSELING

The many ways in which early morbidity and mortality may be ameliorated in SS disease imply that early diagnosis is essential to implement educational and preventive programs. Diagnosis at birth is a simple cost-effective exercise and should be the objective in all communities. Only then can penicillin prophylaxis, parental education about ASS, complete immunization, better management of the aplastic crisis, and general education about disease management have their full potential impact on improving survival of the patient with SS disease.

Counseling services should explain the basic genetics of the disease and the chances that another child of parents with an SS child will be affected. Prenatal diagnosis should be available for couples who wish to make informed decisions about whether to complete an affected pregnancy. Social and general support services can help patients and their families find solutions to the social and other problems that are so often manifest in symptoms of the disease.

NEW APPROACHES TO TREATMENT

There have been many attempts to find effective antisickling agents, on the assumption that inhibition of sickling may ameliorate manifestations of the disease. Inducing higher levels of fetal hemoglobin has been achieved by hydroxyurea, with significant reductions in the prevalence of painful crises and transfusion requirements in a selected group of severely affected adults. Long-term transfusion programs have been grossly overutilized and, although leading to some short-term benefits, have often induced serious iatrogenic pathology. In Jamaica, no patients receive regular transfusion with the exception of a small group with chronic renal failure, and no patients are receiving hydroxyurea for prevention of painful crises. There seem to be other, more appropriate ways of preventing and managing painful crises, and because a high hemoglobin level is a clearly documented risk factor, venesection is currently being assessed by controlled trial. Currently, our knowledge of the natural history of sickle cell disease is not sufficiently detailed to be able to predict the most appropriate forms of intervention. Bone marrow transplantation may represent a treatment option in the prevention of stroke recurrence. However, the cost, the short-term mortality of 10%, the limited availability of suitable compatible donors, and the long-term risks of sterility mandate a cautious approach.

OPTIMAL CARE

Care is best provided in specialized centers with extensive experience with the disease and familiar, competent staff in whom the patient has confidence. Patients should be regularly reviewed every 3 to 6 months when clinically well and should be encouraged to visit the center at any time if ill. Steady-state hematologic assessments are performed in Jamaica every 2 years, or more frequently if clinically indicated, and allow earlier detection of problems such as chronic renal failure. Counseling and other support services should be available within the center. A day care approach to pain management for the painful crisis may provide a more acceptable alternative to frequent emergency room attendance or hospital admission. The average survival of patients with SS disease is currently approximately 50 years and will continue to improve with better medical and social care.

NEUTROPENIA

method of
ROBERT L. BAEHNER, M.D.
University of Southern California School of Medicine
Los Angeles, California

Neutropenia is defined as an absolute granulocyte count (AGC) of less than 1500 granulocytes per mm³. The AGC is calculated as AGC = neutrophils + bands × total white cell count.

Depending on the AGC, neutropenia may be noted during evaluation for severe infection or may be an isolated laboratory finding. Neutropenia can occur alone or in combination with other hematologic abnormalities suggestive of more generalized marrow disease, such as aplastic anemia and leukemia. The family history, association with other disease or cancer therapy, degree and duration of neutropenia, and ability to handle infection should be considered in the evaluation and management of neutropenia.

CLINICAL PRESENTATION

In the absence of infection, there are no signs or symptoms associated with neutropenia itself. The degree of neutropenia determines the probability of infectious complications, such as sepsis, periodontal disease, mouth infection, gastrointestinal ulceration, and perirectal or skin cellulitis. A history of recurrence of fever every 19 to 30 days is suggestive of cyclical neutropenia.

DIFFERENTIAL DIAGNOSIS

Isolated neutropenia can be either acquired or congenital. Certain congenital neutropenias are due to marrow failure, but most are benign and immune in origin. Patients with the latter type do well despite quite low absolute neutrophil counts. Acquired neutropenia can be due to marrow failure, as in the case of drug or chemotherapy toxicity; to increased margination of neutrophils to the microvasculature, as in complement activation or severe burns; or to peripheral destruction, as in hypersplenism or immune neutropenia. A correctable, although rare, cause of neutropenia is vitamin B_{12} or folate deficiency. In the newborn, neutropenia may be a sign of sepsis. Primary or metastatic bone marrow malignancy can present with neutropenia; however, other hematologic abnormalities are usually present as well. Transient neutropenia can follow viral infection or immunization.

EVALUATION

In the absence of any clinical findings or history, isolated mild neutropenia requires only observation. Medications known to be associated with neutropenia should be stopped. Most postviral neutropenias resolve within 4 to 8 weeks. The blood count should be followed weekly until recovery and with each subsequent febrile episode until it is clear that the neutropenia is not recurrent. If anemia or thrombocytopenia develops in conjunction with the neutropenia, bone marrow aspiration should be performed immediately. If the neutropenia is persistent, bone marrow aspiration and biopsy, determination of vitamin B_{12} and folate levels, evaluation for collagen-vascular disease, and a serum antineutrophil antibody assay should be performed. Twice-weekly blood counts for 6 weeks are required to rule out cyclical neutropenia. Epinephrine or steroid stimulation tests and serum lysozyme determinations are sometimes done but are of no help in establishing a diagnosis or selecting treatment.

TREATMENT

Supportive Management

Supportive management of the neutropenic patient depends on the degree of neutropenia, the cause, and the patient's previous history of ability to handle infection. Because it is not possible to predict the duration or progression of neutropenia at first presentation, management must be much more aggressive than in the case of chronic neutropenias. The AGC can be used as a guide (Table 1). There is rarely room for clinical judgment in the management of patients with absolute neutrophil counts below 250 per mm.[3] If these patients have significant fever (temperature higher than 38.5°C [101.3°F]), they must be admitted to the hospital. Then, after appropriate cultures are obtained, they should receive empirical broad-spectrum parenteral antibiotic therapy. Common bacterial causes of febrile episodes in neutropenic patients are gram-negative bacilli and cocci (*Pseudomonas aeruginosa*, *Escherichia coli*, *Klebsiella* species, *Salmonella*, *Shigella*) and gram-positive bacilli and cocci (*Staphylococcus aureus*, *Staphylococcus epidermidis*, *Streptococcus pneumoniae*, *Streptococcus pyogenes*, viridans streptococci, *Enterococcus faecalis*, *Corynebacterium* species). In the clinical setting of prolonged periods of neutropenia, concomitant polymicrobial and sequential infections are not uncommon. Systemic fungal infections, especially candidiasis and aspergillosis, often occur during the course of broad-spectrum antibiotic therapy, and the risk increases beyond the first week of sustained neutropenic fever. Such a large armamentarium of highly effective antibiotics is currently available that it is difficult to recommend a specific antibiotic or combination of antibiotics. The following regimens are suggested on the basis of the Guidelines for the Use of Antimicrobial Agents in Neutropenia Patients with Unexplained Fever formulated by the Infectious Disease Society of America (these guidelines will be updated in late 1997).

Empirical antibiotic regimens should be selected on the basis of knowledge about local predominant pathogens and antibiotic susceptibilities. In patients without renal impairment, combinations of an aminoglycoside (gentamicin, tobramycin, or amikacin, 2.5 mg per kg every 8 hours) and an antipseudomonal carboxy- or ureidopenicillin (piperacillin

TABLE 1. **Clinically Significant Absolute Neutrophil Counts**

Neutrophil Count (Granulocytes/mm³)	Significance
>1000	Normal host defenses against infection.
500–1000	At some increased risk; patient will still show signs of infection and may have chronic periodontal disease.
200–500	Some protection but at great risk for infection; patient may not show signs of infection; usually treated with antibiotics parenterally in the hospital.
<200	At marked risk of overwhelming infection; patient has few signs of inflammation; patient must be hospitalized and empirically treated with antibiotics.

[Pipracil], ticarcillin with [Timentin] or without [Ticar] clavulanic acid, azlocillin [Azlin],* or mezlocillin [Mezlin]), 350 mg per kg per day divided every 4 hours, or an aminoglycoside with a third-generation antipseudomonal cephalosporin (ceftazidime [Fortaz, Tazidime] or cefoperazone [Cefobid]), 30 to 50 mg per kg every 8 hours, are effective. Serum levels of the aminoglycoside should be monitored and doses adjusted as needed to achieve the following therapeutic concentrations: peak, 5 to 8 μg per mL; trough, 2 μg per mL or less.

In patients with renal impairment, combinations of a third-generation cephalosporin, such as ceftazidime or cefoperazone, 30 to 50 mg per kg every 8 hours, and a ureidopenicillin, such as piperacillin or mezlocillin, 350 to 500 mg per kg every 4 hours, are effective.

In patients in whom coagulase-negative staphylococci, methicillin-resistant *S. aureus*, *S. epidermidis*, *Corynebacterium* species, or alpha-hemolytic streptococci are suspected (e.g., those with indwelling central venous catheters), vancomycin can be added later if gram-positive bacteria are isolated in culture or if no response is obtained from the initial antibiotics after a few days. In the author's opinion, this approach limits the number of patients receiving the drug therapy, reduces the costs of treatment, and minimizes adverse drug reactions and the development of antimicrobial resistance. If the cultures are negative and the fever has resolved, antibiotics can be discontinued after 3 to 5 days. If a source of infection is documented, specific therapy should be instituted and should continue longer than in the non-neutropenic patient. Granulocyte transfusions may be of limited use in patients who have blood culture–proven gram-negative sepsis. For patients who remain febrile and neutropenic for more than a week, a systemic fungal infection should be diligently sought: common sites are the lower esophagus, chest, and sinuses. Amphotericin B infusions, starting at 0.1 mg per kg per dose in 5% dextrose water (to a maximum of 1 mg per kg per dose), should be infused during 2 to 6 hours on a daily basis. Lipid emulsion amphotericin is now available and is better tolerated, is equally effective, and has decreased renal toxicity. Serum creatinine levels should be monitored during treatment. If a systemic fungal infection is identified, the course of antifungal therapy will be determined by the extent and response of disease. It is suggested that if after 2 weeks of daily doses of amphotericin B, no discernible lesions can be found by clinical evaluation, chest radiography, endoscopy, and computed tomography of abdominal organs, the drug can be stopped.

In treating patients with benign congenital neutropenia, it is not always necessary to be as aggressive as one would be for neutropenias due to other causes. The patient should be hospitalized and treated with parenteral antibiotics during the first few episodes of fever. If the patient responds well to therapy, hospitalization is not mandatory for future episodes, even though the granulocyte count may be below 500 per mm³. Because most of these patients have immune-mediated neutropenia, a trial of high-dose intravenous immune globulin, 1 gram per kg per day for 1 or 2 days, may result in a transient increase in the neutrophil count. Intravenous immune globulin is indicated for more serious infections, such as pneumonia, osteomyelitis, and cellulitis.

Standard reverse isolation procedures are of no benefit in these patients and probably hinder good care. Rectal examination and rectal thermometers should be avoided. Insistence on excellent dental care with regular professional cleaning and good oral hygiene is important.

Specific Treatment

During the past several years, remarkable progress has been made in the use of recombinant human colony-stimulating factors (CSFs). Granulocyte colony-stimulating factor (G-CSF) and granulocyte-macrophage colony-stimulating factor (GM-CSF) are currently approved for use in the treatment of neutropenia associated with cancer chemotherapy, chronic forms of neutropenia, acquired immune deficiency syndrome, and bone marrow transplantation. Patients with a variety of malignancies who receive GM-CSF after standard doses of chemotherapy have demonstrated significant reductions in the duration of leukopenia. Use of GM-CSF after high-dose chemotherapy with or without bone marrow rescue appears to hasten return of a normal white blood count and to reduce infective complications.

Definitive data are not yet available to guide dosage for most potential indications, but a range of 0.3 to 10 μg per kg per day of GM-CSF appears appropriate. Subcutaneous injection is convenient and generally tolerated except for local site inflammation. However, the intravenous route may be used and is preferred for bone marrow transplantation enhancement. The doses recommended for adults in the 1994 American Society of Clinical Oncology Clinical Practice Guidelines are 5 μg per kg per day for G-CSF and 250 μg per m² per day for GM-CSF. These guidelines recommend that administration of these agents be reserved for patients in whom the intensity of chemotherapy engenders a risk for febrile neutropenia of at least 40%. Existing clinical data suggest that starting G-CSF or GM-CSF between 24 and 72 hours subsequent to chemotherapy may provide optimal neutrophil recovery. Generally, doses of G-CSF or GM-CSF are not required after the AGC rises above 500 per mm³.

In cases of severe congenital forms of neutropenia resulting in significant clinical morbidity, such as congenital neutropenia (Kostmann's syndrome), cyclical neutropenia, and acquired idiopathic neutropenias, G-CSF administration has resulted in a dose-dependent increase in the levels of circulating neutrophils and a significant reduction in the number of infections. Dose levels of G-CSF required to achieve

---

*Not available in the United States.

clinical success vary from 1 to 20 μg* per kg per day given either intravenously or subcutaneously. Generally, a dose of 5 μg per kg per day is effective. Sequential combinations of other bone marrow growth factors, such as interleukin-3 and GM-CSF, appear to have synergistic action in some cases of bone marrow failure, reducing the risk of neutropenia, associated infections, and thrombocytopenic bleeding. Clinical trials employing other combinations of bone marrow growth factors are under way.

Side effects of G-CSF include bone pain, which can be controlled by analgesics, and increased spleen size. G-CSF is contraindicated in patients with known hypersensitivity to *E. coli*–derived proteins. Caution should be exercised in using G-CSF in any malignancy with myeloid characteristics. To avoid potential complications of excessive leukocytosis, a twice-weekly complete blood count is recommended during therapy. Side effects of GM-CSF include fever, fluid retention, pleural effusion, pericardial effusion, respiratory symptoms, cardiac arrhythmias, and renal and hepatic dysfunction. Although rare, these side effects are potentiated by pre-existing organ dysfunction. GM-CSFs are contraindicated in patients with excessive leukemic myeloid blasts in the bone marrow (10% or higher) or peripheral blood and in those with known hypersensitivity to yeast-derived products. Transient rashes and local injection site reactions have occasionally been observed, but no serious allergic or anaphylactic reactions have been reported. If the absolute neutrophil count exceeds 20,000 per mm³ or if the platelet count exceeds 500,000 per mm³, GM-CSF administration should be stopped. Biweekly monitoring of the complete blood count with differential should be performed to preclude development of excessive cell levels.

G-CSF is marketed as filgrastim (Neupogen) by Amgen; GM-CSF is marketed as sargramostim (Leukine) by Immunex and distributed by Hoechst-Roussel Pharmaceuticals.

---

*Exceeds dosage recommended by the manufacturer.

HEMOLYTIC DISEASE OF THE NEWBORN
(Red Cell Alloimmunization)

method of
JAMES W. KENDIG, M.D.
University of Rochester School of Medicine and Dentistry, Children's Hospital at Strong, and Rochester General Hospital
Rochester, New York

Hemolytic disease of the fetus and newborn refers to a spectrum of problems that were formerly classified as four separate entities: erythroblastosis fetalis, congenital anemia, icterus gravis neonatorum, and hydrops fetalis. Further studies demonstrated that these entities are all manifestations of a single disease caused by red blood cell isoimmunization (alloimmunization).

The major red blood cell surface antigen responsible for this process is the RhD antigen. Because there is no corresponding "d" antigen, the term d refers only to the absence of the RhD antigen. RhD-negative individuals (dd) have no RhD antigens on their red blood cells. RhD-positive individuals may be homozygous (DD) or heterozygous (Dd) for the RhD gene, which is located on the short arm of chromosome 1. In addition to the RhD gene, the Rh blood group system includes the related Cc Ee structural gene, which encodes four specific antigens (C, c, E, and e) on the red blood cell surface. Zygosity for RhD may be predicted on the basis of classic serologic tests for the antigens C, c, D, E, e, and the known incidence of various phenotypes in different racial and ethnic groups.

RhD alloimmunization occurs when fetal RhD-positive red blood cells (inherited from the father) cross the placenta and enter the circulation of an RhD-negative (dd) mother. The maternal immune system is stimulated to produce RhD antibodies (IgG). ABO incompatibility (mother O and fetus A or B) helps to protect against the RhD sensitization of the RhD-negative mother.

The maternal RhD antibodies cross the placenta of the current or a subsequent pregnancy and cause the destruction of the RhD-positive fetal red blood cells. The fetus responds to this hemolytic anemia with extramedullary hematopoiesis involving the liver and spleen. The hepatic production of fetal albumin is compromised, leading to hydrops with edema, ascites, and pericardial and pleural effusions. Bilirubin, produced by the hemolysis of fetal red blood cells, readily crosses the placenta and is excreted by the maternal liver. After delivery, however, neonatal hyperbilirubinemia develops, which may lead to an acute encephalopathy (kernicterus). Other red blood cell antigen-antibody systems (Kidd, Kell, Duffy, the C/c and E/e alleles of the Rh system, and, rarely, the ABO system) may occasionally result in hemolytic disease of the fetus and newborn.

PREVENTION OF RhD ALLOIMMUNIZATION

The development, commercial production, and widespread use of commercially prepared RhD immune globulin for the prevention of RhD alloimmunization represents one of the greatest scientific and medical achievements of the 20th century. This is an example of passive immunization's preventing active immunization, but the precise mechanism by which the administration of the RhD antibody blocks the mother's production of the same antibody is still not fully understood. RhD immune globulin is not beneficial to the RhD-negative woman after alloimmunization has taken place, and it does not prevent sensitization due to the C/c and E/e antigens of the Rh blood group system. Table 1 gives a list of events and procedures that may lead to the RhD alloimmunization of the RhD-negative woman. An intramuscular dose of RhD immune globulin (300 μg) should be administered after these events and procedures. In the event of a severe fetal-to-maternal hemorrhage at delivery, more than 300 μg of RhD immune globulin may be required.

Blood type (ABO and RhD) and an antibody screen

TABLE 1. **Reproductive Events and Procedures That May Lead to Alloimmunization of the RhD-Negative Woman**

Events

Threatened abortion and antepartum hemorrhage
Spontaneous abortion
Delivery at any gestational age
Ectopic pregnancy
Hydatidiform molar pregnancy
Abdominal trauma and motor vehicle accidents during pregnancy
Inadvertent transfusion with Rh-positive blood

Procedures

Chorionic villous sampling
Induced abortion
Amniocentesis any time during pregnancy
External cephalic version
Delivery at any time

(the indirect Coombs test) should be obtained on the first prenatal visit. The antibody screen detects RhD antibodies as well as antibodies directed against the other red blood cell antigens such as Kell, Duffy, C/c, and E/e. If the antibody screen is positive, alloimmunization has already occurred, and serial titers should be obtained. If the antibody titer is 1:16 or greater by 20 weeks' gestation, further testing is necessary.

Antepartum Prevention

At 28 weeks' gestation, all RhD-negative mothers should have an antibody screen (indirect Coombs' test). If the test is negative, a prophylactic intramuscular dose of RhD immune globulin (300 µg) should be administered, unless the father of the infant is definitely known to be RhD-negative (dd). The purpose of this prophylactic antepartum dose is to prevent alloimmunization during the pregnancy. The half-life of this dose is 12 weeks. This antepartum dose may lead to a weakly positive indirect Coombs' test in the mother at the time of delivery and a weekly positive direct Coombs' test in the infant.

Postpartum Prevention

Every RhD-negative mother who has not undergone RhD alloimmunization should receive an intramuscular dose of *at least 300* µg of RhD immune globulin after the delivery of an RhD-positive newborn. This critical step in the prevention of RhD disease requires careful communication among the labor and delivery area, the hospital blood bank, and the postpartum floor. These communication issues are particularly important when early discharge from the hospital is being considered and when the birth has occurred outside the hospital.

A single dose of RhD immune globulin (300 µg) neutralizes approximately 30 mL of RhD-positive fetal whole blood or 15 mL of packed fetal red blood cells. If a large fetal-to-maternal transfusion should occur at the time of delivery, a single dose of RhD

immune globulin may be inadequate to prevent alloimmunization. Because of this possibility, the hospital blood bank should check the mother's blood after delivery to determine the presence and the magnitude of a fetal-to-maternal bleed. The rosette test is used to screen maternal blood for the presence of fetal red blood cells, and the Kleihauer-Betke stain is used to evaluate the magnitude of a fetal-to-maternal bleed. This information is used to determine the need for a larger (more than 300 µg) dose of intramuscular RhD immune globulin. RhD immune globulin should be administered within 72 hours of delivery. If administration has been inadvertently omitted, it may still be given up to 4 weeks after delivery. The RhD-negative mother who is already RhD alloimmunized at the time of delivery will not benefit from the administration of RhD immune globulin.

OBSTETRIC MANAGEMENT OF THE MOTHER WITH A POSITIVE INITIAL ANTIBODY SCREEN

All pregnant women should have an antibody screen (indirect Coombs' test) at the first prenatal visit. If the result is positive, the blood bank identifies the antibody and determine its titer. The blood bank examines the father's red blood cells for the corresponding antigen. If the father's result is negative for the antigen, and if the mother has absolutely no doubts regarding paternity, no further studies are required. If the father's result is positive for the involved antigen, the mother should have serial antibody titers at 1-month intervals. Early ultrasonography should also be done for gestational age assessment. If a critical antibody titer of 1:16 is reached, there is a risk of the development of erythroblastosis fetalis and hydrops, and further investigation and interventions are required (Figure 1).

The RhD-alloimmunized mother with a history of a previous pregnancy requiring an intrauterine transfusion or a neonatal exchange transfusion is at a high risk for hydrops. With this history, serial delta O.D. 450 evaluations of amniotic fluid are recommended, starting at 20 to 22 weeks' gestation, even if the antibody titer has not reached the critical level of 1:16.

Paternal Zygosity

If the maternal antibody is RhD and the father has the corresponding RhD antigen, the blood bank determines whether he is homozygous (DD) or heterozygous (Dd). This prediction is based on the classic serologic tests for the C, c, E, and e antigens and the known incidence of various phenotypes in different racial and ethnic groups. If the father is heterozygous, there is a 50% chance that the fetal red blood cells are RhD-negative (dd) and that the fetus is not at risk for the development of erythroblastosis fetalis. If the father is heterozygous, it is useful to determine the fetal blood type.

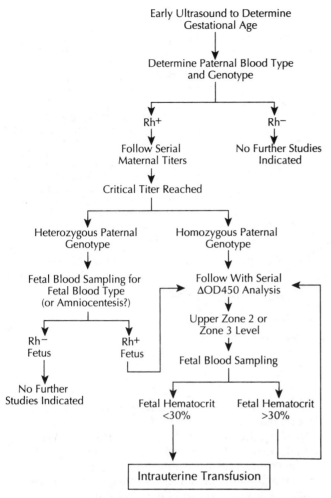

Figure 1. Algorithm used at Baylor College of Medicine, Houston, for the management of newly diagnosed red blood cell RhD alloimmunization in pregnancy. (From Moise KJ: Changing trends in the management of red blood cell alloimmunization in pregnancy. Arch Pathol Lab Med *118*:421–428, 1994. Copyright 1994, American Medical Association.)

Determination of Fetal Blood Type

Techniques for obtaining samples of fetal blood from the umbilical vessels, using ultrasound guidance, have been perfected and are available at large regional perinatal centers. This procedure, known as cordocentesis, involves obvious risks and should be performed only by specialists experienced in fetal and maternal medicine. Several centers have used the polymerase chain reaction (PCR) to identify the fetal RhD genotype. This new technique is based on the amplification of the DNA from a few fetal red blood cells found in a centrifuged sample of amniotic fluid. If the mother has RhD antibodies and the fetus is RhD-negative (by cordocentesis of a fetal blood sample or by PCR of fetal red blood cells from amniotic fluid), no further studies are indicated.

Amniotic Fluid Delta O.D. 450 Measurements

If the maternal antibody titer reaches a critical titer of 1:16 and if there is a possibility that the fetal red blood cells are positive for the corresponding antigen, serial measurements of amniotic fluid delta O.D. 450 should be done every 10 to 14 days to evaluate the level of bilirubin in the amniotic fluid. These values are plotted on the modified Liley curve (Figure 2).

Intrauterine Fetal Transfusion

When delta O.D. 450 values climb to the upper indeterminate zone or anywhere in the RhD-positive (affected) zone on the modified Liley curve, cordocentesis should be done to measure the fetal hematocrit. If this value is less than 30%, an intravascular fetal transfusion (via cordocentesis) of packed red blood cells should be carried out at a regional perinatal center by specialists experienced in maternal and fetal medicine. For severe hydrops, more than one intrauterine transfusion may be required. The timing of delivery should be based on gestational age estimates and the determination of fetal lung maturity.

DELIVERY ROOM MANAGEMENT OF THE NEWBORN WITH ERYTHROBLASTOSIS FETALIS AND HYDROPS

With advances in the field of maternal-fetal medicine and the use of intravascular fetal transfusions, it is unusual for an infant to be delivered with severe erythroblastosis and hydrops secondary to RhD. When this does occur, however, three teams of neonatologists, pediatricians, and nurse practitioners must be immediately available to initiate multiple interventions.

One team is responsible for airway management, including intubation, and the initiation of positive-pressure ventilation. This team also monitors the heart rate and initiates chest compressions, if needed. A second team is responsible for securing immediate intravascular access, usually via the umbilical vein. A hematocrit value is obtained immediately, and if it is below 30%, a partial exchange transfusion using 25 to 80 mL per kg of packed red blood cells is carried out within 30 minutes of birth to raise the hematocrit to 40% or higher. A third team should be available to perform paracentesis and thoracentesis, if needed. With severe hydrops, effective pulmonary ventilation frequently cannot be achieved until large collections of pleural and ascitic fluid have been removed.

Immediately after umbilical cord clamping, the obstetric team should obtain a sample of cord blood, which is sent to the laboratory for a direct Coombs test and determination of hematocrit, reticulocyte count, total and direct bilirubin levels, cord pH, and blood gas tension values.

NEONATAL DOUBLE-VOLUME EXCHANGE TRANSFUSION

With the widespread use of RhD immune globulin to prevent the alloimmunization of RhD-negative

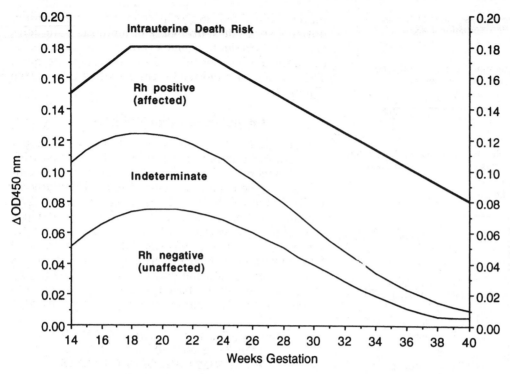

Figure 2. Amniotic fluid optical density (delta O.D. 450) zones for management of pregnancy complicated by RhD alloimmunization. (From Queenan JT, Tomai TP, Ural SH, King JC: Deviation in amniotic fluid optical density at a wavelength of 450 nm in Rh-immunized pregnancies from 14 to 40 weeks' gestation: A proposal for clinical management. Am J Obstet Gynecol *168*:1370–1376, 1993.)

women, coupled with advances in fetal intravascular transfusion therapy, neonatal double-volume exchange transfusions are becoming rare procedures. When neonatal exchange transfusions are required, they should be done by experienced neonatologists and pediatricians working in neonatal centers that are prepared to deal with the various complications of the procedure, which include hypoglycemia, thrombocytopenia, necrotizing enterocolitis, and infection.

After the delivery of an infant with erythroblastosis fetalis, serial serum bilirubin values (total and direct) should be obtained at 2- to 3-hour intervals to establish the rate of rise. A serum indirect bilirubin level that is climbing by more the 0.5 mg per dL per hour indicates that there is a relatively brisk hemolytic process that may require a double-volume exchange transfusion within the first 12 hours after birth. In addition to lowering the serum bilirubin level, an early double-volume exchange transfusion helps to correct the fetal anemia and removes a significant portion of the antibody-coated red blood cells before they hemolyze. The blood sample for routine metabolic screens for hypothyroidism, inborn errors of metabolism, and hemoglobinopathies should be drawn before the exchange transfusion is performed.

Serial serum bilirubin levels should be continued even if an early double-volume exchange transfusion is not mandated by the rate of rise. It is impossible to determine exactly what level of indirect bilirubin constitutes a risk for encephalopathy (kernicterus on neuropathology) in any given infant at any given time. Prematurity, hypoxia, asphyxia, acidosis, sepsis, and hypoalbuminemia may increase the risk of bilirubin encephalopathy. Various drugs, such as the sulfa preparations and ceftriaxone, displace bilirubin from albumin-binding sites and increase the risk for encephalopathy.

In the otherwise healthy full-term newborn with hemolytic disease, the indirect bilirubin level should not be permitted to climb above 20 mg per dL. With prematurity and hemolytic disease, lower threshold levels for exchange transfusion, based on gestational age, birth weight, chronologic age in days, and the presence or absence of other risk factors for bilirubin encephalopathy, are recommended. Premature newborns with hemolytic disease should be managed by experienced neonatologists working in regional perinatal centers. Phototherapy may be used as an adjunct to exchange transfusion, and in the case of mild hemolytic disease, phototherapy alone may be sufficient to control the bilirubin level.

DELAYED NEONATAL RED BLOOD CELL TRANSFUSIONS

A slow hemolysis frequently continues for up to 6 to 8 weeks after delivery in those infants who received a fetal intravascular transfusion or an exchange transfusion after delivery and in those infants with a mild hemolysis requiring only phototherapy. These infants should be followed up with serial hematocrit determinations at 1- to 2-week intervals during the first 6 to 8 weeks after birth. A transfusion of packed red blood cells (10 to 15 mL per kg) may be necessary to correct severe anemia. With severe hemolytic anemia, particularly in infants who received intrauterine transfusions, fetal and neonatal iron stores are elevated. Neonatal iron therapy should be withheld until the serum ferritin level returns to normal.

HEMOPHILIA AND RELATED CONDITIONS

method of
W. KEITH HOOTS, M.D.
Gulf States Hemophilia Center
Houston, Texas

Hemophilia A (factor VIII deficiency) and hemophilia B (factor IX deficiency) are X-linked hereditary bleeding disorders. By contrast, von Willebrand's disease (vWD) is autosomally inherited so that males and females are affected equally. Hemophilia A and hemophilia B present as clinically identical conditions, with joint bleeding (hemarthrosis) and joint destructions constituting the primary morbid manifestation. The reason that the clinical findings are indistinguishable is that factor VIIIc (hemophilia A) and factor IX (hemophilia B) are essential cofactors for activating factor Xa in the intrinsic clotting pathway. Each of these factors is primarily produced in the liver. Factor IX is a serine protease and factor VIII is a large glycoprotein essential for configuring the clotting enzymes on the platelet surface so that enzyme-substrate reactions occur at optimal maximal kinetics.

Both hemophilia A and B exhibit a range of clinical severities that correlate fairly well with assayed factor levels. Specifically, severe disease is defined as less than 1% assayed clotting factor in plasma; approximately 1 to 5% and more than 5% of normal are defined as moderate and mild disease, respectively. Males within a family almost always have the same degree of impairment because they share the same defect in the DNA coding for the clotting protein.

Both hemophilia A and B are coded for by DNA on the long arm (q) of the X chromosome. The factor VIII gene, coding as it does for a glycoprotein that is substantially larger than the factor IX protein (approximately 340,000 daltons versus approximately 70,000 daltons), has been demonstrated to be highly susceptible to mutation events including deletions, insertions, and missense and nonsense mutations. In addition, an inversion sequence of intron 22 of the gene encoding factor VIII is now known to account for more than 34% of mutations giving rise to hemophilia A. This inversion involves a crossover between the intragenic and extragenic copies of factor VIII on the X chromosome (the so-called flip-tip inversion).

Although significantly smaller than the gene encoding factor VIII, the gene encoding factor IX also has been shown to be prone to new mutation events, particularly of the missense and nonsense type. In practical terms, this results in approximately 25 to 30% of newly diagnosed cases of either hemophilia A or B representing a *new* mutation event within a family previously unaffected by hemophilia. This also accounts for the exceptional consistency of prevalence and incidence of both hemophilia A and B across all racial and ethnic groups.

The incidence of hemophilia A and B together is between 1 in 5000 and 1 in 10,000 live male births. Approximately 80 to 85% of these affected neonates have hemophilia A. Approximately two thirds of those with hemophilia A have severe or moderately severe ($\leq$1% factor VIII) disease. By contrast almost half of hemophilia B individuals have factor IX levels of more than 1%. Hemophilia A and B of comparable severities bleed with similar frequency.

vWD results when there is a defect in the gene for von Willebrand factor (vWF), which is located on chromosome 12. The disease is among the most prevalent of genetic diseases. As high of 1% of certain cohort studies using molecular biologic analyses for gene mutation have shown abnormalities. The glycoprotein coded for by the vWF gene is a large subunit of approximately 226,000 daltons that multimerizes into large cell-adhesive molecules that are essential both for platelet aggregation by cross-linking of glycoprotein Ib receptors between platelets and for platelet adhesion at the site of blood vessel endothelial cell injury. In addition, these vWF multimers, which are secreted from both endothelial cells and platelets, are essential for stabilizing factor VIIIc from proteolysis in the circulating plasma. This explains the low level of factor VIIIc seen in several types of vWD (see later) despite the fact that both the factor VIIIc gene and its coded protein are entirely normal.

Unlike hemophilia A and B, the clinical bleeding pattern for vWD is primarily localized to mucous membrane surface. Hence, epistaxis, menorrhagia, post–dental surgical bleeding, and gastrointestinal bleeding are common manifestations for individuals with vWD. Postsurgical bleeding or hemorrhage secondary to significant trauma occurs to varying degrees, depending on the qualitative or quantitative defect or deficiency in the circulating vWF molecule.

Despite the heterogeneity of the molecular defects of vWF, the categorization of clinical vWD is based on the amount and the functional capacity of the vWF protein in the plasma. Abnormalities have been divided into three major types on the basis of the specific laboratory tests that assess both quantity and function of vWF in the plasma of an affected individual.

Type 1 vWD (formally type I) is a heterozygous state in which the genetic defect inherited from one parent (or representing a new mutation) is partially compensated for by normal vWF production directed by the normal gene from the other parent. This type or classic vWD is the clinical state most commonly diagnosed. Laboratory studies that measure *quantitative* vWF protein immunologically (factor VIII–related antigen) are abnormal. *Functional* studies that measure qualitative function of vWF (factor VIII van Willebrand factor:ristocetin cofactor activity [VIII vWF:RCoF]) are proportionally reduced in the plasma. Further, as noted before, the factor VIIIc level in the plasma is frequently abnormal as well because the diminished VIII vWF:RCoF results in a decreased plasma half-life for the factor VIIIc molecules produced by the hepatocyte.

Type 2 vWD consists of multiple genetic defects sharing one common defining characteristic: there is normal production of vWF protein, which is measured by protein antigen assays in the plasma; however, these vWF molecules are defective to varying degrees in their function. A comprehensive discussion of all the type 2 variants of vWD is beyond the scope of this article. Nonetheless, several distinct categories of these that create the heterogeneity can be listed; examples include abnormalities in the multimerization of the vWF subunits, a defective factor VIIIc binding site, and a defective secretion of vWF from platelets despite normal plasma vWF structure and function. Any and all may produce clinical bleeding syndromes. Further, as with vWD in general, there is often substantial clinical heterogeneity between individuals of the same type 2 variant.

Persons with type 3 vWD have a defect in the vWF genes of both chromosomes 12. In many cases, neither parent will have a clinically significant bleeding history because subclinical disease among type 1 heterozygotes is common. By contrast, the individual with type 3 homozygous vWD will have severe clinical bleeding because he or she has little if any vWF protein or circulating factor VIIIc. The latter is deficient because a paucity of vWF in plasma results in rapid proteolysis of the factor VIIIc even though its production is normal. Hence, individuals with type 3 vWD may experience both the mucous membrane hemorrhage pattern seen with vWD as well as the bleeding into deep tissue or organs (e.g., hemarthroses) seen more commonly in hemophilic persons. Further, chronic morbidity is much more commonly observed in these individuals.

Inherited bleeding diatheses secondary to other plasma proteins, platelets, or blood vessels are much less common than either hemophilia or vWD. Genetic defects in factors XI, prekallikrein, and high-molecular-weight kininogen will result in prolongation of the activated partial thromboplastin time (APTT) and may cause clinical bleeding syndromes, although usually less severe than hemophilia A or B. By contrast, inherited factor XII deficiency, although prolonging the APTT, produces no clinical bleeding.

Autosomally inherited factors VII, V, and X and prothrombin deficiencies are rare. When diagnosed, they may produce a significant hemorrhagic state the severity of which correlates inversely with the circulating plasma concentration of the deficient protease (factors II, VII, and X) or glycoprotein (factor V).

Factor VII deficiency is suggested when the prothrombin time (PT) is prolonged but the APTT is normal. Homozygous factor VII deficiency is exceedingly rare and may suggest consanguinity. However, the clinical course is often quite severe, and infants are at significant risk for intracranial hemorrhage. Homozygous autosomal afibrinogenemia, the clinical incidence of which is approximately 1 in 1 million live births, may present in the neonatal period with life-threatening hemorrhage necessitating emergent and aggressive replacement therapy with cryoprecipitate. Abnormalities of factors II, V, and X and fibrinogen prolong both the PT and the APTT.

Two inherited protein deficiencies are notable for their likelihood for producing hemorrhagic syndromes despite normal PT and APTT screening test results. The first, factor XIII deficiency, frequently presents with an indicative clinical history: delayed bleeding after initial adequate hemostasis. This occurs because factor XIII is required for clot stabilization. The second is homozygous deficiency of the inhibitor α_2-antiplasmin, which also produces a bleeding diathesis. Deficiency of this natural inhibitor for the fibrinolytic protein plasmin permits exaggerated clot lysis, thus producing clinical bleeding after tissue injury. Inherited disorders of platelet and endothelial cell function do, in a number of circumstances, cause clinical bleeding. These are discussed elsewhere.

TREATMENT

Hemostatic Abnormalities

Replacement Therapy

For the majority of inherited coagulation disorders, primary therapy consists of infusing a protein product that repletes the deficient clotting component. The source for these replacement clotting proteins has historically been human plasma. The majority of these clotting proteins have their hemostatic activity defined as unit of clotting activity per milliliter of pooled normal human plasma. Hence, the blood banking and pharmaceutical strategy for improving

the replacement capacity for the specific deficient factor has been to concentrate the specific protein. In some cases, similar proteins co-purify in the concentration process from the source plasma. An example is cryoprecipitate, which results from the slow thawing of fresh-frozen plasma (FFP) and results in a severalfold concentration of the following clotting proteins: factor VIIIc, factor VIII vWF, fibrinogen, factor XIII, and fibronectin.

Commercial fractionation of cryoprecipitate yielded the first generation of lyophilized factor VIII concentrates, which resulted in an approximate 100-fold increase per mL of infusate in the concentration of factor VIII. This commercial scale-up resulted when source plasma from 5000 to 25,000 donors was converted into lyophilized vials of factor VIII. These vials range in potency from 200 to 1500 units (20 to 35 units per mg of protein) per vial. For the first time, convenient home infusion of hemophilia-associated hemorrhage was feasible. Unfortunately, because of the number of donors contributing to the commercial plasma pool, transfusion-transmitted viral disease (particularly transfusion-associated hepatitis and human immunodeficiency virus [HIV] infection) became a common complication in the hemophilia A population. Purification strategies to alleviate or ultimately eliminate this viral risk required advances in technology. A discussion of this evaluation in purity follows.

Similar viral transmission risk existed for the fractionated therapeutic clotting factor produced for hemophilia B. Because cryoprecipitation does not enrich factor IX, the initial step in fractionation of factor IX clotting factor products has traditionally been barium or aluminum sulfate absorption followed by further column fractionation. For therapies used in the 1970s and 1980s, this resulted in co-purification of all the molecularly similar vitamin K–dependent factors (II, VII, IX, and X), yielding a final product called prothrombin complex concentrates (PCCs). Like factor VIII products, production of PCC yielded a final concentration of 200 to 1500 units (20 to 40 units per mg of protein) per vial. Like the factor VIII products, these commercially produced factor concentrates, in the years before more effective viral attenuation techniques, almost invariably had viral contamination, notably several species of hepatitis and HIV (after 1979).

The co-purification of factors II, VII, and X in the preparation of factor IX concentrates sometimes resulted in selective conversion of one or more of these zymogen proteases to its active enzyme (e.g., factor VII is converted in trace amounts to factor VIIa). This trace contamination with active proteases creates a thrombogenic potential for PCCs. Indeed, PCCs given therapeutically in high and recurrent dosing schedules have produced significant and sometimes fatal clotting events in patients with hemophilia B, particularly among individuals receiving the PCCs to provide hemostasis in association with orthopedic surgery. Other clinical situations in which thrombogenesis may be associated with the infusion of PCCs include (1) sustained crush injuries; (2) large intramuscular bleeds, e.g., psoas or thigh; (3) treatment of neonates with hemophilia B who have immature natural anticoagulation; and (4) hemostatic therapy given to individuals with severe chronic hepatitis (because this may adversely affect their ability to make antithrombin III and the vitamin K–dependent inhibitors protein C and protein S in their hepatocytes). In its most severe manifestations, dosing with PCCs has produced acute myocardial infarction and disseminated intravascular coagulation. The risk for disseminated intravascular coagulation may be mitigated by not infusing more than 50 to 75 units per kg per 24 hours when recurrent dosing is required (e.g., after surgery or to treat life-threatening hemorrhage) and by adding small amounts of heparin to each infusate. Fortunately, as discussed subsequently, more advanced purification technologies have resulted in the production of single-component factor IX products that are free of any significant trace activated proteases. These now provide the mainstay of therapy for hemophilia B patients and are obligatory when high-dose, recurrent infusion therapy is required.

Later Generation Clotting Factor Concentrates

THERAPEUTIC OPTIONS FOR TREATMENT OF HEMOPHILIA A AND B IN THE MID-1990s

Factor VIII Products. Because of the high frequency and profound clinical impact of transfusion-associated transmission of the hepatitis virus and HIV in the hemophilia population during the 1970s and 1980s, there were exigent and profound advances in the attenuation (and even elimination) of these and other viral contaminants. The first step in this evolution was heat treatment of factor VIII products first licensed for use in 1983. Subsequent advances included the following: pasteurization; solvent detergent treatment to eliminate lipid envelope viruses; advanced Sepharose chromatography; affinity chromatography with monoclonal antibodies directed against the factor VIIIc–factor VIII vWF complex or against factor IX; and most recently, the commercial production of a recombinant factor VIIIc product in transfected mammalian cell systems. Each non-recombinant clotting factor concentrate presently produced in the United States is made from a donor pool screened for HIV, hepatitis B virus, and hepatitis C virus. In addition, each of the currently marketed products undergoes either heating to high temperatures and of long duration or solvent detergent treatment. Both processes appear sufficient to remove the risk for HIV transmission. Hepatitis risk is further reduced when concomitant donor screening is employed.

This degree of confidence of safety from HIV infection does not exist for cryoprecipitate and FFP, which typically undergo no viral attenuation other than donor screening (an exception is the investigational pasteurized FFP product made by the New York Blood Center). Efficient donor screening has reduced the relative risk from either of these single-donor products to between 1 in 40,000 and 1 in 100,000 per donor unit for HIV infection and to 0.03% or less per donor unit for hepatitis C. Even though the risk for hepatitis B from single-donor cryoprecipitate or FFP is similarly low, anyone likely to be treated with *any* plasma-derived product (whether single-donor or pooled, attenuated product) *should* receive a full three-inoculation course of the hepatitis B vaccine.

Each one of the factor VIII concentrates available at this time is considered safe from HIV and similar retroviral transmission. However, not all are free of hepatitis C virus transmission risk. Fortunately, the relative risk that any single lot of any of the products will transmit hepatitis C appears low. Nonetheless, transmissions of hepatitis C virus, hepatitis A virus, and human parvovirus B19 from some existing factor VIII products have been documented. A product–by-product comparison of the relative risk for transmission of these viruses is beyond the scope of this discussion and would quickly become outdated as technology advances. However, a basic stratification of relative product purity is discussed by the following product groupings after a definition of each is provided: (1) intermediate-purity products; (2) high-purity products; (3) ultra-high-purity products.

The intermediate-purity factor concentrates are so designated because even though they undergo aggressive viral inactivation with heat (even pasteurization) and/or solvent detergent, the final concentration of factor VIII in the end product represents a small percentage of the total heterogeneous plasma proteins present (6 to 10 units of factor VIIIc per mg of total protein excluding albumin).

High-purity products are factor concentrates that have at least 50 units (range, 50 to 150) of factor VIIIc per mg of protein (excluding albumin for stabilization). In the majority of cases, specialized column chromatographic techniques (e.g., heparin Sepharose) result in the significantly higher purity, although there still is trace contamination with immunoglobulins or other plasma proteins. The chromatographic technique provides some viral attenuation, but enhanced viral safety is dependent on postchromatographic pasteurization or solvent detergent treatment. These products are considered safe from HIV in the end product and relatively but not absolutely safe for hepatitis C.

Ultra-high-purity products are the monoclonal antibody affinity–purified plasma-derived factor concentrates and the recombinant factor VIII products. For the former, the affinity chromatography step not only is efficient at removing all non–factor VIIIc protein but also is an efficient viral attenuation process. Nonetheless, effective elimination of hepatitis C from the monoclonal products has required subsequent treatment with either pasteurization or solvent detergent. The specific activity of the monoclonal preparations (before the addition of human serum albumin) is 3000 units of factor VIIIc per mg of protein. This is essentially identical to the effective purity of the licensed recombinant products, which also require comparable dilution with albumin to maintain stability after lyophilization.

There is a notable distinction with regard to theoretical viral safety to be made between the monoclonal and the recombinant products. Because the recombinant factor VIII products are affinity purified from the cell culture of transfected hamster-derived cell lines, there is no requirement for any further viral attenuation. The addition of human serum albumin constitutes the sole theoretical source for human viral contamination. There remains a theoretical risk for other nonhuman, mammalian viruses or other infective species.

Frequent infusions of ultrapure products (specifically the monoclonal products) have been shown in scientific studies to produce a stabilization of the CD4+ cell count in HIV-infected hemophiliacs compared with chronic infusion of similar amounts of intermediate clotting factor concentrates. It is suspected that this results from the absence of other protein contamination in these ultrapure products rather than from greater purity from viral contamination. Nonetheless, most physicians treating hemophilia have opted to use one of these products to treat their HIV-infected patients. Many have also chosen to treat their previously untreated hemophilia A patients (particularly the young children) with these products because of a perceived theoretical viral safety. This safety margin is inferred from (1) studies showing enhanced capacity to remove surrogate viruses during the monoclonal processing and (2) the bypassing of a human plasma source (with the exception of the added human serum albumin) from the recombinant products.

Clinical trials are ongoing at this time of a recombinant factor VIIIc preparation from which the B domain of the gene has been removed before transfection of the hamster cell lines. The protein portion of factor VIII coded for by the B domain of the gene is not required for efficient clotting function; further, its deletion confers greater stability on the resultant smaller factor VIIIc molecule. Hence, there is no requirement for human serum albumin to stabilize the final lyophilized product. This may provide a higher level of confidence against any future microbiologic contamination. It is not yet apparent when this product will be available for clinical use.

Factor IX Products. The clotting factor products available for treating hemophilia B must be assessed for two potential complications: (1) theoretical viral safety and viral purity (activity per mg protein) and (2) thrombogenicity. The factor IX products determined to be free of thrombogenic potential are those preparations that have effectively purified the factor IX protein from the other prothrombin complex proteins (factors II, VII, and X). Two technical strategies have been employed to purify factor IX from the other vitamin K factors and thereby to remove the thrombogenic risk: (1) chromatographic partitioning followed by solvent detergent treatment and (2) monoclonal affinity purification of factor IX. The

product produced by the former process contains some residual nonclotting plasma proteins. By contrast, the monoclonal product is free of other plasma proteins. Viral attenuation to remove HIV appears effective for both processes. The hepatitis virus risk is significantly reduced by both processes. However, studies using surrogate viruses imply greater safety from hepatitis C or similar viruses with the monoclonal factor IX concentrate.

The other plasma-derived clotting factor concentrates available for treating hemophilia B patients are PCCs. They can, therefore, produce thrombotic complications when given in high dose or after repeated sequential dosing. Viral attenuation strategies for PCCs are either solvent detergent treatment or heating to 80°C for more than 10 hours. PCCs using the heat process may provide a greater viral attenuation for some viruses, although this has not been proved scientifically. As discussed later, either of these PCCs may prove efficacious for treating moderate bleeding (e.g., hemarthrosis) in individuals with high responsive factor VIII inhibitors for whom factor VIIIc concentrates are nonhemostatic because of the factor VIII antibody.

Recombinant factor IX clotting factor concentrate has recently been licensed. Unlike the presently licensed recombinant factor VIII preparations, recombinant factor IX has no human albumin in the viral product. The theoretical advantages of this are discussed earlier with the B domain–deleted recombinant factor VIII. The in vivo half-life of recombinant factor IX concentrate is identical to that of plasma-derived monoclonal factor IX concentrate. Because of a slightly different volume of distribution, recombinant factor IX recovery may vary a small amount from monoclonal factor IX.

Anti-inhibitor Clotting Preparations. Because PCCs are thrombogenic owing to their trace contamination with the active proteases (e.g., factor VIIa or factor Xa), they have been used for nearly 2 decades to treat bleeding in factor VIII–deficient patients with high responsive (i.e., anamnestic) factor VIII antibodies. Later manufacturers of PCCs increased the trace amounts of these active proteases to produce activated prothrombin complex concentrates (APCCs). There is no in vitro assay for either of the two licensed APCC products that correlates with in vivo hemostatic efficacy. Hence, it is often difficult to predict the hemostatic efficacy of APCCs. Both individual response and therapeutic efficacy for specific hemorrhagic episodes vary widely. Stated another way, it is a problem, if not impossible, to predict a priori whether a given dose (units per kilogram of body weight) will provide the necessary hemostasis after a single infusion in a patient with no prior use of APCC. This is true even though the factor VIIIc "bypassing" activity of APCCs is supplied according to units of hemostatic activity per vial and is dosed accordingly. (Typical dosing for hemarthroses is 75 to 100 units per kg per dose.) To further complicate the issue, there are two APCC preparations. One may be ineffective in an individual, whereas the other may provide effective hemostasis for an acute bleeding episode. Because of this capriciousness of the use of APCC in individuals with inhibitors, an individualized therapeutic plan needs to be established empirically. However, certain principles generally apply. (1) Effective dosing of APCCs is minimally 75 to 100 units per kg. (2) Dosing frequency more often than every 6 hours predisposes to significant thrombogenicity, particularly after the third to fourth consecutive dose. (Hence, monitoring for markers of disseminated intravascular coagulation is warranted when sequential dosing for several days is required.) (3) Because the activated proteases that account for the procoagulant activity of APCCs are short-lived, initial hemostasis may be followed by breakthrough bleeding between doses that may create difficulty for maintenance hemostatic therapy. Therapy with APCCs is expensive, is less than reliable, and carries risk for significant complications. Experience and expertise in their use help to mitigate these risks and to differentiate the appropriate use of APCCs from the other alternatives for inhibitor therapy cited in the following.

One alternative therapy for treating patients with inhibitors is porcine factor VIII. This product is produced from porcine plasma by use of a polyelectrolyte resin separation technology. The residual nonhuman protein is relatively low, although this does not completely eliminate the anaphylactoid potential of this product. Another characteristic of porcine factor VIII will often limit its efficacy in many individuals with inhibitors. In many cases, the specific anamnestic antibody directed against the human factor VIIIc glycoprotein cross-reacts with shared epitopes on the porcine molecule. Therefore, before the therapeutic efficacy of the product of porcine factor VIII can be assessed in an individual, it is necessary to quantitate the neutralizing capacity of the antibody against both the porcine and the human factor VIII product by use of the Bethesda assay. In those instances in which the antiporcine Bethesda unit titer is significantly lower (<10 Bethesda units) than the corresponding antihuman Bethesda titer, therapy with porcine factor VIII may be the therapy of choice. Before the first dose of porcine factor VIII is infused at a starting dose of approximately 100 units per kg, there is need to infuse a test dose of approximately 100 units to ensure that there is no immediate hypersensitivity reaction. If none occurs, a slow infusion during 20 to 30 minutes with careful monitoring for allergic symptoms can proceed. Further, because the porcine Bethesda unit inhibitor assay provides only an in vitro estimate of the neutralizing capacity of the anti–factor VIII antibody against porcine factor VIII, it is essential to monitor factor VIII levels in these patients. As with most therapies for hemophilia A patients with inhibitors, therapy with porcine factor VIII is costly.

The indications for use of other more esoteric and experimental therapies for factor VIII inhibitors (e.g., factor VIIa, immune tolerance induction, or antibody depletion using a staphylococcal protein A Sepharose chromatographic column) are beyond the scope of this discussion. Comprehensive hemophilia treatment centers provide expertise for these specialized therapeutic procedures. Further, because optimal methodologies are still to be determined by collaborative research protocols, discussion with physician-scientists at these centers offers the best prospect for providing clinicians with up-to-date information about therapeutic options for treating complex inhibitor patients.

Therapies for von Willebrand's Disease

Patients with type 1 and most with type 2 vWD may often be treated with desmopressin acetate (DDAVP), a synthetic analogue of the antidiuretic hormone 8-arginine vasopressin. Similarly, because of its efficacy in inducing release of vWF multimers from endothelial cells, it results in a concomitant rise in factor VIIIc (because vWF spares the latter molecule from rapid proteolysis in plasma). Desmopressin at a dose of 0.3 µg per kg (maximal dose is 25 µg per dose) by slow intravenous infusion will increase circulating vWF by approximately 250% in the average individual and factor VIIIc approximately 300%. Therefore, it becomes a treatment of choice for mild to moderate bleeding in most individuals with both mild hemophilia A (e.g., >5% factor VIII activity) and types 1 and 2 vWD. (Note: In type 2B vWD in which the largest vWF multimers are missing from plasma but are released in excess after desmopressin use, there is a theoretical risk for thrombocytopenia from excessive platelet aggregation. Hence, its use in this subgroup must be evaluated on an individual case basis.) Because a 2.5- to 3-fold increase in both factor VIIIc and factor VIII vWF is often sufficient to raise both to normal ranges in vWD patients, many such individuals may never require any other type of therapy for either acute hemorrhage or prophylaxis for surgical or dental procedures. Tachyphylaxis after repeated dosing with desmopressin can occur because of depletion of the vWF stores in the endothelial cells. Therefore, monitoring of levels in those individuals requiring frequent dosing (e.g., daily or more often) is indicated.

A highly concentrated (150 µg per spray = 1.5 mg per mL) intranasal form of desmopressin is also available for use in vWD and mild hemophilia A. Two inhalations in a single nostril acutely in adults and one in children will typically achieve approximately two thirds of the intravenous dosing. As with the intravenous preparation, facial flushing, mild to moderate blood pressure elevation, and antidiuretic side effects are expected.

For individuals with type 3 vWD, for those with types 1 and 2 who either fail to respond to desmopressin or respond to a degree inadequate to achieve complete and predictable hemostasis, and for those vWF patients who experience tachyphylaxis precluding required repeated therapy, other therapeutic options are needed. Cryoprecipitate administered in a dose calculated to elevate factor VIIIc or factor VIII vWF or both to the normal range has traditionally been the most effective means for achieving hemostasis in such patients. However, as noted previously, single-donor cryoprecipitate has a small but finite risk for hepatitis and even HIV infection, and for this reason caution must be exercised before cryoprecipitate is administered. Accordingly, most coagulationists have chosen one of three intermediate- or high-purity factor VIII concentrates that have been demonstrated to have most sizes of vWF multimers present after reconstitution to treat vWD patients when desmopressin is deemed inadequate for hemostasis. Unlike cryoprecipitate, these concentrates may not have the ideal ratio of vWF multimers compared with the physiologic state. Nonetheless, the theoretical viral safety conferred by the attenuation they undergo in preparation more than compensates for this theoretical hemostatic deficit. Several studies have shown clinical efficacy to be good even when individuals with severe disease (type 3) have experienced potential or actual life-threatening hemorrhage.

Antifibrinolytic Agents

Tranexamic acid and ε-aminocaproic acid (EACA) act by inhibiting plasminogen activation, thereby enhancing clot stability. These two agents are useful therapeutic adjuncts to stabilize clots that have formed after therapy in individuals with underlying hemostatic defects. For patients with inherited clotting disorders, they have proved particularly efficacious for bleeding in the oral cavity (e.g., after dental or oral surgical procedures or trauma to the mouth) and for epistaxis. Dosing for tranexamic acids is 25 mg per kg per dose every 6 to 8 hours; for EACA, it is 75 to 100 mg per kg per dose every 6 hours (maximal dose, 3 to 4 grams every 6 hours). For patients with hemophilia and vWD, treatment may be required for 7 to 14 days, depending on the amount of tissue injury. In hemophilia B, it is prudent to use a purified factor IX preparation rather than PCC when concomitant antifibrinolytic therapy is contemplated because of the added thrombotic risks of the PCC and antifibrinolytic agents together.

PREVENTIVE CARE

Male infants born to known or suspected hemophilic carrier mothers should not be circumcised until hemophilia in the infant has been excluded by laboratory testing. Blood for assay for APTT and factor VIII or factor IX assay (or both if family history is uncertain) should be obtained from cord blood. When a cord blood sample is not available, venipuncture should be performed from a superficial limb vein to lessen the likelihood of producing a hematoma that might then require replacement therapy. Femoral and jugular sites must be avoided.

Routine immunizations requiring injection, such as diphtheria-pertussis-tetanus or measles-mumps-rubella vaccines, may be given in the deep subcutaneous tissue (rather than by deep intramuscular injection as is the usual practice), using the smallest gauge needle that is feasible. Hepatitis B vaccine should be given as soon after birth as possible to all infants with confirmed diagnosis of hemophilia. The live attenuated oral poliovirus vaccine should not be given to an infant whose hemophilic older brother (or grandfather in the household) is known to be HIV immune suppressed; Salk vaccine may be substituted. Hepatitis A vaccine should also be administered to those individuals with hemophilia who have no hepatitis A virus antibody in their serum.

Early dental examination of the infant is recommended to teach proper tooth-brushing and to ensure adequate household water fluoridation. In addition to education about hemophilia, both genetic counseling and psychosocial counseling are important for the mother of a newborn with hemophilia. This is particularly true for the approximately 30% for whom hemophilia represents a new mutation and for whom there is no previous family experience with the disease. Reluctance to clean the teeth routinely should be dispelled early, and anticipated problem areas for causing bleeding should be discussed.

Both parents should be encouraged to participate intensively in every part of the infant's care. Further, normal socialization opportunities must not be limited because of the hemophilia. Experienced personnel should discuss specifically what minimal limitations are reasonable versus what constitutes overprotection and, therefore, may jeopardize the child's normal development.

An appropriate exercise regimen that excludes "contact" sports (e.g., tackle football) should be encouraged as a daily routine. Further, the role of such a program for the child and adult after episodes of hemarthrosis is best discussed before the child has a joint bleed.

SPECIAL CONSIDERATION FOR HEMOPHILIC BLEEDING

Early treatment improves the quality of life. It is not only necessary but will in many cases diminish the ultimate duration of therapy. For example, infusion for an acute hemarthrosis with an appropriate dose of factor concentrate (generally 15 to 25 units per kg of body weight) immediately on recognition of pain may often obviate the need for a second infusion by forestalling the inflammatory response in the joint. This may curtail the predisposition for rebleeding in the same joint. Appropriate dosage is chosen to ensure some circulating factor level for at least 48 hours. The strategy for maintaining such a minimal level always is known as prophylaxis and has been demonstrated to be efficacious in preventing essentially all joint bleeding in patients with both hemophilia A and B. A decision to undertake primary prophylaxis requires extensive prospective evaluation and is best done in close consultation between the parent of the hemophilic child and professionals in the comprehensive hemophilia treatment center.

For life-threatening bleeding in a hemophiliac, the exigency for immediate infusion is superseded only by resuscitative requirements. Every effort should be made to keep the factor level in this normal range (e.g., >50%) until this bleeding emergency has passed. Further, an acutely hemorrhaging hemophiliac should be transported, if at all possible, to an emergency center that stocks appropriate clotting factor products. All head injuries must be considered nontrivial unless proved otherwise by observation and computed tomography or magnetic resonance imaging. Late bleeding after head trauma can occur as long as 3 to 4 weeks after the injury. Hence, patients with head and neck injuries should be infused immediately unless one is totally convinced that the injury is insignificant. In addition, if the patient is not hospitalized, the patient and his or her family should be instructed in the neurologic signs and symptoms of central nervous system bleeding so that the patient will return for reinfusion, clinical and radiologic reassessment, and hospitalization at the earliest manifestation of bleeding.

Bleeding from the floor of the mouth or the pharynx or epiglottic region frequently results in partial or complete airway obstruction. Therefore, such bleeding should be treated with an aggressive infusion program with extended clinical follow-up to ensure resolution. Such bleeding may be precipitated by coughing, tonsillitis, oral or otolaryngologic surgery (e.g., extraction of wisdom teeth, tonsillectomy, adenoidectomy), or regional block anesthesia. For surgery and anesthesia, prophylaxis with appropriate infusion therapy before the procedure usually obviates the need for further treatment.

Patients with hemophilia who have gastrointestinal lesions, such as ulcers, varices, or hemorrhoids, must be managed with an appropriate continuous infusion regimen that maintains nearly normal circulating levels for factor VIIIc or factor IX until some healing has been achieved. Concomitant transfusion with packed red blood cells may also be required.

Selected types of hemarthroses may be a particular problem. Hip joint or acetabular hemorrhages can be dangerous because increased intra-articular pressure from bleeding and the associated inflammation may lead to aseptic necrosis of the femoral head. Twice-daily infusion therapy designed to sustain a factor level above 10 units per dL for at least 3 days should be given, along with enforced bed rest that includes Buck's traction for immobilization.

A hemarthrosis of the hip joint may, at first appearance, be difficult to differentiate from a bleed in the iliopsoas muscle. The iliopsoas bleed limits primary hip extension, whereas a bleed in the joint makes any motion of the hip excruciatingly painful. Further, an iliopsoas bleed may decrease sensation over the ipsilateral thigh because of compression of the sacral plexus root of the femoral nerve. Ultrasonography may demonstrate a hematoma in the iliopsoas region. Treatment of the two is similar, although rehabilitation from the hip bleed is more protracted. Both will benefit from a physical therapy regimen that strengthens the supporting musculature while slowly mobilizing the affected area. Closed compartment muscle and soft tissue hemorrhages are dangerous because they frequently impinge on the neurovascular bundle. These can occur in the upper arm, forearm, wrist, and volar aspect of the hand as well as in the anterior or posterior filial compartments. Swelling and pain precede tingling, numbness, and loss of distal arterial pulses. Infusion must maintain an adequate hemostatic level of factor VIIIc or factor IX. Other possible therapeutic maneuvers include elevation to enhance venous return and, as a last resort, surgical decompression if medical therapy fails to forestall progression.

COMPREHENSIVE CARE

Special treatment centers have been established in the United States and many other countries to provide multidisciplinary care of hemophilia and related disorders. Many patients infused with plasma-derived factor concentrates before 1984 to 1985 were infected with HIV and/or one of the hepatitis viruses. The comprehensive hemophilia centers provide voluntary testing for these viruses, counseling of patients found seropositive for previous infection, and access to appropriate care and therapy. Risk reduction counseling and education are essential elements of comprehensive treatment centers, as is repeated testing for evidence of hepatitis infection.

Comprehensive hemophilia treatment centers are also the mainstay for ongoing education of patients and families about the management of their bleeding disorder. The centers coordinate home therapy and preventive services and work closely with hemophilia consumer organizations to advocate advances in therapy and care.

Further information about hemophilia care, hemophilia centers, and HIV infection risk reduction and counseling is available through the National Hemophilia Foundation, The Soho Building, 110 Green Street, Suite 303, New York, NY 10012 (telephone, 212-219-8180) or from its local chapter.

PLATELET-MEDIATED BLEEDING DISORDERS

method of
ROBERT McMILLAN, M.D.
Scripps Clinic
La Jolla, California

Platelets are necessary to prevent leaking of blood from the blood vessels. After vascular injury, platelets adhere to the subendothelium and form a platelet plug. This plug serves subsequently as a scaffold to allow clot formation and, ultimately, healing. Initially, the GPIb/IX/V platelet glycoprotein complex binds to exposed subendothelium, primarily to von Willebrand factor, although other proteins also contribute. Platelet activation follows adhesion and is due to multiple stimuli, especially thrombin and components of the subendothelial matrix (particularly collagen). Once activated, the platelet undergoes many changes, including the release of agents, such as adenosine diphosphate, serotonin, and thromboxane A_2, that recruit and activate surrounding platelets, leading to formation of the platelet plug. Stabilization of the platelet plug is mediated by binding of adhesive proteins, primarily fibrinogen and von Willebrand factor, to the now-activated GPIIb/IIIa receptor. Platelet plug formation is a necessary protective event that prevents bleeding and allows healing of injuries. Bleeding due to platelet problems may be due to insufficient platelet numbers or abnormally functioning platelets.

CLINICAL PRESENTATION AND EVALUATION

This discussion of treatment involves only adult patients. Because the treatment of some of these disorders in children may differ (e.g., chronic idiopathic thrombocytopenic purpura [ITP]), the reader should seek another source for their treatment. In thrombocytopenic patients, the symptoms and signs are similar regardless of the disorder. Patients may be asymptomatic, with thrombocytopenia being noted during routine blood studies. However, most patients seek medical attention because they develop a rash (petechiae or purpura) or have mucosal bleeding from the nose or gastrointestinal or genitourinary tract. Women often note prolonged or heavy menstrual bleeding. Occasionally, central nervous system bleeding occurs, but only as a late manifestation in conjunction with severe mucosal bleeding. Platelet-related symptoms and signs are rare if the platelet count is more than 50,000 per mm³. Purpura with minor trauma is noted with platelet counts of 30,000 to 50,000 per mm³, and spontaneous purpura with counts less than 30,000 per mm³. Serious mucosal bleeding is rare unless the platelet count is less than 5000 to 10,000 per mm³. Symptoms may be exaggerated by certain medications (e.g., aspirin). If thrombocytopenia is associated with another disease process, symptoms and physical findings of the primary disease may dominate. Patients with platelet function defects have similar platelet-related symptoms but may have normal or near-normal platelet counts.

The common platelet-mediated disorders are listed in Table 1. Thrombocytopenia has three causes: decreased production, abnormal distribution (splenomegaly with pooling of platelets), and increased destruction. In some disorders (e.g., lymphomas), more than one cause may be involved. Few laboratory studies are required to evaluate these possibilities: complete blood count, platelet count, and bone marrow examination. Aside from alcohol-induced and some drug-induced thrombocytopenias, diseases associated with decreased platelet production can be diagnosed from the physical examination, the complete blood count, or the marrow examination (e.g., leukemias, lymphomas, aplastic anemia, myelodysplasia). Thrombocytopenia due to splenic pooling (e.g., congestive splenomegaly) requires the presence of splenomegaly. Disorders causing increased destruction usually manifest as isolated thrombocytopenia with increased numbers of megakaryocytes in the bone marrow.

Platelet disorders, due to abnormally functioning platelets, usually occur in the setting of normal or near-normal platelet counts. Abnormal platelet function can be demonstrated by a prolonged bleeding time and by abnormalities of platelet aggregation.

TABLE 1. Platelet-Mediated Disorders

Decreased Platelet Production

Aplastic anemia or marrow hypoplasia
Myelodysplastic syndrome
Myeloproliferative disorders (acute leukemias, myeloma, chronic granulocytic leukemia)
Lymphoproliferative disorders
Myelophthisis (solid tumors: prostate, breast, lung, gastrointestinal)
Drugs (e.g., chemotherapy, thiazides, alcohol)

Platelet Redistribution (Enlarged Splenic Pool)

Congestive splenomegaly (cirrhosis)
Others (e.g., lymphoma, Gaucher's disease)

Platelet Destruction

Nonimmune
  Infection
  Disseminated intravascular coagulation
  Hemangiomas
  Platelet loss (massive bleeding with only red blood cell replacement)
Immune
  Autoimmune (chronic idiopathic thrombocytopenic purpura)
  Alloimmune (post-transfusion purpura)
  Drug-dependent antibodies (e.g., quinine, quinidine, sulfas, heparin)
  Disease associated
    Collagen disease (e.g., systemic lupus erythematosus)
    Lymphoproliferative disorders
    Infection
      Viral (e.g., human immunodeficiency virus, cytomegalovirus, Epstein-Barr virus)
      Bacterial

Qualitative Platelet Defects

Hereditary defects
  Glanzmann's thrombasthenia
  Bernard-Soulier syndrome
  Storage pool deficiency
  Alpha granule deficiency
Acquired defects
  Drug induced (e.g., aspirin, nonsteroidal anti-inflammatory drugs, ticlopidine)
  Renal disease
  Liver disease

NONSPECIFIC THERAPY

Platelet Transfusion

Regardless of the cause of platelet-mediated bleeding, the presence of severe mucosal bleeding is an indication for platelet transfusion. In this setting, a single plateletpheresis or 6 to 8 units of random platelets are given. Transfusion should be repeated as needed. In some disorders (e.g., chronic ITP), the transfused platelets may be rapidly destroyed. However, transfusion should be continued until the bleeding is controlled by specific treatment.

Aminocaproic Acid

In severely thrombocytopenic patients in whom specific therapy is ineffective and bleeding continues (e.g., those with myelodysplasia or refractory leukemia), aminocaproic acid (Amicar) can prevent bleeding to a remarkable extent. The dose is 0.1 gram per kg orally (PO) or intravenously (IV) during 30 to 60 minutes followed by 6 grams PO or IV every 6 hours. Once bleeding is controlled, the dose is tapered to 1 to 3 grams every 6 hours.

SPECIFIC THERAPY

It must be understood that platelet counts higher than 25,000 to 30,000 per mm^3 are sufficient for hemostasis (unless the platelets are qualitatively defective), and that severe bleeding rarely occurs unless the platelet count is lower than 10,000 per mm^3. Treatment plans must be based on these facts. Table 2 lists the commonly used agents (alphabetically) with their doses, time to response, and expected side effects.

Disorders of Platelet Production

If the reduced platelet production is due to alcohol or a drug (e.g., thiazides), the offending agent should be stopped. However, control of thrombocytopenia due to decreased platelet production requires suc-cessful therapy of the primary disease. Until the primary disease is controlled, nonspecific measures are indicated.

Disorders of Platelet Distribution

The platelet count is usually not low enough to require therapy for disorders of platelet distribution. However, if the thrombocytopenia is symptomatic and surgery is not contraindicated, splenectomy is usually successful.

Disorders of Platelet Destruction

Drug-Induced Thrombocytopenia

Most drugs destroy platelets through immune mechanisms that are not fully understood but usually involve drug-dependent antiplatelet antibodies. The most common drugs are quinidine, quinine, sulfa, sulfa derivatives, valproic acid, procainamide, and gold. The treatment involves stopping the drug and supporting the patient with nonspecific therapy

TABLE 2. **Treatments Used in Platelet-Mediated Disorders**

Therapy	Dose	Response	Common Side Effects
Aminocaproic acid	Initial: 0.1 gm/kg PO/IV, then 6 g PO or IV q 6 h	Few days	Dizziness, hypotension, abdominal discomfort, GI symptoms, headache, arrhythmias, rash, delirium, myopathy, seizures, thrombogenic phenomena
Azathioprine	150 mg PO qd	2–10 mo	Cytopenias, GI symptoms, secondary malignancies*
Colchicine	0.6 mg PO tid	4–8 wk	Diarrhea (may limit therapy), nausea, vomiting
Corticosteroids			
Dexamethasone	40 mg PO qd × 4 d; repeat every 4 wk (6 cycles)	1–4 wk	Hypokalemia, gastric upset, sodium and fluid retention, weight gain, hyperglycemia, hypertension, myopathy, osteoporosis, increased infection risk, psychosis
Prednisone	1 mg/kg PO qd	1–4 wk	Same as for dexamethasone
Cyclophosphamide			
Standard dose	150 mg PO qd	6–8 wk	Cytopenias, hemorrhagic cystitis, GI symptoms, sterility, secondary malignancies*
High dose	1.0–1.5 gm/m^2 IV every 4 wk	1–4 wk	Cytopenias, hemorrhagic cystitis, GI symptoms, alopecia, sterility, myocardiopathy, secondary malignancies*
Cyclosporine	1.25–2.5 mg/kg PO bid	Variable	Renal insufficiency, hepatotoxicity, hypertension, tremor, hirsutism, gum hyperplasia, hypomagnesemia, secondary malignancies*
Danazol	200 mg PO qid	3–6 mo	Weight gain, fluid retention, seborrhea, hirsutism, vocal changes, amenorrhea, acne, headache, liver toxicity, thrombocytopenia
Dapsone	75–100 mg PO qd	4–8 wk	Hemolysis, agranulocytosis, aplastic anemia, exfoliative dermatitis, toxic hepatitis, cholestatic jaundice, peripheral neuropathy
Desmopressin (DDAVP)	0.3 µg/kg IV	30–60 min	Water intoxication, blood pressure changes, rare thrombotic events
Immune globulin	0.5–1.0 gm/kg IV	7–10 d	Headache, fever, rare fatal thrombosis in elderly patients; no AIDS or HIV seroconversion; although hepatitis C is reported, this is an unlikely future problem with solvent- or detergent-treated products
Interferon	3 million units SC 3 times/wk for 12 doses	Variable: during or after therapy	"Flulike" symptoms, fever, cytopenias, cardiomyopathy, hypotension, tachycardia, depression, confusion, hepatotoxicity, respiratory insufficiency
Staphylococcal-A Immunoadsorption Column	6 treatments	1–2 wk	Generalized pain, fever, chills, rash, nausea, vomiting, respiratory distress, hives, diarrhea, dizziness, tachycardia, severe generalized vasculitis
Vinca alkaloids			
Vinblastine	5–10 mg/wk IV	7–10 d	Leukopenia, alopecia, constipation, local corrosive effects if extravasated
Vincristine	1–2 mg/wk IV	7–10 d	Peripheral neuropathy, alopecia, constipation, local corrosive effects if extravasated

*Lymphoproliferative disorders or acute leukemia has occurred in patients receiving this drug.
Abbreviations: AIDS = acquired immune deficiency syndrome; GI = gastrointestinal; HIV = human immunodeficiency virus.

until the platelet count recovers (usually within 10 days). If severe mucosal bleeding occurs, corticosteroids, immune globulin intravenous (IGIV), and platelet transfusions may be needed until recovery occurs. The exception to this rule is thrombocytopenia due to gold. This agent remains in the tissues for several months, and successful therapy requires chelation with dimercaprol.

Thrombocytopenia due to heparin is rarely severe enough to require therapy. However, the danger associated with the heparin-induced thrombocytopenia syndrome is thrombosis. The mortality and morbidity rates for this syndrome (caused by, for example, myocardial infarction, cerebrovascular accidents, peripheral artery occlusions) are substantial. For this reason, the heparin should be stopped immediately, and another form of treatment should be substituted.

Post-Transfusion Purpura

The transfusion of platelets containing a surface antigen (usually the Pl^{A1} antigen) into a recipient who lacks the antigen leads to post-transfusion purpura. Antiplatelet antibody is formed, and for reasons that are poorly understood, the patient's platelets (which are antigen-negative) are also destroyed. The disorder is self-limited, but thrombocytopenia may be severe, with associated mucosal bleeding. The treatment of choice is IGIV. Patients for whom this treatment fails should undergo plasmapheresis.

Chronic Immune Thrombocytopenic Purpura

Chronic ITP is the most common cause of thrombocytopenia in adults. It is due to platelet destruction by an autoantibody usually directed against antigens on one of the major platelet glycoprotein complexes (GPIIb/IIIa or GPIb/IX/V).

INITIAL TREATMENT

No treatment is indicated unless the platelet count is less than 25,000 to 30,000 mm^3. Patients are treated initially with prednisone; if there is no response or relapse occurs on tapering of the prednisone, splenectomy is indicated. Patients should be immunized with pneumococcal, meningococcal, and *Haemophilus influenzae* vaccines before surgery to prevent subsequent severe infections with these organisms, which occur more commonly in splenectomized patients. Therapy with corticosteroids and splenectomy results in the cure of about 70% of patients.

REFRACTORY CASES

The treatment of ITP that is refractory to prednisone and splenectomy is more complex. Therapy can be arbitrarily divided into four levels according to the severity of the disease, the side effects associated with the treatment, and the evidence that the treatment might work. The treatments should generally be given in the order and for the indications given here. In the event of severe mucosal bleeding, concurrent therapy with IGIV plus platelets or high-dose methylprednisolone plus platelets may be required (see "Emergency Treatment").

Level 1 Treatments

INDICATION. These treatments should be tried for a platelet count less than 30,000 per mm^3.

STANDARD-DOSE PREDNISONE. Give 1 mg per kg PO daily; taper to the lowest dose allowing a platelet count higher than 30,000 per mm^3. Continue if that dose is 10 mg or less per day.

VINCRISTINE (ONCOVIN).* Give 2 mg IV every week. Stop if there is no response after the second dose. Do not give more than 4 to 6 doses, or peripheral neuropathy will occur.

PULSED DEXAMETHASONE. Give 40 mg PO daily for 4 days; repeat every 4 weeks for a total of six courses. Stop after three courses if there is no response or if relapse occurs during treatment.

DANAZOL (DANOCRINE)* PLUS PREDNISONE. Give danazol, 200 mg PO four times a day, with prednisone, 1 mg per kg PO daily. Taper the prednisone when the platelet count reaches safe levels or after 6 weeks. The danazol should be continued for at least 4 to 6 months before it is abandoned. If the platelet count becomes normal, continue danazol at full doses for 1 year, and then taper by 200 mg per day every 3 months to the lowest dose allowing safe platelet counts.

DAPSONE.* Give 75 to 100 mg PO daily. Continue for 8 weeks, and then stop if there is no response. In responsive patients, therapy must be continued or relapse will occur. Dapsone may cause severe hemolysis in glucose-6-phosphate dehydrogenase (G6PD)–deficient patients, so G6PD status should be tested before this agent is used.

COLCHICINE.* Give 0.6 mg PO daily, and increase the dose every 2 weeks to a maximum of 0.6 mg PO three times daily. Diarrhea often limits dosage. Continue for 3 months, and stop if there is no response. In responsive patients, therapy must be continued, or relapse will occur.

Level 2 Treatments

INDICATION. Because the toxicities are greater, these agents should be used only if the platelet count is less than 10,000 to 15,000 per mm^3 or if mucosal bleeding is present.

STAPHYLOCOCCAL-A IMMUNOADSORPTION COLUMN. Give a maximum of six treatments (three times a week for 2 weeks) per the manufacturer's instructions. Toxicity may be substantial, and some experts do not recommend this treatment.

CYCLOPHOSPHAMIDE (CYTOXAN).* Give 150 mg PO daily for 8 weeks; adjust the dose if neutropenia occurs. The patient must drink 2 quarts of fluid daily to prevent hemorrhagic cystitis. If a complete response occurs, continue at the full dose for 3 months, and then stop the drug. If no response occurs within 8 weeks, stop the drug.

AZATHIOPRINE (IMURAN).* Give 150 mg PO daily for 6 months (responses often occur slowly). If a complete response occurs, continue at full doses for 18 months,

---

*Not FDA approved for this indication.

and then stop therapy. If no response occurs in 6 months, stop therapy.

Level 3 Treatments

INDICATION. Because of the more serious side effects, these treatments are reserved for patients whose ITP is refractory to the level 1 and 2 treatments and who have life-threatening symptoms or extremely low platelet counts (less than 5000 per mm³).

PULSED CYCLOPHOSPHAMIDE (CYTOXAN).* Give 1.0 to 1.5 grams per m² IV every 4 weeks for a total of four courses. The patient must drink at least 2 quarts of fluid daily for the 3 days after each treatment or must receive comparable fluids IV to prevent hemorrhagic cystitis. Antinauseants should be given.

COMBINATION CHEMOTHERAPY. Several "lymphoma-type" regimens have been used. This treatment should be given after consultation with a hematologist or oncologist familiar with such regimens. No specific regimen has been found superior.

Level 4 Treatments

INDICATION. These treatments are in the "when all else fails" category, because experience with them is limited, response rates are low, or their expense and frequency of administration weigh against their use.

INTERFERON ALFA-2B (INTRON A).* Give 3 million units subcutaneously three times a week for 4 weeks. Responses may occur during therapy or after the drug is stopped. For patients showing response, consideration should be given to long-term treatment, although there is minimal experience with this approach.

IMMUNE GLOBULIN. Some patients in whom all other treatments fail show response to IVIG. Give 0.5 to 1.0 gram per kg IV. Responses are temporary, lasting 1 to 6 weeks. This therapy is extremely expensive and inconvenient but may be the only option in some patients.

VINBLASTINE (VELBAN).* Some patients with ITP who respond to vincristine also respond to this agent; responses are temporary, however, and the treatment is inconvenient. Give 5 to 10 mg IV weekly. Peripheral neuropathy is rare, and this drug can be given for long periods to patients who show response.

CYCLOSPORINE (SANDIMMUNE).* Give 1.25 to 2.5 mg per kg PO twice daily. Kidney damage may occur, so serum creatinine and cyclosporine levels must be monitored. Reported responses have been short despite continued treatment.

EMERGENCY TREATMENT

In patients with severe mucosal bleeding, give one of the following: (1) IGIV, 1.0 gram per kg IV, followed by a platelet transfusion (a single plateletpheresis or 6 to 8 units of random platelets) or (2) methylprednisolone (Solu-Medrol), 1.0 gram IV daily for 3 days, and give platelets after the first dose. These treatments may be repeated, although osteoporosis may be a problem if methylprednisolone is used on multiple occasions.

---

*Not FDA approved for this indication.

Qualitative Platelet Disorders

Disorders of platelet quality may be inherited (Glanzmann's thrombasthenia, Bernard-Soulier syndrome, storage pool deficiencies, alpha granule deficiency, and other poorly characterized disorders with prolonged bleeding time or aggregation abnormalities) or acquired (drug induced, such as from aspirin, nonsteroidal anti-inflammatory drugs, or antiplatelet drugs such as ticlopidine [Ticlid]; chronic renal failure; liver disease; myeloproliferative disorders; and paraproteinemias). The reader is referred to other sources for a description of the clinical pictures of and the diagnostic approaches to these disorders.

Treatment

Obviously, if drugs that affect platelet function are involved, they should be discontinued.

Platelet Transfusion. As noted previously, platelet transfusion is indicated in the case of severe mucosal bleeding or in situations in which bleeding may occur (e.g., major surgery, tooth extractions).

Empirical Therapy. The use of desmopressin (DDAVP),* 0.3 μg per kg IV, has been found useful in some of the acquired disorders (liver disease, renal disease) and the inherited disorders, particularly the platelet release defects (e.g., storage pool defects). There is also evidence that conjugated estrogens (Premarin)* are useful in patients with renal disease.

---

*Not FDA approved for this indication.

DISSEMINATED INTRAVASCULAR COAGULATION

method of
PETER E. BRAVERMAN, M.D.
The Johns Hopkins University School of Medicine
Baltimore, Maryland

Disseminated intravascular coagulation (DIC) is an acquired coagulopathy that is best understood as an epiphenomenon of a broad variety of disease states. The effects of this clinicopathologic entity range along a spectrum from asymptomatic laboratory abnormalities, through "chronic compensated" coagulopathies, to acute and fulminant catastrophic bleeding and thrombosis. The diagnosis and especially the management of this disorder remain controversial topics, but progress has been made in the appreciation that this is really a group of disorders of heterogeneous etiology and expression, and that treatment may differ greatly depending on the clinical circumstances.

The first experimental demonstration of DIC was described in 1834, when intravenous injection of solubilized brain tissue into animals induced lethal clotting. If the infusion was given more slowly, thrombi did not develop, but the blood became incoagulable. Since then, further studies have implicated many "triggering" factors that disrupt the complex homeostatic mechanisms of activation and inhibition in the coagulation system, but a detailed review of the pathogenesis is beyond the scope of this discussion.

The recognition of the DIC syndrome is obvious when unusual bleeding or thrombosis occurs in the appropriate clinical settings, such as those listed in Table 1. Confirming laboratory features include newly prolonged prothrombin time and activated partial thromboplastin time (APTT), thrombocytopenia, hypofibrinogenemia, and elevated fibrinogen-fibrin degradation (or split) products. Other assays that may add specificity to the diagnosis include those for antithrombin III (AT-III), α_2-antiplasmin, D dimer, and fibrinopeptide A. Work from Japan shows that a soluble fibrin monomer assay may eventually prove to be the most sensitive and specific indicator of DIC activity. Some investigators have developed scoring systems that quantify the severity of the coagulopathy, adding points for lower platelet counts, lower fibrinogen levels, higher fibrinogen-fibrin degradation product titers, and so on.

TREATMENT

There are three general elements in the management of DIC: treatment of the underlying cause or trigger, replacement of depleted platelets and/or procoagulation factors, and use of inhibitors of coagulation and/or fibrinolysis. By far the most important of these remains the first—the prompt identification, reversal, and eradication (or at least control) of the condition that caused the coagulopathy. If this cannot be accomplished, all other treatment modalities are only temporizing and doomed to failure. In some situations, control or reversal of the underlying trigger alone will be sufficient (e.g., abruptio placentae), but in others, replacement and inhibitor therapy may significantly reduce morbidity and mortality. This discussion emphasizes that management must be individualized to the particular setting and circumstances in which the coagulopathy is occurring, but certain general guidelines are appropriate.

TABLE 1. **Conditions Associated with Disseminated Intravascular Coagulation**

Any cause of extensive tissue damage and necrosis (resulting in massive release of tissue factor)
 Shock, burns, trauma, brain injury
 Heat stroke, acidosis, rhabdomyolysis
Infections, especially
 Sepsis (gram-negative *and* gram-positive)
 Rickettsia infection (Rocky Mountain spotted fever)
 Postsplenectomy bacteremia
Malignancies, especially
 Leukemias (promyelocytic *and* others)
 Mucin-producing adenocarcinomas *and* others
Obstetric complications, especially
 Abruptio placentae
 Retained dead fetus
 Amniotic fluid embolism
 Toxemia of pregnancy
Vascular diseases, especially
 Giant hemangiomas
 Aortic aneurysm
Miscellaneous
 Hemolytic transfusion reactions
 Hyperacute allograft rejection
 Venomous snake bites
 Peritoneovenous shunts
 Liver disease

Along with prompt treatment of the underlying trigger, general supportive care is crucial, especially with regard to limiting further tissue damage, infarction, or any complication that may release more tissue factor and contribute to further progression of the coagulopathy. This includes maintenance of circulatory volume, sufficient blood pressure for organ perfusion, correction of hypoxemia, and prevention of venous stasis. Whenever possible, and especially when peripheral ischemia and thrombosis are in evidence (e.g., purpura fulminans), aggressive volume support should be given in preference to adrenergic pressors, to limit vasoconstriction in the acral distribution.

There is little evidence to support the long-held notion that factor replacement in DIC "fuels the fire" and worsens outcome. In general, if platelet or fibrinogen levels are dangerously low and hemorrhage is occurring, replacement attempts should be made. However, postinfusion increments in platelet or fibrinogen level must be demonstrated (5000 to 10,000 platelets per mm^3 for each unit, and 10 mg of fibrinogen per dL for each unit of cryoprecipitate); if such increments are not observed, no further replacement should be given. When such immediate "consumption" is evident, repeated infusions after the start of low-dose heparin (500 to 800 units intravenously per hour) may, in some circumstances, produce more sustained increments. When bleeding is a problem, the approximate goal for platelets is a count of at least 50,000 per mm^3, and for fibrinogen, at least 50 to 75 mg per dL. When there is no bleeding, my colleagues and I attempt to give replacement therapy "prophylactically" for platelet levels below 10,000 to 20,000 per mm^3, and for fibrinogen levels less than 50 mg per dL. Effective replacement therapy is more important in conditions in which insufficient production is a large part of the problem (e.g., platelets in leukemic patients and coagulation factors in cirrhotic patients).

Bleeding is often the most salient and dramatic feature of the DIC syndrome, but in our experience, thrombosis produces most of the end-organ damage and morbidity, including renal and respiratory failure, stroke, and gangrene. Although the use of heparin in situations involving factor consumption and bleeding remains controversial, its use is clearly indicated in any setting of DIC complicated by large-vessel thromboembolism or by the dermal necrosis of purpura fulminans. In these situations, if hemorrhage is not a problem, full-dose heparin therapy (1000 to 1600 units per hour) should be given. If the APTT is already prolonged by the DIC, we either estimate appropriate infusion rates from published weight tables or mix the patient's plasma 1:1 with normal control plasma and adjust for a target of 1.5 to 2.0 times the APTT control. To reiterate, these are guidelines only, and it is more informative to consider the efficacy of different treatment modalities for DIC in each etiologic context.

When DIC accompanies septic shock, survival is probably more directly related to the severity of the infection and hypotension than to the complications of DIC. Nevertheless, the question of the value of coagulation inhibitors in these situations remains the most heated controversy in this disease and has historically been dominated more by anecdote and dogma than by data. Even now, despite accumulating publications on the possible efficacy of heparin and AT-III in these patients, there is still no prospective controlled trial with the power to demonstrate a survival advantage. Work with AT-III is promising but typically shows far greater improvements in laboratory abnormalities than in clinical outcomes. A French study of AT-III in sepsis showed a trend toward improved survival but did not have the numbers to show statistical significance. Nevertheless, some experts in the field now tout AT-III therapy as their treatment of choice for fulminant DIC in septic shock, given in an intravenous dose of approximately 100 IU per kg per day. Our experience with this therapeutic modality is limited.

For the subset of septic patients with features of classic purpura fulminans, we almost always advocate the use of heparin. (Caution must be exercised if there is a suggestion of possible central nervous system hemorrhage.) Studies clearly support its efficacy in pediatric patients, but we continue to see this catastrophe in adult asplenic patients and support its use in them as well. Unfortunately, we are usually called after the patient has progressed to full gangrene of digits. It must be emphasized that heparin should be started at the very first sign of dermal or acral ischemia, such as livedo reticularis, and as long as there are no contraindications, such as excessive or central nervous system bleeding, it should be given at full dose (1000 to 1600 units per hour).

Certain malignancy states deserve special mention. When DIC complicates acute promyelocytic leukemia (APL), it is usually manifested more by hemorrhage than by thrombosis, perhaps as a consequence of more fibrinolytic activity. Many still use heparin prophylactically before chemotherapy in this disease, but without the support of good data. A few studies have documented a reduction in hemorrhagic events with the use of inhibitors of fibrinolysis, such as tranexamic acid (Cyklokapron),* used alone in a dose of 2 grams every 8 hours intravenously, or ε-aminocaproic acid (EACA) combined with heparin. It should be noted that DIC has been less of a problem in APL with the introduction of all-*trans*-retinoic acid induction therapy for APL.

In the special circumstance of malignancy-associated chronic compensated DIC described by Armand Trousseau, heparin therapy is absolutely essential. Heralded by migrating superficial recurrent thrombophlebitis, and complicated by large-vessel venous and arterial thromboembolism, this syndrome responds only to heparin. Indeed, failure of warfarin treatment in any hypercoagulable state should immediately suggest the Trousseau syndrome, and the search for an occult malignancy should begin. Heparin should be given in full dose, either intravenously

*Not FDA approved for this indication.

to achieve an APTT of 1.5 to 2.0 times control, or in equivalent low-molecular-weight subcutaneous form, such as enoxaparin (Lovenox),* at 30 mg every 12 hours.

Obstetric complications associated with DIC should also be addressed individually. In the case of abruptio placentae, heparin therapy has no role. In this situation, bleeding predominates over thrombosis. Cryoprecipitate should be given to maintain a fibrinogen level above 150 mg per dL if hemorrhage begins, but nothing should delay evacuation of the uterus, which is the only and assured way to arrest the coagulopathy. In the case of a retained dead fetus, a low-grade chronic hemorrhagic diathesis may ensue, and heparin is often effective in raising fibrinogen levels and improving hemostasis in preparation for evacuation. If delivery is already under way and hypofibrinogenemia is present, cryoprecipitate, not heparin, should be given. In the unusual circumstance of a twin fetal death, subcutaneous heparin can control the consumption of fibrinogen while the living twin matures. In amniotic fluid embolism, survivors develop excessive bleeding related to uncontrolled fibrinolysis, and EACA may be useful in this circumstance.

Those entities causing a "local" vascular coagulation also require separate consideration. In the Kasabach-Merritt syndrome, characterized by giant hemangiomas and a bleeding tendency secondary to local platelet and fibrinogen consumption, the use of EACA has proved successful, inducing local thrombosis in the hemangiomatotic tissue and normalizing counts. In some cases of aortic aneurysm, a compensated form of DIC with low fibrinogen levels and thrombocytopenia may occur. In preparation for surgery, if vessel leaking is ruled out, low-dose heparin often stops the consumption process and returns reduced clotting factors to normal levels.

*Not FDA approved for this indication.

PLATELET-MEDIATED THROMBOSIS: HEPARIN-INDUCED THROMBOCYTOPENIA AND THROMBOTIC THROMBOCYTOPENIC PURPURA

method of
THEODORE E. WARKENTIN, M.D.
*Hamilton Health Sciences Corporation and
    McMaster University
Hamilton, Ontario, Canada*

Heparin-induced thrombocytopenia (HIT) and thrombotic thrombocytopenic purpura (TTP) share a striking characteristic: both of these thrombocytopenic disorders are strongly associated with *thrombosis* rather than bleeding. However, HIT and TTP are distinct with respect to their clinical and pathologic profile of thrombosis, pathogenesis, and treatment approaches. Clinicians must be familiar with both disorders, as prompt recognition and appropriate treatment significantly affect mortality and morbidity.

HEPARIN-INDUCED THROMBOCYTOPENIA

HIT is characterized by thrombocytopenia that begins 5 to 10 days after starting heparin therapy. Sometimes, patients develop thrombocytopenia immediately on receiving heparin for clinically suspected thrombosis; typically, these patients have recently received heparin (usually within 2 months). The explanation for this characteristic temporal profile of thrombocytopenia is related to the immune pathogenesis of HIT: (1) the formation of heparin–platelet factor 4 (PF4) complexes shortly after heparin therapy is started triggers the formation of pathogenic anti–heparin-PF4 IgG antibodies (HIT-IgG); (2) immune complexes form on the platelet surface; (3) HIT-IgG binds to the platelet Fc receptors, which leads to (4) potent platelet activation. It takes a minimum of 5 days for the pathogenic IgG antibodies to achieve clinically significant platelet-activating levels. Intriguingly, the HIT-IgGs are transient and usually become undetectable within 2 months. This explains why patients who develop abrupt thrombocytopenia on re-exposure to heparin usually have recently received heparin.

There are several reasons besides IgG-mediated platelet activation per se that explain why HIT is associated with thrombosis, including (1) activation of coagulation via triggering of the platelet procoagulant response; (2) activation of endothelium via cross-reactivity of HIT-IgG for PF4–(endothelial) heparan sulfate complexes; and (3) release of PF4 from activated platelets leading to neutralization of the anticoagulant effect of heparin (heparin "resistance"). The importance of coagulation activation and thrombosis in HIT has led to an increased focus on treatment approaches that emphasize indirect or direct thrombin inhibition (e.g., danaparoid, hirudin, argatroban).

Functional and antigen assays are available to help diagnose HIT. The most reliable functional assays measure activation of washed platelets by the patient's serum in the presence of heparin (e.g., platelet serotonin release assay). In contrast, widely used assays that measure aggregation of platelets in citrated plasma are not reliable for diagnosis of HIT. Antigen assays detect the presence of immunoglobulin reactive against the heparin-PF4 complex, e.g., by the enzyme-linked immunosorbent assay. It is now recognized that some patients receiving heparin form HIT-IgG without developing thrombocytopenia or thrombosis; thus, laboratory tests for HIT must be interpreted in the clinical context.

Venous thrombosis complicates HIT more often than does arterial thrombosis (approximately a 4:1 ratio; Table 1). Arterial thrombi typically involve

TABLE 1. **Clinical Sequelae of Heparin-Induced Thrombocytopenia**

Venous thrombosis
  Deep venous thrombosis, pulmonary embolism
  Venous limb gangrene (likely caused by warfarin treatment of HIT)
  Cerebral sinus thrombosis
  Adrenal hemorrhagic infarction (likely related to adrenal vein thrombosis)
Arterial thrombosis
  Lower limb major vessel and distal aortic occlusions
  Thrombotic stroke
  Myocardial infarction
  Miscellaneous (e.g., upper limb, renal, or mesenteric arterial thrombosis)
Heparin-induced skin lesions at subcutaneous heparin injection sites*
  Erythematous plaques
  Skin necrosis
Acute reactions described after intravenous heparin bolus
  Inflammatory reaction (e.g., fever, chills, flushing)
  Respiratory reaction (e.g., acute dyspnea)
  Cardiac arrest
  Transient global amnesia

*The majority of patients with heparin-induced skin lesions do not develop thrombocytopenia, although HIT-IgG is typically present in these patients' sera.

large vessels (macrovascular thrombosis; see the discussion of TTP) and are characteristically platelet rich ("white clot syndrome"). Venous thrombi are not distinct pathologically, except that a minority of patients with deep venous thrombosis (DVT) and HIT can develop limb gangrene requiring amputation because of warfarin treatment (discussed subsequently). About 2% of HIT patients develop adrenal hemorrhagic infarction, which can be bilateral and therefore result in acute and chronic adrenal insufficiency.

The frequency of HIT is variable and depends on the type and dose of heparin used; the population of patients receiving the heparin; duration of heparin administration; and definition of thrombocytopenia used. Clinically significant HIT (i.e., associated with thrombosis) occurs in approximately 1 to 3% of high-risk patients, e.g., postoperative orthopedic and cardiovascular patients who receive unfractionated heparin for more than 1 week. The risk of HIT and HIT-IgG seroconversion is lower in orthopedic patients given low-molecular-weight heparin prophylaxis.

Treatment (Table 2)

Commonly used treatment approaches for HIT are often ineffective. For example, simple discontinuation of heparin was associated with a subsequent 50% risk for thrombosis at 30-day follow-up in patients with serologically confirmed HIT in one study. Also, the use of warfarin to treat HIT complicated by DVT has been linked to a devastating syndrome of venous limb gangrene (necrosis complicating DVT despite palpable or Doppler-identifiable arterial pulses). Affected patients characteristically have an

TABLE 2. **Summary of Treatment Approach to Heparin-Induced Thrombocytopenia and Thrombotic Thrombocytopenic Purpura***

Disorder	Primary Therapy	Adjunctive Therapy	Special Situations	Avoid
HIT	Anticoagulant that inhibits thrombin generation: danaparoid or hirudin (or argatroban)	Aspirin (intravenous IgG, plasmapheresis)	*Selected arterial occlusions*: surgical thromboembolectomy; thrombolytic therapy	Warfarin† Ancrod Low-molecular-weight heparin Platelet transfusions
TTP	Plasma, preferably cryosupernatant plasma given by exchange	Corticosteroids (antiplatelet agents: e.g., aspirin and dipyridamole)	*Refractory patients*: (vincristine; splenectomy; solvent-detergent–treated plasma)	Platelet transfusions

*I consider the efficacy of treatments listed in parentheses to be less well established.

†Warfarin is not advised for treatment of acute HIT until there is adequate control of thrombin generation (e.g., with danaparoid or hirudin) and substantial resolution of the thrombocytopenia.

elevated International Normalized Ratio (INR) (usually >4.0) that coincides with the onset of necrosis. I believe that warfarin is a plausible explanation for this syndrome because plasma from affected patients showed marked depletion of protein C activity but persisting thrombin generation (shown as elevated thrombin-antithrombin complexes). Thus, there is evidence for a warfarin-induced disturbance in procoagulant-anticoagulant balance.

The primary treatment for HIT is an anticoagulant agent that inhibits thrombin generation. However, the most promising agents are not approved to treat HIT in most countries. Thus, clinicians must often obtain these agents via compassionate release programs, or use them for a nonapproved indication. For example, danaparoid sodium (Orgaran) is a mixture of anticoagulant glycosaminoglycans with predominant anti–factor Xa activity that is effective in more than 90% of HIT patients (Table 3). Danaparoid is approved in both Canada and the United States for use in DVT prophylaxis; however, its major clinical use is for the treatment of HIT (an unapproved indication). Approximately 10 to 20% of HIT sera cross-react with danaparoid in vitro; however, in vitro cross-reactivity is usually not associated with clinically significant in vivo cross-reactivity, which occurs in less than 5% of patients overall.

Recombinant hirudin (e.g., Refludan) is approved to treat HIT-associated thrombosis in the European community (see Table 3). Hirudin* is a natural antithrombin derived from the medicinal leech that can be conveniently monitored by using the activated partial thromboplastin time. Hirudin undergoes renal metabolism, and the drug must be used cautiously (if at all) in patients with moderate to severe renal impairment. A potent, synthetic antithrombin known as argatroban (Novastan) is undergoing investigation in the United States; anecdotal reports describing the use of argatroban for HIT in Japan suggest that this agent is likely to be effective in HIT.

I do not recommend the use of ancrod (a defibrinogenating snake venom) or low-molecular-weight heparin to treat HIT. Ancrod does not inhibit thrombin generation in HIT, nor does it prevent platelet aggregation in vitro by HIT-IgG. Further, warfarin-induced venous limb gangrene has occurred in patients who were also receiving ancrod. Low-molecular-weight heparin is essentially 100% cross-reactive with HIT-IgG. This is consistent with clinical experience suggesting that the risk of clinically significant cross-reactivity is higher with low-molecular-weight heparin than with danaparoid. Prophylactic platelet transfusions are contraindicated in HIT because bleeding is uncommon, and platelet transfusions could contribute to thrombosis.

TABLE 3. **Treatment of Thromboembolic Complications of Heparin-Induced Thrombocytopenia**

Danaparoid Sodium (Orgaran)

Loading dose: 2250 U intravenous bolus,* followed by 400 U/h for 4 h, then 300 U/h for 4 h. Then *maintenance*: 150–200 U/h, with subsequent dose adjustments made using anti–factor Xa levels (target range, 0.5–0.8 anti–Xa U/mL), if assay available.†

or

Recombinant Hirudin‡

Loading dose: 0.4 mg/kg bolus, followed by *maintenance*: 0.15 mg/kg/h infusion, with dose adjustments to maintain APTT 1.5–3.0 times the mean of the normal laboratory APTT range.

*Adjust bolus for body weight: <60 kg, 1500 U; 60–75 kg, 2250 U; 75–90 kg, 3000 U; >90 kg, 3750 U. The recommendations are based on 750-U ampule availability; for 1250-U ampules, the loading dose would be 2500 U, and so forth.

†Therapeutic anticoagulation is generally achieved with this protocol, and thus the unavailability of an anti–factor Xa assay should not necessarily prevent the use of danaparoid to treat HIT. The calibration curve for anti–factor Xa levels should be derived using danaparoid rather than low-molecular-weight heparin.

‡Not available in the United States.

Abbreviation: APTT = activated partial thromboplastin time.

THROMBOTIC THROMBOCYTOPENIC PURPURA

TTP is a clinicopathologic syndrome characterized by microangiopathic hemolysis, thrombocytopenia, and a high frequency of organ dysfunction, particularly brain and kidneys, caused by microvascular thrombosis. The term "microangiopathy" indicates

*Not available in the United States.

the presence of highly characteristic red blood cell fragments (schistocytes), such as helmet and triangular red blood cells, together with thrombocytopenia. In contrast, the term "macroangiopathy" suggests the presence of red blood cell fragments alone, without thrombocytopenia, as can be observed in some patients with regurgitant valvular heart disease; this latter syndrome is not associated with microvascular thrombosis. The possibility of TTP is an important reason why the clinician must carefully examine the blood films of all patients with thrombocytopenia and/or anemia.

Organ dysfunction in TTP is related to platelet–von Willebrand factor (vWF), or "hyaline," microthrombi that are especially likely to form within the cerebral and renal arterioles (microvascular thrombosis; see the discussion of HIT). Although the pathogenesis of TTP remains uncertain, both a platelet-activating factor and vWF may participate in the pathogenesis. For example, TTP plasma contains an enzyme (calcium-dependent cysteine proteinase) that activates platelets as well as proteolyzes vWF into a form that potentiates platelet aggregation. Large multimers of vWF circulate in the plasma of patients with chronic relapsing TTP in remission, suggesting that the disappearance of the largest multimers during active disease is related to participation of the vWF multimers in the formation of microthrombi. Although many patients with TTP have a flulike prodrome, the etiologic trigger of TTP is a mystery.

The clinical presentation of TTP is highly variable. Patients are most frequently middle-aged; there is a female predominance (3:2 ratio). Neurologic symptoms can range from headache and mild confusion to slurring of speech and focal neurologic deficits to seizures and coma. Renal involvement can range from microscopic hematuria without azotemia to severe oliguric or anuric renal failure. Fever is commonly observed in TTP. Less common complications include myocardial infarction and abdominal pain secondary to gastrointestinal ischemia or acute pancreatitis.

TTP is usually idiopathic. In contrast, a related entity known as the hemolytic-uremic syndrome (HUS) is often triggered by certain gastrointestinal infections, e.g., with verocytotoxin (Shiga-like toxin)–producing enterohemorrhagic *Escherichia coli* in Western populations; with *Shigella* in certain Third World populations. HUS can be considered a nephrotropic variant of TTP that is most common at the extremes of age (young children and elderly persons). Other clinical settings that are sometimes associated with clinical syndromes or conditions that resemble TTP or HUS include vasculitis (e.g., systemic lupus erythematosus); infections, including human immunodeficiency virus infection; after bone marrow or solid organ transplantation; pregnancy (HELLP syndrome: hemolysis, elevated liver enzymes, low platelets; postpartum HUS); and familial TTP or HUS. Rarely, TTP or HUS may be caused by certain drugs (e.g., mitomycin, ticlopidine, quinine).

Routine coagulation tests are usually normal in TTP, although a subset of patients with severe TTP can exhibit coagulopathy including positive testing for disseminated intravascular coagulation. However, the clinician should consider occult malignancy in patients who present with laboratory evidence of disseminated intravascular coagulation and microangiopathy on the peripheral blood film. Of the various laboratory markers of intravascular hemolysis observed in TTP, lactate dehydrogenase serum levels are most useful in following the clinical course of TTP.

Treatment (see Table 2)

Treatment with plasma has dramatically altered the natural history of TTP, lowering the untreated mortality rate from greater than 80 to less than 20%. I recommend as optimal treatment the administration of cryosupernatant plasma, given by plasma exchange (apheresis). A multicenter Canadian trial showed that plasma exchange is more effective than plasma given by infusion, likely because of the larger amounts of plasma that can be administered by pheresis. Although the additional clinical benefit of using cryosupernatant plasma is unproved, there are good reasons for preferring this blood product, including (1) the lack of vWF in cryosupernatant plasma; (2) anecdotal reports of refractory TTP patients whose condition remitted when cryosupernatant plasma was substituted for frozen plasma; and (3) the fact that cryosupernatant plasma is now widely available. Whenever possible, aggressive plasmapheresis should be performed (1.5 times the estimated patient plasma volume exchanged daily for 5 days, then one patient plasma volume exchanged daily if the patient is improving). Plasma exchange is usually tapered over 5 to 10 days after clinical and laboratory remission to try to reduce the risk for early relapse.

Many physicians use additional treatment for TTP, including corticosteroids (e.g., prednisone 100 to 200 mg once daily initially with subsequent tapering) and antiplatelet agents (e.g., aspirin 325 mg per day and dipyridamole 400 mg per day were given routinely in the Canadian multicenter plasmapheresis study). Although the efficacy of corticosteroids is unproved, I recommend that they be given in addition to intensive plasma exchange therapy. However, I usually avoid antiplatelet agents until the platelet count is greater than 50,000 per mm^3.

Some patients are refractory to exchange therapy. It is important to maintain aggressive apheresis in these patients because the therapy may be preventing further organ injury and may be lifesaving until the TTP eventually remits. Refractory TTP sometimes responds to vincristine infusion or splenectomy. Solvent-detergent–treated plasma, which also lacks large multimers of vWF, has been reported to be effective in TTP refractory to exchange with cryosupernatant.

There is a 20 to 30% risk of late recurrence of TTP in patients who recover fully from acute TTP, and this should be treated as primary TTP, i.e., with plasma exchange as primary therapy. Splenectomy may reduce the risk for subsequent relapse in patients with recurrent TTP. Some patients with frequent episodes of TTP or HUS may require prophylactic monthly plasma administration by infusion or exchange to prevent recurrences.

HEMOCHROMATOSIS

method of
LAWRENCE RICE, M.D.
Baylor College of Medicine
Houston, Texas

Astounding is the prevailing ignorance of hereditary hemochromatosis in the general medical community. Why do medical students and practitioners confidently exclaim, "Rare," when asked about its prevalence and demonstrate no shame when unable to recite common manifestations? One would expect that this disease would be intimately familiar to every practitioner given that (1) the disease is actually quite common, (2) it produces severe morbidity and mortality, yet (3) all manifestations are potentially preventable or treatable.

Close to 10% of whites may be carriers of the hemochromatosis gene; thus, close to 1 million Americans may be affected homozygotes. Tragically, more than 90% are unaware of their problem and continue to accumulate iron until organ damage occurs. Fortunately, this situation may be changing. In 1996, the hemochromatosis gene was isolated and its protein product characterized, and a genetic test should be widely available soon. The Centers for Disease Control and Prevention has begun to promote efforts to increase awareness of the disease and has promulgated recommendations for routine population screening.

This discussion focuses on hereditary hemochromatosis and then briefly considers "secondary" disorders in which there is a similar pattern of iron-induced organ dysfunction (Table 1). Underlying these disorders is the fact that the body's protection against excessive iron accumulation is by limiting absorption. If the absorptive barrier is dysfunctional or is bypassed, no physiologic processes can eliminate the excess iron.

HEREDITARY HEMOCHROMATOSIS

Clinical Features

Affected homozygotes hyperabsorb iron from birth. In a normal adult, total body iron is regulated at just below 4.0 grams, whereas iron accumulates in hemochromatosis over decades to 15 to 50 grams, causing oxidative damage to susceptible body tissues. The onset of clinically apparent disease is variable but most often strikes men in their forties or fifties and women a decade or two later. Not only does menstrual iron loss delay the onset of clinically apparent disease in women, but indeed, men predominate in any series of clinically afflicted patients. There is a relatively rare juvenile form of hemochromatosis in which more severe iron hyperabsorption

TABLE 1. **Organs Affected by Iron Overload**

Liver	Pancreas (diabetes)
Cirrhosis	Pituitary (hypogonad)
Hepatoma	Joints (arthropathy)
Heart	Skin (color)
Congestive cardiomyopathy	
Heart block and/or	
arrhythmia	

leads to clinical manifestations near age 20 years; this form affects males and females equally.

Organs affected are listed in Table 2. Common presenting symptoms include fatigue and generalized weakness as well as symptoms related to specific affected organs (e.g., arthritis, heart failure, and diabetes). Most deaths are attributable to liver or heart involvement. The liver is enlarged in 90% of cases. Death ensues not only from the encephalopathy and portal hypertension (variceal hemorrhage) that complicate other forms of cirrhosis, but also from an exceedingly high incidence of hepatocellular carcinoma. Heart disease manifests as congestive cardiomyopathy or conduction system disturbances.

Hemochromatosis does not necessarily present as a multisystem disease. Rather, it should be considered whenever there is disease of a typically affected organ. This issue is important, because hemochromatosis is generally the most treatable possibility in the differential diagnosis.

Diagnosis

Screening of asymptomatic individuals is by serum transferrin saturation measurements. In normal adults, transferrin saturation (the serum iron divided by the total iron-binding capacity) is 20 to 45%, but in patients with hemachromatosis, it is greater than 60% in men and greater than 50% in women. Actually, affected individuals frequently have transferrin saturations of 90 to 100%. An abnormal result precipitates an evaluation, which includes repeated transferrin saturation measurement (ensuring that iron supplements are not being taken), complete blood count (with attention to possible "iron-loading" anemias), serum ferritin level, and blood tests of

TABLE 2. **Iron Overload States**

Disorder	Examples	Behavior of "Intestinal Barrier"
Hereditary hemochromatosis (primary; idiopathic)	Autosomal recessive HLA linked Juvenile form African form	Intrinsically dysfunctional
Chronic, excessive iron ingestion	Bantu siderosis	Overwhelmed
Iron-loading anemias	Thalassemias Sideroblastic anemia	Fooled
Chronic transfusion therapy	Transfusion-dependent anemia	Bypassed

glucose and liver function (although these may be abnormal only quite late in the course of the liver injury). For evaluation of possible hemochromatosis in symptomatic patients, the same tests are recommended. Detailed endocrine testing is warranted for some.

Liver biopsy is the traditional way to establish a definitive diagnosis, and many authorities continue to recommend this for all suspected cases. The biopsy shows impressive iron deposition in hepatocytes (preferentially over Kupffer cells) and determines the presence and degree of cirrhosis. Special handling of the specimen for quantitative iron determination is mandatory. The hepatic iron index (quantitative liver iron corrected for age) affords more precise separation of affected individuals from heterozygous carriers, in whom there may be some increase in stainable hepatic iron, and from patients with other liver diseases, in whom there can be secondary iron deposition (see later). In straightforward cases, I have not found liver biopsy necessary. The procedure is offered and discussed, and the results always convey added information, but only one third of my hemochromatosis patients have undergone liver biopsy in recent years.

Radiologic imaging studies can be helpful. Computed tomography may show abnormal liver density, but not reliably. Single photon emission computed tomography may be most accurate but is not generally available. Because of the powerful and unique paramagnetic properties of iron, magnetic resonance imaging of iron-loaded organs demonstrates sensitive and specific changes in signal intensity on T2-weighted images. While efforts to better quantitate these changes are ongoing, magnetic resonance imaging can be a useful confirmatory test in patients who do not have liver biopsy.

A genetic test for hemochromatosis will have an impact on screening and evaluation of suspected cases. Liver biopsy will likely become less necessary. Preliminary studies find that 82 to 83% of patients with hemochromatosis in the United States are homozygous for the mutated gene. One implication is that other mechanisms (other genetic abnormalities) can give rise to the iron hyperabsorption syndrome. Thus, a negative genetic test will not rule out some form of hemochromatosis, and transferrin saturation and serum ferritin measurements will continue to have utility in diagnosis and follow-up.

It is worth noting that in some patients, it is impossible to be sure whether hemochromatosis is present (see later). Such patients (one every few years in a referral practice) should be treated as if they have hemochromatosis. It can be determined in retrospect whether they actually have hemochromatosis from the number of phlebotomies required to exhaust iron stores.

Problems in Diagnosis

Diagnosis is simple and straightforward in most cases. For example, an asymptomatic, healthy, nonal-coholic individual with persistent elevated serum ferritin levels and transferrin saturation of 90% could have nothing else. Additional testing would be ancillary, and therapy is mandated.

On the other hand, a definitive diagnosis can be extraordinarily difficult in some cases because of the limitations of available tests and because other clinical situations can mimic hemochromatosis. A genetic test would improve the situation but would not completely eliminate problems. Some more important diagnostic problems are as follows:

1. Heterozygote carriers absorb more iron than normal persons but not enough to cause organ dysfunction. They tend to have transferrin saturation and serum ferritin levels that overlap with those of homozygous, affected patients. This problem is exacerbated by the large number of heterozygotes in the general population. (Not completely resolved is whether heterozygote carriers could develop clinically significant iron overload if subjected to stresses such as alcoholism or some types of anemia.)

2. Serum iron, total iron-binding capacity, and serum ferritin levels are influenced by intercurrent inflammatory, infectious, and neoplastic diseases. These diseases tend to mask the high transferrin saturation of hemochromatosis and to increase ferritin levels. Experimentally, measuring the iron content of ferritin is helpful.

3. Chronic liver disease, especially that due to alcohol, can lead to the same abnormalities in transferrin saturation and serum ferritin levels that characterize hemochromatosis, making it difficult to distinguish cause and effect. With advanced cirrhosis, even a liver biopsy may be unable to differentiate these processes, although the hepatic iron index may help. When the diagnosis is unsure, quantitative phlebotomy therapy is prudent.

4. Not all homozygous individuals with classic abnormalities of iron studies are destined to develop clinically significant organ damage. Although this phenomenon has been little discussed or studied, some authorities estimate that almost half of genetically affected men and three fourths of genetically affected women may never manifest disease. Is this situation due mainly to inadequate evaluation? Given our current level of understanding, it is prudent to treat all genetically affected individuals.

Treatment

The treatment of hemochromatosis is phlebotomy. Period. There is 1 mg of iron in 1 mL of packed red blood cells, so the removal of 1 unit (500 mL) of whole blood removes about 200 mg of iron. Phlebotomies are performed about once a week and are continued until iron deficiency is apparent from serum ferritin and transferrin saturation studies. The duration of therapy is several months to few years. Weekly phlebotomies are well tolerated by most patients, with little or no anemia developing. Therapy is generally postponed if the hematocrit is less than 34%. A daily multivitamin containing 1 mg of folic acid should be administered to help meet the metabolic demands of chronic reticulocytosis. Once iron deficiency has been induced, maintenance phlebotomies are required approximately every 4 months to keep the serum ferritin and transferrin saturation levels low.

Dietary manipulations and proscriptions are misguided, because it is the iron that has accumulated over decades that is the problem, not the iron currently coming in. The main dietary sources of iron are red meat and organ meat. Consider that a thick steak contains 3 mg of iron, of which about 1 mg may be absorbed. If one consumed steak every day of the year, that iron one had absorbed from the steak and more would be removed by two phlebotomies. Unfortunately, some patients are subjected to unpalatable and non-nutritious iron-poor diets, frequently including obsessions about the iron content of foods from which iron is poorly absorbed (e.g., spinach).

There is ordinarily no role for iron chelation therapy with deferoxamine (Desferal) in hereditary hemochromatosis, because of the issues of toxicity, cost, convenience, and efficacy. Deferoxamine would be reasonable if a superimposed refractory anemia prohibits phlebotomies. (I have never encountered such a patient.) Erythropoietin (Procrit, Epogen) injections would be an alternative that, if effective, could permit phlebotomies.

The treatment of hemochromatosis obviously includes management of complications. Examples include insulin for diabetes, nonsteroidal anti-inflammatory agents for arthropathy, pacemakers for heart block, and hormone replacement for gonadal failure. For patients with cirrhosis, some authorities recommend periodic screening for hepatoma. The hope that early diagnosis would facilitate curative surgery remains unproven. A mandatory ancillary step in the care of patients with hemochromatisis is the screening of their relatives for the disease.

The efficacy of phlebotomy treatment and thus the overall prognosis in hemochromatosis depend on the extent of disease at diagnosis. Therapy begun in a presymptomatic stage is highly effective in preventing disease manifestations. Once organ damage has occurred, therapy is effective in arresting progression. Therapy is less reliably effective in reversing already present organ dysfunction, but sometimes the degree of organ functional recovery may be surprising. Problems not reversible are arthropathy and the risk of hepatocellular carcinoma once there is cirrhosis.

SECONDARY IRON OVERLOAD

It is difficult if not impossible for a normal person to develop clinical iron overload from long-term excessive iron ingestion. An exception may be African Bantus, who habitually consume large quantities of beer brewed in iron vessels. Even in that group, however, studies implicate an autosomal dominant, non–HLA-linked genetic cofactor. In African-Americans hereditary hemochromatosis is less common than in whites, but cases that do occur may be related to this different iron hyperabsorption gene.

In chronic anemias in which there is erythroid hyperplasia and ineffective erythropoiesis, iron hyperabsorption and clinical iron overload may develop in the absence of transfusion therapy. This applies mainly to thalassemia intermedia and hereditary sideroblastic anemia, and less to acquired refractory anemias. Some iron hyperabsorption may occur with hemolytic and megaloblastic anemias.

In transfusion-dependent anemias, clinically important iron overload can develop within several months. Each unit of red blood cells delivers 225 to 250 mg of iron, which cannot be eliminated. Iron overload was the major cause of morbidity and mortality in transfusion-dependent patients before effective chelation therapy.

Treatment

Phlebotomy remains the preferred treatment when possible. In iron-loading anemias of moderate degree, modified phlebotomy regimens may remove adequate amounts of iron without worsening the anemia.

Iron chelation with deferoxamine is the therapy for transfusion-dependent patients. Such therapy has proved dramatically effective in reducing morbidity and mortality in patients receiving long-term transfusion therapy, such as those with thalassemia major. In older patients with acquired transfusion-dependent anemias, the clinician must judge whether the iron loading versus other aspects of the disease is likely to be limiting to health and longevity. For example, transfusion-dependent patients with severe problems related to neutropenia or thrombocytopenia or with factors predicting rapid evolution to leukemia are unlikely to benefit from iron chelation.

There is no consensus on exactly when to initiate chelation therapy or how best to monitor and adjust dosage. One authority recommends beginning therapy when measured hepatic iron exceeds 7 mg per gram of dry weight, another when transferrin saturation is elevated and a deferoxamine test shows high urinary iron excretion, and still others simply use serum ferritin levels. Deferoxamine is more toxic when the body's iron burden is low, so there is harm in treating too early as well as too late. The goal of therapy differs from that in hereditary hemochromatosis. One does not strive to induce iron deficiency but rather to stabilize iron burden at a moderate level that produces no organ damage.

Deferoxamine is generally given by 12-hour infusions either subcutaneously or intravenously every other day, or as often as needed. We measure 24-hour urinary iron excretion to determine the optimal dose in a given patient, usually 1 to 2 grams per infusion. Problems with deferoxamine include the inconveniences of parenteral infusions, high cost of the drug (and the infusion pump and appliances), inflammation at injection sites, infection (the drug predisposes to unusual infections, such as mucormycosis), auditory and ocular effects, and, in children, skeletal abnormalities. Compliance problems are common. Ascorbic acid given with deferoxamine increases iron excretion, but high doses are associated with acute cardiac decompensation. If ascorbic acid is given, the dose should not exceed 100 to 200 mg daily.

The search for an oral iron chelator has stretched more than 2 decades. Deferiprone (L1)* removes adequate amounts of iron for clinical benefit. The drug induces a high incidence of agranulocytosis and arthritis, and good outcome data proving clinical benefit are lacking.

---

*Not available in the United States.

HODGKIN'S DISEASE: CHEMOTHERAPY

method of
GEORGE P. CANELLOS, M.D.
*Harvard Medical School and Dana-Farber
   Cancer Institute
Boston, Massachusetts*

The systemic therapy of malignancy with cytotoxic chemotherapeutic agents received a vital injection of enthusiasm after the demonstration that advanced Hodgkin's disease (HD) could be cured by that approach. The model for the management of HD was also applied, with some success, to non-Hodgkin's lymphoma and other cancers.

The most useful diagnostic test in the assessment of the patient with presumed HD is a review of the histopathology by a hematopathologist. The basic division of histologic subgroups includes lymphocyte-predominant (LP) HD, which is relatively rare (<10% of cases) and has been defined as a B cell malignancy with immunophenotypically unique Reed-Sternberg (R/S) cells, so-called (L/H) cells, and extremely favorable prognosis. The more common nodular sclerosis (70 to 80% of cases) and mixed cell histology (30%) have classic R/S cells and associated normal reactive fibrosis and T lymphocytes. The immunophenotype of the R/S cells is usually (but not always) devoid of B or T cell markers but is frequently reactive with antibodies to CD30 (Ki-1) and CD15 (Leu-M1), except in LP HD. The diagnosis can occasionally be difficult to differentiate from the non-Hodgkin's lymphoma variants: T cell–rich B cell lymphoma; Ki-1 anaplastic large cell lymphoma; and mediastinal large cell lymphoma with sclerosis. Immunophenotypic studies of paraffin-embedded tissue can greatly assist in the diagnostic process, because the tumor cells of these non–Hodgkin's lymphomas react with markers for B cell differentiation and/or leukocyte common antigen. The R/S cells usually lack the former and almost always the latter.

There is no specific molecular marker or accompanying cytogenetic abnormality. The role of chemotherapy has expanded since the early days, when MOPP (mechlorethamine [Mustargen], vincristine [Oncovin], prednisone, and procarbazine) was used primarily for advanced HD stage IIIB/IV disease. In the subsequent years, systemic therapy has improved survival and progression-free survival by virtue of (1) its application with radiation therapy (combined modality) for poor-risk localized or stage III disease; (2) its use, where appropriate, as sole modality for patients with nonbulky, localized, or early stage III disease; (3)

as systemic salvage for patients who have relapses after primary radiation therapy; and (4) as second- or third-line systemic therapy after relapse from primary chemotherapy either as salvage or as preparation for high-dose therapy with bone marrow or peripheral stem cell support.

Prognostic factors likely to exclude chemotherapy from the primary management are those that predict a favorable outcome with localized radiation therapy. They include extremely favorable presentations: clinical stage IA; female patient younger than 40 years; no bulky disease; favorable histology, LP or nodular sclerosis or a somewhat more advanced localized nonbulky disease at stage IIA with fewer than four sites involved; and an erythrocyte sedimentation rate less than 50 mm per hour and/or a negative staging laparotomy. In almost all other presentations, systemic or combined modality therapy is often required. The European Organization for Research and Treatment of Cancer (EORTC) has defined prognostic features for combined modality therapy in localized HD. The risk criteria are shown in Table 1.

CLINICAL FACTORS THAT PREDICT OUTCOMES OF CHEMOTHERAPY

Assessment of the patient includes appropriate staging of extent and bulk of disease and evaluation of the impact of disease on performance status. Bone marrow biopsy is useful but not essential, because (1) it is rarely positive in limited asymptomatic stage I/IIA diseases and (2) in more advanced localized or advanced disease, it will not influence choice of therapy or predict the degree of myelosuppression. Important negative prognostic factors from various series include age greater than 50 years; hematocrit less than 38% in men or 34% in women; stage; number of extranodal sites; extent of the response to chemotherapy; bulk greater than 10 cm or mediastinal/thoracic ratio greater than 0.35 or 0.45 (depending on series); and reduction of dose administered. The literature contains a large number of factors that were considered negative for overall survival when systemic therapy with or without radiation was used for advanced disease; they are shown in Table 2.

The basic staging studies are thoracic and abdominal computed tomography, upright chest film, and bone scan if the bone marrow assay is positive or if there is bone pain.

TABLE 1. **Prognostic Features and Therapy for Localized Hodgkin's Disease (EORTC Criteria)**

Very Favorable

CS IA, female, age <40 y, favorable histology (lymphocyte predominant, no NS), ESR <50 mm/h, no bulk
Therapy: Mantle RT

Favorable

No unfavorable features (i.e., CS IIA, 3 sites, NS histology)
Therapy: Laparotomy, if negative mantle/para-aortic RT or chemotherapy and involved-field RT without laparotomy

Unfavorable

Age ≥50 y or unfavorable histology (mixed cellularity) or ESR > 50 mm/h with no symptoms or ESR >30 mm/h with symptoms or bulky disease, mediastinal/thoracic ratio ≥0.35 in CS II with four or more sites
Therapy: Combined modality or chemotherapy alone in selected patients

---

Abbreviations: CS = clinical stage; EORTC = European Organization for Research and Treatment of Cancer; ESR = erythrocyte sedimentation rate; NS = nodular sclerosis; RT = radiation therapy.

TABLE 2. **Advanced Hodgkin's Disease: Features Indicating Poor Prognosis After Systemic or Combined Modality Therapy (Various Publications)**

Age >45 or 50 y
Elevated lactate dehydrogenase
Mediastinal mass (mediastinal/thoracic ratio >0.45)
Low hematocrit
Inguinal involvement
Lymphocyte count $<0.75 \times 10^3/mm^3$
Multiple extranodal sites
Dose of chemotherapy
Advanced stage IV
Erythrocyte sedimentation rate >80 mm/h
Low serum albumin

A gallium 67 radionuclide scan at diagnosis can be useful as a baseline assessment for subsequent follow-up. The evaluation of residual masses is greatly enhanced by the ^{67}Ga scan, because residual positivity due to tumor is usually associated with early relapse and because necrotic and fibrotic residual masses can become ^{67}Ga-negative and predict a durable remission. The current Ann Arbor staging system (Cotswolds' modification) is shown in Table 3.

Staging laparotomy is now rarely performed except when clinical factors are such that a negative laparotomy would allow for limited radiation therapy alone or when the toxicity of systemic therapy is to be avoided.

TREATMENT PROGRAMS

There are a number of variants of the two basic regimens, MOPP and ABVD (doxorubicin [Adriamycin], bleomycin, vinblastine, and dacarbazine). Table 4 outlines the MOPP regimen and its variants, and Table 5 lists non–alkylating agent regimens such as ABVD. The hybrid MOPP-ABV is also widely used and similar in outcome to that of MOPP alternating with ABVD.

TABLE 3. **The Cotswolds Staging Classification**

Stage I	Involvement of a single lymph node region or lymphoid structures (e.g., spleen, thymus, Waldeyer's ring)
Stage II	Involvement of two or more lymph node regions on the same side of the diaphragm (the mediastinum is a single site, hilar lymph nodes are lateralized)
	The number of anatomic sites should be indicated by a suffix (e.g., II3)
Stage III	Involvement of lymph node regions or structures on both sides of the diaphragm
III1	With or without splenic hilar, celiac, or portal nodes
III2	With para-aortic, iliac, and mesenteric nodes
Stage IV	Involvement of extranodal site(s) beyond that designated "E"
A	No symptoms
B	Fever, drenching sweats, weight loss
X	Bulky disease: >one-third widening of mediastinum >10 cm maximal dimension of nodal mass
E	Involvement of a single extranodal site, contiguous or proximal to known nodal site
CS	Clinical stage
PS	Pathologic stage

Prospective randomized trials have confirmed that ABVD alone with or without radiation therapy offers an equivalent if not superior progression-free survival compared with MOPP with or without radiation therapy or even MOPP alternating with ABVD. The current Intergroup trial comparing the MOPP-ABV hybrid with ABVD alone has been completed and is currently under analysis. Thus, ABVD is the most commonly used first regimen either in combined modality or alone. ABVD does not appear to have the associated myelodysplasia or leukemia and sterility that are associated with alkylating agents, nor does it seem to be as myelosuppressive. Among the unknowns are (1) the optimal number of cycles of chemotherapy when combined with radiation therapy for localized disease, (2) the minimal size of bulk sites that require complementary radiation therapy after chemotherapy, and (3) which of the newer chemotherapy approaches, if any, is superior to ABVD. The newer approaches include hybrid regimens such as MOPP-ABV, concentrated 12-week regimens such as Stanford V and VAPEC-B (doxorubicin, cyclophosphamide, vincristine, bleomycin, etoposide, prednisolone; Christie Hospital, Manchester, UK), and even early high-dose intensification.

UNIQUE TOXICITY

As with other chemotherapy regimens, myelosuppression, anorexia, nausea and vomiting, and hair loss characterize the side effects of MOPP, ABVD, and their variants. The toxicity effects associated more or less uniquely with the various agents include vincristine, peripheral neuropathy; vinblastine, autonomic neuropathy, especially in the intestine; procarbazine, flushing with alcohol use; bleomycin, pulmonary toxicity; doxorubicin, cardiac muscle damage; and prednisone, aseptic osteonecrosis.

SALVAGE REGIMENS

Patients whose disease is refractory to MOPP and ABVD generally require third-line regimens, which usually contain etoposide, a nitrosourea, methyl GAG (mitoguazone),* mitoxantrone, and melphalan in various mixtures. Patients who have a relapse but are not necessarily refractory may be retreated with MOPP-ABVD, especially if the duration of the first remission was longer than 12 months and the patient has an asymptomatic, localized recurrence of disease.

In the setting of true refractoriness, partial response, or early generalized relapse after chemotherapy, patients are candidates for high-dose therapy with bone marrow or peripheral stem cell support. Persistence of residual masses as radiographic abnormalities that are negative for gallium avidity in asymptomatic patients is not necessarily reflective of refractory disease and should be followed up rather than considered evidence of therapy failure.

---

*Not available in the United States.

TABLE 4. **Alkylating Agent–Containing Regimens Active in the Treatment of Hodgkin's Disease**

Regimen	Contents	Dosage (mg/m²/d)	Days Given
MOPP	Mechlorethamine	6	1, 8
	Vincristine	1.4	1, 8
	Procarbazine	100 PO	1–14
	Prednisone	40	1–14 q 28 d
ChlVPP	Chlorambucil	6 (10 max.) PO	1–14
	Vinblastine	6 (10 max.)	1, 8
	Procarbazine	100	1–14
	Prednisone	40	1–14 q 28 d
LOPP	Chlorambucil	6 (10 max.)	1–10
	Vincristine	1.4	1, 8
	Procarbazine	100 PO	1–10
	Prednisone	40 PO	1–14 q 28 d
MOPP-ABV hybrid	Mechlorethamine	6	1
	Vincristine	1.4	1
	Procarbazine	100 PO	1–7
	Prednisone	40 PO	1–14
	Doxorubicin	35	8
	Bleomycin	10	8
	Vinblastine	6	8
Stanford V (per cycle)	Doxorubicin	25	1, 15
	Vinblastine	6	1, 15
	Mechlorethamine	6	1
	Etoposide	60 IV	15, 16
	Vincristine	1.4 (max. 2.0)	8, 22
	Bleomycin	5 U/m²	8, 22
	Prednisone	40 qod	
	Prophylactic co-trimoxazole, ketoconazole, acyclovir	Total of 3 cycles over 12 wk	

CURRENT THERAPEUTIC OPTIONS

Radiation Therapy Alone

1. Very favorable clinical stage IA (mentioned previously) may be treated with mantle radiation therapy alone.

2. Pathologic stage I/IIA or B disease in patients younger than 50 years in the *absence* of unfavorable features such as mixed cellularity histology, bulk disease, or multiple (four or more) sites above the diaphragm may be considered for radiation therapy alone if the laparotomy is negative. Alternatively, the patient may opt for subtotal nodal irradiation, including the splenic field.

Combined Modality

1. All other localized presentations with unfavorable features (as mentioned previously). Also, patients with predominantly favorable features who elect to avoid a laparotomy and/or prefer not to receive subtotal nodal irradiation. In the absence of bulk disease, systemic chemotherapy alone may be an option for the uncommon patient who refuses radiation.

2. Clinical stage IA/IIA bulky mediastinal disease (10 cm or larger or with mediastinal/thoracic ratio 0.35 or higher) requires combined modality therapy and no laparotomy. The numbers of cycles of chemotherapy, usually ABVD, administered before radiation can vary from two to six.

Combination Chemotherapy

1. All presentations of clinical stage IIB to IVB disease require systemic therapy. Usually, six to eight cycles are required, but maintenance chemotherapy does not improve the results. The most commonly used regimen is ABVD. No scientific evidence indicates that the MOPP-ABVD hybrid should be used in preference, but this issue is currently under analysis in another Intergroup trial that addresses this form.

2. With rare exceptions, all patients with stage I/II disease in relapse after primary radiation therapy and all patients with stage III/IV disease in relapse

TABLE 5. **Combination Chemotherapy Regimens Without Alkylating Agents**

Regimen	Contents	Dosage (mg/m²/d)	Days Given
ABVD	Doxorubicin (Adriamycin)	25 IV	1, 15 q 28 d
	Bleomycin	10 U	1, 15
	Vinblastine	6	1, 15
	Dacarbazine	375	1, 15
EVA	Etoposide	100 IV	1, 2, 3
	Vinblastine	6	1 q 28 d
	Doxorubicin	50	1
VEEP	Vincristine	1.4 (2.0 max.)	1, 8
	Epirubicin*	50	1 q 21 d
	Etoposide	100	1–4
	Prednisolone	100 PO	1–8
NOVP	Mitoxantrone (Novantrone)	10	1
	Vincristine (Oncovin)	1.4	8
	Vinblastine	6	1 q 21 d
	Prednisone	100 PO	1–5

*Not available in the United States.

after primary chemotherapy require salvage chemotherapy and possibly high-dose therapy consolidation.

It is less certain whether radiation therapy must be given to patients with stage III/IV disease after clinical complete remission with combination chemotherapy. The Southwest Oncology Group (SWOG) conducted randomized trials to test whether involved-field radiation therapy to previous masses (>6 cm) after chemotherapy offered a survival advantage. It did not improve the survival with chemotherapy alone. Extensive bulky sites (>10 cm) with a mediastinal/thoracic ratio of 0.35 or greater in patients with known stage III/IV disease are usually treated with complementary radiation therapy after chemotherapy.

Long-term Complications of Chemotherapy

The most significant long-term complication of systemic chemotherapy is the alkylating agent–associated myelodysplasia and acute leukemia that occur in about 3% of patients treated with MOPP or its variants. Myelodysplasia usually appears between 3 and 8 years after therapy, and the likelihood of its appearance may be enhanced by extensive radiation therapy. Alkylating agent–containing regimens given in the full dose and for six cycles will result in long-term male and female sterility. There is a rare recovery of spermatogenesis in time, and young women (younger than 25 years) usually retain normal reproductive function. Sperm banking should be recommended to all men who are to receive chemotherapy until more data are available. It is advisable to consider sperm banking even with chemotherapy regimens that do not contain alkylating agents.

Chronic compromise of pulmonary function secondary to bleomycin is rare. It has been noted to be enhanced by radiation therapy, but the likelihood of severe or life-threatening lung toxicity is low, as it occurs in less than 3% of patients. Similarly, long-term cardiac toxicity due to doxorubicin is rare after ABVD, but again, radiation therapy delivered to the left ventricle may contribute to a higher likelihood of cardiac toxicity, especially in children. Variants of ABVD that omit bleomycin may be required in the special circumstance of severe chronic lung disease. It is uncertain whether late-appearing non-Hodgkin's lymphoma is related to therapy or is more associated with the natural history of HD, especially the lymphocyte-predominant variant, which is a B lymphocyte tumor. Late-appearing solid tumors have been noted to occur 10 to 20 years after treatment, but in almost all instances, these tumors occur in the field of irradiation. They include breast cancer (especially in young women), mesothelioma or sarcoma, lung cancer, and head or neck cancer. Chemotherapy alone or combined with radiation therapy may result in subtle long-term immunosuppression, which can lead to unusual secondary infections such as herpes zoster.

HODGKIN'S DISEASE: RADIATION THERAPY

method of
NANCY PRICE MENDENHALL, M.D.
University of Florida College of Medicine
Gainesville, Florida

Radiation is the single most effective agent available in the treatment of Hodgkin's disease (HD). It may be used as the sole treatment in early-stage patients; in combined-modality treatment regimens for patients of all stages; as the sole salvage therapy in patients with nodal recurrence after chemotherapy; as part of salvage regimens that include standard or high-dose chemotherapy; and for palliation or in situations requiring rapid tumor response. Successful radiation treatment requires appropriate equipment, an experienced radiation oncologist, and adequate imaging to define the limits of disease.

RADIOTHERAPY TECHNIQUE

Treatment Volume

"Involved-field irradiation" refers to treatment of only the region(s) of clinical involvement. "Extended-field irradiation" refers to treatment of region(s) of clinical involvement plus elective treatment of contiguous, clinically uninvolved lymph node regions at risk for subclinical disease. "Total nodal irradiation" (TNI) refers to treatment of all nodal and extranodal areas commonly involved in HD, including the mantle, spleen, para-aortic, and pelvic nodal fields; in some clinical settings, the liver and lung may also be treated. "Subtotal nodal irradiation" (STNI) differs from TNI in that the pelvis is not irradiated.

The *mantle* is an irregularly shaped volume that includes the cervical, supraclavicular, infraclavicular, axillary, mediastinal, and hilar lymph nodes. When indicated (because of large mediastinal adenopathy; hilar or subcarinal disease; pleural effusion or involvement; pericardial effusion or involvement), treatment of the whole lung, hemilung, or heart may be incorporated into treatment of the mantle. Opposed anterior and posterior fields are used. The lower border of the mantle is approximately at the bottom of T-10 when there is either minimal or no mediastinal disease. The upper border is at midtragus. Custom blocks made of Lipowitz's metal shield the lung parenchyma, larynx, humeral heads, and portions of the mandible and parotid glands. In patients with middle or upper cervical lymph nodes, the preauricular nodes are treated with separate preauricular fields. In patients with bulky upper neck adenopathy, it may be necessary to treat a *Waldeyer ring* field, which includes not only the preauricular nodes but also the deep upper cervical, occipital, and submental nodes as well as the lymphoid tissue in Waldeyer's ring. The mantle field may be combined with the spleen and para-aortic fields. The advantages of the combined field are a shorter treatment time and better dose distribution in the area of field junction. The disadvantage is increased acute toxicity.

The *spleen* field includes the spleen and the splenic hilar nodes. If the spleen has been removed, the splenic hilar nodes may be treated through a small field if the splenic pedicle is clipped by the surgeon at the time of splenectomy. If there is extensive splenic involvement, consideration is given to elective irradiation of the liver because of the high risk for subclinical involvement.

The *para-aortic* field includes all para-aortic and paracaval lymph nodes between the aortic bifurcation and the bottom of the mantle field. The celiac axis nodes are incidentally covered. The para-aortic volume is treated through opposed anterior and posterior fields, matched (with an appropriate gap) to the mantle fields superiorly, the pelvic fields at the bottom of L-4 inferiorly, and the spleen field laterally. The spleen and para-aortic fields may be treated in a single combined field.

The *pelvic* field includes the femoral nodes and the common, external, and internal iliac nodes. The pelvic volume is treated through opposed anterior and posterior fields. The superior border is at the bottom of L-4, matched, with an appropriate gap, to the bottom of the para-aortic fields. A customized block made of Lipowitz's metal shields the iliac wings and the midline structures not at risk, including the ovaries after transposition at laparotomy or laparoscopy. In male patients, special testicular shielding is required to decrease indirect exposure by radiation scattered from the pelvic field, which could otherwise cause azoospermia. An *inverted Y* field combines the pelvic and para-aortic fields. A *spade* field is similar to the inverted Y but does not include the femoral or pelvic lymphatics below the level of the common iliac nodes.

Time-Dose Factors

The doses used at the University of Florida for treatment of adults with radiotherapy alone are 35 Gy for clinically involved sites and 30 Gy for sites suspected of harboring subclinical disease. The dose for elective treatment of the lung or liver is 10 to 15 Gy. After a complete response to six cycles of chemotherapy, doses are reduced to 30 Gy for previously involved sites and 25 to 30 Gy for sites suspected of harboring subclinical disease. Dose reductions are not typically made after only two or three cycles of chemotherapy or in patients whose response to chemotherapy is poor. In children, after four or more cycles of chemotherapy, the dose to clinically involved sites is 25 Gy. In sites of nodal disease, the dose per fraction is 1.5 to 1.8 Gy. The dose per fraction is limited to 1.5 Gy or less when the entire cardiac silhouette is included in the field. When hemilung or whole lung is treated, the dose per fraction must be limited to 1 Gy per day or less. Thin lung transmission blocks in place during mantle irradiation allow delivery of a lower dose per day to lung parenchyma than the remainder of the treatment volume.

Patients are treated once a day 5 days a week. In the rare patient with rapidly progressive disease, it may be necessary to treat twice a day. Occasionally, the treatment course may be split with a 2-week break to allow tumor shrinkage and field reduction for the high-dose area. This schema of split-course radiotherapy in HD (in contrast to split-course radiotherapy for carcinomas) has no detrimental effect on the probability of disease control.

Sequencing in Combined-Modality Therapy

In combined-modality therapy, chemotherapy is delivered first. Chemotherapy treats all sites of clinical and subclinical disease in nodal and extranodal sites at once, whereas typically only one region may be treated at a time with radiotherapy. In addition, the response to chemotherapy typically results in tumor shrinkage that permits reduction in the radiation field size and consequently less exposure to normal tissue.

TREATMENT RECOMMENDATIONS

Cure is achieved in approximately three quarters of patients treated for HD, and attention must be paid to sequelae of successful treatment. Treatment goals are not only survival and freedom from relapse but also survival without complications of treatment. Treatment alternatives include radiation therapy alone, chemotherapy alone, and a combination of the two modalities. Treatment selection depends on stratification of patients into prognostic groups and consideration of the late sequelae of available treatment options. Patients may be grouped into low-, intermediate-, and high-risk groups on the basis of the Ann Arbor stage and other prognostic factors such as tumor bulk (more than 6 cm or mediastinal mass greater than one third the maximal intrathoracic diameter), number of sites involved (greater than three or four), and presence and extent of splenic disease. Because of the possibility of salvage after first-treatment failure, it is occasionally appropriate to select an initial management approach that results in a lower probability of freedom from relapse but a higher probability of freedom from treatment sequelae. The results achieved with the approach used at the University of Florida are shown in Table 1.

Adults

Low Risk

Patients with stage IA or stage IIA disease with fewer than three or four sites of involvement and no bulky disease are at low risk for treatment failure

TABLE 1. **Hodgkin's Disease Treatment Recommendations and Results at the University of Florida**

Stage	Treatment	10-Year Survival Rates (%)		
		Relapse Free	*Overall*	*Cause Specific*
Low risk				
IA, IIA with small-volume disease and <4 sites involved	STNI or TNI	84	85	95
Intermediate risk				
IB, IIB; IA, IIA with bulky disease or ≥4 sites involved; IIIA	Chemo × 2–3 and STNI	92	85	93
High risk				
IIIB	Chemo × 6 and IF RT*	60	40	43
IVA, B	Chemo × 6 and IF RT*	53	64	64

*Usually STNI or TNI.
Abbreviations: STNI = subtotal nodal irradiation; TNI = total nodal irradiation; chemo = chemotherapy; IF = involved field; RT = radiation therapy.

with radiotherapy alone. If the patient is clinically staged, the radiotherapy volume should be STNI or TNI. The 10-year relapse-free, cause-specific, and absolute survival rates approach 85, 95, and 85%, respectively. If the patient has undergone staging laparotomy and has a lymphocyte-predominant or nodular sclerosis histologic type and a normal erythrocyte sedimentation rate, mantle irradiation alone may be considered. Relapse-free and absolute survival rates approach 75 and 85%, respectively.

Intermediate Risk

Patients with stage IA or stage IIA disease with more than three or four sites of involvement or bulky disease, or those with stage IIIA, stage IB, or stage IIB disease, are at intermediate risk of treatment failure and may be treated with radiotherapy alone or with combined-modality therapy. With radiotherapy alone, the relapse-free and overall survival rates are approximately 50 and 80%, respectively, at 10 years. Two basic combined-modality approaches are commonly used in patients with intermediate-risk disease: two or three cycles of chemotherapy followed by standard irradiation (usually STNI) and four to six cycles of chemotherapy followed by irradiation of involved fields. Our institutional preference is two cycles of chemotherapy followed by radiotherapy, except in the patient with extensive subcarinal involvement that would require more cardiac irradiation. With combined-modality therapy using two or three cycles of chemotherapy, the relapse-free, cause-specific, and overall survival rates are approximately 92, 93, and 85%, respectively.

High Risk

Patients with stage IIIB or stage IV disease are usually treated with combined-modality therapy or chemotherapy alone. If combined-modality therapy is used, the role of radiation may be to treat all areas of clinical involvement, only areas of bulky involvement, or only areas of incomplete response to chemotherapy. The radiation volume and dose vary with the role of radiotherapy in a particular combined-modality approach. There is a low probability of salvage after initial treatment with chemotherapy. Free-

dom from relapse, cause-specific, and absolute survival rates have been 60, 40, and 43%, respectively, for stage IIIB and 53, 64, and 64%, respectively, for stage IV at 10 years.

Children

Because of the musculoskeletal hypoplasia after radiation doses greater than 25 Gy, chemotherapy is used more extensively in children, even in the early stages of disease. When radiation is used in children who have not reached growth potential, doses are generally limited to 25 Gy or less. Children may be treated with chemotherapy alone, but the doses required are six or more cycles, even in early-stage disease; alternatively, they may be treated with combined-modality therapy using low-dose irradiation to involved fields as a means of limiting the chemotherapy dose. In early-stage disease, a common approach is three or four cycles of chemotherapy followed by irradiation with 25 Gy to involved fields. In intermediate and advanced disease, a common approach is four to six cycles of chemotherapy followed by involved-field radiotherapy to 20 to 25 Gy.

POTENTIAL SIDE EFFECTS AND COMPLICATIONS

Acute Side Effects

Acute side effects occur during therapy and are usually resolved within 2 to 3 weeks after treatment. Expected side effects of mantle and Waldeyer's ring irradiation include transient hair loss, xerostomia, and an erythematous skin reaction. Hair loss is particularly noticeable in the occipital region and preauricular regions in all patients and in the beard and anterior chest of men. Partial regrowth is usually observed within 2 to 4 months of treatment. Transient xerostomia occurs in many patients because of incidental parotid irradiation. Recovery of normal salivary function is related to the patient's pretherapy salivary output and age; young patients usually recover full salivary function, and older patients occasionally retain some mild xerostomia. The skin reaction is usually most prominent on the neck and over the shoulders and may be tender or pruritic. Lotions based on petrolatum (Aquaphor), lanolin, vitamin E, or aloe provide symptomatic relief and promote skin healing.

Nausea is frequently associated with splenic and para-aortic irradiation and may be controlled with standard antiemetics such as prochlorperazine maleate (Compazine), promethazine HCl (Phenergan), metoclopramide HCl (Reglan), chlorpromazine HCl (Thorazine), or ondansetron HCl (Zofran).

Bone marrow suppression may occur with TNI or irradiation preceded by chemotherapy. Thrombocytopenia is usually the first and most significant cytopenia resulting from irradiation. Treatment interruption may be required to allow bone marrow recovery. Generally, radiation therapy is withheld until the platelet count is greater than 50,000 per mm^3 and the white blood cell count is greater than 2000 per mm^3.

Subacute Side Effects

Fatigue and loss of energy are common complaints during and after irradiation. Although most patients continue their routine activities during treatment, it may be 4 to 6 months after completion of treatment before the patient is back to a normal baseline energy level.

Within 1 to 4 months after completion of mantle irradiation, some patients experience Lhermitte's syndrome, usually characterized by an electric shock sensation associated with neck flexion; this may last from several weeks up to 9 months and is not associated with late or permanent neurologic sequelae of treatment.

Patients with HD have a propensity to develop herpes zoster. The outbreak usually occurs within 2 years of treatment; later outbreaks may be associated with recurrence of HD. Typically the outbreak is restricted to a single dermatomal distribution and is self-limited. The pain may be excruciating and the pruritus may be unrelenting. The symptoms and course may be ameliorated by acyclovir (Zovirax). Disseminated disease should be treated in the hospital.

Radiation pneumonitis occurs in less than 5% of patients, primarily in patients with extensive mediastinal disease, 2 to 4 months after mantle irradiation. The syndrome is characterized by a dry, hacking cough with an infiltrate confined to the radiation portals on chest radiographs. Symptoms may also include dyspnea, chest tightness, and fever. Occasionally, the radiographic changes may extend outside the radiation portals. Although the condition is usually self-limited, severe cases may be fatal if not managed aggressively and expeditiously. If the patient has a cough without dyspnea, close observation is appropriate. If dyspnea is present, pulmonary function studies are helpful in assessment. If there is significant clinical pulmonary dysfunction or evidence of compromise on pulmonary function testing, patients are treated with prednisone (40 to 100 mg per day). With mild compromise, outpatient treatment is adequate with close surveillance, but if there is significant compromise, patients are hospitalized. It is important to rule out other processes such as *Pneumocystis* pneumonia. In the immunocompromised patient, however, steroid therapy initiation should not be delayed for biopsy. Once steroid therapy is initiated, the treatment is continued until the patient is asymptomatic, and then steroids are tapered slowly, usually over 1 to 2 months.

Acute pericarditis occurs in 1 to 2% of patients (usually those who had extensive mediastinal and pericardial disease) 2 to 6 months after mantle irradiation. Most patients are asymptomatic, and the diagnosis is made from plain chest radiography. The amount of effusion present can be assessed with echocardiography. Symptomatic patients report fatigue, dyspnea, chest pain, and/or chest tightness and may show signs of pericardial friction rub or paradoxical pulse and electrocardiographic changes. Nonsteroidal anti-inflammatory medications such as indomethacin (Indocin) and ibuprofen are usually effective at relieving symptoms. The patient should be observed for increasing pericardial effusion and possible tamponade, in which case emergent pericardiocentesis may be indicated.

Late Complications

Potential late complications include hypothyroidism, sterility, pulmonary fibrosis, cardiac damage, transverse myelitis, nephritis, growth abnormalities, and second malignancies.

Because thyroid dysfunction develops in 25 to 50% of patients, symptoms are routinely assessed, and annual thyroid function tests are obtained in asymptomatic patients. Estrogen replacement is instituted in women if ovarian ablation occurs as a result of radiotherapy or chemotherapy. No effective treatment is known for mediastinal or pulmonary fibrosis, but pericardiectomy can be performed for symptomatic constrictive pericarditis. Hyperbaric oxygen is used but is of limited value in transverse myelitis.

The use of doses greater than 25 Gy in preadolescent children results in hypoplastic development of the irradiated tissues. Musculoskeletal deformities detract from the child's sense of well-being and may contribute to psychosocial dysfunction. The younger the child and the higher the dose of radiation, the more significant the subsequent growth abnormality will be. Common sequelae include a "skinny neck" and shortened interclavicular distance secondary to mantle irradiation, a posterior left abdominal wall deficit from the spleen field, and shortened sitting height secondary to irradiation of the mantle and para-aortic fields.

Survivors of HD have an increased risk of second malignancy. In particular, an increased frequency of leukemia, non-Hodgkin's lymphoma, and breast, lung, and thyroid cancer has been observed. Some of the increased risk is related to the use of alkylating agent chemotherapy, some to radiation therapy, and some to host factors. Although the leukemias usually appear between 2 and 8 years after treatment, the solid malignancies may occur 20 or more years after treatment. In addition, an increased frequency of cardiac disease, particularly coronary artery disease, has been noted in HD survivors. Patients should be advised of the risk of late effects and counseled with respect to other risk factors such as smoking, high blood cholesterol levels, obesity, and stress. Women should be advised to do breast self-examinations and receive routine mammography; surveillance begins at or before the age of 30 years, as many of the breast cancers have been observed in women in their early thirties.

NEW DIRECTIONS

With the high survival rates currently achieved in HD and the variety of effective treatment approaches, attention is focused on reducing the late effects of treatment. As most serious late effects from both chemotherapy and radiation are dose related, combined-modality therapy is being used as a means not only of reducing the risk of relapse associated with single-modality therapy, but also of limiting the doses of each modality. In children, the use of chemotherapy has permitted a lowering of the radiation dose so that little if any hypoplasia is expected. In adults, combined-modality therapy has been used with only two or three cycles of chemotherapy, producing a lower relapse rate than single-modality therapy as well as a lower risk of leukemia, sterility, and cardiac and lung problems than expected with six cycles of chemotherapy.

ACUTE LEUKEMIA IN ADULTS

method of
HANS W. GRÜNWALD, M.D.

Queens Hospital Center
Jamaica, New York
Mount Sinai School of Medicine
New York, New York

The prognosis of acute leukemia in adults is not yet as good as that achieved by newer treatments in children. However, enormous strides have been made in adults in the last few years with intensive induction and postremission combination chemotherapy and with the use of bone marrow transplantation in selected patients. With currently available therapeutic measures, the projected cure rate of acute leukemia (predicted from rate of the freedom from relapse in the first 3 years) is expected to be 30 to 40% of all adults, and in selected subsets of patients with good prognostic features, the cure rate may be as high as 50 to 60%. In addition to more intensive regimens of treatment, the reason for improved results can be ascribed to better supportive care and the increasing use of newer methods for the identification of characteristics of the disease, which better guide therapeutic decisions. Nowadays, it is essential to obtain not only cytochemical markers of the leukemic cells but also their biochemical, immunologic,

and, especially, cytogenetic characteristics. These may frequently be complemented by the investigation of molecular alterations at the DNA level utilizing well-defined probes.

The use of growth factors (colony-stimulating factors) in the management of patients with acute leukemia is still under investigation. On the one hand, they may prove beneficial in enhancing recovery from severe cytopenias induced by cytotoxic chemotherapy. On the other hand, they could stimulate regrowth of the leukemic cells that carry receptors for such growth factors, a feature of greatest concern in the acute myeloid leukemias and less so in the lymphoid leukemias. Major scientific advances that may yield a higher proportion of cures of acute leukemia in the future include the identification of minimal residual disease after completion of intensive postremission therapy using immunologic and/or molecular markers, and the potential for eradication of the residual disease by the use of biologic response modifiers (interleukins, interferons, growth factors, and other cytokines) singly, in combination, or even combined with cytotoxic chemotherapeutic agents, or by the use of monoclonal antibodies either alone or attached to either toxins or radioisotopes. These investigational advances require that as many patients as possible participate in clinical trials. All new patients with acute leukemia should first be evaluated for eligibility for investigational protocols. Any patient can be treated off-protocol who is proved not to be eligible or who refuses to participate. The intensive therapy needed both during remission induction and during postremission consolidation is associated with a high rate of complications and even a significant mortality. Therefore, all patients should be treated in a major medical center capable of providing the needed supportive measures for such critically ill patients.

ACUTE MYELOID LEUKEMIA

Presentation

The clinical manifestations of acute myeloid leukemia (AML) are related mostly to bone marrow failure. The lack of erythropoietic activity, manifested by anemia of varying severity, causes fatigue, palpitations, lightheadedness, and dyspnea on exertion. The lack of megakaryocytic activity, manifested by thrombocytopenia, leads to purpura and mucosal bleeding. The lack of normal myeloid maturation, manifested by granulocytopenia, frequently leads to infections, often of life-threatening nature. Common infections at presentation include pneumonia, perirectal abscesses, sinusitis, and otitis, but fever and bacteremia without a localizing site of infection are also common.

Some patients with hyperleukocytosis (more than 80,000 myeloblasts per mm³) can have mental symptoms, characterized by confusion and even loss of consciousness (cerebral leukostasis), or pulmonary symptoms, characterized by dyspnea and inadequate gas exchange (pulmonary leukostasis). Caution must be used in the interpretation of the results of an arterial blood gas specimen obtained in a patient with high leukocyte counts: the laboratory report may suggest extreme hypoxia in the patient; this pseudohypoxia is due to in vitro oxygen consumption by the white blood cells ("leukocyte oxygen larceny"). This laboratory abnormality can be avoided by adding fluoride to the heparin in the syringe loaded with arterial blood, thus arresting glycolysis. Many patients with high leukocyte counts have been inappropriately intubated and placed on respirators for this reason.

Some patients with the myelomonocytic or monocytic variety of AML may present with severe gingival hyperplasia, marked tendency to gum bleeding, and skin and/or subcutaneous infiltrates.

Patients with the promyelocytic variant of AML commonly present with serious hemorrhagic manifestations and are found to have consumption coagulopathy (disseminated intravascular coagulation [DIC]) due to release of proteolytic (thrombin-like) enzymes into the circulation. These patients require close monitoring, including all of their coagulation parameters. Such patients benefit from the administration of heparin in addition to fresh-frozen plasma and/or cryoprecipitate.

Prognostic Factors

Patients with a history of cytopenias due to marrow dysplasia (myelodysplastic syndrome), of exposure to aromatic hydrocarbons such as benzene, or of treatment with alkylating chemotherapeutic agents (secondary myeloid leukemias) have a low remission induction rate (approximately half the complete remission rate of comparable patients with de novo AML). These remissions, when achieved, are rarely durable. Thus, in younger patients (younger than 40 years) with secondary AML and an HLA-matched sibling donor, early bone marrow transplantation should be considered.

Age is the second important prognostic factor in AML. The complete remission rate and the cure rate are higher in younger patients. In spite of the poorer prognosis of AML in the elderly, complete remission can be achieved even in patients in the eighth and ninth decades of life, and treatment with curative intent should always be offered to the elderly, provided that they understand the risk involved. The risk/benefit ratio must be clearly presented so the patient can make an informed decision concerning treatment.

Certain subsets of patients with AML identified by using the FAB (French-American-British) classification (based on morphology and cytochemical features of the leukemic cells) are associated with a better prognosis (e.g., M4 with marrow eosinophilia, M3 hypergranular promyelocytic). These rare patients can often be better identified from their characteristic cytogenetic abnormality. Therefore, it is better to rely on the karyotype for therapeutic decisions after complete remission has been achieved (postmission therapy). The chromosome analysis (karyotype) is one of the best methods of identifying subsets of patients with AML who have a higher probability of prolonged remissions and cures. Such subsets include those with chromosomal inversions and translocations such as inv 16, t(15;17), and t(8;21). Chromosome analysis is also the best method of identifying subsets of AML patients with a poor prognosis, such as those with trisomy 8, abnormalities or loss of chromosome 5 or 7, abnormalities of chromosome 11q, or multiple translocations or trisomies. These abnormalities predict not only a short remission duration but also refractoriness to standard remission induction chemotherapy. More intensive regimens incorporating high-dose cytarabine may be warranted for such patients.

Finally, immunophenotypic markers can identify patients with poorer prognosis. In patients whose blasts have the CD34 antigen (an antigen of early hematopoietic progenitors) on their surfaces, there is a high probability of refractoriness to conventional induction chemotherapy, warranting trials with a more intensive regimen.

ACUTE LYMPHOBLASTIC LEUKEMIA

Presentation

Most patients with acute lymphoblastic leukemia (ALL) present with manifestations of bone marrow failure: ane-

mia, thrombocytopenia (with the characteristic purpura and mucosal bleeding), and granulocytopenia (with infections of all kinds). In addition, such patients often have bone pain and tenderness, generalized lymphadenopathy, and/or splenomegaly. Fever at presentation can be due to the high leukemic cell turnover but should always be considered to be of infectious origin until exhaustive investigations prove negative.

Prognostic Factors

Age is an extremely important prognostic factor in ALL. Young adults have a cure rate of about 70%, whereas in the elderly, the prognosis of ALL is not much better than that for AML (i.e., 20%).

The initial white blood cell count is a major prognostic factor in ALL. Patients with leukocytosis above 50,000 cells per mm^3 readily achieve a complete remission but usually have an early relapse. Such patients warrant more intensive postremission therapy or bone marrow transplantation.

The morphologic characteristics of the leukemic blasts in peripheral blood and bone marrow smears can identify the Burkitt type (FAB L3) of ALL. Such blasts are characteristically large, with deep blue cytoplasm and cytoplasmic vacuoles. This type of leukemia has a much lower complete remission rate than the L1 and L2 varieties of ALL and warrants the use of different, more intensive therapeutic regimens. The Burkitt type of leukemia can also be identified from the surface immunoglobulin of the blast cells, a characteristic of B cells, and from the characteristic chromosomal translocations—t(8;14) or t(8;22) —involving the c-*myc* oncogene on chromosome 8.

Chromosome analysis in ALL can also yield important prognostic clues. One or more translocations, especially t(4;11) and t(9;22), predict for a high probability of early relapse after a remission has been attained. This justifies more intensive postremission chemotherapy or allogeneic bone marrow transplantation if a suitable donor is available.

INITIAL EVALUATION IN THE PATIENT WITH ACUTE LEUKEMIA

Initial evaluation of the patient begins with a complete history and physical examination. Next is a careful and accurate evaluation of the peripheral blood and bone marrow smears for the morphology and classification of the leukemia. The bone marrow aspirate and biopsy specimen stained with Wright-Giemsa stains yield the exact cytologic type and subtype (AML or ALL and its FAB class) in 80 to 90% of patients. It is also essential to perform a full cytochemical panel on the blood and marrow smears, assay for terminal deoxynucleotidyltransferase, immunophenotyping, and cytogenetic analysis on the bone marrow cells. These analyses serve not only to confirm the morphologic classification but also to identify the prognostic subtypes mentioned previously.

Also part of the initial evaluation of the patient is a careful analysis of the coagulation system, including prothrombin time (PT), activated partial thromboplastin time (APTT), plasma fibrinogen level, and serum fibrin degradation product (FDP) assay. These tests can identify the consumption coagulopathy (DIC) present in most patients with acute promyelocytic leukemia (AML FAB M3) and in some patients with myelomonocytic and monocytic leukemia (FAB M4 and M5).

Renal, hepatic, pulmonary, and, especially, cardiac functions should also be assessed, because most antileukemic drugs are excreted by the kidneys and/or detoxified by the liver and therefore are potentially toxic to these organs. Cardiac dysfunction diagnosed before treatment is begun can prevent the use of anthracyclines, which may lead to potentially fatal cardiac insufficiency in patients with poor cardiac function.

Multiple cultures should be obtained from blood and excreta, and also from various mucosae prone to colonization by bacteria, fungi, and viruses (pharynx, nose, and rhinopharynx). Such cultures should be obtained not only in patients with suspected infection and fever but also in asymptomatic and afebrile patients, to predict the possible microorganism responsible for an infection that occurs later in the patient's course ("surveillance" cultures).

Finally, histocompatibility (HLA) typing should be performed in every new patient, not only to identify potential bone marrow donors among the patient's siblings (or even from the unrelated donor data banks) but also to provide HLA-matched platelet transfusions if and when the disease becomes refractory to unmatched platelet transfusions due to alloimmunization. It is usually not possible to determine HLA type in the patient at the time alloimmunization is detected, because there usually are few or no leukocytes in the peripheral blood to type as a result of the cytotoxic chemotherapy.

TREATMENT

Chemotherapeutic drugs should be started as soon as possible after the diagnosis of AML or ALL is made. There is rarely a need to initiate such treatment as an emergency, and there is usually sufficient time to perform all the aforementioned pretreatment evaluations. Biochemical, hemostatic, or other abnormalities should be corrected before initiation of cytotoxic chemotherapy. Hyperleukocytosis (more than 80,000 blast cells per mm^3), however, constitutes a medical emergency requiring immediate leukapheresis (removal of leukocytes by blood centrifugation at the bedside) and the rapid initiation of the cytotoxic chemotherapy to avoid pulmonary and/or cerebral leukostasis, which may be fatal.

Before chemotherapy, patients with acute leukemia should be hydrated and given allopurinol (Zyloprim), 300 mg per day orally, to avoid the development of hyperuricemia and urate nephropathy. Optimally, the allopurinol should be started 36 hours before the initiation of cytotoxic chemotherapy and continued for a total of 10 days. Thereafter, the risk of urate nephropathy is minimal, and the frequency of cutaneous hypersensitivity to the drug increases.

Venous access for the duration of treatment and the period of severe cytopenias that follows should be ensured before initiation of the treatment. Many patients have adequate peripheral veins to permit administration of all required drugs and blood products. However, some patients eventually develop venous access problems during induction chemotherapy. Therefore, it is common to centrally implant a Silastic catheter (Hickman's or Broviac's) that is exposed to the outside. Alternatively, a port may be attached to the catheter and remain permanently under the skin (requiring a noncoring needle to ac-

cess). Another method of achieving venous access is by means of a peripherally inserted central line (PIC line), which does not require use of operating room facilities for insertion but can remain in place for only 3 to 6 weeks.

Another important issue to address before the initiation of cytotoxic chemotherapy is the control of infections. Appropriate bactericidal antibiotic, antiviral, and/or antifungal agents are used as needed. The use of bacteriostatic antibiotics *must* be avoided, because they are ineffective in a granulocytopenic patient and may antagonize bactericidal antibiotics.

Finally, severe anemia and thrombocytopenia are corrected by packed red blood cell and platelet transfusions, and fresh-frozen plasma and heparin are given to correct the hemostatic abnormalities of the consumption coagulopathy. All blood cell transfusions (red blood cells and platelets) should incorporate a white blood cell–retaining filter to minimize the exposure to allogeneic HLA antigens and thus reduce the risks of eventual platelet refractoriness and presensitization for an eventual bone marrow transplant. For the same reason, family members of a patient who are deemed suitable as allogeneic bone marrow donors should *not* be used as donors for red blood cell or platelet transfusions.

If evidence of a consumption coagulopathy is detected (prolonged PT and APTT, increased FDP, prolonged thrombin time, decreased factors I, II, V, and VIII), prompt heparinization in addition to administration of fresh-frozen plasma and/or cryoprecipitate reduces the incidence of fatal hemorrhage. Heparin should be started with a bolus of 8000 to 10,000 units intravenously, followed by a continuous intravenous infusion of 1000 units per hour during the first 48 hours, which is thereafter reduced to 700 units per hour. The heparin infusion is continued until all evidence of intravascular coagulation activity disappears (normalization of FDP and factors I, II, V, and VIII).

Acute Myeloid Leukemia

The majority of patients with AML of all types (FAB M1 through M7) respond to the standard induction combination chemotherapy of cytarabine (Cytosar) and an anthracycline given in the "7 + 3" regimen. Cytarabine (Cytosar-U) is given as a continuous intravenous infusion of 100 to 200 mg per m^2 per day for 7 days, and daunorubicin (Cerubidine), 45 mg per m^2 per day, as a slow intravenous bolus for the first 3 days. An alternative anthracycline with a therapeutic spectrum similar to that of daunorubicin is idarubicin (Idamycin), given at a dose of 12 mg per m^2 per day as a slow intravenous bolus for 3 days. These doses are given regardless of the initial blood count, because the goal is to achieve temporary marrow aplasia to be followed by normal marrow regeneration (achievement of a complete remission). However, if initial liver function tests demonstrate major impairment (bilirubin level more than 3 mg per dL, alanine aminotransferase [ALT] level more than three times normal), the doses of both drugs should be reduced to half and the cytarabine infusion stopped after 5 days if the liver function tests have not improved by then. Antiemetics such as ondansetron (Zofran), metoclopramide (Reglan), and prochlorperazine (Compazine) may be used liberally.

In patients older than 70 years, the anthracycline dose should be decreased by 33% (30 mg per m² per day for 3 days of daunorubicin or 8 mg per m² per day for 3 days of idarubicin). Patients who have a history of coronary artery disease or heart failure or have a decreased cardiac ejection fraction at multigated angiography can be given mitoxantrone (Novantrone) instead of daunorubicin, because of a lower risk of heart failure. The dose is 12 mg per m² per day, given as a 1-hour intravenous infusion for the first 3 days, and the mitoxantrone is given together with the 7-day cytarabine infusion. A bone marrow examination is performed on the day immediately after the conclusion of the cytarabine infusion, to assess the extent of cytoreduction. If the marrow cellularity on biopsy has not decreased to 20% or less and the proportion of leukemic blasts has not decreased by 80% or more, it is improbable that a complete remission will result. Additional chemotherapy, consisting of 3 days of mitoxantrone, etoposide (VePesid),* or high-dose cytarabine (at dosages discussed later for refractory or recurrent AML), may then be considered, but at the cost of increased toxicity (e.g., mucositis, pancytopenia of greater duration).

An exception to the preceding recommendations is acute promyelocytic leukemia (FAB M3) with the t(15;17) translocation, in which the ability of the leukemic blast cells to differentiate when exposed to retinoids has led to the use of all-trans-retinoic acid (ATRA [Vesanoid]) as the mainstay of remission induction therapy. This has yielded not only an increase in the rate of complete remissions but also a dramatic prolongation of survival and a significant increase in the number of long-term disease-free surviving patients (projected to exceed 60%). The treatment with ATRA is given orally, 45 mg per m² per day (divided in 2 doses), until a complete remission is achieved; if, during treatment with ATRA, the white blood cell count starts to rise over 10,000 per mm³, or if a remission is not attained within 90 days of ATRA treatment, it is advisable to add standard 7 + 3 treatment with cytarabine and daunorubicin (or idarubicin) as described previously for myeloblastic leukemia. A not uncommon complication of ATRA administration is the development of the "retinoic acid syndrome," consisting of dyspnea, fluid retention, pleural and/or pericardial effusions, and occasionally even pulmonary edema. The retinoic acid syndrome usually improves with the administration of corticosteroids. Dexamethasone (10 mg orally twice daily for 3 to 5 days) should be initiated as soon as the first symptoms of the syndrome appear.

Daily blood count monitoring during and after induction chemotherapy is essential as a measure of the cytoreduction induced. Close platelet count monitoring guides the administration of platelet transfusions. Hemoglobin levels influence the administration of packed red blood cell transfusions. Frequent monitoring of serum electrolyte levels is needed to detect the occurrence (fortunately rare) of a tumor lysis syndrome.

A second postinduction bone marrow aspiration and biopsy should be performed 1 week after completion of the course of chemotherapy, to help the decision regarding the need for a second course. If the proportion of leukemic blasts in the aspirate remains above 5% and the cellularity on biopsy is more than 10%, a second course of the same drugs used initially should be given. However, the duration of the second chemotherapy course should be shorter, with a 5-day infusion of cytarabine and 2 daily doses of the anthracycline at the same daily doses given for the first course (5 + 2). If the bone marrow shows a cellularity of less than 10% but the majority of cells are blasts, it is advisable to wait 3 to 5 days and repeat the bone marrow aspiration and biopsy, because it is virtually impossible to differentiate between residual leukemia and very early marrow regeneration. A subsequent marrow aspiration can reveal further lineage differentiation (appearance of promyelocytes, myelocytes, and even metamyelocytes) if it is early regeneration. A persistently leukemic marrow shows a further increase in blasts. If, after a second course of cytarabine plus anthracycline (5 + 2) the marrow remains leukemic, one has to characterize the patient as refractory to the induction chemotherapy.

Refractory or Relapsed AML

Patients whose disease is refractory to induction chemotherapy or relapses after a complete remission is attained require more intensive induction chemotherapy, usually the high-dose cytarabine (HIDAC) regimen consisting of 1 to 3 grams of cytarabine per m² every 12 hours for 6 days (a total of 12 doses) given as 75-minute infusions. Because cytarabine at these high doses concentrates in tears and can cause keratitis, it is important to wash the eyes with saline or artificial tears at least six times per day. Patients must also be closely monitored for cerebellar toxicity involving coordination and speech. The drug must be discontinued at the first sign of ataxia or slurred speech. Less common toxicities of high-dose cytarabine include hemorrhagic enterocolitis and noncardiac pulmonary edema (adult respiratory distress syndrome).

After completion of the 6 days of cytarabine infusions, bone marrow aspiration and biopsy are performed: if the marrow still shows more than 20% leukemic blasts, it is advisable to give 3 days of mitoxantrone, 12 mg per m² per day as a 1-hour infusion.

An alternative regimen for refractory or relapsed AML is the use of mitoxantrone and etoposide; etoposide is given as a 5-day continuous infusion of 150 mg per m² per day, and mitoxantrone is given as a 1-hour infusion of 12 mg per m² per day for the first 3

---

*Not FDA approved for this indication.

days. If, after completion of this 5-day regimen, the marrow shows reduction but not disappearance of the leukemic blasts, a second 5-day course of these two drugs can be administered. These drugs require hepatic function for detoxification and thus should not be used if the patient has abnormal liver function tests (ALT value more than three times normal, bilirubin value more than 3 mg per dL).

Postremission Consolidation

Once complete remission has been achieved (normal bone marrow and reticulocyte, platelet, and granulocyte counts), and the patient is deemed free of infections and aftereffects of the induction chemotherapy (attainment of a near-normal performance status), postremission therapy is planned. A significant advance has been the attainment in some patients of long relapse-free survival (and thus possible cure of the leukemia) by the institution of intensive postremission consolidation chemotherapy. The intensity of treatment is similar to or greater than that used for remission induction. Such treatment, however, may produce life-threatening toxicities. Most patients can be treated on an ambulatory basis (provided that they live at a reasonable distance from the hospital). The regular need for platelet transfusions requires an ambulatory transfusion center. Furthermore, because most patients remain markedly neutropenic for periods ranging from 10 to 30 days after each consolidation course, they are advised to avoid external sources of infection (e.g., crowds, animals, vases with stagnant water) and to come to the hospital for prompt initiation of antibiotic therapy at the first evidence of fever or infection. Complete blood counts to monitor hemoglobin level and leukocyte and platelet counts are performed every other day (until recovery of adequate granulocyte and platelet counts), and blood biochemical monitoring is done weekly.

Drugs used for consolidation are the same as those used in induction, and at doses similar to or higher than those used for induction. Thus, a first consolidation course may consist of cytarabine and an anthracycline used in the 7 + 3 induction regimen. The patient should also receive at least one course of the high-dose cytarabine regimen. A third consolidation course might consist of the combination of etoposide and mitoxantrone (as described for refractory or relapsed AML). The total number of consolidation courses ranges between three and six, depending on the patient's tolerance to the drugs, the rate of recovery from each course of consolidation (if the hematologic depression from a course is longer than 3 weeks, the probability for prolonged or even irreversible cytopenias after an ensuing course increases), and the initial prognostic category (patients with high relapse risk should receive the highest possible number of consolidation courses).

Patients at extremely high risk for early relapse (high initial white blood cell count or other sign of high leukemic burden such as a very high lactate dehydrogenase value, trisomy 8, and abnormalities

of chromosome 5 or 7) should be considered for bone marrow transplantation if they attain a complete remission. Young patients (younger than 45 years) with an HLA-matched sibling should receive an allogeneic transplant from that sibling. For patients between 45 and 60 years of age or for patients without an appropriately matched sibling, autologous marrow transplantation should be considered. This procedure involves harvesting bone marrow shortly before a planned consolidation chemotherapy course. The marrow is subjected to in vitro purging (using either drugs or antibodies with complement) and is frozen. Peripheral blood stem cell harvesting may also be done when the white blood cell count is increasing after a course of chemotherapy. In this case, the patient is subjected to repeated blood cell pheresis. Thereafter, the patient is given the preparative regimen of high-dose cyclophosphamide plus total body irradiation (or busulfan) followed by infusion of the thawed marrow (and peripheral blood, if available) cells.

Acute Lymphoblastic Leukemia

The majority of patients with ALL achieve a remission after vincristine and prednisone therapy. Significant increases in both remission rate and duration can be attained by the addition of anthracyclines, L-asparaginase, and alkylating agents. The currently recommended remission induction regimen for adults with ALL consists of the following drugs: cyclophosphamide (Cytoxan), 1 gram per m^2 by slow intravenous injection, once; vincristine (Oncovin), 2 mg by slow intravenous injection weekly for 4 doses; prednisone, 100 mg per day orally for 21 days (no need to taper); daunorubicin (Cerubidine), 45 mg per m^2 per day by slow intravenous injection for 3 days; and L-asparaginase (Elspar), 6000 units per m^2 intramuscularly (subcutaneously if the platelet count is below 50,000 per mm^3) every 4 days for 6 doses. For patients older than 65 years, the cyclophosphamide dose is reduced to 700 mg per m^2, the daunorubicin dose to 30 mg per m^2, and the duration of prednisone administration to 10 days. The administration of filgrastim (Neupogen), a granulopoiesis stimulant, at the dose of 5 μg per kg of body weight, may be initiated on day 5 and continued until a granulocyte count of 10,000 per mm^3 is attained. Blood counts are performed daily to monitor cytoreduction and to evaluate the need for red blood cell and platelet transfusions. Bone marrow aspiration and biopsy are performed 4 weeks after the start of chemotherapy. If the leukemic blasts have not disappeared, an alternative induction regimen with teniposide, cytarabine, and prednisone should be initiated. If the marrow on day 28 shows disappearance of the leukemic blasts but is not yet normal, an additional 7 to 10 days without chemotherapy may lead to the signs of remission (normalization of marrow and of reticulocyte, granulocyte, and platelet counts).

Once remission has been documented, central nervous system prophylaxis is given with 15 mg of intrathecal methotrexate (with care taken to use preservative-free drug) every week for 4 weeks combined with cranial radiation (24 Gy). During this 4-week period, the patient is also given 6-mercaptopurine (6-MP) (Purinethol), 60 mg per m^2 daily by mouth, and methotrexate, 20 mg per m^2 weekly by mouth. Blood counts are obtained at least twice weekly, and the dosages of 6-MP and methotrexate are reduced if cytopenias occur. Liver function tests should also be closely monitored, and the dosage of both drugs reduced if abnormalities occur.

After completion of the central nervous system prophylaxis, and only if and when the blood counts and blood chemistry parameters are normal, an intensive 2-month consolidation chemotherapy is initiated as follows: cyclophosphamide, 1 gram per m^2 intravenously during weeks 1 and 5; cytarabine, 75 mg per m^2 per day subcutaneously for 4 days during weeks 1, 2, 5, and 6; 6-MP, 60 mg per m^2 per day orally during weeks 1, 2, 5, and 6; vincristine, 2 mg intravenously per week during weeks 3, 4, 7, and 8; and L-asparaginase, 6000 units intramuscularly (subcutaneously if the platelet count is below 50,000 per mm^3) twice weekly during weeks 3, 4, 7, and 8. Patients usually require frequent platelet and occasional red blood cell transfusions during this period of consolidation, but the treatment can be accomplished on an ambulatory basis if an ambulatory transfusion and chemotherapy unit is available. If, at the start of week 5, there is persistent thrombocytopenia (less than 50,000 cells per mm^3) and/or neutropenia (less than 1000 cells per mm^3), the scheduled chemotherapy should be postponed for 1 week.

After completion of this intensive consolidation chemotherapy, repeated bone marrow aspiration and biopsy are performed to confirm continued remission. Then the 2-year maintenance phase is initiated, consisting of 6-MP, 60 mg per m^2 by mouth daily; methotrexate, 20 mg per m^2 by mouth weekly; vincristine, 2 mg intravenously monthly; and prednisone, 80 mg per day for 5 days every month (starting on the day of vincristine administration). Blood counts are performed weekly, and blood chemistry evaluations biweekly. If significant cytopenias or liver disfunction occurs, the maintenance chemotherapy doses are reduced or the chemotherapy is temporarily withheld until acceptable values are achieved.

Patients with prognostic indicators for early relapse, such as initial white blood cell count of 50,000 per mm^3 or higher, or t(9;22) or t(4;11) translocations, may be considered for allogeneic bone marrow transplantation after achieving a remission, if an HLA-compatible sibling is available.

Patients with B cell ALL (Burkitt type, FAB L3) may be treated with a more intensive, shorter, more aggressive lymphoma-like induction chemotherapy followed by central nervous system prophylaxis, without a prolonged maintenance phase. The regimen includes the use of high doses of cyclophosphamide and methotrexate (with leucovorin reversal) plus vincristine, dexamethasone, cytarabine, etoposide, and doxorubicin.

Supportive Care

In addition to the proper chemotherapeutic agents, all other aspects of the patient's care must be optimal. The major reason for failure to achieve complete remission is the death of the patient due to complications of the disease and/or the chemotherapy. Primary resistance to chemotherapy is uncommon.

A most important clinical consideration is the assurance of adequate hemostasis; thrombocytopenia either associated with acute leukemia or resulting from the use of cytotoxic drugs is the most common cause of hemorrhage. Platelet transfusions have markedly reduced morbidity and mortality from bleeding. Platelets should be given whenever the platelet count is 20,000 per mm^3 or less, although hemorrhage can occur even with higher levels. Some patients may have very low platelet counts (less than 10,000 per mm^3) without bleeding. In patients who require an invasive intervention (e.g., insertion of a Hickman catheter, performance of a spinal tap), the platelet count should be increased to 50,000 per mm^3 with platelet transfusions. The presence of signs of consumption coagulopathy (DIC), that is, prolonged PT and APTT, elevated FDP, and/or decreased fibrinogen in addition to thrombocytopenia, mandates the administration not only of platelet transfusions (to bring the platelet count above 30,000 per mm^3) but also of fresh-frozen plasma and/or cryoprecipitate to restore the hemostatic function to normal. In addition, heparin given to such patients (as described previously) has proved helpful in this situation. Finally, prolongation of PT and/or APTT well into the course of treatment may occur in some patients, probably as a consequence of vitamin K deficiency. The deficiency may be due to poor oral food intake and to prolonged antibiotic therapy, which alters the intestinal flora. Hemostatic function must thus be monitored, and supplementary vitamin K given as needed.

After a few weeks of treatment, some patients become totally refractory to platelet transfusions, as shown by a lack of increase in platelet count 1 hour after completion of the transfusion. This situation is usually due to HLA alloimmunization and can be overcome if one obtains HLA-matched platelets for transfusion. The use of filters that remove white blood cells from all transfused blood products (red blood cells and platelets) from the start of therapy reduces (but does not eliminate) the incidence of HLA alloimmunization. This benefit not only decreases the incidence of platelet refractoriness but also reduces the risk of an eventual graft rejection after bone marrow transplantation.

The main cause of morbidity and mortality in patients with acute leukemia is infection, both during induction chemotherapy and later during the intensive consolidation phases of treatment. Prophylactic antibacterial therapy with a quinolone such as ciprofloxacin (Cipro) or with trimethoprim-sulfamethoxazole (Bactrim) and/or antifungal prophylaxis with fluconazole (Diflucan) have not yet been proved to decrease the risk of such infections. However, it is advisable to initiate such therapy as soon as the granulocyte count is less than 500 per mm³, in spite of the risk of the development of an infection resistant to these drugs.

Fever in the neutropenic patient requires prompt and intensive attention: specimens for culture for bacteria, fungi, and viruses should be obtained from all potential sites of infections. Immediately thereafter, treatment with broad-spectrum bactericidal antibiotics, for example, a semisynthetic penicillin such as piperacillin (Pipracil) and an aminoglycoside such as gentamicin (Garamycin), should be initiated. For the possible cutaneous entry of hospital bacteria such as methicillin-resistant *Staphylococcus aureus*, or for catheter colonization by *Corynebacterium* of the JK subtype, the addition of vancomycin (Vancocin) is recommended. If the patient remains febrile after 72 hours of such triple-antibiotic therapy, antifungal therapy with amphotericin B (Fungizone) should be started on an empirical basis. Therapy of infections is guided and modified by results of cultures obtained before the initiation of the antibiotic therapy.

Viral infections, although uncommon, must also be addressed. Serologic tests for herpes simplex virus and cytomegalovirus should be done before the start of induction chemotherapy. Changes are then monitored during febrile episodes if mucosal lesions suggesting herpes simplex appear. Treatment with intravenous acyclovir (Zovirax) may be highly effective. Cytomegalovirus can cause interstitial pneumonia as well as esophagitis, enterocolitis, and hepatitis, all of which can be treated with ganciclovir (Cytovene).

Psychosocial Aspects

Great caution has to be used in addressing the patient with acute leukemia and his or her family. They are not prepared for the major alterations in lifestyle that the disease and its treatment will cause. In addition to calm counseling and explanation of all planned phases of treatment, it is important to reinforce these concepts repeatedly. An excellent source of information for both patient and family is a patient with a similar diagnosis who has already undergone a treatment similar to the one planned and who can discuss the information in terms easily understood by lay people.

Once the induction chemotherapy has led to a complete remission and the patient has returned home, the availability of a group of patients with successfully treated hematologic neoplasms (such as Candlelighters) has proved valuable in helping the patient make the adjustments required by the disease and its therapy more tolerable. These groups are led by a trained professional and offer the wherewithal for physical and psychologic adjustment. The availability of a social worker and a psychiatrist with oncologic orientation as team members helps greatly in care of patients.

ACUTE LEUKEMIA IN CHILDREN

method of
BRUCE M. CAMITTA, M.D.
*Midwest Children's Cancer Center, Medical
  College of Wisconsin
Milwaukee, Wisconsin*

Leukemias, accounting for 30% of all diagnoses, are the most common type of cancer in children. One child in 3000 will develop leukemia before age 15 years. Most of these are "acute" leukemias: 80% acute lymphocytic leukemia (ALL) and 15% acute nonlymphocytic leukemia (ANLL). Chronic myelogenous leukemia represents only 2 to 5% of childhood leukemias, and well-documented cases of chronic lymphocytic leukemia are almost nonexistent.

There is increasing evidence that numerical or structural chromosome changes play an important role in leukemogenesis. These abnormalities cause a gain or loss of cellular functions, including, in most cases, a decreased ability of the cell to mature. The net result is an accumulation of immature blood cells in the bone marrow, blood, and other organs. The chromosome changes that cause leukemia are usually acquired. However, patients with Down syndrome and inherited diseases associated with abnormal chromosome fragility (e.g., ataxia telangiectasia, Bloom's syndrome, Fanconi's anemia) have high risks of developing leukemia.

There are many effective therapy protocols for childhood leukemias. However, treatment of these diseases involves more than simply following a recipe. Outcomes for children with leukemia are optimal when care is coordinated by an oncologist with specific expertise in treating children, in a setting where subspecialty consultation is readily available. In addition, enrollment of patients into cooperative trials facilitates the development of more effective, less toxic treatments.

DIAGNOSIS

Work-up for a child with suspected leukemia has two components: (1) determining the presence and type of leukemia and (2) assessing the functional status of organ systems before the start of therapy. The studies listed in Table 1 should be considered a minimum. Other tests may be indicated by the patient's clinical condition or by results of the initial studies.

CLASSIFICATION

The acute leukemias can be divided into subcategories on the basis of clinical and laboratory findings. This classification allows treatment trials to evaluate relatively homogeneous groups of patients. It also permits tailoring of the intensity of treatment to pharmacologic characteristics or to the risk of relapse. Finally, accurate classification enables investigators to compare outcomes between trials.

ALLs are divided into broad classes according to their cell surface and cytoplasmic antigens (immunophenotype). Cell types are B precursor–early pre-B (64% of cases), pre-B (20%), transitional pre-B (1%), B cell (1%), T cell (13%), and other (1%). B precursor ALL may be further subcategorized by the criteria listed in Table 2. Most infants have B precursor ALL but are considered separately because of their poor prognosis and their need for distinct treatment.

ANLLs are initially classified according to morphologic characteristics (Table 3). Chromosome data provide addi-

TABLE 1. **Initial Diagnostic Studies for Leukemia in Children**

History and physical examination
Complete blood count with differential
Examination of the peripheral smear
Blood chemistries: electrolytes, calcium, phosphorus, uric acid, BUN, creatinine, ALT, bilirubin
Coagulation studies: PT, PTT, fibrinogen
Quantitative immunoglobulins
Titers for cytomegalovirus and varicella
Chest radiograph
Assessment of urinary output
Bone marrow aspirate: morphology, cytochemistry, chromosomes, DNA index,* cell surface markers and cryopreservation (for future studies)
Lumbar puncture: glucose, protein, cell count, and cytocentrifuge differential

*DNA index (DI) = DNA content in leukemic cell/DNA content in normal cell.
Abbreviations: ALT = alanine aminotransferase; BUN = blood urea nitrogen; PT = prothrombin time; PTT = partial thromboplastin time.

tional prognostic information. Cell surface marker analyses have not been as useful as in ALL.

SUPPORTIVE CARE

Transfusion

Transfusions of packed red blood cells and platelets should be based on the complete clinical status rather than on fixed cutoff points. Because many children with acute leukemia may eventually require bone marrow transplantation, cytomegalovirus-negative blood products should be used if the patient's cytomegalovirus titer is negative or unknown.

Anemia is well tolerated by children in the absence of other clinical stresses. Indications for packed red blood cells include symptomatic anemia, ongoing

TABLE 2. **Risk Group Classification of B Precursor Acute Lymphocytic Leukemia**

Consensus Risk Definitions
Standard: WBC <50,000/mm³ *and* age 1.00–9.99 y
High: WBC ≥50,000/mm³ *or* age ≥10 y

Modifying Prognostic Factors*

Better Risk	Factor	Worse Risk
Female	Gender	Male
>1.16	DNA index	≤1.16
Hyperdiploid	Chromosomes	Hypodiploid
Trisomy 4 *and* 10		Translocation (9;22)
Translocation (12;21)		MLL gene (11q23) disruption
No blasts	CSF status	Blasts present
Present	CALLA	Absent
Rapid	Treatment response†	Slow or absent

*Most of these (except CNS status) do not apply to T cell or B cell ALL. T cell ALL and B cell ALL used to be considered poor risk, but with modern therapy, this is no longer so.
†Measured by peripheral blood status at day 7 or bone marrow at day 8 or 15.
Abbreviations: CALLA = common acute lymphocytic leukemia antigen; CNS = central nervous system; CSF = cerebrospinal fluid; MLL = Motatedin lymphocytic leukemia; WBC = white blood cell count.

TABLE 3. **Classification of Acute Nonlymphocytic Leukemias**

Morphologic

M1	Myelocytic–no differentiation
M2	Myelocytic—with differentiation
M3	Promyelocytic
M4	Myelomonocytic
M5	Monocytic
M6	Erythroleukemia
M7	Megakaryocytic

Modifying Prognostic Factors

Better Risk	Factor	Worse Risk
Lower	White blood cell count	Higher
Translocation (8;21) Translocation (15;17)* Inversion 16	Chromosomes	Deletion of 5 or 7
Down syndrome	Other	Secondary leukemia† Prior myelodysplasia

*Seen exclusively in M3 (promyelocytic) leukemia.
†Leukemia caused by chemotherapy for prior malignancy.

hemorrhage, a need for increased oxygen-carrying capacity, and exchange transfusion. A packed red blood cell transfusion of 10 mL per kg raises the hemoglobin value by 2.4 grams per dL.

In the absence of other problems, platelet counts may be allowed to fall to 5000 per mm³. If fever, bleeding, or a coagulopathy is present, platelet counts should be kept above 20,000 per mm³. A dose of one platelet unit per 6 to 10 kg raises the platelet count by 50,000 per mm³.

Hyperleukocytosis

Leukostasis (increased blood viscosity and intravascular clumping of leukemic blasts) may occur when the white blood cell count is greater than 150,000 per mm³, especially when this cell count is rapidly rising. The risk is greater in ANLL than in ALL. Lung involvement results in tachypnea and hypoxemia. Central nervous system (CNS) involvement may cause mental status changes, visual abnormalities, and stroke. Infarction in other organs is less common. Exchange transfusion or leukapheresis rapidly lowers the white blood cell count. Prompt initiation of chemotherapy is also important.

Tumor Lysis Syndrome

Rapid lysis of leukemic cells during the first several days of treatment may cause tumor lysis syndrome, which consists of hyperkalemia, hyperphosphatemia, hyperuricemia, and disseminated intravascular coagulation. Secondary hypocalcemia and renal failure may also occur. The risk of tumor lysis syndrome is greatest in patients with a high tumor burden (massive organomegaly, high white blood cell count). Intravenous fluids *without potassium* should be given at two to three times the calculated maintenance rate. Electrolytes, calcium, phosphorus, creatinine, and uric acid levels should be followed closely. Urine alkalinization (with intravenous bicarbonate) and allopurinol (Zyloprim), 10 mg per kg per 24 hours divided three times daily, are also helpful for control of uric acid levels. Enzymatic lysis of uric acid is currently being investigated.

Fever and Infection

Fever is present at diagnosis in 50% of children with acute leukemias. A specific source is found in only half of these individuals. In the absence of a known cause of infection, empirical broad-spectrum antibiotic coverage should be given until cultures are negative and the patient has defervesced. Documented infections should be treated with specific antibiotics.

Infection is common during treatment of acute leukemias, especially in patients with neutrophil counts less than 500 per mm^3 and in patients with central venous access lines regardless of the white blood cell count. Febrile neutropenic patients and patients with central venous lines should receive empirical broad-spectrum antibiotic therapy after appropriate cultures have been obtained. The choice of antibiotics depends on the patient's clinical status, suspected sites of infection, and local antibiotic susceptibility patterns. Antibiotics should be continued until the patient is afebrile, with negative cultures and with evidence of returning marrow function (absolute phagocyte count greater than 200 per mm^3 and rising). Antibiotic choices should be adjusted as indicated for positive cultures.

Patients receiving intensive chemotherapy are at increased risk for developing *Pneumocystis carinii* pneumonia. Co-trimoxazole (Bactrim, Septra) prophylaxis, 25 to 30 mg per kg per day of the sulfa component (divided twice daily) on 3 consecutive days each week, markedly decreases this risk. Some centers recommend prophylactic fluconazole (Diflucan), 5 mg per kg per day, for patients expected to have periods of marked and prolonged neutropenia.

Venous Access

Modern treatment regimens require repeated venous access for testing, chemotherapy, and treatment of complications. Implantable venous access devices decrease the trauma associated with frequent venipunctures. We routinely implant an external (Hickman's or Broviac's catheter) or subcutaneous (Port-A-Cath) central access device at the time of initial diagnosis. In the absence of complications, this line remains in place at least until the end of the intensive phase of chemotherapy.

TREATMENT
Acute Lymphocytic Leukemia

The treatment strategy listed in Table 4 is "risk adapted": the intensity of chemotherapy is directly proportional to the risk of relapse. Thus, chemotherapy regimens with the greatest potential for both acute and long-term toxicities are reserved for those patients with the highest risk of relapse. With this strategy, long-term event-free survival rates according to ALL class are B precursor, low risk, 95%; B precursor, standard risk, 80 to 85%; B precursor, higher risk, 65%; infants, 50 to 60%; T cell, 75%; and B cell, 80%.

Induction Therapy

More than 95% of children enter complete remission using the strategies listed in Table 4. Patients who do not enter remission with these regimens may respond to teniposide (VM-26, Vumon) plus cytosine arabinoside (Cytosar-U) or to etoposide (VP-16, VePesid)* plus 2-chlorodeoxyadenosine (Leustatin).* Even if remission is achieved, initially nonresponding patients are at extremely high risk for eventual relapse and should be considered for early bone marrow transplantation or other intensified treatment.

Intensive Therapy

The goal of the intensive phase of therapy is to rapidly eliminate as many residual leukemic cells as possible. This decreases the chance that one or more leukemic cells will mutate to resistance or that these cells might enter an area of the body relatively inaccessible to chemotherapy (a pharmacologic "sanctuary"). In addition, the use of intensive drug doses may effectively treat cells that are already relatively resistant or that have entered pharmacologic sanctuaries. An intensive phase appears to be an important component of treatment for all risk groups of children with ALL.

Continuation Therapy

Continuation therapy, less intense than previously discussed phases of treatment, is used to eliminate small numbers of residual leukemic cells. When cure was rare, treatment duration was often indefinite. As long-term event-free survival improved, randomized studies showed that 2.5 to 3 years of treatment after attainment of remission was adequate for patients with B precursor and T cell ALL. Patients with B cell ALL require only 4 to 6 months of total chemotherapy (no continuation phase). The optimal treatment duration for infants is not certain.

Central Nervous System Protection

In the absence of specific therapy directed at the CNS, meningeal leukemia developed in 70% of children with ALL. A combination of cranial irradiation plus intrathecal methotrexate or the use of craniospinal irradiation alone was found to decrease the incidence of CNS leukemia to 3 to 8%. However, significant long-term morbidity was associated with irradiation (especially in children younger than 6 years). There is now general agreement that CNS leukemia can be prevented with intrathecal medica-

---

*Not FDA approved for this indication.

TABLE 4. **Treatment Strategy for Acute Lymphocytic Leukemias***

Risk Group	Treatment Phase			
	Induction	*Intensive*	*Continuation*	*CNS Protection*
B precursor	PRED	IDMTX (6)	MTX	IT MTX
Low risk‡	VCR		MP	
	ASP		VCR + PRED	
Standard risk	PRED	IDMTX (12)	MTX	IT MTX
	VCR		MP	
	ASP			
Higher risk	PRED	IDMTX + IDMP (6)	MTX	IT MTX + AraC + HDC
	VCR	VM-26 + AraC (3)	MP	
	ASP	DAUNO + AraC + PRED + VCR + ASP (3)		
	DAUNO			
Infants	DEX	HDMTX (4)	VCR + DEX;	IT MTX + AraC + HDC
	VCR	CYCLO + VP-16 (2)	MTX + MP;	
	ASP	Repeat induction (1)	CYCLO + VP-16	
	DAUNO			
	CYCLO			
T cell	PRED	CYCLO + AraC + MP;	MTX	IT MTX + Cranial XRT
	VCR	VCR, DEX, ASP	MP	
	ASP	DOXO, CYCLO	VCR + PRED	
	DAUNO	AraC, TG		
B cell	CYCLO	CYCLO, VCR, IDMTX, HDAraC (2); DOXO (2)	None	IT MTX + AraC
	DOXO			
	VCR			
	IDMTX			
	HDAraC			

*Recommendations are based on the following protocols: B precursor, low risk, Pediatric Oncology Group (POG) 9201; B precursor, standard risk, POG 9005; B precursor, higher risk, POG 9006; infants, POG 9407; T cell, Children's Cancer Group (CCG) 106 and 123; B cell, POG 9317.

†Numbers in parentheses indicate number of cases.

‡Low-risk definition: standard risk (by age and white blood cell count) *plus* trisomies of both chromosomes 4 and 10 (or, if chromosomes not available, DNA index >1.16).

Abbreviations: AraC = cytosine arabinoside (Cytosar-U); ASP = asparaginase (Elspar); CYCLO = cyclophosphamide (Cytoxan); DAUNO = daunorubicin (Cerubidine); DEX = dexamethasone (Decadron); DOX = doxorubicin (Adriamycin); HDAraC = high-dose cytosine arabinoside; HCD = hydrocortisone (Solu-Cortef); HDMTX = high-dose methotrexate (Methotrexate); IDMP = intermediate-dose mercaptopurine (Purinethol); IDMTX = intermediate-dose methotrexate (Methotrexate), IT = intrathecal; MP = mercaptopurine (Purinethol); MTX = methotrexate (Methotrexate); PRED = prednisone (Deltasone); TG = thioguanine (6-TG); VCR = vincristine; VM-26 = teniposide (Vumon); VP-16 = etoposide (VePesid); XRT = irradiation.

tion alone in most children. It should be noted, however, that some treatment centers still utilize 1800 cGy of cranial irradiation as part of the CNS protection strategy for children with higher risk B precursor and T cell ALL.

Treatment of Relapse

BONE MARROW RELAPSE

Patients who have relapse in the bone marrow during or within 6 months of completing treatment do poorly. With chemotherapy alone, only 80% achieve a second remission, and long-term event-free survival for such patients is less than 10%. These individuals should be treated with an allogeneic bone marrow transplant shortly after achieving a second remission (or the best marrow status possible). Event-free survivals of 30 to 60% have been reported for patients with second-remission bone marrow transplants using an allogeneic (related or unrelated) donor in this "early relapse" group.

Patients who have bone marrow relapse more than 6 months after completing chemotherapy have a better outcome with chemotherapy: at least 90% achieve a second remission, and 35% may be cured. About 50% of these patients may be cured by an allogeneic bone marrow transplant in second remission. However, decision analysis suggests that the use of che-

motherapy alone followed by bone marrow transplantation in third remission (for those who have relapse) results in long-term survival equivalent to that for marrow transplantation in second remission. Both options should be explained to families.

CNS RELAPSE

Treatment of isolated CNS relapse should comprise (1) reinduction followed by intensive chemotherapy with agents that have good penetration into the cerebrospinal fluid and (2) intrathecal medications until the cerebrospinal fluid has cleared, followed by cranial irradiation plus intrathecal medication or craniospinal irradiation alone. Because irradiation (especially craniospinal) may depress bone marrow function, it should be delayed for at least 6 months to permit full-dose chemotherapy during that time. Event-free survival using this approach depends on the time of CNS relapse: it is 80% if relapse occurs at least 18.0 months after initial remission, but 45% if relapse occurs less than 18 months after initial remission.

TESTICULAR RELAPSE

Since the introduction of more intensive chemotherapy, the incidence of testicular relapse has fallen from 20% to less than 5%. There is a high frequency

TABLE 5. **Treatment Strategy for Acute Nonlymphocytic Leukemias**

Subtypes	Induction	Consolidation	CNS Protection
M1, M2, M4–M7*	DAUNO AraC VP-16 TG DEX (days 0, 10, 42, 52)	HDAraC + ASP AraC + TG + VCR + CYCLO + AZA (2)†; AraC + DAUNO + VP-16 + TG + DEX	IT AraC
M3‡	Retinoic acid	DAUNO + AraC; DAUNO + HDAraC ± retinoic acid	None

*Based on Children's Cancer Group protocol 2891.
†(2) = number of cycles.
‡Based on European APL (acute promyelocytic leukemia) 91 protocol.
Abbreviations: AZA = azacitidine; see Table 4 for others.

of bilateral disease even when only one testicle is enlarged clinically. Optimal treatment includes intensified chemotherapy and bilateral testicular irradiation (2400 cGy). Once again, event-free survival depends on the time of relapse: it is 65% for overt relapse that occurs after treatment has stopped and for occult disease detected at the time treatment is stopped, but 35% for overt relapse that occurs during treatment.

Acute Nonlymphocytic Leukemia

Patients with ANLL should receive an induction phase of treatment followed by intensive consolidation. There is little evidence that a period of less intensive continuation treatment is necessary. Except for promyelocytic leukemia (M3), all other morphologic subtypes may be treated similarly (Table 5). With this strategy, long-term event-free survival rates are for M3, 70 to 80%; for all others, 40 to 60%.

Induction Therapy

Eighty to 85% of children achieve remission with one or two courses of chemotherapy. Increasing the doses of induction drugs does not raise the percentage of patients who enter remission but may reduce the risk of later relapse. Data suggest that giving the second course of chemotherapy at a fixed time is superior to waiting for evidence of bone marrow recovery or persistent leukemia before giving the second course of treatment. Regardless of the induction strategy, patients with ANLL usually have prolonged bone marrow aplasia, requiring antibiotics and transfusion support. Half of induction failures are due to resistant disease; the other half are due to complications of treatment.

Patients with M3 leukemia achieve remission with all-*trans*-retinoic acid (ATRA) (Vesanoid),* as frequently as those treated with chemotherapy. If retinoic acid syndrome (fever, respiratory distress, pulmonary infiltrates, weight gain) develops, temporary cessation of retinoic acid and treatment with dexamethasone (Decadron) plus chemotherapy is recommended.

---

*Investigational drug in the United States.

Consolidation Therapy

Induction is followed by intensive courses of chemotherapy at 3- to 4-week intervals designed to eradicate residual leukemic cells. There is no consensus on the number of courses or the optimal drug combinations. However, high-dose cytosine arabinoside appears to be the single most active drug.

At some treatment centers, bone marrow transplantation from a histocompatible related or unrelated donor is the treatment of choice for children with ANLL in first remission. However, decision analysis suggests that the use of chemotherapy alone followed by bone marrow transplantation in second remission (or in first relapse) results in long-term survival equivalent to that for marrow transplantation in first remission. Both options should be explained to families.

Retinoic acid alone is inadequate therapy for M3 leukemia. If retinoic acid is used alone for induction therapy, chemotherapy should be included in consolidation therapy. The converse is also true. The combination of ATRA plus chemotherapy significantly improves event-free survival compared with chemotherapy alone for patients with M3 ANLL.

Central Nervous System Prophylaxis

In the absence of specific therapy directed at the CNS, 20 to 40% of patients with ANLL develop meningeal leukemia. Intrathecal chemotherapy provides adequate protection against this complication but has not conclusively improved event-free survival.

Chloroma

Chloromas (solid masses of ANLL cells) usually respond to chemotherapy. The addition of local irradiation (2400 to 3000 cGy) may be indicated for incompletely responding lesions.

Treatment of Relapse

BONE MARROW RELAPSE

Bone marrow transplantation is the treatment of choice for bone marrow relapse of ANLL. Patients with early relapse may proceed directly to bone marrow transplantation. Patients with florid relapse and those in whom a prolonged donor search is necessary may benefit from chemotherapy to lessen their body burden of leukemia. Achieving a second remission should not be a prerequisite for proceeding to marrow transplantation.

RELAPSE AT OTHER SITES

Isolated CNS relapse should be treated with intrathecal medication to clear the cerebrospinal fluid, followed by cranial or craniospinal irradiation. Isolated relapse in other sites during initial chemotherapy also may be treated with local radiation therapy. When isolated relapse occurs after completion of treatment, induction chemotherapy should also be given. The choice between consolidation chemotherapy and bone marrow transplantation must then be made on an individual basis.

LONG-TERM COMPLICATIONS

As treatment of acute leukemias becomes more successful, we must be increasingly alert to potential complications of treatment. These include organ dysfunction and a higher risk of developing a second malignancy. True cure of leukemia is tripartite:

1. Biologic cure: eradication of disease with minimal risk of relapse
2. Functional cure: absence of complications from the original disease or the treatment thereof
3. Emotional cure: acceptance by the patient and society of the patient's status as a cancer survivor

CHRONIC LEUKEMIAS

method of
ARTHUR SAWITSKY, M.D.
Long Island Jewish Medical Center
New Hyde Park, New York

CHRONIC LYMPHOCYTIC LEUKEMIA

During the past 20 years, clinical observations of patients with chronic lymphocytic leukemia (CLL) have demonstrated that after definition of the patient's clinical stage and biologic disease activity, treatment that induces a significant clinical remission prolongs survival. Studies also indicate that supportive therapy directed at reducing infectious episodes and promoting the patient's general well-being are associated with an increased quality of life.

In the Western world, CLL is diagnosed in about 30% of all leukemia patients, with an overall incidence of 3 per 100,000 population. In addition, in medical practice an increase in the use of laboratory procedures, especially complete blood counts, has led to an increase in the diagnosis of CLL in otherwise asymptomatic patients. Both black and white populations are equally affected. In Asia, however, CLL is much less frequently diagnosed and accounts for only 2.5% of all leukemias. CLL is a disease of the elderly,

unusual in persons younger than 40 years, rare below the age of 20 years, and more common in male than in female patients. A demonstrable family incidence of both CLL and chronic myeloid leukemia (CML) has been described, but studies of consanguinity, blood groups, and HLA haplotypes have shown no consistent association with family incidence.

The cause of CLL is not known, and no relationship has yet been made between the incidence of the disease and environmental factors. Exposure to drugs, chemicals, or radiation does not appear to be directly involved. The role of repeated antigenic stimuli is not clear, and a role for virus exposure, especially to retroviruses and DNA viruses such as human T cell lymphotropic virus type I and the Epstein-Barr virus, has been postulated. Current research activity includes studies of virus exposure, gene rearrangement, and chromosomal translocation. Overexpression of Bcl-2 protein and an inhibition of programmed cell death (apoptosis) have been demonstrated. Cell proliferation is thought to play an important adjunct role.

The leukemia cells in CLL are functionally inactive and characteristically poorly responsive or nonresponsive to the common well-defined B cell mitogens. Nevertheless, in vitro culture studies with various cytokines, phorbol esters, or lipopolysaccharides show that CLL cells can be costimulated to undergo mitosis or further differentiation even to plasmacytic-type cells. Under these conditions, chromosomal studies can be carried out, and these have delineated various chromosomal aberrations such as trisomy 12, structural abnormalities of the long arms of chromosomes 6 and 14, and a t(11;14) translocation involving the *bcl*-1 and immunoglobulin genes.

The normal T cell/B cell ratio is reversed, and the immunophenotype of B cell CLL (B-CLL) cells defines the clone to be $CD19^+$, $CD20^+$, and usually $CD21^+$, $CD24^+$, and $CD23^+$ with coexpression of $CD5^+$. The absolute number of T lymphocytes in B-CLL is variable and is frequently within the normal range, but a reversal in the helper ($CD4^+$)/suppressor ($CD8^+$) cell ratio is usual. Early in CLL the immune status of the patient is intact, but with progressive disease an immune-deficient state develops and diminished serum levels of IgG, IgA, and IgM are noted, with an associated increase in the frequency of bacterial and opportunistic viral and fungal infections.

Autoimmune complications are frequent in this group of patients, and a Coombs-positive red blood cell population is present in about 20 to 30% of patients. About 10 to 15% of B-CLL patients have an active hemolytic syndrome with anemia requiring therapy at some phase of their disease. Immune thrombocytopenia is much less common (2 to 5%).

Clinical Features

The most frequent presenting complaints of CLL patients are weakness, easy fatigability, fever, night sweats, weight loss, recurring or unexpectedly long bouts of respiratory or urinary infections, and an

TABLE 1. **National Cancer Institute Working Group Guideline for Diagnosis of Chronic Lymphocytic Leukemia**

Absolute peripheral blood lymphocytosis	≥5000 lymphocytes/mm³
B cell markers	CD19 and CD20, with coexpression CD5
Bone marrow lymphocytosis	≥30% of all nucleated bone marrow cells
Cell surface membrane immunoglobulin	Faint low-intensity staining, IgM, or IgG with or without IgD
Monoclonality	One light chain, either κ or λ

exaggerated response to insect bites. More recently, asymptomatic peripheral lymphocytosis or the incidental finding of peripheral lymphocytosis during an annual medical checkup discloses the diagnosis in an increasing number of CLL patients. Physical examination of these patients when positive identifies a minor but significantly enlarged multiple-site peripheral adenopathy not necessarily in a generalized distribution. The lymph nodes when enlarged are nonpainful, discrete, and firm but not stony hard. A palpable spleen and/or liver of variable size may be present. Pruritus may be present, but a skin infiltrate is unusual. A small number of patients present with autoimmune anemia and/or thrombocytopenia.

Diagnosis

Recently published (1996) and updated International Workshop on CLL and National Cancer Institute–sponsored Working Group (NCI-WG) guidelines for the diagnosis of CLL follow (Table 1):

1. Peripheral blood must show an absolute lymphocyte number greater than 5000 cells per mm³ with a morphologically well-differentiated lymphocyte.

2. The lymphocyte immunophenotype must show a predominant population of B cells that are CD19+, and CD20+ with coexpression CD5+; there must be monoclonality of the light chain (either κ or λ); surface immunoglobulin must be with faint expression, i.e., low intensity.

3. Bone marrow aspirate and biopsy are not necessary if the first two criteria are met and the absolute peripheral lymphocyte count is well above 5000 cells per mm³. It is recommended for future comparison should serial bone marrow examinations be required. Bone marrow aspirate must show greater than 30% of all nucleated bone marrow cells to be lymphocytes in the presence of a normal or hypercellular marrow. In addition, the bone marrow biopsy provides prognostic information because a diffuse lymphocytic infiltrate pattern has been correlated with active and progressive disease in contrast to the nondiffuse (interstitial or nodular) patterns that are associated with a better prognosis.

Differential Diagnosis

Although we think of B-CLL as a single disease entity, we have learned over the years that peripheral blood lymphocytes may at first glance look alike but in fact show distinct variation both in morphology and in the pattern of lymphocyte immunophenotype that requires recognition and a differential separation into individual clinical entities, each of which has its own clinical course, prognosis, and treatment needs. Such differentiation and clinical separation require determination of the lymphocyte immunophenotype; light microscopy of bone marrow aspirates and biopsy material; and occasionally electron microscopic study. In other circumstances, lymph node biopsy may be needed to differentiate hairy cell leukemia from splenic lymphoma with villous lymphocytosis. Other lymphoproliferative disorders to be considered are large granular lymphocytosis, Sézary cell leukemia, the leukemia phase of well-differentiated lymphocytic lymphoma, and adult T cell leukemia/lymphoma. The clinical prognosis of each of these lymphocyte malignancies is unique, and the indication for treatment or continued observation as well as the choice of chemotherapeutic or radiologic treatment is quite different.

Clinical Staging Systems and Clinical Disease Prognosis

Clinical staging of CLL, by both the Rai and the Binet systems, has been shown to be a useful predictor of short-term prognosis and the need for treatment. My colleagues and I use the NCI-WG modification of the three-risk group modification of our original five-stage schema (Tables 2 and 3). The median life expectancy of patients has been revised and extended. The low-risk group median survival is greater than 14 years; the intermediate-risk group is at 8 years, and the high-risk group has increased its median survival time from 18 months to about 4 years.

We also find the prognosis criteria of Montserrat and Rozman for lymphocyte doubling time to be helpful; a doubling time greater than 12 months is found to be a favorable omen of more stable disease. Other helpful criteria consistent with a more favorable disease course are a bone marrow biopsy pattern of nondiffuse lymphocyte infiltration, low serum beta₂-microglobulin levels, low serum levels of soluble D23

TABLE 2. **Criteria for Clinical Staging of Chronic Lymphocytic Leukemia**

Stage	Criteria
0	Lymphocytosis in blood and bone marrow only
I	Lymphocytosis with palpable adenopathy
II	Lymphocytosis with hepatic and/or splenic enlargement
III	Lymphocytosis with anemia (hemoglobin <11 g/dL)
IV	Lymphocytosis with thrombocytopenia (platelet count <100,000/mm³)

TABLE 3. **Staging Systems and Risk Prognosis in Chronic Lymphocytic Leukemia**

Stage	Risk	Criteria	Survival in Years
0	Low	Only PB and BM lymphocytosis	12+
I	Intermediate	Plus lymphadenopathy	8.5
II		Hepatosplenomegaly	6.0
III	High	<11 gm of Hgb/dL	2.0
IV		Thrombocytopenia (<100,000 platelets/mm³)	

Those patients with proven B-CLL and with only mild to moderate splenomegaly and no lymphadenopathy may prove to be low-risk stage patients.

Abbreviations: PB = peripheral blood; BM = bone marrow; B-CLL = B cell chronic lymphocytic leukemia; Hgb = hemoglobin.

antigen, and a normal bone marrow cytogenetic pattern.

Clinical Course

B-CLL is characterized by a highly variable clinical course and survival time. Some patients live 20 years or longer, whereas others die of the disease within the year of diagnosis. This variability in survival led us to offer our clinical staging system as a means of identifying survival prognosis and thereby the need for treatment. We believe that the need for treatment is established after a short period of observation of 8 to 12 weeks during which time clinical and laboratory features disclose the presence or absence of active disease.

The clinical stage remains the strongest predictor of survival, but even in any one stage, variability of survival exists so that additional prognostic features have been proposed without complete unanimity of opinion but with general acceptance of a poorer prognosis in the presence of a number of these factors (Table 4).

In patients showing advanced disease, about 5 to 10% evolve to a more serious form of disease. These changes may take one of three forms: (1) a prolymphocytoid type of cell may become predominant in the peripheral blood; (2) a second form of disease may present with unexplained fever, weight loss, and a single-site lymph node enlargement that on biopsy

TABLE 4. **Factors Associated with Poorer Prognosis in Chronic Lymphocytic Leukemia**

1. Signs and symptoms of active disease
2. Shortening of lymphocyte doubling time (<12 mo)
3. Bone marrow biopsy infiltrative pattern nondiffuse becoming diffuse
4. Developing or worsening anemia and/or thrombocytopenia
5. Repeated infectious episodes
6. High serum beta₂-microglobulin levels
7. Chromosomal abnormalities (when tests are available)
8. High level of serum-soluble CD23

discloses a histologic pattern of a large cell lymphoma (Richter's syndrome); (3) the least frequent type of progression is to blast transformation, acute leukemia that is usually resistant to all treatment schedules.

An important feature of CLL is the presence of autoimmune and hyperimmune manifestations. These include hypersensitivity to insect bites or newly acquired allergies, or acute hemolytic anemia with a positive direct antiglobulin (a direct Coombs) test. A positive direct Coombs test is found in about 20% of CLL patients, but only about 10% develop anemia. Immune thrombocytopenia is less frequently encountered.

Hypogammaglobulinemia, although unusual in patients with early disease, is almost universal in all patients as disease progression becomes evident. In about 10% of patients hypergammaglobulinemia may be present.

Treatment

Once the diagnosis is made and the clinical stage of patients with CLL is established, a visit with the patient and his or her family is required for full discussion of the disease, its prognosis, and the initial phase of observation. Future treatment options and schedules should be outlined. In the initial phase we observe all patients for 8 to 12 weeks to assess disease activity; for this we use the criteria listed in Table 5. Exceptions are those patients with disease-related symptoms at diagnosis, those with anemia or thrombocytopenia, and those with an absolute peripheral blood lymphocytosis greater than 15,000 per mm³.

We do not treat patients in stage 0 (low-risk category). We do start treatment of patients who are deemed to be stage III or IV (high-risk category). Patients classified as stage I or II disease (intermediate-risk group) are observed for evidence of progression of disease (see Table 4).

Our initial treatment choice is a single alkylating agent, most commonly oral chlorambucil (Leukeran) and less frequently cyclophosphamide (Cytoxan), with regular monitoring of the peripheral blood count. The ease of administration and tolerability of

TABLE 5. **Indications for Treatment of Chronic Lymphocytic Leukemia**

Treatment reserved for patients manifesting disease-related symptoms:
  Increasing and/or extreme fatigue
  Fever, night sweats
  Developing or worsening anemia
  Developing or worsening lymphadenopathy or hepatosplenomegaly
  Repeated infectious episodes, especially bacterial infections
  Hyperlymphocytosis in excess of 150,000 lymphocytes/mm³

Most patients at time of diagnosis have stable disease, and the need for treatment should be based on clinical indications of active or progressive disease.

chlorambucil without chemical cystitis, a major side effect of cyclophosphamide, weigh in favor of that drug.

The chlorambucil administration schedule may be a daily oral dose of 0.07 mg per kg with adjustment as required by peripheral blood monitoring at weekly or biweekly intervals. Our present preference is the use of an intermittent bolus oral dose (0.7 mg per kg) taken over 10 to 30 minutes, at intervals of 3 to 4 weeks with adjustment as required by peripheral blood monitoring at 2 weeks and before each 3 to 4 week dose. Nausea and vomiting are not a major problem and when present are readily controlled by an antiemetic.

Cyclophosphamide and chlorambucil are equal in effectiveness, but when chlorambucil is initial therapy, should the patient become refractory to the chlorambucil, cyclophosphamide may be given with an anticipated good response. Cyclophosphamide is given as a daily oral dose of 2.5 to 3.0 mg per kg, or if an intermittent schedule is desired, the dose is 15 to 20 mg per kg at 4-week intervals. With the higher dosage, a high urinary flow to limit urinary cystitis is advised. Patients with large lymphoid masses, not readily irradiated, may be treated with intravenous single-agent cyclophosphamide with good response. Cyclophosphamide is often used in combination with prednisone or in combination with doxorubicin (Adriamycin) and prednisone. Although vincristine (Oncovin) is frequently recommended as part of such a chemotherapy combination, the threat of peripheral neuropathy with vincristine in the elderly population makes us wary of its use in these patients. Other treatment schedules that are temporarily successful in patients with CLL are variations and/or modifications of chemotherapy schedules recommended for treatment of non-Hodgkin's lymphoma.

There is no evidence that maintenance therapy is of benefit for CLL-responsive patients; therefore, therapy is discontinued once a maximal response has been obtained. It is important, on the other hand, to be sure that a maximal response has been obtained because past studies indicate that a better response status correlates with better survival. When possible, chronic bone marrow toxicity with potential stem cell reduction is to be avoided.

For second-line treatment, we use fludarabine monophosphate (Fludara). The agent is a fluorinated analogue of adenosine that is resistant to deamination by the cellular enzyme adenosine deaminase. In patients resistant to alkylating agents, fludarabine given intravenously as a course, at a dosage of 25 mg per m^2 per day for 5 days every 4 weeks, has proved to be effective. Usually four to six courses produce maximal response. The major difficulty with this drug is an associated immunosuppression after the early courses. The risk for *Pneumocystis carinii* and *Listeria monocytogenes* infection is high. If the patient is taking concomitant prednisone therapy or recently had full-dose prednisone therapy, opportunistic infection is a real threat. In addition, courses of fludarabine given after the patient has achieved a maximal response risk serious cumulative myelotoxicity and infectious complications. A fludarabine response can be precipitous, and precautions against tumor lysis syndrome should be instituted. The nucleoside cladribine (2-CdA)* is currently not used except in an occasional patient relapsing from a previous response to fludarabine. This drug has a toxicity profile similar to that of fludarabine and in our hands has been a little more immunosuppressive. Combinations of fludarabine with an alkylating agent can be quite toxic and require more study.

Corticosteroids

Corticosteroids (prednisone and dexamethasone) are frequently used as single agents for the treatment of patients with complicating autoimmune hemolytic anemia and/or immune thrombocytopenia or as adjuncts to combination chemotherapy schedules. In CLL, an initial increase in peripheral blood lymphocytosis may be noted with the institution of corticosteroid therapy. Lympholysis occurs with gradual resolution of the initial increase in lymphocytosis. The side effects of steroid treatment are well known, and in view of the age of the treatment population, side effects are frequent, i.e., diabetogenesis, salt retention, psychiatric reactions, and immunosuppression.

Radiotherapy

Radiotherapy can be an effective modality and in selected patients with single-area lymphadenopathy, or marked splenomegaly, may be a treatment of choice.

Splenectomy

In special situations, patients with little or no adenopathy and only splenomegaly with significant anemia and/or thrombocytopenia attributable to hypersplenism, and patients who have manifested an unsatisfactory response to steroid or local radiotherapy, should be considered candidates for splenectomy. Pneumococcal vaccine and immune prophylaxis concepts must be instituted before and after such splenectomy.

Supportive Treatment

All infectious episodes in patients with CLL are treated vigorously. We culture blood, urine, and sputum as indicated and have high suspicions for associated opportunistic infections, i.e., oral candidiasis, *Pneumocystis* infection, and tuberculosis. Even minor respiratory infections are monitored carefully because this event may progress rapidly to become one of major proportions.

We give intravenous immune globulin (IGIV) at 3- to 4-week intervals to patients with increased frequency of infections and serum hypogammaglobulinemia. The IGIV is effective in reducing the frequency and severity of bacterial infections. IGIV is administered at a dose of 400 mg per kg every 3 to 4

---

*Not FDA approved for this indication.

weeks. In general we do not use prophylactic antibiotics. In patients with early-stage disease we give pneumoccal vaccine and influenza vaccine.

Packed red blood cell transfusions and platelet transfusions are prescribed for patients who show no peripheral blood response to chemotherapeutic agents or oral prednisone. Patients with low baseline serum erythropoietin levels or those who manifest inadequate low-normal levels are given a trial of subcutaneously administered recombinant erythropoietin.

For our younger CLL patients (<50 years), bone marrow transplantation, although currently a research option, is discussed with the patient and a bone marrow transplant service recommended for consultation and further discussion and consideration.

CHRONIC MYELOID LEUKEMIA

In the past, a variable number of neoplastic diseases of myeloid tissue have been called CML. These have included both Philadelphia chromosome–positive and –negative CML, juvenile CML, chronic myelomonocytic leukemia, and eosinophilic leukemia. In this chapter the most common form of these leukemias, Philadelphia chromosome–positive CML, is discussed. In these leukemias there is leukocytosis of myeloid cells with predominance of the granulocyte population in which all stages of maturation are discernible. Not only are the peripheral white blood cells increased in numbers, but immature granulocytic cells are also present. Blast cells in the peripheral blood may be seen even in early CML but not in excess of 3 to 5%. If the blood film shows an excess or predominance of eosinophils and no Philadelphia-positive chromosome, the leukemia is not CML. A synonym for CML is chronic granulocytic leukemia. The overall incidence of CML is 1 in 100,000, and CML is found in about 15% of all patients with the diagnosis of leukemia.

In 90 to 95% of CML patients, a classic Philadelphia-positive chromosome is identified in the myeloid cells. The Philadelphia-positive chromosome is the result of a reciprocal translocation between the long arms of chromosomes 9 and 22 (t9;22). A new fusion protein, p210, is produced with a cellular increase in tyrosine kinase activity. About 5% of CML patients may show varied forms of a Phildelphia-positive chromosome translocation, i.e., translocation of the distal arm of chromosome 22 to a chromosome other than number 9; complex translocations involving numbers 9 and 22 with a third chromosome; or other complex translocations involving chromosome 22.

Clinical Features

The most frequent presenting symptoms of CML patients have been weakness, easy fatigability, marked lethargy, anemia, weight loss, and on physical examination, splenomegaly. Anorexia and abdominal fullness mirror the degree of splenomegaly noted in at least 50% of patients. As with CLL patients, an increasing number of asymptomatic patients are being diagnosed because of an annual routine physical examination that includes a complete blood count. Easy bruisability and nose and gum bleeding are also not uncommon complaints. Other symptoms include visual disturbances, headaches, bone pains, and occasionally priapism. The patient's symptoms reflect the marrow hypercellularity with resultant overabundance of white blood cells and occasionally platelets. In some patients anemia or thrombocytopenia may present at diagnosis.

The clinical disease course progresses through three clinical phases: an initial chronic relatively indolent phase, in which fatigability is the most prominent feature; a second phase of accelerated disease marked by unexplained fever and increasing leukocytosis with resistance to the initial treatment drug; and the third phase or blast phase characterized by fever, progressive anemia, a high peripheral blood blast count, and incomplete or no response to aggressive chemotherapy. Persistent progressive disease is followed by death, usually within the year. These disease phases are of variable duration. The chronic phase has a median duration of 2 to 5 years, with occasional patients remaining in the chronic phase for even 8, 12, or 15 years. The accelerated disease phase may last between 6 and 18 months, but patients who have entered the blast phase, also called blast crisis, rarely live for more than 6 to 10 months. The increased frequency of diagnosis in asymptomatic patients has largely influenced and lengthened the duration of the chronic phase. Better supportive care has had a small but real positive influence on the duration of the accelerated phase but only a small influence in prolonging the life of patients with blast crisis.

The greatest incidence of CML is in the 40- to 60-year age group. This type of leukemia has been related to radiation exposure. Japanese survivors of the atomic bomb explosions were found to have an increased incidence of CML and acute myeloid leukemia directly related to the degree of radiation they were exposed to. The relationship of other leukemia risk factors such as viruses has not been demonstrated.

Although no generally accepted clinical staging schema is in use, the following clinical factors have been proposed as prognostic criteria:

1. Chronic phase (good prognosis)
   a. Patients are asymptomatic, or there is disappearance of significant symptoms after a response to initial treatment. In these patients there are no features of an accelerated or a blast phase.
2. Accelerated phase (guarded prognosis)
   a. The white blood cell count is difficult to control with the initial or standard therapy.
   b. Anemia and thrombocytopenia become unresponsive to chemotherapy.
   c. There is persistent thrombocytosis in spite of therapy.

d. A changing chromosomal pattern (clonal evolution) may become apparent.

e. There is usually progressive splenomegaly, and the peripheral leukocyte doubling time is shortened and is usually less than 5 to 7 days.

f. There are increasing numbers of basophils and/or eosinophils in the peripheral blood. In this phase increasing numbers of blasts and promyelocytes are seen in the peripheral blood or bone marrow and may reach 10 to 25%.

3. Blast phase (poor prognosis)

a. The proportion of blast cells in peripheral blood and/or bone marrow continues to increase and becomes equal to or greater than 30% of the total cell population.

Treatment

Although various cooperative group clinical chemotherapeutic trials have resulted in improvement in the duration of survival of CML patients compared with historical controls, the most significant and "curative" modality now more and more frequently used is bone marrow transplantation with normal allogeneic donor marrow. Autologous bone marrow transplantation using harvested peripheral blood progenitor cells is under active investigation.

The conventional past and current therapy for chronic phase CML are the oral agents busulfan (Myleran) and hydroxyurea (Hydrea). We favor the use of hydroxyurea, an inhibitor of DNA synthesis. Hydroxyurea suppresses bone marrow activity within 24 to 72 hours with the potential for rapid reversal of toxicity on withdrawal of the drug. On the other hand, busulfan may show little or no reduction in leukocytosis for 7 to 14 days and has cumulative and potentially nonreversible marrow hypoplasia effects. When given long term, busulfan has been associated with pulmonary fibrosis, skin pigmentation, and an Addison disease–like wasting syndrome.

The initial goal of treatment of chronic phase CML is rapid reduction of leukocytosis by chemotherapy or mechanical leukapheresis to prevent organ damage especially to the lung and brain. Attention must also be paid to a potential tumor lysis syndrome and uric acid stone precipitation when chemotherapy is used. Adequate hydration and oral allopurinol (Zyloprim) are necessary for the prevention of such an episode.

We start treatment with oral hydroxyurea, about 50 mg per kg or a single dose of 3 to 5 grams in two or three divided doses given daily, along with a high volume of oral liquids to promote urine dilution. At the same time or a day before, allopurinol is given at a dose of 300 mg per day. If peripheral blood cell counts are above 100,000 cells per mm³, we start treatment with leukapheresis before initiating chemotherapy. Careful monitoring of peripheral blood white blood cells, either daily or weekly, is then continued until the peripheral white blood cell counts fall below 50,000 cells per mm³. Peripheral blood monitoring is carried out at weekly or biweekly inter-vals. When the peripheral white blood cell count is reduced and becomes equal to or less than 30,000 cels per mm³, we reduce and adjust the hydroxyurea dose accordingly.

After the peripheral white blood cell count falls to 20,000 cells per mm³ or less, we start interferon alfa-2 (IFN-α-2) therapy. The aim of this therapy is total reduction in the percentage of Philadelphia-positive CML cells. This reduction in such Philadelphia-positive CML cells is thought to be a reflection of overall tumor load and is associated with better duration of survival. Early adverse effects of IFN-α-2 may include fever, malaise, fatigue, and emotional depression and may limit the use of interferon in some patients. These side effects tend to be ameliorated with continued treatment, and patients should be encouraged to persist with the interferon treatment. We start IFN-α-2 therapy at a dose of 3×10^6 units subcutaneously given daily for 7 to 10 days and then escalate the dose to 5.0×10^6 units daily and if that is tolerated maintain the dose at that level. Acetaminophen may be given to improve tolerance of the treatment. Should an increase in toxicity ensue with longer treatment, re-evaluation of the patient's clinical status may require discontinuance of IFN-α-2 therapy and/or reinitiation or the addition of hydroxyurea.

Allogeneic bone marrow transplantation is the treatment of choice in younger patients (younger than 50 years), especially patients with available and HLA-compatible normal siblings. Patients potentially eligible for bone marrow transplantation should be referred to transplant centers even as initial therapy is being prescribed and carried out.

All patients with CML should be considered for and encouraged to enroll in clinical research studies where available. Although the chemotherapy and IFN-α-2 therapy are initially largely successful for 80 to 90% of patients, the remission achieved is highly variable, as is the patient's remission duration. The disease is always ultimately characterized by progression to an accelerated phase in which only transient benefit may be obtained in spite of more aggressive chemotherapy utilizing schedules that include anthracycline and cytarabine. Ultimate progression to the blast phase is unavoidable.

The blast phase is treated as an acute myeloblastic leukemia, and unfortunately death is the end point. In this phase, approximately 30% of patients may show transformation of the cell type to that of a lymphoblastic cell. Such transformation may allow for a little better, but again only temporary, response by the patient to anti–acute lymphoblastic leukemia therapy. Survival with either acute myeloblastic leukemia or acute lymphoblastic leukemia is usually less than 1 year.

NON-HODGKIN'S LYMPHOMA

method of
AUAYPORN NADEMANEE, M.D.
City of Hope National Medical Center
Duarte, California

Non-Hodgkin's lymphoma (NHL) represents 4.0% of all cancer deaths in the United States. The incidence of NHL has been increasing during the past 2 decades. The increase has been disproportionately in elderly white men, in extranodal presentations, and in lymphomas of high-grade malignancy. Lymphomas associated with acquired immune deficiency syndrome are responsible for some new lymphomas seen in young and middle-aged men in urban areas since 1982 but represent only a few percent of the total increase. Occupational and environmental exposure to herbicides, solvents, and other potential etiologic factors can account for a small fraction of the observed increase.

ETIOLOGY AND RISK FACTORS

NHLs constitute a diverse group of malignancies of the lymphoid system and represent a clonal malignant expansion of lymphocytes that appear to be arrested at a specific stage of normal lymphocytic differentiation. The precise etiology of NHL is unknown, despite considerable advances in understanding the biology and molecular genetics of this disorder during the past decade.

Chromosomal Translocations and Molecular Rearrangement. Nonrandom chromosomal and molecular rearrangements play an important role in the pathogenesis of many lymphomas and correlate with the histologic findings and immunophenotype. The most commonly associated chromosomal abnormality in NHL is the t(4;18)(q32;q21) translocation, which is found in 85% of follicular lymphomas, although it may be seen in multiple histologic subtypes of NHL. This translocation results in the juxtaposition of the *bcl*-2 apototic inhibitor "oncogene" at chromosome band 18q21 to the heavy chain region of the immunoglobulin locus within chromosome band 14q32, leading to altered *bcl*-2 expression and accumulation of clonal lymphoid cells susceptible to additional transforming events, such as p53 mutation.

The t(11;14)(q13;q32) translocation results in overexpression of *bcl*-1 (cyclin D1/PRAD 1), a cell cycle–control gene on chromosome 11q13, and has a strong, nonrandom association with centrocytic, or mantle cell, lymphoma. The gene product of *bcl*-1, cyclin D, is directly involved in the regulation of cell division.

Chromosomal translocations involving band 24 on the long arm (q) of chromosome 8 (8q24) lead to c-*myc* deregulation and are frequently seen in high-grade small noncleaved lymphomas (Burkitt's and non-Burkitt's types), including those associated with human immunodeficiency virus (HIV) infection.

Rearrangement of *bcl*-6, a gene located at band 3q27, has been reported in a third of diffuse large cell lymphomas. The product of *bcl*-6 resembles a class of zinc finger transcription factors that regulate cell proliferation and differentiation, as well as organ development.

The spectrum of cytogenetic and molecular genetic abnormalities of T cell lymphoma differs from that of B cell neoplasms. Translocation frequently involves T cell receptor genes on the long arm of chromosome 14 and on the short arm of chromosome 7. A translocation involving chromosomes 2 and 5, t(2;5)(p23;q35), is characteristic of anaplastic large cell lymphoma.

Environmental Factors. Environmental factors may play a role in the development of NHL. Certain workers have an increased risk of developing NHL, including farmers, pesticide applicators, grain (flour) millers, meat workers, wood and forestry workers, chemists, painters, machinists, printers, and workers in the petroleum, rubber, plastics, and synthetics industries.

Certain chemicals have also been linked to the development of NHL, including a variety of pesticides and herbicides (2,4-D, organophosphates, chlorophenols), solvents, and organic chemicals (benzene, carbon tetrachloride), wood preservatives, and some components in hair dye.

Patients who receive cancer chemotherapy and/or radiation therapy are also at increased risk of developing NHL.

Viruses. Several viruses have been implicated in the pathogenesis of NHL including Epstein-Barr virus (EBV), human T cell lymphotropic virus type I (HTLV-I), HIV, Kaposi's sarcoma–associated herpesvirus (or human herpesvirus 8), and hepatitis C virus.

Immunodeficiency. Patients with congenital or acquired immunodeficiency are at increased risk for NHL. EBV is regularly associated with NHL, which occurs in a variety of primary and secondary immunodeficiency states. These EBV-associated NHLs vary from polyclonal B cell proliferations to monoclonal large cell lymphomas of B lineage, usually immunoblastic lymphomas. EBV has also been isolated from the NHL that follows radiation treatment of Hodgkin's disease.

DIAGNOSIS AND STAGING

A definitive diagnosis can be made only by excisional biopsy of pathologic lymph nodes or tumor tissues. A needle biopsy is generally not adequate because it may not provide sufficient information about the malignant cells or the architecture of the lymph node. Determining the extent of disease in patients with NHL provides prognostic information and is useful in treatment planning; however, histologic subclassification is the primary determinant of survival and potential for cure.

The Ann Arbor system, although initially devised for Hodgkin's disease, has been routinely applied for staging of NHL (Table 1). The Ann Arbor system does not reflect

TABLE 1. **Ann Arbor Staging Classification for Non-Hodgkin's Lymphoma***

Stage	Area of Involvement
I	One lymph node region
IE	One extralymphatic organ or site
II	Two or more lymph node regions on the same side of the diaphragm
IIE	One extralymphatic organ or site (localized) in addition to criteria for stage II
III	Lymph node regions on both sides of the diaphragm
IIIE	One extralymphatic organ or site (localized) in addition to criteria for stage III
IV	One or more extralymphatic organs with or without associated lymph node involvement (diffuse or disseminated): involved organs should be designated by subscript letter (P, lung; H, liver; M, bone marrow)

*Class A patients experience no symptoms; class B patients experience unexplained fever (temperature of >101.5°F); unexplained, drenching, night sweats; or loss of >10% body weight within the previous 6 mo.

420

TABLE 2. Staging Evaluation for Non-Hodgkin's Lymphoma

Careful history (night sweats, weight loss, fever; neurologic, musculoskeletal, or GI symptoms)

Physical examination (lymph nodes, including submental, infraclavicular, epitrochlear, iliac, femoral, and popliteal nodes; pericardial rub, pleural effusion, distended neck and/or upper extremity veins in superior vena cava syndrome; breast masses; hepatosplenomegaly, bowel obstruction, renal mass, and testicular or ovarian mass; focal neurologic signs, such as plexopathy, spinal cord compression, nerve root infiltration, and meningeal involvement; skin lesions)

CBC with differential and platelet count examination of peripheral blood smear for lymphoma cells

Liver and renal function tests; lactate dehydrogenase level; alkaline phosphatase level; calcium level; beta$_2$-microglobulin assay; and serum protein electrophoresis

Chest radiograph (mediastinal or hilar adenopathy, pleural effusions, parenchymal lesions)

CT of the chest (mediastinal, hilar, or parenchymal pulmonary disease)

CT of the abdomen and pelvis (enlarged lymph nodes, splenomegaly, filling defects in the liver and spleen)

Bilateral bone marrow biopsies

Gallium scan (selected cases)

Bone scan (selected cases) if musculoskeletal symptoms are present or alkaline phosphatase level is elevated

HIV testing for patients with intermediate- or high-grade NHL

Abbreviations: GI = gastrointestinal; CBC = complete blood count; CT = computed tomography; HIV = human immunodeficiency virus; NHL = non-Hodgkin's lymphoma.

the noncontiguous nature of disease spread in NHL and fails to take tumor bulk or the number of extranodal sites into consideration.

The diagnostic evaluation of patients with NHL is designed to establish the stage of the disease and to specify sites of tumor involvement to best assess the patient's response to treatment. The appropriate evaluation of a patient with NHL is outlined in Table 2. Serum lactate dehydrogenase (LDH) levels are important because they correlate with tumor burden. Serum beta$_2$-microglobulin levels should be measured because of their prognostic value. A staging laparotomy is generally not performed in NHL because the diseases are often disseminated at presentation and most require chemotherapy as part of their treatment. A lymphangiogram, although useful in Hodgkin's disease, is not recommended in NHL. A gallium scan is useful for assessing the response to therapy and determining the disease activity in a residual enlarged mass or nodes in patients who present with bulky mediastinal or abdominal disease but is not part of the routine evaluation for NHL. Lumbar puncture and cerebrospinal fluid examination should be done in patients with lymphoblastic lymphoma and small noncleaved cell lymphomas and in those with peripheral blood, bone marrow, testicular, paranasal sinus, or nasopharyngeal involvement by intermediate- or high-grade lymphoma because of the high incidence of central nervous system (CNS) involvement. HIV serologic testing should be done in patients with diffuse large cell, immunoblastic, or small noncleaved lymphomas.

PATHOLOGY AND CLASSIFICATION

Despite an improvement in immunologic, cytogenetic, and molecular techniques, the pathologic classification of the NHLs continues to be problematic. The Working Formulation (Table 3) proposed in 1982 as a modification of the Rappaport classification has been established as a tool for the correlation of several histologic classifications and the natural history of NHLs. This classification is based on the morphology (growth pattern and cytologic features) and biologic aggressiveness (low, intermediate, and high grade) of neoplastic cells.

Unfortunately, the Working Formulation has a multitude of problems. For example, immunoblastic lymphomas, a morphologic variant of diffuse large cell lymphoma, and diffuse small noncleaved non-Burkitt's lymphoma are classified as high grade, yet their clinical courses and survivals are not different from those of DLCs. In addition, the Working Formulation does not distinguish between neoplasms of B and T cell lineage or recognize several subtypes of lymphoma that have unique clinical and biologic features (Table 4). These include mantle cell lymphomas (MCLs), also known as intermediate lymphocytic lymphomas. Some that are of either the diffuse or the mantle zone type were called "diffuse small cleaved cell lymphoma" in the Working Formulation. B lymphocytes in the mantle zone of the lymphoid follicles express CD5 and have a characteristic t(11;14) translocation involving *bcl*-1 rearrangement. MCL is derived from these B cells. MCL has an aggressive clinical course, often with extranodal involvement and a low potential for cure with standard treatments. Marginal zone lymphomas were mostly previously considered to be small lymphocytic lymphomas in

TABLE 3. Working Formulation and Rappaport Classification Equivalents for Non-Hodgkin's Lymphoma

Working Formulation	Rappaport Equivalent
Low Grade	
A. Small lymphocytic	Diffuse, well-differentiated, lymphocytic (DWDL)
B. Follicular, predominantly small cleaved cell	Nodular, poorly differentiated, lymphocytic (NPDL)
C. Follicular, mixed, small cleaved and large cell	Nodular, mixed (NM)
Intermediate Grade	
D. Follicular, predominantly large cell	Nodular, histiocytic (NH)
E. Diffuse, small cleaved cell	Diffuse, poorly differentiated, lymphocytic (DPDL)
F. Diffuse, mixed small and large cell	Diffuse, mixed (DM)
G. Diffuse, large cell	Diffuse, histiocytic (DH)
High Grade	
H. Large cell, immunoblastic	Diffuse, histiocytic (DH)
I. Lymphoblastic	Lymphoblastic (LL)
J. Diffuse, small noncleaved cell	Diffuse, undifferentiated (DU) (Burkitt's and non-Burkitt's types)

TABLE 4. **Lymphomas and Atypical Lymphoproliferative Disorders**
Not Recognized by the Working Formulation

Mantle cell lymphoma*
   Resembles follicular small cleaved cell non-Hodgkin's lymphoma (NHL) but derived from a different B cell found in the mantle zone
      surrounding B cell follicles; propensity for extranodal involvement and aggressive behavior; low potential for cure with standard
      treatments; t(11;14) translocation involving *bcl*-1 rearrangement frequently detected
Monocytoid B cell lymphoma
   Low-grade NHL; extremely indolent course; predominant lymph node involvement
Lymphoma of mucosa-associated lymphoid tissue (MALT)
   Tends to have an indolent natural history; primarily affects organs containing epithelial cells, such as the gastrointestinal tract,
      lung, breast, thyroid, and salivary glands
Anaplastic large cell lymphoma (Ki-1 lymphoma)
   Commonly infiltrates the sinusoids of lymph nodes; frequently misdiagnosed as Hodgkin's disease (HD), malignant histiocytosis, or
      metastatic carcinoma; skin often involved; most cases are of T cell origin and are characterized by the detection of t(2;5)
      translocation
Mycosis fungoides
   Indolent cutaneous T cell lymphomas with CD4+ phenotype; initially involve the skin but disseminated into lymph nodes and
      visceral organs in many patients; more advanced form (leukemic peripheral blood involvement and generalized erythroderma)
      known as Sézary syndrome; ulcerated lesion commonly complicated by bacteria, involvement of viscera (usuall lung and liver)
      associated with very poor prognosis
Angiocentric lymphoma
   T cell neoplasm with propensity to invade and destroy blood vessels
   T cell–rich B cell lymphoma
   Previously classified as a subset of diffuse lymphocyte-predominant HD; usually aggressive, response to multiagent chemotherapy
      and outcome similar to those of other large B cell lymphomas
Angiotropic (intravascular) large cell lymphoma
   Usually of B cell lineage; characterized by diffuse intravascular proliferation of neoplastic cells within capillaries, arterioles, and
      venules
Angioimmunoblastic lymphadenopathy (AILD)
   Lymphoproliferative disorder characterized by diffuse lymphadenopathy, hepatosplenomegaly, rash, systemic symptoms, cytopenias,
      and polyclonal hypergammaglobulinemia; frequently evolves into T cell lymphoma, but Epstein-Barr virus–related B cell
      lymphomas can also develop
Divergent or discordant lymphoma
   Large cell histologic findings in a lymph node with low-grade small cleaved cell lymphoma in bone marrow; histologic transformation
      of low-grade NHL into a more aggressive lymphoma occurs at annual rate of 32–34% and is associated with increased morbidity
      and mortality
Composite lymphoma
   Two histologic subtypes in the same lymph node, sometimes with coexistent HD
Castleman's disease
   Lymphoproliferative disorder associated with both immunodeficiency (human immunodeficiency virus infection) and increased rate of
      malignancy (lymphoma, HD, and Kaposi's sarcoma); associated with human herpesvirus 8 infection
Adult T cell leukemia/lymphoma
   Aggressive T cell malignancy with unique clinical features, including skin infiltration, lytic bone lesions, and hypercalcemia;
      associated with human T cell lymphotropic virus type I infection

*Also known as mantle zone or lymphocytic lymphoma of intermediate differentiation.

the Working Formulation. When marginal zone lymphomas involve the nodes, they are called "monocytoid B cell lymphomas"; when they involve extranodal sites, they are called "mucosa-associated lymphoid tissue (MALT) lymphomas." The monocytoid B cell lymphomas have an extremely indolent course and typically present with disseminated disease in elderly women. MALT lymphomas commonly involve extranodal tissue such as gastrointestinal tract, lung, breast, thyroid, and salivary glands. In addition, more than 90% of gastric MALT lymphomas have been associated with *Helicobactor pylori* infection; approximately one half of gastric MALT lymphomas completely regress when infection is eradicated.

The Working Formulation applies poorly to T cell lymphoma and does not include the new clinical and pathologic entities that have been identified. One example is anaplastic large cell lymphoma, which is usually of T cell origin, expressing CD30 (Ki-1) antigens on its surface and sometimes exhibiting a t(2;5) chromosomal translocation. The diagnosis may be confused with Hodgkin's disease and anaplastic carcinoma. This lymphoma is relatively common in children and usually presents with skin involvement; most patients have stage III or IV disease at diagnosis. It

has an aggressive course but appears to respond to therapy similar that for DLC. Several other T cell lymphomas do not fit well into the classification, including adult T cell leukemia/lymphoma, which is associated with HTLV-I infection; mycosis fungoides and Sézary's syndrome; peripheral T cell lymphoma; angiocentric lymphoma; and T cell–rich B cell lymphoma.

Because of the deficiency in the Working Formulation, a new classification, the Revised European-American Lymphoma (REAL) classification, was proposed in 1994 by the International Lymphoma Study Group, which consisted of a large group of pathologists from all over the world who were experts in lymphomas. The REAL classification groups diseases on the basis of the cell of origin, B cell versus T cell. The proposal has been criticized as being inadequate for clinical use. Therefore, until a more accurate, scientifically defined classification is established, the Working Formulation should be used for prognostication and therapeutic decisions.

PROGNOSTIC FACTORS

Several clinical pretreatment characteristics are consistently associated with a poor prognosis in aggressive NHL, including features that reflect the growth and invasive potential of the tumor (Ann Arbor stage, high LDH level, large tumor bulk, and number of extranodal sites), the patient's response to tumor (B symptoms, poor performance status), and the patient's ability to tolerate therapy (age, performance status, bone marrow involvement). An international prognostic model has been developed based on age, tumor stage, serum LDH level, performance status, and number of extranodal sites. This International Index separates patients at the time of diagnosis into four risk groups with predicted 5-year survival rates of 73, 51, 43, and 26%. For patients 60 years of age or younger, the age-adjusted model based on stage, LDH level, and performance status identified four other risk groups with predicted 5-year survival rates of 83, 69, 46, and 32%. The International Index and the age-adjusted International Index can be used to identify specific risk groups and to compare different treatment modalities in patients with aggressive NHL.

In addition to the clinical features described, an elevated serum beta$_2$-microglobulin level and a high Ki-67 proliferative index have both been reported to be associated with a poor prognosis. The prognostic significance of B versus T cell lymphoma remains controversial; in some studies, the prognosis of T cell lymphomas is worse than that of B cell lymphomas.

Similar clinical characteristics have been identified as prognostic factors in low-grade lymphomas. The International Index also appears to be useful in predicting the outcome in patients with low-grade lymphomas; however, the most predictive prognostic factors in these patients are the response to initial treatment, age, and duration of response.

TREATMENT (Table 5)

In general, the treatment of NHL is combination chemotherapy with or without radiation therapy. Radiation therapy alone as primary treatment has been limited to a small subset of patients with NHL. An appropriate treatment plan is selected based on the histologic type (low, intermediate, and high grade) and the disease stage; therefore, it is important to have an accurate histologic diagnosis and appropriate clinical staging evaluation before the initiation of therapy.

TABLE 5. **Treatment of Non-Hodgkin's Lymphoma**

Category	Option
Low Grade	
Stage I or II	Radiation therapy
Stage III or IV	Watch and wait or combination chemotherapy ± interferon
Intermediate Grade	
Stage I or II	CHOP ± radiation therapy
Stage II, bulky, III, IV	CHOP
High Grade	
Lymphoblastic	Combination chemotherapy + CNS prophylaxis ± radiation therapy
Small noncleaved (Burkitt's and non-Burkitt's)	Combination chemotherapy + CNS prophylaxis

Abbreviations: CHOP = cyclophosphamide, vincristine, prednisone, doxorubicin; CNS = central nervous system.

Stages I and II Low-Grade Lymphoma

Patients with early-stage low-grade lymphoma have a better prognosis than patients with more advanced disease. After staging evaluation, about 10 to 15% of patients with low-grade lymphoma are found to have localized disease that may be curable with radiation therapy. All patients should undergo thorough staging evaluation; however, staging laparotomy is not recommended routinely. Radiation therapy is the standard treatment, with an approximately 50% overall probability of cure. Recommended radiation therapy fields include involved field for stage I disease and extended field or total lymphoid irradiation for stage IIA disease. Patients younger than 40 years with nonbulky, contiguous disease have a better prognosis.

Stages III and IV Low-Grade Lymphoma

Most patients with low-grade lymphoma have advanced-stage disease at the time of diagnosis, and their median survival has been reported to be 8 to 10 years. Because the natural history of low-grade lymphoma has not been significantly altered by the use of single-agent or multiagent chemotherapy, the treatment options have been varied from no therapy (watch and wait) to more aggressive therapy similar to that of DLC. Many of the regimens produce a 60 to 75% complete remission rate; however, remissions are usually of short duration, and the likelihood of cure is low. Most patients experience relapses and die of complications related to the disease or its treatment. Therefore, the choices of therapy should be individualized and based on the patients' age, their ability to tolerate therapy, their symptoms, and whether they have features of poor prognosis. Asymptomatic patients with nonbulky disease should be observed closely, and treatment should be initiated when clinically indicated. In a study reported from Stanford University, the median time before therapy was required was approximately 3 years, and approximately 20% of patients did not require therapy for up to 10 years. However, the watch and wait approach may be inadequate for younger patients who are almost certain to have their life span shortened by the disease and therefore are candidates for aggressive chemotherapy protocols, autologous bone marrow transplantation, or other innovative treatment protocols. A similar approach should also be offered to those patients who present with poor-risk features in an effort to enhance disease-free survival and overall survival.

The commonly used chemotherapy regimens for low-grade lymphoma include single alkylating agents (chlorambucil [Leukeran] or cyclophosphamide [Cytoxan]) and combination chemotherapy regimens: CVP (chemotherapy regimens are described in Table 6), C-MOPP, CHOP, and CHOP-Bleo. Oral single-agent alkylating therapy is generally recommended for older patients because the acute toxicities are relatively low, whereas combination therapy regi-

TABLE 6. Common Chemotherapy Regimens for Non-Hodgkin's Lymphoma

CVP	Cyclophosphamide, vincristine, prednisone
CHOP	CVP + doxorubicin
m/M-BACOD	Methotrexate, bleomycin, doxorubicin (Adriamycin), cyclophosphamide, vincristine (Oncovin), dexamethasone
MACOP-B	Methotrexate, doxorubicin, cyclophosphamide, vincristine, prednisone, bleomycin
ProMACE/cytaBOM	Prednisone, methotrexate, doxorubicin, cyclophosphamide, etoposide, cytarabine, bleomycin, vincristine
CHOP-BLEO	CHOP + bleomycin
C-MOPP	Cyclophosphamide, mechlorethamine, vincristine (Oncovin), procarbazine, prednisone

Salvage Chemotherapy Regimens for Relapsed Non-Hodgkin's Lymphoma

DHAP	Dexamethasone, high-dose cytarabine, cisplatin (Platinol)
ESHAP	Etoposide, Solu-Medrol, high-dose cytarabine, cisplatin
EPOCH	Infusional etoposide, doxorubicin, vincristine with bolus cyclophosphamide and prednisone
CEPP	Cyclophosphamide, etoposide, procarbazine, prednisone
MINE	Mesna, ifosfamide, mitoxantrone (Novantrone), etoposide
FND	Fludarabine, mitoxantrone, dexamethasone

mens are recommended for younger and symptomatic patients, or patients who require a more rapid response.

Two new and promising chemotherapeutic agents, purine analogues fludarabine (Fludara) and 2-chlorodeoxyadenosine (2-CdA), have been shown to be active agents in the treatment of low-grade lymphoma, and further studies are in progress to determine the role of these purine analogues either alone or in combination with other agents, i.e., mitoxantrone (Novantrone), in untreated patients with low-grade lymphoma.

Another promising approach to the treatment of low-grade lymphoma is the administration of recombinant human interferon alfa (rHuIFN-α). The addition of IFN-α to the standard chemotherapeutic regimens in the treatment of low-grade NHL prolongs the duration of remission but does not provide a significant improvement in survival. These results suggest that IFN-α has a significant role in maintenance therapy for low-grade NHL, and it is reasonable to offer maintenance IFN-α at 2 to 3 million units per m² three times per week to those patients who do not suffer from toxicity associated with IFN-α.

Relapsed Low-Grade Lymphoma

Although many patients with advanced low-grade NHL may achieve a complete remission (CR) with standard treatment, the median duration of the first CR is often short (ranging from 12 to 36 months). Patients who present with advanced-stage disease or with poor-risk factors are at very high risk for relapse with a disease-free survival of only 25% at 5 years. Even though salvage chemotherapy may remain effective, the overall response rate declines with successive recurrences, and the duration of subsequent responses progressively decreases. Moreover, 15 to 70% of low-grade NHLs undergo histologic transformation to a higher grade lymphoma, which has been associated with a poor prognosis.

Several salvage combination chemotherapy regimens utilized for aggressive lymphoma (i.e., DHAP, ESHAP, EPOCH; see Table 6) have also been shown to be effective in low-grade NHL. Encouraging results have been reported with purine analogues, fludarabine and 2-CdA alone or in combination with other chemotherapeutic drugs. Despite these encouraging results, relapse remains a problem with salvage regimens.

High-dose therapy and autologous bone marrow transplantation (ABMT) have been shown to induce a complete remission in a high proportion of patients with recurrent low-grade NHL. A 2-year disease-free survival of 67% was reported from the Dana-Farber Cancer Institute. Although cure is difficult to document because of the long, indolent natural history and the late relapse in low-grade NHL, the remission after ABMT remains durable for several years in several reported series. One major obstacle to ABMT in low-grade NHL is bone marrow involvement with lymphoma. About 80% of patients with low-grade NHL have histologic evidence of bone marrow involvement at diagnosis, and virtually all patients have marrow involvement at the time of relapse. Because of the potential problem of marrow contamination with lymphoma cells, most of the studies of high-dose therapy and ABMT in low-grade NHL have utilized anti–B cell monoclonal antibody–purged marrow. Peripheral blood stem cells have been used as an alternative to marrow purging in some studies. Alternative therapy with radiolabeled monoclonal antibodies given in conjunction with the conventional myeloablative regimen and ABMT may increase the efficacy of high-dose therapy and improve the outcome of bone marrow transplantation (BMT).

Allogeneic BMT has been performed in a limited number of patients with low-grade NHL. The obvious benefit is the use of healthy and uncontaminated marrow, but the major drawbacks are the lack of a suitable donor for most patients and the higher treatment-related mortality associated with graft-versus-host disease. Nevertheless, allogeneic BMT should be considered in young patients with relapsed low-grade NHL who have persistent bone marrow and peripheral blood involvement after salvage therapy.

Stages I and II Aggressive Lymphoma

The treatment of limited-stage aggressive NHL has evolved from radiation therapy alone, producing

5-year relapse-free survivals of 25 to 50%, to the current practice of combination chemotherapy and involved field radiotherapy, which produces a CR rate of 98% and a 5-year relapse-free survival of 83%. Many patients with stage I or II disease have microscopic evidence of disease at distant sites; therefore, combination chemotherapy is considered standard treatment. Systemic therapy with doxorubicin-containing regimens has resulted in cures in approximately 95% of stage I patients and 75% of stage II patients. The additional benefit of adjuvant radiotherapy has been confirmed in several randomized studies that show a significant improvement in both disease-free survival and overall survival in those receiving combination chemotherapy with adjuvant radiotherapy compared with chemotherapy alone. In addition, a shorter course (three or four cycles instead of six to eight cycles) followed by involved field radiotherapy has been proved to be highly effective and curative in most patients, and this approach has been recommended as standard therapy for patients with limited-stage aggressive NHL.

Advanced-Stage Aggressive Lymphoma

Since the introduction of the CHOP regimen in 1975, it has remained the best available treatment for patients with advanced-stage aggressive NHL. Several generations of combination chemotherapy programs utilizing six to eight chemotherapeutic drugs have been developed and shown to produce higher CR and survival rates in pilot trials. However, when these regimens were compared with CHOP in prospective, randomized trials, there were no statistical differences in the response rate or survival. The CR rates were 44 to 56% and the estimated 3-year disease-free survival was 41 to 46%. Newer approaches to improve the response rate and survival are being investigated. High-dose CHOP with growth factor support has produced encouraging results. High-dose therapy and ABMT as consolidation therapy during first remission has been shown to improve survival and prognosis of patients with poor-risk aggressive lymphoma in several pilot trials and in some randomized studies.

Relapsed Large Cell Lymphoma

Patients who have achieved an initial CR but relapse have an extremely poor prognosis, with an expected survival rate of less than 15% at 3 years. Both conventional-dose salvage chemotherapy regimens and high-dose intensive therapy with autologous marrow or peripheral blood stem cell transplants have been extensively explored in this group of patients. Although objective response rates of greater than 50% have been reported in several salvage combination chemotherapy regimens, remission durations are usually brief and the majority of patients fail to attain a CR. The benefit of ABMT in relapsed lymphoma has been confirmed in a randomized study that showed higher cure rates and freedom from progression with ABMT compared with salvage therapy. Therefore, high-dose therapy with ABMT has been accepted as the "gold standard" for treatment of relapsed NHL. However, patients with lymphoma resistant to primary or secondary chemotherapy are unlikely to benefit from ABMT. Currently, high-dose therapy and ABMT have been applied mostly to a selected group of patients with relapsed lymphoma who are young with good performance status and chemosensitive disease. Thus, the majority of relapsed lymphoma patients who are old (>60 years), debilitated (poor performance status), or with bulky disease are usually not considered eligible for ABMT. Alternative salvage strategies need to be developed for these patients.

Despite the favorable outcome of high-dose therapy and ABMT, relapse occurs after transplantation in a significant proportion of patients. Therefore, new therapeutic approaches to intensify the regimen and to prevent relapse are needed. Radioisotope-labeled monoclonal antibodies are quite attractive as they provide a mechanism by which radioactivity can be directly targeted to tumor sites while sparing normal tissues. The role of radiolabeled monoclonal antibody with or without ABMT for treatment of lymphoma is currently being investigated. Studies to determine the role of cyclosporine after ABMT to induce autologous graft-versus-host disease and the graft-versus-lymphoma effect are under way. The role of post-transplant interleukin-2 to prevent relapse is being investigated.

High-Grade Lymphoma

Long-term survival among adults with these rapidly growing lymphomas was uncommon before the use of intensive combination chemotherapy and CNS prophylaxis. Although relatively infrequent in adults, these malignancies constitute the majority of NHLs in children. Generally, patients can be divided into good- or poor-risk groups based on the extent of disease as defined by the presence or absence of bone marrow or CNS involvement, tumor mass greater than 10 cm, and LDH levels greater than 1.5 times normal. The Ann Arbor staging system is inadequate but unfortunately is still used in this population of patients.

Lymphoblastic Lymphoma

Lymphoblastic lymphomas were previously included in the diffuse, poorly differentiated category of the Rappaport classification and are sometimes misdiagnosed. These malignancies are histologically and cytologically indistinguishable from the lymphoblasts of acute lymphoblastic leukemia. Most cases are of T cell phenotype. Bone marrow involvement is common, with clinical features of both leukemia and lymphoma at presentation or in the course of the disease. Criteria to distinguish between these diseases are arbitary, such as the presence or absence of greater than 25% involvement of bone marrow, which is used by some pediatric oncologists. Mediastinal masses are seen in 50 to 70% of patients at presentation. Because of a propensity for CNS relapse, CNS prophylaxis with intrathecal chemotherapy and/or irradiation is part of all successful treatment regimens. Currently, acute lymphoblastic leukemia–like regimens utilizing multiple drug combinations in alternating fashion with intrathecal chemotherapy and maintenance therapy for 2 to 3 years have demonstrated CR rates of up to 80% with 45% long-term survival. Patients with adverse prognostic features (stage IV, high LDH levels, bone marrow or CNS involvement) are candidates for consolidation with ABMT or allogeneic BMT after completion of induction therapy.

Small Noncleaved Cell Lymphoma (Burkitt's and Non-Burkitt's Types)

These neoplasms are the fastest growing and most aggressive of all the lymphomas. Prolonged staging procedures should be avoided because these neoplasms can double in size in a matter of days. High-risk features include elevated LDH levels, bone marrow involvement, and unresectable tumor masses greater than 10 cm. A CHOP-like regimen (Stanford University) with midcycle high-dose methotrexate for CNS prophylaxis results in 70 to 80% durable complete remissions in patients without high-risk features but only 20 to 30% of patients with adverse prognostic features. A brief, high-intensity, cyclophosphamide-based regimen (Vanderbilt University) results in more durable responses in about 50% of high-risk patients. Selected patients with high-risk features are candidates for ABMT or allogeneic BMT in first complete or partial remission.

Human Immunodeficiency Virus–Related Lymphoma

Most lymphomas seen in patients with HIV infection are of high-grade histologic type (immunoblastic and small noncleaved cell) and advanced stage at presentation. Extranodal disease is commonly seen, with unusual sites of presentation, including rectum, CNS, and multiple soft tissue masses. Factors related to poor risk include high LDH levels, large tumor bulk, extranodal disease, and low CD4+ cell counts (<100 cells per mm^3).

Because of the increased risk of opportunistic infections and impaired hematologic reserve, many patients are unable to tolerate aggressive chemotherapy regimens. Attenuated-dose regimens with growth factor support have been well tolerated, although hematologic toxicity remains problematic in some patients. CNS prophylaxis is necessary to prevent leptomeningeal disease.

MULTIPLE MYELOMA

method of
ROBERT A. KYLE, M.D.
Mayo Clinic and Mayo Foundation and Mayo Medical School
Rochester, Minnesota

Multiple myeloma is characterized by the neoplastic proliferation of a single clone of plasma cells producing a monoclonal (M) protein in the serum or urine. The plasma cell proliferation in the bone marrow frequently invades the adjacent bone, resulting in skeletal destruction producing bone pain or fractures. Anemia, hypercalcemia, and renal insufficiency are important features. In the United States, multiple myeloma constitutes 1% of all malignant diseases and slightly more than 10% of hematologic malignancies. The annual incidence is 4 to 5 per 100,000; the incidence in African-Americans is twice that in whites. The apparent increase in rates in more recent years is probably due to increased availability and utilization of medical facilities and improved diagnostic techniques, particularly in the older population. The median age at diagnosis is approximately 65 years. Only 3% of patients are younger than 40 years.

Weakness, fatigue, bone pain, recurrent infections, and symptoms of hypercalcemia or renal insufficiency should alert the physician to the possibility of multiple myeloma. Anemia is present in two thirds of patients at the time of diagnosis. An M protein is found in the serum or urine in 99% of patients with multiple myeloma. Lytic lesions, osteoporosis, or fractures are present at diagnosis in 75%. Technetium Tc 99m bone scanning is inferior to conventional radiography and should rarely be used. Magnetic resonance imaging or computed tomography is helpful in patients who have skeletal pain but no abnormality on radiographs or when spinal cord compression occurs. Hypercalcemia is present in 20% of patients, and the serum creatinine value is 2 mg per dL or greater in one fifth of patients at diagnosis.

DIAGNOSIS

If multiple myeloma is suspected, the patient should have, in addition to a complete history and physical examination, the following: determinations of hemoglobin levels, leukocyte levels with differential count, and platelet levels; measurements of serum creatinine, calcium, and uric acid levels; a radiographic survey of bones, including humeri and femurs; serum protein electrophoresis with immunoelectrophoresis or immunofixation; quantitation of immunoglobulins; bone marrow aspiration and biopsy; routine urinalysis; and electrophoresis, immunoelectrophoresis, and immunofixation of an adequately concentrated aliquot from a 24-hour urine specimen. Determination of the plasma cell labeling index, beta$_2$-microglobulin, thymidine kinase, C-reactive protein, and lactate dehydrogenase values is helpful for prognosis. Patients with a low labeling index and normal beta$_2$-microglobulin level have a median survival of 6 years when treated with conventional chemotherapy.

Minimal criteria for the diagnosis of multiple myeloma consist of more than 10% plasma cells in the bone marrow or a plasmacytoma and one of the following: (1) M protein in the serum (usually more than 3 grams per dL), (2) M protein in the urine, or (3) lytic bone lesions. These findings must not be related to metastatic carcinoma, connective tissue disease, chronic infections, or lymphoma. Patients with multiple myeloma must be differentiated from those with monoclonal gammopathy of undetermined significance (MGUS; benign monoclonal gammopathy) and smoldering multiple myeloma (SMM) because they should not be treated. The plasma cell labeling index is helpful in differentiating MGUS or SMM from multiple myeloma. The patient's symptoms, physical findings, and all laboratory and radiographic data must be considered in the decision to begin chemotherapy. If there are doubts about whether to begin treatment, therapy should be withheld and the patient re-evaluated in 2 or 3 months.

THERAPY

If the patient is younger than 65 years, the physician should discuss the possibility of autologous peripheral blood stem cell transplantation. Ideally, this should be done as part of a prospective study. The peripheral stem cells should be collected before the patient is exposed to alkylating agents. Most investigators prefer vincristine (Oncovin), doxorubicin (Adriamycin), and dexamethasone (VAD) as the initial chemotherapy. Patients older than 65 years should be treated with melphalan (Alkeran) and prednisone or a combination of chemotherapeutic agents.

Radiotherapy

Palliative radiation in a dose of 20 to 30 Gy should be limited to patients with disabling pain who have a well-defined, focal process that has not responded to chemotherapy. Analgesics in combination with chemotherapy can usually control the pain. This approach is preferred to local radiation because pain frequently occurs at another site and local radiation does not benefit the patient with systemic disease. In addition, the myelosuppressive effects of radiotherapy and chemotherapy are cumulative; if possible, the palliative radiotherapy should be completed 3 weeks before starting chemotherapy.

Chemotherapy

Oral administration of melphalan and prednisone produces an objective response in 50 to 60% of patients. We prefer to give melphalan orally in a dosage of 8 to 10 mg daily for 7 days and prednisone in a dosage of 20 mg three times a day orally for the same 7 days. The dosage of melphalan should be calculated on the basis of the patient's ideal body weight. Melphalan should be given when the patient is fasting because absorption is reduced after food is eaten. Leukocyte and platelet counts must be determined at 3-week intervals after the start of therapy, and the melphalan dosage should be altered until midcycle cytopenia (neutrophil count of 1000 to 1500 per mm^3 or platelet count of 100,000 per mm^3) occurs. The melphalan and prednisone regimen should be repeated every 6 weeks. The patient should avoid alcohol and caffeine-containing products and take an H_2

antagonist while receiving the prednisone. If the neutrophil count is less than 1500 per mm^3 or the platelet count is lower than 100,000 per mm^3 at 6 weeks, chemotherapy should be delayed and the counts determined at weekly intervals until the pretreatment level is reached. If the neutrophil and platelet counts remain low or if the counts are unduly low at 3 weeks, the melphalan dose in the next 7-day course must be reduced. Unless the disease progresses rapidly despite adequate therapy, at least three courses of melphalan and prednisone should be given before this therapy is discontinued. An objective response may not be achieved for 6 to 12 months or longer in some patients.

Because of the obvious shortcomings of melphalan and prednisone, various combinations of therapeutic agents have been tried. One of the best-known combinations is the M2 protocol, which includes vincristine, carmustine (BCNU), melphalan, cyclophosphamide (Cytoxan), and prednisone (VBMCP). This regimen produces an objective response in about 70% of patients. Patients with renal insufficiency should have a 50% reduction in the amount of BCNU and cyclophosphamide. In a meta-analysis of 18 published trials, no difference in efficacy was shown between melphalan-prednisone and combination chemotherapy, except in two studies. Thus, there is little evidence that combinations of chemotherapy are efficacious.

Chemotherapy should be continued for at least 1 year or until the patient is in a plateau state. This is defined as stable serum and urine M-protein levels and no evidence of progression. Continued chemotherapy may lead to the development of a myelodysplastic syndrome or acute leukemia. Interferon alfa-2b (Intron A)* appears to prolong the duration of the plateau but does not significantly influence survival. Patients should be followed closely during the plateau state, and the same chemotherapy should be reinstituted when relapse occurs.

Allogeneic or Syngeneic Bone Marrow Transplantation

Bone marrow transplantation from an identical twin donor (syngeneic) has been associated with occasional prolonged survival, but most patients ultimately die of their multiple myeloma. Allogeneic bone marrow transplantation is advantageous in that the graft contains no tumor cells that can subsequently lead to a relapse. However, there is a mortality rate of 20 to 25% within 100 days, the risk of graft-versus-host disease is significant, and most patients ultimately have a relapse. In addition, only 5 to 8% of patients with multiple myeloma are eligible for allogeneic transplantation because an HLA-compatible donor is available in only one third of patients, 80% are older than 50 years, and renal insufficiency occurs in 20%.

---

*Not FDA approved for this indication.

Autologous Peripheral Stem Cell Transplantation

Autologous peripheral blood stem cell transplantation has virtually replaced autologous bone marrow transplantation because there is less contamination with myeloma cells and engraftment is more rapid. Autologous peripheral stem cell transplantation is applicable to more patients than is allogeneic transplantation because the age limit is higher (65 to 70 years) and a matched donor is unnecessary. However, two major problems exist: (1) eradication of myeloma from the patient usually does not occur even with large doses of chemotherapy and radiation, and (2) reinfusing autologous peripheral blood stem cells contaminated by myeloma cells or their precursors may contribute to relapse.

A study from France reported that peripheral stem cell transplantation was superior to combination chemotherapy. Currently, a large prospective study comparing autologous peripheral stem cell transplantation and combination chemotherapy is well under way in the United States. Prior treatment with alkylating agents reduces the number of granulocyte-macrophage colony-forming units and results in delayed engraftment. Thus, peripheral blood stem cells should be collected before alkylating agents are given. Selection of CD34+ stem cells may be a useful approach.

It is essential to develop more sensitive techniques for determination of residual myeloma with the advent of more aggressive therapy with autologous and allogeneic transplantation. When an M protein is not detected in the serum and urine with immunofixation and the bone marrow contains no identifiable myeloma cells with immunofluorescence, the patient still frequently has a relapse with myeloma of the same isotype that was present initially. Oligonucleotide primers to amplify regions of rearranged heavy chain alleles with the polymerase chain reaction can detect 1 myeloma cell in 100,000 cells.

Treatment for Refractory Multiple Myeloma

Almost all patients with multiple myeloma who respond to chemotherapy eventually have a relapse. The highest response rates for patients resistant to alkylating agents have been with VAD. Much of the activity of VAD is from dexamethasone. Methylprednisolone (2 grams intravenously three times weekly for a minimum of 4 weeks) is helpful for patients with pancytopenia, and we find fewer side effects than from dexamethasone. If there is a response, the administration of methylprednisolone is reduced to once or twice weekly. VBAP (vincristine, carmustine [BCNU], and doxorubicin [Adriamycin]) intravenously on day 1 and prednisone daily for 5 days every 3 to 4 weeks benefits 30% of patients. We begin with a total dose of 30 to 40 mg of BCNU and 30 to 40 mg of doxorubicin if leukopenia or thrombocytopenia is present. Interferon alfa-2 produces an objective response in 10 to 20% of patients with myeloma refractory to alkylating agents. Cyclophosphamide (600 mg per m² intravenously daily for 4 days) plus prednisone followed by granulocyte colony-stimulating factor has been helpful in patients with refractory, advanced disease.

The reversal of resistance to chemotherapeutic agents is an important area of research. The use of verapamil (Isoptin)* or quinine* to reverse the resistance to doxorubicin has been disappointing. PSC-833, an analogue of cyclosporine, is being investigated in an effort to reduce multidrug resistance to vinca alkaloids and anthracyclines. It appears to be a much more effective inhibitor of multidrug resistance than cyclosporine.

Supportive Therapy

Hypercalcemia

Hypercalcemia must be suspected if the patient has anorexia, nausea, vomiting, polyuria, increased constipation, weakness, confusion, stupor, or coma. If it is untreated, renal insufficiency usually develops. Hydration, preferably with isotonic saline, and prednisone (25 mg orally four times daily) relieve the hypercalcemia in most cases. The dosage of prednisone must be reduced and the use of the agent discontinued as soon as possible. After hydration has been achieved, furosemide (Lasix) may be helpful. If these measures fail, pamidronate (Aredia), etidronate (Didronel), or gallium nitrate (Ganite) is useful.

Renal Insufficiency

Twenty percent of patients with multiple myeloma have a serum creatinine concentration more than 2 mg per dL at diagnosis. Hypercalcemia, protein casts in the proximal and distal tubules (myeloma kidney), hyperuricemia, and deposition of amyloid may all contribute to renal insufficiency. Maintenance of a high fluid intake producing 3 liters of urine per 24 hours is important for preventing renal failure in patients with Bence Jones proteinuria. Intravenous pyelography or preparation for barium enema may precipitate renal failure, but these tests can be performed with little risk if dehydration is avoided. If hyperuricemia occurs, allopurinol (Zyloprim) (300 mg daily) provides effective therapy.

Acute renal failure must be treated promptly with the maintenance of fluid and electrolyte balance. Hemodialysis may be necessary. Plasmapheresis may be helpful for regaining renal function, but patients with severe myeloma cast formation or other irreversible changes are unlikely to benefit from plasmapheresis. Peritoneal dialysis is useful for patients with hypotension from hemodialysis. Renal transplantation for myeloma kidney has been followed by prolonged survival.

---

*Not FDA approved for this indication.

Infections

Bacterial infections are more common in patients with myeloma than in the general population. Pneumococcal and influenza immunizations should be given to all patients despite their suboptimal antibody response. Intravenously administered immune globulin may be helpful for patients with recurrent infections, but it is too expensive for long-term therapy. Prophylactic daily oral penicillin often benefits patients with recurrent pneumococcal infections. The greatest risk for infection is during the first 2 months after the initiation of chemotherapy. Prophylactic trimethoprim-sulfamethoxazole (Bactrim, Septra) may be useful during the first 2 months. Significant fever is an indication for appropriate cultures, chest radiography, and consideration of antibiotic therapy.

Skeletal Lesions

Bone lesions manifested by pain and fractures are a major problem. Patients should be encouraged to be as active as possible because confinement to bed increases demineralization of the skeleton. Trauma must be avoided because even mild stress may result in a fracture. Fixation of long-bone fractures or impending fractures with an intramedullary rod and methyl methacrylate has given excellent results. Bisphosphonates such as pamidronate may be of benefit for reduction of skeletal complications.

Anemia

Almost every patient with multiple myeloma eventually becomes anemic. An increase of plasma volume from the osmotic effect of the M protein may produce hypervolemia and spuriously lower the hemoglobin concentration and hematocrit. Transfusion of packed red blood cells may be necessary. Successful therapy of myeloma often improves erythropoiesis. Erythropoietin (Epogen) is helpful for many patients with symptomatic anemia when the plateau state has been reached.

Hyperviscosity Syndrome

The symptoms of hyperviscosity may include oronasal bleeding, blurred vision, neurologic symptoms, and congestive heart failure. Most patients have symptoms when the relative serum viscosity reaches 6 or 7 centipoises (normal, less than 1.8), but the relationship between serum viscosity and clinical manifestations is imprecise. Hyperviscosity is more common in IgA myeloma than in IgG myeloma. Plasmapheresis promptly relieves the symptoms of hyperviscosity.

Extradural Myeloma

The possibility of extradural myeloma must be considered if weakness of the legs or difficulty in voiding or defecating occurs. The sudden onset of severe radicular pain or severe back pain is suggestive of compression of the spinal cord. Magnetic resonance imaging is most helpful for diagnosis. Radiation therapy in a dose of approximately 30 Gy is beneficial.

Dexamethasone should be administered during radiation therapy to reduce the edema.

VARIANT FORMS OF MYELOMA

Solitary Plasmacytoma (Solitary Myeloma) of Bone

The diagnosis of solitary plasmacytoma is based on histologic evidence of a tumor consisting of plasma cells identical to those seen in multiple myeloma. In addition, complete skeletal radiographs must show no other lytic lesions, the bone marrow aspirate must contain no evidence of multiple myeloma, and immunoelectrophoresis or immunofixation of the serum and concentrated urine should show no M protein. Some exceptions to the last-mentioned criterion occur. The most uncertain criterion for the diagnosis is the length of observation necessary before it can be ascertained that the disease will not become generalized. The disease-free survival rate at 10 years ranges from 15 to 25%, and about 50% of patients survive 10 years. Treatment consists of radiation in the range of 40 to 50 Gy. Myeloma occurs within 3 years in two thirds of patients who have progression. There is no evidence that adjuvant chemotherapy influences the incidence of conversion to multiple myeloma. Electrophoresis and immunoelectrophoresis or immunofixation of serum and urine are essential for following the course of a patient with a solitary plasmacytoma.

Extramedullary Plasmacytoma

Extramedullary plasmacytoma is a plasma cell tumor that arises outside the bone marrow, most frequently in the upper respiratory tract, including the nasal cavity, sinuses, nasopharynx, and larynx. Extramedullary plasmacytomas may occur in the gastrointestinal tract, central nervous system, urinary bladder, thyroid, breast, testis, parotid gland, and lymph nodes. The diagnosis is based on the finding of a plasma cell tumor in an extramedullary site and the absence of multiple myeloma at bone marrow examination, radiography, and appropriate studies of blood and urine. Treatment consists of tumoricidal radiation. The prognosis is favorable, although experience is limited. In approximately 25% of patients, the extramedullary plasmacytomas spread to the adjacent lymph nodes, but typical multiple myeloma is uncommon.

Osteosclerotic Myeloma (POEMS Syndrome)

The osteosclerotic myeloma syndrome is characterized by polyneuropathy, organomegaly, endocrinopathy, M protein, and skin changes (POEMS). The major clinical features are a chronic, inflammatory-demyelinating polyneuropathy with predominantly motor disability and sclerotic skeletal lesions. Hepatosplenomegaly, lymphadenopathy, hyperpigmentation, hypertrichosis, gynecomastia, and testicular atrophy may occur. The hemoglobin level is usually normal or increased, and thrombocytosis is common. The bone marrow usually contains less than 5% plasma cells, and hypercalcemia and renal insufficiency rarely occur. Most patients have a λ light chain type of M protein. Evidence of Castleman's disease may be present. If the lesions are in a limited area, radiation produces substantial improvement in more than half of patients. If the patient has widespread osteosclerotic lesions, chemotherapy with melphalan and prednisone may be helpful.

Plasma Cell Leukemia

Plasma cell leukemia is characterized by more than 20% plasma cells in the peripheral blood and an absolute plasma cell count of at least 2000 per mm^3. It is classified as primary when it is diagnosed in the leukemic phase (60%) and as secondary when there is leukemic transformation of a previously recognized multiple myeloma (40%). Patients with primary plasma cell leukemia are younger and have a greater incidence of hepatosplenomegaly and lymphadenopathy, a higher platelet count, fewer bone lesions, a smaller serum M-protein component, and a longer duration of survival than patients with secondary plasma cell leukemia. Treatment with VAD followed by peripheral stem cell transplantation may be a helpful aggressive approach. The use of combination chemotherapy or melphalan and prednisone may produce remission. Patients with secondary plasma cell leukemia rarely respond to chemotherapy because they have already received alkylating agents and are resistant to them.

POLYCYTHEMIA VERA

method of
STEVEN M. FRUCHTMAN, M.D.
Mount Sinai Medical Center
New York, New York

DIAGNOSIS

The most crucial aspect of managing patients who present with erythrocytosis, and possibly polycythemia vera (PV), is to establish the correct diagnosis by using appropriate diagnostic studies. The original Polycythemia Vera Study Group (PVSG) diagnostic criteria (Table 1) were important in establishing parameters to help investigators confirm or exclude the diagnosis of PV. Although these parameters are helpful to the clinician in arriving at the correct diagnosis, they were designed to create a relatively uniform population of patients who could be entered into study protocols. Thus, patients with erythrocytosis who do not meet these diagnostic criteria may have PV on the basis of newer techniques and a greater understanding of the pathophysiology of the disorder.

A powerful tool, now widely available to clinicians, is the measurement of the erythropoietin level by using a sensitive and accurate radioimmunoassay. This assay was not

TABLE 1. Diagnostic Criteria* for Polycythemia Vera (Adapted from Eligibility Criteria of the Polycythemia Vera Study Group)

Category A (Major)	Category B (Minor)
A1 Red blood cell mass Male ≥36 mL/kg Female ≥32 mL/kg A2 Normal arterial oxygen saturation ≥92% A3 Splenomegaly	B1 Thrombocytosis, platelet count >400,000/mm^3 B2 Leukocytosis, count >12,000/mm^3 (no fever or infection) B3 ↑ Leukocyte alkaline phosphatase >100 (no fever or infection) ↑ Serum vitamin B$_{12}$ (>900 pg/mL) or unbound B$_{12}$-binding capacity (>2200 pg/mL)

*Diagnosis is acceptable if the following combinations are present: A1 + A2 + A3 or A1 + A2 + any two from category B.

From Fruchtman SM: Polycythemia vera and agnogenic myeloid metaplasia. *In* Handin RI, Lux SE, Stossel TP (eds): Blood: Principles and Practice in Hematology. Philadelphia, JB Lippincott Co, 1995, p 416.

available at the initiation of the PVSG studies and thus could not be included in the diagnostic criteria. Patients who present with an elevated hematocrit and an increased red blood cell mass and normal plasma volume, the secondary causes of erythrocytosis (Table 2), can be excluded if the serum erythropoietin level is low. Thus, by measuring the erythropoietin level, one may be able to avoid an expen-

TABLE 2. Erythrocytosis Associated with an Elevated Red Blood Cell Mass (Absolute Polycythemia)

Secondary Polycythemia

Increased erythropoietin production (physiologically appropriate)
  High altitude
  Cardiopulmonary disease
  Decreased blood oxygen-carrying capacity due to carboxyhemoglobin
  Impaired oxygen delivery, hemoglobin with increased oxygen affinity, or congenital decreased red blood cell 2,3-diphosphoglycerate
  Renal artery stenosis
  Familial elevated erythropoietin level with appropriate physiologic response
Autonomous erythropoietin production
  Tumors
    Hypernephroma
    Cerebellar hemangioblastoma
    Hepatoma
    Uterine fibroids
    Pheochromocytoma
    Adrenocortical adenoma
    Ovarian carcinoma
  Renal disorders
    Cysts
    Hydronephrosis
    Bartter's syndrome
    Transplantation
  Familial polycythemia due to autonomous erythropoietin production

Polycythemia Vera

From Fruchtman SM: Polycythemia vera and agnogenic myeloid metaplasia. *In* Handin RI, Lux SE, Stossel TP (eds): Blood: Principles and Practice in Hematology. Philadelphia, JB Lippincott Co, 1995, p 419.

sive and potentially invasive series of laboratory and radiologic studies. For instance, in the absence of evidence of lung disease and the presence of a low erythropoietin level, perhaps an arterial oxygen saturation determination is not required to evaluate the possibility of hypoxemia as a cause of erythrocytosis. If hypoxemia is the cause of erythrocytosis, the erythropoietin level should be high.

Although a bone marrow evaluation is not one of the initial diagnostic criteria, this test may prove important in cases in which the cause of erythrocytosis remains uncertain. Approximately 50% of patients with erythrocytosis secondary to PV have a clonal cytogenetic abnormality. Thus, a clonal cytogenetic abnormality confirms the diagnosis of PV if the cause of erythrocytosis remains problematic. In addition, in the presence of thrombocythemia, it is important to perform cytogenetic studies to be certain that a Philadelphia chromosome–positive chronic myelogenous leukemia is not the cause.

At initial presentation, some patients with PV may have only a high-normal hematocrit because of concomitant iron deficiency. This is especially true in women, due to menstrual blood loss, or in either sex if recent acute bleeding occurred and may obscure the diagnosis. For problematic cases, the presence of endogenous erythroid colonies can be studied. Patients with PV may have endogenous in vitro erythroid colony formation, without the need for additional exogenous erythropoietin added to the culture system. Thus, tests such as the leukocyte alkaline phosphatase assay score and vitamin B_{12} levels are less informative than these newer tools.

CLINICAL FEATURES

Patients with PV have a multitude of possible presentations. Many have no complaints and are found to have abnormalities on routine complete blood counts. Others present with nondescript complaints such as headache, generalized itching, malaise, bone and epigastric pain, visual disturbances, and tingling or pain in the digits of the hands and feet. Some patients may present with a complication of PV, such as hemorrhage or thrombosis. The thrombosis may be in an unusual site, such as the hepatic circulation. More typically, thrombosis may involve the myocardium, central nervous system, or venous circulation. The diagnosis of a myeloproliferative disorder must be considered in the setting of a thrombosis in an unusual location, or in a young patient. The most important finding on physical examination can be the presence or absence of splenomegaly. One should be careful, however, not to be misled by patients with chronic liver disease, portal hypertension, and splenomegaly. They may have an erythropoietin-secreting tumor causing an elevated hematocrit, specifically, a hepatoma. Other abnormalities on physical examination in patients with PV may be a ruddy complexion, congested conjunctiva, and hypertension. Evaluation of the peripheral blood smear may reveal a thrombocytosis, although the smear can be completely normal. In patients with fibrosis and extramedullary hematopoiesis, nucleated red blood cells and teardrop red blood cell forms may be found in the peripheral blood. A bone marrow evaluation typically reveals hypercellularity with evidence of a panmyelosis and decreased to absent iron stores. Megakaryocytes may be increased in number and found in clumps, especially in the spicule. There may be an increase in reticulin fibers, although these may not be seen early in the natural history of PV. The longer a patient has had PV, the greater the tendency to have increased fibrosis on bone marrow examination. As mentioned, there are no characteristic cytogenetic abnormalities associated with PV, but a clonal cytogenetic abnormality may be found in a significant number of patients.

TREATMENT

The optimal therapy for PV remains controversial. However, as a result of studies conducted by the PVSG, a significant improvement in both diagnosis and management has occurred. Treatment of PV must be individualized, with the guidelines of the patient's age, presenting complaints, and risk factors for both hemorrhage and thrombosis considered.

Phlebotomy Therapy

Patients with PV have an elevated hematocrit. Once the diagnosis of PV has been established with certainty, the hematocrit should gradually be brought into the normal range. To minimize the risk of an elevated red blood cell mass, the patient should have adequate phlebotomies to maintain the hematocrit at less than 45%. Typically, this can be done by subjecting the patient to 500-mL phlebotomies once or twice weekly as tolerated, until the therapeutic goal is met. After this initial phase, the patient should be seen approximately every 4 to 6 weeks, and if the hematocrit is above 45%, additional phlebotomies are prescribed as guided by the degree of hematocrit elevation.

Phlebotomy is the mainstay of therapy for patients younger than 60 years and for women of childbearing age. However, patients older than 60 years, especially those with a prior history of thrombosis, have a greater incidence of thrombotic complications when managed with phlebotomy alone. Thus, investigators continue to study other therapeutic modalities. Antiplatelet agents have been studied in this disorder, in an attempt to minimize thrombotic complications. Aspirin at a dose of 325 mg orally three times daily and dipyridamole (Persantine) were shown not to be efficacious in the doses studied in preventing thrombosis and resulted in a greater bleeding tendency. Some clinicians prescribe low-dose aspirin to patients with PV managed with phlebotomy alone in an attempt to minimize the thrombotic complications of this disorder.

Myelosuppression

Myelosuppressive therapy is recommended for patients who are at considerable risk for thrombotic complications. Hydroxyurea (Hydrea)* is a myelosuppressive agent extensively studied in the management of PV. Hydroxyurea is a ribonuclease reductase inhibitor, and thus its mechanism of action is different from that of alkylating agents. Alkylating agents, such as chlorambucil (Leukeran), should be avoided in the management of PV, as they have been shown to be leukemogenic when used in this setting. To

---

*Not FDA approved for this indication.

date, with the longest follow-up of more than 15 years, patients treated with hydroxyurea in this study do not have a significantly greater incidence of acute leukemic transformation than a historical cohort of PV patients treated with phlebotomy alone. However, further study is ongoing to ensure the safety of this agent.

Myelosuppressive therapy in this disorder should be reserved for patients with the appropriate indications. The initial dose is typically 1.0 to 1.5 grams per day orally. Phlebotomy must be used as an adjunct to maintain the hematocrit below 45% and to minimize the dose of hydroxyurea required to suppress marrow function. The dose of hydroxyurea is adjusted depending on the response of the leukocyte and platelet counts. Many patients require daily therapy, but some require minimal doses of hydroxyurea, such as 1 tablet three times per week, to maintain the peripheral blood count in an acceptable range. Patients who respond need the dose of hydroxyurea to be continuously scrutinized. A complete blood count should be done approximately every 6 weeks and the dose of hydroxyurea adjusted as needed for cytopenias. If a severe cytopenia should develop, the drug should be withheld and reinstituted at a much lower dose. Clinically the drug is well tolerated, although some patients report rashes, oral ulcerations, nail changes, and gastrointestinal disturbances. Some clinicians prescribe allopurinol (Zyloprim) 300 mg per day orally, along with hydroxyurea, to prevent complications of hyperuricemia.

Radioactive Phosphorus

Phosphorus 32 is a well-tolerated agent that is easy to administer. Unfortunately, many clinicians do not have experience using this agent, and a nuclear medicine license is required. ^{32}P is leukemogenic. Approximately 10% of patients with PV treated with ^{32}P develop leukemia. Therefore, ^{32}P should be reserved for use only in the elderly, with a life expectancy of less than 5 years. It is an excellent agent for elderly patients who are at risk for thrombosis, who cannot tolerate routine phlebotomy, or who have poor venous access and thus require myelosuppression.

Interferon Alfa

Interferon alfa is a newer addition to the myelosuppressive armamentarium for patients with PV who require marrow suppression. It can normalize blood counts and diminish organomegaly. However, it must be administered subcutaneously and is expensive, and many patients have difficulty tolerating this agent because of a flulike syndrome it may be associated with. To minimize this side effect, patients can be premedicated with acetaminophen. Its long-term safety in the management of PV needs to be established. However, it is a therapeutic option for patients who require myelosuppressive therapy but cannot tolerate hydroxyurea, or are too young to be treated with ^{32}P.

COMPLICATIONS OF PV

Leukemia

PV must be considered a preleukemic condition. In the long-term follow-up of PV patients treated with phlebotomy only, the PVSG reported a 2% incidence of leukemic transformation. The therapy chosen influences the natural history of developing acute leukemia. Thus, ^{32}P and chlorambucil were shown to increase the tendency to leukemic transformation in this cohort of patients. Therefore, chlorambucil is no longer recommended for use in the management of patients with PV. Acute leukemia developing as a complication of PV is more refractory to induction chemotherapy than is de novo acute leukemia.

Thrombosis

Patients with PV have a propensity to develop thrombosis. Typically, these are life-threatening and can involve the myocardium or pulmonary and cerebral circulations. Unusual thromboses are also seen, such as in the hepatic circulation. Thrombosis can be the first presentation of PV. Although phlebotomy is instrumental in minimizing thrombosis by decreasing the red blood cell mass, patients with PV managed with phlebotomy alone for the first 3 years after diagnosis have a higher incidence of thrombotic complications when compared with patients managed with hydroxyurea or ^{32}P. Patients with a normal hematocrit and/or platelet count may still experience thrombotic complications. Some investigators believe that this is related to abnormalities of platelet function and thus the rationale for the addition of antiplatelet agents to the management of PV.

Spent Phase

A significant number of patients with PV develop the spent phase, also referred to as agnogenic myelofibrosis with myeloid metaplasia. This manifests itself by increasing fibrosis of the bone marrow as seen by bone marrow biopsy, in association with progressive hepatosplenomegaly. Nucleated red blood cells and teardrop red blood cell forms may be seen in the peripheral blood. Some patients go on to develop an apparent bone marrow failure syndrome, requiring transfusional support of red blood cells and/or platelets. Effective therapy to improve peripheral blood counts can be problematic, and the mainstay of therapy has been transfusional support. Androgens, steroids, and more recently growth factors such as erythropoietin (Epogen, Procrit) have been utilized in an attempt to minimize transfusional requirements. For young patients with spent phase PV who require transfusional support, and for those who develop acute leukemia and have an HLA-identical sibling, an allogeneic stem cell transplant is being studied as a therapeutic option.

Pruritus

A frequent clinical complaint is generalized pruritus, which may be exacerbated after baths or showers. Some patients improve with antihistamines; others remain refractory. If pruritus remains severe and poorly controlled, the addition of myelosuppressive therapy to phlebotomy may prove beneficial.

Surgery

Because patients with PV tend to be elderly, not infrequently they require coincidental surgical procedures. Patients with PV requiring surgery are at greater risk because of excessive bleeding and thrombosis. To minimize surgical risk, it is imperative that PV be well controlled, with blood counts approaching the normal level. Postoperatively, early ambulation is an important measure to prevent thrombosis.

Pregnancy

Female patients of childbearing age with PV should be managed with phlebotomy alone. For patients who do become pregnant, because of changes in plasma and red blood cell volumes, the hematocrit tends to normalize. However, because of the increased incidence of thrombosis and bleeding in patients with PV, women of childbearing age must be counseled regarding the risks of pregnancy, and they should be considered at high risk and managed accordingly.

THE PORPHYRIAS

method of
CLAUS A. PIERACH, M.D.
University of Minnesota and Abbott
Northwestern Hospital
Minneapolis, Minnesota

The porphyrias are a group of at least eight individual types of enzymatically caused metabolic disturbances along the heme biosynthetic pathway (Figure 1), mostly inherited but also acquired. There are some chemical and symptomatic overlaps and also many similarities among various types; for example, the acute neurologic manifestations are identical in all four types exhibiting prophyric neuropathies as are many of the dermatologic abnormalities in porphyrias with porphyric skin. The prevalence of the porphyrias is not known and varies: for example, variegate porphyria is rare in the United States and common in South Africa, where it can be found in a frequency of 3 per 1000 inhabitants.

The main manifestations of the porphyrias are neurologic and cutaneous, sometimes affecting both systems simultaneously or in sequence. Liver disease can be caused by protoporphyria and often accompanies porphyria cutanea tarda. Liver cancer seems to be more common in some porphyrias, but the exact prevalence is not known. The clinical picture can vary widely, and porphyria is included with some frequency among a wide variety of symptoms.

Waldenström called porphyria *la petite simulatrice* (whereas syphilis was *la grande simulatrice*). Thus, it is not surprising that clinicians may often think of porphyria when encountering a set of fitting symptoms, but no matter how well the diagnosis might seem established at the bedside, *biochemical proof is required*. This is particularly important when small elevations of porphyrin levels, often coproporphyrin, are found, clearly outside the normal range but often too low to permit the diagnosis of porphyria.

Unfortunately, there is not a single all-encompassing test to determine whether or not porphyria is present. A high index of suspicion is required to diagnose patients with these rare diseases. Patients with porphyria may obtain explanatory information from a self-help group: American Porphyria Foundation, PO Box 22712, Houston, TX 77227.

In patients suspected of having a porphyric attack with neurologic symptoms, a screening test such as the Watson-Schwartz or the Hoesch test for elevated urinary porphobilinogen levels is of great help (Figure 2), whereas patients with porphyric skin disease should be subjected to porphyrin measurements (strictly speaking, porphobilinogen is not a porphyrin). In any event, when the initial test for porphyria is positive, detailed studies are always required in new cases to establish the precise type of porphyria (see Figure 1). Ideally one would like to have genetic testing, but this is not yet clinically available. Even the next best test, enzyme measurements along the heme biosynthetic pathway, are not yet a clinical routine (except for acute intermittent porphyria), and one has to rely on assays for porphyrins and their precursors, best done in a specialized laboratory with subsequent expert interpretation of the results.

Although one may divide the porphyrias into hepatic and erythropoietic according to the predominant site of the porphyric disturbance, a clinically more useful separation is into acute and nonacute porphyrias.

THE ACUTE PORPHYRIAS

All signs and symptoms of the acute attack are attributable to neurologic disturbances, the cause of which is not completely elucidated. Two hypotheses are frequently discussed: (1) a toxic phenomenon due to an excess of porphyrins and/or their precursors; and (2) an intracellular deficiency of heme. Four types of porphyria have to be considered here: (1) plumboporphyria (from latin *plumbum* meaning lead, because it resembles lead poisoning); (2) acute intermittent porphyria (the most common acute porphyria in the United States); (3) hereditary coproporphyria (often misdiagnosed when small, clinically unimportant elevations of coproporphyrin are found); and (4) variegate porphyria (also called South African porphyria). The acute attack and its management are the same in all four acute, inducible (drug-sensitive) types (see Figure 2). The background is always genetic, and a positive family history can be of immense value. Precipitating factors must be searched for and, if found, at once eliminated. The past clinical abundance of barbiturates and sulfonamides made these common culprits and should be avoided in all patients with an acute porphyria. Nowadays a wide variety of different drugs and circumstances must be considered (Table 1), but in a sub-

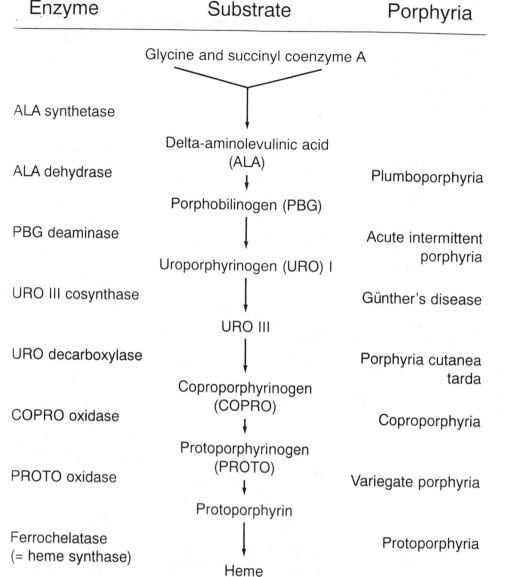

Enzyme	Substrate	Porphyria
	Glycine and succinyl coenzyme A	
ALA synthetase		
	Delta-aminolevulinic acid (ALA)	
ALA dehydrase		Plumboporphyria
	Porphobilinogen (PBG)	
PBG deaminase		Acute intermittent porphyria
	Uroporphyrinogen (URO) I	
URO III cosynthase		Günther's disease
	URO III	
URO decarboxylase		Porphyria cutanea tarda
	Coproporphyrinogen (COPRO)	
COPRO oxidase		Coproporphyria
	Protoporphyrinogen (PROTO)	
PROTO oxidase		Variegate porphyria
	Protoporphyrin	
Ferrochelatase (= heme synthase)		Protoporphyria
	Heme	

Figure 1. Heme biosynthetic pathway. Enzymes whose defects or deficiencies cause the different porphyrias are listed on the corresponding left side.

stantial number of attacks no inducer can be found. Although these porphyrias are inherited autosomally, women, especially of childbearing age, suffer more frequently from attacks, pointing toward the importance of the hormonal background and suggesting great caution with hormonal manipulation such as with oral contraceptives and menopausal estrogen (best given in a low dose as a transdermal application). The list of so-called safe (Table 2) and unsafe (see Table 1) drugs (and other inducing circumstances) can never be complete because new drugs are frequently introduced and because no infallible test exists to address their potential porphyrogenicity. If no alternative drugs exist, even unsafe drugs may have to be used in life-threatening situations because little is gained by endangering a patient's life out of fear that the porphyria might be exacerbated. Furthermore, it is not possible to predict how a given patient might react to a drug, safe or unsafe.

Cardinal findings in a porphyric attack include otherwise unexplained, often colicky abdominal pain and an at times disproportional tachycardia in which a pulse of about 140 beats per minute might be seen in an afebrile patient at rest and without a cardiac history. Previous abdominal surgeries are not infrequent. A screening test for excessive amounts of porphobilinogen such as the one described by Watson and Schwartz or by Hoesch should be available in every hospital and emergency room where acute care is delivered. A random urine sample and a few chemicals, mainly Ehrlich's aldehyde, are needed, and the interpretation of the test is visual. If properly executed, the test takes about 10 minutes and if negative rules out a porphyric attack (with the exception of the extremely rare plumboporphyria, in which no elevation of porphobilinogen levels is found; a clinically useful rapid screening test for excessive amounts of δ-aminolevulinic acid is not yet available). Spontaneous darkening of the urine when exposed to light and to air (due to transformation of

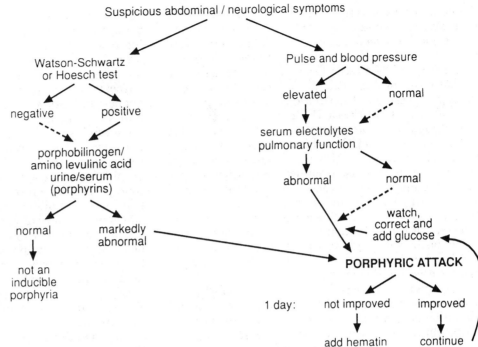

Figure 2. Algorithm for the diagnosis and therapy of a porphyric attack

porphobilinogen to porphobilin) is a helpful hint of an acute porphyria.

The porphyric neuropathy resembles the Guillain-Barré syndrome, and the much-feared ascending paralysis with respiratory insufficiency has to be carefully watched for with frequent assessment of the patient's respiratory function. Intubation and ventilator support may become necessary. Seizures occur not infrequently, facilitated by the often-present syndrome of inappropriate secretion of antidiuretic hormone, inducing sometimes extremely low serum sodium levels (as low as about 100 mEq per liter). Anticonvulsive therapy is difficult in this setting because only bromides can be considered safe (among newer anticonvulsants, gabapentin [Neurontin] seems promising). Clonazepam (Klonopin) seems the least porphyrogenic of the more commonly used anticonvulsants, but frequent monitoring of urinary porphyrin precursor excretion is mandatory, as it is for the use of all drugs not listed as safe (see Table 2).

The acute porphyric attack is a medical emergency requiring swift and decisive action (see Figure 2). Discontinuation of as many drugs as possible is necessary. A negative caloric balance can be an inducer and is best reversed with daily administration of 400 grams of carbohydrate, either by mouth or intravenously (total parenteral nutrition is less suitable and at least initially not necessary). In addition to carbohydrates, hematin should be given as soon as the porphyric attack is established beyond doubt. This lyophilized drug can be obtained as hemin (Panhematin) from the manufacturer (Abbott Laboratories, 800-255-5162, or after hours, 847-937-7970) and should be given in a dose of 2 to 4 mg per kg twice daily* for 3 days. Longer administrations have not been shown to offer substantial additional benefit. Hematin regularly causes a coagulopathy of at least a mild degree, necessitating daily measurements of

*Exceeds dosage recommended by the manufacturer.

TABLE 1. **Unsafe Drugs and Inducers of Porphyric Attacks (Selected List)**

Infections	Meprobamate
Weight loss (starvation!)	Chloramphenicol
Alcohol	Chloroquine
Stress?	Danazol
Pregnancy	Ergot
All inducers of cytochrome P-450	Eucalyptus oil
and of heme turnover	Glutethimide
Sulfonamides	Imipramine
Barbiturates	Methyldopa
Estrogens*	Phenylbutazone
Griseofulvin	Theophylline
Phenytoin	Tolbutamide

*Considered safe in small replacement doses.

TABLE 2. **Safe Drugs for Patients with an Inducible Porphyria (Selected List)**

Aspirin	Labetalol
Atropine	Meperidine (Demerol)
Bromides	Methadone
Bupivacaine	Morphine
Buserelin*	Nitrous oxide
Chloral hydrate	Paraldehyde
Chlorpromazine	Penicillin
Corticosteroids	Propranolol
Digoxin (Lanoxin)	Succinylcholine
Gallamine	Tetracycline
Fentanyl	D-Tubocurarine
Isoflurane	Vitamins

*Not available in the United States.

platelets and prothrombin time. Concomitant use of anticoagulants should be avoided. A thrombophlebitis is sometimes seen, especially if the hematin preparation is not reconstituted immediately before administration. The newer form of hematin as heme arginate (Normosang) is better tolerated but at present only available in the United States as an investigational drug (409-772-4661). Early therapeutic interventions with carbohydrates and, if necessary, with hematin are mandatory because porphyric damage must be avoided. Although a good biochemical response is always seen, clinical remission hinges on early employment of these interventions. A good response can be expected within a day. Long-term disabilities are rare once the acute attack is survived, especially if rehabilitation is offered. Anesthesia can nowadays be safely administered, if barbiturates are avoided. Pregnancy poses an only slightly increased risk for a porphyric attack.

Prevention of attacks is of great importance. Patients should be instructed about their porphyria and should be encouraged to seek consultations with experts. Abrupt weight loss (crash diets), smoking, and alcohol ingestion are to be avoided by patients with an acute type of porphyria because these are known inducers. Once an inherited porphyria has been diagnosed, family studies are of great importance. Identification of patients and carriers with an appropriate bracelet is advisable.

THE NONACUTE PORPHYRIAS

Among the nonacute porphyrias, porphyria cutanea tarda is by far the most common, never leading to attacks or other neurologic symptoms and mainly a cutaneous problem, fairly easily handled with phlebotomies, in which in approximately 2-week intervals 300 to 400 mL of blood is withdrawn (the beneficial effect is due to the removal of iron). A total of up to 10 liters might be necessary over time with careful attention to the hematocrit. Improvement in the skin condition should be expected in approximately half a year. Once remission has been attained, the skin appearance dictates the frequency of subsequent phlebotomies (porphyrin measurements are not necessary). Should phlebotomies fail or be contraindicated in patients with anemia or cardiovascular or pulmonary compromise or those undergoing dialysis, small doses of chloroquine* (125 mg twice weekly) can be used. The skin shows varied degrees of blistering and fragility, mostly on sun-exposed areas. Even after healing, a mild discoloration and scleroderma-like plaques may remain, as do milia, small whitish intradermal inclusions. Patients are sensitive to alcohol and estrogens, but this sensitivity should not be confused with that in the acute porphyrias. Facial hypertrichosis and a violaceous hue are often seen. There are two forms of porphyria cutanea tarda, the inherited (familial) type and the sporadic form, both clinically indistinguishable. The

---

*Not FDA approved for this indication.

enzymatic defect alone does not seem sufficient to bring out the clinical picture, but revealing or unveiling factors must be present, most commonly alcohol (even in small amounts) and now also hepatitis C and the acquired immune deficiency syndrome. Hepatocellular carcinomas are seen with some frequency in patients with porphyria cutanea tarda, and periodic measurements of alpha-fetoprotein seem advisable. Among the acute porphyrias, variegate as well as hereditary coproporphyria can at times have skin manifestations resembling those in porphyria cutanea tarda but not requiring specific therapy besides protection of the skin from sunlight and from even minor trauma. In these cases, phlebotomies and chloroquine are contraindicated.

Protoporphyria can at times be seen early in childhood, occasionally diagnosed as exquisite sun sensitivity or as allergy. Diagnosis is made by measurement of protoporphyrin in stool (because it is so poorly water soluble that it is not found in urine). The skin manifestation (photosensitivity with often instant and severe itching, blistering, and ulcerations) usually responds well (in about 80% of patients) to β-carotene (up to 400 mg orally per day for adults), but porphyrin production is not affected by this therapy. A more frequently found manifestation of protoporphyria is liver involvement, in which the hepatocytes become choked by protoporphyrin. Therapeutic interventions with hematin, colestyramine, bile salts, or charcoal have been disappointing, and liver transplantation seems to be the only reasonable therapy should liver failure be present or imminent. Because the erythron is the main production site for protoporphyrin, bone marrow transplantation seems to hold some promise.

Günther's disease (congenital erythropoietic porphyria) is quite rare (approximately 100 cases have been reported worldwide) and often severe with profound photosensitivity and subsequent mutilations of ears, nose, and fingers. A hemolytic anemia may require frequent blood transfusions. The often enlarged spleen makes splenectomy attractive, but the benefits of this intervention have been short-lived and often disappointing. Again, bone marrow transplantation and genetic engineering seem to hold some promise.

THERAPEUTIC USE OF BLOOD COMPONENTS

method of
CATHY CONRY-CANTILENA, M.D.
National Institutes of Health
Bethesda, Maryland

Transfusion therapy has changed over the last decade since the acquired immune deficiency syndrome (AIDS) was determined to be transmissible by transfusion. The general public and the average physician appear more aware of the risks of blood transfusion despite the fact that blood is safer than ever before. With the exception of emergency transfusions, signed informed consent before transfusion is now required in many hospitals. Caution is desirable if it means that more thought is given to the appropriate use of blood components and to suitable alternatives, but concerns should not interdict or delay transfusion when it is indicated. Judicious use of blood and blood products is also important, for the demand for blood can exceed the supply, with resultant blood shortages.

The calculated risk for exposure to the human immunodeficiency virus (HIV) via blood transfusion in the United States is small, approximately 1 case per 460,000 units transfused (Table 1). Improvements in blood screening tests for the hepatitis C virus since testing began in 1990 have resulted in a large reduction in the risk for acquiring hepatitis from transfusion compared with the early 1980s. The potential for exposure to a variety of other organisms (such as malarial parasites and trypanosomes) exists, but fortunately, life-threatening infection as a result of blood transfusion in the United States is rare.

Other adverse effects of blood transfusion include a variety of allergic reactions and volume overload. Red blood cell (RBC) alloimmunization occurs with a frequency of approximately 1% per unit transfused. Febrile transfusion reactions, although common, are of limited clinical importance. Hemolytic transfusion reactions occur infrequently (1 per 6000 units transfused). Fatal transfusion reactions are even less likely (1 per 600,000); most are the result of clerical error, especially in emergency situations.

Transfusion must be justified on an individual basis to minimize risk and maximize benefit. Suitable alternatives and adjunctive therapy should be sought for specific clinical situations to avoid unnecessary blood use.

BLOOD COLLECTION AND STORAGE

Almost all blood in the United States is collected from volunteer donors who undergo direct oral questioning before donation to exclude donors at increased risk of harboring blood-borne pathogens. All components are tested for HIV (with two different screening assays), hepatitis viruses B and C, human T cell lymphotropic virus (HTLV), and syphilis to minimize the risk of transfusion-transmitted disease. Compared with the rate of viral contamination, there is a slightly greater rate of bacterial contamination in blood, particularly platelet concentrates, which may be stored for up to 5 days at room temperature.

TABLE 1. **Estimated Infectious Risk per Unit of Blood, 1997**

Infectious Agent	Risk
Human immunodeficiency virus (HIV)	1/460,000
HIV (using HIV antibody plus antigen screening)	1/676,000
Hepatitis C virus	1/103,000
Hepatitis B virus	1/63,000
HTLV type I/II	1/641,000
Hepatitis A virus	<1/1,000,000
Bacteria (sepsis)	1/25,000*

*Risk per platelet unit, lower in red blood cell units in refrigerated storage.
Abbreviation: HTLV = human T cell lymphotropic virus.

Volunteer donors provide approximately 450 mL of whole blood (WB) collected into sterile plastic bags containing a citrated anticoagulant-preservative solution. Blood clots if calcium-containing solutions are mixed with stored blood. To simplify separation, WB is collected into a system of sterile bags, and components are prepared by centrifugation. Fresh WB is separated into RBCs, platelets, and plasma. RBCs can be stored for up to 42 days or further processed (see later). Platelets from single units of blood are referred to as "random donor" platelets and can be pooled with other units to provide a dose immediately before transfusion. Plasma can be refrigerated as liquid plasma or frozen (−18°C) within 6 hours of collection for future use to provide fresh-frozen plasma (FFP). Cryoprecipitate (antihemophilic factor, or cryo) can subsequently be harvested from FFP. Derivatives of plasma, such as albumin and immune serum globulin, are prepared by commercial manufacturers from pools of thousands of plasma units using cold ethanol precipitation.

WHOLE BLOOD AND RED BLOOD CELLS

WB is indicated for actively bleeding patients who have lost 30% or more of their blood volume. It provides both oxygen-carrying capacity by the RBCs and intravascular volume expansion through plasma. The platelets and granulocytes collected with WB are not clinically functional in stored, refrigerated WB. Nearly all WB collected is separated into components for their specific uses. Obtaining WB for transfusion may be difficult, because more than 90% of RBC units in the United States are available as packed cells only and not as part of an integrally related WB unit.

WB can be used in massive transfusion settings such as severe trauma or rapid, unanticipated operative blood loss. In emergency situations or exsanguination in which the patient's blood type is unknown, uncrossmatched group O WB can be administered while crossmatching of compatible units is under way. Crystalloid and colloid infusions should be started immediately to support intravascular volume expansion and tissue perfusion. Rapid infusion of refrigerated RBCs can lower the body temperature; therefore, the use of an in-line blood warmer may be advisable.

In addition to providing intravascular volume expansion, the plasma portion of WB generally contains therapeutic doses of most clotting factor proteins except for the labile factors V and VIII; however, even these proteins are present in reduced amounts. Although massive transfusion with banked blood dilutes out platelets, the use of WB can retard the loss of plasma coagulation factors by dilution. Fresh WB (less than 7 days old) can be employed for neonatal exchange transfusion to minimize potassium load and provide adequate RBC 2,3-diphosphoglycerate content for better oxygen off-loading. There are few other indications for fresh WB. One unit of

WB should increase the hemoglobin level 1 gram per dL in the average adult. For pediatric patients, 3 mL of WB per kg should produce an incremental increase in hemoglobin of 1 gram per dL.

RBCs (given with or without crystalloid colloid solutions) increase the oxygen-carrying capacity and are indicated for most situations in which blood loss results in symptomatic anemia. The hemoglobin threshold at which a patient should be transfused (or the transfusion trigger) should be tailored to an individual patient's needs and depends on the clinical circumstances. Caution is warranted in regard to the level of hemoglobin at which a transfusion should be ordered because ischemic damage to organ systems must be avoided. Yet a hemoglobin level of 7 grams per dL may be adequate, provided there is no impairment of tissue oxygenation or signs of ongoing blood loss. In young individuals or those with chronic anemias, compensatory physiologic mechanisms such as increased cardiac output and improved oxygen delivery to tissues can reduce the need for transfusion of additional RBCs. However, patients who cannot appropriately increase cardiac output due to underlying disease may require transfusion to raise the hemoglobin level enough to ensure adequate tissue oxygenation. Pharmacologic interventions to stimulate erythropoiesis (such as erythropoietin) or to enhance hemostasis (such as desmopressin or ϵ-aminocaproic acid) may reduce allogeneic blood requirements.

The usual dose for RBCs is the same as that for WB, and an incremental increase in the hemoglobin level or hematocrit should be expected and checked after each transfusion episode. One unit of RBCs is infused through a 170-μm filter to remove particulate debris, generally over 1 to 2 hours or as tolerated with careful monitoring for adverse effects. If RBC transfusion therapy does not satisfactorily provide sustained increases in hemoglobin levels, and immune RBC destruction is a diagnostic consideration, radiolabeling selected RBCs to study their recovery may be clinically helpful in influencing decisions for further transfusions.

Acetaminophen can be given to the patient as premedication to prevent nonhemolytic febrile reactions. The addition of solutions other than normal saline can cause hemolysis or agglutination of RBCs and should be undertaken with caution. Chronic transfusion therapy results in iron overload, and chelation therapy should be considered for patients who have received more than 50 RBC transfusions.

Saline-Washed Red Blood Cells

The purpose of washing RBCs with normal saline is to remove plasma. As an added benefit, washing reduces the number of white blood cells (WBCs) by about 80%. Although washing is not the most efficient method of leukocyte removal, it can help to prevent both febrile and allergic transfusion reactions. Saline washing of RBCs using automated equipment can remove 99% of the plasma with a small amount of RBC loss. RBCs used for intrauter-

ine exchange transfusion should be type O, Rh-negative, and washed to decrease potentially high levels of potassium, lactate, and ammonia. Because washing of RBCs violates the sterility of the closed storage system, washed RBCs must be transfused within 24 hours. Transfusion of blood or components that contain IgA can cause anaphylaxis in IgA-deficient recipients. Therefore, washed RBCs may be indicated in this situation if IgA-deficient or autologous blood is unavailable. Washed RBCs for patients with paroxysmal nocturnal hemoglobinuria have been advocated, but group-specific RBCs transfused through a leukocyte reduction filter (as described later) are sufficient in most cases.

Leukocyte-Reduced Red Blood Cells

Leukocyte-reduced (leukoreduced) RBCs by definition contain less than 80% of the original WBC content and specifically must contain less than 5×10^8 WBCs in the product, which is usually sufficient to prevent febrile reactions. Leukocyte-poor products can be achieved by removal of a buffy coat layer by centrifugation, saline washing, or microaggregate filtration. The most effective method of leukoreduction is by way of leukoreduction filters. Newly developed RBC and platelet leukoreduction filters can effect a greater than 3-log reduction in the number of WBCs per unit while retaining more than 85% of the RBCs in the original unit. The use of such leukoreduced RBCs appears to decrease the rate of HLA alloimmunization and may eliminate transmission of such cell-associated viruses as HTLV type I and cytomegalovirus (CMV) by reducing the number of WBCs in the products to levels that are far below 5×10^6 per bag. Unless leukoreduction filters are used to prevent febrile, nonhemolytic reactions, there is generally no reason to use them in transfusion recipients with pre-existing antibodies to HLA antigens or CMV.

Because leukocytes in stored blood products can produce cytokines in sufficient amounts to cause nonhemolytic transfusion reactions in recipients, the use of blood products whose WBCs are removed before storage should decrease the number of transfusion reactions related to cytokines. Although leukoreduction of RBC and platelet concentrates at the bedside is permissible, proper technique in the preparation of a blood product to meet standards set for quality control is probably best achieved by blood bank personnel having expertise in leukoreduction filter use. If bedside leukoreduction is performed, health care personnel should be specifically trained and a quality control program implemented to monitor the process.

Leukoreduced components may also be advantageous for previously minimally transfused patients who will require lengthy transfusion support during chemotherapy or for transplant patients. Unintentionally transfused leukocytes appear to have no advantage for patients, yet the expense of leukoreduction filters limits more widespread use.

Frozen, Deglycerolized Red Blood Cells

RBCs can be frozen using glycerol as a cryoprotectant and stored at temperatures below $-65°C$ for 10 years or longer. After being thawed and washed to remove glycerol, these frozen RBCs are essentially plasma-free and leukopoor. In addition, freezing does not alter their survival or functional characteristics. Freezing, thawing, and washing must be performed by trained staff to prevent hemolysis and maximize recovery of frozen RBCs. Thawed and washed units should be used within 24 hours of deglycerolization. If post-thaw washing is incomplete, osmotic lysis of transfused cells can result in hemoglobinuria. Indications for using deglycerolized RBCs are limited to patients with rare blood types or multiple alloantibodies; autologous storage; and neonatal transfusion.

PLATELETS

Platelets are transfused to effect hemostasis or to prevent bleeding in patients with low levels of circulating platelets or qualitative platelet dysfunction. An individual "unit" of platelets is prepared from WB and contains at least 5.5×10^{10} platelets in 50 to 70 mL of plasma. Transfusing 1 unit of platelets per 10 kg of recipient weight is a useful rule for ordering platelets. Six to 8 units can be pooled to provide a standard dose of random donor platelets for administration to an average adult. Platelets should be administered within 4 hours of pooling. Single-donor apheresis platelets collected with automated instruments should contain more than 3×10^{11} platelets in 200 to 300 mL of donor plasma. A variety of apheresis instruments can collect platelets by centrifugation with little WBC contamination but not with sufficient reliability to prevent alloimmunization to HLA antigens. HLA-compatible single-donor platelets are the components of choice for patients who have acquired HLA alloantibodies and immune platelet refractoriness (see later).

Platelets are generally indicated when thrombocytopenia is due to decreased platelet production in the setting of bleeding (Table 2). With platelet counts of less than 10,000 per mm³, the risk of serious spontaneous hemorrhage is great and prophylactic platelet transfusion is often prudent. Patients with platelet counts of 10,000 to 20,000 per mm³ may be predisposed to bleeding. Platelet concentrate transfusion is advisable in such patients, especially if the patient is actively bleeding, febrile, or septic or if the platelet count has been falling rapidly. Excessive bleeding during invasive procedures may be prevented by prophylactic use of platelet concentrates. For major operative procedures, platelet counts in the 50,000 to 100,000 per mm³ range are desirable and should be maintained for several days. During massive transfusion, platelets may be required to thwart the dilutional "washout" of platelets; 6 units of platelets for every 10 to 20 units of RBCs is a useful rule of thumb, but usage should be monitored with platelet counts. For patients with adequate platelet numbers but qualitative platelet defects, platelets can be administered along with pharmacologic therapy (such as desmopressin [DDAVP] for uremic patients) for bleeding episodes. Rough guidelines to gauge platelet therapy are as follows: for an adult, 1 unit of random donor platelets should increase the platelet count 5000 to 10,000 per mm³. For infants and small children, the same dose should increase platelet counts by 75,000 to 100,000 per mm³. More precise response to platelet transfusions can be calculated with the following formula, often called the "corrected count increment":

$$\frac{\text{Postplatelet count} - \text{preplatelet count}}{\text{Number of units transfused}} \times \text{body surface area (m}^2)$$

A patient can be considered platelet refractory when a fresh (less than 24 hours old), ABO-compatible platelet concentrate fails to result in a corrected increment of greater than 5000 per mm³ on two occasions. Good practice includes monitoring the effectiveness of platelet transfusions with a post-transfusion platelet count drawn 15 to 60 minutes after platelets are given. Factors that contribute to poor platelet increments include fever, sepsis, disseminated intravascular coagulation, hypersplenism, platelet autoantibodies, poor-quality platelet concentrates, and platelet and HLA alloimmunization to HLA- and platelet-specific antigens. If immune platelet refractoriness is evident with a serum screen that is positive for HLA alloantibodies, subsequent avoidance of these HLA antigens using HLA-typed, single-donor apheresis platelet concentrates can improve platelet increments. Platelet crossmatching, although employed in some centers, is not yet a standardized laboratory technique. Out-of-group plasma in which the platelets are suspended can be minimized by volume reduction of the platelet concentrate, albeit this can result in a 10 to 15% loss in the number of platelets administered in the transfusion.

Rh₀D sensitization can occur if Rh-positive platelets are given to an Rh-negative recipient as a result of the small number of RBCs that are transfused in each bag. Anti-Rh₀D hyperimmune globulin (RhoGAM) can be given in standard doses (300 μg per 15 mL of RBCs transfused) to prevent the formation of anti-D in Rh-negative recipients. This is especially important in Rh-negative women of childbearing age.

TABLE 2. **Indications for Platelet Transfusion**

Platelet Count (1000/mm³)	Indications for Platelet Concentrate
<10	Risk of spontaneous hemorrhage
10–50	Perioperative bleeding, fever, infection, rapid decline in platelet count
>50	Bleeding in the presence of platelet dysfunction

The design of platelet collection systems in the latest apheresis devices allows the collection of a highly pure platelet product, with few RBCs and contaminating leukocytes. Pooled platelets or pheresis platelets with greater numbers of leukocytes can be leukoreduced by high-efficiency filters to remove leukocytes and thus decrease the rate of HLA alloimmunization and circumvent potential CMV infection if CMV-negative donors are unavailable for CMV-negative recipients. Platelets can be washed and frozen, but these are not standard techniques for platelets as they are for RBCs.

GRANULOCYTES

Granulocytes are collected by apheresis and have traditionally been used for severely granulocytopenic patients with gram-negative infections. One "unit" of granulocytes contains approximately 0.8 to 3.5 × 10^{10} granulocytes, about one fortieth the number of cells a normal individual mobilizes for infection. Because granulocyte concentrates contain a large number of RBCs (hematocrit, 20 to 30%), the granulocyte unit must be crossmatched and compatible with recipient serum. Because granulocytes lose function rapidly after procurement, they should be transfused as soon as possible after collection, and certainly within 24 hours.

Modern antibiotics have made granulocyte transfusions less valuable, although they are still useful for patients with severe neutropenia (absolute neutrophil count less than 500 per mm^3) and sepsis or continued fever despite appropriate antibiotic therapy or for progressive local infection. They are also used as adjunctive therapy in neonatal sepsis. The utility of granulocyte therapy in fungal infections is unknown. Prolonged courses (weeks) of granulocyte therapy reportedly help patients with chronic granulomatous disease and documented infection. One unit of granulocytes should be infused over 2 to 4 hours. Once begun, daily infusions are given for a minimum of 4 days.

Adverse effects of granulocyte transfusions are common and include fever, chills, and shortness of breath. Respiratory distress can be related to HLA alloimmunization with pulmonary sequestration of granulocytes. In view of the severe reactions and the likelihood that granulocytes will not migrate to sites of infection in an alloimmune recipient, the development of HLA alloimmunization is a contraindication to further granulocyte transfusion therapy unless donors can be found that are HLA matched to the recipient. If amphotericin B therapy is also required, it should be temporally separated from granulocyte transfusion, because pulmonary compromise has been reported with their concomitant administration. WBC concentrates from CMV-positive donors are likely to transmit CMV. The large number of lymphocytes in the granulocyte concentrate poses a risk for transfusion-associated graft-versus-host disease, and these should be irradiated for susceptible recipients (see later). Although irradiation of granulocytes obviates this risk of transfusion-associated graft-versus-host disease, some research has suggested that it impairs granulocyte function. Because hazards of granulocyte transfusion can be significant, the potential benefits should be weighed carefully before a course of therapy is undertaken.

There has been renewed interest in granulocyte therapy with the availability of agents such as granulocyte colony-stimulating factor (G-CSF) that allow the collection of granulocyte products containing approximately fourfold more granulocytes than those harvested from donors stimulated by dexamethasone. Clinical studies using G-CSF–stimulated granulocyte concentrates to demonstrate their survival, functional characteristics, and efficacy may alter indications and the dosing schedule for granulocyte use in antibiotic-refractory infections for selected patients.

PLASMA

Refrigerated liquid plasma contains all the stable clotting factors. Labile clotting factors V and VIII (FVIII), and von Willebrand factor diminish in plasma that is stored at 1 to 6°C beyond 6 hours. Clotting factors are present at an average level of 1 unit per mL, and fibrinogen levels average 1 to 2 mg per mL. The indications for liquid plasma transfusion are similar to those for FFP, except for states in which the labile factors are deficient. FFP contains factors V and VIII and all clotting factors (also at concentrations of approximately 1 unit per mL); levels of all the coagulation proteins can vary somewhat with each unit of FFP. A hemostatic dose for infusion is 10 to 15 mL per kg. To prevent allergic responses to plasma infusion, particularly urticaria, diphenhydramine (Benadryl), 25 to 50 mg, can be used as premedication.

Neither plasma nor FFP should be used for the sole purpose of volume expansion, wound healing, or nutritional supplementation. Indications for appropriate use include specific clotting factor deficiencies when specific concentrates are unavailable or unsafe; traumatic or operative blood loss requiring massive transfusion with documented coagulopathy and bleeding; bleeding or invasive procedures when a coagulopathy exists as a result of liver dysfunction; rapid reversal of warfarin therapy; and treatment of thrombotic thrombocytopenic purpura in conjunction with plasma exchange. Plasma therapy should be monitored by assessment of prothrombin time, partial thromboplastin time, or specific factor levels when appropriate. Plasma infusions will not reverse the anticoagulation induced by heparin.

Advances in techniques to improve blood safety to inactivate lipid-enveloped viruses such as HIV and hepatitis B and C viruses using a solvent-detergent method to treat FFP may soon be available. This will certainly assuage the practitioner's concerns over transmission of these particular viruses but it is hoped not result in overuse or misuse of this precious medical commodity.

CRYOPRECIPITATED ANTIHEMOPHILIC FACTOR

Cryo, the cold-insoluble portion of plasma remaining after FFP is thawed, contains FVIII, von Willebrand factor, factor XIII, fibrinogen, and fibronectin. The yield of FVIII is 40 to 60%, providing 80 to 120 units per bag of cryo with fibrinogen levels usually 150 to 250 mg per bag. Fibronectin has no practical uses yet and is therefore not quantitated for clinical use. Each "bag" has a volume of 15 to 20 mL. The usual therapeutic dose of cryo requires thawing and pooling of 10 to 20 bags to provide an average adult with approximately 2 grams of fibrinogen and 2000 units of the other coagulation proteins. Nowadays, given the availability of safer, virally inactivated or recombinant clotting factor concentrates, cryo is used almost exclusively for its fibrinogen content.

Historically, cryo has been used to control bleeding in patients with hemophilia A, but safer factor concentrates have largely replaced its use in these patients except in dire emergencies. For patients with von Willebrand's disease whose response to desmopressin is insufficient, pasteurized clotting factor concentrates that contain hemostatically effective, high-molecular-weight multimers of von Willebrand factor (such as Humate-P) may be used for large bleeding episodes and in the perioperative setting. However, no clotting factor concentrates are "labeled" for use in von Willebrand's disease. In the future, solvent-detergent treatment of plasma should make cryo safer for use in von Willebrand's disease. Factor XIII and fibrinogen deficiencies, although rare, respond to cryo replacement. Cryo has also been reported to be effective in controlling bleeding in uremic patients with platelet dysfunction. Many physicians use a combination of cryo and platelet transfusion to support patients with disseminated intravascular coagulation until the underlying disease process is controlled. Cryo does not contain factor IX (FIX) and is ineffective for patients with hemophilia B (Christmas disease). "Fibrin glue" is prepared for topical hemostasis by mixing cryo with thrombin directly at the site of bleeding.

COAGULATION PROTEINS (FACTORS VIII AND IX)

Although cryo contains concentrated FVIII, the protein can be further purified. However, yield is sacrificed at the expense of purity. There is evidence to suggest that the cellular immunity may be better preserved in hemophilic patients who receive FVIII concentrates of higher purity. FVIII concentrate is commercially available as a lyophilized product. It is obtained by fractionation of pooled plasma from thousands of donors, and in the past, recipients had a high risk of contracting a transfusion-transmitted disease. Current manufacturing processes, including heat treatment, have probably eliminated the risk of HIV and hepatitis B and C virus transmission. Using recombinant FVIII, licensed and available in the early 1990s, obviates any remaining concerns over transmission of blood-borne viruses. Recombinant FVIII products are the most costly of the available preparations.

FVIII content is expressed as units per milligrams of protein on the label. After reconstitution, FVIII concentrate is administered at 10 to 20 units per kg for episodes of acute bleeding or for bleeding prophylaxis in hemophilia A. Specific doses can be adjusted based on the clinical need, degree of deficiency, and plasma level to be obtained. The FVIII half-life is approximately 10 hours. It can be given as a constant infusion perioperatively. Approximately 10% of patients with hemophilia A who have been treated with clotting factors (including recombinant FVIII) develop FVIII antibodies that can inhibit the activity of FVIII concentrate. Immunosuppression and desensitization strategies have had limited success in these patients. Commercially available anti-inhibitor complex has been effective in some patients with FVIII antibodies who require treatment.

FIX concentrate or prothrombin complex (PTC) is available as the lyophilized preparation of vitamin K–dependent clotting factors II, VII, IX, and X as well as proteins C and S. The units for each protein are specified on the label. PTC is used in congenital clotting factor deficiencies with clinical bleeding and, specifically, FIX deficiency (hemophilia B). The half-life of FIX is 18 to 24 hours. PTC has been associated with thrombosis. As with FVIII concentrate, the risk of acquiring HIV infection or hepatitis is diminished by heat treatment of this blood product. Like preparations for FVIII therapy, high-purity, plasma-derived, virally attenuated FIX concentrates are now available. Further, clinical trials of recombinant FIX are complete, and it has been licensed for use in hemophilia B.

IRRADIATION OF BLOOD

Transfusion of immunologically competent T lymphocytes can initiate a graft-versus-host reaction in susceptible patients. Transfusion-associated graft-versus-host disease (TA-GVHD) has a reported mortality exceeding 90%. TA-GVHD has been reported after infusion of very small numbers of lymphocytes; therefore, leukoreduction alone is probably insufficiently reliable in preventing this potential complication of transfusion. Irradiation of blood or blood components with 25 Gy (2500 rad) is sufficient to inactivate immunocompetent donor lymphocytes. Once the blood is irradiated, the refrigerated storage time for RBCs is reduced to 28 days. Patients at high risk for the development of TA-GVHD whose cellular blood components should be irradiated before transfusion include bone marrow transplant recipients; premature neonates; premature fetuses for intrauterine transfusion; patients with congenital immunodeficiency syndromes (subacute combined immunodeficiency disease and Wiskott-Aldrich syndrome), acute and chronic leukemias, lymphomas, and several other malignancies; and patients receiving directed blood donations from blood relatives. Irradiation does not prevent febrile reactions or transfusion of infectious agents, nor do the blood components carry a risk of radiation injury to the recipient. Despite severe immune compromise, AIDS patients have not yet been reported to develop TA-GVHD and are not currently restricted to receiving irradiated blood components.

ALTERNATIVES TO ALLOGENEIC TRANSFUSION

Autologous (the patient's own) blood is the safest blood. Predonation of the autologous WB is desirable when an elective operative procedure is planned and the patient's health does not preclude blood donation. If a patient is unable to donate a sufficient number of autologous units before elective surgery, using erythropoietin and oral iron therapy to enhance the number of autologous RBC units collected may be worthwhile when there is a high likelihood that more than 3 units of allogeneic blood will be transfused. Alternatively, erythropoetin might be of use perioperatively without collection of autologous blood when the patient refuses blood transfusion. Autologous blood may be refrigerated or stored frozen for future use for rare donor types. Autologous blood should not be transfused simply because of its availability but should be used as indicated just as allogeneic transfusions are.

Several studies suggest that "directed" blood donation (blood from friends and relatives of a specific patient) may carry a greater risk of infectious complications than donations from volunteers because the directed donor is motivated to give blood for specific reasons and thus less likely to self-exclude during donor screening. Directed donations are a form of allogeneic donation and should not be confused with autologous blood. Other methods used to minimize perioperative allogeneic blood use are intraoperative blood salvage, preoperative hemodilution, and postoperative blood salvage techniques. Intraoperative salvage is most useful when a large-volume loss is anticipated (open heart surgery, orthopedic procedures), and postoperative salvage may not save enough to be practical.

Human serum albumin is a plasma fractionation component. Viral inactivation is accomplished by treating this product for 10 hours at 60°C. Albumin is available as 5 and 25% solutions and is the active component of plasma protein fraction. Approximately 96% of the albumin solution is albumin; the remaining 4% is globulin. In contrast, plasma protein fraction contains approximately 83% albumin, the rest consisting of alpha and beta globulins. Albumin is responsible for providing the majority of plasma's colloid oncotic pressure and remains predominantly in the intravascular space after administration; therefore, its primary use is as a volume expander. Support of intravascular volume is particularly important in burn patients and in patients with hypo-

tension and shock. Albumin can be used as a replacement solution after plasmapheresis. Crystalloid solutions are usually used as adjunctive therapy when albumin is administered. Plasma protein fraction has been reported to cause hypotensive reactions thought to be secondary to the presence of prekallikrein activator, and there is no reason to prefer it to albumin.

Blood substitutes are commonly used in clinical practice to provide volume expansion and intravascular oncotic pressure. Most often, albumin solutions are used for this purpose. Hydroxyethyl starch, pentastarch, and low-molecular-weight dextran are less frequently used colloids. Dextrans interfere with platelet function and have been associated with an increased bleeding tendency. Perfluorochemicals are efficient oxygen carriers, but their use in severely anemic patients failed to produce any significant increase in survival of patients in clinical trials, although newer formulations are undergoing testing in clinical trials. Older hemoglobin-based oxygen solutions have been fraught with toxicities such as vasoconstriction as well as renal and gastrointestinal dysfunction. Modified hemoglobin solutions are under clinical study, but such solutions are not yet available to the general practitioner. No RBC substitute has thus far proved safe and effective.

ADVERSE REACTIONS TO BLOOD TRANSFUSIONS

method of
GERALD L. LOGUE, M.D.
*VA Western New York Healthcare System and
State University of New York at Buffalo
Buffalo, New York*

Although of empirical origins, transfusion medicine has emerged as a clinical discipline with a strong scientific base. Advancement in immunology, blood resource management, and organization of services have allowed transfusion therapy to become standard treatment for a large number of medical conditions. Adverse reactions to blood transfusion therapy range from severe life-threatening emergencies to those posing only minor inconvenience. These reactions may be immediate, occurring during or within hours of transfusion, or delayed, occurring days to months after transfusion.

IMMEDIATE TRANSFUSION REACTIONS

Immediate Hemolytic Transfusion Reactions

Transfusion of ABO-incompatible red blood cells, such as type A cells into a type O recipient, results in the most dangerous and most preventable of immediate reactions. Naturally occurring complement-activating antibodies usually cause rapid intravascular hemolysis producing hemodynamic shock, disseminated intravascular coagulation, and acute renal failure. The prevention of acute hemolytic reactions requires special care to identify the blood drawn from the patient for analysis by the blood bank as well as the blood products to be transfused. These identification procedures should be taken seriously, because clerical errors account for the majority of acute hemolytic transfusion reactions.

Effective therapy requires rapid diagnosis. Because symptoms of an acute hemolytic reaction overlap those of a nonhemolytic reaction, all transfusions must be stopped immediately if there is a suspicion of such a reaction. Steps should be taken to identify the cause of this reaction.

Signs and symptoms of an acute hemolytic reaction in a conscious patient include fever, chills, pain at the site of infusion, back or chest pain, flushing, and generalized bleeding. In an unconscious patient, a falling blood pressure, increased bleeding or oozing, and hemoglobinuria may be the presenting signs. When an immediate hemolytic transfusion reaction is expected, labeling of the donor blood and identification of the patient should be immediately confirmed. A sample of blood should be drawn from the patient and sent immediately to the blood bank with the donor blood. After infusion of incompatible blood, the plasma is usually red. Fresh urine should be examined for hemoglobin.

If an acute hemolytic reaction is verified, therapy must begin immediately to maintain blood pressure, intravascular volume, blood pH, urine alkalinity, and urine output. Hypotension should be treated with volume replacement, and a screen for disseminated intravascular coagulation should be ordered. If the patient has overt disseminated intravascular coagulation, therapy with cryoprecipitate, 2 to 4 units, should be given if the fibrinogen level is less than 100 mg per dL; platelets, 4 to 6 individual units, should be given if the platelet count is less than 50,000 per mm^3 and fresh-frozen plasma, 1 to 3 units as tolerated by fluid volume status, given if the partial thromboplastin time is elevated. Mannitol or furosemide (Lasix) should be used as necessary to prevent acute tubular necrosis. Urine output and serum electrolyte and creatinine levels should be monitored closely. Immediate hemodialysis may be required.

Acute Febrile Reactions

Febrile nonhemolytic reactions are characterized by fever and tachycardia. These reactions occur in previously transfused or multiparous patients and are caused by antileukocyte antibodies. When fever occurs during a blood transfusion, the transfusion should be stopped and the patient studied for a hemolytic reaction. If a hemolytic reaction has not occurred, antipyretics such as acetaminophen may be administered. If recurrent febrile reactions occur, it may be necessary to premedicate the patient with antipyretics before the transfusion. Associated white blood cell antibodies can rarely produce a transfu-

sion-associated acute respiratory distress syndrome that is characterized by acute pulmonary edema with normal cardiac function. Microaggregate filters are useful to prevent febrile transfusion reactions as well as transfusion-associated acute respiratory distress syndrome.

Rarely, blood products become contaminated with bacteria. Some gram-negative organisms such as species of *Yersinia* and *Pseudomonas* can survive and multiply under refrigerated conditions. The recipient has fever and signs and symptoms of sepsis. If this complication is suspected, the transfusion must be discontinued and the blood product must be cultured and gram stained immediately. If a contaminated transfusion is suspected, therapy should include support of the patient's blood pressure, kidney function, and tissue oxygenation. Shock, if present, is caused by infusion of endotoxin, but broad-spectrum antibiotics should also be started pending the results of culture.

Acute Urticarial Reactions

Hives occur in approximately 3% of patients receiving blood transfusions and usually are caused by a reaction to plasma antigens present in the transfused blood. Such reactions are rarely serious. To treat this reaction, the transfusion is stopped and an antihistamine such as diphenhydramine administered. The patient is then watched carefully for 10 to 30 minutes. If further signs and symptoms of allergic reactions such as dyspnea, wheezing, chills, or fever ensue, epinephrine may be given.

Anaphylactic Reactions

Patients who are IgA deficient may experience anaphylactic reactions after receiving blood products. These reactions are caused by antibodies against IgA, usually in individuals previously exposed to blood products. The incidence of severe IgA deficiency in the general population is approximately 0.1%. If an anaphylactic reaction to blood products is suspected, the patient should have quantitation of serum IgA levels before further transfusion therapy is attempted.

Congestive Heart Failure

Hypervolemia may occur when blood is rapidly given to patients with compromised cardiovascular status. Such patients should obviously receive packed red blood cells rather than whole blood. For patients with severe chronic anemia who have evidence of congestive heart failure, packed red blood cells should be infused slowly with the patient in a semiupright position. Packed red blood cell transfusions are usually well tolerated, and the increased oxygen-carrying capacity of the blood hastens the patient's overall improvement.

Complications of Massive Blood Product Transfusion

Other immediate reactions include the potential for citrate toxicity. With massive infusions of large volumes of blood products containing citrate, it is potentially possible to decrease ionized calcium levels. When massive transfusions are being given, it is important to continue careful cardiac monitoring, and if arrhythmias related to calcium occur, it is important that intravenous calcium be administered. Also, hypothermia can be produced with massive blood transfusions of cold blood. Acute vascular hypothermia may affect platelet function and produce cardiac arrhythmias. In all situations of massive transfusion, temperature-controlled warming devices should be used to warm blood before its infusion. With large-volume transfusion it is also theoretically possible to produce hyperkalemia by potassium leakage from stored red blood cells. Transfusion-associated hyperkalemia is rare, but in large-volume transfusion situations, careful monitoring for cardiac arrhythmias related to hyperkalemia is also essential. Dilutional coagulopathy and thrombocytopenia are occasionally seen when massive transfusion requirements are met by transfusion of packed red blood cells alone. It is useful to transfuse fresh-frozen plasma and platelets along with red blood cells if the blood loss exceeds an entire blood volume.

DELAYED TRANSFUSION REACTIONS

A variety of complications may occur days to months after transfusion of blood products. Some of these reactions are immune, but the largest number of reactions occurs as the result of the transfusion of infectious agents.

Delayed Hemolytic Transfusion Reactions

Delayed hemolytic reactions occur in patients who have previously been sensitized to minor blood group antigens but whose antibody levels have fallen below detectability by routine screening procedures. After transfusion, an anamnestic antibody response occurs, usually within 2 weeks after transfusion of red blood cells containing the offending antigen. These reactions are characterized by a falling hemoglobin level and hematocrit and a rise in the bilirubin concentration. The direct antiglobulin test may or may not become positive transiently, but plasma antibody against the antigen usually becomes detectable in 1 to 2 weeks. Although the hemolysis remains limited to the transfused cells that possess the antigen, delayed transfusion reactions may rarely produce abrupt intravascular hemolysis with the risk of renal failure. It is important to identify delayed hemolytic transfusion reactions because on subsequent transfusion the antibody may again have disappeared, and blood bank records are the only method of identifying the antibody and preventing recurrent delayed hemolytic transfusion reactions.

Post-transfusion Purpura

Post-transfusion purpura is a rare, delayed reaction of blood transfusion that occurs most commonly after packed red blood cell transfusions. Patients with post-transfusion purpura usually lack a common "public" platelet antigen such as PL[A1] (HPA-1A). When these individuals are transfused with the antigen, an immune thrombocytopenic syndrome that destroys the patient's own platelets is triggered. The reaction is characterized by the abrupt onset of severe thrombocytopenia, usually with bleeding, 3 to 14 days after the transfusion of blood products. Treatment is empirical and includes the use of high-dose intravenous immune globulin (2 grams per kg) and plasmapheresis.

Transfusion-Associated Graft-Versus-Host Disease

Because blood products contain circulating stem cells, a transfusion recipient, especially if immunocompromised, may be inadvertently engrafted with the donor stem cells and develop graft-versus-host disease. The clinical complex of rash, mucositis, diarrhea, and abnormal liver functions from this disease may not be recognized in transfusion recipients. Although such complications usually occur in patients with recognized immunosuppression, they have been described in patients with no known predisposing conditions. Clinical symptoms usually occur 1 to 2 weeks after transfusion and are almost invariably fatal. Thus, it is extremely important that patients with known or suspected immunodeficiency syndromes receive irradiated blood products. It is also recommended that blood irradiation be used for directed donations from first-degree relatives.

Viral Agents

Hepatitis Viruses

Three of the hepatitis viruses, hepatitis B, C, and D viruses, are transmitted by transfusion of blood products. The infectious hepatitis agents A and E are rarely transmitted and only in certain unique clinical circumstances. Screening of blood for hepatitis B virus is well characterized and effectively eliminates the transfusion of this agent by blood products. There are rare mutant forms of hepatitis B virus that apparently do not express antigens recognized by the viral screening procedures. Hepatitis C testing for transfusion products now involves "third-generation" anti–hepatitis C antibody testing that eliminates the vast majority of hepatitis C transmissions. Thus, with the advent of rigorous testing for the various hepatitis viruses, the likelihood of transmitting viral hepatitis has been reduced to the range of 1% or less in most areas.

Retroviruses

Human immunodeficiency virus types 1 and 2 (HIV-1 and HIV-2) and human T cell lymphotropic virus types I and II (HTLV-I and HTLV-II) may be transmitted by blood products. Prevention of transmission of HIV in blood products is accomplished by several mechanisms. The first includes rigorous questioning to exclude individuals likely to be infected with the virus and immunologic screening, including testing for HIV antibodies and most recently HIV antigen testing in transfusion products. These testing procedures make the transmission of HIV by transfusion extraordinarily rare. HTLV screening also occurs, although debate continues as to the value of such screening. As in other situations described previously, leukodepletion may markedly reduce the transmissibility of agents such as HTLV.

Herpesvirus

The herpesviruses cytomegalovirus and Epstein-Barr virus are known to be transmitted by blood products. Most individuals receiving transfusion therapy are immune to Epstein-Barr virus, so the significance of transmission of this virus is questionable. Cytomegalovirus can also be transmitted by transfusion of blood products, and cytomegalovirus-negative blood is used in certain restricted situations such as for low-birth-weight infants and bone marrow transplant recipients. It is also clear that leukodepletion of blood products markedly reduces the transmissibility of cytomegalovirus infection.

Parvovirus

Parvovirus, an agent that produces erythroid hypoplasia, may be transmitted by transfusion. Parvovirus-induced aplastic anemia is a risk in patients with underlying hematologic diseases with increased red blood cell production such as patients with sickle cell disease. There is no effective method to screen transfusion products for this virus.

Transmission of Other Infections

Rare diseases transmitted by transfusion therapy include malaria, trypanosomiasis, babesiosis, and syphilis. Transmission of falciparum, vivax, and ovale malaria has been controlled by deferring the donation of blood by potentially exposed individuals for 6 months. Persons who have been infected with *Plasmodium malariae* are excluded from blood donation because of the high incidence of asymptomatic carriers of this disease. *Trypanosoma cruzi* causes Chagas' disease in Latin America. Transmission in developed countries has occurred through blood donations from immigrants from areas endemic for this agent. Creutzfeldt-Jakob disease could theoretically be transmitted by transfusion, but no cases of such transmission have been clearly proved. Epidemiologic studies continue in this area. Finally, transmission of *Treponema pallidum,* the causative agent of syphilis, is possible through blood transfusion. Current serologic testing includes studies to detect circulating antibodies to these agents. Although some have suggested that syphilis screening is no longer necessary for blood products, it is likely that identifying individuals who have been exposed to syphilis is also a surrogate marker for other sexually transmitted infections and therefore a useful means of excluding blood donors who are potentially infectious with retroviruses.

Immune Modulation

Controversy exists regarding the role of transfusion of blood products in modulation of the recipient's immune system. This immune modulation probably occurs through exposure of the individual to donor leukocytes. Some retrospective clinical studies suggest that recurrence of tumors is increased after resection in individuals who have received blood products. Also, both retrospective and prospective human studies have found an increase in postoperative bacterial infections in individuals receiving transfusion therapy. This increased risk of bacterial infection appears to be reduced with leukodepleted blood products. Clinical studies in this area are continuing. Leukoreduced blood products are also useful for reducing primary HLA alloimmunization in transfusion recipients. Leukoreduction is clearly most beneficial for prevention of recurrent febrile nonhemolytic transfusion reactions as described previously.

Iron Overload

Chronic transfusion therapy carries the long-term risk of iron overload. Transfusions in the range of 50 to 100 units of red blood cells carry the risk of tissue damage similar to that seen with idiopathic hemochromatosis, including endocrine, hepatic, and cardiac failure. Symptoms of iron overload may be insidious, and the clinical diagnosis may not be established early. The iron chelation agent deferoxamine (Desferal) is available but difficult to use. Clearly, the judicious use of chronic transfusions is indicated, including erythropoietin administration whenever possible.

Section 6

The Digestive System

CHOLELITHIASIS AND CHOLECYSTITIS

method of
DAVID L. NAHRWOLD, M.D.
Northwestern University Medical School
Chicago, Illinois

An estimated 25 million people in the United States harbor gallstones. Less than half of these develop symptoms, and 500,000 to 700,000 cholecystectomies are performed annually. Epidemiologic studies clearly show that only symptomatic patients should be treated.

SYMPTOMATIC CHOLELITHIASIS

Cholelithiasis, the presence of gallstones, may become manifest by an episode of pain in the area of the gallbladder, which includes the right upper quadrant and epigastrium. These episodes, called biliary colic, often occur after large meals and result from cholecystokinin-induced contraction of the gallbladder during obstruction of its outlet by a stone. The pain characteristically radiates around the right side toward the tip of the right scapula, but radiation is to the substernal region in some patients. The pain typically increases in intensity during 10 to 15 minutes and remains steady for approximately 30 minutes to 5 hours, subsiding rapidly. Nausea and vomiting are the only other frequent symptoms. Systemic signs and symptoms of inflammation are absent.

Physical examination reveals tenderness and guarding localized to the right upper quadrant and epigastrium but no signs of acute inflammation or peritonitis, such as involuntary guarding and rebound or percussion tenderness. The intensity of the pain varies greatly. Some patients seek immediate medical attention because of the pain or fear that they are having a heart attack. The differential diagnosis includes gastroesophageal reflux, esophageal spasm, angina or myocardial infarction, and right-sided pneumonia. Other acute abdominal conditions such as pancreatitis and acute duodenal or gastric ulcer must be considered. The diagnosis of gallstones is best made by gallbladder ultrasonography, which demonstrates the stones in more than 95% of patients who harbor them. Cholescintigraphy, or nuclear scanning after injection of technetium Tc 99m

bound to an iminodiacetic acid, does not demonstrate gallstones and should be used only in cases of suspected acute cholecystitis (described later).

Repeated attacks of biliary colic and acute cholecystitis lead to chronic cholecystitis, characterized by chronic inflammation and fibrosis of the gallbladder wall, dysfunction of the gallbladder, fatty food intolerance, nausea, vomiting, belching, and episodes of upper abdominal discomfort.

Treatment of Biliary Colic and Chronic Cholecystitis

Laparoscopic cholecystectomy should be recommended in patients who do not have significant risk factors to prevent future attacks and the morbidity associated with the development of acute cholecystitis. The operation should be performed electively. The frequency of subsequent attacks of gallbladder colic is reduced in patients who avoid all forms of fat in their diets, but this is not always effective and is impractical long-term therapy. Medical therapy with gallstone dissolution agents, gallstone lithotripsy, and instillation of methyl *tert*-butyl ether are safe but not as effective as cholecystectomy because of gallstone recurrence, which approximates 50% within 5 years.

ACUTE CHOLECYSTITIS

Approximately 20% of cholecystectomies are performed for acute cholecystitis, an acute inflammation of the gallbladder that, left untreated, can lead to complications including gangrene and perforation of the gallbladder, pericholecystic abscess, and cholecystoenteric fistula with or without gallstone ileus.

Acute Calculous Cholecystitis

Approximately 95% of patients with acute cholecystitis have gallstones. They develop constant right upper quadrant pain with radiation to the right scapula that becomes progressively severe. Nausea, vomiting, and fever are often present. Patients usually seek medical attention because of the severity of the pain. On physical examination, they have voluntary and involuntary guarding in the region of the gallbladder and, if localized peritonitis has developed, rebound and percussion tenderness. The differential diagnosis includes perforated peptic ulcer and acute pancreatitis. Objective signs of inflammation including fever, elevated white blood cell count, and a shift to immature leukocytes on the differential count are usually present. Biliary scintigraphy is the specific test for acute calculous cholecystitis, because obstruction of the cystic duct, a sine qua non of the disease, prevents the nuclide from entering the gallbladder.

Treatment

Initial therapy should be intravenous fluids, nothing by mouth, and administration of a broad-spectrum antibiotic. Cholecystectomy should be performed when the condition of the patient is optimized. Most surgeons experienced in laparoscopic cholecystectomy prefer this method. However, the edema and inflammation may make identification of important structures difficult, so that the rate of conversion to the open procedure is higher than when the operation is performed electively. Formerly, patients were kept in the hospital and treated medically until the inflammation subsided, with the plan to remove the gallbladder 6 weeks later when the procedure would be easier. This is no longer necessary. Immediate cholecystectomy reduces the pain and suffering, shortens the length of hospitalization, eliminates the possibility of another episode after recovery from the first, and permits a more rapid return to normal activity.

Acute Acalculous Cholecystitis

Acute inflammation of the gallbladder in the absence of stones is found in approximately 5% of cholecystectomies. A majority of patients with this condition have had a recent unrelated operation, burns, or a serious concomitant medical problem. Acute acalculous cholecystitis often occurs in the intensive care unit setting, which makes diagnosis and treatment difficult. The diagnosis is suspected when the patient has unexplained upper abdominal pain and tenderness or unexplained fever and other signs of infection. Ultrasonography and biliary scintigraphy are often helpful. Ultrasonography demonstrates a thick gallbladder wall, pericholecystic fluid, and sometimes air in the gallbladder wall or lumen. Scintigraphy demonstrates the absence of nuclide in the gallbladder, but this test has a high false-positive rate in acalculous cholecystitis because the oral intake of these severely ill patients has not been sufficient to contract the gallbladder and the outlet is occluded by thick bile, called sludge, which prevents the nuclide from entering the gallbladder.

Treatment

The treatment of acute acalculous cholecystitis is cholecystectomy. The risk of operation in patients who have serious concomitant conditions may be too high. These patients should be treated by ultrasonography-guided percutaneous drainage of the gallbladder, which can be performed at the bedside with use of local anesthesia, if necessary. They should be monitored carefully for gallbladder perforation from gangrene, and the abdomen should be explored if perforation is suspected.

Complications of Acute Cholecystitis

Untreated, progressive acute cholecystitis may result in perforation of the gallbladder. This complication may lead to bile peritonitis; a pericholecystic or subhepatic abscess; or a fistula into the abdominal wall, bile duct, or intestine. The discharge of gallstones through an enterocutaneous fistula may lead to obstruction of the small intestine in its narrowest portion, the ileum, by a stone, a condition called gallstone ileus.

LAPAROSCOPIC CHOLECYSTECTOMY

The standard method for removal of the gallbladder is the laparoscopic technique. The procedure is performed by creating a pneumoperitoneum with carbon dioxide, which creates a space within the abdomen for visualization and manipulation of its contents. This gas is nonflammable and quickly absorbed through the peritoneal surfaces into the circulation. Most surgeons insert four trocars 5 or 10 mm in diameter through the abdominal wall. One is used for a small camera mounted on an endoscope for visualization of the abdominal contents on a video screen, and the others are used for instruments for dissection, cauterization, cutting, and retraction. Small clips are used to occlude vessels and the cystic duct. The gallbladder is dissected free from its attachments and brought out through a trocar site after the bile is suctioned from it and, when necessary, the stones are crushed within it. The operation takes less than 90 minutes in experienced hands.

Many surgeons perform operative cholangiography through the cystic duct before the gallbladder is removed. This permits detection of unsuspected bile duct stones, which are managed postoperatively by endoscopic extraction unless they are less than 5 mm in diameter, in which case they will pass spontaneously. On occasion, large stones or a large number of stones are found, necessitating conversion to an open procedure and removal of the stones. Advocates of operative cholangiography believe that the procedure also confirms the anatomic arrangement of the important identified structures and therefore reduces the risk for inadvertent bile duct injury. Others perform operative cholangiography only in patients who are at high risk for bile duct calculi. They believe that operative cholangiography does not prevent bile duct injury, citing cases in which bile ducts were injured after operative cholangiography was performed.

The laparoscopic approach is abandoned when the anatomy of the biliary tract is not clearly evident, when bleeding is excessive and cannot be controlled safely, or when a bile duct or other organ is injured and laparoscopic repair is not feasible. Conversion to the open technique is necessary in approximately 5% of cases.

Open cholecystectomy is preferred in patients who will not tolerate pneumoperitoneum, usually because of severe pulmonary disease, and in patients who need concomitant procedures that cannot be performed laparoscopically. Although pregnancy was a contraindication to laparoscopic cholecystectomy when the procedure was introduced, many reports have documented its safety and efficacy.

Some surgeons discharge patients on the evening of the operation, but most send them home on the first postoperative day. Overnight monitoring in the hospital reduces the remote risk for death due to undetected intra-abdominal hemorrhage or sepsis at home.

Results

Complications unique to the laparoscopic technique include injury to the intestine, great vessels, ureter, or mesentery during insertion of the first trocar. The proved advantages of laparoscopic cholecystectomy over the open procedure are less postoperative pain, shorter length of hospitalization, and more rapid return to normal activity. Several studies show lower rates of wound infection and other complications than previous reports of open cholecystectomy. Overall mortality rates are quite low, in the range of 0.0 to 0.3%, rates achieved for open cholecystectomy before introduction of the laparoscopic technique.

The most frequent serious complication of cholecystectomy is injury to the bile duct system. Whereas the injury rate for open cholecystectomy was approximately 0.2%, rates for laparoscopic cholecystectomy are approximately 0.4%. Experience and improvements in technique may eliminate this problem. Injuries not recognized at the time of operation become manifest by the presence of biliary ascites, drainage of bile from a trocar site, or sepsis. Excision of portions of the common hepatic and the common bile ducts is the most frequent serious error. To rectify this, a biliary-enteric anastomosis, usually a hepaticojejunostomy, must be performed. Some injuries can be treated endoscopically by inserting a stent into the bile duct system through the sphincter of Oddi.

CHOLEDOCHOLITHIASIS

Bile duct stones are present in 5 to 15% of patients who are considered for cholecystectomy. The stones presumably migrate from the gallbladder. Primary bile duct stones occur in patients who have had cholecystectomy and form de novo in the duct system. Patients may be asymptomatic, especially if the stones are small. Symptoms result from bile duct obstruction and typically include upper abdominal pain, transient jaundice or dark urine, and chills and fever (Charcot's triad). Patients may manifest only one or two of these symptoms, which may be transitory or intermittent.

Cholangitis

Cholangitis, inflammation of the bile ducts, results from bile duct obstruction in the presence of bacterbilia, the presence of bacteria in bile. The symptoms include Charcot's triad, but sepsis and shock supervene when ductal obstruction is complete and the biliary system is, in effect, a tense, undrained abscess. This constellation of symptoms is referred to as acute toxic cholangitis.

Diagnosis

When obstruction is present, the liver function tests show increases in bilirubin, predominantly the direct fraction, and alkaline phosphatase. However, results of these tests are usually normal in the absence of obstruction. Ultrasonography is performed to detect cholelithiasis and enlarged bile ducts. Although bile duct stones may be detected, the sensitivity of ultrasonography for them is less than 80%. Computed tomography and magnetic resonance imaging have no role except to rule out other conditions, when necessary. The definitive tests are endoscopic retrograde cholangiography and operative cholangiography.

Treatment of Acute Toxic Cholangitis

Patients who have severe cholangitis and sepsis should receive intravenous antibiotics, intravenous fluids, and cardiopulmonary care in the intensive care unit. The primary treatment, however, is emergency drainage of the biliary duct system. This should be performed even when attempts to resuscitate the septic patient are not completely successful, because sepsis will progress and multiorgan failure will supervene unless the duct system is decompressed. The most frequently used methods are endoscopic sphincterotomy and stone extraction or insertion of a nasobiliary drainage catheter into the duct system. Percutaneous transhepatic biliary drainage can be done under the guidance of ultrasonography if endoscopic methods are unsuccessful or unavailable. If neither of these therapies is successful or available, emergency laparotomy and insertion of a T tube in the common bile duct must be carried out. Stones are removed endoscopically or surgically at the time of drainage if the patient's condition permits or later if it does not.

Elective Management of Choledocholithiasis

Bile duct stones found during investigation for symptoms of biliary tract disease should be managed by endoscopic sphincterotomy and stone extraction. Rarely, large stones require the adjunctive use of extracorporeal lithotripsy. Open choledocholithotomy is occasionally necessary. The treatment of the postcholecystectomy patient who has primary common duct stones is endoscopic sphincterotomy and stone extraction. Open choledochoduodenostomy or sphincterotomy is performed in patients who have multiple large stones not amenable to endoscopic removal.

Management of Stones Found at Cholecystectomy

Stones detected by palpation or cholangiography during open cholecystectomy are removed by choledocholithotomy. Small stones detected by operative cholangiography during laparoscopic cholecystectomy can be removed by special techniques, but large or multiple stones require conversion to an open procedure or postoperative endoscopic sphincterotomy and stone extraction.

CIRRHOSIS

method of
TELFER B. REYNOLDS, M.D.
University of Southern California School of Medicine
Los Angeles, California

Cirrhosis is a pathologic process characterized by diffuse hepatic fibrosis with nodular regeneration of hepatocytes. The normal architecture of the organ is markedly disturbed. The liver is firmer than normal and has a rounded leading edge, and the surface is irregular or frankly nodular. The size of the nodules has some but limited value in indicating the cause of the cirrhosis. Micronodular (<3 mm in diameter) cirrhosis is usually due to chronic alcoholism, whereas macronodular (3 to 20 mm in diameter) cirrhosis is more likely due to chronic viral or autoimmune hepatitis. However, many cirrhotic livers show a mixture of large and small nodules, which makes assignment of etiology from the gross appearance unreliable.

The physiologic consequences of cirrhosis are multiple. Increased resistance to blood flow through the fibrotic liver leads to portal hypertension, which in turn leads to portal collateral flow, reduction of nutrient portal blood flow, esophageal and gastric varices, bypass of the metabolic action of the liver on ammonia and other toxic substances absorbed from the colon, and altered pharmacokinetics of ingested drugs that are metabolized by the liver. The total number of functioning hepatocytes is reduced as cirrhosis progresses, leading to reduced synthetic and excretory functions.

In patients with chronic liver disease, the physical findings that suggest the development of cirrhosis are loss of flesh and muscle tissue in the upper part of the body, development of vascular spiders, marked firmness of the liver edge to palpation, and any finding that suggests the presence of portal hypertension. These include splenomegaly, ascites, and dilated tortuous superficial abdominal collateral veins. Other physical findings such as parotid enlargement, palmar erythema, opaque white fingernails, and gynecomastia are less frequent and less specific.

The various known causes of cirrhosis in adults in the United States are listed in Table 1 in descending order of frequency. In approximately 10% of cases ("cryptogenic cirrhosis"), the cause remains unknown in spite of thorough evaluation. Those causes that are specifically treatable, in the present state of our knowledge, are indicated

TABLE 1. **Causes of Cirrhosis in Adults**

**	Chronic alcoholism
*	Chronic viral hepatitis (B, C, and D)
*	Primary biliary cirrhosis
****	Autoimmune hepatitis
*	Primary sclerosing cholangitis
****	Hemochromatosis
****	Wilson's disease
*	Hepatic vein occlusion
*	Secondary biliary cirrhosis
	Nonalcoholic steatohepatitis
****	Therapeutic drugs (methotrexate, amiodarone, nitrofurantoin, vitamin A)
	Alpha$_1$-antitrypsin deficiency
*	Glycogen storage disease
	Cystic fibrosis
	Sarcoidosis
**	Jejunoileal bypass

*Those disease causes that have specific treatments are indicated by asterisks; the number of asterisks reflects increasing effectiveness of treatment.

by asterisks in Table 1 and should be the major focus of our diagnostic effort. These specific treatments are discussed under separate headings; treatment of the consequences of cirrhosis are reviewed in a general sense.

TREATMENT

General Measures (Table 2)

Vaccination against hepatitis A and B should be undertaken in nonimmune patients at risk for either of these infections. Acute viral hepatitis can be fatal if it is superimposed on already existing liver cirrhosis. Annual influenza vaccination is useful in reducing morbidity.

Ingestion of raw seafood, particularly oysters harvested from warm-water areas such as the Gulf of Mexico, should be forbidden because of the risk for *Vibrio vulnificus* infection, which is often catastrophic in patients with chronic liver disease.

Elective surgery carries only minimally increased risk in patients with compensated cirrhosis (Child-Pugh score less than 8; Table 3), but the risk for a poor outcome or prolonged convalescence increases substantially with decompensated liver disease. This scoring system (see Table 3) was developed to predict the mortality risk from major surgery (portosystemic shunt) but is useful in rating the relative risk for any surgical procedure requiring general anesthesia. Minimally invasive surgery is better tolerated, but in the peritoneal cavity there is a risk for trauma to dilated portal collateral vessels.

Coagulopathy is present in most patients with cir-

TABLE 2. **General Measures for Cirrhosis**

Vaccination for hepatitis A and B and influenza
Avoid raw seafood (*Vibrio vulnificus*)
Limit acetaminophen to 3 gm in 1 d
Check pharmacokinetics of all drugs prescribed
Test for primary fibrinolysis if large hematomas appear
Monitor for hepatocellular cancer

TABLE 3. **Child-Pugh Staging Score**

Parameter	Points		
	1	2	3
Ascites	None	Easily controlled	Difficult to control
Encephalopathy	None	Mild	Severe
Albumin (gm/dL)	>3.5	2.8–3.5	<2.8
Bilirubin (mg/dL)	<2.0	2.0–3.0	>3.0
Prothrombin time* (seconds prolonged)	1.0–4.0	4.0–6.0	>6.0

Class A: 5–6 points; class B: 7–9 points; class C: 10–15 points

*The scores for prothrombin time prolongation are approximate because we do not know the characteristics of the thromboplastin used in Pugh's hospital laboratory.

rhosis with decreased levels of prothrombin and, often, of platelets. Ordinarily, this does not cause spontaneous bleeding. Infusions of fresh-frozen plasma and/or platelets are not indicated except, on occasion, to precede an invasive procedure. Development of a large subcutaneous hematoma spontaneously or after mild trauma suggests the possibility of enhanced primary fibrinolysis that can cause catastrophic bleeding. This calls for testing of either euglobulin lysis time or dilute whole-blood clot lysis time. If this time is substantially shortened, then all invasive procedures, including tooth extraction and arterial puncture for blood gas analysis, should be avoided until treatment has been instituted with ε-aminocaproic acid (Amicar).

Vitamin K administration is unlikely to improve prothrombin time unless there is a possibility of vitamin K deficiency (poor diet plus inhibition of gastrointestinal bacterial production of vitamin K by antibiotic treatment). If vitamin K is administered to patients with cirrhosis, a single injection of 5 mg is sufficient to overcome any deficiency. Vitamin K has no effect on prothrombin time if the abnormal value is due to liver disease. On occasion, intramuscular vitamin K administration causes a delayed, erythematous, tender skin reaction 3 to 5 cm in diameter. Three skin reactions appear if the widespread practice of giving three vitamin K injections is followed.

Cirrhosis can markedly affect the pharmacokinetics of many therapeutic drugs. Current alcohol ingestion with accompanying poor nutrition and glutathione deficiency can enhance the toxicity of some therapeutic drugs by increasing the activity of certain cytochrome P-450 enzymes. Examples are acetaminophen and isoniazid. Reduced functioning liver mass can delay the metabolism of many drugs, leading to higher than expected blood levels for a given dose. One example is phenytoin (Dilantin), an overdose of which can cause a syndrome resembling hepatic encephalopathy with disequilibrium, confusion, and asterixis. Another is chlordiazepoxide (Librium), whose half-life is increased to approximately 40 hours with advanced liver disease. Marked accumulation and prolonged coma can result from 1 to 2 days of 4-hourly administration.

When liver disease has advanced to the stage of cirrhosis, there is a substantially increased risk for development of hepatocellular cancer. This is particularly true for chronic viral hepatitis. The most effective treatment of hepatocellular carcinoma is resection, which can be accomplished successfully only if a minimal amount of functioning liver tissue is removed with the tumor. Regular monitoring (every 4 to 6 months) of serum alpha-fetoprotein levels allows detection of many of the 50 to 75% of primary liver cancers that secrete this protein if ultrasonography or computed tomography is used to follow steadily rising alpha-fetoprotein levels.

Drugs that prevent hepatic collagen formation or enhance lysis of collagen should be helpful for treatment of early cirrhosis. The only such drug currently in use is colchicine.* One encouraging long-term study from Mexico City has been published, using 0.5 mg twice daily. A large-scale, multicenter study in patients with alcoholic liver disease is currently being conducted by the Veterans Administration. Because colchicine is inexpensive and has few side effects, many clinicians are prescribing it for patients with cirrhosis of various causes.

Disease-Specific Treatments

Alcoholic Liver Disease

Many patients with alcoholic liver disease will have substantial improvement with cessation of alcoholism. This is true even when the liver disease has advanced to the point of cirrhosis. This, then, is the primary objective in the treatment of alcoholic liver disease. Unfortunately, only a minority of patients, particularly those in the lower socioeconomic class, can achieve long-term sobriety. Social and family supports are often lacking. Joining a support group such as Alcoholics Anonymous can be helpful, as can long-term supervision by an empathetic physician. Failure to improve in spite of sobriety can be due to progression of coexisting chronic hepatitis C (nearly one third of patients with alcoholic liver disease in the United States have hepatitis C) or may be unexplained.

Long-term treatment with propylthiouracil* has shown benefit in a large, well-designed, randomized

*Not FDA approved for this indication.

controlled trial conducted in Toronto by Orrego and colleagues. The hypothesis of these investigators is that alcohol consumption causes perivenular hepatic hypermetabolism and hypoxic hepatocellular damage and that the hypermetabolism is counteracted by propylthiouracil. The majority of their patients continued to ingest alcohol to some degree during the trial, so another possible explanation for the apparent benefit of propylthiouracil is direct interference in some manner with the toxic action of alcohol on the liver. Propylthiouracil treatment for alcoholic liver disease has not been widely adopted. A second confirmatory trial is certainly indicated but has not been accomplished as yet.

Acute alcoholic hepatitis is commonly a precirrhotic lesion but can be superimposed on chronic alcoholic cirrhosis. It is an inflammatory state characterized by hepatocyte swelling and necrosis; numerous Mallory's bodies; polymorphonuclear infiltrate in the hepatic parenchyma, especially adjacent to Mallory's bodies; and diffuse, mostly perivenular, intrasinusoidal collagen formation. Clinically, there is often jaundice, fever, leukocytosis, and sometimes pain and tenderness over the liver. Numerous treatments aimed at suppressing inflammation and collagen deposition have been tested in randomized controlled trials, all with negative results. These include propylthiouracil, colchicine, insulin plus glucagon, penicillamine, and parenteral nutrition. Corticosteroid therapy has been tried extensively. Results of 13 randomized controlled trials have been published, mostly with negative results. Meta-analysis of a subgroup of patients in these trials with severe disease, i.e., those having spontaneous hepatic encephalopathy or a Maddrey index of greater than 32 (Maddrey index = serum bilirubin concentration [mg per dL] + prothrombin time prolongation in seconds $\times$ 4.6), has suggested some benefit. In three such trials in the University of Southern California liver unit, two published and one unpublished, virtually identical mortality was found in treated and control patients, including many patients with a high Maddrey index. Pentoxifylline is currently under trial in our liver unit because it has been shown to suppress formation of tumor necrosis factor, which is substantially elevated in acute alcoholic hepatitis.

Autoimmune Liver Disease

Autoimmune liver disease presents as chronic active hepatitis with elevated serum transaminase levels, variable degrees of jaundice, raised gammaglobulin levels (polyclonal IgG), and presence of autoimmune markers (nuclear and smooth muscle antibodies). Four fifths of patients are female ranging in age group from children to the elderly. Most often there are chronic features at presentation (amenorrhea, vascular spiders, splenomegaly), suggesting that the earlier stages of this mysterious disorder are often asymptomatic. Extrahepatic manifestations like those seen in systemic lupus erythematosus (Coombs' test–positive hemolytic anemia, arthritis, pleuritis, glomerulonephritis, false-positive serologic test result for syphilis) are present in occasional patients and are responsible for the original name "lupoid hepatitis." Liver biopsy often shows substantial numbers of plasma cells in the portal infiltrate as well as the usual features of chronic active liver disease.

With rare exceptions, such patients respond well to corticosteroid therapy (20 to 30 mg of prednisone daily) with improvement in all liver tests to nearly normal levels within 3 to 6 weeks. If cirrhosis is already present, the serum albumin and prothrombin levels may not become normal, but bilirubin usually returns to a nearly normal level and transaminases to less than 100 units per liter. As transaminase levels improve, the dose of corticosteroid can be tapered to a maintenance level, usually 10 to 15 mg per day. After improvement is evident, most hepatologists add azathioprine* (Imuran), 100 mg daily. With addition of azathioprine, the corticosteroid dose can be tapered further, sometimes to as low as 7.5 mg per day of prednisone. Therapy should be long term (several years), with monitoring of serum transaminase levels to judge efficacy and periodic blood counts to assess possible hematopoietic toxicity from azathioprine (rarely seen at this dosage level). Long-term prednisone toxicity can be manifested as obesity, diabetes, and/or osteoporosis. Exacerbation of active liver disease commonly occurs with treatment withdrawal, even after several years. There is no consensus as to how long treatment should be continued. In our liver unit, we have gradually increased treatment duration to 5 to 10 years because of a high frequency of relapse to active disease after treatment withdrawal. There is published evidence that long-term maintenance of azathioprine at 100 to 150 mg per day will prevent reactivation after withdrawal of prednisone. Lymphoproliferative malignant disease is a potential complication of long-term azathioprine treatment, although we have not encountered this in our liver unit.

Measurement of serum transaminase values at regular intervals, i.e., every 3 months, after treatment withdrawal is important because disease reactivation is often asymptomatic for a prolonged period and it is presumed that active hepatic inflammation can promote fibrogenesis during such periods.

Rarely, a patient with seemingly typical autoimmune liver disease will fail to respond to corticosteroid therapy. This should prompt reconsideration of diagnosis, and if no other diagnosis seems likely, a trial of cyclosporine (Sandimmune)* is indicated and frequently successful in suppressing the hepatic inflammation.

Hemochromatosis

Treatment by iron removal is highly effective in hemochromatosis, particularly if it is carried out before the development of cirrhosis, which usually occurs in the thirties or forties in men and 10 to 15 years later in women. Early case finding, therefore,

---

*Not FDA approved for this indication.

becomes important. One should not wait for a presentation as bronzed diabetes. Fasting serum iron concentration with transferrin saturation and serum ferritin determinations are suitable screening tests with good sensitivity but poor specificity. Liver disorders with substantial transaminase elevation will often result in raised serum iron concentration and transferrin saturation, and serum ferritin behaves like an acute phase reactant and rises in many inflammatory disorders. Although liver density at computed tomography and the appearance of the liver at magnetic resonance scanning can be highly suggestive of hemochromatosis, the "gold standard" is liver biopsy, preferably with accompanying quantitative determination of hepatic iron content. Because the findings on biopsy vary directly with the duration of time of iron accumulation, the iron index (quantitative iron divided by age) is the most reliable parameter for diagnosis. In patients who refuse liver biopsy, serial phlebotomy treatment to the point of anemia allows retrospective calculation of body iron excess.

The most effective method for depletion of excess body iron stores is serial phlebotomy. Most patients tolerate 500-mL phlebotomy every 1 to 2 weeks. Each phlebotomy removes approximately 250 mg of iron; most adult patients with hemochromatosis need 40 to 80 phlebotomies before iron depletion is evident. The only serial measurement needed is hemoglobin; a fall of 2 grams per dL suggests that readily available iron stores have been depleted. If, subsequently, the hemoglobin level rapidly returns to baseline, it is likely that there is still excess iron to be removed. A small folate supplement, 1 mg three or four times weekly, guards against folate deficiency during serial phlebotomy treatment. After depletion of excess iron stores, serum transferrin saturation and ferritin values should return to normal. Because abnormal iron absorption continues throughout life, three or four phlebotomies yearly are needed to maintain normal iron stores. Supplemental iron, as in some multivitamin preparations, should be avoided. Patients who already have cirrhosis at the time of discovery of hemochromatosis are at increased risk for hepatocellular carcinoma, even with iron depletion therapy, so they should have surveillance with serum alpha-fetoprotein determinations every 4 to 6 months with hepatic ultrasonography if there is a suspicious rise in alpha-fetoprotein level. Effective oral iron chelators are being developed with the potential for greatly simplifying treatment.

Hereditary hemochromatosis is an autosomal recessive disease. When an index patient is identified, there should be a search for unidentified cases among siblings and first-degree relatives. Fasting serum iron concentration and transferrin saturation are suitable screening tests. The identification of the abnormal gene for hemochromatosis will greatly simplify case finding when practical tools for gene analysis become available.

Wilson's Disease

Normal copper balance is maintained by secretion of excess copper in bile. Wilson's disease is caused by a genetic defect in copper transport from hepatocytes into bile that reduces copper excretion and causes a build-up of copper in liver, kidney, and brain. The gene responsible for the copper transport enzyme has now been determined, and a number of mutations have been identified.

The disease can present as fulminant hepatic failure, chronic active hepatitis, or cirrhosis. Often there are accompanying neurologic abnormalities resembling parkinsonism. Diagnostic features are Kayser-Fleischer rings on the iris and low serum ceruloplasmin (95% of cases), elevated serum free copper, and elevated urine copper levels. The gold standard for diagnosis is markedly increased quantitative copper content on hepatic biopsy; this is not pathognomonic because hepatic copper content can be considerably increased in chronic cholestatic disorders.

Treatment of Wilson's disease, except for cases presenting as fulminant hepatitis, consists of depletion of excess body copper stores by reducing copper intake and enhancing either intestinal or renal excretion of copper. The most effective means of increasing renal copper excretion is with the chelating agent D-penicillamine (Cuprimine) taken orally at 250 to 500 mg three times daily. This results in cupriuresis of 1000 to 2000 μg per 24 hours in the first few months of treatment. As readily available copper stores are reduced, the amount of urinary copper usually decreases to somewhere between 500 and 1000 μg per day. D-Penicillamine has a number of potential side effects including allergic skin reactions, proteinuria (sometimes to the point of nephrotic syndrome), fever, arthralgias, and a systemic lupus erythematosus–like syndrome. These reactions can usually be overcome by temporary discontinuance of penicillamine; treatment is resumed with small doses initially accompanied by a corticosteroid, which is gradually decreased during a 30-day period while the dose of penicillamine is increased. If this approach is unsuccessful, a second-line chelating agent, trientene (Syprine), can be used at 750 to 1250 mg per day. Treatment must be lifelong.

An alternative treatment, favored by some authorities, is oral zinc sulfate 250 mg or zinc acetate 50 mg three times daily. Zinc acts by preventing gastrointestinal copper absorption. It does this by preferentially occupying the intestinal metallothionine that is the transport mechanism for absorption of both zinc and copper. Negative copper balance is achieved, without any increase in urinary copper, through the gastrointestinal tract. Biliary copper excretion, although reduced in Wilson's disease, is not absent and this, without any intestinal reabsorption, provides the negative copper balance. Zinc plus penicillamine is not a useful combination because the penicillamine preferentially chelates the excess zinc instead of copper. Zinc treatment is much less costly than penicillamine and has no important side effects. However, it takes longer to remove the excess copper. My preference is to use penicillamine for the first few years of treatment, provided that it is well tolerated, and then switch to zinc when readily available copper stores have been substantially diminished, as indicated by 24-hour urine copper values less than 500 μg while the patient is receiving 1.5 grams of penicillamine daily.

When Wilson's disease presents as fulminant hepatic failure, chelation therapy is ineffective and urgent liver transplantation is required for survival.

Primary Biliary Cirrhosis

This progressive liver disease is eight times more common in women than in men. Its onset is usually in the third to sixth decade, and it is often asymptomatic for 5 to 10 years before development of pruritus, jaundice, and fatigue. Extrahepatic manifestations occurring in subsets of patients include osteopenia, thyroid disease, increased pigmentation, elements of the CREST syndrome, and xanthomatous skin deposits. Progression to a fatal termination is consistent enough that a reasonably reliable "risk score" has been developed; duration of survival is predicted from a formula that includes serum bilirubin, albumin, and prothrombin levels and age. Etiology is unknown and presumed to be autoimmune in nature. Diagnostic aids include a moderately consistent histologic change on liver biopsy, presence in serum of mitochondrial antibody (90%), elevated serum IgM level (80%), and a characteristic "cholestatic" pattern of liver test abnormalities with markedly elevated serum alkaline phosphatase and serum bile acids. Treatment is symptomatic and supportive. Vitamin D and calcium supplementation are of some but limited value for prevention of bone disease, which is chiefly osteoporosis. Supplemental fat-soluble vitamins (A, E, and K) in aqueous-soluble form should be given when jaundice appears. Cholestyramine (Questran, 4 grams with each meal) or colestipol (Colestid, 5 grams with each meal) often relieves the pruritus. If it fails to do so, then rifampin* (10 mg per kg per day) and/or bedtime phenobarbital (60 to 120 mg) may be helpful. Ursodiol (Actigall),* 600 to 900 mg daily, has been shown to improve biochemical test results and is widely used, but it remains uncertain whether it prolongs life or increases the time to liver transplantation. Ursodiol is a non human, hydrophilic bile salt intended to partially replace, in the bile salt pool, the normal human hydrophobic bile salts that are hypothesized to be potentially hepatotoxic during cholestasis. Low-dose methotrexate treatment is undergoing a controlled trial on an empirical basis as a result of its demonstrated benefit in other diseases with a presumed autoimmune component, such as rheumatoid arthritis.

Estrogen probably exacerbates primary biliary cirrhosis, so postmenopausal estrogen should be administered by skin patch to minimize the amount that reaches the liver.

Primary Sclerosing Cholangitis

This biliary tract disorder is characterized by irregular fibrosis and stricture formation in the extrahepatic and/or intrahepatic bile ducts. There is episodic jaundice and pruritus and a liver test pattern emphasizing alkaline phosphatase increase. Seventy-five percent of patients have concomitant chronic ulcerative colitis that may either precede or follow the biliary disease. The etiology is unknown. It is not likely to be a direct result of the colitis because removal of the colon does not affect the course of the biliary disorder, which is slowly progressive to cirrhosis, although often with prolonged remissions. Diagnosis is made by cholangiography, which may show areas of extrahepatic biliary narrowing or, more commonly, irregular beading and narrowing of the intrahepatic bile ducts. There are frequently episodes of right upper quadrant pain and fever that resemble acute bacterial cholangitis. Blood cultures are sometimes positive for intestinal organisms during such episodes, so it is customary to treat with antibiotics that are effective against gram-negative organisms, even though blood cultures are often negative.

Supportive treatment for sclerosing cholangitis is similar to that used for primary biliary cirrhosis. Although ursodiol* is widely used, there is less objective evidence of benefit than in primary biliary cirrhosis. Extrahepatic or "dominant" intrahepatic biliary strictures are treated by surgery or endoscopic balloon dilatation, with variable results.

Cholangiocarcinoma is a relatively common complication of long-standing sclerosing cholangitis. Concern regarding the development of this complication leads to relatively early referral for liver transplantation.

Treatment of the Complications of Cirrhosis

Ascites

Ascites in liver disease is caused primarily by portal hypertension with raised pressure in the hepatic sinusoids. The sinusoidal walls are highly fenestrated to facilitate passage of plasma ultrafiltrate into the space of Disse for interaction with hepatocyte microvilli. Raised sinusoidal pressure causes more fluid to accumulate in Disse's space than can be accommodated by the hepatic lymphatic drainage system. The surplus fluid drips from the liver surface into the peritoneal cavity. As this occurs, plasma volume decreases somewhat and plasma oncotic pressure rises. Portal pressure is highly related to plasma volume and decreases with ascites formation. The combination of a slight fall in portal pressure and a slight rise in plasma oncotic pressure brings the splanchnic bed back into balance again, with ascites reabsorption now equaling formation. However, the small decrease in plasma volume results in retention of sodium and water by the kidneys with restoration of plasma volume when sodium ingestion occurs. The original imbalance in Starling's forces then recurs, with formation of more ascites.

*Not FDA approved for this indication.

*Not FDA approved for this indication.

Presence of ascites is usually recognizable by physical examination. In addition, the 24-hour urinary excretion of sodium is low (<20 mEq). To the degree that the dietary sodium intake exceeds the renal output there will be weight gain, approximately 1 kg for each 130 to 140 mEq. Ascites is easily detected by ultrasonography if there is doubt about its presence. Diagnostic paracentesis can be safely performed with a 21-gauge needle inserted in the left lower quadrant, outside the span of the rectus muscle. If ascites is due to portal hypertension, the gradient between serum and ascitic fluid albumin level should be greater than 1.1 grams per dL. This test has a sensitivity of 97% and specificity of 92% for indicating that portal hypertension is the cause of the ascites. Somewhat less sensitive and less specific, but nevertheless useful, is the finding of a total protein level of less than 3 grams per dL in the ascitic fluid.

Management of ascites in portal hypertension consists of managing sodium balance. The sodium concentration of ascitic fluid is similar to that in the plasma. Most patients who form ascites have small amounts of sodium, regardless of their sodium intake, in their urine (usually less than 20 mEq in 24 hours). A positive or negative sodium balance of 130 to 140 mEq will result in an increase or decrease of 1 liter in the amount of ascites present. Sodium intake consists of that taken by mouth or by vein. Sodium output, in the absence of diarrhea, is that present in the urine. Sodium balance can be rendered negative by limiting dietary sodium intake (1 to 2 grams or 44 to 88 mEq daily) and enhancing renal sodium output with diuretic drugs. Because of the hyperaldosteronism present in most patients with cirrhosis, the use of loop diuretics alone (furosemide [Lasix], bumetanide [Bumex], ethacrynic acid [Edecrin]) will result in hypokalemia and metabolic alkalosis. I prefer, therefore, to use combinations of a loop diuretic and a distally acting antikaliuretic diuretic. My usual combination is furosemide, 80 mg, and amiloride (Midamor), 20 mg given once daily, with proportional increases in each drug if there is insufficient natriuresis. Diuretic efficacy is monitored by daily weight recording. Measurement of 24-hour urinary sodium output is often essential in patients who fail to lose weight. The purpose of this measurement is to differentiate between excessive sodium intake (either accidental or deliberate) and inadequate natriuresis. Thoroughness of the 24-hour urine collection should be evaluated by its creatinine content. For those who prefer spironolactone (Aldactone), one 5-mg amiloride tablet is approximately equivalent in natriuretic effect to one 25-mg tablet of spironolactone. In patients with renal impairment, i.e., serum creatinine concentration above 1.5 mg per dL, the distally acting diuretics should be used with caution, if at all, because of concern about dangerous hyperkalemia.

In patients who have peripheral edema as well as ascites, it is safe to pursue rapid diuresis and weight loss. However, in patients with no peripheral edema, diuresis and weight loss should be limited to 0.75 kg per day to avoid hypovolemia and renal impairment.

Nonsteroidal anti-inflammatory drugs, including aspirin, should be avoided in patients who are receiving diuretics because they markedly interfere with natriuretic action by reducing intrarenal production of prostaglandin E.

Many patients with ascites have hyponatremia and excessive output of vasopressin. Fluid restriction in addition to sodium restriction in such patients is indicated.

Approximately 8% of patients with cirrhosis and ascites will develop serious complications with the use of diuretics and are said to be refractory to diuretics. These complications include renal impairment (rise in serum creatinine concentration to 2 mg per dL), hepatic encephalopathy, or a fall in serum sodium concentration to less than 120 mEq per liter in spite of fluid restriction. Diuretics should be discontinued if any of these events occur. In the case of hepatic encephalopathy, it would be wise to exclude unsuspected spontaneous bacterial peritonitis by diagnostic paracentesis. After correction of the complication, some hepatologists would resume diuretic use, hoping that the complication was a coincidental event rather than being diuretic related. Four options are available for management of truly refractory ascites. One is liver transplantation, if the patient is an otherwise suitable candidate. Refractory ascites implies a poor prognosis with less than 50% 1-year survival. A second option is the transjugular intrahepatic portosystemic shunt (TIPS) procedure. In most cases, ascites becomes easier to manage after TIPS placement, but there is an approximately 25% frequency of new-onset or worsening hepatic encephalopathy from this procedure. In addition, the reduction in transhepatic portal blood flow seems to lead to hepatic failure in occasional patients. A third option, peritoneovenous shunt, allows constant replenishment of plasma volume, which seems to facilitate diuretic action and prevent diuretic-induced renal impairment. Disseminated intravascular coagulation is common after placement of this device but can be combated by replacement of ascites fluid with saline at the time of shunt insertion and by use of antiplatelet drugs such as dipyridamole (Persantine) 100 mg every 6 hours during the first 2 to 3 weeks after insertion. Peritoneovenous shunt devices contain a one-way valve to prevent backflow of blood in the tubing, and this valve often becomes occluded with debris or fibrin after several weeks or months and has to be replaced.

The simplest solution to the problem of refractory ascites is repeated, as needed, large-volume paracentesis. Paracentesis is no longer regarded as a highly dangerous procedure. With 2-liter vacuum bottles, it is not as tedious a procedure as it has been in the past, although it is still labor-intensive for the physician. Most patients with refractory ascites have virtually zero urinary sodium output, so the frequency of paracentesis depends directly on sodium intake. A 7-liter paracentesis will have to be repeated every 26 to 28 days, if the patient adheres to a 1-gram (44 mEq) daily sodium intake, compared with every 13 to 14 days if the intake is 2 grams (88 mEq) per day. An unsettled issue about large-volume paracentesis is the need for albumin replacement accompanying the procedure to prevent hypovolemia. In the liver unit at the University of Southern California, our experience leads us to believe that albumin infusion is not needed, whereas members of a highly respected liver unit in Barcelona have data convincing them that 6 to 8 grams of albumin should be infused for each liter of ascites removed. The current high cost of albumin ($3 to $5 per gram) makes this more than a trivial issue.

Spontaneous Bacterial Peritonitis

Patients with chronic liver disease and ascites are at risk for the development of bacterial infection of the ascitic fluid. This may occur at any time and often without the usual symptoms of peritonitis. It is frequently the reason that patients become ill enough for hospitalization, and its onset is often the explanation for an unexplained deterioration in condition of a patient already hospitalized for chronic liver disease. Predisposing factors are advanced and severe liver disease, recent variceal hemorrhage, and low opsonic activity in ascitic fluid. The last is correlated with low ascites total protein levels (<1 gram per dL). Patients with spontaneous bacterial peritonitis may have pain, fever, and leukocytosis, but these are not invariably present. Recognition of spontaneous bacterial peritonitis is achieved by diagnostic paracentesis with the ascitic fluid showing a low total protein level (usually <1 gram per dL) and a polymorphonuclear cell count of more than 250 per mm³. Because of a low density of organisms, ascites culture may be negative in the presence of active infection. If two blood culture bottles are inoculated with 10 mL of ascitic fluid in each, at the bedside, culture will be positive in approximately 90% of cases. Blood culture is sometimes positive as well. Gram's stain of the ascitic fluid is rarely helpful because of the low concentration of bacteria. The most common organisms causing the infection are gram-negative intestinal aerobes, but occasionally *Streptococcus pneumoniae* is present. Anaerobic infections are rarely if ever found. "Secondary" bacterial peritonitis due to gut perforation or adjacent abscess is suspected if more than one organism is cultured, the glucose level in the ascitic fluid is low, and the ascites total protein level is greater than 2 grams per dL (i.e., not at the low level usually found in spontaneous bacterial peritonitis).

Antibiotic therapy should be started when an elevated ascites polymorphonuclear cell count is reported, without waiting for the culture result. A third-generation cephalosporin gives satisfactory coverage. A large study by Runyon and colleagues showed that 5 days of treatment is usually sufficient. The ascites polymorphonuclear cell count should fall exponentially with successful treatment. Repeated diagnostic paracentesis 48 hours after initiation of treatment is useful in that failure to find the expected fall in polymorphonuclear cell count should lead to re-evaluation for secondary bacterial peritonitis or inappropriate choice of antibiotic.

Patients who develop spontaneous bacterial peritonitis have advanced liver disease with limited survival and are potential candidates for liver transplantation. Recurrence of spontaneous bacterial peritonitis is sufficiently common in such patients to justify use of prophylactic oral antibiotics. Randomized trials have shown benefit with norfloxacin* (400 mg daily) and trimethoprim-sulfamethoxazole* (1 double-strength tablet daily). Other randomized trials have shown that prophylactic antibiotic treatment is also useful in patients with ascites total protein level of less than 1 gram per dL, because they are predisposed to have low ascites opsonic activity and a relatively high frequency of the infection.

Hepatic Hydrothorax

In 1966, Lieberman and colleagues from the University of Southern California liver unit showed that the occurrence of massive right-sided pleural effusion in patients with ascites is due to rupture of a tiny hernia located near the dome of the right diaphragm, in a small area where the diaphragm has few muscle fibers. With each inspiration, the negative intrathoracic pressure sucks a small amount of ascitic fluid into the pleural cavity. In some patients, the hernial sac collapses around the tiny perforation during expiration, preventing any of the fluid from returning to the peritoneal cavity. Such patients may have a huge pleural effusion in the absence of any detectable ascites. On rare occasions, hepatic hydrothorax may develop in the left side of the chest. Many patients with liver disease and ascites have pleural effusions of mild to moderate size on one or both sides in the absence of any diaphragmatic perforation.

Management of hepatic hydrothorax is similar to management of ascites. Diagnostic thoracentesis should be done to demonstrate the transudative nature of the fluid to exclude pleural tuberculosis, which is an occasional complication of alcoholic liver disease. With restricted sodium intake and use of diuretics and careful attention to sodium balance, most patients with hepatic hydrothorax can be managed without need for more than an occasional thoracentesis. Should the sodium retention prove refractory to diuretics, management becomes a problem. Peritoneovenous shunt is rarely helpful, presumably because ascitic fluid encounters less resistance in entering the pleural cavity directly than in traversing the long plastic tube. Repeated paracentesis is often not helpful in reducing the pleural fluid accumulation, presumably owing to the valvelike action of the small hernia. Repeated thoracentesis is somewhat more traumatic for the patient than is repeated paracentesis. Attempts to obliterate the pleural space (pleurodesis) with tetracycline instillation are often unsuccessful because of difficulty in attaining

---

*Not FDA approved for this indication.

a "dry" pleural cavity, even with a chest tube in place. The TIPS procedure is effective in most patients with refractory hepatic hydrothorax. Other options are liver transplantation and either thoracotomy or thoracoscopy to find and close the diaphragmatic defect.

Renal Impairment

Creatinine production is reduced in cirrhosis so that normal serum levels are usually less than 1.0 mg per dL. Patients with cirrhosis are subject to several types of renal disease that can lead to renal impairment. Chronic viral hepatitis B or C can cause membranous or membranoproliferative glomerulonephritis associated with cryoglobulinemia or with immune complex deposition on the glomerular basement membrane. Liver disease seems to confer increased susceptibility to the nephrotoxic effects of the aminoglycosides, especially gentamicin, so I avoid this antibiotic as much as possible. Diuretics often cause renal impairment, either by hypovolemia or by systemic hemodynamic effects. This type of renal impairment is functional and disappears soon after diuretics are discontinued or after saline is administered. Cirrhotic patients with ascites frequently develop renal impairment during administration of nonsteroidal anti-inflammatory drugs, probably because of reduction of renal prostaglandin E production. Natriuresis from diuretics is greatly impaired by these drugs even when the increase in serum creatinine concentration is minimal. Patients with cirrhosis may be more susceptible than others to contrast-induced acute tubular injury during radiologic procedures. However, the most common reason for renal impairment in cirrhosis is the hepatorenal syndrome, characterized by intense constriction of the renal microvasculature, oliguria, low sodium excretion, and poor short-term prognosis. It occurs only in severe liver disease—advanced cirrhosis, severe acute alcoholic hepatitis, or fulminant acute hepatic failure. There is little or no proteinuria; microscopic findings on urinalysis are minimal; urinary osmolality is somewhat higher than serum osmolality; and urinary sodium concentration is low, usually less than 25 mEq per liter. The original term for this disorder was "functional renal failure," which better describes the pathophysiologic process. The cause for the intense renal microvascular constriction remains elusive.

Treatment is supportive. The presence of hepatorenal syndrome is a sign of severe liver disease; renal impairment is unlikely to improve, or the patient to survive, unless there is improvement in the liver disease. In severe acute alcoholic hepatitis, I find that about 10% of my patients with hepatorenal syndrome survive, concomitantly with slow spontaneous improvement in liver function. After liver transplantation in cirrhotic patients, improvement in renal function occurs within a few days.

Numerous treatments have been used for hepatorenal syndrome. They include vigorous volume expansion, peritoneovenous shunt, prostaglandin analogues such as misoprostol* and prostaglandin A, intravenous felypressin (Octapressin), various vasodilator drugs including dopamine, vasoconstrictor drugs, and calcium channel blockers. No treatment has been consistently effective. A major concern is the role of hemodialysis. Many believe that it should not be employed unless there is a possibility that an acute renal insult is responsible for the renal impairment or there is a reasonable likelihood of improvement in liver disease. The TIPS procedure seems to have been helpful in a few reported cases, and further trials will no doubt be reported.

Hepatic Encephalopathy

There are several competing theories for the pathogenesis of hepatic encephalopathy, which seems to be the result of some toxic substance originating in the bowel and acting on the brain. Ammonia intoxication is the simplest of the theories—ammonia is produced from protein or urea in the colon, bypasses the liver through portal collaterals or fails detoxification to urea as it passes through the sick liver, and ultimately reaches the brain where it is detoxified to glutamine by combining with α-ketoglutarate. Depletion of α-ketoglutarate reduces the energy metabolism of the brain. Whatever the agent or agents responsible, it is clear that hepatic encephalopathy can occur in the absence of liver disease if the portal circulation completely bypasses the liver (e.g., after portacaval shunt surgery) or in the absence of portal collateral circulation if the liver is severely damaged (e.g., in fulminant hepatic necrosis). In most patients with hepatic encephalopathy, there is a variable combination of portal collateral circulation and liver dysfunction.

In patients with cirrhosis, hepatic encephalopathy can be obvious or subtle, continuous or episodic, severe or mild. Recognition is by behavioral change, lethargy progressing in some cases to coma, asterixis, and difficulty with calculation and number connection. Helpful test findings are the electroencephalographic pattern, a characteristic pattern of low *myo*-inositol and elevated glutamine concentration on magnetic resonance spectroscopy of the brain, increased blood ammonia level, and elevated cerebrospinal fluid glutamine concentration. Potential precipitating factors should be looked for. These include gastrointestinal bleeding, spontaneous bacterial peritonitis, constipation, and use of diuretics. Patients who have had a surgical portosystemic shunt or a TIPS procedure or who have a large spontaneous splenorenal shunt often have no recognizable precipitating factor.

For treatment, the precipitating factor, if recognizable, should be dealt with as rapidly as possible. Measures designed to reduce colonic production of ammonia are instituted. These include enemas to empty the colon and lactulose administration by nasogastric tube or by enema to acidify the stool to diminish ammonia absorption and to enhance the

---

*Not FDA approved for this indication.

growth of ammonia-consuming bacteria. Overadministration of lactulose to a comatose or semistuporous patient can result in serious hypernatremia from osmotic diarrhea, so dosage should be adjusted to produce three to five loose stools daily. Oral or nasogastric tube administration of neomycin, 1 gram every 8 hours, poses a small risk of interfering with the action of lactulose by inhibiting the growth of the bacteria that cause stool acidification, but in most cases, its action is complementary to that of lactulose by reducing growth of urease-producing bacteria. Nutrition should be supplied parenterally because of the risk for aspiration. Some believe in the use of parenteral branched chain amino acids. Some use the benzodiazepine receptor antagonist flumazenil (Romazicon)* on the basis of the theory that endogenous benzodiazepines may contribute to hepatic encephalopathy.

Patients who have recurrent hepatic encephalopathy without an obvious precipitating factor are usually those with large surgically created or spontaneous portosystemic venous shunts. Standard prophylactic treatment measures in such patients include a low-protein (<40 grams per day) or totally vegetarian diet and daily lactulose or lactilol in a quantity sufficient to result in two or three loose stools daily. Low-dose neomycin (1 gram twice daily) is less costly than lactulose and is preferred by some hepatologists. Other treatment agents not in general use include sodium benzoate, zinc, and metronidazole.

Pulmonary Hypertension with Cirrhosis

Approximately 5% of patients with cirrhosis are found to have a "primary" type of pulmonary hypertension when right-sided heart catheterization is performed. Clinical clues to this complication are a loud pulmonary second sound and rightward deviation of the electrocardiographic axis. Pulmonary pressure sometimes reaches systemic levels and can be the cause of much disability and even death from right-sided heart failure. The hypertension is unresponsive to most antihypertensive medications but does respond to continuous intravenous infusion of prostacyclin, which is largely inactivated in the lungs after its relaxing effect on the pulmonary vascular smooth muscle. The cause of this complication of cirrhosis is unknown. In advanced cases, there is marked increase in morbidity and mortality from liver transplantation with no assurance of relief of the pulmonary hypertension.

Hepatopulmonary Syndrome

Approximately 5 to 10% of patients with advanced cirrhosis are found to have marked hypoxemia (PaO_2 <70 mm Hg), cyanosis, clubbing of the fingers, and higher than expected hematocrits. The hypoxemia worsens in the erect position (orthodeoxia). Some patients have radiologic abnormalities in the hands and distal ends of the radius and ulna (pulmonary

osteoarthropathy). Pulmonary angiography shows moderate-sized arteriovenous connections at the alveolar level that have been called "pulmonary vascular spiders." These abnormal communications can be recognized by contrast-enhanced echocardiography or by demonstration of radioactive macroaggregated albumin particles in the brain or kidney after they are injected into a peripheral vein.

Although the hepatopulmonary syndrome has long been recognized, the cause remains elusive and there is no effective treatment known. There are a few single case reports of improvement in oxygenation after the TIPS procedure. Oxygen inhalation is of limited benefit because the hypoxemia is due to shunting of blood past the alveoli. This syndrome increases morbidity and mortality from liver transplantation, but there are sporadic examples of improvement in hypoxemia after successful transplantation.

Liver Transplantation

The time to consider transplantation is when quality of life is poor and when the natural history of the disease indicates that there is little likelihood of survival for more than 1 to 2 years.

Because there are many more candidates for liver transplantation than there are available organs, some degree of selection of those candidates most likely to benefit is justified. Those most likely to benefit have good family and social support and a high likelihood of compliance with post-transplantation therapeutic regimens. They should be free of serious co-morbid disorders such as coronary artery disease, chronic pulmonary insufficiency, and chronic renal impairment. They should have liver diseases not likely to recur in the transplant. Advanced age is a problem, particularly with primary biliary cirrhosis. A patient who, absent the liver disease, has a 10-year life expectancy is a suitable transplant candidate, in my opinion.

Waiting for terminal hepatic failure before considering transplantation is a mistake, I believe, because operative mortality, cost of hospitalization, and 1-year survival are all substantially worse in patients who go to transplant surgery from an intensive care unit setting compared with those who are ambulatory at the time of the operation.

BLEEDING ESOPHAGEAL VARICES

method of
CHRISTOPHER J. GOSTOUT, M.D.
Mayo Clinic
Rochester, Minnesota

The patient with acute bleeding from esophagogastric varices demands prompt attention to reduce the extent of hemorrhage and potentially fatal complications. Most patients with bleeding varices have a known history of liver disease. Occasional patients present with bleeding

---

*Not FDA approved for this indication.

TABLE 1. **Child's Classification of Cirrhosis**

Measure	Class A	Class B	Class C
Bilirubin (mg/dL)	<2	2–3	>3
Albumin (gm/dL)	>3.5	3–3.5	<3.0
Ascites	None	Easily controlled	Poorly controlled
Encephalopathy	None	Minimal	Advanced (coma)
Nutrition	Good	Good	Wasting

due to late sequelae from portal, splenic, or superior mesenteric venous thrombosis. These patients are most often bleeding from gastric varices. Unlike acute gastrointestinal bleeding from other causes, e.g., peptic ulcers, Mallory-Weiss tears, and colonic diverticula, variceal bleeding carries a higher risk for death directly due to hemorrhage. This risk increases with the severity of liver disease as measured by Child's criteria (Table 1).

Patients with acute gastrointestinal bleeding at the Mayo Clinic in Rochester, Minnesota, are evaluated and managed by the GI Bleeding Team. A review of the GI Bleeding Team's prospective database from 1990 through 1995 revealed a total of 268 patients with acute variceal bleeding. Seventy-four percent of these patients bled from esophageal varices. The rebleeding rate during the hospitalization for these patients was 27%. The rebleeding rate for gastric varices was 41%. Rebleeding has been noted to be more common in patients with alcoholic cirrhosis. Rebleeding is greatest within 48 to 72 hours. The overall hospital mortality rate due to esophageal variceal bleeding was 16%, with 76% of deaths directly due to bleeding. For gastric variceal bleeding, the overall hospital mortality rate was 9%, with two thirds of deaths directly due to bleeding. Overall mortality rates based on Child's criteria in the Mayo population of patients were 12% for Child's class A, 33% for Child's class B, and 83% for Child's class C patients. Mortality is the greatest within a 6-week period of the acute bleeding event.

Management of acutely bleeding esophagogastric varices is associated with substantial cost (estimated annual cost of $30,000 per patient) and has improved with the potential to reduce these costs. Once patients with acute bleeding have survived the acute event and related hospitalization, major rebleeding episodes are uncommon. The improvements in management include endoscopic variceal ligation, acute and chronic pharmacotherapy, the transjugular intrahepatic portosystemic shunt (TIPS), and liver transplantation.

WHO WILL BLEED FROM VARICES?

The presence of varices in patients with cirrhosis varies from 20 to 70% and is dependent on the severity of the liver disease. Approximately one third of patients with varices and cirrhosis will experience acute bleeding. The first episode of bleeding will occur within 2 years of identifying varices in the majority of cirrhotic patients. Varices that have the greatest tendency to bleed are large, are under excessive portal pressure (>12 mm Hg; normal, <6 mm Hg), and can be identified endoscopically by their appearance. Portal pressures demonstrate a circadian rhythm with a peak around midnight, suggesting why patients seem to present with variceal bleeding at inconvenient times. Red signs—red wales involving esophageal varices (thin, short, serpiginous mucosal vessels overlying the variceal trunk) and hemocystic spots (small, red, and sometimes raised spots) involving gastric varices—are the

specific endoscopic observations that carry increased risk for bleeding. Varices that bleed most often are located in the distal 5 cm of the esophagus and at the esophagogastric junction. Large gastric varices within the fundus present with the most difficult form of acute variceal bleeding. Gastric varices within the body and antrum of the stomach typically lie deeper beneath the mucosa and rarely bleed.

Other factors that influence the risk for bleeding (Table 2) include Child's C classification of advanced disease, continued alcohol use, presence of gastric varices, changes in velocity or reversal of portal blood flow (by Doppler examination), and persistent ascites.

MANAGEMENT OF ESOPHAGEAL VARICEAL BLEEDING

The main areas discussed in this section include assessment and resuscitation of the patient, pharmacotherapy, endoscopy, balloon tamponade, and refractory bleeding.

Assessment and Resuscitation of the Patient

General Assessment

Several critical and immediate observations must be made. These observations are directed at globally estimating the patient's stage of liver disease, the status of the bleeding, and the bleeding symptoms. Confusion, obtundation, jaundice, and ascites indicate advanced liver disease with decompensation and a high risk for complications, especially sepsis but also encephalopathy, renal failure, and an uncorrectable coagulopathy. Repeated and large-volume hematemesis as well as hematochezia would suggest, in the absence of the vitals signs, active bleeding. Repeated hematemesis and large-volume hematemesis additionally increase the risk for aspiration during endoscopy. Isolated orthostatic symptoms with anemia are less suggestive of active bleeding and supportive of volume loss only.

Variceal bleeding is abrupt and involves rapid loss of a large volume of blood. Coffee-ground hematemesis and melena are not strongly supportive of variceal bleeding. These symptoms may indicate nonvari-

TABLE 2. **Factors That Influence Esophageal Variceal Bleeding**

Physiologic

Portal pressure >12 mm Hg
Altered velocity or reversal of portal blood flow

Anatomic

Large varices*
Red wale markings*
Fundal gastric varices

Clinical

Child's C classification*
Ongoing alcohol use
Ascites

*Independent risk factors for an initial bleeding event.

ceal bleeding. The most common form of nonvariceal upper gastrointestinal bleeding is due to portal hypertensive gastropathy. Bleeding in this setting is subacute and involves oozing from multiple mucosal sites during a prolonged time from days to months. Some patients may have bleeding from mucosal angiectasis scattered throughout the antrum, the cardia, and less often the body of the stomach. Patients may also develop bleeding from erosions and ulcers related to their underlying portal hypertensive gastropathy.

Laboratory Tests

The hemoglobin level (or hematocrit), platelet count, prothrombin time, electrolyte determinations, glucose level, and creatinine concentration are the key laboratory tests that should allow a complete assessment of the patient's status and predict potential problems that may arise. A platelet count above 40,000 per mm^3 is satisfactory and can be observed. With active bleeding, an effort should be made to correct an abnormal prothrombin time with a minimum of 2 units of fresh-frozen plasma.

Resuscitation

Intravenous access is mandatory and should be established promptly. Peripheral sites are satisfactory. Central venous access is a consideration if close monitoring of cardiac and pulmonary hemodynamics is needed and is an issue during intensive care management. Fluid resuscitation should be carefully monitored to avoid fluid overload, exacerbation of portal pressure, and the introduction or exacerbation of ascites. Blood transfusion with packed red blood cells is satisfactory. Fresh-frozen plasma should be given when more than 4 units of blood are consecutively transfused to replete clotting factors.

One of the most critical decisions is whether to proceed with endotracheal intubation. Endoscopy plays a pivotal role in the assessment of and therapy for the variceal bleeder. Inherent with this procedure is a risk for aspiration. Endotracheal intubation should therefore be performed in the setting of active hematemesis and especially if obtundation is present. Endotracheal intubation should also be considered in the patient for whom balloon tamponade is performed.

Because endoscopy is an integral component of the patient's assessment and therapy, some administer prophylactic antibiotics to the patient with Child's class C disease or lesser classes but with ascites. This practice remains controversial and is more of an issue when injection sclerotherapy will be used.

Triage (Table 3)

The admission of the patient to the intensive care unit or to a standard hospital room, or even dismissal from the emergency unit, depends mostly on the endoscopic findings. Evidence of massive bleeding, active bleeding, Child's class C disease, endotracheal intubation, balloon tamponade, and the use of intravenous pharmacotherapy require an intensive care

TABLE 3. Triage of the Patient with Bleeding from Portal Hypertension

Triage Decision	Clinical Problem
Intensive care unit	Massive bleeding
	Actively bleeding varix
	Child's class C cirrhosis
	Endotracheal intubation
	Balloon tamponade
	Intravenous pharmacotherapy (vasopressin)
Hospital room	Less than severe bleeding (e.g., melena)—endoscopic therapy performed
	Less than severe bleeding (e.g., melena)—no endoscopy available
Outpatient care	Melena and/or anemia and portal hypertensive gastropathy
	Coffee-ground hematemesis—no change in hemoglobin level
	Hematocrit; stable vital signs

unit. Lesser bleeding, if it is variceal and if it is effectively treated immediately with endoscopic therapy, can be observed in a non–intensive care unit setting. If endoscopy is not available, then admission to the hospital is advisable for observation of all acute bleeding events. Patients will occasionally present to the emergency room with a history of melena that has been present for days (or even weeks) and anemia. These patients are probably bleeding from portal hypertensive gastropathy that is unassociated with major acute bleeding events. Once the diagnosis is evident during endoscopy, this group of patients may be managed as outpatients. Coffee-ground hematemesis in the absence of significant changes in the hemoglobin level (or hematocrit) and the vital signs is not an indicator of a major bleeding event. Patients with this presentation can be managed electively.

Pharmacotherapy

The pharmacologic agents used in the management of varices can be segregated into those drugs given during acute bleeding and those used prophylactically. The former drugs include vasopressin, terlipressin,* somatostatin,* octreotide, and nitroglycerin. The latter drugs include nonselective beta blockers (propranolol and nadolol) and the long-acting nitrates isosorbide mononitrate and dinitrate. These agents can be divided further by their effects of creating vasoconstriction or vasodilatation. The vasoconstrictors (vasopressin, terlipressin, somatostatin, octreotide, propranolol, and nadolol) induce splanchnic vasoconstriction with a reduction in portal blood flow and pressure. The vasodilators (nitroglycerin and isosorbide mononitrate or dinitrate) lower portal blood flow and pressure by means of peripheral vasodilatation and a subsequent reflex

---

*Investigational drug in the United States.

TABLE 4. **Pharmacotherapy for Variceal Bleeding**

Drug	Dosing Schedule
Acute Therapy	
Vasopressin	20-U slow IV bolus in 20 min
	0.3–0.6 U/min constant infusion
Terlipressin	1–2 mg IV q 4–6 h
Nitroglycerin*	40–400 μg/min IV constant infusion
	Given in conjunction with vasopressin
	and terlipressin
Somatostatin	250 μg IV bolus
	250–500 μg/h constant infusion
Octreotide*	50 μg IV bolus
	25–50 μg/h constant infusion†
Prophylaxis	
Propranolol*‡	80 mg PO (long-acting) initial dose
	320 mg maximal daily dose
Nadolol*‡	20 mg PO initial dose
	240 mg maximal daily dose
Isosorbide mononitrate*	20 mg PO bid (7 h apart)
Isosorbide dinitrate*	10–20 mg PO qid
	Increase dose 10 mg as tolerated

*Not FDA approved for this indication.
†Exceeds dosage recommended by the manufacturer.
‡Reduction of resting heart rate by 25%; lower limit 55 bpm.

splanchnic vasoconstriction. They also reduce intrahepatic vascular resistance.

In the setting of acute bleeding, pharmacotherapy is useful as initial adjunctive treatment, as a supplement to balloon tamponade, and as a temporizing measure until endoscopic therapy can be performed. These drugs are also useful for continuation as adjunctive therapy to endoscopic therapy, especially when there is uncertainty regarding hemostasis. Table 4 lists these medications and their common dosages.

Acute Bleeding

VASOPRESSIN

Arginine vasopressin (Pitressin) is a potent vasoconstrictor with the ability to reduce portal venous pressure approximately 30%. It can be administered initially in a 20-unit slow infusion bolus during 20 minutes followed by a constant infusion of 0.3 unit per minute. The constant infusion dosage may be increased up to 0.6 unit per minute, after which tolerance of the vasoconstrictive effects is poor and little additional therapeutic benefit is gained.

Vasopressin is associated with significant side effects and complications warranting close monitoring of its use. Cardiovascular problems include coronary vasoconstriction with myocardial ischemia and infarction; reduced cardiac output; arrhythmias, especially ventricular; and hypertension with reflex bradycardia. Peripheral arterial vasoconstriction may create mesenteric ischemia, ischemia of the extremities, and cerebrovascular accidents. Vasopressin affects the kidney, impairing excretion of free water, which can cause fluid overload, hyponatremia, and worsening of ascites. The drug must be discontinued in approximately 30% of patients. Interest in the use of this medication has waned.

TERLIPRESSIN

Terlipressin (Glypressin)* is a synthetic derivative of vasopressin with a longer duration of action. In vivo, the drug is cleaved into vasopressin. Terlipressin is administered by bolus intravenous injection of 1 to 2 mg every 4 to 6 hours. There is evidence suggesting that terlipressin is more effective than vasopressin.

NITROGLYCERIN

Nitroglycerin should be used routinely in combination with vasopressin and terlipressin to reduce the cardiovascular side effects described before. The vasodilatation properties associated with this medication cumulatively add to the control of bleeding provided by vasopressin and terlipressin. The preferred route of administration of nitroglycerin is intravenous rather than transdermal (50 mg) and sublingual (0.6 mg every 30 minutes). The last two routes of administration will not effectively counter the adverse cardiovascular side effects of vasopressin. Dosing with nitroglycerin is accomplished with an initial dose of 40 μg per minute; additional increments in dosage are given if the blood pressure remains above 100 mm Hg systolic. Although the upper limit is considered to be 400 μg per minute, most patients will not tolerate more than 100 μg per minute. The combination of vasopressin with nitroglycerin has been shown to be more effective than vasopressin alone in controlling bleeding.

SOMATOSTATIN

Somatostatin (Zecnil)* is a naturally occurring 14–amino acid peptide with a range of inhibitory effects in the gastrointestinal tract. It decreases splanchnic blood flow by a direct effect on mesenteric vascular smooth muscle and also by reducing glucagon levels (which increase portal blood flow). It has a major advantage over vasopressin by the absence of systemic vasoconstriction. Somatostatin has a short half-life of approximately 2 minutes and requires continuous intravenous administration. It is given as an initial intravenous bolus of 250 μg followed by continuous infusion of 250 to 500 μg per hour. In direct comparative studies, it has been shown to be equal to or better than vasopressin in reducing rebleeding. It is a drug of choice in patients who have known ischemic heart disease, peripheral vascular disease, and cardiac dysrhythmias.

OCTREOTIDE

Octreotide (Sandostatin) is a long-acting octapeptide analogue of somatostatin. A half-life of 2 hours has made it the preferred drug to use over somatostatin in the acute setting. It reduces portal blood flow, has little effect on systemic vascular resistance, and dramatically reduces azygos blood flow. Octreotide also reduces postprandial splanchnic hyperemia in cirrhotic patients by direct vasoconstriction and

*Investigational drug in the United States.

inhibiting glucagon. Clinical trials have shown octreotide to be more effective than placebo, vasopressin, or balloon tamponade in controlling acute bleeding with minimal side effects. It has been shown in conjunction with sclerotherapy to reduce bleeding-related mortality during a 5-day period of infusion. The drug is administered as a 50-μg bolus followed by a constant infusion of 25 to 50 μg per hour. The efficacy and low rate of side effects have made octreotide the drug of choice for the management of bleeding varices.

Prophylaxis

NONSELECTIVE BETA-ADRENERGIC BLOCKERS

The two drugs in use for control of portal hypertensive bleeding are propranolol and nadolol. Beta blockers reduce cardiac output and induce splanchnic vasoconstriction by reflex activation of alpha-adrenergic receptors in the splanchnic circulation. Peripheral vasoconstriction is caused by eliminating beta$_2$-receptor–mediated vasodilatation and allowing unopposed alpha-adrenergic–mediated vasoconstriction. The result of these effects is a decrease in gastroesophageal collateral blood flow measurable by azygos venous blood flow.

The two main issues regarding the use of these medications are the prevention of initial bleeding and the prevention of rebleeding. It has been demonstrated and accepted that nonselective beta-adrenergic blockers should be used as standard prophylaxis against initial bleeding. Reductions in portal pressures below 12 mm Hg are associated not only with a lower risk for bleeding but also with a decreased mortality. Patients who have large varices benefit the most from beta-blocker therapy. There is also evidence that the initiation of beta-blocker therapy in concert with endoscopic therapy after an initial bleed is associated with a significant reduction in rebleeding. These medications fail to reduce portal pressure in 25% of patients. Beta blockers are most effective in patients with Child's class A and B cirrhosis.

The goal of prophylactic therapy with nonselective beta-adrenergic blockers is to reduce portal pressure as much as possible. Ideally, portal pressures should be monitored before and during therapy. Alternatively, the resting heart rate is used to accomplish this goal. The target reduction is a decrease in the resting heart rate by 25% with a lower limit of 55 beats per minute. Propranolol should be used as a long-acting formulation with readjustments in the dosage made weekly. The maximal dose is 320 mg per day with a mean dose of 160 mg per day and a starting dose of 80 mg per day. Nadolol (Corgard) is another longer acting nonselective beta-adrenergic antagonist that can be administered once daily. It is excreted primarily by the kidneys; for this reason, dosage adjustments are more reliable. It also does not cross the blood-brain barrier, which minimizes central nervous system side effects. The initial dose of nadolol is 20 mg with a maximal dose of 240 mg.

Once initiated, these drugs should be used indefinitely. There is no evidence to suggest that beta blockers interfere with reflex circulatory responses to acute hemorrhage and impair management of patients in this setting.

The contraindications to the use of propranolol and nadolol are congestive heart failure, atrioventricular block, dysrhythmias, severe chronic obstructive pulmonary disease, asthma, psychosis, and insulin-dependent diabetes. The major side effects include fatigue, depression, hypotension, bradycardia, impotence, sleep disruption, and cardiac failure. These side effects occur in 10 to 25% of patients. Nadolol is more commonly used in place of propranolol if it is not tolerated.

To receive prophylactic therapy with either propranolol or nadolol, the patient should ideally be compliant, have Child's class A or B cirrhosis, and have a high risk for bleeding with the presence of large esophageal varices containing red wale marks or large gastric varices with hemocystic spots.

LONG-ACTING NITRATES

There is limited experience with these medications with evidence that portal pressure can be reduced by either isosorbide mononitrate (Ismo) or dinitrate (Isordil). These drugs are used as supplements to beta-blocker therapy or in replacement of beta-blocker therapy when it is poorly tolerated. Long-acting nitrates have been anecdotally useful as adjunctive therapy to beta blockers and endoscopic therapy in patients with extensive extrahepatic venous occlusive disease and recurrent bleeding from gastric varices who are not candidates for shunt surgery or the TIPS procedure. Isosorbide mononitrate is orally administered in 2 doses of 20 mg in the morning followed by a second 20-mg dose 7 hours later. Isosorbide dinitrate can be initiated in a 10- to 20-mg four-times-daily dosing schedule with 10-mg increments as tolerated.

Endoscopy

The main goal in management of acute esophageal variceal bleeding is to control bleeding as expeditiously as possible within the shortest hospitalization and with the least morbidity. The endoscopic examination is critical in providing the diagnosis, directing management, and providing therapy. If endoscopy is unavailable, the clinician must act on a presumptive diagnosis based on a history of known liver disease or other conditions giving rise to portal hypertension (e.g., portal and splenic venous thrombosis).

Endoscopy should be performed promptly once signs of stabilization are evident during the resuscitative effort. Torrential bleeding in an occasional patient will prevent a successful examination. It may be reattempted after a short period (1 to 2 hours) of balloon tamponade and pharmacotherapy. Large-diameter-tube gastric lavage is needed on occasion to ensure complete endoscopy when excessive clots and pooled blood are encountered. Although controversial, antibiotics should be considered to avoid bacteremic sepsis in Child's class C patients who are likely to undergo endoscopic sclerotherapy.

The major challenge for the endoscopist is to determine whether the bleeding is arising from esophageal, esophagogastric, or isolated gastric varices or another problem, such as portal hypertensive gastropathy that can additionally be complicated by ulceration. In the absence of active bleeding or an obvious adherent or protruding clot, large distal (within 5 cm of the esophagogastric squamocolumnar junction) varices with red wale markings should be interpreted as the cause of esophageal variceal bleeding. Endoscopic therapy should be initiated and directed at these varices. If the varices continue into the cardia, i.e., are esophagogastric varices, endoscopic therapy should begin on the cardia side of the squamocolumnar junction because the gastric component of these varices can be eliminated by this approach. Once initiated, endoscopic therapy should be resumed with the eventual goal of eradication. After the initial endoscopic therapy, it is usually repeated in 5 to 7 days, then every 1 to 2 weeks until the distal esophageal varices are obliterated or else reduced to a small size. The interval between follow-up procedures tends to be longer (i.e., 2 weeks) in patients who undergo variceal band ligation. Once eradicated, varices are typically re-examined for recurrence in 6-month periods.

Although the focus of this chapter is on esophageal variceal bleeding, a diagnosis of gastric variceal bleeding is important to exclude. Gastric variceal bleeding can be established with the following observations in addition to the presence of gastric varices:

1. Active bleeding: spurting; focal oozing; pooling of fresh blood within the proximal stomach with no pathologic process evident in the esophagus and stomach

2. Adherent clot resistant to washing: fresh and of varying size; minute, protruding, and fibrinous

3. Absence of esophageal varices, small esophageal varices, and no esophageal red wale markings

4. A red hemocystic spot confined to the varix

Endoscopic therapy, by means of sclerotherapy, band ligation, or a combination of both techniques, remains the mainstay of medical management. It is successful in controlling acute bleeding in 60 to 85% of patients in a single session and in 70 to 95% of patients in two sessions. If rebleeding occurs after two endoscopic treatment sessions, alternative therapy should be sought.

Sclerotherapy is the most common endoscopic therapy performed worldwide. Each varix (variceal trunk) is directly injected with a sclerosant, or else the sclerosant is injected alongside the varix (paravariceal). A variety of sclerosants are available (sodium tetradecyl sulfate, morrhuate sodium, ethanolamine, ethanol). There does not appear to be any advantage of one over the others. Sclerotherapy may also be performed with a cyanoacrylate glue. This adhesive is not available in the United States. It has proved to be valuable in the treatment of fundal varices.

Complications from injection sclerotherapy include deep injection site ulceration with the potential for serious bleeding, necrosis with perforation, and stricture. A self-limited fever, mediastinitis, and pleural effusion can occur within hours of injection. Adult respiratory distress syndrome, local and distant abscesses, and bacterial peritonitis have occurred in association with sclerotherapy. Sclerotherapy remains a major indication for bacterial endocarditis prophylaxis in select patients.

Variceal band ligation is a newer technique with the potential to eradicate distal esophageal varices sooner and with less morbidity. Similar to injection sclerotherapy, each varix or variceal trunk is treated by applying minute rubber bands to a portion of a varix that has been suctioned into a cylinder affixed to the end of the endoscope. The banded portion of varix is strangulated by the band and sloughs during an average period of up to 1 week. A residual shallow ulcer is left at the banding site. Multiple bands are typically placed in a single session; evidence suggests that the more bands placed, the faster the eradication of the varices. Band ligation may be performed with two techniques. One technique employs an overtube that has the added advantage of protecting the airway. Bands are placed one at a time; the endoscope banding apparatus is refitted with a new band after each placement. The newest method uses a multiband device; during a single intubation of the esophagus, five or six bands may be placed. An overtube is not needed with the newer multiband ligators. Complications from variceal band ligation are predominantly short term and include transient dysphagia, odynophagia, and chest pain. Mild mucosal strictures have developed. Variceal band ligation has become the preferred method of endoscopic esophageal variceal therapy.

Balloon Tamponade

Balloon tamponade remains an important treatment option. Its role in therapy has become adjunctive rather than primary with the exception of bleeding from gastric fundal varices. As a primary therapy, balloon tamponade has been demonstrated to control 70 to 90% of bleeding. Early rebleeding remains a significant problem after the balloons are deflated. Balloon tamponade should be attempted in patients with torrential bleeding. Once bleeding has ceased, the patient should undergo repeated endoscopy with the intent of initiating endoscopic therapy. Balloon tamponade is typically performed with inflation of the gastric balloon first, using 250 to 300 mL of air. If bleeding continues as determined by continued aspiration of bloody gastric and esophageal contents, the esophageal balloon is inflated to a pressure of 40 mm Hg. Complications associated with balloon tamponade include aspiration, esophageal rupture, mucosal and nasal necrosis, asphyxiation from airway occlusion, and chest pain. Placement of the gastric balloon is critical for avoiding traumatic injury of the esophagus during inflation of this balloon. Traction and position of the balloon tamponade device are equally important to avoid inadvertent displacement of the inflated esophageal balloon or partially deflated gastric balloon and impairment of the patient's airway. The risk for aspiration has been reduced by the addition of the esophageal aspiration port in the redesigned Sengstaken-Blakemore tube (Minnesota tube). Endotracheal intubation will also reduce the frequency of aspiration. Experience and a deliberate effort at short-term use (≤2 days) will otherwise minimize complications.

Refractory Bleeding

Patients who continue to bleed while hospitalized or have recurrent bleeding episodes with persistent varices are potential candidates for portosystemic shunt surgery, liver transplantation, or the TIPS procedure. Logistics, such as time for an evaluation before transplantation and the availability of a compatible donor organ, make transplantation less desirable on an emergency basis. Urgent liver transplantation has been shown to be most effective in patients with Child's class C cirrhosis.

Shunt surgery is an alternative that has appeal for the patient with Child's class A cirrhosis (good liver function) and who may live long distances from tertiary care centers. The type of shunt operation that can be performed depends on the venous vascular anatomy and the urgency of the operation. There are three basic types of shunts. Nonselective shunts, e.g., portacaval, completely decompress the portal venous system and divert all portal blood away from the liver. Portacaval shunts should be avoided in patients who may be eventual candidates for liver transplantation. Selective shunts, e.g., distal splenorenal, compartmentalize the portal venous system, diverting blood flow from the esophagogastric vasculature and allowing the liver to be perfused by the superior mesenteric and portal venous compartment. Partial shunts, e.g., calibrated portacaval, partially decompress the portal venous system while permitting flow of portal venous blood into the liver. Shunt surgery is the most effective treatment to reduce the risk for rebleeding. The decrease in hepatic perfusion and portosystemic shunting can result in the development of hepatic encephalopathy and reduced long-term survival because of deteriorated liver function. Encephalopathy occurs less in patients who receive a distal splenorenal shunt and who have nonalcoholic liver disease. Esophageal transection offers an alternative to surgical shunting. It is less efficacious in preventing rebleeding and has been found to be comparable to endoscopic therapy in preventing rebleeding and mortality.

The TIPS procedure involves the creation of an intrahepatic fistula between the portal and hepatic (systemic) veins. This angiographic procedure employs a self-expanding metal stent to maintain the patency of the fistula. The technique effectively decompresses varices. Encephalopathy occurs in up to 25% of patients, but overall, it is less than with shunt surgery and is usually mild. Rebleeding occurs in approximately 10% of patients. This is typically due to shunt occlusion, which approaches 40% by 2 years and is a major drawback to the procedure. Revision of the shunt is possible. TIPS is regarded as a bridge to transplantation but is also a consideration in the patient with refractory bleeding who is not a candidate for surgery.

TABLE 5. Treatment of Bleeding Esophageal Varices

Management Problem	Therapy		
	Primary	*Adjunctive*	*Secondary*
Prophylaxis	Beta blockers		
Acute bleeding	Endoscopy	Octreotide Balloon tamponade	TIPS Surgery
Prevention of rebleeding	Endoscopy	Beta blockers	Child's A: shunt surgery Child's B: shunt surgery versus TIPS Child's C: TIPS, transplantation

Abbreviation: TIPS = transjugular intrahepatic portosystemic shunt.

SUMMARIZED MEDICAL MANAGEMENT (Table 5)

1. Prompt endoscopy on presentation with acute bleeding
   a. Performed after resuscitation efforts have been initiated
   b. Endotracheal intubation with large-volume and repeated hematemesis and/or obtunded patient
   c. Includes endoscopic therapy
2. Octreotide infusion
   a. Initiate before endoscopy in all patients with acute bleeding
   b. As adjunctive therapy if bleeding (oozing) continues after endoscopic therapy, especially if varices are large or as a supplement to balloon tamponade
3. Balloon tamponade
   a. With torrential bleeding
   b. Failure to control bleeding with endoscopic therapy
   c. Unavailability of endoscopic therapy
   d. Adjunctive endotracheal intubation
4. Repeated early endoscopic therapy
   a. Within 5 to 7 days after initial therapy
   b. With rebleeding event
   c. For esophageal and esophagogastric varices
5. Nonselective beta-blocker therapy
   a. After stabilization of bleeding and progression to oral intake
   b. During endoscopic therapy for variceal eradication

c. In patients with gastric variceal bleeding not amenable to endoscopic therapy
6. Long-acting nitrates
   a. Patients intolerant of beta blockers
   b. As supplemental therapy in patients at maximal doses of beta blockers or with gastric varices not amenable to shunt surgery or TIPS
7. Refractory bleeding
   a. Shunt surgery, preferably distal splenorenal, in Child's class A patients
   b. Liver transplantation
   c. TIPS in patients who are liver transplant candidates but do not satisfy criteria for transplantation, or in a patient who is not a surgical candidate

DYSPHAGIA AND ESOPHAGEAL OBSTRUCTION

method of
PETER J. KAHRILAS, M.D.
Northwestern University Medical School
Chicago, Illinois

Dysphagia implies difficulty in swallowing. As generally interpreted, this encompasses any difficulty in the passage of a solid or liquid bolus from the mouth, through the esophagus, into the stomach. Odynophagia is a related symptom indicating pain on deglutition. Both dysphagia and odynophagia occur only during the act of swallowing, distinguishing themselves from globus hystericus (globus sensation), which is the continuous sensation of a lump in the throat. In the case of oropharyngeal dysphagia, the patient's perception of the problem is highly accurate. Patients usually recognize that food accumulates in the mouth; that they are unable to control a food bolus within the oral cavity; that they are unable to initiate a swallow; or that they aspirate food before, during, or after a swallow. The patient's localization of the problem corresponds closely to the radiographic verification of the cause in almost all instances. The situation is different in the case of esophageal dysphagia, in which a patient's identification of the locus of bolus hang-up is of limited accuracy. The actual level of bolus hang-up or obstruction observed radiographically occurs at or below the level of hang-up identified by the patient. Thus, it is often the case with a distal esophageal obstruction or an esophageal motor disorder that the sensation of dysphagia is referred to the level of the neck. In such instances, identification of associated symptoms such as aspiration, neurologic symptoms, nasopharyngeal regurgitation, hoarseness, esophagopharyngeal regurgitation, weight loss, drooling, heartburn, chest pain, or intermittent esophageal obstruction is of great value in localizing the problem to the oropharynx or esophagus.

OROPHARYNGEAL DYSPHAGIA

Tumors of the oral cavity, pharynx, hypopharynx, or tongue can present with dysphagia. Dysphagia is also a common consequence of radiation therapy for tumors in these regions as a result of either radiation injury to the musculature or stricturing in the retro-cricoid region, effectively narrowing the esophageal inlet. Postcricoid webs can also occur congenitally or, perhaps, in association with iron deficiency. Because of these possibilities and the importance of early detection of mass lesions, the initial evaluation of oropharyngeal dysphagia must be a careful oral examination and laryngoscopy. If a mass lesion is discovered, biopsy and appropriate surgical-oncologic treatment are initiated. Benign strictures or webs of the retrocricoid area are treated with dilation, regardless of the cause. In most instances, this can be done by endoscopically placing a guide wire through the stricture and threading it distally into the stomach under fluoroscopic guidance. It is desirable to achieve and maintain dilatation to a 15-mm diameter. Restricturing is often a problem, and repeated dilations are required at intervals defined by the natural history of the stricturing process.

Cervical osteophytes are also sometimes invoked as a cause of dysphagia. Because the posterior wall of the pharynx is so closely apposed to the anterior aspect of the cervical vertebrae, cervical osteophytes result in an anterior bulging into the pharynx that can make passage of a normal-sized bolus difficult. It is unusual for an osteophyte to warrant surgical management, although removal of the osteophyte is helpful in extreme cases. An analogous situation can arise as a result of edema that follows the surgical stabilization of the vertebral column, from the implantation of metal stabilization devices, or after cervical laminectomy.

Neuromuscular Diseases

Once anatomic causes of oropharyngeal dysphagia have been excluded, neuromuscular causes of swallow dysfunction should be considered. The most common neurologic problem resulting in dysphagia is a cerebrovascular accident. Either extreme difficulty in initiating the swallow response or complete absence of the swallow response can be observed after a brain stem infarct. Similar problems can arise as a result of brain stem tumors or head trauma. The abnormality with anterior cortical strokes is of a significant delay in the triggering of the pharyngeal swallow response or, in severe instances, a complete absence of the pharyngeal swallow response. This probably reflects damage to the afferent neural pathway with a resultant increased triggering threshold for the initiation of the swallow. The motor cortex governing the tongue can also be affected, resulting in poor oral control of the bolus. With cortical strokes, lingual or pharyngeal paresis is often unilateral, a situation that lends itself to the compensatory strategy of swallowing with the head turned toward the paretic side to favor the more functional side.

Other central nervous system diseases characteristically causing some degree of dysphagia are amyotrophic lateral sclerosis (ALS), multiple sclerosis, and Parkinson's disease. Of these, ALS is the most severe, associated with a predictable decline in swallow function that invariably ends with gastrostomy feeding. The progression starts with reduced tongue control and weakened pharyngeal contraction resulting in poor clearance of food from the pharynx and, eventually, postswallow aspiration of the residua. Swallowing is no longer practical when swallowing deteriorates to the point of an inability to protect the airway. Dysphagia associated with multiple sclerosis or Parkinson's disease is more variable in severity and progression. Muscular diseases can also affect the pharyngeal musculature. Myasthenia gravis is initially characterized by subtle fatigue that may require 15 to 20 minutes of exercise before it manifests itself. In more advanced cases of myasthenia gravis, dysphagia can be profound, even to the extent of being confused with bulbar ALS. Dermatomyositis, muscular dystrophy, and dystonia also cause oropharyngeal dysphagia, depending on the degree of involvement of the pharyngeal musculature.

The evaluation of oropharyngeal dysphagia is aimed at identifying the neuromuscular disorder (which is not addressed here) and characterizing the oropharyngeal dysphagia mechanistically. Functional characteristics of the oropharyngeal swallow are best evaluated with a cineradiographic or videofluoroscopic swallowing study to adequately detail the motor events of the swallow for analysis during slow-motion playback. A swallowing study (done upright with recording of 30 frames per second or more) is not synonymous with a barium swallow x-ray examination, which focuses on the esophagus, is done in a supine position, and usually has only a few static images of the oropharynx recorded on film.

Regardless of the particular cause, dysphagia due to neuromuscular disease results in characteristic dysfunction. Nasal voice and nasopharyngeal regurgitation reflect impairment of soft palate musculature. Poor oral control of the bolus results from impaired lingual function. Postswallow residua in the valleculae or hypopharynx reflect an ineffective pharyngeal contraction. Aspiration suggests either weakened laryngeal elevators with impairment of laryngeal closure or a swallow so defective as to result in a postswallow residuum that is then aspirated after the swallow sequence is completed. As the ability of swallowing is progressively compromised, patients first take longer to eat and then change the foodstuffs that they eat. Data from patients with surgically induced lesions suggest that if a given food consistency cannot be swallowed within 10 seconds, the patients either discontinue eating that particular consistency of food or reduce their intake to the extent of being unable to maintain their weight. A similar relationship was seen with aspiration. If patients aspirate more than 10% of each bolus of a given consistency swallowed and are aware of the aspiration, they eliminate that food consistency from the diet. If they are unable to swallow any consistency with less than 10% aspiration, they discontinue eating altogether. In instances of marginal dysfunction, swallow therapy may be effective in compensating for the dysfunction and allowing the patient to continue with oral intake that would otherwise not have been possible.

Xerostomia

Xerostomia (oral dryness) is almost always associated with reduced salivary secretion. This is a relatively common problem present in up to 16% and 25% of elderly men and women, respectively. The problem is also present in an estimated 50% of patients with rheumatoid arthritis. Symptoms associated with xerostomia are (1) difficulty in mastication, swallowing, and speech; (2) pain, burning, and soreness of the oral mucosa, especially the tongue; (3) impairment of taste; (4) painful oral ulcers; (5) difficulty wearing dentures; (6) increased dental caries; and (7) increased frequency of and/or total fluid intake. The dysphagia associated with xerostomia is primarily attributable to the absence of lubricating properties of saliva.

The most common causes of xerostomia are drugs, autoimmune diseases (including Sjögren's syndrome and rheumatoid arthritis), and radiation therapy. More than 400 pharmacologic agents have been identified that can limit salivary flow; anorectics, anticholinergics, antidepressants, antipsychotics, sedatives and hypnotics, antihistamines, antiparkinsonian agents, antihypertensives, and diuretics are the common classes involved. Radiation therapy for head and neck tumors results in a predictable decline in salivary function. The initial effect is evident within a matter of days and probably results from damage to blood vessels and nerves. The later histologic effects are of profound parenchymal destruction. Salivary flow is reduced by about 50% after exposure to 1000 to 2000 cGy and to nearly zero after 3000 to 5000 cGy.

Evaluation of salivary function begins with measurement of resting salivary flow rate. Normal, unstimulated salivary flow rate should be 0.3 to 0.5 mL per minute; flow rates of less than 0.1 mL per minute are consistent with xerostomia. Ancillary tests that can be useful in selected circumstances include sialography and salivary scintigraphy. Finally, to investigate possible autoimmune destruction of the salivary glands, biopsy of the labial salivary glands is the "gold standard." Therapy for hyposalivation depends on whether the salivary glands are capable of secretory function when they are stimulated. Stimulated flow is determined by measuring salivary secretion either during paraffin chewing or after the instillation of 2% citric acid solution into the mouth. If normal rates of salivation are still not achieved, there is no merit to mechanical, gustatory, or pharmacologic therapy. If stimulation results in adequate salivary secretion, then treatment with sugarless gum, sour-tasting lozenges, or, in rare instances, pharmacologic agents should be initiated. Effective medications include pilocarpine and cholinergic agonists, although the latter should be used with care because of gastrointestinal, pulmonary, urinary tract, and cardiac side effects. Individuals without stimulated salivary response can try commercially available saliva substitutes, although the experience with these agents has not been good, primarily because they lack the lubrication properties of native saliva that aid in swallowing.

ESOPHAGEAL DYSPHAGIA

Similar to the case with oropharyngeal dysphagia, the evaluation of esophageal dysphagia begins with examination for structural lesions. Esophageal strictures, rings, or webs can cause an impediment to bolus transit. Esophageal strictures or webs can be congenital or malignant, or they can be the result of benign processes, most commonly reflux esophagitis. Rings formed at the gastroesophageal junction, described by Schatzki, are generally symptomatic when the internal diameter of the ring is less than 13 mm. Dysphagia secondary to mechanical obstruction typically occurs on swallowing solid food, especially meat or bread, and is often intermittent. Dysphagia can also result from external structures impinging on the esophagus or limiting the distensibility of the esophagus. Dysphagia lusoria is caused by compression of the esophagus by an anomalous right subclavian artery arising from the descending aorta and passing behind the esophagus. Hilar adenopathy or a mediastinal tumor can similarly result in dysphagia by compression of the esophagus.

A carefully done barium swallow x-ray examination is the most sensitive method for detecting structural abnormalities of the esophagus. Appreciation of external compression requires that the esophagus be demonstrated in relation to external structures in the mediastinum in a way that is best achieved on a radiograph. However, fluoroscopy is a relatively insensitive method for detecting the most common esophageal lesions encountered clinically, subtle mucosal lesions characteristic of peptic or infectious esophagitis. Endoscopy, with use of either fiberoptic or video-type endoscopes, provides a means for direct inspection of the mucosal lining of the pharynx, esophagus, and stomach. Because the endoscopic examination is the most sensitive method for detecting the mucosal lesions of peptic or infectious esophagitis, it should be considered as the initial evaluation and usually obviates the need for a subsequent radiographic examination. The added strength of endoscopy is that it provides a simple means of obtaining directed biopsy specimens, microbiology culture specimens, or cytology specimens.

Nearly all esophageal webs, rings, and strictures can be successfully managed by endoscopically or fluoroscopically guided dilation. In each case, the technique of dilation is determined by the specific stricture. For strictures 10 mm in diameter or larger, rubber mercury-filled dilators with a tapered or blunt tip are suitable. For tighter, longer, or tortuous strictures, hard plastic dilators that are passed over endoscopically or fluoroscopically positioned guide wires or hydraulic dilators passed through the instrumentation channel of an endoscope and positioned under

direct visualization are often necessary. The frequency with which dilation must be repeated is a function of the stricturing process. Complex strictures secondary to ischemia, radiation injury, pill esophagitis, caustic ingestion, or malignant neoplasm predictably require repeated dilations for extended periods. Peptic strictures also tend to recur, but the restricturing process can be minimized with adequate control of reflux by either antireflux surgery or continuous suppression of gastric secretion with a proton pump inhibitor (omeprazole [Prilosec] $\geq$20 mg per day or lansoprazole [Prevacid] $\geq$30 mg per day). In every case, the end point of dilation is either the elimination of dysphagia or, if this is not possible, attainment of maximal swallowing function.

When dysphagia occurs as a result of malignant obstruction, the disease is usually advanced with little chance of curative resection. Regardless, therapy has two distinct elements: staging and treatment of the neoplastic process (not discussed here) and amelioration of the obstruction itself. Similar to the case with benign obstructing lesions, dysphagia associated with malignant strictures involves peroral dilation. However, because of the exophytic nature of these lesions, adjunct therapy is often necessary. Cautery, laser ablation, and sclerosis by intralesional alcohol injection are effective at necrosing the malignant tissue, and all have been used with reasonable palliative success. However, as with dilation of malignant strictures, these increasingly invasive procedures are associated with an increased risk for perforation or formation of tracheoesophageal fistulas. In such instances, or with extremely stenotic tumors, wire mesh wall stents can be endoscopically placed as palliative therapy.

Neuromuscular Diseases

In the absence of mechanical obstruction or mucosal inflammation as an explanation for esophageal dysphagia, neuromuscular disease should be considered. If there is a physiologic correlate of dysphagia, unrelated to a luminal narrowing from within or without, it relates to a peristaltic defect. This may relate to disordered peristalsis of the esophagus such as achalasia or diffuse esophageal spasm (DES), or it may result from absent peristalsis as in severe reflux disease or scleroderma (not discussed here). These contractile abnormalities are optimally evaluated by esophageal manometry. Although, in principle, manometry can be used to study contractile activity of any region of the alimentary canal, the test is most commonly employed clinically in the esophagus primarily because of its accessibility and because excellent normative data are available.

Achalasia

Achalasia is the best defined motor disorder of the esophagus with an estimated incidence of about 1 per 100,000 population per year. Achalasia is characterized by (1) failure of the lower esophageal sphincter (LES) to relax completely with swallowing and

(2) aperistalsis in the distal esophagus. If there are spasmotic contractions in the esophageal body, the disease is referred to as vigorous achalasia. Achalasia results from destruction of the myenteric plexus within the smooth muscle esophagus either as a result of parasitic infestation as in Chagas' disease or as an idiopathic entity. It is unclear whether the disease selectively affects inhibitory neurons; functionally, it is clear that the inhibitory neurons are necessarily impaired as an early manifestation of the disease and that these neurons use nitric oxide as a neurotransmitter. Clinical manifestations of achalasia may include dysphagia, regurgitation, chest pain, weight loss, and aspiration pneumonia. Achalasic patients can often sense passage of material from the esophagus into the stomach and augment this by drinking a lot while eating or applying maneuvers such as straightening the back, raising their arms over their heads, or standing while eating. Regurgitation can be a problem when large amounts of food are retained in the dilated esophagus; patients often note regurgitant on their bed sheets when they sleep supine and elect to sleep with several pillows or upright. Chest pain is a frequent complaint early in the course of the disease; its etiology is unclear.

Achalasia is diagnosed by barium swallow x-ray examination or esophageal manometry. The characteristic radiographic appearance is of a dilated intrathoracic esophagus with an air-fluid level. The LES tapers to a point giving the distal esophagus a beak-like appearance. The beak does not open with swallowing but will open after the inhalation of amyl nitrite (a smooth muscle relaxant). The defining manometric features of achalasia are aperistalsis and incomplete LES relaxation. Neither the radiographic nor the manometric features of achalasia are specific for idiopathic achalasia; tumor-related pseudoachalasia accounts for up to 5% of cases with manometrically defined achalasia. Pseudoachalasia is more likely with progressive age, abrupt onset of symptoms, and early weight loss. Tumor infiltration (especially carcinoma in the gastric fundus) can completely mimic the functional impairment seen with idiopathic achalasia. It is because of this potential pitfall that a thorough anatomic examination including endoscopy should be done as part of the evaluation of every new case of achalasia.

The treatment of achalasia is either to incapacitate the LES pharmacologically or to disrupt it mechanically. Pharmacologic treatments, on the whole, are not effective. Smooth muscle relaxants such as isosorbide dinitrate (Isordil),* 10 mg orally before meals, or nifedipine (Procardia),* 10 mg administered sublingually immediately before eating, may offer partial relief of dysphagia. Experimental approaches to therapy for achalasia include the local injection of botulinum toxin into the sphincter muscle. However, definitive treatment of achalasia is still disruption of the LES either surgically (Heller's myotomy) or by the use of a pneumatic dilator. Pneu-

matic dilation of the esophagus is done with inflatable balloon dilators that forcefully stretch the LES to a diameter of about 3 cm and in so doing incur a 1 to 5% risk for perforation. This is completely different from the type of dilation done as therapy for peptic strictures. Pneumatic dilators are either radiographically (Rigiflex dilator) or endoscopically (Witzel dilator) positioned across the gastroesophageal junction and inflated to 6 to 9 pounds per in² for a period of 30 to 60 seconds. Many practitioners routinely obtain a fluoroscopic examination of the esophagus with water-soluble contrast enhancement after pneumatic dilation to make sure that perforation has not occurred. If perforation has occurred, surgical repair should be pursued quickly.

The standard surgical approach to the treatment of achalasia is the Heller myotomy done by thoracotomy. Once exposed, the circular muscle layer of the esophagus is cut from the distal esophagus to the proximal stomach. Some surgeons perform an antireflux procedure concurrently with the myotomy; others reserve this added manipulation for patients with an associated hiatal hernia. Although clearly efficacious, a Heller myotomy is associated with considerable morbidity, which has led most patients to pursue pneumatic dilation as the initial intervention. However, new surgical approaches to achalasia using laparoscopic or thoracoscopic techniques may tip the balance toward surgery as an initial intervention because these techniques have substantially reduced morbidity.

Spastic Disorders

Abnormal peristalsis can cause dysphagia and chest pain that may mimic angina pectoris. An esophageal cause of chest pain should be considered only after careful consideration of potential cardiopulmonary causes. However, even within the spectrum of esophageal diseases, neither chest pain nor dysphagia is specific for a spastic disorder because both symptoms are also characteristic of peptic, pill, or infectious esophagitis. After these more common diagnostic possibilities have been excluded by appropriate radiographic evaluation, endoscopic evaluation, and, in some instances, a therapeutic trial of antisecretory medications, spastic disorders should be considered the cause of the still unexplained symptoms.

Unlike with achalasia, the esophagus usually retains its ability to propagate peristaltic waves the majority of the time in patients with esophageal spasm. Thus, defining radiographic and manometric criteria vary. In the unequivocal case, nonperistaltic, high-amplitude, prolonged contractions are seen during esophageal manometry, and these are associated with the patient's experiencing chest pain. These unequivocal cases are probably associated with damage to the myenteric plexus, in the continuum of vigorous achalasia and achalasia. DES may appear radiographically as a "corkscrew esophagus."

Ironically, the medical therapies for esophageal spasm are similar to those for coronary artery dis-

---

*Not FDA approved for this medication.

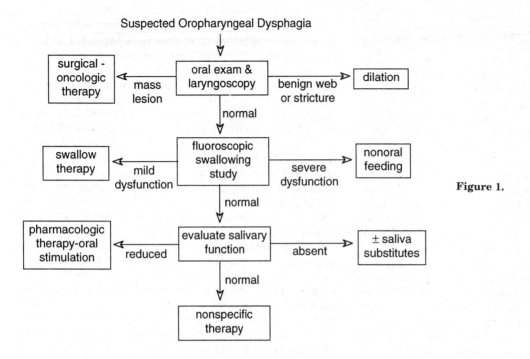

Figure 1.

ease, a disease with which it can be confused. However, despite the dogma of treatment with smooth muscle relaxants, there are few controlled data on the medical treatment of esophageal spasm. Long-term outcome studies of the medical treatment of DES with smooth muscle relaxants are not available, and the entire basis for this therapy remains at an anecdotal level. Likewise, there are no controlled studies of treatment of well-defined patients with DES with pneumatic dilatation or myotomy. Some DES patients have been observed to evolve into achalasia, for which there are defined treatment strate-

gies. However, at this time, therapy for esophageal spastic disorders is typically a trial-and-error experience reflecting the inhomogeneity of this population of patients.

CLINICAL EVALUATION OF DYSPHAGIA

After this review of the varied causes of dysphagia, it should be obvious how important it is to obtain a detailed history from the patient, exploring related symptoms such as heartburn, drooling, aspiration,

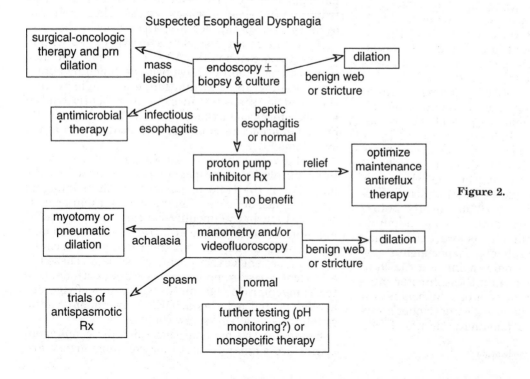

Figure 2.

voice changes, regurgitation, bolus impaction, dry mouth, odynophagia, additional neurologic symptoms, and chest pain. The history should initially guide the clinician to pursue a diagnosis of oropharyngeal versus esophageal dysphagia (Figures 1 and 2). Within each algorithm, the logic is similar. First pursue anatomic causes, then functional causes. In most instances, the cause of dysphagia can be well defined and corrective therapy rendered. The clinician should define the likely cause of the dysphagia and then tailor the examination to the individual patient in terms of both the sequence of tests used and the emphasis placed on obtaining a definitive diagnosis.

DIVERTICULA OF THE ALIMENTARY TRACT

method of
ANTHONY ALBRIGHT, M.D.
St. Tammany Parish Medical Society and
Affiliated Hospitals
St. Tammany Parish, Louisiana

Diverticula are epithelium-lined mucosal pouches of the intestinal tract and may be categorized as true or false. True diverticula contain all layers of the intestinal wall, including the mucosa, submucosa, and muscle, whereas false diverticula contain only the mucosal and submucosal layers. Diverticula may result from congenital abnormalities, motility disorders, or traction and pulsion forces. Although usually asymptomatic, diverticula may bleed, perforate, or become infected. Excessive numbers of bacteria may colonize diverticula, leading to malabsorption.

ESOPHAGEAL DIVERTICULA

Hypopharyngeal Diverticula

The hypopharyngeal diverticulum (Zenker's) is the most common diverticulum of the esophagus. It is located posteriorly in the midline, protruding between the cricopharyngeus and inferior constrictor muscles. It is found in approximately 2% of patients presenting with dysphagia. It is rarely seen in patients younger than 30 years, and most patients present in the sixth or seventh decades of life. As the diverticulum enlarges, it dissects toward the left side and downward into the superior mediastinum. Its cause has long been debated. Some investigators suggest that high-amplitude pressures in the cricopharyngeus muscle, along with poor compliance of the upper esophageal sphincter, lead to its development. Symptoms are usually classic, with transient dysphagia early in the course. However, once the pharyngeal sac becomes large enough to retain contents, the patient may complain of progressive cervical dysphagia, gurgling, regurgitation, nocturnal wheezing from aspiration, or a palpable mass in the neck. Rarely, the sac becomes so large that it pushes anteriorly

and causes obstruction. Squamous cell carcinoma has been reported in less than 1% of these diverticula.

The diagnosis is suspected by the patient's history and confirmed by an esophagogram. Upper endoscopy is not necessary for diagnosis and may be contraindicated, owing to the risk of perforation. This demonstrates the necessity of obtaining an esophagogram in patients with dysphagia before undertaking endoscopy.

Treatment

Patients with asymptomatic diverticula do not require treatment; however, surgical treatment is indicated for symptomatic diverticula. If the diverticulum is small, it can be treated with a cricopharyngeal myotomy; otherwise, a diverticulectomy is the surgery of choice.

Midesophageal Diverticula

Midesophageal diverticula were once called traction diverticula because they were thought to be secondary to mediastinal granulomatous disease (tuberculosis, histoplasmosis). The mediastinal adhesions were thought to have pulled on the esophagus, causing a traction diverticulum. It is now believed that these diverticula are secondary to an underlying motility disorder. They are usually small and wide mouthed and are found incidentally on upper gastrointestinal studies and require no treatment. If the patient has symptoms of chest pain, a work-up for a motility disorder should be considered.

Epiphrenic Diverticula

Epiphrenic diverticula occur in the distal esophagus and are believed to be caused by motor abnormalities of the esophagus. One study demonstrated that 75% of patients with epiphrenic diverticula had an underlying motor disorder. Symptoms usually relate to the motor disorder, but some patients regurgitate massive amounts of fluid while recumbent. This is thought to be due to food trapped in the diverticulum during waking hours. Although extremely rare, squamous cell carcinoma has been reported in epiphrenic diverticula.

Treatment

Asymptomatic diverticula require no treatment. Therapy for symptomatic diverticula associated with esophageal spasm or achalasia should be directed toward the underlying motility disorder, using oral nitrates* or calcium channel blockers.* Progressive enlargement of the diverticulum or aspiration of food is an indication for surgery. Diverticulectomy, together with a procedure directed at the underlying motility disorder, such as a lower esophageal myotomy, is the surgery of choice.

---

*Not FDA approved for this indication.

Intramural Diverticulosis

Intramural diverticulosis is a rare condition associated with an upper esophageal stricture, and numerous 1- to 3-mm outpouchings of the esophagus are demonstrated on upper gastrointestinal barium studies. Pathologically, these are not true diverticula but represent dilated ducts arising from submucosal glands. The vast majority of patients present with dysphagia. The cause remains obscure, although previous corrosive injury may be implicated. Esophageal candidiasis has been reported in 50% of patients, although it is not known whether it is a causative agent. Treatment consists of dilatation of the associated stricture. After dilatation, the pseudodiverticula remain but may be less prominent.

GASTRIC DIVERTICULUM

Gastric diverticulum is a rare entity that generally does not produce symptoms. The diagnosis is usually made by radiographic studies that show a true diverticulum near the posterior gastric wall. It may also occur near the pylorus, in association with previous peptic, granulomatous, or neoplastic disease. Rare cases of bleeding and perforation have been reported. Gastric diverticula are not thought to be prone to carcinogenesis, nor is there any correlation between these diverticula and other diverticula of the intestinal tract. Specific treatment is rarely indicated.

SMALL INTESTINAL DIVERTICULA
Duodenal Diverticula

Duodenal diverticula occur in approximately 10 to 20% of the population, with an increasing incidence in older patients. They have a 2:1 predilection for females and are usually periampullary. Most are asymptomatic but remain clinically important because they can cause obstruction of the common bile duct. This may also lead to pancreatitis, cholangitis, and recurrent common bile duct stones even after cholecystectomy. Complications of the biliary tract are thought to be caused by an enlarged diverticulum that is impacted with food and debris, causing mechanical distortion of the common bile duct. This results in stasis, proliferation of bacteria, and dysfunction of the choledochal sphincter. Bleeding and perforation of duodenal diverticula have been reported but are rare.

Treatment

The diagnosis of bleeding duodenal diverticulum should be made endoscopically. Its management is similar to that of other causes of upper gastrointestinal bleeding, with institution of supportive care and fluid and blood replacement, and monitoring of hemodynamic status. Surgical resection of the diverticulum is indicated when supportive measures fail.

Biliary disease is more complicated, and even in jaundiced patients most duodenal diverticula are incidental findings. Duodenal diverticulum as a cause of obstructive jaundice is a diagnosis of exclusion. It requires an endoscopic retrograde cholangiogram to evaluate the biliary tract and rule out other causes, along with the presence of an enlarged diverticulum. When definite proof implicates the diverticula, a choledochoduodenostomy or Roux-en-Y choledochojejunostomy is the surgical treatment of choice.

Jejunal and Ileal Diverticula

Jejunal and ileal diverticula are uncommon and are considered to be acquired diverticula. They are found along the mesenteric border of the intestine where vessels penetrate into the intestinal wall. They are associated with motility disorders of the intestine such as degenerative visceral myopathy and neuropathy, pseudo-obstruction, and more generalized motility disorders such as scleroderma. They may lead to bacterial overgrowth within the diverticula.

The symptoms are those of malabsorption with steatorrhea, weight loss, and associated fat-soluble vitamin deficiencies. Diagnosis is made by an abnormal urinary D-xylose test and the absence of mucosal disease on small bowel biopsy. The Schilling test, performed with and without intrinsic factor, shows malabsorption of vitamin B_{12}. Small bowel radiographs demonstrate the diverticula, and a careful history may reveal dysphagia or previous obstructions that may indicate scleroderma or intestinal pseudo-obstruction, respectively. Aspiration and culture of small bowel contents confirm overgrowth when organisms exceed 10,000 per mL. Hydrogen and carbon dioxide breath tests can also be used to diagnose bacterial overgrowth.

Treatment

Bacterial overgrowth responds to antimicrobial therapy. One should choose agents that are effective against both aerobic and anaerobic bacteria. A 10-day course of a cephalosporin such as cephalexin (Keflex), 250 mg by mouth four times a day, or metronidazole (Flagyl), 250 mg three times a day by mouth, is quite effective. Tetracycline, 250 mg four times a day by mouth, is also effective, although resistance has been reported, especially with *Bacteroides*. Vitamin B_{12} and folic acid should be provided as supplements, as well as other fat-soluble vitamins. Relapse is common, and repeated treatment is often necessary. Surgery should be performed only for bleeding, perforation, or volvulus.

Meckel's Diverticulum

Meckel's diverticulum is the most common true diverticulum of the gastrointestinal tract, with a reported incidence of 2% in autopsy series. It arises from the antimesenteric border of the ileum, usually within 100 cm from the ileocecal valve. Meckel's diverticula have a wide-open mouth, are about 5 cm long, and result from the incomplete closure of the omphalomesenteric duct. Most are asymptomatic.

About 45% of Meckel's diverticula contain gastric mucosa. An additional 45% contain normal mucosa, and the remaining 10% have duodenal, pancreatic, colonic, and endometrial mucosa. *Helicobacter pylori* has been shown to be present in those diverticula having active gastritis.

Complications include hemorrhage, obstruction, diverticulitis, intussusception, and perforation. Bleeding is the most common complication and is due to acid production of the ectopic gastric mucosa that results in subsequent ulceration. The bleeding may arise within or adjacent to the diverticulum and is usually painless. It occurs mostly in children younger than 2 years. The stools are usually dark red and may have a "currant jelly" appearance, although occasionally they may be tarry.

Intestinal obstruction is caused by intussusception or volvulus around persistent fibrous remnants of the vitelline duct. Diverticulitis of Meckel's diverticulum may produce a clinical picture indistinguishable from that of acute appendicitis. Failure to find an inflamed appendix warrants a search for a Meckel diverticulum.

Treatment

Meckel's diverticular bleeding should be suspected in young patients especially but must be considered in the differential diagnosis of all patients. Once the condition is suspected, a technetium Tc 99m scan should be performed before any barium studies to determine the presence of any ectopic gastric mucosa. Pentagastrin (Peptavlon) may be used to stimulate the uptake of technetium by gastric mucosa and reduce the number of false-negative studies. Enteroclysis studies have been shown to demonstrate a Meckel diverticulum in adults. Diverticulectomy is recommended for patients with a bleeding diverticulum, as well as those with diverticulitis and bowel obstruction. A Meckel diverticulum discovered incidentally during surgery should not be removed, because the morbidity of the operation is greater than the likelihood of the diverticulum's becoming symptomatic.

DIVERTICULAR DISEASE OF THE COLON

The colon is the most common site of diverticular formation in the gastrointestinal tract, with greater than 50% of patients older than 50 years having colonic diverticula. These are not true diverticula but rather are herniations of the mucosa and submucosa. They occur in rows between the circular muscle layers at the point where the nutrient arteries penetrate the wall of the colon. They vary in number from one to several hundred and may be several centimeters in diameter. Most are found in the sigmoid colon; if they exist throughout the colon, they are usually in continuity with the sigmoid.

Diverticulosis

Diverticulosis usually refers to the presence of diverticula in the colon. These are generally discovered incidentally by barium studies or flexible sigmoidoscopy. Uncomplicated diverticulosis is asymptomatic and requires no treatment. Spastic colon diverticulosis is the most common form, associated with marked thickening of the sigmoid wall. A second type is simple massed diverticulosis that involves extensive, numerous diverticula without the circular muscle hypertrophy. Solitary diverticula are usually in the ascending colon and cecum and are true diverticula, thought to be congenital and not related to diverticulosis.

The cause of diverticulosis is unknown, although weakness in the colonic wall clearly plays a role and is thought to be secondary to deposition of elastin with aging. Diverticulosis is more common in Western societies, which prompts the "fiber hypothesis." This suggests that a low-fiber diet reduces stool bulk and leads to extensive colonic motility and increased intraluminal pressure, resulting in herniation of the mucosa. Others believe that diverticulosis is the end stage of the irritable bowel syndrome, although the different natural histories and myoelectric activities suggest otherwise. Colonic diverticula may be complicated by infection, perforation, or bleeding.

Diverticular Bleeding

Diverticular bleeding usually occurs as massive, painless bleeding in an elderly patient. The patient may feel a sudden urge to defecate, and the stools are usually red to maroon but may be black. Bleeding is thought to be due to the erosion of an artery into a diverticulum and is not related to inflammation, e.g., diverticulitis. Most bleeding occurs on the right side of the colon and in 80% of patients stops spontaneously. The incidence of rebleeding approaches 25%. However, once bleeding recurs, the risk of subsequent hemorrhage increases dramatically.

Treatment

Localization of the bleeding site is imperative for treatment of hematochezia. An upper source must be ruled out and can be excluded by nasogastric aspiration of gastric contents, or more effectively, by endoscopic examination. As with all gastrointestinal bleeding, the patient must be made hemodynamically stable with fluids and blood products, and a surgical consultation should be obtained. Once an upper gastrointestinal site has been excluded, the lower tract should be evaluated. If the rectal bleeding is severe or continuous, angiography of the celiac and mesenteric arteries should be the first approach to diagnosis. Once a bleeding site is located, selective intra-arterial vasopressin at 0.3 unit per minute should stop the bleeding. If there is a contraindication to angiography, or if the patient is intermittently bleeding, a nuclear medicine bleeding scan may be the first choice for localization. If the bleeding has stopped or slowed significantly, a colonoscopic examination should be performed. This may be an examination without bowel preparation or preferably done after cleansing the bowel with an agent such as Go-

LYTELY or Colyte. Colonoscopy can help define the location and source of bleeding, e.g., a diverticulum or arteriovenous malformation. The colonoscope may also be used for therapeutic treatment of bleeding. If medical support including intravascular vasopressin has failed, surgical resection of the portion of colon containing the bleeding diverticulum is indicated. A subtotal colectomy should only be performed in patients with recurrent bleeding in whom the specific bleeding site has not been identified, as this procedure has a much higher morbidity.

Diverticulitis

Diverticulitis is the most common complication of diverticulosis, occurring in up to 20% of patients. It results from a microperforation of a diverticulum, thought to be brought on by the presence of inspissated fecal material. Usually this occurs in the sigmoid colon and involves only one diverticulum. This perforation is walled off and becomes a localized phlegmon or abscess. Only rarely is there free perforation of a diverticulum into the abdominal cavity, causing peritonitis.

Left lower quadrant pain and fever are the most common presenting symptoms. The pain is usually sudden in onset and constant and may radiate to the back. The patient may also experience nausea and vomiting or a change in bowel habits. Occasionally, dysuria and frequent urination are present, indicating bladder irritation.

Physical examination reveals tenderness in the left lower quadrant. Abdominal guarding and frequently rebound tenderness may be present. Bowel sounds are usually hypoactive, although with obstruction they may be hyperactive, with rushes and tinkles. Rectal examination may reveal tenderness or a mass in the cul-de-sac. An elevated white blood cell count and fever help to differentiate between diverticulitis and symptomatic diverticulosis or irritable bowel syndrome.

Diagnosis is usually clinical and is based on the presenting picture as described. Flexible sigmoidoscopy with minimal air insulation and preparation is relatively safe and is helpful to rule out an obstructing carcinoma or inflammatory bowel disease. Inability to pass the sigmoidoscope because of edema and angulation is consistent with, but not pathognomonic of, diverticulitis. Diagnostic use of barium or diatrizoate (Hypaque) radiography is controversial, as this may cause a localized perforation to progress. It is probably wise not to perform either sigmoidoscopy or barium studies unless the diagnosis is in doubt. Computed tomography of the abdomen and pelvis is a noninvasive and accurate tool for diagnosing the presence of diverticula and recognizing changes consistent with acute diverticulitis.

Treatment

Patients with pain and fever who require analgesics should be admitted to the hopsital. They should be put at bed rest and given intravenous fluids, and their oral intake should be restricted to rest the bowel. Nasogastric suction should be used in patients with nausea and vomiting or evidence of obstruction. Surgical consultation should be made, although 80% of patients can be managed medically. Parenteral broad-spectrum antibiotics should provide coverage against gram-negative and anaerobic organisms. Most authors recommend an aminoglycoside such as gentamicin (Garamycin), 1.5 mg per kg every 8 hours with doses adjusted for renal insufficiency, along with clindamycin (Cleocin), 600 mg every 6 hours. Aztreonam (Azactam), 500 mg to 1 gram every 8 hours, may be substituted for aminoglycosides in patients with renal insufficiency. Single-drug therapy with cefoxitin (Mefoxin), 2 grams every 8 hours, is also effective. Other antibiotic combinations, or β-lactamase antibiotics (in particular ticarcillin [Timentin] or imipenem-cilastatin [Primaxin]), are effective. The careful monitoring of aminoglycoside levels is imperative. The patient should be followed up frequently with abdominal examinations and appropriate laboratory and radiographic studies. Most patients improve after 3 to 4 days, whereas others may require 1 to 2 weeks of medical therapy. Surgical intervention is usually reserved for patients who fail to improve, develop a free perforation, or have a persistent small bowel obstruction. Commonly, a one-stage procedure, with resection of the involved area of the colon and a primary reanastomosis, is all that is necessary. A staged operation with a diverting colostomy is performed if significant peritonitis or infection is present. Elective surgical treatment is appropriate in patients with recurrent bouts of diverticulitis, in the presence of fistulas, or in cases of partial obstructions, when carcinoma cannot be excluded.

Patients without peritoneal signs may be treated at home with oral ciprofloxacin (Cipro), 500 mg by mouth every 12 hours, along with metronidazole, 250 mg by mouth every 8 hours for 10 days. Patients should be informed that if their condition does not improve or worsens, they need to notify their physician immediately. Follow-up examination is mandatory.

Methods of prevention are controversial, although it is generally recommended that patients follow a high-fiber diet, along with psyllium or cellulose products, after the acute episode has subsided. The effectiveness of avoiding seeds, nuts, corn, and other hard particles that may have an impact on diverticula has not been demonstrated empirically.

ULCERATIVE COLITIS

method of
STEPHEN B. HANAUER, M.D.
University of Chicago Pritzker School of Medicine
Chicago, Illinois

ETIOLOGY

Ulcerative colitis and Crohn's disease encompass the most common of the idiopathic inflammatory bowel diseases. Inherent in the definition and diagnosis is the absence of known causes of colonic inflammation, including enteric pathogens, drug-induced colitis (e.g., chemotherapy, nonsteroidal anti-inflammatory drugs [NSAIDs]), ischemia, and radiation. The etiopathogenesis of ulcerative colitis has not been discovered. Current research is exploring a mechanism by which the enteric mucosal immune system fails to down-regulate an acute inflammatory reaction induced by an as yet unknown stimulus or stimuli, leading to an overexuberant chronic inflammatory response in genetically predisposed individuals.

Clues to the genetic underpinnings include the identification of multiply affected family members with inflammatory bowel disease and a concordance among identical twins compared with dizygotic twins. In comparison to the predominant TH_1 cytokine profile in Crohn's disease, the cytokine profile in ulcerative colitis is directed more toward the TH_2 spectra of mediators with increased production of IgG1, and there is preliminary evidence for increased representation of allele 2 of the gene encoding the interleukin-1 receptor antagonist in patients with ulcerative colitis. Patients with ulcerative colitis are also more likely to have circulating perinuclear antineutrophil cytoplasmic antibodies (pANCA), which may reflect a genetic disposition or a response to colonic luminal contents that identify a subgroup of patients more likely to develop pouchitis after undergoing colectomy and ileoanal anastomosis.

Environmental factors that initiate ulcerative colitis have been sought in the diet and intestinal flora without success. It has been observed that many patients develop ulcerative colitis after traveler's diarrhea, upper respiratory infections, or a course of antibiotics, suggesting that an alteration in colonic microflora may initiate the disease. However, no specific pathogen has been identified to date, and antibiotic therapy has been uniformly unsuccessful. The only environmental factors that have a predictable impact on the disease are NSAIDs and cigarette smoking. As with other forms of intestinal inflammation and ulceration, NSAIDs are well recognized to exacerbate inflammatory bowel disease, most likely owing to the inhibition of prostaglandins that are necessary to promote mucosal repair. Conversely, cigarette smoking has a protective effect against ulcerative colitis. One of the few detrimental aspects of smoking cessation is the development of ulcerative colitis after quitting. The smoking history is one of the few epidemiologic clues that differentiate ulcerative colitis from Crohn's disease because nonsmokers (or ex-smokers) are more likely to develop ulcerative colitis, and smokers are more likely to develop Crohn's disease.

We now anticipate that ulcerative colitis (and Crohn's disease) will encompass a spectrum of colonic inflammatory diseases on the basis of disease location, systemic complications, and response to therapy. Investigators are currently attempting to correlate genotypic data with clinical subgroups to identify specific patterns of presentation, natural history, and therapeutic responsiveness.

DIAGNOSIS

Patients present with a spectrum of symptoms and signs, depending on the extent and severity of mucosal disease and associated extraintestinal complications. Bowel movements are most often affected, but the pattern may range from normal or even constipated stools with blood or mucopus to bloody diarrhea. Abdominal cramping and rectal urgency and tenesmus are more common than localized abdominal pain. Early morning rectal urgency and nocturnal bowel movements with the presence of rectal bleeding discriminate between inflammatory disease and irritable bowel syndrome. Patients may also present with fever, weight loss, anemia, hypoproteinemia, and abnormal liver enzyme activities. Potential extraintestinal symptoms include peripheral arthritis (typically pauciarticular involving larger joints), central arthritis (ankylosing spondylitis or sacroiliitis), iritis or episcleritis, erythema nodosum or pyoderma gangrenosum, or sclerosing cholangitis.

The presence of rectal bleeding alone is sufficient to warrant a flexible sigmoidoscopic or colonoscopic examination to define the cause. Ulcerative colitis manifests as diffuse, contiguous, and superficial ulceration beginning at the anorectal verge and extending proximally in a diffuse pattern, usually to a distinct cutoff to normal mucosa. The extent is variable among patients but tends to remain constant for individuals. Some proximal or distal change in the extent of colitis can occur, typically within the first years of disease. The histologic features of ulcerative colitis are superficial inflammation limited by the muscularis mucosae with crypt architectural distortion, crypt abscesses, and a nonspecific acute and chronic inflammatory infiltrate of the lamina propria and epithelium. As the acute inflammation remits, there may be endoscopic evidence of mucosal vascular distortion, postinflammatory polyps (pseudopolyps), and an atrophic appearance where prior ulcerations occurred. With mucosal regeneration and healing, residual histologic features include atrophic and distorted glands and resolution of the neutrophilic infiltration of epithelial crypts. Proximal to the upper margin of disease, the mucosa is endoscopically and histologically normal.

The primary consideration in the differential diagnosis is to determine whether the presentation is acute and likely to be infectious (self-limited colitis due to a bacterial pathogen such as *Escherichia coli, Campylobacter jejuni, Salmonella, Shigella*) or caused by *Clostridium difficile*. The overlap in presentation and the potential for infectious colitis to coexist with or exacerbate quiescent disease requires stool cultures and *C. difficile* toxin assays in new patients and during hospitalization or atypical flare-ups. Amebic colitis occasionally presents with a diffuse, continuous pattern of inflammation but more often with a focal, deeply ulcerating pattern. In the elderly population, ischemic colitis should be considered, but it more typically spares the rectum and involves the sigmoid colon in a more "necrotizing," ulcerated appearance. The main confounding chronic and idiopathic disease to be differentiated is Crohn's disease, which can mimic ulcerative colitis but more often presents in a focal, asymmetrical pattern with aphthoid or linear ulcerations separated by normal-appearing mucosa. Crohn's disease commonly spares the rectum and may be associated with perianal manifestations (such as protuberant skin tags, abscesses, or fistulas) and more proximal inflammation in the colon or ileum or with aphthous stomatitis. On histologic examination, Crohn's disease is also more focal with similar crypt abscesses in active disease and architectural distortion in quiescent disease. Noncaseating granulomas are useful, when present, to differentiate Crohn's disease from ulcerative colitis, but because of their infrequency (15 to 40%), other signs of microscopic focality of inflammation or deeper inflammation into the submucosa associated with focal lymphoid aggregates may be more helpful. In about 10 to 20% of patients, the pattern of colitis may be indeterminate between "classic" ulcerative colitis and Crohn's disease with some degree of patchiness or focality, often occurring in partially treated colitis. Determination of pANCA may be useful as a marker of ulcerative colitis, although it is now recognized that pANCA-positive Crohn's disease patients may have a pattern of left-sided colitis similar to that of patients with ulcerative colitis. The pANCA status has not been evaluated as a discriminant feature in patients with indeterminate colitis.

Since the availability of flexible sigmoidoscopes and colonoscopes, the diagnosis of ulcerative colitis is more readily at hand. Because of the virtual omnipresence of rectal inflammation in ulcerative colitis, a proctoscopic examination usually demonstrates inflammation, and a flexible sigmoidoscope can reveal the proximal extent and pattern of colitis in a majority of patients. Mucosal biopsies may be helpful in excluding acute self-limited colitis (more superficial inflammation without crypt architectural distortion) and Crohn's disease (focal inflammation with the occasional presence of granuloma), but findings are typically nonspecific. At some point in the course of the disease, a colonoscopy is warranted to define the proximal extent (if it has not been determined at sigmoidoscopy), which will be useful from the standpoints of prognosis and therapeutic alternatives.

Barium contrast studies are no longer used as a standard for the diagnosis of ulcerative colitis owing to the lack of sensitivity at defining mild or quiescent inflammation and the inability to obtain a biopsy specimen of the mucosa. In severe or fulminant colitis (patients who are febrile, have distention, or have rebound tenderness), invasive diagnostic procedures run the risk of inducing toxic megacolon or perforation. In this setting, plain abdominal radiographs often define the proximal extent of disease by the absence of stool in the inflamed lumen and an ahaustral-appearing, edematous colonic wall, often with thumbprinting of the mucosa. Technetium- or indium-labeled leukocyte scans may occasionally be useful to define the extent of colitis in patients with severe disease.

Before initiating therapy, it is useful to define the extent and severity of colitis as well as the presence of extraintestinal manifestations and the response to prior treatment approaches. The proximal extent of ulcerative colitis is relevant to therapeutic delivery of drug by oral or rectal administration and the formulation of topical drug (suppository, foam, or enema). In addition, the long-term risk for developing dysplasia or cancer is related to the duration of disease, the mucosal extent, and the presence of sclerosing cholangitis. The severity of the attack will determine the potency of the initial therapeutic strategy, as will the presence of inflammatory extraintestinal symptoms such as pyoderma gangrenosum or severe arthritis. Finally, the responsiveness to different therapeutic classes, or lack thereof, will predict the subsequent efficacy of treatment.

Classifying patients into distal or extensive disease categories with mild to moderate, moderate to severe, or fulminant-toxic colitis may be the most facile way of approaching therapy:

Distal colitis (proctitis, proctosigmoiditis): mild-moderate; moderate-severe
Extensive colitis: mild-moderate; moderate-severe
Fulminant colitis–toxic megacolon

Severity criteria include the number of trips to the toilet (not necessarily number of stools), rectal bleeding, rectal urgency (or incontinence), abdominal pain, fever, tachycardia, anemia, and hypoalbuminemia. The erythrocyte sedimentation rate is an unreliable indicator of inflammation in ulcerative colitis aside from the more severe situations. Patients with mild disease usually have fewer than 6 to 10 bowel movements daily without abdominal pain, incontinence, fever, or anemia. Patients with more than 10 bowel movements per day associated with fever, tachycardia, anemia, or hypoalbuminemia are considered to have severe disease. Fulminant colitis occurs in the setting of toxic manifestations such as high fever, abdominal tenderness, orthostatic hypotension, and leukocytosis. If any segment of the colon is dilated greater than 8 to 10 cm in the setting of severe symptoms, the condition is termed "toxic megacolon"; this is a medical and potentially surgical emergency that can be induced in patients with severe disease who develop hypokalemia or are treated with antimotility agents (including narcotic analgesics or antidiarrheals such as diphenoxylate or loperamide) or who have had invasive procedures such as colonoscopic examinations or contrast-enhanced radiography. These individuals are at significant risk for colonic perforation because of marked thinning of the colonic wall and a virtual "melting away" of the muscle layers due to transmural extension of the usually superficial inflammatory process.

TREATMENT

The goal of therapy in ulcerative colitis is to induce and then maintain remission. Remission is defined by the absence of inflammatory symptoms (bleeding, urgency, tenesmus, and diarrhea) with healing or regeneration of the colonic mucosa. Endoscopic confirmation is not usually required, although follow-up sigmoidoscopic examinations may help to clarify whether persisting symptoms are due to residual inflammation or colonic irritability. Four basic classes of therapy are applicable to ulcerative colitis: supportive-symptomatic therapies, aminosalicylates, corticosteroids, and immunomodulators.

Supportive Therapies

Although no dietary factors have been identified that have an impact on the inflammatory reaction in ulcerative colitis, it is unrealistic to ignore the role of diet in controlling symptoms. Patients with distal colitis (especially ulcerative proctitis) are often constipated and may benefit from the addition of fiber to their diet, whereas patients with more extensive disease and diarrheal stools feel better with less fiber and the avoidance of highly spicy foods that stimulate motility. Lactose intolerance should be considered a contributing factor to diarrhea or flatus, and adequate calcium supplementation should be ensured for these individuals, especially for patients receiving systemic corticosteroids. Iron supplementation is commonly required for patients with longer histories of bleeding or anemia. Because of protein loss from the inflamed colon, patients need to have adequate calories and protein in their diet to maintain muscle stores.

In addition to fiber supplements for constipated patients, many individuals with mild disease or irritable bowel symptoms in addition to their colitis benefit from antispasmodics such as dicyclomine (Bentyl) or hyoscyamine (Anaspaz, Levsin) to reduce cramping or antidiarrheal preparations such as diphenoxylate or loperamide. The antidiarrheal preparations should be avoided in patients with more severe symptoms who are at risk for developing toxic megacolon. Use of narcotics should be avoided in patients with ulcerative colitis because significant abdominal pain or tenderness implies transmural inflammation and a risk for perforation or megacolon.

Aminosalicylates

The 5-aminosalicylic acid (5-ASA, mesalamine [Asacol, Pentasa, Rowasa]) derivatives of sulfasalazine are the most commonly used agents to induce remission in mild to moderate ulcerative colitis and to maintain remissions after inductive therapy. Sulfasalazine (Azulfidine) has been employed for more than 50 years in ulcerative colitis. It is now recognized that sulfasalazine, composed of sulfapyridine linked to 5-ASA by an azo bond, is primarily an oral delivery formulation that releases the 5-ASA (mesalamine) into the colonic lumen. Because unprotected mesalamine is rapidly absorbed and metabolized by the proximal small bowel, it is necessary to formulate the drug for release into the colon. The exact therapeutic mechanisms are not known, although virtually every mediator that has been identified to contribute to inflammation in ulcerative colitis (leukotriene production, platelet-activating factor, reactive oxygen species, interleukin-1, and nitric oxide) is inhibited to some degree by 5-ASA. Sulfasalazine uses an azo linkage to sulfapyridine, which acts as a carrier for colonic delivery. The dose-response effect of sulfasalazine is compromised by both a dose-related intolerance to the sulfapyridine (producing headaches, nausea, and myalgias in many patients) and sulfa-related hypersensitivity reactions, bone marrow suppression, and sperm abnormalities in up to 80% of men. Olsalazine (Dipentum) is an alternative azo bond preparation linking two molecules of 5-ASA for similar colonic delivery. Olsalazine has been a useful alternative to sulfasalazine for maintenance therapy in patients with sulfa-related intolerance, although the compound has not been as beneficial in active disease owing to the potential to induce small bowel secretion and watery diarrhea.

Mesalamine preparations have become the most commonly prescribed therapies for mild to moderate ulcerative colitis and as maintenance agents. Several oral formulations are now available that have similar dose-related efficacy and minimal dose-related side effects (see "Medical Treatment"). These agents are therapeutically equivalent to sulfasalazine when equimolar amounts of 5-ASA are delivered but have the advantage of higher dosing because of the absence of dose-related intolerance or sulfahypersensitivity. In addition, topical formulations of mesalamine are extremely useful for patients with distal colitis. Mesalamine suppositories are effective for inducing and maintaining remission in ulcerative proctitis; mesalamine enemas are effective for the treatment of ulcerative proctosigmoiditis and left-sided colitis extending up to the splenic flexure.

Corticosteroids

Glucocorticosteroids are used to treat moderate to severe colitis and are effective with oral, parenteral, or topical administration. These agents should be reserved for the induction of remission and treatment of active disease but are not effective or indicated as maintenance agents. Unfortunately, up to one third of patients may become steroid dependent, and the disease may flare with tapering of the drug. This is not the same as having a maintenance role but instead is an indication for colectomy if the patient cannot be successfully weaned from steroids. Corticosteroids also have many anti-inflammatory activities, including a direct effect on lymphocyte trafficking, leukocyte adherence, and chemotaxis; the reduction of arachidonic acid metabolites; the inhibition of cytokines and nitric oxide; and a diminished expression of adhesion molecules.

Rectal administration of corticosteroids is useful to treat distal disease and as an adjunct to parenteral or oral steroids to treat rectal symptoms (urgency, tenesmus) in patients with more severe disease. Prednisone is the most common oral preparation for moderate to severe symptoms in outpatients; parenteral formulations of hydrocortisone, prednisolone, and methylprednisolone are reserved for hospitalized patients. Adrenocorticotropic hormone administered by intramuscular injection or continuous intravenous infusion is favored by some clinicians.

Pharmaceutical development has produced more potent steroids with topical (mucosal) activity and a rapid first-pass hepatic metabolism. These compounds are becoming available in different international markets and may have a therapeutic advantage over the more systemically active steroids. Budesonide enemas* have been introduced, and an oral colonic delivery system is under development. Budesonide has nearly 200 times the potency of hydrocortisone but with little systemic availability or adrenal suppression when it is administered as a 2-mg enema.

Immunomodulators

Both azathioprine† and its active metabolite 6-mercaptopurine† have been used for decades in steroid-dependent or steroid-refractory ulcerative colitis. These agents have been demonstrated to be useful in steroid weaning and maintaining remissions in ulcerative colitis but require 3 to 6 months for efficacy to be ascertained and steroid weaning to be achieved. Toxicity has not been a major issue, although these drugs require regular monitoring (at least every 3 months) of the complete blood count to avoid leukopenia. Up to 10 to 15% of patients may also develop an allergic pancreatitis or, less commonly, another systemic hypersensitivity reaction (fever, arthralgias, hypotension). It remains to be

---

*Not available in the United States.
†Not FDA approved for this indication.

TABLE 1. **Management of Distal Colitis**

Oral	Topical
Sulfasalazine (Azulfidine) 2–4 gm/d	Mesalamine suppository (Rowasa)* 500 mg bid to tid
Mesalamine (Asacol, Pentasa) 1.5–5 gm/d	Mesalamine enema (Rowasa) 1–4 gm/hs
	Hydrocortisone foam (Cortifoam)* 90 mg hs to bid
	Hydrocortisone enema (Cortenema) 100 mg/hs
	Budesonide enema† 2 mg/hs

*Ulcerative proctitis.
†Not yet FDA approved.

determined whether the induction of leukopenia hastens or improves the therapeutic efficacy of these agents. The potential of increasing the risk for colonic cancer has not been confirmed in case-control series, and it is anticipated that these agents will require long-term administration (i.e., years).

The long-term efficacy of azathioprine and 6-mercaptopurine and the lag time toward effects have led to the use of cyclosporine* in the setting of acute, steroid-unresponsive ulcerative colitis. In this setting, up to 80% of patients who failed to improve with intravenous steroids responded to the addition of intravenous cyclosporine. This potent immunosuppressive agent has a narrow therapeutic margin, creating controversy regarding its ultimate utility. The drug has "salvaged" colons from colectomy and may serve as a "bridge" to long-term immunosuppressive therapy with azathioprine or 6-mercaptopurine, which appear to be required (in addition to aminosalicylates) to maintain remissions after cyclosporine.

MEDICAL TREATMENT

Distal Colitis

Mild to moderate distal ulcerative colitis can be approached from either oral or topical routes. The choice of initial therapy depends on the patients' desires and lifestyles. There is evidence that topical treatment with mesalamine suppositories (for proctitis) administered two or three times daily or enemas (for disease up to the splenic flexure) administered nightly offers faster symptom improvement than does treatment with an equal dose of an oral aminosalicylate. Nevertheless, many patients will prefer oral therapy to repeated rectal dosing. Conversely, patients who have not responded to initial oral aminosalicylate therapy tolerate rectal therapy well.

Thus, the initial management of distal colitis includes the options listed in Table 1. Patients should be treated with full doses until they achieve a complete remission (complete relief of symptoms). Combination therapy with an oral aminosalicylate and topical treatment with either mesalamine or a corticosteroid is acceptable and may hasten the clinical response. The dose-response effect for oral therapy

*Not FDA approved for this indication.

must be considered in patients who fail to respond to introductory therapy. Increasing the dose to the maximal tolerated is more efficacious but compromised by side effects with sulfasalazine and primarily by cost with the mesalamine formulations.

Once patients improve, maintenance therapy is continued with either the same inductive dose of the oral aminosalicylate or with topical mesalamine. Most patients prefer substitution of long-term oral treatment for continuous topical therapy. However, recognize that patients who require topical treatment to respond are more likely to require long-term intrarectal mesalamine to maintain remissions. Again, dose is a consideration. There is a documented dose-response effect for both oral and topical aminosalicylate therapy. With intrarectal treatments, the dose-response effect is related to applications per week (i.e., at bedtime, every other day, every third day, and so on). Individuals who develop side effects from sulfasalazine can be treated with an alternative aminosalicylate (olsalazine or mesalamine). In this situation, it may be necessary to titrate up the dose of 5-ASA to achieve or maintain remission. Patients who have received topical corticosteroids to induce remission should be transferred to maintenance therapy with an aminosalicylate.

Refractory distal colitis that has not responded to either an oral aminosalicylate or topical corticosteroid still has a high likelihood of responding to topical mesalamine. Patients should be instructed to continue with daily intrarectal therapy until they have a complete response. Withdrawing treatment before remission increases the chance for creating an even less responsive state. Combination therapy with intrarectal corticosteroids and mesalamine is also effective in refractory disease. Only rarely will resistant disease require a course of systemic steroids to induce remission. These patients usually require a combination of oral and rectal aminosalicylates to maintain well-being. Ex-smokers may also respond to the reintroduction of cigarettes or the addition of a nicotine patch.

Extensive Colitis

Mild to moderate ulcerative colitis extending proximal to the splenic flexure requires therapy with an oral aminosalicylate. There is therapeutic equivalence between sulfasalazine and the oral mesalamine formulations when equal amounts of 5-ASA are provided, although the non–sulfa-containing formulations offer improved tolerance and the ability to provide higher doses of the active component without the dose-related side effects from sulfasalazine. In patients who tolerate sulfasalazine, this is the more cost-effective therapy. Dosing is the same as for distal disease (see earlier), and if patients are not responding to introductory therapy at the lower end of the dose range, the dosage is increased until there is a therapeutic response.

Patients who fail to improve with aminosalicylates at the optimal end of the dose range or individuals with moderate to severe symptoms (e.g., more than 10 bowel movements daily, fevers, weight loss, extraintestinal symptoms) require inductive therapy with an oral corticosteroid such as prednisone. The introductory dose is 40 to 60 mg per day, and this should be maintained until the patient is asymptomatic. Initiating therapy with lower doses or tapering before complete remission jeopardizes the ultimate benefits of inductive therapy or initiates maintenance treatment before the patient is in remission. If the patient had not been receiving an aminosalicylate, one is added and the steroids are tapered in a schedule according to the time required to achieve a full response. In general, it may require a few weeks for the patient to fully respond to the introduction of prednisone, after which the dose may be tapered by 5 mg weekly down to 10 to 20 mg per day and then by 2.5 mg per week. Tapering should proceed only as long as the patient remains asymptomatic.

Patients who become steroid dependent with flareups of disease activity with tapering should receive an aminosalicylate at the upper end of the dose range (e.g., sulfasalazine 4 to 6 grams per day or mesalamine 4 to 5 grams per day) after reinduction of remission. The tapering process is then resumed at a more gradual rate. Exogenous factors should be reconsidered if the patient remains steroid dependent or steroid refractory (e.g., concurrent NSAID use, intercurrent infection, or *C. difficile*). If patients remain dependent on or refractory to steroids, then either azathioprine or 6-mercaptopurine can be added as long as the patient is not at risk for modest immunosuppression (e.g., elderly, chronic infections, poorly compliant, or with long-standing colitis or evidence of dysplasia or prior neoplastic polyps). Azathioprine or 6-mercaptopurine is added (in addition to the steroids and aminosalicylate) initially at 50 mg per day, and the dose is titrated upward every 2 weeks with monitoring of the white blood cell count. Initially, I attempt to get the white blood cell count below 8000 to 10,000 per mm^3 and anticipate that it may require 3 to 6 months to achieve steroid weaning. An alternative approach for outpatients who are refractory to the introduction of oral prednisone is to admit the patient into the hospital for a course of intravenous steroids (see later).

Remission should be maintained with an oral aminosalicylate. Because of the documented dose-response effect with mesalamine, the optimal maintenance dose is the same as the inductive dose. However, from the standpoint of cost and compliance, the maintenance dose is sometimes reduced after a year but should not be lowered below 2 grams per day of sulfasalazine or 800 mg per day of mesalamine. If patients have a flare-up at a less than optimal dose of the aminosalicylate, reinduction should proceed as described and the maintenance dose increased to prevent subsequent relapse. It is often easier to maintain remissions than to reinduce remission. Exogenous factors, as before, should be considered in patients at the time of relapse, particularly NSAID use, which is so common with over-the-counter formulations.

Severe Colitis

Patients with severe colitis should be hospitalized to receive parenteral steroids, the equivalent of hydrocortisone 300 to 400 mg per day or methylprednisolone 40 to 60 mg per day. I prefer a continuous intravenous infusion to intermittent bolus administration. Aminosalicylates are withheld until the patient is markedly improved, feeling well, and tolerating a full diet. Patients who are hungry and able to eat can continue a low-residue diet. If they have severe cramping, tenesmus, nausea, or vomiting, solid foods should be withheld temporarily. Parenteral nutrition should be provided for patients unable to eat or with evidence of malnutrition or hypoproteinemia. Transfusion or parenteral iron infusion may be required, depending on the hematocrit and iron stores.

The continuous intravenous steroid regimen is continued until the patient is having formed bowel movements without blood or urgency. This generally requires 5 to 10 days. Withdrawing therapy before a complete response compromises the ultimate response. After resolution of diarrhea, bleeding, and abdominal cramps, a full diet is resumed and the steroid is changed to an oral form at the same daily dose (e.g., prednisone 40 to 60 mg). An aminosalicylate is then added, and the steroids are tapered after discharge.

Fulminant Colitis or Toxic Megacolon

Fulminant colitis, with or without colonic dilatation, is a medical emergency. Patients presenting with fever, abdominal tenderness (with or without rebound), marked hemorrhage, or anemia and leukocytosis should be co-managed with a surgical team. Patients should be rapidly resuscitated with fluids, electrolytes, and blood transfusion to maintain the hematocrit above 30%. An abdominal flat plate is necessary to rule out colonic dilatation or intraperitoneal air. Patients should receive nothing by mouth, and parenteral nutrition should be administered after the initial resuscitative efforts. Intravenous corticosteroids are administered as for severe colitis. In addition, broad-spectrum antibiotics (e.g., third-generation cephalosporin, or a combination of metronidazole and an aminoglycoside) are added because of the transmural nature of the progressive colitis and the possibility of walled-off perforation or impending colectomy. In the setting of colonic dilatation, patients should be encouraged to roll from side to side to redistribute the colonic gas. Some clinicians advocate a rectal tube or "knee-chest" position to assist in decompressing the colon. A nasogastric tube is placed in patients with small bowel ileus. Failure to rapidly respond with defervescence and reduced abdominal tenderness or evidence of progressive colonic dilatation or rebound tenderness requires emergent colectomy.

In the setting of a partial response or persisting symptoms in the absence of "toxicity," intravenous cyclosporine can be added after discussions with the patient and family regarding the potential benefits and risks and the need for long-term maintenance therapy and surveillance. Cyclosporine is added at an initial dose of 2 to 4 mg per kg as a continuous infusion. I do not use cyclosporine in patients with cholesterol levels below 100 mg per dL because of the risk for seizures. Whole-blood cyclosporine levels are monitored along with the blood pressure, blood urea nitrogen and creatinine concentrations, and magnesium levels with attempts to maintain monoclonal cyclosporine assays between 200 and 400 μg per mL. Intravenous therapy is maintained until the patient has a complete response, at which point the cyclosporine and steroids are administered orally.

Oral cyclosporine is initiated at twice the intravenous dose in two divided doses, and the same trough levels are monitored on a weekly basis. I usually add azathioprine or 6-mercaptopurine to the regimen as soon as the patient responds along with a maintenance aminosalicylate and trimethoprim-sufamethoxazole three times weekly owing to the risk of *Pneumocytis carinii* pneumonia in patients with "triple immunosuppression." The steroids are tapered as described for severe colitis and the cyclosporine is maintained for approximately 3 months, giving time for the azathioprine or 6-mercaptopurine to take effect.

SURGERY

Removal of the colonic mucosa cures ulcerative colitis. This can be accomplished by a proctocolectomy and ileostomy or with sphincter-saving procedures such as subtotal colectomy and ileoanal anastomoses. Partial or segmental colectomy is contraindicated because of the high likelihood of relapse. Indications for surgery in ulcerative colitis include failure to improve with medical therapy, complications of medical treatment, perforation or progressive toxic megacolon (not responding within 24 hours), intractable hemorrhage (rare), or evidence of confirmed dysplasia or cancer. The sphincter-saving procedures offer an excellent "escape" option from a chronic disease and should be considered in patients with compromised quality of life due to ulcerative colitis or the medical therapy. The major risks of the ileoanal procedures are the requisite for several staged surgeries (colectomy with diverting ileostomy, then ileostomy "takedown"), bowel obstruction (usually during the time of ileostomy diversion), and pouchitis. Pouchitis is probably a recurrence of colitis within the surgically formed ileal pouch. Although common, pouchitis is usually responsive to a course of an antibiotic such as metronidazole. Most episodes of pouchitis are acute and limited, although a small percentage of patients require long-term antibiotic therapy.

LONG-TERM MANAGEMENT

Cancer Surveillance

Ulcerative colitis is recognized as a risk factor for colorectal cancer. Despite the small absolute risk (3 to 4%), the risk for developing cancer increases in time such that after 20 to 40 years of disease, the risk for cancer or dysplasia approaches 10% per decade of disease. In addition to the duration of disease, the risk for cancer is increased according to the amount of colon involved and the presence of sclerosing cholangitis. The age at onset and the severity of disease are not independent risk factors. Epithelial dysplasia, defined as an "unequivocal neoplastic change," is a risk factor for cancer, and the presence of confirmed dysplasia on mucosal biopsy is sufficient indication for colectomy because of the high risk of a coexisting or impending cancer. Patients with ulcerative colitis for more than 8 to 10 years should be entered into a surveillance program with pancolonic biopsies at a regular interval according to the duration. I survey patients every 2 to 3 years between 10 and 20 years of disease and every year after a 20-year history of ulcerative colitis. Random biopsy specimens are obtained at least at 10-cm intervals throughout the colon. Dysplasia diagnosed by an experienced gastrointestinal pathologist is sufficient to recommend colectomy no matter what the disease activity or grade of dysplasia. Carcinoembryonic antigen detection, barium enema examinations, and sigmoidoscopic screening are not sufficient screening examinations.

Fertility and Pregnancy

Ulcerative colitis commonly occurs during the reproductive years of men and women. In men, ulcerative colitis does not affect fertility. Sulfasalazine impairs sperm number and morphologic features and can be a cause of reversible infertility in men, a side effect that is reversed by substituting an alternative aminosalicylate. In women, the impact of ulcerative colitis on pregnancy is less than the impact of pregnancy on ulcerative colitis. Most women with ulcerative colitis have a normal pregnancy potential as long as their disease remains under control. There may be a slight increase in spontaneous abortions when patients with active disease become pregnant, but most pregnancies are unaffected by ulcerative colitis. The current armamentarium of medical therapies for ulcerative colitis is safe for use in pregnancy, despite the ambiguous regulatory labeling. In most situations, the pregnant patient should be treated in the same manner as if she were not pregnant. The aminosalicylates and corticosteroids have had a long empirical use without significantly enhanced fetal risk. Immunomodulators or cyclosporine can be used in exceptional circumstances. Careful attention to the nutritional status of the pregnant woman and supplementation with iron and folic acid are essential.

Conversely, there may be an impact of pregnancy on ulcerative colitis. Approximately one third of women have a flare-up during pregnancy; another third may improve and notice a remission in disease activity. The postpartum period is another vulnerable time for flare-ups. I recommend continuing maintenance therapy throughout pregnancy and breast-feeding.

Social Support

Ulcerative colitis is a chronic medical illness that typically affects young individuals who must learn to live with the uncertainties of embarrassing symptoms and side effects of medications (steroids). Diarrhea and rectal bleeding, the need for immediate toilet access, and cushingoid side effects can be socially disabling. Careful attention to the patient and family support systems is important for the long-term management. This is not a stress-induced disease. However, it is a stressful illness. A supportive medical and ancillary environment is essential for the patient and family. Additional information for the patient and about support groups is available from the Crohn's and Colitis Foundation of America.

CROHN'S DISEASE

method of
MARK A. PEPPERCORN, M.D.
Beth Israel–Deaconess Medical Center and
Harvard Medical School
Boston, Massachusetts

Crohn's disease is a recurrent segmental inflammatory condition of unknown etiology that may affect the gastrointestinal tract from the mouth to the anus. Fifty percent of patients have involvement of both the small intestine and colon, whereas one third have disease limited to their small intestine and the remaining 20% have inflammation in the colon only. Perianal lesions and inflammatory conditions involving the skin, eyes, joints, and liver are common. The transmural inflammatory process and variable anatomic extent of disease contribute to diverse clinical presentations with unpredictable spontaneous exacerbations and remissions.

DRUG THERAPY
Aminosalicylates

Sulfasalazine

Introduced into clinical medicine in the early 1940s, sulfasalazine (Azulfidine)* has since become a mainstay in the therapy for inflammatory bowel disease. Controlled trials have shown its efficacy for active Crohn's disease involving the colon, and although the studies have not uniformly demonstrated the drug's benefit in isolated ileitis, there appears to be a subset of patients with Crohn's ileitis who benefit from its use. It has not been shown to be useful

in maintaining remission in Crohn's disease and in preventing recurrence after operation. In any patient with mild to moderately active Crohn's disease, the drug should be considered and given initially at a dose of 500 mg orally twice daily with advancement if tolerated to 3 to 4 grams per day. Folic acid, 1 mg per day, should be added because sulfasalazine may interfere with dietary folate absorption. Responses are usually seen within 4 weeks, and the drug should be continued at the level that achieved the clinical response for 4 to 6 months. If relapse occurs quickly on stopping of the agent, then reinstitution and long-term maintenance at a dose of 3 to 4 grams per day should be considered.

Adverse effects with sulfasalazine may be seen in as many as 20% of patients receiving the drug. Anorexia, nausea, and dyspepsia may be overcome by lowering the dosage and/or using an enteric-coated preparation. The complete blood count should be monitored carefully during the initial few weeks of therapy, because neutropenia and hemolysis may occur and be reversed by lowering the dose. Although a process of gradual desensitization may overcome minor allergic reactions such as fever and rash, almost all patients experiencing such a reaction will be switched to one of the new oral aminosalicylate agents. Serious adverse reactions such as agranulocytosis, severe hemolysis, pancreatitis, hepatitis, pneumonitis, pericarditis, neuropathy, alteration of sperm counts and morphologic features with reversible male infertility, and exacerbation of colitis mandate stopping the drug.

Sulfasalazine links sulfapyridine to 5-aminosalicylic acid (5-ASA) by an azo bond. The azo bond is first reduced by intestinal bacteria with release of the two moieties. The sulfapyridine is largely absorbed and excreted in the urine and accounts for most of the drug's toxicity. The 5-ASA component stays largely within the lumen of the intestinal tract and is excreted with the feces. Observations on the distribution of the metabolites of sulfasalazine led to investigations of the 5-ASA moiety itself, in both topical and oral formulations.

Topical 5-Aminosalicylic Acid Agents

Controlled trials confirmed the hypothesis that 5-ASA might be the active moiety in sulfasalazine. Moreover, 80 to 90% of patients intolerant of or allergic to sulfasalazine tolerate the 5-ASA derivative. Although not well studied in controlled trials in Crohn's disease, the enema and suppository forms of 5-ASA, known generically as mesalamine (Rowasa),* should be used for patients with Crohn's disease involving the distal colon or rectum alone. A response is usually seen within 6 weeks, at which point maintenance therapy can be attempted on an every-other-night or every-third-night basis.

Oral 5-Aminosalicylic Acid Agents

For the patient with small bowel Crohn's disease or with colonic disease above the rectosigmoid, oral

*Not FDA approved for this indication.

*Not FDA approved for this indication.

5-ASA agents can be considered an alternative to sulfasalazine. Available oral forms include mesalamine (Pentasa)* encapsulated in ethylcellulose microspheres, mesalamine (Asacol)* coated with an acrylic resin that dissolves at pH greater than 6, and olsalazine (Dipentum) that links 5-ASA to itself by an azo bond requiring bacterial metabolism as in sulfasalazine. Although controlled trials in active disease have given conflicting results, it is reasonable to consider oral mesalamine as a first-line agent for any patient with mild to moderately active Crohn's ileitis, ileocolitis, or colitis, using the drugs in doses up to 4.8 grams per day. If remission is achieved, long-term maintenance therapy at a dosage of 3 grams per day should be considered because there is evidence to suggest the benefit of these drugs in preventing relapse. Their use should also be considered in the patient undergoing resection and anastomosis because doses of 3 grams per day have been shown to delay endoscopic and clinical recurrence up to 3 years.

Although 5-ASA agents are well tolerated, adverse effects have been reported and include serum sickness–like reactions, pericarditis, pneumonitis, exacerbation of colitis, and nephritis. Because of nephritis, periodic monitoring of the urine sediments and the blood urea nitrogen and creatinine concentrations should be done.

Antibiotics

Metronidazole (Flagyl)* is the best studied of the antimicrobial agents and has been shown in controlled trials to be effective in active Crohn's colitis and ileocolitis but not in isolated ileitis. A largely uncontrolled experience suggests utility in perianal disease as well. Although there are no trials investigating its use in relapse prevention in Crohn's disease, a 3-month course of the drug after ileal resection and anastomosis was more effective than placebo at preventing endoscopic and clinical recurrence up to 1 year.

For patients with colonic disease who are unresponsive to or intolerant of one of the aminosalicylates, metronidazole should be considered at a dose of 10 mg per kg per day. A therapeutic response is usually seen in 2 to 4 weeks, and the drug can be continued for 3 to 6 months, at which point it is usually stopped. Patients with severe perianal disease, however, often require the agent for indefinite periods and at least initially may require doses of 20 mg per kg per day. Side effects are common and include nausea, anorexia, tongue discomfort, and paresthesias. Paresthesias are usually dose dependent and reversible but may be prolonged.

Great enthusiasm has recently emerged for other antimicrobial agents as primary therapy for Crohn's disease, although they are less well tested. The history of the use of broad-spectrum antibiotics, including cephalosporins and tetracycline, in the management of active Crohn's disease goes back 25 years, but new agents such as ciprofloxacin (Cipro)* and clarithromycin (Biaxin)* have rekindled interest in their use. Open trials have suggested impressive efficacy for ciprofloxacin alone and in combination with metronidazole* in active Crohn's ileitis and colitis. A small controlled trial and one large open trial gave similar results for clarithromycin. Clarithromycin may work through its effects on an atypical mycobacterium reported to be causally important in Crohn's disease. Other trials of multiple antituberculous agents have given conflicting results in both active and remitted Crohn's disease. However, further controlled data are awaited with regard to these agents. It is currently reasonable to consider the use of ciprofloxin, clarithromycin, and metronidazole as primary therapy; response is usually seen within 2 to 3 weeks. For responders, continuation of therapy for up to 6 months may provide prolonged remissions.

Corticosteroids

For patients not responding to or intolerant of the preceding measures, and for those presenting with severe manifestations of disease activity, corticosteroids need to be considered. Hydrocortisone enemas (Cortenema) can be used in patients with active proctosigmoiditis; foam preparations (Cortifoam) are available for those with proctitis. One preparation should be given every night for 2 to 3 weeks and then tapered to every other night during the subsequent 2 weeks.

For patients with mild to moderate symptoms and with colonic disease proximal to the rectosigmoid, and for those with small bowel involvement, prednisone 40 to 60 mg per day is initiated and continued at the initial dose for 10 days to 2 weeks. If a desired response is obtained, the dosage should be tapered by 5 mg every 7 to 10 days. Once remission is achieved, there is no benefit of continued steroid therapy as prophylaxis against relapse of disease activity. However, some patients with mild smoldering activity as the dose is tapered may benefit from continued low-dose therapy in the range of 5 to 10 mg per day. Alternate-day steroid therapy should be considered for such patients, in whom the risks of such long-term steroid therapy have to be weighed against the benefit and treatment alternatives.

More rapidly metabolized forms of steroids have emerged as efficacious in short-term trials with considerably fewer side effects than standard preparations. Budesonide enemas† have proved to be as effective as hydrocortisone and 5-ASA enemas in ulcerative proctosigmoiditis but have not been formally studied in distal Crohn's colitis. A slow-release oral preparation of budesonide has been shown to be more effective than placebo and as effective as oral prednisolone in active Crohn's ileitis with or without right colon involvement. Preparations are now being

---

*Not FDA approved for this indication.

*Not FDA approved for this indication.
†Not available in the United States.

studied in more distal disease. Although budesonide taken chronically by patients in remission delayed the onset of relapse of activity, the relapse rate after 1 year was no different in patients taking or not taking the drug. The ultimate role of this agent, not yet approved for use in the United States, is not clear, but its high benefit/side effect ratio suggests that it may replace standard steroids in the management of some patients with active disease.

Parenteral corticosteroids are indicated for patients with severe symptoms of Crohn's disease requiring hospitalization. Such patients in addition usually receive parenteral nutrition and broad-spectrum antibiotics. Intravenous hydrocortisone (Solu-Cortef) 300 mg per day, or the less salt-retaining and less potassium-wasting preparations methylprednisolone (Solu-Medrol) or prednisolone 48 to 60 mg per day, should be administered. Some prefer intravenous adrenocorticotropic hormone, 120 units* per 24 hours as a continuous infusion, although no benefit of this agent over standard preparations for Crohn's disease patients has been shown. For patients responsive to such therapy, oral prednisone should be substituted for the parenteral agent initially at a dose of 40 to 60 mg per day with subsequent gradual tapering.

Immunomodulators

6-Mercaptopurine (Purinethol)† and azathioprine (Imuran)* have emerged as important agents in the management of Crohn's disease patients dependent on steroids and refractory to other agents and with nonhealing fistulas. In more seriously ill patients, their use adjunctively with steroids as initial therapy should be considered. The drugs can be used interchangeably and should be started at 50 mg per day with advance to 1.5 mg per kg per day for 6-mercaptopurine and 2.5 mg per kg per day for azathioprine, depending on the clinical response and effects on bone marrow. Careful monitoring of a complete blood count will usually avoid problems with bone marrow depression, although some believe that achievement of mild leukopenia may be necessary to obtain a maximal benefit of the drugs. The mean onset of action is 3 months; some patients do not show benefit for 6 to 9 months. The use of azathioprine intravenously to induce a more rapid response is under study.

Ten percent of patients will experience irreversible adverse hypersensitivity reaction including fever, rash, pancreatitis, and hepatitis. An increased risk for malignant neoplasm, especially lymphoma, has been of concern with use of these drugs, but studies of large numbers of patients with inflammatory bowel disease receiving 6-mercaptopurine and azathioprine suggest that the risk is minimal and may not be increased above that of patients with Crohn's disease not receiving the drugs. The patient should

attempt to stop the agents before conception, although the emerging experience is that the risk for fetal abnormalities in those becoming pregnant and carrying to term is extremely low.

These drugs are effective at maintaining remission in Crohn's disease. Their long-term use for a period of at least 4 years should be considered in those patients who have flare-ups frequently while receiving 5-ASA agents, who are steroid dependent, and who have had recurrence early after resection.

For patients refractory to or intolerant of 6-mercaptopurine or azathioprine, methotrexate* has emerged as a useful alternative. The drug may be especially useful at inducing remission in patients who are steroid dependent. Its long-term efficacy as a remission agent is under study. Administration intramuscularly at a dose of 25 mg per week should be initiated and continued for 3 months in those responding, and an attempt to convert to oral administration can be made with gradual reduction of dosage. However, in patients with prior small bowel surgery, the variability in absorption after oral administration may mandate its continued use intramuscularly. Folic acid at 1 mg per day should be administered concomitantly to avoid side effects. Adverse reactions include leukopenia, abnormalities of liver function, and a hypersensitivity pneumonitis. Liver biopsy should be performed to exclude the development of fibrosis in those who have taken a cumulative dose of 1500 mg.

For patients refractory to these therapies and for those with nonhealing fistulas, cyclosporine (Sandimmune)* therapy should be considered. In hospitalized patients with severe active disease or those with refractory fistulas, the drug should be used intravenously as a continuous infusion at a dose of 2 to 4 mg per kg per 24 hours with careful monitoring of blood levels. A response can be expected within 7 to 10 days. Once a response is achieved, oral administration of the drug at a dose of 6 to 8 mg per kg per day should be tried. For less severely ill patients with refractory disease, initial therapy with cyclosporine orally can be attempted. Adverse effects may include hirsutism, paresthesias, seizures, hypertension, irreversible renal dysfunction, and predisposition to infection. Long-term studies of low-dose oral cyclosporine have not shown efficacy over placebo for Crohn's disease patients, so the use of this drug as a remission agent cannot be recommended.

Modifications of the immune system with interferon* and T lymphocyte apheresis have been of use in patients with refractory disease, although their use has not been supported by placebo-controlled trials. A promising alternative may emerge from studies of monoclonal antibodies directed at T cells and proinflammatory cytokines. An initial short-term placebo-controlled trial of anti–tumor necrosis factor-α showed great promise, but more studies will be needed before this class of agents becomes available for routine use.

---

*Exceeds dosage recommended by the manufacturer.
†Not FDA approved for this indication.

---

*Not FDA approved for this indication.

Nonspecific Antidiarrheal Drugs and Cholestyramine

For patients with mild chronic symptoms, agents such as loperamide (Imodium), diphenoxylate with atropine (Lomotil), codeine, and deodorized tincture of opium may be of use. Given their addictive potential, except for loperamide, their use should be limited, and they should be avoided as drugs to control pain in patients with acute severe symptoms because of the risk for precipitating ileus. Fiber in various forms including bran and psyllium (Citrucel, Metamucil, Perdiem) may be of use in decreasing watery diarrhea and in treating those with constipation alternating with diarrhea.

Cholestyramine (Questran) can be of major benefit in the patient with nonstenosing ileitis or in one who has had an ileal resection. In such patients, watery diarrhea due to bile acid malabsorption can usually be controlled with 1 scoop or packet (4 grams) in a glass of juice taken once or twice daily.

NUTRITIONAL SUPPORT

General Dietary Instructions and Nutritional Supplements

Food is the best source of nutrition, and the emphasis for most patients should be on normalization of the diet and adequate caloric intake. Patients with intestinal strictures and partial obstruction may benefit from a low-residue diet. Those patients with calcium oxalate stones associated with steatorrhea and hyperoxaluria should be instructed in a low-oxalate diet. In patients with extensive ileal resection and steatorrhea, a low-fat diet with medium chain triglyceride supplementation should be considered. These patients need replacement of calcium, vitamin D, and vitamin K as well. Lactose intolerance can mimic the symptoms of Crohn's disease and should be documented or excluded if there is any question of its existence. A lactose-free diet with calcium supplementation can be offered if appropriate. In addition, patients with evidence of malabsorption, those with a low-calcium intake, and those receiving long-term steroid therapy are at risk for osteoporosis and osteomalacia. Bone density studies and referral for possible therapy with agents to prevent bone disease should be considered. Finally, vitamin B_{12} replacement may be necessary for patients with moderate or extensive ileal resections or those with chronic extensive ileal disease. A Schilling test should be performed several months postoperatively to document the need in those patients undergoing resection, and routine vitamin B_{12} levels should be obtained in those with long-standing active ileal disease.

Enteral and Parenteral Diets

Although there is some debate about their actual utility, both enteral diets and total parenteral nutri-

tion have been shown to be useful as primary therapy in inducing remissions in certain patients with Crohn's disease. This should be considered in particular in patients refractory to pharmacologic therapy, especially in poor operative risk candidates. Such diets can also be used in an attempt to heal fistulas as adjuncts to drug therapy and in helping to prepare patients for surgery. Growth failure in children with Crohn's disease can often be overcome by increasing caloric intake with elemental diets. Finally, total parenteral nutrition given at home is often a necessity for patients with severe short-bowel syndrome, usually resulting from multiple resections.

PSYCHOSOCIAL CONSIDERATIONS

Although there is no evidence to support the concept that psychologic factors are etiologic in Crohn's disease, there is no question that psychosocial pressures can influence the course of the patient's illness and have to be addressed. The caring physician who is willing to answer questions and be available at all times is often all that is needed. At other times, mild psychotropic agents in conjunction with behavior modification and support groups are of enormous benefit. In this regard, the Crohn's and Colitis Foundation of America can be extremely helpful in providing patients with emotional support and educational materials.

IRRITABLE BOWEL SYNDROME

method of
RAY E. CLOUSE, M.D.
Washington University School of Medicine
St. Louis, Missouri

Treatment of irritable bowel syndrome (IBS) is not standardized because of several important facts. First, the clinical syndrome undoubtedly represents more than one underlying disorder. Second, the neuromuscular dysfunction responsible for the manifestations, even in the most typical case, is not well understood. In addition, psychologic factors play variable roles in affecting the presentation, possibly more so than in most other medical conditions. It is not surprising, therefore, that a single class of medications or narrow management approach is not effective for all patients.

There are probably as many management algorithms for IBS as there have been authors writing on this topic. I have found a three-component process to be useful for the majority of patients (Figure 1). Effective treatment ultimately emanates from securing the correct diagnosis, determining the psychologic factors that may be influencing presentation, and carefully characterizing the specific gastrointestinal complaints.

SECURING THE DIAGNOSIS OF IRRITABLE BOWEL SYNDROME

Unfortunately, the term IBS has been applied loosely to many different unexplained abdominal syndromes. Pa-

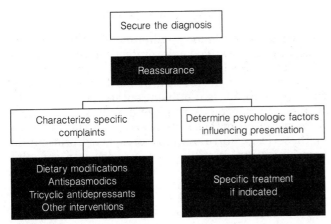

Figure 1. A three-component process useful in managing irritable bowel syndrome. Attention is given to all components in each patient.

tients with poorly defined abdominal pain or simple derangements in bowel habit (e.g., chronic diarrhea) are not infrequently included under this rubric, but such presentations are more likely to represent an underlying organic disease and deserve more extensive diagnostic evaluation. In contrast, patients who fulfill criteria as outlined in Table 1 require a limited exclusionary evaluation, primarily of the colon, and have less than 5% likelihood of receiving an alternative diagnosis during a 5-year observation period. The individual symptoms also occur with structural disorders of the gastrointestinal tract, but their clustering strongly suggests the diagnosis of IBS. Note that the diagnosis relies on the type of gastrointestinal complaints and not on their possible relationship to stress or dietary factors.

The criterion symptoms are often not volunteered by the patient and must be extracted during a thorough history and physical examination. Tenderness over the colon and other parts of the gastrointestinal tract, the only abnormal physical finding, is thought to represent increased sensitivity by the patient to visceral distention or stretch. The office examination is otherwise used to exclude disorders

TABLE 1. **Criteria Used for Establishing the Diagnosis of Irritable Bowel Syndrome*

1. Abdominal pain or discomfort
   - Relieved with defecation, and/or
   - Associated with change in stool frequency, and/or
   - Associated with change in stool consistency

2. Two or more of the following (at least a quarter of occasions or days)
   - Altered stool frequency
   - Altered stool form
   - Altered stool passage (straining, urgency, feeling of incomplete evacuation)
   - Passage of mucus
   - Bloating or feeling of abdominal distention

3. ≥3 mo of continuous or recurrent symptoms

4. Symptoms not attributable to other gastrointestinal disease

*All four criteria are required for diagnosis.
Adapted from Thompson WG, Creed F, Drossman DA, et al: Functional bowel disorders and functional abdominal pain. Gastroenterol Int 5:75–91, 1992.

that might be mimicking the diagnosis. Laboratory and imaging studies should be limited in the face of typical IBS symptoms and no other objective abnormalities.

PROVIDING REASSURANCE

Reassurance that emanates from a secure diagnosis remains an essential aspect of IBS management, and reassurance alone is sufficient treatment for some patients. It informs the patient of the physician's familiarity with the disorder while setting the stage for discussions regarding a good prognosis, no matter how ill the patient feels at the time of presentation. Six sequential steps have been recommended for effective reassurance therapy.

The first is to elicit a detailed description of the gastrointestinal symptoms. Rushing through a history suggests the predetermined notion of exaggerated or unimportant complaints. The second step requires a conscious attempt to allow the patient to describe his or her feelings associated with the symptoms, a step that is useful in modeling the approach to reassurance for the individual patient. For example, the patient who describes pain as frightening may need reassurance that acute pain will not lead to a morbid outcome (e.g., surgery or death) or that chronic pain will not lead to cancer. Examining the patient is the next step. Not only is this required for securing the diagnosis, it also reflects the physician's serious attitude toward the complaints. The fourth step is to make the diagnosis, a step that may take more than one visit if an exclusionary evaluation is required. The physician should keep the sequence in mind and not reassure prematurely if a comfortable diagnosis requires further investigation. The fifth step involves explaining the symptoms to the patient using the best information available as to the pathogenesis of the disorder. The final step is to reassure the patient of the disorder's favorable course and good prognosis.

DETERMINING PSYCHOLOGIC CONTRIBUTIONS TO CURRENT SYMPTOMS

It is well established that psychiatric diagnoses are more common in patients seeking medical care for IBS than for other structurally defined gastrointestinal diseases, but the importance of co-morbid psychiatric disorders with regard to the gastrointestinal syndrome remains debated. Clinical experience indicates that the psychiatric disorders and other psychologic factors have variable relevance from patient to patient. Nevertheless, the interaction is sufficiently important that exploring the psychologic meaning of symptoms and determining presence of co-morbid psychiatric disease are essential components of the management process.

Psychologic factors can modify physical symptoms, turning low-grade feelings of chronic bowel dysfunction into high-grade symptoms that prompt medical attention. Fear of cancer or other serious gastrointestinal illness may be sufficient for this conversion; depressed mood in response to a stressful life event can also be responsible for symptom amplification. Psychologic amplification of complaints is not unique to IBS or to the gastrointestinal tract. For example, the reporting of diabetes symptoms in type II diabetic patients is more closely associated with current mood than with objective measures of metabolic control.

Three types of psychologic dysfunction have been most commonly observed in IBS patients seeking medical attention: anxiety, depression, and somatization. Anxious patients tend to misinterpret symptom significance. Mild, chronic rectal urgency might be suddenly interpreted as a sure sign of rectal cancer by the anxious patient. Depression results in a tendency to focus on unpleasant experiences or situations. The newly depressed patient with background chronic bowel dysfunction and discomfort may become preoccupied with abdominal complaints and thereby now desire medical attention. Somatization results in an uninhibited inclination to report symptoms. Somatization tendencies alone can result in health care–seeking behavior, and compounding the process, inability to discriminate significant from insignificant gastrointestinal sensations becomes an additional stressor.

Although these psychologic mechanisms may influence symptom reporting in IBS patients, the interaction of psychologic and physical complaints is multidimensional. Acute stress, for example, has well-defined effects on gastrointestinal motor and sensory functions. Consequently, psychologic disturbances may directly feed into the abnormal processes responsible for gastrointestinal dysfunction. Likewise, gastrointestinal symptoms can be anxiety provoking. Reassurance therapy alone may help break the vicious circle, but patients who manifest criteria for psychiatric diagnoses are likely to have better outcome with therapy directed at the specific disorder.

At least 70% of patients meeting criteria for IBS who are actively seeking medical attention will fulfill criteria for an axis I psychiatric diagnosis. Not unexpectedly, the most common diagnoses are anxiety states, major depressive disorder, and somatization disorder. The anxiety and affective disorders represent the majority of patients in most series. Fortunately, these diagnoses are responsive to psychopharmacologic and behavioral treatment approaches. I recommend looking for the criterion symptoms of these disorders in the initial office visits of a patient with IBS symptoms. Emphasize the multidimensional interaction of psychiatric phenomena with the gastrointestinal syndrome to avoid the patient's hostility. If it is explained early to the patient that psychiatric or psychologic management sometimes provides an important avenue for treatment, the physician can prevent the appearance of desertion if no organic disease is detected during the diagnostic evaluation.

Most primary care physicians today are comfortable with using anxiolytic and antidepressant agents. Generalized anxiety disorder and panic disorder may be managed with benzodiazepines, buspirone, or tricyclic antidepressants. Major depressive disorder is now most commonly managed with selective serotonin reuptake inhibitors, but tricyclic antidepressants may have additional utility in the case of IBS, as discussed in the next section. Referral to a mental health professional can be of important help if the patient seems encumbered by a co-morbid psychiatric illness that cannot be managed without referral or if a psychiatric disorder or psychologic factors seem relevant and the gastrointestinal syndrome remains refractory to management efforts.

MANAGING SPECIFIC GASTROINTESTINAL COMPLAINTS

No single dietary or pharmacologic intervention is helpful in all patients with this syndrome. The specific complaints should have been carefully elicited and characterized in the first steps of the management process. Dominant complaints can be manipulated in most cases.

Altered Bowel Habit

Diarrhea is a common symptom of many gastrointestinal processes. The gastrointestinal tract handles as much as 9000 mL of fluid on a daily basis, yet produces less than 300 mL of fecal material. More than 1000 mL of ileal effluent enters the colon daily. Although we normally think of diarrhea as resulting from secretion or absorption errors in the handling of these large intraluminal volumes, alterations in gastrointestinal motility as seen with IBS can also dramatically alter normal bowel habit. Diarrhea in this syndrome can be managed with antispasmodic or antidiarrheal medications (Table 2) on an as-needed basis. Chronic use of opiate antidiarrheals has traditionally been discouraged, but chronic use in IBS is normally not required and is not of conspicuous concern.

Dietary manipulations for diarrhea in IBS focus primarily on a reduction of incompletely absorbed dietary carbohydrates. An initial 2-week trial of a lactose-free diet is recommended for patients with symptoms suggesting carbohydrate malabsorption (diarrhea, gaseousness). Although lactose malabsorption may be only a contributing factor, dietary restriction may be helpful in long-term management. Patients with a symptomatic response to lactose restriction may use lactase tablets or drops while lactose is reintroduced into the diet. Other incompletely absorbed carbohydrates include fructose (fruits, soft drinks, honey), sorbitol (certain diet candies and foods), and dietary fiber. For this and other reasons, not all patients with IBS benefit from dietary fiber supplementation. It is advisable to inform patients that a fiber trial may exacerbate this specific symptom.

Constipation and feelings of incomplete evacuation are also common in IBS. Constipation associated with hard, scybalous stools yet relatively frequent evacuation (e.g., daily) often responds well to antispasmodics (see Table 2). This "spastic constipation" differs from constipation characterized by infrequent bowel movements. Other functional or organic disturbances of colonic function may be responsible for the infrequent bowel habit pattern, and antispasmodics may actually prolong transit time and worsen constipation. This group of patients may benefit from osmotic laxatives (e.g., lactulose syrup, milk of magnesia) or prokinetic agents, such as cisapride (Propulsid), 10 to 20 mg before meals and at bedtime. One must assume in these cases that the IBS symptom complex is superimposed on a background disorder of constipation. As for diarrhea, the response to dietary fiber supplementation for constipation is heterogeneous. A therapeutic trial is often worthwhile, starting with 1 or 2 teaspoons of commercial fiber supplement per day and escalating the dose weekly.

Bloating, Flatulence

Abdominal bloating, often without any visible distention, is a common IBS complaint. This symptom

TABLE 2. **Antispasmodic Medications for Irritable Bowel Syndrome**

Type	Medication	Active Ingredients*	Usual Adult Dose†
Short acting	Belladonna tincture	Belladonna alkaloids	6–12 drops before meals and at bedtime
	Bellatal	Hyoscyamine sulfate	1–2 tablets
		Atropine sulfate	
		Scopolamine hydrobromide	
		Phenobarbital (16.2 mg)	
	Bentyl	Dicyclomine hydrochloride	1 capsule (10 mg) or tablet (20 mg)
	Donnatal	Hyoscyamine sulfate	1 tablet or capsule
		Atropine sulfate	
		Scopolamine hydrobromide	
		Phenobarbital (16.2 mg)	
	Levsin	Hyoscyamine sulfate	0.125 mg
	Librax	Clidinium bromide	1 or 2 capsules
		Chlordiazepoxide (5 mg)	
	Pro-Banthīne‡	Propantheline bromide	7.5–15 mg
	Quarzan‡	Clidinium bromide	2.5–5 mg
	Robinul‡	Glycopyrrolate	1 mg
Long acting	Donnatal Extentabs	Hyoscyamine sulfate	1 tablet q 8–12 h (each is equivalent to 3 Donnatal tablets)
		Atropine sulfate	
		Scopolamine hydrobromide	
		Phenobarbital (48.6 mg)	
	Levbid	Hyoscyamine sulfate	1 capsule (0.375 mg) q 8–12 h (each is equivalent to 3 Levsin tablets)
	Levsinex Timecaps	Hyoscyamine sulfate	1 tablet (0.375 mg) q 8–12 h (each is equivalent to 3 Levsin tablets)

*Antimuscarinic anticholinergic agents, some in conjunction with anxiolytic-sedatives (milligrams of the latter provided for reference).
†Given before meals and at bedtime unless otherwise specified. Some of these medications are not approved by the FDA for use in irritable bowel syndrome.
‡Not FDA approved for this indication.

presumably results from abnormal sensitivity to normal degrees of gastrointestinal distention. The treatment approach includes attempts to reduce gastrointestinal gas or to reduce gastrointestinal sensitivity to normal distention through a trial-and-error process. The former, also employed for excessive flatulence, is accomplished by dietary restriction of the previously mentioned carbohydrates as well as legumes, beans, and starches. Activated charcoal* administered before a meal reduces intestinal complaints resulting from consumption of indigestible carbohydrates, an approach that is helpful for some patients. Few data support the use of simethicone in reducing gaseousness, flatulence, or bloating.

Bloating can also result from an abnormal sensitivity to normal amounts of gastrointestinal gas. Consequently, this symptom may respond to approaches used for abdominal pain in IBS. Therapeutic trials are often required.

Abdominal Pain

Pain is the dominant symptom in the IBS cluster, is required for diagnosis according to the international criteria, and is most often the symptom that brings the patient to medical attention. Pain in IBS is no longer thought to result solely from intestinal spasm or similar motor activity. Rather, it is considered an outcome of increased sensitivity to visceral distention. Although the amount of pain reported by IBS patients is much greater in the sample seeking health care, the increase cannot be attributed to psychologic factors alone.

Maneuvers used to improve bowel habit or reduce bloating or flatulence also improve abdominal pain. Short-acting antispasmodics given before meals may be helpful in patients who have a dependable onset of symptoms in the postprandial period. Antispasmodics are better used for prophylaxis than after the pain has begun. If short-acting antispasmodics are effective, preparations with extended duration (see Table 2) may be substituted in patients who need treatment on more than an as-needed basis.

Tricyclic antidepressants* appear to have particular utility in IBS patients. Symptom improvement is not related solely to anticholinergic effects of these drugs but may result from nonspecific analgesic effects as are presumably operational when tricyclic antidepressants are used for other chronic pain conditions. Pain reduction is also independent of changes in mood. Response of IBS symptoms to tricyclic antidepressants occurs in more than 80% of patients, and complete symptomatic remission is seen in the majority of subjects. The response may be superior in patients without overt psychiatric disorder; other clinical features (duration of symptoms, age, gender) are not as predictive of outcome.

If tricyclic agents are used for IBS symptoms, a low-dose treatment regimen is usually effective (e.g., amitriptyline 50 mg orally at bedtime). Starting at a lower dosage for the first few days of therapy is recommended to avoid discontinuation because of un-

*Not FDA approved for this indication.

*Not FDA approved for this indication.

TABLE 3. **Side Effect Profiles of Tricyclic Antidepressant Medications Used in Managing Symptoms of Irritable Bowel Syndrome***

Medication	Anti-cholinergic	Drowsiness	Insomnia and/or Agitation	Orthostatic Hypotension	Cardiac Arrhythmia	Weight Gain
Tertiary Amines						
Amitriptyline (Elavil)	+ + + +	+ + + +	0	+ + + +	+ +	+ + + +
Doxepin (Sinequan)	+ + +	+ + + +	0	+ +	+ +	+ + +
Imipramine (Tofranil)	+ + +	+ + +	+	+ + + +	+ +	+ + +
Trimipramine (Surmontil)	+	+ + + +	0	+ +	+ +	+ + +
Secondary Amines						
Nortriptyline (Pamelor)	+	+	0	+ +	+ +	+
Desipramine (Norpramin)	+	+	+	+ +	+ +	+
Protriptyline (Vivactil)	+ +	+	+	+ +	+ +	0

*Not FDA approved for this indication. Rated from 0 (absent) to + + + + (relatively common).

Adapted from U.S. Department of Health and Human Services, Public Health Service: Depression in Primary Care: Detection, Diagnosis, and Treatment, Vol 5. Rockville, MD, Agency for Health Care Policy and Research, 1993. AHCPR publication 93-0552.

pleasant side effects. The full advantage of tricyclic antidepressant therapy in this dosage range probably results from multiple effects of the drugs. For example, sleep restoration from histamine$_1$-receptor blockade may be beneficial rather than an adverse reaction. Likewise, the anticholinergic effects of the tricyclic antidepressants may contribute to response.

Side effect profiles are important in choosing the initial tricyclic agent for a patient deemed eligible for this approach, and these same profiles are important when switching to an alternative medication if the first choice is poorly tolerated (Table 3). In contrast to the antidepressant response from these drugs, IBS improvement occurs promptly after the initiation of a successful tricyclic agent. Selective serotonin reuptake inhibitors do not appear as effective as tricyclic agents when they are used for this purpose but may be helpful if active major depression is a contributing factor toward presentation. Tachyphylaxis is uncommon in patients treated successfully with low-dose tricyclic antidepressants for IBS. The medications are withdrawn when successful and sustained symptom remission occurs and are reinstituted for symptom relapses.

HEMORRHOIDS, ANAL FISSURE, AND ANORECTAL ABSCESS AND FISTULA

method of
RICHARD P. BILLINGHAM, M.D.
University of Washington
Seattle, Washington

HEMORRHOIDS

Hemorrhoids are enlarged veins in the anal area, similar to varicose veins in the legs. Internal hemorrhoids are located inside the anal canal, above the dentate line, where the veins are covered with mucosa of the rectum; external hemorrhoids are located on the perianal skin. Whereas some authorities maintain that such structures represent "vascular cushions," contain arterioles, or contribute somehow to continence, such concepts are irrelevant from the standpoint of practical management. Humans are born with such submucosal rectal veins or other blood vessels, but these are considered to be hemorrhoids only when they become enlarged or otherwise symptomatic.

Hemorrhoids usually occur in three areas: the right posterior, the right anterior, and the left lateral areas of the anus. People may be bothered by internal hemorrhoids only, by external hemorrhoids only, or by both. Symptomatic hemorrhoids may develop in response to chronic constipation and straining at stool, presumably owing to pulsion forces, or there may be a familial tendency. However, for the majority of people with such symptoms, no definite cause can be determined. Despite popular folklore, there is no evidence that the development of hemorrhoids is related to prolonged sitting, heavy lifting, or other work-related activities, although these situations may exacerbate the symptoms of hemorrhoids that are already present.

It is important to question patients carefully regarding the specific symptoms that they may attribute to hemorrhoids, because most people are unaware of the possible existence of any other name for perianal disease. Inquiry should be made regarding pain (character, location, and association with bowel movements or other activity), bleeding (color; whether it occurs just with bowel movements or at other times; and whether it is noticed on the toilet paper, in the toilet bowl, on the outside of the stools, mixed in with the stools, or on underclothing), protrusion (if present, whether it is just with bowel movements or all the time; if associated with defecation, whether the swelling goes away spontaneously or requires manual reduction), and itching (called pruritus ani; rarely related to hemorrhoids) as well as the patient's normal bowel pattern and any recent alteration thereof.

Internal hemorrhoids may cause bleeding and/or prolapse but are almost never associated with pain.

Prolapse associated with bowel movements may resolve spontaneously or may require manual reduction in more severe cases. Blood is characteristically bright red and seen in the toilet bowl as well as on the toilet paper. External hemorrhoids are generally asymptomatic when small and may appear as skin tags; as they enlarge, they may cause some difficulty cleaning after bowel movements. Thrombosis of one or more external hemorrhoids may occur suddenly and is associated with an acutely painful perianal nodule. Bleeding rarely occurs with such thrombosis unless the clot erodes through the perianal skin after a few days, in which case the resulting blood is usually dark red and may be seen on underclothes.

Examination of the patient with "hemorrhoid symptoms" should include external anal inspection, digital anorectal examination, anoscopy, and, ideally, sigmoidoscopy. Other causes of similar symptoms must be ruled out, including neoplasms, which may cause increased straining; inflammatory bowel disease, which may cause bleeding; perianal tumors, which may be confused with external hemorrhoids; anal fissure, the most common cause of perianal pain; and anorectal abscesses, which are also painful and may occasionally be confused with thrombosed external hemorrhoids.

Treatment

Treatment of hemorrhoids depends on the severity of symptoms. If these are mild or infrequent, bulk laxatives and topical hydrocortisone cream are often sufficient. Topical cream is most effectively applied with a finger cot inside the anus; suppositories are almost never helpful.

Office Procedures

Thrombosed external hemorrhoids are of sudden onset and are associated with varying degrees of pain. For patients in whom pain is severe and/or does not rapidly resolve, office excision of the involved hemorrhoid with use of local anesthesia is well tolerated and associated with rapid resolution of pain. Local anesthetic agents containing epinephrine 1:100,000 are often helpful in achieving spontaneous hemostasis after such excision as well as in prolonging anesthesia. Usually, 2 to 3 mL of 1% lidocaine with epinephrine, administered with a 30-gauge needle, is well tolerated. Electrical cautery, if necessary, can be easily used in the office setting without additional anesthetic. Sutures are occasionally necessary for hemostasis but the wounds heal well without them, even with the excision of larger external hemorrhoids, and there is less pain afterward if no sutures are used.

After such treatment, sitz baths in warm water, 15 to 20 minutes at a time, three times daily, often give further symptomatic relief; medications for pain relief are occasionally helpful. Incision of the involved hemorrhoid, with an attempt at clot evacuation, is less than adequate therapy. Not only is it often unsuccessful in relieving symptoms because of the multiloculated nature of the clots, but it leaves the hemorrhoid to continue to hurt for several days as well as to remain to cause similar symptoms in the future.

For internal hemorrhoids that bleed but do not prolapse (first-degree internal hemorrhoids), injection sclerotherapy is usually both effective and painless. This is performed through an anoscope using approximately 1 mL of an agent such as 1% sodium tetradecyl sulfate for each of the friable internal hemorrhoids. Such injection should be done only above the dentate line, where there is generally no sensation to pain; three hemorrhoids can be done at one session, if necessary. For second-degree internal hemorrhoids (prolapsing, but with spontaneous reduction) or third-degree internal hemorrhoids (prolapsing but requiring manual reduction), rubber band ligation is usually helpful. This technique uses an applicator to place a tiny rubber band around the base of an internal hemorrhoid, devascularizing the prolapsing tissue and causing it to slough within 3 to 10 days. Care must be taken to place the band sufficiently above the dentate line to avoid pain. When the rubber band is properly placed, most people feel minimal or no discomfort. After proper placement, approximately 15% of patients have a sensation of having to have a bowel movement, and 5 to 10% have a mild aching sensation, lasting in both cases for a day or two. Such treatments are usually best performed by ligating only one hemorrhoid at a time and done at 3-week intervals. Complications include bleeding at the time of sloughing in 0.5 to 1% and thrombosis of adjacent external hemorrhoids in 1 to 2% of patients.

Rarely, life-threatening infections have been reported after rubber banding, without known precipitating factors. Such infections are always heralded by the development of severe local pain and inability to urinate, occurring within 24 to 72 hours of the application of a band. Prompt, aggressive treatment of such problems may be lifesaving. Although such incidents have occurred, their frequency is less than 1 in 10,000; as such, rubber banding is far safer than operative hemorrhoidectomy.

Internal hemorrhoids may recur after rubber banding in 15 to 20% of patients within 5 years, but such patients can usually be treated again with rubber band ligation without the necessity of surgery.

Other methods of office treatment include cryotherapy, infrared photocoagulation, laser, and electrical coagulation, but these techniques have not been demonstrated to have any advantage over the use of the rubber banding technique and are generally more expensive to the patient.

Operative Measures

Surgical hemorrhoidectomy is reserved for those with advanced third-degree (prolapsing, requiring manual reduction) and fourth-degree (prolapsing and irreducible) internal hemorrhoids and for those with both symptomatic internal hemorrhoids and symptomatic external hemorrhoids. Hemorrhoidectomy does not generally require an overnight hospital stay, and modern techniques have markedly decreased the discomfort as well as other postoperative morbidity commonly associated with this procedure. The procedure can be performed with the use of local, regional, or general anesthesia. The recurrence rate after surgical hemorrhoidectomy is 1 to 2%.

Other therapies for hemorrhoids gain popularity from time to time, such as electrocautery, cryotherapy, laser therapy, and anal dilatation. These techniques have not been shown to have the permanence offered by surgical hemorrhoidectomy, and claims of diminished pain have not been substantiated.

ANAL FISSURE

An anal fissure is a crack or tear, sometimes referred to as an ulcer, in the lining of the anus. This is associated with pain, particularly during and after bowel movements, as well as with a small amount of bright red bleeding, which is usually noted only on the toilet paper after bowel movements. A fissure may occur after a hard dry stool, after diarrhea, and with inflammatory bowel disease or other cause of local inflammation, or the specific event or cause may be undiscoverable. Most persistent fissures are associated with increased tone or spasm of the internal sphincter muscle; whether this is a cause or an effect of fissures is not known. More than 90% of anal fissures are located in the midline of the body, 60% posteriorly and 30% anteriorly. Fissures not in the midline should raise suspicions of other systemic disease, such as inflammatory bowel disease or blood dyscrasias, although such conditions may not be found.

Many fissures may heal by themselves, often within a day or so; of those that are seen by physicians, about 50% will heal with the combination of topical steroid cream, bulk laxatives, and sitz baths. Suppositories, foams, and topical pads containing witch hazel and other nostrums are generally ineffective. Topical cream is best applied by the patient, using a finger cot to place a small amount of cream directly into the anal canal and onto the painful area; the fenestrated applicators supplied with such preparations are, surprisingly, much less effective. In general, fissures that are going to heal by such conservative means will do so within 1 month.

For those patients whose fissures remain symptomatic after a month of such treatment, outpatient surgery is effective and gives rapid relief. Excision of the fissure with suturing of the resultant defect is associated with a 90% success rate and moderate postoperative pain for several days. However, another procedure, lateral internal sphincterotomy, divides the internal anal sphincter laterally in the anal canal, without removing the fissure. This procedure is effective in about 98% of cases, and most patients are able to return to normal activity the day after surgery, without discomfort. Because the internal anal sphincter is not under voluntary control and is not an important determinant of fecal continence,

the procedure is rarely associated with transient incontinence of flatus and almost never with stool incontinence. After such surgery, recurrence of anal fissure is extremely uncommon.

PERIANAL ABSCESS AND FISTULA

Abscesses and fistulas of the perianal area are different phases of the same basic process: the abscess is the acute stage, and the fistula is the chronic aspect. The process almost always originates from an otherwise useless anal gland, of which there are 6 to 12 arranged radially around the anus. The opening of each gland is located in the base of one of the anal crypts at the dentate line; the body of each gland is thought to lie between the internal and external sphincters. When the neck or opening of a gland becomes occluded, whether by inflammation, inflammatory bowel disease, or unknown causes, the bacteria and secretions within the gland proliferate. This causes the body of the gland to swell and fester, producing pus. Symptoms at this stage include perianal pain, which is constant and increasing during hours or days and unaffected by bowel movements and may be associated with fever or other evidence of systemic infection. Pain can sometimes occur initially in the absence of perianal induration, erythema, or other physical findings. When an abscess is suspected in such instances, repeated examination of the patient within 24 hours is warranted.

As the process continues, the abscess either ruptures spontaneously, through the perianal skin, or is drained by a physician before the time of such rupture. This is usually accompanied by a dramatic improvement in symptoms.

After rupture or spontaneous drainage, about 50% of all such abscesses rapidly resolve spontaneously, without sequelae; the other 50% go on to the stage of fistula. This is caused by the reopening of the original ostium and neck of the anal gland and by the persistence of an external opening at the site of abscess drainage. Symptoms of a fistula are usually limited to the drainage of small amounts of mucus or purulent material from time to time throughout the day, with rare small amounts of blood. The external opening of a fistula will occasionally epithelialize and heal over, with the reaccumulation of pus and the return of abscess symptoms. This resolves either spontaneously or after repeated surgical drainage.

Other causes of perianal inflammation and superficial abscess include hidradenitis suppurativa, pilonidal cyst and abscess, inflammatory bowel disease (most commonly Crohn's disease), foreign bodies, and Bartholin's abscess.

Treatment

Treatment of an abscess consists of incision and drainage. This may be done in the office with use of local anesthesia in most situations, but larger and more complex abscesses should be drained in the operating room. Antibiotics are generally neither necessary nor helpful in this setting; exceptions may include the diabetic patient, the presence of a prosthetic joint or heart valve, or extensive associated cellulitis. Drainage of the abscess is rapidly followed by resolution of associated signs and symptoms without further medications. Principles of such drainage include making the incision as close to the anal verge as possible (to reduce the length of any possible fistula) and the removal of an ellipse of skin, rather than making a small slit, to keep the skin opening from prematurely closing before the resolution of the abscess. Cultures of the abscess fluid universally show mixed aerobic and anaerobic bowel flora and are not helpful.

The practice of using gauze packing to "encourage drainage" is oxymoronic; it is uncomfortable and actually discourages drainage and, therefore, the rapid resolution of the underlying process. It is unnecessary to "break up loculations" within the abscess cavity itself; if these even actually exist, they seem to manage themselves. Sitz baths in comfortably warm water, three times daily for 20 minutes each time, are helpful in encouraging rapid healing as well as in giving symptomatic relief.

Management of perianal fistulas is complex and requires a thorough knowledge of relevant anatomy and fistula types. A surgical approach is almost always required, unroofing the entire extent of the fistula tract from external to internal opening; this requires division of the internal anal sphincter and usually a portion of the external anal sphincter. After such unroofing, or fistulotomy, a careful search must be made for additional fistula tracts, and the granulation tissue in the bed of the fistula must be removed. Curettage is almost always sufficient for this purpose, rather than removal of the fistula tract itself, or fistulectomy. An alternative to fistulotomy, used when preservation of a maximal amount of sphincter muscle is critical, is the use of an endorectal advancement flap to cover the internal opening of a fistula.

Such procedures can almost always be done in an outpatient setting, with only a few days of moderate postoperative discomfort. Complete healing may take 6 to 12 weeks but without interfering with normal function and lifestyle.

Some authors advocate fistulotomy at the time of incision and drainage of an abscess, for those abscesses that must be treated in the operating room. With increased appreciation that office management is effective for the abscess itself, as detailed before, and with the consideration that only 50% of all those with abscesses will develop fistulas, most specialists now advocate a delayed approach to fistula repair. The specific management of complex anorectal fistulas (such as horseshoe fistulas, suprasphincteric or extrasphincteric fistulas) or the role of setons is beyond the scope of this discussion.

ACUTE AND CHRONIC VIRAL HEPATITIS

method of
GEOFFREY C. FARRELL, M.D.
*The Storr Liver Unit, University of Sydney at
    Westmead Hospital*
Sydney, Australia

ACUTE VIRAL HEPATITIS

Acute viral hepatitis is a syndrome characterized by anorexia, malaise, nausea, low-grade fever, tender hepatomegaly, and a 10-fold or greater elevation of the serum alanine aminotransferase (ALT) levels. Jaundice is a common but variable feature. The syndrome results from hepatic inflammation and liver cell necrosis, and it may be caused by any of the known human hepatitis viruses, A, B, C, D, E, and possibly G. The Epstein-Barr virus in infectious mononucleosis, cytomegalovirus, and Q fever are occasional causes of acute hepatitis but are not discussed further. Viral hepatitis must be distinguished from autoimmune hepatitis, hepatic drug reactions, veno-occlusive disease, and ischemic hepatitis. The diagnosis can often be suspected on the basis of relevant risk factors and is confirmed by use of the specific serologic and molecular tests detailed in Table 1. Identification of the causative agent is important for predicting outcome and is the first step toward prevention of transmission of infection. Two types of hepatitis, hepatitis A and B, can now be prevented by vaccination (Table 2).

Hepatitis A

The hepatitis A virus (HAV) is a small, nonenveloped RNA virus that is enterically transmitted. It causes acute but not chronic hepatitis; chronic carriage of HAV has not been described. The incubation period is 3 to 6 weeks, and the virus is shed in stools for up to 2 weeks after the onset of jaundice. Recent infection is indicated by the presence in serum of IgM anti-HAV; antibody is detectable at the onset of symptoms. IgG anti-HAV indicates past infection. It also confers immunity to reinfection, and this is the basis for an effective hepatitis A vaccine (see Table 2). Hepatitis A is endemic in countries with poor sanitation and hygiene. In industrialized nations, miniepidemics occur in association with contaminated food and water supplies; shellfish are a common source. Sexual transmission occurs in relation to oral-anal practices. Parenteral transmission of HAV is rare.

Children and young adults are most often affected by hepatitis A, but the disease is more severe in older persons. Illness is mild in most cases, and return of appetite and well-being are evident after 2 to 3 weeks. Management is generally symptomatic. A carbohydrate-rich low-fat diet is better tolerated in the early stages, and attention to fluid intake is appro-

TABLE 1. **Diagnostic Tests for Acute and Chronic Viral Hepatitis**

Virus	Diagnostic Test	Comment
HAV	IgM anti-HAV IgG anti-HAV	Recent infection Past infection, immunity
HBV	HBsAg Anti-HBs IgM anti-HBc IgG anti-HBc HBeAg; anti-HBe HBV DNA	Acute or chronic hepatitis B Past infection, immunity Active infection (acute or chronic) Past infection Viral replication active; inactive Active viral replication
HCV	Anti-HCV HCV RNA (by RT-PCR)	Always positive in chronic hepatitis C, may be negative in acute hepatitis Usually positive in chronic hepatitis, useful in seronegative cases of acute hepatitis
HDV	IgM anti-HDV IgG anti-HDV	Active infection Past infection
HEV	Anti-HEV	Reference laboratory—consider in travelers with acute hepatitis
HGV	HGV RNA (by RT-PCR)	Research test; HGV rarely responsible for hepatitis

Abbreviations: HAV = hepatitis A virus; HBV = hepatitis B virus; HCV = hepatitis C virus; HDV = hepatitis D virus; HEV = hepatitis E virus; HGV = hepatitis G virus; anti-HAV = antibody to HAV; HBsAg = hepatitis B surface antigen; anti-HBs = antibody to HBsAg; anti-HBc = antibody to HBV core antigen; HBeAg = hepatitis B e antigen; anti-HBe = antibody to hepatitis B e antigen; anti-HCV = antibody to HCV; anti-HDV = antibody to HDV; anti-HEV = antibody to HEV; RT-PCR = reverse transcription–polymerase chain reaction.

priate. Bed rest is unnecessary. The patient need refrain from alcohol only until recovery is evident and liver test results have returned to normal. Drugs are best avoided, but severe nausea or vomiting may be relieved by prochlorperazine (Compazine), 5 to 10 mg orally or 12.5 mg by intramuscular injection, two or three times daily, or metoclopramide (Reglan), 10 mg three times daily. Acetaminophen can be used for hepatic pain (maximal dose, 2 grams per day) and is preferred over aspirin, but repeated doses should be avoided if the patient has been fasting for more than a few days because of the heightened risk for acetaminophen-induced hepatotoxicity. In cases of severe hepatitis, drug metabolism may be impaired. Thus, patients taking regular medications such as anticonvulsants, antidepressants, oral hypoglycemic agents, and anticoagulants should have blood drug levels monitored.

Relapse is an uncommon and usually benign complication of hepatitis A. It requires only simple supportive therapy. Cholestasis complicates recovery in 5 to 10% of cases; persistent jaundice and pruritus are the main features. The liver tests reflect cholestasis (disproportionate elevation of serum alkaline phosphatase), but ultrasonography will indicate bile ducts of normal caliber. If necessary, a liver biopsy can be performed; laparotomy should be avoided.

Cholestyramine (Questran), 4 grams orally up to four times daily with meals, is effective against itch in two thirds of cases. Local therapies (tepid baths, calamine lotion) and a nonsedating H_1-receptor blocker such as terfenadine (Seldane, 60 mg once daily) may also be tried. Corticosteroids have been recommended for refractory cases of cholestasis after viral hepatitis but should be reserved exclusively for hepatitis A cases with cholestasis failing to resolve after 6 weeks.

The most serious complication of acute hepatitis is acute liver failure, indicated clinically by the onset of hepatic encephalopathy. Acute liver failure complicates about 0.2% of cases of hepatitis A. It is designated fulminant if onset is within 3 weeks and subfulminant between 3 and 8 weeks. The warning signs are repeated vomiting, deepening jaundice, and prolongation of the prothrombin time. These are indications for admission to the hospital for intravenous hydration, correction of hypoglycemia, and observation of mental status. Transfer of the patient to a liver transplant center is appropriate at the onset of liver failure. Aplastic anemia is a rare complication of acute viral hepatitis.

Transmission of HAV to others is avoided by simple enteric precautions of hand washing, use of one's own eating utensils, and correct disposal of feces. Strict

TABLE 2. **Immunization Against Viral Hepatitis**

Virus	Type of Immunization	Efficacy
HAV	Passive: ISG Active: hepatitis A vaccine	>70% effective if given within 2 wk of exposure Highly effective after 3 injections
HBV	Passive: HBIG Active: hepatitis B vaccine	Highly effective, temporary immunity after exposure 95% effective, postexposure efficacy, long-standing immunity
HCV	Passive: ISG	Ineffective

Abbreviations: HAV = hepatitis A virus; HBV = hepatitis B virus; HCV = hepatitis C virus; ISG = immune serum globulin; HBIG = hepatitis B immune globulin.

isolation is not required. Acute contacts, particularly family members, should be passively immunized by injection of pooled immune serum globulin (ISG) (0.02 mL per kg body weight), preparations of which contain high titers of anti-HAV; this is at least 70% protective when given early. ISG also conveys short-term (4- to 6-month) protection to travelers to endemic regions. Active immunization against hepatitis A is achieved with hepatitis A vaccine (Havrix or Vaqta), which is a formalin-killed preparation from whole HAV propagated in tissue culture. The vaccination schedule is composed of a 1-mL dose by intramuscular injection at the indicated time and repeated 4 weeks later; a booster is required at 6 to 12 months to provide lasting immunity. The indications include impending travel to an endemic region (at least 4 weeks before departure), high-risk occupation (sewerage workers, child care workers), male homosexuals with multiple sexual partners, and children living in communities with frequent outbreaks of hepatitis A. Patients with pre-existing liver disease should also be vaccinated because of the severity of acute hepatitis in the presence of cirrhosis. Hepatitis A vaccination is safe. The incidence of local complications is 20 to 50%. There have been rare reports of anaphylaxis, Guillain-Barré syndrome, and other obscure neurologic complications.

Hepatitis B

The hepatitis B virus (HBV) is a DNA virus composed of a lipoprotein envelope; the hepatitis B surface antigen (HBsAg); and a core containing HBV DNA and several proteins, including the DNA polymerase, the core antigen (HBcAg), and the hepatitis B e antigen (HBeAg) (see Table 1). The presence of "core markers" in peripheral blood, such as HBV DNA and HBeAg, indicates active viral replication and high infectivity of patients. Their absence, particularly in the presence of anti-HBe, indicates relatively inactive viral replication and lower (but not necessarily zero) infectivity. Anti-HBc occurs in both acute and chronic infection (both characterized by IgM anti-HBc) and persists indefinitely after recovery (IgG anti-HBc). Anti-HBs is a neutralizing antibody that together with loss of HBsAg indicates recovery from hepatitis B with lasting immunity. Pure preparations of HBsAg provide an effective hepatitis B vaccine (see Table 2).

Hepatitis B is contracted parenterally, by sexual transmission or other intimate contact, and by vertical transmission (mother to newborn) but not by oral ingestion. The incubation period is 6 weeks to 6 months. The major risk factors for acute hepatitis B are sexual contact (homosexual or heterosexual), injection drug use (IDU), and needle stick injury to health care workers. As discussed later, chronic hepatitis B may follow acute hepatitis B but is more often the consequence of asymptomatic infection acquired at the time of birth from an HBsAg-positive mother. Acute hepatitis B tends to be more severe than hepatitis A, and 0.5 to 1% of cases lead to acute

liver failure. One to 6 weeks before the onset of symptoms typical of hepatitis, there may be a prodromal illness. This resembles serum sickness and is characterized by fever, rash, arthralgia, arthritis, and occasionally hematuria; glomerulonephritis may complicate hepatitis B.

Management of acute hepatitis B is along symptomatic lines. Cholestasis is less common than with hepatitis A and should not be treated with corticosteroids because immunosuppression predisposes to chronicity. Cases of acute liver failure should be transferred to a liver transplant center. The results of orthotopic liver transplantation (OLT) for acute hepatitis B are excellent (as opposed to chronic hepatitis B, discussed later). The main limitation is donor availability. Liver support systems, such as the extracorporeal liver assist device, are a promising adjunct for management of acute liver failure, although they are not yet generally available.

Hepatitis B is an important public health problem principally because chronic hepatitis B leads to cirrhosis and hepatocellular carcinoma (HCC). Universal childhood vaccination against hepatitis B is therefore recommended for both high-risk and low-risk countries; implementation will be facilitated by extended immunization programs and reduction of cost. Persons at high risk for acquiring hepatitis B should be vaccinated. These include health care workers (before they enter the work place for the first time), those with multiple sexual partners (heterosexual or homosexual), injection drug users, and patients with chronic renal failure or recipients of clotting factors.

Hepatitis B vaccines (including currently used recombinant and the original plasma-derived products) are safe. The incidence of sore arm is low, and serious complications such as anaphylaxis and Guillain-Barré syndrome, although reported, are rare. Injections should be made into the deltoid muscle because gluteal injections have been associated with suboptimal immunogenicity. The standard schedule of vaccination with hepatitis B vaccine (Recombivax HB, or Engerix-B) is three intramuscular injections (20 μg) at designated times, 4 to 6 weeks and 4 to 6 months. The pediatric dose is 10 μg. Approximately 95% of recipients will develop protective levels of anti-HBs (>10 mIU per mL). Titers of anti-HBs wane to nonprotective levels in 50% of recipients after 5 to 10 years, but despite this, hepatitis B vaccination confers long-standing efficacy against clinically relevant HBV infection. For practical reasons, the antibody response needs to be verified only in subjects at high risk for hepatitis B. A low titer is an indication for a further course of vaccination. About 5% of the normal population are unable to mount any immune response to HBsAg and therefore do not respond to current hepatitis B vaccines; such persons remain at risk for hepatitis B. It is recommended that children who have been vaccinated against hepatitis B receive a booster injection at adolescence (e.g., age 12 years) because of heightened risk during the early years of sexual activity. Patients likely to have a suboptimal immunologic response, such as those with renal failure, should be given double-dose (40 μg) vaccination and should be monitored for anti-HBs.

Two additional measures may be appropriate after acute exposure to hepatitis B (see Table 2). The first is administration of hepatitis B immune globulin (0.05 mL per kg), ideally within the first 48 hours after exposure. Vaccination should commence at the same time. HBIG is also indicated for infants of HBeAg-positive mothers. The second measure is an accelerated vaccination schedule, with doses administered immediately and then at 4 weeks and 8 weeks; this should be followed by a booster at 6 to 12 months to ensure sustained high-titer anti-HBs. The incubation period of hepatitis B is long, and postexposure vaccination can protect against clinical infection with HBV.

Hepatitis C

The hepatitis C virus (HCV) is an enveloped RNA flavivirus-like agent. It is responsible for at least 95% of parenterally transmitted non-A, non-B hepatitis and also accounts for about 25% of cases of community-acquired sporadic acute hepatitis. The incubation is between 2 weeks and 3 months. Current (second- or third-generation) serologic tests for anti-HCV have high sensitivity (>99%) for chronic hepatitis C but may not become positive in the first 6 weeks of HCV infection. Thus, some cases of acute hepatitis C may be associated with a negative anti-HCV, and once other causes of acute hepatitis have been excluded, reverse transcription–polymerase chain reaction (RT-PCR) for HCV RNA is indicated as an alternative diagnostic test.

HCV is spread parenterally. Thus, the main risk factors are IDU and transfusion of blood products before 1990 when screening of blood donors with anti-HCV was introduced. Other risk factors include tattooing, nosocomial transmission other than by transfusion of blood products, and occupational exposure to needle stick injuries; approximately 10% of health care workers exposed to HCV through needle sticks become infected. The high prevalence of chronic HCV infection in some countries is thought to be related to medical or paramedical use of unsterilized needles 20 to 50 years ago. Sexual transmission of HCV is possible but accounts for relatively few cases; it is more likely after contact with a person with acute hepatitis C than with chronic HCV infection. Likewise, vertical transmission of HCV occurs with 5% of pregnant women who have hepatitis C, being related to a high circulating titer of HCV RNA or co-infection with the human immunodeficiency virus (HIV).

Acute hepatitis C tends to be less severe than hepatitis A or B; jaundice occurs in only 25%, and acute liver failure is less common than for hepatitis B. Only 15% of patients recover completely from acute hepatitis C, and chronic hepatitis C is the leading cause of viral hepatitis in the United States (see later). There is no hepatitis C vaccine. ISG has been recommended but is not effective as passive immunoprophylaxis. Enteric precautions are not required. Corticosteroids should be avoided because they may be associated with worsening of the disease. Transmission within hospitals requires careful attention to possible blood contamination during surgery, anesthesia, and other invasive procedures such as therapeutic endoscopy, in which appropriate cleansing, sterilization, and use of disposable biopsy devices will prevent infection.

Hepatitis D (Delta Hepatitis)

The hepatitis D virus (HDV) is a small RNA agent. It is not infectious unless it is encapsulated within the HBsAg, so that hepatitis D occurs only as a co-infection with HBV infection or as a superinfection in a chronic HBV carrier. Both circumstances can result in acute hepatitis. The clinical course is often severe and may result in liver failure. A chronic course is also common, and this results in cirrhosis in about two thirds of cases. Diagnosis of hepatitis D is by the presence of anti-HDV; IgM anti-HDV indicates recent or continuing infection, IgG anti-HDV indicates previous infection. The most important risk factor for HDV is IDU, although HDV is relatively common in some geographic areas, such as Italy and parts of South America. Prevention of co-infection is by immunization against hepatitis B. Chronic HBV carriers cannot be immunized against HDV; thus, harm reduction behavior (especially not sharing needles or injection devices) is essential for persons engaging in IDU.

Hepatitis E

The hepatitis E virus (HEV) is a calicivirus, like HAV a nonenveloped RNA virus that is enterically transmitted. It is responsible for both epidemic and sporadic outbreaks of hepatitis in Mexico, Central and South America, western China, parts of the Indian subcontinent, North Africa, and the Middle East. It is contracted from heavily contaminated drinking water; secondary cases are uncommon. In the United States, hepatitis E may be a cause of acute hepatitis in persons who have recently traveled to an endemic region. Serologic diagnosis (positive anti-HEV) can be performed by reference laboratories. Acute hepatitis E is clinically similar to hepatitis A, with the exception that 20% of women develop fulminant and subfulminant hepatic failure, and fetal loss is common. Other types of acute viral hepatitis are not more severe during pregnancy. There is no specific treatment for hepatitis E. To date, development of a vaccine has not reached the stage of clinical testing. ISG is unlikely to be protective.

Hepatitis F and Hepatitis G–Related Agents

The Sentinel Counties Study of the Centers for Disease Control and Prevention indicated that hepatitis A, B, and C viruses together account for 97% of cases of community-acquired hepatitis in the United States. However, there remains interest in the possibility that occasional cases of acute or chronic hepatitis may be caused by other human hepatitis viruses. In particular, the rare condition of fulminant hepatitis is often not due to known viruses. An agent designated hepatitis F virus was ascribed to some cases of sporadic hepatitis in India, but its existence has not been verified independently. In contrast, the genome for the hepatitis G virus (HGV) has been partly characterized. It is a flavivirus-like agent that is about 25% similar to HCV. The hepatitis GB virus type C (GBV-C) is either similar to or identical with HGV.

Chronic HGV infection is more common than with HCV, and the virus is transmitted by the same parenteral modes of spread. Hepatitis G may exist on its own or as a co-infection with hepatitis B or C. To date, however, there is no convincing evidence that HGV (or GBV-C) causes either acute or chronic hepatitis. At worst, HGV and related agents are rare causes of mild hepatitis. A serologic diagnostic test has not been devised, and diagnosis rests on determination of HGV RNA by RT-PCR (see Table 1). Because of the dubious pathogenicity of HGV, screening of blood donors is not currently conducted, and there are no measures advocated for prevention.

CHRONIC VIRAL HEPATITIS

HBV, HDV, HCV, and HGV infections can persist for more than 6 months. Thus, each agent can cause chronic hepatitis, as characterized by raised serum ALT levels and liver histology. However, chronic hepatitis virus infections are not always associated with severe or progressive types of liver disease. Co-infections with hepatitis viruses include HBV with HDV, HBV and HCV, and HBV plus HDV plus HCV; such co-infections are particularly likely to result in progressive chronic liver disease. In contrast, co-infection with HGV does not worsen the clinical course, histologic severity, or outcome of interferon treatment in hepatitis C.

Management of chronic viral hepatitis involves general measures to ameliorate morbidity, antiviral therapy, and interventions for complications. In general, antiviral therapy is directed at interrupting the natural history of the progressive forms of the disease that lead to cirrhosis and thereafter carry a high risk for liver failure and HCC. A secondary benefit of treatment may be to render individuals noninfectious to others through sexual spread or professional activity in the case of infected health care workers.

Chronic HBV Infection and Chronic Hepatitis B

Chronicity complicates 5% of HBV infections in adults, but it is the usual outcome of infection in the perinatal period or in early childhood. The natural history of neonatally acquired chronic HBV infection

evolves in 20 to 40 years. In brief, the initial phase is one of active viral replication and complete immune tolerance. Such "HBV carriers" (chronic HBV infection is a better term) are asymptomatic, have normal liver test results, and are HBeAg- and HBV DNA–positive as well as HBsAg-positive. The second phase is one of "immune elimination," in which immune tolerance to HBV has waned, viral replication persists (HBV DNA–positive, HBeAg-positive), and a cytotoxic T cell–mediated attack on infected liver cells results in hepatic inflammation and raised ALT. The resulting hepatitis may continue as chronic hepatitis B, but it more often ends when HBV replication is arrested during the process termed seroconversion in which HBV DNA becomes undetectable, HBeAg reverts to negative, and anti-HBe becomes positive. Seroconversion often happens without the patient's experiencing symptoms. Liver test results are then normal, and so the patient appears healthy, the so-called healthy hepatitis B carrier. However, in some instances, seroconversion may be delayed for years after the onset of chronic hepatitis. In such cases, the patient may actually have developed cirrhosis and remains at risk for HCC.

The management of chronic HBV infection varies according to the stage of the natural history and the state of viral replication. However, all individuals should be counseled about the risks of sexual, household, and occupational (in the case of health care workers) transmission. This is highest among HBeAg-positive individuals. Vaccination of at-risk contacts should include household members and sexual partners. General measures include reduction of harmful drinking, although it is not necessary for patients to avoid alcohol entirely unless liver function is poor or there is a history of lack of self-control with alcohol intake. General health advice should be given, such as the benefits of smoking cessation, a balanced diet, and moderate exercise. There is much interest in dietary therapy, homeopathy, and other alternative therapies for chronic viral hepatitis. For those who believe in alternative medicine, this approach may improve well-being, but there is no evidence that such measures affect the natural history of chronic viral hepatitis. Likewise, use of vitamins C and E and other antioxidants is an unproven approach. Many patients will inquire about herbal remedies, vitamins, and liver tonics; some of these may contain antioxidants, such as silimarin in extracts of St. Mary's thistle. Most herbal remedies are not toxic provided that recommended doses are observed, but Chinese herbal medicines such as *jin bu huan* and *syo-saiko-to* (popular in Japan) have been associated with idiosyncratic (dose-independent) hepatotoxicity. For these reasons, I do not recommend herbal remedies. Their use should be discussed openly with the patient, and it is encouraged that both physicians and patients keep an open mind on the subject.

Management of Apparently Healthy HBV Carriers

Antiviral therapy is not indicated and in any case is not effective in eliminating HBV among apparently

TABLE 3. **Interferon and Other Antiviral Therapy for Chronic Viral Hepatitis**

Disease	Interferon Dose and Course	Indications	Unsuitable Cases	Results
Hepatitis B	5 million U 3 times/wk, 4–6 mo	Histology—chronic hepatitis, ALT >120 IU/L, HBeAg-positive, HBV DNA–positive	Severe cirrhosis HBeAg-negative, HBV DNA–positive (precore mutant) Co-infection with HDV (see text)	30–45% lose HBeAg 10–15% lose HBsAg ALT returns to normal Histology improved
Hepatitis C	3 million U 3 times/wk, 12 mo	Histology—chronic hepatitis, particularly of moderate severity by fibrosis score	Cases with cirrhosis are less responsive (not absolute contraindication) Co-infection with HBV (see text)	End-treatment response in 35–60% Sustained response 20–35% (10–20% with 6 mo of treatment) Improved liver histology RT-PCR negative for HCV RNA

Abbreviations: ALT = alanine aminotransferase; HBV = hepatitis B virus; HBeAg = hepatitis B e antigen; HCV = hepatitis C virus; HDV = hepatitis D virus; RT-PCR = reverse transcription–polymerase chain reaction.

healthy carriers (those with normal ALT levels). Patients who are HBeAg-positive should be monitored a little more closely than HBeAg-negative patients because of the risk for developing chronic hepatitis. It is appropriate to perform liver tests and virus serology (especially HBeAg and anti-HBe) every 6 months.

Among HBeAg-negative patients, yearly monitoring of liver tests is all that is required until 40 years of age. After this, screening for HCC may be warranted, with measurements of serum alpha-fetoprotein every 6 months and hepatic ultrasonography each 12 months. Screening for HCC in this group remains contentious, as opposed to those known to have cirrhosis who are at higher risk, but it is particularly recommended in those with a family history of HCC. Conversely, it is not appropriate to screen HBV carriers if other medical disorders would contraindicate a curative procedure for HCC.

Interferon for Chronic Hepatitis B

The only licensed treatment of chronic hepatitis B is interferon alfa-2b (Intron A). The indication is histologically confirmed chronic hepatitis B with raised ALT levels and positive HBeAg and HBV DNA. Treatment is most strongly indicated in those with hepatic fibrosis; it is most likely to be effective if disease is of short duration, ALT levels are high (greater than three times the upper limit of normal), and HBV DNA levels are low (less than 200 pg per mL). Interferon is less effective if ALT is mildly elevated (i.e., to less than twice the upper limit of normal or 100 IU per liter). It is also relatively ineffective in the presence of infection with HIV, particularly if the CD4+ cell count is low. Interferon is contraindicated in patients with hepatitis B and cirrhosis who have poor liver function, as indicated by ascites, muscle wasting, coagulation disorder, or reduction of serum albumin concentration to below 32 grams per liter and elevation of serum bilirubin concentration above 1.5 mg per dL. This is because the seroconversion illness that accompanies a response to interferon can precipitate fatal liver failure in those with poor hepatic "reserve" function and also

because hematologic adverse effects are more severe in patients with cirrhosis.

The usual treatment course is 5 million units of recombinant interferon alfa-2b by subcutaneous injection three times a week for 16 to 24 weeks (Table 3). Outside the United States, treatment with similar doses of interferon alfa-2a (Roferon-A) or interferon beta, as well as cell line–derived "natural" interferon products such as lymphoblastoid interferon alfa-n1, has produced similar results. The patient should be monitored every 4 weeks for efficacy and safety. The best efficacy tests are HBV DNA, HBeAg, and anti-HBe. If HBV DNA is still present in serum after 8 weeks of interferon, the dose should be increased to 10 million units and treatment continued for another 8 to 16 weeks. The end point of treatment is loss of HBeAg with formation of anti-HBe. This is achieved in 30 to 45% of cases. In the absence of interferon treatment, spontaneous loss of HBeAg occurs in 10 to 15% of patients during the first year of observation. Seroconversion (whether spontaneous or interferon induced) is preceded by a rise in ALT level (and rarely bilirubin concentration) and is followed by reduction in enzyme values toward normal. If HBeAg has not been lost at 24 weeks, there is no value in continuing treatment. Loss of HBV DNA and HBeAg after interferon treatment is permanent in most cases, but about 10% will relapse with reversion to HBeAg positivity and raised ALT levels. Conversely, about 30% of patients who lose HBsAg after a course of interferon treatment subsequently lose HBsAg and develop anti-HBs; this amounts to 10 to 15% of all treated subjects.

Interferon treatment is associated with a number of adverse effects; most are uncomfortable and transient, and it is uncommonly necessary to stop treatment. On the other hand, some adverse effects can be life-threatening or permanent. In the early stages of treatment, patients usually experience an influenza-like reaction, with fever, myalgia, headache, sweating, rigors, and occasionally delirium. These symptoms begin about 2 hours after the interferon injection; they may be partly ameliorated by acetaminophen (1 gram) taken 2 hours before the injection and repeated once or twice as required. After 2 to 4 weeks, tachyphylaxis to these adverse effects develops, although intermittent or persistent headache and myalgia may occur. The most common complaint during interferon treatment is fatigue, usually a minor reduction of physical and psychologic energy and well-being. However, more severe psychologic symptoms can occur and include profound lethargy and malaise, depression, irritability, and uncontrolled behavior. Counseling patients and their partners about psychologic adverse effects is important before embarking on interferon treatment. Those with a past history of depression or violent behavior may be at particular risk; if at all possible, interferon should be avoided in patients being treated with antidepressants.

The other adverse effects of interferon treatment include weight loss, diarrhea, rash (including severe exacerbations of psoriasis), pruritus, hair loss, bad taste, paresthesias, neutropenia, leukopenia, and thyroid disorders. Interferon predictably lowers both the leukocyte and platelet counts; patients with pre-existing abnormalities, such as those with advanced cirrhosis, are particularly at risk. Interferon should be stopped if the platelet count falls to below 50,000 cells per mm^3 or if the neutrophil count is below 1000 cells per mm^3. Values will return to pretreatment levels within days. Thyroid disease occurs in up to 0.5 to 2% of cases; it is more common with prolonged interferon treatment and in those with pre-existing thyroid autoantibodies. The functional abnormalities include hypothyroidism and hyperthyroidism; these conditions can resolve after stopping interferon but may be permanent. Other rare adverse effects of interferon include precipitation or exacerbation of other autoimmune diseases, including autoimmune hepatitis, worsening of epilepsy, diabetes mellitus, or unstable coronary heart disease. Older patients should be subjected to ophthalmoscopic examination before treatment because of the suspicion that interferon may exacerbate some forms of retinopathy.

Use of Interferon for Hepatitis B in Special Situations (Including Hepatitis D)

Re-Treatment. Among patients who fail to respond to interferon or who respond and then relapse, few will respond to re-treatment. Should there be a change in disease activity (e.g., increase in ALT levels, decrease in HBV DNA), re-treatment may be contemplated in selected cases, but other therapeutic strategies are generally more desirable. These include use of "steroid priming" or nucleoside analogues (discussed later).

Children. Children with histologically proven chronic hepatitis B can be treated with interferon. Provided that the ALT level exceeds 100 IU per liter, there is the same chance of response as for adults. On a dose per body weight basis, children appear to tolerate interferon at least as well as adults do.

Chronic Hepatitis B with Lesser Elevation of ALT (<100 IU per Liter). The chance that such cases will respond to interferon alone is less than 20%. Pretreatment with steroid priming may be tried if the liver disease warrants treatment or the patient has disabling symptoms. A recommended regimen is prednisone 60 mg daily for 2 weeks, then 40 mg daily for 2 weeks, and finally 20 mg for 2 weeks. Prednisone is then stopped for 2 weeks (washout phase), after which interferon is administered in the same dose and schedule as for high-level ALT cases.

Chronic Hepatitis B with Positive HBV DNA but Negative HBeAg (Precore Mutant HBV). HBV may undergo many mutations, but one that affects the natural history of chronic hepatitis B and the response to interferon treatment is the precore mutant, in which the capacity to clip a peptide from the core protein is lost; this step converts the core protein to HBeAg. Precore mutants may arise during chronic HBV infection, but their emergence may be accelerated by interferon treatment. Although ALT levels may fall during therapy, patients with the precore mutant HBV do not usually have a permanent response to interferon. They are candidates for nucleoside analogue antivirals (see later).

Chronic Hepatitis B in HIV-Infected Persons. The response to interferon is suboptimal except in cases with a good CD4$^+$ cell count (>400 cells per mm^3). Because HIV and HBV both respond to the (−) enantiomer of 3-thiacytidine (lamivudine), this is now the preferred treatment if the hepatitis B is symptomatic or associated with progressive liver disease.

Chronic Hepatitis B and Renal Failure. Renal failure is not an absolute contraindication to interferon, although the associated immunosuppression reduces the chance of a satisfactory response. Interferon is cleared partly by renal excretion, so that the dose used in renal failure or dialysis patients should be halved to avoid profound weight loss. Interferon can precipitate graft rejection and should therefore be avoided or used with caution in patients who have undergone renal transplantation.

Treatment of Hepatitis D. High-dose interferon for prolonged courses (at least 1 year) has been advocated for hepatitis D, but there are doubts about the efficacy of this approach, and adverse effects usually restrict treatment. It should be reserved for severely progressive cases.

Hepatitis B with Severe Cirrhosis. Interferon treatment is hazardous for patients with hepatitis B–related cirrhosis and poor liver function. Borderline cases should be treated only under the supervision of a unit experienced with this disease and with ready access to hepatic transplantation. Lower doses of interferon may be preferred. In my view, use of nucleoside analogues is preferable in these cases (see the following).

Nucleoside Analogue Antivirals for Hepatitis B

Several nucleoside analogues are potent antiviral agents against HBV and related animal viruses both in vitro and in vivo. Earlier agents such as adenine arabinoside monophosphate and fialuridine proved toxic; the latter was associated with several deaths from a form of hepatorenal failure that appears attributable to mitochondrial toxicity. Experience with lamivudine (Epivir)* 100 mg once daily and famciclovir (Famvir),* the oral prodrug of penciclovir, 500 mg three times a day indicates that these agents can suppress HBV replication for prolonged periods. Such suppression is associated with control of hepatitis, as indicated by a fall in ALT levels and improved liver histology. The agents have good oral availability, are well tolerated, and have few serious adverse effects. However, the occurrence of mutations in the HBV polymerase has led to the emergence of drug-resistant strains in a small proportion of cases, particularly after hepatic transplantation and prolonged treatment.

Lamivudine and famciclovir are not yet licensed for use in hepatitis B in the United States, and the precise indications and duration of the treatment course are currently being defined in clinical trials. They may be available from the manufacturers for compassionate use in clinical trial protocols. This should be considered in patients with early liver failure from either wild-type or precore mutant forms of HBV as well as before and after OLT (see following).

Liver Transplantation for Hepatitis B and D

Chronic hepatitis B is a common cause of end-stage cirrhosis with liver failure, but treatment by OLT has been associated with poor results because of recurrence of hepatitis B in the engrafted liver. For this reason, some units no longer perform transplantation for hepatitis B patients. HBV reinfection often causes severe liver disease; the mortality is 50% at 2 years. It may involve the pattern of fibrosing cholestatic hepatitis that is different from hepatitis B under most other circumstances. It carries a poor prognosis and fails to respond to interferon treatment. The risk for HBV reinfection can be reduced by administration of hepatitis B immune globulin during and after OLT, but efficacy is limited and large intravenous doses and prolonged courses of treatment are required. Studies have indicated that lamivudine administered 4 weeks or more before OLT can prevent reinfection of the transplanted liver. Likewise, nucleoside analogues have proved lifesaving in fibrosing cholestatic hepatitis B after OLT. These agents are likely to revolutionize the approach to liver transplantation in hepatitis B.

Contrary to earlier reported experiences, the outcome of liver transplantation for patients with HBV and HDV co-infection is actually superior to that of uncomplicated hepatitis B. This is because the rate of HBV reinfection is less with HDV co-infection, presumably because viral interference reduces the replication activity of HBV.

Chronic Hepatitis C

Hepatitis C is a common chronic disease that may extend for 40 to 50 years without adverse clinical events, but liver failure or HCC occurs in 5 to 15% of cases. Thus, management of individuals involves assessment of the severity of liver disease, reduction of co-morbidity, consideration of antiviral treatment with interferon, adjunctive therapies, relief of symptoms, and psychosocial support of the patients and their families. Histologic assessment of disease severity is vital, preferably with the grading of fibrosis that allows staging of the disease. Thus, milder disease (typified by absence of fibrosis in asymptomatic patients) need not necessarily be treated with interferon. Conversely, the presence of cirrhosis indicates that a sustained response to interferon is less likely. Symptoms and ALT levels correlate poorly with histologic severity of disease, but the presence of symptoms may influence whether to use interferon.

General Measures

Excessive alcohol ingestion allows more active replication of HCV and is associated with adverse clinical outcomes. Patients should therefore be advised to abstain or considerably reduce intake of alcoholic beverages; a safe threshold of alcohol intake has not been defined for chronic viral hepatitis. Vaccination against hepatitis A and B is recommended, as are the general health measures in relation to diet and lifestyle mentioned in the section on chronic hepatitis B. Likewise, many patients with chronic hepatitis C take or consider taking alternative medicines; this issue was discussed earlier for hepatitis B. Individual counseling involves sharing of information about the virus, the infectivity of individuals, and prevention of transmission in the home. As well, knowledge is conveyed about the indolent nature of the liver disease; the relatively low frequency of adverse outcomes; and the need to remain active, optimistic, and attentive to health issues that are equally or more important, such as cigarette smoking. Self-help groups are of considerable value for patients with hepatitis C, particularly in their pursuit of information and mutual support.

Interferon for Hepatitis C

In the United States, interferon alfa-2b (Intron A) is the only licensed treatment of hepatitis C, but other interferon alfa and beta products have been shown to have similar efficacy and are used elsewhere. The goals of treating hepatitis C are to prevent end points of the disease, to arrest progression of hepatic fibrosis, and to improve liver function and well-being; the best way to achieve these goals is to eliminate HCV infection. The optimal dose of interferon is 3 million units administered by subcutaneous injection three times a week; 5 million units may be tried in refractory cases, but it has a less favorable profile of adverse effects. About 50% of patients will normalize ALT levels during and at the end of treatment (end-treatment response). The licensed duration of treatment is 6 months, but this is not optimal because the relapse rate after end-treatment response is 70%. Extending treatment to 12 or 18 months reduces the chance of relapse to 40%, thereby

---

*Not FDA approved for this indication.

increasing the sustained response from about 10 to 20% up to 20 to 35%. I recommend initial treatment with 3 million units for 12 weeks. Should the ALT level normalize, treatment should be continued for a total of 12 months. If initial response is incomplete and tolerance is good, the dose of interferon can be increased to 5 million units in a further attempt to achieve response.

Monitoring of patients receiving interferon treatment includes safety testing (as for hepatitis B) and ALT determinations at 4-week intervals. Should an initial good response be followed by a rise in ALT level on more than one occasion, the patient has breakthrough of HCV replication and either the dose of interferon should be increased to 5 million units or treatment discontinued; the latter course is my preference. Should the platelet or neutrophil counts fall to unacceptable levels or the patient experience other significant adverse effects (e.g., reduction of body weight by more than 10%), the dose of interferon should be reduced to 2 million units or treatment temporarily discontinued. It is advisable to determine serum thyroid-stimulating hormone levels at 6 months to detect possible thyroid dysfunction.

Correlates of Response to Interferon. The personal factors associated with response to interferon treatment include age, sex, country of birth, and route of acquisition of the disease. However, disease-related factors and virus determinants are more important primary "predictors" (correlates is a more accurate term) of treatment outcome. Thus, response to interferon is least likely when cirrhosis is present and most likely in cases with minimal hepatic fibrosis. It remains my view that some patients with cirrhosis and active hepatitis C should be offered interferon treatment, but any features of hepatic decompensation (Child-Pugh class B or C categories) are a contraindication, whereas patients with cirrhosis caused by HCV genotypes 1 and 4 are highly unlikely to respond. The presence of excessive iron staining on liver histology is a negative correlate of interferon treatment outcome, but there is no evidence to date that such patients should be subjected to phlebotomy for removal of iron overload before starting interferon treatment.

HCV genotype and load (indicated by serum titer of HCV RNA) are independent correlates of sustained response to interferon. Thus, response is at least twice as likely with genotypes 2 and 3 as with genotypes 1 and 4; genotypes 1 and 4 are predominant among HCV isolates in the United States. Patients with a lower HCV RNA titer (absolute titers depend on the method used) are twice as likely to have a sustained response to interferon as are those with higher titer. Whereas laboratory methods for HCV genotyping and quantification are now reliable, testing is expensive and not always available. In my view, genotyping is particularly important in making individual decisions about interferon treatment.

Assessment of Treatment Response, Post-Treatment Monitoring, and Re-Treatment. The assessment of response to interferon treatment is made principally by monitoring liver test results, particularly ALT. A liver biopsy is not required at the end of treatment. However, it is highly desirable to make a virologic assessment of treatment response using RT-PCR for HCV RNA. Positive RT-PCR at the end of treatment indicates a high probability of relapse, although negativity at that time does not correlate with sustained response. However, a negative RT-PCR at 12 months after interferon treatment, together with normal ALT levels, is a reliable indicator of sustained response with histologic and functional improvement of the liver disease; relapse after this time can occur but is rare.

The post-treatment management of hepatitis C includes reassurance of the patient, the frequency of visits depending largely on the severity of liver disease. Patients with mild disease who elect not to be treated with interferon should be subjected to a progress liver biopsy after 3 to 5 years. Patients with cirrhosis or grade 3 fibrosis (cirrhosis in evolution) are at risk for HCC and can be offered screening with alpha-fetoprotein and hepatic ultrasonography, as discussed for hepatitis B. Re-treatment can be considered if the first course of interferon was for only 6 months. A subsequent 12-month course of treatment can be associated with permanent clearance of HCV. Trials are under way to assess whether prolonged or repeated suppression of hepatitis C with interferon alters the natural history of the disease. Given the extended nature of the natural history in the majority of cases of hepatitis C, it is often appropriate to encourage patients to wait for more acceptable and effective therapies (see the following).

Adjunctive Therapies and Future Antivirals

Several agents appear to improve biochemical abnormalities in hepatitis C without a demonstrable effect on HCV replication. Among others, these include ursodeoxycholic acid (ursodiol [Actigall]), cyclosporine (Sandimmune), Chinese herbal medicines, phlebotomy, N-acetylcysteine, and cysteamine (Cystagon). The value of such adjunctive therapies on their own or in combination with interferon is unknown, and they are not currently recommended outside the context of clinical trials. Ribavirin (Virazole) is a guanosine analogue that is effective against the respiratory syncytial virus. In early trials, it improved liver test results without altering serum HCV RNA; liver histology improved after prolonged (2 years) treatment. A more impressive effect of ribavirin is to improve the rate of sustained response to interferon treatment when used in combination, including among patients who have relapsed after an end-treatment response. Large trials are in progress. Patients who failed to respond to interferon seem to have little likelihood of response to re-treatment with interferon and ribavirin.

Much work is now going into developing new antivirals against HCV, based on the enzymes encoded by the HCV genome, such as the protease, polymerase, and internal ribosomal entry site. Given the protracted nature of hepatitis C, most patients who have failed interferon treatment or who have contraindications to interferon can be advised that the next 3 to 5 years should bring more satisfactory treatments. As for HIV, combination antiviral therapy is likely to become the optimal approach.

HCV with HBV Co-infection

HCV with HBV co-infection is usually associated with HBeAg and HBV DNA negativity. One might therefore predict that the resultant hepatitis would respond to doses of interferon directed at HCV. Unfortunately, this is not the case, with few if any responses to interferon. The exceptions are rare cases of HBeAg positivity, which respond to interferon in the same way as other cases of HBeAg-positive chronic hepatitis B. The majority of co-infected patients have severe liver disease, and the risk for HCC is accentuated. Thus, closer monitoring and screening for HCC are indicated.

Liver Transplantation for Hepatitis C

Hepatitis C is the most common indication for liver transplantation among United States adults. The results are the same as for other disorders and differ from those with hepatitis B. This is despite the almost universal finding of recurrence of hepatitis C in the transplanted liver. To date, 5-year follow-up studies indicate no excess mortality attributable to hepatitis C. Treatment remains a problem because of concern that interferon would stimulate graft rejection.

MALABSORPTION

method of
DAVID H. ALPERS, M.D.
Washington University School of Medicine
St. Louis, Missouri

GENERAL CONSIDERATIONS

The usual manner of considering malabsorption syndromes is to provide an algorithm for the differential diagnosis and to list the specific treatments for each cause. Unfortunately, patients present not with a diagnosis of malabsorption but with chronic diarrhea, with or without weight loss. Moreover, many of the available treatment modalities are designed to deliver macronutrients or micronutrients, regardless

of the cause or when the cause of the malabsorption cannot be reversed. Thus, the patient with possible malabsorption should be approached with four questions in mind: (1) Is the diarrhea secondary to malabsorption, or is it secretory or inflammatory? (2) Is the cause of the malabsorption amenable to specific therapy? (3) If weight loss or steatorrhea-diarrhea is a major problem, how should the energy sources be provided when the cause of malabsorption cannot be treated? (4) If malabsorption or a low body store of a specific micronutrient is a major problem, how can these nutrients be provided efficiently? The basis for many of the answers to these questions will reside in a careful nutritional history (Table 1). Such a history suggests the presence of various nutrient deficiencies and, as a result, directs the work-up of the patient with chronic diarrhea.

IS THE DIARRHEA SECONDARY TO MALABSORPTION?

The causes of chronic diarrhea can be classified as malabsorptive, secretory, and inflammatory. Most of the findings thought to be characteristic of malabsorption are in fact due to steatorrhea. When symptoms (foul smell, gray color, coating of the toilet bowl, passage of undigested food, weight loss in the face of increased or constant intake) and signs (gray pasty stool strongly positive for Sudan III stain, documented weight loss) suggest energy deficit and/or steatorrhea, the diagnosis of malabsorption is clear. However, some secretory causes (e.g., Zollinger-Ellison syndrome, carcinoid syndrome) and some inflammatory conditions (e.g., *Mycobacterium avium-intracellulare* complex infection, Crohn's disease) can cause malabsorption. Moreover, some malabsorptive states (e.g., carbohydrate malabsorption) can cause watery diarrhea without steatorrhea. Steatorrhea can be detected (if it is not apparent from the history and stool examination) by a 72-hour stool fat collection. In practice, this is not frequently necessary. Watery diarrhea can be detected (other than by history and stool examination) by 24-hour stool frequency and weight. Inflammation can be detected by the presence of abnormal findings on endoscopy or by white blood cells in the stool. Thus, it is more practical to classify chronic diarrhea as steatorrheic, watery, or inflammatory, recognizing that overlap can still exist for a single cause. In general, further work-up for malabsorption is indicated if steatorrhea is

TABLE 1. **Nutritional Screening History for Patients with Suspected Malabsorption**

Mechanism of Deficiency	If History of	Suspect Deficiency of
Inadequate intake	Anorexia, alcohol intake, dental disease, taste disturbance	Calories, protein, most vitamins and minerals
Inadequate absorption	Diarrhea, weight loss, gastrointestinal surgery, acquired immune deficiency syndrome, ileal disease or resection	Especially vitamins A and D, folate, vitamin B_{12}, calcium, magnesium, iron
Increased losses	Blood loss	Iron
	Diarrhea	Sodium, potassium, zinc
Increased requirements	Fever, surgery, infection	Calories, protein

TABLE 2. **Clues to the Diagnosis of Common Malabsorptive Disorders for Which Specific Therapy May Be Available**

Disorder	History and Symptoms	Signs and Laboratory Findings
Celiac sprue	Family history, age at onset <3 y or 20–40 y, aphthous oral ulcers, absence of abdominal pain, nocturia, weight loss	Small spleen and lymph nodes, edema, abdominal distention, peripheral neuropathy, abnormal findings on small bowel biopsy
Tropical sprue	Adults living >1 y in Puerto Rico, Cuba, Haiti, Dominican Republic	Glossitis, stomatitis, abnormal findings on small bowel biopsy
Whipple's disease	Male >> female; fever, weight loss, slow onset; involvement of central nervous system, eye, heart, joints	Fever, lymphadenopathy, neurologic findings, cardiac murmur, abnormal findings on small bowel biopsy
Giardiasis	Subacute course (weeks to months), weight loss, intermittent symptoms, recent travel to endemic area	Stool for ova and parasites, duodenal aspirate, small bowel biopsy
Bacterial overgrowth	Condition favoring small bowel stasis: stricture (Crohn's, external beam radiation), blind pouch (jejunoileal bypass, Billroth's II), hypomotility (scleroderma, diabetes mellitus)	Vitamin B_{12} deficiency, abnormal hydrogen breath test result
Pancreatic insufficiency	Alcoholism >6 y, weight loss, abdominal pain, prominent symptoms of steatorrhea, diabetes mellitus	Epigastric tenderness, calcified pancreas, pseudocyst, malodorous stools, glucose intolerance, abnormal secretin test result
Zollinger-Ellison syndrome	Prior peptic disease, thyroid nodule, family history	Elevated serum gastrin
Lymphoma	Progressive history, weight loss, abdominal pain, onset 2nd-3rd decade (IPSID), or <10 y and >50 y (Western type)	Small bowel mass, heavy chain paraprotein (IPSID), abnormal small bowel biopsy
Mastocytosis	Abdominal pain, skin lesions, headache, pruritus, flushing, wheezing	Urticaria pigmentosa, elevated urine histamine
Lactase deficiency	Nonwhite patient, milk product intolerance, response to restriction	Abnormal hydrogen breath test or lactose tolerance test result
Hyperthyroidism	Temperature intolerance, enlarged thyroid, tachycardia	Tremor, thyroid enlargement, TSH and/or T_4
Crohn's disease	Perianal disease, prior surgery, abdominal cramps, altered bowel pattern after intestinal resection	Abdominal mass or tenderness, anemia, abnormal findings on colonic or small bowel radiography and/or endoscopy

Abbreviations: IPSID = immunoproliferative small intestinal disease; TSH = thyroid-stimulating hormone; T_4 = thyroxine.

present or if no obvious cause for watery diarrhea is evident after initial studies are completed.

IF MALABSORPTION IS SUSPECTED OR DEMONSTRATED, IS IT AMENABLE TO SPECIFIC THERAPY?

Specific causes of malabsorption are often suggested by the history or physical examination findings (Table 2). For example, clues to the presence of celiac sprue, tropical sprue, acquired immune deficiency syndrome (AIDS), pancreatic insufficiency, lactose intolerance, Zollinger-Ellison syndrome, bacterial overgrowth, liver disease, hyperthyroidism, or Whipple's disease may be evident with this information. Thus, the work-up can be targeted to the tests most likely to provide a definitive diagnosis. Treatment should then be directed to the specific cause of the malabsorption (Table 3). In a real sense, then, the treatment of malabsorption depends on establishment of the correct diagnosis. A more complete outline of such a work-up can be found in many standard texts, and it is not covered here to allow more space for discussion of management. Some more detailed (but still not comprehensive) comments follow on the wide variety of causes of malabsorption. An expanded discussion of many of these areas is provided elsewhere.*

*See Alpers DH, Stenson WF, Bier DM: Manual of Nutritional Therapeutics, 3rd ed. Boston, Little, Brown, 1995.

Malabsorptive Conditions Primarily Presenting with Steatorrhea

Celiac Sprue

Glutens found in wheat, rye, oats, barley, and buckwheat should be eliminated as much as possible using a gluten-restricted diet. The diet should be maintained throughout life. Packaged foods that contain an unspecified flour, starch, emulsifiers, stabilizers, and hydrolyzed plant or vegetable protein should be avoided. These products may not contain gluten,

TABLE 3. **Specific Treatment of Diseases Presenting with Malabsorption**

Disorder	Treatment
Celiac sprue	Gluten-restricted diet
Tropical sprue	Folate, tetracycline
Whipple's disease	Antibiotics
Giardiasis	Metronidazole, quinacrine
Bacterial overgrowth	Antibiotics
Small bowel lymphoma	Chemotherapy, surgery
Crohn's disease	Corticosteroids, 5-aminosalicylates
Zollinger-Ellison syndrome	Proton pump inhibitors, surgery
Lactose intolerance	Low-lactose diet
Glucose/galactose malabsorption	Glucose- and galactose-free diet
Pancreatic insufficiency	Pancreatic enzymes
Thyrotoxicosis	Thyroid ablation or resection
Mastocytosis	H_1-receptor antagonists, disodium cromoglycate

but the company should be contacted to verify that fact. Full information about the diet can be obtained from the Celiac Sprue Association (P.O. Box 31700, Omaha, NE 68131-0700) or from The Gluten Intolerance Group of North America (P.O. Box 23053, Seattle, WA 98102-0353).

Tropical Sprue

Administration of oral folate (5 mg per day) and subcutaneous cyanocobalamin (1000 µg per week) for a few weeks is used to treat the anemia. In conjunction with this treatment, tetracycline (250 mg per day orally) is given to alter the bacterial flora.

Whipple's Disease

Although many antibiotics have been used, initial treatment should employ double-strength trimethoprim-sulfamethoxazole (twice daily) for 1 year, because this antibiotic crosses the blood-brain barrier and can treat the central nervous system as well as intestinal involvement. Penicillin is used for those allergic to sulfa.

Giardiasis

Metronidazole (Flagyl) 250 mg three times per day orally for 1 week is preferred initially, because of its lower side effect profile. An alternative therapy is quinacrine (100 mg three times per day orally).

Bacterial Overgrowth

Numerous antibiotics have been used, most of them with success. Tetracycline (250 mg four times daily) is inexpensive, well tolerated, and active against the mixture of aerobes and facultative anaerobes found in this syndrome. For long-term use, it is unclear whether it is better to use antibiotics cyclically, to rotate different antibiotics, or to use nonabsorbable antibiotics for at least part of the time. In many conditions predisposing to bacterial overgrowth (e.g., scleroderma), the cause of the overgrowth cannot be addressed, and antibiotic treatment must be continual.

Pancreatic Insufficiency

Sufficient doses of pancreatic enzymes should be used with each meal to significantly decrease steatorrhea and symptoms. Symptomatic relief for most patients will follow the use of 24,000 to 28,000 IU of lipase per meal. Most preparations of enzymes are therapeutically equivalent. If good control cannot be achieved by increasing the doses, an H_2-receptor antagonist can be added to decrease gastric acid secretion and deliver more functional enzyme to the small intestine. This approach is counterproductive if the enzyme preparation coated with a pH-dependent polymer (Pancrease) is used, because increased gastric pH would cause the release of pancreatic enzymes in the stomach. Even under the best circumstances, enzyme replacement therapy will not completely eliminate steatorrhea. Thus, in some patients, specific therapy (enzyme replacement) must

be combined with nonspecific treatment (e.g., low-fat diet).

Zollinger-Ellison Syndrome

The malabsorption is secondary to acid inactivation of pancreatic lipase and acid-induced precipitation of bile salts. Therapy is directed toward complete suppression of acid secretion with proton pump inhibitors. An average dose of 60 mg per day for omeprazole (Prilosec) has been suggested as effective for maintenance, but titration of acid secretion during therapy may be needed to ensure control of gastric pH.

Lymphoma

When the lymphoma is generalized in the small bowel as primary B cell (Mediterranean) lymphoma, non–T cell lymphoma (immunoproliferative small intestinal disease), or enterocyte-associated T cell lymphoma, malabsorption is common. The B and T cell lymphomas respond to chemotherapy; immunoproliferative small intestinal disease responds to antibiotics and/or chemotherapy.

Malabsorptive Conditions Primarily Presenting with Watery Diarrhea

Mastocytosis

This uncommon condition presents more with watery diarrhea, which can be controlled in some patients with a combination of H_1-receptor antagonists and disodium cromoglycate.

Lactase Deficiency

Watery diarrhea, cramps, and bloating is the common presentation. The symptoms are dose related; about half the patients note symptoms after 12 grams of lactose (the content of an 8-ounce glass of milk). Skim milk contains added lactose; creamed cheeses contain more lactose than hard cheeses, which contain about 0.5 to 1.0 gram of lactose per ounce. Ice cream contains about 9 grams per cup, and sherbet about half that amount. Only sorbets and ices are free of lactose. Yogurt is often tolerated because the fermentation of lactose continues in the intestine. Treatment uses a low-lactose diet, avoiding all milk products except perhaps yogurt made with live yeast cultures. Symptoms can often be controlled by the use of lactase-containing tablets or capsules derived from crude yeast preparations (1 to 3 tablets or capsules taken before food ingestion). Occasionally, patients are sufficiently sensitive that they must avoid ingested material containing lactose only as an added sweetener (e.g., cordials, dietetic preparations, instant potatoes, salad dressings, pie crusts and fillings, liquid antibiotics). In the rare disorder glucose-galactose malabsorption, it is essential that *all* glucose and galactose be removed from the diet and replaced with fructose. Because lactose is nearly the only source of dietary galactose, such a diet then becomes a lactose-free diet.

Hyperthyroidism

Treatment is usually ablative, with either surgery or radioiodine.

Malabsorptive Conditions in Which Inflammation Is a Major Factor

Crohn's Disease

Corticosteroids and 5-aminosalicylate preparations are the mainstays for treatment of active disease. When malabsorption is due to the short-bowel syndrome, after resection, then nonspecific therapy (e.g., modified fat diet, vitamin and mineral replacement) must be used, either alone or in combination with specific drug therapy. In most patients, the colon is retained and a low-fat diet is important in the control of symptoms. Those patients with a jejunostomy often do better symptomatically with a high-fat, low-carbohydrate diet, because the source of fermentation of fat (the colon) is not present.

IF WEIGHT LOSS OR STEATORRHEA-DIARRHEA IS A MAJOR PROBLEM, HOW SHOULD ENERGY SOURCES BE PROVIDED WHEN THE CAUSE OF MALABSORPTION CANNOT BE TREATED?

Many causes of the malabsorption syndrome cannot be treated. Moreover, in some cases, the cause cannot be established with certainty or is multifactorial. In such circumstances, a variety of nonspecific dietary manipulations can be introduced to minimize the symptoms of steatorrhea and/or diarrhea and to prevent further weight loss. These are outlined in Table 4. To these dietary maneuvers can be added the use of antidiarrheal or antispasmodic agents to prolong small intestinal transit, allowing more time for absorption. In addition, a decrease in stool frequency may be beneficial for the patient's long range coping skills. Finally, additional chronic supplementation with micronutrients when applicable (see later) is often indicated, when the cause of the malabsorption cannot be treated.

TABLE 4. **Use of Modified Diets in Nonspecific Treatment of Malabsorption**

Diet	Possible Indication
Low fat	Steatorrhea, especially when colon is present
High fat	Steatorrhea, when colon is absent
Low oxalate	Steatorrhea, moderate to severe
Medium chain triglyceride oil	Steatorrhea, as calorie supplement
Low fiber	Diarrhea, especially with bloating and increased flatus
Comprehensive	Acquired immune deficiency syndrome, debilitating disease
Enteral supplements	Inadequate oral intake

Low-Fat Diet

The objective is to lower fat intake enough to decrease the symptoms of steatorrhea to manageable proportions. Average fat intake for adults in the United States is about 40% of total caloric intake (or 110 grams of fat with a 2500-kcal intake). When diarrhea is decreased, absorption of protein and carbohydrate may also be improved. Because the diet is used to improve symptoms, there is no single level of restriction appropriate for all patients. For purposes of this diet, fat means triglycerides and not cholesterol. Almost all dietary sources of triglyceride are also rich sources of protein. The major exceptions are all oils and fats and shellfish. Thus, when fat restriction must be severe, protein supplements may need to be provided. The basic principle for a low-fat diet is to avoid the use of fats and oils and to eliminate all easily removable portions of fat from foods. The general outlines of the low-fat diet can be initiated by the physician, but the dietitian can play a key role in fine-tuning the diet and in ensuring compliance.

Broil, bake, or boil all meats and fish.

Use skim milk and cheeses, and avoid cream sauces.

Remove skin from poultry; trim fat from all meats; and use flat, not steaklike, fish fillets.

Avoid most desserts.

Understand the new labeling categories. *Low fat* means 3 grams or less per serving. *Lean* means less than 10 grams of fat per serving; *extralean* means less than 5 grams of fat per serving. By comparison, most meat choices contain 15 to 20% fat content.

The problems sometimes encountered with use of a low-fat diet are related to the fact that it is also a high-carbohydrate, high-osmolarity diet, if it is to remain isocaloric. Thus, carbohydrate-induced diarrhea, bloating, or excess flatus may occur. When the benefit of reducing symptoms from steatorrhea greatly exceeds any carbohydrate-induced symptoms, there is no need to modify the diet. However, one should restrict fat only up to therapeutic tolerance. Because fat restriction is not complete, supplementation with fat-soluble vitamins is not always indicated. However, if deficiency of vitamin A, D, E, or K was present before initiation of a low-fat diet, then supplements should be given.

Low-Oxalate Diet

When steatorrhea is clinically significant, it is usually accompanied by increased oxalate absorption from the intestine and by hyperoxaluria (>40 mg per day), a significant risk factor for kidney stones. This complication is due to the removal of calcium in the form of calcium–fatty acid complexes, thus preventing the formation of the relatively insoluble calcium oxalate in the lumen. The much more soluble sodium oxalate is then formed, and it is absorbed not only in the small intestine but in the colon, which is made more permeable by the action of unabsorbed bile salts. A low-oxalate diet is helpful in reducing the hyperoxaluria due to steatorrhea but creates dietary restrictions that are added to those of the low-fat diet. Certain carbohydrate-containing snack foods that are often helpful in the low-fat diet are not allowed on a low-oxalate diet. These include chocolate-containing foods, cola beverages, nuts (especially peanuts and pecans), and tea. Other high-oxalate foods (>10 mg per serving) are spinach, rhubarb, beer, green beans, beets, Swiss chard, collards, kale, eggplant, sweet potatoes, blueberries, strawberries, raspberries, and tomato soup.

High-Fat Diet

Patients with short-bowel syndrome and total colectomy have been reported to benefit by this diet, which is a variant of the low available carbohydrate diet (see later). Such patients are limited in the amount of intestinal secretion produced in response to unabsorbed lipid; rather, their diarrhea is largely due to unabsorbed carbohydrate and osmotically active metabolites. Moreover, the symptoms of steatorrhea are produced by the action of colonic flora on the malabsorbed fat. In selected patients without a colon, the high-fat diet may be useful.

Medium Chain Triglyceride Supplements

Medium chain triglyceride (MCT) supplementation is indicated if fat restriction must be so severe and carbohydrate-induced symptoms prevent addition of extra carbohydrate such that caloric intake is impaired. MCTs contain fatty acids of 6 to 12 carbon residues and are found in coconut and kernel oils. MCT is available commercially as MCT oil and contains 8.3 kcal per gram. One tablespoon weighs 14 grams and contains 116 kcal. MCTs are especially useful in conditions in which luminal bile salts and/or pancreatic enzymes are limited, because MCTs can be hydrolyzed in the presence of limited lipase and in the absence of bile salts. The use of more than 3 to 4 tablespoons per day of MCT oil can produce osmotic diarrhea, particularly in patients with short-bowel syndrome, so high doses should be used only if they are tolerated.

Low Available Carbohydrate Diet

This diet restricts low-molecular-weight compounds (e.g., glucose, fructose, lactose, sucrose) that are more osmotically active than larger carbohydrates (e.g., maltodextrins, starches). Thus, the diet is useful for patients with short-bowel syndrome and with dumping syndrome. The general outlines of this diet are as follows:

Avoid alcohol, carbonated beverages, sweetened drinks and prepared foods, milk and milk products, juices, jams, and jellies.

Divide intake into smaller portions during the days.

Take liquids separately to allow the potential osmotic load in solids to be emptied more slowly from the stomach.

Limit intake of fruits, but do not exclude them.

Low-Lactose Diet

From the large number of patients who are lactase deficient, about half will be symptomatic when lactose is ingested. Because the degree of sensitivity varies greatly, the degree to which lactose intake must be limited also varies. In general, about half the patients become symptomatic on ingestion of 12 grams of lactose (included in 8 ounces of milk). However, when milk is included in a meal with other foods, gastric emptying is delayed more than with milk alone, and symptoms may not occur. Thus, the patient is counseled to eliminate all milk and milk products and then to add back foods to the amount that can be tolerated. Liquid milk and ice cream produce the most symptoms. Yogurt (containing active culture of lactase-producing yeast) and small amounts of hard pressed cheeses are the best tolerated. Patients who are sensitive to small amounts of lactose should be cautioned to avoid prepared foods that contain milk products, milk solids, whey, casein, curd, lactose, galactose, or milk sugar. Because milk is the best source of bioavailable calcium, patients on a low-lactose diet who are at risk for osteopenia should have calcium supplements added to their diet (see later).

Low-Fiber Diet

This diet is used when decreased fecal bulk is desired or when high-fiber intake as part of a low-fat diet leads to increased colonic fermentation with bloating and increased flatus. Short-bowel syndrome is the malabsorption syndrome most likely to benefit from such a dietary modification, but as with the low-oxalate diet, one must remember that its restrictions are grafted onto the basic low-fat diet. Sometimes a modified low-fiber diet is useful for patients with Crohn's disease who have small intestinal strictures that lead to food-induced episodes of partial obstruction. To avoid making the diet too restrictive, fiber restriction is usually partial when it is used chronically for these malabsorptive syndromes.

Dietary Considerations in AIDS

Weight loss and malnutrition are important complications of AIDS. There are many infectious causes of chronic diarrhea in AIDS, and the treatable ones should be addressed initially, especially *Giardia lamblia* infection. Oral or esophageal pain due to herpesvirus, cytomegalovirus, or *Candida* and AIDS enteropathy should be appropriately treated. Weakness, anorexia, and nausea are the major symptoms left that determine the selection of nutritional support for patients with weight loss. If oral feeding is possible, attention must be given to preparing attractive meals with variety but low fat, if steatorrhea is present. Avoidance of alcohol and heavily spiced foods is helpful for someone with anorexia. Providing limited liquids with the meals aids in reducing satiety. Vitamin supplements should be provided (see later), especially for vitamin B_{12} and folate, because levels of these vitamins can be low in up to one third of patients. Some patients may need supplementation with commercial products. It may be important to balance the carbohydrate and fat content of these supplements with the rest of the diet to avoid worsening of the diarrhea. Some patients with AIDS will not be able to ingest adequate nutrients by oral feedings and will require enteral tube feedings or total parenteral nutrition.

Enteral Nutrition Support

Many of the disorders that lead to malabsorption cause anorexia, and for some patients, the intake of table food in quantities large enough to maintain weight is not easy. Commercially available complete enteral nutrition products are useful in these patients as a supplement, providing perhaps up to 25% of their total caloric intake. The same considerations should be given to the type of macronutrient emphasized as in the use of diets (e.g., low fat, low carbohydrate). Most patients are able to use products with intact protein. Most products are isosmolar, because they contain lipid. Thus, some of these supplements may not be compatible with a low-fat diet or may have to be used in small amounts. The supplements provided with fiber, or those that are milk based, are frequently not so helpful in managing the patient with steatorrhea and diarrhea. The need for high protein content is also infrequent in the chronic management of malabsorption. Most of the standard products (those without special features) contain about 1 kcal per mL and have an osmolarity from 290 to 470 mOsm per kg. Forced enteral feeding or total parenteral nutrition is sometimes necessary when patients are acutely ill to preserve lean body mass.

General Support Measures

Because malabsorption is often associated with some degree of diarrhea, antidiarrheal therapy can be useful. Frequent small meals may be better than large ones. Commercially available agents such as diphenoxylate-atropine (Lomotil) 1 or 2 tablets before meals or loperamide (Imodium) 4 mg before meals can be tried. Some patients are more responsive to deodorized tincture of opium (5 to 15 drops before meals) to decrease stool frequency and/or tincture of belladonna (5 to 15 drops before meals) to reduce meal-induced cramping. If dehydration occurs chronically and signs of volume depletion occur, sodium and fluid can be replaced orally by use of an oral rehydration solution. The one recommended by the World Health Organization is useful because it can be made at home and is inexpensive. To 1 liter of

water add ¾ teaspoon of table salt, ½ teaspoon of baking soda or 1 teaspoon of baking powder, 1.5 grams of KCl (½ tablespoon of 20% solution) or 1 cup of orange juice, and 4 tablespoons of cane or table sugar (sucrose) or 2 tablespoons of honey. This can be flavored as needed, and 2 to 3 liters per day can be ingested to maintain extracellular fluid volume. Use of multivitamin preparations (with or without minerals) containing water- and fat-soluble vitamins is often helpful to ensure that vitamin and mineral stores are maintained. In general, the prenatal preparations contain the highest levels of these nutrients. In many patients, however, these levels are insufficient as maintenance therapy for specific nutrient supplementation. The most important of these supplements are described in the following section.

IF MALABSORPTION OR A LOW BODY STORE OF A MICRONUTRIENT IS A MAJOR PROBLEM, HOW CAN THESE NUTRIENTS BE PROVIDED EFFICIENTLY?

Many micronutrients (vitamins and minerals, e.g., calcium, iron, folate, vitamin B_{12}) are concentrated more in certain groups of foods. Thus, intake can become limited when the diet is not balanced with samples from all food groups (Table 5). Moreover, many micronutrients either undergo enterohepatic circulation or are secreted into the lumen, and losses from the endogenous body stores are added to the loss produced by malabsorption of dietary nutrients. Therefore, malabsorption syndromes frequently produce deficiency of micronutrients. Those nutrients whose absorption is inefficient (e.g., iron, calcium, magnesium), whose body stores are low (e.g., folate, vitamin B_{12}), whose rate of turnover is rapid (e.g., sodium, potassium, folate), or for which the enterohepatic circulation represents a major source of potential loss from the body (e.g., folate, vitamins A and D) are most likely to become deficient during the course of a malabsorption syndrome. The symptoms and signs of deficiency of these nutrients are included in Table 6. When the cause of malabsorption is reversible, treatment may be necessary only initially to replete the body stores. When the cause of malabsorption cannot be treated, long-term replacement therapy is necessary. Only the micronutrients most

TABLE 5. **Pathophysiologic Mechanism of Vitamin and Mineral Deficiency in Malabsorption**

Physiologic Factor	Vitamins and Minerals Affected
Decreased intake	All vitamins except K, B_6, biotin Calcium and iron
Enterohepatic circulation	Retinoic acid (vitamin A), folate, vitamin B_{12}, 1,25-dihydroxyvitamin D
Enteric secretion	Calcium, potassium, sodium
Increased loss from body	All vitamins and minerals

TABLE 6. **Micronutrient Deficiencies Commonly Associated with Malabsorption**

Nutrient	Clinical Setting	Clinical Signs	Test	Treatment
Folate	Anorexia, diffuse small bowel disease	Anemia, glossitis, sore tongue	Red cell folate	Folate PO daily
Vitamin B_{12}	Ileal disease or resection	Anemia, long tract signs	Serum vitamin B_{12}, methylmalonic acid, homocysteine	Vitamin B_{12} SC monthly
Vitamin A	Steatorrhea, liver disease	Night blindness, hyperkeratosis	Serum vitamin A	Vitamin A PO daily
Vitamin D	Steatorrhea, decreased sun exposure	Bone tenderness	25-Hydroxyvitamin D	Vitamin D, 25-hydroxyvitamin D, 1,25-dihydroxyvitamin D PO
Sodium	Watery diarrhea, dehydration	Thirst, lethargy	Urinary sodium	NaCl IV or PO
Potassium	Watery diarrhea	Weakness, electrocardiographic changes, paresthesias	Serum potassium	Potassium bicarbonate, citrate, gluconate PO
Calcium	Steatorrhea, lactose intolerance	Tetany, arrhythmias, electrocardiographic changes	Urinary calcium, bone density	Calcium carbonate, citrate, glubionate PO daily
Iron	Duodenal disease or bypass, gastrointestinal bleeding	Anemia, pallor	Serum ferritin, mean corpuscular volume, transferrin saturation	Ferrous sulfate PO daily

commonly deficient in patients with malabsorption are discussed, but any vitamin or mineral deficiency can be present if the malabsorption is severe or prolonged.

Folate

Folate is ingested largely as the polyglutamate and must be hydrolyzed to the monoglutamate for absorption. Moreover, its bioavailability in foods varies because of binders and inhibitors. Enterohepatic circulation of 5-methyltetrahydrofolic acid is significant, and tissue stores are small relative to daily intake. A number of drugs can interfere with folate absorption, especially alcohol, sulfasalazine, and anticonvulsants. All these factors make the patient with malabsorption at risk for deficiency. Specific diagnosis is best with red blood cell folate, which correlates with tissue stores. Treatment is with the unreduced pteroylglutamic acid (usually at doses of 1 mg per day), which is not so efficiently metabolized as the natural reduced compound. Thus, doses needed for maintenance are higher than the recommended daily allowance and exceed that available in most multivitamin preparations.

Vitamin B_{12} (Cyanocobalamin)

The ileum is required for active transport, but the body pool size, although small, is large compared with the maximal daily loss in the stool. Thus, deficiency takes months to years to develop, usually in short-bowel syndrome when the ileum is lost. Diagnosis is made by screening with serum vitamin B_{12} levels. If deficiency is suspected clinically, but the serum level is above 180 pg per mL, serum levels of methylmalonic acid and of homocysteine can be measured, because these compounds require vitamin B_{12}–dependent enzymes to be converted to their products in the face of vitamin B_{12} deficiency. Symptoms

and signs may not include the classic long tract signs and/or anemia; only fatigue or macrocytosis may be present. Patients with human immunodeficiency virus infection or with ileal resection are especially subject to deficiency. Treatment should be with parenteral (subcutaneous) vitamin, 1000 µg per month.

Vitamin A

Dietary vitamin A is lost when steatorrhea is present. Moreover, one of its major metabolites, retinoic acid, undergoes extensive enterohepatic circulation. Detection of deficiency should rely only on vitamin A, not on carotene levels, because carotene is not stored in the body, being converted to vitamin A after ingestion. Treatment should be with retinol at doses of at least 5000 IU per day. When steatorrhea is present, this supplement is malabsorbed, even though it is supplied as the water-miscible form, so that higher doses may be necessary. In the face of malabsorption, there should be little fear of producing hypervitaminosis A, provided that megadoses (50,000 IU per day) are not used and that the serum vitamin A level is monitored to document adequate replacement.

Vitamin D

Like vitamin A, vitamin D is lost in the stool when steatorrhea is present because of both intraluminal sequestration with unabsorbed fat and the enterohepatic circulation of 1,25-dihydroxyvitamin D. Mild to moderate malabsorption could be counteracted by production of 25-hydroxyvitamin D from the skin, which normally accounts for more than 90% of the circulating vitamin. However, when patients are feeling ill, they may stay indoors much of the time and thus lose this potential benefit. Patients at risk for osteopenia should be especially considered for deficiency, including postmenopausal women, smokers, and alcohol abusers. Serum levels of 25-hydroxyvitamin D can be used to screen for deficiency, but levels can be falsely low when protein deficiency or severe liver disease is present. Assessment of vitamin D function can be obtained by serum alkaline phosphatase activity (elevation) or by bone densitometry, although these become abnormal late in the course of deficiency. Moreover, they can be abnormal with calcium deficiency and normal vitamin D stores. Treatment in patients with steatorrhea should use one of the forms of vitamin D that is not completely water insoluble, either 25-hydroxyvitamin D or 1,25-dihydroxyvitamin D, provided daily. Alternatively, the much larger formulation (50,000 IU) can be used once or twice weekly, because fat malabsorption is rarely complete and some absorption will occur with such a large dose. Intoxication is unusual in patients with malabsorption, but the effect of the treatment can be monitored with either serum 25-hydroxyvitamin D levels or 24-hour urinary calcium concentration.

Sodium

Sodium deficiency is not often considered in chronic steatorrhea-diarrhea, but it may account for some of the fatigue noted by patients. Because sodium in intestinal fluid is isotonic, large-volume diarrhea can lead to chronic intravascular dehydration, further contributing to potassium loss in the kidneys. Thus, some patients need NaCl tablets (1 gram) once or twice a day to avoid intermittent depletion. Alternatively, more salt can be added to the food.

Potassium

Potassium is lost when excess sodium-rich fluid is presented to the aldosterone-responsive portions of the intestine, i.e., ileum and colon. Moreover, intravascular depletion and acidosis (due to bicarbonate loss) increase renal potassium loss. Thus, deficiency should be considered in patients with moderate to large-volume diarrhea. In some patients, food sources can provide the added potassium, e.g., milk, fruits or fruit juices (not only bananas), vegetables, fish, and nuts. Many preparations of supplemental potassium are available, but most are designed to replete potassium deficiency due to diuretic therapy and thus are provided as KCl. With intestinal loss, $KHCO_3$ is the principal form, so it makes sense to replace when possible with one of the forms in which HCO_3^-, citrate, or gluconate is the anion.

Calcium

Absorption of calcium is only about 30% efficient, and the most bioavailable dietary source is milk products, which are often restricted in the diet of patients with malabsorption. Moreover, there are obligatory calcium losses into the intestinal lumen from internal secretions, so that negative calcium balance is possible when intake is restricted, even in patients with normal absorption. When steatorrhea is present, not only is vitamin D malabsorbed, but calcium is sequestered in the lumen by its association with unabsorbed fatty acids. Thus, low 24-hour urinary calcium excretion (which at steady state correlates with absorption) is common in malabsorptive states. The urinary calcium concentration should be used to assess current intake, and bone densitometry should determine whether body stores are low. In patients at risk for calcium (and vitamin D) malabsorption and especially if other risk factors for osteopenia are present, these tests should be used for screening purposes. The time to detect calcium malabsorption is before body stores are low and certainly before symptoms (e.g., tetany, fracture) occur. Long-term supplementation with calcium is essential to preserve bone mass in these patients. Calcium carbonate is poorly soluble, but it is generally used because it is inexpensive and large doses can be delivered in a small number of pills. However, some patients will absorb better when they are ingesting a more soluble form of calcium (e.g., citrate, glubionate). Patients should be followed up with 24-hour urinary calcium determinations until the amount excreted reaches normal levels. This will not be possible to achieve in some cases, and supplemental vitamin D will be necessary, even in the absence of vitamin D deficiency.

Iron

The dietary sources of bioavailable iron are restricted (nuts, seeds, red meat, egg yolks), the mineral has limited solubility from other sources, and absorption is restricted largely to the upper small intestine. Moreover, many intestinal disorders that lead to malabsorption also produce blood loss (e.g., Crohn's disease). Thus, iron deficiency is common. It must be distinguished from the anemia of chronic inflammation that also accompanies many of the same disorders that produce malabsorption. Unfortunately, the tests available to detect deficiency are neither sensitive nor specific. Serum ferritin levels are proportional to marrow iron levels but can be elevated in acute or chronic inflammatory diseases. Low transferrin saturation correlates with iron deficiency when the total binding capacity is elevated. Serum iron levels can be variable and are not by themselves a good determinant of deficiency. Treatment with iron that raises the hemoglobin level is often the best proof of deficiency. Oral iron is available in a bewildering array of forms. The sulfate or fumarate preparations are usually used, because they contain the highest percentage of elemental iron. Gastrointestinal side effects may be somewhat less common with slow-release forms of oral preparations, but these forms may delay release of iron until it is beyond the most efficient sites of absorption in the duodenum. The addition of vitamin C may enhance absorption by maintaining the reduced form of the mineral. In unusual cases, parenteral (intravenous) iron may be necessary to overcome the malabsorptive defect.

ACUTE PANCREATITIS

method of
JON M. BURCH, M.D.
*Denver Health Medical Center and University of
Colorado Health Sciences Center
Denver, Colorado*

Eighty to 90% of all cases of acute pancreatitis are caused either by gallstones or by alcohol abuse. Other known factors include hyperparathyroidism, hyperlipemia, postoperative states, trauma, hereditary conditions, drugs, and infectious diseases. In about 10% of cases, the cause is not clear, and these are referred to as idiopathic. The frequency with which a particular etiologic factor is noted depends on the population of patients in question.

In the United States, gallstones are the most common cause of acute pancreatitis. Although the relationship between gallstones and the development of pancreatitis is clear, the mechanism is not well understood. At the turn of the century, Opie hypothesized that a stone could occlude the ductal ampulla distal to the junction of the common bile duct and pancreatic duct, thereby permitting bile to flow into the pancreatic duct and activate pancreatic enzymes. Subsequent experiments have shown that this is unlikely to occur. It has been demonstrated that patients with gallstone pancreatitis have a high rate of gallstones that can be recovered in the feces. These stones appear to either transiently obstruct the pancreatic duct or create a temporary path that permits duodenal contents to enter the pancreatic duct and induce the development of pancreatitis.

The mechanism by which alcohol causes acute pancreatitis is also unknown. Current theories have incriminated an alteration of the normal constituents of pancreatic secretions resulting in concretions in the pancreatic ducts. It is also possible that alcohol exerts a direct toxic effect on the pancreatic parenchyma as it does in the liver.

DIAGNOSIS

Patients usually give a history of progressive epigastric or right upper quadrant pain that radiates in a bandlike distribution or straight through to the back. The pain is sharp and stabbing or boring in nature, and nothing the patient can do will ameliorate the discomfort. Nausea and vomiting almost always accompany the pain.

On physical examination, the patient appears acutely ill and dehydrated. Fever is not uncommon but is usually of low grade; tachycardia and tachypnea may be present. Blood pressure is normal except in a few patients with severe disease who may be in shock. Bowel sounds can be absent because of ileus, and the abdomen may be distended. Palpation reveals epigastric tenderness with voluntary or involuntary guarding. True abdominal rigidity is rare. A mass may be palpable in the upper abdomen, suggesting a pseudocyst, an abscess, or a diffuse enlargement of the pancreas.

The laboratory hallmark of acute pancreatitis is elevation of the serum amylase level, in most cases to three or more times the upper limit of normal. Patients with gallstone pancreatitis tend to have higher peak amylase levels than those with alcohol pancreatitis. Regardless of etiology, the serum amylase value falls to nearly normal levels within 2 to 3 days in most patients. A persistently elevated amylase level suggests the development of pseudocyst.

Unfortunately, serum amylase alone is neither sensitive nor specific for acute pancreatitis. Indeed, some of the most critically ill patients with pancreatitis have a normal serum amylase level when they are first seen by a physician. Furthermore, many other abdominal and extra-abdominal diseases may be associated with hyperamylasemia. Alternative available enzyme analyses include measurement of urinary amylase and serum lipase. Urinary amylase concentration parallels serum amylase and does not enhance the accuracy of diagnosis. Serum lipase does improve specificity, although it may not be elevated in all cases.

Because of the difficulties with serum amylase interpretation, two modifications have been proposed. The ratio of amylase clearance to creatinine clearance yields a percentage that, if greater than 5, is said to be compatible with acute pancreatitis. Although the test is more precise than serum amylase alone, it is not uniquely specific for pancreatitis. Furthermore, the sensitivity of the test is diminished in patients with near-normal serum amylase levels. Preliminary evidence suggests that isoenzyme determinations of pancreatic amylase may improve specificity. Pancreatic isoamylase levels are not currently available for routine use in many hospitals.

An upright chest film and plain abdominal radiographs should be obtained in all patients suspected of having acute pancreatitis. Although such films may not aid in diagnosis of pancreatitis, they do help to avoid missing other diseases that can mimic pancreatitis, such as a perforated ulcer.

Ultrasonography is a valuable screening test because it is both sensitive and specific for identifying concomitant gallstones, and it is inexpensive. It can also detect the presence of associated fluid collections. The major disadvantage of ultrasonography is its inability to consistently image the pancreas, especially in obese individuals or when surrounding gas shadows prevent penetration of the beam.

Computed tomography (CT) can be used to identify gallstones, masses within the pancreas, fluid collection, and diffuse enlargement of the gland. The advantages of CT over ultrasonography are that the overlying gas shadows do not obscure the pancreas, and anatomic relationships can be precisely defined. The major disadvantage of CT is its cost. For this reason, CT is not recommended for early diagnostic use in uncomplicated cases. The primary role of CT is to clarify the diagnosis in questionable cases and to survey for septic intra-abdominal complications in patients with severe disease.

In making the diagnosis of acute pancreatitis, the clinician must always be on guard for the possibility that the diagnosis is in error. Several abdominal surgical emergencies can resemble acute pancreatitis, including perforated ulcer without free intraperitoneal air, bowel obstruction (especially closed loop obstructions), acute cholecystitis, and small bowel infarction. At times, patients with persistent severe symptoms may require diagnostic laparotomy with the knowledge that the cause could be acute pancreatitis. However, CT has reduced the need for exploratory laparotomy to a low level.

TERMINOLOGY

The most important development in the management of acute pancreatitis during the past decade has been the creation and acceptance of a consistent terminology (Table 1). Note that the term hemorrhagic pancreatitis is no longer used. Formerly, hemorrhagic pancreatitis and necrotizing pancreatitis were used interchangeably. Another important step has been the abandonment of the Marseille classification. The original system described the course of some patients with alcoholic pancreatitis but in no way

TABLE 1. **Terminology in Acute Pancreatitis**

Term	Definition
Acute interstitial pancreatitis	Sterile inflammation and edema of the pancreas
Necrotizing pancreatitis	Same as above but with necrosis of peripancreatic fat (mostly transverse mesocolon) and/or pancreas
Infected pancreatic necrosis	Necrotizing pancreatitis that has become infected
Pancreatic abscess	A collection of peripancreatic pus surrounded by an inflammatory wall; includes "infected pseudocysts"
Pseudocyst	A collection of sterile peripancreatic fluid, high in amylase, which is surrounded by an inflammatory wall
Fat sequestra	A collection of sterile necrotic fat surrounded by an inflammatory wall

described the course of patients with gallstone pancreatitis. Even the simplified revised version is largely ignored.

TREATMENT

Mild to Moderate Disease

All patients with a tentative diagnosis of acute pancreatitis should be hospitalized for observation and supportive care. Patients with mild to moderate disease can be cared for on a general ward provided that close observation is maintained. Because of the capricious nature of the disease, some patients who appear well when they are first seen may deteriorate rapidly; therefore, vigilant observation should be maintained for 24 to 48 hours.

Most patients demonstrate some degree of dehydration, and all should receive intravenous fluids. This can be accomplished with 2 liters of D5 half-normal saline with 30 mEq potassium chloride per liter each day. In addition, nasogastric losses should be replaced on a volume-per-volume basis with normal saline to prevent alkalosis. Patients who are seriously dehydrated require resuscitation with isotonic fluids such as lactated Ringer's. In this situation, serum electrolyte levels should be obtained and the hourly urine output monitored with a Foley catheter. When the urine output reaches 0.5 mL per kg per hour, routine fluid orders can be resumed.

The patient should take nothing by mouth, and a nasogastric tube should be inserted. Prospective studies in patients with mild to moderate pancreatitis have shown that the use of a nasogastric tube does not significantly alter the course of the disease. However, I continue to recommend this therapy because it effectively relieves nausea and vomiting.

Acute pancreatitis causes severe pain, and the use of parenteral narcotics is an important adjunct to general supportive care. The selection of a specific narcotic agent is not important. Patient-controlled analgesia pumps have become increasingly popular. Reasonable starting doses for an alert and competent adult receiving intravenous morphine sulfate are a basal rate of 1 mg per hour and a patient-controlled

additional dose of 1 mg every 15 minutes. Dosage should be adjusted according to the patient's age, weight, general condition, and response to the medication.

The prophylactic use of antibiotics is controversial. Prospective studies have suggested that antibiotics do not help prevent the septic complications of acute pancreatitis in patients with mild or moderately severe disease.

Many other medications have been employed in an attempt to alter the course of acute pancreatitis, but virtually all have been ineffective to date. Parasympatholytic drugs such as atropine have had little effect in improving the course of the disease and because of their unpleasant side effects are not recommended. H$_2$ blockers have been used to reduce the secretin-mediated stimulation of the pancreas by decreasing gastric acid secretion. Unfortunately, these drugs have not been effective. Either H$_2$ blockers or antacids should be used in critically ill patients with necrotizing pancreatitis to reduce the possibility of acute gastric mucosal hemorrhage. The enzyme inhibitor aprotinin (Trasylol)*† has been shown to improve the course of acute pancreatitis in laboratory animals if the drug is administered before the induction of pancreatitis. In humans, aprotinin has not been shown to be beneficial and is not recommended. Somatostatin† and gabexate mesylate (the latter being a protease inhibitor similar to aprotinin but much lower in molecular weight) can now be added to the long list of medications that have been shown in clinical trials to be ineffective in altering the course of acute pancreatitis.

When patients begin to recover from the acute attack as evidenced by the return of bowel function and disappearance of epigastric pain and tenderness, oral feedings should be resumed. The diet should be low in fat and other gastropancreatic secretagogues. Some patients will have a prolonged ileus, and parenteral hyperalimentation should be employed if they are unable to eat by the fifth to seventh day after admission.

Severe Disease

Virtually all patients who become critically ill with pancreatitis have necrotizing pancreatitis, infected necrosis, or pancreatic abscess. All patients with potentially severe pancreatitis should be admitted to an intensive care unit for careful monitoring and prompt intervention if necessary. Life-threatening complications include shock, respiratory failure, renal failure, infection, and hemorrhage. Invasive monitoring with an arterial line, a Foley catheter, and a central venous catheter is essential in these patients.

Patients with severe pancreatitis may experience hypotension or shock soon after admission. The shock is primarily hypovolemic and is due to the sequestration of fluid in the abdominal cavity. Because several

---

*Not available in the United States.

†Not FDA approved for this indication.

liters of crystalloid solution may be required for volume resuscitation, isotonic solutions such as lactated Ringer's or Plasma-Lyte should be used to avoid acute hyponatremia. The end point for resuscitation is a clear sensorium and normal urine output. For patients who fail to respond to the usual regimen of fluid resuscitation, a Swan-Ganz catheter should be inserted and intravenous fluids administered until the pulmonary artery wedge pressure reaches approximately 15 to 18 mm Hg. If oliguria or anuria persists, acute renal failure has almost certainly occurred and appropriate consultations should be sought. Some authorities advocate the addition of albumin to resuscitation solutions for patients with severe disease. I subscribe to this view although I acknowledge the lack of supporting data.

When fluid resuscitation is completed, some patients may remain hypotensive. Mild hypotension, systolic blood pressure of 90 to 100 mm Hg, does not necessarily require further blood pressure support if urine output is good and the patient's sensorium is clear. For patients with severe hypotension (systolic blood pressure less than 80 mm Hg) and oliguria, inotropes to enhance cardiac output and/or vasomotor tone are indicated. The preferred drug in this circumstance is dopamine, which should be started at 3 to 5 μg per kg per minute. Further adjustments should be made according to hemodynamic parameters and urine output.

Respiratory failure is common in patients with severe pancreatitis and is indistinguishable from adult respiratory distress syndrome of other causes. For this reason, at least one determination of arterial blood gases should be made for all patients admitted with acute pancreatitis. Those with persistent tachypnea require frequent blood gas measurements. A falling Po_2 is an ominous sign, and endotracheal intubation and mechanical ventilation may be required. Positive end-expiratory pressure is helpful in maintaining an adequate Po_2 in hypoxemic patients who require high fractional inspired oxygen concentrations (FIO_2 more than 50%).

Renal failure may occur and is usually related to hypovolemia and shock. Although azotemia is often prerenal in nature, acute tubular necrosis or cortical necrosis can occur if the early prerenal phase is not treated aggressively. This requires careful monitoring of urine output, suitable administration of crystalloid solutions, and avoidance of nephrotoxic medications.

Potentially severe metabolic complications include hypocalcemia and hyperglycemia. A falling serum calcium level is a sign of poor prognosis, and treatment may be required to prevent tetany. Calcium gluconate should be administered by careful intravenous infusion with electrocardiographic monitoring if the patient becomes symptomatic or if the serum calcium reaches levels inappropriately below 8 mg per dL. Hyperglycemia is also a serious sign in patients who are not already diabetic and suggests extensive damage to the pancreas. A sliding scale of regular insulin based on the patient's serum glucose level can be used to treat this problem. In a few patients, continuous insulin infusion (insulin drip) may be necessary.

Evidence is slowly accumulating that the broad-spectrum antibiotic imipenem-cilastatin (Primaxin) may reduce the rate of septic complications for patients with necrotizing pancreatitis and perhaps improve survival. This drug has the ability to penetrate both pancreatic and necrotic peripancreatic tissue while retaining activity against organisms usually found in infected necrosis. Doses in the literature are in the range of 0.5 gram intravenously every 8 hours. The drug is begun when the diagnosis is made. The appropriate duration of treatment is unknown; it varies in the literature from 3 to 14 days.

COMPLICATIONS REQUIRING SURGICAL TREATMENT

The most serious of all complications is the development of intra-abdominal infection. This may take the form of a pancreatic abscess or infection of necrotic peripancreatic tissue (infected necrosis). Patients with continued elevation of the white blood cell count or persistent unexplained fever should be suspected of having intra-abdominal infection. CT is the most reliable test for diagnosing this condition. It may reveal abnormal lucencies, suggesting gas accumulation within necrotic tissue or well-delineated fluid collections. If the patient appears septic, CT-directed percutaneous aspiration of suspicious fluid collections is an effective method for the surveillance of intra-abdominal infection. This procedure can be repeated as often as necessary. If pus is aspirated or if enteric bacteria are grown on culture, laparotomy is indicated.

Proper therapy for intra-abdominal infection includes laparotomy with débridement of necrotic tissue, adequate drainage, and culture-specific antibiotics. Attempts to treat infected necrosis or pancreatic abscesses with percutaneous drainage have been largely unsuccessful because of necrotic debris and multiple loculations that are often present.

The necrotizing nature of severe pancreatic inflammation renders patients susceptible to the development of enteric fistulas. These may involve the colon, stomach, or small intestine. Treatment consists of establishing adequate drainage and general supportive care until the fistula heals. Persistent fistulas may require operative intervention as the patient's condition permits.

Life-threatening hemorrhage is uncommon. If it occurs, it is usually related to bleeding into a pseudocyst or erosion of a necrotizing process into an adjacent blood vessel. A falling hematocrit, unexplained shock, or sudden bleeding from surgical drains may be the first signs of severe hemorrhage. Profuse bleeding is best controlled by immediate laparotomy and oversewing of the offending vessel. The use of arteriography with embolization of the bleeding site should be reserved for patients who cannot tolerate laparotomy.

Pancreatic pseudocyst is another complication of acute pancreatitis. The diagnosis should be considered in all patients with pancreatitis whose serum amylase levels remain elevated for more than a few days. Ultrasonography is the most cost-effective technique for the diagnosis and surveillance of a pseudocyst. If this study is obtained early in the course of acute pancreatitis, peripancreatic fluid collections are often visualized. These collections tend to come and go and are seen at different times in different areas juxtaposed to the pancreas. This phenomenon has led to a misunderstanding that pseudocysts frequently resolve without surgical treatment. True pseudocysts do not disappear and are consistently found in the same location. In general, a pseudocyst requires 4 to 6 weeks from the onset of symptoms of acute pancreatitis to develop. These rare and potentially lethal cysts require treatment once the diagnosis is made. The timing of invasive intervention is based on the natural history of the disease or evidence of maturation (a thickened capsule) on ultrasound or CT examination. Ideal management consists of internal drainage, usually into the stomach. Complications of pseudocyst include hemorrhage, infection, or rupture, all of which can be prevented by timely invasive intervention.

Endoscopists are now performing transgastric endoscopic drainage, and interventional radiologists are treating pseudocysts by percutaneous drainage. The role of these new procedures remains to be determined, but they are reasonable options in patients who are poor operative candidates.

ADDITIONAL INDICATIONS FOR SURGERY

It is clear that cholecystectomy in patients with gallstone pancreatitis will prevent further attacks. It has been demonstrated that the gallbladder can be safely removed during the initial hospitalization. This can be accomplished within a few days of admission when the patient shows signs of clinical improvement.

Emergency endoscopic sphincterotomy has been advocated as an alternative to cholecystectomy for definitive treatment of gallstone pancreatitis. At present, there is no evidence that this procedure alters the course of the disease. Because cholecystectomy will still be necessary, needless risk and expense are incurred by patients so treated. This technique may have a place in those patients who also have obstructive jaundice or cholangitis.

A few patients with necrotizing pancreatitis who are not infected experience progressive systemic failure in spite of intensive support and should be considered candidates for surgical exploration. Laparotomy under these conditions is hazardous, and expert judgment is essential. At the time of surgery, extensive necrosis of the pancreas and peripancreatic tissue may be found. Appropriate treatment includes resection of all necrotic tissue. Understandably, the

TABLE 2. **Ranson's Criteria for Prognosis in Acute Pancreatitis**

At Admission

Age > 55 y
White blood cell count > 16,000/mm³
Blood glucose level > 200 mg/dL
Serum lactate dehydrogenase level > 350 U/L
Serum aspartate aminotransferase level > 250 U/dL

Within 48 Hours

Hematocrit value decrease > 10%
Blood urea nitrogen level rise > 5 mg/dL
Serum calcium level > 8 mg/dL
Arterial Po_2 < 60 mm Hg
Base deficit > 4 mEq/L
Estimated fluid sequestration > 6 L

mortality rate for these patients is high, but some may be saved.

PROGNOSIS

Overall, acute pancreatitis in my institution is associated with a mortality rate of less than 4%. Many factors influence prognosis, including etiology, history of previous attacks, age, and pre-existing comorbidity. It is generally recognized that most patients who die of acute pancreatitis do so with the first attack. The natural history of alcoholic pancreatitis is one of frequent recurrences. The mortality rate for each subsequent attack is less than for the previous one. Consideration should be given to performing endoscopic retrograde cholangiopancreatography for any patient who requires repeated admissions to the hospital for pancreatitis. In some of these individuals, surgically correctable lesions, such as pancreatic ductal strictures, may be identified.

The prognosis for gallstone pancreatitis during the first attack is similar to that for the first attack of alcoholic pancreatitis. Recurrent attacks of pancreatitis or biliary tract disease can occur in as many as 50% of patients if the gallbladder is not removed. Once the gallbladder has been removed and the common duct is noted to be free of stones, recurrent pancreatitis is rare.

As noted earlier, the course of acute pancreatitis is difficult to predict when patients are first seen. To address this problem, early clinical and laboratory prognostic indicators of the severity of disease have been developed. The most popular of these is Ranson's criteria (Table 2). This system contains 11 elements, some of which are determined at the time of admission and others 48 hours later. Patients with fewer than three positive criteria almost always have mild disease. Those with three or more criteria may have severe disease with a significantly higher mortality rate; patients in this category deserve early admission to an intensive care unit and careful monitoring.

CHRONIC PANCREATITIS

method of
RICARDO L. ROSSI, M.D.
Pontificia Catholic University of Chile
Santiago, Chile

RODRIGO L. VALDERRAMA, M.D.
University of Chile
Santiago, Chile

and

GUILLERMO S. WATKINS, M.D.
Pontificia Catholic University of Chile
Santiago, Chile

Chronic pancreatitis (CP) implies irreversible and usually progressive changes in the pancreas, whereas the acute forms imply reversible changes. The Marseille-Rome classification of 1988 defined acute pancreatitis as a spectrum of inflammatory lesions in the pancreas and in the peripancreatic tissues (edema, necrosis, hemorrhagic necrosis, fat necrosis). CP was defined as the presence of chronic inflammatory lesions characterized by the destruction of exocrine parenchyma and fibrosis and, at least in the later stages, the destruction of endocrine parenchyma. This classification is not always easy to apply clinically because of the overlap that frequently occurs on clinical presentation, especially in the early stages of CP, in which acute attacks of pain may be the only clinical symptom. Because biopsy specimens are not readily available, attempts have been made to classify pancreatitis according to clinical or radiologic criteria. For example, the Cambridge classification uses changes in the pancreatic ducts as seen by endoscopic pancreatography. The incidence and prevalence of CP are not well known. The prevalence is estimated to be 4 in 100,000 inhabitants older than 20 years, according to studies in Sweden and the United States. In autopsy reports, the ranges are from 0.04 to 5%.

The natural history of CP is not well known. A French study of 240 patients with CP of any etiology, with a 9-year follow-up, observed that this disease is more frequent in men and that alcohol is the main cause. About 50% of the patients developed diabetes, 40% presented some kind of associated liver disease, most of them showing pancreatic calcifications, and 40% required surgical treatment. The mortality rate reached 24%, and the probability of staying alive after 20 years was 70%, this probability being significantly lower than that of the reference population.

ETIOLOGY

Many causative factors have been identified in pancreatitis (Table 1). Alcohol consumption is the main factor, associated with up to 70% of the cases of CP in developed countries. It has been suggested that the use of alcohol to produce CP should be of more than 100 grams a day for more than 6 years, associated with a diet rich in fats. The obstruction of pancreatic drainage (by trauma, tumors, pancreas divisum) can be associated with CP. Other causes

TABLE 1. **Causative Factors of Chronic Pancreatitis**

Alcohol	Congenital abnormalities
Obstruction	Autoimmune
Trauma	Idiopathic

TABLE 2. **Presenting Features of Chronic Pancreatitis**

Pain
Exocrine or endocrine insufficiency or both
Complications
   Pseudocyst
   Infection
   Biliary or duodenal obstruction or both
   Fistula (ascites, pleural effusion)
   Obstructed splenic (left-sided) portal hypertension

include cystic fibrosis, autoimmune diseases (Sjögren's syndrome), and hyperparathyroidism. Gallstone disease has not been proved as a definitive cause of CP. Up to 40% of cases fall into the group of idiopathic CP.

The basic pathogenic mechanism remains obscure, and in most instances, management continues to be empirical and directed to the treatment of symptoms, sequelae, and complications. Our limited knowledge of the mechanisms of pain and of the natural history of the disease hampers successful treatment. Longitudinal studies suggest that pain is completely relieved in more than 60% of the patients when the follow-up period is long enough, regardless of cause. It has been shown that at least half of the patients became diabetic and that one third of the patients with alcohol-induced pancreatitis had nonprogressive disease with preservation of endocrine function. However, the concept that the disease may "burn itself out" may be flawed by a methodologic bias, because the higher earlier mortality in patients with severe disease may reduce the incidence of pain in the late follow-up groups. Other studies have not clearly shown this "burnout" phenomenon. Unifactorial and multifactorial analyses of death associated with CP in a series of 240 French patients showed that the mortality rate after 20 years of illness was 35.8% higher than the mortality rate of the matched population. The main causes of death were alcoholic liver disease, carcinoma, and postoperative complications. That CP was less frequently the direct cause of death contrasted with the multivisceral consequences of alcoholism and smoking. It was suggested, but not well documented, that abstinence from alcohol improved long-term survival.

DIAGNOSIS

Pain is the most common symptom (Table 2). The diagnosis of CP relies on a clinical history of characteristic pain and some objective evidence of disease, which includes elevation in the level of serum amylase, the presence of calcifications, abnormalities of the pancreas seen by computed tomography (CT), ductal changes consistent with pancreatitis seen at retrograde pancreatography, or the presence of a firm, fibrotic white pancreas found at previous abdominal exploration with or without biopsy of the pancreas. The presence of endocrine or exocrine insufficiency strengthens the diagnosis. A small number of patients with the characteristic pain of pancreatitis fail to have objective signs of disease, although these patients have an abnormal pancreas at the time of exploration and biopsy.

Clinical Findings

Abdominal pain is the main and commonly the first symptom. It is characterized by recurrent pain attacks in the upper abdomen, occasionally radiated to the back, often exacerbated with meals, at intervals of months or years.

These attacks tend to become more frequent until pain becomes persistent. The incidence of pain ranges between 70 and 90% of the diagnosed cases, being severe in 50% of them. This disease starts clinically with an episode of acute pancreatitis in approximately 50% of patients, whereas in 40% of cases the onset of pain is quite insidious. Painless CP accounts for 10 to 20% of patients and is more likely to present in older patients. In advanced stages of the disease, when exocrine function is reduced by 90%, diarrhea and weight loss may appear. Diabetes may also occur in these stages as a manifestation of endocrine insufficiency, with a prevalence ranging between 28 and 70%. Other manifestations of CP are cholestasis caused by common bile duct stenosis, occurring in 27% of cases; duodenal stenosis; ascites, described in 3% (commonly from a ruptured pseudocyst or pancreatic duct); and associated liver disease, described in about 40% of cases.

For assessment of pancreatic disease there are two main groups of studies: imaging techniques and functional tests.

Imaging Techniques

The development of imaging techniques, such as ultrasonography, CT, and endoscopic retrograde cholangiopancreatography (ERCP), has allowed better morphologic evaluation of the pancreatic gland.

Plain abdominal radiography shows pancreatic calcifications in 30 to 50% of patients. Abdominal ultrasonography is often the first study to be carried out for suspected CP, because of its efficacy and low cost. We are interested in the size of the pancreas, its characteristics, peripancreatic changes, calcifications, cysts, fluid collections, biliary tree, pancreatic duct, and portal system. For these changes, ultrasonography has a sensitivity ranging between 60 and 70% and a specificity between 75 and 90%. The role of endoscopic ultrasonography is being evaluated.

Abdominal CT is today the favored imaging technique for pancreatic pathology. Although more expensive and requiring radiation, it provides the most reliable overall assessment of the pancreas and peripancreatic area in CP with a sensitivity between 75 and 90% and a specificity between 94 and 100%. It should be considered for all patients for whom surgery is contemplated. Additional data are necessary to define the role of magnetic resonance imaging in the evaluation of CP and pancreatic masses.

Finally, ERCP allows visualization of the papilla of Vater and the opacification of the common bile duct and pancreatic ducts. ERCP is useful in evaluating the state of the CP, outlining the ductal morphology when considering surgery, and in some cases helping to differentiate CP from a neoplasm. The sensitivity of ERCP in the diagnosis of CP is 71 to 93% and its specificity 81 to 100%. It is abnormal in most of the cases with calcifications, and an inverse correlation between the degree of ductal alterations and the exocrine pancreatic function has been observed. However, there is a poor correlation between the degree of ductal changes and pain.

Functional Tests

It is rare that one requires functional studies of the pancreas for the diagnosis of CP. One possible case is that of the patient with chronic pain suggestive of pancreatic origin but with negative imaging studies.

Pancreatic Exocrine Function Tests

TESTS REQUIRING DUODENAL INTUBATION. These tests involve stimulating exocrine pancreatic secretion through the intravenous administration of secretin, cholecystokinin, or cerulein. The concentrations of the pancreatic enzymes amylase, lipase, trypsin, and chymotrypsin and of bicarbonates are quantified from the drainage collected from the duodenum. These concentrations are significantly reduced in advanced stages of CP. However, in early disease, a decrease in only one or two enzymes may be detected, with lipase being the first one to drop. The sensitivity and specificity are higher than 90%. Nevertheless, these studies are invasive, expensive, and performed only in highly specialized centers.

ORAL TESTS. These are based on use of a test meal to stimulate pancreatic secretion, as well as administration of a synthetic pharmaceutical preparation that requires the action of certain pancreatic enzymes to be hydrolyzed. Part of the hydrolyzed product is absorbed by the intestine and excreted through the kidney. The proportion of the synthetic preparation in the urine reflects the intraluminal pancreatic enzyme activity.

The most widely used techniques are those measuring urinary excretion of p-aminobenzoic acid (N-benzoyl-L-tyrosyl-p-aminobenzoic acid [NBT-PABA] test) and fluorescein (pancreolauril test). These substances are released from substrates within the intestinal lumen through the action of chymotrypsin and esterase, respectively. Both tests have a high accuracy in detecting pancreatic exocrine insufficiency, but their value decreases in mild pancreatic disease. Malabsorption and renal failure may interfere with the results. The sensitivity and specificity of the described oral tests in severe pancreatic insufficiency range from 70 to 90% and from 72 to 80%, respectively, similar to those for tests by direct stimulation.

SERUM PANCREATIC ENZYME QUANTIFICATION. Serum quantification of some pancreatic enzymes (P-isoamylase and trypsin) is highly specific but has a low sensitivity for CP. Abnormally low values appear when there is an important functional deterioration of the gland. High values reflect a reduction in the flow of pancreatic secretion to the duodenum. Serum levels of trypsin associated with the NBT-PABA test have allowed distinction of three different secretor patterns in CP: normal NBT-PABA and serum trypsin, low NBT-PABA and serum trypsin, and low NBT-PABA and normal or high serum trypsin. Serum levels of trypsin are directly correlated with the functional pancreatic reserve. An abnormal NBT-PABA test associated with low serum trypsin has been suggested to be predictive of the nonreversibility of pancreatic exocrine function, whereas low values of NBT-PABA together with normal or high trypsin levels suggest a possible improvement of the pancreatic function, especially in relation to alcohol abstinence and surgical treatment.

FECAL FAT QUANTIFICATION. The fecal fat content is useful only in the final stages of pancreatic exocrine insufficiency, because it appears when 90% of the exocrine function is lost. Typical values in steatorrhea are those over 7 grams per 24 hours. This test may be useful in control of the therapeutic effect of oral administration of substitutive pancreatic enzymes in pancreatic exocrine insufficiency. A breath test with ^{14}C-labeled triolein has been introduced. This test consists of measuring the proportion of ^{14}C exhaled after the ingestion of ^{14}C-marked triolein. It is a sensitive, simple, and noninvasive technique, but, like fecal fat determination, it does not distinguish between different etiologies of steatorrhea. The main disadvantage of this test is that it is qualitative, so it does not determine the amount of fat loss.

Pancreatic Endocrine Function Tests.

Endocrine pancreatic function abnormalities are frequently observed in advanced CP stages. Plasma levels of glucagon after arginine infusion are useful for distinguishing primary from secondary diabetes in CP, as they are decreased in secondary diabetes. On the other hand, the integrated response of plasma pancreatic polypeptide to a meal, secretin, or cerulein seems to be a reliable test in the diagnosis of CP and also in distinguishing mild and severe stages of the disease. However, the sensitivity of this test is low in early disease.

THERAPY

Medical therapy, for the most part, is limited to control of the pain, removal of a causative factor when identified (e.g., alcohol), and management of diabetes or exocrine insufficiency when present (pancreatic enzymes). Behavioral modifications and personal and family support are crucial in the management of related alcoholism and drug addiction and in facilitating control of pain and rehabilitation.

Etiologic Factors

Alcohol is the main etiologic factor in CP. Therefore, it is important that the patients be managed by a multidisciplinary group that includes a comprehensive program for alcoholism. In areas of the world (South India, Indonesia) where nutritional deficiencies appear to play a role in the pathogenesis, adequate nutrition should be a goal. The role of antioxidant agents (selenium, β-carotene, vitamins C and E, methionine) and the use of zinc supplements remain controversial and under evaluation.

Pancreatic Endocrine Insufficiency

Vascular complications of diabetes are infrequent; however, neuropathy can be seen more often, probably because of the associated effects of alcohol and malnutrition. Treatment of diabetes in CP does not differ substantially from that of diabetes mellitus. Oral hypoglycemic agents are usually not effective. Patients may require low doses of exogenous insulin and are more susceptible to developing hypoglycemia because of inappropriate insulin release, glucagon deficiency, and a low hepatic glycogen reserve.

Pancreatic Exocrine Insufficiency

A major loss of exocrine function is required for malabsorption of pancreatic origin to occur. Steatorrhea appears when pancreatic function has been reduced to less than 10 to 15% of its capacity. The end points of treatment are fitting the diet to the digestive capacity and metabolic requirements; supplementing fat-soluble vitamins (e.g., vitamin B_{12}) and trace elements such as zinc, selenium, and folic acid if required; and, finally, treating protein, carbohydrate, and fat malabsorption with administration of exogenous pancreatic enzymes. It is advisable to restrict fats and vegetable fiber; in severe cases, medium chain triglycerides should be used. The end point of the substitutive therapy with exogenous pancreatic enzymes is restoration of the physiologic intraluminal digestion.

The result of pancreatic enzyme administration depends on several intraluminal factors: (1) gastric pH, (2) appropriate mixture of the alimentary bolus (granules give better results than tablets), (3) duodenal pH, and (4) appropriate enzymatic concentration in the intestinal lumen, the concentration of lipase being especially important. It is well known that pancreatic enzymes given orally, and especially lipase, are inactivated at a pH lower than 4. To avoid this effect, a histamine H_2-receptor antagonist can be added to increase gastric as well as duodenal pH. It is important to use preparations high in lipase concentration. A minimum of 11,000 to 30,000 lipase units per meal is recommended, adjusting the dose to the clinical improvement of the steatorrhea. Pancreatic enzymes are supplied as conventional tablets, as enteric-coated pills, or as microspheres. Microspheres are the most suitable presentation, because they mix better with the alimentary bolus and have greater gastric pH resistance.

Finally, for some selected patients, such as those with severe malnutrition or with complications, total parenteral nutrition may be required.

Pain Management

Increased ductal and interstitial pressure, perineural fibrosis, an increase in the number and diameter of pancreatic nerves, the role of various neuropeptides in processing the information concerning pain, and the possibility of a neuroimmunologic disorder have all been suggested as mechanisms for pain. The first step in pain management is to exclude any complication as responsible for this symptom, such as an acute exacerbation of the pancreatitis, a pseudocyst, or biliary obstruction. Often a computed tomogram gives this information. It is important to insist on alcohol abstinence, because it has been proved that such abstinence can relieve pain. A retrograde pancreatogram can suggest a possible pathogenic mechanism (e.g., pancreas divisum, ampullary stenosis, ductal dilatation with pancreatic stones). A negative feedback mechanism between the duodenal trypsin content and the pancreatic exocrine secretion has been suggested. This phenomenon justifies a trial of exogenous pancreatic enzyme preparations high in trypsin. They would decrease intraductal pressure in these patients through inhibition of the exocrine pancreatic secretion. Significant relief of pain after exogenous pancreatic enzyme administration in comparison with placebo has been proved.

When pain does not respond to analgesics and/or enzyme administration, a celiac plexus block by percutaneous alcohol injection may be tried. However, the benefits may last only a few months, and repeated injections tend to be less effective.

Early results of endoscopic removal of pancreatic stones and the use of stents in main pancreatic ducts in selected cases appear good. Nevertheless, longer follow-ups are required and a critical analysis of the cases is needed.

TABLE 3. **Indications for Surgery in Chronic Pancreatitis**

Disabling pain
Multiple relapses during year
Considerable lost time from work during year
Prevention of drug addiction
Complications
 Pseudocyst
 Gastrointestinal tract obstruction or biliary tract obstruction
  or both
 Fistula
 Infection
 Left-sided portal hypertension
Inability to rule out neoplasm

Surgery

The indications for surgery are summarized in Table 3. Severe intractable pain, complications of the disease that require surgical management, and the inability to rule out a neoplasm are some of these reasons.

The factors that should be considered in the assessment of a patient as a possible candidate for operation are listed in Table 4. The first category, clinical information, deals with the severity of the pain, previous treatments, the presence of drug or substance abuse, the presence or absence of diabetes, and estimation of the patient's willingness and ability to manage the condition postoperatively, which may include the apancreatic state. In the second category are studies to define the morphologic characteristics of the pancreas and the surgical options available. ERCP and imaging techniques, such as CT and ultrasonography, are helpful in obtaining information.

In general, for patients with severe disabling disease and dilated pancreatic duct, side-to-side pancreaticojejunostomy is the procedure of choice; for patients with a pseudocyst, internal drainage is recommended; and for the rare instance of ampullary stenosis, sphincterotomy is recommended. For patients with a nondilated pancreatic duct in whom previous decompressive operations have failed, when a mass effect is present, or when the disease appears to be lateralized, therapy usually entails some form of pancreatic resection.

No standard protocol for assessing and reporting results of the various surgical treatments exists.

TABLE 4. **Basic Considerations for Surgical Therapy in Chronic Pancreatitis**

Clinical information
 Symptoms
 Personality
 Addiction to drug or substance abuse
 Diabetes
 Associated diseases
 Previous operations
Structural changes found on
 Pancreatography
 Computed tomography or ultrasonography or both
 Operative finding

TABLE 5. **Surgical Procedures**

Direct to pancreas
 Anastomosis to intestinal tract (jejunum, stomach,
  duodenum)
 Drainage of cysts and abscesses
 Resection
  Distal
  Subtotal
  Pancreatoduodenectomy
  Duodenum preserving
  Total
 Resection and autotransplantation (islet cells, segmental)
 Occlusion of pancreatic duct (surgical, endoscopic)
Indirect to pancreas
 Sphincterotomy, sphincteroplasty
 Biliary enteric anastomosis
 Gastroenterostomy
 Nerve interruption

Comparison of the results reported in the literature is difficult because frequently the population of patients, type of disease, length of follow-up study, and criteria for improvement vary. However, relief of pain cannot be the only criterion for success, especially when the results of pancreatic resection are reviewed. The metabolic consequences of the therapy (i.e., endocrine and exocrine insufficiency), the related late morbidity and mortality, and the possibility for rehabilitation with return to a productive life should be considered. To optimize results, a multidisciplinary team approach that includes gastroenterologists, consultants in behavioral medicine, nutritionists, and surgeons is preferable.

The surgical procedures available in the management of patients with CP are listed in Table 5.

Pancreaticojejunostomy

This procedure is indicated for patients with a dilated pancreatic duct and usually requires a duct 8 mm or more in diameter. The technique requires extensive opening of the pancreatic duct from the tail to the head of the pancreas. When present, calculi should be removed.

The operative risk associated with the procedure is low, and the remaining glandular tissue is preserved. At 5 years after operation, about two thirds of all patients experience relief of pain. Some reported results are included in Table 6. The proportion of patients who achieved relief of pain is inversely related to the length of the postoperative period. In our experience, only 54% of patients had improvement of pain at 5 years. Good results after pancreaticojejunostomy have been reported in the management of patients with chronic relapsing pancreatitis and in children with an associated dilated pancreatic duct. In this latter group, CP has increasingly been recognized as a cause of abdominal pain, and in children, unlike adults, alcoholism is rarely the cause of the disease.

If pain recurs, endoscopic retrograde pancreatography is indicated to assess the patency of the anastomosis. When the anastomosis is obstructed, a re-

TABLE 6. **Results of Pancreaticojejunostomy for Relief of Pain**

		Pain	Operative	
Author, Date	No. of Patients	Improvement (%)	Follow-up (y)	Mortality (%)
Prinz, 1981	86	71	24.0	4
Taylor, 1981	20	54	5.0	0
Hart, 1983	75	63	4.0	0
Morrow, 1984	46	80	6.6	0
Holmberg, 1985	51	72	8.2	0
Crombleholme, 1990*	10	80	4.0	0

*In children.

peated pancreaticojejunostomy can result in improvement of pain in about half the patients.

Sphincterotomy and Sphincteroplasty

In the past, patients who had disabling pain and laboratory findings suggestive of pancreatitis, often with minimal evidence of pancreatic parenchymal or ductal disease, frequently underwent ampullary procedures because of the belief that impaired outflow of pancreatic secretions was responsible for the disease. This procedure is used rarely now for the management of patients with CP because the true incidence of ampullary stenosis is thought to be extremely small.

A study from the Lahey Clinic reported that by 6 months after operation, more than 60% of patients had improvement of pain, but by 5 years after operation, only 40% of the patients noted some degree of relief of pain. The more complex sphincteroplasty appeared to offer no advantage over the simpler sphincterotomy and, in patients who were alcoholic, avoidance of alcohol appeared to be the major determinant of a better outcome after operation.

Sphincteroplasty of the minor papilla in patients with CP and pancreas divisum offers no benefit. Successful results are seen with recurrent acute pancreatitis and a normal gland. Some endoscopists use endoscopic papillotomy and stenting in patients with CP. This procedure is likely to reproduce the limited results associated with open sphincteroplasty.

Cystogastrostomy, Cystoduodenostomy, and Cystojejunostomy

Pancreatic cysts associated with chronic pancreatitis are unlikely to resolve spontaneously and in most instances have mature walls that permit internal drainage. Therefore, it is usually not necessary to delay resolution for pseudocysts in patients with chronic pancreatitis. Operation is delayed for 4 to 6 weeks only in selected patients—specifically, in patients with a recent identifiable acute relapse. Although internal drainage of a pseudocyst usually results in resolution of the cyst, persistent or recurrent pain is common in patients with chronic pancreatitis because of persistence of the underlying disease. In our experience, only one third of patients with cysts in the head of the pancreas achieved long-term pain improvement. Therefore, retrograde pancreatogra-

phy is performed preoperatively to assess the pancreatic ductal system. This procedure identifies patients who are candidates for more definitive treatment, such as concomitant drainage of a dilated main pancreatic duct or pancreatic resection.

When the cyst is in the retrogastric position, cystogastrostomy is the treatment of choice. With cysts in the head of the gland, Roux-en-Y cystojejunostomy or transduodenal drainage is preferred. Endoscopic transgastric and transduodenal drainages have been performed; however, perforation and bleeding have been described. The long-term results after these procedures require further assessment. In our experience, external drainage performed for selected cysts in the head of the pancreas and in difficult locations has been associated with resolution of the cysts in most patients and with minimal morbidity and mortality. The high morbidity and mortality associated with external drainage reported by surgeons may be in part the result of treating patients with acute pseudocysts.

Not all cysts need to be treated. When a patient is asymptomatic or has minimal symptoms and the cyst is small (5 cm or less), treatment is probably unnecessary. Follow-up study with serial ultrasonography is advisable. When cystic neoplasms are suspected, resection is required.

Pancreatic Resection

Resection is indicated in patients with disabling disease and a small pancreatic duct, in patients in whom previous decompression operations have failed, in patients with disease that is lateralized or dominant in the head or the tail of the gland, in some patients with pseudocysts or pancreatic fistulas, and in patients in whom a neoplasm cannot be ruled out.

Pancreatic resections consist of standard distal resection, in which the pancreas is divided at the level of the superior mesenteric vessels and approximately 60% of the gland is removed; near-total or 80 to 95% resection, in which the pancreas is divided to the right of the superior mesenteric vessels, leaving a rim of tissue of variable size attached to the duodenum to preserve the pancreaticoduodenal vessels and common bile duct; and pancreatoduodenectomy, in which the head of the gland and the duodenum are removed, leaving the pancreas in place distal to the superior mesenteric vessels. We prefer the pylorus-preserving technique. Total pancreatectomy removes the entire gland.

In the assessment of the results of resective operations, one has to consider that removal of pancreatic tissue can precipitate or accelerate the development of endocrine or exocrine insufficiency and therefore increase the morbidity and mortality associated with the procedure. The surgical treatment of patients with pancreatitis is based on the preservation of as much pancreatic function as possible while attempting to improve the patient's symptoms. It must be kept in mind, however, that diabetes mellitus eventually occurs in about 40% of patients with chronic pancreatitis even without surgery. Therefore, the incidence of diabetes after resection should be compared with the incidence in medically treated patients and patients who have undergone decompression procedures and not with members of the population at large. On occasion, in patients whose personality may preclude the management of an apancreatic state, it is better to accept some degree of pain and disability rather than the metabolic complications.

Distal Resection

Usually, lesser forms of distal resection are associated with a lower incidence of endocrine (30%) and exocrine insufficiency but tend to achieve less pain relief (50%). With maximal distal resection (90 to 95% of the gland), the pain is relieved more often (90%), but the incidence of metabolic complications increases substantially (70%). Limited distal resection achieved relief of pain by 5 years in only 20% of our patients. Other surgeons have reported better results, perhaps because of a different or better selection of patients. When we extended resection to near-total pancreatectomy, long-term improvement of pain occurred in approximately two thirds of patients but with an appreciable rise in metabolic complications. Distal resection appears to be best suited for patients with disease lateralized to the tail of the gland, for some patients with cysts in the body and tail, for patients with severe disease in the body and tail with ductal obstruction at the neck of the gland, and for patients with previous ductal injury resulting from blunt abdominal trauma with fracture of the pancreas and stenosis of the duct at the midbody level. When the pancreatic duct is patent toward the head of the gland, the transected surface of the pancreatic duct is managed by suture ligation. When the pancreatic duct is obstructed proximally, pancreaticojejunostomy to the transected pancreas is favored. The patency of the duct can be assessed by retrograde pancreatography before operation or at the time of operation either by operative pancreatography or by probing the duct, preferably with a Fogarty catheter. Of patients who underwent 80 to 95% resection, those with simultaneous segmental pancreatic autotransplantation had the lowest incidence of insulin-dependent diabetes in the late postoperative period.

Total Pancreatectomy

Complete removal of the pancreas is associated with pain relief in 60 to 100% of patients. However, exocrine and endocrine insufficiency occurs in all these patients. Most total pancreatectomies are staged and are done in patients who previously underwent partial resection. Although the operative mortality is low, the late mortality in the Lahey Clinic experience was 46% at the median follow-up time of 5 years and in the Mayo Clinic series was 40% with a median follow-up time of 9 years. The short- and long-term morbidity was significant. In the Lahey Clinic experience, 24 of 26 patients required multiple readmissions, uncontrolled diabetes being the most common reason. Related late operations were common. Causes of death included cardiovascular problems, carcinoma at other sites (esophagus, larynx), hypoglycemia, suicide, complications of narcotic addiction, and alcohol-related death and disease. Because of the appreciable morbidity and mortality that result from an apancreatic state, especially in a patient with substance addiction or alcoholism, total pancreatectomy should be performed only as a last resort in patients whose previous operations have failed and who appear capable of managing their apancreatic state. In patients who already have insulin-dependent diabetes, indications for extensive pancreatectomy can be less rigid. When total pancreatectomy is performed, the pylorus-preserving technique is used. In postoperative management, we avoid the strict regulation of glucose levels and favor levels between 150 and 200 mg per dL to decrease the number of hypoglycemic episodes. All patients require exocrine pancreatic replacement therapy.

Proximal Pancreatic Resection

Increasing evidence in the literature suggests that resection of the head of the pancreas and uncinate process results in a higher degree of relief of pain than does distal resection. The better results obtained with proximal resection, together with the gradual decrease in the operative mortality associated with pancreatoduodenectomy and the realization of the limited results of distal resection, explain the increase in the frequency of proximal pancreatic resection in the management of patients with CP. This procedure is advocated for patients with severe disabling pain and a pancreatic duct of small diameter, for patients with a mass in the head of the pancreas with or without biliary and duodenal obstruction, and when the possibility of a neoplasm cannot be ruled out. The procedure is also used for patients in whom previous decompression operations and ampullary procedures have failed. In the Lahey Clinic experience, approximately 80 to 90% of patients continued to have relief of pain 5 years after the procedure. Of the insulin-independent patients before operation, 40% required insulin within 5 years after operation. However, the diabetes was stable and easy to control in most instances. Although the late mortality was 26%, only in 5.4% of patients was it related to the underlying pancreatic disease. By 5 years after operation, half the patients were maintaining a normal lifestyle and an additional 30% claimed to do so intermittently. The use of narcotics had decreased from 85% before operation to 28% by 5 years after operation.

Pylorus-preserving pancreatoduodenectomy has been used extensively because it facilitates the procedure, avoids gastric resection, preserves gastric capacity, minimizes postgastrectomy syndromes, and may be associated with better absorption of fat than if gastric resection had been performed. Beger and coworkers have reported extensively on the technique of duodenum-preserving resection of the head of the pancreas with pain relief in 89% of the patients with a median follow-up time of 3.6 years; confirmatory data from other centers are required to determine the value of this procedure.

Techniques of Preservation of Endocrine Function

Implantation of islet cells into the portal system after extensive pancreatic resection has been reported. However, the low yield of isolation of islet cells in a fibrotic and calcified pancreas and the decreased mass of islet cells in these patients are in part responsible for the fact that in most of these patients, insulin is required within a few months after operation. Our experience with extensive distal pancreatic resection and segmental autotransplantation suggests that this technique is effective in preventing or delaying the onset of diabetes in these patients. However, because of the limited relief of pain provided by distal resection, in most of these patients we favor initial pancreatoduodenectomy, and we defer distal resection and autotransplantation for the patients whose proximal resection would fail.

Nerve Interruption Techniques

Relief of pain is the main goal of therapy for most patients with CP. Mallet-Guy reported extensive experience with splanchnicectomy and celiac ganglionectomy in 127 patients, with a minimal follow-up time of 5 years. Mallet-Guy's preferred method is a lumbar approach with resection of the 12th rib, followed by removal of the great splanchnic nerve and celiac ganglion. Poor results were reported in only 10% of his patients. These results, however, have not been duplicated. Leger and associates reported relief of pain in only about one third of patients during a 2-year period of observation. White and associates achieved long-term reduction of pain in only 4 of 27 patients. The good initial results reported by Stone and associates for bilateral vagotomy with left splanchnicectomy through a thoracic approach need confirmation by other groups. Anesthetic agents, alcohol, or phenols have achieved relief of pain in up to half of patients with CP; however, this relief lasts for only a couple of months after performance of this technique. For the most part, nerve ablation

procedures have a minimal role in the management of patients with CP.

ASSOCIATED PROBLEMS

Pancreatic Ascites and Pancreatic Pleural Effusion

Pancreatic ascites and pancreatic pleural effusion result from disruption of the pancreatic duct either into the peritoneal cavity or through the retroperitoneum to the chest. Patients with pancreatic ascites present with a distended abdomen. A history of alcoholism or previous abdominal pain from pancreatitis may occasionally be absent. Patients with pleural effusion of pancreatic origin present with the nonspecific symptoms common to patients with pleural effusion, the severity of which depends on the accumulation of fluid in the chest. Analysis of fluid in these patients discloses whether the ascitic or pleural fluid has a high concentration of amylase and protein (2.5 grams per dL). Medical therapy for patients with this condition includes the usual measures for ascites plus somatostatin, total parenteral nutrition, paracentesis, and no oral intake. Although a trial of this therapy is probably justifiable, failure is common in more than half of patients. Because medical therapy is accompanied by serious morbidity and mortality, perseverance is not justified when the patient's condition is failing and no progress is noted.

Retrograde pancreatography is essential in the work-up of these patients before operation because it permits determination of the site of leakage in the pancreatic ductal system and thus facilitates surgical exploration and selection of therapy. Depending on the location of the leakage and the characteristics of the ductal system, Roux-en-Y anastomosis to the site of the fistula or pancreatic resection, with or without pancreaticojejunostomy, may be selected for treatment. The placement of an endoscopic stent has been reported to be useful in selected cases.

Biliary Obstruction in Patients with Chronic Pancreatitis

Obstruction of the distal biliary tree may be the result of progressive fibrosis, formation of a pseudocyst, acute inflammatory changes, common bile duct calculi, or underlying carcinoma. An elevated level of alkaline phosphatase, which precedes jaundice, appears to be the most sensitive assay in detecting such obstruction. The incidence of stenosis of the distal bile duct in alcoholic pancreatitis has been reported to be at least 8%.

Obstruction of the biliary tree can be transient, recurrent, or persistent, depending on the basic mechanism causing the obstruction. The characteristics of the clinical course, results of cholangiography, and characteristics of the head of the pancreas, such as the presence of a pseudocyst, are factors that determine the need for therapy. Because fibrosis is the most common cause of distal biliary stricture in these patients, it should not be assumed that drainage of a cyst in the head of the gland will necessarily relieve the obstruction. Patients with a severely dilated common duct, recurrent or persistent obstruction as determined by continued elevation in the level of serum alkaline phosphatase, persistent jaundice, or recurrent episodes of cholangitis benefit from biliary enteric anastomosis. A patient with transient obstruction during an episode of acute relapse may be observed. Operative cholangiography after drainage of a cyst in the head of the pancreas can help assess the role of the cyst in the obstruction of the distal common duct. In well-selected patients with disabling pain and with disease lateralized to the head, pseudocyst in the head, and biliary obstruction, pancreatoduodenectomy may be the procedure of choice. Chronic stenosis of the common bile duct can cause cholangitis and biliary cirrhosis.

TRENDS

The management of patients with CP continues to achieve limited success. The diagnosis is usually based on a history of classic pain and some objective finding of pancreatic disease. Morphologic information provided by ERCP and ultrasonography or CT is essential in selecting the procedure that may achieve the result with the lowest morbidity and mortality. Other than morphologic data, clinical information regarding characteristics of personality, drug or substance abuse, presence of exocrine and endocrine insufficiency, and the patient's ability to manage the disease is essential in determining who is a surgical candidate and what procedure to perform. The basic surgical principles are to be conservative and to try to preserve as much pancreatic tissue as possible. The operation should be tailored to each patient according to the clinical and morphologic characteristics. Although management of pain is the primary goal of treatment in most patients, the morbidity and late mortality that can result from different procedures must be a major consideration in the selection of therapy. Pancreaticojejunostomy is the procedure of choice at this time for patients with a dilated pancreatic duct and internal drainage for a pseudocyst. Different forms of pancreatic resection are indicated for patients with severe disease and small pancreatic ducts, for patients in whom decompression operations have failed, for patients with lateralized disease to the tail of the gland, for some patients with pseudocysts or pancreatic fistulas, and for some patients when carcinoma cannot be ruled out. Procedures on the ampulla (sphincterotomy, sphincteroplasty) are now rarely performed. Of the resective procedures, operations that remove the head of the pancreas and uncinate process appear to achieve the best long-term results. This result, plus the decreased operative morbidity and mortality associated with operations on the head of the pancreas, explains the increase in use of these procedures. Endoscopic procedures are being used more often, and their results need further evaluation.

GASTROESOPHAGEAL REFLUX DISEASE

method of
ADRIAN P. IRELAND, M.D., and
TOM R. DeMEESTER, M.D.
University of Southern California School of Medicine
Los Angeles, California

Gastroesophageal reflux disease is the spectrum of diseases related to excess reflux of gastric content into the esophagus. Diagnostic testing is required to confirm the diagnosis and plan the optimal mode of therapy. In up to 25% of patients with esophagitis the disease follows a recurrent, progressive course necessitating lifelong therapy. The reasons for this are that acid suppression therapy may fail to suppress acid production owing to inadequate dosage or poor compliance and does not address the nonacid components of the disease. The most effective treatment in these patients is a technically adequately performed antireflux operation that eliminates esophageal exposure to all refluxed material.

The role of the physician is to identify the patients at highest risk of recurrent or progressive disease and to halt the disease process before the point of end-stage disease when medical therapy is considered a failure and surgical therapy gives less satisfactory results. This approach should reduce the prevalence of complications, in particular specialized intestinal metaplasia, a premalignant condition that may progress to esophageal adenocarcinoma.

MAGNITUDE OF THE PROBLEM

Gastroesophageal reflux disease is the most common disease of the foregut in the Western Hemisphere. There is a wide spectrum of disease, from patients with occasional symptoms without mucosal damage to patients with complications. More than 30% of the population experience heartburn on a frequent basis, and 10% experience heartburn daily. Results from a long-term follow-up of a group of 701 adult patients with esophagitis in Lausanne, Switzerland, were reported in 1993 and give the best available information on the natural history of reflux esophagitis. This "natural history" is in patients treated with a variety of medical agents such as antacids, H_2-receptor antagonists, omeprazole, and prokinetic agents and as such represents the course of the patients undergoing medical therapy. Seventy-seven percent of patients have an isolated episode of esophagitis or have recurrent, nonprogressive disease. These patients may be viewed as having a "benign" form of reflux disease in that they have only one episode of esophagitis, or when they do have a relapse they do so to the same or a less severe grade of esophagitis. The remaining 23% of patients have recurrent, progressive disease. These have a more severe form of reflux disease, because the degree of esophagitis worsens despite medical therapy.

Specialized intestinal epithelium (Barrett's esophagus) develops in 10 to 18% of patients with chronic gastroesophageal reflux disease. A postmortem study has shown that the age- and sex-adjusted prevalence of Barrett's esophagus is 376 per 100,000 population, compared with the clinically diagnosed prevalence of 22.6 per 100,000. This represents a 20-fold increase and indicates that the majority of patients with reflux never seek medical attention. Concomitantly and for unknown reasons, the incidence of esophageal adenocarcinoma is increasing faster than that of any other cancer, and in many centers esophageal adenocarcinoma outnumbers squamous cancer.

Several investigators have reported an increase in the incidence of reflux esophagitis. It was thought that this reflected an increase in the availability of endoscopy, but deaths resulting from nonmalignant esophageal disease are also on the increase. These data indicate that reflux disease is becoming more common. This is reflected in drug sales, with a large share consisting of sales of antacids and acid suppressants. Most who suffer with symptoms of gastroesophageal reflux disease treat themselves before seeking the advice of a physician. This self-treatment has been confined to the use of antacids in the past, but H_2-receptor antagonists have become available as over-the-counter medications. Fewer patients are expected to seek medical attention for reflux symptoms because of this.

MANIFESTATIONS

The physician suspects that gastroesophageal reflux disease may be present when the patient presents with reflux symptoms or investigation reveals complications of the disease. Typical symptoms of reflux include heartburn (sensation of retrosternal discomfort related to the reflux of gastric content into the esophagus), regurgitation (reflux of gastric content into the mouth), and dysphagia (sensation of swallowed material sticking in the esophagus). Regurgitation of gastric content into the mouth must be differentiated from regurgitation of bland material that has never reached the stomach. This may be seen in patients with esophageal motility disorders or a pharyngeal (Zenker's) diverticulum. The typical patient with gastroesophageal reflux disease complains of heartburn and regurgitation that are aggravated by a large meal (especially fatty) and by lying down. The patient has usually noted that antacids partially relieve heartburn but have less effect on regurgitation. Some patients experience excess salivation (waterbrash). The atypical presentations of reflux include dental erosions, chronic cough, hoarseness, asthma, and noncardiac chest pain. Eighty percent of patients with asthma or chronic hoarseness have reflux. Reflux is present in 50% of patients with noncardiac chest pain. It has been noted that gastroesophageal reflux disease is frequently present in patients who present with Zenker's diverticulum and cricopharyngeal dysphagia. In some patients, reflux is precipitated by exercise, which may lead to diagnostic confusion. The sensation of postprandial abdominal bloating, often described as a complication of antireflux surgery, is as common in patients treated with medication as in those who have undergone surgery. Complications of reflux disease include ulceration, stricture, short esophagus, Barrett's epithelium, high-grade dysplasia, and esophageal adenocarcinoma.

DIAGNOSTIC INVESTIGATION

Patients who have just one episode of heartburn and respond to lifestyle modification and a course of acid suppressant therapy require no further investigation or treatment. Indications for investigation are summarized in Table 1. Investigation should be tailored to the patient and available resources along the following guidelines.

Barium Esophagogram

If dysphagia is a primary symptom, a barium esophagogram should precede endoscopy. Barium esophagography

TABLE 1. Indications for Investigation of the Patient with Suspected Gastroesophageal Reflux Disease

Before surgery
Incomplete response to treatment, recurrent disease, or prolonged acid suppressant therapy
Atypical symptoms; laryngeal, pulmonary, or noncardiac chest pain
Idiopathic pulmonary fibrosis or recurrent aspiration pneumonia
Presence of complications before or during therapy

provides information complementary to that provided by stationary esophageal motility and endoscopy. The anatomy of the pharynx and esophagus is outlined so that there is less chance of iatrogenic injury upon instrumentation. It permits assessment of esophageal motility and demonstrates the presence and reducibility of a hiatal hernia. Provocative testing for the presence of reflux at barium esophagography is often positive in normal subjects and should not be used. Video recording of the study increases usefulness to the clinician and provides a basis for the radiologist to compare studies.

Endoscopy and Biopsy

Endoscopy reveals the presence of esophagitis and permits acquisition of tissue for histologic examination. All patients with dysphagia should have endoscopy with biopsy of mucosal abnormalities to rule out cancer. The degree of esophagitis should be classified using one of the published systems. Our preferred grading system is given in Table 2. Biopsy is essential to diagnose specialized intestinal epithelium that may be invisible on endoscopy or interpreted as esophagitis. In cases of macroscopic Barrett's esophagus, four-quadrant biopsies every 2 cm and biopsy of any mucosal abnormality should be done to confirm the diagnosis and sample for the presence of high-grade dysplasia or cancer. In view of the rising incidence of adenocarcinoma of the cardia and the reports of specialized intestinal epithelium on biopsy specimens taken from this location, we advocate routine biopsy of the cardia in all patients undergoing endoscopy for the investigation of foregut symptoms. The detection of specialized intestinal metaplasia at this location may be associated with an increased risk of malignant degeneration as it is in the esophagus. Patients with this finding should be enrolled in a surveillance program so that dysplasia or early cancer in the cardia may be detected and cured by surgical resection.

Histologic examination of squamous epithelium may show signs associated with reflux disease, such as basal cell hyperplasia (>15% of the thickness of the epithelium comprising the basal zone where cells are separated by less than one nuclear diameter), increase in the number of papillae, and papillary elongation (papillae extending >65% of the thickness of the epithelium). These changes indicate irritation of the squamous epithelium and are

TABLE 2. Endoscopic Grading of Esophagitis

Grade	Endoscopic Findings
I	Erythema and friability
II	Linear erosions
III	Deeper and wider erosions with islands of edematous mucosa between erosive furrows
IV	Fibrous stricture or large ulcer

not specific for reflux disease. The presence of microscopic ulceration or an intraepithelial accumulation of neutrophils or eosinophils is more specific for reflux but may be due to other causes of esophageal inflammation. Further, these changes are not found in equal intensity in adjacent biopsy specimens, which may range from normal to inflamed.

Manometry and pH Testing

All patients should undergo stationary esophageal motility testing before ambulatory pH testing to ensure accurate placement of the pH probe. The motility test also provides information on the characteristics of the lower esophageal sphincter and function of the esophageal body, which are important in ruling out achalasia and planning the optimal mode of surgical repair.

Ambulatory pH monitoring detects pathologic reflux in the majority of patients with reflux disease. False-negative results are rare. Technical failures may cause a false-negative test. The pH probe should be calibrated in suitable buffers both before and after the test to ensure that there has been no electrode drift. The physician should check the pH tracing for evidence of technical failure. Misplacement of the pH probe at too high a position may cause a false-negative result. Rarely the probe is displaced after initial satisfactory placement by an episode of coughing or vomiting. Low acid content in the stomach, resulting from medication or chronic gastric atrophy, in pernicious anemia, and after surgery, may result in a negative pH test in a patient with reflux. Antacids and H_2-receptor antagonists should be discontinued at least 48 hours and proton pump inhibitors at least 2 weeks before the test. In some patients, a marked degree of duodenogastric reflux may be increasing gastric pH. This would require a large amount of duodenogastric reflux such that 40 to 70% of gastric content would have to consist of duodenal juice to maintain gastric pH greater than 4. It is possible that a patient may eat a smaller amount and therefore reflux less, or the tubing may cause an increase in salivation so that the esophageal pH profile is shifted to the alkaline range. Strictures may cause false-negative tests and should be dilated before the test. The stricture may prevent reflux of gastric content into the esophagus, and with associated poor contractility pooling of saliva shifts the pH profile in the alkaline direction.

If the patient's symptoms are typical for reflux disease and the pH test is negative, then the physician should search for causes of false-negative results. If the investigator suspects that there is hypochlorhydria, this can be assessed with gastric secretion studies. If there is hypochlorhydria, then an alternative to pH monitoring, such as ambulatory monitoring for the presence of duodenal juice using the Bilitec device, should be considered. The pH test should be repeated if there has been an avoidable failure or when there are no reasons for a false-negative test in a patient with esophagitis or typical symptoms. If the second test is negative, a nonreflux cause for the patient's symptoms or esophagitis should be sought.

Bilitec Device

The Bilitec device combines a data logger with a spectrophotometer that is carried on the patient's belt. The probe consists of a white Teflon reflector, a sampling area, and a bundle of optical fibers that carry alternating light signals (blue reference and green sampling) to the device. The light signal travels down the probe through the sampling area (and any material in it) and is reflected by the Teflon back up the probe, where the intensity of the reflected signal is measured. Absorbance at a wavelength of 453 nm is compared with the absorbance of the reference light to ensure that a reduction in absorbance is not due to blockage of the sampling area or loss of light from another cause. The maximal absorbance of bilirubin is close to 453 nm, which is used as a marker for the presence of duodenal juice in the same way as pH is used as a marker for the presence of gastric content. The Bilitec device is useful for detecting increased esophageal exposure to duodenal juice and may help predict the patients at greatest risk of progression to Barrett's esophagus. The role of this device in clinical decision-making is under evaluation.

Other Investigations

In certain circumstances, other tests may be added to these basic investigations to provide additional information. Ambulatory pH monitoring with dual pH probes placed in the proximal and distal esophagus can provide objective evidence of reflux into the upper esophagus in patients with laryngeal and pulmonary symptoms. Some investigators have shown drops in tracheal pH in association with pulmonary symptoms. Assessment of esophageal motility over the circadian cycle permits correlation of motility abnormalities with symptoms in patients with noncardiac chest pain. It also shows the response of the esophagus to a meal, which is a more physiologic situation than the conventional assessment using swallows of water in the supine position.

The acid perfusion test lacks the sensitivity and specificity of ambulatory pH monitoring and for this reason has fallen out of favor. A worrying aspect of this test is that it may be negative in patients with Barrett's esophagus who have a reduced sensitivity to acid. As part of the ambulatory pH test, the examiner may look for correlation between symptoms noted in the patient's diary and reflux episodes on the pH record; this is the essence of the Bernstein test. A standard or modified acid reflux test similarly lacks the sensitivity and specificity of ambulatory pH monitoring. This test may be useful in cases of decreased acid content of the stomach when pH testing is likely to give a false-negative result and ambulatory monitoring for duodenal juice using the Bilitec device is not available.

MEDICAL THERAPY

The nonsurgical therapies for gastroesophageal reflux disease are lifestyle modifications and drugs to neutralize acid, suppress acid secretion, or enhance motility in the foregut. It is conventional to start with lifestyle modifications and add the minimal drug therapy that keeps the patient free from symptoms and complications.

Lifestyle modifications form part of conservative management of the patient. Advice may be given to lose weight, stop smoking, elevate the head of the bed, avoid recumbency for 3 hours after eating, and avoid fat, chocolate, peppermint, and onions. Treatment with medication should be accompanied by advice on lifestyle modifications.

Histamine-receptor antagonists were the first drugs to have a marked impact on gastroesophageal reflux disease. Results of trials are variable, with about 60% amelioration of symptoms and 50% initial healing in esophagitis. However, relapse is common on cessation of therapy. Lifelong maintenance therapy is required for a group of patients. The efficacy of maintenance therapy with ranitidine (Zantac), 150 to 300 mg daily, in maintaining the patient free from esophagitis varies between 10 and 83%.

Proton pump inhibitors are more effective than H_2-receptor antagonists and give symptom relief and initial healing of esophagitis in 80% of patients. Discontinuation of omeprazole (Prilosec) is frequently followed by return of the patient's symptoms. In patients who have been free from heartburn, the return of symptoms is less tolerable. In these patients and in those whose esophagitis relapses on cessation of therapy, lifelong maintenance therapy is required. Maintenance therapy with omeprazole, 20 mg daily, is associated with a relapse rate in esophagitis of 11 to 33% within 1 year. A higher dose of 40 mg a day gives better results, with a relapse rate of 0 to 14%.

The main prokinetic agent in clinical use for the treatment of gastroesophageal reflux disease is cisapride (Propulsid), 10 mg 15 to 30 minutes before meals and at bedtime. Cisapride is superior to placebo for the relief of symptoms and healing of esophagitis. The effect of cisapride is comparable to that of cimetidine or ranitidine. When used in conjunction with cimetidine, there is a 46 to 70% improvement in the rate of healing of esophagitis. It is unknown whether the addition of cisapride to omeprazole increases symptom relief and healing of esophagitis.

Acid suppressant medications have their beneficial effects in gastroesophageal reflux disease by reducing the volume of gastric secretion and increasing gastric pH so that pepsin's activity is minimized. This reduces the injurious effects of the acid-peptic component of the refluxate and the volume of gastric content refluxed. Heartburn appears to be largely due to the effects of acid in the esophagus. Long-term acid suppressant therapy effectively relieves heartburn in the majority of patients. This lulls the patient and physician into a false sense of security while the reflux of gastric juice with a higher pH continues. Duodenal components of gastric juice have most of their deleterious effects in a nonacid pH range and as a consequence may be potentiated by acid suppressant therapy. In addition, acid may protect the esophagus against the effects of bile salts by causing their irreversible precipitation. Consequently, some patients progress to Barrett's esophagus while taking acid suppressant medication. Other patients remain symptomatic, and esophagitis persists despite increasing doses of acid suppressant medications.

SURGICAL THERAPY

The prerequisites for surgical therapy in a patient with suspected gastroesophageal reflux disease are objectively proven reflux, a mechanically defective lower esophageal sphincter, and proof that the patient's symptoms are caused by increased esophageal exposure to gastric content. The patient should have had a course of medical therapy, consisting of lifestyle modifications and acid suppressant therapy, for at least 8 to 12 weeks.

In patients with these prerequisites whose symptoms and esophagitis are controlled by medication, there is a choice between continued maintenance medical treatment and surgery. If the patient shows an incomplete response to medication with continued symptoms or persistent esophagitis, then surgery should be considered. When complications develop in a patient receiving medical therapy, there is clearly a treatment failure and surgery is indicated.

It is unfortunate that the patient is referred to surgery at this late stage, because the results are less satisfactory than for disease without complications. How can one tell which patients will go on to develop complications? Indications for surgery that are too liberal result in unnecessary operations with a small but significant morbidity and perhaps mortality. Too restrictive a policy results in many missed opportunities to prevent the complications of chronic gastroesophageal reflux disease. This is a difficult balance and more research is needed. From the data available at present, the following risk factors appear to be important.

Male Sex. There is a marked male preponderance in esophageal adenocarcinoma, with a slightly less marked male preponderance in Barrett's esophagus. Men are also more likely to have erosive esophagitis than women.

Family History. There are several reports in the literature of Barrett's esophagus or esophageal adenocarcinoma in many members of the same family. This may be due to a hereditary factor or to similar lifestyles or both. It is prudent to investigate and treat aggressively patients with such a family history.

Mechanical Defect in the Lower Esophageal Sphincter. The presence of a mechanically defective sphincter is a well-recognized indicator of poor prognosis. These patients respond less well to medical therapy and commonly have relapses.

Presence of Severe Esophagitis. Patients with Savary-Miller grade 3 or 4 esophagitis respond less well to medical therapy than patients with lesser grades of esophagitis. If the esophagitis does not heal after 4 weeks of medical therapy, then consideration should be given to surgery.

Pattern of Reflux. A combined upright and supine reflux pattern on ambulatory pH monitoring is associated with more advanced disease. Some investigators have reported that an isolated upright reflux pattern is associated with early disease. Caution should be observed in offering surgery to patients with a competent sphincter. If the patient has an incompetent sphincter, then the pattern of reflux is unimportant when there is increased esophageal exposure to acid.

Composition of the Refluxate. Increased esophageal exposure to duodenal juice is associated with advanced disease. Experimental evidence and clinical observation link esophageal exposure to duodenal juice to Barrett's esophagus and esophageal adeno-carcinoma. It is possible that patients without complications who have increased esophageal exposure to duodenal juice are more likely to develop progressive disease.

In patients with these risk factors, the choice between continued medical therapy and surgery should be swayed in the direction of surgery. It is wise to ask specifically about symptoms of gastric dysfunction in a patient being considered for antireflux surgery; if the patient complains of nausea, early satiety, or postprandial abdominal bloating, then preoperative assessment should include gastric emptying studies and an assessment for the presence of duodenogastric reflux.

Patients with extraesophageal manifestations of reflux disease, particularly pulmonary ones, are best managed by surgery.

THE TAILORED APPROACH TO SURGERY

With the wide spectrum of pathology in gastroesophageal reflux disease, no single operation is suitable for all cases (Figure 1). Factors to consider in the selection for the best operation in the patient with gastroesophageal reflux disease are the presence of complications, force of esophageal contraction, acid hypersecretion or history of peptic ulcer disease, duodenogastric reflux, delay in gastric emptying, and presence of hiatal hernia. Patients who have had previous gastric or antireflux surgery present especially complex cases and should be treated in a center with the facilities for complete assessment of foregut physiology and the expertise to apply the optimal surgical procedure tailored to the patient's pathophysiology. The chance of a satisfactory result in this group of patients is indirectly related to the number of previous attempts at repair. A thoracic approach should be considered when there has been previous gastric or antireflux surgery, severe stricture, short esophagus, obesity, or when thoracic access is required to deal with concomitant pulmonary pathology.

The transabdominal Nissen fundoplication is the procedure of choice for the straightforward patient with gastroesophageal reflux disease. The long-term results for this procedure in appropriately selected patients show that the actuarial success rate is greater than 90% at up to 10 years. These results are for the open procedure with an upper midline incision. Provided the operative indications are the same and that the operation is performed in the same manner, the newer laparoscopic Nissen fundoplication should have the same long-term results. Early reports are encouraging, but long-term results are not yet available.

The main contraindication to the abdominal Nissen fundoplication is poor motility in the esophageal body. In our laboratory, this is assessed from 10 wet swallows performed with the patient supine. Sensors are placed 1, 6, 11, 16, and 21 cm below the lower border of the upper esophageal sphincter. A median contraction amplitude less than the 2.5th percentile of normal (20 mm Hg) in any of the sensors placed at 11, 16, or 21 cm is used to define poor contractility. If there is greater than 20% simultaneous waves (peak-to-peak velocity greater than 20 cm per second) between these levels or poor contractility in all three sensors, then the patient has poor motility. Patients with poor motility have an inadequate force of esophageal contraction to overcome the resistance of a full fundoplication. If a full fundoplication is applied in this situation, there is a risk of dysphagia. A transthoracic Belsey partial fundoplication, along with full mobilization of the esophageal body to reduce tension

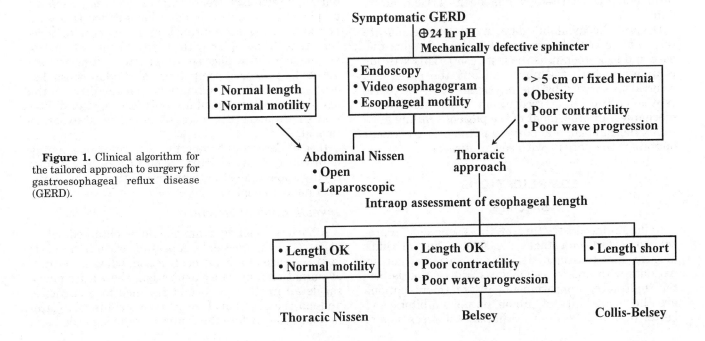

Figure 1. Clinical algorithm for the tailored approach to surgery for gastroesophageal reflux disease (GERD).

on the repair, gives a good result in most of these patients, but the procedure is not as effective in eliminating reflux as a complete fundoplication.

Esophageal shortening is defined as the presence of greater than 5 cm between the crura and the gastroesophageal junction on endoscopy or an irreducible hiatal hernia on a barium esophagogram. In this situation, an attempt to perform an abdominal Nissen fundoplication results in a plication placed around the proximal stomach ("slipped Nissen") or around the esophagus under undue tension; the result is a failed antireflux procedure. A thoracic approach is necessary first to mobilize the esophagus. If the repair can easily be placed within the abdomen, a transthoracic Nissen is the best option, provided esophageal contractility is adequate. If the repair cannot easily be placed in the abdomen, then a lengthening procedure in the form of a Collis gastroplasty is needed. After the new distal esophagus is constructed from the proximal stomach, a partial fundoplication is used to halt further reflux.

COMPARISON OF MEDICAL AND SURGICAL THERAPY

Many reports of long-term follow-up of patients undergoing antireflux surgery are a testament to its effectiveness. Such reports on the long-term follow-up of medically treated patients are lacking. There have been two trials of medical therapy compared with surgical therapy for chronic reflux disease. In the first, which compared the then optimal medical therapy of lifestyle modifications and antacids with a Nissen fundoplication, surgery was clearly superior. When H_2 blockers were introduced, the trial was repeated and surgery was again superior. A cost-benefit analysis showed that surgery was cheaper than medical therapy for patients younger than 49 years. No comparison of surgical therapy with long-term omeprazole therapy has been carried out to date.

Despite the available data, many physicians are reluctant to consider surgery for chronic reflux disease and look upon it as the last resort. This attitude is unfair to both the physician and the patient. A referral to surgery by the physician does not represent a failure but a recognition of the need for a mechanical improvement of the patient's failing antireflux mechanism, and surgery is the best treatment option for the patient with severe disease.

COMPLICATIONS

Stricture

Reflux-induced stricture of the esophagus represents one of the end stages of gastroesophageal reflux disease, and treatment is less satisfactory than for patients with erosive esophagitis. Prevention is better than cure. Improvements in treatment options are the availability of proton pump inhibitors and better dilatation systems. Schatzki's ring consists of mucosal hyperplasia and is not a true stricture. It is associated with reflux disease and may progress to stricture, particularly in patients who have esophagitis. Stricturing occurs when healing is accompanied by fibrosis. In most patients, fibrosis is confined to the submucosa, but in others it extends into the muscularis propria. Besides the depth of fibrosis, other important characteristics of reflux-induced strictures are their location in the esophagus, luminal diameter, and length. The lower border of the stricture is located just above the squamocolumnar junction, so when the junction is displaced orally, as in Barrett's esophagus, the stricture is found at a more proximal location. The internal luminal diameter of the stricture may be measured endoscopically and classed as mild (12 mm), moderate (10 to 12 mm), and severe (<10 mm). An open biopsy forceps (7.5 mm diameter for the 2.5-mm forceps) or the size of the endoscope may be used to measure the diameter of the stricture. Most reflux-induced strictures are short, less than 1 cm in length, but may be longer, particularly when associated with a superimposed drug injury.

In some patients there is no history of gastroesophageal reflux disease; instead, the history may be that after taking some medication for a headache the patient lay down to sleep and the next day had some chest pain that resolved but was followed by dysphagia. The pill usually lodges at one of the narrow areas in the esophagus such as the aortic arch, the level of the left main bronchus, or the gastroesophageal junction. The history and location of the stricture may suggest the possibility of pill injury to the clinician. Esophageal function testing may reveal an esophageal motor disorder and show no evidence of increased esophageal exposure to acid on ambulatory pH testing.

Associated pathologies include Zollinger-Ellison syndrome (10% of patients have strictures), scleroderma, previously treated achalasia, and Barrett's esophagus. Some patients develop a stricture after a period of nasogastric intubation. Patients with stricture tend to be older with a long history of gastroesophageal reflux disease. Diagnostic testing reveals markedly impaired competence of the lower esophageal sphincter and subnormal contractility in the distal esophagus. Ambulatory pH testing after dilatation shows markedly increased esophageal exposure to acid.

It is of paramount importance to rule out a malignant cause of any stricture regardless of how benign it may appear. Most patients presenting with a stricture have a neoplasm.

Investigation of Stricture

A barium esophagogram should be obtained before endoscopy when possible. A possible exception to this is in the case of a bolus obstruction, when a contrast examination may cause aspiration, show little mucosal detail in the presence of retained food particles, and make extraction of the bolus more difficult. Careful endoscopy before the contrast study is needed and should be therapeutic and diagnostic. In cases of mild stricture it is necessary to distend the esophagus to identify the stricture. This may be accomplished by asking the patient to swallow solid contrast agents ("barium burgers and marshmallows") or by positioning the patient prone and asking him or her to swallow liquid barium while esophagus is fluoroscoped. The barium study may overestimate the length of tight strictures because of streaming of the barium below the stricture.

All patients with a stricture should have urgent endoscopy to ensure that there is not an underlying malignancy. This may require several attempts at dilatation and biopsy. More biopsy specimens should be taken if there is a suspicion that this is a malignant stricture. Brush cytology is a useful adjuvant to forceps biopsy. Clues to a malignant stricture are abnormal location, long length, asymmetry on endoscopy, and heaped-up margins on the contrast study.

Management of Reflux-Induced Stricture

In the elderly frail patient, the best course of action is dilatation accompanied by maximal medical therapy. Dilatation needs to be repeated on a regular basis in most of these patients. Placement of an endoprosthesis across the stricture is contraindicated; reflux continues and the patient develops esophagitis and a further stricture proximal to the prosthesis, which becomes stuck and cannot be removed.

The optimal operative intervention must be tailored to the patient, depending on the underlying pathophysiology. The best predictor of the patient's response to surgery is dilatation. When possible the esophagus should be preserved, as the function of the natural esophagus is better than that of a substitute. Esophagectomy is required when there is transmural esophageal fibrosis, indicated by an undilatable stricture or persistent dysphagia after dilatation. If there is associated Barrett's epithelium, then all the esophagus containing Barrett's epithelium should be resected to eliminate the possibility of subsequent adenocarcinoma. A short distal esophagectomy with gastric pull-up into the left chest provides only temporary relief of dysphagia, as reflux is aggravated with early restricturing at the esophagogastrostomy. In this situation we prefer a colon interposition.

For the dilatable stricture, progressive preoperative dilatation to a No. 60 French bougie is recommended. Coexisting pathophysiology includes esophageal foreshortening and poor motility in the esophageal body. In these circumstances, an abdominal Nissen fundoplication is contraindicated. The mission of the surgeon is to safely restore swallowing and prevent restricturing by eliminating further reflux. There are two surgical strategies in this situation. The first, favored by many European surgeons, is to dilate the stricture and leave the esophagus alone but eliminate injurious agents by suppressing acid and diverting duodenal content. Acid suppression is accomplished by vagotomy and antrectomy, duodenal juice diversion by a Roux-en-Y reconstruction. The second approach, preferred by us, is to operate on the esophagus and tailor the repair to the underlying pathophysiology, as previously discussed.

The results of surgery for stricture are more effective and durable than continued medical therapy. With continued medical therapy, there is usually a need for repeated dilatations. With each dilatation there is a risk of perforation and other complications. Antireflux surgery is followed by excellent results in 65 to 92% of patients, with a rate of repeated dilatations (usually only once) of 1 to 30%. When esophageal resection is required for advanced disease, results are not as good, indicating the need for earlier effective treatment.

BARRETT'S ESOPHAGUS

Barrett's esophagus is an acquired condition that represents a peculiar form of healing that occurs at any stage in reflux disease. The squamous epithelium of the terminal esophagus is replaced by a columnar epithelium containing goblet cells. This specialized intestinal epithelium warrants special attention because it is the initiating step in a sequence of metaplasia to dysplasia to carcinoma. Barrett's metaplasia is accepted to be a complication of gastroesophageal reflux disease and links this common malady to one of the most lethal cancers.

The relative risk of a patient with benign Barrett's esophagus progressing to esophageal adenocarcinoma is 30 to 125 times the risk in the general population. The actual risk is about 500 adenocarcinomas per 100,000 patients with Barrett's esophagus per year.

Dysplasia and Barrett's Esophagus

Histologically, Barrett's epithelium may be classified as without dysplasia, indefinite for dysplasia, low-grade dysplasia, and high-grade dysplasia. An experienced pathologist is required to make the diagnosis. There is good pathologic agreement for the presence of high-grade dysplasia (86%), but for the lower grades of dysplasia agreement is less, with 75% for low-grade dysplasia and 58% for indefinite dysplasia. The main diagnostic difficulty for the pathologist regarding the presence of dysplasia is differentiation of the findings from those related to inflammation and regeneration. High-grade dysplasia looks like cancer but there is no evidence of invasion beyond the basement membrane of the epithelium. Some investigators refer to high-grade dysplasia as intraepithelial cancer.

Dysplasia is the best marker for the risk of progression to adenocarcinoma. Innovations such as cell flow cytometry to search for aneuploidy and immunohistochemistry to look for overexpression of tumor suppressor gene *p53* have not been shown to have greater predictive benefit than high-grade dysplasia. In patients who undergo esophagectomy for high-grade dysplasia, adenocarcinoma is present in the resected specimen in 50% of cases.

Role of Surgery in Patients Free of Dysplasia

Many patients with Barrett's esophagus seen in our surgical clinic have developed Barrett's epithelium while receiving medical therapy. Experimental evidence supports a pathogenetic role for duodenal juice in the genesis of Barrett's esophagus and esophageal adenocarcinoma. Reflux of duodenal content into the esophagus continues despite medical therapy aimed at acid suppression. There are no prospective trials that compare the prognosis of patients with Barrett's esophagus randomized to receive either medical or surgical therapy, but one report has shown a lower rate of progression to cancer in patients with Barrett's esophagus after surgery than in those who continue with medical therapy. For these reasons, we recommend that patients with Barrett's esophagus should be considered for antireflux surgery rather than being managed by continued medical therapy. Surgery restores lower esophageal sphincter function and abolishes reflux of both gastric and duodenal juice into the esophagus. This eliminates further damage to Barrett's epithelium and normal esophageal mucosa. It is still recommended that after surgical therapy the patient should continue with annual endoscopic surveillance.

Management of the Patient with Low-Grade Dysplasia

Low- or indefinite-grade epithelial dysplasia means that the pathologist cannot be sure whether the changes in the specimen represent a neoplastic process or are due to regeneration and inflammation. If medical therapy was not previously used, the patient should receive an intensive course of medical therapy, and the endoscopy should be repeated, with biopsy of the four quadrants of the esophagus every 2 cm of macroscopic Barrett's epithelium and areas of mucosal abnormality. If there is no evidence of high-grade dysplasia, the patient should be treated with an antireflux procedure followed by surveillance every 6 months until the low-grade dysplasia regresses.

Management of the Patient with High-Grade Dysplasia

Management decisions about a patient with high-grade dysplasia should not be made until two experienced pathologists have reviewed the slides and agreed on the diagnosis. Some investigators believe that the patient with high-grade dysplasia can be safely followed up with repeated biopsy and referred for esophagectomy when adenocarcinoma develops. The idea behind this approach is that some patients do progress to adenocarcinoma or die of another cause before adenocarcinoma develops.

Another approach is to treat all patients with high-grade dysplasia and who are fit for surgery with an esophagectomy. We reviewed our own experience with 17 patients referred from surveillance programs. Seven of 11 patients referred with the diagnosis of high-grade dysplasia had adenocarcinoma in the resected specimen. The tumor was intramucosal in five and submucosal in one, and in one patient who had ulceration the tumor reached the muscularis propria. None of these patients had lymph node metastases. The patients were all alive and well at follow-up, a median of 12 (range, 4 to 66) months. Aggressive rebiopsy of these patients before surgery revealed only two of the seven adenocarcinomas found in the surgical specimen. For this reason we believe that it is not possible to be sure that there is no adenocarcinoma when the patient has high-grade dysplasia.

Because of the difficulty in ensuring that a patient with high-grade dysplasia does not have adenocarcinoma, the future risk of the patient developing adenocarcinoma if it is not present, and the relative safety with which elective esophagectomy can be performed in expert hands, we advocate esophagectomy for the patient with high-grade dysplasia. A careful continued surveillance policy should be adopted only for the patient who is judged unfit for surgery. The aim of surveillance in patients with Barrett's esophagus is to detect adenocarcinoma at an early curable stage. Once high-grade dysplasia is found, surveillance has served its purpose and has detected the patient who will benefit from esophagectomy.

GASTRITIS AND PEPTIC ULCER DISEASE

method of
MICHAEL B. KIMMEY, M.D.
University of Washington Medical Center
Seattle, Washington

Medical practitioners consider the diagnoses of gastritis and peptic ulcer disease together in several clinical situations. Whereas there is overlap between these two diagnoses, they are different pathologically. In many cases, pathologic and diagnostic tests are not available, so a diagnosis is given on the basis of symptoms alone. The astute clinician should distinguish symptoms from a specific diagnosis and tailor therapy for the individual patient on the basis of a current knowledge of the pathophysiologic mechanisms of these diverse conditions.

In this article, the treatment of several upper gastrointestinal problems is divided into categories based on what information is known to the treating clinician. In some instances, this is only symptoms; in other situations, specific diagnostic information is available. An effort to separate these different situations is made because the best prescribing will be done by the clinician who can separate symptoms from diagnosis.

DYSPEPSIA

Dyspepsia is a term used to describe a range of symptoms that originate in the upper gastrointestinal tract. Epigastric pain or discomfort, usually of mild to moderate severity, is the predominant component of dyspepsia. Nausea, vomiting, a sense of indigestion, and anorexia may also be present. The relationship of the symptoms to eating is variable but should be sought. The pain may be relieved, exacerbated, or unaffected by all or only certain types of food.

There are numerous causes of the symptom dyspepsia. It is a common symptom of patients with peptic ulcer disease (see later); however, only about 20% of patients with dyspepsia have an ulcer. On evaluation with endoscopy or radiographic contrast-enhanced studies, those without an ulcer are often said to have "nonulcer dyspepsia." This term is also not a specific diagnosis and refers to patients with the symptom of dyspepsia in whom no organic cause can be found. It is usually not possible to distinguish patients with nonulcer dyspepsia from those with an ulcer by symptoms alone. Histologically confirmed gastritis and *Helicobacter pylori* infection (see later) are infrequent causes of dyspepsia.

Several other gastrointestinal conditions may present with dyspepsia as the predominant symptom. Gastroesophageal reflux disease is probably the most common cause when one is identifiable (see the article on gastroesophageal reflux disease). These patients often describe a burning retrosternal discomfort and regurgitation of stomach contents into their mouths or throats. Motility disturbances of the stomach or upper intestine may also cause dyspepsia. Nausea, bloating, and early satiety are other frequent complaints of patients with motility disorders. These patients may also have other intestinal complaints such as diarrhea and/or constipation and are probably afflicted with a variant of the irritable bowel syndrome (see the article on irritable bowel syndrome). Lactose intolerance may also cause dyspepsia along with more typical symptoms of bloating and diarrhea.

Dyspepsia may also be a side effect of several medications, including some antibiotics, medications for osteoporosis, and nonsteroidal anti-inflammatory drugs (NSAIDs). Drugs in this class more commonly cause dyspepsia than ulcers, and most patients with NSAID-associated dyspepsia do not have ulcers.

Cholelithiasis and chronic pancreatitis can sometimes present with dyspepsia, although other features usually suggest these diagnoses. Cholelithiasis generally results in severe epigastric pain with radiation to the back or right scapula that lasts for several hours after being precipitated by eating. Pain from chronic pancreatitis may also be precipitated by meals and radiates to the back but is more of a dull, boring pain and is often accompanied by nausea or vomiting.

Evaluation of the Dyspeptic Patient

A complete history and physical examination should be performed to recognize possible causes of dyspepsia and also to identify patients with findings that cause concern for the presence of a more serious problem. Simple laboratory tests such as a blood count, liver enzyme activities, and a serum amylase determination can also be helpful in this regard. Abdominal ultrasonography is an effective screening test when considering gallstones or pancreatitis as a cause of the symptoms. An aggressive diagnostic evaluation is recommended for patients with fever, weight loss, dysphagia, new onset of dyspepsia in individuals older than 45 years, anemia, melena, and hematemesis. Other patients may be candidates for empirical treatment, with further evaluation reserved for those patients whose symptoms are refractory to empirical therapy.

Treatment

Symptoms of dyspepsia usually resolve with effective treatment of its underlying cause (see later). When the cause of dyspepsia is not known, empirical treatment may be attempted if there are no findings to suggest the presence of a serious underlying disease. Reassurance and alleviation of anxiety are sometimes the only intervention required. Some patients may also benefit from treatment with medications, however.

Drugs that reduce gastric acid are used most commonly for this purpose. In fact, patients often have treated themselves with antacids or over-the-counter (OTC) histamine H_2-receptor blockers before they see a physician. The response to antacids may be of limited duration or associated with side effects of diarrhea when these agents are taken in sufficient quantity. If the response to the OTC H_2 blockers is partial, then prescribing prescription doses of the same medication (two times greater than the OTC dose) will often be effective. A 6-week course of therapy is usually prescribed if there is a beneficial response to allow time for healing of undiagnosed ulcers.

When the patient's dyspepsia is associated with significant heartburn and regurgitation, use of a proton pump inhibitor may be necessary to control symptoms. Cisapride (Propulsid) may also be useful if the reflux occurs primarily at night or after late evening meals. Cisapride may also be useful for the dyspeptic patient with an underlying motility disorder.

Empirical treatment of dyspepsia with antibiotics is discouraged. Serologic diagnosis of *H. pylori* infection is inexpensive, sensitive, and specific and should be pursued before antibiotics are prescribed (see later). Other medications that have been used with variable success in the treatment of dyspepsia include sucralfate (Carafate) and anticholinergic drugs with or without a sedative or benzodiazepine (Levsin, Donnatal, Librium, others). When nausea is a prominent symptom, use of cisapride, metoclopramide (Reglan), or phenothiazine-type antiemetics (prochlorperazine [Compazine], others) can be helpful.

The empirical treatment of dyspepsia without a firm diagnosis has its drawbacks. The duration of therapy, what to do with relapses on discontinuation of therapy, and how closely to observe the patient all become potential problems for the clinician. Many of these patients ultimately undergo further diagnostic testing including upper endoscopy such that the cost savings from avoiding endoscopy in the short term may not be realized in the long term.

GASTRITIS

The correct definition of gastritis is "inflammation of the stomach." This can be detected reliably only with histologic evaluation of the gastric mucosa. Symptoms of dyspepsia should not be called gastritis. Endoscopic and radiographic appearances are also unreliable and should not be used to make the diagnosis of gastritis.

The main cause of true gastritis is *H. pylori* infection. This common infection causes gastric inflammation but is asymptomatic in the overwhelming majority of those who have it. NSAIDs and bile reflux, especially after gastric surgery, also cause gastritis. Other less frequent causes of gastritis include autoimmune disease associated with vitamin B_{12} deficiency, Crohn's disease of the stomach, sarcoidosis, and rarely syphilis and other infections. Other manifestations of these diseases are usually present that direct the alert physician to the correct diagnosis.

Treatment

Effective treatment of *H. pylori* infection causes resolution of gastric inflammation. The presence of gastritis alone, however, is not an indication for antibiotic treatment. Specific treatment of other causes of gastritis (e.g., avoidance of NSAIDs, prednisone for Crohn's or eosinophilic gastritis, antibiotics for syphilitic gastritis) usually leads to resolution of gastric inflammation.

PEPTIC ULCER DISEASE

Ulcers are breaks or defects in the gastrointestinal mucosal lining that extend into deeper parts of the gastrointestinal wall. They may occur in the esophagus, usually caused by gastroesophageal reflux disease, or in the stomach or duodenum. The latter ulcers have traditionally been called peptic ulcers, although this term implies nothing about etiology. The majority of these ulcers are benign and heal with medical treatment. Duodenal ulcers are rarely malignant; however, between 2 and 4% of otherwise benign-appearing gastric ulcers are really ulcerated adenocarcinomas. This risk for malignant change mandates that all gastric ulcers either be examined by biopsy at the time of diagnosis or have healing confirmed with follow-up imaging studies.

There are other less dramatic differences between gastric and duodenal ulcers. Duodenal ulcers are associated with *H. pylori* infection 95% of the time, whereas only 70% of patients with gastric ulcers have this infection. The remainder of gastric ulcers are caused predominantly by NSAIDs, medications that have a greater effect on the stomach than on the duodenum. Gastric ulcers are also more difficult to treat than duodenal ulcers, often requiring longer courses of more potent medications.

Cigarette smoking is another factor that contributes to ulcer disease. Smokers have a twofold greater risk for developing an ulcer than do nonsmokers. Smokers are also more likely to have an ulcer complication and have delayed ulcer healing with standard medications. The problem of delayed healing is less pronounced if concomitant *H. pylori* infection is treated. Stress and diet do not contribute significantly to ulcer development. Other rare causes of ulcers include gastric acid hypersecretion (e.g., gastrinoma) and Crohn's disease.

The typical symptoms of a duodenal ulcer are a burning epigastric pain without radiation that is most apparent a few hours after eating or at night. The pain is usually relieved by eating or taking antacids. Gastric ulcers may cause similar symptoms or may be associated with pain that is increased by eating and may be located in the left upper quadrant. Nausea or vomiting may accompany the pain. Ulcers associated with NSAID use are often painless.

Ulcers can also cause life-threatening problems. Bleeding is the most common ulcer complication and may present with anemia, melena, or hematemesis. Prompt gastrointestinal endoscopy is desirable to accurately diagnose and often treat the cause of bleeding. Endoscopic findings also assist in the decision on whether to hospitalize the patient. Perforated ulcers can cause peritonitis and require emergency surgery. Chronic recurrent ulcers can also lead to strictures of the pylorus or duodenum, resulting in gastric outlet obstruction.

The diagnosis of an ulcer is usually made with an upper gastrointestinal x-ray study or with endoscopy. Endoscopy is more sensitive than radiography and allows biopsy of gastric ulcers to exclude malignant disease. However, endoscopy is more expensive than radiography. Upper gastrointestinal x-ray studies are less useful in detecting ulcer recurrences and ulcers after gastric surgery because of scarring and other anatomic alterations.

Treatment

The goals of treating the patient with peptic ulcer disease are the alleviation of symptoms, the avoidance of complications, and the prevention of ulcer recurrence. Pain usually responds within 1 week of beginning medications that inhibit acid secretion (Table 1). Breakthrough pain can be managed with antacids as needed; liquid antacids may be more effective than tablets. Avoiding ulcer complications requires ulcer healing. This is also usually achievable with the same antisecretory medications given for 4 to 12 weeks. Proton pump inhibitors heal most ulcers an average of 2 weeks (for duodenal ulcers) to 4 weeks (for gastric ulcers) faster than H_2 blockers.

Other treatments that promote ulcer healing are also available. Sucralfate is an organic complex of

TABLE 1. **Drugs Used for Ulcer Healing**

Agent	Dose	Duration (wk) Duodenal Ulcer	Gastric Ulcer
Antacids			
Magnesium-aluminum hydroxides (Mylanta, Maalox, Riopan, others)	30 mL qid	6	Not advised
Aluminum hydroxides (Amphojel, ALternaGEL)	30 mL qid	6	Not advised
Calcium carbonates (Tums, others)	1500 mg qid	6	Not advised
H₂-Receptor Antagonists			
Cimetidine (Tagamet)	400 mg bid	6	8–12*
Ranitidine (Zantac)	150 mg bid	6	8–12*
Nizatidine (Axid)	150 mg bid	6	8–12*
Famotidine (Pepcid)	20 mg bid *or* 40 mg hs	6	8–12*
Proton Pump Inhibitors			
Omeprazole (Prilosec)	20 mg qd	4	—
	20 mg bid	—	4–8*
Lansoprazole (Prevacid)	30 mg qd	4	—
	30 mg bid	—	4–8*
Others			
Sucralfate (Carafate)	1 gm qid	8	8–12*

*Longer durations are recommended for large (>2 cm) ulcers.

aluminum that binds to ulcers and promotes healing through several potential mechanisms. The prostaglandin analogue misoprostol (Cytotec)* also promotes ulcer healing, but medication-related side effects limit compliance with this drug. Stopping NSAIDs and treating *H. pylori* infection also have beneficial effects on ulcer healing that are independent of the prevention of recurrence. Diet and reduction in activity have no role in the treatment of peptic ulcer disease.

Surgery for uncomplicated ulcer disease is fortunately only of historical interest. Vagotomy with or without antrectomy cured ulcers but at the expense of numerous side effects, such as dumping syndrome and bile reflux gastritis. Surgery is now reserved for ulcer complications: bleeding ulcers that cannot be stopped with endoscopy, perforated ulcers, and gastric outlet obstruction that is not adequately treated with endoscopic balloon dilatation.

Approximately two thirds of ulcers recur within 1 year of ulcer healing, and about half of these recurrences are symptomatic. Successful treatment of *H. pylori* infection reduces annual ulcer recurrences to less than 5%. *H. pylori* infection should be sought and treated if it is present in all patients with ulcers. Even if the patient has another potential reason for ulcers, such as NSAID use, the *H. pylori* infection should still be treated.

The majority of ulcer patients without *H. pylori* infection are taking NSAIDs. These drugs should be

*Not FDA approved for this indication.

avoided if possible and less ulcerogenic medications substituted (Table 2). When NSAIDs are required for inflammatory-type pain, cotherapy with misoprostol has been shown to reduce the frequency of recurrent ulcers and ulcer complications. When misoprostol is not tolerated owing to side effects of diarrhea and abdominal cramping, use of a proton pump inhibitor may also reduce the frequency of ulcer recurrence. Avoidance of NSAIDs is the best strategy because none of the prophylactic regimens completely eliminates the risk for recurrent ulcers and ulcer complications.

Patients who do not have *H. pylori* infection and who are not taking NSAIDs require special consideration. Serum gastrin levels should be checked to detect the rare patient with gastrinoma. In this condition, ulcers are typically multiple and may be associated with diarrhea caused by the high levels of acid secretion. Long-term treatment of ulcer patients who do not have an underlying cause identified has not been well defined. Those without ulcer complications can be followed up after ulcer healing. If they have recurrent ulcers or if an ulcer complication is present, maintenance therapy should be considered. Full doses of H₂ blockers, twice-daily sucralfate, or single doses of a proton pump inhibitor are all reasonable options for these infrequent patients.

HELICOBACTER PYLORI INFECTION

H. pylori selectively colonizes gastric-type epithelium, leading to a local inflammatory reaction (gastri-

TABLE 2. **Ulcer Risk of Analgesic and Anti-inflammatory Drugs**

No risk
  Acetaminophen (Tylenol)
  Tramadol (Ultram)
  Narcotics (numerous agents)
Low risk
  Nonacetylated salicylates
    Salsalate (Disalcid)
    Choline-magnesium trisalicylate (Trilisate)
Moderate risk
  Low-dose aspirin (<325 mg/d)
  Etodolac (Lodine)
  Nabumetone (Relafen)
Higher risk
  Aspirin (in higher doses)
  Diclofenac (Voltaren, Cataflam)
  Diflunisal (Dolobid)
  Fenoprofen (Nalfon)
  Ibuprofen (Motrin, Advil,* Nuprin*)
  Indomethacin (Indocin)
  Ketoprofen (Orudis, Oruvail, Actron*)
  Ketorolac (Toradol)
  Mefenamic acid (Ponstel)
  Meclofenamate
  Naproxen (Naprosyn, Aleve*)
  Oxaprozin (Daypro)
  Piroxicam (Feldene)
  Tolmetin (Tolectin)
Highest risk for ulcer bleeding
  NSAIDs plus steroids or oral anticoagulants

*Available without a prescription in the United States.
Abbreviation: NSAIDs = nonsteroidal anti-inflammatory drugs.

tis) and a systemic immune response. This is probably the most common bacterial infection of humans. Most evidence suggests that it is transmitted between humans by the fecal-oral or oral-oral routes. It is more common in developing than in developed countries and is more prevalent in lower socioeconomic groups. In developed countries, infection is much more common in those born before World War II than in those born later.

Acute infection with *H. pylori* causes abdominal pain and a temporary reduction in acid secretion by the stomach. Chronic infection with its resultant gastritis is usually asymptomatic, however. As discussed before, *H. pylori* is associated with most cases of ulcers, probably through a variety of mechanisms. These include increased levels of acid secretion and reduced mucosal defenses caused by the infection. *H. pylori* infection is also associated with gastric cancer and gastric lymphoma, although other factors are likely to play a role in the pathogenesis of these malignant neoplasms.

There are several ways to diagnose *H. pylori* infection. All of the available tests have sensitivities and specificities above 90% for detecting *H. pylori* infection. The choice of test depends primarily on the specific clinical situation. Detection of antibodies to *H. pylori* in either serum or whole blood is the least invasive and least expensive. Serology should be used for diagnosis of infection when endoscopy is not required. Serology is less useful for documenting treatment response because antibodies persist for years after successful treatment. When endoscopy is being done for other reasons, three biopsy specimens should be taken from the gastric antrum. One of the biopsy specimens can be placed into one of several available rapid urease tests, which may give a positive result within 1 hour. If the rapid urease test result is negative, the other two biopsy specimens can be sent for histologic evaluation of the presence of gastritis and for special stains that demonstrate *H. pylori*. Confirmation of effective *H. pylori* treatment, when needed (see later), is best achieved by a carbon-labeled urea breath test administered at least 1 month after antibiotics have been stopped.

Treatment

The primary indication for treating *H. pylori* is current or past ulcer disease. Other less common indications include the rare patient who has gastric mucosa-associated lymphoid tissue lymphoma and possibly the patient who has a first-degree relative with gastric cancer. Less accepted indications are patients with nonulcer dyspepsia. Most double-blind, placebo-controlled studies in *H. pylori*–positive dyspeptic subjects have not shown a significant advantage to *H. pylori* eradication.

Numerous antibiotic regimens have been proposed for the treatment of *H. pylori* infection (Table 3). Combinations of two or three antibiotics are required to eradicate this organism. Adding an agent that reduces gastric acid secretion (e.g., omeprazole [Prilo-

TABLE 3. **Treatment Regimens for *Helicobacter pylori***

Agent	Dose	Duration (d)
Bismuth-Based Therapy		
Triple therapy*		14
Bismuth subsalicylate (Pepto-Bismol)	525 mg qid	
Tetracycline†	500 mg qid	
Metronidazole (Flagyl)	250 mg qid	
Triple therapy + proton pump inhibitor	(see above)	
Omeprazole (Prilosec)	20 mg bid	7
or		
Lansoprazole (Prevacid)	30 mg bid	7
Ranitidine bismuth citrate (Tritec)	400 mg bid	14‡
plus		
Clarithromycin (Biaxin)	500 mg tid	14
Dual Therapy		
Omeprazole (Prilosec)	20 mg bid	14
or		
Lansoprazole (Prevacid)	30 mg bid	14
plus		
Clarithromycin (Biaxin)§	500 mg tid	14
Proton Pump Inhibitor with Two Antibiotics		
Omeprazole (Prilosec)	20 mg bid	7
or		
Lansoprazole (Prevacid)	30 mg bid	7
plus		
Clarithromycin (Biaxin)	500 mg bid	7
plus		
Metronidazole (Flagyl)‖	500 mg bid	7

*Also available in a prepackaged multidose form (Helidac).

†Amoxicillin (500 mg qid) can be substituted for tetracycline, but efficacy is reduced by about 20%.

‡Can be continued for an additional 2 wk to achieve duodenal ulcer healing.

§Use of amoxicillin instead of clarithromycin has unacceptably low success rates and should not be a first-line regimen.

‖Amoxicillin (1 gm bid) can be substituted for metronidazole, especially if there is a history of significant metronidazole exposure.

sec], lansoprazole [Prevacid], or ranitidine [Zantac]) improves eradication rates and reduces the upper gastrointestinal side effects that are associated with the antibiotics. When an ulcer is present, these drugs also reduce ulcer pain and speed ulcer healing. Compliance with these often complicated multidrug regimens is also important. All of the regimens listed in Table 3 should achieve eradication of *H. pylori* in more than 80% of patients if they are compliant with taking the medications.

Several factors should be considered in selecting an *H. pylori* treatment regimen for the individual patient. Up to one third of isolates of *H. pylori* are resistant to metronidazole (Flagyl), so this antibiotic should not be used if the patient has had significant metronidazole use in the past. Resistance to clarithromycin (Biaxin) is less common (less than 10%), and resistance to amoxicillin (Amoxil) is nonexistent currently. Reliability and compliance of the patient, cost of the treatment regimen, and whether a coexisting ulcer is present are other factors that affect treatment choice. For most patients, the 1-week, twice-daily regimen of a proton pump inhibitor (omeprazole or lansoprazole) with two antibiotics (clarithromycin and either metronidazole or amoxicillin) is the treatment of choice because it is simple and effective in more than 90% of patients.

Recurrence of infection after successful treatment is uncommon. Recurrence rates of about 2% in the first year and less than 1% annually in subsequent years have been reported. Routine surveillance for recurrent infection and even for the effectiveness of eradication is not advised for most patients. The main exception is patients who have had ulcer complications. Eradication should be confirmed in these patients by repeated endoscopy and biopsy or the urea breath test before antisecretory therapy is discontinued.

SUMMARY

A knowledge of the differences and overlaps between dyspepsia, gastritis, and peptic ulcer disease will lead to more effective prescribing practices. These conditions are common, so diagnostic testing is used selectively. However, widespread treatment of *H. pylori* infection is not advocated because of limited information about the effectiveness and consequences of this treatment except in patients with ulcer disease. In these patients, *H. pylori* eradication can produce a dramatic reduction in health care costs and improvement in the quality of the patient's life.

TUMORS OF THE STOMACH

method of
FRANK L. LANZA, M.D.
Baylor College of Medicine
Houston, Texas

Despite its rapidly decreasing incidence in the United States, gastric cancer is still the second most common cause of death from cancer worldwide. Adenocarcinoma represents 95% of all gastric malignant neoplasms. Of the remainder, 4% are gastric lymphoma and 1% are various sarcomas. The etiology of gastric cancer is unknown. However, many epidemiologic factors have been identified that are of considerable interest. The incidence of gastric carcinoma is higher in countries in which smoked or salted fish or meat constitutes a high proportion of the diet. Underdeveloped and developing countries have a much higher incidence of cancer of the stomach than do Western nations, especially the United States. A link has recently been found between *Helicobacter pylori* infection and gastric adenocarcinoma. *H. pylori* is thought to be the major cause of chronic, superficial gastritis, which leads to atrophic gastritis, intestinal metaplasia, and ultimately gastric cancer. This may explain the increased incidence of gastric cancer in undeveloped nations that also have the highest prevalence of *H. pylori* infection. There is also a link between *H. pylori* infection and B cell mucosa-associated lymphoid tissue (MALT) tumors. Although gastric cancer in general has decreased in incidence in North America during the past several decades, there has been a relative increase in the number of cases of adenocarcinoma of the cardia of the stomach. Whether this is truly a gastric lesion or an adenocarcinoma of the distal esophagus arising from specialized columnar epithelium, known as Barrett's mucosa, that is found in patients with severe gastroesophageal reflux disease is unknown.

ADENOCARCINOMA

Diagnosis

Because gastric cancer can be cured only by complete surgical excision of all neoplastic tissue, it becomes critically important to diagnose this disease early in its course. In countries such as Japan where the incidence of gastric cancer is high, screening programs, much like those for colon cancer in the United States, are in place. Many asymptomatic patients with early gastric cancer are diagnosed in that country by surveillance with upper gastrointestinal endoscopy or radiography. Endoscopy is a much more accurate technique and has a far higher yield than radiography, even when good double-contrast air and barium upper gastrointestinal radiography is employed. All symptomatic patients should definitely undergo endoscopy. Unfortunately, by the time gastric cancer is symptomatic, the disease has usually progressed to an incurable state. The Japanese have classified early gastric cancer into three types, some of which are difficult to recognize even endoscopically. Application of Congo red–methylene blue dye to the gastric mucosa during endoscopy can aid in the early diagnosis of small lesions. Biopsy of all gastric lesions should be performed. Six to eight biopsy specimens are optimal, and in the case of ulcerating lesions, they should be obtained from the edge of the crater. Cytologic examination is less often used today because biopsy techniques have been shown to be extremely accurate. Cytology is probably best used in follow-up examinations in patients in whom malignant disease is suspected but prior biopsy results have been negative. In these cases, brush or salvage cytology is preferred to gastric washing.

Treatment

The only curative treatment for adenocarcinoma of the stomach is gastric resection. It is extremely important to define the extent of tumor before surgery. The old Borrmann classification for gastric cancer has been largely replaced by the newer TNM classification. This system assesses tumor by its degree of invasion (T), nodal involvement (N), and presence or absence of distant metastasis (M). Patients with stage I cancer confined to the mucosa and not penetrating into the muscularis propria have a 5-year survival rate of almost 90%. Preoperative methods of assessment include computed tomography (CT) of the abdomen and endoscopic ultrasonography (EUS). However, final staging of gastric cancer can be made only after exploratory laparotomy. Nodal metastases are especially difficult to detect with both EUS and CT. It was previously thought that the only adequate operation for the cure of gastric cancer was total gastrectomy. The reason for this recommendation was that most series of surgeries for gastric cancer were reported from the United States and western Europe, where this disease, unfortunately, presents late in its clinical course. It is now recognized that lesser surgical procedures are adequate for earlier and more localized gastric cancers. The Japanese in particular, using their surveillance techniques, are finding many early stage I adenocarcinomas of the stomach. In many cases, these are being successfully treated by local excision, sometimes with use of strip mucosal resections and suction and ligation techniques that can be performed through the endoscope. In Western countries, traditional gastric resection is usually still performed. The surgery of choice for carcinoma confined to the gastric antrum with or without nodal metastasis is distal subtotal gastrectomy. For lesions of the cardia and upper stomach, total gastric resection is still the preferred procedure. Proximal hemigastrectomies lead to significant postoperative morbidity and are generally unsatisfactory. The value of extensive regional lymphadenectomy is still controversial. Reports from Japan would seem to indicate that this does improve survival, but this may also reflect diagnosis of an earlier stage of disease. Splenectomy is a consideration when tumor is located along the greater curvature of the upper stomach and there are nodal metastases in this area.

Palliative resection should be considered in those cases in which there is extensive nodal involvement, large bulky tumor with penetration into adjacent tissues, and liver or other distant metastasis. Palliation is indicated when gastric outlet obstruction is present or if there is significant hemorrhage from an ulcerated lesion. If it is technically feasible to remove tumor in these situations, it is probably advisable to do so. There is no real value in second operations for anastomotic recurrences, nor is there any good indication for resection of metastatic disease.

Radiotherapy alone has not been shown to be effective in improving cure rates. Intraoperative adjuvant radiation may show some promise, but this technique has not been thoroughly evaluated. Radiation combined with chemotherapy has shown little benefit.

Chemotherapy for the treatment of metastatic disease produces generally low response rates. The most commonly used agents are 5-fluorouracil (5-FU), mitomycin C (Mutamycin), and doxorubicin (Adriamycin), which are much more effective in combination than singularly and when used in this manner are referred to as FAM. Response rates, i.e., a 50% decrease in the size of measurable tumor, are in the range of 30 to 35%. Postsurgical adjuvant chemotherapy with various agents has been proved to be of no significant value.

GASTRIC LYMPHOMA

The gastrointestinal tract is the most common site for extranodal occurrence of lymphoma. Sixty percent of these lesions occur in the stomach and are often associated with chronic gastritis. They are clinically indistinguishable from gastric carcinoma and the various sarcomas. The most common histologic type is diffuse histiocytic lymphoma. B cell–type MALT lymphoma has been associated with H. pylori infection in populations remarkably similar to those at risk for gastric carcinoma. The clinical symptoms and diagnostic techniques referable to gastric lymphoma do not differ from those for gastric carcinoma.

Gastric lymphoma is often treated surgically; however, in these cases, staging is extremely important because chemotherapy and radiotherapy play a large role in treatment when there is disease beyond the confines of the stomach. When extragastric disease is diagnosed preoperatively, the patient may be better treated with various standard chemotherapeutic protocols normally used in the treatment of the various lymphomas. Radiation may also play a role in these cases, especially when there is retroperitoneal nodal involvement.

There have been numerous reports of cures of B cell–type MALT lymphomas by treatment of H. pylori infection with triple-antibiotic therapy and acid suppression.

OTHER GASTRIC MALIGNANT NEOPLASMS

Sarcomas of the stomach are quite rare. The most common of these is leiomyosarcoma, which cannot be distinguished clinically from gastric cancer or lymphoma. Other exceedingly rare gastric cancers include liposarcoma, fibrosarcoma, choriocarcinoma, and adenosquamous carcinoma. Diagnosis and treatment of these lesions do not differ from those for gastric carcinoma.

GASTRIC POLYPS

Gastric polyps are of two principal types, hyperplastic and adenomatous. Hyperplastic polyps are far more common and present little risk for malignant change. Some large hyperplastic polyps can contain mixed adenomatous elements. Adenomatous polyps are often premalignant and are more common in patients with atrophic gastritis and pernicious anemia.

Gastric polyps are usually asymptomatic. However, large polyps can be associated with iron deficiency anemia; in some cases, if they are located in the prepyloric antrum, they can produce obstructive symptoms by prolapsing into and intermittently obstructing the pylorus. The treatment of choice for most gastric polyps is endoscopic polypectomy. This is a relatively simple technique and allows retrieval of the entire polyp for histologic examination.

Adenomatous polyps usually occur singularly or in small numbers and can be easily managed endoscopically. Patients with proven adenomatous polyps should undergo surveillance endoscopy at least every 3 to 5 years. Patients with large numbers of polyps usually have hyperplastic lesions. The largest of these should be removed endoscopically and examined carefully for adenomatous elements. Patients with large numbers of hyperplastic polyps present a slightly different clinical problem. As noted previously, the largest of these should be removed and several others should be sampled by biopsy. If all lesions are completely hyperplastic, the patient should have surveillance endoscopy every 3 to 5 years. Biopsies and/or polypectomy should be performed when appropriate. All patients with familial polyposis syndrome should undergo at least one surveillance endoscopy.

CARCINOIDS

Carcinoid tumors usually occur in the upper stomach, are usually single, but in approximately 15% of the cases may be multiple. They are often asymptomatic or are found incidentally at endoscopy. Carcinoids are difficult to differentiate from other submucosal tumors in the upper stomach. They are rarely associated with the carcinoid syndrome; however, when this is the case, hepatic metastases are usually present. Carcinoids occur more commonly in patients with clinical entities associated with increased serum gastrin levels. These include Zollinger-Ellison syndrome, atrophic gastritis, and pernicious anemia. These lesions can usually be easily removed endoscopically, by either the snare and cautery or hot biopsy forceps techniques.

BENIGN GASTRIC TUMORS

Most benign gastric tumors are of mesenchymal origin and present as submucosal lesions. The most common of these is leiomyoma, which is usually found in the fundus and occasionally in the antrum. Other benign submucosal lesions include lipoma, fibroma, ectopic pancreas, eosinophilic granuloma, and glomus tumors.

It is extremely difficult to obtain diagnostic tissue from these lesions. The usual forceps biopsy is productive only of normal overlying mucosa. Various other biopsy techniques have been devised. These include the "lift and cut" technique, needle biopsies, and large loop cautery biopsies. EUS has been used to further define the nature of these lesions. This technique has been accurate in excluding malignant neoplasia in many of these patients. Lipomas and leiomyomas in particular can often be accurately diagnosed with EUS.

Except in the case of leiomyoma, which may ulcerate and hemorrhage extensively because of its vascularity, these lesions rarely require treatment. If they appear benign to an experienced endoscopist and results of both biopsy and ultrasound examination are negative, they may be followed up by interval endoscopy. If there is any change in size or appearance, surgical removal is advisable. If there is no change in the appearance of the lesion after 6 months and 1 year, no further follow-up is indicated.

TUMORS OF THE COLON AND RECTUM

method of
SIDNEY J. WINAWER, M.D.
Memorial Sloan-Kettering Cancer Center
New York, New York

Adenocarcinoma accounts for nearly 98% of the malignant tumors arising in the colon and rectum. The three most common nonadenocarcinoma cancers at these anatomic sites are carcinoids, lymphomas, and sarcomas. The colon and rectum can also be the site of metastatic cancer and a variety of benign tumors, the most common of which is the adenomatous polyp. This article focuses on adenocarcinoma of the colon and rectum, commonly called colorectal cancer. The most frequent cancers in patients in the United States and most Western countries are cancers of the breast, lung, colon, rectum, and prostate. The number of new colorectal cancer cases in the United States this year will be 135,000, and the number of deaths 50,000, making colorectal cancer the second leading cause of cancer death in the United States after lung cancer. The incidence of and death rate from this cancer are the same for women as for men. The mortality has been gradually declining during the last few years, attributable to improved therapy and earlier diagnosis. The incidence has also shown a downward trend, the reason as yet being unclear but possibly the result of increasingly widespread use of colonoscopy and polypectomy with removal of the premalignant stage of this disease.

PATHOLOGY

Adenocarcinoma of the colon is almost always preceded by a precursor lesion, the benign adenomatous polyp. The concept of the adenoma as a precursor of adenocarcinoma of the colon is strongly supported by epidemiologic and pathologic studies. In addition, clinical studies have provided evidence that polypectomy dramatically reduces the risk of subsequent colorectal cancer. Approximately two thirds of polyps encountered in the clinical setting are adenomas. These are classified histologically as tubular, tubulovillous, and villous and according to whether high-grade dysplasia is present. The most prevalent histologic growth pattern is tubular. Adenomas with a villous pattern are more likely to show high-grade dysplasia and transform into invasive malignant tumors. Other colorectal polyps include hyperplastic polyps, mucosal tags, inflammatory polyps, juvenile polyps, hamartomas, and a variety of nonmucosal lesions. Adenomas represent a monoclonal proliferation of stem cell progeny. The acquired mutation that underlies sporadic adenoma formation is not known, but it is speculated that it may be related to the familial adenomatous polyposis (FAP) gene locus. Two thirds of the adenomatous polyps are distal to the splenic flexure in clinical studies. This parallels the distribution of adenocarcinoma of the colon.

Colorectal cancer can be tiny to massive. The size is not predictive of metastatic potential. The tumors can be exophytic and polypoid with variable extension into the lumen or endophytic with little luminal involvement. The exophytic tumors can be broad based and sessile or, less commonly, pedunculated. New tumors tend to grow circumferentially, especially in the distal colon, producing obstruction, and often have ulcerations with associated bleeding. Staging is based on the degree of penetration into the bowel wall, the presence or absence of lymph node metastases, and the presence or absence of distant metastases (Table 1). The tumor can spread by direct extension to involve not only lymph nodes and mesentery but adjacent organs, and it can spread through vascular and lymphatic routes to distant sites, the most common of which are the liver and lung. Direct extension to surrounding pelvic tissues is especially seen with rectal cancers. Synchronous lesions are seen in about 3 to 5% of patients. The majority of these tumors are moderately well differentiated gland-forming adenocarcinomas with typical characteristic histologic features. Tumors that have abundant mucin in the cytoplasm, especially when forming a "signet cell" appearance, are usually aggressive tumors with poor prognosis. Residual adenomatous tissue is often seen, especially when the cancers are small.

A number of genetic abnormalities have been demonstrated in adenomatous polyps and cancers as adenomas form, grow, and transform to cancer and the cancer advances. The most common genetic abnormalities are mutations and deletions in chromosomes 5 (APC [adenomatous polyposis coli] genes), 17 (p53 genes), and 18 (DCC [deleted in colorectal cancer] genes) and mutations in the K-ras oncogene. In a small percentage of colorectal cancers, a "mutator" phenotype has been demonstrated that is characterized by genomic instability at simple repeated sequences in DNA, thought to be a consequence of a mutation in genes involved in DNA repair. This abnormal phenotype is commonly seen as a germline or inherited abnormality in hereditary nonpolyposis colorectal cancer (HNPCC or the Lynch syndrome). Growth factors, immunologic factors, and factors associated specifically with invasiveness and metastatic potential have also been described.

ETIOLOGY

Colorectal cancer is associated with age; more than 90% occur in men and women older than 50 years (Table 2). Rectal cancer, in contrast to colon cancer, is more common in men than in women. Lifestyle factors have been shown to be important in the causation. A positive association has been demonstrated with a diet high in fat and low in fiber, fruits, and vegetables; sedentary lifestyle; lack of exercise; cigarette smoking; and excess alcohol consumption.

Individuals with a prior history of colorectal cancer or

TABLE 2. **Risk Factors for Colorectal Cancer**

Average Risk
Age 50 y and older, asymptomatic
High Risk
Inflammatory bowel disease
  Chronic ulcerative colitis
  Chronic granulomatous colitis
Familial adenomatous polyposis
  Familial polyposis
  Gardner's syndrome
Turcot's syndrome
Oldfield's syndrome
Juvenile polyposis
Hereditary nonpolyposis colorectal cancer
  Family cancer syndrome
  Site-specific inherited colorectal cancer
Family history
  Colorectal adenomas
  Colorectal cancer
Past history
  Colorectal adenomas
  Colorectal cancer
  Breast, ovarian, and uterine cancer

adenomatous polyps have a higher risk of subsequent colorectal cancer if their colon has not been cleared of polyps. Individuals with inflammatory bowel disease (IBD) are at increased risk, which is related to the length of time of their ulcerative or granulomatous colitis and the extent of the anatomic involvement. IBD accounts for 1% of the new cases of colon cancer in this country each year, usually in those who have involvement of the entire bowel 8 years or longer or involvement of the distal bowel 15 years or longer. Women with a prior cancer of the endometrium, breast, or ovary may have an increased risk of colorectal cancer, the magnitude of which is unclear but may be related to the age at diagnosis and family history of cancer.

There is an increased susceptibility to colorectal cancer with a family history of colorectal cancer, especially when the diagnosis of colorectal cancer is made before the age of 55 years or adenomatous polyps are diagnosed before the age of 60 years. The overall increased risk for first-degree relatives (siblings, parents, children) of these patients is twofold. A greater increase in risk for colorectal cancer is present in individuals who are in families demonstrating a strong pattern of inheritance based on transmission of germline mutations. The two major inherited genetic syndromes are FAP and Gardner's syndrome, which is a full expression of FAP, and HNPCC. FAP accounts for approximately 1% and HNPCC for approximately 5% of the new cancers diagnosed each year (Figure 1). Both are inherited in an autosomal dominant pattern. In FAP, the colon is studded with thousands of adenomatous polyps throughout, beginning in adolescence, with cancers being seen in the twenties and thirties. In HNPCC, the polyps are fewer and are found mostly on the right side of the colon, with cancer occurring in the forties and fifties compared with the average age at diagnosis of colorectal cancer in the general population of 67 years. FAP is associated with inheritance in gene carriers of mutations on chromosome 5; HNPCC is associated with mutations on chromosomes 2, 3, and 7. FAP is associated with other cancers, including those of the stomach and duodenum, and with desmoid tumors. HNPCC is associated with a variety of tumors including stomach, pancreas, uterus, melanoma, and others.

TABLE 1. **Comparison of TNM and Dukes' Staging Systems for Colorectal Cancer**

Stage	TNM Designation			Dukes' Designation
0	Tis	N0	M0	—
I	T1	N0	M0	A
	T2	N0	M0	
II	T3	N0	M0	B
	T4	N0	M0	
III	Any T	N1	M0	C
	Any T	N2, N3	M0	
IV	Any T	Any N	M1	D

Abbreviations: Tis = in situ; T1 = tumor invades submucosa; T2 = tumor invades muscularis propria; T3 = tumor invades through muscularis propria; T4 = tumor invades serosa ± adjacent organs; N0 = negative lymph nodes; N1 = one to three positive nodes; N2 = more than three positive nodes; N3 = positive nodes on vascular trunk; M0 = no distant metastases; M1 = distant metastases.

Colorectal Cancer Cases

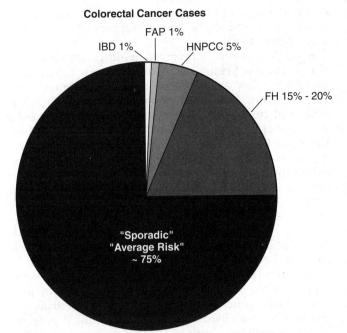

Figure 1. Factors associated with annual new cases of colorectal cancer. Sporadic = men and women age 50 years and older with no special risk factors; IBD = inflammatory bowel disease; FAP = familial adenomatous polyposis; HNPCC = hereditary nonpolyposis colorectal cancer; FH = positive family history. (From Winawer SJ, Schottenfeld D, Flehinger BJ: Colorectal cancer screening. J Natl Cancer Inst *83*:243–253, 1991.)

SYMPTOMS, SIGNS, AND DIAGNOSIS

Symptoms occur after an adenoma has formed, grown, and transformed into cancer and the cancer has advanced. It has been estimated that this takes on the average 10 to 15 years. The earliest symptoms may be fatigue as a result of anemia, especially from right-sided lesions. Changes in bowel habits with constipation and irregularities may occur especially from left-sided lesions, which may also be associated with abdominal discomfort, mild distention, and cramps. Rectal lesions may be associated with tenesmus, rectal bleeding, and pelvic discomfort. Any of these symptoms requires a diagnostic work-up, which would include a digital rectal examination and either flexible sigmoidoscopy and double-contrast barium enema examination or colonoscopy. If a cancer is not found in the lower bowel by sigmoidoscopy, the remainder of the bowel needs to be evaluated. One should not be satisfied with a diagnosis of hemorrhoids in a patient with bright red rectal bleeding. The advantage of the endoscopic methods are biopsy for tissue diagnosis of observed abnormalities and the ability to remove polyps, which are found more commonly than cancer in symptomatic patients, especially those with rectal bleeding.

SCREENING

Although it is important to perform an aggressive work-up for individuals with symptoms suggestive of neoplasia, the diagnosis of cancer in asymptomatic patients as a result of screening more often results in an earlier diagnosis, with a much higher probability of survival, and will be associated with less morbidity and a much lower likelihood of additional treatment with radiation and chemotherapy. Screening approaches should be divided into those for average-risk men and women with no other risk factors and for

high-risk individuals who have factors that increase their risk, including familial factors, IBD, or prior history of polyps or colorectal cancer.

There is strong evidence now that screening with fecal occult blood testing (FOBT) annually and flexible sigmoidoscopy every 5 years reduces the mortality from colorectal cancer. This should be offered to all men and women older than 50 years with no other risk factors. Other options for screening average-risk individuals include colonoscopy or double-contrast barium enema examination with flexible sigmoidoscopy. There are good reasons to consider these other options in individual people but insufficient evidence to recommend them as general guidelines.

Individuals who have one or two first relatives with colorectal cancer particularly before the age of 55 years or adenomatous polyps before the age of 60 years should be encouraged to have the same screening as the average-risk individuals but starting at age 40 years because there is evidence that a family history is associated with younger age at onset of the cancer or adenomatous polyps. Many physicians and patients prefer either colonoscopy or double-contrast barium enema examination and flexible sigmoidoscopy rather than FOBT and flexible sigmoidoscopy in these families. I recommend colonoscopy every 5 years for these people. Individuals and families identified as having either FAP or HNPCC need to have individualized screening at a young age and should be referred to genetic counselors for full discussion of their risk, age at which they should start screening for colorectal cancer, and recommendations for other cancer screening. Genetic testing is of value only in these families at present. Obtaining a family history is a powerful clinical tool for identifying those at increased risk for these syndromes as well as those at increased risk because of one or two first relatives with colorectal cancer or adenomatous polyps. The latter accounts for 15 to 20% of individuals destined to develop colorectal cancer each year.

People with IBD need to be examined by colonoscopy every 1 to 2 years after disease for 8 years involving the entire colon or 15 years involving the distal colon. The search for early cancer and the premalignant dysplasia in the colon is the goal of these examinations. Prophylactic colectomy is an alternative approach that should be seriously considered, especially in young individuals.

People who have their colon cancer resected need to have periodic follow-up to search for additional adenomatous polyps. I prefer a complete colonoscopy before surgery, if it is possible to pass the endoscope beyond the cancer, a second complete examination or colonoscopy 1 year later, and less frequent colonoscopies thereafter. Individuals who have had adenomatous polyps removed from their colon can have their first follow-up colonoscopy 3 years later provided that their first colonoscopy completely removed all polyps from rectum to cecum, unless there were numerous polyps, malignant polyps, or a large sessile polyp, in which case an earlier examination is in order. At the 3-year follow-up, there is little in the way of significant disease found. Subsequent follow-ups can be at 5 years.

MANAGEMENT

Surgical resection provides the best opportunity for cure. This can be done as the sole modality of treatment or in conjunction with radiation or chemotherapy. There is evidence that colon cancer involving lymph nodes is associated with better survival in patients who are treated with a course of postoperative chemotherapy with a combination of either 5-

fluorouracil and levamisole (Ergamisol) or 5-fluorouracil and leucovorin (Wellcovorin). The survival of patients with rectal cancer that has penetrated through the bowel wall with or without lymph node involvement is improved with a combination of radiation therapy and chemotherapy postoperatively. This is considered to be adjuvant treatment of patients with no known residual disease. In some patients, radiation therapy given preoperatively may convert a potentially unresectable rectal cancer into one that is resectable. The approach to each patient is individualized and is based on physical examination, digital rectal examination, imaging with computed tomography (CT), and in the case of rectal cancer, endoscopic ultrasonography. The standard treatment of resectable colon cancer is a hemicolectomy and a regional lymphadenectomy based on the regional vascular supply. Rectal cancers can usually be resected by an abdominal approach (low anterior resection) even when the cancers are within 3 to 4 cm of the anal verge. Permanent colostomies are necessary in few patients today. Laparoscopic colectomy is being evaluated within the framework of clinical studies as an alternative to open laparotomy.

There are special considerations for the surgical approach in some patients. Patients with IBD having prophylactic colectomy can now have the option of either an ileostomy or a pouch reconstruction. Individuals with FAP need a total colectomy, and patients with HNPCC who are having surgery for colorectal cancer, usually on the right side of the colon, should have a subtotal colectomy at that time if possible to reduce their future risk for additional cancers. Patients having had a polyp removed that histologically is found to have an invasive cancer will require follow-up surgical intervention only if the malignant tumor has encroached on the cautery line or involved vascular spaces or lymphatic spaces. The location of the polyp and co-morbidity are other factors that need to be considered in this decision.

After curative resection, I usually follow-up patients with office visits, carcinoembryonic antigen (CEA) determination, and other blood tests every 3 months, and chest radiography and CT of the abdomen annually in patients who are at high risk for recurrence because of the stage of the disease at the time of surgery.

TREATMENT OF RECURRENT AND METASTATIC DISEASE

At the time of surgery, it will usually be clear whether the patient has gross residual disease after the resection. This will commonly be in the form of nodules on the liver or peritoneal surface that are too small to have been detected by preoperative imaging. A solitary implant or a small number of implants in the liver can be resected at that time or subsequently. A single pulmonary nodule is usually resected because it may be a new primary cancer of the lung rather than a metastatic focus from the colon. Residual disease after surgery may also be suspected if a preoperative CEA level has not fallen to normal in spite of the absence of gross residual disease observed at the time of surgery or on postoperative imaging.

Recurrent colon cancer is usually outside the bowel. Rarely, primary anastomotic recurrences are found after low anterior resections. Anastomotic recurrences are usually secondary to intra-abdominal recurrent tumor. Recurrent cancer that is nonresectable is usually treated with 5-fluorouracil, which is the most active agent, in combination with another agent, usually leucovorin. Other agents are used less successfully. Direct infusion into the liver of fluorodeoxyuridine (floxuridine, FUDR) has been shown to have significant response rates compared with systemic chemotherapy, but it is not clear whether survival is better. Radiation therapy is usually reserved for painful pelvic or bone disease and for the less common brain metastases. Patients who present initially with metastatic incurable disease may nevertheless have surgery offered, especially if the primary colon cancer is associated with bleeding or obstruction, provided that the patient has a reasonable performance status.

CONCLUDING COMMENTS

It is clear that colorectal cancer is a highly curable disease when it is detected at an early stage. This can be accomplished in a high percentage of people in the general population by use of FOBT and flexible sigmoidoscopy. More aggressive screening with colonoscopy has the potential for being highly effective in individuals at high risk for colorectal cancer, especially in those with a family history. In all of these patients, adenomatous polyps are often identified and removed with a dramatic reduction in the likelihood of developing colorectal cancer. This is a unique opportunity for cancer prevention. Thus, cancer deaths can be prevented not only by detecting the cancer at an earlier stage but by finding the precursor lesions, the adenomatous polyps, and removing them, thus avoiding the occurrence of cancer. In addition, we know much about lifestyle and its relationship to colorectal cancer, modification of which can dramatically reduce the probability of developing colorectal cancer and precursor adenomatous polyps. At present, we can identify genetic syndromes in only 5 or 6% of the people who are destined to get colorectal cancer. With future advances in molecular genetics, the percentage of individuals who will be identified as being susceptible to colorectal cancer may increase considerably. We will then be able to target a smaller subset of the general population for colonoscopy and polypectomy to reduce colon cancer incidence. There is also considerable interest in research into better methods for screening, including more sensitive FOBT and noninvasive means of examining the colon in the general population by "virtual colonoscopy." While we await results regarding these promising developments, we need to aggressively increase the participation of people in techniques now available that can dramatically reduce the incidence, morbidity, and mortality of this disease.

INTESTINAL PARASITES

method of
RICHARD D. PEARSON, M.D.
University of Virginia School of Medicine
Charlottesville, Virginia

Enteric parasites are prevalent among residents of developing areas of the world where sanitation is poor, and they also pose a risk for international travelers. Some enteric parasites are endemic in North America. Several have merged as important pathogens in persons with the acquired immune deficiency syndrome (AIDS). Enteric parasites can be divided into two groups, protozoa and helminths. Protozoa are single-celled organisms with the capacity to multiply by simple division. Theoretically, infection with even one protozoan can lead to life-threatening disease. Helminths, in contrast, are multicellular worms with internal organs and complex life cycles. With two important exceptions, *Strongyloides stercoralis* and *Hymenolepis nana,* which are capable of autoinfection, helminths cannot multiply in their human hosts. The severity of helminthic diseases is usually correlated with the magnitude of the worm burden, but on occasion a single adult worm or larva can cause serious, life-threatening disease, such as when an adult *Ascaris lumbricoides* migrates into the pancreatic duct and causes acute pancreatitis.

In most instances, the diagnosis of an intestinal parasitic infection is made by identifying trophozoites or cysts of protozoa or ova, larvae, or adult helminths in the stool. Eosinophilia is common when helminths migrate through tissue during the initial stages of infection, but it is often absent when adult worms reside in the gastrointestinal tract during established infections. Eosinophilia is not typically a feature of protozoal infections. In some parasitic diseases, the finding of antibodies in serum allows a presumptive diagnosis. Techniques for detecting coproantigens are available for *Giardia lamblia* and are being developed for other enteric parasites.

Effective drugs are available for the treatment of all but a few enteric parasites. Specific recommendations for protozoal infections are listed alphabetically in Table 1 and for helminthic diseases in Table 2. They are based on the consensus recommendations of the *Medical Letter on Drugs and Therapeutics* (37:99–108, 1995). In many instances, the drugs of choice for parasitic diseases have been licensed by the Food and Drug Administration (FDA) and are commercially available. In others, the drugs have not been licensed but can be obtained from the Centers for Disease Control and Prevention, CDC Drug Service. It is possible to provide only an overview of therapeutic issues in this chapter. A full description of the life cycles, clinical manifestations, and methods used to identify enteric parasites is available elsewhere.* Detailed information on the administration, pharmacology, and side effects of licensed drugs can be found in *Drug Information for the Health Care Professional,* 17th ed. (USP DI, Rockville, MD, The United States Pharmacopeial Convention, 1997).

INTESTINAL PROTOZOA

G. lamblia is an important cause of diarrhea in North America. Large water-borne outbreaks have been reported from communities in the Rocky Mountains and Appalachian Mountains. Infection is also acquired by hikers who drink contaminated surface water, children in day care centers, and international travelers. Giardiasis has historically been a problem among Americans who visit major cities in Russia. Although *G. lamblia* is prevalent among residents of many developing areas, it is not a significant cause of diarrhea in them.

Metronidazole (Flagyl), administered at the relatively low dose of 250 mg three times a day for 5 days (all dosages in the text are for adults; pediatric doses are summarized in Tables 1 and 2), is the treatment of choice for giardiasis, although it has not been approved by the FDA for that specific indication. Gastrointestinal disturbances, headache, dry mouth, and a metallic taste are relatively frequent side effects. On rare occasions, metronidazole has been associated with seizures, encephalopathy, peripheral neuropathy, ataxia, or pancreatitis. Patients must be warned against the use of alcohol while taking metronidazole because of its disulfiram-like effects. Although not available in the United States, another nitroimidazole, tinidazole (Fasigyn), administered as a single dose of 2 grams, is equally effective and better tolerated. On occasion, it too causes nausea, vomiting, rash, or a metallic taste.

Furazolidone (Furoxone) is available in liquid form for the treatment of giardiasis in children. Side effects include nausea and vomiting. Allergic reactions with fever, pulmonary infiltrates, urticaria, vesicular rash, or hypotension occur on occasion, as does headache or hypoglycemia. Rare side effects include hemolytic anemia in persons with glucose-6-phosphate dehydrogenase deficiency, disulfiram-like reactions with alcohol, polyneuritis, or adverse interactions with monoamine oxidase inhibitors. Paromomycin (Humatin), 25 to 35 mg per kg per day in three divided doses for 7 days, is not always effective against *G. lamblia,* but it has been used to treat giardiasis during pregnancy. It is a poorly absorbed aminoglycoside and is discussed in detail later. Quinine (Atabrine) was once widely used for the treatment of giardiasis, but it is associated with frequent

---

*See Pearson RD: Parasitic diseases: Helminths. *In* Yamada T, Alpers DH, Owyang C, et al (eds): Textbook of Gastroenterology, 2nd ed. Philadelphia, JB Lippincott Co, 1995, pp 2362–2379 (the third edition is in press); Hill DR, Petri WA Jr, Guerrant RL: Parasitic diseases: Protozoa. *In* Yamada T, Alpers DH, Owyang C, et al (eds): Textbook of Gastroenterology, 2nd ed. Philadelphia, JB Lippincott Co, 1995, pp 2343–2361 (the third edition is in press).

TABLE 1. **Drugs for the Treatment of Protozoal Infections**

Infection	Drug	Adult Dosage	Pediatric Dosage
Amebiasis (*Entamoeba histolytica*)			
Asymptomatic			
Drug of choice	Iodoquinol	650 mg tid × 20 d	30–40 mg/kg/d in 3 doses × 20 d
	or		
	Paromomycin	25–35 mg/kg/d in 3 doses × 7 d	25–35 mg/kg/d in 3 doses × 7 d
Alternative	Diloxanide furoate*	500 mg tid × 10 d	20 mg/kg/d in 3 doses × 10 d
Mild to moderate intestinal disease			
Drug of choice	Metronidazole	750 mg tid × 10 d	35–50 mg/kg/d in 3 doses × 10 d
	or		
	Tinidazole†	2 gm/d × 3 d	50 mg/kg (maximum 2 gm) qd × 3 d
Followed by paromomycin, iodoquinol, or diloxanide furoate as above			
Severe intestinal disease			
Drugs of choice	Metronidazole	750 mg tid × 10 d	35–50 mg/kg/d in 3 doses × 10 d
	or		
	Tinidazole†	600 mg bid or 800 mg tid	50 mg/kg or 60 mg/kg (maximum 2 gm) qd × 3 d
Followed by paromomycin, iodoquinol, or diloxanide furoate as above			
Blastocystis hominis infection			
Drug of choice	See text		
Cryptosporidiosis (*Cryptosporidium parvum*)			
Drug of choice	Paromomycin (see text)	500–750 mg qid	
Cyclospora species infection			
Drug of choice	Trimethoprim-sulfamethoxazole	TMP 160 mg, SMZ 800 mg bid × 7 d	TMP 5 mg/kg, SMZ 25 mg/kg bid × 7 d
Dientamoeba fragilis infection			
Drug of choice	Iodoquinol	650 mg tid × 20 d	40 mg/kg/d in 3 doses × 20 d
	or		
	Paromomycin	25–30 mg/kg/d in 3 doses × 7 d	25–30 mg/kg/d in 3 doses × 7 d
	or		
	Tetracycline	500 mg qid × 10 d	40 mg/kg/d (maximum 2 gm/d) in 4 doses × 10 d (not recommended for children younger than 8 y)
Entamoeba polecki infection			
Drug of choice	Metronidazole	750 mg tid × 10 d	35–50 mg/kg/d in 3 doses × 10 d
Giardiasis (*Giardia lamblia*)			
Drug of choice	Metronidazole	250 mg tid × 5 d	15 mg/kg/d in 3 doses × 5 d
Alternatives	Tinidazole†	2 gm once	50 mg/kg once (maximum 2 gm)
	or		
	Furazolidone	100 mg qid × 7–10 d	6 mg/kg/d in 4 doses × 7–10 d
	or		
	Paromomycin	25–35 mg/kg/d in 3 doses × 7 d	
Isosporiasis (*Isospora belli*)			
Drug of choice	Trimethoprim-sulfamethoxazole	160 mg TMP, 800 mg SMZ qid × 10 d, then bid × 3 wk	
Microsporidiosis			
Intestinal (*Enterocytozoon bieneusi, Septata intestinalis*)			
Drug of choice	See text		

*Available from the CDC Drug Service, Centers for Disease Control and Prevention, Atlanta, GA 30333; 404-639-3670 (evenings, weekends, or holidays, 404-639-2888).

†Not available in the United States.

Modified from Drugs for parasitic infections. Med Lett Drugs Ther *37*:99–108, 1995.

side effects and is no longer available in the United States.

Entamoeba histolytica is an important cause of colitis and extraintestinal disease, primarily liver abscesses, in developing areas where sanitation is poor. The stool is almost always positive for gross or occult blood in persons with amebic colitis, but fecal leukocytes may be absent or pyknotic because they are lysed by *E. histolytica* trophozoites. In North America, amebiasis is most likely to be encountered among immigrants, returning American travelers, or institutionalized psychiatric patients with no history of travel. Asymptomatic *E. histolytica* infections are treated with a luminally active agent: paromomycin, iodoquinol, or diloxanide furoate. Paromomycin is given orally, 25 to 35 mg per kg per day in three

TABLE 2. **Drugs for the Treatment of Helminth Infections**

Infection	Drug	Adult Dosage	Pediatric Dosage
Angiostrongyliasis (*Angiostrongylus costaricensis*) Drug of choice	Thiabendazole	75 mg/kg/d in 3 doses × 3 d (maximum 3 gm/d); toxicity may require dosage reduction	75 mg/kg/d in 3 doses × 3 d (maximum 3 gm/d); toxicity may require dosage reduction
Anisakiasis (*Anisakis* and other genera) Treatment of choice	Surgical or endoscopic removal		
Ascariasis (*Ascaris lumbricoides*) Drug of choice	Albendazole	400 mg once	400 mg once
	or Mebendazole	100 mg bid × 3 d	100 mg bid × 3 d
	or Pyrantel pamoate	11 mg/kg once (maximum 1 gm)	11 mg/kg once (maximum 1 gm)
Capillariasis (*Capillaria philippinensis*) Drug of choice	Mebendazole	200 mg bid × 20 d	200 mg bid × 20 d
Alternative	Albendazole	200 mg bid × 10 d	200 mg bid × 10 d
	or Thiabendazole	25 mg/kg/d in 2 doses × 30 d	25 mg/kg/d in 2 doses × 30 d
Cysticercosis; see Tapeworm infection			
Enterobius vermicularis (pinworm) infection Drug of choice	Pyrantel pamoate	11 mg/kg once (maximum 1 gm); repeat after 2 wk	11 mg/kg once (maximum 1 gm); repeat after 2 wk
	or Mebendazole	A single dose of 100 mg; repeat after 2 wk	A single dose of 100 mg; repeat after 2 wk
	or Albendazole	400 mg once; repeat in 2 wk	400 mg once, repeat in 2 wk
Flukes (intestinal infection) *Fasciolopsis buski* Drug of choice	Praziquantel	75 mg/kg/d in 3 doses × 1 d	75 mg/kg/d in 3 doses × 1 d
Heterophyes heterophyes Drug of choice	Praziquantel	75 mg/kg/d in 3 doses × 1 d	75 mg/kg/d in 3 doses × 1 d
Metagonimus yokogawai Drug of choice	Praziquantel	75 mg/kg/d in 3 doses × 1 d	75 mg/kg/d in 3 doses × 1 d
Nanophyetus salmincola Drug of choice	Praziquantel	60 mg/kg/d in 3 doses × 1 d	60 mg/kg/d in 3 doses × 1 d
Flukes (liver infection) *Clonorchis sinensis* (Chinese liver fluke) Drug of choice	Praziquantel	75 mg/kg/d in 3 doses × 1 d	75 mg/kg/d in 3 doses × 1 d
	or Albendazole	10 mg/kg × 7 d	
Fasciola hepatica (sheep liver fluke) Drug of choice	Bithionol	30–50 mg/kg on alternate days × 10–15 doses	30–50 mg/kg on alternate days × 10–15 doses
Metorchis conjunctus (North American liver fluke) Drug of choice	Praziquantel	75 mg/kg/d in 3 doses × 1 d	75 mg/kg/d in 3 doses × 1 d
Opisthorchis viverrini Drug of choice	Praziquantel	75 mg/kg/d in 3 doses × 1 d	75 mg/kg/d in 3 doses × 1 d
Hookworm infection (*Ancylostoma duodenale, Necator americanus*) Drug of choice	Albendazole	400 mg once	400 mg once
	or Mebendazole	100 mg bid × 3 d	100 mg bid × 3 d
	or Pyrantel pamoate	11 mg/kg/d (maximum 1 gm) × 3 d	11 mg/kg (maximum 1 gm) × 3 d
Oesophagostomum bifurcum Drug of choice	See text		
Schistosomiasis (bilharziasis) *Schistosoma haematobium* Drug of choice	Praziquantel	40 mg/kg/d in 2 doses × 1 d	40 mg/kg/d in 2 doses × 1 d
Schistosoma japonicum Drug of choice	Praziquantel	60 mg/kg/d in 3 doses × 1 d	60 mg/kg/d in 3 doses × 1 d
Schistosoma mansoni Drug of choice	Praziquantel	40 mg/kg/d in 2 doses × 1 d	40 mg/kg/d in 2 doses × 1 d
Alternative	Oxamniquine	15 mg/kg once (higher doses are used in some areas)	20 mg/kg/d in 2 doses × 1 d
Schistosoma makongi Drug of choice	Praziquantel	60 mg/kg/d in 3 doses × 1 d	60 mg/kg/d in 3 doses × 1 d

Table continued on following page

TABLE 2. **Drugs for the Treatment of Helminth Infections** *Continued*

Infection	Drug	Adult Dosage	Pediatric Dosage
Strongyloidiasis (*Strongyloides stercoralis*)			
Drug of choice	Ivermectin or	200 µg/kg/d × 1–2 d	200 µg/kg/d × 1–2 d
	Thiabendazole	50 mg/kg/d in 2 doses (maximum 3 gm/d) × 2 d; ≥5 d for hyperinfection	50 mg/kg/d in 2 doses (maximum 3 gm/d) × 2 d; ≥5 d for hyperinfection
Tapeworm infection—adult (intestinal stage) *Diphyllobothrium latum* (fish), *Taenia saginata* (beef), *Taenia solium* (pork), *Dipylidium caninum* (dog)			
Drug of choice	Praziquantel	5–10 mg/kg once	5–10 mg/kg once
Hymenolepis nana (dwarf tapeworm)			
Drug of choice	Praziquantel	25 mg/kg once	25 mg/kg once
Cysticercus cellulosae (cysticercosis)			
Treatment of choice	Albendazole or	15 mg/kg/d in 2 or 3 doses × 8–28 d, repeated as necessary	15 mg/kg/d in 2 or 3 doses × 8–28 d, repeated as necessary
	Praziquantel	50 mg/kg/d in 3 doses × 15 d	50 mg/kg/d in 3 doses × 15 d
Echinococcus granulosus (hydatid cyst)			
Treatment of choice	Drainage and instillation of a scolicidal agent		
Alternative	Albendazole	400 mg bid × 28 d, repeated as necessary	15 mg/kg/d × 28 d, repeated as necessary
Echinococcus multilocularis			
Treatment of choice	Surgery		
Alternative	Albendazole for inoperable disease (see text)		
Trichinosis (*Trichinella spiralis*)			
Drug of choice	Mebendazole plus steroids for severe symptoms	200–400 mg tid × 3 d, then 400–500 mg tid × 10 d	
Alternative	Albendazole (see text) plus steroids for severe symptoms		
Trichostrongylus infection			
Drug of choice	Pyrantel pamoate	11 mg/kg once (maximum 1 gm)	11 mg/kg once (maximum 1 gm)
Alternative	Mebendazole or	100 mg bid × 3 d	100 mg bid × 3 d
	Albendazole	400 mg once	400 mg once
Trichuriasis (*Trichuris trichiura*, whipworm)			
Drug of choice	Mebendazole or	100 mg bid × 3 d	100 mg bid × 3 d
	Albendazole	400 mg once; may require 3 d for heavy infection	400 mg once; may require 3 d for heavy infection

Modified from Drugs for parasitic infections. Med Lett Drugs Ther *37*:99–108, 1995.

divided doses for 7 days. Side effects include gastrointestinal disturbances. Although it is poorly absorbed from the gastrointestinal tract, paromomycin can cause eighth nerve and kidney damage in persons with pre-existing renal insufficiency. Iodoquinol (Yodoxin), 650 mg three times a day for 20 days, is another luminally active agent. It can cause rash, slight thyroid enlargement, or gastrointestinal side effects. It is contraindicated in persons with known iodine sensitivity. Rarely, iodoquinol has been associated with optic neuritis, optic atrophy, or loss of vision after prolonged use at high doses. To avoid these complications, the recommended dose and duration of treatment should never be exceeded. Diloxanide furoate (Furamide),* although not licensed for use in the United States, is a well-tolerated alternative. It is administered at a dose of 500 mg three times a day for 10 days. Flatulence is relatively frequent, and on rare occasions it is associated with diplopia, dizziness, urticaria, or pruritus.

Intestinal amebiasis and amebic liver abscesses are treated with high-dose metronidazole, 750 mg

---

*Available through the CDC.

three times a day for 10 days. Although metronidazole at this dose eradicates *E. histolytica* cysts in some patients, a course of one of the luminally active agents already discussed should also be administered. Outside the United States, tinidazole is often used; it is at least as effective as metronidazole and less toxic. In persons with mild to moderate intestinal amebiasis, 2 grams of tinidazole is administered daily for 3 days. In those with severe intestinal disease or hepatic abscesses, 600 mg twice a day or 800 mg three times a day is administered for 5 days. Treatment should be followed by a course of a luminally active agent.

Other intestinal protozoa are occasionally identified in the stools of persons with diarrhea. The significance of *Blastocystis hominis* is controversial, but clinical responses have been anecdotally reported with metronidazole, 750 mg three times a day for 10 days, or iodoquinol, 650 mg three times a day for 20 days. The finding of *B. hominis* suggests that the person has been exposed to fecally contaminated food or water. *G. lamblia* is easily missed on microscopic examination of the stool and may be present concomitantly with *B. hominis*. The administration of metronidazole for *B. hominis* has the advantage of eradicating concurrent, occult *G. lamblia* infection, should it be present.

Dientamoeba fragilis responds to paromomycin, 25 to 35 mg per kg per day in three divided doses for 7 days; tetracycline, 500 mg four times a day for 10 days; or iodoquinol, 650 mg three times a day for 20 days. Tetracycline is usually well tolerated but can cause gastrointestinal disturbances, photosensitivity dermatitis, vaginal candidiasis, and on rare occasion pseudomembranous colitis. In addition, it should not be used for children younger than 8 years or women who are pregnant.

In the past decade, *Cryptosporidium parvum* has been increasingly recognized as a cause of enteric disease among children in developing areas where sanitation is poor. It has also been responsible for water-borne outbreaks in the United States; a major epidemic occurred in Wisconsin. *Cryptosporidium* causes acute or subacute, self-limited diarrhea in immunocompetent persons, but it can cause severe, chronic diarrhea in those with AIDS. Despite extensive studies of a large number of antimicrobial agents, none has emerged as universally effective against *Cryptosporidium*. Paromomycin has been shown to have limited effectiveness in some patients.

Isospora belli is prevalent in many tropical areas but is encountered infrequently in the United States. It produces self-limited diarrhea in immunocompetent patients but can cause severe, chronic diarrhea in persons with human immunodeficiency virus (HIV) infection. *I. belli* disease is treated with 160 mg of trimethoprim and 800 mg of sulfamethoxazole (Bactrim DS) four times a day for 10 days, then twice a day for 3 weeks. Relapses are common in persons with HIV infection, and it may be necessary to continue therapy indefinitely. In sulfonamide-allergic individuals, pyrimethamine, 50 to 75 mg daily, has been used effectively.

Microsporidiosis caused by *Enterocytozoon bieneusi* or *Septata intestinalis* has been identified in HIV-infected persons with diarrhea. Although the pathogenic role of the microsporidians has been questioned, albendazole, which is discussed in detail later in relation to the treatment of nematode infections, has been used effectively for the treatment of *S. intestinalis* at a dose of 400 mg twice a day, and it may be helpful for those infected with *E. bieneusi*.

Cyclospora species, coccidian parasites previously known as cyanobacterium-like bodies, cause diarrhea in normal as well as immunocompromised persons in the United States and abroad. North American outbreaks of *Cyclospora cayetanensis* infection have been traced to contaminated raspberries imported from Central America. Trimethoprim (160 mg)–sulfamethoxazole (800 mg) given twice a day for 7 days is effective in the treatment of immunocompetent patients. HIV-infected patients may require a higher dose and long-term maintenance therapy.

INTESTINAL NEMATODES

Intestinal helminths are classified as nematodes (roundworms) or platyhelminths (flatworms), which are subdivided into trematodes (flukes) and cestodes (tapeworms). This classification is helpful not only in organizing the parasites but also in discussing chemotherapy, because members of these groups are frequently susceptible to the same drugs or family of drugs.

A. lumbricoides, the hookworms *Necator americanus* and *Ancylostoma duodenale,* and *Trichuris trichiura* are prevalent throughout the world in areas where sanitation is poor. Residents, particularly children, frequently have heavy worm burdens and are infected with more than one species. In North America these intestinal nematodes are most frequently encountered among immigrants, but on occasion they are diagnosed in returning international travelers or in residents of the southern United States who have not traveled abroad.

The benzimidazoles, albendazole and mebendazole, are used for the treatment of these intestinal nematodes. Albendazole (Zentel) has the advantage that it is effective when administered as a single dose of 400 mg, although in heavy *T. trichiura* infections it may be necessary to extend therapy for 3 days. Albendazole has been administered as a single dose in mass treatment programs in Africa, where it has been shown to improve weight gain and performance in children infected with *A. lumbricoides,* hookworms, and/or *T. trichiura*. It is generally well tolerated, although sometimes it is associated with diarrhea, abdominal pain, or migration of *A. lumbricoides*. Albendazole and other benzimidazoles are potentially genotoxic and are contraindicated during pregnancy. High-dose therapy, which is used for the treatment of echinococcal disease and neurocysticercosis, has been associated, on occasion, with neutropenia, alopecia, or elevated serum transaminase levels. Mebendazole (Vermox) has a spectrum of activity similar to that of albendazole, but it is administered at a dose of 100 mg twice a day for 3 days. It is generally well tolerated, but on occasion it too is associated with diarrhea, abdominal pain, or migration of *A. lumbricoides*. Rarely, it is associated with leukopenia, agranulocytosis, or hypospermia, particularly when administered at high doses for prolonged periods to treat persons with echinococcosis. Pyrantel pamoate (Antiminth), administered at a dose of 11 mg per kg of body weight to a maximum of 1.0 gram, is a depolarizing neuromuscular blocking agent that is effective against *A. lumbricoides* as a single dose and the hookworms when administered once a day for 3 days, but not *T. trichiura*. It is usually well tolerated, although gastrointestinal disturbances, headache, dizziness, rash, and fever occur on occasion. Pyrantel pamoate should not be given concurrently with piperazine,* a hyperpolarizing neuromuscular blocking agent, because the two drugs are mutually antagonistic.

Enterobius vermicularis, the pinworm, is prevalent in North America and other industrialized countries among children from all socioeconomic classes. The diagnosis is usually made by finding ova or dying adult female worms in the perianal region. On occasion, ova are identified in the stool or in ectopic sties in the urogenital tract of females. Pinworms can be treated with a dose of pyrantel pamoate, 11 mg per kg to a maximum of 1 gram; mebendazole, 100 mg; or albendazole, 400 mg followed by a second dose of the same drug 2 weeks later. Pyrantel pamoate is available over the counter in the United States for the treatment of pinworms. If infections recur and there is more than one young child in the household, empirical therapy of all children should be considered. In addition, clothing and bedding must be washed and the house thoroughly cleaned.

S. stercoralis is endemic in many developing areas of the world and in some regions of the southern United States. It may be diagnosed in immigrants, returning travelers, military personnel including former prisoners of war from Southeast Asia, and residents of endemic areas of North America. *S. stercoralis* is important because it is capable of autoinfection. It can persist for decades after a person leaves an endemic area, and it can cause life-threatening disseminated hyperinfection in those who become immunocompromised. The hyperinfection syndrome may occur after organ transplantation, in persons taking corticosteroids or other immunosuppressive agents, or in malnourished residents of endemic, developing areas. It has not been as prevalent among HIV-infected persons as might have been predicted on the basis of their CD4+ T cell defects.

Ivermectin (Mectizan), which is widely used for the treatment of onchocerciasis, is effective against *S. stercoralis* when administered at a dose of 200 μg

per kg for 1 or 2 days. Ivermectin is likely to emerge as the treatment of choice for strongyloidiasis because it is as effective as the alternative, thiabendazole, but much better tolerated. Thiabendazole (Mintezol) has been the treatment of choice for *S. stercoralis* for many years. It is administered at a dose of 50 mg per kg (maximum 3 grams) per day in two divided doses for 2 days for intestinal disease or for at least 5 days in persons with the hyperinfection syndrome. Thiabendazole is well absorbed after oral administration. Nausea, vomiting, and vertigo are common, and rash, erythema multiforme, leukopenia, hallucinations, and olfactory disturbances occur occasionally. Rare side effects include shock, tinnitus, intrahepatic cholestasis, convulsions, angioneurotic edema, and the Stevens-Johnson syndrome.

Trichinella spiralis is acquired through ingestion of inadequately cooked or raw pork, bear, walrus, or other contaminated meat. Abdominal pain and diarrhea occur during the early phases of infection. Later, invading larvae produce the classic picture of myalgia, periorbital edema, and eosinophilia. Chronic diarrhea caused by *Trichinella nativa* has been reported among Inuit populations in Canada who have had prior *Trichinella* infection. Mebendazole, 200 to 400 mg three times a day for 3 days followed by 400 to 500 mg three times a day for 10 days, is recommended. It eradicates adult *Trichinella* in the intestinal tract, and animal studies suggest that it has activity against invading larvae in muscle as well. Albendazole may also be effective. Steroids are frequently used to reduce the symptoms that accompany larval invasion.

A number of other intestinal nematodes are encountered less frequently. *Trichostrongylus* species are important pathogens of cattle. They are periodically acquired by people living in cattle-raising areas through fecal contamination of food or water. Human infection is usually mild or asymptomatic. The treatment of choice is pyrantel pamoate, 11 mg per kg to a maximum of 1 gram. Mebendazole, 100 mg twice a day for 3 days, and albendazole, 400 mg, are alternatives. *Oesophagostomum* species, common parasites of monkeys and gorillas, have been reported to cause intestinal disease in humans in Africa and Indonesia. They may be susceptible to albendazole or pyrantel pamoate.

Capillaria philippinensis is acquired by ingestion of incompletely cooked or raw contaminated fish in the Philippines or other endemic regions. Infection can result in malabsorption, diarrhea, and severe weight loss. High-dose, prolonged treatment with mebendazole, 200 mg twice a day for 20 days, has been recommended. Albendazole, 200 mg twice a day for 10 days, and thiabendazole, 25 mg per kg daily in two divided doses for 30 days, are alternatives.

Angiostrongylus costaricensis, which is endemic in scattered areas of Latin America, is acquired through ingestion of raw snails or snail-contaminated food. *A. costaricensis* invades mesenteric arterioles and results in the formation of granulomatous, eosinophilic, inflammatory masses. Patients are often initially

---

*Not available in the United States.

thought to have appendicitis or a neoplasm. The diagnosis is frequently made at the time of surgical exploration when involved tissue is resected. Thiabendazole, 75 mg per kg per day (maximum 3 grams) given in three divided doses for 3 days, is the treatment of choice. This dose of thiabendazole is likely to be toxic, and the dosage may have to be decreased. Mebendazole, 200 to 400 mg three times a day for 10 days, is an alternative.

Anisakiasis follows ingestion of raw or inadequately cooked fish that are infected with larvae of *Anisakis* species or related genera. The larvae can elicit painful, inflammatory responses when they attempt to invade the wall of the stomach, small intestine, or colon. On some occasions, invading larvae can be visualized and removed endoscopically from the stomach or duodenum.

SCHISTOSOMA AND OTHER TREMATODES (FLUKES)

Trematodes, or flukes, have complex life cycles involving snails as intermediate hosts. In schistosomiasis, adult blood flukes live in mesenteric venules. *Schistosoma mansoni*, which is endemic in many areas of Africa, Latin America, and the Middle East, and *Schistosoma japonicum* and *Schistosoma mekongi*, which are endemic in Southeast Asia, are the major intestinal pathogens. They produce ova that result in mucosal inflammation, hypertrophy, and ulceration before they reach their destination of the lumen of the intestine. Other ova are swept back through the portal circulation to the liver, where they elicit granulomatous inflammatory responses and scarring that can result in hepatic enlargement, portal hypertension, splenomegaly, and esophageal varices. *Schistosoma haematobium* typically resides in the vesical venous plexus, where ova produce inflammation and scarring in the bladder and lower ureters, but on occasion *S. haematobium* involves the appendix or other parts of the intestinal tract.

All of the *Schistosoma* species that infect humans are susceptible to praziquantel (Biltricide). *S. mansoni* and *S. haematobium* can be treated with 40 mg per kg per day in two divided doses, whereas *S. japonicum* and *S. mekongi* require 60 mg per kg daily in three divided doses. Although associated with mild, transient side effects, praziquantel is without serious long-term sequelae. Malaise, headache, and dizziness are common; sedation, abdominal pain, sweating, fever, nausea, and fatigue occur occasionally. Abdominal pain and gastrointestinal symptoms have been reported in some patients with heavy *S. mansoni* infections, possibly because of the inflammatory response that accompanies the release of antigens from dying flukes. On rare occasions, rash or pruritus is encountered. Oxamniquine (Vansil) is an alternative for the treatment of *S. mansoni*; a single dose of 15 mg per kg is generally recommended, but higher doses may be necessary to treat *S. mansoni* infections acquired in East Africa, South Africa, or Egypt. On occasion oxamniquine is associated with

headache, fever, dizziness, somnolence, insomnia, nausea, diarrhea, hepatic enzyme elevations, or electrocardiographic changes. Seizures and neuropsychiatric disturbances are rare side effects. Oxamniquine can produce orange-red discoloration of the urine.

Several trematodes reside in the lumen of the human gastrointestinal tract. They include *Fasciolopsis buski*, which is acquired by eating contaminated water plants such as bamboo shoots, water chestnut, or caltrop; *Heterophyes heterophyes* and *Metagonimus yokogawai*, which are acquired from contaminated, inadequately cooked fish; and *Nanophyetus salmincola*, which is acquired by eating raw or uncooked salmon or other fish. Other trematode genera infect the liver. They include the Chinese liver fluke *Clonorchis sinensis*, and the closely related species *Opisthorchis viverrini*, which are acquired from raw or inadequately cooked freshwater fish that are grown in water contaminated with human feces, and the North American liver fluke *Metorchis conjunctus*, which caused an outbreak of acute illness in a group of people in Montreal, Canada, who ate raw fish (sashimi) prepared from white suckers. The sheep liver fluke *Fasciola hepatica* is contracted when humans eat contaminated watercress. All of these trematodes, with the exception of *F. hepatica*, appear to be susceptible to praziquantel, although data on its efficacy are limited in some instances. The dose is 75 mg per kg daily given in three divided doses, except for *N. salmincola*, which is treated with 60 mg per kg daily in three divided doses. *F. hepatica* should be treated with bithionol (Bitin),* 30 to 50 mg per kg per day on alternate days for 10 to 15 doses. Photosensitivity reactions, diarrhea, abdominal pain, and urticaria are common; leukopenia and hepatitis are rare untoward effects with bithionol.

CESTODES (TAPEWORMS)

Humans are the definitive host for a number of tapeworm species; that is, adult tapeworms reside in the human gastrointestinal tract. *Diphyllobothrium latum* and other *Diphyllobothrium* species, fish tapeworms, are acquired by eating raw or inadequately cooked contaminated freshwater fish. They compete with their human host for vitamin B_{12}. The adult tapeworms of *Taenia saginata*, which is acquired from contaminated beef, and *Taenia solium*, from pork, grow to great lengths in the lumen of the human intestine, but they produce few, if any, symptoms. *H. nana*, the dwarf tapeworm, is acquired through the ingestion of ova originating in the feces of infected humans and is capable of autoinfection. On rare occasions, the dog tapeworm, *Dipylidium caninum*, is acquired by young children when they inadvertently ingest infested fleas from dogs, the usual definitive host.

Praziquantel is the treatment of choice for adult tapeworm infections. Most cestode species can be treated with 5 to 10 mg per kg given in a single dose,

---

*Available through the CDC.

but *H. nana* requires 25 mg per kg. Niclosamide (Niclocide)* is also effective against intestinal tapeworms. A single dose of 2 grams chewed thoroughly is recommended for *T. saginata* and *Diphyllobothrium* species. A 7-day course with 2 grams the first day and 1 gram per day thereafter is required for *H. nana*; a single dose of praziquantel is preferable.

With *T. solium,* humans serve as the definitive host when they consume cysticerci in contaminated pork. Adult tapeworms develop in the gastrointestinal tract. If humans ingest *T. solium* ova in food or water contaminated with human feces, invading larvae can encyst in their brains, producing neurocysticercosis, in other organs, or in subcutaneous tissue. Most physicians prefer to treat persons with adult *T. solium* in their intestines with praziquantel, which has larvicidal activity, rather than niclosamide, because of the theoretical concern that adult tapeworms killed by niclosamide might release ova in the small intestine that could excyst, invade, and result in cysticercosis.

The treatment of neurocysticercosis is more complicated. Persons with single parenchymal cysts have been reported to do well even without therapy. For patients with multiple parenchymal cysts, many physicians prefer albendazole, 15 mg per kg per day in 3 doses for 8 to 28 days; treatment with praziquantel is 50 mg per kg per day in three divided doses for 15 days. Albendazole should be administered with fatty meals to maximize absorption. There is marked first-pass metabolism. The major metabolite albendazole sulfoxide is responsible for the anthelmintic activity and reaches good levels in the central nervous system. Side effects of high-dose, prolonged albendazole therapy include neutropenia, alopecia, and liver enzyme elevations. Dying cysticeri release antigens that can trigger local inflammatory responses resulting in increased intracranial pressure, which on rare occasions has been fatal. Corticosteroids are usually administered concurrently to prevent or limit increased intracranial pressure. Anthelmintic drugs should not be used in patients with intraocular or spinal cord cysticeri because of the local inflammatory damage that can follow the release of parasite antigens.

In echinococcosis, humans serve as an intermediate host for *Echinococcus* species; dogs or other canines are the definitive hosts. The World Health Organization Working Group on Echinococcosis has recommended surgery as the treatment of choice for *Echinococcus granulosus* and *Echinococcus multilocularis.* Percutaneous drainage followed by instillation of a scolicidal agent, such as hypertonic saline, and then by aspiration, or laparoscopic approaches have been advocated as alternatives for patients with *E. granulosus* cysts. Treatment with albendazole before surgery can reduce the risk of peritoneal implants. Albendazole, three or more cycles of 400 mg twice a day for 28 days, each followed by a 2-week rest period, cures approximately one third of those infected with *E. granulosus* and is the treatment of choice for patients with inoperable *E. granulosus* or *E. multilocularis* disease. Mebendazole is an alternative for the treatment of echinococcosis, but it is not as well absorbed as albendazole.

SUMMARY

A diverse array of parasites can produce intestinal disease in humans. *E. histolytica* and *G. lamblia* are well-known protozoal pathogens. In the past decade, increasing attention has been paid to the importance of *Cryptosporidium*. It has been responsible for water-borne outbreaks in the United States, it is a major cause of childhood diarrhea in developing areas, and it is responsible for severe, chronic diarrhea in persons with HIV infection. Reports have focused on the emergence of *Cyclospora* species in immunocompetent and immunocompromised persons and on microsporidians as a cause of diarrhea in those with AIDS. With the important exception of *Cryptosporidium,* effective chemotherapy is available for the treatment of enteric protozoal diseases.

The benzimidazoles albendazole and mebendazole are active against a number of intestinal nematodes (roundworms). They are effective for the treatment of *A. lumbricoides,* the hookworms, *T. trichiura, E. vermicularis, Trichostrongylus* species, and other nematodes. Albendazole has the advantage of being effective when administered as a single dose. It has been widely used in mass treatment programs in developing areas. Pyrantel pamoate is available over the counter in the United States for the treatment of the pinworm *E. vermicularis,* and it has activity against *A. lumbricoides,* hookworms, and *Trichostrongylus* species. *S. stercoralis* should be treated with either ivermectin or thiabendazole. Both are effective, but ivermectin is much better tolerated.

Praziquantel is the treatment of choice for schistosomiasis and other trematode (fluke) infections with the exception of *F. hepatica* infection, which should be treated with bithionol. Praziquantel is also recommended for the treatment of adult cestode (tapeworm) infections of the intestinal tract. Although mild side effects are common, praziquantel is relatively well tolerated, and there are no long-term effects. Niclosamide, which is poorly absorbed, offers an alternative for the treatment of adult tapeworms of several species including *T. saginata* and *D. latum,* but praziquantel is preferred for the treatment of *T. solium* and *H. nana* infections.

Albendazole or praziquantel at high doses can kill cysticerci of *T. solium* in persons with parenchymal neurocysticercosis. Corticosteroids are usually administered concurrently to minimize the effects of inflammation and the potential for increased intracranial pressure that accompanies the release of cysticercal antigens. Surgery is the treatment of choice for *E. granulosus* and *E. multiloculiaris.* Percutaneous drainage followed by instillation and aspiration of a scolicidal agent or laparoscopic approaches have been advocated as alternatives for patients with *E.*

---

*Not available in the United States.

granulosus cysts. Treatment with albendazole before surgery can reduce the risk of peritoneal implants. Albendazole cures approximately one third of those infected with *E. granulosus* and is the treatment of choice for patients with inoperable *E. granulosus* or *E. multilocularis* infections. In summary, safe, effective drugs are available for the treatment of most of the major intestinal helminths that infect humans.

Metabolic Disorders

DIABETES MELLITUS IN ADULTS

method of
HAROLD E. LEBOVITZ, M.D.
*State University of New York Health Science
Center at Brooklyn
Brooklyn, New York*

EPIDEMIOLOGY

Non–insulin-dependent diabetes mellitus (NIDDM; type 2 diabetes mellitus) will continue to be one of the major health care problems well into the 21st century. This heterogeneous disorder accounts for between 90 and 97% of the diabetes cases that occur in various populations. It is increasing in prevalence because of aging of the population, elevated population growth rates of high-risk racial groups, and worldwide adoption of Western diets and cultural patterns. Diabetes and its complications are responsible for more than 10% of inpatient hospital use and one seventh of the health care budget of the United States. It is clear that unless the epidemic of NIDDM can be stopped and/or its complications prevented, the cost in human life and suffering as well as the economic burden will seriously handicap all societies.

In the United States, there are currently 16,000,000 diabetic patients (6.2% of the population). One half of these individuals are virtually asymptomatic and are undiagnosed. Approximately 625,000 new cases of diabetes are diagnosed each year, which means that 1.25 million people or 0.5% of the population develop diabetes each year. Nonwhite Americans have from a twofold to a fivefold greater prevalence of NIDDM than white Americans (5% of whom have diabetes). The average age at diagnosis of symptomatic NIDDM in white individuals is approximately 53 years and that in nonwhite individuals is about 43 years. Nonwhite individuals not only have a higher prevalence of NIDDM than whites but also develop clinical disease about 8 to 10 years earlier.

Diabetic retinopathy is the leading cause of new blindness in the United States (12% of all cases). Diabetic nephropathy accounts for 35% of all new cases of end-stage renal disease. Lower extremity arterial disease is 10 times more common in diabetic patients than nondiabetic patients, and half of all lower extremity amputations in the United States occur in diabetic patients. Diabetic men have two times and diabetic women three times the rate of coronary heart disease of nondiabetic individuals. Diabetic subjects also have a poorer prognosis after myocardial infarction than subjects without diabetes. It is the complications of diabetes that account for most of the excessive use of health care resources by diabetic patients.

Therapeutic approaches to diabetes management in the adult should therefore be focused in the following areas:

1. Preventive measures to decrease the development of diabetes in populations at high risk

2. Early diagnosis when diabetes does develop
3. Treatment regimens to prevent acute complications
4. Glycemic control to prevent microvascular complications
5. Metabolic control to reduce the increased risk of macrovascular disease
6. Early treatment of complications when they do occur

PATHOPHYSIOLOGY

To prevent the development of NIDDM in populations at risk, it is necessary to understand the pathophysiology of the disorder. Patients who develop NIDDM have an underlying genetic predisposition to develop the disease (Figure 1). This has been ascertained by the high concordance rate in monozygotic twins in contrast to dizygotic twins and the fourfold higher prevalence of NIDDM in individuals with two or more first-degree relatives with diabetes in contrast to those with no first-degree relative with diabetes. Environmental factors, however, play a major role in bringing about the expression of the clinical disease (see Figure 1). Racial populations who express a high prevalence of NIDDM do so only in an environment of high-calorie diets, decreased physical activity, stress, and obesity. Black, Hispanic, Asian, and Indian populations have a low prevalence of NIDDM in their native cultures but develop a 5- to 10-fold increase in prevalence after migrating to the United States or Western Europe or adopting a Western culture in their native land.

The genetic predisposition appears to manifest itself in limited beta cell insulin secretory reserve and perhaps a propensity for disproportionately increased intra-abdominal fat. The environmental factors may include intrauterine malnutrition leading to a decreased number of beta cells, but most important are an increase in high-fat and high-calorie diets and decrease in physical activity (both of which lead to obesity) and increased levels of stress. These cause insulin resistance at the level of muscle and increase the individual's requirement for insulin four- to sixfold. This combination of increased insulin requirement (insulin resistance) and limited beta cell insulin secretion causes the hyperglycemia of most persons with NIDDM. Individual patients vary in the proportions in which insulin resistance and insulin deficiency dominate the metabolic abnormality. The ultimate effect of the combined abnormalities is to cause insulin insufficiency, either absolute or relative.

As an individual becomes insulin deficient, the initial alteration in glucose metabolism is a rise in the postprandial blood glucose value. This occurs because postprandial blood glucose is taken up by muscle under the influence of high concentrations of insulin and either stored or utilized (Table 1). When postprandial levels of plasma insulin are inadequate to utilize the glucose load, the postprandial plasma glucose levels rise excessively and remain high for long periods. Initially with insulin deficiency, the 2-hour postprandial plasma glucose level is borderline (140 to 199 mg per dL). This is called impaired glucose tolerance (IGT).

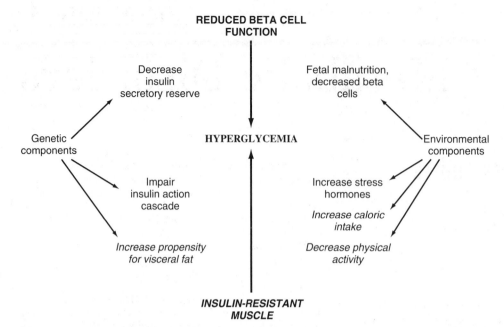

Figure 1. Pathogenesis of hyperglycemia in NIDDM. Hyperglycemia results from inadequate insulin secretion relative to the individual's insulin requirement. In any individual, increased requirements or inadequate beta cell function may be the predominant abnormality. Both reduced beta cell function and increased insulin requirements have genetic and environmental components. See text for further details.

Thirty to 40% of such individuals progress to NIDDM in 5 to 10 years. As insulin deficiency becomes greater, the 2-hour postprandial plasma glucose level exceeds 200 mg per dL, and that defines diabetes mellitus. At this stage the fasting plasma glucose level is minimally if at all elevated.

Fasting plasma glucose is regulated by the balance between hepatic glucose production and brain glucose utilization. The brain is insulin independent and uses 5 grams of glucose per hour. During fasting that glucose comes from hepatic glucose production. The rate of hepatic glucose production is controlled by plasma insulin and glucagon levels. As the plasma insulin level falls, hepatic glucose production increases. As the plasma insulin level rises, hepatic glucose production is suppressed. When insulin deficiency becomes severe, there is not enough insulin to suppress the fasting hepatic glucose production normally (see Table 1), and fasting hyperglycemia occurs because production exceeds utilization. The sequence of events observed in the evolution of diabetes as insulin insufficiency progresses is IGT, then postprandial hyperglycemia, and finally fasting hyperglycemia. Ketoacidosis occurs only when little or no insulin is available.

PREVENTION OF DEVELOPMENT OF NIDDM

Strategies for preventing the development of NIDDM focus on reducing the environmental factors that lead to insulin resistance or treating patients at high risk of developing diabetes with pharmacologic agents that decrease the individuals' requirements for insulin.

The most effective means of reducing insulin resistance are dietary modification, increased physical activity, and weight loss. A reduction to near-ideal body weight frequently reduces postprandial hyperglycemia, restores IGT to normal, and/or prevents its progression to NIDDM. This has been shown in several prospective studies. Unfortunately, the majority of individuals in a Western society are unable to change their lifestyle sufficiently to achieve these goals.

In the event that patients cannot maintain dietary interventions and achieve weight loss with traditional methods including behavior modification, several appetite suppressant drugs are available to help achieve those ends. These drugs include the serotonin reuptake inhibitor dexfenfluramine (Redux) and the combined serotonin and norepinephrine reuptake inhibitor sibutramine (Meridia).* Dexfenfluramine is administered at 15 mg twice a day. Sibutramine is given as 15 or 20 mg once a day. Both drugs are adjuncts to a weight-reducing diet. Weight losses of 10% or greater may be expected in 40 to 50% of patients. Weight loss is usually maximal at 6 months and can be maintained if drug therapy is continued. Discontinuation of drug treatment is usually accompanied by weight gain back toward the baseline weight. Side effects of norepinephrine reuptake inhibition are increased blood pressure, tachycardia, dry mouth, and insomnia. Side effects of dexfenfluramine are loss of concentration, memory impairment, fatigue, drowsiness, and rarely primary pulmonary hypertension.

Currently, a reasonable recommendation is to use these agents in conjunction with a low-calorie diet

TABLE 1. **Relative Tissue Sensitivity to Insulin**

Tissue	Dose Range of Effect (µU/mL)	Relative Requirement
Brain glucose uptake and utilization	None	—
Muscle glucose uptake and utilization	25–500	25
Suppression of hepatic glucose production	2.5–25	2.5
Inhibition of adipose tissue release of free fatty acids	1–10	1

*Investigational drug in the United States.

and increased physical activity to enhance weight loss in the short term in high-risk patients with IGT. Therapy should be stopped after 6 months and attempts to keep weight down with continued diet and increased physical activity pursued. Such a preventive program is particularly beneficial for an individual with IGT who has associated metabolic problems such as hypertension, central obesity, and/or diabetic dyslipidemia.

The use of pharmacologic therapy to decrease requirements for insulin in patients with IGT and insulin resistance for the purpose of preventing progression of IGT to NIDDM is being tried in several large multicenter controlled studies. In the United States, Diabetes Prevention Trial II has both a metformin and a troglitazone arm. A large Canadian-European study is evaluating the effect of the α-glucosidase inhibitor acarbose to prevent the progression from IGT to NIDDM. The results of these studies will not be available for 3 to 5 years. Small preliminary studies with all three agents have yielded results which show short team improvement in IGT with treatment (metformin [Glucophage], 850 mg twice daily; troglitazone [Rezulin], 200 to 400 mg once daily; acarbose [Precose], 50 mg three times daily).

EARLY DIAGNOSIS OF NIDDM

The evolution of metabolic abnormalities in patients with NIDDM obscures the early diagnosis. Individuals in whom insulin resistance is a major contributor to the development of NIDDM frequently start with an increase in body fat (particularly visceral fat). Associated with this central obesity and insulin resistance are an increase in blood pressure, an increase in plasma triglycerides, a decrease in plasma high-density lipoprotein (HDL) cholesterol, and the development of a procoagulant state (increased plasma fibrinogen and increased plasminogen activator inhibitor type 1). The fasting plasma glucose level is usually normal but IGT is common. This so-called insulin resistance syndrome or syndrome X usually persists for several years before the postprandial blood glucose becomes elevated sufficiently for the individual to develop asymptomatic NIDDM. The postprandial blood glucose elevation characteristic of the early stages of NIDDM is not ordinarily accompanied by a significant rise in fasting plasma glucose (FPG < 125 mg per dL) or a significant increase in hemoglobin A_{1c} beyond the normal range (hemoglobin A_{1c} < 6.2%). After 4 to 7 years of postprandial hyperglycemia, the fasting plasma glucose level becomes elevated (greater than 140 mg per dL) and the individual develops the classic symptoms of diabetes.

Complications of diabetes occur at all stages of the evolution of NIDDM. Individuals with IGT, although not at risk for microvascular disease, are twice as likely as normal individuals to die with coronary heart disease. Individuals with undiagnosed NIDDM (those with primarily postprandial hyperglycemia) develop the early stages of microvascular as well as macrovascular disease.

Significantly decreasing the morbidity and mortality in NIDDM requires early diagnosis and initiation of appropriate treatment. An individual with a random plasma glucose level of 200 mg per dL or greater and symptoms is easily recognized as having diabetes mellitus. In the past, a fasting plasma glucose level of 140 mg per dL or greater on two occasions was sufficient to make the diagnosis of diabetes mellitus. This level has a sensitivity of only 31% but a specificity of approximately 100%. It is likely that a fasting plasma glucose level of 125 mg per dL or greater will be recommended for the diagnostic criterion. This value has a specificity of 99%, but the sensitivity is increased to approximately 50%. The most sensitive and specific test for diabetes mellitus in nonpregnant adults is a plasma glucose value 2 hours after 75 g of oral glucose equal to or greater than 200 mg per dL.

The use of hemoglobin A_{1c} for diagnosis of diabetes is not recommended for two reasons. It is determined by a variety of techniques with different normal ranges. It is not as sensitive as the 2-hour postprandial plasma glucose value in making the diagnosis.

When early diabetes or its associated abnormalities are detected, they should be treated according to the goals described in subsequent sections. The initial approach to treatment should be lifestyle modifications. If that does not achieve the target goals, pharmacologic agents should be added to the regimen.

TREATMENT REGIMENS TO PREVENT ACUTE COMPLICATIONS

Acute complications resulting from poor metabolic control still cause significant morbidity and mortality in NIDDM patients. Diabetic ketoacidosis (DKA) has a reported incidence in the United States of 4.6 to 8.0 cases per 1000 diabetic persons per year. Twenty to 30% of DKA cases occur as the initial presentation of diabetes. The reported mortality rate for DKA ranges from as low as 2 to 3% to as high as 9 to 14%. Data are not available on the percentage of DKA cases that occur in NIDDM patients compared with patients with autoimmune insulin-dependent diabetes mellitus. However, ketoacidosis occurs not infrequently as the initial presentation for black and Hispanic Americans with NIDDM. Approximately 34% of cases of DKA occur in adults older than 45 years and 49% occur in those 18 to 44 years old.

Hyperosmolar nonketotic coma (plasma glucose level of >600 mg per dL; plasma osmolality of >320 mOsm per liter) occurs predominately in NIDDM patients. It is much less common than ketoacidosis (about one tenth as common) but the mortality rate associated with it is quite high, varying from 10 to 50%.

An important clinical issue is that acute complications can be prevented by education of patients, early diagnosis, and effective initial treatment. Morbidity and mortality resulting from the acute metabolic complications of diabetes are directly related to the severity of the metabolic derangement and the time between the onset of the derangement and the initiation of effective treatment. Patients who are at high risk for acute metabolic complications should be educated about the early symptoms and measures that can be used to avoid the severe metabolic derangements. When patients present initially for hyperglycemia, their evaluation must include estimates of the state of hydration, acid-base balance, and ketosis. Hospitalization or more intensive treatment or both are indicated if significant dehydration, acidosis, or ketosis is present. Similarly, whether the patient requires insulin therapy or oral antihyperglycemic agents can be tried is determined by the presence or absence of these severe associated metabolic abnormalities.

Obviously, if a patient presents with DKA or hyperosmolar nonketotic coma, immediate treatment with fluids, electrolytes, and intravenous regular insulin is indicated.

GLYCEMIC CONTROL TO PREVENT MICROVASCULAR COMPLICATIONS

Data indicating that diabetic microvascular and neuropathic complications are directly related to the magnitude and duration of hyperglycemia are incontrovertible. Multiple mechanisms have been proposed to explain how hyperglycemia causes these complications. They include glycosylation of proteins and the generation of advanced glycosylation end products, an exaggeration of flux through the aldose reductase pathway, changes in cellular oxidative stress, and alterations in the protein kinase C regulatory system.

Glycemic control of the diabetic is monitored by blood glucose measurements by the patient and measurements of hemoglobin A_{1c} or glycosylated hemoglobin by the laboratory. Self-monitoring of blood glucose by patients is done occasionally (one to four times per week) to ensure that control is stable, to check whether an acute illness has caused an exacerbation of hyperglycemia, to clarify whether symptoms are truly due to hypoglycemia, or to give the patient feedback about the influence of his or her behavior on the diabetic regulation. More frequent self-monitoring of blood glucose (before meals and at bedtime for several days) is useful when the therapeutic regimen is being changed.

Hemoglobin A_{1c} or glycosylated hemoglobin should be measured every 3 to 4 months. This measurement assesses the mean blood glucose level for the preceding 6 to 8 weeks, and it is essential for the management of all diabetics. The development and progression of microvascular and neuropathic complications are highly correlated with long-term hemoglobin A_{1c} measurements. In an assay in which the normal range of hemoglobin A_{1c} is 4.0 to 6.0%, microvascular and neuropathic complications can be minimized if the hemoglobin A_{1c} level is maintained at 7.0% or

less. At levels of hemoglobin A_{1c} greater than 8% microvascular complication rates and severity increase remarkably with time. Table 2 defines the goals of chronic glycemic treatment for NIDDM patients. It also gives an estimate of the plasma glucose levels that correlate with the various levels of hemoglobin A_{1c} control. The goals of glycemic control must be individually defined and depend on the age of the patient, years of expected functional survival, presence of diabetic complications or other complicating illnesses, and the patient's willingness to comply. It is irrational to strive to achieve excellent glycemic control for an individual who will not survive long enough to benefit from it.

The first step in achieving chronic glycemic control in NIDDM patients is to modify the lifestyle that has contributed to the development of the hyperglycemia in most of the patients. A diet is tailored to the appropriate caloric and nutritional requirements for the particular individual. An obese individual (greater than 120% ideal body weight) should be given a restricted calorie diet to achieve some weight reduction if possible. It is recommended that the diet contain 50 to 60% carbohydrates, mostly complex carbohydrates. Fat should not make up more than 30% of calories, and saturated fats should be kept to less than 10%. Protein content is recommended to be 10 to 20%. In some individuals, a high-carbohydrate diet causes a significant rise in plasma triglycerides, in which case some of the carbohydrate should be replaced by monounsaturated fats. If compliance is to be achieved, a dietary regimen must be designed and continually reinforced by a nutritionist who takes into account the patient's cultural and personal background.

An increase in physical activity must accompany the dietary program. The increase in physical activity must again be tailored to the individual. Walking is good exercise if there are no lower extremity contraindications. A planned exercise regimen should

TABLE 2. **Goals of Treatment for NIDDM Patients**

Treatment Aim	Normal	Goal	Unacceptable
Glucose regulation			
Fasting plasma glucose (mg/dL)	≤115	80–125	>140 <80
2-h postprandial plasma glucose (mg/dL)	≤150	100–160	>200 <80
Hemoglobin A_{1c} (%)	<6.0	<7.0	>8.0
Blood pressure regulation			
Systolic BP (mm Hg)	≤120	≤130	>140
Diastolic BP (mm Hg)	≤80	≤85	>90
Lipid regulation			
Plasma LDL cholesterol (mg/dL)	≤140	100–130	>130
Plasma HDL cholesterol (mg/dL)	35–60	>35	<35
Fasting plasma triglyceride (mg/dL)	≤150	≤150	>200

Abbreviations: NIDDM = non–insulin-dependent diabetes mellitus; BP = blood pressure; LDL = low-density lipoprotein.

TABLE 3. **Oral Antidiabetic Agents in Common Use**

Agent	Mechanism of Action	Dose Range (mg)	Major Side Effects
Sulfonylureas	↑ Endogenous insulin		Hypoglycemia Weight gain
Long acting			
Chlorpropamide (Diabinese)		100–500/d	
Glyburide (DiaBeta, Micronase)		1.25–20/d	
Glyburide, micronized (Glynase PresTabs)		0.75–6/d	
Glipizide (Glucotrol XL)		5–10/d	
Intermediate acting			
Glipizide (Glucotrol)		2.5–25/d	
Glimepiride (Amaryl)		4–8/d	

Metformin (Glucophage)	↓ Hepatic glucose production
	↑ Insulin action on muscle glucose
	  uptake
		500–2500/d	Diarrhea
			↓ Serum vitamin B_{12}
			Lactic acidosis if
			  inappropriately
			  prescribed

α-Glucosidase inhibitors	Delay carbohydrate digestion and decrease postprandial glycemia		Flatulence Abdominal discomfort
Acarbose (Precose)		25–100 with meals	
Miglitol (Glyset)		25–50 with meals	

Troglitazone (Rezulin)	↑ Insulin action on muscle and fat
	  glucose uptake
		200–600/d	Slight decrease in red
			  blood cell count

always be preceded by an appropriate evaluation of the cardiovascular and musculoskeletal systems.

The combination of dietary management and increased physical activity, if effective, results in decreased insulin resistance and improved glycemic control. For patients presenting with fasting plasma glucose values less than 180 mg per dL and hemoglobin A_{1c} value less than 7.5%, this lifestyle modification therapy may be sufficient to restore normal glycemia. Unfortunately, the majority of NIDDM patients are unable to effect these lifestyle changes or are not sufficiently responsive to them to achieve the target glycemic control. In such cases, pharmacologic therapy must be added to their regimen. Pharmacologic therapy does not obviate the need for continued dietary and physical activity programs. The drugs are additive.

Pharmacologic therapies for hyperglycemia (Tables 3 and 4) address one of three major targets: (1) reducing appetite and thereby decreasing obesity, (2) increasing insulin availability, or (3) decreasing insulin requirements. The appetite suppressant drugs were discussed in the previous section on prevention of NIDDM. Drugs to increase insulin availability include all of the sulfonylureas, insulin preparations, and the newer insulin analogues such as insulin lis-

TABLE 4. **Insulin Preparations in Common Use**

Preparation	Onset of Action	Duration of Action (h)
Regular	30–60 min	4–6
Lispro	5–10 min	3–4
NPH	2–3 h	9–12
Lente	2–3 h	9–12
Premixed (70:30)	30–60 min	9–12
Ultralente	2–3 h	18–24

Abbreviation: NPH = neutral protamine Hagedorn.

pro (Humalog). These agents decrease glycemia by improving the insulin deficiency state. The sulfonylureas do so by potentiating endogenous glucose-mediated insulin secretion from beta cells. Insulin injections do so by adding exogenous insulin to the endogenous insulin pool.

Sulfonylureas differ in their actions primarily on the basis of their pharmacokinetics (see Table 3). Long-acting drugs are generally given once a day and have an effect that lasts 24 hours or longer. The intermediate-acting drugs can be given once or twice a day. They have a duration of action of 12 to 16 hours. Sulfonylureas lower the fasting plasma glucose by a mean of 60 mg per dL and decrease the hemoglobin A_{1c} value 1.0 to 2.0%. About 15% of NIDDM patients are initially unresponsive to sulfonylureas (primary failure). Among those who respond well (50%) or partially (35%), a secondary failure rate of 3 to 5% per year occurs. The major side effects of sulfonylurea drugs are hypoglycemia and weight gain. The long-acting sulfonylureas are more likely to cause severe hypoglycemia than the intermediate-acting ones. Sulfonylureas are contraindicated for patients with significant liver disease or impaired renal function.

Administration of insulin to control hyperglycemia in NIDDM patients frequently requires large doses and multiple injections and is limited by the development of hypoglycemia and weight gain. There is little advantage to using insulin in treating NIDDM patients who are still responsive to oral antihyperglycemic agents because the degree of glycemic control is comparable.

The newest additions to the pharmacologic agents for treating hyperglycemia in NIDDM patients are several classes of drugs that decrease insulin requirements. Two, biguanides and thiazolidinediones, decrease insulin resistance. α-Glucosidase inhibitors lower the need for insulin by decreasing the rate of postprandial glucose absorption.

Metformin is a biguanide and acts predominantly by decreasing the overproduction of glucose by the liver that is responsible for the fasting hyperglycemia. It also improves the action of insulin on muscle glucose uptake to a modest degree. An occasional patient also experiences anorexia when taking metformin. The net result of these actions in NIDDM patients is a decrease in mean fasting plasma glucose of 60 mg per dL and a decrease in hemoglobin A_{1c} of 1 to 2%. Accompanying metformin therapy are a small weight loss and small decreases in serum low-density lipoprotein (LDL) cholesterol and triglycerides. Metformin should not be given to patients with impaired renal function or significant hypoxic states.

Troglitazone is a thiazolidinedione. It acts by binding to a nuclear receptor in the genome (peroxisome proliferator-activated receptor $PPAR_x$) and influences the transcription of a number of gene products in adipose tissue and perhaps muscle. Among the observed effects are increases in insulin-responsive and non–insulin-responsive glucose transporter molecules in fat cells and muscle. The net effect is a potentiation of insulin-mediated glucose utilization in muscle and fat cells. This drug action is called insulin sensitization. The decrease in insulin resistance is seen in other insulin-resistant states as well as NIDDM. Troglitazone is effective in reducing hyperglycemia in patients with IGT. It lowers fasting plasma glucose in NIDDM patients about 40 mg per dL and hemoglobin A_{1c} 0.5 to 0.8%. It decreases serum triglyceride and plasma free fatty acid levels 15 to 20%.

The alpha-glucosidase inhibitors (acarbose and miglitol [Glyset]) lower insulin requirements by decreasing peak postprandial plasma glucose rises. These drugs are competitive inhibitors of the α-glucosidase enzymes located in the brush border of the cells of the small intestine, which are responsible for the digestion of oligosaccharides and disaccharides. Ordinarily, carbohydrate is completely digested in the upper jejunum and immediately absorbed, giving rise to the rapid and marked rise in plasma glucose after a meal. When the enzymes in the upper jejunum are blocked, the carbohydrate has to be digested and absorbed throughout the small intestine. This delays digestion and thus decreases the rate of glucose absorption. The effect of these drugs in NIDDM patients is to lower peak postprandial plasma glucose by 45 to 60 mg per dL and decrease hemoglobin A_{1c} 0.5 to 1.0%. Because they are competitive inhibitors, they must be taken at the beginning of each meal. Drug dosage should be low initially and increased slowly to minimize gastrointestinal symptoms.

The availability of so many drugs with different modes of action to treat hyperglycemia provides tools for adequately controlling glycemia in most NIDDM patients. It has, however, also added considerable complexity to determining how to develop treatment strategies.

An NIDDM patient who presents with symptoms, has a random plasma glucose level less than 400 mg per dL, and does not have evidence of dehydration, acidosis, or marked ketosis can be started on a program consisting of diet, increased physical activity, and monotherapy with an oral antihyperglycemic agent. If the plasma glucose level is less than 250 mg per dL and symptoms are mild, diet and exercise may be tried alone. If the plasma glucose value is above 400 mg per dL and/or the patient has evidence of dehydration, acidosis, or marked ketosis, insulin therapy should be initiated as two or three injections a day unless the patient is ketoacidotic or hyperosmolar, in which case hospital admission and intensive therapy are indicated.

For monotherapy with an oral antihyperglycemic agent, the following issues should be considered. An individual who is normal in weight or only mildly obese with a fasting plasma glucose level greater than 240 mg per dL is likely to be more insulin deficient than insulin resistant and to benefit from an agent that increases insulin availability. Obese individuals with fasting plasma glucose values of 240 mg per dL or less are probably more insulin resistant than insulin deficient and would benefit from a drug that decreases insulin requirements, such as metformin or troglitazone. A patient with mild fasting hyperglycemia (<165 mg per dL) and predominantly postprandial hyperglycemia would be a good candidate for therapy with acarbose or miglitol.

Monotherapy, either initially or eventually, may not achieve the glycemic goal. In that case, a combination of oral antihyperglycemic agents has been shown to be quite effective provided the drugs combined have different modes of action. The most logical approach is to combine a drug that increases insulin availability with a drug that decreases insulin requirements. Such combinations as sulfonylureas plus metformin, sulfonylureas plus acarbose, and sulfonylureas plus troglitazone achieve a 0.8 to 1.5% further decrease in hemoglobin A_{1c}. Combinations of drugs that lower insulin requirements (metformin plus acarbose, metformin plus troglitazone) are being evaluated.

As endogenous insulin secretion further decreases in NIDDM patients, even combinations of oral agents become inadequate. At that stage neutral protamine Hagedorn (NPH) insulin or insulin zinc (Lente Insulin) at 10 PM can be added to the regimen. The intermediate insulin dose (starting dose is usually 5 to 10 units) is adjusted to achieve a fasting plasma glucose level of 120 mg per dL and the combined oral agents are continued during the day. Multiple insulin injections (NPH and Regular Insulin before breakfast, Regular Insulin before the evening meal, and NPH insulin at 10 PM) are introduced when the previous regimen is inadequate. Data show that addition of troglitazone at 200 to 600 mg per day for NIDDM patients inadequately controlled with insulin improves glycemic control by a decrease in hemoglobin A_{1c} of 0.8 to 1.4% and lowers insulin requirements.

Glycemic control is achieved by defining the target

value and then developing a strategy using a combination of lifestyle changes and pharmacologic agents to achieve that target.

METABOLIC CONTROL TO REDUCE MACROVASCULAR DISEASE

Macrovascular disease occurs more commonly and is more severe in diabetic than in nondiabetic patients. A multitude of factors are responsible for the increase in morbidity and mortality. Among them are central obesity, increased prevalence of hypertension, diabetic dyslipidemia, a diabetic procoagulant state, and hyperglycemia. The relative risk attributed to each of these factors is unclear and quite complicated. When death resulting from coronary artery disease is expressed in terms of known cardiovascular risk factors, the diabetic patient has a threefold higher death rate than the nondiabetic for comparable risk factors. This suggests a specific diabetic risk factor or a multiplier effect of risk factors in the diabetic.

The role of hyperglycemia itself as a cause of increased macrovascular disease has been clarified. Each 1% increase in hemoglobin A_{1c} increases the risk of coronary heart disease by approximately 10%. This is only about one fourth to one fifth of the effect of hyperglycemia on the risk of microvascular disease in the retina. Poorly controlled glycemia in NIDDM patients is associated with more coronary heart disease events and deaths than well-controlled glycemia (hemoglobin A_{1c} value of <8.0%). Thus, hyperglycemia contributes to but is not the major component in the increased macrovascular disease of the diabetic.

A major influence can be attributed to the diabetic dyslipidemia and the interaction of plasma lipoprotein particles with the blood vessels. The insulin-resistant state with its central obesity is associated with increased plasma triglycerides and decreased plasma HDL cholesterol levels (diabetic dyslipidemia). Although plasma LDL cholesterol levels are not different in diabetic and nondiabetic persons, the composition of the lipoprotein particles is different. Diabetic patients tend to have an increase in small, dense LDL particles (B pattern). The interaction of the lipoprotein particles with the vessel walls (abnormal endothelial function), the procoagulant state (increased plasma fibrinogen and increased plasminogen activator inhibitor type 1), and the increase in blood pressure, which occurs in 60 to 70% of NIDDM patients, all contribute to the increased macrovascular disease of the diabetic patient.

Clinical data support the hypothesis that treatment of diabetic patients with lipid-lowering agents reduces coronary heart disease morbidity and mortality. The data arise from secondary analyses of diabetic patients who found their way into the various studies rather than from studies designed specifically for diabetic patients. Decreases in elevated plasma triglycerides and increases in depressed plasma HDL cholesterol caused some reduction in coronary heart disease risk and death in the diabet-

ics treated with gemfibrozil (Lopid) in the Helsinki Heart Study. The 4S study (Scandinavian Simvistatin Survival Study) showed that decreasing the plasma LDL cholesterol level by 37% and the plasma triglyceride level by 11% and raising the plasma HDL cholesterol level by 7% reduced the risk of death or an additional myocardial infarction by 54% for 6 years in diabetic patients who had a myocardial infarction and were treated with simvastatin. Similarly, results of the CARE (cholesterol and recurrent events) study showed a 25% reduction in coronary heart disease events in diabetic patients whose plasma LDL cholesterol value was lowered from a mean of 139 mg per dL to a mean of 98 mg per dL with pravastatin (Pravachol) after an initial myocardial infarction.

Because NIDDM patients have such a high prevalence of coronary heart disease, frequently present with atypical symptoms, have such poor outcomes after myocardial infarction, and are likely to benefit from lipid-lowering agents, more aggressive and earlier treatment of plasma lipid abnormalities in NIDDM patients is indicated. Table 5 lists the lipid-lowering agents that are likely to be most beneficial in NIDDM patients. They are classified according to their specific lipid effects. Table 2 gives reasonable goals for lipid regulation in NIDDM patients. Most NIDDM patients should be treated for plasma LDL cholesterol levels greater than 130 mg per dL and triglyceride levels greater than 200 mg per dL. Nicotinic acid must be used with caution in diabetic patients because it frequently worsens glycemic regulation. Because NIDDM patients frequently have diabetic dyslipidemia as well as serum LDL cholesterol levels greater than 130 mg per dL, they have been treated with both a fibrate and an hydroxymethylglutaryl–coenzyme A (HMG-CoA) reductase inhibitor. The availability of more potent HMG-CoA reductase inhibitors such as atorvastatin (Lipitor), which is effective in lowering both serum triglycerides and LDL cholesterol, may obviate the need for combination drug therapy, with which a side effect of myopathy is a concern. Side effects to be monitored for are gallstones and liver function abnormalities with gemfibrozil and liver function abnormalities with HMG-CoA reductase inhibitors.

Pharmacologic therapy for plasma lipid abnormalities in NIDDM patients should be implemented only after step 1 and step 2 National Cholesterol Education Program diets have failed. NIDDM patients are more likely than nondiabetics to need pharmacologic therapy.

Hypertension is another major risk factor for macrovascular disease in NIDDM patients. Sixty to 70% of NIDDM patients have hypertension, and the treatment regimen must be designed to achieve the target blood pressure control (see Table 2) without detrimental effects on glycemic and lipid regulation. Calcium channel antagonists, angiotensin-converting enzyme (ACE) inhibitors, and alpha-adrenergic antagonists have no detrimental effects on plasma lipoprotein profiles and either do not influence (calcium

TABLE 5. **Lipid-Lowering Drugs**

Effect	Mechanism	Effect on HDL Cholesterol	Daily Dose
Decrease LDL cholesterol and triglycerides			
Atorvastatin (Lipitor)	↓ Cholesterol synthesis	Variable	10–40 mg
Nicotinic acid	↓ VLDL synthesis	↑	1–3 gm
Decrease LDL cholesterol			
Simvastatin (Zocor); pravastatin (Pravachol)	↓ Cholesterol synthesis	Variable	10–40 mg
Lovastatin (Mevacor); fluvastatin (Lescol)			
Cholestyramine (Questran); colestipol (Colestid)	Promotes sterol excretion	0	4–24 gm
Decrease triglycerides			
Gemfibrozil (Lopid)	↓ VLDL synthesis		
	↑ Lipoprotein lipase	↑	1.2 gm

Abbreviations: HDL = high-density lipoprotein; LDL = low-density lipoprotein; VLDL = very-low-density lipoprotein.

channel antagonists) or may improve (ACE inhibitors, doxazosin [Cardura]) glucose metabolism.

Diuretics in high doses can lead to deterioration of glucose control, hypokalemia, and increases in plasma LDL cholesterol and triglyceride levels. Beta-adrenergic antagonists can worsen glycemic regulation by interfering with insulin secretion, can block the counter-regulatory responses to hypoglycemia, and may increase plasma LDL cholesterol and triglyceride levels. The latter two classes of antihypertensives may, however, be useful in NIDDM patients with certain restrictions. Thiazide diuretics in doses of 12.5 to 25 mg of hydrochlorothiazide are useful adjuncts to other agents for nonedematous hypertensive diabetics as they potentiate blood pressure lowering effects and are without detrimental effects on glucose and lipid metabolism at these doses. Selective beta$_1$-adrenergic antagonists may be useful for NIDDM patients with significant coronary heart disease, as several studies have shown as much as a 40 to 50% reduction in mortality in diabetic patients with coronary heart disease treated with these drugs during a 2- to 3-year period.

ACE inhibitors, in addition to their antihypertensive effects, have specific renal protective actions in diabetes as well as beneficial actions in congestive heart failure.

A reasonable approach to blood pressure regulation after the effects of diet have been maximized would be to add an ACE inhibitor. This could be combined with a low-dose calcium channel antagonist and/or low-dose hydrochlorothiazide. Patients with significant coronary artery disease should probably have a selective beta$_1$-adrenergic receptor antagonist as part of their antihypertensive regimen. Vasodilators and central alpha$_2$ antagonists may be needed for selected patients.

EARLY TREATMENT OF COMPLICATIONS

Diabetic Retinopathy

Diabetic retinopathy is the leading cause of new-onset blindness in the United States. The two components of diabetic retinopathy that lead to blindness are macular edema and hemorrhage resulting from proliferative retinopathy. Macular edema cannot be diagnosed by routine direct ophthalmoscopy, but it can be suspected if hard exudates are seen close to the macula. Proliferative retinopathy (neovascularization) and preproliferative changes such as soft exudates, dilated and tortuous capillaries, and beaded retinal veins can be seen by careful direct ophthalmoscopy through adequately dilated pupils. The extent of retinopathy and the necessity for intervention can be determined only by a thorough examination by a trained retinal specialist.

The major responsibilities of the primary care physician in management of retinopathy are (1) to educate the patient about the symptoms and cause of retinopathy, (2) to maximize glycemic and blood pressure control, (3) to see that the patient is examined by a competent retinologist yearly, and (4) to refer the patient to the ophthalmologist immediately for acute visual symptoms, remembering, however, that blurring of vision can occur solely as a result of fluctuating blood glucose levels.

When macular edema and preproliferative or proliferative retinopathy occur, laser photocoagulation treatment is indicated. Such treatment reduces visual loss in 50 to 60% of eyes for 3 to 5 years or longer. For nonproliferative retinopathy without macular edema, there is no specific treatment other than glycemic control, which can decrease progression to macular edema by 30% and to proliferative retinopathy by 50%.

Diabetic Nephropathy

End-stage renal disease occurs in 4 to 20% of NIDDM patients. Whites have a lower prevalence and nonwhite populations such as black Americans, Mexican Americans, and Native Americans a higher prevalence. The most effective methods of screening for the development of diabetic nephropathy are blood pressure measurements every 6 months and urinary albumin excretion rate determinations yearly. Urinary albumin excretion rates can be determined from a random urine sample by measuring the albumin/creatinine ratio. A value less than 30 µg of albumin per mg of creatinine is normal, 30 to 300 μg per mg represents microalbuminuria, and greater than 300 μg per mg indicates clinical proteinuria. An abnormal screening test should be confirmed by at least two 24-hour urinary albumin excretion measurements (microalbuminuria, 30 to 300 mg per 24 hours; clinical proteinuria, >300 mg per 24 hours). The development of microalbuminuria signifies early diabetic nephropathy. About 35% of NIDDM patients with microalbuminuria progress to end-stage renal disease. A somewhat larger percentage develop clinically significant macrovascular disease. Decreasing renal function is followed by measuring serum creatinine levels every 6 months.

The development of microalbuminuria and/or increasing blood pressure is an indication for treatment with an ACE inhibitor. Both captopril and enalapril have been shown to decrease progression from microalbuminuria to clinical diabetic nephropathy. All ACE inhibitors decrease urinary albumin excretion rates. Captopril has been shown to reduce progression of clinical nephropathy to end-stage renal disease. The effects of ACE inhibitors are due to a specific renal protective action independent of their blood pressure lowering effect.

Progression of diabetic nephropathy is slowed by aggressive blood pressure control (mean arterial pressure 92 to 94 mm Hg). The antihypertensive regimen should include drugs that do not interfere with glycemia and lipid control as described previously. Low-protein diets (0.8 g per kg of body weight) have some beneficial effects in slowing the rate of deterioration of renal function.

When the serum creatinine level exceeds 3 mg per dL, the patient should be referred to a nephrologist for initiation of renal replacement therapy.

Diabetic Neuropathy

Diabetic neuropathy occurs as sensorimotor peripheral neuropathies and autonomic neuropathies. Mononeuropathies such as those involving cranial nerves III and VI resolve spontaneously in 3 to 6 months. Diabetic amyotrophy of the lower extremities usually resolves in 6 to 12 months after intensification of glycemic control and physical therapy. Symmetrical distal sensorimotor neuropathy with severe dysesthesias, anorexia, and weight loss does not respond uniformly to any specific therapy. Analgesics and antidepressants are occasionally effective.

Autonomic neuropathies may involve, for example, the heart, stomach, colon, bladder, and peripheral blood vessels. Treatment is symptomatic. Impotence is quite common. Its cause (atherosclerosis versus neuropathy) needs to be determined. Medical therapy includes intracavernosal injections of prostaglandins. Various external and implantable penile devices are now available through urologic consultation.

Diabetic Foot Problems

Foot problems in the diabetic patient result from anatomic deformities, neuropathy that reduces pain and pressure perception, and vascular insufficiency. One half of all lower extremity amputations in diabetic patients can be eliminated by proper prophylactic foot care. Education about foot care is essential. Routine care by a podiatrist can treat minor problems before they become major. High-risk characteristics need to be identified and treated if possible. Once a foot lesion has developed, débridement, antibiotic therapy, and alleviation of pressure must be instituted. Vascular insufficiency may require intervention by a vascular surgeon.

DIABETES MELLITUS IN CHILDREN AND ADOLESCENTS

method of
JOSEPH I. WOLFSDORF, M.B., B.Ch., and
CHRISTINA LUEDKE, M.D., Ph.D.
Children's Hospital
Boston, Massachusetts

Type I diabetes mellitus, or insulin-dependent diabetes mellitus (IDDM), results from insulin deficiency caused by chronic progressive autoimmune destruction of the insulin-producing beta cells of the islets of Langerhans. In the United States, the prevalence of IDDM in people younger than 20 years is about 1.7 cases per 1000; it is estimated that there are about 125,000 children and teenagers with IDDM.

Hyperglycemia occurs when at least 90% of the beta cell mass has been destroyed. The most common symptoms are polyuria, polydipsia, and weight loss. Dehydration results from the osmotic diuresis induced by hyperglycemia. More severe insulin deficiency causes unrestrained lipolysis and ketoacid production that leads to an anion gap acidosis characterized by nausea, vomiting, abdominal pain, and hyperpnea (Kussmaul's respiration).

At diagnosis, most children have residual beta cells whose function is impaired by hyperglycemia. Reversal of the metabolic derangements restores function of the remaining beta cells for months to years until they are destroyed by progression of the autoimmune process. Similarly, correction of hyperglycemia restores tissue sensitivity to insulin. These two factors account for the period of partial remission, often called the "honeymoon," during which normal or nearly normal glycemic control is easily maintained with a relatively low dose of insulin, on the order of less than 0.3 to 0.5 unit per kg per day. After destruction of the remaining beta cells, the insulin dose gradually increases until the full replacement dose is reached.

At our center, most children are briefly hospitalized to initiate therapy. Even when the child is not gravely ill, the emotional impact of the diagnosis on the child and family often causes great distress. Therefore, we prefer to begin the program of diabetes education and self-care training in a safe and supportive environment. This enables grieving and overwhelmed parents to acquire survival skills while they are coping with the emotional upheaval caused by the crisis resulting from the discovery of this incurable disease in their child.

The initial goals of therapy are to stabilize the metabolic state with insulin, fluid, and electrolyte replacement and to provide basic diabetes education and self-care training to the patient, in an age-appropriate fashion, and to parents and other important caregivers.

DIABETIC KETOACIDOSIS

Approximately one-third of newly diagnosed children referred to Children's Hospital in Boston arrive in diabetic ketoacidosis (DKA). The principles of the treatment protocol used at this center are presented here.

Initial Evaluation

1. Perform a clinical evaluation to establish the diagnosis and determine its cause (especially any evidence of infection) and to assess the patient's degree of dehydration. Weigh the patient and measure height or length.
2. With a glucose meter, determine the blood glucose concentration at the bedside.
3. Obtain a blood sample for measurement of plasma glucose, electrolytes, total carbon dioxide, blood urea nitrogen, serum osmolality, arterial or venous pH, partial pressure of carbon dioxide (PCO_2) and of oxygen (PO_2), hemoglobin, hematocrit, white blood cell count and differential, calcium, magnesium, and phosphorus. Calculate the anion gap.
4. Perform a urinalysis and obtain appropriate specimens for culture (blood, urine, throat) even if the patient is afebrile.
5. Obtain an electrocardiogram for baseline evaluation of potassium status.
6. Determine baseline neurologic status.

Supportive Measures

1. In semiconscious or unconscious patients, secure the airway and empty the stomach by nasogastric suction to prevent aspiration.
2. Give supplementary oxygen to patients who are cyanosed or in shock or when the arterial PO_2 is less than 80 mm Hg.
3. Measure urine output accurately; use bladder or condom catheterization if necessary.
4. Record in a flow-chart the patient's clinical and laboratory data, details of fluid and electrolyte therapy, administered insulin, and urine output. Successful management of DKA requires meticulous monitoring of the patient's clinical and biochemical response to treatment so that timely adjustments in the treatment regimen can be made when necessary.
5. Measure plasma glucose, serum electrolytes (and corrected sodium), pH, PCO_2, total carbon dioxide, anion gap, calcium, and phosphorus every 2 hours for the first 8 hours and then every 4 hours until the values are normal.
6. Admit to an intensive care unit infants, toddlers, and severely ill older children with DKA, especially those with central nervous system obtundation or cardiovascular instability.
7. Administer broad-spectrum antibiotics to febrile patients after appropriate culture specimens of body fluids have been obtained.

Fluid and Electrolyte Treatment

All patients with DKA are dehydrated and suffer total body depletion of sodium, potassium, chloride, phosphate, and magnesium. Patients with mild to moderate DKA are usually about 5% (50 mL per kg) dehydrated, and those with severe DKA are up to 10% (100 mL per kg) dehydrated.

1. Start an intravenous infusion using a large-bore cannula and infuse 10 mL per kg of isotonic saline solution (0.9%) within 60 minutes. In the severely dehydrated patient or the patient in shock, initially give 20 mL per kg followed by an additional 10 mL per kg in 60 minutes if hypotension or shock persists.
2. Once the circulation has been stabilized, change to half-normal saline solution and aim to replace the calculated fluid deficit at an even rate during 24 to 36 hours. Aim to achieve slow correction of the serum hyperosmolality and to avoid a rapid shift of water from the extracellular to the intracellular compartment. The sodium concentration of the solution should be increased to 100 to 130 mEq per liter if the corrected serum sodium concentration fails to rise as the plasma glucose concentration decreases. The corrected sodium is calculated as

$$Na^+ + (1.6 \times [\text{plasma glucose mg per dL} - 100]/100)$$

3. Maintenance fluid is given as half isotonic saline solution at a rate of 1500 mL per m² per day.
4. Add 5% dextrose to the infusion fluid when the plasma glucose concentration reaches 300 mg per dL and attempt to maintain the plasma glucose concentration at approximately 200 mg per dL for the first 36 to 48 hours. To avert hypoglycemia, 10% dextrose may be needed.
5. Continue intravenous fluid administration until acidosis is corrected and the patient can eat and drink without vomiting.

Insulin

Regular insulin is diluted in normal saline (50 units in 50 mL). After an intravenous priming dose of 0.1 unit per kg, insulin is given at a rate of 0.1 unit per kg per hour, controlled by an infusion pump. Insulin has a serum half-life of approximately 5 to 7 minutes; therefore, insulin deficiency develops rapidly if the insulin infusion is interrupted. Intravenous insulin therapy should not be used unless it can be closely supervised.

When DKA has resolved (venous pH greater than 7.32, total carbon dioxide greater than 18 mEq per liter) and the change to subcutaneous insulin is planned, the first injection should be given 60 to 120 minutes before stopping the infusion, to allow sufficient time for the injected insulin to be absorbed.

Potassium Replacement

All patients with DKA are potassium depleted (4 to 6 mEq per kg) despite an initial serum potassium concentration that may be normal or increased. With the administration of fluid and insulin, serum potassium may decrease abruptly, predisposing the patient to cardiac arrhythmias. Patients whose serum potassium level is initially low are the most severely depleted. They should receive potassium after urination, and the serum potassium concentration should be measured hourly. The serum potassium level should be maintained in the normal range. Half the potassium is given as potassium acetate and the other half as potassium phosphate; this reduces the total amount of chloride administered and partially replaces the phosphate deficit.

Acidosis

Routine administration of bicarbonate neither hastens resolution of acidosis nor improves survival and may impair tissue oxygenation and cause hypokalemia. Its routine use is not recommended. However, when acidosis is severe (arterial pH less than 7.0) or there is hypotension, shock, or an arrhythmia, sodium bicarbonate, 1 to 2 mEq per kg or 40 to 80 mEq per m², is infused over 2 hours.

Cerebral Edema

This uncommon complication of DKA can cause acute brain herniation and death. It typically develops abruptly within 2 to 12 hours of starting treatment and manifests as headache, vomiting, altered level of consciousness, delirium or restlessness, incontinence, bradycardia, increased blood pressure, unequal pupils, papilledema, respiratory arrest, and sudden onset of polyuria from acute diabetes insipidus. Computed tomography of the brain confirms brain swelling. When cerebral edema is suspected, the following steps should be taken immediately: administer mannitol, 1 gram per kg intravenously, and repeat as necessary; reduce the rate of fluid administration; insert an endotracheal tube; and hyperventilate the patient.

INSULIN THERAPY

The three major categories of insulin preparations differ in their absorption kinetics (Table 1). Several

TABLE 1. Insulin Preparations*

Action	Type	Onset of Action (h)	Peak Action (h)	Duration of Action (h)
Short acting	Lispro	<0.25	0.5–1.5	3–4
	Regular	0.5	2–4	6–8
Intermediate acting	NPH (isophane)	1–3	6–12	18–24
	Lente	1–3	6–12	18–24
Long acting	Ultralente	4–6	8–20	24–28

*These figures are for human insulins and are approximations from laboratory studies in test subjects. The times of onset, peak, and duration of action vary greatly within and between patients and are affected by many factors, including size of dose, site of injection, exercise of the injected area, temperature, and insulin antibodies.

TABLE 2. Insulin Regimens

Doses	Breakfast	Lunch	Dinner	Bedtime
Two	R + NPH/L		R + NPH/L	
	R + NPH/L		R + UL	
	R + UL		R + UL	
Three	R + NPH/L	R	R	NPH/L
	R + UL	R	R + UL	
Four	R	R	R	NPH/L
	R + NPH/L	R	R	NPH/L

Abbreviations: R = regular (or lispro) insulin; NPH = neutral protamine Hagedorn insulin; L = Lente insulin; UL = Ultralente insulin; NPH/L = either intermediate-acting insulin may be selected for use with this regimen.

insulin regimens can be used; each has the same goal, namely, to provide basal insulin throughout the day and more with meals (Table 2). The most commonly used regimen consists of a combination of short- and intermediate-acting insulin given twice daily, before breakfast and before the evening meal. A modification of this regimen that involves 3 doses per day, with intermediate-acting insulin given at bedtime instead of before supper, is especially recommended for adolescents. The child's age, weight, and pubertal status guide the initial choice of dose.

Subcutaneous insulin is started in a newly diagnosed child who is not significantly dehydrated, is not vomiting, and either does not have ketoacidosis or has mild ketoacidosis (arterial pH greater than 7.25, venous pH greater than 7.20). In a child diagnosed early with moderate hyperglycemia and no ketonuria, the recommended starting dose of insulin is 0.3 to 0.5 unit per kg per day. When metabolic decompensation is more severe (ketonuria but without acidosis or dehydration), the initial dose is 0.5 to 0.75 unit per kg, supplemented, if necessary, with 0.1 unit per kg of regular insulin subcutaneously at 4- to 6-hour intervals. The upper end of each suggested range is used for pubertal patients and for those who are physically inactive and overweight. The total daily dose is divided so that two thirds is given before breakfast and one third in the evening. The ratio of short- to intermediate-acting insulin at both times is 1:2. Target blood glucose levels for different ages are shown in Table 3. The insulin dose is adjusted until satisfactory blood glucose control is achieved.

For toddlers and young children, we use U10 (U100

TABLE 3. Target Blood Glucose Levels for Children and Adolescents*

Age Group	Fasting (mg/dL)	Premeal (mg/dL)	2–4 AM (mg/dL)
Infant or toddler	80–180	100–200	80–180
School age	80–150	80–180	80–150
Adolescent	70–120	70–180	70–150

*Target blood glucose levels for patients with normal counter-regulatory mechanisms who practice intensive insulin therapy are 70–120 mg/dL fasting and before meals, <180 mg/dL 90–120 min after meals, and 70–100 mg/dL at 2–4 AM.

insulin diluted 1:10) regular insulin; children of this age typically require a smaller fraction of regular insulin (10 to 20%) with proportionally more intermediate-acting insulin.

The optimal ratio of rapid- to intermediate-acting insulin for each patient is determined empirically, guided by the results of frequent blood glucose measurements. Five measurements daily: before each meal, before the bedtime snack, and at 2 to 4 AM, are initially required to determine the effects of each prescribed dose. Adjustments are made to each dose at 3- to 5-day intervals, usually in 10% increments or decrements, in response to patterns of consistently elevated or low blood glucose levels, respectively. The daily insulin requirements of patients with complete insulin deficiency is 0.5 to 1.0 unit per kg before puberty and 0.8 to 1.5 units per kg during puberty.

Good glycemic control is impossible to achieve without strict attention to the other important factors that influence blood glucose levels, namely, diet and physical activity.

NUTRITION

Attention must be paid to the timing and content of meals to match food intake with the availability of injected insulin. The registered dietitian is an important member of the diabetes treatment team. Starting with the initial hospitalization and continuing with intermittent visits in the outpatient setting, the dietitian is responsible for instructing patients on the principles of nutritional management of diabetes and formulating an individualized meal plan that attempts to minimize postprandial hyperglycemia and avoid hypoglycemia between meals.

General Principles

The nutritional needs of children with diabetes do not differ from those of healthy children. Newly diagnosed children, however, typically have lost weight, and the initial diet prescription aims to restore a desirable weight for height. Once this has been achieved, the total intake of calories and nutrients must be sufficient to balance the daily expenditure of energy and satisfy the requirements for normal growth and development. A method commonly used to estimate energy requirements is based on age and is useful as a crude approximation for children up to 12 years of age: to 1000 kcal, add 100 × the patient's age in years.

The American Diabetes Association currently recommends that carbohydrate provide 50 to 60% of the total calories, with protein and fat making up 15 and 30%, respectively. The diet prescription has to be periodically adjusted to achieve an ideal or desirable body weight and to maintain a normal rate of physical growth and maturation. The main objective of dietary therapy in obese patients is to lose weight.

People with diabetes are predisposed to atherosclerosis and should follow a prudent diet with regard to fat content; the amount of fat should not exceed 30% of the total daily calories. Dietary cholesterol is reduced to 300 mg per day or less and saturated fat to less than 10% of calories by consumption of less beef and pork and leaner cuts of meat, chicken, turkey, fish, low-fat milk, and vegetable proteins.

Dietary fiber may benefit the diabetic patient by blunting the rise in blood glucose after meals. Unrefined or minimally processed foods, such as grains, legumes, and vegetables, should replace highly refined carbohydrates. To avoid abrupt increases in blood glucose, children should eat fruit whole and avoid fruit juices, which should be reserved for treating episodes of hypoglycemia.

Because insulin is released continuously from the injection site, hypoglycemia, exacerbated by exercise, may occur if snacks are not eaten between the main meals. Hence, most children who receive twice-daily injections of insulin (split-mixed insulin regimen) have a snack between each meal and at bedtime; adolescents usually prefer to omit the midmorning snack. Meals and snacks should be eaten at approximately the same time each day, and the total consumption of calories and the proportions of carbohydrate, protein, and fat in each meal and snack should be consistent from day to day.

Exchange System

The meal plan is formulated using the system of food exchanges and is individualized to meet the ethnic, religious, and economic circumstances of each family and the food preferences of the individual child. The diet prescription must take into account the child's school schedule, gym classes, and after-school physical activity. The exchange system is based on six food groups—milk, fruit, vegetable, bread/starch, meat/protein, and fat—and the meal plan contains the number of exchanges from each food group to be included in each meal and snack. Parents should learn to calculate exchanges from the information on food labels.

EXERCISE

Exercise acutely lowers the blood glucose concentration by increasing utilization of glucose to a variable degree, depending on the intensity and duration of physical activity and the concurrent level of insulinemia. Children and teenagers with diabetes are encouraged to participate in sports and to exercise throughout the year. In addition to normalizing the child's life and promoting a positive self-image, exercise promotes good health practices, facilitates weight control, and may improve glycemic control.

Young children's activities tend to be spontaneous; bursts of activity are covered with a snack before and, if the exercise is prolonged, during the activity. A useful guide is to provide 15 grams of carbohydrate (one bread or fruit exchange) per 30 to 60 minutes of vigorous physical activity. Strenuous exercise in the afternoon or evening should be followed by a 10 to 20% reduction in the presupper or bedtime dose of intermediate-acting insulin and a larger bedtime snack, to reduce the risk of nocturnal or early-morning hypoglycemia from the lag effect of exercise.

Acute vigorous exercise in the face of poorly controlled diabetes can aggravate hyperglycemia and ketoacid production. Therefore, a child with ketonuria should not exercise. Exercising the limb into which insulin has been injected accelerates the rate of insulin absorption. If exercise is planned, it is recommended that the preceding insulin injection be given in a site that is least likely to be affected by exercise. Youngsters who participate in organized sports are advised to reduce the dose of insulin, which is predominantly active during the period of sustained physical activity. The size of such reductions is determined by measuring blood glucose levels before and after exercise and are generally in the range of 10 to 30% of the usual insulin dose.

DIABETES CARE IN THE OUTPATIENT SETTING

The child is discharged from the hospital as soon as she or he is medically stable and the parents (or other care providers) have learned the essentials of diabetes management: insulin administration, self-monitoring of blood glucose (SMBG), urine ketone measurement, basic meal planning, and recognition and treatment of hypoglycemia. Frequent telephone contact, often daily, is initially needed to help parents interpret SMBG data and adjust insulin dose(s) necessitated by the home schedule of activity and meals. Within the first few weeks of diagnosis, two thirds of children enter partial remission, and the dose of insulin usually has to be reduced considerably.

The patient is seen frequently in the first month, primarily by the nurse specialist educator and dietitian, to review and consolidate the skills and principles taught in the hospital. Thereafter, follow-up visits with members of the diabetes team occur every 3 months. The purpose of regular clinic visits is to ensure that the child's diabetes is being appropriately managed at home and that the goals of therapy are met. A focused history should obtain information about self-care behaviors; the child's daily routines; the frequency, severity, and circumstances surrounding hypoglycemic events; and evidence of hyperglycemia (polyuria, polydipsia, nocturia, weight loss, blurry vision, perineal candidiasis).

At every visit, height and weight are measured and plotted on a growth chart. The weight curve is especially helpful in assessing adequacy of therapy, because a significant weight loss usually indicates that the prescribed dose is insufficient or the patient is omitting injections. A physical examination should be performed at least twice per year and includes measurement of blood pressure, pubertal staging, signs of thyroid disease, skin examination, and an evaluation of the organs most affected by long-standing diabetes. The injection sites are inspected for evidence of lipohypertrophy from overuse of the site.

Insulin therapy must be viewed as a dynamic process that takes into account growth and development, changes in lifestyle and activity, intercurrent illness, and other factors that influence insulin requirements. Doses are adjusted with the goal of maintaining blood glucose levels within the target range as much as possible. The target range varies with the age of the patient (see Table 3). For infants and toddlers, who cannot understand or easily express symptoms of hypoglycemia, the target range is higher to minimize the risk of severe hypoglycemia.

Regular clinic visits are opportunities to reinforce and expand on the diabetes self-care training that began in the hospital. Optimal care of diabetes depends on the patient's intimate understanding of the interplay of medication and lifestyle. At each visit, the goal is to increase the patient's and family's understanding of diabetes management, so that as the child becomes more independent, he or she can assume increasing responsibility for daily self-care. Mature and motivated teenagers are encouraged to use intensified insulin management techniques that involve multiple daily insulin injections, use of algorithms for insulin dose selection, and target blood glucose levels in or near the normal range (see Table 3).

Self-Monitoring of Blood Glucose

This technique is routinely taught to all patients with IDDM, and the ability of patients to obtain accurate results is confirmed at clinic visits, when patients are asked to compare results obtained with their meters with simultaneous blood glucose determinations in the clinical chemistry laboratory. SMBG is the cornerstone of any intensive diabetes management program, and frequent SMBG in conjunction with urine tests for ketones is essential to manage intercurrent illnesses and prevent ketoacidosis. A variety of meters with a digital display are available that enable the user to obtain measurements of blood glucose concentration within 10% of the value obtained in a clinical chemistry laboratory.

Patients ideally should test before each meal and at bedtime. If this is impractical or intolerable, patients should be encouraged to test before each dose of insulin and perform additional tests before lunch and at bedtime at least twice each week. Alternatively, for patients who cannot tolerate such frequent monitoring or who cannot afford the cost of the reagent strips, a period of intensive monitoring before each meal, at bedtime, and between 2 and 4 AM for several consecutive days before an office visit often provides sufficient information to confirm satisfactory control or serve as a basis for modifying the insulin regimen.

Urine should be tested for the presence of ketones whenever the child is sick, when the blood glucose level exceeds 250 mg per dL, and when blood glucose levels are high before breakfast and the possibility of unrecognized nocturnal hypoglycemia is suspected.

Glycosylated Hemoglobin (Hemoglobin A₁ or A₁c). The level of glycosylated hemoglobin, formed when glucose is bound nonenzymatically to the hemoglobin molecule, is directly proportional to the time-integrated mean blood glucose concentration during the preceding 2 to 3 months. Quarterly determinations of glycosylated hemoglobin should be used to provide an objective measure of average glycemia in the intervals between office visits.

PSYCHOSOCIAL ISSUES

A social worker performs a psychosocial assessment on all newly diagnosed patients and their families. Thereafter, patients are referred to the mental health specialist on the diabetes team when emotional, social, or financial concerns are identified that may be obstacles to achieving and maintaining acceptable glycemic control. Common problems encountered in a diabetes clinic are financial hardship affecting the ability to purchase costly supplies, parental guilt, the child's rebellion against treatment, noncompliance with medication, family adjustment problems, and frequently missed appointments. Recurrent ketoacidosis is the most extreme indicator of psychosocial stress.

HYPOGLYCEMIA

Occasional episodes of hypoglycemia are an unavoidable consequence of insulin therapy aimed at maintaining blood glucose levels near normal. The goal is to minimize the frequency and severity of hypoglycemia while maintaining blood glucose levels as close to normal as possible.

Patients and family members must be taught to recognize the early symptoms of hypoglycemia and to treat it promptly with a suitable form of concentrated carbohydrate. Because infants and toddlers may be unable to recognize the symptoms of hypoglycemia and cannot verbalize their symptoms, parents are advised to measure the blood glucose concentration whenever the child's behavior is unusual. Most episodes of hypoglycemia are satisfactorily treated with 10 to 20 grams of glucose; 5 grams is sufficient for an infant or toddler. Suitable forms of rapidly absorbed carbohydrate for treatment of hypoglycemia are glucose tablets (each contains 5 grams of glucose), Lifesavers candy (3 grams each), granulated table sugar (4 grams per teaspoon), and orange or apple juice (10 to 12 grams per 120 mL). Family members are taught to use glucagon (which should be available at home) to treat an episode of severe hypoglycemia in which the child is unconscious or unable to swallow or retain ingested carbohydrate. Glucagon (0.02 to 0.03 mg per kg, maximal dose 1.0 mg) is injected intramuscularly or subcutaneously and raises the blood glucose level within 5 to 15 minutes. Nausea and vomiting may follow the administration of glucagon. After consciousness has been regained, oral carbohydrate should be given to prevent further hypoglycemia. If the patient cannot take it orally or retain

sugar-containing fluids, glucose, 0.5 gram per kg, is injected intravenously followed by a continuous infusion at a rate that maintains a normal blood glucose concentration.

A Medic Alert bracelet or necklace should always be worn to identify the patient as having diabetes mellitus.

SCREENING FOR COMPLICATIONS

The organs most affected by diabetes are the eyes, kidneys, circulatory system, and peripheral nervous system. Diabetic complications develop insidiously but can be detected years before they become symptomatic. Systematic screening is performed to detect abnormalities early, when intervention to arrest, reverse, or retard complications is most beneficial. Both diabetic retinopathy and nephropathy are rare before puberty and in patients who have had IDDM for less than 5 years. Therefore, beginning 5 years after diagnosis, patients should have an annual dilated retinal examination and measurement of albumin and creatinine concentrations in a timed overnight or first-morning urine specimen to detect microalbuminuria. Circulatory and neurologic complications of diabetes are seldom clinically significant in the pediatric and adolescent population.

CONCLUSION

Advances in the treatment of diabetes in children in the past 2 decades now make it possible to ensure normal growth and development and safely achieve a level of blood glucose control that was previously unattainable. It is reasonable to expect that the benefits of sustained improvement in glycemic control will prevent, or at least delay, the appearance of the chronic complications of diabetes. It is important, however, to remember that the arduous task of controlling blood glucose in a child is difficult and frustrating. The members of the diabetes team must set realistic and attainable goals for each patient and constantly provide encouragement and support. The resources of a multidisciplinary health care team—physician, nurse educator, dietitian, mental health specialist, and ophthalmologist—are essential for the successful management of IDDM by the child or adolescent and family.

DIABETIC KETOACIDOSIS

method of
SEAN F. DINNEEN, M.D., M.Sc.
Mayo Clinic
Rochester, Minnesota

Diabetic ketoacidosis (DKA) is a state of altered carbohydrate, fat, and protein metabolism that results from a complete or relative lack of insulin. It is most commonly seen in patients with insulin-dependent diabetes mellitus

(IDDM) and represents a hallmark of this form of diabetes. It can, however, occur in patients with non–insulin-dependent diabetes mellitus, although hyperosmolar nonketotic coma is the hyperglycemic emergency most characteristic of this group of patients.

Despite advances in our understanding of the pathophysiology and optimal management of DKA, the condition is still associated with a significant mortality. These deaths frequently result from complications of DKA management rather than the altered metabolic state itself. In this chapter are reviewed the principles of optimal management of DKA, recognizing that treatment needs to be modified for individual patients.

INITIAL ASSESSMENT (Table 1)

Certain clinical findings should raise the suspicion of DKA in an obtunded patient. These include the presence of a bracelet identifying the patient as having diabetes, evidence of subcutaneous injection sites on skin examination, and the combination of dehydration, Kussmaul-type respirations, and acetone-scented breath. In the majority of cases, the patient is not obtunded and may give a history of decompensation of glucose control (in the setting of known IDDM) due to an intercurrent illness and/or inadvertent omission of insulin. Abdominal pain, nausea, and vomiting, if present, may be features of the DKA itself rather than an indication of an acute abdomen. This distinction may be difficult to make, however, as DKA can lead to a leukocytosis and hyperamylasemia, both of which are typically mild and resolve with treatment of the altered metabolic state.

Accurate recording of body weight and vital signs (including postural blood pressure change) is important at baseline and can help in estimating the total body and intravascular fluid deficits. The presence of a fever should instigate a thorough search (by history, physical examination, and targeted laboratory investigations) for an underlying infectious process. Infections can be unmasked by rectal (prostatitis), pelvic (abscess), and ear (mucormycosis) examinations. Myocardial or cerebral infarction should be considered in the older patient, in whom an electrocardiogram is mandatory. Identification and treatment of a precipitating cause of DKA are important aspects of overall management. If the metabolic derangements are slow to improve with appropriate fluid and insulin therapy, a renewed search should be undertaken for an unidentified precipitating cause of the DKA.

Confirmation of the diagnosis of DKA requires laboratory results including (1) a pH less than 7.3, (2) a plasma bicarbonate level less than 15 mEq per liter, (3) a plasma glucose level greater than 250 mg per dL, and (4) elevated urine or plasma ketone levels. In some cases, one or more of these diagnostic criteria may be absent; for example, cases of DKA have been reported in which associated vomiting or hyperventilation has led to a mixed acid-base disturbance rather than a pure metabolic acidosis. Although an anion gap acidosis is typical at presentation, a mixed hyperchloremic–anion gap acidosis or even a frank hyperchloremic acidosis can occur. The degree of hyperglycemia may be attenuated by partial treatment before presentation or by the suppressive effects of alcohol on hepatic gluconeogenesis. Finally, in the presence of an elevated creatinine level, certain plasma ketone assays can be falsely low.

Once the diagnosis of DKA has been established, the next step is to obtain intravenous access and commence therapy. Frequently, this process takes place in the emergency department before hospital admission. A safe approach is to infuse isotonic saline at 1 liter per hour and write subsequent fluid orders when baseline electrolyte levels are available. An intramuscular and/or intravenous bolus of short-acting (regular) insulin (0.15 unit per kg) would also be appropriate in the emergency department. The decision about where to transfer the patient for inpatient management depends on several factors including the patient's degree of obtundation; the need for airway protection, cardiac monitoring, and central venous pressure monitoring; the existence of protocols for the management of DKA; and (possibly) the turnaround time for laboratory results in different units of the hospital. It is essential that the medical and nursing personnel involved in caring for the patient be experienced with DKA management.

ONGOING MANAGEMENT (Table 2)
General

The combination of acidosis and major fluid and electrolyte shifts during therapy makes frequent clinical assessment of the patient with DKA most important. A flow-sheet can facilitate this by providing a summary at a glance of changes in the key clinical and laboratory parameters. A list of the more important items to include in a DKA management flow-sheet is provided in Table 3. There are several ongoing controversies surrounding the optimal management of DKA. Rather than presenting the pros and cons of each management issue, I have opted to emphasize the approach to DKA management used at our institution.

Intravenous Fluid Therapy

The initial choice of intravenous fluid should reflect the needs of the majority of patients. Because intra-

TABLE 1. **Initial Assessment of Diabetic Ketoacidosis**

Confirm the diagnosis
  pH < 7.3
  HCO_3^- < 15 mEq/L
  Glucose > 250 mg/dL
  Urine or plasma ketone levels elevated
Consider other causes of acidosis and/or coma
  Lactic acidosis
  Drug-induced metabolic disturbance
  Alcohol-related problem
Identify a precipitating cause
  Infection (e.g., pulmonary, genitourinary, gastrointestinal)
  Infarction (e.g., myocardial, cerebral)
  Insulin omission
Decide where to manage the patient (ward vs. ICU)
  Severity of acidosis, obtundation, and so forth
  Existence of management protocols for DKA
  Physician and nursing experience with DKA management
  Turnaround time for laboratory results
Begin therapy
  Intravenous access (peripheral vs. central)
  Saline infusion
  Regular insulin intravenous bolus and infusion
  Urinary catheter

Abbreviations: DKA = diabetic ketoacidosis; ICU = intensive care unit.

TABLE 2. **Ongoing Management Guidelines for Diabetic Ketoacidosis**

Intravenous fluid therapy
  Begin with isotonic fluid
  Change to hypotonic fluid when laboratory results are available
  Use colloid if necessary for severe hypovolemia and/or hypotension
  Change to dextrose-based fluid when glucose value < 250 mg/dL
  Aim to replenish estimated fluid deficit of 3.5–7.0 L
Insulin therapy
  Intravenous route is preferable for initial management
  Use only short-acting insulin
  Flush intravenous infusion sets before commencing infusion
  Bolus with 0.15 U/kg
  Infuse at 0.1 U/kg/h
  Continue until acidemia and ketosis are resolved
  Adjust rate by 50% based on clinical and laboratory response
Potassium therapy
  Electrocardiogram may be used as initial assessment for hypo- or hyperkalemia
  If initial K^+ is

<3.0 mEq/L	give 40 mEq/h by infusion
3.0–5.0 mEq/L	give 20 mEq/h
5.0–5.9 mEq/L	give 10 mEq/h
≥6.0 mEq/L	withhold intravenous K^+ until serum K^+ < 6.0 mEq/L

  Give K^+ as KCl (two thirds) and KPO_4^{2-} (one third) unless initial serum PO_4^{2-} is elevated
Bicarbonate therapy
  Consider only if (a) severe acidosis (pH < 7.0)
               (b) poor response to standard therapy
               (c) refractory hypotension
  Give HCO_3^- as 1–2 mEq/kg during 2 h
  Intensify serum K^+ monitoring if HCO_3^- is administered
Other considerations
  Look for and treat precipitating cause(s) of DKA
  Use nasogastric suctioning for severe vomiting
  Consider central venous pressure monitoring if there is tenuous cardiopulmonary or renal reserve
  Continue Ultralente insulin on routine schedule if used before admission

Abbreviation: DKA = diabetic ketoacidosis.

vascular volume replacement is the immediate priority in most patients, an isotonic crystalloid solution such as normal saline is a reasonable first choice. If significant hypotension is present, a colloid solution may be necessary. Once the patient has received 1 to 2 liters of isotonic fluid (usually during the first 1 to 2 hours), the replacement fluid can be changed to a hypotonic fluid such as half-normal saline. This facilitates repletion of the large intracellular fluid deficit present in DKA. As outlined in the next section, when the plasma glucose level decreases to less than 250 mg per dL, glucose should be added to the replacement fluid. Use of either 5% dextrose in half-normal saline or 5% dextrose in water depends on the plasma sodium concentration at the time of this transition. Although several formulas exist for estimating a patient's total body fluid deficit, a more pragmatic approach is to establish the patient's usual dry weight and use this, along with an accurate admission weight, to estimate the fluid needs. Most

patients have deficits amounting to 5 to 10% of their body weight. Remember to include the urine output in the assessment of net volume replaced.

Insulin Therapy

The amount of insulin required to treat a patient with DKA is that which will correct the acidosis and ketosis and not just the hyperglycemia. A common mistake is to assume that correction of the hyperglycemia equates to correction of the overall metabolic disturbance. Although some authorities still recommend intramuscular delivery of insulin in DKA, at our institution we favor the intravenous route. The half-life of insulin in the circulation is short (approximately 6 minutes); however, its biologic half-life (at the cellular level) is considerably longer. Steady-state plasma concentrations can be reached quickly, although it may take several hours to reach a true steady state for insulin action. These observations suggest that a bolus injection is unlikely to have a major impact on overall management. However, boluses of insulin are still widely used, with a typical dose of 0.15 unit per kg. An intravenous infusion at a rate of 0.1 unit per kg per hour is a widely accepted

TABLE 3. **Items to Include in a Diabetic Ketoacidosis Management Flow-sheet**

	Suggested monitoring frequency
Clinical and nursing parameters	
Vital signs	
Mental status	
Cumulative fluid intake and output	
Fluid therapy	
Maintenance intravenous infusion	
Type	
Hourly rate	
Cumulative total	
Supplemental intravenous infusion(s), e.g., for intravenous patency, "piggyback" for K^+, insulin, and so forth	
Type	
Hourly rate	
Cumulative total	
Insulin therapy	
Mode of administration (intravenous, subcutaneous, intramuscular)	
Hourly rate	
Cumulative total	
Potassium therapy	
Type	
Hourly rate	
Cumulative total	
Bicarbonate therapy	
Cumulative total	
Laboratory parameters	Suggested monitoring frequency
Glucose (reflectance meter)	B; q 1 h × 6 h; 2 h × 6 h
Glucose (plasma)	B; q 12 h
K^+, Na^+, and Cl^-	B; q 4 h × 12–24 h
HCO_3^- pH (venous)	B; q 6 h
Urine and plasma ketones	B; q 6 h
PO_4^{2-} and Ca^{2+}	B; q 12 h
Creatinine and urea	B; q 12 h
CBC	B; q 24 h
ECG, CXR, and urine culture	B; as indicated clinically

Abbreviations: B = baseline; CBC = complete blood cell count; ECG = electrocardiogram; CXR = chest radiograph.

starting dose of insulin in DKA. This dose is usually associated with a safe rate of decline of the plasma glucose concentration. If the plasma glucose concentration falls by more than 50 mg per dL in 1 hour and/or when the plasma glucose concentration falls below 250 mg per dL, the insulin infusion rate should be reduced by 50%. At this time the replacement intravenous fluid should be changed to a dextrose-based fluid to enable continuation of the insulin infusion until the acidosis and ketosis have resolved. Rapid rates of decline in the plasma glucose concentration have been associated with the development of cerebral edema, particularly in children (see later). Occasionally, the insulin infusion rate has to be increased above 0.1 unit per kg per hour because of an inadequate plasma glucose response. There is no role for intermediate-acting insulin in the initial management of DKA. Patients using subcutaneous long-acting insulin (i.e., Ultralente) before admission should have this continued on schedule during hospitalization for DKA to avoid interruption of the basal insulin effect. Short-acting insulin analogues, such as insulin lispro (Humalog), have not been studied in the management of DKA but are unlikely to offer any major advantage over conventional short-acting insulin if the intravenous route of delivery is used.

Potassium Therapy

Although the plasma potassium concentration in patients with DKA may be low, normal, or high at presentation, overall body potassium stores are invariably depleted. The baseline electrocardiogram can suggest the presence of hypokalemia (U waves and/or low-voltage T waves) or hyperkalemia (peaked T waves). However, therapeutic decisions about potassium replacement should be guided by careful monitoring of the plasma level and its response to the initiation of fluid, insulin, and potassium therapy. Although the algorithm outlined in Table 2 represents a reasonable approach to initial replacement, ongoing needs may call for modification of this algorithm. In particular, rapid correction of acidosis (e.g., by the administration of bicarbonate therapy) is associated with an increase in potassium requirements. Potassium is generally replaced as potassium chloride, although some authorities recommend administering part (usually one third) of the required potassium as potassium phosphate. This has theoretical advantages, although a clinical benefit remains to be demonstrated.

Bicarbonate Therapy

The majority of patients with DKA have acidosis corrected with intravenous fluids and insulin therapy alone. In a minority of patients, in whom the degree of acidosis is severe (pH less than 7.0) or in whom more rapid correction of acidosis is deemed necessary (because of deleterious effects of the acidosis on, e.g., cardiac function), intravenous bicarbonate therapy is a consideration. This is most often administered as sodium bicarbonate and infused at 1 to 2 mEq per kg during 2 hours. If bicarbonate is administered, the frequency of potassium monitoring needs to be intensified.

SPECIAL CONSIDERATIONS

Cerebral Edema

Cerebral edema is the most dreaded complication of DKA management and occurs more frequently in children than in adults. Its cause remains uncertain, although the production of so-called idiogenic osmoles by brain cells appears to be important. These represent a protective response of the brain against intracellular volume depletion. A major factor in the development of cerebral edema is the rate at which the total body fluid deficit and the hyperglycemia are corrected. For this reason, great caution needs to be taken to avoid being overly aggressive in management. The ideal treatment of cerebral edema in DKA is to avoid its occurrence.

Cardiac or Renal Failure

Management of DKA is greatly facilitated by the ability of the cardiovascular and renal systems to handle the large volume loads required during treatment. If a patient is known to have acute or chronic renal failure or be at risk for congestive heart failure, serious consideration should be given to hemodynamic monitoring in conjunction with DKA management. Hemodialysis may be necessary to deal with volume overload, hyperkalemia, or acidosis when DKA occurs in the setting of renal failure. When DKA is precipitated by a myocardial infarction, the possibility that pulmonary edema will develop during treatment must be considered. Such patients are best managed in a unit with facilities for hemodynamic monitoring.

Insulin Resistance

There have been reports of patients with DKA that is resistant to the standard therapeutic approaches just outlined. In such cases, before rare syndromes of insulin resistance are invoked, a thorough review of the management plan should be undertaken with particular reference to (1) an unrecognized (and therefore untreated) precipitating cause of DKA, (2) the appropriateness of the net fluid balance achieved with therapy, and (3) whether insulin was administered appropriately (e.g., with flushing of the intravenous tubing system before administration). If a true state of insulin resistance does exist, such rare patients may benefit from infusion of insulin-like growth factor I* instead of insulin.

---

*Not available in the United States.

TRANSITIONING AND DISCHARGE PLANNING (Table 4)

After correction of the acute metabolic derangements associated with DKA, the next step in management is to make the transition from inpatient therapy to a treatment program suitable for discharge. Oral intake can be cautiously resumed once the patient is alert and free of nausea or vomiting. If the body fluid and potassium deficits have not been corrected by the intravenous route, the patient will gradually replace the remainder over several days by the oral route.

Subcutaneous insulin should be introduced only after the acidosis and ketosis have resolved. The insulin infusion should be continued for 2 (short-acting) or 4 (intermediate-acting) hours after the first subcutaneous insulin injection to avoid a period of insulinopenia. If the patient was receiving an adequate subcutaneous insulin program before admission, it is reasonable to resume insulin therapy at the preadmission doses. If the patient's diabetes is newly diagnosed, insulin requirements can be assessed by administering subcutaneous short-acting insulin every 4 hours for 24 hours to maintain glucose levels close to a predetermined goal range. By using this estimate of the patient's 24-hour insulin needs, a program based on intermediate-acting insulin alone or intermediate- and short-acting insulin can be constructed.

Many patients admitted to the hospital with DKA are poor attenders at diabetes outpatient clinics. For this reason, it is important to assess the patient's overall diabetes management skills during the DKA hospitalization. In particular, a review of the principles of outpatient sick day management may be beneficial and may prevent future admissions with DKA. If necessary, further outpatient diabetes education should be scheduled. A pattern of recurrent admissions with DKA should raise the suspicion of an underlying social or psychologic problem requiring the input of a medical social worker and/or clinical psychologist. Such problems could include eating disorders, chemical dependency, or financial constraints limiting the patient's ability to obtain diabetes supplies. Given the current emphasis on early discharge of patients from the hospital, it is most unlikely that all aspects of diabetes care can (or should) be addressed during an admission for DKA. It is essential, therefore, to arrange outpatient follow-up to optimize the patient's diabetes management and thereby prevent future admissions with DKA.

TABLE 4. **Transitioning and Discharge Planning**

Transition from intravenous to oral fluid intake
  Nausea and/or vomiting resolved
  Estimated fluid deficit >50% replenished by intravenous route
Transition from intravenous to subcutaneous insulin
  Acidosis and ketosis resolved
  Continue intravenous insulin for 2 h after first subcutaneous regular insulin injection
  Use regular insulin every 4–6 h based on bedside glucose levels
  Use intermediate-acting insulin based on preadmission regimen or based on per kilogram estimated needs
Assess diabetes education
  Assess need for outpatient review by diabetes nurse educator
  Review sick day management guidelines
Assess social history relevant to diabetes management
  If pattern of recurrent episodes of DKA, consider input from medical social worker and/or clinical psychologist
Establish diabetes follow-up
  Physician
  Diabetes nurse educator
  Others as needed

HYPERURICEMIA AND GOUT

method of
W. NEAL ROBERTS, M.D.
The Medical College of Virginia
Richmond, Virginia

Gout is a heterogeneous group of diseases in which monosodium urate crystals precipitate into tissues. In more than 90% of patients, renal tubular defects prevent normal excretion of uric acid. Hypertension treated by thiazide diuretics, inducing iatrogenic hyperuricemia and symptomatic gout, may be responsible for the increase (10.9%) in gout found among black men. Gout also has an increased frequency of about 3% in the older age groups, again predominantly in men. Drug toxicities from medication used to treat gout are also more common in the older age group, and the potential for these toxicities creates difficult management choices. Uncertainties of gout management revolve around three problematic areas: (1) the use of allopurinol and alternatives to it; (2) treatment when renal insufficiency coincides with gout; and (3) the roles of diagnostic maneuvers, including polarized light microscopy of joint fluid for crystals, radiographs, 24-hour urine determination of uric acid, and colchicine trials.

FACTORS CONFOUNDING TREATMENT DECISIONS

Treatment is designed to avoid harmful outcomes in the natural history of gout, including tophi; uric acid nephrolithiasis; erosive disease of the joint; least commonly, urate nephropathy; and most commonly, acute painful gout attacks. The main significance of urate nephropathy is that it is sometimes invoked as a reason for treating moderate (7 to 10 mg per dL) asymptomatic hyperuricemia with allopurinol (Zyloprim)—a clinical decision that is usually incorrect. Almost all cases of urate nephropathy occur in patients with overt gouty arthritis, usually with tophi, instead of in asymptomatic hyperuricemia. In fact, 85% of patients with tophaceous *gout* have renal ultrasound studies with echogenic lesions suggesting urate nephropathy. In contrast, correction of hyperuricemia in *nongouty* subjects did not favorably affect renal function in a 2-year randomized, placebo-controlled trial.

In addition, there are several confusing clinical presentations of acute crystal deposition in and around joints. The joint affected by a typical gout attack resembles a septic joint, and both can occur together in the same joint, but some attacks appear clinically more like cellulitis over a joint. Joints in the hand, multiple joints, or joints exhibiting only moderate pain may represent gout. Sixty percent of first attacks are in the first metatarsophalangeal joint and resolve in days, leaving only reddened desquamating skin. However, in postoperative gout the knee and ankle are more common sites of disease. In elderly patients, tophi without acute gout can be the first presentation, particularly over the distal interphalangeal joints.

Finally, the conventional classification into four related phases—asymptomatic hyperuricemia, acute arthritis, intercritical gout between attacks, and chronic tophaceous gout—does not imply progression between phases. More than 80% of patients with hyperuricemia never have gout, and most patients with gout never develop tophi. One third of acute attacks occur in people with normal serum uric acid levels; the percentage of patients with near-normal values doubles in alcoholic patients. Despite the epidemiologic association between the two, a serum urate value is a poor predictor of a clinical event in the individual patient, and hyperuricemia by itself is not a disease.

MANAGEMENT OF ASYMPTOMATIC HYPERURICEMIA

Several times more allopurinol is sold in the United States and Canada than would be used by every symptomatic gout patient taking 300 mg daily. These epidemiologic figures are consistent with case series showing that more than half of the rare deaths from the hepatotoxicity or exfoliative dermatitis due to allopurinol occur among patients who did not really need hypouricemic therapy but received it for asymptomatic hyperuricemia. Therapy is indicated only for a few patients with asymptomatic hyperuricemia who meet criteria for a greater than 50% risk of nephrolithiasis and acute gout: greater than 1100 mg of uric acid in a 24-hour urine collection; greater than 13 mg per dL serum urate on repeated measurements in men; greater than 10 mg per dL in women; or anticipated lysis of cells due to cytotoxic chemotherapy or radiation of lymphoma or leukemia.

MANAGEMENT OF ACUTE GOUT

Acute gout can be treated with nonsteroidal anti-inflammatory drugs (NSAIDs), corticosteroid injection, oral corticosteroids, oral colchicine, intravenous colchicine, combinations of these agents, and avoidance of alcohol (Table 1). The most widely used regimen for acute gout is a double dose of indomethacin (Indocin) (50 mg three or four times daily) for 2 days followed by a 2-day transition to a usual dose of 25 mg three times a day. Such a regimen permits the

TABLE 1. Drug Treatments for Acute Gout in Order of Benefit/Risk Ratio and Convenience

Very Close, Overall

NSAIDs (but these drop off the list with renal insufficiency)

Intra-articular corticosteroid (triamcinolone acetonide [Kenalog], dose 10–40 mg depending on joint size)

Intramuscular corticosteroid (60 mg of triamcinolone acetonide or equivalent)

ACTH gel, 40–80 U (intramuscularly)

More Difficult to Manage

Oral prednisone

Oral colchicine (not in renal failure, not dialyzable)

Intravenous colchicine (with rheumatology consultation)

Abbreviations: ACTH = corticotropin; NSAIDs = nonsteroidal anti-inflammatory drugs.

Adapted from Agudelo CA: Crystal deposition diseases. *In* Weisman MH, Weinblatt ME (eds): Treatment of the Rheumatic Diseases. Companion to the Textbook of Rheumatology. Philadelphia, WB Saunders Co, 1995, pp 271–285.

patient to avoid both prolonged high-dose NSAID treatment, with its increased risk of gastrointestinal bleeding, and high doses of oral colchicine, which 50% of the time leads to diarrhea just at the dose that is effective in controlling the gout. Four days of treatment is often sufficient; the earlier treatment begins, the less prolonged it must be.

Alternative treatment employing oral colchicine alone calls for up to 6 mg in the first 24 hours and a dose limit of 8 mg during the first 3 days. An important difference between the NSAID protocol and the colchicine protocol is that the former relies on a rigid schedule, whereas colchicine is titrated against the pain within strict limits on the total dose to keep to the minimal effective dose. Caution particularly applies to intravenous colchicine given as 1 to 3 mg diluted in 30 mL of normal saline over 30 minutes. A scalp vein needle (butterfly) should not be used as the intravenous access, because extravasation of the colchicine leads to painful local inflammation. Intravenous colchicine has the advantage of being the most rapidly effective of all drugs used against acute gouty arthritis. This feature makes it particularly useful in the emergency department. Intravenous colchicine carries the disadvantage of having the smallest therapeutic index of any drug used in acute gout. Intravenous colchicine bypasses gastrointestinal side effects; a two- or threefold dosage error by this route may lead to neutropenia, sepsis, and death without preceding nausea. Intravenous colchicine should be reduced according to the percentage of renal function remaining by using the assumption that a young person with normal renal function will get a maximum of a 4-mg total dose with no repeat course within 2 weeks. For the elderly patient, 3 weeks should elapse between courses of intravenous colchicine. For older people, the upper limit calculated in proportion to renal function is often about 2 mg of intravenous colchicine per attack. A creatinine clearance less than 10 mL per minute is an absolute contraindication to colchicine by any route.

For acute gout, then, NSAIDs are the most frequently used agents. Indomethacin is the most common individual agent, but any nonsteroidal agent will work. Intravenous colchicine is the single most effective agent but also the most dangerous if a dosage error should occur. Oral or intra-articular corticosteroids for treatment of acute gout are often overlooked. Their disadvantage is said to be that gout symptoms rebound on the third or fourth day after treatment, especially if corticotropin (ACTH) gel, given intramuscularly, is the chosen agent. As with NSAID therapy, initial corticosteroid treatment can be supplemented by maintenance oral colchicine (0.6 mg orally twice per day) as prophylaxis against recurrent gout after the initial 72 hours.

MANAGEMENT OF INTERCRITICAL GOUT

The decision to treat intercritical gout is usually made either to treat tophi, to prevent subsequent kidney stones in a patient who has already experienced one, or to prevent subsequent acute attacks of gouty arthritis in a patient who is experiencing attacks at a rate of four or more per year. Fewer debilitating and prolonged attacks can justify lowering the serum uric acid level. The dollar cost of lowering the serum urate level with allopurinol and preventing one attack per year is less than the cost of a few days of missed work. A more important determinant of the decision to start allopurinol is the patient's answer to the question "Is it worth it to you to take a pill daily and indefinitely, to avoid attacks?" If not, compliance over the longer term and impact on the disease will be minimal, regardless of the number of attacks. People who start allopurinol therapy for tophi or frequent attacks, the two usual indications, and attempt to discontinue it in subsequent years are usually unable to do so without eventual return of the original problem.

There are two approaches to preventing attacks of arthritis. Prophylaxis against attacks of arthritis can be achieved conveniently with 0.6 mg of oral colchicine twice daily, or with relatively low doses of NSAIDs such as 25 mg of indomethacin twice daily if colchicine is inappropriate. The second approach is to lower the serum uric acid level with allopurinol or probenecid. Indications for choosing the uricosuric approach (probenecid [Benemid]) or xanthine oxidase inhibition (allopurinol) are listed in Table 2. About 75% of patients receiving allopurinol have no further attacks of gout even with prolonged follow-up.

If the patient does not meet the criteria for hypouricemic therapy described in Table 1, if the acute attacks of gouty arthritis are not disabling, and if radiographs of the most frequently involved joint show no erosions, a more convenient and less expensive approach is to allow the patient to treat attacks at home. At the earliest perception of pain the patient uses a standby supply of an NSAID or colchicine. Gout manifested as only two or three manageable attacks per year may not justify a lifelong commitment to daily medication as long as radiographs shows no erosion. A poorly understood feature of treatment with hypouricemic agents is the propensity of the patient to develop more frequent acute gout attacks during the first 6 months of hypouricemic treatment; prophylaxis with daily oral colchicine may be needed while the serum urate level is declining toward a plateau in the patient receiving therapy. Once the serum value stabilizes, prophylaxis can be discontinued. Up to 2 years of colchicine prophylaxis can be necessary for some patients with severe tophaceous gout. Because allopurinol can exacerbate an acute attack, it should be added only during an intercritical period. The dose range for allopurinol is 100 to 600 mg daily in a single dose. The usual dose is 300 mg per day. An effective policy is to use the minimal dose that keeps the serum uric acid to a level between 6 and 7 mg per dL. The dose is adjusted every 2 weeks, to find the correct level for the individual patient. With both allopurinol and probenecid, beginning at the lowest dose and increasing it avoids wide swings in serum urate levels, which tend to bring on attacks.

Probenecid inhibits renal tubular uric acid reabsorption and can be used to reduce the serum uric acid level. The side effects of probenecid include rash and gastrointestinal upset. Gastric intolerance is less common at lower doses. Sulfinpyrazone (Anturane) has a similar mechanism but carries greater risk of bone marrow suppression. The starting dose of probenecid is 250 mg twice daily, increasing to 1 gram per day during 2 weeks. Up to 3 grams per day is sometimes tolerated, but gastrointestinal side effects can limit the total dose and leave the patient with an overall decrement in uric acid of only 2 mg per dL. This practical limitation of efficacy to 2 mg per DL makes the simpler allopurinol regimen more applicable to most patients. Forced fluids up to 3 liters per day initially, alkalinization of urine to pH 6.5 with Shohl's solution, and perhaps prophylactic oral colchicine therapy are necessary adjuncts to the use of uricosuric treatment in tophaceous gout to prevent nephrolithiasis and acute attacks.

MANAGEMENT OF TOPHACEOUS GOUT

Tophaceous gout is the strongest indication for hypouricemic treatment (see Table 1). Tophi are crystallized deposits of urate and imply risk of joint and renal damage; joint erosions on radiographs also represent crystalline deposits and are equally strong indications. Every effort should be made to reduce the serum uric acid level to 7 mg per dL to mobilize urate in tophaceous gout. Because practical use of probenecid often results in only a 2 mg per dL decrement in the serum uric acid level, probenecid is often insufficient for patients with tophaceous gout. Specific indications for choosing allopurinol over probenecid include a creatinine clearance less than 80 mL per minute, stones, or a 24-hour urinary uric acid level greater than 800 mg.

TABLE 2. **Indications for Hypouricemic Treatment of Gout**

Indication	Explanation
Frequent (2–4/y) and disabling attacks of gouty arthritis	How frequent and how disabling vary according to patient's inclination to comply with a daily medication schedule.
Tophaceous deposits in soft tissues	These imply high total body stores and more potential for joint and renal damage.
Destructive gouty joint disease	Erosions on radiograph, crystal-proven gout.
Recurrent urolithiasis; most recent stone within last 2 y	One stone and severe hyperuricemia or urinary uric acid level >800 mg/d is sufficient if the patient can be convinced to take daily medication.
Severe hyperuricemia (>13 mg/dL in men; >10 mg/dL in women; >15 mg/dL in renal failure)	Risk of arthritis and stones is quite high; the theoretical risk of urate nephropathy is unquantified.
Severe uric acid overproduction (urinary uric acid excretion >1100 mg/d)	There is a high risk of nephrolithiasis.
Gout with renal damage, urate nephropathy	Most patients considered for this criterion qualify because of severe hyperuricemia or tophi. Control of any associated hypertension is critical.
Prevention of acute uric acid precipitation in renal tubules in patients with high tumor burden of leukemia-lymphoma about to receive cytotoxic treatment	Allopurinol may potentiate toxic effects of cyclophosphamide.

Rarely, a patient with a strong indication for lowering of the serum uric acid level exhibits hypersensitivity to allopurinol. Oral allopurinol desensitization may be the safest method of avoiding hypersensitivity reactions if probenecid therapy is not applicable. Oxypurinol is the active metabolite of allopurinol but 40% of patients sensitive to allopurinol exhibit the same T cell–mediated hypersensitivity to oxypurinol. Oral desensitization to allopurinol requires cooperation of a pharmacist, a patient fully informed of potentially fatal reactions, and close follow-up. The protocol begins at 0.008 mg in an oral solution and advances to 8 mg a day at day 10 accelerating to reach 20 mg at day 20 and 300 mg at day 30.

MANAGEMENT OF GOUT IN RENAL INSUFFICIENCY

Clinical gout occurs in less than 1% of uremic patients, but doses of every drug used for gout, except corticosteroids, are affected by renal function. The allopurinol dosage needs to be drastically reduced in the presence of diminished renal function. For an anephric patient, the dose can go as low as 100 mg every third day. A creatinine clearance of 10 mL per minute implies an allopurinol dose of 100 mg every other day; 20 mL, 100 mg daily; and 40 mL, 200 mg daily. In patients with renal insufficiency, 0.6 mg of colchicine by mouth twice daily occasionally leads to a myopathy with elevated creatine kinase levels or to a peripheral neuropathy. These cases are diagnostic problems mimicking polymyositis and uremic neuropathy. Patients with creatinine clearances less than 50 mL per minute should try gout prophylaxis with 0.6 mg only once per day. Probenecid is not able to increase uric acid excretion substantially in patients with renal insufficiency; it should not be used. Sulindac probably has the least effect on intrarenal prostaglandin production and glomerular filtration pressure. However, every nonsteroidal agent can result in a decrease in glomerular filtration. De-

hydrated patients who already exhibit some decrement in creatinine clearance are the most vulnerable to NSAID-induced acute renal failure. Prominent in this latter group are older patients exhibiting serum creatinine levels within normal limits but who have small muscle masses and actual creatinine clearances of 30 to 40 mL per minute.

The least problematic regimen for acute gout in renal insufficiency begins with oral or injectable corticosteroid (10 or 15 mg of prednisone orally for 3 days is often adequate), accompanied by an optional reduced regimen of oral colchicine (0.6 mg daily) to prevent the rebound sometimes seen after corticosteroid treatment of gout. Corticotropin (ACTH gel [H.P. Acthar Gel] intramuscularly) produces rebound in two thirds of patients, but rebound occurs in only about one third of patients using other corticosteroid regimens. Moderate doses of prednisone produce surprisingly little perturbation in glucose control in most forewarned diabetic patients. Rebound after steroid treatment may not occur, especially if injectable steroids have been used, and in any case rebound can be avoided with reduced doses of nonsteroidal agents or oral colchicine that would, by themselves, be inadequate to control the acute attack. The feared complications of corticosteroids rarely occur, owing to the short courses of treatment needed for gout.

GOUT AFTER TRANSPLANTATION

Azathioprine (Imuran), must be reduced to one quarter of its original dose if allopurinol, which blocks its metabolism, is added. Because cyclosporine (Sandimmune) induces a major defect in renal tubular urate secretion, the prevalence of gout can be as high as 50% in heart transplant patients followed up for 5 years or longer, much lower among recipients of liver transplants, and intermediate in kidney transplant patients.

POSTOPERATIVE GOUT

Postoperative gout may be precipitated by blood loss and fluid shifts brought on by large volumes of intravenous infusion. Fifteen percent of postoperative attacks are first-ever attacks. They occur on postoperative day 4 on average, typically involve the knee or ankle in a monoarticular distribution, and can confound diagnosis because of accompanying fever and peripheral blood leukocytosis. A steroid regimen (see Table 1) is often the best choice in postoperative or other hospital gout. In one center fully atuned to the potential toxicities of the various choices, only 20% of hospitalized patients experiencing gout received NSAIDs.

EMERGENCY DEPARTMENT SETTING

In the emergency department when a quick resolution of gout symptoms is important, narcotic analgesia may play a role. Narcotics are particularly helpful when angina or myocardial infarction occurs with acute gout. A 2-mg infusion of intravenous colchicine can produce a rapid analgesia (usually within 3 hours) through its specific anti-inflammatory effect. A rapid response to intravenous colchicine serves a diagnostic function as well. Safe use of intravenous colchicine in the emergency department requires that the drug not be given in doses above 1 or 2 mg and until renal function has been assessed. An initial trial of 1 mg intravenously is appropriate for older patients. ACTH gel, and by extension other steroid regimens, have proved less toxic than NSAIDs in the emergency department setting (see Table 1).

DIAGNOSTIC PROBLEMS AFFECTING THERAPY

Several diagnostic questions frequently affect treatment choices in acute and intercurrent gout. These questions include the following: (1) when to omit arthrocentesis with crystal diagnosis and substitute another method such as radiographs, a colchicine trial, or assessment of the general clinical picture; (2) when to obtain a radiograph; (3) when to obtain a 24-hour urine collection for uric acid measurement; (4) when to revise the diagnosis and consider entirely different monoarticular diseases such as peripheral arthritis of ankylosing spondylitis, psoriatic arthritis, or Reiter's syndrome.

When urgent diagnosis is needed, usually to help rule out a septic joint, there is no substitute for arthrocentesis, Gram stain, culture, and examination for crystals under polarized light. In particular, patients who have fever and uncertain follow-up, uncertain compliance, or diabetes and an inflamed joint in the foot need arthrocentesis. Patients whose attacks elude crystal-proven diagnosis and respond to treatment slowly may have another type of monoarthritis. A radiograph is rarely helpful in the few years of the course. If there have been multiple attacks for several years, then one should order a radiograph to look for the characteristic erosion with an overhanging edge. In contrast, when there have been only one or two attacks, a radiograph ordered in the emergency department is of little value. In particular, an acute septic joint cannot be ruled out by radiograph. A 24-hour urinary uric acid measurement is most useful in resolving indecision about starting uricosuric therapy or xanthine oxidase inhibition, especially if renal function is abnormal. For a patient whose stone history and frequency and severity of attacks of arthritis are almost sufficient to justify a lifelong prescription, hyperexcretion (a 24-hour urine collection with a uric acid level above 800 mg per day) sways the decision in favor of starting allopurinol therapy. Patients about to receive probenecid should have a 24-hour urine collection to confirm uric acid excretions less than 800 mg per dL per day and a creatinine clearance greater than 80 mL per minute, to preclude giving a uricosuric agent to someone predisposed to form uric acid stones.

CAUTIONS REGARDING INDIVIDUAL AGENTS

NSAIDs can cause perforations in patients with peptic ulcer disease or inflammatory bowel disease. Other pitfalls in the treatment of gout are outlined in Table 3. From the public health standpoint, the greatest impact comes from the excessive use of allopurinol for asymptomatic hyperuricemia. Adjustments of colchicine and allopurinol dosages for renal insufficiency are also important. Serious allopurinol toxicity characterized by eosinophilia, exfoliative dermatitis, fever, hepatocellular damage, acute renal failure, and vasculitis occurs more often in patients taking thiazide diuretics and patients with renal insufficiency. From 10 to 20% of these are idiosyncratic reactions that are fatal. Allopurinol is the agent for gout that exhibits the most interaction with other drugs. Warfarin (Coumadin), azathioprine

TABLE 3. **Errors in Gout Management**

Prescription of allopurinol for asymptomatic hyperuricemia, or for hyperuricemia due to diuretics (most common error; more than half of U.S. allopurinol usage falls into this category)

Failure either to adjust doses of colchicine or allopurinol for renal insufficiency or to substitute corticosteroid

Prescription of allopurinol and an interacting drug such as azathioprine, cyclophosphamide, or warfarin without reduction in dosage

Daily intravenous colchicine for patients unable to take medication by mouth

Failure to recognize gouty erosions on radiographs as equivalent to tophi as indications for hypouricemic treatment (most common omission)

Failure to reconsider the diagnosis when treatment fails and gout is not crystal-proven (alternative diagnoses include Reiter's syndrome, psoriatic arthropathy, peripheral joint involvement in spondyloarthropathy)

Arthrotomy for a presumed septic joint, especially in the hand, in a setting compatible with gout, before arthrocentesis and examination for crystals (which is metabolized by xanthine oxidase), and cyclophosphamide are all potentiated by allopurinol. When azathioprine is prescribed with allopurinol, the azathioprine should be reduced to one quarter dosage. Allopurinol and ampicillin prescribed together frequently cause a rash.

With one exception, deaths from colchicine have been described only in patients who received at least some of the drug intravenously and in whom a dosage error was made. Sources of dosage errors are (1) the assumption that patients who can take nothing by mouth can have oral colchicine replaced milligram for milligram with intravenous colchicine over a period of days; (2) failure to follow the total dosage guidelines; (3) the impression that a 4-mg course of intravenous colchicine can be repeated for the same attack if unsuccessful the first time; (4) overestimation of an elderly patient's creatinine clearance; and (5) the prescription of intravenous colchicine in unusual situations that exacerbate cochicine's toxicity or interfere with its metabolism. These unusual situations include inflammatory bowel disease; combined liver and renal disease; and a pre-existing regimen of a drug such as cyclophosphamide, which suppresses bone marrow and potentiates the capacity of an overdose of colchicine to produce neutropenia and sepsis. Some successful experimental approaches to treating and preventing drug toxicity have been developed. Antibody fragments can bind colchicine in cases of colchicine toxicity. Uricase can lower the serum urate level in patients not able to take allopurinol.

HYPERLIPIDEMIA

method of
ANTONIO M. GOTTO, JR., M.D., D. PHIL.
Cornell University Medical College
New York, New York

In the last 5 years, epidemiologic, genetic, laboratory, and clinical data have convincingly demonstrated that lowering cholesterol levels by a variety of lipid-regulating interventions results in improvement in angiographic end points, cardiac morbidity and mortality rates, and all-cause mortality rates in different primary and secondary prevention clinical settings. The National Cholesterol Education Program and its second Adult Treatment Panel (ATP II) have established guidelines for risk stratification and interventions based on the lipid profile and associated risk factors.

GUIDELINES FOR THERAPY

The ATP II has specifically described risk stratification criteria and algorithms for implementation of both dietary and pharmacologic therapy. The intensity of treatment is focused on the patient's total risk factor profile for coronary heart disease (CHD); the most important factor is the presence of established atherosclerosis as manifested by known CHD, prior

myocardial infarction, peripheral vascular disease, or cerebrovascular disease. Individuals who have documented atherosclerosis are thought to be at the highest risk for either progression or a recurrent event and are considered candidates for more intensive interventions.

Primary preventive measures are directed at people without definite evidence of CHD, and the cumulative risk is stratified by the number of other risk factors present. The ATP II has designated five positive risk factors and one negative risk factor in considerations for primary prevention (Table 1). The presence of symptomatic CHD is the major risk factor consideration in secondary prevention.

Primary Prevention

In primary prevention, the total number of risk factors together with the cholesterol concentration is assessed to determine treatment. The ATP II recommends screening of all adults after the age of 20 years, using total cholesterol (TC) and high-density lipoprotein cholesterol (HDL-C) determinations to stratify patients initially (Table 2). An individual whose TC value is below 200 mg per dL and HDL-C value exceeds 35 mg per dL is considered to be at low risk. No specific intervention other than general education regarding the benefits of increased physical activity and other lifestyle measures is provided. Another cholesterol determination is recommended in 5 years.

A TC concentration in the borderline high range (200 to 239 mg per dL) with a satisfactory HDL-C value that is not accompanied by more than two other risk factors is also thought to suggest low risk, and lifestyle information is provided to the patient

TABLE 1. **Other Risk Factors in Evaluating Coronary Heart Disease Risk**

Positive risk factors	
Age	Men, age of ≥45 y
	Women, age of ≥55 y
Family history of CHD	Premature CHD in first-degree family members are considered to constitute an increased risk for atherosclerosis (e.g., definite MI or sudden death without a noncardiac cause younger than 55 y in father or other first-degree male relative; younger than 65 y in mother or other first-degree female relative)
Hypertension	Blood pressure 140/90 mm Hg or higher with the concomitant use of antihypertensive agents even if blood pressure is normalized
Current tobacco use	
Low HDL-C	HDL-C < 35 mg/dL
Negative risk factor	
HDL-C ≥60 mg/dL	Also, inverse coronary risk associated with hyperalphalipoproteinemia

Abbreviations: CHD = coronary heart disease; MI = myocardial infarction; HDL-C = high-density lipoprotein cholesterol.

TABLE 2. **Risk Stratification Based on Lipid Concentration**

Category	Lipid Concentration (mg/dL)		
	Undesirable	Borderline	Desirable
Primary Prevention			
Initial stratification			
TC	≥240	200–239	<200
HDL-C	<35	—	≥35
			(≥60 is a negative risk factor)
Fasting lipid profile			
LDL-C	≥160	130–159	<130
Secondary Prevention			
LDL-C	>100	—	≤100

Abbreviations: TC = total cholesterol; HDL-C = high-density lipoprotein cholesterol; LDL-C = low-density lipoprotein cholesterol.

with this profile. However, in this group, another cholesterol level should be obtained in 1 to 2 years.

Patients who have either borderline high TC levels accompanied by two or more other risk factors, low HDL-C (<35 mg per dL) levels, or TC levels in excess of 240 mg per dL are recommended to have a fasting lipoprotein analysis with further stratification by the concentration of low-density lipoprotein cholesterol (LDL-C) (see Table 2). On the basis of data taken from a fasting sample, LDL-C is estimated by use of the Friedewald equation:

$$LDL\text{-}C = TC - HDL\text{-}C - (triglycerides/5)$$

The proper use of this equation requires not only that a fasting specimen be taken, but also that triglyceride concentrations be under 400 mg per dL to prevent miscalculation due to very-low-density lipoprotein (VLDL) particles with abnormal composition.

Risk stratification in subjects with a borderline high LDL-C value requires the tabulation of the number of other CHD risk factors present (Table 3). A borderline high LDL-C level accompanied by fewer than two other risk factors requires lifestyle instruction concerning diet and physical activity, and a lipoprotein determination should be repeated in 12 months. An elevated or borderline LDL-C level accompanied by more than two risk factors requires intervention to return the LDL-C concentration to a desirable range.

Secondary Prevention

Patients with documented CHD are recommended to undergo a complete fasting lipoprotein analysis. TC and LDL-C concentrations may fall in the acute recovery phase of an ischemic event, thus leading to a false value if measurements are made during this period. However, there is evidence to suggest that TC and LDL-C measurements at the time of admission or within the first 24 hours of an acute event may be reliable. Secondary prevention requires more stringent stratification, and an LDL-C level of less than 100 mg per dL is considered to be desirable in patients with known coronary or peripheral atherosclerosis.

DIETARY THERAPY

Dietary therapy should be considered the primary line of intervention in addressing hyperlipidemia and should be continued even if subsequent pharmacologic therapy is required. Dietary therapy is directed at caloric restriction to optimize weight, and reduction of saturated fat and cholesterol intake. Dietary therapy should be initiated in primary prevention in subjects who have fewer than two other risk factors if the LDL-C level exceeds 160 mg per dL, with a treatment goal to reduce LDL-C levels below this threshold. Subjects without documented disease who have two or more other risk factors are recommended to begin dietary therapy with an LDL-C value of

TABLE 3. **Treatment Targets Based on Concentration of Low-Density Lipoprotein Cholesterol**

Category of Patients	Initiation Level of LDL-C (mg/dL)		LDL-C Goal (mg/dL)
	Dietary Therapy	Drug Therapy	
Primary Prevention			
Without CHD, <2 other risk factors	≥160	≥190	<160
Without CHD, ≥2 other risk factors	≥130	≥160	<130
Secondary Prevention			
With CHD	>100	≥130	≤100

Abbreviations: CHD = coronary heart disease; LDL-C = low-density lipoprotein cholesterol.
Adapted from Expert Panel on Detection, Evaluation, and Treatment of High Blood Cholesterol in Adults. Summary of the second report of the National Cholesterol Education Program (NCEP) Expert Panel on Detection, Evaluation, and Treatment of High Blood Cholesterol in Adults (Adult Treatment Panel II). JAMA *269*:3015–3023, 1993. Copyrighted 1993, American Medical Association.

greater than 130 mg per dL, with a treatment goal to reduce LDL-C levels below this value. Secondary prevention has more stringent guidelines, with the goal for dietary therapy of an LDL-C level of less than 100 mg per dL.

The step I diet of the National Cholesterol Education Program recommends restriction of the percentage of dietary calories derived from fat to less than 30% of the total caloric intake, with a goal of 8 to 10% of total calories from saturated fat. Polyunsaturated fats should not exceed 10% of total calories, and monounsaturated fats should not exceed 15%. Carbohydrates should be at least 55% of the total calories with an emphasis on complex carbohydrates as found in grains and fruits. The amount of protein in the diet should approximate 15%, and cholesterol should be restricted to 300 mg per day. Three months are allowed to assess the effect of diet. Lifestyle measures as monotherapy may be extended in patients who are considered to be at low risk, such as younger patients and premenopausal females.

If dietary goals are not achieved, the step II diet may be initiated; this consists of further restriction of cholesterol to less than 200 mg per day in addition to a further reduction of saturated fats.

PHARMACOLOGIC THERAPY

Pharmacologic intervention should be considered in subjects whose LDL-C concentrations remain above the recommended treatment guidelines after an adequate trial of lifestyle interventions (Table 4). Drug therapy may be considered earlier if patients suffer from severe genetic disorders such as familial hypercholesterolemia that fail to respond to lifestyle interventions. Dietary therapy should be continued even if pharmacologic interventions are instituted because of the diminishing of drug efficacy under the challenge of a high-fat diet.

In primary prevention, drug therapy with a goal of an LDL-C level of 160 mg per dL or less should be considered if the LDL-C level continues to exceed 190 mg per dL after an adequate dietary trial (usually 6 months, during which both step I and step II diets should be tried). In primary prevention, subjects who have two or more other risk factors should be considered for drug therapy at lower LDL-C levels. Pharmacologic therapy may be instituted in patients in this group whose LDL-C concentrations exceed 160 mg per dL, with a treatment goal of 130 mg per dL.

In secondary prevention, patients may be considered candidates for drug therapy if dietary measures do not reduce circulating LDL-C levels lower than 100 mg per dL after 3 months. A growing number of cardiologists now recommended that dietary measures and drug therapy be instituted simultaneously in individuals at the time of an acute event, rather than delaying 3 to 6 months to determine the response to dietary therapy.

Agents That Predominantly Influence Low-Density Lipoprotein Cholesterol

Bile Acid Sequestrants (Resins)

A large body of clinical experience has accumulated regarding the resins' lipid-lowering efficacy, tolerability, and impact on clinical end points. The currently available resins, cholestyramine (Questran) and colestipol (Colestid), are highly charged polycationic compounds that differ in chemical structure but share a common mechanism of action. The clinical use of the bile acid sequestrants has declined in the past decade because of the introduction of agents that achieve greater cholesterol reductions with relatively fewer side effects.

MECHANISM OF ACTION

The major mechanism of action of the bile acid sequestrants is to interrupt the normal physiologic recirculation of the cholesterol-rich bile acid pool. After hepatic synthesis, bile acids are secreted via the biliary tract. Under normal physiologic conditions, approximately 3% of the bile acid pool is excreted; the remainder undergoes enterohepatic recirculation after absorption in the distal ileum. The fecal excretion of bile acids is generally less than 0.2 to 0.6 gram, which may be increased 2- to 10-fold after the administration of the maximal dose of cholestyramine. Administration of bile acid sequestrants results in an enhanced conversion of cholesterol into bile acids. In addition to increasing the fecal loss of bile acids, resin therapy results in an up-regulation of the LDL receptor, which allows lipoproteins containing apolipoproteins B and E (apo B and apo E) on their surface to be removed from the plasma compartment to a greater extent. The resins thus exhibit a dual mechanism of action, with a resultant lipid reduction due to increased plasma clearance of cholesterol-rich lipoproteins coupled with in-

TABLE 4. **Metabolic Effects of Major Available Lipid-Regulating Drug Classes***

Drug Class	LDL-C	HDL-C	TG
Bile acid sequestrants	↓ 15–30%	↑ 5%	⟷
HMG-CoA reductase inhibitors	↓ 20–60%	↑ 5–15%	↓ 10–37%
Fibric acid derivatives	⟷, ↓ 10–15%	↑ 5–20%	↓ 20–50%
Nicotinic acid	↓ 20–30%	↑ 15–35%	↓ 20–50%

*↓ = decrease; ↑ = increase; ⟷ = variable.
Abbreviations: LDL-C = low-density lipoprotein cholesterol; HDL-C = high-density lipoprotein cholesterol; TG = triglyceride; HMG-CoA = 3-hydroxy-3-methylglutaryl coenzyme A.

terrupted intrahepatic circulation of bile acids. The long-term efficacy of resin therapy is blunted by a secondary stimulation of 3-hydroxy-3-methylglutaryl coenzyme A (HMG-CoA) reductase activity in the liver, which increases cholesterol synthesis.

DOSAGE AND EFFICACY

Cholestyramine and colestipol are administered as a powdered resin, which may be mixed with liquids or combined with food to increase palatability. The compliance rates for resin therapy are increased if the initial dose is low and then slowly advanced to the maximal level of 24 grams per day of cholestyramine and 30 grams per day of colestipol. These levels are rarely achieved or sustained for long periods. The predominant therapeutic effect of resin therapy is the lowering of TC and LDL-C levels, and the expected reductions range from 15 to 30%. HDL-C has been reported to increase by up to 5%, although the mechanism underlying this potentially beneficial increase has not been determined. The effects on triglyceride levels are variable, and an increase in VLDL may be documented after the administration of resins. The risk for this potentially adverse effect is increased when the pretreatment triglyceride level is elevated. The resins have no demonstrable effect on chylomicrons.

SIDE EFFECTS

Resin therapy is attractive because these compounds are not absorbed by the body, thus resulting in no significant direct systemic side effects. However, the chemical composition of the resins frequently renders these compounds unpalatable, and the side effects include bloating, nonspecific abdominal pain, and gastroesophageal reflux. Constipation is a common side effect and may be disabling in elderly patients. The impact of resin therapy on bowel function may be ameliorated by increasing fluid and fiber intake or using stool softeners. Resins also tend to raise triglyceride levels, and this may be a problem in patients with significant baseline hypertriglyceridemia.

The cationic nature of these compounds results in nonspecific binding of a large number of coadministered drugs such as thyroxine, digoxin, warfarin, diuretics, beta blockers, and various antibiotics. The nonspecific binding and reduced absorption of concomitant medications may be minimized by administering these drugs 1 hour before or 4 to 6 hours after the ingestion of the bile acid resins.

The resins prolong bowel transit time, thus potentially increasing the exposure to a variety of toxins. The question of the carcinogenic potential of these drugs has been raised from an observed increase in the frequency of 1,2-dimethylhydrazine–related gastrointestinal tumors in experimental animals. Despite the theoretical concern for increased neoplasms, no clinical trial in humans has documented an increase in malignancy after prolonged administration of these agents.

HMG-CoA Reductase Inhibitors (Statins)

The advent of the HMG-CoA reductase inhibitors into clinical practice approximately 10 years ago marked a major advance in the pharmacologic management of dyslipidemias. The original HMG-CoA reductase inhibitors were isolated from cultures of microorganisms and were subsequently found to partially inhibit the rate-limiting enzyme in cholesterol synthesis (HMG-CoA reductase). The five currently available statins are atorvastatin (Lipitor), fluvastatin (Lescol), lovastatin (Mevacor), pravastatin (Pravachol), and simvastatin (Zocor).

MECHANISM OF ACTION

Although the HMG-CoA reductase inhibitors differ in chemical structure, they share a common dual mechanism of action that alters the relative proportion of circulating lipid subfractions. The statins induce the partial inhibition of the rate-limiting enzyme in cholesterol synthesis, resulting in a decrease in the cellular production of cholesterol. The resultant decrease in intracellular cholesterol levels causes a secondary up-regulation of the LDL receptor. Thus, the administration of HMG-CoA reductase inhibitors results in an increased rate of removal of apo B– and apo E–containing lipoproteins—namely LDL and, to a lesser extent, VLDL and intermediate-density lipoprotein—caused by a decline in intracellular cholesterol synthesis. The statins may also have effects on the hepatic synthesis and production of apo B–containing particles such as VLDL. Atorvastatin has been reported to decrease LDL-C levels by 22% in receptor-negative homozygotes with familial hypercholesterolemia, possibly through a mechanism that involves decreasing VLDL synthesis or secretion.

EFFICACY

The established dosing ranges for the HMG-CoA reductase inhibitors and their expected maximal LDL-C reduction is variable. The synthesis of cholesterol follows a diurnal pattern, and the administration of the statins in the evening is thought to result in increased efficacy, because maximal cholesterol synthesis occurs at approximately midnight. Fluvastatin, which is synthetic, is given at 20 to 80 mg per day (the 80-mg-per-day dose is approved as 40 mg twice daily) and may result in an LDL-C reduction of approximately 20 to 35%. Lovastatin is given in the range of 10 to 80 mg per day in divided doses and results in LDL-C reductions of approximately 30 to 35% at the maximal dose. Pravastatin is given at 10 to 40 mg per day and also results in a 30 to 35% reduction in circulating LDL-C levels. The dosing range of simvastatin is 5 to 40 mg per day at bedtime, and approximately a 35 to 40% reduction in LDL-C levels may be achieved. The administration of these statins is generally associated with a modest but predictable increase in HDL-C levels that ranges from 5 to 15%. VLDL, which contains both apo B and apo E on its surface, may be cleared by the hepatocyte or peripheral tissues that have undergone up-regulation of the LDL receptor, and circulating triglyceride levels may fall approximately 10 to 20%. The most recently available statin, atorvastatin, has been shown to lower LDL-C levels by 39 to 60% and triglyceride levels by 19 to 37%, and to raise HDL-C levels by 5 to 9%. The dosing range of atorvastatin is 10 to 80 mg per day. Lipoprotein Lp(a) does not appear to be significantly altered by any of the statins.

SIDE EFFECTS AND DRUG INTERACTIONS

Because of their relatively facilitated clinical release, the statins have been intensively evaluated in the past 10 years for potential side effects. The major clinically encountered abnormalities associated with the use of these agents are alteration of liver function and myositis.

The potential for hepatic toxicity as indicated by elevations of transaminase levels has been prospectively evaluated in several large clinical trials. All the statins appear to be associated with some degree of transaminitis, although the incidence of elevations of liver enzymes in excess of three times normal is generally less than 2%. Hepatic failure and progression to cirrhosis have not been reported with the statins. Liver function abnormalities appear to be most common in the first 4 to 12 months of therapy, and it is recommended that liver function tests be intermittently monitored.

Clinically significant myopathy is uncommon with the statins, and definite rhabdomyolysis (defined as a 10-fold elevation of creatine kinase levels associated with a compatible symptom complex and myoglobinuria) occurs in approximately 0.1% of patients who receive statin monotherapy. The mechanism by which the statins cause muscle toxicity has not been clearly elucidated but may be the result of an alteration of membrane structural stability due to reduced cholesterol availability or of decreases in the production of ubiquinone, which the mitochondria use for electron transport. The incidence of significant muscle toxicity is increased when the statins are combined with agents such as cyclosporine, gemfibrozil, erythromycin, or nicotinic acid. The incidence of significant muscle toxicity with combination therapy may also be enhanced if baseline renal insufficiency is present. The statins have been used in combination therapy for hyperlipidemic patients in an attempt to maximize the lipid response or to use different mechanisms of action to obtain a synergistic effect on circulating lipid subfractions. The combination of a statin and a resin has been utilized because of their complementary mechanisms of action. Patients may better tolerate combination therapy of a resin at lower doses with a statin. Statins have been combined with fibrates in patients with mixed dyslipidemia. However, the combination of a fibrate and statin is associated with an approximately 1 to 5% rate of myositis and should be used with caution. Statin therapy in combination with nicotinic acid also has the potential to increase the incidence of significant muscle toxicity.

Estrogen

Estrogen replacement therapy (ERT) has not been traditionally considered an intervention for treating dyslipidemia. However, the increased prevalence of CHD in postmenopausal women and data from epidemiologic studies that correlate decreased rates of CHD in postmenopausal women using hormone replacement therapy has increased interest in the use of ERT in postmenopausal women to decrease the subsequent risk for atherosclerosis.

MECHANISM OF ACTION

The role of ERT as a means of decreasing the risk for CHD is complicated, and the beneficial effect may not lie totally in improvement in the lipid profile associated with ERT. Endothelial dysfunction has been restored to normal by ERT, and a variety of beneficial effects on the clotting mechanism, including alteration of platelet aggregation, has been attributed to estrogen use. Estrogen therapy activates a promoter region on the LDL receptor gene that increases the number or activity of the LDL receptors. Estrogen also increases the secretion of VLDL and may thus have variable effects on triglyceride levels depending on the capacity to catabolize the increased circulating levels of VLDL effectively. HDL-C levels are generally increased by ERT, although the mechanism involved is complex. Lp(a) levels are also effectively lowered by estrogen therapy.

EFFICACY

The effects of estrogen therapy on circulating lipid levels are variable, but oral estrogens are generally associated with an approximately 15% decrease in circulating LDL-C levels. Transcutaneously administered estrogen may have a less dramatic effect on circulating lipid levels because of the elimination of the first-pass effect. The effects of estrogen on triglyceride levels are at least partially dependent on the pretreatment triglyceride levels combined with the functional activity of the apo B/E receptor.

SIDE EFFECTS

Estrogen therapy has a variety of potential side effects including induction of uterine malignancies when hormone replacement therapy is administered as unopposed estrogen. The addition of progesterone generally counteracts the adverse effect of estrogen on uterine carcinogenesis without affecting the beneficial lipid effects of estrogen therapy. The potential effects of estrogen on breast cancer are controversial. ERT may also raise triglyceride levels appreciably, especially in female patients who are already hypertriglyceridemic.

Probucol

Probucol is an agent with structural similarities to the powerful antioxidant butylated hydroxytoluene. Its use has declined in the past several years.

Agents That Predominantly Influence Triglyceride and High-Density Lipoprotein Cholesterol

Nicotinic Acid

Nicotinic acid (niacin) is an essential B vitamin that has been determined to alter the lipid profile at dosage levels that far exceed the amounts necessary to prevent deficiency. Nicotinic acid exhibits beneficial effects on multiple lipoprotein subclasses and has been extensively tested in primary and secondary prevention trials using both combination and monotherapy regimens.

MECHANISM OF ACTION

Nicotinic acid should not be confused with nicotinamide, which is also sometimes called niacin but has not been demonstrated to exert significant lipid-lowering effects as a potential pharmacologic intervention. Nicotinic acid exerts beneficial effects on the lipid profile and is effective in all lipid disorders with the exception of Fredrickson's type I hyperlipidemia, which is characterized by increased levels of chylomicrons. The major lipid-lowering activity of nicotinic acid results in a decrease in the production and release of VLDL. The formation of VLDL is the first step in the endogenous lipid cascade, and reduced synthesis or release of this initial lipoprotein results in decreased levels of all subsequent particles, including VLDL remnants and LDL. Nicotinic acid also has major beneficial effects on HDL-C levels, and the increase in circulating HDL-C is most marked in patients whose pretreatment triglyceride levels were elevated. Nicotinic acid therapy results in significant lowering of Lp(a) by a mechanism that is complex and not completely delineated but does not apparently involve increased receptor-mediated clearance of this particle from the plasma compartment.

EFFICACY

The nicotinic acid administered as a vitamin to prevent deficiency requires a dosing level of 1 to 5 mg per day, whereas significantly higher doses are required to exert a hypolipidemic effect. One gram of niacin per day may increase HDL-C concentrations, but dosing ranges of 2 to 6 grams of crystalline nicotinic acid per day are necessary to attain the maximal expected benefit of nicotinic acid on other lipoprotein subfractions. LDL-C may be expected to decline by approximately 20 to 30%, and triglyceride levels may fall in the 20 to 50% range. The response of HDL-C to nicotinic acid therapy is variable and may range from 15 to 35% depending on pretreatment triglyceride levels. Nicotinic acid therapy may also be beneficial in the treatment of familial defective apo B-100, a dyslipidemia in which the circulating levels of LDL-C are increased because an abnormality in the apo B-100 structure impairs receptor-mediated removal of LDL.

SIDE EFFECTS AND DRUG INTERACTIONS

The use of nicotinic acid has been limited because of a variety of side effects that frequently result in decreased compliance by patients. The majority of side effects associated with nicotinic acid, although troublesome, may be self-limited or minimized with effective counseling of patients and dosing regimens. The most common side effect associated with nicotinic acid is cutaneous flushing that is prostaglandin mediated and may be severe enough to cause hypotension. The flushing is frequently accompanied by severe pruritus and may be minimized by beginning at low doses (50 mg three times daily) and increasing the administered dose at intervals of 4 to 7 days. Pretreatment with aspirin may blunt the prostaglandin-mediated vasodilatation and should be considered to be a necessary concomitant medication if there are no contraindications.

The other effects of nicotinic acid are considerably more problematic and include potentially fatal complications such as fulminant hepatic failure (more commonly associated with sustained-release preparations of nicotinic acid). Abnormalities in circulating transaminase levels above the upper limits of normal are seen in approximately 5% of patients whose dosing ranges of nicotinic acid exceed 3 grams per day. The transaminase elevations are generally asymptomatic and thus require intermittent monitoring of liver function tests. A sudden, unexplained fall in circulating cholesterol levels may herald impending severe hepatic dysfunction, and this complication may be more common when switching from crystalline nicotinic acid to the sustained-release forms. Mild, asymptomatic, and persistent elevations of liver enzyme values are not an absolute indication to terminate nicotinic acid therapy, and dose reductions of up to 50% may be beneficial in an attempt to determine if the liver function will return to normal. However, persistent transaminitis in excess of three times the normal levels should result in discontinuation of the drug.

A variety of adverse metabolic effects may also be associated with nicotinic acid therapy including alteration of glucose tolerance (which may occur in up to 10% of patients). Diabetes is not an absolute contraindication to the use of nicotinic acid therapy, but this agent should be used with caution in individuals with a history of documented diabetes or insulin resistance. Lifestyle measures or alterations of the dosing levels of insulin or oral hypoglycemic medications would be required to minimize the potential adverse effects on the long-term development of atherosclerosis due to worsening of diabetes.

Myositis is uncommon with nicotinic acid monotherapy but the prevalence is increased when niacin is combined with other agents such as the HMG-CoA reductase inhibitors or fibric acid derivatives. It is not necessary to monitor creatine kinase elevations routinely in patients receiving nicotinic acid, except when a symptom complex compatible with myositis is reported.

Hyperuricemia and precipitation of gouty arthritis have been reported with nicotinic acid therapy. Uric acid elevations may occur in 5 to 10% of patients receiving nicotinic acid, and patients who are predisposed to gout should be informed of this potential complication.

Gastrointestinal symptoms are common with nicotinic acid monotherapy, and exacerbation of peptic ulcer disease may be encountered. Nonspecific symptoms such as nausea or mild abdominal discomfort may occur in up to 20% of patients receiving nicotinic acid therapy, and this may be further exacerbated by the concomitant administration of aspirin in an attempt to minimize the cutaneous complications. Acanthosis nigricans and toxic ambylopia have been described in rare instances.

Fibric Acid Derivatives (Fibrates)

A variety of fibric acid derivatives are available worldwide, but in the United States, clofibrate (Atromid-S), whose clinical use has declined markedly in the past 2 decades, and gemfibrozil (Lopid) are the currently available agents of this class, although fenofibrate has been approved for use but is currently not marketed.

MECHANISM OF ACTION

The mechanism of action of the fibric acid derivatives is complex and involves multiple effects on both the synthetic and the catabolic pathways of triglyceride-rich particles. Lipoprotein lipase, which is the key enzyme in VLDL and chylomicron catabolism, is a ubiquitous endothelium-bound enzyme that is normally activated by apo C-II on the surface of these lipoproteins. The predominant effect of the fibric acid derivatives is to increase the catabolism of triglyceride-rich lipoproteins by the activation of this enzyme. Lipoprotein lipase activation catalyzes the hydrolysis of chylomicrons and VLDL into remnant particles and intermediate-density lipoprotein, respectively. The activation of lipoprotein lipase also results in the transfer of cholesterol-rich surface lipids from VLDL into HDL, resulting in the frequently observed inverse relationship between triglyceride and HDL-C levels. There is also evidence that gemfibrozil may affect hepatic lipase activity. The effect of fibric acid derivatives on LDL is complex and is a function of the relative activity of the LDL receptors and the pretreatment triglyceride levels. Activation of lipoprotein lipase in a hypertriglyceridemic patient with defective or reduced activity of the apo B/E receptor may increase the catabolic pathway of VLDL, with a resultant increase in LDL particles that cannot be cleared effectively from the circulation. Hypertriglyceridemic patients frequently have increased concentrations of atherogenic small, dense LDL, and fibric acid derivative therapy may result in the remodeling of LDL into a larger, buoyant, and potentially less atherogenic form.

EFFICACY

Fibric acid derivatives are predominantly used in patients with elevated triglyceride and/or low HDL-C levels. A dose of 1200 mg daily administered as 600 mg twice a day may decrease triglyceride levels by 20 to 50%, with an accompanying increase in HDL-C values of 5 to 20%. LDL-C levels are unpredictable after the administration of the fibric acid derivatives but may be expected to decrease by 10 to 15% in normotriglyceridemic subjects. Fibric acid derivatives may have effects beyond altering the circulating lipid concentrations, including reductions in fibrinogen, factor VII phospholipid complex, and plasminogen activator inhibitor 1 levels. Fibric acid derivatives may also have beneficial effects on epinephrine-induced platelet aggregation. No substantial effect on Lp(a) levels has been demonstrated consistently with administration of the fibrates. Data from the primary prevention Helsinki Heart Study demonstrated that gemfibrozil treatment was associated with the greatest benefit in the subgroup of patients with elevated LDL-C and triglyceride and low HDL-C levels.

SIDE EFFECTS AND DRUG INTERACTIONS

Fibric acid derivatives are generally free of clinically significant side effects, although earlier intervention trials implied an increase in noncardiac morbidity and mortality after the use of clofibrate. The impact of clofibrate on noncardiac morbidity has been controversial; no definite adverse effects have been documented with the other fibric acid derivatives. The major side effects of fibric acid derivatives are gastrointestinal and may be noted to occur in up to 5% of patients receiving these agents. Clofibrate was documented to be associated with an increased prevalence of cholelithiasis, although this has not been convincingly demonstrated with the other agents. Liver function abnormalities may occasionally be noted, but hepatic failure or progression to chronic liver disease has not been documented with these compounds. Myositis is uncommon with the use of fibric acid derivatives as monotherapy but may increase to an incidence rate of approximately 5% when these agents are combined with the statins. The adverse interaction between the fibrates and the statins with the induction of myositis is especially accentuated in subjects with renal insufficiency. The fibrates potentiate the action of warfarin, and the prothrombin time should be monitored while these drugs are being administered.

SUMMARY

The National Cholesterol Education Program recommends the identification of patients at risk for a coronary event based on the stratification of their overall risk factor profile. Subjects who are considered to be at high risk for an adverse outcome are patients with multiple risk factors, including most especially the presence of established atherosclerosis. A conservative approach can be recommended in people who are considered to be at low risk or who are young, and dietary and other lifestyle measures should be emphasized in these patients. However, subjects requiring more aggressive intervention now have available a large number of potential interventions, and significant progress has been made in the pharmacologic management of dyslipidemia. Pharmacologic therapy should be tailored to address the predominant underlying lipid phenotype. Bile acid sequestrants and the HMG-CoA reductase inhibitors are the most commonly used LDL-C–lowering agents. These compounds may be combined in severe cases in an attempt to obtain a synergistic effect on the lipid profile. Nicotinic acid, gemfibrozil, and atorvastatin are the major agents for influencing VLDL, with consequent effects on LDL-C, HDL-C, and triglyceride levels. ERT is currently not indicated by the Food and Drug Administration for either lipid lowering or reduction of cardiac end points but should be considered in postmenopausal women who do not have a contraindication to its use.

OBESITY

method of
F. XAVIER PI-SUNYER, M.D.
*Columbia University College of Physicians and
   Surgeons
New York, New York*

The treatment of obesity is difficult and often discouraging because the failure rate is extremely high. The primary emphasis must be on self-control, and what must be recognized by both patient and physician is that the primary agent for change is the patient rather than the physician. Self-motivation and commitment of the patient are required, and the support, understanding, and knowledge of the physician are quite helpful.

Because physicians are accustomed to giving pharmacologic agents to treat most diseases that they see, they are often not attuned to the tedious task of slow, difficult weight loss, with its relapses, plateaus, and disappointing statistics. Because of this, other health professionals have become involved in treatment. Many dietitians, psychologists, social workers, and nurses advise and treat patients who want to lose weight and can be helpful. Nevertheless, a physician should monitor the weight loss program and treat any health problems that may develop.

Obesity is extremely common in the United States, and a physician usually requires nothing more than a quick look to determine the need for weight loss. However, because there is much preoccupation with overweight and because social, psychologic, and economic rewards are perceived to be derived from a trim look, patients who are not truly obese may wish to lose weight. This should not be allowed. A table of healthy weight ranges for height has been published by the U.S. Department of Agriculture (Table 1). The percentage of body fat can also be calculated and followed during weight loss by using the sum of four subcutaneous skinfolds (Table 2), or a bioimpedance instrument can be used.

Another guideline that can be used is the body mass index (BMI), calculated by dividing the weight in kilograms by the height in meters squared (kg/m²). Such guidelines have been recommended by the 1985 National Institutes of Health Consensus Development Conference Statement on the Health Implications of Obesity. Recommended guidelines for the BMI in the population are as follows: younger than 35 years, a BMI of 20 to 25 is a good

TABLE 1. **Healthy Weight Ranges
for Men and Women**

Height*	Weight (lb)†
4'10"	91–119
4'11"	94–124
5'0"	97–128
5'1"	101–132
5'2"	104–137
5'3"	107–141
5'4"	111–146
5'5"	114–150
5'6"	118–155
5'7"	121–160
5'8"	125–164
5'9"	129–169
5'10"	132–174
5'11"	136–179
6'0"	140–184
6'1"	144–189
6'2"	148–195
6'3"	152–200
6'4"	156–205
6'5"	160–211
6'6"	164–216

*Without shoes.
†Without clothes.

value for most people, a BMI of 25 to 27 may lead to some health problems, and one greater than 27 presents an increasing risk of developing health problems.

How the fat is distributed on the body is also important to the risk of morbidity. An excessive amount of fat in the trunk (central fat, upper body fat) carries more risk than fat on the lower body (peripheral fat, lower body fat), is a better indicator of the presence of risk factors such as hypertension and hyperlipidemia, and is a better predictor of some diseases, such as coronary heart disease and diabetes.

Obesity aggravates or precipitates a number of other diseases, including diabetes mellitus, hypertension, dyslipidemia, coronary heart disease, congestive heart failure, thromboembolic disease, restrictive lung disease, sleep apnea, gout, degenerative arthritis, gallbladder disease, and infertility. In cases in which one or more of these conditions are present, more stringent standards of weight seem appropriate, such as those of the 1983 Metropolitan Life Insurance Company weight tables. In any case, the physician must recognize that although the loss of weight is likely to ameliorate any associated conditions, therapy targeted specifically for these disorders may also be necessary.

Obesity develops because energy intake exceeds energy expenditure. Once obesity has been attained, however, there may be a new weight plateau at which intake is equivalent to expenditure and weight is stable. To lose weight, energy intake must be decreased and energy expenditure increased to disequilibrate the energy balance equation and create a caloric deficit.

The three approaches to weight reduction, in order of importance, are diet, exercise, and drugs.

TREATMENT

Goals of Therapy

It is common for patients beginning a weight-loss program to have faulty and unrealistic beliefs about

TABLE 2. **Equivalent Fat Content, as a Percentage of Body Weight, for a Range of Values for the Sum of Four Skinfolds (Biceps, Triceps, Subscapular, and Suprailiac) of Males and Females of Different Ages**

Skinfolds (mm)	% of Body Weight for Males of Age (y)				% of Body Weight for Females of Age (y)			
	17–29	30–39	40–49	50+	16–29	30–39	40–49	50+
15	4.8				10.5			
20	8.1	12.2	12.2	12.6	14.1	17.0	19.8	21.4
25	10.5	14.2	15.0	15.6	16.8	19.4	22.2	24.0
30	12.9	16.2	17.7	18.6	19.5	21.8	24.5	26.6
35	14.7	17.7	19.6	20.8	21.5	23.7	26.4	28.5
40	16.4	19.2	21.4	22.9	23.4	25.5	28.2	30.3
45	17.7	20.4	23.0	24.7	25.0	26.9	29.6	31.9
50	19.0	21.5	24.6	26.5	26.5	28.2	31.0	33.4
55	20.1	22.5	25.9	27.9	27.8	29.4	32.1	34.6
60	21.2	23.5	27.1	29.2	29.1	30.6	33.2	35.7
65	22.2	24.3	28.2	30.4	30.2	31.6	34.1	36.7
70	23.1	25.1	29.3	31.6	31.2	32.5	35.0	37.7
75	24.0	25.9	30.3	32.7	32.2	33.4	35.9	38.7
80	24.8	26.6	31.2	33.8	33.1	34.3	36.7	39.6
85	25.5	27.2	32.1	34.8	34.0	35.1	37.5	40.4
90	26.2	27.8	33.0	35.8	34.8	35.8	38.3	41.2
95	26.9	28.4	33.7	36.6	35.6	36.5	39.0	41.9
100	27.6	29.0	34.4	37.4	36.4	37.2	39.7	42.6
105	28.2	29.6	35.1	38.2	37.1	37.9	40.4	43.3
110	28.8	30.1	35.8	39.0	37.8	38.6	41.0	43.9
115	29.4	30.6	36.4	39.7	38.4	39.1	41.5	44.5
120	30.0	31.1	37.0	40.4	39.0	39.6	42.0	45.1
125	31.0	31.5	37.6	41.1	39.6	40.1	42.5	45.7
130	31.5	31.9	38.2	41.8	40.2	40.6	43.0	46.2
135	32.0	32.3	38.7	42.4	40.8	41.1	43.5	46.7
140	32.5	32.7	39.2	43.0	41.3	41.6	44.0	47.2
145	32.9	33.1	39.7	43.6	41.8	42.1	44.5	47.7
150	33.3	33.5	40.2	44.1	42.3	42.6	45.0	48.2
155	33.7	33.9	40.7	44.6	42.8	43.1	45.4	48.7
160	34.1	34.3	41.2	45.1	43.3	43.6	45.8	49.2
165	34.5	34.6	41.6	45.6	43.7	44.0	46.2	49.6
170	34.9	34.8	42.0	46.1	44.1	44.4	46.6	50.0
175	35.3				44.8	47.0	50.4	
180	35.6				45.2	47.4	50.8	
185	35.9				45.6	47.8	51.2	
190					45.9	48.2	51.6	
195					46.2	48.5	52.0	
200					46.5	48.8	52.4	
205						49.1	52.7	
210						49.4	53.0	

From Durnin JVGA, Womersley J: Body fat assessed from total body density and its estimation from skinfold thickness. Br J Nutr 32:77–97, 1974. Reprinted with the permission of Cambridge University Press.

how rapidly they can lose weight. It is important to instruct them in this regard to prevent disappointment and attrition.

One pound of fat is equivalent to 3500 to 4000 kcal. A caloric deficit of 350 kcal per day causes a 1-pound weight loss in 10 days; if the caloric deficit is 700 calories, it will take 5 days. (It may be a bit faster because, particularly initially, a water diuresis also occurs.) A regimen of diet and exercise that creates a deficit of 700 to 1000 kcal per day seems reasonable. Thus, a man weighing 100 kg whose caloric intake to maintain weight is 2800 kcal needs to reduce his intake to between 1800 and 2100 kcal. Such a diet should enable him to lose between 1 and 2 pounds per week, assuming that there is no increase in activity. It is clear that if this man's ideal body weight is 73 kg, it will take him between 30 and 60 weeks to reach this weight. At the start a clear realization of the amount of time of sustained effort required to reach the goal that is set is important for keeping a patient motivated and positively reinforced. Also, the goal need not be set at the ideal weight but at a certain percentage from the present baseline such as 10 to 15%, weight that is known to improve co-morbid conditions.

Diet

The most important component of a weight-loss program is the diet. To lose weight successfully, obese persons must lower their caloric intake and sustain such a reduced intake for a prolonged period. It is important to develop a diet program within the framework of a patient's current food habits and preferences. This is sometimes impossible when dietary habits are so poor that a radical restructuring must take place. However, better compliance occurs in patients for whom it can be done, because such patients are familiar and comfortable with the foods that they are already eating. Factors such as available cooking facilities, ethnic background, and economic background cannot be ignored. Documentation of food intake (e.g., diet records) is a good method of tracking dietary pitfalls, patterns, and progress, but physicians must beware of perfect records unaccompanied by weight loss. These should serve as a signal that a patient may not be ready to accept the weight problem or be willing to work seriously on improving it.

When available, the resting metabolic rate (RMR) should be measured and used to establish a reasonable caloric restriction. Alternatively, a formula such as the Harris-Benedict equation can be used. The RMR multiplied by 1.4 gives a reasonable approximation of 24-hour energy expenditure. For example, a 120-kg male with a measured 24-hour RMR of 2500 and a calculated 24-hour expenditure of 3500 kcal may choose to lose 1 kg per week on 1500 kcal per day rather than 1.5 kg per week on 1000 kcal per day because the quantity of food takes priority over the rate of weight loss. Such decisions should be made jointly by the patient and dietitian and/or physician to help promote long-term compliance. A diet should be adequate nutritionally, and this is possible without supplements only in diets of 1100 to 1200 kcal per day or more. To achieve this, patients must be taught to eat certain micronutrient-rich foods that they may not be used to eating. With very hypocaloric diets, the nutrients most likely to be in deficit are iron, folacin, vitamin B_6, and zinc. If kilocalorie values fall below 1100, vitamin and mineral supplements become necessary and should be prescribed by the physician; a multivitamin-multimineral tablet once a day is enough. Extra macrominerals (sodium, potassium, calcium) are usually not necessary unless subjects go on very-low-calorie diets (300 to 800 kcal), which are not recommended for long-term use.

During weight loss, the emphasis should be on the reduction of adipose (rather than lean) tissue.

Although there is some obligate loss of lean body mass, it should be kept to a minimum. Lean body mass can generally be spared during weight loss with a protein intake of 1.0 to 1.5 grams per kg of ideal body weight (calculated from Table 1). The dietary sources of protein should be of high biologic value (e.g., egg whites, fish, poultry, lean beef, and low-fat dairy products). A vegetarian diet is perfectly acceptable, but the concept of protein complementing must be explained and encouraged. The remainder of calories should come from carbohydrates (preferably high-fiber foods) and fat. Although the macronutrient ratio can vary according to the patient's needs and preferences, it is important to obtain some of the antiketogenic and digestive high-fiber benefits of carbohydrate and to get adequate amounts of fat-soluble vitamins and essential fatty acids from the dietary fat.

In all cases of weight reduction, the emphasis should be on micronutrient-dense food choices and away from empty calorie selections. A brief discussion of basic nutrition should help alert the patient to the most appropriate food choices to maximize the caloric restriction. A patient must be taught that alcohol and sweets are not sources of any essential micronutrients. These should therefore be avoided, especially in the early stages of weight reduction, because they provide little more than excess calories. It should be made clear that although some fats are less atherogenic than others, all fats are high-energy, low-micronutrient foods and should be restricted to less than 30% of the total daily calories. Gram for gram, pure fat has more than double the caloric concentration of carbohydrate or protein (9 calories per gram vs. 4 calories per gram). Because carbohydrate often absorbs water on cooking, the actual caloric density of hydrated carbohydrate on the plate may be as low as 1 to 2 calories per gram. Thus, eliminating high-fat foods from the diet should provide a substantial caloric decrease, even if pure carbohydrate foods are substituted. In general, high-fat spreads, condiments, sauces, and gravies are far more detrimental in a weight-reduction program than are bread, potatoes, pasta, and rice.

Many of the more popular media-touted diets have no scientific basis and simply play on vulnerable persons' desperation to lose weight. They often completely ignore the concept of balanced nutrition by totally eliminating or providing insufficient amounts of a particular macronutrient (e.g., protein, carbohydrate, or fat). In time this can result in a concurrent micronutrient imbalance. Such diets are clearly unsound, and if they are followed for any significant time period, serious health consequences such as electrolyte imbalances, deficiency syndromes, or protein malnutrition can ensue.

Very-low-calorie diets (300 to 500 kcal per day) are counterproductive and potentially dangerous. Although weight loss can be large on such diets, the results are often short-lived. A return to prediet weight after solid foods are resumed is the rule. Unless such diets are undertaken in the context of a complete medically supervised, stepwise program in which the very-low-calorie diet is replaced after a few weeks by a high-calorie balanced diet and intensive behavior modification program, they accomplish little except for periodic loss of water and electrolytes.

To help the patient adhere to a diet balanced in micronutrients and vitamins, it is wise to introduce the concept of the basic six food groups and the food pyramid. These consist of the following, with suggested numbers of servings in a regular diet: (1) bread, cereal, rice, and pasta (6 to 11 servings); (2) fruits (2 to 4 servings); (3) vegetables (3 to 5 servings); (4) meat, poultry, fish, dry beans, eggs, and nuts (2 to 3 servings); (5) milk, yogurt, and cheese (2 to 3 servings); (6) fats, oils, and sweets (use sparingly). By selecting judiciously from these groups, cutting down on the number of servings, and being especially careful of groups 4 to 6, patients can obtain adequate nutrients. Group 1 provides carbohydrate, protein, thiamine, niacin, vitamin E, iron, phosphorus, magnesium, zinc, and copper; groups 2 and 3 provide carbohydrate, vitamins A and C, iron, and magnesium; group 5 provides protein, fat, vitamins A and D, magnesium, calcium, phosphorus, and zinc; and group 6 provides essential fatty acids and fat-soluble vitamins.

Dieters should be encouraged to select a wide variety of food choices within these basic six food groups to help alleviate a lack of compliance caused by boredom or monotony. The number of servings per day from each group will vary according to the individual's caloric restriction and macronutrient breakdown. Because portion sizes are crucial, they should be explained in terms of common household measures (e.g., cups, ounces) and with the aid of food models.

Behavioral Therapy

The traditional technique of handing a patient a printed description of a 1200- or 1500-kcal diet, complete with specific menus and specific portion sizes, has generally been unsuccessful. Because of inadequate education and support, patients quickly dispensed with it.

As an outgrowth of that failure, behavioral therapy has been increasingly employed. The goal of behavioral therapy is twofold: to decrease food intake and to increase physical activity. The behavior of a patient is changed in ways that are possible and in reasonable steps, in concert with a physician or group therapy leader, who helps one patient or, preferably, a group of patients.

The first step in such therapy is to describe the behavior to be controlled. This means helping the patients in self-monitoring to become aware of the amount, time, and circumstances of their eating and their activity (or inactivity) patterns. This increases awareness, which is required before corrective measures can be instituted. The second step is to practice control over stimuli that affect eating behavior. Typical stimuli would be persons or situations that increase stress, anxiety, or hostility. The particular stimuli need to be identified, and the patient needs to make an effort to distance himself or herself from them. The third step is to develop techniques to control the act of eating. These include the places where the patient eats, the speed of eating, the size of mouthfuls, the number of times that eating occurs, and the attention paid to eating. It also includes learning the differences in the caloric value and nutrient content of foods, which is of great importance. Some therapists have suggested that prompt reinforcement of behaviors that delay or control eating is quite helpful. This would mean setting up some reward system (e.g., money, entertainment) as positive reinforcement for improved behavior.

The program is adapted to a patient's goals and skills rather than to a physician's idea of how a patient should behave. This individualization of treatment enhances the chances for success in a motivated person.

The advantage of a behavioral approach is that both the patient and the therapist (which may include the group) focus on the specific environmental variables that seem to govern a particular person's behavior. As A. Stunkard has suggested, "Central to a behavioral analysis is the search by patient and therapist for solutions to problems which are at the same time both relatively modest and potentially soluble." This simplifies and focuses therapy. It has been the experience in the weight-control program at St. Luke's–Roosevelt Hospital Center that conducting behavioral therapy in a group setting is highly efficacious. The group setting leads to inquiry and mutual support and encouragement that are conducive to success.

Another advantage of a behavioral approach is that when patients are given the major responsibility for the weight-loss strategy, they can attribute increased power to themselves. This tends to reinforce the treatment, inasmuch as when patients believe that the positive results are attributable to their own efforts, they gain confidence and a desire to continue.

The final and most important advantage of a behavioral approach is that it allows patients to learn to eat under the natural social and environmental conditions with which they live day to day. Thus, the habits learned during the weight loss can be continued during the difficult period of weight maintenance. This is not possible in programs of very-low-calorie formula diets, in which the patient avoids natural foods for a period of time and then is suddenly confronted with returning to regular food and having to modify behavior at that point. The learning then comes too little and too late and most often leads to failure and weight regain. It must be remembered that a behavioral program produces the slowest initial weight loss because calorie reduction is not radical and patients are encouraged to eat a hypocaloric but balanced and sensible diet. Patients must be advised to develop a long-term view. A goal weight should be set and perseverance encouraged. Also of importance is that the goal weight is often higher than the normal weight. It is imperative that the patient remain in the treatment program not only until the goal weight is achieved but also well into the weight-maintenance period.

Exercise

Because exercise expends calories, it is a logical part of any weight-loss program. Overweight persons are generally inactive, spending much of their day sitting or lying down. Many of them, particularly the heavier ones, have a real problem walking even short distances and climbing steps and tend to avoid situations that require these activities. By staying as sedentary as they do, they are essentially almost at their resting metabolic rate for most of the day. These persons must be taught first to walk, then to walk faster, and then to run or bicycle or do aerobic dance. An exercise program must start slowly. If an obese person is pushed too rapidly, discomfort and avoidance occur. Careful observation for treatment of skin intertrigo, dependent edema, and foot or joint injuries is mandatory.

It is helpful to educate the patient about how many calories are spent in an individual exercise activity (Table 3). Most tables of calorie expenditure with given levels of activity have been compiled to reflect total caloric expenditure, not the amount over the basal metabolic rate. As a result, the caloric contribution of exercise must be calculated as the difference between the calories expended per minute during exercise and the calories that a person would have expended just sitting. It is instructive and often disappointing to patients to discover just how much exercise they must do to expend a significant number of calories. For instance, if an overweight woman's basal metabolic rate is 1400 kcal per day, lying down awake she expends 1.1 kcal per minute; sitting, about 1.2 kcal per minute; walking slowly, about 1.9 kcal per minute; and walking a treadmill at 4.0 miles per hour, 7.2 kcal per minute. Thus, the difference in caloric expenditure between sitting quietly and walking fast on a treadmill (at 4.0 miles per hour) is 6.0 kcal per minute. In an hour, therefore, the energy expended by walking 4 miles is only 360 calories higher than the subject would have expended just quietly sitting. It is important to emphasize that a significant and persistent commitment to exercise must be present for exercise to have any substantial effect on caloric balance and weight loss.

Drugs

Drugs have a definite role in weight-loss programs, but they are often overused and abused. Drug therapy is never primary but always adjunctive. It should under no circumstances ever be the sole therapy but should always be used in conjunction with diet and exercise.

The anorectic drugs presently available are presumed to act on hypothalamic brain centers. They have either adrenergic or serotonergic effects. The

TABLE 3. **Approximate Energy Expenditure in Selected Activities for People of Different Weights**

	Energy Expenditure in Kilocalories per 30 Minutes for Weight of					
Activity	110 lb	130 lb	150 lb	170 lb	190 lb	210 lb
Aerobic dancing						
Walking pace	99	114	132	150	168	186
Jogging pace	159	186	213	243	270	300
Running pace	204	240	276	315	351	387
Basketball	207	243	282	318	357	396
Canoeing—leisure	66	78	90	102	114	126
Canoeing—racing	156	183	210	237	267	294
Carpentry	78	93	105	120	135	147
Cycling—5.5 mph	96	114	132	147	165	183
Cycling—9.4 mph	150	177	204	231	258	285
Dancing—ballroom	78	90	105	117	132	144
Dancing—disco	156	183	210	237	267	294
Gardening	150	177	204	231	258	285
Golf	129	150	174	195	219	243
Judo	294	345	399	450	504	558
Lying or sitting down	33	39	45	51	57	63
Mopping floor	96	105	120	138	153	171
Running						
11.5 min/mi	204	240	276	315	351	387
9 min/mi	291	342	393	447	498	552
7 min/mi	366	417	468	522	573	624
5.5 min/mi	435	513	591	669	747	828
Skiing, cross-country	216	252	291	330	369	408
Standing quietly	39	45	51	57	66	72
Swimming						
Backstroke	255	300	345	390	435	486
Crawl	192	228	261	297	330	366
Table tennis	102	120	138	156	174	195
Tennis	165	192	222	252	282	312
Walking						
3 mph	102	114	126	138	153	165
4 mph	120	141	162	186	207	228

Adapted from The High Energy Factor by Bernard Gutin and Gail Kessler. Copyright © 1983 by Bernard Gutin and Gail Kessler. Reprinted by permission of Random House, Inc.

adrenergic (also called sympathomimetic) drugs, except for mazindol (Mazanor), share a phenethylamine group and exert anorexia via a catecholaminergic or dopaminergic effect. Amphetamine and its analogues (methamphetamine and phenmetrazine) are no longer used because of their abuse potential. Phendimetrazine, benzphetamine, and chlorphentermine are schedule II drugs and are also little used. Diethylpropion (Tenuate), phentermine (Fastin, Ionamin), and phenylpropanolamine (Acutrim, Dexatrim) are widely used. Side effects of the adrenergic drugs include insomnia, excitement, agitation, headache, tremor, dizziness, dry mouth, impotence, hallucinations, confusion, palpitations, and tachycardia. Serotonergic agents include fenfluramine (Pondimin) and dexfenfluramine (Redux). Their mechanism of action is mediated via central serotonergic satiety systems. They are not stimulants but, in fact, sedatives. Side effects include drowsiness, depression, abdominal discomfort, and diarrhea. There are reports of memory impairment. A new drug, sibutramine, has both adrenergic and serotonergic effects.

Both adrenergic and serotonergic drugs have been implicated in the development of primary pulmonary hypertension. The risk is 23 to 46 cases per million per year, compared with 1 to 2 cases per million in the general population. Because this condition is lethal within 5 years in half the patients, it cannot be taken lightly. The risk is quite small, but, being present, makes judicious use of these pharmacologic agents especially important. The guidelines outlined by the Food and Drug Administration should be followed. They should be used for those with a BMI of 27 or higher with co-morbid conditions, or those with a BMI of 30 or above without co-morbid conditions. For those below the weights outlined, diet and exercise programs alone should be used.

The average weight loss has been compared in long-term studies (1 year) with the combination of fenfluramine plus phentermine, and with dexfenfluramine. The weight loss improvement over placebo in a year is of the order of 6 to 10 kg. Thus, the effect is significant but not enormous. Some patients respond well and others get little effect. It is not possible to predict who will or will not have side effects of drug therapy and what those side effects will be. Good therapeutic practice mandates that an appetite suppressant not be prescribed without a careful explanation of potential side effects. Careful monitoring of the patient is necessary, and, if the drug is ineffective, it should be stopped.

Thyroid preparations, digitalis, and diuretics

should not be used for weight loss. Inhibitors of carbohydrate absorption (α-amylase, α-glucosidase, and sucrase inhibitors) have not been successful as weight-reduction agents. Interest in possible thermogenic agents is growing, but no satisfactory one is available as yet.

Weight Maintenance

Maintaining reduced weight once a loss has been achieved is most difficult. There is a persistent tendency to regain the weight, and there is experimental evidence, particularly in animal models, that the metabolic rate is abnormally depressed after weight loss and that lipogenic pathways enhancing the reaccretion of fat may be particularly efficient. Although diet may be liberalized after the goal weight has been reached, it must be done gradually with daily weight monitoring. It is likely that a limitation of caloric intake will be required indefinitely. All the lifestyle changes learned during the weight-loss period should be continued, including a continuation of the exercise program. More long-term experience with the efficacy and safety of drugs (longer than 2 years of use) is necessary before chronic use can be recommended.

Surgery

Surgery may be indicated in patients who are massively obese and who have tried all other forms of therapy and have failed. Because of the significant rates of morbidity and even mortality from the procedure, however, it is indicated only in patients in whom the obesity itself or an associated condition is life-threatening. The surgery should be performed only in centers with adequate support from anesthesia, pulmonary, cardiac, and metabolic divisions. Lifelong follow-up is essential, and the surgeon must truly be interested in such follow-up. The surgery must be considered experimental, because no wholly adequate operation has yet been developed.

The initial procedure was jejunoileal bypass, but it has been abandoned because its side effects were such that the benefit/risk ratio was unacceptable. Problems included electrolyte and vitamin depletion, hepatic toxicity, renal stones, and polyarthritis. As a result, interest has moved to gastric procedures. In gastric bypass, a small 30- to 60-mL pouch is made in the proximal stomach with a small outlet into the small intestine, so that only a very small amount of food can be eaten at any one time. In gastroplasty, a staple line partitions the stomach into two segments, which are connected by a narrow outlet. This staple line can be horizontal or vertical. The side effects are less common and less serious than those in the intestinal operations. However, this operation is technically more difficult. Also, success rates vary, and there have been quite a few failures. These are generally related to poor operative technique or to a patient's eating around the procedure by frequent ingestion of small meals that include high-calorie fluids.

VITAMIN DEFICIENCY

method of
RICHARD S. RIVLIN, M.D.
*Memorial Sloan-Kettering Cancer Center and
New York Hospital–Cornell Medical Center
New York, New York*

Before beginning to treat any suspected vitamin deficiencies, the physician must first consider all the factors that may have contributed to this condition and how they can be prevented in the future. Certain general considerations should be taken into account:

1. The impact of a poor diet is greatly intensified by the prolonged use of certain medications, such as laxatives and diuretics, particularly in older individuals.
2. Alcohol has specific and selective effects on vitamin metabolism that may become overt when the diet is also compromised.
3. The presence of so-called classic features of vitamin deficiency, such as the petechiae and curly hairs of scurvy, indicates that the disorder is far advanced and requires prompt intervention.
4. Vitamin deficiencies are rarely encountered singly; clusters of multiple deficiencies are usually the rule.
5. Deficiencies develop gradually, and symptoms may be nonspecific in their early stages.

When a poor dietary pattern develops, the deficiencies of the vitamins emerge in an ordered manner. Thus, water-soluble vitamin stores may be seriously depleted in a matter of weeks. Longer periods are needed for major depletion of fat-soluble vitamin stores (see the article on vitamin K deficiency). Several years of seriously inadequate vitamin B_{12} intake are necessary before there is clinically apparent deficiency of this vitamin.

In the process of correction of vitamin deficiency, the physician must remember that large doses of vitamins are in reality drugs, with a toxic/therapeutic ratio. Some vitamins, particularly A and D, have a real potential for causing untoward effects. Thus, both the prevention and the treatment of vitamin deficiency require a knowledge of physiology and nutrition.

In recent years increasing attention has been directed toward detecting relative or marginal vitamin deficiency early in an effort to maximize the benefits of nutrition. For example, folic acid deficiency leads to elevated blood levels of homocysteine, an amino acid that is suspected of being a risk factor for cardiovascular disease. When serum levels of homocysteine are stratified according to the serum folic acid levels within the so-called normal range, individuals at the lower end of normal have been shown to have higher blood levels of homocysteine than persons at the higher end of normal. Possible health benefits may derive from elevating the lower levels of folic acid within the normal range through diet, food fortification, or supplementation.

THIAMINE DEFICIENCY (BERIBERI)

In the United States at present, overt thiamine deficiency is often encountered in the setting of chronic alcohol ingestion. Drinking portions of alcohol throughout the day prevents most of the dietary thiamine from being absorbed. It is for this reason that a proper clinical history tries to ascertain not only how much the patient drinks but also when the drinking occurs. It has been estimated that about one quarter of alcoholic patients admitted to hospitals in the United States show some evidence of thiamine deficiency. It is likely that alcohol has deleterious effects on thiamine metabolism as well as on its absorption. When alcohol abuse of long duration is superimposed on a dietary inadequacy of this vitamin, serious neurologic consequences may result.

Beriberi due to dietary thiamine deficiency is encountered more frequently in developing countries than in the United States, particularly where polished rice is a dietary staple. This food contains little thiamine. Whole-grain, unprocessed rice is much more nutritious. Thiamine deficiency may be encountered from time to time under conditions in which the metabolic requirement is increased, as in severe diabetes, far-advanced cancer, or pregnancy and lactation. Early features of the deficiency state are relatively nonspecific and include anorexia, irritability, weight loss, and weakness. Later there is prominent involvement of two major organ systems in the classic syndrome: (1) the cardiovascular system with beriberi heart disease, exhibiting high-output failure and features suggestive of thyrotoxic heart disease, and (2) the central and peripheral nervous systems, with peripheral neuropathy and the Wernicke-Korsakoff syndrome.

Prevention

With a diet containing adequate amounts of thiamine-rich sources, such as red meat, whole grains, legumes, and nuts, and with avoidance of milled or polished rice, beriberi should be preventable. Thiamine is unstable at alkaline pH and is also heat sensitive except under acidic conditions below a pH of 5. Thus, cooking may compromise thiamine sources to some degree.

The Food and Nutrition Board of the National Research Council, National Academy of Sciences, has established a recommended dietary allowance (RDA) that ranges from 1.2 to 1.5 mg per day for males 11 years of age and older, and 1.0 to 1.1 mg per day for women, depending on age, with an increase of 0.5 mg during pregnancy and lactation. For infants the RDA is 0.3 to 0.4 mg per day and for children 1 to 10 years of age it is 0.7 to 0.9 mg per day. Such figures are intended to meet the needs of nearly all healthy persons and would need to be higher under conditions of increased metabolic requirements.

Treatment

The physician must keep a high index of suspicion in mind that thiamine deficiency may be present when heart disease or neurologic manifestations are prominently displayed in a patient who chronically abuses alcohol. In case of doubt the physician should err on the side of treatment, because little harm would result from thiamine injection when it is not needed. If thiamine deficiency is likely, prompt administration of 50 to 100 mg* intramuscularly or intravenously is indicated. Such large doses should be continued for 3 to 4 days, after which 5 to 10 mg can be given orally or intramuscularly.

As noted earlier, in far-advanced beriberi it is highly likely that other significant deficiencies in vitamins and minerals coexist and will also necessitate vigorous treatment. Continued alcohol abstinence is absolutely crucial to prevent recurrence, and the diet must be adequate in calories and nutrients.

Peripheral neuropathy in thiamine deficiency, manifested by numbness, tingling, and burning in the extremities, may be debilitating and responds poorly to analgesics. It is suggested that patients be kept active and that physiotherapy be instituted early. Recovery from the neurologic disorder may be quite prolonged, and patients are often discouraged by the slow rate of progress.

Cardiovascular symptoms of beriberi often resemble those of hyperthyroidism, as noted previously. Heart failure may develop and necessitate therapy with digitalis, diuretics, and other drugs. A brisk response to thiamine may obviate or reduce the need for diuretics. Thiamine alone may result in significant improvement in cardiovascular function, with a prompt diuresis in cases of heart failure, but the use of standard cardiac medications is generally required for an optimal response and full recovery. The possibility that other forms of heart disease, such as alcoholic cardiomyopathy, may be present as well must be considered, as they may be masked by the hyperkinetic state.

Rarely, one may encounter genetic disorders of thiamine metabolism, such as congenital lactic acidosis, Leigh's disease, and maple syrup urine disease, in which large doses of thiamine (100 to 500 mg) are necessary to achieve some benefit.

RIBOFLAVIN (VITAMIN B$_2$) DEFICIENCY

In understanding the pathogenesis and treatment of riboflavin (vitamin B$_2$) deficiency, it is essential to realize that the metabolic action of riboflavin resides largely in its role as a precursor of the coenzymes riboflavin-5'-phosphate (flavin mononucleotide [FMN]) and flavin adenine dinucleotide (FAD), and of flavins bound covalently to tissue proteins. All these derivatives of riboflavin are widely involved as coenzymes in intermediary metabolism. More recently, it has been suggested that riboflavin may provide antioxidant activity in its role as the precursor of flavin adenine dinucleotide, the cofactor for glutathione reductase. This enzyme generates reduced glutathione, which is the substrate for glutathione peroxidase, a powerful enzyme that degrades reactive lipid peroxides.

Dietary deficiency of riboflavin is nearly always encountered in the setting of multiple deficiencies. It is important to remember that in addition to being

---

*Exceeds dosage recommended by the manufacturer.

caused by a poor diet, riboflavin deficiency may also result from the effects of hormones, drugs, or diseases that impair the body's utilization of this vitamin and its conversion to active derivatives. Phototherapy of newborn infants for elevated serum bilirubin concentrations may provoke riboflavin deficiency because the vitamin is light sensitive. Alcohol may also cause riboflavin deficiency by interfering with the digestion and absorption of the vitamin. There are conditions, such as severe burns, trauma, surgery, dialysis, and others, in which vitamin B_2 deficiency may also result from increased demands on tissue stores. Psychotropic drugs, antimalarial agents, and some cancer chemotherapeutic drugs impair the conversion of riboflavin into its active coenzyme derivatives.

Early in the course of riboflavin deficiency, the patient may exhibit burning and itching of the eyes and mouth as well as personality disturbances. Subtle manifestations of early deficiency, such as weakness and fatigue, may be difficult to distinguish from those of many other causes. Later on, angular stomatitis, seborrheic dermatitis, glossitis, and other epithelial abnormalities are found. Cheilosis and angular stomatitis are no longer believed to be specific for riboflavin deficiency. With further progression of the deficiency state, anemia and corneal neovascularization may develop.

Prevention

Riboflavin deficiency should be preventable if the diet contains an adequate supply of milk and dairy products, meat, and green, leafy vegetables. In the United States, dairy products are the most important sources of the vitamin, and the riboflavin nutritional status is generally correlated quite closely with that of calcium. Low-fat dairy products remain excellent sources of riboflavin as well as calcium. In developing countries, vegetable sources predominate. The RDA for riboflavin is 1.4 to 1.8 mg for males 11 years of age and older and 1.2 to 1.3 mg for women, with an increase of 0.5 mg during pregnancy and lactation. The RDA for infants is 0.4 to 0.5 mg per day and that for children of ages 1 to 10 years is 0.8 to 1.2 mg per day.

Treatment

Riboflavin deficiency can be treated with the previously mentioned food sources that are rich in this vitamin. Riboflavin can also be administered as a component of a multivitamin tablet. For rapid treatment of riboflavin-deficient patients, doses in the range of 10 to 15 mg per day are recommended. The poor solubility of riboflavin in aqueous solution limits its feasibility for intravenous administration and this formulation is seldom used.

NIACIN DEFICIENCY (PELLAGRA)

The well-described deficiency disease pellagra was quite common in the United States when corn was a dietary staple. Corn is relatively poor in tryptophan, the essential amino acid that serves as a precursor of niacin. At present, niacin deficiency in the United States largely results from prolonged alcohol abuse under conditions in which multivitamin deficits prevail. In rare instances, some degree of niacin deficiency may occur after the use of specific drugs that interfere with niacin metabolism, such as isoniazid (INH) or 6-mercaptopurine. In the malignant carcinoid syndrome, dietary tryptophan is diverted from the synthesis of niacin to that of serotonin, and some patients may exhibit signs of pellagra, particularly if they are also malnourished. In the autosomal recessive disorder Hartnup's disease, pellagra may develop because of a deficit in the absorption of tryptophan and other amino acids from the intestinal tract.

Prevention

Niacin deficiency is preventable by a diet that is high in proteins of animal origin, which have a high tryptophan content. Some vegetable proteins also have tryptophan but at lower amounts. The best sources of niacin besides meats are yeast, cereals, legumes, and seeds. Some newer varieties of corn have higher tryptophan and niacin concentrations than those prevalent earlier. Grain products often contain niacin but of relatively lower bioavailability. The RDA is expressed in terms of niacin equivalents; 60 mg of dietary tryptophan yields about 1 mg of niacin synthesized endogenously. Expressed in this manner as niacin equivalents, the RDA for niacin is 15 to 20 mg in males 11 years of age and older and 13 to 15 mg in women, with an additional 5 mg recommended during pregnancy and lactation. The RDA for infants is 5 to 6 mg per day, and for children of ages 1 to 10 years the RDA is 9 to 13 mg per day.

Treatment

Advanced pellagra is a serious life-threatening disorder, classically known by the four *d*'s: diarrhea, dermatitis, dementia, and death. Doses in the form of niacinamide (nicotinamide) in the range of 50 to 150 mg have generally been given to ill patients; marked clinical improvement is demonstrable within several days. Once these large doses have been administered, maintenance levels of several times the RDA together with satisfactory diet should be given to the patient. Other measures involved in supportive care include correction of acid-base imbalance, treatment of the skin disease, and recognition that the neurologic impairment may follow a prolonged course before recovery occurs.

Niacin in the form of nicotinic acid in much larger doses (3 to 6 grams per day) is a first-line drug for management of an elevated serum cholesterol level. Niacinamide, another form of niacin, does not cause the flushing symptoms associated with nicotinic acid, nor does it lower the serum cholesterol level.

PYRIDOXINE (VITAMIN B₆) DEFICIENCY

Vitamin B_6 is found in dietary sources primarily in three forms, as pyridoxal, pyridoxamine, and pyridoxine. Animal foods contain predominantly pyridoxal and pyridoxamine, whereas the predominant form in plants is pyridoxine. As an important coenzyme, pyridoxal phosphate participates in a wide range of reactions. Although best known for its involvement in transamination, pyridoxal phosphate also catalyzes decarboxylation, side chain cleavage, and dehydratase reactions. These functions are central to glucogenesis, lipid metabolism, central nervous system functioning, the immune system, nucleic acid synthesis, and endocrine function as well as synthesis of certain other vitamins (e.g., niacin).

Dietary deficiency of pyridoxine occasionally occurs in the United States but almost never as an isolated entity. It is sometimes observed after prolonged therapy with certain pharmacologic agents, such as INH or cycloserine for tuberculosis, both of which are pyridoxine antagonists. Deficiency of pyridoxine occurs commonly in severe alcoholism in association with deficiencies of the other vitamins, as noted earlier.

Prevention

Deficiency of pyridoxine should be preventable by a diet that contains adequate amounts of meat, wheat, nuts, vegetables (particularly beans and potatoes), fruits, cereals, and grains. Some amount may be lost during pressure cooking and storage. The bioavailability of pyridoxine from food sources varies widely. The RDA for vitamin B_6 is 1.7 to 2.0 mg for males 11 years of age and older and 1.4 to 1.6 mg for women and is increased another 0.5 to 0.6 mg during pregnancy and lactation. The RDA for infants is 0.3 to 0.6 mg per day and that for children of ages 1 to 10 years is 1.0 to 1.4 mg per day.

Treatment

The dietary deficiency of pyridoxine can generally be treated with doses in the range of 2 to 10 mg per day. In more severe cases, particularly those occurring during pregnancy, doses in the range of 10 to 20 mg have generally been administered. In the event that deficiency has resulted from a drug inhibiting vitamin B_6 metabolism, somewhat higher doses may be needed, in some instances up to 50 to 100 mg per day. It is advisable to initiate pyridoxine therapy concomitantly when certain drugs are prescribed, a practice that is generally followed with INH treatment for tuberculosis but should be applicable more widely with vitamin B_6 antagonists. With respect to L-dopa, however, vitamin B_6 is generally not prescribed because it is believed by some authorities to interfere with therapeutic efficacy.

Rare cases of a pyridoxine-dependency syndrome, such as pyridoxine-responsive anemia, have been treated with doses in the 300- to 500-mg range. It is important to remember that peripheral neuropathy has been reported as a side effect of vitamin B_6 ingestion when 2 grams or more has been used in treatment. It is possible that lower doses, in the neighborhood of 200 to 500 mg, may also cause some degree of peripheral neuropathy.

FOLIC ACID DEFICIENCY

Folic acid and related compounds all have a pteroylglutamic acid structure and participate in many important reactions, including the synthesis of serine and methionine, purines, and thymidylate. Folic acid together with vitamin B_{12} is central to maintaining normal hematologic function. Attention has recently focused on folic acid as a methyl donor involved in the formation of methionine from homocysteine, the latter a compound associated with accelerated development of coronary, cerebrovascular, and peripheral vascular disease. The vital role of folic acid in the nervous system is exemplified by the association of its deficiency with formation of neural tube defects.

Dietary deficiency of folic acid occurs in people who do not consume adequate amounts of sources, such as meat, legumes and other vegetables, and fruits. The bioavailability of folates from food sources differs widely, and cooking destroys significant amounts. For individuals who shop infrequently and obtain out-of-date produce, there is some risk of folate deficiency because food folic acid is sensitive to processing, preparation, and storage. Alcohol intake damages the intestinal mucosa, and prolonged abuse, often of an episodic nature, is associated with folate deficiency. The first indication of folate deficiency is usually a macrocytic anemia, and later megaloblastosis may become more widespread throughout the gastrointestinal tract. Drugs that interfere with folate metabolism, the classic example of which is methotrexate, also produce manifestations of folic acid deficiency. Other important drugs causing folic acid deficiency are diphenylhydantoin and sulfasalazine.

Prevention

The current RDA for folic acid is 150 to 200 μg per day in men and 150 to 180 μg per day in women, figures that are considerably lower than the 400 μg previously recommended for adults, both male and female. Furthermore, it is recommended that during pregnancy and lactation, the allowance be increased to 400 and 280 μg, respectively. During pregnancy the blood volume is greatly increased and folate reserves may be strained, and for this reason folate intake should be greatly increased. For infants the RDA is 25 to 35 μg per day and for children of ages 1 to 10 years it is 1.0 to 1.4 μg per day.

A new dimension to the role of folic acid during pregnancy has been the recognition that the frequency of neural tube defects, such as spina bifida and anencephaly, may be reduced by daily consumption of 400 μg of folic acid. The folic acid must be consumed during the first 4 weeks of pregnancy to be effective, a period of time in which most women are unlikely to be aware of being pregnant. Furthermore, in the United States, approximately 50% of pregnancies are unplanned. With these considerations in mind, the Centers for Disease Control and Prevention recommended that "all women of childbearing age in the United States who are capable of becoming pregnant should consume 400 µg of folic acid per day for the purpose of reducing their risk of having a pregnancy affected with spina bifida or other NTDs (neural tube defects)."

Folic acid fortification of foods will be mandated in the United States beginning in 1998. Improvements in diet, food fortification, and the appropriate use of vitamin supplements should all help to prevent folic acid deficiency from becoming widespread. Increased folic acid intake, in turn, may be beneficial not only in the prevention of neural tube defects, but also possibly in diminishing the prevalence and severity of atherosclerosis in all of its manifestations. There is now evidence that folic acid may also have a protective role in preventing certain forms of cancer, such as those involving the epithelium of the uterine cervix, upper airway, breast, and colon.

Treatment

Folic acid deficiency can be treated by consistently adhering to a diet rich in folate-containing items, such as liver; yeast; green, leafy vegetables; legumes; and fruits. Care must be taken not to destroy food folates during food preparation and storage.

Therapeutic doses in the range of 1 to 2 mg per day can be administered to correct folate deficiency rapidly. In patients receiving anticonvulsant drugs, larger doses may be required to reverse the megaloblastic anemia that may result. One potential risk in administering excessive amounts of folic acid is that it may interfere with the diagnosis of vitamin B_{12} deficiency. At dose levels in excess of 1 mg per day, folic acid may correct the anemia due to the deficiency of vitamin B_{12} but not delay the progression of neurologic deterioration. Thus, in cases in which combined vitamin deficiency is suspected, vitamin supplementation should include both vitamin B_{12} and folic acid.

VITAMIN B_{12} DEFICIENCY

Vitamin B_{12} deficiency is discussed in the treatment section in the article on pernicious anemia.

VITAMIN A DEFICIENCY

The best known function of vitamin A is in vision; a cascade of reactions involving vitamin A and its derivatives, particularly retinal has been clearly defined. Vitamin A has important functions in other areas, including cellular differentiation, e.g., embryogenesis and spermatogenesis; sensations (taste); immunity; and growth.

Deficiency of vitamin A is of crucial importance as a worldwide nutritional problem because it is a cause of blindness in approximately half a million preschool children each year in the developing countries. In these areas the diet is composed primarily of such items as rice, wheat, maize, and tubers that contain far from adequate amounts of vitamin A precursors. The World Health Organization and other foundations and groups have made great efforts to plan programs to identify people at risk and to institute appropriate preventive measures on a broad scale.

Clinical deficiency of vitamin A may be overt or subclinical. In either instance, deficient children manifest increased incidence of serious and life-threatening infections and elevated mortality rates. It has been recognized that deficient vitamin A status is a risk factor for the maternal-to-fetal transmission of human immunodeficiency virus: the relative risk of transmission of this virus is fourfold greater in vitamin A–deficient than vitamin A–sufficient mothers.

Vitamin A deficiency in the United States is identified largely with certain risk groups: the urban poor; elderly persons, particularly those living alone; abusers of alcohol; patients with malabsorption disorders; and other persons with a poor diet. Vitamin A deficiency is generally found in a setting in which there are multiple vitamin and mineral deficiencies. Special attention must be paid to deficiency of zinc, a frequent finding in alcoholism, which interferes with the mobilization of vitamin A from its storage sites in liver. This effect is achieved by blocking the release of holo–retinol-binding protein from the liver.

The physician must keep in mind that deficiency of vitamin A in the United States may also develop after the long-term use of several medications. Drug-induced nutritional deficiencies in general, particularly those involving vitamin A, occur most frequently among elderly persons because they use medications in the largest number and for the most prolonged duration and may have borderline nutritional status to begin with. Among the drugs that are most relevant to compromising vitamin A status are mineral oil, which dissolves this nutrient; other laxatives, which accelerate intestinal transit and may diminish the rate of vitamin A absorption; cholestyramine and colestipol, which bind vitamin A; and, under certain conditions, neomycin and colchicine.

Prevention

Deficiency of vitamin A can be prevented by a diet high in carotenes, which serve as precursors to vitamin A. The carotenes, particularly β-carotene, are derived from plant sources, the richest of which are palm oil; carrots; sweet potatoes; dark-green, leafy vegetables; cantaloupe; oranges; and papaya. Vitamin A itself (preformed vitamin A) is derived from animal sources, such as dairy products, meat, and fish. The commercial preparations of fish oils are rich, sometimes too rich, as sources of preformed vitamin A.

The RDA for vitamin A is expressed in terms of retinol equivalents (RE): i.e., 1 RE is equal to 1 µg of all-*trans*-retinol or 6 µg of β-carotene. The RDAs are 1000 µg RE for males and 800 µg RE for females from ages 11 to 51+ years. For infants the RDA is 375 µg RE and for children 1 to 10 years of age it is 400 to 700 µg RE. This standard nomenclature is nevertheless rarely found on vitamin bottles, on which the former system of IU is used. Expressed in this manner, the RDAs for vitamin A are 5000 IU for men and 4000 IU for women. Some authorities believe that because currently 1 IU of vitamin A is equal to 0.3 µg of all-*trans*-retinol, the RDA is actually 3333 IU for men and 2667 IU for women.

The nutritional value of dietary sources of vitamin A may be compromised when the food items are subject to oxidation, particularly in the presence of light and heat. Antioxidants, such as vitamin E, may prevent the loss of vitamin A activity.

Treatment

Vitamin A deficiency has been treated worldwide with single injections of massive amounts (100,000 to 200,000 IU) repeated at intervals of approximately 6 months to 1 year. Such doses have been effective and are associated with remarkably little toxicity, perhaps because body stores are so depleted at the time of therapy. These doses may, however, produce acute toxic symptoms in well-nourished persons.

Clinical vitamin A deficiency in the United States can be treated with either β-carotene, if there is normal body conversion to vitamin A, or vitamin A itself. Daily doses in the range of 25,000 IU of β-carotene are being consumed by many healthy individuals without apparent toxicity of any kind. The yellowish discoloration of the skin associated with prolonged use of β-carotene is not harmful. Vitamin A, in contrast, is quite toxic when ingested in amounts considerably higher than the RDA, especially for prolonged periods. It is probably advisable not to exceed two to three times the RDA for vitamin A in planning a treatment program. Congenital malformations, a particularly disturbing consequence of vitamin A overdosage, have been reported in women consuming 25,000 to 50,000 IU daily during pregnancy. It is not known with certainty what the lowest dose of vitamin A that would be completely safe as a supplement for pregnant women is. Therefore, it is not a good idea for pregnant women to take supplementary vitamin A unless there are specific indications, such as malabsorption, or proven deficiency. Many advisory groups caution that the maximal intake of preformed vitamin A consumed during pregnancy should not exceed 10,000 IU.

At present, there is widespread interest in other therapeutic applications of vitamin A and its derivatives. Large doses of vitamin A have been found to reduce morbidity and mortality rates among children suffering from severe cases of measles. Certain forms of leukemia have been found to respond to derivatives of vitamin A. The therapeutic potential of this vitamin is being expanded greatly in studies of the chemoprevention and treatment of cancer. The toxicity of large doses of vitamin A itself places important limits on its feasibility in cancer prevention. Attention has turned to β-carotene and related agents, which in addition to their role as precursors of vitamin A have strong antioxidant activity and other effects as well.

Diminished prevalence of certain cancers has been found among people whose intake of fruits and vegetables is quite high; this finding has been attributable at least in part to the high content of carotenoids in the diet. There is some evidence that a combination of antioxidants (i.e., vitamin E, vitamin C, and β-carotene) may be more effective in chemoprevention than any of these agents singly. This area of research is innovative and exciting, but it is still too early to make firm recommendations for cancer prevention in the general public in the United States, particularly because prospective trials of β-carotene in cancer prevention have yielded disappointing results. There are many other substances in fruits and vegetables that appear to hold promise for cancer prevention.

VITAMIN D DEFICIENCY

Vitamin D occurs in two major forms, vitamin D_2 (ergocalciferol), a compound that is produced by irradiation of plant sterols, and vitamin D_3 (cholecalciferol), which is produced in the skin. Scientists are becoming increasingly aware of the important nutritional role of the skin in manufacturing vitamin D_3 under the influence of solar ultraviolet light.

Vitamin D_3 itself is relatively inert biologically and must be converted into active metabolites to exert its major effects. In the liver, vitamin D is converted to 25-hydroxyvitamin D_3, $25(OH)D_3$. Subsequently, in the kidneys, $25(OH)D_3$ is converted to 1,25-dihydroxyvitamin D_3, $1,25(OH)_2D_3$, the most important and active derivative. A less active vitamin D derivative, the 24,25-dihydroxy form, $24,25(OH)_2D_3$, is also produced from $25(OH)D_3$ in the kidney and other tissues. $1,25(OH)_2D_3$ is a secosteroid, and it has many properties of a steroid hormone. Indeed, vitamin D is considered to have hormonal properties.

There are three major sites of action of vitamin D in regulating calcium metabolism. Its best known action is to increase the absorption of calcium, both dietary and secreted, from the intestinal tract. At low doses of vitamin D, the amount of calcium absorbed is linear to the dose given. The second major site of action is bone, where together with parathyroid hormone it stimulates osteoclastic bone resorption. Under a wide variety of conditions, both physiologic and pathologic, the serum calcium level can be maintained within a narrow range at the expense of the calcium derived from bone. The third major site of action of vitamin D is the kidney tubule, where it increases the reabsorption of calcium.

Deficiency of vitamin D occurring in infancy and childhood is manifested as rickets, with severe developmental abnormalities. Vitamin D deficiency occurring during adult life is central to the pathogenesis of osteomalacia. In a general way, deficiency of vitamin D can result from inadequate intake from dietary sources; diminished synthesis in the skin; intestinal malabsorption, as occurs in a variety of diseases; accelerated catabolism, as caused by certain drugs; and defects in the conversion of vitamin D into its active derivatives. In a rare genetic disorder, vitamin D–resistant rickets, type II, the abnormality appears to reside not in the synthesis of the active derivatives but in target organ resistance to their action.

Prevention

Deficiency of vitamin D can be prevented by an adequate diet, conditions favorable to skin synthesis of the vitamin, or both. Studies suggest that exposure of small amounts of skin (i.e., the hands and face), for several minutes to the summer sun is enough to meet the nutritional needs of the body. Thus, prolonged exposure of the body to sunlight is not necessary to achieve optimal vitamin D synthesis. The goal of preventing skin cancer by avoiding excessive skin exposure to sunlight and consequent sunburn remains compatible with the goal of exposing enough skin to sunlight to achieve adequate synthesis of vitamin D. In northern cities, such as Boston, winter sun appears to be ineffective in promoting vitamin D synthesis in the skin. Furthermore, the ability of the skin to synthesize vitamin D is diminished with aging.

In the United States, where some foods, particularly milk, are fortified with vitamin D, sources of calcium and vitamin D often become consumed together. In children as well as in adults, having a quart of skim milk per day, with its 10 μg of cholecalciferol (400 IU), is a good way to ensure satisfactory vitamin D intake. If adequate amounts of dairy products are not consumed, a good case can be made, especially for older people, for the consumption of an additional 400 to 800 IU in the form of a supplement together with calcium. With persons exposed to abundant sunlight, dietary sources become less important nutritionally, and it is difficult to set an RDA for vitamin D in such persons. Nevertheless, many conditions often prevail that limit the optimal synthesis of vitamin D in the skin. Air pollution and sunscreens prevent ultraviolet light from reaching the skin. Staying indoors or walking in shaded areas precludes any beneficial effects of sunlight. In addition, as noted previously, exposure to winter sun in northern cities does little to enhance vitamin D synthesis in skin. The amount of 10 μg of cholecalciferol has been set as the RDA in males from 6 months of age until the age of 24 years, after which 5 μg is advised. For females, similar recommendations are made except that all pregnant and lactating women are advised to consume 10 μg of cholcalciferol. For infants 0 to 6 months of age the RDA is 7.5 μg per day.

Treatment

The goal in the treatment of vitamin D deficiency is to restore bone structure and function to normal and to correct serum concentrations of calcium if inadequate. Rickets, the form of vitamin D deficiency in infants and children, as well as osteomalacia, the manifestation of vitamin D deficiency in adults, responds to the administration of vitamin D if calcium intake is also adequate. For this reason, the physician must first determine that calcium intake is at the level of 1 to 2 grams per day as elemental calcium, in the form of either food sources rich in calcium or supplementation.

The initial doses of vitamin D to be administered in either rickets or osteomalacia are in the general range of 400 to 4000 IU per day. Most authorities recommend 2000 to 4000 IU with supplementary calcium. As a frame of reference, a quart of milk is supplemented with 400 IU of vitamin D. Thus, consuming a diet high in milk and dairy products is a good way to treat vitamin D deficiency if continued consistently for an adequate time. Probably several months of treatment at these high doses is needed, after which daily doses in the range of 400 to 800 IU are generally adequate. During the treatment period, it is essential to provide exposure to sunlight and to encourage physical exercise of a weight-bearing nature that will facilitate the normal mechanisms of bone renewal.

In the event that the deficiency of vitamin D is complicated by intestinal malabsorption, larger doses of vitamin D in the range of 10,000 to 25,000 IU or higher may be required. Water-soluble preparations of vitamin D are now available and can be administered parenterally if necessary. More calcium, in the range of 2 to 3 grams per day, is also needed. An important consideration to keep in mind is that in some instances of hypocalcemia associated with malabsorption, the provision of supplementary magnesium renders the hypocalcemia more sensitive to treatment with calcium and vitamin D. If severe liver disease is present in association with vitamin D deficiency, larger doses of vitamin D are also needed because, as mentioned earlier, the initial conversion of vitamin D to $25(OH)D_3$ occurs in liver. If the patient requires certain drugs that bind bile salts (such as cholestyramine) or that increase vitamin D catabolism (such as phenytoin), larger doses are required for adequate therapy of the vitamin D deficiency.

Vitamin D deficiency complicated by renal disease is only poorly responsive to treatment with vitamin D, because the $1,25(OH)_2D_3$ derivative is formed inadequately from precursor in the renal parenchyma. For this reason, $1,25(OH)_2D_3$ (calcitriol [Rocaltrol]) must be given. Most patients respond quite satisfactorily to doses in the 0.5- to 1.0-μg range per day. A similar strategy of treatment is required in autosomal recessive vitamin D–dependent rickets, type I, in which there is a selective genetic defect in the conversion of $25(OH)D_3$ to $1,25(OH)_2D_3$. Much higher doses than these must be tried in the case of vitamin

D–dependent rickets, type II, in which the defect is in the receptor response to $1,25(OH)_2D_3$. Patients with renal disease complicating the vitamin D deficiency also require other ancillary measures, such as phosphate restriction.

VITAMIN E DEFICIENCY

The most widely recognized role for vitamin E is as a scavenger of free radicals, and in this capacity it protects cell membranes from damage. It has many other properties as well. Vitamin E is essential for the immune system, particularly T lymphocytes, and has a role in DNA repair. Interest is growing in the effect of vitamin E on inhibiting oxidation of low-density lipoprotein (LDL): oxidized LDL is quite atherogenic. The neuromuscular system and the retina also require vitamin E for optimal function. The role of vitamin E as an antioxidant in health and disease is under intensive study at present.

Dietary vitamin E deficiency tends to be unusual under ordinary circumstances, as sources of vitamin E are widely available from the food supply. The recognizable cases of vitamin E deficiency tend to arise in debilitated patients who have had severe and prolonged periods of fat malabsorption. The reason is that vitamin E is incorporated into chylomicrons with other products of fat absorption. Any process that interferes with fat digestion and absorption also impairs absorption of vitamin E.

Other disorders in which symptomatic vitamin E deficiency may develop include cystic fibrosis, celiac disease, cholestatic liver disease, short-bowel syndrome of any cause, and unusual genetic disorders mentioned later. Major abnormalities of neurologic function are observed in severe and prolonged vitamin E deficiency with evidence of involvement of the posterior column and spinocerebellar tract. Patients display areflexia, ophthalmoplegia, and disturbances of gait, proprioception, and vibration. In premature infants, vitamin E deficiency results in hemolytic anemia, thrombocytosis, edema, and intraventricular hemorrhage. There is increased risk of retrolental fibroplasia and bronchopulmonary dysplasia.

In hemolytic anemia, such as glucose-6-phosphate dehydrogenase deficiency and sickle cell anemia, vitamin E levels in blood tend to be decreased. Inborn errors of vitamin E metabolism have been identified. In one disorder, familial isolated vitamin E deficiency, there are severe neurologic abnormalities. Because of a genetically determined defect in incorporation of dietary vitamin E into the lipid transport protein very-low-density lipoprotein, vitamin E is cleared rapidly from plasma. In another genetic disorder, abetalipoproteinemia, there is a defect in the serum transport of vitamin E. A hallmark of this disease is the finding of an extremely low serum cholesterol level together with a very low serum level of vitamin E.

Prevention

Deficiency of vitamin E can be avoided by regular consumption of the many sources of this vitamin in the food supply. The richest sources of vitamin E in the U.S. diet are vegetable oils, including corn, cottonseed, safflower, and soybean oils, and the margarines and other products made from these oils. Green, leafy vegetables are also good sources of vitamin E. In evaluating the adequacy of any given dietary regimen, one should keep in mind that losses of the vitamin occur during storage, cooking, and food processing, particularly with exposure to high temperatures and oxygen.

Because vitamin E deficiency occurs as a result of severe intestinal malabsorption, it is essential to identify this condition early and to avoid measures that may intensify the degree of malabsorption. For example, cholestyramine (Questran) and colestipol (Colestid), resins used in the treatment of hypercholesterolemia, cause malabsorption of vitamin E and should be used only when strictly indicated.

The RDA for vitamin E has been set at 10 mg α-tocopherol equivalents (TEs) per day for males aged 11 years and older and at 8 mg α-TEs per day for females aged 11 years and older. It is recommended that women consume 10 mg α-TEs per day during pregnancy and 11 to 12 mg α-TEs during lactation. The RDA for infants is 3 to 4 mg α-TEs per day and for children 1 to 10 years of age it is 6 to 7 mg α-TEs per day. The storage capacity of the body for vitamin E is quite considerable.

There is a great deal of contemporary interest in the potential role of vitamin E in the prevention of heart disease, one mechanism of which may be the inhibition of LDL oxidation described previously. Studies are actively being pursued to determine whether vitamin E alone or in combination with other agents is effective not only in the prevention of heart disease, but also in the prevention of cataract, cancer, and other disorders of aging.

Treatment

Vitamin E deficiency can be treated satisfactorily with oral preparations of the vitamin. There is a wide margin of safety in the therapeutic administration of the vitamin. Daily doses of vitamin E in the range of 100 to 800 mg can be given safely to nearly all deficient patients. This dose range can be used appropriately in those patients with vitamin E deficiency diagnosed in association with celiac disease, inflammatory bowel disease, or other chronic and prolonged forms of intestinal malabsorption. In such instances, many other nutrient deficiencies are likely to be found in association with that of vitamin E, and they too necessitate treatment.

In the genetic disorders of vitamin E metabolism, such as isolated vitamin E deficiency, higher doses of the vitamin, in the range of 800 to 1000 mg and higher, must be taken. Large doses of vitamin E given therapeutically can be quite safe. Some investigators have suggested that pharmacologic doses of vitamin E may possibly interfere with the intestinal absorption of vitamins A and K, but there are few data with which to evaluate this potential risk. There are reports that doses of vitamin E in excess of 1200 mg per day may interfere with the action of vitamin K and intensify the actions of anticoagulant drugs.

VITAMIN C DEFICIENCY (SCURVY)

Vitamin C is a powerful water-soluble antioxidant, and there is much contemporary interest in this action of the vitamin. Vitamin C is involved in lipid and vitamin metabolism, facilitates the intestinal absorption of nonheme iron, and is involved in collagen metabolism, biosynthesis of neurotransmitters, wound healing, immune function, and many other aspects of normal health. Vitamin C is a cofactor or substrate for eight known enzymes. Important physical properties of vitamin C include its sensitivity to prolonged storage and cooking at high temperatures, common events that greatly decrease biologic potency. As an antioxidant, vitamin C is destroyed by oxidation, as in exposure to air.

Vitamin C deficiency in its early stages gives rise to fatigue and lethargy, followed by petechiae and ecchymoses, follicular hyperkeratosis, and swollen and bleeding gums. Later there are arthralgias and joint effusions. Corkscrew hairs may be recognizable characteristics. Wounds heal poorly, and healed wounds have been observed to reopen.

Prevention

The best dietary sources of vitamin C are citrus fruits and green, leafy vegetables, particularly broccoli, green peppers, and cabbage. Tomatoes are also a good source. As noted earlier, care must be taken in proper food preparation and storage.

Vitamin C deficiency is common among urban poor persons, who may not be able to afford the fresh fruits and vegetables that constitute important sources. Vitamin C deficiency is also common among elderly persons, who may shop infrequently and allow produce to be stored longer than optimal. Food faddism, particularly the macrobiotic diet, adherents of which regularly subject food to pressure cooking, results in serious vitamin C deficiency. A "tea and toast" diet is virtually devoid of sources of vitamin C. Scurvy develops in alcoholic patients if their diet is deficient in food items containing vitamin C. Thus, much vitamin C deficiency could be prevented by making good dietary sources available to urban poor, elderly, and other persons on a subsistence economy; by ensuring that prolonged storage is avoided; by preventing alcohol abuse; and by learning proper food habits generally.

The RDA has been established at 50 to 60 mg per day in both males and females 11 years of age and older, at up to 70 mg per day in pregnancy, and at 90 to 95 mg per day during lactation. These estimates are considered generally to be quite generous, as doses as low as 10 mg per day have been adequate in treating scurvy. It has been suggested that a new RDA of 200 µg per day more accurately reflects the amounts needed to saturate tissue stores. The RDA for infants is 30 to 35 mg per day and it is 40 to 45 mg per day for children 1 to 10 years of age.

Treatment

In approaching the treatment of scurvy, it is essential to recognize the nutritional deficiency before it becomes extreme. Early symptoms and signs, such as weakness, lethargy, and general malaise, are nonspecific. Pain in the bones and joints, perifollicular hemorrhages, and petechiae should alert the physician to the strong likelihood of scurvy. Swollen, bleeding gums indicate advanced disease, as does edema, oliguria, and peripheral neuropathy.

As noted earlier, as little as 10 mg per day of vitamin C can treat scurvy satisfactorily, but it is advisable to begin with larger amounts, in the range of 100 to 200 mg per day. Significant improvement should be noted within several days. A good diet is obviously crucial for recovery and for maintenance of health. Such doses should be safe to administer for weeks to months if necessary to restore health to normal.

Rare inborn errors of metabolism, including osteogenesis imperfecta, tyrosinemia, and Chédiak-Higashi syndrome, have in case reports been ameliorated by doses in the range of 50 to 200 mg per day. Further experience is needed in the management of these disorders before guidelines can be definitive. Vitamin C at the level of 0.5 to 2 or 3 grams per day has been used to acidify urine. In smaller amounts (40 to 100 mg), ascorbic acid is recommended to increase the intestinal absorption of nonheme iron. Patients following a strict vegetarian diet should be encouraged to consume orange juice with their meals, because the 40 to 50 mg contained in a glass of orange juice increases the bioavailability of iron from vegetable sources significantly. However, ascorbic acid decreases the absorption of copper. Care must be taken to avoid giving potentially toxic doses of vitamin C, and restricting therapeutic doses to the 1- to 2-gram range should minimize this possibility.

Inasmuch as vitamin C is widely used as a supplement by the general public, a word of caution is indicated. The gene for hemochromatosis is widely prevalent, and in individuals who have this gene, there may be a tendency to absorb excessive amounts of iron. Measurements of serum ferritin levels readily identify a state of excess iron stores.

There is great contemporary interest in the potential use of vitamin C alone or in combination with the other antioxidant vitamins, β-carotene and vitamin E, in the possible prevention of cancer, heart disease, certain manifestations of aging, and other conditions. This is an active area of research, and further investigations are necessary before recommendations for the general public as well as for the management of specific disorders can be advanced.

VITAMIN K DEFICIENCY

method of
JAMES J. CORRIGAN, JR., M.D.
Tulane University Medical Center
New Orleans, Louisiana

Vitamin K_1 (phylloquinone), the most biologically active of the naturally occurring vitamin Ks, is fat soluble and found in leafy vegetables and some meats. It is a required vitamin for the maintenance of normal hemostasis. The minimal daily requirement of vitamin K is estimated to be between 1 and 2 µg per kg of body weight per day, which is mainly provided by diet. Because body stores are limited, a deficiency can occur within days to several weeks in circumstances of reduced intake or absorption. After oral ingestion, the vitamin binds to bile salts and is absorbed into the lymphatics and transported and stored in the liver. The serum level of vitamin K (e.g., phylloquinone) correlates poorly with vitamin K stores in the liver and with dietary intake.

Vitamin K is a carboxylase cofactor for the gamma carboxylation of glutamic acid residues of specific proteins, especially the procoagulants factor II (prothrombin), factor VII, factor IX, and factor X; and the anticoagulant protein C and protein S. These carboxylated glutamic acid residues (called Gla proteins) are found in other proteins (such as protein Z, osteocalcin, nephrocalcin, and others), bind calcium ions, and are the biologically active proteins. The precursor proteins (the non–Gla-containing proteins) have no biologic activity. They are also called PIVKA, i.e., protein induced by vitamin K absence or antagonists.

CLINICAL FEATURES

The only clinical manifestation of vitamin K deficiency is excessive hemorrhage after local trauma. Spontaneous bleeding can occur in severe cases. The signs of bleeding include easy bruising, mucosal bleeding (epistaxis, gastrointestinal hemorrhage, menometrorrhagia, and hematuria), and oozing from puncture sites, cutdowns, and surgical incisions. Intracranial bleeding can cause severe morbidity.

The causes of vitamin K deficiency are shown in Table 1. The major reason for vitamin K deficiency is decreased intake of the vitamin, as seen in patients with anorexia,

TABLE 1. **Causes of Vitamin K Deficiency**

Reduced intake and/or absorption
  Dietary
  Small bowel abnormalities
    Fat malabsorption
    Short-bowel syndrome
    Diffuse inflammatory diseases
  Pancreatic insufficiency
    Cystic fibrosis
  Hepatobiliary diseases
    Obstructive jaundice
    Prolonged T tube drainage
    Internal biliary fistula
  Total parenteral nutrition
Impaired utilization
  Antibiotics
  Anticonvulsants
  Oral anticoagulants
  Superwarfarins (brodifacoum)

TABLE 2. **Laboratory Findings in Vitamin K Deficiency**

Test	VKD	DIC	LD
Partial thromboplastin time	P	P	P
Prothrombin time	P	P	P
Platelet count	N	R	N or R
Fibrinogen level	N	R	R
PIVKA-II	+	0	0
FSPs (D dimer)	0	+	0

Abbreviations: VKD = vitamin K deficiency; DIC = disseminated intravascular coagulation; LD = liver disease; PIVKA-II (precursor factor II) = protein induced by vitamin K absence or antagonists; FSPs = fibrinolytic split products; P = prolonged; N = normal; R = reduced; + = present; 0 = not present.

those recovering from major gastrointestinal surgery, patients using exclusively total parenteral nutrition (TPN), normal newborns, and newborns and infants fed exclusively breast milk. Vitamin K deficiency may also result from diminished absorption from either diffuse intestinal mucosal disease and/or pancreatic insufficiency (e.g., fat malabsorption conditions including cystic fibrosis) or diminished flow of bile (e.g., obstructive jaundice). Impairment of vitamin K utilization can also produce the clinical picture of vitamin K deficiency with bleeding. This occurs with the therapeutic use of an antagonist (e.g., warfarin or indanedione anticoagulants), certain β-lactam antibiotics (e.g., cefamandole, moxalactam,* cefoperazone, mezlocillin, and others), and rarely, in newborns of mothers receiving anticonvulsants, certain antibiotics, and vitamin K antagonists.

Vitamin K deficiency bleeding in the newborn is classified as early, classic (so-called hemorrhagic disease of the newborn), and late onset. The early form appears during or shortly after birth and is due to drug-induced activity of vitamin K. The classic form develops at ages 3 to 5 days in newborns with delayed or inadequate feeding. The late form occurs after the first week of life (range 2 to 12 weeks); the majority of these infants have been exclusively breast-fed.

DIAGNOSIS

The laboratory manifestations of vitamin K deficiency are characteristic and include a prolonged prothrombin time (PT) and partial thromboplastin time (PTT). The platelet count and plasma fibrinogen level are normal. If needed, specific assays for factors II, VII, IX, and X or laboratory tests for detecting the noncarboxylated protein precursors of the vitamin K–dependent procoagulants can be performed. This coagulopathy can be differentiated from other acquired defects such as severe liver disease and disseminated intravascular coagulation (Table 2).

TREATMENT

Therapeutic approaches include prevention and the treatment of clinical bleeding due to vitamin K deficiency. Replacement of the vitamin can be accomplished with the lipid-soluble phytonadione preparations (AquaMEPHYTON, Konakion, Mephyton) and with menadiol (Synkayvite) a water-soluble agent.

*Not available in the United States.

Prevention

All newborns should receive vitamin K_1 (phytonadione) at birth. The use of 0.5 to 1.0 mg intramuscularly or 2 to 5 mg orally has significantly reduced the frequency of the classic form of vitamin K deficiency bleeding. Repeated doses may be necessary in those infants who are exclusively breast-fed.

Patients with reduced intake of vitamin K (e.g., anorexia, TPN, major gastrointestinal surgery) and those with impaired absorption of the vitamin should also receive vitamin replacement therapy. This could be by periodic administration of vitamin K_1 intramuscularly, subcutaneously, or orally, daily or three times a week using 2.5 or 5.0 mg. A water-soluble preparation may be used depending on the clinical circumstances.

Vitamin K Deficiency Bleeding

Patients with striking laboratory abnormalities or clinical bleeding manifestations are best treated with parenteral vitamin K. This is most usually the natural derivative vitamin K_1 (such as AquaMEPHYTON). The dose varies with the size of the patient; 0.5 to 1.0 mg is adequate for premature and term infants; 2 to 3 mg for infants and 5 to 10 mg for children after 1 year of age to adults. The route of administration is dictated by the severity of the clinical picture. In severe cases it is best to avoid intramuscular injections because this causes hematoma formation and delayed absorption. The subcutaneous and intravenous routes are acceptable. The intravenous administration has the advantage of prompter delivery of the vitamin to the hepatocytes, resulting in a more rapid onset of carboxylation of the precursor proteins and, thus, correction of the coagulopathy. The slow intravenous infusion is only rarely associated with hypotension and anaphylaxis. In most instances, vitamin K therapy is followed in the next 12 to 24 hours by cessation of hemorrhage and normalization of the PT and PTT. The usual practice is to repeat these studies 24 hours after parenteral therapy. If a decrease in bleeding and improvement in the laboratory studies have not occurred, the diagnosis is incorrect or the patient has other associated coagulation disturbances.

In patients with clinically significant bleeding manifestations (e.g., severe anemia, shock, intracranial bleeding), the immediate correction of the coagulation defects is needed. In addition to replacement of the vitamin, such patients can be treated with fresh-frozen plasma (10 to 20 mL per kg of body weight), or, rarely with a prothrombin complex concentrate (Konȳne, Proplex). Fresh-frozen plasma usually suffices. The use of blood products carries the risk of viral transmission and with the prothrombin complex concentrates, thrombosis, especially in patients with associated liver disease.

OSTEOPOROSIS

method of
SUNDEEP KHOSLA, M.D.
Mayo Clinic and Mayo Foundation
Rochester, Minnesota

Osteoporosis is defined as a metabolic bone disease characterized by low bone mass and microarchitectural deterioration of the skeleton, leading to enhanced bone fragility and a consequent increase in fracture risk. To define more fully the prevalence and incidence of osteoporosis, the World Health Organization convened an expert panel to define osteoporosis on the basis of bone mineral density (BMD). The definition is based on T scores, or the number of standard deviation units a given individual is below the young adult reference mean (Table 1). On the basis of these criteria, it has been estimated that there are approximately 9.4 million white women in the United States with osteoporosis and 16.8 million with osteopenia (comparable estimates for other ethnic groups and for men are not yet available). In addition, recent estimates indicate that more than 1.5 million Americans have fractures related to osteoporosis each year, and the annual cost to the United States health care system is at least $13 billion. Moreover, as the population ages, these figures are likely to continue to increase into the foreseeable future, unless widespread preventive measures are implemented.

CLINICAL SPECTRUM

Bone is limited in the ways it can respond to disease processes. A common skeletal response is bone loss, and it is not surprising that what we call "osteoporosis" is actually a syndrome, with many causes and a number of clinical forms. Table 2 provides a classification of the clinical spectrum of generalized osteoporosis. Osteoporosis is categorized as primary or secondary by the absence or presence of associated medical diseases, surgical procedures, or medications known to be associated with accelerated bone loss. Involutional osteoporosis is the most common form of the disease, and this chapter focuses on the prevention and treatment of this important disorder. It is further divided into type I, or postmenopausal osteoporosis, and type II, or age-related osteoporosis. Type I osteoporosis typically affects women within 15 to 20 years after the menopause and is characterized by fractures that occur at sites rich in cancellous bone, "crush fractures" of the vertebrae, Colles' fracture of the distal forearm, and fractures of the ankle. In contrast, type II osteoporosis can occur at any age but is the predominant form in both men and women aged 70 years and older; it is twice as common in women. It is characterized by fractures at sites containing substantial

TABLE 1. **Diagnostic Criteria for Osteoporosis**

Normal	BMD within 1 SD of the young adult reference mean
Low bone mass (osteopenia)	BMD between −1.0 and −2.5 SD below the young adult reference mean
Osteoporosis	BMD −2.5 SD or more below the young adult reference mean
Severe (established) osteoporosis	Osteoporosis with one or more fragility fractures

Abbreviations: BMD = bone mineral density; SD = standard deviation.

TABLE 2. Classification of Generalized Osteoporosis

Primary
    Idiopathic juvenile osteoporosis
    Idiopathic osteoporosis in young adults
    Involutional osteoporosis
        Type I (postmenopausal osteoporosis)
        Type II (senile osteoporosis)
Secondary (partial listing)
    Hypercortisolism
    Hypogonadism
    Hyperthyroidism
    Hyperparathyroidism
    Seizure disorder (anticonvulsants)
    Malabsorption syndrome
    Rheumatoid arthritis
    Connective tissue disease
    Chronic neurologic disease
    Chronic obstructive lung disease
    Malignancy

From Khosla S, Riggs BL, Melton LJ III: Clinical spectrum. *In* Riggs BL, Melton LJ III (eds): Osteoporosis: Etiology, Diagnosis, and Management, 2nd ed. Philadelphia, Lippincott-Raven, 1995, pp 205–223.

proportions of both cortical and cancellous bone. The main manifestations are hip and vertebral fractures, although fractures of the proximal humerus, proximal tibia, and pelvis are also common. The vertebral fractures often are of the multiple wedge type and lead to painless dorsal kyphosis (dowager's hump).

DIAGNOSTIC APPROACH

The initial history and physical examination should focus on assessing the possible risk factors for osteoporosis as well as searching for potential secondary causes. The history should include previous fractures; age at menopause; lifestyle factors such as smoking, alcohol intake, and exercise habits; and an assessment of dietary calcium intake. A family history of osteoporosis is an additional risk factor for developing the disease and should be documented.

Spine radiographs are too insensitive a tool for diagnosing osteoporosis and should be obtained only to define the number and extent of vertebral fractures or deformities. All patients suspected of having osteoporosis, with or without fracture, should have a BMD measurement. This is generally most reliably obtained by using dual-energy x-ray absorptiometry, and, in general, it is preferable to measure both the spine and the proximal femur sites. The spine, which is rich in cancellous bone, is often the most sensitive site for assessing early postmenopausal bone loss; with advancing age, however, aortic calcifications and osteoarthritis tend to falsely elevate the spine BMD, and the hip site may give a more accurate measure of the extent of bone loss.

Most patients should also have a biochemical profile to further exclude potential secondary causes of bone loss. This helps to exclude diagnoses such as primary hyperparathyroidism and hepatic or renal dysfunction. A hematologic profile might also provide clues to the presence of myeloma or other hematologic disorders. A sensitive thyroid-stimulating hormone level test helps exclude hyperthyroidism, which may accelerate bone loss. A 24-hour urine collection for calcium excretion is helpful because hypercalciuria, if present, may require modification of the prescription for calcium supplementation and may in itself warrant therapy. Conversely, a low 24-hour urinary cal-

cium level (i.e., 50 mg per day or less) may provide a clue to the presence of vitamin D malnutrition or malabsorption. Other studies, such as a 24-hour urine test for free cortisol, should be obtained depending on the clinical index of suspicion for Cushing's syndrome or other secondary causes of osteoporosis.

A number of biochemical markers for bone resorption and formation have now become available (Table 3) and have the potential to provide prognostic information on rates of bone loss. Thus, although measuring the BMD remains the method of choice for making a diagnosis of osteoporosis, it represents a static measurement and cannot predict the rate at which a given individual may lose bone. It does appear that increased levels of resorption and formation markers are predictive of increased rates of bone loss when groups of individuals are studied; however, the ability of these markers to accurately predict rates of bone loss for the individual patient remains to be established. At present, therefore, the most practical use of these markers is to monitor the response to therapy. Thus, the changes in markers after just 3 months of therapy have been shown to correlate with changes in bone mass after 2 years of therapy. In addition, although the changes in the bone biochemical markers occur after weeks or a few months of initiating therapy, the changes in BMD may not be discernible for 1 to 2 years after initiating therapy.

THERAPEUTIC PRINCIPLES

Once the appropriate evaluation has been completed, the therapeutic approach consists of both nonpharmacologic and, if needed, pharmacologic therapy. Nonpharmacologic measures, which are clearly essential as both a preventive and a therapeutic strategy, consist of lifestyle changes, such as smoking cessation and moderation of alcohol intake. Excessive caffeine or sodium intake may adversely affect calcium balance and should be avoided. Regular weight-bearing exercise has also been shown to have at least modest skeletal benefits and should be encouraged. When back deformity or pain is present, a program of physiotherapy, emphasizing in particular back extensor exercises, should be initiated, preferably under the supervision of a trained physiotherapist.

MEDICAL THERAPY

Theoretical Background

Bone is constantly being remodeled at discrete foci in the skeleton called bone-remodeling units. At each site, bone resorption is initiated by osteoclasts, which

TABLE 3. Biochemical Markers of Bone Remodeling

Bone formation (serum)
    Osteocalcin (OC)
    Bone-specific alkaline phosphatase (BSAP)
    Carboxy-terminal extension peptide of type I procollagen (PICP)
Bone resorption (urine)
    Pyridinoline (Pyd)
    Deoxypyridinoline (Dpd)
    N telopeptide of the cross-links of collagen (NTx)
    C telopeptide of the cross-links of collagen (CTx)

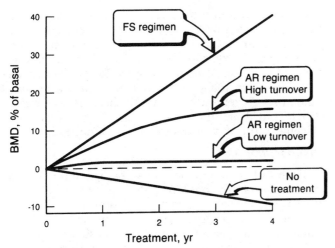

Figure 1. Patterns of change in bone mineral density (BMD) in the lumbar spine of women with osteoporosis during various treatment regimens. When an antiresorptive (AR) drug is given, the response varies directly with the rate of bone turnover at baseline. When the turnover rate is high, gains of 8 to 20% may be achieved but plateau after 2 to 3 years. The mechanism for the waning of the therapeutic effect is unknown; the magnitude and duration of the initial increase in BMD seem to be too great to be explained entirely by refilling of increased numbers of resorption cavities present when the bone turnover rate is high. When the turnover rate is normal or low, bone mass is stabilized but does not increase. With no treatment, bone loss continues, although its rate varies among individual patients. When a formation-stimulating (FS) drug, such as fluoride, is given, BMD increases linearly up to 10% annually for at least 4 years. The dashed line represents no change in BMD. (With permission from Riggs BL, Melton LJ III: The prevention and treatment of osteoporosis. N Engl J Med 327:620–627, 1992. Copyright 1992 Massachusetts Medical Society. All rights reserved.)

are subsequently replaced by osteoblasts, which in turn refill the space excavated by the osteoclasts. When bone resorption exceeds bone formation, bone loss ensues. Drugs used to treat osteoporosis can be grouped into those that decrease bone resorption and those that increase bone formation. Figure 1 summarizes the differences in bone response between antiresorptive and formation-stimulating drugs and also illustrates the point that the antiresorptive drugs are most effective when bone turnover is increased. The drugs commonly used in the treatment of osteoporosis are calcium, vitamin D, estrogen, bisphosphonates, and calcitonin. All these drugs are in the anti-

resorptive class and thus can be expected to maintain bone mass or transiently increase it. Thus far, no formation-stimulating drug has been approved by the Food and Drug Administration (FDA), although sodium fluoride is currently under review.

Antiresorptive Drugs

Calcium

Several studies now indicate that calcium supplementation can retard the rate of postmenopausal bone loss, although the effect of calcium intake on the rate of fracture has not been evaluated in a controlled clinical trial. As per a National Institutes of Health consensus panel recommendation on optimal calcium intake, the total intake of calcium in postmenopausal women should be in the range of 1000 to 1500 mg per day. Typical dietary intakes of calcium range from 500 to 1000 mg per day, so calcium supplements are often required to achieve optimal calcium intake. A variety of calcium preparations are available; the most commonly used are given in Table 4. Calcium carbonate is the most widely used preparation and is generally well tolerated. In some patients, however, it can cause constipation or abdominal discomfort. Also, calcium carbonate is poorly absorbed in the absence of stomach acid. Because a significant percentage of postmenopausal and elderly women have relative achlorhydria and generate free stomach acid only during meals, it is best to give the calcium supplement with meals. For those patients with absolute achlorhydria, calcium citrate is the preferred option.

Vitamin D or Vitamin D Analogues

Vitamin D is usually given with calcium therapy to increase the fractional absorption of calcium. For most patients, 400 to 800 IU of vitamin D (amounts in most over-the-counter multivitamin preparations) is sufficient to ensure adequate vitamin D status. In some patients, however, despite calcium and this vitamin D supplementation, calcium absorption remains low. Thus, for patients with persistently low urinary calcium values of less than 100 mg per day, higher doses of vitamin D (50,000 IU every 7 to 10 days) may be appropriate. In addition to the tablet form, vitamin D is available in a liquid preparation

TABLE 4. **Commonly Used Calcium Preparations**

Trade Name	Type of Salt	Elemental Calcium per Tablet (mg)	Cost of 1500 mg ($)
Os-Cal* (SmithKline Beecham)	Carbonate	250	0.54
Os-Cal 500 (SmithKline Beecham)	Carbonate	500	0.30
Generic oyster shell calcium	Carbonate	500	0.15
Tums (SmithKline Beecham)	Carbonate	200	0.29
Posture (Whitehall)	Phosphate	600	0.38
Citracal (Mission)	Citrate	200	0.70

*Contains 125 IU of cholecalciferol.

From Riggs BL, Khosla S: Practical clinical management. In Riggs BL, Melton LJ III (eds): Osteoporosis: Etiology, Diagnosis, and Management, 2nd ed. Philadelphia, Lippincott-Raven, 1995, pp 487–502.

(Calciferol drops) providing 8000 IU per mL or calcifediol (25-hydroxyvitamin D) (Calderol). A dose of 50 μg of calcifediol is approximately equivalent to 50,000 IU of vitamin D. Another alternative is calcitriol (1,25-dihydroxyvitamin D) (Rocaltrol), which has been shown to decrease vertebral fracture rates by 50%. When calcitriol is used with calcium supplementation, no more than 0.25 μg per day should be used. With all high-dose vitamin D supplements, monitoring of serum and urine calcium levels is required.

Estrogen

Estrogen remains the best current option for the prevention and treatment of osteoporosis. Numerous studies have now established that, in general, estrogen increases the mean vertebral bone mass by more than 5% and reduces the vertebral fracture rate by half. Estrogen can be prescribed either as an oral preparation or as a transdermal patch. The most commonly used estrogen preparations in the United States are shown in Table 5.

In addition to reducing fracture rates, long-term estrogen therapy may decrease the occurrence of coronary disease by up to 50%. Preliminary studies suggest that long-term estrogen replacement therapy may also reduce the risk of Alzheimer's disease, although much more work needs to be done in this area before this can be considered a definite benefit of therapy. For the individual patient, the benefits of estrogen replacement therapy should be weighed against the possible risks. For women with an intact uterus, the potential increased risk of endometrial cancer is eliminated by the concurrent administration of a progestin, either cyclically (i.e., medroxyprogesterone acetate [Provera], 10 mg per day for 12 to 14 days each month) or continuously (2.5 mg daily). The most controversial issue is the possible increase in breast cancer risk with estrogen therapy. A meta-analysis of the existing literature suggests that there may be a 30% increase in risk after long-term estrogen therapy for 10 years or more. This issue is far from resolved, however, as evidenced by two recent publications that arrived at conflicting conclusions. In one study, an approximately 30 to 40% increase in breast cancer risk was found among current estrogen users, whereas in another study, no increase in breast cancer risk could be demonstrated in estrogen users. On the basis of the cumulative body of evidence, the beneficial effects of estrogen replacement in terms of the skeleton and cardiovascular disease generally outweigh the potential risks; clearly, however, the decision regarding estrogen replacement therapy needs to be individualized.

Bisphosphonates

Bisphosphonates are carbon-substituted analogues of pyrophosphate that are potent inhibitors of bone resorption. These drugs have the potential to become attractive alternatives to estrogen for women in whom estrogen is contraindicated or those who are intolerant of the side effects of estrogen therapy. The first bisphosphonate to be used in the treatment of osteoporosis was etidronate (Didronel). Initial data indicated that the intermittent use of etidronate* (400 mg daily for 2 weeks followed by 11 to 13 weeks of calcium supplementation) decreased the vertebral fracture rate. This was not confirmed, however, by further follow-up. Because of the potential for therapeutic doses of etidronate for impairing mineralization and the long retention of bisphosphonates in bone, there is concern that etidronate could have adverse long-term effects such as increasing the incidence of hip fracture. Second- and third-generation bisphosphonates such as tiludronate,† alendronate (Fosamax), and risedronate† are much more potent and have a greater therapeutic window between inhibition of bone resorption and inhibition of mineralization than does etidronate. Alendronate is the first of these second-generation bisphosphonates to be approved by the FDA for the treatment of osteoporosis. In a large-scale clinical trial, there was a progressive increase in spine and hip BMD during 3 years of daily therapy with alendronate at a dose of 10 mg per day. This, in turn, resulted in significantly fewer spinal fractures in patients receiving alendronate compared with those receiving placebo. Preliminary data indicate that alendronate therapy may also decrease the rate of hip fracture. The drug is generally well tolerated, although there does appear to be a low but significant rate of gastrointestinal side effects, including gastroesophageal discomfort and, of greater concern, widespread esophageal ulcerations in some patients. Thus, pre-existing upper gastrointestinal symptoms are a relative contraindication to the drug. In addition, the absorption of most bisphosphonates is poor, and the drug needs to be administered at least 30 minutes before breakfast or other medications, with the patient instructed to remain upright and not lie down after taking the drug.

Calcitonin

Calcitonin is also an option for the patient in whom estrogen is contraindicated or who is unwilling to

TABLE 5. **Comparable Dosages of Estrogen Preparations**

Preparation	Trade Name	Dosage (mg/d)
Tablets		
Conjugated estrogen	Premarin (Wyeth-Ayerst)	0.625
Estropipate	Ogen (Abbott)	0.75
Ethinyl estradiol	Estinyl (Schering)	0.02
Dermal patch		
Transdermal estradiol	Estraderm (Ciba-Geigy)	0.05 (1 patch every 3.5 d)

From Riggs BL, Khosla S: Practical clinical management. *In* Riggs BL, Melton LJ III (eds): Osteoporosis: Etiology, Diagnosis, and Management, 2nd ed. Philadelphia, Lippincott-Raven, 1995, pp 487–502.

*Not FDA approved for this indication.
†Not yet approved for use in the United States.

take estrogen. The disadvantages of calcitonin had been the expense ($1500 to $3000 per year) and the requirement for parenteral administration. However, intranasally administered calcitonin has now been approved by the FDA for the treatment of osteoporosis and is available in the United States at a significantly lower cost than the parenteral preparation.

Calcitonin has been shown to transiently increase vertebral bone mass in women with postmenopausal osteoporosis, particularly those with increased rates of bone turnover. Side effects include nausea and flushing. Also, some patients may develop resistance to calcitonin because of the development of neutralizing antibodies. The usual dosage is 0.5 mL (100 units) of salmon calcitonin (Calcimar or Miacalcin) daily by subcutaneous injection or one spray (200 units) per day of nasal calcitonin (Miacalcin nasal spray). Because of the possibility of inducing secondary hyperparathyroidism, calcium supplements should always be given with calcitonin.

Estrogen Analogues

Tamoxifen (Nolvadex)* is a triphenylethylene derivative that is an antiestrogen for breast tissue but appears to have an estrogen agonist effect on bone tissue. However, the use of tamoxifen is limited because of its side effects, which include a partial agonist effect on the uterus. Another estrogen analogue, raloxifene,† appears to have estrogen agonistic effects on bone with antiestrogenic effects on breast and uterine tissue. Thus, it could be given without a progestin and may become a useful alternative to estrogen in the management of patients with osteoporosis.

Regimens That Stimulate Bone Formation

Sodium Fluoride*

Sodium fluoride is the only formation-stimulating drug that has been widely tested. In two major adequately controlled clinical trials, fluoride at a dose of 75 mg per day‡ substantially increased bone mass but did not significantly decrease the rate of vertebral fractures. In contrast, studies using a lower dose (50 mg per day‡) in a delayed-release form did indicate a reduction in vertebral fracture rates. However, these early results need to be confirmed, and it is likely that the therapeutic window of fluoride will be small. Further, direct studies of bone from patients treated with a dose of 50 mg per day‡ indicate increased fragility of the fluoride-treated bone. Thus, the future role of sodium fluoride in the treatment of osteoporosis remains unclear at present, and the FDA is currently reviewing the status of sodium fluoride as a possible treatment for osteoporosis.

Parathyroid Hormone and Growth Factors

Several studies suggest that the intermittent use of low doses of parathyroid hormone† may be ana-

bolic for bone. In addition, several growth factors with potential anabolic effects on bone, such as insulin-like growth factors I and II* and transforming growth factor-β,* are available in highly purified or recombinant form. Although theoretically attractive, clinical application of these agents in the treatment of osteoporosis remains highly investigational at this point.

SELECTION OF THERAPY

All patients, regardless of whether the goal is the prevention or the treatment of osteoporosis, should be advised on the nonpharmacologic measures noted previously. Similarly, unless there is a specific contraindication, such as the presence of renal nephrolithiasis, they should be advised on adequate calcium and vitamin D supplementation. In terms of pharmacologic therapy, the mainstay for both prevention and treatment remains estrogen replacement, for both its skeletal and its nonskeletal benefits. This is likely to be the case from medical and overall cost-effectiveness standpoints. For those women who cannot tolerate estrogen or in whom estrogen is contraindicated, and if they are at high risk of fracture or have progressive bone loss, either calcitonin or alendronate is an available option for therapy. Finally, it is likely that the additional therapeutic options are likely to continue to increase in the next several years, particularly in the area of newer bisphosphonates and estrogen analogues.

---

*Orphan drug.

PAGET'S DISEASE OF BONE

method of
WILL G. RYAN, M.D.
Rush–Presbyterian–St. Luke's Medical Center
Chicago, Illinois

Paget's disease of bone is a disorder that usually manifests itself in middle or old age. It is estimated that about 3% of the U.S. population older than 40 years have some evidence of the disease, although likely only about 10% of these individuals will ever become symptomatic as a result.

The skeleton is normally remodeled at a rate of about 10% per year under the control of the osteoclasts and osteoblasts. In Paget's disease in the areas of the skeleton involved, the osteoclasts are excessively numerous and active, resulting in initial excessive lytic activity, followed by compensatory osteoblastic repair resulting in a markedly increased bone turnover rate. This abnormally rapid turnover results in normally lamellar bone's being replaced by embryonic nonlamellar or "woven" bone that is structurally inferior. There is some evidence that this process may be induced by a virus or viruses, but this is not established. The advancing wall of disease activity tends to progress at a rate of about 1 cm per year. As the disease progresses, varied degrees of deformity of long bones or of the other involved bones appear. The extent of disease may range

---

*Not FDA approved for this indication.
†Not yet approved for use in the United States.
‡Exceeds dosage recommended by the manufacturer.

from a single small bone's being detected incidentally on a bone scan to one of virtually every bone in the skeleton being involved and producing marked deformities.

The manifestations of the disease are largely related to its strategic location in the skeleton. Large areas of the pelvis, ilium, or calvaria may be involved and yet produce few or no symptoms. However, if bone adjacent to a hip or knee joint is involved, it tends to cause degenerative disease with attendant mild to marked disability. Basilar skull disease tends to cause mild to marked nerve deafness. Involvement of other cranial nerves occurs but is much less common. Extensive basilar skull disease results in platybasia and if severe may on occasion produce medullary compression or hydrocephalus by mechanical interference with the flow of cerebrospinal fluid. Involvement of facial bones sometimes results in grotesque facial deformity. Long-bone involvement, particularly of the lower extremities, usually results in considerable bowing and easy fracture. Upper extremity involvement may produce deformity and easy fracturability, but usually not significant disability, presumably because of lack of weight bearing. Finally, involvement of one or multiple vertebrae may cause sufficient neural compression (or on occasion a vascular steal syndrome) to result in paraparesis or paraplegia. Patients with extensive disease and with already compromised myocardial function may develop congestive heart failure because of increased blood flow through pagetic bone. Osteogenic sarcoma is the most dreaded complication but fortunately occurs in less than 0.1% of patients with Paget's disease.

DIAGNOSIS

Paget's disease is characterized by having at least five useful objective parameters of the disease process. The serum alkaline phosphatase level, reflecting increased osteoblastic activity, is the most useful of these for routinely assessing activity of the disease. Specific immunochemical methods for measuring bone alkaline phosphatase levels are now available. Specific assays for bone matrix collagen degradation reflecting osteoclastic activity have become available and are known by a variety of names (cross-links, pyridinolines, deoxypyridinolines, N telopeptides [NTx], and so forth) and are useful in diagnosis and monitoring of disease activity as well. Small amounts of disease may be detectable only by bone scan, and it is the only reliable means of assessing the distribution throughout the skeleton. Less expensive (except for total body survey) than bone scanning is radiography of involved areas, and its images are also usually sufficiently characteristic for diagnosis. Computed tomography and magnetic resonance imaging may also be useful on occasion, particularly when occult sarcoma is suspected, but are unnecessary as routine diagnostic methods. Bone biopsy is rarely if ever indicated but may be mandatory when osteosarcoma or other malignant degeneration is suspected. In the initial phases of therapy (with calcitonin or bisphosphonates), obtaining a serum alkaline phosphatase level at about monthly intervals is sufficient to determine the response in most cases.

In later stages of monitoring treatment, the determinations may be extended to 3- to 12-month intervals depending on the response obtained.

TREATMENT

Many patients with Paget's disease have only mild symptoms of bone pain or arthritis and can be treated with simple analgesics or the nonsteroidal anti-inflammatory agents. Before the late 1960s, there were no specific effective antipagetic (antiresorptive) agents; now there are several, which fall into three general classes—calcitonins, bisphosphonates (formerly called diphosphonates), and plicamycin (formerly called mithramycin). It is estimated that 80% of patients are elderly and asymptomatic. If the disease is in a location likely to produce complications at a later time (such as near but not yet involving the acetabulum or cochlea), early antiresorptive therapy is indicated, whereas if the disease involves the wing of the ilium or a small part of the calvaria, such treatment is probably not urgently needed. It is also important, particularly in treating back pain, to determine if the site of the disease is likely to be related to the patient's symptoms. However, with the development of new, more potent and safer agents (the newer bisphosphonates), it is likely that physicians will be treating virtually all patients early to prevent progression or possibly cure the disease before it has a chance to produce significant disability.

Bisphosphonates

Bisphosphonates are compounds structurally related to pyrophosphate but are resistant to destruction by pyrophosphatase. They have a great avidity for the actively metabolizing areas of the skeleton, and it is this type of compound, with radioactive technetium attached, that is used in performing bone scans. Also, because of the markedly increased metabolic activity in the areas involved with Paget's disease, these compounds are highly concentrated in such areas. Although it is not known with certainty, it seems likely that the high concentration in these areas results in the compounds' being ingested by the pagetic osteoclasts, resulting in toxicity to them and thus accounting for the therapeutic effect.

Alendronate

Alendronate (Fosamax) is the most useful approved bisphosphonate for treatment of Paget's disease, although several other similar agents, such as ibandronate and zoledronate, are in various stages of investigation and some will likely be approved shortly (risedronate); tiludronate (Skelid) has now been approved. As these agents are potent inhibitors of normal osteoclast activity as well, they have a major role in the treatment of osteoporosis. Alendronate is used in a dose of 40 mg per day orally, but because of its poor absorption and potential for upper gastrointestinal irritation it must be taken precisely as directed.

The patient takes the drug on an empty stomach 30 to 60 minutes before breakfast, with water only until breakfast, and remains upright for at least 30 minutes after taking the drug. If these precautions are taken, gastrointestinal side effects are minimized. An occasional patient has musculoskeletal pain of unexplained origin. Courses of 40 mg per day are usually given for 6 months, and during that time most patients' levels of serum alkaline phosphatase (and urinary collagen excretion products) normalize. Courses longer than 6 months could be given if necessary because the drug does not cause osteomalacia, but experience is limited. Repeated courses may be given if the serum alkaline phosphatase level increases.

Pamidronate

Intravenous pamidronate (Aredia), a less potent bisphosphonate than alendronate, was initially approved for treatment of hypercalcemia but was subsequently approved for Paget's disease treatment as well. Given orally, it produces too many gastrointestinal side effects. Given intravenously (60 mg* in 250 to 500 mL of D5W) over a 2- to-4-hour period, usually on an outpatient basis, it is an effective suppressor of Paget's disease activity. Although many regimens have been used, the most common one is 60 mg per day* for 3 days, repeated as necessary depending on the serum alkaline phosphatase response. Caution must be taken not to let it infuse too rapidly as it may cause renal damage.

Etidronate

Etidronate (Didronel) has been available in the United States for general therapeutic use in Paget's disease for almost 2 decades. Although etidronate is an effective agent in the treatment of Paget's disease, it has the side effect of inhibiting crystallization of hydroxyapatite, the major mineral component of bone. Thus, if used at a high dose or for prolonged (>6 months per course) periods it tends to cause clinically significant osteomalacia, resulting sometimes in increased bone pain and/or susceptibility to easy fracture. Compounded by the already structurally inferior pagetic bone, this may result in extremely adverse consequences, and I tend to avoid its use in patients with disease in weight-bearing long bones (femur and/or tibia). The usual dose is 400 mg per day orally with nothing but water by mouth for 2 hours before and after taking the drug. Six-month courses may be repeated after a 3- to 6-month interruption, and many patients have been managed in this manner for several years.

The newer therapeutic bisphosphonates are characterized by an increased antiresorptive effect and by lessened or virtual abolishment of the inhibition of crystallization of hydroxyapatite, and unless unexpected consequences occur it is likely that they will replace etidronate for use in Paget's disease.

Calcitonins

Two forms of calcitonins are available in the United States—salmon calcitonin in injectable form and as a nasal spray, although the latter is useful only in treating osteoporosis. At pharmacologic doses the calcitonins have a potent osteoclast inhibitory

activity, and this property makes them effective in the treatment of Paget's disease. They may be the safest agents to use for long-term treatment, although this impression may change as more experience is gained with the newer bisphosphonates. Unfortunately, they tend to be the least effective and the most expensive, they have to be given by subcutaneous injection, and there is often loss of effectiveness over time. A few patients have a sustained response for the duration of therapy. Salmon calcitonin (Calcimar or Miacalcin) is packaged as 2-mL vials containing 200 IU per mL. It should be refrigerated or at least kept cool for the short periods when refrigeration might not be possible. The usual starting dose is 100 IU per day (0.5 mL), but this may later be reduced to as little as 50 IU subcutaneously three times a week. Injection using insulin syringes is a convenient mode of administration. Because a foreign peptide is being injected, it is advisable that the patient have a skin test for possible allergenicity by using the directions in the package insert. Severe anaphylactoid reactions are unusual but do occur sometimes after institution of therapy, although I am not aware of any resulting in death.

Calcitonins have associated side effects, the most troublesome of which is nausea, occurring in up to 10% of patients. This may be minimized by having patients take the dose at bedtime. Flushing also occurs but is not often troublesome enough to discontinue therapy. Local skin reactions are usually minor, and other side effects are infrequent.

Plicamycin

Plicamycin (Mithracin)* is a cytotoxic antibiotic originally used in cancer chemotherapy. Why it particularly has osteoclast toxicity is unknown, but it must have such activity because it is useful in therapy in any form of life-threatening hypercalcemia.

Although plicamycin is a potent agent against Paget's disease (but not officially approved by the Food and Drug Administration for this indication), because of its toxicity, it should be used exclusively in patients who have failed to respond to other therapies or in whom a rapid response is required, such as patients with neural compression syndromes. Also, because of its toxicity (hepatic, renal, platelet), it should be used only by physicians thoroughly familiar with the principles of chemotherapy. It is generally given as 10-day courses infused intravenously at a dosage of 15 to 25 μg per kg of body weight per day with careful daily monitoring. Physicians contemplating its use may receive detailed information from me by calling 312-942-6163 or writing to me.† The drug may also be given as 3- to 4-hour infusions on an outpatient basis.

Another major side effect is nausea; the nausea (sometimes anticipatory) may limit prolonged use,

---

*Exceeds dosage recommended by the manufacturer.

*Not FDA approved for this indication.

†Rush–Presbyterian–St. Luke's Medical Center, 1653 West Congress Parkway, Chicago, IL 60612.

although granisetron (Kytril) is quite useful for its treatment. It can, however, be a valuable therapy when used in patients with appropriately severe problems resistant to other therapies.

General Comments

Obviously, orthopedic or neurosurgical intervention is appropriate in certain situations (e.g., hip replacement), and pagetic bone usually heals well. If there is time, suppression of disease activity with alendronate before surgery is likely of value. I tend to avoid the use of etidronate for several months perioperatively. Unless neural compression syndromes require urgent intervention, a trial of medical therapy is indicated and is often gratifying, particularly in those with extensive vertebral disease. Other investigators have indicated that antiresorptive agents may be useful in therapy for nonunion fractures of pagetic bone, and although I have had no experience with this type of treatment, it seems worthy of consideration.

PARENTERAL NUTRITION IN ADULTS

method of
MARK J. KORUDA, M.D.
University of North Carolina
Chapel Hill, North Carolina

PREOPERATIVE NUTRITIONAL SUPPORT

It has been more than 50 years since H. Studley's landmark study defining the relationship between preoperative weight loss and adverse operative outcome. The mechanisms whereby malnutrition predisposes patients to complications are quite varied. Efforts have been made toward enhancing the perioperative nutritional status of malnourished patients by using total parenteral nutrition (TPN). The presumption is that by improving the nutritional state of the patient, postoperative outcome will improve.

In the past 15 years, numerous reports evaluating the effectiveness of preoperative TPN have been published. These data show that the use of preoperative TPN reduced postoperative complications in only the severely malnourished. In summary, the use of preoperative TPN should be based on an evaluation of nutritional status and an assessment of the degree of malnutrition. If there is no evidence of severe malnutrition (80% of usual body weight or serum albumin levels less than 3.0 grams per dL), there is little compelling evidence to support the routine use of preoperative parenteral nutrition. However, patients who are severely malnourished probably benefit from nutritional supplementation, although the evidence for this remains inconclusive. Table 1 out-

TABLE 1. Indications and Contraindications for Perioperative Total Parenteral Nutrition

Indications
  Short-bowel syndrome
  High-output enterocutaneous fistula
  Prolonged postoperative ileus
  NPO status for more than 1 wk during medical management or preoperative work-up
  Severe malnutrition (80% of usual body weight or serum albumin levels of <3.0 gm/dL)
Relative indications
  Low-output enterocutaneous fistula
  Moderate malnutrition (80–90% of usual body weight or serum albumin level 3.0–3.5 gm/dL)
Contraindications
  Ability to be fed enterally
  Terminal disease with poor prognosis
  Adequate nutritional status

Abbreviation: NPO = nil per os (nothing by mouth).

lines relative indications and contraindications for the use of TPN in surgical patients.

Parenteral Nutrition Access

To avoid phlebitis and thrombosis, it is necessary to infuse hypertonic nutrient solutions into a large-diameter, high-flow vein, typically the superior vena cava and less frequently the inferior vena cava. Access to the superior vena cava for the purpose of intravenous nutrient administration is best accomplished by percutaneous cannulation of the subclavian vein. Alternatively, a cannula may be directed into the superior vena cava via the internal or external jugular vein, but the location of the catheter exit site in the neck makes it more difficult to secure the catheter and cover the exit site with a sterile dressing. Thus, a long-term catheter with the exit site located in the neck is more susceptible to potential contamination and catheter sepsis than is a catheter exiting from the skin of the upper chest.

The introduction of the multilumen catheter, notably the triple-lumen catheter, in the mid-1980s responded to the need in the critical care setting to deliver a variety of medications, blood, blood products, and infusions to patients with limited venous access. The administration of parenteral nutrition through these multiport catheters has challenged the traditional practice mandating TPN delivery through an inviolate line in an effort to reduce catheter-related sepsis.

Consensus in the catheter-related infection literature remains an elusive goal. Catheter care protocols should differentiate between the various purposes for catheterization, such as dialysis, parenteral nutrition, and pressure monitoring. *Parenteral nutrition infusion should be performed through a dedicated, inviolate port.* Although varied clinical circumstances dictate different insertion sites, a higher incidence of catheter infection has been observed with (1) peripheral versus central lines, (2) lower limb versus upper limb catheterization, and (3) internal jugular versus subclavian vein catheterization. Most important, the risks and benefits of ongoing catheterization must be reassessed daily and the catheter promptly removed when no longer indicated.

Nutrient Requirements

In the hospitalized patient, the issue of total nutrient intake, enteral and parenteral, is crucial. Too few calories allow excessive catabolism, whereas too many calories impose added cardiopulmonary stress. In addition, the amounts of carbohydrate, fat, amino acids, and protein required to fulfill nutrient requirements are important.

Five basic steps form the framework of the essentials of nutritional support:

1. Prevent malnutrition.
2. Establish energy goals.
3. Select, establish, and maintain feeding access.
4. Choose and design the optimal formula.
5. Monitor the patient to ensure safe and effective results.

The memory aids KCALS and FACE MTV are useful for remembering the components of these basic steps (Table 2).

Energy Requirements

The number of calories that should be prescribed to hospitalized patients who require nutritional support is controversial. Just as inadequate caloric prescription can be detrimental to the patient, excessive caloric administration can produce serious metabolic complications.

Energy requirements can be predicted with reasonable accuracy in normal patients by the Harris-Benedict equations:

Males: kcal per 24 hours = 66.473 +
13.756 (body weight in kg) +
5.0033 (height in cm)
− 6.755 (age in years)

Females: kcal per 24 hours = 655.0955 +
9.5634 (body weight in kg) +
1.8498 (height in cm)
− 4.6756 (age in years)

These equations calculate the expected *basal* energy expenditure in kilocalories per 24 hours. To obtain the actual energy expenditure, various coefficients must then be added to the basal energy expenditure to account for activity and the level of stress. In early recommendations, it was estimated that injury, sepsis, and burns increased energy requirements by 30, 60, and 100%, respectively. However, recent reviews question this concept of hypermetabolism; injury and sepsis have been found to increase the metabolic rate only 15 to 20% above normal. Whenever possible, it is desirable to measure resting energy expenditure by indirect calorimetry. If indirect

TABLE 2. **KCALS and FACE MTV: Essentials of Nutritional Support**

K: Keep the patient nourished
C: Calculate the energy and protein goals
A: Access
L: List (or think about) the components of the formula and choose amounts best suited for the patient as follows:

F: Fluids: Should fluids be restricted?
A: Amino acids and protein: Are special formulas indicated?
C: Calories: What are the goals and what is the most appropriate mix of carbohydrate and fat calories?
E: Electrolytes: Are there special electrolyte considerations?
M: Miscellaneous: Should heparin, insulin, and so forth be added?
T: Trace elements: Are the standard amounts adequate?
V: Vitamins: Are the standard amounts adequate?

S: Special monitoring to ensure safe and effective nutritional support

calorimetry is unavailable, energy requirements should be satisfactorily met by estimating basal energy expenditure by the Harris-Benedict formula with the use of premorbid body weight and the addition of the appropriate stress factor (Table 3). Even more simply, caloric goals can be approximated by providing a calorie load of approximately 30 kcal per kg per day.

Protein Requirements

Activation of the metabolic response to injury produces a rapid mobilization of body nitrogen, a process called "autocannibalism," with resultant large increases in urinary nitrogen excretion that are proportionate to the degree of metabolic stress. The requirement for protein is dependent on a variety of metabolic factors, such as the patient's premorbid nutritional status, the amount of nonprotein energy provided, the degree of hypercatabolism, renal function, liver function, and the amount of excessive nitrogen losses in urine, stool, and drainage.

TABLE 3. **Stress Factors**

Condition	Stress Factor*
Uncomplicated, semistarvation	0.8
Well nourished, unstressed	1.0
Multiple trauma (acute phase)	
Normotensive	1.1–1.5
Hypotensive	0.8–1.0
Multiple trauma (recovery)	1.0–1.2
Sepsis (acute phase)	
Normotensive	1.2–1.7
Hypotensive	0.5
Sepsis (recovery)	1.0
Burn 20–40% BSA	
Before skin grafting	1.5–2.0
After skin grafting	1.0–1.3

*Multiply the estimated basal energy expenditure by the stress factor to yield an estimated resting energy expenditure.
Abbreviation: BSA = body surface area.

The protein requirement for nitrogen equilibrium in stable adults is 0.8 gram per kg per day. Nitrogen retention increases with increases in either protein or total energy intake. The higher the nitrogen intake, the less dependent is the balance on energy intake. Exogenously administered nitrogen is not very effective in reducing the rate of catabolism. It can, however, increase the rate of protein synthesis and therefore reduce net protein loss. The administration of substantial amounts of amino acid nitrogen must be tempered by the status of hepatic and renal function, which may reduce tolerance to nitrogen loads. Table 4 outlines guidelines for protein administration under a variety of clinical conditions.

Energy Source: Glucose Versus Fat

In general, glucose and lipids are interchangeable as a source of nonprotein calories. Although the cellular uptake of glucose is increased with increasing infusion rates, glucose oxidation plateaus at a maximal infusion rate of 5 to 7 mg per kg per minute (400 to 500 grams per day for a 70-kg patient) in stressed patients. Higher infusion rates stimulate lipogenesis and not glucose oxidation. In addition, fat oxidation persists in trauma patients despite adequate glucose infusion, and in septic patients, a metabolic preference for fat may exist. These factors therefore emphasize the provision of a mixed substrate (glucose and fat) fuel source for critically ill patients.

Fat emulsions are cleared by either lipoprotein lipase activity or the macrophage. If enzyme clearance is reduced, macrophage clearance seems to compensate. Excessive doses of lipid emulsions (2 to 3 grams per kg per day) have been associated with impaired reticuloendothelial function and interference with polymorphonucleocyte and monocyte migration, chemotaxis, and antigen-induced blastogenesis.

If triglyceride clearance is adequate, lipid emulsions are generally a safe and effective caloric and essential fatty acid source. It is generally recommended to provide 25 to 30% of nonprotein calories as fat (<1.0 gram per kg per day), to administer the emulsion continuously in a 24-hour period, and to maintain a triglyceride level of less than 350 mg per dL.

TABLE 4. **Guidelines for Protein Administration**

Condition	Protein (gm/kg/d)*
Renal failure, not undergoing dialysis	0.8
Renal failure, undergoing dialysis	2.0
Renal failure, undergoing peritoneal dialysis	1.2
Malnourished, not metabolically stressed	1.0–1.2
Postoperative, no organ failure	1.2–1.5
Severely catabolic, no renal or organ failure	1.5–2.0

*Based on current dry weight unless patient is >140% of desirable weight, in which case use the mean of actual and desirable weights.

Electrolyte and Vitamin Supplementation

It is difficult to define standard electrolyte requirements for hospitalized patients requiring nutritional support. Factors such as perioperative fluid shifts and drainage from nasogastric tubes, biliary drains, fistulas, and wounds mandate close monitoring of fluid and electrolyte changes and tailoring each patient's requirements accordingly.

Although standard electrolyte mixtures are suitable for most patients receiving parenteral nutrition, it is not uncommon for patients to require a specialized electrolyte prescription. Special considerations of individual electrolytes are as follows.

Sodium. Most TPN patients do well after receiving 30 to 50 mEq of sodium per liter of TPN solution. Ongoing fluid losses from ileostomies, gastric drainage, diarrhea, fistulas, or urine necessitate additional supplementation and careful monitoring. Hepatic, renal, and cardiac failure may be indications for sodium restriction.

Potassium. Supplementation of potassium to patients receiving nutritional support is based, in part, on the amount of carbohydrate calories delivered. Typically, 30 to 40 mEq of potassium is required for every 800 kcal. The coupled glucose-potassium transport system shifts potassium rapidly into cells. A significant fall in serum potassium concentration may result if TPN solutions contain an insufficient amount of this cation.

Chloride and Acetate. As with sodium, 30 to 50 mEq of chloride per TPN liter is sufficient under most circumstances. Amino acid mixtures are typically buffered with significant quantities of acetate to prevent the acidosis that results from arginine and lysine metabolism. Acetate, in addition to that present in amino acid solutions, is commonly added. Careful electrolyte monitoring is especially indicated in patients at risk for metabolic alkalosis as a result of drainage losses, because supplemental acetate in the TPN exacerbates this alkalosis.

Phosphorus. As with potassium supplementation, phosphorus dosing is related to the amount of glucose administered. In general, 15 mmol of phosphorus should be added per 800 glucose calories. Insufficient phosphorus supplementation produces hypophosphatemia, usually between 2 and 4 days after TPN is started. Severe hypophosphatemia (<1.0 mg per dL) should be corrected *before* TPN begins.

Calcium and Magnesium. Although the quantity of calcium necessary for adult patients receiving nutritional support is not established, 5 to 10 mEq per liter of TPN is recommended. Renal wasting of magnesium as a result of diuretics, cisplatin, or amphotericin usage frequently produces hypomagnesemia, which necessitates supplementation.

Trace Elements. It is difficult to assess trace element status clinically, and serum levels are not correlated with other measures of deficiency. The typical prescription of trace elements includes zinc, 5.0 mg; copper, 1.0 mg; manganese, 500 µg; chromium, 10 µg; and selenium, 60 µg. Zinc is the only trace element for which extra supplementation is likely to be needed. Zinc losses in upper gastrointestinal tract fluid reach 17 mg per liter. Therefore, supplementation of additional zinc, up to 25 mg per day, is indicated in patients with large intestinal fluid losses.

Vitamins. Specific vitamin requirements for critically ill patients have not been determined, and the current dosage of intravenous vitamins is based on diverse information. Current recommendations for therapeutic doses of vitamins stipulate that they not exceed 10 times the recommended daily allowance. These guidelines may still be somewhat liberal for fat-soluble vitamins, which are stored in body fat and thus may become toxic at high levels of intake.

METABOLIC MONITORING AND COMPLICATIONS

Periodic nutritional assessment is required to evaluate the adequacy of the nutritional support. Unfortunately, there is no optimal way of evaluating the adequacy of a patient's nutritional support. Body weight changes over ensuing weeks are useful. However, in the day-to-day management of hospitalized patients, short-term changes in body weight reflect more the variations in fluid status than the direct result of nutritional intervention. Changes in the plasma concentration of proteins with short half-lives such as transferrin, retinol-binding protein, and transthyretin (prealbumin) are commonly used to test the adequacy of nutritional intervention. None of these is truly a sensitive or specific indicator of nutritional repletion, inasmuch as each is subject to non-nutritional influences on synthesis and degradation.

Nitrogen balance is considered the most consistent and practical method for estimating the adequacy of nutritional support. A nitrogen balance assessment compares the amount of nitrogen a patient receives (generally 1 gram of nitrogen for every 6.25 grams of protein) with the amount of nitrogen lost (urine, stool, integument, drainage).

A wide variety of metabolic complications may occur during parenteral feeding. These can be minimized by frequent monitoring and appropriate adjustments of nutrients in the infusion. Table 5 summarizes many of the potential metabolic complications that may arise during the administration of TPN.

SPECIAL PROBLEMS AND REQUIREMENTS

High–Branched Chain Amino Acid Solutions

The hormonal response to stress (trauma, burn, sepsis) promotes early, increased proteolysis and hydrolysis of branched chain amino acids (BCAAs) (leucine, isoleucine, valine) in skeletal muscle. This process leads to irreversible combustion of BCAAs, which the skeletal muscle oxidizes for energy, mak-

TABLE 5. **Metabolic Complications of Parenteral Nutrition**

Glucose
Hyperglycemia
Hypoglycemia
Amino acids
Hyperchloremic metabolic acidosis
Azotemia
Hyperammonemia
Fats
Hypertriglyceridemia
Essential fatty acid deficiency
Impaired immune function*
Electrolytes
Hypo-, hypernatremia
Hypo-, hyperkalemia
Hypo-, hypercalcemia
Hypo-, hyperphosphatemia
Hypo-, hypermagnesemia
Miscellaneous
Anemia
Bleeding
Liver-associated enzyme elevations

*Possible complication, not verified.

ing available other amino acids (alanine and glutamine) for gluconeogenesis, enzyme synthesis, wound healing, and immune function. Exogenous administration of BCAAs as part of TPN or special enteral diets has been proposed to compensate for the altered protein metabolism and blood amino acid levels in stressed patients with a resultant reduction in skeletal muscle catabolism and an increase in protein synthesis. Solutions containing 40 to 50% of the BCAAs are now available.

In numerous clinical studies, investigators have examined the effect of BCAA administration to critically ill patients. The results are controversial. Well-done randomized, prospective, and controlled studies have demonstrated that BCAA-enriched formulas improve nitrogen retention, visceral protein status, and glucose homeostasis in moderate to severely stressed patients. There has been no significant demonstrable improvement in morbidity, length of hospital stay, or mortality. Therefore, the use of these products should be restricted to the highly catabolic patient, as documented by markedly negative nitrogen balance, increasing blood urea nitrogen, or intolerance to standard diets.

Acute Renal Failure

Patients with renal failure are unable to excrete the end products of nitrogen metabolism, primarily urea, from the body. Urea is generated from dietary amino acids or protein and from endogenous protein. Urea generation can be modulated in part by nutrient intake: decreasing dietary nitrogen intake decreases urea production, and the provision of calories limits the breakdown of endogenous protein and hence lowers urea generation. In general, the goal in the nutritional management of critically ill patients with renal failure is to optimize energy balance but avoid symptoms of uremia, volume overload, and metabolic complications.

The specialized amino acid formulas for renal failure contain essential amino acids as the nitrogen source. In theory, by supplying only essential amino acids, one can decrease urea production by recycling nitrogen into the synthesis of nonessential amino acids. In clinical trials, these products have not shown clinical superiority over products containing essential and nonessential amino acids. Although survival and improvement in renal function are not enhanced with the use of these products, dialysis requirements may be reduced. Because of the lack of demonstrable clinical efficacy, coupled with the high cost of these formulas, it is recommended that renal failure formulations be used only during the course of *acute* renal failure during attempts to avoid dialysis or decrease dialysis requirements.

Hepatic Failure and Hepatic Encephalopathy

Protein intake must be altered in patients with advanced hepatic failure and impending encephalopathy. In general, amino acids given intravenously are better tolerated than the equivalent quantity of enteral protein. Patients with hepatic failure have elevated blood levels of the aromatic amino acids and low levels of the BCAAs. Possible therapeutic approaches in the nutritional management of these patients are to reduce the quantity of dietary amino acids to 20 to 40 grams per day or to administer special amino acid solutions designed to correct the altered concentrations of blood amino acids. The specialized formulas for hepatic encephalopathy contain high quantities of BCAAs and low quantities of the aromatic amino acids and methionine. The prospective randomized studies evaluating the efficacy of intravenous hepatic formulations in patients with hepatic encephalopathy suggest that these diets have a beneficial effect on the resolution of encephalopathy and nutritional status and perhaps even an improvement in survival. It is recommended that these preparations be restricted to those patients who exhibit hepatic encephalopathy and not be used in those with nonencephalopathic manifestations of liver disease.

Pulmonary Insufficiency

Nutrition is an important consideration for critically ill patients with respiratory insufficiency, because the maintenance of nutritional status is associated with enhanced ability to wean patients from ventilatory support. High-carbohydrate diets, either parenteral or enteral, and overfeeding have been shown to increase carbon dioxide production, oxygen consumption, and ventilatory requirements. Glucose infusion rates greater than the maximal oxidation rate of glucose, 5 to 7 mg per kg per minute, result in glycogen and fat synthesis and rather dramatic increases in carbon dioxide production and respiratory quotient (RQ). In patients with compromised

pulmonary function, these sequelae can precipitate respiratory failure or complicate weaning from mechanical ventilation. The complete oxidation of fat produces less carbon dioxide than does either glucose or protein on a per calorie basis. Replacing carbohydrate calories with fat calories in enteral or parenteral feeding has resulted in reductions in carbon dioxide production, oxygen consumption, and minute ventilation.

The approach to patients with pulmonary compromise should be on an individual basis. Initially, energy requirements should be reassessed to avoid feeding excessive calories by providing maintenance levels or even reducing calories to provide only 80 to 90% of maintenance. Glucose and/or carbohydrate dosing should be adjusted to 4 to 5 grams per kg per day to avoid carbohydrate-driven increases in RQ. For patients receiving TPN, providing 60 to 70% of energy requirements as carbohydrate and 30 to 40% as lipid suffices in most instances. In practice, the increment in carbon dioxide production from an RQ of 0.7 (all fat) to an RQ of 1.0 (all carbohydrate) is only 25% and not likely to be of major consequence in the patient to be weaned from ventilatory support. More important, it is during *overfeeding* when the RQ exceeds 1.0 (net lipogenesis) that substantial increases in carbon dioxide production become clinically important.

Glutamine and Parenteral Nutrition

Glutamine (GLN) is classically considered a nonessential amino acid. It is a constituent of peptides and the precursor for many molecules including purines and pyrimidines, and ultimately DNA and RNA. The latter function of GLN may partly explain the high GLN requirements of rapidly dividing tissues such as lymphocytes, tumor cells, and intestinal epithelial cells.

As a nonessential amino acid, GLN has not been used as a nutritional supplement. It has a short shelf life in aqueous solution and is therefore not a component of standard parenteral nutrition amino acid formulations. When it is not ingested in the diet, the sources of GLN to the host are skeletal muscle and the lungs. These organs release large amounts of GLN into the blood. Under conditions that induce net protein catabolism, such as starvation, trauma, or sepsis, skeletal muscle levels of free GLN fall and remain low for up to 30 days. Studies suggest that endogenous GLN synthesis and storage mechanisms may not be sufficient to meet the needs of the individual during periods of severe metabolic stress. This has led many to consider GLN a "conditionally essential" amino acid.

Animal and clinical studies have attempted to delineate those conditions under which GLN may be an essential amino acid. GLN supplementation to parenteral nutrition has demonstrated improved outcome in animal models of sepsis, tolerance to chemotherapy, and radiation therapy, and adaptation to intestinal resection. In randomized, controlled clinical trials of short-term morbidity in adult allogeneic bone marrow transplant recipients, GLN-supplemented parenteral nutrition has demonstrated some clinical benefit. When coupled with the supplementation of human growth hormone and fiber, GLN enhanced parenteral nutrition and improved intestinal adaptation in patients with TPN-dependent short-bowel syndrome.

Although the importance of GLN in the metabolic response to critical illness has been recognized, the role of GLN supplementation in the nutritional and metabolic management of patients has yet to be realized. Additional clinical supporting studies are necessary before the widespread application of GLN supplementation to parenteral nutrition can be endorsed. Until these confirmational studies are done, GLN-supplemented TPN should be considered only a research tool.

INTRAVENOUS FLUID THERAPY IN INFANTS AND CHILDREN

method of
L. LEIGHTON HILL, M.D.
Baylor College of Medicine
Houston, Texas

It is essential that any physician who cares for infants and children, even in a limited capacity, have some knowledge of fluid and electrolyte therapy in this age group. At the very least the physician should understand maintenance salt and water requirements and be able to recognize and treat dehydration, which is by far the most common fluid and electrolyte disorder seen in infants and young children. The focus of this discussion is therefore maintenance fluid requirements and the management of dehydration. Although the title of this article refers to *intravenous* fluid therapy, the principles discussed as well as many of the details of management apply equally well to oral maintenance and rehydration therapy.

MAINTENANCE WATER AND SALT REQUIREMENTS

Maintenance requirements for water and salt depend on ongoing losses of water and salt from the body.

Water Losses

Insensible Water Losses. Insensible water loss is a means of eliminating from the body the heat produced by metabolism. This loss, which is obligatory, occurs from the lungs (one third) and skin (two thirds) and is essentially water without salt. The metabolic rate is high in infants compared with adults when corrected for body weight. This is because the infant's body weight is made up to a greater extent of organs with a high metabolic rate and high oxygen requirement, such as the brain, lungs, heart, liver, and kidneys. In contrast, the adult's body weight is made up to a greater extent of tissues such as muscle and the skeletal system, which have a lower metabolic rate. Anything that increases the metabolic rate such as elevated body temper-

TABLE 1. Obligatory Renal Water Requirement Related to Solute Load and Ability to Concentrate Urine

Solute Load, SL (mOsm/24 h)*	Maximal Ability to Concentrate, C (mOsm/kg)	V = SL/C†	Obligatory Renal Water (L)
600	1200	600/1200	0.5
600	600	600/600	1.0
600	300	600/300	2.0
600	100	600/100	6.0
300	600	300/600	0.5
300	300	300/300	1.0
300	100	300/100	3.0

*An average diet might yield 600 mOsm of solute to be excreted by the kidney each day.
†V = SL/C, where V = obligatory urine volume in L, SL = 24-h renal solute load, and C = concentration of urine in mOsm/kg.

ature,* elevated environmental temperature, increased activity, and increased pulmonary ventilation (e.g., with metabolic acidosis or primary respiratory alkalosis) increases insensible fluid losses and therefore increases maintenance requirements. On the other hand, greatly reduced physical activity or subnormal body temperature, and so forth, have the opposite effect, that is, to reduce insensible fluid losses. Under normal hospital conditions, insensible water losses average about 45 mL per 100 calories expended.

Sweat Water Losses. Sweat water losses may occur either from increased body temperature or from increased environmental temperature. This amount varies greatly depending on the rate and duration of sweating. These losses can usually be diminished or eliminated under hospital conditions.

Renal Water Losses. The obligatory water loss in urine depends on the solute load (resulting from intake and metabolism) presented to the kidneys for excretion and on the ability of the kidney to concentrate urine (Table 1). The renal solute load includes urea and other nitrogenous substances and electrolytes. Urea, sodium, and chloride, under most circumstances, make up the bulk of the renal solute load. Young infants may not concentrate solutes as well as older infants and children, especially under circumstances of stress, so that their obligatory renal water losses may be greater. An increased renal solute load such as from glucosuria also increases obligatory renal water losses. The usual allowance for urinary water losses is 55 mL per 100 calories metabolized.

Gastrointestinal Water Losses. Although 80 to 90% of stool volume is made up of water, the total loss by this route in the absence of diarrhea is usually quite low (about 10 mL per kg of body weight per day in infants and toddlers and negligible in older children). In children with absorptive-type diarrheas, stool losses may go up to as much as five to six times normal; however, when infants with absorptive-type diarrheas are given nothing by mouth, stool losses quickly drop off in the majority of cases. With secretory diarrheas, stool volume may increase 6 to 20 times or more over normal and losses may continue even though the patient is without oral intake. Vomiting may also contribute to gastrointestinal losses, although in the patient before therapy, vomiting is probably more important in that it cuts off intake.

---

*For each °C elevation in body temperature above normal, a 10% increase in caloric expenditure occurs and therefore a 10% increase in sensible water loss.

Salt Losses

Insensible fluid contains no electrolytes, so there is no sodium or chloride loss from this source. Sweat losses are also quite hypotonic, that is, much more water than salt is lost. Three possible exceptions to this are patients with adrenal insufficiency, those with hypoalbuminemia, and those with cystic fibrosis of the pancreas. Normal stools have a relatively low concentration of electrolytes, with the sodium concentration usually less than 30 mEq per liter of stool water. With absorptive-type diarrhea, the stool sodium concentration is usually in the range of 30 to 60 mEq per liter of stool water. However, with secretory diarrheas stool sodium concentrations greater than 60 mEq per liter are seen and may be as high as 130 to 150 mEq per liter of stool water. Renal salt losses depend on the status of volume of the body fluids and the status of renal function. Under conditions of dehydration or impending dehydration, sodium and chloride are conserved by the kidney so that concentrations are low in the urine even though the urine is concentrated. With upper gastrointestinal losses of fluid such as with nasogastric suction, the fluids do contain considerable electrolyte concentrations and must therefore be considered nearly isotonic or only mildly hypotonic. Concentrations of electrolytes should be measured in the laboratory if the losses from nasogastric suction are large and/or prolonged.

THERAPY TO REPLACE LOSSES

Average Normal Maintenance Requirements

The average normal maintenance requirements are not basal, but rather the requirements under usual hospital conditions. Water requirements are probably best expressed on the basis of body weight as calculated from calories consumed. This is the most physiologic way to express water requirements and is shown in Table 2. Under most circumstances, maintenance fluid is calculated by using the average amounts shown in Table 2 and then adjusted as indicated. Deviations from the average to a lower value (average to −25% of average) may be indicated in the patient with hypothermia, the patient with greatly decreased activity (e.g., the comatose infant), and the patient who is hypoventilating. On the other hand, maintenance fluids may be prescribed on the high side of average (average to 50% above average) in the patient who remains febrile or continues to be in an environment with a high ambient temperature. Higher maintenance estimates may also be indicated in the infant who cannot concentrate urine appropri-

ately, the patient taking diuretics, and, most important, the infant or child who continues to have significant diarrheal water losses even though the oral intake has been temporarily suspended. Maintenance fluid can also be calculated by routinely using the average amounts and then adding in an additional amount for abnormal continuing losses such as diarrheal losses, insensible losses, sweat losses, and so forth. Obviously these two ways of looking at maintenance requirements are essentially the same. Because ongoing losses of water via the kidney, gastrointestinal tract, skin, and lungs continue each day that the patient is hospitalized, it is obvious that maintenance fluids must be provided each 24 hours.

The maintenance requirement for sodium is 2 to 3 mEq per kg per day. Potassium requirements may vary depending on age and size. Infants require 2.0 to 2.5 mEq of potassium per kg per day, whereas the toddler and young child probably require 1 to 2 mEq per kg per day. Adolescents require about 1 mEq of potassium per kg per day and adults, 0.5 to 1.0 mEq per kg per day.

Composition of Maintenance Intravenous Fluids

From the previous discussion it is apparent that more water than salt is lost in the normal ongoing losses (losses are for the most part dilute). Therefore, the maintenance fluids should be dilute. The usual fluid used for maintenance is D5 in 0.15 to 0.3% saline, which would have a sodium and chloride content of between 25 and 50 mEq per liter. Because of the way intravenous fluids are prepared and marketed, D5 in 0.225% saline is a popular choice (39 mEq of sodium and chloride per liter). Potassium is added to the dilute saline solution at a concentration of 15 to 20 mEq per liter.

During the perioperative period and in the patient with moderate to severe continuing emesis, more sodium and chloride should be in the maintenance fluids, so that D5 in 0.45% saline is a better solution to use under these circumstances. The increase in sodium and chloride in the maintenance intravenous fluids in these two clinical situations is because of the associated high antidiuretic hormone output and the possibility of encountering clinically significant hyponatremia.

DEHYDRATION

Factors Producing Dehydration

Dehydration or contraction of the body fluid compartments occurs whenever the loss of water and salt exceeds the intake. If intake increases, dehydration may not occur despite increased losses. Infants and young children frequently have poor intake of fluids or may vomit what they take in. This severely compromises water balance. In fact, because of their high metabolic rate, infants may become dehydrated just from poor intake without increased losses. For exam-

---

TABLE 2. **Maintenance Fluid Requirements Using Body Weight as Calculated from Calories Consumed**

Average
  100 mL/kg for first 10 kg
                plus
  50 mL/kg for next 10 kg
                plus
  20 mL for each kilogram over 20 kg
Range
  From 25% below to +50% above the average
    totals shown

ple, the 10-kg infant with no intake would have ongoing losses of 100 mL per kg per day (see Table 2), which is 10% of the body weight. At the end of 24 hours, the infant would have lost up to 1 liter of fluids (100 mL per kg times 10). Even with compensatory mechanisms being brought into play, the infant would still be moderately to severely dehydrated (8 to 10% dehydration) just from no or little intake. Increased losses of fluids leading to dehydration include diarrhea, increased insensible losses, sweat losses, vomiting, intestinal obstruction, and increased suction of gastrointestinal secretions. Increased renal losses can occur because of a decrease in renal function, diuretic use, diabetes insipidus, diabetes mellitus (osmotic diuresis), and adrenal insufficiency. In the majority of infants and children reaching degrees of dehydration that require intravenous fluid treatment, a combination of increased losses and decreased oral intake is seen.

Types of Dehydration

The type of dehydration seen depends on the relative losses of salt and water from the body as a result of the volume and composition of intake and the volume and composition of ongoing losses during the days immediately before admission.

Isotonic Dehydration (Normonatremic). In isotonic dehydration the losses of water and electrolytes have been proportional and the ratio between solute and water in the body fluids remains normal even though the total amounts of both salt and water are reduced. Because there is no change in the osmolality in the extracellular fluid space, there is little or no osmotic shift of water between body water compartments. The serum sodium concentration is essentially normal (between 132 and 148 mEq per liter). This is the most common type of dehydration and the type with the best prognosis. The cumulative losses come mostly from the extracellular fluid space, so this type of dehydration should be treated fairly rapidly.

Hypotonic Dehydration (Hyponatremic). In hypotonic dehydration the loss of salt exceeds the loss of water over the days leading up to the presentation with dehydration. This again depends on the volume and composition of the intake and the volume and composition of losses in this period. The serum sodium level is less than 132 mEq per liter. Because the tonicity of the extracellular fluids is reduced, there is a shift of fluid from the extracellular fluid space into the intracellular fluid space until equilibration of tonicity is reached. This leads to a marked decrease in the extracellular and blood vascular volume and a higher incidence of peripheral vascular insufficiency then in the other types of dehydration. Fluid is lost not only to the outside of the body, but also from the extracellular fluid space to the intracellular space. These patients must be treated rapidly to reverse the hypovolemia and poor tissue perfusion often seen in this type of dehydration. This type of dehydration is more dangerous than isotonic

dehydration. The causes of hyponatremic dehydration include secretory diarrheas, intake of very-low-sodium–containing fluids such as tap water or rice water, adrenal insufficiency, renal salt wasting, and excess use of diuretics.

Hypertonic Dehydration (Hypernatremic). Hypernatremic dehydration occurs when the volume and composition of intake and the volume and composition of ongoing losses result in a greater loss of water than of solute. The serum osmolality is in excess of 300 mOsm per kg, and the plasma sodium level is greater than 148 mEq per liter. Factors contributing to the development of this type of dehydration include young age; elevated environmental and/or body temperatures; heating systems in dwellings producing an extremely low humidity; intake of high-electrolyte solutions; and, probably most important, markedly reduced oral intake of fluids. With the increase in extracellular tonicity there is movement of water from the intracellular fluid space to the extracellular fluid space until equilibration of tonicity between the two fluid compartments is reached. This movement of fluid gives good support to the extracellular fluid and blood vascular volume but leads to intracellular dehydration. The intracellular dehydration of the brain results in central nervous system (CNS) signs and symptoms such as lethargy, stupor, coma, neuromuscular hypertonicity, and seizures. The shrinkage of the brain may lead to rupture of bridging blood vessels with CNS hemorrhage. This type of dehydration is treated much more slowly than isotonic or hypotonic dehydration to avoid overshoot, that is, going from a dehydrated brain to cerebral edema. There are several reasons for this tendency to overshoot. First, the dehydration of the brain cells has usually occurred during 2, 3, or 4 or more days, bringing into play compensatory mechanisms by the brain cells to defend against a reduction in brain cell volume. This includes the movement of some sodium into the cells, but, more important, the use by the brain of some amino acids such as taurine to serve as idiogenic substances to increase osmotic pressure in the brain cells. Slow rehydration during 2 to 3 days allows the brain cells to reverse the compensatory mechanisms and avoid superimposing edema on the formerly dehydrated brain. The sodium concentration should not be lowered faster than 0.5 mEq per hour. This is the least common type of dehydration but probably has the highest morbidity and mortality rate.

Determination of the Type of Dehydration (Tonicity of Body Fluid)

The history may provide a clue to the type of dehydration, e.g., the volume and composition of the patient's intake, the characteristics of the diarrhea, the prior environmental and body temperatures, and so forth. The physical examination may also suggest one type of dehydration or another. Patients with classic findings of extracellular volume depletion are more likely to have isotonic (normonatremic) or hypotonic (hyponatremic) dehydration, whereas patients with CNS signs and symptoms are more likely to have hypertonic (hypernatremic) dehydration.

The most reliable and widely used determinant is the serum sodium level, which should of course be obtained in any patient sick enough with dehydration to require intravenous fluid therapy. Rarely, a serum osmolality determination is necessary.

Estimation of the Antecedent Deficit

Before the beginning of therapy for dehydration, an estimation of the deficit of body fluids must be made (Table 3). If the patient has had a recent accurate weight determination when hydrated, then a correct deficit can be calculated by the determination of an additional accurate body weight and subtracting the dehydrated weight from the hydrated weight. For example, if the patient was seen the day before while still well hydrated and weighed 10 kg, and then the next day in a dehydrated state weighing 9 kg, the deficit would be 1 liter of fluids (10 − 9 kg = 1 kg or 1 liter) and the patient would be 10% dehydrated based on total body weight (1/10 = 10%). However, in the great majority of instances no recent hydrated weights are available, and unfortunately no laboratory tests are available to tell a physician what the antecedent deficit is. Therefore, the clinician must rely on the physical examination to estimate the deficit of fluids.

A patient with mild dehydration, defined as 4 to 6% body weight loss (4 to 6% dehydration), may have dry skin and slightly dry mucous membranes. The pulse rate may be up slightly, and the patient may be thirsty and have some physiologic reduction in urine output. There is usually no loss of skin turgor or skin elasticity, and if there is, it is minimal. The infant who is moderately dehydrated (7 to 9% dehydration) has all the signs of mild dehydration but more so. The infant usually has a body temperature elevation. The fullness (turgor) of the skin is definitely reduced in moderate dehydration, and similarly the skin elasticity is reduced. Elasticity is checked by pulling up 1 to 2 inches of skin and subcutaneous tissue over the abdomen between the index finger and thumb and then quickly releasing it. If the crease does not disappear instantly, a loss of elasticity has occurred. The fontanels may be mildly depressed and the eyes may appear sunken. Capillary refill time may be slightly prolonged. Capillary refill time is generally tested using the toe- or fin-

gernails. Pressure on the nails squeezes the blood under the nails out. Normally these capillaries should refill in less than 2 seconds. If it takes longer than this for the blood to reappear under the distal end of the nails, it is said that capillary refill time is prolonged.

The child with severe dehydration has lost 10 to 12% of body weight as water. All the signs of mild and moderate dehydration are present but are exaggerated further. Skin turgor and elasticity are poor, and capillary refill time is definitely prolonged. The tongue and mucous membranes are "parched." The depression of the fontanel and retraction of the eyeballs may be marked. Patients with this degree of dehydration may not have had urinary voidings for 12 to 24 hours. Extreme dehydration (13 to 16%) is associated with very poor tissue perfusion and peripheral vascular collapse. CNS signs such as coma may be present. All the signs of severe dehydration are heightened. These infants and children are usually oliguric or anuric, and the prognosis is guarded.

Acidosis of Dehydration

Most cases of dehydration in infants and children are due to diarrheal disease. With significant diarrhea there are rather large losses of bicarbonate in the stools. The loss may be obscured to some extent by the intraluminal lactic acid production by bowel bacteria. The loss of bicarbonate in stools leads to a hyperchloremic (non–anion gap) metabolic acidosis. Diarrhea is the most common cause of this type of metabolic acidosis. In patients with severe to very severe dehydration, i.e., 12% or greater body weight loss, there may be a significant reduction in renal blood flow leading to an impairment in the ability of the kidney to excrete hydrogen ions. In extreme degrees of dehydration, there may also be a reduction in peripheral vascular perfusion resulting in increased tissue lactic acid production. In such circumstances, a mixed hyperchloremic and anion gap type of metabolic acidosis may be seen.

Recommended Laboratory Work

The pediatric patient dehydrated enough to require intravenous fluid therapy should at the minimum have a complete blood count, a routine urinalysis, and determination of levels of blood urea nitrogen, serum creatinine, and electrolytes. A blood pH may be indicated in the patient with severe and extreme dehydration. Material for cultures is obtained as indicated. The electrolyte determinations should be repeated at 4- to 6-hour intervals depending on the severity of the illness until near normalization has occurred. A blood urea nitrogen and creatinine determination should be repeated the next day if initially or subsequently elevated.

Fluid Therapy of Dehydration

The following sections discuss the total volume of fluids required (maintenance plus deficit), the compo-

TABLE 3. **Calculation of Antecedent Deficit**

% Body Weight Loss	Degree of Dehydration	Replacement Range (mL/kg)	Average Replacement (mL/kg)
4–6	Mild	40–60	50
7–9	Moderate	70–90	80
10–12	Severe	100–120	110
13–15	Extreme	130–150	140

sition of the fluids, and their rate of administration. It should be emphasized that this outline of management is not intended to be a cookbook approach, but rather a suggested framework of therapy. Clinical judgment remains paramount, and deviations from the treatment outline are often necessary and are encouraged should the clinical course suggest that a change may be necessary.

Volume of Fluids

The volume of fluids includes the fluids for maintenance to replace the ongoing losses (see Table 2) and the volume of fluids required for deficit replacement (see Table 3). Maintenance fluids must be provided for each day of therapy. The deficit fluids are, of course, only replaced once. Fluid orders are written for each 24-hour period, but with the infant and small child, frequent re-evaluations are made and adjustments in the fluid plan carried out as indicated. The deficit replacement fluids can be calculated from body weights if a recent hydrated weight is available to go with the admission (dehydrated) weight. Most often the deficit is estimated from the physical examination expressing it as percentage of body weight loss (see the section on estimation of the antecedent deficit and Table 3).

Example. A 13-kg child is estimated to be severely dehydrated (10 to 12% dehydration) and to have roughly average ongoing maintenance requirements.

Maintenance (see Table 2):

$$10 \text{ kg} \times 100 \text{ mL/kg} = 1000 \text{ mL}$$
$$3 \text{ kg} \times 50 \text{ mL/kg} = 150 \text{ mL}$$
$$\text{Total maintenance} = 1150 \text{ mL}$$

Deficit (see Table 3):

$$13 \text{ kg} \times 110 \text{ mL/kg} = \text{total deficit} = 1430 \text{ mL}$$

Total fluids:

$$1150 \text{ mL} + 1430 \text{ mL (maintenance + deficit)}$$
$$= 2580 \text{ mL}$$

It should be apparent in this method that the deficit fluids are not given first followed by the maintenance fluids, but rather the maintenance and deficit volumes are added together and are administered as the total fluids (see the next section).

Rate of Administration

The patient who is judged to be in preshock or shock or who is experiencing peripherovascular insufficiency or who has a degree of dehydration in excess of 10% should be treated with an intravenous bolus of normal saline or its equivalent at a dose of 10 to 15 mL per kg. This should be given as fast as the intravenous access will bear and can be repeated at least once if indicated by the severity of the situation.

Isotonic (normonatremic) dehydration and hypotonic (hyponatremic) dehydration are treated rapidly, the isotonic dehydration because the losses are borne entirely by the extracellular fluid space and the patients with hypotonic dehydration because the patient has lost fluid from the extracellular fluid space both to the outside of the body and into the intracellular fluid space. As far as the rate of fluid administration is concerned, isotonic dehydration and hypotonic dehydration are treated the same. The total fluids are calculated by adding the maintenance fluids and the deficit, and one third of this total is given in the first 4 hours, one third in the next 8 hours, and one third in the next 12 hours. The period of rapid replacement is the first 12 hours, when the patient gets two thirds of the total fluids for the day. Any fluid given as a bolus can be subtracted from the total fluids.

Example. Return to the example started in the previous section. We can see that the total fluids (maintenance plus deficit) required by the 13-kg infant with severe dehydration was calculated to be 2580 mL. The serum sodium level of this patient is reported to be 136 mEq per liter. Because this patient's degree of dehydration as judged by the physical examination was thought to be severe (in excess of 10% body weight loss), the patient was given a bolus of 14 mL per kg, or roughly 180 mL.

$$\text{Total fluids calculated } 2580 - 180 \text{ mL (bolus)} =$$
$$2400 \text{ mL still to be given}$$

The rate of administration is calculated as

$$\frac{1}{3} \text{ of total fluids first 4 h} = \frac{1}{3} \text{ of 2400 or 800 mL}$$
$$\div 4 \text{ h} = 200 \text{ mL/h}$$
$$\frac{1}{3} \text{ of total fluids next 8 h} = \frac{1}{3} \text{ of 2400 or 800}$$
$$\text{mL} \div 8 \text{ h} = 100 \text{ mL/h}$$
$$\frac{1}{3} \text{ of total fluids next 12 h} = \frac{1}{3} \text{ of 2400 or 800}$$
$$\text{mL} \div 12 \text{ h} = 67 \text{ mL/h, rounded off to 70 mL/h}$$

The treatment of all patients with dehydration is started as if they have isotonic or hyponatremic dehydration because these types of dehydration account for more than 90% of the total cases of dehydration in infants and children. If it is discovered from the electrolyte determinations that the patient has hypernatremic dehydration (serum sodium level in excess of 148 mEq per L), the treatment program is recalculated and orders rewritten, greatly slowing down the rate of correction. If the hypernatremia is mild to moderate (149 to 165 mEq per liter), then 2 days are used for rehydration: maintenance $\times$ 2 + deficit given evenly in a 48-hour period. If the hypernatremia is severe (>165 mEq per L), then the rehydration is carried out over 3 days: maintenance $\times$ 3 plus the deficit = total fluids given evenly over a 72-hour period. It is absolutely essential that the intracellular fluid space be rehydrated very slowly to avoid overshoot and to avoid cerebral edema replacing brain cell dehydration.

Example. A 6-kg infant is estimated to have 9% dehydration from his physical examination. His maintenance fluid requirements are judged to be average (see Table 2). One hour after intravenous fluid therapy is started, a serum sodium level of 162 mEq per liter is reported. Because almost all patients are initially treated as if they have isotonic or hypotonic dehydration, the infant received 80 mL of fluids in the first hour. This patient has a moderate hypernatremia and therefore is corrected over a 48-hour period.

Fluid requirements for maintenance:

$$100 \text{ mL/kg} \times 6 \text{ kg} = 600 \text{ mL/24 h}$$

Deficit:

$$9\% \text{ dehydration or } 90 \text{ mL/kg } 90 \text{ mL/kg} \times 6 \text{ kg} = 540 - 80 \text{ mL} = 460 \text{ mL}$$

Total fluids:

$$\text{Maintenance} \times 2 \text{ d} = 600 \times 2 = 1200 \text{ mL}$$
$$\text{Deficit} = 460 \text{ mL}$$
$$\text{Total} = 1660 \text{ mL}$$
$$1660 \text{ mL} \div 48 \text{ h} = 35 \text{ mL/h}$$

Composition of Fluids in Different Types of Dehydration

The recommended composition of the intravenous fluids is shown in Table 4. Initial fluids should be isotonic saline or its equivalent and are given during the first hour or two until the laboratory work is reported. Once the serum sodium level is known, the intravenous fluids are changed depending on the type of dehydration. Half-normal saline is the fluid of choice for isotonic dehydration. The maintenance fluids are dilute and the deficit fluids are roughly isotonic. Because the maintenance fluids and deficit fluids are usually of the same order of magnitude in regard to volume, a D5 in half-normal solution of saline (0.45%) provides about what is needed for maintenance and deficit. This fluid is used during

TABLE 4. **Composition of Intravenous Fluids in Different Types of Dehydration**

Starting fluids (first 1–2 h)
  Isotonic saline
Follow-up fluids
  For isotonic dehydration
    D5 in 0.45% saline* (during period of rapid dehydration, first 12 h)
             then
    D5 in 0.225% saline* (for balance of fluids)
  For hypotonic dehydration
    D5 in 0.9% saline* (first 12 h)
             then
    D5 in 0.45% saline* (for balance of fluids)
  For hypertonic dehydration
    D5 in 0.225% saline* (throughout treatment)

*Add 20–30 mEq of NaHCO$_3$ per liter; also add approximately 30 mEq of potassium per liter when patient has voided and it is known that blood potassium levels are not elevated. In hypernatremic dehydration, the physician may want to use 40 mEq of potassium per liter.

the period of rapid rehydration (first 12 hours), and then D5 in one fourth normal saline (0.225% saline) is used for the balance of the fluid administration.

Patients with hypotonic or hyponatremic dehydration require more sodium to raise the serum sodium concentration; therefore, D5 in 0.9% saline solution is used during the period of rapid rehydration (first 12 hours), and then D5 in one half normal saline (0.45% saline) is used for the balance of the fluids required.

In hypernatremic dehydration the fluid used should be D5 in 0.225% saline. It is desirable to have some sodium in the intravenous fluids as an additional measure to avoid the rapid correction of the elevated serum sodium concentration, although this is not as important as using 2 to 3 days to achieve rehydration. Because of the shift of fluids from the intracellular to the extracellular fluid space in hypernatremic dehydration, most of the fluid loss is from the intracellular fluid space. Potassium is the principal intracellular cation, so it is essential to administer adequate amounts of potassium as the intracellular fluid space is rehydrated.

Sodium bicarbonate is added at physiologic amounts (20 to 30 mEq per liter of fluids). This is added so that the patient's kidneys do not have to make new bicarbonate for the fluid that is being replaced into the body pool. It may not be necessary to add bicarbonate if the total carbon dioxide level is greater than 10 mmol per liter and the infant is older than 6 months. In patients with isotonic or hypotonic dehydration, potassium is added as the chloride salt at about 30 mEq per liter of fluids. In infants with hypernatremic dehydration, a higher concentration of potassium is often used, i.e., in the range of 32 to 40 mEq per liter. Potassium is not added until the patient is voiding and it is known that the potassium level is not elevated.

Therapy of the Acidosis of Dehydration

If intravenous fluids are used, the patient will likely receive nothing by mouth for 8 to 24 hours, which will almost invariably cut down on stool losses and therefore bicarbonate losses. In patients with severe to very severe dehydration, peripheral circulation may be diminished and renal function may be impaired, but rapid rehydration should reverse these tendencies and thereby reduce lactic acid production and enhance renal acid excretion. The use of chloride-bicarbonate mixtures provides a more physiologic fluid. This is achieved by the addition of 20 to 30 mEq of sodium bicarbonate to the intravenous saline solutions. Intravenous pushes of bicarbonate are not desirable unless the acidosis is very severe (blood pH <7.00)

Evaluation of the Adequacy of Therapy

Constant re-evaluation of the infant and small child is indicated as rehydration proceeds. Clinical improvement should occur, particularly in regard to the general appearance, skin color, activity, mental status, and vital signs. The patient should be weighed at least daily. Adequate urine output should be achieved within 6 to 8 hours of beginning intravenous therapy. Electrolyte levels and other laboratory studies should be followed and improvement in these studies expected. A failure of clinical response may suggest that the deficit or the maintenance requirements have been underestimated or that the patient may have associated metabolic, renal, adrenal, or pituitary dysfunction or associated diseases such as sepsis or meningitis. Re-evaluation becomes imperative when clinical response to rehydration is less than expected.

Section 8

The Endocrine System

ACROMEGALY

method of
SHLOMO MELMED, M.D.
*Cedars-Sinai Research Institute–UCLA School of
    Medicine*
Los Angeles, California

The anterior pituitary consists of at least five differentiated cell types secreting specific trophic hormones, including growth hormone (GH), prolactin, thyroid-stimulating hormone, luteinizing hormone, follicle-stimulating hormone, and the corticotropin-related pro-opiomelanocortin peptides. Functional hypersecretory pituitary adenomas may develop from any of these cells, giving rise to a pituitary adenoma with peripheral endocrinopathy depending on the tumor cell type. GH-secreting tumors causing acromegaly account for about one third of the functional pituitary adenomas. Gigantism occurs when these tumors occur before epiphyseal closure.

The hypothalamus controls GH secretion by two regulatory hormones: growth hormone–releasing hormone (GHRH), which stimulates GH secretion, and somatostatin, which inhibits GH secretion. GH secreted from the pituitary stimulates peripheral hepatic and extrahepatic synthesis of insulin-like growth factor I (IGF-I), which in turn stimulates bone chondrocytes, skeletal growth, and replication of epithelial cells. GH also has direct anti-insulin actions and affects carbohydrate and fat metabolism. In the treatment of acromegaly, the concern, in addition to suppressing GH levels, is lowering IGF-I levels that contribute to many of the somatic and acral changes seen in acromegaly.

More than 95% of patients with acromegaly harbor pituitary tumors that express either GH alone or GH with prolactin (Table 1). Others have extrapituitary causes of acromegaly as a result of ectopic tumor production of GHRH or, rarely, ectopic GH. Tumors elaborating GHRH include bronchial and abdominal carcinoids and, rarely, tumors of other endocrine organs, including the pancreas and adrenal glands.

TABLE 1. Causes of Acromegaly

Cause	Estimated Relative Frequency (%)
Excess growth hormone secretion by tumor	
Pituitary	95
Abdomen or chest	<1
Excess growth hormone–releasing hormone secretion by tumor	
Carcinoid	5
Other abdominal tumor	<1

DIAGNOSIS

Establishing the Biochemical Diagnosis

Because GH secretion is pulsatile, a high random GH determination may reflect normal physiologic variation. Uncontrolled diabetes, liver disease, and malnutrition may also be associated with elevated GH levels. Therefore, an oral glucose tolerance test is most specific for establishing the diagnosis of acromegaly. In normal subjects, GH levels are suppressed to less than 2 μg per liter within 2 hours of oral glucose ingestion. The diagnosis of acromegaly is therefore established by failure of GH suppression to less than 2 μg per liter after a glucose load (Figure 1). In some patients with acromegaly, GH levels may actually be paradoxically stimulated by glucose. If a newer ultrasensitive chemiluminescence assay is employed, GH levels should drop to less than 1 μg per liter after a glucose load.

Circulating IGF-I and IGF-BP3 (the major carrier protein for IGF-I) levels are a valid and precise reflection of integrated GH secretion. Measuring random IGF-I levels is therefore a precise screen for GH hypersecretion (see Figure 1).

Establishing the Source of Excess GH

Imaging techniques are utilized to anatomically localize the source of GH hypersecretion. Pituitary magnetic resonance imaging is the most sensitive technique for accurately diagnosing the presence of a pituitary adenoma (>2 mm in diameter) as well as its anatomic extent.

Most GH-secreting adenomas are more than 10 mm in diameter and may impinge on adjacent parasellar structures at the time of diagnosis. The presence of a clearly documented pituitary adenoma together with dynamic biochemical evidence for GH hypersecretion thus confirms the diagnosis of acromegaly.

Rarely, extrapituitary imaging reveals an ectopic source of excess GHRH or GH. In such cases, invasive studies may be required to demonstrate an arteriovenous concentration gradient over the tumor; ultimately, tumor excision is required to confirm the diagnosis.

TREATMENT

Besides the physical disfigurement of acromegaly and the local pressure effects of the tumor, the effects of elevated GH and IGF-I levels contribute to a significantly increased morbidity and mortality. Cardiovascular and respiratory disease and malignancies occur with increased prevalence, resulting in a 30% enhanced mortality rate. Highly significant determinants of mortality are now clear from several studies: the level of GH; the presence of hypertension, cardiac disease, or diabetes mellitus; and the duration of the disease (Table 2). Clearly, to reverse the enhanced

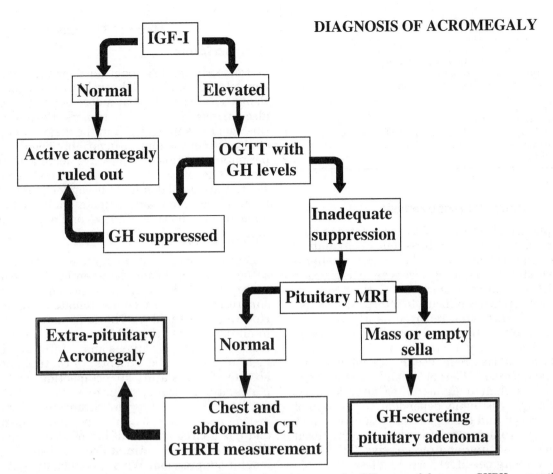

DIAGNOSIS OF ACROMEGALY

Figure 1. Diagnosis of acromegaly. *Abbreviations:* CT = computed tomography; GH = growth hormone; GHRH = growth hormone–releasing hormone; IGF-I = insulin-like growth factor I; MRI = magnetic resonance imaging; OGTT = oral glucose tolerance test. (Adapted from Melmed S: Anterior pituitary. *In* Bone CC [ed]: Current Practice of Medicine, Vol 1. Churchill Livingstone, New York, 1996, pp 2.1–2.12.)

mortality in acromegaly, GH levels should be maximally suppressed. In fact, true normalization of GH levels may actually reduce mortality for patients with acromegaly to that of an age-matched population.

The deleterious systemic effects of hypersomatotropism include diabetes mellitus, hypertension, ischemic heart disease, hypercalcemia, renal dysfunction, arthritis, and nerve entrapments. Increased prevalence of benign and malignant neoplasms, including skin tags, lipomas, colon polyps, and colon carcinoma, further emphasizes the importance of attaining a sustained suppression of GH secretion in these patients.

The criteria to be fulfilled to effectively treat the patient with acromegaly are listed in Table 3. First, unrestrained GH secretion should be abolished, and the tumor mass itself should be ablated or reduced.

The latter is particularly important, because the critical location of the pituitary may lead to local pressure effects of a tumor, including visual field defects, cranial nerve palsies, cavernous sinus invasion, internal hydrocephalus, and invasion of temporal or frontal lobes. Therapy should correct visual or neurologic dysfunction caused by the tumor. Successful treatment should preserve residual pituitary trophic hormone function and prevent development of pituitary failure. Effective therapy should also prevent recurrence of the tumor and hypersecretion of GH. These criteria have, unfortunately, not been fulfilled satisfactorily with available surgical, radiation, or medical modes of management (Table 4).

TABLE 3. **Criteria for Effective Management of Growth Hormone–Secreting Anterior Pituitary Adenomas**

Suppression of autonomous GH secretion
Ablation or reduction of pituitary tumor mass
Correction of visual and neurologic defects
Preservation of pituitary trophic hormone function, especially adrenal, thyroid, and gonadal axes
Prevention of biochemical or local recurrence

TABLE 2. **Determinants of Mortality in Acromegaly**

GH levels	Diabetes mellitus
Hypertension	Symptom duration
Cardiac disease	

TABLE 4. **Acromegaly: Management Options**

Surgical ablation of excess GH or GHRH source
   Trans-sphenoidal pituitary adenomectomy
   Extrapituitary tumor resection
Irradiation of source of excess GH secretion
   Conventional external radiation therapy
   Proton beam
   Gamma knife
Functional suppression of excess GH or GHRH secretion
   Bromocriptine
   Octreotide

Surgical Management

Trans-sphenoidal resection of the somatotroph adenoma invariably results in a brisk fall in circulating GH levels, improvement in well-being, and amelioration of symptoms including excessive perspiration and soft tissue swelling. Unfortunately, the results of most surgical series are difficult to interpret, because criteria for cure are often reported as a percentage fall in GH levels. Alternatively, random GH levels less than 10 or 5 μg per liter, respectively, are reported. These criteria are inadequate to define a true "cure" of the disorder. About 60% of all patients have GH levels less than 5 μg per liter after surgery. Success of surgery is highly dependent on the skill of the neurosurgeon and the expertise of the treatment center. Larger tumors (greater than 5 mm), local invasiveness, and higher preoperative GH levels (higher than 50 μg per liter) portend a less favorable surgical outcome (30% remission rate).

Side effects of surgery include new pituitary failure, diabetes insipidus, cerebrospinal fluid leaks, and meningitis. These complications are seen in 5 to 15% of patients undergoing trans-sphenoidal surgery but are rarely encountered by experienced neurosurgeons. Long-term biochemical and/or clinical recurrence rates are difficult to assess from the literature. It would appear that recurrence rates are low in patients who are initially truly cured as defined by strict biochemical criteria.

Radiation Therapy

Two modes of irradiation of GH-secreting tumors are employed. Conventional external irradiation (4 to 6 cGy) is administered over 6 weeks. GH levels fall slowly, often taking up to 10 years to normalize. The tumor mass invariably shrinks. Unfortunately, about 50% of patients develop some degree of hypopituitarism within 10 years and require replacement of adrenal hormones, thyroid hormone, and/or sex steroids. Furthermore, cranial nerve damage, visual defects, cerebral radionecrosis, and personality disturbances are rare but serious side effects. Proton beam irradiation causes a more rapid reduction in GH levels but is associated with a higher incidence of cranial nerve damage and should be reserved for intrasellar tumors only. The introduction of stereotactic gamma knife surgery will offer another therapeutic option.

Medical Therapy

Bromocriptine

Bromocriptine (Parlodel), a dopamine agonist, effectively normalizes GH levels in about 20% of patients. The drug, given at a dose of up to 20 mg daily, also shrinks about 10% of tumors. Despite failure of this agent to suppress GH in the majority of patients, clinical benefit is almost invariably noted, with most patients reporting a subjective feeling of improvement. Side effects of bromocriptione include transient nausea, abdominal discomfort, and hypotension. Uncommon side effects include Raynaud's phenomenon, nasal stuffiness, and depression.

Octreotide Acetate

Because somatostatin suppresses GH secretion, it seemed a natural candidate peptide for treatment of acromegaly. GH secretion in acromegaly is indeed suppressed by intravenous somatostatin infusions. However, the rapid half-life of somatostatin results in an immediate rebound hypersecretion of GH, precluding the use of native somatostatin for the treatment of acromegalic patients. In contrast, octreotide acetate (Sandostatin) an octapeptide synthetic somatostatin analogue, suppresses elevated GH levels for 8 to 10 hours after subcutaneous injection. The drug is relatively resistant to peripheral degradation and has a circulating half-life of about 2 hours. Unlike native somatostatin, it does not cause significant insulin suppression. When acromegalic patients are treated with a 50-μg single injection of octreotide, 95% exhibit lower GH levels, which in two thirds of patients fall to less than 2 μg per liter. Long-term subcutaneous injection (100 to 300 μg every 8 hours) or continuous subcutaneous infusion of octreotide normalizes GH and IGF-I levels in up to 60% of patients. Octreotide also shrinks pituitary tumors in up to half of patients with acromegaly. These patients experience marked symptomatic improvement. Arthralgias, soft tissue swelling, facial coarsening, paresthesias, and tiredness all improve. The excessive perspiration peculiar to acromegaly is diminished. Most patients report improvement of acromegaly-related headache within minutes of the injection. The cardiac failure and renal disturbances seen in acromegaly are also improved by the medication. Patients resistant to octreotide treatment after surgery or irradiation have benefited from a combined regimen of bromocriptine and octreotide, which appears to have an additive effect in suppressing GH secretion.

Octreotide is a safe and effective treatment for acromegaly (Table 5). The drug suppresses unrestrained GH secretion and may reduce the tumor mass and correct visual and neurologic defects without altering residual pituitary function. Insufficient data are available on long-term recurrence of acromegaly during octreotide treatment. The potential for gallstone development in the long term will require further studies using prophylactic measures to prevent gallstone formation. As a primary agent or an adjuvant to currently available surgical and radio-

TABLE 5. Actions of Octreotide

Long-acting suppression of GH (8–10 h) with no rebound hypersecretion and no residual pituitary damage
Improvement of soft tissue swelling, hyperhidrosis, headaches, menstrual disturbances, paresthesias, glucose intolerance, impotence, hypertension, cardiac failure, and sleep apnea
Optimal dosage for GH suppression and tumor shrinkage: 100–500 μg q 8 h as subcutaneous injection
Maximal effects seen with more frequent injections or continuous subcutaneous infusion

logic therapeutic modalities, octreotide represents a major therapeutic advance.

EFFICACY OF OCTREOTIDE IN EXTRAPITUITARY ACROMEGALY

Ectopic secretion of GHRH by carcinoid tumor may cause acromegaly by stimulating the pituitary to produce excessive amounts of GH. Octreotide simultaneously suppresses both GHRH and GH levels in these patients. The high correlation between suppression of GHRH and GH levels in response to octreotide indicates that the drug acts both on the ectopic GHRH secreted by the carcinoid tumor and on the GH secreted by the pituitary. Octreotide is therefore useful in management of patients with carcinoid and chronic hypersomatotrophism.

SIDE EFFECTS

About 30% of patients receiving octreotide experience abdominal discomfort, loose stools, and transient glucose intolerance. Because the drug attenuates gallbladder motility, asymptomatic cholelithiasis may develop in up to 30% of patients with long-term treatment. The occurrence of echogenic particles appears to be limited to the first 2 years of therapy.

Novel Drugs

Several exciting new therapeutic agents are currently not yet approved for clinical use or are currently in development. Two long-acting somatostatin analogues requiring either every-2-week or once-a-month injection suppress GH for several weeks after a depot injection. GH antagonists, blocking GH action at the level of its peripheral receptor, may also be available in ensuing years.

An Integrated Approach to Management
(Figure 2)

The currently available data indicate that in patients in whom there is no medical contraindication, trans-sphenoidal surgery by a skilled neurosurgeon is the preferred primary treatment. If the adenoma is larger than 5 mm, a preoperative course of octreotide may be helpful in shrinking the tumor mass. Octreotide may be offered as primary therapy for patients who are elderly or who decline surgery for medical or other reasons. Octreotide may also be used for urgent control of symptoms in patients awaiting surgery or with recurrent disease. Residual biochemical or local disease after surgery warrants an initial trial of bromocriptine, which is relatively inexpensive and has few major side effects. Because only about 20% of patients respond to bromocriptine, most patients with clinical or biochemical recurrence require octreotide. Although octreotide requires subcutaneous injection and the drug is relatively costly, compliance by the patient is remarkably high, owing to the symptomatic relief provided. Some patients who fail to respond to octreotide may benefit from a combined regimen of octreotide with bromocriptine. Patients who are resistant to medical management

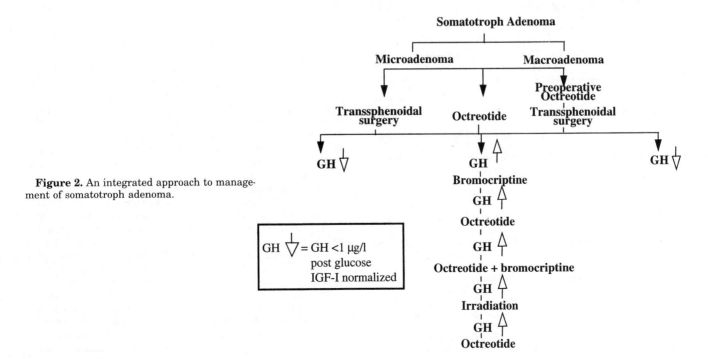

Figure 2. An integrated approach to management of somatotroph adenoma.

should be referred for irradiation. If, however, disease recurrence is associated with extrasellar extension, additional surgery may be warranted.

Long-term Follow-up

Regardless of the treatment mode employed, long-term follow-up is imperative for these patients. After initial treatment, examination of these patients should include pituitary magnetic resonance imaging and measurements of serum GH levels 2 hours after an oral glucose load and of the circulating IGF-I level. Anterior pituitary reserve, including adrenal, gonadal, and thyroid axes, should also be tested. Because reduced quality of life and shorter life expectancy are associated with acromegaly, these patients require several specific medical evaluations and therapies in addition to their neuroendocrine management (Table 6). Physical examination should carefully note new soft tissue growths, including skin tags, lipomas, and nerve entrapments. Gastrointestinal neoplasms, including benign and premalignant polyps and colon carcinoma, occur at a significantly higher frequency, so patients should be offered prospective colonoscopy at the time of diagnosis. More frequent follow-up colonoscopy is indicated for male patients older than 50 years, patients with a family history of colon polyps, and all patients who have more than three skin tags.

Because cardiovascular mortality is so high in acromegaly (approaching 100% within 15 years), extremely aggressive management of hypertension and cardiac failure is indicated. Echocardiography at the time of diagnosis establishes a baseline of cardiac structural and functional status. The treating physician should also be sensitive to the anxiety and depression generated by the patient's self-image perception. Psychologic counseling, reparative maxillofacial surgery, and fertility advice are important therapeutic approaches that should be considered.

Conclusion

It is clear that no single mode of therapy is ideally effective in the therapy of this chronic, debilitating disorder. Thus, an integrated, patient-focused approach is recommended (see Table 6). Development of new and safe long-term neuropeptide preparations will certainly contribute to successful biochemical and clinical management of acromegaly.

ADRENOCORTICAL INSUFFICIENCY

method of
ROBERT J. ANDERSON, M.D.
*Creighton University School of Medicine and
  VAMC
Omaha, Nebraska*

Adrenal insufficiency encompasses endocrine disorders of high morbidity that are fatal if the patient is undiagnosed and untreated. Patients' dramatic responses to treatment underscore the necessity for accurate and timely diagnosis and treatment. Adrenal insufficiency is divided into two categories on the basis of the anatomic location of the deficit in the hypothalamic-pituitary-adrenal axis. Primary adrenal insufficiency refers to the loss of cortisol and mineralocorticoid due to destruction or drug-induced dysfunction of the adrenal gland. Secondary adrenal insufficiency refers to lack of corticotropin (adrenocorticotropic hormone, ACTH) due to pituitary damage or destruction. Hypothalamic etiologies that lead to loss of corticotropin-releasing hormone (CRH) (tertiary insufficiency) are included in the secondary group for convenience, because the differentiation is often difficult and the treatment is the same.

PRIMARY ADRENOCORTICAL INSUFFICIENCY

Etiology

Primary adrenocortical insufficiency (Addison's disease) is an uncommon but urgent clinical problem that has multiple causes (Table 1). The most common cause (approximately 80% of cases) is autoimmune destruction of the adrenal glands. The autoimmune disease can occur as an isolated disorder, or it can be associated with other autoimmune deficiencies in polyglandular failure syndrome type I (primary adrenal insufficiency, hypoparathyroidism, chronic mucocutaneous candidiasis, and pernicious anemia) and polyglandular failure syndrome type II (primary adrenal insufficiency, primary hypothyroidism, type I diabetes mellitus, and vitiligo). The second most common cause is infection (approximately 20% of cases). Within this group, tuberculosis and histoplasmosis are the most frequent. Fungal infections—blastomycosis, cryptococcosis, and coccidioidomycosis—have also been reported as causes. With the resurgence of tuberculosis today, the classic presentation of primary adrenal insufficiency described by Addison in 1855 may be more frequent. The adrenal necrosis commonly seen in patients with acquired immune deficiency syndrome is usually caused by associated oppor-

---

TABLE 6. **Patient-Focused Management of Acromegaly**

Problem	Management
GH hypersecretion and tumor mass	Surgery, medical therapy, or irradiation
Cardiovascular morbidity	Aggressive hypertension and cardiac failure therapy
Diabetes mellitus	Appropriate oral or insulin therapy
Sleep apnea	Sleep studies
	Respiratory therapy
Colon polyps	Colonoscopy and biopsy
Arthritis	Rheumatologic or orthopedic therapy
Side effects of pituitary-directed therapy	Specific endocrine replacement; neuro-ophthalmologic evaluation
Patient's anxiety and self-image	Counseling
	Maxillofacial surgery
	Balanced interpretation of laboratory test results
	Supportive evaluation of management options

TABLE 1. **Causes of Primary Adrenal Insufficiency**

Autoimmune adrenalitis—up to 80% of cases

Infectious—up to 20% of cases
  Tuberculosis
  Histoplasmosis
  Blastomycosis
  Cryptococcosis
  Coccidioidomycosis
  Bacterial
  AIDS-associated opportunistic infections

All other causes
  Bilateral adrenal hemorrhage—postoperatively, trauma, heparin
  Surgical—bilateral adrenalectomy
  Metastatic disease—lung, breast, gastric
  Congenital adrenal hyperplasia
  Adrenoleukodystrophy (X linked)
  Drugs—*decreased cortisol biosynthesis:* mitotane (Lysodren), ketoconazole (Nizoral), aminoglutethimide (Cytadren), metyrapone (Metopirone); *accelerated cortisol metabolic clearance:* rifampin (Rifadin), phenytoin (Dilantin), phenobarbital

Abbreviation: AIDS = acquired immune deficiency syndrome.

tunistic infections, especially cytomegalovirus and tuberculosis. Numerous other causes of primary adrenal insufficiency exist, and each is potentially fatal if unrecognized (see Table 1). Increased awareness and better imaging techniques have led to more frequent reports of bilateral adrenal hemorrhage in patients after abdominal surgery or trauma. Table 1 includes drugs that may lead to partial or complete cortical dysfunction and adrenal insufficiency either by decreasing cortisol biosynthesis (metyrapone, mitotane [Lysodren], aminoglutethimide [Cytadren], ketoconazole [Nizoral]) or by enhancing cortisol catabolism via induction of hepatic microsomal enzymes (rifampin [Rifadin], phenytoin [Dilantin], phenobarbital). Patients taking corticosteroid replacement have increased corticosteroid requirements when treated with rifampin or similar agents.

Clinical Presentation

Acute and chronic courses are the major modes of presentation of adrenal insufficiency. The presentation may be confusing if it is acute primary (e.g., disseminated histoplasmosis or postoperative bilateral adrenal hemorrhage), before the typical features of chronic primary adrenal insufficiency have had time to develop. A patient with a rapid onset of primary adrenal insufficiency is usually ill enough with the underlying disease to present in adrenal crisis. Major manifestations are dehydration, fever, and hypotension, with cardiovascular collapse associated with hyponatremia, hyperkalemia, and hypoglycemia. The patient responds to fluid resuscitation, glucose, and blood pressure maintenance initially but often expires if the cortisol lack is unrecognized. If acute primary adrenal insufficiency is suspected, it should be treated first, and the diagnostic testing completed when the patient's condition is stable.

Chronic primary adrenal insufficiency, the second major mode of presentation, may include more clues to the diagnosis. Such patients decline in health over months, with gradual weakness, fatigue, anorexia, weight loss, and postural hypotension. They develop hyperpigmentation of the skin (described by Addison as "a dingy or smokey appear-ance of various tints or shades of deep amber or chestnut brown"), especially at the palmar creases, extensor surfaces (particularly the knuckles, elbows, and knees), buccal mucosa, recent scars, and sun-exposed areas. Vitiligo that is either stippled or expansive in confluent areas may be present. These findings, together with hyperkalemia, hyponatremia, fasting hypoglycemia, possible hypothyroidism, pernicious anemia, and other deficiencies, assist in the diagnosis. Patients may have difficulty with minor illnesses. They are always at risk for the third major mode of presentation—catastrophic acute adrenal crisis concomitant with the underlying chronic insufficiency—if the stress is severe enough. Vigilance, early diagnosis, and timely treatment are lifesaving for these patients.

SECONDARY ADRENOCORTICAL INSUFFICIENCY

Etiology

Causes of secondary adrenal insufficiency commonly involve hypothalamic-pituitary tumors and accompanying anatomic and therapeutic sequelae (Table 2). Other causes include trauma, infarction, infiltrative and infectious diseases, and autoimmune disease. The most common cause of secondary adrenal insufficiency is iatrogenic—the use and withdrawal of exogenous glucocorticoid preparations. Patients who have received a course of high-dose glucocorticoids for a month or more within the previous year can have variable degrees of suppression and recovery of the hypothalamic-pituitary-adrenal axis. The possibility of secondary adrenal insufficiency must be considered in these individuals.

Clinical Presentation

General malaise, fatigue, weakness, hypotension, and lack of skin hyperpigmentation are suggestive findings. Hyponatremia can occur, and some patients may present with symptomatic hypoglycemia as the main finding. Female patients may have loss of pubic and axillary hair because of the lack of adrenal androgens. Patients may

TABLE 2. **Causes of Secondary Adrenal Insufficiency**

Iatrogenic causes
  Discontinuation of exogenous glucocorticoid treatment or inadequate coverage during stress in patients given long-term or intermittent glucocorticoids by any route
Tumor
  Pituitary adenoma—functioning plus nonfunctioning
  Craniopharyngioma
Isolated ACTH deficiency
Trauma
Infarction or vascular
  Ischemic necrosis
  Sheehan's syndrome (postpartum pituitary necrosis), diabetes mellitus, sickle cell disease
  Pituitary apoplexy—necrosis of tumor
Radiation of pituitary
  Usually gradual and progressive decline in function
Infiltrative and infectious disease
  Sarcoidosis
  Hemochromatosis
  Meningitis
  Tuberculosis
Autoimmune disease
  Lymphocytic hypophysitis
Idiopathic causes

also present with other manifestations of pituitary disease, such as mass effect of the lesion with headache and cranial nerve paralysis. The loss of growth hormone (GH), thyroid-stimulating hormone (TSH), follicle-stimulating hormone, luteinizing hormone, and antidiuretic hormone leads to the accompanying lack of GH effects, hypothyroidism, hypogonadism, and diabetes insipidus, respectively. Hyperfunctioning tumors may produce excess GH, prolactin, TSH, gonadotropins, or their subunits. The combined effects of one or more overproduced hormones may occur with variable pituitary hormone losses due to tumor compression or destruction of normal pituitary cells. Patients given exogenous glucocorticoids may be cushingoid but may present in the interesting situation of having secondary adrenal insufficiency with clinical Cushing's syndrome if the corticosteroid is withheld or withdrawn. Careful review of the patient's history and drug records should help avoid secondary adrenal insufficiency due to the patient's non-compliance or inadvertent omission of corticosteroids in the perioperative period or in the intensive care unit.

DIAGNOSIS

Clinical Features

Typical skin hyperpigmentation and vitiligo help establish the diagnosis of chronic primary adrenocortical insufficiency or acute adrenal crisis if they occur in a patient with underlying chronic primary insufficiency. Because isolated ACTH deficiency is rare, the diagnosis of chronic secondary adrenal insufficiency can be assisted by the finding of accompanying pituitary hormone hypofunction and/or hyperfunction. Skin hyperpigmentation is not present. Diagnosis of acute adrenal crisis, whether due to the rapid onset of primary disease or to decompensated secondary adrenal insufficiency, depends on laboratory results. A careful history is useful to detect exogenous glucocorticoid administration and subsequent interruption of treatment. Exogenous glucocorticoid suppression of the hypothalamic-pituitary-adrenal axis is the most common cause of secondary adrenal insufficiency.

Laboratory Tests

In primary adrenal insufficiency, the simultaneous serum cortisol and ACTH levels are diagnostic. The serum cortisol value is low (usually <10 μg per dL), and the ACTH level is high (>200 pg per mL). If it is possible to draw these values in the acute situation or before treatment is initiated in chronic disease, the diagnosis can be documented. Treatment should not be withheld if the diagnosis is suspected, however. Frequently, further testing with ACTH stimulation is required (see the later discussion). The presence of hyponatremia, hyperkalemia, and hypoglycemia adds to the diagnostic information. The usual findings in secondary hypoadrenalism are a low or "normal" ACTH level (0 to 50 pg per mL) in association with a serum cortisol level of less than 10 μg per dL in the morning or during severe stress. The patient may present in an acute crisis with cardiovascular collapse. A serum cortisol level of less than 20 μg per dL in this situation is highly suggestive of adrenal dysfunction.

To evaluate any patient suspected of having adrenal insufficiency when the ACTH value is not immediately available, a rapid adrenocortical screen with the synthetic α_{1-24}-ACTH (cosyntropin [Cortrosyn]) should be done. A baseline plasma cortisol value is obtained, 250 μg of ACTH is given intravenously, and cortisol levels are drawn at 30 and 60 minutes. A normal response is a cortisol level of at least 18 μg per dL at 30 minutes. Cortisol levels show little or no response in primary adrenal insufficiency. Simultaneous aldosterone levels do not rise to 16 ng per dL at 30 minutes. In secondary adrenal insufficiency, the response of cortisol is usually less than 18 μg per dL at 30 and 60 minutes. A normal response excludes primary, but does not exclude secondary adrenal insufficiency. If the patient has already been treated with glucocorticoids and the clinical picture is not clear, the use of a 1- to 3-day intravenous ACTH infusion documents a rise in cortisol and the presence of adrenal cortical function in secondary adrenal insufficiency. There is no cortisol response or only a minimal response in primary adrenal insufficiency. The metyrapone test or insulin-induced hypoglycemia test may be needed to confirm secondary adrenal insufficiency by demonstrating a lack of cortisol response associated with low ACTH. Both tests entail risks and can precipitate an adrenal crisis. They should be used only with appropriate precautions. Ovine CRH (corticorelin [Acthrel]) will probably play a more prominent role in the evaluation of the pituitary-adrenocortical axis in patients who are not candidates for metyrapone or insulin hypoglycemia testing. The reader is referred to standard endocrinology texts for detailed protocols of these tests.

Computed tomography or magnetic resonance imaging of the adrenals can be helpful in the differential diagnosis of primary adrenal insufficiency. In autoimmune adrenalitis, the glands are small, atrophied, and difficult to visualize, whereas chronic granulomatous adrenal disease and hemorrhage are associated with high-density areas or calcifications. Bilateral enlarged adrenals are present in hemorrhage, metastases, and subacute granulomatous diseases. Magnetic resonance imaging is equally informative in hemorrhage and may be superior in differentiating inflammatory from metastatic disease.

TREATMENT

Acute Adrenal Crisis

The treatment for acute adrenal insufficiency is the same whether it is primary or secondary (Table 3). Hydrocortisone sodium succinate (Solu-Cortef) 100 mg intravenously every 6 hours should be given for the first 24 hours, with full fluid resuscitation with dextrose and normal saline. Mineralocorticoid replacement is not needed because of the adequate mineralocorticoid effect with a glucocorticoid dose of 100 mg per day or greater. The dose of hydrocortisone can be reduced by half each day as the patient improves. Oral treatment can be resumed rapidly once the patient has recovered. An aggressive review is required to define and treat the precipitating event and associated illnesses.

Chronic Primary and Secondary Adrenal Insufficiency

Corticosteroid replacement in both chronic disorders is the same. The major goal in treatment is to restore normalcy by attempting to reproduce the diurnal rhythm of cortisol production with a glucocorticoid preparation. ACTH is not used in secondary insufficiency because it is parenteral and immunogenic, and it is more difficult to mimic the diurnal pattern. I prefer to use cortisone acetate (Cortone)

TABLE 3. **Treatment of Adrenal Insufficiency**

Type of Insufficiency	Treatment	Items to Monitor
Acute		
Primary and secondary	Hydrocortisone sodium succinate (Solu-Cortef) 100 mg IV q 6 h Dextrose 5% in normal saline Treat underlying illness, precipitating event	Blood pressure, electrolytes, glucose
Chronic		
Primary	Cortisone acetate 25 mg PO, AM, 12.5 mg PO, PM or Prednisone 5.0 mg PO, AM, 2.5 mg PO, PM or Hydrocortisone 20 mg PO, AM, 10 mg PO, PM	Sense of well-being, strength, blood pressure, electrolytes Avoid cushingoid changes Skin pigmentation
	and Fludrocortisone 0.05–0.2 mg/d (usual dose 0.1 mg/d)	Blood pressure, electrolytes
Secondary	Same as primary except no fludrocortisone	Same as primary except skin changes do not occur and potassium value is usually normal

25 mg in the morning and 12.5 mg in the late afternoon or prednisone (Deltasone) 5 mg in the morning and 2.5 mg in the late afternoon. Hydrocortisone (Hydrocortone tablets) at a dose of 20 mg in the morning and 10 mg in the late afternoon can also be used. The standard hydrocortisone replacement dose is 12 to 15 mg per m² per day. I avoid longer acting preparations, such as dexamethasone (Decadron, Hexadrol), because of the higher occurrence of exogenous Cushing's syndrome. In primary adrenal insufficiency, the mineralocorticoid preparation fludrocortisone (Florinef) is used at a dose of 0.05 to 0.2 mg per day (usual dose, 0.1 mg per day). Too little fludrocortisone leads to hyperkalemia, hyponatremia, and dehydration. Too much causes upright and supine hypertension and hypokalemia. Rarely, a patient does not require the mineralocorticoid because of an adequate effect from the glucocorticoid or residual adrenal mineralocorticoid production. In most cases of secondary adrenal insufficiency, a mineralocorticoid preparation is not required, because the renin-angiotensin system is intact.

How do we know how much glucocorticoid replacement is enough? Urine free cortisol or serum cortisol measurements are not reliable indicators of adequate cortisol replacement. In primary adrenal insufficiency, progressive increases in the skin hyperpigmentation may serve as an indication of inadequate replacement. The ACTH level is not a good measure of adequate replacement because it may not be suppressed into the normal range in some patients with primary adrenal insufficiency. Likewise, in secondary insufficiency, there are no special laboratory tests for defining the adequacy of replacement. In both primary and secondary adrenal insufficiency, the best approach is to follow the clinical examination and history for a sense of well-being and good appetite and to monitor blood pressure and serum electrolyte

levels. The peripheral tissue response is helpful. Occasionally, patients become cushingoid with the estimated doses and require a smaller twice-per-day dose or a once-per-day dose. In some situations, the afternoon dose has to be given earlier or later in the day to allow the patient to function as normally as possible. In secondary adrenal insufficiency, the corticosteroids may unmask underlying mild diabetes insipidus in some patients.

The patient must understand the need to increase the glucocorticoid dose during sick days. Each patient receives a detailed sheet that lists how to adjust the medicine. The patient should double the dose during the 1 to 3 days of a moderate illness such as the flu with a low-grade fever (temperature ≤ 100°F) and triple the dose if fever (temperature > 100°F) is present. Patients are given 1.0-mL vials with injectable dexamethasone (Decadron Phosphate 4 mg per mL in 1.0-mL vials) to use if they are vomiting and cannot get to medical care quickly. Patients administer the dose intramuscularly (4 mg) and repeat if necessary every 12 hours before arriving at the hospital. They frequently keep one vial at work and one in the car, taking care to renew them as needed. Patients must get medical information bracelets or necklaces that detail their need for cortisol (Medic Alert Foundation International, 2323 Colorado Avenue, Turlock, CA 95382; telephone 1-800-432-5378).

Glucocorticoid Coverage

Glucocorticoid coverage for surgery and stressful procedures is the same for primary and secondary adrenal insufficiency. I give a depot of 100 mg hydrocortisone sodium succinate intramuscularly on call to surgery and then 50 to 100 mg hydrocortisone intravenously every 6 hours (starting in surgery) the first 24 hours. The intramuscular dose is given to ensure a depot in case the intravenous access is interrupted. The dose is decreased by 50% each postoperative day as indicated by patient progress until the oral glucocorticoid (and mineralocorticoid for primary adrenal insufficiency) can be resumed. An intravenous preparation of prednisolone sodium phosphate (Hydeltrasol) can be used if less mineralocorticoid effect is desired. Prednisolone 40 mg intramuscularly is given on call, then 20 to 40 mg intravenously every 8 hours for the first 24 hours. The dose is tapered to 50% of the previous day's dose as tolerated and is given every 8 to 12 hours until oral glucocorticoids can be used.

CUSHING'S SYNDROME

method of
PAUL C. CARPENTER, M.D.
Mayo Clinic and Mayo Foundation
Rochester, Minnesota

Cushing's syndrome is caused by prolonged exposure to excess levels of exogenous or endogenous glucocorticoid hormones. The excess can result from exogenous administration of adrenocorticotropic hormone (ACTH; corticotropin) or glucocorticoids, or from endogenous increased secretion of cortisol, ACTH, or corticotropin-releasing hormone (CRH). Other forms of physiologic and pathophysiologic endogenous hypercortisolism are not termed Cushing's syndrome (Table 1).

ACTH-dependent Cushing's syndrome, which accounts for 85% of endogenous cases, is caused by excessive pituitary ACTH secretion (80% of cases) or by ectopic ACTH or CRH secretion (20%) from nonpituitary neoplasms. The pituitary ACTH-dependent form is designated Cushing's disease. ACTH-independent Cushing's syndrome is caused by benign or malignant adrenocortical neoplasms in most instances. A minority of cases are caused by ACTH-independent micronodular or macronodular adrenocortical disease in which the adrenals contain multiple, autonomous, cortisol-secreting adenomas. The micronodular form may be a familial disease.

Pseudo–Cushing's syndrome is a term often used to describe the physiologic or pathophysiologic hypercortisolism seen in various psychiatric diseases, metabolic disorders, and pregnancy that resolves with the control of the primary condition.

DIAGNOSTIC STRATEGY

It cannot be overly stressed that the appropriate treatment of Cushing's syndrome relies on accurate diagnosis. The majority of cases can be precisely diagnosed by combining clinical and laboratory assessments. However, in some cases of pseudo–Cushing's syndrome and ACTH-dependent Cushing's syndrome, the differential diagnosis is challenging.

All forms of endogenous Cushing's syndrome have in common increased secretion of cortisol. The first step in diagnosis is the establishment of hypercortisolism. The single best laboratory test for this purpose is measurement of the urinary free cortisol level, preferably performed with a chromatograph-purified assay and normalized according to body surface area. Virtually all patients with Cushing's syndrome have increased urinary free cortisol excretion. Measurement of urinary 17-ketogenic steroid or 17-hydroxysteroid excretion, corrected for daily creatinine excretion, is useful but has more false-negative results than measurement of urinary free cortisol. Plasma cortisol determinations have limited precision because of the wide normal range and the pulsatile nature of cortisol production. Sensitivity is heightened by use of the 1-mg overnight dexamethasone suppression test. If results are inconclusive, a CRH stimulation test after dexamethasone suppression may increase precision in differentiating endogenous Cushing's syndrome from pseudo–Cushing's syndrome.

When hypercortisolism has been demonstrated, tests are done to establish the diagnosis and differential diagnosis of Cushing's syndrome. These tests consist of (1) static and dynamic tests to determine the condition of the pituitary-adrenal axis and (2) imaging techniques to find pituitary neoplasms, define adrenal shape and size, and search for ectopic ACTH- or CRH-secreting neoplasms.

A diagnostic algorithm is used to establish the cause of Cushing's syndrome. Some components of biologic diagnostic testing have existed for more than 25 years, including low-dose dexamethasone, high-dose dexamethasone, and metyrapone testing. ACTH concentration identifies subtypes of the ACTH-dependent (ACTH normal or elevated) and ACTH-independent (ACTH undetectable) types. CRH stimulation testing and inferior petrosal venous sampling for ACTH levels have now been added to improve diagnostic precision. Advances in computed tomography and magnetic resonance imaging have improved the ability to detect neoplasms in adrenal and pituitary glands.

TREATMENT
Surgical Therapy

The primary definitive therapy of the various endogenous forms of Cushing's syndrome is currently

TABLE 1. **Causes of Hypercortisolism**

Exogenous glucocorticoid administration (most common cause)
Endogenous causes
  ACTH dependent
    Physiologic
      Major stress
      Severe malnutrition
      Last trimester of pregnancy
      Regular strenuous exercise
    Pathophysiologic
      Psychiatric (CNS mediated)
        Acute and chronic alcoholism
        Panic attacks
        CNS-active drug withdrawal
        Depression, melancholic
        Anorexia nervosa
        Obsessive-compulsive disorder
      Glucocorticoid resistance syndrome
      Severe central obesity
      Cushing's disease
      Ectopic ACTH syndrome
      Ectopic CRH syndrome
  ACTH independent
    Unilateral adrenal disease
      Adenoma
      Carcinoma
    Bilateral adrenal disease
      Primary pigmented nodular disease
      Macronodular hyperplasia

Abbreviations: ACTH = adrenocorticotropic hormone; CNS = central nervous system; CRH = corticotropin-releasing hormone.

surgical. Trans-sphenoidal surgery for removal of pituitary microadenomas by experienced neurosurgeons generally produces a remission in Cushing's disease (>90%) and minimizes the chance of recurrent disease (4 to 8%). Failure to obtain remission generally results from the presence of minuscule or invasive pituitary tumor, or instances of anterior pituitary corticotroph hyperplasia. Postoperative CRH stimulation testing predicts persistent disease. Repeated trans-sphenoidal surgery for persistent or recurrent disease carries a 50% success rate.

Complete extirpation of adrenocortical neoplasms is the preferred therapy for ACTH-independent forms of Cushing's syndrome. Unilateral adrenalectomy cures benign adrenocortical adenomas that cause Cushing's syndrome. The advent of laparoscopic adrenalectomy has offered the advantage of lowered surgical morbidity, avoidance of rib resection, short hospitalizations, and earlier recovery. An anterior abdominal surgical approach should be used when adrenocortical carcinoma is suspected. Unfortunately, many individuals in whom adrenocortical carcinoma is the origin of Cushing's syndrome have distant metastatic spread of disease at the time of the original diagnosis. Bilateral adrenalectomy is used to manage ACTH-independent bilateral nodular adrenocortical hyperplasia. The laparoscopic approach is quite feasible for this procedure as well.

Removal of the neoplastic tissue secreting CRH or ACTH eliminates the ectopic forms of Cushing's syndrome. However, as with adrenocortical malignancy, metastatic spread of the sources of ectopic peptides can make surgical cure untenable.

Radiation Therapy

As primary therapy, conventional x-rays, gamma knife, or proton beams can be used to treat pituitary neoplasms or corticotroph hyperplasia causing Cushing's disease. These modalities produce 40, 60, and 70% success rates, respectively. Remission rates are somewhat higher if radiation therapy is used adjunctively after failed trans-sphenoidal pituitary surgery. Disease remission rates after conventional x-ray therapy are also higher in children. Pituitary irradiation carries significant risk for anterior pituitary hormonal function losses. Adrenocortical malignancies are generally radiation resistant, but there is some success in the palliation of bone pain from metastases. Radiation can be used as augmentative therapy for some forms of ectopic ACTH-producing tumors.

Medical Therapy

Pharmacologic therapy of Cushing's syndrome has had limited use, but in some instances it can become an important component in the management of hypercortisolism. The agents used are of three types: (1) those that modify pituitary ACTH release, (2) those that interfere with the production of adrenocortical hormones, and (3) those that modify the cellular effects of glucocorticoids (cortisol) or mineralocorticoids (aldosterone, deoxycorticosterone).

The various drugs cited here should always be used under the supervision of an experienced physician, because significant toxicity can occur with each. Some of these agents are considered investigational and are therefore used only under established research therapeutic protocols. Many clinicians routinely administer small doses of dexamethasone (0.25 to 0.75 mg per day) when using these drugs to avoid clinical adrenocortical insufficiency if the drug therapy is highly effective.

Table 2 lists some of the drugs that are used in the adjunctive management of Cushing's syndrome. The antiserotonergic properties of cyproheptadine and metergoline appear to be the origin of the effect of these agents. Both have been used in the short-term and long-term management of selected cases of Cushing's disease, but with minimal success; even when such treatment is successful, remissions have generally been incomplete. Cyproheptadine and metergoline have generally not been effective in altering secretion of ACTH from ectopic sources. Bromocriptine (Parlodel),* may lower ACTH production from the pituitary in a few patients with Cushing's disease. It has been suggested that the pituitary neoplasm in these patients is derived from neural elements in the pars intermedia of the pituitary, as opposed to the much more common eosinophilic corticotroph adenomas of the anterior pituitary. This group of patients represents less than 10% of all patients with Cushing's disease, which explains the limited utility of bromocriptine. On an investigational basis, somatostatin and some of the longer acting somatostatin analogues have also been noted to diminish ACTH production in Cushing's disease after repeated subcutaneous administration. These agents are also under investigation for the adjunctive management of ectopic ACTH production.

There is a large experience with drugs that interfere with adrenocortical steroid production and release. Metyrapone, aminoglutethimide (Cytadren), and ketoconazole diminish adrenocortical steroid production by interfering with one or more of the enzymatic steps involved in adrenocortical steroid biosynthesis. Mitotane (o,p'-DDD; Lysodren) is an adrenal cytolytic agent that inhibits adrenal steroid synthesis and destroys normal and neoplastic adrenocortical cells.

The best tolerated of these drugs is ketoconazole, which is currently the most popular one for the management of hypercortisolism, particularly because it is relatively free of side effects. Individual sensitivity to ketoconazole varies widely, necessitating close monitoring of steroid production and dose adjustment. Substantial hepatic toxicity is noted, particularly when high doses are used. This effect is generally reversible when the dosage is lowered or the

---

*This use of bromocriptine is not listed in the manufacturer's official directive.

TABLE 2. **Drugs Used for Medical Therapy of Cushing's Syndrome***

Drug	Daily Dose	Complications and Restrictions
Inhibits Pituitary ACTH Release		
Cyproheptadine (Periactin)†	12–24 mg	Drowsiness, weight gain Very limited efficacy
Inhibits Cortisol Production		
Ketoconazole (Nizoral)†	200–1200 mg‡	Liver toxicity, nausea, oligospermia Incomplete absorption without gastric acid
Mitotane (*o,p'*-DDD) (Lysodren)	2–10 gm	Gastrointestinal disturbances (80%); central nervous system depression, somnolence, dizziness (30%); rash (15%)
Aminoglutethimide (Cytadren)	1–2 gm	Drowsiness (35%); rash (16%); postural hypotension, dizziness (6%); headache (5%); hypothyroidism (5%)
Metyrapone (Metopirone)†	1–4 gm‡	Hypokalemia, virilization, gastrointestinal disturbances
Inhibits Steroid Receptor		
RU 486 (mifepristone)	10–20 mg/kg	Low yield ? Effect overridden by increased ACTH production in Cushing's disease Limited by inability to monitor efficacy, as it does not lower blood or urine cortisol levels

*These drugs should be used only by those experienced with them, and any use must be closely monitored.
†Not FDA approved for this indication.
‡Drug dosages are higher than those conventionally recommended.

drug is discontinued. The starting dose is 200 mg daily.

Large doses of metyrapone can cause gastrointestinal upsets. Its major effect is the inhibition of 11β-hydroxylation in the adrenal cortex. Diminished cortisol production is achieved at the expense of accumulation of 11-deoxy steroids, which include androgenic cortical products, resulting in virilization in women, and excess deoxycorticosterone, resulting in hypertension and hypokalemia. Some patients with Cushing's disease respond to the diminished cortisol levels created by metyrapone with increased ACTH production, resulting in effective override of the competitive enzymatic blockade. This phenomenon is seen less often when ketoconazole, aminoglutethimide, or mitotane is used.

The primary problems with mitotane use are gastrointestinal, manifested as anorexia, nausea, and vomiting. Rashes are common. Symptoms of depression, excessive somnolence, and lightheadedness occur in one third of patients. The drug may affect the zona glomerulosa in the adrenal cortex, leading to mineralocorticoid deficiency that may require replacement with oral fludrocortisone (Florinef), in doses of 50 to 150 μg daily. Mitotane can be used as an adjunct to pituitary irradiation because clinical and biochemical improvement can be delayed for several months and incomplete to even 2 years after radiation therapy. The drug may be used in divided doses ranging from 1 to 4 grams daily to gain more rapid control of the hypercortisolism. The dose is diminished as the effects of pituitary irradiation become more prominent with the passage of time.

Aminoglutethimide also has significant gastrointestinal side effects. For many patients, the most bothersome side effects are significant lethargy and sedation. Aminoglutethimide has the peculiar side effect of causing hypothyroidism in a small number of patients. A maculopapular rash is often seen during the first 2 weeks of therapy, but it generally resolves despite continuation of treatment. Similar problems were observed with the use of trilostane when it was under investigation.

There has been a long search for agents that specifically interfere with the glucocorticoid effect on target cells. The focus has been predominantly on drugs that block the cortisol receptor. Most of those developed in the past had limited success and were abandoned. Currently, mifepristone (RU 486) is being used in some clinical trials of hypercortisolism in children and adults, with limited success. The efficacy of therapy is difficult to monitor, because plasma and urine cortisol levels are not lowered (and may, in fact, rise). Modification of the steroid-receptor complex interactions with the nuclear proteins is another area of research.

Many individuals with severe hypercortisolemia, particularly those with adrenocortical malignancy or ectopic ACTH syndrome, may have substantial hypertension and severe hypokalemia as a result of overproduction of mineralocorticoid in the form of deoxycorticosterone, aldosterone, or even cortisol. Spironolactone (Aldactone) interferes with the renal mineralocorticoid effect, and its use is often necessary and efficacious. In addition, spironolactone is known to partially block androgen receptors, an action that helps to minimize the skin oiliness, acne, and hirsutism that occur in Cushing's syndrome accompanied by androgen excesses. Most individuals require 100 to 200 mg per day to achieve significant benefit, and as much as 400 mg per day in divided doses may be necessary. In severe cases, potassium supplementation may still be used, but the need for it is markedly diminished when spironolactone is used.

All of the preceding agents are used in the various forms of Cushing's syndrome predominantly as adjunctive or temporizing therapy. In some instances, the drugs that diminish steroid production, either by interfering with ACTH or by their direct adrenocortical effect, are used to try to improve the patient's condition before surgery. It should be stressed that delaying definitive surgical intervention carries significant risks, probably greater than those associated with having the patient go to surgery with full-blown Cushing's syndrome. Therefore, preoperative normalization of cortisol levels should not be a major focus. Preoperative normalization of serum potassium level, however, does have significant value.

These adjunctive agents are also used on a short-term basis until in Cushing's disease pituitary irradiation takes effect. In inoperable adrenocortical carcinoma with Cushing's syndrome, mitotane is the only drug shown to have relatively consistent antitumor effects, but even then it does not significantly alter the long-term survival of patients with this malignancy. The use of mitotatane as a single agent for 6 to 12 months in patients who have undergone resection of adrenocortical malignancy, even in those with no apparent residual disease, has not given improved long-term survival; this approach was an attempt to alter the poor long-term prognosis in those patients who initially seemed to be cured. Other chemotheraputic agents (e.g., cisplatin, interleukin-2) may offer therapeutic benefit for inoperable adrenocortical carcinoma. The rare nature of this malignancy restricts chemotherapeutic trials.

In some cases of Cushing's syndrome, combined therapy using adrenolytic agents and steroidogenic enzyme inhibitors may be of benefit, and results of long-term clinical trials are pending. Because metyrapone, mitotane, and aminoglutethimide inhibit different steroidogenic enzymes and have different side effects, combinations using low doses of these drugs may lead to effective therapy with diminished side effects as a result of the low doses.

Therapeutic Goals

The goals of therapy in Cushing's syndrome, similar to the goals in other therapeutic endeavors, are to treat the patient with modalities that involve minimal risk, to obtain complete remission from the hypercortisolism or other steroid excesses, and ideally to allow the patient to lead a medication-free life. Selective trans-sphenoidal adenomectomy for Cushing's syndrome generally yields these results. After pituitary surgery, patients are ACTH deficient, because of the chronic hypercortisolism suppressing normal CRH production and directly inhibiting normal anterior pituitary corticotroph function. These patients require glucocorticoid but not mineralocorticoid replacement.

Intraoperatively and during the first 2 or 3 postoperative days, parenteral glucocorticoid is given at a rate equivalent to 100 mg per m² per day of hydrocortisone or a comparable water-soluble steroid. This agent can be given by continuous intravenous infusion or by intramuscular injection every 12 hours. My colleagues and I routinely use methylprednisolone perioperatively, giving 40 mg parenterally every 12 hours on the day of surgery. We then taper the dosage rapidly over 2 or 3 days by halving the dose daily and then starting oral replacement with hydrocortisone or cortisone (12 to 15 mg per m² per day) or oral prednisone (5 mg per m² per day) in divided doses. This regimen is maintained for 1 month, and then tapering begins. The dose can be diminished by discontinuing the lower evening doses of glucocorticoid replacement for 1 or 2 months and then tapering the morning doses, or the daily doses can be doubled but given on an every-other-day basis for 1 or 2 months.

Recovery of the pituitary-adrenal axis can be monitored by measuring the morning plasma cortisol level before administering morning steroid doses or by monitoring the response to a short ACTH stimulation test (cosyntropin [Cortrosyn], 250 μg intramuscularly, with cortisol measurements at 0 and 30 minutes). If the response to stimulation is normal (absolute values above 18 μg per dL), replacement steroid therapy can be discontinued. If suboptimal plasma levels are noted or there is insufficient ACTH stimulation, steroid therapy can be continued for another 1 or 2 months, and testing repeated. In our experience, the majority of patients are able to stop glucocorticoid replacement therapy in 3 or 4 months, but some require therapy for as long as 1 year. During recovery time, illnesses that cause stress should be treated by doubling the daily dose of glucocorticoid, and severe stresses, such as major trauma, substantial body burns, or surgery with general anesthesia, should be supported with parenteral steroid injections at 4 to 10 times the daily replacement levels. After extirpation of unilateral benign, cortisol-secreting adenomas, a similar tapering glucocorticoid schedule and testing can be used.

In cases of ectopic ACTH or CRH production causing Cushing's syndrome, complete surgical extirpation of the neoplasm is the preferred therapy. If the tumor is completely removed, the patient generally undergoes prompt remission of Cushing's syndrome or returns to good health. Again, glucocorticoid replacement therapy on a tapering schedule is necessary for several weeks to months after curative surgical therapy. Replacement mineralocorticoid therapy is not necessary.

When faced with the problem of an incompletely resectable tumor, the physician must choose from among a variety of adjunctive therapies. Pharmacologic therapy, as noted earlier, can be used to control hypercortisolism, mineralocorticoid excess, or androgen excess. Embolization of residual tumor, particularly hepatic metastases, has also been used to diminish ectopic peptide production. Intraoperative focal radiation therapy and direct organ infusion chemotherapy are other options for some neoplasms.

When laboratory evaluation indicates the diagnosis of ectopic ACTH syndrome and no tumor is found with imaging or localization techniques, the patient is periodically re-evaluated, with attempts to find the source of the occult tumor. If cortisol overproduction causes significant Cushing's syndrome, bilateral adrenalectomy can be considered. Adrenalectomy is also warranted when long-term survival is anticipated in unresectable malignancies causing ectopic ACTH syndrome. This is again an optimal occasion to consider laparoscopic adrenalectomy because of the minimal morbidity involved for these chronically ill patients.

DIABETES INSIPIDUS

method of
ARNOLD M. MOSES, M.D.
SUNY Health Science Center
Syracuse, New York

GENERAL PRINCIPLES OF TREATING DIABETES INSIPIDUS

The hormonal treatment of diabetes insipidus is accomplished by use of synthetic peptides (arginine vasopressin [AVP], desmopressin, and, rarely, lypressin). AVP is the natural hormone of humans. Desmopressin (DDAVP) is a synthetic analogue of AVP that does not constrict smooth muscle and has a longer antidiuretic action than the natural hormone. Because of its lack of vasoactivity, desmopressin can be used without fear of precipitating angina or of causing abdominal cramps or headaches. It can also be used to treat diabetes insipidus during pregnancy, because it resists inactivation by placental vasopressinase. The available preparations of vasopressin and the antidiuretic responses are listed in Tables 1 and 2.

For most patients with diabetes insipidus, the treatment of choice is intranasal administration of desmopressin (100 µg per mL). Two delivery systems are available: a nasal (rhinal) tube, which the patient uses to blow measured amounts (0.05 to 0.2 mL) into the nose, and a compression pump system, which delivers 0.1 mL. Table 2 shows the duration of action of the nasal preparation in the adult when 10-, 15-, and 20-µg doses of the drug (0.1 to 0.2 mL) are instilled.

Treatment of the adult is usually initiated with 10 µg of nasal desmopressin, and patients are instructed to repeat this dose when they note the reappearance of polyuria. Some patients do better if instructed to take the hormone on a more defined schedule. The dose administered can be increased or decreased in accordance with the patient's response. Patients should be told to drink only when thirsty.

Some patients prefer to start therapy with the oral form of desmopressin, and others may be switched to the oral preparation when absorption of the nasal form of desmopressin is decreased in the presence of upper respiratory infection or nasal congestion or blockage. The starting dose of the tablet is usually 0.05 mg (half of a 0.1-mg tablet) twice a day. The maintenance dose is gradually adjusted to provide an adequate rhythm of water turnover, which may range from 0.1 to 1.2 mg divided two or three times daily. Now that the nasal spray and oral forms of desmopressin have become available, I do not recommend the use of lypressin nasal spray or of nonhormonal oral agents such as chlorpropamide, clofibrate, or carbamazepine.

In the uncooperative or unconscious patient with diabetes insipidus, desmopressin should be given by subcutaneous or intravenous injection, usually starting with 1 µg. The duration of action in adults given various forms and amounts of desmopressin is noted in Table 2. The major clinical effect of raising the dose is to increase the duration of antidiuresis (the increase in urinary concentration between low-dose and high-dose therapy is less important). The main use of subcutaneous AVP is in the initial management of patients with acute onset of diabetes insip-

TABLE 1. **Vasopressin Preparations Available to Treat Diabetes Insipidus**

Trade Name	Chemical Composition	Concentration	Size	Pharmaceutical Company
Intranasal Preparations				
Desmopressin Rhinal Tube	Desmopressin acetate	100 µg/mL	2.5-mL bottle	Ferring
DDAVP Rhinal Tube	Desmopressin acetate	100 µg/mL	2.5-mL bottle	Rhône-Poulenc Rorer
DDAVP Nasal Spray (Spray Pump)	Desmopressin acetate	100 µg/mL	5.0-mL bottle	Rhône-Poulenc Rorer
Diapid Nasal Spray (Squeeze Bottle)	Lypressin (lysine vasopressin)	50 USP U (185 µg)/mL	8.0-mL bottle	Sandoz

Caution: Stimate (desmopressin acetate) is marketed by Armour Pharmaceutical Co. in a 2.5-mL nasal spray bottle. It is designed for treating bleeding disorders and contains 1.5 mg/mL desmopressin. Stimate can be confused easily with the less concentrated preparations of desmopressin acetate that are used for treating diabetes insipidus.

Oral Preparation				
DDAVP Tablets	Desmopressin acetate	—	0.1-mg, 0.2-mg tablets	Rhône-Poulenc Rorer
Injectable (SC, IV) Preparations				
Pitressin	Arginine vasopressin	20 USP U (50 µg)/mL	0.5-mL, 1.0-mL ampules	Parke-Davis
DDAVP Injection	Desmopressin acetate	4 µg/mL	1.0-mL, 10.0-mL vials	Rhône-Poulenc Rorer

TABLE 2. **Mean Time That Urine Remains Hypertonic After Administration of Vasopressin to Adults with Diabetes Insipidus***

Chemical Composition	Route of Administration	Amount Administered	Mean Duration of Action (h)
Desmopressin acetate	Intranasal	10 μg (0.1 mL)	12
Desmopressin acetate	Intranasal	15 μg (0.15 mL)	16
Desmopressin acetate	Intranasal	20 μg (0.2 mL)	20
Lypressin	Intranasal	2 sprays in each nostril (about 10 U)	6
Desmopressin acetate	Subcutaneous, intravenous	0.5 μg	10
Desmopressin acetate	Subcutaneous, intravenous	1.0 μg	14
Desmopressin acetate	Subcutaneous, intravenous	2.0 μg	18
Desmopressin acetate	Subcutaneous, intravenous	4.0 μg	22
Arginine vasopressin	Subcutaneous	12.5 μg (5 U)	4
Desmopressin acetate	Oral	0.1 mg	6–8
Desmopressin acetate	Oral	0.2 mg	8–12
Desmopressin acetate	Oral	0.4 mg	16–20

*Note: Onset of the antidiuretic action of the subcutaneous and intravenous preparation is 30–45 min. Onset of antidiuretic effect with tablets is about 60 min.

idus after head trauma or neurosurgical procedures. Its short duration of action allows prompt recognition of the recovery of neurohypophysial function and helps prevent the development of water intoxication in patients receiving intravenous fluids. As with desmopressin, it is safest to administer subsequent doses of subcutaneous AVP when polyuria reappears.

As long as untreated patients with diabetes insipidus are conscious, retain normal thirst, and have enough fluid to drink, they seldom allow themselves to become more than mildly dehydrated. However, severe dehydration with extremely high serum sodium concentrations may occur acutely when patients with untreated diabetes insipidus cannot or do not drink adequate fluids and intravenous fluids are inadequate.

The most common and clinically most important problem in the hospitalized patient with diabetes insipidus is iatrogenic hyponatremia. Particularly when it occurs rapidly, hyponatremia may cause neurologic problems (see later). Hyponatremia in this setting is caused by overhydration (rarely, sodium loss may contribute) in patients being treated with vasopressin. The overhydration is almost always due to excessive amounts of intravenous fluids and can be avoided by allowing patients to self-regulate their oral intake of fluids whenever possible. When such self-regulation is not feasible because a patient is obtunded, has a defective thirst mechanism, or cannot swallow fluids, extreme care must be taken in ordering the intravenous fluids to prevent hyponatremia. The patient should be kept in an antidiuretic state with desmopressin, 0.5 to 1.0 μg every 12 hours subcutaneously or when the urine becomes dilute. The intravenous fluid should consist largely of 5% dextrose in water with amounts of normal saline gauged to replace daily urinary sodium losses. The amount of intravenous fluid for every 8-hour period should replace 8-hour urine volumes plus estimated 8-hour insensible losses and fluid losses by way of perspiration and other routes. The amount of intravenous fluid should be adjusted according to plasma sodium, blood urea nitrogen, and creatinine levels. If hypernatremia occurs, the amount of intravenous fluid should be increased accordingly.

If a major decrease in serum sodium concentration occurs, intravenous fluids should be temporarily discontinued, and if necessitated by clinical manifestations, the patient should be given 200 to 300 mL of 3% saline, perhaps along with 40 mg of furosemide (Lasix) intravenously. Temporary discontinuation of desmopressin should also be considered. To emphasize, the patient with central diabetes insipidus whose fluid intake is maintained intravenously presents a major medical problem and must be followed up carefully to maintain normonatremia.

PRINCIPLES OF TREATING SPECIFIC PROBLEMS

The Alert Patient with Intact Thirst

When antidiuretic therapy is initiated in the alert patient with diabetes insipidus, the patient must consciously avoid excessive drinking for at least several days. By that time, the thirst mechanism usually adapts to the consequences of the more normal urine volume. However, some patients with diabetes insipidus must be reminded constantly to avoid excessive drinking, which results in water intoxication with a disorder much like the syndrome of inappropriate antidiuretic hormone. Thirst may be perceived with normal or low plasma sodium concentrations because of a dry mouth such as might occur with mouth breathing, anticholinergic drugs, beta-adrenergic blockers, or cigarette smoking. An occasional patient is hyperdipsic because of increased circulating angiotensin II levels or from hypothalamic involvement such as may occur with sarcoidosis involving the hypothalamus. In some patients, education about water intake must constantly be reinforced to prevent hyponatremia from drinking fluids such as beer when they are not thirsty.

The Alert Patient with Adipsia

The alert patient with adipsia presents a difficult management problem in the hospital and particularly after being discharged from the hospital. Because of the loss of thirst perception, normal serum sodium concentration is maintained only with the greatest difficulty. The patient and family must closely and continuously monitor the patient's intake and output of fluids, body weight, and vital signs. Plasma sodium concentration and blood urea nitrogen, uric acid, and creatinine levels should be checked often. Such a patient must always relate fluid intake to volume of urine plus fluid losses in perspiration and via the gastrointestinal tract. The patient may fail to experience thirst despite the development of hypovolemic shock with extremely high serum sodium concentrations.

The Confused, Obtunded, or Unconscious Patient

When confused, obtunded, or unconscious, such as postoperatively or after head trauma, the patient with diabetes insipidus is monitored in the same way as previously described for the alert patient with adipsia. Urine should be measured frequently for volume and osmolality monitoring, and fluid losses should be replaced with intravenous fluids to match urinary losses plus insensible (and other) fluid losses. The patient's serum sodium concentration should be monitored at least daily, along with body weight, vital signs, and renal function studies. These measurements provide worthwhile supportive information. In the presence of hypernatremia, normal saline is required only to help restore pulse and blood pressure to normal in hypovolemic patients. Otherwise, patients with hypernatremia should be treated with dextrose in water (see later) while appropriate antidiuretic therapy is instituted and maintained.

Postoperative hypernatremia should be prevented by the early recognition of diabetes insipidus before and during, as well as after, surgery and by avoidance of the use of osmotic diuretics during surgery. The patient should be changed to oral fluids as soon as possible, and the adequacy of the patient's thirst mechanism to control fluid intake appropriately should be evaluated. Diabetes insipidus that occurs postoperatively or after head trauma may be variable (biphasic or triphasic), and frequently, the diabetes insipidus is transient. Therefore, hormonal treatment should be withheld periodically to determine whether the diabetes insipidus recurs. Symptoms may be ameliorated for up to 6 months and even longer.

SPECIAL PROBLEMS OF FLUID BALANCE

The Hypernatremic Patient

Hypernatremia in patients with diabetes insipidus is usually associated with normal total body sodium.

The hypernatremia is due to loss of free water by way of the kidneys, but losses from the skin and lungs can aggravate the problem. When hypernatremia is severe, there may be clinical evidence of dehydration, including dry skin and mucous membranes, along with postural hypotension and/or tachycardia. Infants with acute hypernatremia commonly have a depressed sensorium, fever, and labored respiration. Grand mal seizures and coma are common. The symptoms in adults with hypernatremia are often masked by other associated medical conditions. They may not perceive thirst because of depressed sensorium or because of specific thirst center abnormalities. Lethargy, stupor, coma, and convulsions may be present to varying degrees. Neurologic sequelae, particularly in children, are not uncommon. The cause of the neurologic changes includes the shrinkage of brain cells, tearing of cerebral vessels, and intracranial bleeding. Alterations in the composition of water and solutes in brain cells may contribute to the symptoms of hypernatremia. An abrupt increase in plasma sodium concentration causes more severe symptoms than a gradual rise to the same level of sodium.

The goal of treating hypernatremia in patients with diabetes insipidus is the restoration of normal plasma volume and tonicity. Desmopressin should be injected to maintain a concentrated urine. If there are circulatory disturbances due to hypovolemia, isotonic saline should be given until systemic hemodynamics are stabilized. In fact, isotonic saline is relatively hypotonic to plasma in patients with severe hypernatremia and simultaneously corrects both volume and water deficits. After volume deficits are corrected, the hypernatremia should be treated intravenously with 5% dextrose in water. Water can be given by mouth if the patient is conscious and able to drink.

The water deficit in these patients can be calculated on the basis of the serum sodium concentration and on the assumption that 60% of body weight is water. For example, if the patient's usual weight is 75 kg, total body water would normally be 75 kg × 0.6 = 45 liters. If the serum sodium value is 154 mEq per liter, the patient has a 10% deficit of water—(154 − 140) ÷ 140—and requires 4.5 liters of water to correct the deficit. Obviously, continuing losses of water must also be replaced. Despite inaccuracies, including the assumption that body water is always 60% of the body weight and the postulate that water is lost uniformly throughout all body cells, this approach provides an approximate value that can be used in planning therapy. The major problem is to determine the appropriate rate at which to lower serum sodium concentration to normal, although there are few hard data on how rapidly serum sodium concentration can be lowered safely in patients with hypernatremia. Because seizures or even fatal cerebral edema may occur when serum sodium concentration is lowered rapidly, the best estimate is that hypernatremia should be corrected over 48 to 72 hours and at a rate not to exceed 0.5 to 2.0 mEq per liter per hour. As total body water expands, the serum sodium concentration may fall proportionately. Serum electrolyte values should be monitored frequently to ensure an appropriate response.

Treatment of the hypernatremia due to water loss such as occurs in untreated patients with diabetes insipidus must also address associated electrolyte abnormalities and underlying medical and surgical conditions. A special example of this would be the patient with diabetes insipidus who has coexisting hyperglycemia. When marked hyperglycemia exists, the "corrected" serum sodium value should be used to calculate the water deficit. Slightly low or normal serum sodium concentrations in the presence of high serum glucose concentrations often result, when corrected, in hypernatremic values. The corrected serum sodium concentrations can be calculated by increasing the serum sodium concentration by 1.5 mEq per liter for every 100 mg per dL increment in the serum glucose concentration above 100 mg per dL. For example, in a patient with a sodium level of 138 mEq per liter and a glucose level of 700 mg per dL the corrected serum sodium would be 138 + (1.5 × 6), or 147 mEq per liter.

The Hyponatremic Patient

Hyponatremia in patients with diabetes insipidus occurs almost exclusively in patients who are overhydrated orally or parenterally while they are being treated with desmopressin. The severity of hyponatremia closely correlates with the extent of water overload. The magnitude of the excessive body water can be calculated by use of the same approach as described for hypernatremia. Occasionally, hyponatremia is aggravated by large amounts of sodium in the urine, probably related to increased levels of atrial natriuretic peptide, inhibition of aldosterone, and an increased glomerular filtration rate. Random measurements of urine sodium concentrations should be obtained to determine whether they are in the usual range (20 to 40 mEq per liter), high (about 100 mEq per liter), or extremely high (about 180 mEq per liter). The hyponatremia due to natriuresis in the water-overloaded patient can be corrected only partially with saline infusions, because the natriuresis continues until the hypervolemic state is corrected. Hyponatremia can be caused or aggravated by thyroid or adrenal insufficiency.

The symptoms of hyponatremia depend on the acuteness and degree of the condition. Neurologic manifestations of acute water intoxication are usually not observed until the plasma sodium concentration has fallen to less than 125 mEq per liter. They include nausea, emesis, muscular twitching, grand mal seizures, and coma. Acute water intoxication, which causes plasma sodium concentration to fall below 125 mEq per liter in less than 24 hours, carries substantial morbidity and mortality rates. When plasma sodium is lowered slowly to the same level, patients are usually less symptomatic.

There is a large body of literature on the appropriate rate at which to correct hyponatremia. Rapidly occurring (acute) and marked hyponatremia can be lethal and should be treated urgently. Under these conditions, and when neurologic symptoms are severe, initial therapy should raise the serum sodium concentration by 1 to 2 mEq per liter per hour regardless of the duration of the electrolyte abnormality. Most authorities agree that the rate of change in serum sodium concentrations should not exceed 12 to 20 mEq per liter per day. However, in patients with chronic hyponatremia, correction of serum sodium approximating this rate can occasionally cause serious, even fatal, complications by inducing the central pontine myelinolysis syndrome.

In the treatment of the asymptomatic mildly hyponatremic patient, fluid restriction is adequate. Urine should be analyzed every 4 to 8 hours for volume and osmolality, and fluid replacement should be ordered in relation to *urine volume*. Remember also that insensible fluid losses of about 600 mL of free water per day occur in the usual adult. *It is inappropriate to write for a fixed amount of fluid replacement.* Plasma sodium concentration should be checked frequently, and fluid replacement adjusted accordingly. The complaint of thirst by a water-restricted patient should never be ignored. Long-term management is usually less disrupted by adjusting fluid intake than by discontinuing hormonal therapy and allowing the patient to "break through." In severe situations, however, interruption of hormonal therapy may be justified with close monitoring. Alternatively, when the patient has symptomatic or severe hyponatremia (serum sodium value less than 115 mEq per liter in chronic hyponatremia or 125 mEq per liter in acute hyponatremia), the patient should be treated with intravenous furosemide and hypertonic saline (even in the presence of vasopressin, furosemide causes the excretion of urine that is slightly hypotonic or isotonic). After the injection of 40 mg or more of furosemide, 100 mL of 3% saline should be infused in the first hour. This rate should be decreased or discontinued subsequently if symptoms have ameliorated or if the plasma sodium concentration has increased by more than 2 mEq per liter in that hour. It is rarely necessary to infuse more than a total of 250 to 300 mL of 3% saline.

Preparation for Diagnostic Tests or Treatment

Special care must be taken when patients with treated diabetes insipidus are subjected to certain "standard protocols" associated with many diagnostic and therapeutic procedures. These protocols require the patient either to be fluid restricted, as for preparation for intravenous pyelography, or to be hydrated, as for the intravenous administration of chemotherapy. Tests that require a patient to have no oral fluids should not be performed without adequate intravenous hydration matched to the patient's urine output. Intravenous fluids should be started from the time the patient is no longer able to take oral fluids and may be discontinued when oral fluids are again allowed. In contrast, patients receiving antidiuretic therapy for diabetes insipidus should not be made to "force fluids" beyond the amounts determined by thirst or to have hydration orders at rates not related to urine output. If high urine flow rates are desired, the patient's antidiuretic therapy should be discontinued so that polyuria results. Oral or intravenous fluids can then be given to match the large urine volumes. Sometimes, it may be appropriate (to obtain more precise timing of a diuresis) to continue antidiuretic therapy and administer intravenous furosemide. The close monitoring of serum sodium levels will greatly assist in determining the status of fluid balance in these situations.

HYPERPARATHYROIDISM AND HYPOPARATHYROIDISM

method of
LAWRENCE E. MALLETTE, M.D., Ph.D.
*Baylor College of Medicine and Veterans Affairs
Medical Center
Houston, Texas*

DIAGNOSIS

Primary Hyperparathyroidism

Primary hyperparathyroidism arises from the intrinsic hyperfunction of one or more of the parathyroid glands. Its hallmark is hypercalcemia, but the elevation in total serum calcium may be borderline or intermittent in mild cases or early in the course of severe cases. Total serum calcium values that lie near the upper limit of normal should be checked by direct estimation of the free calcium ion concentration with an ion-selective electrode (ionized calcium measurement). In primary hyperparathyroidism, the ionized calcium value can be clearly elevated when the total serum calcium value is near the upper limit of normal.

To confirm that the cause of hypercalcemia is parathyroid hyperfunction, serum parathyroid hormone (PTH) can be measured. The availability of biterminal, or sandwich, assays that measure only the intact PTH molecule (and not the circulating catabolic fragments of PTH that are devoid of calcemic activity and are normally cleared by the kidney) has simplified diagnosis. Renal dysfunction has only a slight effect on the intact PTH value, and false-positive elevations are rare. The normal range for intact PTH is from 10 pg per mL to 55 to 65 pg per mL (the upper limit increases with age). Normal PTH values can be higher in the afternoon or evening, so morning samples are preferred for diagnosis. Approximately 80% of patients with primary hyperparathyroidism have intact PTH values above 65 pg per mL, and values in the remainder fall between 25 and 65 pg per mL. A normal intact PTH value thus does not exclude the diagnosis of primary hyperparathyroidism. In nonparathyroid hypercalcemia, the intact PTH value is usually suppressed below 20 pg per mL unless renal dysfunction is present, in which case the intact PTH value may be as high as 25 pg per mL.

When the intact PTH value of a hypercalcemic patient lies between 25 and 65 pg per mL, presumably signaling a lack of suppressibility of PTH secretion, it may be helpful to measure the midregion PTH value by radioimmunoassay (RIA), as long as renal function is normal. Parathyroid adenomas secrete, in varying proportions, the intact PTH molecule and noncalcemic fragments of the hormone, and both contain the midregion epitopes read by the RIA. Thus, midregion PTH values may be elevated when the intact PTH value is normal. Two factors must be borne in mind when one is interpreting midregion PTH RIA values, however. First, nonparathyroid hypercalcemia does not suppress serum midregion PTH values as fully as it does the intact PTH value, because the parathyroid cell continues to release hormone fragments even when intact PTH secretion is inhibited by hypercalcemia. Second, midregion PTH fragments are cleared largely by the kidneys, so that renal failure can increase the midregion PTH value even in patients with nonparathyroid hypercalcemia.

Secondary Hyperparathyroidism

Secondary hyperparathyroidism represents the expected physiologic response of the parathyroid glands to hypocalcemia, a decrease in vitamin D metabolites, or a long-term rise in serum phosphate. All three factors have been shown independently to increase PTH secretion and/or to produce parathyroid hyperplasia. The most common settings for clinically evident secondary hyperparathyroidism are renal failure and intestinal malabsorption of fat-soluble vitamins. An increasingly common cause of subtle or subclinical secondary hyperparathyroidism is a failure of adequate vitamin D nutrition in the confined geriatric population, in whom risk factors include little sun exposure, an inefficient cutaneous formation of vitamin D, an age-related inefficiency of intestinal absorption of vitamin D and its metabolites, and decreased renal 1α-hydroxylation of 25-hydroxyvitamin D, due to the age-related decline in renal function. Secondary hyperparathyroidism increases fracture risk by accelerating bone loss and producing muscle weakness, and preventive measures can lower the incidence of fractures.

As vitamin D deficiency develops, serum calcium tends to be well maintained by the secondary rise in PTH. Serum phosphate values fall in response to the increase in PTH. At this stage, the patient may show only an increase in serum PTH, with normal total calcium values, low-normal ionized calcium values, and a drop in serum phosphate within the normal range. Serum 25-hydroxyvitamin D values are usually below 15 ng per mL but are often above the formal lower limit of normal. Serum 1,25-dihydroxyvitamin D values are often normal or even slightly increased, because renal formation of this metabolite, although limited by a low substrate (25-hydroxyvitamin D) concentration, is stimulated by the increase in PTH and the decline in calcium and phosphate. Bone remodeling is accelerated by the increase in PTH, but bone synthesis and mineralization are inhibited by the falls in vitamin D metabolite levels and in serum calcium-phosphate product. Patients may be largely asymptomatic at this stage but show accelerated bone loss. This is the ideal time for diagnosis and intervention, but this stage of the disease can be detected only by measurement of PTH values (with support for the diagnosis by ionized calcium and 25-hydroxyvitamin D measurements). As the vitamin D deficiency worsens, serum phosphate and calcium values eventually fall below normal. By this stage of the deficiency, histologic evidence of osteomalacia is present, and the patient often has bone pain, muscle weakness, an increase in serum alkaline phosphatase, and hyperchloremic acidosis due to the proximal renal tubular effects of the hypocalcemia and increased PTH. Intervention is also rewarding at this stage, but the goal should be earlier diagnosis.

Secondary hyperparathyroidism occurs in renal failure as a function of the drop in serum 1,25-dihydroxyvitamin D values engendered by the rise in serum phosphate, by the decline in functional renal mass, and perhaps by the acidosis. Hyperphosphatemia and hypocalcemia, produced by the decline in intestinal calcium absorption, make additional contributions to parathyroid growth. By the time the renal patient has developed symptomatic hyperparathyroid bone disease, intact PTH values are usually above 300 pg per dL, and midregion PTH values are elevated more than 40-fold.

Tertiary Hyperparathyroidism

Tertiary hyperparathyroidism is defined as hypercalcemia produced by parathyroid autonomy that develops on a background of long-standing secondary hyperparathyroidism. Tertiary hyperparathyroidism most often occurs in the setting of long-term dialysis therapy but may also affect patients with a malabsorption syndrome. It often manifests clinically as severe hyperparathyroid bone disease, but in renal patients it may be associated with widespread focal cutaneous calcification and infarction (calciphylaxis). Hypercalcemia can also be superimposed on secondary parathyroid hyperplasia by overtreatment with a vitamin D congener, excess oral calcium supplements, the sudden institution of effective restriction of intestinal phosphate absorption, or a concomitant disease such as sarcoidosis. These parathyroid-independent hypercalcemias can be confused with tertiary hyperparathyroidism. In these cases, the serum PTH value is less elevated than it was just before the hypercalcemia developed, usually lying in the lower or middle part of the expected range for secondary hyperparathyroidism. In contrast, PTH values in tertiary hyperparathyroidism are even more elevated than those in secondary hyperparathyroidism.

Hypoparathyroidism

Hypoparathyroidism is characterized by hypocalcemia and hyperphosphatemia with inappropriately low or undetectable serum PTH values. When the hypoparathyroidism is complete, serum PTH is undetectable in the face of hypocalcemia. In partial hypoparathyroidism, serum PTH is inappropriately normal or is minimally elevated despite hypocalcemia. Parathyroid loss can be due to autoimmune attack, surgery or other cervical trauma, infiltrative diseases, or congenital deficiency. Functional hypoparathyroidism also occurs in magnesium depletion, which is known to inhibit both PTH secretion and PTH action. Measurement of serum PTH before and after magnesium administration can help establish the diagnosis of hypocalcemia due to magnesium depletion.

Pseudohypoparathyroidism

Hypocalcemia and hyperphosphatemia also occur in pseudohypoparathyroidism, but serum PTH values are increased (by the hypocalcemia and low 1,25-dihydroxyvitamin D values). Only two other situations can give this biochemical picture. The first is renal failure, which is easy to exclude. The second is true hypoparathyroidism with an erroneous PTH RIA result. False elevations of PTH RIA values can occur (in less than 2% of subjects), probably arising from antibodies in the patient's serum that inter-fere with binding of tracer to the assay (anti-PTH) antibody. Thus, an increased PTH RIA value should be confirmed in a second assay system, such as a biterminal assay for intact PTH. Approximately 70% of pseudohypoparathyroid patients have type 1 pseudohypoparathyroidism and manifest brachydactyly and/or subcutaneous ossifications. PTH infusion with measurement of urinary phosphate and cyclic AMP responses is needed, however, for the formal differentiation of type 1 from type 2 pseudohypoparathyroidism.

TREATMENT

Primary Hyperparathyroidism

Selection of Therapy

Surgical intervention is safe and effective, producing a permanent cure in more than 95% of patients, with few complications. On the other hand, mild primary hyperparathyroidism may cause minimal morbidity that for some patients may not outweigh the cost and risk of surgery. Because we have no randomized prospective studies to guide our recommendations, the selection of optimal therapy remains an art as well as a subject for future scientific inquiry.

I usually recommend surgical treatment when the patient's serum calcium values average more than 1.0 mg per dL above the upper normal limit, because the risk of complications is increased. Patients with mild hypercalcemia present a more difficult decision, as many seem to be asymptomatic, and there is little evidence for major long-term morbidity. Factors favoring surgical intervention include a younger age (more years over which morbidity might accumulate); a low bone mass, especially at the hip; and the presence of symptoms (even nonspecific ones). Parathyroid surgery has been shown, unlike thyroid surgery, to produce an improvement in neuromuscular and psychologic symptoms. A diagnosis of asymptomatic hyperparathyroidism can be incorrect. I have observed patients who initially reported no symptoms but who experienced a remarkable improvement in well-being, mood, or stamina after successful parathyroid surgery.

Before medical follow-up is chosen, the hyperparathyroidism must first be demonstrated to be of the stable variety shown by perhaps 95% of patients, with serum calcium and PTH values remaining stable for years. Most of these patients have an adenoma that arose from a set point error in calcium detection in the clone of cells that now constitutes the tumor. This abnormal cell misinterprets a normal calcium value as too low and responds by producing more PTH and by dividing. Eventually this clone expands enough to produce sufficient PTH to increase the serum calcium value to the clone's new inhibitory set point. This removes the stimulus to growth of the tumor, and tumor size and serum calcium value remain stable indefinitely.

Approximately 5% of parathyroid tumors arise on a different basis and produce a slow but steady increase in serum calcium and PTH values that becomes evident over weeks or months. These tumors are analogous to other endocrine neoplasms and grow steadily regardless of the ambient calcium value. Serial measurements of serum calcium and PTH (which I make at progressively longer intervals) identify these patients (both calcium and PTH should tend to increase). At the far end of this tumor spectrum is the rare (less than 0.5% of all cases) parathyroid carcinoma, which grows rapidly enough that the patient usually has a serum calcium level above 13.5 mg per dL by the time the tumor is discovered.

Patients who otherwise seem to be candidates for medical management should be screened for cortical bone loss (measurement of bone mass at the forearm or femoral neck). Mild primary hyperparathyroidism does not decrease spinal bone mass significantly but does reduce cortical bone mass. Patients with a critically low bone mass may benefit from parathyroidectomy, because a moderate increase in bone mass (10 to 15%) occurs during the first 6 months after parathyroidectomy. The added bone mass may protect against fracture in patients whose skeleton is nearing their own "fracture threshold."

A radiographic or ultrasonographic examination of the kidneys should also be done before medical management is elected as the long-term strategy. Nephrocalcinosis, nephrolithiasis, or even a staghorn calculus can develop without symptoms and must be excluded before the election to delay surgery.

I regard the development of pancreatitis as a strong indication for parathyroidectomy. It is true that further attacks still occur in some patients despite the normocalcemia, the illness in these cases being ascribed to another cause. There is, however, no method to determine whether hypercalcemia has been an important contributor in a given case, and pancreatitis is such a painful and life-threatening disease that any and all potential causes should be removed.

Medical Management

As yet, no medication can attack the parathyroid tumor or hyperplasia itself. Medical therapy is therefore intended simply to minimize the complications of long-term PTH excess in patients who are poor surgical candidates, who refuse surgery, or in whom surgery fails.

Measures can be designed to minimize the rise in either serum calcium or PTH. A basic problem is that PTH excess and hypercalcemia probably contribute independently to symptoms and morbidity. Steps to reduce one factor often increase the other, because most parathyroid tumors remain sensitive to ambient calcium values, albeit at the higher set point. Hypercalcemia predisposes to ectopic calcification, renal stones, pancreatitis, and gastric hypersecretion and possibly to chondrocalcinosis and accelerated development of atherosclerosis. Increased PTH levels are probably responsible for the neurologic complications of hyperparathyroidism, including decreased memory, depression, and muscle weakness. For this reason, I avoid steps that tend to lower serum calcium values (and increase PTH values) in patients with neurologic or muscular symptoms or signs.

In the past, it was traditional to restrict dietary calcium intake for primary hyperparathyroidism. This is a reasonable measure to minimize hypercalcemia in preparation for surgery or to reduce urinary calcium excretion in a patient with nephrolithiasis. Long-term restriction of calcium intake might, however, accelerate bone loss. The higher serum PTH values would increase bone resorption, and the secondary decrease in serum phosphate would tend to slow bone formation. Until long-term studies of the relationship of dietary calcium to skeletal health in chronic hyperparathyroidism are available, it would seem prudent for patients with mild hyperparathyroidism to maintain the calcium intake that would normally be recommended for their age.

A feared complication of primary hyperparathyroidism is the hypercalcemic crisis, which can develop even in patients who initially have minimal symptoms and modest hypercalcemia. A crisis is most likely to occur when an intercurrent illness decreases renal perfusion (decreased renal calcium clearance) and immobilizes the patient in bed (increased bone resorption). Examples of such intercurrent illnesses are myocardial infarction, diarrheal illness with vomiting, cholecystitis, and automobile accident with multiple fractures. Patients must be educated to report to an emergency facility if, during the course of their diagnostic evaluation or medical follow-up, a severe bout of gastroenteritis or other illness predisposing to dehydration should occur, or if significant lethargy or somnolence develops. Dehydration may occur more often in elderly patients because of their impaired thirst mechanism, combined with the decreased renal concentrating ability produced by the hypercalcemia. These patients need a system for ensuring adequate fluid intake on a daily basis.

Another potential cause of severe hypercalcemia is the overuse of calcium carbonate antacids to produce the equivalent of the milk-alkali syndrome. Primary hyperparathyroidism may predispose to this complication, because it can produce dyspeptic symptoms and it increases intestinal calcium absorption. Patients who are to be followed up medically should be educated to avoid over-the-counter antacids that contain calcium.

Estrogen replacement therapy has been advocated for postmenopausal women with primary hyperparathyroidism, because it lessens the degree of hypercalcemia engendered by a given excess of PTH, probably by blunting bone resorption. The effect on serum calcium values is not a large one, however, and there are no long-term studies to confirm the expected skeletal protective effect in hyperparathyroidism. Nevertheless, the antiatherogenic effects of estrogen replacement can easily justify its use, and any beneficial effect on the skeleton can be considered a bonus.

Other antiresorptive agents, such as calcitonin and bisphosphonates, have been advocated for their skeletal protective effects. I generally use these agents only for the hypercalcemic emergency or for the rare patient with severe hyperparathyroidism who is not a surgical candidate because of a concomitant serious illness. An example is a patient with terminal rheumatic heart disease and severe obstructive pulmonary disease whose serum calcium values tended to average 13.5 mg per dL, but in whom lethargy developed when the value was 13 mg per dL. My colleagues and I successfully managed the patient's hyperparathyroidism for more than 18 months with intermittent infusions of pamidronate (Aredia) given on an outpatient basis whenever the serum calcium value exceeded 12.5 mg per dL.

Oral administration of one of the newer and more potent bisphosphonates would seem to be a reasonable alternative to estrogen replacement, when it is contraindicated, or perhaps to intravenous pamidronate for severe hypercalcemia. I have no personal experience with oral bisphosphonates in these settings, however.

Neutral phosphate taken orally has been proposed as a treatment to minimize the risk of nephrolithiasis. Few patients with primary hyperparathyroidism are candidates for this therapy, because nephrolithiasis is a strong indication for parathyroid surgery. Use of neutral phosphate in an attempt to prevent formation of a first kidney stone is probably unnecessary, because most hyperparathyroid patients who are predisposed to stone formation have already formed a stone by the time their hypercalcemia is discovered. Preventive therapy is important, however, for patients with known stone disease who are not surgical candidates. Neutral potassium phosphate (NeutraPhos-K) in divided doses (at a level of 750 to 1500 mg per day) can be used to decrease serum 1,25-dihydroxyvitamin D values, intestinal calcium absorption, and urinary calcium excretion. I prefer the potassium salt to the mixed sodium/potassium salt, because sodium has a calciuric effect. If the serum calcium value exceeds approximately 11.5 mg per dL, oral phosphate therapy should be undertaken only with great caution, because the calcium-phosphate product can increase enough to cause ectopic calcification in the kidney and elsewhere. Renal insufficiency is also a contraindication to neutral phosphate therapy for two reasons: no additional renal injury can be tolerated, and the poor renal clearance of phosphate can predispose to hyperphosphatemia and ectopic calcification.

Surgical Treatment

Surgical treatment of hyperparathyroidism is the chosen therapy for most patients with primary (and tertiary) hyperparathyroidism. The risk of parathyroid surgery is essentially the risk of a general anesthetic, with the added small risks of recurrent laryngeal nerve injury and hypoparathyroidism. For patients who are not good candidates for inhalation anesthesia but are cooperative and relaxed about the idea of surgery, parathyroidectomy can be carried out with regional (cervical block) anesthesia.

When the operation is performed by a surgeon experienced in parathyroid surgery, the cure rate is approximately 95%, and damage to the recurrent laryngeal nerve is rare in the absence of prior neck surgery. Preoperative assessment and preparation are the same as for any general anesthesia, except that the patient should usually be given intravenous hydration during the "nothing per os" period before surgery. If serum calcium values are above 13 mg per dL or there is a history of pancreatitis, I often choose to give intravenous pamidronate 2 or 3 days before surgery, so the patient enters the operation with a lower serum calcium value. Mobilization after the procedure and recovery from the procedure itself are usually rapid, because the patient is not handicapped in the postoperative period by a painful thoracic or abdominal incision.

Although relatively safe and easy for the patient, parathyroid surgery can be quite involved and complicated for the surgeon. The parathyroid glands lie ectopically in a fairly high percentage of cases. Knowledge of the common "hiding places" and experience in approaching and exploring them are essential. Accurate assessment of parathyroid gland size at the operating table is essential to the differentiation of adenoma from hyperplasia but requires experience. The parathyroid carcinoma must be recognized at the time of surgery and treated properly, by en bloc resection of the parathyroid tumor and surrounding tissues, if the patient is to have any chance of cure. Thus, parathyroid surgery should be undertaken only by those experienced in the procedure. The surgeon should have "scrubbed" with a more experienced parathyroid surgeon many times before attempting to carry out the procedure on his or her own.

The use of preoperative localization studies is an evolving area of practice. For patients without prior neck surgery, localization studies in general are not necessary, because the surgical success rate is already 95% without such studies. Thus, I reserve the use of nuclear thyroid scanning, computed tomography, magnetic resonance imaging, arteriography, or venous sampling procedures for patients with prior cervical surgery or with persistent or recurrent hyperparathyroidism.

The exception to this general rule is ultrasonography of the thyroid region, which either should be performed preoperatively or should be available intraoperatively in all cases. The procedure is painless, relatively inexpensive, and risk free. If the preoperative ultrasonogram fails to show a candidate lesion, the surgeon may elect to set aside more time for the procedure, because a prolonged exploration may be needed. Also, it is wise to know the internal details of thyroid anatomy when embarking on a cervical exploration, for several reasons. First, a parathyroid adenoma or one or more hyperplastic glands can be located within the thyroid gland. When exploration of the neck fails to uncover an adenoma, the hypoechoic lesion found on thyroid ultrasonogram becomes the next candidate for resection. Fifteen percent of subjects have five or more parathyroid glands, and a fifth hyperplastic gland located within the thyroid could be missed if ultrasonography is not performed.

A thorough family history concerning parathyroid disease and other endocrine disorders can be important to the surgical management of the patient, because surgical treatment of the hyperparathyroidism is often modified for familial parathyroid disease. Total parathyroidectomy with autogenous parathyroid grafting is favored by many specialists for the patient with multiple endocrine neoplasia type 1 or type 2. Another well-characterized familial parathyroid disease is the hereditary cystic parathyroid adenoma–fibro-osseous jaw tumor syndrome, a dominant trait that is carried on chromosome 1. In this syndrome, bilateral inferior parathyroidectomy may be favored, because the adenomas tend to occur most often in the inferior parathyroid glands, and metachronous second adenomas are common. Parathyroid tissue from familial cases should be preserved for possible use in future autotransplantation or for genetic studies of the mechanisms of tumorigenesis.

POSTOPERATIVE COURSE

After resection of a parathyroid tumor, the serum calcium level usually falls slowly and steadily, either back to or below normal, generally reaching a nadir on the evening of surgery or 1 to 4 days later. An occasional patient may develop a positive Chvostek sign or circumoral paresthesias even before serum calcium value has reached normal, perhaps because of a rapid fall in calcium. These symptoms need not be treated with intravenous calcium and will resolve spontaneously without tetany. Serum magnesium values are low in some of these patients, in which case parenteral magnesium is indicated.

Postoperative pancreatitis has been reported after general anesthesia for many procedures, but it may be more common after parathyroid surgery. Its management is the same as for pancreatitis of other causes. Postoperative flares of gout or pseudogout can also occur but respond well to anti-inflammatory agents.

The serum calcium value falls below normal in less than half the patients. Hypocalcemia indicates either transient or permanent hypoparathyroidism or the "hungry bones" syndrome: the skeleton goes into strong positive balance, because the osteoclast count returns rapidly to normal but the osteoblasts continue to synthesize bone for several weeks. The serum phosphate value remains low in the hungry bones syndrome but increases in hypoparathyroidism. Measurement of PTH itself gives a more accurate differentiation, however. The hungry bones syndrome is often accompanied by a transient rise in serum alkaline phosphatase values, and sometimes by an increase in bone pain. A transient rise in serum creatinine is also not unusual in the few days after surgery for moderate or severe primary hyperparathyroidism; its basis is unknown.

The hungry bones syndrome may persist for several weeks. It can usually be treated satisfactorily with calcitriol in doses of approximately 1 μg per day, plus oral calcium supplements. The syndrome may abate rather quickly, however, when the crop of osteoblasts that was recruited by the hyperparathyroidism nears the end of its life span. To avoid iatrogenic hypercalcemia, serum calcium values should be monitored frequently until calcitriol is no longer needed.

After resection of a parathyroid adenoma, the patient is considered cured if serum calcium and PTH values are normal at 6 months. Serum calcium values need to be measured only infrequently (every few years) after this, because the risk of later recurrence is only approximately 0.5%.

Parathyroid Crisis

Primary hyperparathyroidism occasionally manifests as life-threatening hypercalcemia, with serum calcium values above 14.0 mg per dL and nausea and vomiting or major alterations in mentation. The emergent treatment of parathyroid crisis is similar to that for any severe hypercalcemia, except that oral neutral phosphate can be quite effective. To eliminate the element of increased renal calcium retention due to volume contraction, the patient should undergo volume repletion with normal saline, followed by volume expansion to increase proximal tubular rejection of calcium. This may require several liters of fluid. If renal function is adequate, these measures usually stop the upward spiral of calcium values and may lower the serum calcium level significantly.

Oral administration of neutral phosphate is quite effective in parathyroid crisis and can be especially important for patients who do not tolerate intravenous fluids well. Doses of 1000 to 2000 mg per day safely lower serum calcium values in most patients. The dosage must be moderated if renal function is compromised, and phosphate therapy is contraindicated if the serum phosphate value is above the middle of the normal range. Oral phosphate, of course, cannot be used if the patient is vomiting or has depressed mentation. Hypokalemia can complicate oral phosphate therapy, so close monitoring of serum potassium is important.

When oral phosphate therapy cannot be used, I usually begin antiresorptive therapy early during treatment, to eliminate any skeletal contribution to the hypercalcemia, which may have been further increased by immobilization. As soon as I am confident, because of the blood chemistry values and adequate urinary flow, that renal function is not severely compromised, I begin an intravenous infusion of pamidronate (usually 60 mg over 4 to 6 hours). If the serum creatinine value is above 5 mg per dL, I avoid pamidronate and use synthetic salmon calcitonin instead (100 units subcutaneously every 12 hours).

Now that highly effective antiresorptive agents are available, emergency parathyroid exploration is rarely necessary. Older PTH assays required several days to complete, but the intact PTH assay requires only a few hours, so a rapid confirmation of the diagnosis is possible, even when emergency neck exploration is contemplated. To lessen the risk of a recurrent crisis, elective parathyroid exploration should usually be carried out as soon as the hypercalcemia has been controlled.

Secondary Hyperparathyroidism

Secondary hyperparathyroidism is treated by provision of the missing vitamin D metabolite(s). For intestinal malabsorption, ergocalciferol can be given orally in doses that usually range from 50,000 units weekly to the same amount daily. To circumvent potential problems from variable intestinal absorption or to decrease the number of oral medications the patient must contend with, ergocalciferol can be given intramuscularly (500,000 IU in 1 mL given monthly). This substance has been estimated to be about 10% bioavailable, so this dosage amounts to approximately 1500 units daily, well below the usual limit of toxicity. There is no rationale for the use of the more expensive vitamin D congeners (calcifediol, calcitriol, or dihydrotachysterol) in treating malabsorption or vitamin D deficiency.

The skeletal lesions of patients who have symptomatic hypocalcemia and osteomalacia probably heal faster if oral calcium and phosphate supplements are given during the early weeks of treatment, when skeletal remineralization is consuming large amounts of substrate. I usually prescribe 500 mg of calcium as the carbonate with breakfast and supper and 250 mg of neutral potassium and sodium phosphate with lunch and at bedtime. I usually stop the phosphate supplement after 4 to 6 weeks but continue the calcium supplement indefinitely.

Renal hyperparathyroidism can be such a devastating complication that treatment should begin with preventive measures at an early stage in the evolution of renal insufficiency. Dietary protein restriction, now known to slow the progression of chronic renal insufficiency, has the added benefit of decreasing phosphate intake as well. Oral phosphate binders and assurance of adequate calcium and vitamin D nutrition are important in slowing the development of renal secondary hyperparathyroidism but are now known to be inadequate alone. As the renal insufficiency advances and 1,25-dihydroxyvitamin D values decline, an active form of vitamin D must be provided to prevent parathyroid hyperplasia, by keeping the parathyroid glands supplied with an active vitamin D metabolite.

Oral calcitriol (Rocaltrol) has seen heavy use in renal insufficiency and is quite effective in stimulating intestinal calcium absorption. It is not well absorbed, however, and may not reach the parathyroid glands in sufficient amounts. One of four strategies can be used to circumvent this problem. Calcitriol itself can be delivered to the parathyroid glands in increased amounts either by giving it intravenously at the time of each hemodialysis or by giving it intermittently in large oral doses (3 to 5 μg given every 3 to 4 days). The third strategy is to use synthetic 1α-hydroxyvitamin D, currently in use in other countries and undergoing testing in the United States. Itself

biologically inactive, this agent is absorbed and 25-hydroxylated in the liver to produce 1,25-dihydroxycholecalciferol (calcitriol), which then enters the circulation to produce "equal" intestinal and parathyroid effects. The fourth strategy is the use of dihydrotachysterol, which is a by-product of the photoactivation step that forms ergocalciferol. Dihydrotachysterol is formed when the B ring opens differently to rotate the steroid A ring 180 degrees, placing the original 3β-hydroxy group into the 1α steric position. It is thus a congener of 1α-hydroxyvitamin D and need only be 25-hydroxylated in the liver to acquire biologic activity. It likewise has equal intestinal and parathyroid effects. Historically, this was the first vitamin D congener found clinically to have biologic potency in uremia, but for unclear reasons, it seems to have been largely forgotten.

Any of these methods must be monitored carefully to avoid inducing untoward rises in serum calcium and phosphate, with the risk of ectopic calcifications. In some patients, these measures are insufficient to prevent or reverse severe parathyroid hyperplasia, and subtotal parathyroidectomy may become necessary.

Tertiary Hyperparathyroidism

Renal parathyroid hyperplasia can eventually become a nodular hyperplasia, and some of the nodules have been shown to possess a high set point for inhibition by calcium, analogous to the parathyroid adenoma. This produces the syndrome of tertiary hyperparathyroidism, with uncontrollable hypercalcemia and hyperphosphatemia. Tertiary hyperparathyroidism is a state of true parathyroid autonomy and is best managed by parathyroid surgery. During attempts to control the parathyroid hyperfunction by medical means, which are generally unsuccessful, these patients can develop severe skeletal disease or rarely calciphylaxis. The diagnosis should, of course, be confirmed before surgery by demonstrating that serum PTH values are markedly elevated even for a patient with renal failure.

Hypoparathyroidism

Severe Symptomatic Hypocalcemia

Hypocalcemia requires emergency treatment when it produces overt tetany, laryngospasm, or seizures. I use intravenous calcium gluconate as a bolus of 5 mg of elemental calcium per kg of body weight over 3 to 5 minutes, followed by infusion of 5 mg per kg per hour for 3 or 4 hours. This usually raises the serum calcium value by 2 to 3 mg per dL. The infusion without the bolus can be used for severe symptoms without overt tetany. The change in serum calcium is confirmed at 2 hours and intermittently thereafter. I avoid the use of intravenous calcium chloride, which some have advocated as a better treatment because it has more free calcium ion immediately available. Subcutaneous infiltration of calcium chloride may cause skin necrosis, a side effect not seen with the gluconate salt, which itself produces an adequate clinical response. If hypocalcemia is associated with magnesium depletion, parenteral magnesium is mandatory and produces a much better and more complete response than intravenous calcium alone.

Surgical Management

Parathyroid tissue implanted with proper technique into a muscle bed will survive and function well enough to maintain calcium homeostasis. Successful transplantation of parathyroid tissue between identical twins has been reported once, and parathyroid homografts have been carried out successfully in a small number of immunosuppressed renal transplant recipients. For most patients with hypoparathyroidism, however, the complications of immunosuppression are too great to justify parathyroid homografts.

Prevention of hypoparathyroidism during thyroid surgery is important. Muscle implantation of questionably viable parathyroid glands or of glands recovered from the resected thyroid specimen (by dissection in a sterile field under a dissecting microscope) markedly reduces the incidence of hypoparathyroidism. Too few surgeons employ these stratagems, in my opinion.

Medical Therapy

The most important long-term goal of treatment is the prevention of tetany and seizures. It can be accomplished by keeping the serum calcium value above approximately 7.0 to 7.5 mg per dL (unless the patient has an independent seizure disorder that is exacerbated by hypocalcemia). Additional goals are the prevention of premature cataract formation and the prevention of calcifications of the central nervous system, especially the basal ganglia. These goals can be accomplished by keeping serum calcium values between 8.5 and 8.8 mg per dL. Maintenance of *normal* serum calcium values is not necessary and is harmful.

For any given degree of hypocalcemia, the patient with hypoparathyroidism has a greater urinary calcium excretion than the patient with intact parathyroids, because the renal tubular reabsorption of calcium is no longer stimulated by PTH. Returning the filtered calcium load to normal often renders a hypoparathyroid patient hypercalciuric. The therapeutic goal is to keep the serum calcium value as close to normal as possible without producing hypercalciuria. Before this physiology was understood, patients were often overtreated, and many developed the severe complications related to nephrocalcinosis and the resulting high renin hypertension.

An occasional patient has partial hypoparathyroidism and can be maintained with an oral calcium supplement alone (1000 to 2000 mg daily in divided doses). Most hypoparathyroid patients, however, require additional therapy. Until a long-acting and easily administered PTH analogue is available, treatment of hypoparathyroidism will rely on use of vitamin D congeners.

Vitamin D$_2$ itself (ergocalciferol) increases intestinal calcium absorption enough to maintain a satisfactory serum calcium value. Large doses are required, however, because renal 1α-hydroxylation is inhibited by the high serum phosphate and low PTH values. Nevertheless, ergocalciferol is the most economical vitamin D congener for use in hypoparathyroidism. The usual dosage range is 50,000 to 100,000 units per day, although a few patients with partial hypoparathyroidism require less. These doses of ergocalciferol produce a severalfold elevation of serum 25-hydroxyvitamin D, with a 1,25-dihydroxyvitamin D value in the normal range. Doses above 100,000 units per day eventually produce hypercalcemia in most patients, sometimes after a delay of many weeks. Ergocalciferol has a long half-life, so equilibrium is not reached for several weeks after a change in dosage, making management a bit clumsy. An advantage of the long half-life is that if the patient runs out of medication, there is a grace period of several weeks before tetany becomes a risk.

Dihydrotachysterol (DHT, Hytakerol), discussed previously in the renal hyperparathyroidism section, can be used to advantage. Because it does not have to undergo 1α-hydroxylation (inhibited in hypoparathyroidism), its onset of action is earlier than that for ergocalciferol. The polarity (and fat solubility) is similar to that of ergocalciferol, so that dihydrotachysterol still requires many days to reach a new equilibrium after a dosage change, and its effects abate slowly after it is discontinued. The usual dosage range for hypoparathyroidism is 0.125 to 0.50 mg per day.

Calcitriol, or 1,25-dihydroxycholecalciferol, is also effective for hypoparathyroidism. It is not well absorbed orally but increases intestinal calcium absorption well enough to maintain good serum calcium values. The compound has the advantage of a rapid onset of action, and the potential disadvantage of a rapid dissipation of its action. I use it in two ways. It can be used as the long-term maintenance agent, usually in doses of 1 to 2 μg per day. It can also be used as a "bridge" in a newly diagnosed patient for whom the long-term agent will be ergocalciferol: the patient is initially given ergocalciferol, 50,000 units daily, plus calcitriol, 1 μg daily, with an oral calcium supplement. The calcitriol increases blood calcium within just 2 or 3 days, allowing more rapid discharge from the hospital. Close monitoring of serum calcium is mandatory for the first 2 or 3 weeks to avoid hypercalcemia. Starting at about 3 weeks, the calcitriol dosage is tapered, the goal being to discontinue the agent by 12 to 18 weeks. Meanwhile, the ergocalciferol dosage is increased intermittently as needed to eventually stabilize the serum calcium value near the lower limit of normal. The time to equilibrium can be shortened by initially giving a large (loading) dose of ergocalciferol (300,000 units daily for the first 3 days) to "fill up the fat stores of the vitamin" more rapidly. The same bridge and loading strategies can also be used for initiation of therapy with dihydrotachysterol.

I often prescribe a calcium supplement in the range of 1000 to 2000 mg per day in hopes of lowering the requirement for the vitamin D congener. I generally use calcium carbonate and recommend that it be taken with meals to secure a more predictable calcium absorption and maximize the desired phosphate-binding activity of the calcium (see later). The calcium supplement is not essential; a few of my patients have not wished to contemplate a lifetime of taking tablets several times a day and have maintained themselves in stable fashion for many years on ergocalciferol alone, with a normal dietary intake of calcium.

A few women with hypoparathyroidism may show a symptomatic drop in serum calcium values with the onset of menses. The addition of an oral calcium supplement during the menses is a useful means of minimizing this change without varying the dosage of the vitamin D congener.

Once treatment has established the desired serum calcium value, I check urinary calcium excretion. The goal is to show that the fasting morning urinary calcium to creatinine ratio is less than 0.15 or that the 24-hour urine calcium value is less than 4 mg per kg of body weight per day. If hypercalciuria is present even though the serum calcium value is in the desired range, I first prescribe a low-sodium diet. Then, especially if the patient has undergone thyroidectomy, I decrease the amount of calcium supplement while increasing the dosage of vitamin D congener to maintain the same fasting serum calcium value. It has been shown that thyroidectomized patients (lacking calcitonin) show a greater rise in serum calcium after an oral calcium dose than do thyroid-intact subjects. For any given fasting serum calcium value, they thus have a higher filtered load of calcium. Sometimes the calcium supplement must to be discontinued altogether to avoid hypercalciuria. Even then, an occasional patient is able to avoid hypercalciuria only by maintaining a total serum calcium value near 8.0 mg per dL.

The use of a thiazide diuretic has been advocated in an effort to reduce urinary calcium excretion, but thiazides are less effective in lowering urinary calcium in hypoparathyroid patients. The thiazide can also complicate matters by worsening the metabolic alkalosis that these patients usually show (due to loss of the PTH stimulation of renal bicarbonate excretion).

The dosages of vitamin D and calcium that are needed to maintain the desired serum calcium value may vary from month to month, or year to year. Episodes of ethanol abuse can lead to hypocalcemia in an otherwise stable patient, either by producing magnesium deficiency or perhaps by interfering with activation of ergocalciferol. Other reasons for changing dosage requirements have not been identified. Varying potency of the vitamin D congener has been suspected on clinical grounds, but potency comparisons between medication batches or brands have not been reported. To minimize the risk of hypercalcemia, the serum calcium value should be monitored every 6 months, even when the patient appears stable. Even a single bout of hypercalcemia can produce nephrocalcinosis and permanent renal scarring. Hypoparathyroid patients are probably predisposed to developing nephrocalcinosis, because they are often alkalotic. Experiments in laboratory animals have shown that systemic alkalosis predisposes to the development of nephrocalcinosis at any given level of hypercalcemia. Because the damage done by nephrocalcinosis is only partly reversible, hypercalcemia must be avoided.

Serum phosphate values should also be monitored in hypoparathyroid patients. The calcium ion itself stimulates renal phosphate clearance, so serum phosphate declines as serum calcium increases during the early days of treatment. I prefer to maintain serum phosphate values below approximately 5.5 mg per dL. Whereas the cataracts that can complicate hypoparathyroidism are caused by hypocalcemia, central nervous system and other ectopic calcifications are thought to arise from hyperphosphatemia. In a rare patient, it is necessary to prescribe a lower protein diet or to add a phosphate-binding agent (first calcium carbonate, then aluminum hydroxide) to ensure the desired normophosphatemia.

Pseudohypoparathyroidism

Treatment of pseudohypoparathyroidism is similar to that of hypoparathyroidism. The doses of vitamin D that are required are usually less, because the resistance to PTH does not seem to be complete. In type 1 pseudohypoparathyroidism, the renal tubule is usually not resistant to the effects of PTH on renal tubular calcium reabsorption (although there is resistance to its effects on phosphate clearance and 1α-hydroxylation). For patients with this disorder, normal serum calcium values can often be maintained without hypercalciuria, although normal urinary calcium values should, of course, be verified in each individual before he or she embarks on a lifetime of normocalcemia. The advantage of maintaining normocalcemia is that the increase in PTH is minimized (the skeleton can be less resistant to PTH than is the kidney). To further lessen the tendency to parathyroid hyperplasia, I favor the use of ergocalciferol or dihydrotachysterol over oral calcitriol. Patients with pseudohypoparathyroidism should usually be referred to an academic center with interest in the disease and its genetics, so that full characterization of the pathophysiology of the particular family can be accomplished, together with genetic screening and counseling.

PRIMARY ALDOSTERONISM

method of
THEODORE A. KOTCHEN, M.D.
The Medical College of Wisconsin
Milwaukee, Wisconsin

Aldosterone is a potent mineralocorticoid that affects sodium-potassium exchange in all cells. In the kidney, it acts on the distal tubule and collecting duct to increase sodium reabsorption and facilitate potassium secretion. Aldosterone is secreted by the zona glomerulosa of the adrenal cortex and is primarily regulated by the renin-angiotensin system. In patients with primary aldosteronism, however, increased aldosterone production is not regulated by renin-angiotensin, and in these patients the consequences of hyperaldosteronism are sodium retention, hypokalemia, low plasma renin activity (PRA), and hypertension. Most estimates of the prevalence of this disorder range between 0.5 and 2.0% of hypertensive patients; however, this may be an underestimate. Because primary aldosteronism is potentially a surgically curable cause of hypertension, it is important to identify and evaluate patients in whom this diagnosis is suspected. Several different adrenal abnormalities may account for this syndrome, and the appropriate therapy depends on identifying the specific adrenal disorder. A diagnosis of primary aldosteronism can generally be established with relatively simple outpatient testing. Subsequent definition of the specific form of hyperaldosteronism requires additional testing.

SCREENING

The age at the time of diagnosis is generally in the third through fifth decades, and equal numbers of men and women are affected. Hypertension is usually mild to moderate, although occasionally severe, and may be associated with glucose intolerance. Most patients are asymptomatic, although infrequently polyuria, polydipsia, paresthesias, and rarely weakness progressing to tetany or paralysis may occur as a consequence of hypokalemic alkalosis and hypomagnesemia.

Primary aldosteronism is diagnosed in up to 50% of patients with unprovoked hypokalemia (serum K^+ level < 3.5 mEq per liter), profound hypokalemia with diuretic use (serum K^+ level < 3.1 mEq per liter), or hypokalemia resistant to replacement. Inappropriate kalliuresis (urine K^+ level > 30 mEq per 24 hours) in the presence of hypokalemia also suggests mineralocorticoid-induced hypertension. Although the serum potassium concentration is the most practical screening test, based on screening with measurements of renin and aldosterone, it has been estimated that primary aldosteronism may also occur in approximately 10% of normokalemic hypertensive patients. Nevertheless, standardized measurements of renin and aldosterone levels in all hypertensive patients are not practical, particularly in view of the fact that patients with normokalemic primary aldosteronism are more likely to have an adrenal condition with a cause that is not responsive to surgery.

In the hypertensive patient, the finding of hypokalemia unrelated to diuretic use is not specific for primary aldosteronism, and other causes should be considered (Table 1). Hypokalemia may be unrelated to the hypertension, e.g., caused by vomiting; diarrhea; or intracellular shifts due to metabolic alkalosis or treatment with beta-adrenergic agonists or theophylline. In these instances, potassium excretion is generally less than 30 mEq per 24 hours. Several other hypertensive diseases are also associated with hypokalemia. In contrast to low PRA in patients with primary aldosteronism, increased aldosterone secretion in patients with secondary aldosteronism is due to increased activity of the renin-angiotensin system, and PRA is elevated. Secondary aldosteronism should be considered in patients with accelerated or malignant hypertension, patients suspected of having renovascular hypertension, and young patients with severe hypertension (renin-secreting

TABLE 1. Differential Diagnosis of Hypertension Associated with Hypokalemia

Hypokalemia unrelated to hypertension
Diuretic usage
Primary aldosteronism
Secondary aldosteronism
    Malignant hypertension
    Renovascular hypertension
    Renin-secreting tumor
Other mineralocorticoid-producing adrenal tumors
Cushing's syndrome
Pheochromocytoma
Inherited forms of mineralocorticoid hypertension
    11β-Hydroxylase deficiency
    17α-Hydroxylase deficiency
    11β-Hydroxysteroid dehydrogenase deficiency
      (may also be acquired)
    Liddle's syndrome

tumor). Appropriate endocrine screening should be carried out in hypokalemic hypertensive patients suspected of having Cushing's syndrome or pheochromocytoma on the basis of a characteristic clinical presentation. Rarely, hypertension, hypokalemia, and low PRA may be related to adrenal tumors that secrete mineralocorticoids other than aldosterone, e.g., 11-deoxycorticosterone, corticosterone, 18-hydroxycorticosterone (18-OHB), or 21-deoxyaldosterone. Plasma and urine aldosterone levels are not elevated and may be low in these patients.

Several inherited hypertensive disorders are induced by mineralocorticoids other than aldosterone, and consequently each is associated with hypokalemia, low PRA, and low aldosterone levels. The 11β-hydroxylase deficiency causes inappropriate virilization, and the 17α-hydroxylase deficiency induces a failure of sexual maturation. Deficiency of 11β-hydroxysteroid dehydrogenase (syndrome of apparent mineralocortioid excess) results in an impaired ability to metabolize cortisol to cortisone, and cortisol activates the mineralocorticoid receptor. Each of these enzyme deficiencies has an autosomal recessive mode of inheritance. Ingestion of glycyrrhizic acid–containing substances (licorice, chewing tobacco, some antacids) may result in an acquired block of 11β-hydroxysteroid dehydrogenase, producing a syndrome that mimics the inherited disorder.

Liddle's syndrome is an autosomal dominant disorder, and hypertension is related to mineralocorticoid-independent renal sodium retention. PRA and aldosterone levels are low. The syndrome is caused by mutations of genes encoding the beta and gamma subunits of the amiloride-sensitive renal epithelial sodium channel, present in the distal nephron. The described mutations activate this channel, resulting in increased sodium reabsorption and an electrochemical gradient favoring potassium secretion. Patients with this syndrome respond to amiloride, but not to the mineralocorticoid antagonist spironolactone.

As in patients with mineralocorticoid-induced hypertension, PRA is also suppressed in approximately 25 to 30% of patients with essential hypertension. Consequently, low PRA by itself is not sufficiently specific or sensitive to be useful as a screening test. However, when combined with measurements of plasma aldosterone (PA) levels, the finding of an elevated PA/PRA ratio is an appropriate screening test and should be considered in certain groups of hypertensive patients, i.e., those with unprovoked or refractory hypokalemia; profound hypokalemia with diuretic use; onset of hypertension at a young age with no apparent secondary cause; a family history of hypertension associated with hypokalemia; or hypertension refractory to antihypertensive drug therapy.

To maximize the sensitivity of the PA/PRA ratio in patients taking antihypertensive medications, spironolactone should be withheld at least 4 weeks before study, and angiotensin-converting enzyme inhibitors, other diuretics, beta blockers, and calcium antagonists should be withheld for at least 2 weeks. Peripherally acting alpha blockers can be used to control hypertension. Patients should consume a regular salt diet, and hypokalemia should have been corrected with potassium supplementation. Preferably, blood should be drawn early in the day, after the patient has been upright for 2 hours.

The definition of an elevated ratio depends on the method for the PRA measurement and the laboratory's normal values for PRA and PA. In laboratories with a normal PA concentration of 5 to 10 ng per dL and normal PRA of 1 to 3 ng per mL per hour, a ratio greater than 30:1, with an absolute PA concentration greater than 20 ng per dL, has the following test characteristics: sensitivity, 90%; specificity, 91%; positive predictive value, 69%; and negative predictive value, 98%. In patients with renal insufficiency, the ratio may be elevated because of decreased aldosterone clearance. False-positive results may be minimized by repeating measurements 60 minutes after a 25-mg dose of captopril, an angiotensin-converting enzyme inhibitor. In patients with primary aldosteronism, the elevated ratio is unaltered by captopril, whereas the ratio declines in patients with essential hypertension. This additional testing with captopril is generally not necessary.

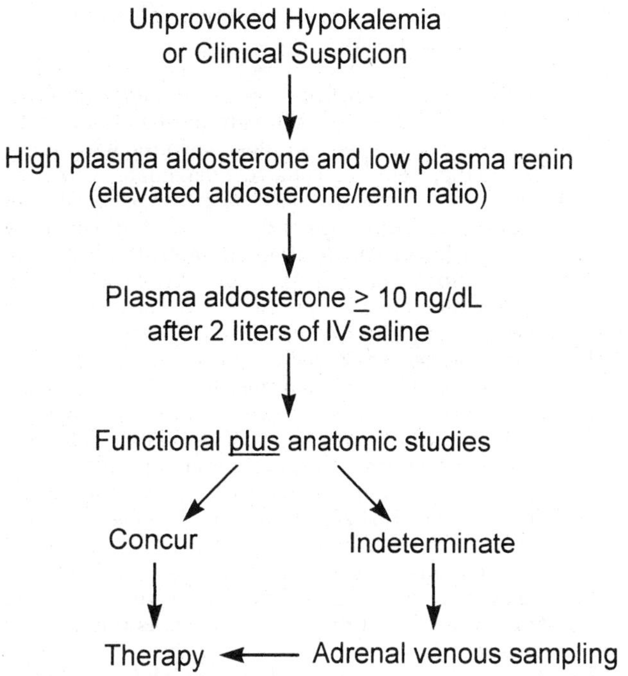

DIAGNOSIS

In patients with an elevated PA/PRA ratio, primary aldosteronism is confirmed by demonstrating the failure to suppress the PA concentration to less than 10 ng per dL after intravenous infusion of 2 liters of isotonic saline over 4 hours. In the presence of low PRA, this is diagnostic of primary aldosteronism.

Several adrenal abnormalities may culminate in the syndrome of primary aldosteronism, and appropriate therapy depends on the specific cause. Consequently, after a diagnosis of primary aldosteronism is confirmed, the next step in the evaluation is to identify its cause (Figure 1). From 60 to 70% of patients have an adrenal aldosterone–producing adenoma (APA). The tumor is almost always unilateral, and most are small, measuring less than 3 cm in diameter. From 20 to 30% of patients have bilateral adrenocortical hyperplasia (idiopathic hyperaldosteronism [IHA]). Although APA and IHA have generally been regarded as distinct adrenal abnormalities, an increasing number of patients with APA have been described who have hyperplastic and/or nodular changes in the "nontumorous" adrenal cortex. Nevertheless, the clinical distinction between APA and IHA provides useful information for outlining therapeutic recommendations.

Hypertension is generally responsive to surgery in patients with APA, but not in patients with IHA, and consequently it is important to distinguish between these two entities. The hormonal and metabolic abnormalities of APA are more marked than those of IHA, and in some patients with IHA, PA levels may be suppressed to levels between 5 and 10 ng per dL after infusion of 2 liters of saline. With increasing awareness that the metabolic alterations may be subtle, and consequently with more extensive screening, the apparent prevalence of IHA is increasing. However, the considerable overlap of serum K^+ levels, PRA, and PA

Figure 1. Clinical approaches for the evaluation of primary aldosteronism.

does not permit reliable discrimination between these two syndromes.

Functional differences in hormone secretion may assist in the differential diagnosis of APA and IHA (Table 2). Aldosterone biosynthesis tends to be more responsive to corticotropin (ACTH) in patients with APA and more responsive to renin-angiotensin in patients with IHA. Renin secretion normally increases in response to upright posture, and patients with IHA tend to have a postural increase in the PA level (e.g., upright posture from 8 AM to noon), whereas in patients with APA, PA tends to decrease during the day (reflecting the circadian rhythm of ACTH). 18-OHB is a by-product of aldosterone biosynthesis, and patients with APA generally have plasma 18-OHB concentrations above 65 ng per dL, whereas those with IHA do

TABLE 2. **Approaches to Differentiate Aldosterone-Producing Adenoma and Idiopathic Hyperaldosteronism**

Approach	Discriminating Value (%)
Functional studies	
Effect of upright posture on plasma aldosterone	85
Decrease—APA	
Increase >30%—IHA	
Plasma 18-OHB	82
>65 ng/dL—APA	
<65 ng/dL—IHA	
Anatomic studies of adrenal	
High-resolution CT or MRI	85
Scintigraphy	90
Adrenal venous sampling	95

Abbreviations: APA = aldosterone-producing adenoma; IHA = idiopathic hyperaldosteronism; 18-OHB = 18-hydroxycorticosterone; CT = computed tomography; MRI = magnetic resonance imaging.

not. By itself, however, the discriminating value of the 18-OHB level is relatively low.

At least two small subsets of patients with primary aldosteronism have been described in whom the adrenal functional abnormality differs from that in most patients with APA and IHA. First, this includes patients with aldosterone-producing, renin-responsive adenomas, who, like patients with IHA, have an increase in PA levels in response to upright posture. Second, patients with primary adrenal nodular hyperplasia, either unilateral or bilateral, have been described. As with APA patients, patients with this latter disorder have an absence of a PA response to upright posture and high plasma 18-OHB concentrations. Both subsets may be considered surgical candidates.

Rarely, primary aldosteronism may be caused by an adrenal carcinoma or an ectopic malignancy, e.g., ovarian arrhenoblastoma. Most patients with carcinoma have excessive production of other adrenal steroids in addition to aldosterone. Although patients with APA may have incomplete suppression of cortisol by dexamethasone and may rarely present with Cushing's syndrome, the finding of elevated 24-hour urine excretion of cortisol or 17-ketosteroids, or elevated plasma dehydroepiandrosterone sulfate levels, strongly suggests adrenal carcinoma as the cause of hyperaldosteronism.

To assist in defining the adrenal disease, abdominal computed tomography (CT) or magnetic resonance imaging (MRI) should be carried out in all patients diagnosed as having primary aldosteronism. These procedures detect unilaterally and bilaterally enlarged adrenals and most adenomas greater that 1.0 cm in diameter. High resolution CT may identify adenomas as small as 0.3 cm. Nevertheless, small tumors may be missed. When a unilateral adenoma is the cause of primary aldosteronism, CT will be positive 90% of the time. If the CT or MRI is not diagnostic,

an adenoma may be detected by adrenal scintigraphy with the isotope 6β-[^{131}I]iodomethyl-19-norcholesterol (NP-59), after dexamethasone suppression (0.5 mg every 6 hours for approximately 7 days). The usefulness of NP-59 scanning, however, is limited by its decreased sensitivity for adenomas smaller than 1 cm.

When results of functional and anatomic studies are in apparent conflict, or the studies are inconclusive, bilateral adrenal venous sampling for aldosterone and cortisol levels in response to ACTH stimulation should be carried out. Ipsilateral/contralateral aldosterone ratios greater than 10, with symmetrical ACTH-stimulated cortisol levels, are considered diagnostic of APA. When technically successful, this results in lateralization in 95% of patients with APA.

Glucocorticoid-remediable aldosteronism (GRA) is an inherited form of primary aldosteronism. This is an autosomal dominant trait characterized by moderate to severe hypertension, often at an early age. Hypokalemia is usually mild or absent. Normally, angiotensin II stimulates aldosterone secretion from the adrenal zona glomerulosa, whereas ACTH stimulates cortisol secretion from the zona fasciculata. The sine qua non of patients with GRA is that ACTH also regulates aldosterone secretion in the zona fasciculata. GRA is linked to a segment of chromosome 8 containing two genes whose products are involved in adrenal and steroid biosynthesis: aldosterone synthase and 11β-hydroxylase. All kindreds studied to date have a novel gene that represents a duplication arising from unequal crossing over between the aldosterone synthase and 11β-hydroxylase genes. The consequences are ACTH-dependent overproduction in the zona fasciculata of both aldosterone and hybrid steroids (18-hydroxycortisol and 18-oxocortisol) due to oxidation of cortisol (Figure 2). Hyperaldosteronism, hypokalemia, and hypertension are corrected by suppression of ACTH with dexamethasone. Although both suppres-

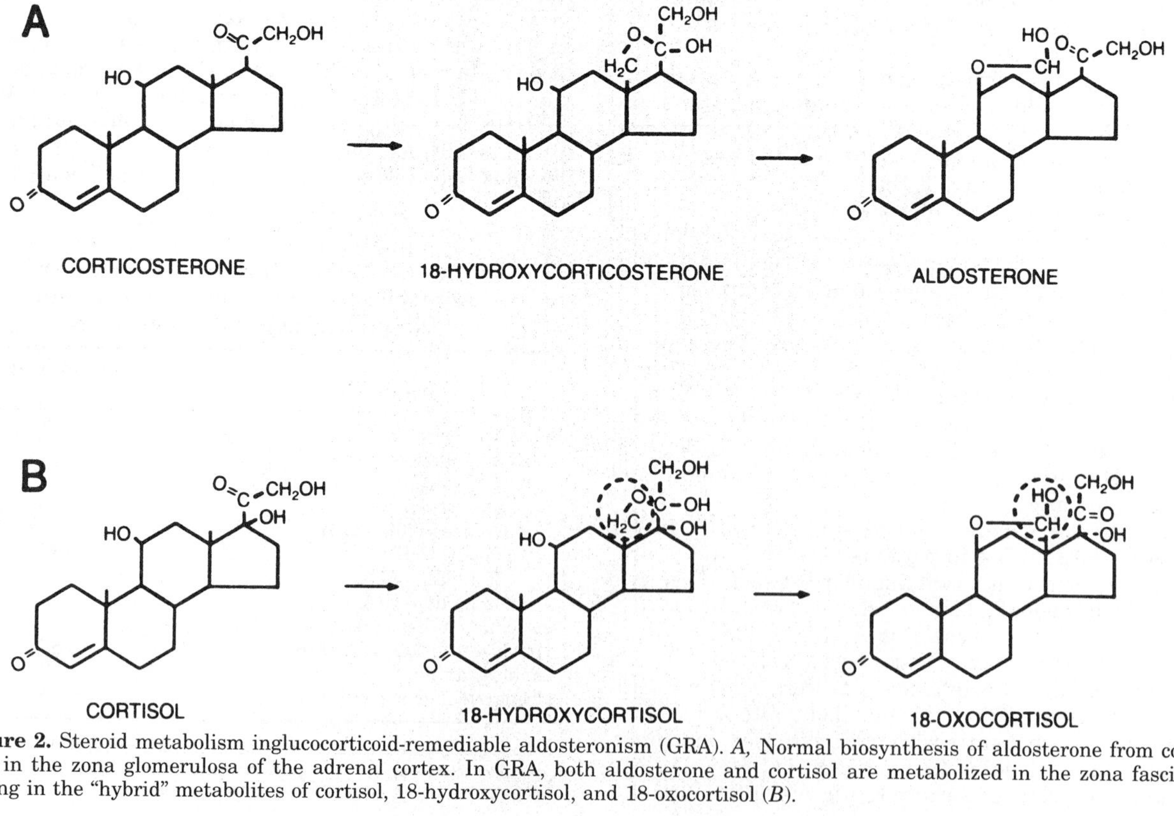

Figure 2. Steroid metabolism inglucocorticoid-remediable aldosteronism (GRA). *A,* Normal biosynthesis of aldosterone from corticosterone in the zona glomerulosa of the adrenal cortex. In GRA, both aldosterone and cortisol are metabolized in the zona fasciculata, resulting in the "hybrid" metabolites of cortisol, 18-hydroxycortisol, and 18-oxocortisol (*B*).

sion of aldosterone secretion with glucocorticoids and familial aggregation have also been reported in patients with APA, this is distinctly unusual.

A diagnosis of GRA may be established in the proband with primary aldosteronism and in family members with biochemical or genetic markers. Urine excretion of 18-hydroxycortisol and 18-oxocortisol is characteristically elevated to 20 to 30 times above normal. Although excretion of these steroids may also be increased in patients with APA, the ratio of urinary excretion of tetrahydro metabolites of these steroids to aldosterone is rarely greater than 1.0 in patients with APA, whereas it exceeds 2.0 in patients with GRA. Direct genetic testing may become a more practical approach than these steroid measurements both for identifying this inherited form of primary aldosteronism and for subsequent screening of family members. The chimeric genes causing GRA can be detected by hybridization to Southern blots of genomic DNA, or they can be specifically amplified with the polymerase chain reaction.

TREATMENT

Appropriate therapy depends on the cause of primary aldosteronism (Table 3). The preferred therapy for patients with APA is unilateral adrenalectomy (either via a flank incision or using a laparoscopic approach), although medical therapy may be indicated for patients who are poor surgical candidates and for patients with bilateral APA (approximately 6% of patients with APA). Adrenal surgery may also be recommended for patients with renin-responsive adenomas and for patients with unilateral nodular hyperplasia.

Laparoscopic adrenalectomy has the potential of shortening the hospital stay, particularly if performed by a surgeon experienced with both adrenal surgical procedures and laparoscopic techniques. Adrenalectomy is curative in 40 to 70% of patients; however, even among "cured" patients, hypertension may persist for several months after surgery. The cure rate in response to unilateral adrenalectomy is higher in younger patients (younger than 50 years) and lower in patients who have either multiple ade-

TABLE 3. **Treatment of Primary Aldosteronism**

Type	Percentage of Cases	Primary Therapy
Common		
APA	60–70	Surgical
Bilateral adrenocortical hyperplasia (IHA)	20–30	Medical
Uncommon		
Unilateral adrenal hyperplasia (primary adrenocortical hyperplasia)	<1	Surgical
Aldosterone-producing renin-responsive adenoma	<1	Surgical/medical
Glucocorticoid-suppressible hyperaldosteronism	<1	Medical
Aldosterone-producing adrenocortical carcinoma	<1	Surgical/medical
Ectopic: ovarian arrhenoblastoma	<1	Surgical

nomas or coexistent macronodules or micronodular hyperplasia in addition to an adenoma in the same gland.

Preoperative management should include correction of hypertension and potassium repletion with the aldosterone antagonist spironolactone (Aldactone), 200 to 400 mg per day, and cautious potassium supplementation, if necessary, for 1 to 2 months. Other metabolic abnormalities, including hypomagnesemia and diabetes, should be treated appropriately. Postoperative hypoaldosteronism, owing to suppression of the contralateral zona glomerulosa, may occur and persist for up to several months. This complication is recognized by hyperkalemia and orthostatic hypotension. Hyperkalemia may be treated with furosemide or thiazide diuretics; occasionally, short-term mineralocorticoid treatment with low doses of fludrocortisone may be required.

Medical therapy is recommended for IHA, because hypertension is cured by surgery, including bilateral adrenalectomy, in only 20% of patients. Potassium-retaining diuretics, either spironolactone or the renal sodium transport inhibitors amiloride (Midamor) and triamterene (Dyrenium), are the cornerstones of drug therapy both for patients with IHA and for patients with APA who are not surgical candidates. Spironolactone is a mineralocorticoid antagonist, whereas amiloride and triamterene are not. Potassium secretion in the distal tubule is linked to sodium reabsorption, and both amiloride and triamterene inhibit distal tubular sodium transport, independent of aldosterone. Both agents cause only modest increases in sodium excretion, but they significantly decrease high rates of potassium excretion.

Treatment with spironolactone may be initiated with relatively high doses (200 to 400 mg per day), and the dose may be reduced after blood pressure is controlled and hypokalemia is corrected. Twice-daily dosing is probably adequate. Similar doses are used in chronic treatment of APA and IHA, and in these disorders, hyperkalemia rarely if ever occurs. In addition to competitive binding to mineralocorticoid receptors, spironolactone exhibits potent antiandrogenic activity at the dihydrotestosterone receptor. This explains the side effects of gynecomastia, decreased libido, and impotence. The combination of spironolactone and a thiazide diuretic may provide better blood pressure control and allow lower doses of spironolactone and hence fewer side effects. Aspirin should be avoided, because it antagonizes the effect of spironolactone. Amiloride may be administered in a once-daily dose of 5 to 20 mg and is about 10 times more potent than triamterene. Both agents may be less effective than spironolactone in controlling hypertension, but they also have fewer side effects and are appropriate alternatives if side effects limit the use of spironolactone.

In the event that blood pressure cannot be adequately controlled with one of the potassium-retaining diuretics alone, a second drug should be added. A long-acting calcium entry blocker, such as nifedipine (Procardia XL, 30 to 90 mg per day) or amlodipine (Norvasc, 5 to 10 mg per day), should be considered. Stimulation of aldosterone biosynthesis is dependent on increases in intracellular calcium, and limited evidence suggests that nifedipine inhibits aldosterone production. Alternatively, in patients with IHA, an angiotensin-converting enzyme inhibitor might be added to the potassium-retaining diuretic. In contrast to most patients with APA, IHA patients have an enhanced aldosterone response to angiotensin II and consequently a greater hypotensive response to captopril.

Surgery is indicated for the treatment of aldosterone-producing adrenocortical carcinomas. Preoperative management is similar to that of patients with APA. Postoperatively, patients may be treated with the adrenolytic agent mitotane (o,p'-DDD). Mean survival for combined surgical resection and mitotane treatment is approximately 6 years, compared with 2 years for patients treated with mitotane alone and less than 1 year for those treated with surgery only. Survival of patients with untreated disease averages less than 3 months.

Patients with GRA usually respond poorly to conventional antihypertensive agents and should be treated with dexamethasone (0.5 to 2 mg per day). Generally, within 2 to 4 days of initiating therapy, aldosterone production is suppressed and PRA and plasma potassium levels increase into the normal ranges. Blood pressure also decreases, although this may require additional time. If hypertension is longstanding, it may not completely respond to glucocorticoids, and rare patients with GRA eventually become resistant to gluocorticoids. To avoid the side effects of higher steroid doses, potassium-retaining diuretics may be useful adjuncts.

HYPOPITUITARISM

method of
BAHA M. ARAFAH, M.D.

Case Western Reserve University School of Medicine and University Hospitals of Cleveland
Cleveland, Ohio

Hypopituitarism is a clinical disorder characterized by diminished secretion of some (partial hypopituitarism) or all (panhypopituitarism) of the hormones secreted by the anterior pituitary gland. Although less frequent, selected deficiency of a single pituitary hormone (monotropic hypopituitarism) can also occur. In most instances, loss of pituitary hormone secretion is a slow and progressive process, occurring over months or years and involving more than one hormonal axis. Often, patients present with several years' history of nonspecific complaints and remain compensated until they experience a major illness, infection, accident, or trauma. Any stressful experience can result in clinical decompensation and the need for urgent medical attention. Occasionally, hypopituitarism develops acutely, leading to a rapid onset of symptoms, as is often seen in patients with pituitary tumor apoplexy.

Hypopituitarism has been considered a permanent and irreversible process that requires lifelong hormone replacement therapy. Although this may be the case in some instances, studies have documented that recovery of pituitary function can be demonstrated in a significant number of patients with hypopituitarism. Furthermore, reversibility of various functional forms of hypopituitarism has been demonstrated repeatedly. For example, recovery of gonadal function after medical or surgical treatment of hyperprolactinemia has been demonstrated.

DIAGNOSIS

Dynamic pituitary hormone testing has been a valuable tool in defining the pathophysiologic mechanisms involved in the development of hypopituitarism. Although dynamic studies are useful in documenting hypopituitarism and demonstrating pituitary hormone reserve, they should be interpreted along with other clinical and/or neuroimaging studies. In some instances, dynamic studies may provide an approximation of the functional reserve of the pituitary gland rather than the site of injury causing impaired hormone secretion. A thorough understanding of the physiology of pituitary hormone secretion and appropriate correlation with additional anatomic and clinical data are essential in the interpretation of dynamic studies.

Although the diagnosis of hypopituitarism can often be made by measurements of basal hormone levels, dynamic studies are sometimes needed for confirmation. Both the target gland hormone product and the pituitary hormone in question should be measured simultaneously to assess the appropriateness of serum values. Each axis should be assessed in patients suspected of having partial or complete loss of pituitary function. The following is a summary of the approach in establishing the diagnosis of hypopituitarism. Evaluation of the function of each axis is presented separately.

Thyroid-Stimulating Hormone (TSH) Secretion. This can be evaluated by measurements of serum thyroxine (total or free) and TSH levels. Deficiency of TSH results in a low serum thyroxine level, associated with a normal or low serum TSH level as well as clinical hypothyroidism.

Corticotropin (Adrenocorticotropic Hormone, ACTH) Function. Measurements of ACTH plasma levels are not helpful in establishing the diagnosis of hypopituitarism or secondary adrenal insufficiency. The levels are, however, useful in differentiating primary from secondary adrenal insufficiency in a patient whose adrenal function is already shown to be impaired. The diagnosis of adrenal insufficiency can be suspected in patients with clinical symptoms who also have low serum cortisol levels (<3 to 4 μg per dL) in the absence of exogenous glucocorticoid intake. In evaluating a single serum cortisol value, one needs to consider many of the known limitations influencing the level, such as the time of the day, degree of stress at the time of measurement, and any other associated illnesses. Patients with borderline serum cortisol levels may need further testing using insulin-induced hypoglycemia. In some instances, the cosyntropin (Cortrosyn) stimulation test is recommended as a screening study. The latter test evaluates adrenal responsiveness to exogenous, synthetic ACTH. Although the test is an excellent screening tool, it is often unreliable in excluding the diagnosis of secondary or tertiary forms of adrenal insufficiency that one would expect to see in patients with hypopituitarism. Many patients with documented ACTH deficiency have "normal" cortisol responses to exogenous ACTH. This is particularly true if the ACTH deficiency is recent in onset or if it is partial rather than complete.

The most reliable test for establishing the diagnosis of ACTH deficiency in patients with borderline serum cortisol levels is the assessment of cortisol or ACTH response to insulin-induced hypoglycemia (0.05 to 0.2 units of insulin per kg intravenously). This test represents the "gold standard" for establishing the diagnosis of adrenal insufficiency. The test should be performed in the presence of an experienced physician to minimize potential side effects. Prolonged hypoglycemia can be avoided if lower doses of insulin are given to patients strongly suspected of having deficiency of growth hormone or ACTH. In centers with experienced staffs and where patients are carefully screened and monitored, the test is rarely associated with complications. The test is generally contraindicated in elderly patients and those with coronary artery disease.

Gonodotropin Secretion. Clinical assessment of gonadal function, particularly in women, is valuable in the proper interpretation of biochemical tests. In a premenopausal, amenorrheic woman, measurements of serum gonadotropins (follicle-stimulating hormone [FSH] and luteinizing hormone [LH]) and estradiol levels can be helpful in establishing the diagnosis of hypogonadotropism. A clinical history of normal, regular menses almost always indicates normal gonadotropin function. In postmenopausal women, in whom serum gonadotropin levels are expected to be high, measurements of the serum FSH and LH levels, in the absence of exogenous estrogen intake, help confirm the diagnosis of impaired gonadotropin function. In men, the simultaneous determination of testosterone and gonadotropin serum levels can establish the diagnosis.

Growth Hormone (GH) Secretion. A single determination of serum GH level is of no clinical significance. Measurements of serum GH levels during insulin-induced hypoglycemia or after an infusion of arginine are the most reliable tests to assess GH secretion. With few exceptions, measurement of plasma levels of insulin-like growth factor I (previously known as somatomedin C) is a reasonably reliable method for the rapid assessment of GH secretion.

Prolactin Secretion. Measurements of basal prolactin levels, on more than one occasion, are often adequate to assess secretion of this lactogenic hormone.

Antidiuretic Hormone (ADH) Secretion. ADH deficiency occurs when the neurosecretory cells of the hypothalamus (supraoptic and paraventricular nuclei) are damaged. Patients with hypopituitarism rarely have ADH deficiency, unless they have hypothalamic disease. Loss of ADH secretion can lead to excessive free water excretion by the kidneys and the clinical diagnosis of diabetes insipidus (DI). Patients with DI have increased free water loss by the kidneys, resulting in dilute urine despite an associated increase in serum sodium concentration and osmolality. Patients with complete loss of ADH secretion (total DI) can lose several liters of water a day in the urine and, in the absence of adequate water intake, may become dehydrated. Diagnosis of DI is established by the presence of dilute urine (low osmolality) despite hypernatremia and/or increased serum osmolality. The diagnosis can be confirmed by measurement of serum ADH levels, although this is not necessary. Instead, one can determine the response to the administration of exogenous ADH or one of its analogues (e.g., desmopressin [DDAVP]). The latter test differentiates patients with central DI, in whom a drop in urinary volume is promptly noted, from those with nephrogenic DI, in whom no such response is expected.

PATHOPHYSIOLOGY

Consideration of the physiology of normal pituitary hormone secretion and its dependence on hypothalamic regulation indicates that at least three different mechanisms can lead to the development of hypopituitarism. Although there are specific examples that apply to each of the three mechanisms, it is important to point out that in most patients, more than one mechanism contributes to the development of hypopituitarism. In each instance, there is often a predominant mechanism that dictates not only the degree of impairment but also whether the process is potentially reversible. Postulated mechanisms include

1. Diminished release and/or secretion of hypothalamic hormone(s). This can be congenital (e.g., gonadotropin-releasing hormone [GnRH] deficiency in Kallmann's syndrome) or acquired as a result of primary or metastatic tumors, inflammation, infection, mass lesions, or ischemia.

2. Interruption of the delivery of hypothalamic hormones to the anterior pituitary. This is commonly seen as a result of parasellar mass lesions such as craniopharyngioma, meningioma, pituitary tumor, and aneurysm. Hypopituitarism in these instances can occur as a result of mechanical compression of the pituitary stalk and portal vessels. In addition, inadvertent damage, injury, or transection of the pituitary stalk can occur intraoperatively and lead to hypopituitarism.

3. Loss or destruction of hormone-producing cells of the pituitary gland. This can occur as a result of an ischemic event (e.g., Sheehan's syndrome), inflammation (lymphocytic hypophysitis), or infiltrative diseases (amyloidosis, hemochromatosis, metastatic cancer) and in response to an expanding pituitary mass lesion such as an adenoma.

CLINICAL MANIFESTATIONS

The clinical manifestations of hypopituitarism are diverse and variable, depending to a large degree on the extent and duration of pituitary hormone deficits. In addition to the signs and symptoms of specific hormone deficits, patients often present with symptoms and signs related to the cause of hypopituitarism. The clinical manifestations in patients presenting with hypopituitarism can therefore be divided into two categories: signs and symptoms of hormone deficits (Table 1) and signs and symptoms related to the etiology of hypopituitarism. Such latter symptoms include headaches and visual disturbances in patients with perisellar mass lesions, as would be expected in patients with pituitary macroadenomas, meningiomas, or craniopharyngiomas. Patients with functioning pituitary adenomas also have clinical manifestations related to and caused by excessive hormone secretion (e.g., signs of acromegaly in a patient with a GH-secreting adenoma presenting with hypopituitarism). Such a patient has signs of hormone excess from the functioning tumor (acromegaly) and signs and symptoms of loss of normal pituitary function, in addition to possible mechanical symptoms such as headache and visual disturbances.

Occasionally, hemorrhage and necrosis (i.e., pituitary tumor apoplexy) are the first reported clinical manifestations of a previously undiagnosed pituitary mass. In this instance, hypopituitarism develops acutely after hemorrhagic infarction of the tumor and often contributes to the associated morbidity of this syndrome.

PRACTICAL MANAGEMENT

Understanding the pathophysiology of hypopituitarism and recognizing the probability for recovery of function are important issues to be emphasized in the management of patients with this disease.

TABLE 1. **Symptoms and Signs of Hypopituitarism**

Axis Deficit	Symptoms	Signs
ACTH	Tiredness; fatigue; low energy, especially in PM; nausea; weight loss	Pale skin, loss of pubic and axillary hair (women)
FSH/LH	In men, loss of libido and potency, infertility, and hot flashes; in women, amenorrhea, hot flashes, dyspareunia, and infertility	In men, loss of facial or body hair, gynecomastia, increased body fat, soft or small testes; in women, vaginal atrophy or dryness
GH	Short stature in children; nonspecific symptoms in adults	Short stature, increased body fat in children; ? increased body fat, ? decreased muscle mass in adults
Prolactin	Absence of lactation in women; no symptoms in men	None
TSH	Cold intolerance, tiredness, slow mentation, constipation, weight gain	Pale, waxy, dry skin; delayed relaxation of tendon reflexes

Patients' education is an essential aspect of the management that is often overlooked. Patients need to understand the impact of pituitary hormone deficiency on their daily lives and activities and must be fully aware that treatment may need to be modified in the event of intercurrent illnesses, accidents, or surgical procedures. Patients should wear Medic Alert bracelets or necklaces identifying them as having hypopituitarism or receiving replacement glucocorticoid therapy. Each patient should, in addition, carry a card providing the diagnosis, list of medications, and name and telephone number of the treating physician. Management of patients with hypopituitarism starts with suspecting the diagnosis and determining the extent of pituitary hormone deficit. The managing physician should appreciate the variable clinical manifestations of the disease and the possible occurrence of other associated neuroendocrine, neurologic, and neuro-ophthalmic signs and symptoms.

HORMONE REPLACEMENT

Hormone replacement should be initiated as soon as the diagnosis of hypopituitarism is made. This is especially true for glucocorticoid replacement, in which a delay in treatment can be life-threatening. Treatment should not be rigid but should always be individualized, taking into consideration the patient's age, sex, education, original disease process, and clinical history. Theoretically, one can provide the deficient hypothalamic or pituitary hormone, which in turn can stimulate other hormones in the periphery and result in clinical benefit. Although this approach may be applicable in certain instances, it is impractical in others. For instance, a patient with central hypothyroidism responds to the administration of thyrotropin-releasing hormone if the cause of hypothyroidism is hypothalamic deficiency and to TSH injections if his or her disease involves the pituitary. Neither approach is as practical as the oral administration of levothyroxine. The same argument can be made for ACTH deficiency, for which oral glucocorticoid therapy is the appropriate choice. The use of hypothalamic hormones in the management of patients with various forms of hypopituitarism has been limited primarily to those with GnRH deficiency. Some patients with GH deficiency secondary to growth hormone–releasing hormone (GHRH) deficiency were similarly treated with the hypothalamic hormone, with reasonable success.

CORTICOTROPIN DEFICIENCY

Either hydrocortisone (cortisol) or cortisone in two or preferably three divided doses, totaling 15 to 30 mg of the former steroid, is the usual glucocorticoid replacement therapy. The dose is titrated individually, using primarily clinical symptoms as a guideline. Measurement of serum or urinary hormone levels is of no clinical value in determining the proper dose unless poor gastrointestinal absorption or poor compliance with drug intake is suspected. In my experience, the vast majority of patients require 20 mg of hydrocortisone or less per day to control symptoms. Although hyponatremia is sometimes seen in patients with ACTH deficiency, mineralocorticoid replacement is rarely, if ever, necessary in patients with hypopituitarism, because the function of the adrenal glomerular zone is maintained. Serum sodium levels return to normal a few days after hydrocortisone therapy is initiated.

THYROID-STIMULATING DEFICIENCY

Levothyroxine (Synthroid) therapy is the preferred replacement therapy in patients with TSH deficiency. Although measurement of total thyroxine and free thyroxine index serum levels is sometimes helpful in determining the optimal dose of levothyroxine in these patients, physicians should rely primarily on clinical signs and symptoms before adjustments are made. In contrast to patients with primary hypothyroidism, in whom serum TSH measurements are used to titrate the dose of thyroid hormone replacement, similar determinations in patients with TSH deficiency are of no value and need not be performed. The optimal dose of thyroxine is variable (0.05 to 0.20 mg per day) and depends on the patients' age, other illnesses, and concurrent medications. It is important to point out that thyroxine replacement therapy in hypopituitary patients can unmask signs of ACTH deficiency that may have been unrecognized previously. Symptomatic patients should be tested and treated appropriately.

DEFICIENCY OF FOLLICLE-STIMULATING HORMONE AND LUTEINIZING HORMONE

Effective treatment of hypogonadism in postpubertal adults can be achieved by giving gonadal steroid replacement. Delay in the treatment of men and women with documented hypogonadism increases the risk for osteoporosis and heart disease. Treatment of such patients is usually oral estrogen with progestin for women and long-acting testosterone for men. Oral equine estrogen preparations are the most widely used form of gonadal steroid replacement in women. The average dose of equine estrogen (Premarin) is 0.625 mg every day. Younger women and those taking antiseizure medications require higher doses of estrogen to provide clinical benefit. Women with intact uteri also need a progestational agent to minimize the development of estrogen-induced endometrial hyperplasia. The latter can be given orally as medroxyprogesterone acetate (Provera) every day (2.5 to 5 mg) or for 12 days of each month. Intermittent spotting often occurs initially in patients using combined daily therapy with estrogen and Provera. This is often followed by the development of amenorrhea, with minimal risk for endometrial cancer. In contrast, women given Provera for 12 days of the month are likely to have a monthly menstrual bleed. Women receiving estrogen replacement therapy should have annual mammograms and Pap smears and should also be educated about routine breast self-examination.

Testosterone therapy in men is often superphysiologic when given in the currently prescribed doses of 200 to 300 mg every 2 to 3 weeks. Such doses provide superphysiologic concentrations of gonadal steroids and are likely to be associated with side effects. A common yet frequently overlooked complication of testosterone therapy is hyperlipidemia, which can increase the risk for cardiovascular disease. Symptoms of prostatism and progression of previously unrecognized prostate cancer can occur with testosterone therapy. For these reasons, particular attention should be paid to any potential abnormalities in the prostate before and during androgen therapy. Similarly, attention should be directed at potential alterations in plasma lipids in treated patients. Excessive snoring and even obstructive sleep apnea can occur after androgen replacement, especially in obese men. Every effort should therefore be made to give the lowest possible dose to minimize these and other potential side effects. In my experience, most men can be adequately replaced with 120 to 150 mg of testosterone enanthate (Delatestryl) or testosterone cypionate (Depotest) intramuscularly every 2 weeks. Testosterone skin patches (Testoderm) that can be applied directly on the scrotum were introduced for clinical use a few years ago. These preparations have been reported to provide a stable and physiologic serum testosterone concentration throughout the day. However, with the increased activity of the enzyme 5α-reductase in the scrotum, higher circulating serum levels of dihydrotestosterone were noted in such patients. These changes have caused some concern among physicians. A more recently introduced preparation of transdermal testosterone, Androderm, appears to be more practical to use, as it can be applied on other areas of the body, such as the thighs and back. When used at the recommended dose of 5 mg per day, these preparations provide stable serum testosterone and dihydrotestosterone levels throughout a 24-hour period. Although these preparations appear to provide testosterone replacement in physiologic doses, there are currently no long-term studies addressing their use, particularly in comparison with other approaches.

Loss of libido is a common symptom in women with hypopituitarism, as a result of diminished adrenal androgen production. Small doses of androgens in the form of parenteral testosterone (15 to 25 mg intramuscularly every 2 weeks) can be used to restore libido in such patients, under strict and careful follow-up.

Male patients desiring the restoration of fertility require a different approach that aims at stimulating intratesticular, endogenous testosterone production using human chorionic gonadotropin (hCG) (A.P.L.). The latter hormone is similar in structure to LH and, at the recommended doses (600 to 1000 units intramuscularly three times per week), can stimulate testosterone secretion by the testes and support spermatogenesis. Often, however, human menopausal gonadotropin (hMG) (menotropins [Pergonal]) also must be used in most of these patients to restore spermatogenesis. This preparation contains equal amounts of human FSH and LH isolated from menopausal women. In many patients in whom the hypogonadism is of recent onset, hCG alone is sufficient to restore fertility. Patients with more prolonged hypogonadism require both hCG and hMG injections to restore fertility.

In both male and female patients in whom the cause of hypopituitarism is a hypothalamic disease process (e.g., Kallmann's syndrome or a hypothalamic disease), the administration of the hypothalamic releasing hormone GnRH can be more effective in restoring fertility and gonadal function. The hypothalamic hormone has to be injected in a pulsatile manner through a portable implantable pump designed to mimic the natural rhythm of GnRH secretion.

GROWTH HORMONE DEFICIENCY

Treatment of GH deficiency is essential in children with documented deficiencies. The availability of synthetic GH has significantly increased its clinical use in children as well as in adults. Although there is extensive experience in the treatment of GH deficiency in children, only limited data are available in adults. Studies have demonstrated the beneficial effects of GH treatment in elderly patients with deficiency. An increase in lean body mass and a decrease in body fat were shown during short-term therapy with exogenous GH. The available studies are primarily short term and should therefore be viewed with caution. An additional issue of concern is the cost of prolonged treatment with GH in adults. It is not clear whether persistent, untreated states of GH deficiency in adults have any impact on the long-term morbidity of patients with hypopituitarism, as has been suggested. If this is confirmed, and if treatment can be given without significant side effects, GH can be offered to all patients with deficits, regardless of age. Additional studies are necessary before a firm recommendation can be given. Treatment of GH deficiency in adults is now approved by the Food and Drug Administration. The drug should be prescribed only after adequate documentation of GH deficiency. Side effects can be minimized by using small doses (4 to 6 μg per kg) and by monitoring plasma levels of insulin-like growth factor I. The goal is to keep these plasma levels in the low- to mid-normal range.

The potential for recovery of pituitary function should always be considered, because it can prevent the unnecessary use of lifelong hormone replacement therapy. This is becoming particularly important in view of data suggesting increased morbidity in treated as well as untreated patients with hypopituitarism. The cause or causes of increased morbidity and mortality in treated patients are not known. It is reasonable to speculate that overtreatment with gonadal steroids, glucocorticoids, and/or thyroid hormone contributes to the increased morbidity. Some reports, however, have implicated persistence of GH deficiency in these patients as a potential cause. Until more firm data are available, treatment with GH should be considered experimental and should be given under specific research protocols. Furthermore, patients with permanent hypopituitarism should be followed regularly, and their hormone replacement doses should be adjusted, as necessary, to avoid overtreatment.

HYPERPROLACTINEMIA

method of
MARK E. MOLITCH, M.D.
Northwestern University Medical School
Chicago, Illinois

PRETREATMENT EVALUATION

Hyperprolactinemia is commonly found, and prolactinoma, one of the major causes of hyperprolactinemia, is the most common of the hormone-secreting pituitary tumors.

Manifestations of Hyperprolactinemia

The presence of even minute amounts of milk expressible from one or both breasts justifies the diagnosis of galactorrhea. Its persistence for more than 1 year after normal delivery and cessation of breast-feeding or its occurrence in the absence of pregnancy is generally considered inappropriate lactation. Galactorrhea may be present in about 5 to 10% of normally menstruating women, and basal prolactin (PRL) levels are abnormal in about 10% of such women.

Hyperprolactinemia suppresses the pulsatile secretion of gonadotropin-releasing hormone and consequent secretion of the gonadotropins. About 10% of women with amenorrhea alone and 75% of women with galactorrhea–oligomenorrhea or amenorrhea are found to have hyperprolactinemia.

Infertility may also be a presenting symptom of patients with hyperprolactinemia and is invariable when gonadotropin levels are suppressed with anovulation. Of women presenting with infertility, 10 to 20% are found to have hyperprolactinemia; many of these women are also found to have oligomenorrhea or amenorrhea, often associated with galactorrhea.

Chronic hyperprolactinemia in males results in decreased testosterone levels, causing impotence and decreased libido in more than 90% of cases. Galactorrhea in men has been reported in 10 to 20% of cases and is virtually pathognomonic of a prolactinoma. Testosterone therapy of hyperprolactinemic men does not usually correct the impotence until PRL levels are brought down to normal.

Hyperprolactinemic hypogonadal patients have a decreased bone mineral density, and correction of the hyperprolactinemia usually results in an increase in bone mass. Hyperprolactinemic women who are not amenorrheic and hypoestrogenemic have normal bone mineral density.

PRL-secreting macroadenomas (>10 mm in diameter) may also cause mass effects such as hypopituitarism, visual field disturbance, and cranial nerve palsies, depending on the extrasellar extent of the tumor.

Diagnostic Evaluation

Because PRL is secreted episodically, when levels are borderline several samples may need to be obtained to determine whether sustained hyperprolactinemia exists. A number of conditions and medications can cause hyperprolactinemia (Table 1). Most of these disorders can be ruled

TABLE 1. **Differential Diagnosis of Hyperprolactinemia**

Pituitary disease	Other
Prolactinomas	Pregnancy
Acromegaly	Hypothyroidism
Empty-sella syndrome	Renal failure
Lymphocytic	Cirrhosis
hypophysitis	Pseudocyesis
Cushing's disease	
Pituitary stalk section	Medications
	Phenothiazines
Hypothalamic disease	Butyrophenones
Craniopharyngioma	Monoamine oxidase inhibitors
Meningioma	Tricyclic antidepressants
Dysgerminoma	Reserpine
Clinically nonfunctioning	Methyldopa
pituitary adenoma	Metoclopramide
Other tumors	Amoxapine
Sarcoidosis	Verapamil
Eosinophilic granuloma	Cocaine
Neuraxis irradiation	
Vascular	Idiopathic
Neurogenic	
Chest wall lesions	
Spinal cord lesions	
Breast stimulation	

out on the basis of a careful history and physical examination and routine chemistry and thyroid blood tests. The most difficult distinctions are in the differentiation between hypothalamic and pituitary diseases. Stimulation and suppression tests with thyrotropin-releasing hormone, hypoglycemia, L-dopa, and so forth give nonspecific results and are not useful in evaluating patients. The basal PRL level suffices. Levels less than 250 ng per mL can be due to any cause. Levels greater than 250 ng per mL are seen only in patients with prolactinomas or in patients with renal failure.

When there is no obvious cause of the hyperprolactinemia from the routine screening, a radiologic evaluation of the hypothalamic-pituitary area is mandatory to exclude a mass lesion. *This includes patients with even mild PRL elevations.* Magnetic resonance imaging (MRI) with gadolinium enhancement delineates structures in the cavernous sinus, vascular structures, and optic chiasm much better than does computed tomography (CT) with intravenous contrast enhancement. It is important to distinguish between a large nonsecreting tumor causing modest PRL elevations (usually <250 ng per mL) from a PRL-secreting macroadenoma (PRL levels usually > 250 ng per mL), as the therapy is quite different. One potential additional problem in investigating patients with mild hyperprolactinemia is a false-positive CT or MRI scan. Because these techniques are now able to detect incidental nonsecreting tumors, cysts, infarcts, and so forth, the finding of a "microprolactinoma" on a scan in a patient with elevated PRL levels may not always be a true-positive finding.

Patients found to have macroadenomas, hypothalamic disease, or empty sellas should have an evaluation of the sufficiency of their other anterior and posterior pituitary hormones. My policy has been to perform visual field testing only in patients whose tumors are adjacent to or pressing on the optic chiasm, as visualized by MRI.

TREATMENT

Idiopathic Hyperprolactinemia

Women in the idiopathic hyperprolactinemia category may require treatment because they wish to decrease troublesome galactorrhea, resume normal cycling, restore libido and normal estrogen status, or become pregnant. In the woman with menses and without bothersome galactorrhea, reassurance may be all that is necessary. In the amenorrheic woman with estrogen deficiency, with its risk of osteoporosis, treatment consists of either lowering PRL levels with a dopamine agonist or estrogen-progestogen replacement. The latter has not been shown to cause the appearance of a tumor. When fertility is an issue, bromocriptine is necessary. With all forms of treatment and also just observation, PRL levels must be monitored to discover that uncertain proportion of patients who ultimately will prove to have a tumor.

Bromocriptine (Parlodel) is the usual dopamine agonist used for treatment, as it has the most extensive safety and efficacy profile, especially for women who desire fertility. Dopamine agonists restore normal ovulatory cycles in about 85% of patients and reduce galactorrhea in more than 90%. Limiting nausea and vomiting occur in 3 to 5% of patients, and digital vasospasm, nasal congestion, and depression occur

in rare patients. Side effects can be minimized by starting with 1.25 mg daily with a snack at bedtime. The dose is gradually increased to 1.25 mg twice daily with meals over 7 to 10 days and PRL levels checked after 1 month; if PRL levels are not normal, the dose is gradually increased further. Most patients respond within 1 to 2 months if they are going to respond. Doses higher than 7.5 mg per day are usually not necessary except in some patients with extremely large tumors. Psychotic reactions and exacerbation of pre-existing schizophrenia have been reported rarely.

Bromocriptine can also be given intravaginally to reduce nausea. Similar reductions of PRL levels are achieved with oral and intravaginal administration of oral bromocriptine tablets, and the drug effect lasts for up to 24 hours with a single intravaginal dose, so once-daily administration is satisfactory.

Pergolide (Permax), another dopamine agonist, has been approved by the Food and Drug Administration (FDA) only for the treatment of Parkinson's disease, but there is considerable, well-documented experience with its use in prolactinoma patients. Hyperprolactinemia can be controlled with single daily doses of 50 to 150 μg, and pergolide is comparable to bromocriptine with respect to tolerance and efficacy. Some patients who do not respond to bromocriptine do so to pergolide and vice versa.

Cabergoline (Dostinex) is different from the other two dopamine agonists in that it has a long half-life and can be given orally once weekly. It is at least as good as if not better than bromocriptine and pergolide with respect to efficacy, and it generally causes substantially fewer side effects in doses of 0.5 to 3.0 mg weekly. At present it is approved by the FDA for the treatment of patients with all forms of hyperprolactinemia.

Prolactinomas

Observation

The indications for therapy in patients with prolactinomas may be divided into two categories: effects of tumor size and effects of hyperprolactinemia. In about 95% of patients, microprolactinomas do not enlarge during a 4- to 6-year period of observation. Thus, the simple argument that therapy is indicated for a microadenoma to prevent it from growing is fallacious. On the other hand, if a documented adenoma exists, it needs to be followed up closely to determine if it is growing. For this purpose, scanning initially at yearly intervals with CT or MRI in patients with microadenomas is carried out for 2 years. It is unlikely that a prolactinoma will grow significantly with no increase in serum PRL levels. Therefore, after perhaps one or two scans at most, most patients can just be followed up with serial PRL levels. If PRL levels rise, additional scanning is indicated. Certainly a microadenoma that is documented to be growing demands therapy for the size change alone, as it may be one of the 5% that will grow to be a macroadenoma.

In patients with macroadenomas, the tumors have already indicated a propensity to grow. Therefore, I am loath to just observe these unless there are specific contraindications to therapy. Local or diffuse invasion and compression of adjacent structures, such as the stalk or optic chiasm, are additional indications for therapy.

Other indications for therapy are relative, being due to the hyperprolactinemia itself. These include decreased libido, menstrual dysfunction, galactorrhea, infertility, hirsutism, impotence, and premature osteoporosis. In a woman with a microadenoma with normal menses and libido and galactorrhea that is not bothersome, there is no specific reason for therapy. The ability to monitor a patient closely with PRL levels, CT or MRI, and estimations of bone mineral density and rather precise estimates of the efficacy of various modes of therapy (see later) allows a highly individualized way of observing patients and choosing the proper timing and mode of therapy.

Surgery

Trans-sphenoidal surgery is the surgical procedure used for microadenomas and most macroadenomas. Rarely is craniotomy performed. In experienced neurosurgical hands, about 70 to 80% of patients with microadenomas and 25 to 30% with macroadenomas can have PRL levels normalized by surgery. In general, the larger the tumor, the lower the success rate. However, there is about a 20% recurrence rate of hyperprolactinemia, bringing the ultimate cure rate as low as 50 to 60% for microadenomas and 10 to 20% for macroadenomas. For virtually all these recurrences, the recurrence is that of hyperprolactinemia and not documented radiologic evidence of tumor regrowth.

Complications from trans-sphenoidal surgery are infrequent. The mortality rate for microadenomas is 0.27% and for macroadenomas is 0.95%, whereas the major morbidity rate for microadenomas is 0.4% and for macroadenomas is 6.5%. Transient diabetes insipidus is quite common with surgery for both micro- and macroadenomas, and permanent diabetes insipidus occurs in about 1% of patients after surgery for macroadenomas. Surgery involving craniotomy is much more hazardous.

Radiotherapy

Because of the excellent therapeutic responses to trans-sphenoidal surgery and medical therapy (see later), radiotherapy is generally not considered to be a primary mode of treatment for prolactinomas. Of patients treated only with radiotherapy, normal PRL levels are achieved in only 38% in 2 to 14 years. When radiotherapy is used alone after noncurative surgery, normalization of PRL levels occurs in only 11% of patients. The major side effect of radiotherapy is hypopituitarism, occurring in more than 50% of patients. Radiotherapy seems best reserved as adjunctive therapy for those patients with enlarging lesions who have not responded to either medical or surgical treatment.

Medical Therapy

BROMOCRIPTINE

Bromocriptine is able to normalize prolactin levels or effect return of ovulatory menses in 80 to 90% of patients. There is little interindividual variability in the absorption and peak blood levels of bromocriptine achieved, but there is considerable interindividual variability in sensitivity to the drug. As with patients with idiopathic hyperprolactinemia, the dose must be started low and gradually increased to reduce side effects. Some patients undergo resolution or reduction of hyperprolactinemia and maintain normal menses after cessation of bromocriptine therapy. In some cases this is associated with a reduction in microadenoma size. In most cases, however, bromocriptine needs to be continued to maintain PRL levels near normal with concomitant resolution of galactorrhea and amenorrhea or impotence. Such long-term therapy appears to be of no harm and of continued benefit.

Macroadenoma size reduction also occurs in response to bromocriptine, 77% of patients having some tumor size decrease. About 40 to 50% have a greater than 50% reduction in tumor size, 25 to 30% have a 25 to 50% reduction, 10 to 15% have a less than 25% reduction, and 10 to 20% have no evidence of any reduction in tumor size. The time course of tumor size reduction is variable. Some patients may experience an extremely rapid decrease in tumor size, significant changes in visual fields being noted within 24 to 72 hours and significant changes noted on scans within 2 weeks. In others, little change may be noted at 6 weeks, but scanning again at 6 months may show significant changes. A progressive decrease is often noted over several years. Visual fields may be expected to improve in 80 to 90% of patients with significant visual field abnormalities.

The extent of tumor size reduction does not correlate with basal PRL levels, nadir PRL levels achieved, the percentage fall in PRL, or whether PRL levels reached normal. Some patients have excellent reduction of PRL levels to normal but only modest changes in tumor size, whereas others have persistent hyperprolactinemia (although >75% suppression from basal values) with almost complete disappearance of tumor. A reduction in PRL levels always precedes any detectable change in tumor size, and PRL nonresponders are also tumor size nonresponders. Once maximal size reduction is achieved, one can often gradually reduce the dose of bromocriptine, following PRL levels and discontinuing the drug only if there are no increases in PRL levels or tumor size on just 2.5 mg per day. Although some tumors expand rapidly when bromocriptine is discontinued in a patient with a macroadenoma that has become reduced in size, this is not usually the case with long-term therapy. About 10 to 20% of patients can maintain normal PRL levels after stopping treatment, and 70 to 80% with marked tumor size reduction do not experience tumor re-expansion with stopping of therapy.

Reduction in tumor size may also cause improvement in other pituitary functions. Normalization of testosterone levels may not occur for 6 to 12 months, however. When the prolactinoma is present prepubertally, improved pituitary function allows resumption of normal growth and pubertal development.

One problem of concern is the tumor that initially shrinks in response to bromocriptine and then enlarges. This is usually due to noncompliance, which is further worsened by the tendency for the patient and physician to resume the full dose instead of gradually restarting. This tends to make side effects worse, further exacerbating the noncompliance. Although extremely rare, tumors that continue to enlarge while being treated with bromocriptine may turn out to be carcinomas.

OTHER DOPAMINE AGONISTS

Pergolide and cabergoline show similar efficacy in reducing tumor size. However, cabergoline tends to be be better tolerated, and its infrequent dosing schedule facilitates compliance.

ESTROGEN REPLACEMENT THERAPY

A limited amount of evidence suggests that estrogen replacement therapy may correct the estrogen deficiency in patients with adenomas without stimulating tumor growth. However, it would be prudent to monitor PRL levels carefully in patients receiving estrogens alone, especially those with macroadenomas, to detect the rare patient who may have an estrogen-responsive tumor that may enlarge.

Recommendations

Medical therapy with dopamine agonists has high efficacy and tolerability and appears to be the primary treatment of choice for prolactinoma. This is particularly true for macroadenomas, in which dopamine agonists usually cause appreciable tumor shrinkage along with normalization of PRL levels, whereas surgery rarely offers a cure.

PREGNANCY

Effects of Bromocriptine on the Developing Fetus

As a general principle, it is advised that fetal exposure to bromocriptine be limited to as short a period as possible. Mechanical contraception should be used after therapy is begun until the first two to three cycles have occurred, so that an intermenstrual interval can be established and a woman will know when she has missed a menstrual period. Thus, bromocriptine can be stopped after having been given for only about 3 to 4 weeks of the gestation. When used in this fashion, bromocriptine has not been found to cause any increase in spontaneous abortions, ectopic pregnancies, trophoblastic disease, multiple pregnancies, or congenital malformations. Long-term follow-up studies of children whose mothers took bromocriptine in this fashion have shown no ill effects.

Limited evidence suggests that cabergoline may have a similar safety profile.

Effect of Pregnancy on Prolactinoma Size

Estrogens have a marked stimulatory effect on PRL synthesis and secretion, and the hormonal milieu of pregnancy can stimulate lactotroph cell hyperplasia and prolactinoma growth. However, review of data for women who became pregnant shows that the risk of significant, symptomatic enlargement of microadenomas is only 1.6% and that of macroadenomas is 15.5%. In comparison, in women with macroadenomas treated with prior surgery and/or irradiation, the risk of significant tumor enlargement is only 4.3%. About 25 to 50% of the patients with symptomatic tumor enlargement required surgery before it was known that bromocriptine could reduce tumor size. Bromocriptine has been used successfully during pregnancy to reduce symptomatic tumor enlargement in a number of cases. No ill effects on the infant were observed in these cases. The use of prophylactic bromocriptine throughout the pregnancy likely prevents tumor regrowth during the pregnancy in most cases, but no formal studies have been carried out.

Recommendations for Management

For the hyperprolactinemic woman with a microadenoma or a macroadenoma that is intrasellar or extends infrasellarly, bromocriptine is preferred as the primary treatment because of its efficacy in restoring ovulation and extremely low (1 to 5%) risk of clinically serious tumor enlargement. Bromocriptine is stopped when pregnancy is diagnosed, and the patient is carefully followed up throughout gestation. PRL levels do not always rise during pregnancy in women with prolactinomas, as they do in normal women. PRL levels may also not rise with tumor enlargement. Therefore, periodic checking of PRL levels is of no benefit. Because of the low incidence of tumor enlargement, routine, periodic visual field testing is not cost-effective. Visual field testing and scanning are performed only in patients who become symptomatic.

In a woman with a larger macroadenoma that may have suprasellar extension, there is a 15% risk of clinically serious tumor enlargement during pregnancy when only bromocriptine is used. There is no clearly best therapeutic approach, and this has to be a highly individualized decision that the patient has to make after a clear, documented discussion of the various therapeutic alternatives. One approach is just to use bromocriptine to allow ovulation, discontinue it when pregnancy is documented, and then observe the patient carefully for evidence of tumor growth. Prepregnancy trans-sphenoidal surgical debulking of the tumor greatly reduces but does not eliminate the risk of serious tumor enlargement. After surgical debulking, bromocriptine is required to restore normal PRL levels and allow ovulation.

A third approach, giving bromocriptine continuously throughout gestation, has been advocated. At this point, however, data regarding the effects of continuous bromocriptine therapy on the developing fetus are still quite meager, and such therapy cannot be recommended without reservation. Should pregnancy at an advanced stage be discovered in a woman taking bromocriptine, the data that exist are reassuring and would not justify therapeutic abortion. For patients with macroadenomas treated with bromocriptine alone or after surgery, careful follow-up with monthly visual field testing is warranted. Repeated scanning is reserved for patients with symptoms of tumor enlargement or evidence of a developing visual field defect, or both and should also be done routinely after delivery to detect asymptomatic tumor enlargement.

Should symptomatic tumor enlargement occur with any of these approaches, reinstitution of bromocriptine therapy is probably less harmful to the mother and child than surgery. Any type of surgery during pregnancy results in a 1.5-fold increase in fetal loss in the first trimester and a fivefold increase in fetal loss in the second trimester, although there is no risk of congenital malformations from such surgery. Thus, bromocriptine reinstitution would appear to be preferable to surgical decompression. However, such medical therapy must be closely monitored, and trans-sphenoidal surgery or delivery (if the pregnancy is far enough advanced) should be performed if there is no response to bromocriptine therapy and vision is progressively worsening.

HYPOTHYROIDISM

method of
INDER J. CHOPRA, M.D.
UCLA Center for the Health Sciences
Los Angeles, California

Hypothyroidism is a result of decreased availability of thyroid hormones to peripheral tissues. Rarely, it is due to resistance to intracellular action of thyroid hormones. The anatomic hallmark of hypothyroidism is the accumulation of hydrophilic glycosaminoglycans, primarily hyaluronic acid, and water in the interstitial tissue of virtually every organ system, leading to mucinous edema (myxedema). Hypothyroidism is insidious in onset and so slowly advancing that its symptoms and signs may be unrecognized or ignored for an extended period.

CAUSES OF HYPOTHYROIDISM

There are multiple causes of hypothyroidism (Table 1), and awareness of them is helpful in the evaluation of patients for hypothyroidism. Primary thyroid failure is a common disorder. Its prevalence has been estimated to approximate 0.8%. It is about seven times more common in women than in men. In patients older than 50 years, up to 10% may demonstrate elevated serum thyroid-stimulating hormone (TSH) levels. Chronic (Hashimoto's or lymphocytic or autoimmune) thyroiditis and spontaneous

TABLE 1. **Causes of Hypothyroidism**

1. Loss of functional thyroid tissue
   a. Idiopathic hypothyroidism: atrophy (probably autoimmune), TSH receptor–blocking antibodies
   b. Thyroiditis: chronic autoimmune (Hashimoto's disease), subacute, postpartum, treatment with cytokines or amiodarone, external irradiation
   c. After ^{131}I treatment
   d. After thyroidectomy
   e. Infiltrating disorders: malignancy, granulomatous disease
   f. Thyroid dysgenesis
2. Biosynthetic defects in thyroid hormone production
   a. Inherited defects in hormone synthesis
   b. Iodine deficiency
   c. Antithyroid agents: thionamides, lithium, iodide
3. Central hypothyroidism
   a. TSH deficiency due to pituitary disease: postpartum infarction, tumors, granulomatous disease (sarcoidosis), irradiation, idiopathic
   b. TRH deficiency due to hypothalamic disease: tumor (e.g., craniopharyngioma), irradiation, and transiently occurring in nonthyroidal illness
4. Peripheral resistance to thyroid hormones

Abbreviations: TSH, thyroid-stimulating hormone; TRH, thyrotropin-releasing hormone.

(idiopathic) thyroid atrophy are the most common causes of hypothyroidism, explaining almost 50% of cases. Iatrogenic hypothyroidism after treatment with radioactive iodine (e.g., for treatment of hyperthyroidism) or surgery (subtotal or total thyroidectomy for hyperthyroidism, thyroid nodules, or carcinoma) is the next most common cause of hypothyroidism, explaining about 30 to 40% of cases. After treatment of Graves' hyperthyroidism with radioiodine (^{131}I), hypothyroidism occurs in about 20% of patients in the first year and in an additional 3% of patients per year thereafter. After subtotal thyroidectomy for Grave's disease, hypothyroidism occurs in about 5 to 10% of patients within 1 year and in an additional 2% of patients per year thereafter. Drugs (antithyroid agents such as propylthiouracil or methimazole [Tapazole], lithium carbonate, iodide or iodine-containing agents like amiodarone [Cordarone]) are also important causes of hypothyroidism. Patients with underlying autoimmune thyroid disease are especially sensitive to iodide-induced inhibition of thyroid hormone synthesis, or the Wolff-Chaikoff effect, and thus are more susceptible to iodide-induced hypothyroidism than normal subjects. Antibodies directed against the TSH receptor may block thyroidal growth and stimulation by TSH; they have recently been implicated in the pathogenesis of hypothyroidism in autoimmune thyroid disease. This form of hypothyroidism may remit or may even be followed by hyperthyroidism when there is concurrence of an excess of thyroid-stimulating antibodies with TSH receptor–blocking antibodies.

Chronic (Hashimoto's) thyroiditis affects 3 to 5% of the U.S. population. Women are affected five to seven times more commonly than men. Typically, it is a progressive disease leading to permanent thyroid failure. There is a genetic predisposition to this disease. What precipitates the actual disease process is not known. Hashimoto's thyroiditis may present as a part of an autoimmune multiple endocrine deficiency syndrome that can also affect the adrenal glands (Addison's disease), parathyroid glands (hypoparathyroidism), pancreas (insulin-dependent diabetes mellitus), and vitamin B_{12} absorption (pernicious anemia).

In subacute thyroiditis and postpartum thyroiditis, hypothyroidism is usually transient, lasting a few weeks to months, and may follow a phase of hyperthyroidism. Hypothyroidism associated with postpartum thyroiditis may recur after subsequent pregnancies. Antithyroid antibodies are usually present in high titers in patients with postpartum thyroiditis but not in those with subacute thyroiditis.

Other thyroid causes of hypothyroidism listed in Table 1 are much less frequent in the United States than those mentioned previously. Worldwide, iodine deficiency remains the most common cause of hypothyroidism. Secondary (or tertiary) causes and peripheral resistance to the action of thyroid hormones are infrequent and explain hypothyroidism in only 1 to 2% of patients. Long-term treatment with lithium carbonate has been observed to cause hypothyroidism in up to 15% of patients in 5 years. These patients should be routinely monitored for hypothyroidism by measuring serum TSH levels every 6 months.

Generalized resistance to thyroid hormones (GRTH) is a rare disorder caused by mutation in one of the two alleles encoding the triiodothyronine (T_3) receptor (TRβ). The abnormal receptor not only binds T_3 poorly but also inhibits, in a dominant fashion, the function of the remaining normal receptor(s). GRTH is inherited, usually as an autosomal dominant disorder. Many patients manifest attention-deficit disorder or a learning disability. Some patients demonstrate tachycardia, suggesting that resistance to tissue effects of thyroid hormones varies among tissues. Treatment of GRTH is still unsatisfactory.

CLINICAL FEATURES

The clinical presentation of hypothyroidism varies with the age at onset, duration, and severity. Hypothyroidism occurs in 1 in 4000 newborns. Many of these newborns show few or no clinical signs of hypothyroidism, and diagnosis requires a routine neonatal screening and/or a high index of suspicion. When the disorder is severe, clinical features of congenital hypothyroidism include respiratory difficulties, cyanosis, persistent jaundice, poor feeding, a hoarse cry, umbilical hernia, and bone retardation. It is extremely important for optimal brain development that the diagnosis be made and treatment instituted as soon as possible. There is evidence that reduction in the intelligence quotient (IQ) is minimal if appropriate treatment is instituted before 3 months of age.

Thyroid hormone deficiency beginning early in infancy and in early childhood is characteristically associated with growth retardation (short stature and delayed bone maturation), mental deficiency, and delayed dentition. Growth retardation is treatable, but mental retardation can persist despite treatment with thyroid hormones. Adolescents with primary hypothyroidism may manifest, in addition to growth retardation, an enlarged sella turcica and rarely precocious puberty.

Clinical features of hypothyroidism in adult patients include lethargy, easy fatigability, diminished energy, dry skin, excessive loss of hair, muscle weakness, sleepiness, impaired memory, weight gain, increased pallor, diminished hearing acuity, paresthesia, and/or menometrorrhagia. In addition, myxedema may result in coarse features, periorbital edema, on enlarged tongue, hoarseness, carpal tunnel syndrome, pleuropericardial effusions, and heart failure. Elderly individuals often demonstrate emotional instability, delusions, hallucinations, and/or frank psychosis. Myxedema coma is a true emergency, and the mortality rate can be quite high (greater than 50%) despite treatment. Usual precipitating factors include some form of severe stress, including infection, trauma, and exposure to cold. The clinical presentation may include hypothermia (temperature as low as 24°C [75°F]); shock; hypoventilation and CO_2 narcosis; severe hyponatremia; and other features suggestive of inappropriate antidiuretic hormone syndrome.

Typical physical findings include absence of palpable thyroid tissue or a firmer than normal, diffusely enlarged thyroid (of chronic thyroiditis), bradycardia, pallor, and characteristic delayed relaxation of deep tendon reflexes.

LABORATORY DATA

Hypothyroidism is characteristically associated with a decreased concentration of serum total and free thyroxine (T_4). It is important to measure the free T_4 concentration (or free T_4 index), because the serum T_4 level may be low in the absence of hypothyroidism when serum binding of T_4 is reduced, as in patients with systemic nonthyroidal illness and those in whom the serum concentration of thyroxine-binding globulin (TBG) is reduced as a result of an inherited disorder, ingestion of some drugs (e.g., androgens), high-dose corticosteroid and asparaginase administration, or loss in urine (e.g., nephrotic syndrome). The serum total T_4 concentration may be normal in hypothyroid patients in whom the serum concentration of TBG is elevated as a result of the ingestion of some drugs (e.g., estrogen), pregnancy, hepatic disorder (e.g., chronic active hepatitis, biliary cirrhosis), acute intermittent porphyria, or an inherited disorder. The free T_4 concentration accurately reflects the thyroid status in all these conditions. I prefer to measure the free T_4 concentration by equilibrium dialysis and radioimmunoassay; cost-effective methods and assay kits are now available commercially for this measurement. Measurement of the free T_4 concentration by dialysis is preferable to the free T_4 index in patients with systemic illnesses; those taking drugs that markedly affect the serum binding of thyroid hormones; patients with inherited abnormalities in thyroid hormone binding (e.g., euthyroid hyperthyroxinemia); and those with thyroid hormone–binding antibodies in circulation. The serum total and free T_3 concentrations are decreased in a majority of hypothyroid patients but are within the normal range in about 15 to 20% of patients. The serum total and free T_3 concentrations are also subnormal in a variety of systemic illnesses, including hepatic and renal diseases. Therefore, low serum T_3 and/or free T_3 concentrations are not helpful in the diagnosis of hypothyroidism.

The serum TSH concentration is typically elevated in primary hypothyroidism. There are now available ultrasensitive immunoradiometric methods of TSH measurement that can easily detect 0.05 µU of TSH per mL or less and clearly differentiate among low, normal, and high values. A normal range of serum TSH in these assays approximates 0.35 to 4.7 µU per mL. An elevated serum TSH level and a low free T_4 level by dialysis are diagnostic of primary hypothyroidism. However, a mildly elevated serum TSH value of up to 15 to 20 µU per mL is transiently seen in some euthyroid patients with systemic illnesses, especially during their recovery phase, and in some acute psychiatric disorders. I prefer to wait about 2 to 3 weeks in these cases of mild TSH elevation and repeat free T_4 and TSH measurements before considering long-term treatment with thyroid hormones. The serum TSH level is low, normal, or mildly elevated in patients with secondary (or tertiary) hypothyroidism. Drugs such as metoclopramide (Reglan) and domperidone (Motilium)* increase the

---

*Investigational drug in the United States.

TSH level, whereas those such as dopamine, glucocorticoids, and somatostatin decrease the TSH level. The serum TSH response to thyrotropin-releasing hormone (TRH) is exaggerated in primary hypothyroidism, decreased (often absent) in secondary (pituitary) hypothyroidism, and normal with a delay in the peak response in tertiary (hypothalamic) hypothyroidism. The availability of ultrasensitive TSH assays has made TRH testing unnecessary or obsolete.

TREATMENT

The daily production rate of T_4 in normal humans approximates 100 µg, and that of T_3 approximates 30 µg. The majority (greater than 75%) of T_3 produced daily derives from conversion of T_4 to T_3 by the action of an enzyme, iodothyronine 5'-monodeiodinase type I (5'-MDI); 5'-MDI is most abundant in liver, followed by kidney and thyroid. 5'-MDI activity is decreased by certain drugs, e.g., oral cholecystography agents (ipodate), glucocorticoids, amiodarone, and propylthiouracil. Normal human thyroid contains little T_3 relative to T_4. The T_4/T_3 ratio in the normal thyroid approximates 15:1 to 20:1. Serum T_4 and T_3 levels in humans show little change in a day. The serum half-life of T_4 approximates 6 to 7 days; that of T_3 is about 1 day.

The treatment that most closely mimics the physiologic situation is administration of synthetic T_4 (levothyroxine [Synthroid, Levothroid, Eltroxin]). Once-daily ingestion of replacement doses of T_4 is associated with normal serum levels of both T_4 and T_3, and there is little ($\leq 20\%$), if any, fluctuation in their levels throughout the day. Absorption of T_4 from the gastrointestinal tract approximates 80 to 90%. The gastrointestinal absorption of T_4 remains essentially normal in systemic illnesses except in patients with severe diarrhea and after a major gut resection. These various considerations suggest that treatment with synthetic T_4 is the treatment of choice for hypothyroidism. The usual daily replacement dose of T_4 in adults is about 75 to 175 µg, approximating 1.6 µg per kg per day. The mean replacement dose of T_4 in an adult human is 0.12 mg per day. The requirement for thyroxine changes with age. It is higher in newborns, infants, and children than in adults, and it decreases with age: it may decrease as much as 50% at 80 years of age compared with the requirement at 20 years of age. The dose of T_4 in infants has been suggested to be 100 µg per m² per day. Alternatively, one may treat term neonates with a daily T_4 dose of 25 µg, and the dose may be increased gradually to 50 µg by 1 year of age. Doses up to 7 µg per kg of body weight have been necessary to achieve clinical euthyroidism in infants. The daily T_4 replacement dose in children is 100 µg per m² or 3 µg per kg of body weight. Some studies suggest that the levothyroxine content of generic preparations can vary considerably, sometimes by as much as 34 to 127% of the stated content.

The adequacy of treatment with T_4 is assessed by clinical examination, coupled with normalization of serum free T_4 and TSH levels. When equilibrium has been reached during replacement T_4 therapy, the serum TSH concentration is normal, the serum free T_4 concentration is high normal or slightly elevated, and the serum free T_3 concentration (or free T_3 index) approximates the mean normal value. Although the elevated serum TSH level of primary hypothyroidism falls steadily soon after T_4 treatment is initiated, it may not normalize for several weeks, sometimes as long as 8 to 12 weeks. Therefore, in the first several weeks of treatment I prefer to gauge the adequacy of T_4 treatment on the basis of serum free T_4 levels. It is, of course, necessary to determine the adequacy of treatment of secondary hypothyroidism on the basis of serum free T_4 levels; serum TSH measurement is not helpful in these patients. It is not necessary or appropriate to continue follow-up of serum T_3 levels during treatment with T_4. Follow-up should be based on serum TSH and serum free T_4 levels. I monitor patients receiving thyroid hormone replacement at 4- to 6-month intervals. In infants, serum TSH levels may not fall to normal despite treatment with adequate doses of T_4. This reflects immaturity of the central nervous system–hypothalamic–thyrotropic axis. Therefore, adequacy of treatment with T_4 in the first 1 to 2 years of life should be based mainly on clinical examination and on rendering serum free T_4 (and free T_3) concentrations to levels that are appropriate for the age of the child.

Thyroid Hormone Preparations Other Than Oral Thyroxine

Besides treatment with T_4, hypothyroidism may be treated with synthetic T_3 (liothyronine [Cytomel]). More than 90% of T_3 is absorbed after oral ingestion. However, T_3 is more expensive than T_4 and results in nonphysiologic levels of serum T_4 and T_3. Thus, the serum T_4 level is subnormal, whereas the serum T_3 level varies markedly during a day. The serum T_3 level during treatment with a replacement dose of T_3 (approximately 50 µg per day) is two to four times the upper limit of normal 2 to 4 hours after ingestion, whereas it is high-normal 24 hours after ingestion. A similar problem of peaking T_3 levels occurs after ingestion of preparations that contain mixtures of synthetic T_4 and T_3 (usually in a ratio of 4:1) (liotrix, Thyrolar, Euthroid) or preparations from animal thyroids (e.g., desiccated thyroid USP and Thyrar, from beef and pork thyroids, respectively, and Proloid from pork thyroglobulin). Animal thyroid preparations, such as desiccated thyroid USP, are not easily available now. The usual replacement dose of desiccated thyroid approximates 65 to 130 mg (1 to 2 grains) per day. The biologic activity of 100 µg of synthetic T_4 approximates that of 25 µg of liothyronine; 65 mg (1 grain) of desiccated thyroid USP, Thyrar, or Proloid; or 1 tablet of a mixture of 50 µg of synthetic T_4 plus 12.5 µg of synthetic T_3 (Thyrolar I or Euthroid I). Among the various thyroid preparations, synthetic T_4 and T_3 are available for parenteral use. They are often used in hypothyroid emergencies (myxedema coma) and in patients not able to swallow or absorb oral preparations of thyroid hormones. The replacement dose for intravenous T_4 is about 70 to 80% that of an oral preparation.

I do not recommend treatment of hypothyroidism with T_3 (liothyronine) except for a short period (about 4 weeks) in patients with thyroid cancer who have already undergone thyroidectomy and are being prepared for thyroid and total body radioiodine scanning. In my experience, symptoms of hyperthyroidism and cardiac aberrations (e.g., worsening of angina, tachyarrhythmias, and congestive heart failure) are more frequent during treatment with T_3 than during treatment with T_4.

Initiation and Assessment of Treatment

In a young patient with mild hypothyroidism and in the absence of cardiac disease, treatment may be started with nearly a replacement dose of about 75 to 100 μg per day. In older patients and in those with known cardiac disease, institution of rapid treatment with a full replacement dose of thyroid hormone may be associated with angina pectoris, tachyarrhythmias, myocardial infarction, and/or congestive heart failure. I prefer to start therapy with a low (usually 50 μg per day and sometimes as low as 25 μg per day) initial dose of T_4; if no adverse effects appear, the dose may be increased gradually in increments of 25 μg per day at about 4-week intervals until a full replacement dose of 0.075 to 0.175 mg per day has been achieved and the adequacy of replacement treatment has been verified by normal serum thyroid hormone and TSH levels. In children, however, appropriate progression of growth (height, weight, and skeletal maturation) should also be monitored periodically. Treatment of hypothyroidism is lifelong in most instances, except in transient hypothyroidism, as noted in patients with subacute or postpartum thyroiditis.

Additional Important Considerations

Risk of Overtreatment

Even mild hyperthyroidism during overtreatment with thyroid hormone may be associated with tachyarrhythmias (especially atrial fibrillation); aggravation of angina; and, over a prolonged period, osteoporosis in elderly individuals. I maintain serum TSH and free T_4 levels in the normal range, usually mid-normal, when T_4 replacement is intended simply to treat hypothyroidism. However, in patients who have had thyroidectomy for thyroid carcinoma or in those receiving T_4 for suppression of goiter, it is desirable to keep TSH suppressed to subnormal levels. Even in these patients, I prefer to maintain the serum TSH concentration near 0.2 to 0.3 μU per mL (normal, 0.35 to 4.7 μU per mL) to minimize hyperthyroidism. I know of no clear evidence that suppressing TSH to undetectable levels offers more benefit than keeping it just below normal, but the difference in the degree of hyperthyroidism may substantially affect the patient's feeling of well-being, cardiac rhythm and function, and osteoporosis.

Associated Adrenal Dysfunction

Treatment of hypothyroidism with thyroid hormones is associated with increased metabolism of hydrocortisone and may precipitate adrenal insufficiency in patients with compromised adrenal function. Severe prolonged hypothyroidism may be associated with reduced adrenal reserve, possibly related to myxedema of the adrenal glands. This form of adrenal insufficiency is temporary and necessitates careful observation and/or temporary treatment with hydrocortisone in the early phase of treatment of hypothyroidism. However, adrenal insufficiency associated with hypothyroidism is permanent in patients with multiple endocrine deficiency syndrome and in most patients with pituitary and/or hypothalamic disease. Adrenal cortical reserve may be tested by using the cosyntropin (Cortrosyn) stimulation test, and if it is compromised, the patient should be treated with replacement doses of glucocorticoids and mineralocorticoids in primary adrenal deficiency and glucocorticoids alone in secondary adrenal deficiency. Hydrocortisone (10 to 20 mg in the morning and 10 mg in the evening) is a reasonable treatment.

Associated Hypoparathyroidism

Hypoparathyroidism in association with hypothyroidism may be observed not just in patients with multiple endocrine deficiency syndrome but also in patients with postsurgical hypothyroidism. Its treatment with calcium and vitamin D should improve the well-being of the patient.

Pregnancy

Studies have demonstrated that women require 25 to 50% more T_4 during pregnancy to maintain serum TSH levels in the normal range. The basis for this increased T_4 requirement is not known but may be related to increased serum TBG levels, passage of T_4 to the fetus, and/or increased metabolism of T_4 by the placenta, which is highly enriched in the type III 5'-MDI, which metabolizes T_4 to reverse T_3 (rT_3) (and T_3 to 3,3'-diiodothyronine). I prefer to follow up patients at about 8-week intervals during pregnancy and adjust their dose of T_4 to maintain the serum concentration of free T_4 (measured by dialysis) and TSH in the normal range.

Allergic Reactions

Allergy to synthetic T_4 is exceedingly rare and manifests as pruritus and rash. These symptoms are most likely a result of an allergic reaction to a dye in T_4 tablets, e.g., tartrazine, or another component of the tablet rather than T_4 per se.

Drug Interactions

Drugs (e.g., iron sulfate, cholestyramine, aluminum hydroxide, sucralfate, fiber, and soybean products) may affect treatment of hypothyroidism by reducing absorption of T_4. I have also observed calcium to affect (increase) T_4 requirements as well. I advise patients to take T_4 2 to 4 hours before or after the drugs that may compromise absorption of thyroxine.

Treatment with thyroid hormones affects metabolism and/or activity of some drugs or biologic factors. Thus, thyroid preparations may potentiate the effects of sympathomimetic agents (e.g., epinephrine), anticoagulants (e.g., warfarin), and tricyclic antidepressants (e.g., imipramine). The dose of warfarin decreases because thyroid hormone enhances the breakdown of vitamin K–dependent clotting factors. Hyperthyroidism caused by high doses of thyroid hormones may aggravate glucose intolerance and may necessitate an increase in doses of hypoglycemic agents.

Effects on Thyroid Function Tests. Drugs may affect thyroid function tests by (1) affecting serum TBG levels, e.g. estrogen, tamoxifen, clofibrate, and methadone (and heroin),* which increase TBG and androgen levels, and glucocorticoids that decrease TBG levels; (2) displacing T_4 from TBG, e.g., phenytoin and salicylate; (3) increasing T_4 metabolism, e.g., phenytoin, rifampin, phenobarbital; (4) inhibiting conversion of T_4 to T_3, e.g., amiodarone, glucocorticoids, sodium ipodate, sodium iopanoate; and (5) affecting TSH levels, e.g., dopamine, glucocorticoids, and somatostatin,† which decrease TSH levels, and metoclopramide, which increases TSH levels. Measurement of the serum concentration of free T_4 and free T_3, preferably by equilibrium dialysis or ultrafiltration, helps one to avoid problems caused by the drugs that affect the serum binding of thyroid hormones. Other drugs may actually affect the thyroid function status of the patient.

Follow-up of Secondary Hypothyroidism

The serum TSH level does not appropriately assist in monitoring thyroid hormone replacement in secondary hypothyroidism. Measurement of the serum concentration of free T_4 (preferably by equilibrium dialysis) is necessary for adjustment of the dose of T_4. As noted previously, the physician must address the issue of adrenal status when treating patients with secondary hypothyroidism.

Diagnosis and Treatment of Hypothyroidism in Patients with Systemic Nonthyroidal Illness

Nonthyroidal illness (NTI) can be associated with many, typically transient, thyroid function abnormalities, including low serum T_3, low free T_3, low total T_4, high severe T_3 (rT_3), and low or high serum TSH levels and it can be difficult to diagnose hypothyroidism in the setting of NTI. I recommend measurement of free T_4 (by dialysis) and TSH. These measurements are normal in most NTI patients. A serum TSH level of greater than 20 μU per mL (normal, 0.35 to 4.7 μU per mL) is strongly suggestive of primary hypothyroidism. The serum rT_3 concentration is not ele-

vated in hypothyroidism (with serum TSH levels of >10 μU per mL). The presence of goiter and antithyroid antibodies favors the diagnosis of hypothyroidism. It is often feasible to wait for 1 to 2 weeks for a recovery from NTI to obtain readily interpretable thyroid function tests before initiating treatment with thyroid hormones. Alternatively, one may initiate treatment of hypothyroidism with replacement doses of T_4 and then discontinue thyroid medication for a month and reassess the situation when the NTI has been corrected.

Subclinical Hypothyroidism

Findings of normal serum total and free T_4 levels, normal total and free T_3 levels, and a high serum TSH level have been referred to as "subclinical hypothyroidism." Many patients with these findings are asymptomatic; others manifest nonspecific symptoms, e.g., fatigue, cold intolerance, constipation, or depression. Enlargement of the thyroid is a common finding. Chronic (Hashimoto's) thyroiditis is a common cause of subclinical hypothyroidism, but the condition is also seen after treatment of hyperthyroidism with radioiodine or partial thyroidectomy. Prospective studies have shown that 5 to 20% of patients with subclinical hypothyroidism develop clinical hypothyroidism annually. I repeat borderline elevated serum TSH tests at 1- to 3-month intervals. If the serum TSH level is persistently elevated, the thyroid is enlarged, and/or antithyroid antibodies are detected, I prefer to treat these patients with T_4 replacement. About half of the patients demonstrate improvement in symptoms, and further enlargement of the thyroid is curtailed. Studies have shown improvement in cognitive function, cardiac indices, and/or serum cholesterol and triglyceride levels in patients with subclinical hypothyroidism treated with T_4.

Patients Receiving Thyroxine for Unknown Reasons

It is not uncommon to see a patient in the clinic who has been taking thyroid hormones for several years but does not know the reason for the treatment. To determine or confirm a diagnosis of hypothyroidism, one should first measure the serum TSH level. If it is elevated, diagnosis of hypothyroidism is evident. If it is normal, thyroid hormone treatment should be discontinued for 4 weeks and serum TSH and free T_4 levels measured. A high serum TSH level and low free T_4 level establish the diagnosis of primary hypothyroidism. Alternatively, one can switch a patient from T_4 to T_3 (liothyronine, 25 μg twice daily) therapy for 20 days and then withdraw T_3 for 10 days only before measuring the serum TSH and free T_4 levels.

Surgery in Hypothyroidism

Surgery in patients with moderate to severe hypothyroidism is associated with an increased incidence of shock, cardiac arrhythmias, congestive heart failure, ileus, electrolyte imbalance (hyponatremia), and

---

*Not available in the United States.
†Orphan drug.

psychiatric difficulties. Hypothyroid patients also demonstrate increased difficulty with mounting a febrile response to infection and increased sensitivity to anesthesia and narcotics. There is also a concern about occurrence of myxedema coma during and after surgery in patients with severe hypothyroidism. Therefore, hypothyroidism should be corrected before an elective surgical procedure. If emergency surgery is needed for a life-threatening condition, patients with severe hypothyroidism should be treated aggressively, as for myxedema coma.

Treatment of Myxedema Coma

Myxedema coma is a serious emergency with a high mortality. It clearly requires aggressive treatment. I usually recommend (1) parenteral (intravenous) T_4: 400 to 500 µg to replace the extrathyroidal pool of T_4 followed by 100 µg daily intravenously for several days when the patient is comatose, followed by 100 µg daily orally when the patient is awake. Some experts favor intravenous T_3 (Triostat). However, we consider T_4 to be more smoothly acting, less toxic, and more easily available. When used, T_3 is given in a dose of 10 to 30 µg every 6 to 8 hours. (2) I recommend treatment of precipitating disorders, if known (e.g., antibiotics for an infection such as pneumonia), and attention to trauma, myocardial infarction, cold exposure, and exposure to narcotics. (3) I also recommend supportive treatment consisting of blankets to reduce heat loss (active warming is not helpful and may lead to peripheral vasodilatation); intravenous fluids and blood transfusion for shock (use of pressor agents requires careful monitoring for cardiac arrhythmias); ventilatory assistance with intubation or tracheostomy for CO_2 retention; fluid restriction and/or hypertonic saline if the serum sodium level is less than 120 mEq per liter; hydrocortisone, approximately 150 mg per day intravenously on the first day (it is to be tapered gradually over 5 to 7 days as the patient improves); attention to the plasma glucose level (which may be low in some cases); and cautious use of diuretics and digoxin for congestive heart failure.

HYPERTHYROIDISM

method of
GILBERT H. DANIELS, M.D.
Massachusetts General Hospital
Boston, Massachusetts

Hyperthyroidism is a clinical *syndrome* due to excess thyroid hormone and its clinical consequences. Symptoms include weight loss with preserved appetite, heat intolerance, fatigue, palpitations, shortness of breath, increased frequency of bowel movements, decreased menstrual flow or irregular menses, weak muscles, tremor, emotional lability, anxiety, and difficulty sleeping. Shortness of breath is common in the absence of congestive heart failure, possibly due to weakness of the respiratory muscles. Weight gain

rather than loss may occur. In the elderly patient, anorexia weight loss, constipation, and a normal heart rate may confuse the clinician. Some patients are surprisingly asymptomatic despite severe chemical hyperthyroidism ("apathetic hyperthyroidism"). Signs include lid lag; widened pulse pressure; tachycardia; hyper-reflexia; tremor; warm, moist skin; oncolysis; and weak muscles. Goiter need not be present. Proptosis, inflammatory eye findings, and pretibial myxedema are specific for Graves' disease. Signs and symptoms of underlying heart disease including angina, tachyarrhythmias, and congestive heart failure are often exacerbated by hyperthyroidism and may dominate the clinical picture.

THYROID FUNCTION TESTING

Sensitive thyroid-stimulating hormone (TSH) measurements have revolutionized thyroid function testing. Except for the rare condition of TSH-induced hyperthyroidism, all hyperthyroid patients have low TSH concentrations. Currently available third-generation TSH assays can measure TSH concentrations as low as 0.01 µU per mL. A clinically useful commercial TSH assay must distinguish hyperthyroid from euthyroid patients; this must be verified with your laboratory. However, a fully suppressed TSH concentration cannot distinguish degrees of hyperthyroidism! Levels of serum free thyroxine (T_4) (or free thyroxine index) and total serum triiodothyronine (T_3) (by radioimmunoassay [RIA]) must be measured when the TSH concentration is low to determine the degree of hyperthyroidism and to monitor therapy.

Subclinical hyperthyroidism is characterized by a consistently low serum TSH concentration with normal free T_4 and total T_3 concentrations, if other causes of the low TSH concentration are excluded. Although patients are variably symptomatic, therapy is often necessary. Nonthyroidal causes of a low TSH concentration include pituitary disease, glucocorticoid or dopamine therapy, and severe illness. In these situations, the free T_4 concentration is often below or at the lower limits of normal and the TSH concentration is not usually less than 0.01 µU per mL (unless glucocorticoids or dopamine is administered to sick patients). The serum TSH concentration alone is less useful as a screening test in the inpatient setting.

Appropriate therapy for hyperthyroidism depends on its cause. The mechanisms and types of hyperthyroidism are summarized in Table 1. The diagnosis is obvious in some patients (e.g., diffuse goiter with a bruit and exophthalmos equals Graves' disease); however, in most cases, the situation is less clear. A 24-hour radioiodine uptake test and a radionuclide (iodine 123 or technetium Tc 99m) scan are helpful in this differential diagnosis. It is most useful to divide patients into those with a near zero radioiodine uptake and those with normal or high uptake (Table 2). For example, hyperthyroidism due to excess thyroid hormone is treated by decreasing or stopping the hormone. Hyperthyroidism due to silent thyroiditis, painful subacute thyroiditis, or amiodarone-induced destructive thyroiditis resolves spontaneously and may not require therapy.

THERAPY

Although indispensable in the diagnosis of hyperthyroidism, sensitive TSH measurements may be misleading during the therapy of hyperthyroidism. Because a suppressed TSH concentration may remain low for weeks to months after achieving the

TABLE 1. **Mechanisms of Hyperthyroidism**

Exogenous Hormone	Thyroid Stimulators	Autonomous Production	Excess Release of Hormone
		Common Mechanisms	
L-T_4	Antibodies (Graves' disease)	Hot nodule	Painful subacute thyroiditis
L-T_3	hCG*	Toxic multinodular goiter	Silent lymphocytic thyroiditis
			Amiodarone-induced destructive thyroiditis
		Rare Mechanisms	
	TSH	Struma ovarii	

*Mild hyperthyroidism due to hyperemesis is common; severe hyperthyroidism due to hydatidiform mole or choriocarcinoma is rare.

Abbreviations: hCG = human chorionic gonadotropin; TSH = thyroid-stimulating hormone; L-T_4 = L-tetraiodothyronine; L-T_3 = L-triiodothyronine.

euthyroid state, serum free T_4 (or index) and T_3 (RIA) concentrations must be monitored during therapy. In some patients, the free T_4 concentration (or index) returns to normal while the T_3 concentration remains elevated ("T_3 toxicosis"). In others, both free T_4 and T_3 (RIA) concentrations return to normal, indicating effective therapy, despite continued TSH suppression.

The choice of therapy for Graves' disease is most problematic and is the major focus of this discussion. Therapeutic choices include inhibition of hormone production (antithyroid drugs), thyroid gland destruction (radioiodine [iodine 131]) or thyroid gland removal (surgery). Graves' hyperthyroidism is due to antibody stimulation of TSH receptors (thyroid-stimulating antibodies). Disease remission due to loss of these antibodies is facilitated by antithyroid drug therapy, whereas the rate of spontaneous remission is only 5 to 10% after 1 year.

Most patients who select antithyroid drugs do so in hopes of a sustained remission and the desire to avoid permanent thyroid damage. After 1 year of therapy, approximately 50% of patients enter a remission of 4 months or longer, particularly those with smaller thyroid glands. Unfortunately, approximately 50% of those in remission have a subsequent relapse. Ultimately, 15% of those in remission after antithyroid drug therapy develop *hypothyroidism*.

Radioiodine is the ultimate therapy for most hyperthyroid adults, based on a 55-year record of safety and efficacy and the overall high relapse rate after

TABLE 2. **Differential Diagnosis of Hyperthyroidism**

Low or Zero RaI Uptake	Normal or High RaI Uptake
Painful subacute thyroiditis	Graves' disease
Silent thyroiditis	Toxic nodular goiter
Factitious (exogenous) hyperthyroidism	Hot nodule
Amiodarone-induced destructive thyroiditis	hCG- or TSH-induced hyperthyroidism
Iodide excess*	
Struma ovarii†	

*Recent exposure to excess iodide may cause a low or normal RaI uptake in all the disorders characterized by normal or high RaI uptake.

†Uptake will be low over the neck but not the pelvis.

Abbreviations: hCG = human chorionic gonadotropin; RaI = radioiodine; TSH = thyroid-stimulating hormone.

antithyroid drug therapy. There is no evidence for increased cancer, infertility, or birth defects after radioiodine therapy of hyperthyroidism. The radiation exposure to the ovaries is comparable to that of many common radiologic procedures including barium enemas, intravenous pyelography, and hysterosalpingography. Most endocrinologists favor antithyroid drugs as the initial therapy for children. However, radioiodine is a safe and effective alternative for those allergic to or poorly compliant with antithyroid drug therapy.

Although surgery is an uncommon therapeutic choice, it remains an important therapeutic alternative, provided a skilled thyroid surgeon is available.

All the therapeutic options are effective, but none are perfect. Therefore, education of and dialogue with the patient are extremely important. Patients must understand their options, be comfortable with their therapeutic choice, and not be coerced into a choice that frightens them.

Older patients with subclinical hyperthyroidism (and TSH concentrations of <0.1 µU per mL) are at high risk for atrial fibrillation, and menopausal women not taking estrogen are at increased risk for bone loss. Persistent subclinical hyperthyroidism should be treated in these populations, even if asymptomatic. Careful observation may be appropriate for young asymptomatic patients.

Adjunctive Therapy

Therapy for hyperthyroidism works slowly. When tachycardia, palpitations, and tremor are disturbing to the patient, long-acting beta blockers provide symptomatic relief. Atenolol (Tenormin),* metoprolol (Lopressor),* nadolol (Corgard),* and long-acting propranolol (Inderal LA) are all effective and probably superior to the shorter acting agents (e.g., propranolol [Inderal]).

Antithyroid Drugs

The antithyroid drugs methimazole (Tapazole) and propylthiouracil (PTU) rapidly block the synthesis of thyroid hormone but do not inhibit the release of

*Not FDA approved for this indication.

thyroid hormone. Therefore, the clinical response and the time to euthyroidism vary greatly (average 6 to 12 weeks) depending in part on thyroid hormone stores. Compliance is extremely important; if 1 to several days of therapy are missed, thyroid hormone stores are replenished, delaying the therapeutic effect. I prefer methimazole because of its longer half-life. Single-daily-dose therapy with methimazole is effective in almost all compliant patients. I generally begin therapy with 30 mg, although lower initial doses may suffice for some patients.

Initially, patients are followed at 6-week intervals. If the 30-mg daily dosage is continued, hypothyroidism usually results. Therefore, as the patients become euthyroid (generally around 6 to 12 weeks), two choices are available. I generally prefer to taper the dosage of methimazole, initially to 15 mg and subsequently to 10 or even 5 mg. Alternatively, a block and replace regimen continues the methimazole at a dose of 30 mg and adds full therapeutic doses of levothyroxine (e.g., 1.7 µg per kg, usually 0.1 to 0.125 mg per day). This latter approach is particularly useful with patients who are away at school or who cannot return for frequent blood studies.

Many endocrinologists prefer PTU because it blocks the peripheral conversion of T_4 to T_3. Unfortunately, in hyperthyroidism, the excess circulating T_3 comes from the thyroid gland, rather than from peripheral conversion. Because of its shorter half-life, PTU may fail to control thyroidal T_3 production unless multiple daily doses are used. PTU is one tenth as potent as methimazole; the usual starting dose is 100 mg three or four times daily. The monthly cost of methimazole 30 mg per day is about $57, and PTU 300 mg per day is about $20. Once maintenance dosages have been established, the cost of the two drugs is comparable.

Side effects of antithyroid drugs are uncommon. Fever, rash, or joint pains occur in 5% of patients and may be more frequent when methimazole doses are greater than 30 mg per day. With these minor allergies, one may switch to the alternative drug with a small risk of cross-reactivity. Agranulocytosis occurs in 0.2 to 0.4% of patients, generally within the first 3 months of starting or restarting therapy. A low white blood cell count (3000 to 4000 per mm³) is common in untreated patients with Graves' disease and is not a contraindication to therapy. I usually check the white blood cell count and differential at each follow-up visit or if symptoms suggestive of agranulocytosis develop (fever, sore throat, mouth ulcerations). Some endocrinologists check the white blood cell count and differential every 2 weeks while the patient is receiving therapy. If agranulocytosis develops, hospitalization is necessary. Granulocyte colony-stimulating factor injections are thought to shorten the recovery period, which is usually 7 to 14 days. Agranulocytosis precludes further antithyroid drug therapy! Less common side effects include toxic hepatitis (methimazole), hepatic necrosis (PTU), and lupus-like reactions (PTU).

Antithyroid drugs are generally prescribed for a period of 1 to 2 years, but there are no absolute time limits. Some patients prefer to continue to take these drugs for much longer periods rather than experience frequent relapses. Relapse after stopping antithyroid drug therapy may be treated by restarting the drug therapy or chosing an alternative therapy such as radioiodine or surgery.

Patients in remission after antithyroid drug therapy need careful, lifelong follow-up. Thyroid function is tested annually or whenever symptoms develop. Relapse of Graves' disease is quite common during the postpartum period.

Patients with "hot" nodules or toxic nodular goiters do not enter remission after treatment with antithyroid drugs. Methimazole or PTU may be used to treat the hyperthyroidism before definitive therapy with radioiodine or surgery.

Radioiodine Therapy

Radioiodine (^{131}I) is administered by mouth as a liquid or a capsule. Pregnancy is a strict contraindication to its use. There are no immediate aftereffects of its administration. Patients do not become ill. Allergy to iodinated contrast materials is not a contraindication to radioiodine use. Radioiodine has a half-life of 8 days; after 40 days virtually no radioactivity remains in the body.

Radioiodine works slowly; thyroidal pain or tenderness is rare. Most patients become euthyroid or hypothyroid 8 to 26 weeks after therapy. During the days or weeks after radioiodine administration, increased release of thyroid hormone may result in worsening hyperthyroidism. Beta blockers are often employed during this time. Some endocrinologists pretreat all patients with antithyroid drugs (weeks to months) to deplete the stores of thyroid hormone and prevent postradioiodine exacerbation of hyperthyroidism. I generally reserve this pretreatment for elderly patients or those with serious heart disease. Antithyroid drug therapy should be stopped for 2 or more days before radioiodine therapy. Approximately 20% of patients require a second dose of radioiodine.

The dose of radioiodine is selected to deliver 5000 to 15,000 rad (50 to 150 Gy) to the thyroid gland. Some physicians use a fixed dosing schedule. I prefer to deliver 160 to 180 microcuries of ^{131}I per estimated gram of thyroid tissue according to the formula

$$^{131}\text{I dose} = \frac{(160-180)\,\mu\text{Ci/gm} \times \text{estimated weight of thyroid (gm)} \times 100}{24\text{-h RaI uptake}}$$

where RaI is either ^{123}I or ^{131}I. Patients previously treated with antithyroid drugs are more resistant to the effects of radioiodine and often require the higher range.

The radioiodine-damaged Graves' thyroid gland is particularly sensitive to inhibition of hormone release when inorganic iodide is administered. When persistent hyperthyroidism is symptomatic or considered dangerous, prescribing a supersaturated solution of potassium iodide (SSKI) 3 drops twice daily, to begin 1 week after radioiodine administration, shortens the average time to euthyroidism from 12 to 6 weeks. Alternatively, methimazole or PTU can be added 4 to 7 days after radioiodine administration.

Hypothyroidism is the expected outcome for most patients with Graves' disease treated with radioiodine, although 20% remain euthyroid. Approximately 50% become hypothyroid at 1 year, with 2 to 3% becoming hypothyroid each additional year. Long-term follow-up of all radioiodine-treated patients is therefore mandatory. I and many other endocrinologists begin levothyroxine therapy as soon as patients become euthyroid, whereas others wait until hypothyroidism develops. If a goiter persists in Graves' disease after radioiodine therapy, hypothyroidism is often transient.

Surgery

Less than 1% of our institution's thyroid unit Graves' patients opt for surgery. Who are these patients? Pregnant women who are allergic to antithyroid drugs, patients who are allergic to antithyroid drugs and afraid of radioiodine, patients with concomitant Graves' disease and suspicious thyroid nodules, and young patients with extremely large goiters who may require multiple treatments with radioiodine after drug failure or allergy make up the bulk of these patients.

A surgeon skilled at performing bilateral thyroidectomy is absolutely necessary. Although a small amount of thyroid remnant can remain, too much residual thyroid tissue results in persistent or recurrent hyperthyroidism, which occurs in 5% or more of patients. Mortality is rare in properly prepared patients. Complications include temporary and permanent hypoparathyroidism hoarseness due to recurrent laryngeal nerve injury, bleeding, wound infection, and keloid or unsightly scar formation. Hypothyroidism occurs in 10 to 60% of patients initially, with 1 to 3% per year thereafter.

It is best to operate on a euthyroid patient, but this is not always possible. In compliant nonallergic patients, methimazole or PTU is prescribed until the patient is euthyroid. SSKI (10 drops twice daily) is added 10 days before surgery to decrease the vascularity of the thyroid gland. When pretreatment is impossible, surgery can be performed under beta-adrenergic blockade. I generally prescribe high-dose propranolol (60 to 240 mg four times daily) for 3 to 4 days before surgery to decrease the resting and postwalking pulse to 70 or less. SSKI (see earlier) can be added as well but is not absolutely necessary. Because of thyroxine's long half-life (7 days), beta blockade must be continued after surgery. In emergency situations, intravenous beta blockers can be given.

When surgery is planned for patients with toxic nodular goiters or hot nodules, iodine is not used for preoperative preparation. I prefer to prepare these patients for surgery with antithyroid drugs or beta blockers, although some major centers choose to operate without preparation.

Effect of Therapy on Graves' Eye Disease

Whether therapy of Graves' hyperthyroidism has an influence on Graves' eye disease is controversial. Some centers report worsening eyes after radioiodine therapy, particularly in patients with severe initial eye disease. Other groups report eye improvement when the thyroid is ablated with radioiodine. For most patients, the choice of therapy can be made independent of the eye findings. For those patients with severe inflammatory eye changes, I generally prefer to start with antithyroid drugs and defer radioiodine therapy until the eyes are quiescent. I occasionally recommend surgery for these patients.

HYPERTHYROIDISM AND PREGNANCY

When hyperthyroidism is mild during pregnancy, including human chorionic gonadotropin–induced hyperthyroidism of hyperemesis gravidarum, no therapy is necessary. When therapy is indicated, antithyroid drugs are the first choice during a hyperthyroid pregnancy; radioiodine is contraindicated, and surgery is best avoided. Antithyroid drugs cross the placenta and inhibit fetal thyroid function. Placental passage is less complete for PTU. PTU is preferred during pregnancy, although methimazole is a reasonable alternative. Maternal thyroid function should be maintained in the high-normal to slightly high range, as low-normal maternal free T_4 concentrations are associated with fetal hypothyroidism. The minimal dose of PTU necessary should be employed; doses less than 150 mg per day rarely cause fetal thyroid dysfunction. The immunosuppressive effects of pregnancy often cause Graves' disease to improve; PTU therapy is progressively tapered and if possible discontinued. In the rare instances when surgery is necessary, it should be delayed until the second trimester, if possible. If necessary, beta-adrenergic blocking agents can be employed for short periods for symptomatic relief. The fetus of mothers previously treated for Graves' hyperthyroidism with radioactive iodine or surgery may be at risk for hyperthyroidism if high titers of TSH receptor–stimulating antibodies are present in the mother.

SEVERE HYPERTHYROIDISM OR THYROID STORM

Thyroid storm, characterized by severe hyperthyroidism, fever, and altered mental status, is rare. However, severe hyperthyroidism may require similar emergency therapy when a complicating illness (e.g., myocardial infarction or sepsis) is present.

Antithyroid drugs in high dosages block thyroid hormone synthesis and are given first, but clinical improvement is slow with this therapy. PTU (200 mg by mouth, nasogastric tube, or rectum every 4 hours) is preferred as it also inhibits conversion of T_4 to T_3. When synthesis is inhibited, thyroid hormone release can be prevented by iodine in several forms (e.g., SSKI 5 drops orally four times a day, iopanoic acid [Telepaque] or ipodate [Oragrafin] 0.5 to 1.5 grams orally twice daily). Iopanoic acid and ipodate are particularly useful as they serve as iodine sources and are potent inhibitors of conversion of T_4 to T_3. Administration of iodine-containing drugs should follow the administration of antithyroid drugs to prevent large increases in thyroid hormone stores. Cholestyramine (Questran),* 4 grams orally three times daily, inhibits enterohepatic circulation of thyroid hormone and is effective in endogenous hyperthyroidism as well as that due to thyroid hormone overdosage.

Beta-adrenergic blocking agents provide the most immediate relief. Oral propranolol in doses of 40 to 160 mg every 6 hours or intravenous propranolol (2 to 5 mg every 4 hours or as an infusion at a rate of 5 to 10 mg per hour) controls the heart rate in most patients. When the blood pressure is low or when there is underlying pulmonary disease, the shorter acting esmolol (Brevibloc)* is the initial therapy of choice. Reserpine,* guanethidine,* and calcium channel blockers* have all been employed in patients intolerant of beta blockers. Stress dosages of glucocorticoids are usually administered, largely based on historical precedent rather than clear rationale. In high doses, glucocorticoids do inhibit the conversion of T_4 to T_3. Plasmapheresis, peritoneal dialysis, and charcoal resin hemoperfusion are rarely necessary.

DESTRUCTIVE THYROIDITIS

Hyperthyroidism due to destructive thyroiditis (painful subacute thyroiditis, silent lymphocytic thyroiditis, amiodarone-induced destructive thyroiditis) is self-limited and can be monitored or treated with beta blockade. When this disorder is severe or with concomitant heart disease, glucocorticoid therapy (e.g., prednisone 40 mg orally per day) shortens the time to euthyroidism and may be lifesaving.

---

*Not FDA approved for this indication.

THYROID CANCER

method of
COLIN G. THOMAS, Jr., M.D.
University of North Carolina School of Medicine
Chapel Hill, North Carolina

Cancer of the thyroid gland is an infrequent neoplasm estimated to account for 16,100 new cases and 1230 deaths in 1997 among the 266 million people in the United States. It is most common in the fourth and fifth decades of life, is the second most prevalent malignant tumor in the second decade, and accounts for 6% of all cancers in individuals younger than 45 years. During the past decade, there has been a 52% increase in the number of new cases, with the number of deaths increasing by 12%. The disease continues to have a greater prevalence in females (70%), although the number of deaths in this group is lower than that in males (37 vs. 63%).

The management of thyroid cancer is related to the identification of thyroid nodules that harbor a malignant neoplasm and recognition that thyroid cancer consists of a spectrum of tumors arising from the cellular components of the thyroid, i.e., follicular epithelium, parafollicular (or C) cells of neural crest origin, and stromal lymphocytes. Rarely, tumors arise from other components. Although surgery is the cornerstone of treatment, there are many controversial aspects relative to the extent of the operation (lobectomy, near-total or total thyroidectomy), the indications for lymph node dissections, and the use of radioactive iodine. Contributing to the problem of management is the markedly different biologic characteristics of these tumors related to the cell of origin, age of the host, and role of adjuvant therapy. The long natural history of differentiated cancers and the frequency of occult disease that has little biologic significance further contribute to the problem of appraising the effectiveness of therapy. Most views are based on retrospective observational studies of patients undergoing a variety of treatments in an uncontrolled fashion. During the last decade, emphasis has been placed on the identification of risk factors that permit patients to be categorized in high- or low-risk groups—critical to the selection of treatment.

CLASSIFICATION

Table 1 provides a histopathologic classification of thyroid cancers; their frequency is seen in Table 2. More than 85% of thyroid cancers are differentiated. Papillary carcinoma includes several variants that may differ in their biologic behavior. Papillary microadenocarcinoma and the diffuse sclerosing type are macroscopic variants. Follicular carcinoma demonstrates variably sized follicle formation and invasion with the absence of any features of papillary carcinoma or its follicular variant. Capsular invasion alone (minimally invasive) is characteristic of a nonaggressive tumor, whereas angioinvasion (highly invasive) reflects a more aggressive neoplasm with a propensity for local invasion and distant metastases. Hürthle cell carcinoma is a variant of follicular thyroid cancer with comparable crite-

TABLE 1. **Classification of Cancers of the Thyroid**

Differentiated (from follicular epithelium)
  A. Papillary adenocarcinoma
    1. Papillary and follicular carcinoma (including mixed papillary-follicular carcinoma)
    2. Variants
      a. Follicular
      b. Oxyphil cell
      c. Tall cell
    3. Papillary microadenocarcinoma (<1 cm)
    4. Diffuse sclerosing type
  B. Follicular adenocarcinoma
    1. Encapsulated (minimally invasive) carcinoma
    2. Angioinvasive (highly invasive) carcinoma
    3. Hürthle cell carcinoma
Medullary thyroid carcinoma (from parafollicular epithelium)
Undifferentiated (spindle cell, giant cell, small cell, insular)
Lymphoma
Others (epidermoid, sarcoma, teratoma, metastatic)

TABLE 2. **Carcinoma of the Thyroid: Frequency Distribution, 1946 to 1971 (1161 Patients)**

Classification	Number	Percentage
Papillary	856	73.7
Follicular	136	11.7
Undifferentiated	82	7.0
Medullary	58	5.0
Hürthle cell	29	2.5
Total	1161	
Metastatic to thyroid	30	

Modified from McConahey WM: Thyroid cancer at the Mayo Clinic. Mayo Clin Proc 59:866, 1984.

ria for malignancy. The carcinomas differ, however, in that only infrequently do they concentrate radioiodine, but they are similar in their ability to produce thyroglobulin. Most differentiated thyroid neoplasms have excitable thyroid-stimulating hormone (TSH) receptors and responsive adenylate cyclase systems that synthesize and secrete thyroglobulin and, when stimulated, thyroxine.

Medullary thyroid carcinoma (MTC) arises from C (calcitonin-secreting), or parafollicular, cells and presents as a sporadic neoplasm or as a component of a familial multiple endocrine neoplasia (MEN) syndrome (20 to 25%). The latter may be expressed as MEN 2A (medullary carcinoma of the thyroid, hyperparathyroidism, and pheochromocytoma); MEN 2B (medullary carcinoma, pheochromocytoma, and mucosal neuromas); or a familial (non-MEN) MTC. Medullary carcinomas in the MEN 2B category are usually more aggressive than those arising sporadically or as a component of MEN 2A. The ability to document the *ret* oncogene in patients with the MEN syndrome should enable differentiation between sporadic tumors and those that have a genetic basis.

Undifferentiated carcinomas are characterized as spindle cell, giant cell, or small cell, with the last needing to be differentiated from lymphomas. These highly aggressive neoplasms commonly arise in patients in the sixth and seventh decades of life, superimposed on a history of long-standing nodular goiter. "Insular" carcinomas, although infrequent, are included in this category.

Primary lymphomas should be distinguished from systemic lymphomas with thyroid involvement (approximately 15%). They should be suspected in patients with a history of chronic lymphocytic thyroiditis and progressive or asymmetrical increase in goiter size. Fine-needle aspiration cytologic examination with associated B cell immunotyping may establish the diagnosis; however, an open biopsy is usually requisite to provide sufficient material for classification.

DIAGNOSTIC EVALUATION OF THYROID NODULES

Fine-needle aspiration biopsy (FNAB) is the key to the cytologic diagnosis of solitary thyroid nodules or a dominant nodule or nodules in a multinodular goiter. It has far greater sensitivity (90%) and specificity (70%) than evaluations by radionuclide scans or ultrasonography, neither of which can distinguish malignant from benign disease. False-positive rates with FNAB have varied from 0 to 1.1% and false-negative rates from 0.7 to 6%. Cytologic studies are usually interpreted as benign (non-neoplastic goiter), papillary carcinoma, follicular neoplasm, other neo-

plasm, indeterminate, or insufficient for diagnosis. The last warrants a repeated FNAB. Fine-needle cytologic examination can identify a follicular neoplasm, but neither architectural nor cytologic atypicality is a reliable criterion of malignancy. The diagnosis of follicular carcinoma requires histopathologic evidence of capsular or vascular invasion by permanent sections. MTC may be suspected on the basis of fine-needle aspiration and confirmed by measuring the serum calcitonin level. In patients with a familial history of disease (MEN syndromes), subclinical disease can be identified with genetic testing for the *ret* oncogene, which has replaced biochemical screening using calcium and pentagastrin stimulation for the release of calcitonin. Palpable cervical lymph nodes are best assessed by aspiration cytologic examination.

After a cytologic diagnosis, radionuclide scans and ultrasound studies are adjuvant and frequently unnecessary. A "cold" nodule by thyroid scan or a solid nodule by ultrasonography does not constitute an indication for thyroidectomy. Radionuclide scans are most often performed with technetium Tc 99m pertechnetate, which measures the "trapping" function of follicular epithelium, in contrast to radioiodine, which measures trapping and organification. Overall, less than 10% of thyroid nodules are "hyperfunctioning" with ^{99m}Tc, of which approximately 10% are nonfunctioning with radioiodine. A hyperfunctioning nodule by a radioiodine test should distinguish a benign (hyperfunction) from a malignant follicular neoplasm as assessed by FNAB. Radionuclide scans are most useful in the patient with a multinodular goiter demonstrating cold, or hypofunctioning, nodules. Ultrasonography is valuable in facilitating fine-needle aspiration of the solid component of cystic nodules and of nodules in patients with chronic thyroiditis, and in appraising the presence of nodules in the contralateral lobe of patients undergoing thyroid lobectomy. Thyroid function is optimally evaluated with a sensitive TSH test, with euthyroidism characteristic of patients with thyroid nodules. An elevated TSH level in a goitrous patient is most consistent with Hashimoto's thyroiditis or thyroid lymphoma.

Preoperative studies unique to patients with suspected thyroid cancer should include chest radiography; measurement of serum calcium, thyroglobulin, and phosphorus levels; and laryngoscopy for vocal cord function. For any patient undergoing thyroidectomy, fine-needle cytologic examination provides information that is valuable in planning the appropriate operative procedure, with the frozen section examination usually complementary to the cytologic diagnosis.

RISK GROUPS

Differentiated thyroid cancers have identifiable biologic characteristics that categorize patients as at high or low risk of dying of their disease. In patients with papillary carcinoma, the most valid predictors are (1) the age of the patient (individuals younger than 20 years despite advanced regional disease have essentially a normal survivorship); (2) the extent of disease, i.e., extracapsular extension with local invasion; (3) the size of the primary tumor—tumors less than 1.5 cm in diameter are associated with an essentially normal survivorship; (4) the completeness of resection; and (5) distant metastasis. Lymph node metastases do not seem to alter survivorship, although they do influence the incidence of recurrent disease in the neck. These prognostic factors have been used in a retrospective manner to develop scoring systems that define risk groups and in turn to design appropriate therapy.

TABLE 3. **MACIS Scoring System for Papillary Carcinoma**

Variable	Score
≤39 y	3.1
>39 y	0.08 × age
Size	0.3 × size (cm)
Incomplete resection	1.0
Locally invasive	1.0
Distant metastases	3.0
Total score	

Abbreviation: MACIS = metastasis, age, completeness of resection, invasion, and size.

Modified from Hay ID, Bergstralh EJ, Goellner JR, et al: Predicting outcome in papillary thyroid carcinoma: Development of a reliable prognostic scoring system in a cohort of 1779 patients surgically treated at one institution during 1940 through 1989. Surgery 114:1050–1058, 1993.

The AMES system from the Lahey Clinic is based on *a*ge, *m*etastasis to distant site, *e*xtra thyroidal extension, and tumor *s*ize and defines high-risk papillary or follicular thyroid cancer by the following criteria: (1) distant metastasis at any age and (2) men older than 40 years or women older than 50 years with (a) extrathyroidal papillary carcinoma and major tumor capsular invasion by follicular carcinoma, and (b) primary tumor diameter 5 cm or larger. The Mayo Clinic scoring system for papillary carcinoma is based on five variables: *m*etastasis, *a*ge, *c*ompleteness of resection, *i*nvasion, and *s*ize (MACIS). The final prognostic score is calculated as in Table 3. Twenty-year cause-specific survival rates are, for patients with scores less than 6, 99%; with scores 6 to 6.9, 89%; 7 to 7.9, 50%, and 8 or more, 24%. Eighty-four percent of patients fell into the lowest risk group (<6.0), and 92% had a score of less than 7.0. Some tumor variants are associated with a higher risk, e.g., carcinoma of the tall or columnar cell type, diffuse sclerosing papillary carcinoma, and focally dedifferentiated carcinomas. Table 4 documents the influence of age on the staging of thyroid cancer—the only malignant tumor in which a nonanatomic factor plays such a role in prognosis.

Follicular adenocarcinoma is less frequent than papillary carcinoma, occurring in a somewhat older age group (mean, 53 years). It is potentially a more aggressive tumor with a median size of 4 cm at diagnosis, a 6% incidence of nodal metastases, and an 8% incidence of multifocal disease with 12% of patients having distant metastases. In reviewing prognostic variables in one representative series,

a high risk was associated with patients older than 50 years, a tumor size greater than 2.5 cm, marked vascular invasion, and metastatic disease at the time of diagnosis. Eighteen percent of patients fell into the high-risk category, of whom 53 and 92% were dead by 5 and 20 years, respectively. Eighty-two percent of the patients were classified in the low-risk category and had a cumulative mortality of 1% at 5 years and 14% at 20 years.

SURGICAL MANAGEMENT

Surgery is the cornerstone of management of patients with differentiated thyroid cancer and is best carried out by an experienced thyroid surgeon. The extent of the operation should reflect the biologic characteristics of a particular neoplasm as indicated by the risk factors, operative morbidity, and mortality. The excellent results of conservative surgery in patients at low risk should temper the surgical approach and use of adjuvant therapies. The minimal treatment for papillary carcinoma is lobectomy, which for tumors 1.0 cm or less in diameter is associated with survival that is not improved by a more extensive operation. Some surgeons recommend total thyroidectomy for all papillary thyroid cancers. This rationale is based on the following: (1) the presence of multifocal disease in the opposite lobe in from 35 to 85% of patients may require additional surgery in approximately 5 to 10% of these patients. (2) The risk for local recurrence in the thyroid bed is reduced. (3) Survival is improved in patients with lesions greater than 1.5 cm in diameter. (4) Treatment of metastatic thyroid cancer and ablation of the thyroid bed with radioiodine is facilitated. (5) The sensitivity of serum thyroglobulin as an indicator of tumor presence and progression is enhanced. (6) The progression of residual disease to an undifferentiated tumor is obviated. (7) Total thyroidectomy by experienced thyroid surgeons is safe and associated with a low morbidity.

Counterarguments for procedures of lesser magnitude are as follows: (1) the biologic significance of microscopic foci in the opposite lobe is uncertain and has not been found to have a deleterious effect on

TABLE 4. **TNM Classification of Papillary or Follicular Thyroid Carcinoma, WHO Revision**

Stage	Age <45 Years			Age >45 Years		
I	Any T	Any N	M0	T1	N0	M0
II	Any T	Any N	M1	T2	N0	M0
				T3	N0	M0
III	—			T4	N0	M0
				Any T	N1	M0
IV	—			Any T	Any N	M1

T1: ≤1 cm
T2: >1–4 cm
T3: >4 cm
T4: extends beyond gland
N1: regional lymph node metastasis
M1: distant metastasis

From Thomas CA Jr: Management of differentiated thyroid cancer. *In* Current Practice in Surgery, Vol 3. London, Churchill Livingstone Medical Division of Longman Group UK Limited, 1991, pp 235–241.

survivorship. (2) Most patients with papillary carcinoma are in a low-risk group and do not require therapy with radioactive iodine. (3) There are no conclusive data indicating that a total, as contrasted with a near-total, thyroidectomy is associated with better survivorship. (4) Progression to a poorly differentiated type of neoplasm is rare. (5) Total thyroidectomy is associated with a higher complication rate. The most compelling argument against routine total thyroidectomy is the morbidity—primarily hypoparathyroidism with a varied incidence, e.g., 2 to 32%, and a definite but low incidence of recurrent nerve paralysis.

SPECIFIC TREATMENT

Papillary Carcinoma

In papillary carcinoma, the operation is tailored to the individual patient based on associated risk factors reflecting the aggressiveness of the disease and the prognosis. As noted, lobectomy is adequate for papillary carcinomas 1 cm or less in diameter. Patients with more extensive disease should undergo near-total or total thyroidectomy contingent on the risk group. Total thyroidectomy is most appropriate for patients at high risk. A near-total or total thyroidectomy is advised for patients who have extracapsular disease or distant metastatic disease requiring therapy with radioactive iodine and for those with a prior history of external radiation indicating the likelihood of significant multifocal disease.

Although total thyroidectomy is considered by many to be superior to near-total thyroidectomy, it is not obligatory and should be tempered by the experience of the surgeon and the need to avoid recurrent nerve injury and hypoparathyroidism. With encasement of a functioning recurrent nerve, the tumor can be usually be removed by "fracture" to preserve nerve integrity, anticipating treatment by radioactive iodine. In patients who are candidates for total thyroidectomy, after a lobectomy has been completed on the side of the primary tumor and the parathyroid glands have not been conserved or when there is concern about the integrity of the recurrent nerve, a near-total lobectomy on the contralateral side seems prudent and is an acceptable operation. The posterior capsule along with a "shell" of thyroid tissue (1 to 2 grams) is preserved to protect the recurrent laryngeal nerve and the parathyroid glands with their blood supply. A near-total thyroidectomy does not compromise subsequent treatment with radioiodine. All vascularized parathyroid tissue is left in situ, and nonviable glands should be diced into fragments approximately 1 mm in diameter and implanted in separate pockets in the sternocleidomastoid muscle. Verification of parathyroid tissue is best done by frozen section.

Excision of cervical lymph node metastases, as demonstrated intraoperatively, is accomplished by a modified anterior neck dissection, with particular attention paid to common sites of metastasis. The internal jugular vein, sternocleidomastoid muscle, and cranial nerve XI are preserved. Involved superior mediastinal lymph nodes can usually be removed through a cervical incision. Although a high incidence of "occult" lymph node metastasis has been demonstrated by some, a "prophylactic" lymph node dissection is not indicated.

Follicular Carcinoma

In patients with high-risk (angioinvasion) follicular carcinoma, total thyroidectomy is warranted, followed by adjuvant radioactive iodine therapy. For patients in the low-risk category (encapsulated, minimally invasive tumors), a lobectomy is adequate with subsequent TSH suppression. Treatment of the opposite lobe by completion thyroidectomy or radiation ablation should not be required.

The recommendations for the treatment of Hürthle cell carcinoma are comparable to those of follicular cancer. Characteristically, these lesions secrete thyroglobulin, which may be used to monitor the course of the disease. The avidity of this neoplasm for radioiodine is low, but approximately 4 to 5% of the neoplasms demonstrate uptake. Many Hürthle cell neoplasms are benign and are adequately treated by lobectomy.

Medullary Carcinoma of the Thyroid

MTC is an aggressive neoplasm, and the only effective form of therapy is surgical excision by total thyroidectomy and meticulous dissection of lymph nodes from the central compartment of the neck. This is the only thyroid neoplasm in which prophylactic dissection is indicated. Because approximately 20 to 25% of these tumors represent a component of the MEN syndrome, type 2A or 2B, preoperative studies should include tests for pheochromocytoma and hyperparathyroidism. Surgical removal of a pheochromocytoma takes precedence over thyroidectomy. The identification of mutations in the *ret* proto-oncogene in a MEN family member constitutes an indication for total thyroidectomy without regard to the plasma calcitonin level. With clinically apparent disease, the serum calcitonin level is a useful index of regional lymph node and systemic involvement.

Anaplastic Carcinoma

Anaplastic carcinomas, aggressive neoplasms that seem to be decreasing in frequency, have a poor prognosis. The role of surgery is primarily to establish an accurate diagnosis and at times an airway. In the patient in whom the lesion is confined to one lobe, radical excision, a near-total or total thyroidectomy, is warranted. External beam radiation is the predominant means of therapy regardless of the extent of surgery. Combining x-ray therapy with chemotherapy has been advantageous in selected patients. Insular carcinoma, a poorly differentiated form of papillary cancer, falls into this group but may respond to excision followed by radioiodine therapy and external radiation.

Thyroid Lymphoma

In thyroid lymphoma, surgery is limited to procuring an adequate specimen for definitive diagnosis. Thereafter, by the use of scans (computed tomography and/or magnetic resonance imaging) the disease is staged as IE confined to the thyroid with or without local invasion, IIE with regional node metastasis, IIIE with distant nodal metastasis, or IVE with systemic disease. Because of the frequency of progression from stage IE and IIE, a combination of external radiotherapy (mantle in type) and systemic chemotherapy has given the best results.

ADJUVANT THERAPY: RADIOACTIVE IODINE, HORMONAL SUPPRESSION, EXTERNAL RADIATION

Radioactive Iodine. Radioactive iodine is intrinsically appealing as an adjuvant to the surgical therapy of differentiated thyroid carcinomas. Distinction should be made between radioiodine ablation, used to destroy normal thyroid tissue after near-total or total thyroidectomy, and radioiodine therapy of persistent or recurrent carcinoma within and outside (metastatic) the thyroid bed. Data are limited with respect to the benefits of postoperative radioactive iodine ablation of thyroid remnants to treat microscopic foci within the remnant and to remove a source of thyroglobulin. Although there does seem to be a decreased incidence of local recurrence, survivorship does not seem to be influenced. Radioiodine ablation is clearly indicated in patients in the high-risk group after a near-total or total thyroidectomy with appraisal of residual disease by whole-body scans in association with an elevated TSH level. Radioiodine therapy is the most effective treatment for nonresectable, residual, recurrent, or metastatic carcinoma that concentrates radioiodine. It has also been used to treat patients in whom the only evidence of disease is an elevated thyroglobulin level.

Hormonal Suppression. Differentiated thyroid cancers contain membrane receptors for TSH and a responsive adenylate cyclase system. This is the rationale for long-term TSH suppression for all patients with tumors arising from follicular epithelium. The differences in numbers as well as sensitivity of TSH receptors may account for the variation in responsiveness. Sufficient thyroid hormone (levothyroxine [Synthroid, Levothroid]) should be administered to suppress TSH to less than 0.1 μIU per mL. The recommended dose is 2.2 μg per kg per day in adults younger than 60 years and 1.5 to 1.8 μg per kg per day in older patients. Hyperthyroxinemia should be avoided. Thyroglobulin levels are also influenced by TSH levels.

External Beam Radiation Therapy. In patients with differentiated cancer, external beam radiation therapy is indicated when the disease is not amenable to surgical excision and when there is no uptake of radioiodine. Its chief role is in the management of thyroid lymphomas and anaplastic carcinoma. The addition of chemotherapy has been of limited value.

FOLLOW-UP

Management of patients with a history of thyroid carcinoma requires continuing evaluation to monitor disease presence by physical examination, thyroglobulin levels, and radioiodine and other scans, and to ensure appropriate TSH suppression. It is highly individualized according to risk groups. For patients at high risk, thyroid hormone may be withdrawn annually to determine thyroglobulin levels and the need for radioiodine scanning. Attention must be paid to the presence of thyroglobulin antibodies, which may give a falsely high or low level. After radioiodine therapy, patients should be re-evaluated for potential treatment at intervals of approximately 1 year until there is no further uptake. In patients with suspected disease that does not concentrate radioiodine, scans with thallium 201 or sestamibi and magnetic resonance imaging may provide alternative diagnostic modalities. Most local recurrences of differentiated carcinoma develop within 5 years; however, because of the long natural history of the disease, a follow-up of 20 years after the last evidence of the disease (residual or recurrent) is advised.

Future developments in the management of thyroid cancer will relate to the role of oncogenes and tumor suppressive genes and more specifically to molecular markers for cells from fine-needle aspirates that indicate invasive behavior; radiolabeled octreotide scintigraphy in localizing MTC and other cancers; recombinant TSH to facilitate radioiodine treatment; and the findings of the National Thyroid Cancer Treatment Cooperative Study Registry formed in 1987.

PHEOCHROMOCYTOMA

method of
LEWIS LANDSBERG, M.D.
Northwestern University Medical School
Chicago, Illinois

Pheochromocytoma is a tumor that arises, most frequently, from chromaffin cells of the adrenal medulla. Tumors arising outside the adrenals are called extra-adrenal pheochromocytomas or paragangliomas. The hallmark of these tumors is the excessive and unregulated release of catecholamines from the tumor. Although many of the clinical manifestations of the disease, including hypertension, are the consequence of the excessive release of catecholamines, pheochromocytomas produce a variety of other biologically active substances that may contribute to the clinical manifestations.

The rarity of pheochromocytoma, which is present in less than 0.1% of unselected hypertensive patients, is in sharp distinction to its importance. With prompt diagnosis and appropriate treatment, the disease is almost always curable; a missed diagnosis or improper treatment, on the other hand, is frequently fatal. Available evidence from unselected autopsy series, moreover, demonstrates that the diagnosis is frequently missed, because as many as 80% of these tumors are found unexpectedly at postmortem examination. Retrospective chart review in these cases indicates that in many of these patients the pheochromocytoma was responsible for the fatal outcome. Many potentially curable cases, therefore, remain undiagnosed.

DIAGNOSIS

Clinical Manifestations

The disease is characterized by hypertension, paroxysmal attacks or crises, and an increase in metabolic rate. Most patients have hypertension, and in most of these the hypertension is sustained although the blood pressure may be more labile than in essential hypertension. Approximately 50% of patients have distinct pressor crises characterized by headache, sweating, palpitations, and chest or abdominal pain. Headaches, diaphoresis, and palpitations are so common that the absence of all three of these manifestations makes pheochromocytoma unlikely. The clinical manifestations, however, are protean, and many unusual presentations have been reported including rhabdomyolysis with myoglobinuric renal failure and unexplained shock with multisystem organ failure. The unexplained bouts of hypotension sometimes seen in patients with pheochromocytoma may be secondary to the production and release of a potent hypotensive peptide, adrenomedullin, from the tumor. Other biologically active substances that may contribute to the clinical manifestations include endothelin and neuropeptide Y (hypertension), erythropoietin (polycythemia, although usually the high hematocrit seen in patients with pheochromocytoma reflects diminished plasma volume), and parathyroid hormone–related peptide (hypercalcemia). Failure to respond to conventional treatment for essential hypertension also suggests the diagnosis, but several of the newer agents, particularly calcium channel blockers and selective alpha$_1$-receptor blockers, are effective at controlling hypertension in patients with pheochromocytoma.

Measurement of Catecholamines and Catecholamine Metabolites

The diagnosis of pheochromocytoma is confirmed by the demonstration of excess catecholamine production by the tumor. This is best done by the demonstration of increased quantities of catecholamines and catecholamine metabolites in urine. There are three commonly employed tests: free (unconjugated) catecholamines, which may be fractionated into norepinephrine and epinephrine; the metanephrines, which may be fractionated into normetanephrine and metanephrine; and 4-hydroxy-3-methoxymandelic acid (VMA or HMMA). The metanephrines are the O-methylated catecholamines, whereas VMA is the O-methylated deaminated metabolite. Recent studies demonstrate the superiority of the catecholamine and metanephrine measurements compared with measurement of VMA. In general, 24-hour urine collections (with a creatinine measurement to ensure adequate collection) are superior to partial collections, although overnight collections normalized for creatinine may be useful when 24-hour urine collections are difficult to obtain. The collection should be obtained with the patient at rest, taking no medication, and without

recent exposure to radiographic contrast media. When it is not practical to discontinue all medications, those drugs known specifically to interfere with the assays used, or to confound the interpretation, should be avoided. The clinician should check with the clinical pathologist at the laboratory used for the determinations for advice appropriate to the determination employed, because interference depends on the specificity of the assays employed. State-of-the-art techniques using high-performance liquid chromatographic separation and electrochemical detection have minimal interference, although exogenous catecholamines and related compounds such as methyldopa, levodopa, and labetalol frequently increase catecholamine measurements, which may stay elevated for up to 2 weeks after the agent is withdrawn. Patients with pheochromocytoma usually have substantial elevations in catecholamine and metanephrine excretion, with values commonly 3 to 10 times the upper limit of normal. The trick is to think of the diagnosis; in the vast majority of cases the diagnosis is confirmed with the first 24-hour urine collection.

Plasma catecholamine determinations have a distinctly limited role in the diagnosis of pheochromocytoma. They are inferior to urinary collections and should not be used as a screening test. Other substances such as chromogranin A and dopamine β-hydroxylase, although measurable in plasma, are not useful for diagnosis.

Familial Pheochromocytoma: Genetic Abnormalities

Pheochromocytoma, inherited as an autosomal dominant trait, is an important component of the multiple endocrine neoplasia (MEN) syndromes (types 2A and 2B), the von Hippel–Lindau syndrome, and a rare component of neurofibromatosis type 1. Pheochromocytoma also occurs in some families as an isolated abnormality. Pheochromocytoma in familial syndromes is frequently bilateral, and a familial syndrome should be suspected in any patient presenting with bilateral tumors. Increases in urinary epinephrine excretion may be the only abnormality early in the course of familial pheochromocytoma; fractionated catecholamine collections, therefore, are the most effective way of establishing the diagnosis in this setting.

The application of molecular biologic techniques has yielded much useful information about the molecular oncogenesis of familial pheochromocytoma. In the MEN 2 syndromes, mutations in the ret proto-oncogene result in the constitutive activation of the ret tyrosine kinase receptor, which renders the affected cells susceptible to malignant transformation. Mutations in the extracellular domain of the tyrosine kinase receptor produce the MEN 2A syndrome, whereas alterations in the intracellular portion of the tyrosine kinase receptor cause the MEN 2B syndrome. Mutations at specific locations in the ret proto-oncogene appear to predispose to pheochromocytoma. The abnormality in the von Hippel–Lindau syndrome has been defined as the loss of one copy of the VHL tumor suppressor gene, which results in the development of the characteristic retinal, cerebellar, and renal tumors as well as pheochromocytoma. Other evidence from molecular genetic studies indicates that specific abnormalities in the VHL gene may be associated with pheochromocytoma without the other manifestations of the von Hippel–Lindau syndrome. Recent studies also demonstrate that somatic mutations in the tumor itself are rarely identified in sporadic cases of pheochromocytoma.

Germline mutations in the familial syndromes can be identified by molecular genetic diagnostic techniques. Within affected kindreds, genetic testing can define those who carry the mutation. Appropriate screening and surgical intervention can be made on the basis of the genetic analysis. Although when applied to patients with apparently sporadic pheochromocytoma, molecular diagnostic methods have occasionally identified familial syndromes that escaped detection by the usual clinical evaluation, there is probably no need to apply molecular diagnostic techniques to the usual case of sporadic pheochromocytoma if careful clinical evaluation does not suggest familial disease.

MANAGEMENT
Localization

Once the diagnosis is confirmed, the tumor is localized by imaging with computed tomography (CT) or magnetic resonance imaging (MRI). In general, localization studies are performed after the biochemical demonstration of increased catecholamine production. Adrenergic blockade (see later) is begun once the biochemical diagnosis is confirmed. Localization studies can be performed as the adrenergic blockade develops. Intravenous contrast medium is safe in patients with pheochromocytoma and can be administered even to "unblocked" patients. Arteriography or aortography, however, should be performed only after adrenergic blockade is well established because the intra-arterial administration of dye may be associated with severe pressor crises.

Eighty-five to 90% of pheochromocytomas are located in or adjacent to the adrenal gland. Because they are usually 3 cm in diameter or greater before they cause symptoms, they are usually well demonstrated by CT with fine cuts through the adrenals. The spatial resolution afforded by current CT technology usually provides excellent visualization of the tumor and its relationship to surrounding structures. MRI is quite useful for demonstrating pheochromocytoma as well, because pheochromocytomas are hyperintense on T2-weighted sequences. Radionuclide scanning with metaiodobenzylguanidine I 131 (MIBG) has limited usefulness in localizing adrenal pheochromocytomas, although theoretically it might be useful in distinguishing pheochromocytomas from incidental nonfunctioning cortical tumors.

Localizing extra-adrenal pheochromocytomas presents more of a challenge. Most extra-adrenal pheochromocytomas are located in or about the sympathetic paravertebral ganglia and preaortic plexes within the abdomen. Less common locations include the thorax, cervical region, and urinary bladder. MRI is frequently useful in localizing extra-adrenal pheochromocytomas. If no tumor can be localized with MRI, scanning with ^{131}I-MIBG should be undertaken. Because extra-adrenal pheochromocytomas are frequently supplied by an aberrant artery of considerable size, angiography involving the abdominal aorta may be useful at delineating elusive lesions, but only after adrenergic blockade is established.

Alpha-Adrenergic Blockade

Once the diagnosis is established, phenoxybenzamine (Dibenzyline) therapy should be started. The long duration of action and the noncompetitive nature of the blockade induced by this agent make it ideal for the preoperative preparation of patients with pheochromocytoma. Because of the long duration of action (greater than 24 hours), the therapeutic effect of phenoxybenzamine is cumulative and the optimal dose must, therefore, be achieved gradually. Ten milligrams every 12 hours is the usual starting dose, with incremental increases of 10 or 20 mg added every few days until the blood pressure is controlled and the paroxysms disappear. The blood pressure must be monitored closely, with the patient supine and upright, several times each day with corresponding measurements of the pulse rate. Dosage adjustment should be made over a 2-week period and is best performed in the hospital. Two weeks of stable alpha-adrenergic blockade allows expansion of the plasma volume and relieves the heart and peripheral organs from the effects of intense vasoconstriction. As the dose of phenoxybenzamine is increased, transient postural falls in blood pressure are common; this does not necessarily mean that an adequate dose has been achieved, especially if the supine pressure remains elevated. As the plasma volume expands during the dosage titration, postural signs tend to diminish. Most patients require between 40 and 80 mg of phenoxybenzamine per day, although some patients may require considerably more. One half of the daily dose should be administered every 12 hours. In patients with paroxysmal hypertension, adjustment of the dose of phenoxybenzamine may be problematic. In these patients, phenoxybenzamine should be titrated to the point at which all paroxsyms cease. When persistent postural signs and symptoms develop, the dose should be stabilized. Nasal stuffiness or diarrhea or both indicate a high degree of adrenergic blockade, but it is not necessary to push alpha-adrenergic blockade until these symptoms appear. Phenoxybenzamine should be continued through the morning of surgery.

Although selective alpha$_1$ antagonists such as doxazosin (Cardura) and terazosin (Hytrin) and the alpha-beta antagonist labetalol (Normodyne) have all been used in treating patients with pheochromocytoma, phenoxybenzamine remains the preferred agent because of its long duration of action and the noncompetitive blockade that it induces.

Hypertensive crises or paroxyms that occur in patients with known or suspected pheochromocytoma may be effectively treated with the intravenous administration of phentolamine. After a secure intravenous route is established, a test dose of 0.5 mg is given as a bolus; if there is no response, 1.0 to 5.0 mg is administered intravenously. The blood pressure should be recorded frequently (every 30 seconds). The response to phentolamine is maximal in 2 or 3 minutes and lasts 10 to 15 minutes. Norepinephrine (Levophed) or phenylephrine (Neo-Synephrine) should be immediately available in case of a severe hypotensive reaction. Phentolamine administration may be repeated as necessary to control the blood pressure. In less urgent situations, oral prazosin

(Minipress) may be administered as needed to control blood pressure before the effect of phenoxybenzamine is established.

Beta-Adrenergic Blockade

Beta blockers should be administered only after alpha-adrenergic blockade is introduced, because the administration of beta-adrenergic blocking agents alone may cause a paradoxical increase in blood pressure due to unopposed alpha-receptor stimulation. As alpha-adrenergic blockade with phenoxybenzamine develops, small doses of propranolol should be administered as significant tachycardia develops. Patients with pheochromocytoma are sensitive to beta-adrenergic blockade, and usually small doses suffice. Ten milligrams three or four times per day is the usual starting dose. The dose is titrated upward to control the pulse rate; only rarely is more than 60 to 80 mg of propranolol required. Beta blockers are quite useful in controlling ventricular and supraventricular arrhythmias, particularly those associated with the administration of anesthetic agents. Intravenous propranolol in doses of 0.5 to 2.0 mg can be used if required for rhythm control and during surgery. Beta blockers should be used cautiously in patients with compromised cardiac reserve.

Inhibition of Catecholamine Biosynthesis

Metyrosine (Demser), an inhibitor of tyrosine hydroxylase, inhibits catecholamine production by 50 to 80% when administered in doses ranging from 0.3 to 4.0 grams per day. In the usual case of pheochromocytoma, this agent is not required, but when catecholamine production is markedly increased by an extremely large tumor, it may be of use in preoperative preparation, along with phenoxybenzamine. The major use of metyrosine is in the long-term treatment of patients with unoperable tumors such as those with malignant pheochromocytoma.

SURGERY

Removal of a pheochromocytoma, the definitive treatment, is technically demanding and should be performed in centers that have experience in the preoperative preparation, anesthesia, and surgical removal of these tumors. As noted previously, successful surgery requires adequate preoperative preparation consisting of a 2-week course of alpha-adrenergic blockade with phenoxybenzamine. Phenoxybenzamine should be administered up to and including the morning of surgery.

Short-acting barbiturates, scopolamine, and succinylcholine are commonly used agents for induction of anesthesia. A combination of anesthetic agents including thiopental, nitrous oxide, narcotics, and enflurane is commonly employed. Narcotics, extremely hazardous in the unblocked patient as noted later, can be safely administered in the well-blocked patient adequately prepared for surgery. All the halogenated hydrocarbon anesthetics (including enflurane) sensitize the heart to the arrhythmogenic properties of catecholamines; because these arrhythmias are effectively antagonized by beta-adrenergic blockade, it is customary to continue beta blockers up to the time of surgery and to administer propranolol during the operative procedure itself if cardiac arrhythmias occur. During the procedure, careful monitoring is of critical importance; continuous assessment of the electrocardiogram and of the intra-arterial and central venous pressures should be carried out. An accurate assessment of blood loss should be recorded from the outset, and saline, albumin, or blood should be administered to replace losses as these occur. Intraoperative hypotension responds better to volume replacement than to vasoconstrictors. The central venous pressure is helpful in estimating the need for volume repletion. If there is a history of impaired cardiac reserve, the pulmonary capillary wedge pressure should be monitored as well.

Increases in blood pressure and cardiac arrhythmias occur most frequently during induction of anesthesia, intubation, and manipulation of the tumor. Hypertension can usually be controlled adequately by the intravenous administration of phentolamine (Regitine) in 1- to 5-mg boluses as needed; large amounts are sometimes required depending on the size of the tumor and the adequacy of preoperative blockade. Nitroprusside (Nipride) is also effective in controlling hypertension and can be used as an alternative to phentolamine during surgery. Sinus tachycardia or ventricular ectopy usually responds promptly to the intravenous administration of propranolol. Lidocaine may be used as well. If a vasopressor is required, norepinephrine or phenylephrine should be used; indirect-acting sympathomimetic amines that release norepinephrine from nerve endings evoke an unpredictable response in these patients and should therefore be avoided.

The choice of the surgical procedure depends on the location of the tumor. Exploratory surgery in which the localization of the tumor has not been accomplished preoperatively is now exceedingly rare. When the tumor has been localized to one adrenal gland, the exploration can be limited to the adrenal gland containing the tumor by a flank or thoracoabdominal incision. These tumors are usually quite vascular, and adequate exposure is required so that the venous drainage may be ligated before manipulation and mobilization of the tumor. The pheochromocytoma should be removed with the capsule intact, including surrounding connective tissue and fat; each tumor should be handled as a potentially malignant lesion. The entire adrenal gland should be removed, because it is usually impossible to remove the tumor and spare the underlying normal adrenal tissue. The blood pressure should fall after the tumor is removed. If hypotension occurs, fluid administration is usually sufficient to maintain blood pressure. If bilateral adrenal pheochromocytomas are being removed, hydrocortisone should be administered, the dose and route of administration being similar to those employed in patients undergoing bilateral adrenal or pituitary surgery for any reason. Laparoscopic removal of pheochromocytoma is being undertaken at some centers but is not appropriate for general application pending further experience.

Hypertension recurring in the immediate postoperative period usually reflects fluid shifts and autonomic instability and does not necessarily indicate residual pheochromocytoma. Loop diuretics may be helpful if large amounts of fluid have been administered and if signs of volume expansion are present. Persistent hypertension may indicate residual tumor or an intraoperative complication such as damage to the kidney or renal artery. Postoperative hypotension may be due to volume depletion, persistent adrenergic blockade, or hemorrhage at the operative site, but the possibility of adrenocortical insufficiency should be considered, particularly if both adrenal glands have been explored.

Postoperative Management and Long-term Follow-up

Two weeks after surgery, urinary catecholamines and metanephrines should be measured to confirm that all functional pheochromocytoma has been removed. These determinations should be repeated on a yearly basis indefinitely because long-term recurrences have been well documented. Obviously, the recurrence of suggestive symptoms or hypertension should prompt an immediate search for recurrent disease.

In those patients in whom operative removal of the tumor is impossible because of either malignancy or concurrent disease that contraindicates surgery, long-term medical management is required. This usually involves the chronic administration of adrenergic blocking agents and, as described earlier, metyrosine.

Malignant Pheochromocytoma

Less than 10% of pheochromocytomas are malignant. Invasive local recurrence and metastases to regional lymph nodes, retroperitoneum, liver, lung, or bone are the usual manifestations of malignant disease. As with most endocrine tumors, malignancy cannot be predicted with confidence on the basis of the histologic appearance of the tumor; the presence of metastatic deposits and unequivocal microvascular invasion are the only reliable microscopic indications of malignant behavior. Recurrence of tumor in the operative site may signify malignancy or incomplete resection. If distal metastases can be excluded, recurrent disease should be surgically resected. Unresectable tumor is difficult to destroy, but some success has been noted with combination chemotherapy including cyclophosphamide (Cytoxan), vincristine (Oncovin), and dacarbazine (DTIC-Dome). Embolization-induced infarction of discrete metastatic deposits may be attempted as well, but only with careful attention to adrenergic blockade. Despite initial enthusiasm, tumor ablation by ^{131}I-MIBG has not been useful clinically, although diminished output of catecholamines and metabolites has been amply demonstrated in many treated patients.

OTHER ISSUES

Adverse Drug Interactions

The clinical course of pheochromocytoma may be complicated by pharmaceutical agents administered for therapeutic or diagnostic purposes. Severe and even fatal crises have been associated with opiates, histamine, corticotropin, saralasin, and glucagon. These agents induce paroxysms by releasing catecholamines directly from the tumor. The importance of opiates, including meperidine (Demerol), has been insufficiently emphasized in the medical literature. The potent opiate fentanyl (Sublimaze) has been implicated in the precipitation of crises during anesthesia induction in patients with unsuspected pheochromocytoma undergoing incidental elective or emergent surgery. When administered intra-arterially, radiographic contrast media also release catecholamines; severe paroxysms, therefore, may result if arteriography is performed in patients with pheochromocytoma before the administration of alpha-adrenergic blocking agents. Intravenous radiographic contrast media, in distinction, are customarily administered without untoward consequences.

Indirect-acting sympathomimetic amines, including intravenously administered methyldopa, may result in an unpredictable increase in blood pressure by releasing catecholamines from the enhanced stores within sympathetic nerve endings. Proprietary cold remedies, which contain sympathomimetic amines as decongestants (phenylpropanolamine and pseudoephedrine) are frequent offenders and may worsen the hypertension and increase the symptoms in patients with pheochromocytoma.

Drugs that block the neuronal uptake of catecholamines, such as tricyclic antidepressants and guanethidine (Ismelin), inhibit a major inactivating process and thereby enhance the physiologic effects of circulating catecholamines. Indeed, suggestive symptoms developing after the administration of tricyclic antidepressants should suggest the possibility of pheochromocytoma. All these drugs should be specifically avoided in patients with known or suspected pheochromocytoma, and all medications should be carefully considered and administered cautiously in this group of patients.

Pheochromocytoma in Pregnancy

Management of pheochromocytoma in pregnancy remains a considerable challenge. Once the diagnosis is established, adrenergic blocking agents should be prescribed as described previously. MRI may be used to localize the tumor. In early to middle pregnancy, the tumor should be removed after suitable preoperative preparation. The pregnancy need not be terminated before surgery, but the risk of spontaneous abortion is high. Spontaneous labor and delivery should usually be avoided. Late in pregnancy, treatment with adrenergic blocking agents should be undertaken until the fetus is of sufficient maturity to sustain viability, when cesarean section followed by tumor resection is undertaken. Although the safety of adrenergic blockade during pregnancy has not been established, in many reported cases these agents have been used without untoward effects.

PROGNOSIS

In experienced hands, surgical mortality should be less than 1%. Postoperative survival for benign lesions approaches the age-related norm. The recurrence rate is usually less than 10%. In approximately 75% of patients with benign pheochromocytomas, the hypertension is completely cured; in the remaining 25% hypertension remains or recurs but is usually well controlled with a standard antihypertensive regimen. Underlying essential hypertension or vascular damage secondary to the pheochromocytoma may contribute to the persistent high blood pressure. In malignant pheochromocytoma, the 5-year survival rate is less than 50%, but occasional long survivals have been noted.

THYROIDITIS

method of
TERRY F. DAVIES, M.D.
Mount Sinai School of Medicine
New York, New York

What is generally meant by the term "thyroiditis" is inflammation of the thyroid gland, whether it is caused by an autoimmune diathesis or viral or bacterial infections or is an accompaniment of neoplasia. Thyroiditis is evidenced by an inflammatory infiltrate on histologic examination, either diffuse or patchy, but it is not necessarily accompanied by thyroid cell dysfunction. Mild degrees of autoimmune thyroiditis are found in many individuals who retain normal thyroid hormone output.

SEQUENTIAL CHANGES IN THYROID FUNCTION CAUSED BY THYROIDITIS

Grades of Hypothyroidism

Patients with autoimmune and nonautoimmune thyroiditis often present with varying degrees of thyroid failure. The term "subclinical hypothyroidism" refers to a condition marked by an increased serum thyroid-stimulating hormone (TSH) level (usually >4 μU per mL depending on the assay and patient's age) but a serum free thyroxine (T_4) level that is within the normal range, often low normal, and with few or no clinical symptoms. Such patients with thyroid autoantibodies are known to progress to thyroid failure at a rate of 3 to 5% per year. In contrast, "mild thyroid failure" refers to patients with increased TSH levels and below-normal serum free T_4 values who complain of a variety of nonspecific symptoms that remit with T_4

replacement therapy. "Overt hypothyroidism" presents with obvious clinical features, a major elevation of serum TSH levels, and a low free T_4 concentration.

Hyperthyroidism in Thyroiditis

Patients with thyroiditis may present with a transient form of hyperthyroidism before the onset of thyroid failure. This is secondary to release of excess thyroid hormone at the time of thyroid cell destruction. Such hyperthyroidism is usually followed by the onset of thyroid failure once most of the thyroid cells are destroyed. Hence, all forms of thyroiditis may present with a sequential clinical pattern of hyperthyroidism followed by hypothyroidism. However, not all patients have a sufficiently vigorous degree of thyroid cell destruction to induce hyperthyroidism. Figure 1 illustates the different possible sequences of events.

AUTOIMMUNE THYROIDITIS

Background

Autoimmune thyroiditis (Hashimoto's disease) results in thyroid decompensation in 1 to 3% of the population. The disease satisfies the classic criteria for an autoimmune disease, including its association with autoreactive T cells and autoantibodies to thyroglobulin and thyroid peroxidase (the microsomal antigen) in more than 90% of patients and, less commonly, autoantibodies to the TSH receptor in 10 to 15% of patients. Because many people with apparently normal thyroid function tests may have detectable thyroid autoantibodies and autoreactive T cells as well as an accompanying lymphocytic infiltration of their thyroid glands, Davies and Amino have reclassified autoimmune thyroiditis into type 1 (euthyroid), type 2 (hypothyroid), and type 3 (hyperthyroid) (Table 1). Type 2 thyroiditis, therefore, includes the three different grades of hypothyroidism—subclinical, mild, and overt.

Patients with autoimmune thyroiditis may present

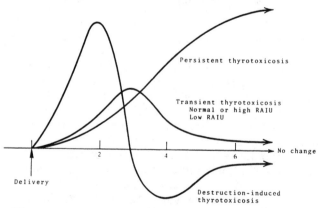

Figure 1. Possible presentations of the postpartum autoimmune thyroid syndromes. Transient hyperthyroidism followed by the onset of hypothyroidism is also seen in other types of thyroiditis, particularly subacute thyroiditis. *Abbreviation:* RAIU = radioactive iodine uptake. (From Davies TF: Autoimmune Endocrine Disease. New York, John Wiley & Sons, 1983, p 255. Copyright © 1983, John Wiley & Sons, Inc. Reprinted by permission of John Wiley & Sons, Inc.)

TABLE 1. **Classification of Human Thyroiditis**

Type 1 Autoimmune thyroiditis (Hashimoto's disease type 1)
  1A Euthyroid—goitrous
  1B Euthyroid—nongoitrous
Type 2 Autoimmune thyroiditis (Hashimoto's disease type 2)
  2A Hypothyroid—goitrous (classic Hashimoto's disease)
  2B Hypothyroid—nongoitrous (primary myxedema, atrophic thyroiditis)
  2C Transient aggravation (postpartum or silent)
Type 3 Autoimmune thyroiditis (Graves' disease)
  3A Hyperthyroid Graves' disease
  3B Euthyroid Graves' disease
  3C Hypothyroid Graves' disease
Type 4 Thyroiditis (nonautoimmune)
  4A Acute thyroiditis
  4B Subacute thyroiditis

with an obvious firm rubbery thyroid enlargement (goitrous thyroiditis, as described by Hashimoto himself) or without a palpable thyroid at all (atrophic thyroiditis, sometimes referred to as primary myxedema). The atrophic variety may be more often associated with TSH-receptor–blocking autoantibodies.

Treatment

In my opinion, all forms of thyroid failure should be treated, including the subclinical variety. An increasing volume of data has suggested that patients with the mildest degree of thyroid failure show, for example, subtle cardiac abnormalities that are corrected with thyroid replacement therapy. Treatment consists of levothyroxine (Synthroid, Levothroid, or Levoxyl) as replacement therapy. This type of replacement treatment must be distinguished from T_4 suppression therapy used in patients with thyroid cancer. The aim in patients with autoimmune thyroiditis and hypothyroidism is to increase their serum T_4 values and lower their increased TSH levels into the mid-normal range (approximately 1 to 3 μU per mL). Such treatment should effectively remove all symptoms related to thyroid disease. Careful follow-up and monitoring of TSH levels also prevent the recurrence of thyroid failure in the future, as any residual thyroid tissue is further destroyed. Treatment should continue to be guided by the normalization of serum TSH levels using a sensitive third-generation immunoassay that is capable of distinguishing normal (>0.4 to 4.0 μU per mL) from suppressed TSH levels. Most patients require less than 150 μg of levothyroxine per day as a once-daily medication for the rest of their lives (1.7 μg per kg of body weight).

To maintain the correct replacement dose as the patient's thyroid reserve diminishes (due to ongoing disease) or as thyroid requirements increase (as in pregnancy), it is important to titrate the patient's levothyroxine dose against the serum TSH level at regular intervals. Any need for increasing the dose should be well documented by evidence of consistent levothyroxine intake in the presence of a persistently raised TSH level. It is wise to allow 4 to 6 weeks for

TSH normalization after a change in the dose of levothyroxine or a change in the brand of levothyroxine preparation being used. There appears to be little to distinguish among the different commercial preparations available, but it is important for the patient to continue with the same reliable preparation rather than switching at random. This is because the patient's serum TSH level should be titrated carefully to avoid the long-term side effects of excessive levothyroxine, including the potential of accelerating bone demineralization in postmenopausal women. The American Thyroid Association has clearly stated that changing the source of the levothyroxine preparation should be followed by a re-evaluation of the patient's thyroid status, and this should be guided by reassessing the serum TSH level. After all, that is what we do when we change the patient's dose of levothyroxine. Generic preparations can be a problem unless the patient can ensure a consistent supply from the same source, a difficult task. Recent studies widely reported in the media do not indicate any change in this long-held recommendation.

Caution should also be exercised when initiating levothyroxine therapy in elderly patients and those with coronary artery disease. The initial dosage should be 12.5 to 25 μg daily for 7 days with a subsequent, very gradual increase to avoid the development of arrhythmias. Thyroid extract preparations should no longer be used. The commonly raised serum triiodothyronine (T_3) levels and suppressed serum TSH levels found in patients taking thyroid extract preparations appear to me to be an unnecessary risk when levothyroxine therapy is available to everyone. Combination preparations of levothyroxine and T_3 (Thyrolar) are also still available, but indications for them are beyond my understanding. Liothyronine (Cytomel) is still used as thyroid replacement therapy, but it has a three-times-daily dosage regimen that makes it unpopular (liothyronine has a shorter half-life than levothyroxine), and it tends to cause tachycardia and arrhythmias in an unacceptably high proportion of patients. I see no reason for its use in such patients.

Surgery is rarely indicated in patients with autoimmune thyroiditis. Particularly firm areas of a goiter may appear as hard nodules and may be a reason in some hospitals for mistaken and unnecessary surgery. This situation is easily avoided by thyroid sonography and, if necessary, aspiration biopsy. Very occasionally, a large goiter due to Hashimoto's thyroiditis causes pressure effects on the trachea that may best be relieved by careful surgery.

POSTPARTUM THYROIDITIS

Background

Pregnancy is associated with a period of generalized immunosuppression. Thyroid antibody titers consistently fall as parturition approaches and then rebound after delivery, sometimes to concentrations greater than those seen before pregnancy. Titers peak at about 3 to 6 months after delivery, and in this period a variety of postpartum thyroid syndromes may be observed in up to 8% of women (see Figure 1). The most common presentation is lethargy in the postpartum period associated with an increased TSH level and high titers of antibodies to thyroid peroxidase (the microsomal antigen), although occasionally hyperthyroid symptoms may be seen. A diagnosis of autoimmune (silent) thyroiditis can be confirmed in the non–breast-feeding mother by a low or absent 24-hour radioiodine uptake. Treatment depends on severity. Most episodes are transient, and rapid recovery can be expected during a 2- to 4-month period.

Treatment

The common symptoms of thyroid failure, combined with reduced serum T_4 levels and raised TSH levels, can be relieved by the administration of 100 to 150 µg of levothyroxine once daily. Thyroid antibody titers should be monitored as well as the TSH level. As antibody titers begin to fall, it should be possible to withdraw the drug completely. However, in some patients such a presentation may indicate the onset of chronic autoimmune thyroiditis. Even the long-term outlook for patients with the transient syndrome is likely to be thyroid failure in a large percentage. It is known that it may recur after a subsequent pregnancy, and data suggest that 20 to 30% of such patients eventually develop permanent thyroid failure. As mentioned previously, the early phase of the disease may be associated with hyperthyroidism because of widespread thyroid cell destruction. This appears to be more common in the postpartum period than in patients with more traditional autoimmune thyroiditis and may be related to the marked immunologic rebound that occurs in such patients. Usually, the mild hyperthyroidism associated with suppressed serum TSH levels (<0.4 µU per mL) settles into thyroid gland failure before treatment is necessary, although propranolol (20 to 40 mg four times per day) may be helpful for tachycardia. It should also be remembered that true Graves' disease may occasionally present in the postpartum period and requires appropriate treatment.

SUBACUTE THYROIDITIS

Background

Subacute (de Quervain's, granulomatous) thyroiditis has a variable prevalence in different countries. It appears to be common in North America, although there are no epidemiologic data. It is associated with HLA-B35 and is more often seen in women than in men (5:1). Often, a prodromal viral type of pharyngitis is rapidly followed by general malaise, headache, fever, and a unique localized, acute tenderness of the thyroid gland. Tenderness usually affects both lobes, but unilateral tenderness may occur and may move sequentially from one side to the other. If the patient allows you to examine the thyroid, you will find that the gland is firm and may be nodular. A lack of radioiodine uptake and a raised erythrocyte sedimentation rate (often >100 mm per hour) and serum thyroglobulin level confirm the diagnosis. It is likely that many individuals experience a mild form of the disease, but only with more severe neck discomfort do they present for treatment. Indeed, a painless variety is sometimes observed and must be distinguished from autoimmune (silent) thyroiditis. The disorder is considered to have a viral cause, and probably many viruses have such a propensity, although there are few data to confirm this.

Treatment

Most patients do not require treatment apart from aspirin to relieve the neck pain. However, severe thyroidal tenderness is sometimes devastating, and in this situation, prednisone, 30 to 40 mg daily for a 5-day period with gradual reduction during the subsequent 2 to 4 weeks, is quite effective. During the period of acute tenderness, massive destruction of thyroid tissue occurs, and biochemical hyperthyroidism is present in more than 50% of patients, requiring beta blockade with propranolol, 20 to 40 mg four times daily or atenolol,* 25 to 50 mg daily. This is followed by a period of euthyroidism, sometimes lasting several weeks, until hypothyroidism appears. This is the period when the gland is undergoing regeneration, and the patient may require levothyroxine supplementation, depending on the patient's clinical status and serum T_4 and TSH values. A dose of 100 µg of levothyroxine daily for a period of 8 weeks should be sufficient to allow subsequent withdrawal and monitoring of the return to normal function. I find that erythrocyte sedimentation rates and serum thyroglobulin levels are effective for monitoring the activity of the thyroiditis. Both may be quite high during the active phase of the disease.

Some patients have a transient thyroid abnormality associated with no thyroid tenderness, the so-called painless thyroiditis. Such a diagnosis can be made during the hyperthyroid phase of the thyroiditis by the absence of radioiodine uptake into the thyroid. Treatment of the hyperthyroid phase is best accomplished with beta blockade using propranolol and then, as the hypothyroid phase ensues, with levothyroxine if it is necessary to replace thyroid function until recovery occurs.

ACUTE (SUPPURATIVE) THYROIDITIS

Background

Now rare, acute (suppurative) thyroiditis, once a more common acute disease, is usually associated with *Staphylococcus aureus, Streptococcus, Klebsiella pneumoniae,* or *Escherichia coli* infection in parallel

---

*Not FDA approved for this indication.

with obvious infective loci elsewhere, often nearby. The gland is generally enlarged and acutely tender, and the patient is ill with fever, tachycardia, and often a septicemia. There may be thrombophlebitis of the external jugular veins. A more chronic course may be seen in patients with immunodeficiency including acquired immune deficiency syndrome and can be associated with infection by actinomyces, mycobacteria, and *Pneumocystis carinii*.

Treatment

Treatment involves high-dose antibiotic therapy and incision and drainage when appropriate. Thyroid function should be monitored throughout the illness and appropriate replacement therapy provided if necessary.

DRUG-ASSOCIATED THYROIDITIS

Autoimmune thyroiditis may be precipitated by iodide-containing drugs or lithium. For example, amiodarone, which can also induce hyperthyroidism, more frequently induces hypothyroidism early in therapy, sometimes accompanied by thyroid tenderness. Interferon alfa is another drug associated with the precipitation of autoimmune thyroiditis in susceptible individuals. Thyroid hormone replacement therapy should be initiated in these patients only as indicated by changes in serum TSH levels. It should also be remembered that thyroid cell destruction induced by radioactive iodine therapy may be accompanied by a painful radiation thyroiditis. This is seen in the first week after high-dose treatment and is a transient phenomenon usually lasting only a few days. Aspirin therapy may be needed for tenderness, but corticosteroids are rarely necessary.

RIEDEL'S THYROIDITIS

Patients with the rare disease Riedel's thyroiditis show replacement of their thyroid with dense fibrous tissue, which may extend locally and even systemically to involve the retroperitoneum, mediastinum, and lungs, with devastating consequences. This presentation may be one end point of chronic autoimmune thyroid disease, and it has become rare because autoimmune thyroiditis is now arrested early by thyroid hormone replacement therapy. Treatment with levothyroxine and corticosteroids does not arrest the development of fibrosis, and any obstruction must be relieved surgically. Although some cases of this disease may be a variant of autoimmune thyroiditis, few cases have been reported with immunologic data.

PERINEOPLASTIC THYROIDITIS

Pathology reports often describe associated thyroiditis adjacent to a benign or malignant thyroid neoplasm. The significance of this is uncertain, although thyroid antibodies have an increased prevalence in patients with thyroid cancer. Such tumors are not tender but rather are firm on examination, but it is unclear whether this firmness is accentuated by the surrounding lymphocytic infiltrate. Similarly, Hashimoto's glands may have areas of more severe infiltrate and even fibrosis and may feel clinically like a suspiciously malignant nodule. Removal of such "autoimmune nodules" is a not uncommon mistake, which can be avoided by performing serum thyroid autoantibody testing, thyroid ultrasonography, and an aspiration biopsy before surgery. Often, thyroid cell aspiration biopsy reveals the diagnosis of thyroiditis. Sometimes, however, lymphoid cells may also appear as atypical, thus confirming the physician's mistake.

Section 9

The Urogenital Tract

BACTERIAL INFECTIONS OF THE URINARY TRACT IN MALES

method of
FREDRIC J. SILVERBLATT, M.D.
Providence VA Medical Center
Providence, Rhode Island

Anatomic differences account for much of the variation in the incidence of urinary tract infections (UTIs) between males and females. Because of the greater frequency of congenital abnormalities of the urogenital tract in male infants, UTIs occur four times more often in infant boys younger than 1 year than in infant girls. Beyond the first year, the greater length of the male urethra protects the male urogenital tract from ascending infection and the relative incidence of UTI between the sexes is reversed. At the other extreme of life, prostatic hypertrophy accounts for the fact that asymptomatic bacteriuria (ABU) is more common in men older than 50 years than in women of the same age.

UTIs are rare among young and middle-aged men, but uncomplicated cystitis occasionally occurs in normal, healthy individuals. More typically, UTIs in men are complicated infections with bacterial invasion of the kidney or prostate. They usually occur in the context of impaired local host defenses, e.g., obstruction of urine flow by a stone or tumor, or in a patient with a neurogenic bladder or diabetes. These complicated infections are caused by antibiotic-resistant organisms that require longer courses of therapy and attention to the underlying disease processes for successful resolution. As a result, recurrent UTIs in men, when they occur, are more often clinical relapses of persistent infections rather than reinfections with new organisms as is common in women.

Escherichia coli is the predominant uropathogen in men, but this species accounts for a smaller proportion of urinary isolates than in women. Other gram-negative organisms, such as *Proteus, Klebsiella,* and *Pseudomonas* species, and gram-positive organisms, such as enterococci and coagulase-negative staphylococci, account for up to 50% of UTIs in men. *Staphylococcus saprophyticus,* the second most common pathogen in women, is rarely the cause of UTI in men.

Because uropathogens in complicated infections are less likely to be susceptible to commonly used oral antibiotics, it is especially important in men to obtain a urine specimen for culture and sensitivity before therapy is started. The presence of 10^4 colonies or more per mL of a single or predominant pathogen in a midstream urine sample and 10 white blood cells or more per high-power field of a drop of unspun urine is good evidence of infection.

TREATMENT

Cystitis can be treated with a number of oral agents such as the combination of trimethoprim and sulfamethoxazole (Bactrim, Septra), amoxicillin, a cephalosporin, or a fluoroquinolone (Table 1). Men with infections of the lower urinary tract do not respond as well as women to short-course therapy and should be treated for 7 to 10 days. Patients with pyelonephritis should be admitted to the hospital for treatment with parenteral antibiotics if sepsis is suspected or if the patient cannot tolerate oral antibiotics. I use gentamicin in addition to ampicillin as empirical therapy. Similar success can be achieved with a single-drug regimen such as a third-generation cephalosporin, an expanded-spectrum β-lactam, a fluoroquinolone, or the combination of trimethoprim and sulfamethoxazole. Blood and urine should be obtained for culture before the initiation of treatment. Once the sensitivity results are known and the patient is afebrile for 24 to 48 hours, an appropriate oral antibiotic can be substituted to complete a course of 2 to 3 weeks. Patients with pyelonephritis who are not vomiting and who have mild disease can be treated at home with an oral third-generation cephalosporin or a fluoroquinolone.

More than 50% of elderly men with UTIs may have a concomitant infection of the prostate gland. It is important to recognize that many agents used for the treatment of UTI, e.g., β-lactam antibiotics such as amoxicillin or cephalosporins, do not penetrate the prostate; thus, prostatitis may go untreated and serve as a nidus for recurrent infection. Chronic prostatitis may be relatively asymptomatic, and its presence should be confirmed by quantitative differential culture of expressed prostatic secretions (see the article on prostatitis). Antibiotics that are known to penetrate the prostate gland, such as the fluoroquinolones and trimethoprim, should be used when chronic prostatitis is suspected. Treatment should be continued for 4 to 6 weeks.

Because of the high likelihood of structural or physiologic abnormalities of the urinary tract, males younger than 1 year and those older than 50 years should be referred to a urologist with their first UTI. Children younger than 1 year are at especially high risk for renal scarring after UTIs. Appropriate treatment of symptomatic episodes and investigation for surgically remedial abnormalities are essential to prevent progressive loss of renal function. It is usually not necessary to investigate the urinary tract of young men presenting with a single episode of UTI; however, recurrent infections or clinical suspicion of a structural abnormality should prompt a urologic evaluation. ABU should be treated if the individual has an abnormal urinary tract, renal insufficiency, or

TABLE 1. **Antibiotic Therapy for Male Urinary Tract Infections**

Antibiotic	Recommended Dose	
	Adult	*Child*
Oral therapy		
Amoxicillin	250 mg orally q 8 h	30 mg/kg/d orally in 3 divided doses
Trimethoprim-sulfamethoxazole (Bactrim, Septra)	1 double-strength tablet (160 mg of trimethoprim and 800 mg of sulfamethoxazole) orally q 12 h	8 mg/kg/d of trimethoprim and 40 mg/kg/d of sulfamethoxazole in 2 divided doses
First-generation cephalosporin (e.g., cephradine [Velosef])	500 mg orally q 6 h	25–50 mg/kg/d orally in 4 divided doses
Second-generation cephalosporin (e.g., cefpodoxime [Vantin])	200 mg q 12 h	
Fluoroquinolone (e.g., ciprofloxacin [Cipro])	250–500 mg orally q 12 h	Not recommended for children
Parenteral therapy		
Gentamicin sulfate*	3–4 mg/kg/d in 2 divided doses	6 mg/kg/d in 3 divided doses
Ampicillin	1–2 gm q 4 h	50–100 mg/kg/d every 6 h
Third-generation cephalosporin (e.g., ceftriaxone [Rocephin])	1 gm q 24 h	50 mg/kg/d once daily
Ciprofloxacin (Cipro)	200–400 mg q 12 h	
Trimethoprim-sulfamethoxazole	160 mg of trimethoprim and 800 mg of sulfamethoxazole q 12 h	Not recommended for children
Ticarcillin-clavulanate (Timentin)	3.1 gm q 4–6 h	Safety and efficacy in children not established
Candida infections of bladder		
Amphotericin B bladder irrigation	50 mg/L, intermittent irrigation for 3 d	Not recommended for children
Fluconazole (Diflucan)	200 mg orally on first day followed by 100 mg qd for 4 d	3–12 mg/kg/d

*Dose must be adjusted with renal failure.

diabetes. There is little evidence, however, to support routine treatment of elderly men with ABU because these episodes are usually self-limited.

URINARY TRACT INFECTIONS IN PATIENTS WITH INDWELLING URINARY CATHETERS

The risk of UTI is increased in patients with indwelling urinary catheters. Although prophylactic antibiotics can prevent the acquisition of bacteriuria in patients with short-term catheterization, it is my practice to try to prevent the acquisition of bacteriuria by minimizing the number of days of catheterization. Newer and more costly methods of preventing nosocomial UTIs, such as silver-impregnated catheters, have not proved to be effective in men. Patients who require prolonged catheterization, such as those with spinal cord injury or with obstructive uropathy, almost invariably develop colonization of their bladder and experience intermittent or recurrent symptomatic infections. Prophylactic antibiotics and treatment of asymptomatic colonization do not reduce the number of symptomatic episodes but do increase the likelihood that a more antibiotic-resistant population will become established. Efforts should be directed at preventing obstruction of the lumen of the catheter. The catheter should be replaced at regular intervals and anatomic obstruction surgically corrected.

For incontinent patients, permanent indwelling catheterization should be instituted only after the cause of the incontinence is fully evaluated and appropriate medical or behavioral methods of management of the incontinence tried (see the article on urinary incontinence). Intermittent self- or assisted catheterization greatly diminishes the incidence of UTI. Patients with indwelling urethral catheters, especially those who have received multiple courses of antibiotics, may develop *Candida* cystitis. Whenever possible, I remove the catheter and stop antibiotic therapy. For those patients in whom conservative measures fail, amphotericin B bladder washouts or oral fluconazole (Diflucan) is effective.

BACTERIAL INFECTIONS OF THE URINARY TRACT IN FEMALES

method of
JOHN A. MATA, M.D.
Louisiana State University Medical Center
Shreveport, Louisiana

Urinary tract infection (UTI) in women is a common problem, accounting for 2 to 5% of primary care visits because of symptoms suggestive of cystitis. Up to 50% of women experience at least one episode of painful voiding (dysuria); half of them have a culture-proven bacterial UTI. The prevalence rate of bacteriuria (2 to 10%) increases with age, but it is known that UTI is a particularly common problem in sexually active women. Contraceptive diaphragm use has been shown to be an independent risk factor for UTI in sexually active females.

The vast majority of UTIs in females are uncomplicated and respond promptly to treatment or resolve spontaneously. However, there is a small cohort of women who have complicating factors (Table 1), such as diabetes, pregnancy, or stone disease, that may create a life-threatening, recurrent, or persistent UTI.

ETIOLOGY AND DIAGNOSIS

The most common cause of UTI in females is bacterial ascent from the periurethral area by organisms that normally constitute the fecal flora. The most common urinary tract pathogens are *Escherichia coli, Klebsiella, Enterobacter, Proteus* species, and *Staphylococcus saprophyticus.* Bacteriuria (presence of 10^5 CFU per mL in an uncontaminated collected urine specimen) is generally preceded by colonization of the periurethral and vaginal mucosa by the infecting organism. The majority of UTIs occur in the lower tract (cystitis, urethritis), not in the upper tract (pyelonephritis), and in more than 90% of the cases the infections are uncomplicated but prone to recurrence. Women with complicated or nosocomial UTIs are more likely to be infected with resistant microorganisms. Studies of host defenses and bacterial virulence factors suggest that many females burdened with recurrent simple UTIs are biologically susceptible to bacteriuria. This can be a frustrating problem for both the patient and the physician. There are vaccines in development to help reduce the incidence of symptomatic UTIs in these patients.

The signs and symptoms of UTI in women are characteristic, but not specific, in that the bladder and urethra respond similarly to a variety of irritative factors. Dysuria, frequency, and urgency are commonly present; however, fever, flank pain, or costovertebral angle tenderness may herald a renal infection in up to 50% of cases. New patients with bladder symptoms should be accurately diagnosed initially, before treatment, to avoid missing other entities that may mimic a UTI (Table 2). After a history and an abdominal and pelvic examination, a properly collected clean-catch or catheterized urine specimen should be analyzed. Urine culture is still considered the "gold standard" for the diagnosis of UTI, but treatment may be initiated with a suspicious urinalysis. New dipstick reagents that test for nitrites and leukocyte esterase are quite accurate in addition to a microscopic examination for confirming the presence of bacteria. Although a urine culture and sensitivity test per se are no longer critical in the majority of females with routine uncomplicated UTIs, these may be prudent on the first visit or in patients with persistent bacteriuria. Up to 30% of women with acute cystitis may have low-colony-count bacteriuria with 10^2 or more CFU per mL and may be treated accordingly on the basis of a well-collected specimen. The presence of two or more bacteria per high-power field in a centrifuged microscopic specimen has a sensitivity and specificity of 90% for the detection of significant bacteriuria.

TREATMENT
Antibiotic Selection

The majority of commonly used antimicrobials in UTI therapy are effective and safe. The duration of antibiotic therapy ranges from single-dose, short-course (3 to 5 days), or standard (7 to 10 days) regimens for cystitis in uncomplicated UTIs to long-term (10 to 14 days) courses for patients with pyelonephritis or complicated UTIs. Because uncomplicated UTIs respond rapidly to treatment, a good compromise is a short-term 3-day regimen (Table 3). The 3-day regimen is cost-effective, minimizes the risk of adverse drug reactions, decreases the chance of a vaginal yeast infection, and decreases the emergence of bacterial resistance. The 3-day regimens promote excellent compliance by the patient, and more than 90% of the cases are cured. Table 3 lists the commonly used oral antibiotics and their dosages and schedules in UTI treatment. A brief review of the drugs and their common side effects follows.

Penicillins. The aminopenicillins such as ampicillin and amoxicillin are commonly prescribed bactericidal agents in nonallergic patients; however, up to 25% of organisms may be resistant. The more expensive β-lactamase inhibitor amoxicillin plus clavulanate (Augmentin) is effective against the majority of isolates resistant to the aminopenicillins. Adverse reactions common to the penicillin family include nausea, diarrhea, rashes, and a propensity for vaginitis due to *Candida* species (10 to 15%).

Sulfonamides. These bacteriostatic agents are effective for more than three quarters of the urinary pathogens. Common agents include sulfisoxazole (Gantrisin) and sulfamethoxazole (Gantanol). They are inexpensive, and side effects include rashes, nausea, and headaches.

Trimethoprim. This bacteriostatic agent is available as a single agent (Trimpex, Proloprim), 100 mg twice daily or 200 mg daily, and is effective for more than 90% of UTI isolates. It is suitable for prophylaxis. Side effects include rash and nausea.

Trimethoprim-Sulfamethoxazole (TMP-SMZ). This synergistic combination available as Bactrim or Septra or in a generic preparation is quite popular because of its effectiveness, low cost, and twice-daily

TABLE 1. **Complicating Factors in Female Urinary Tract Infection**

Diabetes	Pregnancy
Stone disease	Neuropathic bladder
Chronic catheter	Congenital anomalies (reflux)
Urethral diverticulum	Urethral stenosis
Immunosuppression	Urinary tract obstruction

TABLE 2. **Differential Diagnosis of Cystitis Symptoms in Women**

Occult pyelonephritis	Interstitial cystitis
Sexually transmitted diseases	Carcinoma in situ
Vaginitis	Detrusor instability
Urethral syndrome	Neurogenic bladder

dosage. Side effects reflect the component drugs but also include leukopenia and falsely elevated creatinine levels. It is not recommended in the frail, elderly population or in patients with significant renal insufficiency or autoimmune disorders.

Nitrofurantoin. A urinary-specific drug, nitrofurantoin (Macrodantin) is active against gram-negative and gram-positive organisms. Its side effects include nausea, vomiting, and rash. Prolonged therapy may be associated with pulmonary fibrosis. This drug is contraindicated in patients with a glomerular filtration rate less than 40 mL per minute.

Cephalosporins. These are safe, effective antimicrobials with few adverse side effects. There are many preparations now available since the original cephalexin (Keflex), 250 to 500 mg orally four times daily, became available. These include cefaclor (Ceclor), cefuroxime (Zinacef), and cephradine (Anspor, Velosef). Vaginitis due to *Candida* species occurs in up to 15% of women treated with these agents.

Fluoroquinolones. Norfloxacin (Noroxin), 400 mg orally twice daily, and ciprofloxacin (Cipro), 100 to 250 mg orally twice daily, are antimicrobial additions offering oral antipseudomonal coverage. They are more potent than older quinolone nalidixic acid (NegGram), offering a broader gram-negative and gram-positive spectrum. These are generally not first-line drugs for UTI but are welcome antibiotic additions for those women with resistant or complicated UTIs. They are contraindicated in children and in pregnancy. Potential side effects include nausea, vomiting, diarrhea, headache, and vaginitis due to *Candida* species.

Uncomplicated Urinary Tract Infections

The majority of women with UTI have a simple infection that may or may not be recurrent. These infections are most often caused by *E. coli* or *S. saprophyticus* and generally respond rapidly to appropriate antibiotic treatment. Clinically, these infec-

TABLE 3. **Antibiotic Therapy for Female Urinary Tract Infection**

Antimicrobial Agent	Three-Day Oral Regimen (mg bid)
Trimethoprim-sulfamethoxazole	160/800
Nitrofurantoin (Macrobid)	100
Amoxicillin	500
Cephalexin (Keflex)	500
Norfloxacin (Noroxin)	400
Ciprofloxacin (Cipro)	100

tions present with dysuria, frequency, and urgency. These simple infections generally respond to a 3-day course of appropriate antimicrobial agents. TMP-SMZ and nitrofurantoin are commonly used as first-line agents for these infections. Alternatives include the quinilones, cephalosporins, and amoxicillin–potassium clavulanate. Some women may benefit from urinary analgesics or antispasmodics such as phenazopyridine (Pyridium), 100 mg orally three times a day, or flavoxate (Urispas), 100 mg orally twice daily. Rarely in women without UTI risk factors do I need to change antibiotics because of resistant bacteria shown by culture results. In general, patients with uncomplicated infections respond within 1 to 2 days of therapy and their urine becomes sterile. Persistence of symptoms in bacteriuria may be due to a variety of reasons, such as an upper tract infection, bacterial resistance, urinary stones, obstruction, or poor compliance of the patient in taking the medications.

Recurrent Urinary Tract Infections

The greatest risk factors in patients with simple infections include sexual activity (by far the greatest), recent use of a diaphragm contraceptive, and a past history of simple UTI. These patients are prone to recurrences. Recurrence means reinfection with a new organism, although it still may be *E. coli,* but of a different serotype. Plenty of fluids, frequent bladder emptying (especially after intercourse), and occasionally a pericoital antibiotic in patients with recurrent "honeymoon cystitis" are helpful in reducing risks.

The majority (80%) have another symptomatic UTI within a 2-year period. Again, assuming there is no reason to suspect a complicated UTI, treatment is routine. Prophylactic therapy may be indicated in this group of patients, especially if these recurrences are at frequent, closely spaced intervals, such as two or more infections within a 6-month period or less. I tend to use a bedtime dose of nitrofurantoin, 50 to 100 mg; trimethroprim alone, 100 mg; or single-strength TMP-SMZ over a 3- to 6-month period. If these episodes are breakthroughs despite prophylaxis or if they continue, I evaluate the problem with renal and bladder ultrasonography and a voiding cystourethrogram. Occasionally, cystourethroscopy is indicated, but this is generally reserved for patients with abacterial cystitis such as interstitial cystitis or urethral syndrome (these patients by definition do not have culture-proven recurrent UTIs).

Acute Pyelonephritis

"Pyelonephritis" is the term denoting infection in the renal pelvis and parenchyma. Physicians are alert to this diagnosis in patients with UTI symptoms accompanied by flank pain and fever. Approximately one third of women presenting with only symptoms of a lower tract infection may have occult pyelonephritis. Many of these patients can be treated with broad-spectrum outpatient oral antibiotics, depending on the clinical findings and the general condition of the patient. In patients who do not need hospitalization for intravenous (IV) hydration and IV therapy, some may be treated with an intramuscular (IM) dose of ceftriaxone (Rocephin), 500 mg, or gentamicin, 80 mg, before their oral antibiotic regimen. In patients who need to be hospitalized because of high fever, dehydration, nausea, and vomiting, IV antibiotics with hydration can be given for 3 to 5 days until the patient defervesces and can tolerate a culture-specific oral antibiotic. Most patients, however, can be treated with a 10- to 14-day course of therapy with the previously mentioned agents including ciprofloxacin, TMX-SMZ, or cephlasporins. Hospitalized patients, or patients who do not respond promptly to IM and oral antibiotics, benefit from radiographic imaging with a kidney, ureter, and bladder (KUB) film and renal ultrasonography. This imaging rules out kidney stones or obstruction as a complicating factor in the illness. Failure to respond promptly to therapy may indicate a complicated UTI, i.e., lobar nephronia, obstruction, stones, or perinephric abscess. Follow-up urine cultures are generally obtained for patients with upper tract infections.

Urinary Infections in Pregnancy

All asymptomatic bacteriuria in pregnant women must be treated. Safe drugs include the penicillins, cephalosporins, and nitrofurantoin. A 3- to 5-day course suffices for most lower tract infections, followed by another urine culture 2 to 3 days after treatment. Acute pyelonephritis unresponsive to antibiotics quickly mandates that one rule out obstruction. Early on, a KUB and renal ultrasonogram may be diagnostic, but because of the hydronephrosis of pregnancy, often a two- to three-film intravenous pyelogram is required.

Complicated Urinary Tract Infections

A small cohort of female patients may have persistent or unresolved bacteriuria secondary to a complicated UTI. These patients generally have complicating factors (see Table 1) causing these difficult infections (Table 4). Their management generally requires IV antibiotics and uroradiographic and urologic evaluation. Often, endourologic or surgical therapy is necessary. A high index of suspicion is mandatory in these patients to obtain appropriate urologic consultation.

Neurogenic or geriatric patients with long-term Foley's catheters may present special problems with recurrent UTIs secondary to colonization, stones, or candidal overgrowth. Asymptomatic or single-species colonized bacteriuria is not treated unless associated with local or systemic symptoms, or unless stone-producing pathogens such as *Proteus* species are cultured.

Simple candiduria may now be treated with fluconazole (Diflucan), 100 mg orally every day for 3 to 5 days. Alternatively, if an indwelling urethral catheter is present, amphotericin B (Fungizone), 50 mg in 1 liter of sterile water at 40 mL per hour, or 1 liter per day, can be used to clear the lower tract of candiduria over 5 to 7 days. Often, simply discontinuing chronic antibiotic therapy and removing foreign bodies such as catheters, if possible, clear up a noninvasive fungal infection of the urinary bladder.

BACTERIAL INFECTIONS OF THE URINARY TRACT IN GIRLS

method of
LOWELL R. KING, M.D.
Duke University Medical Center
Durham, North Carolina

Most fetuses are now screened by ultrasonography before birth. When hydronephrosis is present, newborns should be given antibacterial prophylaxis until reflux is excluded, as about 40% of such infants have reflux. Twenty percent experience reflux even if the hydronephrosis resolves before birth. If infection is prevented, renal scarring and its long-term sequellae are also prevented.

In infants who are intact neurologically, after birth the bladder and sphincters are synergistic; that is, when the bladder becomes full the bladder contracts as the sphincters open, and voiding is complete. Failure to empty predisposes to urinary tract infection (UTI) from bacteria, which are usually motile and usually from the colon and ascend the short female urethra without difficulty. Residual urine in the bladder then predisposes to bacterial growth, resulting in a UTI 2 to 4 days later.

Probably some bacteria normally, or at least occasionally, ascend the female urethra to the bladder, but the defense mechanisms—antibodies, mucus protection, and complete emptying—are so effective that UTI is uncommon before the child is toilet trained.

A UTI in infants usually presents as a fever. Check for abdominal masses or a palpable bladder. Look at the lower back for a dimple, hairy patch, café au lait spot, or a more overt sign of a tethered spinal cord. The urine can be obtained by bagged sample where

TABLE 4. **Diagnosis in Complicated Urinary Tract Infection**

Upper tract
Renal or perinephric abscess
Pyonephrosis (infected hydronephrosis)
Acute bacterial nephritis (lobar nephronia)
Xanthogranulomatous pyelonephritis
Emphysematous pyelonephritis
Lower tract
Cystitis cystica or glandularis
Malacoplakia
Cystitis emphysematosa
Vesicointestinal fistula
Chronic interstitial cystitis

a clean urinalysis is reliable, but cultures are often positive due to contamination. Because infants with even pyelonephritis may not have adequate generation time in the bladder to produce colony counts in excess of 10^5 on culture, a catheterized or aspirated urine sample should usually be obtained for culture.

About 80% of infant (not yet toilet trained) girls with UTI have a predisposing anatomic anomaly. After the sample for culture is obtained, give gentamicin (Garamycin), 1.5 to 2 mg per kg intramuscularly, and start antibacterial therapy, e.g., trimethoprim-sulfamethoxazole (Bactrim, Septra), until the bacterial sensitivities are available. Sulfa drugs should generally not be used until the patient is 8 weeks of age. Because such a high proportion of infant girls have an anomaly, genitourinary evaluations should virtually always be performed during or after a first infection. Renal and bladder ultrasonography may be done at any time. Reflux should be assumed and the infant continued with prophylaxis until a cystogram (voiding cystourethrogram [VCUG]) is obtained usually about 3 weeks after the infection is cleared. Competent intravesical ureters may reflux during infection because of transient loss of compliance in the overlying flap.

Reflux is the most common anomaly. If it is present, infants should continue antibacterial prophylaxis and VCUG should be repeated every 6 to 12 months. Breakthrough infections are unusual, but because each UTI carries a 2% risk of renal scarring, corrective surgery should usually be elected when this happens. The complication rate from antireflux surgery is about 2% when the bladder is normal. Reflux can also reasonably be corrected surgically when it is quite severe or when secondary to a sizable periureteral diverticulum; obstructions at either end of the ureter and a ureterocele obstruction predispose to UTI and are generally treated surgically soon after diagnosis.

After toilet training, UTI in girls becomes much more common, such that in patients who clear promptly full urologic evaluation is generally omitted after a first infection. Older girls may present with daytime wetting, frequency, or flank pain. The symptoms do not reliably indicate the site of infection, but irritative symptoms without systemic signs are more likely to be due to cystitis than renal infection. Pyelonephritis—renal parenchymal infection—cannot be diagnosed from symptoms, but it is wise to treat children with systemic signs and symptoms with parenteral antibiotics after a sample for culture is obtained. A single dose clears 80 to 85% of non–hospital-acquired UTIs. Trimethoprim-sulfamethoxazole is given until the bacterial sensitivities are known. Treatment is generally continued for 10 days, or, if the infection is recurrent, until reflux is excluded.

Daytime wetting seems to predispose to UTI in some girls. In other words, many if not most girls with UTI have frequency and urgency and urge incontinence, but in some the incontinence antedates the UTI. If wetting is lifelong, an ectopic ureter must be excluded by history (dry sometimes) or an intravenous pyelogram (duplicated collecting system, small bladder), and a cystogram. When incontinence is present, the girl should continue to take antibacterials until she becomes dry. This may occur when the infection clears, but more often bladder retraining is needed. This is most efficiently performed using timed voiding and sphincter (Kegel's) exercises, stopping and starting the stream during voiding several times a day. Persistent wetting has many possible causes, chiefly sphincter dyssynergia, bladder hyperactivity, or inadequate outlet resistance. Urodynamic evaluation is helpful in guiding treatment using anticholinergics for bladder hyperactivity, diazepam (Valium),* more exercises, or intermittent catheterization for sphincter dyssynergia, and pseudoephedrine (Sudafed)* for a weak outlet.

About 6% of school-age girls have one or more UTIs during childhood. About 0.4% have chronic bacteriuria. Conversely, UTIs in such girls may clear spontaneously, and only about 22% have anatomic problems that predispose to infection. VCUG is the cornerstone of investigation, as reflux remains the most common abnormality. Sonography is enough, usually, to evaluate the kidneys and may image a dilated ureter or a ureterocele and allow an estimate of bladder thickness. However, sonography does not replace the cystogram. Even severe reflux may not result in any hydronephrosis except during voiding. Further, the detection of reflux is important because primary reflux, the common cause, is so strongly familial that sibling screening is important. If reflux is severe, the risk in siblings is more than 40%. If one parent had reflux, the risk in a child is more than 50%. Reflux is normally treated by long-term prophylaxis with an antibacterial such as sulfamethoxazole (Gantanol), nitrofurantoin (Macrodantin), or nalidixic acid (NegGram). The risk of renal damage from a breakthrough UTI remains about 2%, and the complication rate of antireflux surgery in school-age children is now less than 2%, so surgery is a good solution in the older child whose reflux is not diminishing with growth. This obviates the need for such surgery during adolescence after full growth has been achieved.

In a subset of girls with UTI, infections recur in spite of normal anatomy and bladder function; in another subset, bladder infections are deep seated and hard to eradicate. They can often be distinguished on the basis of history. Those with cystitis cystica have a recurrence 10 to 14 days after prophylaxis is stopped, whereas more commonly the recurrences are more sporadic. After a third infection, statistics show that subsequent UTIs are more likely than not, and it is reasonable to treat these girls with prophylaxis, just as in the patients with reflux. A trimethoprim-sulfamethoxazole combination may be employed, but the combination has not been shown to be more effective than sulfamethoxazole or nitrofurantoin alone. If trimethoprim is adminis-

---

*Not FDA approved for this indication.

tered, long-term periodic white blood cell counts are recommended, as agranulocytosis may occur. In general, the girls stay well while taking medicine.

UTIs in susceptible but otherwise normal girls may be associated with a failure to secrete antibody into the vagina, bladder, and urethra. As in women, this defect is seldom lifelong, but the period of risk is usually several years. Because hospitalizations for UTIs are more common in the spring and fall, when presumably the susceptible child also has a respiratory infection, I tend to stop prophylaxis in the spring after school is out. If the girl stays well she can continue to not take medicine and simply have her urine checked whenever she is ill. If the infection recurs it is eradicated with antibiotics, and then she resumes taking an antibacterial for another year.

When the infection recurs a week or two after stopping prophylaxis, cystitis cystica is often present. This is a poorly understood deep-seated bladder infection found usually in otherwise healthy girls. Continuous medication is required for 3.5 to 7 years before the tendency to rapid reinfection disappears. Thus, a diagnostic cystoscopy may help to explain the UTIs and helps with compliance in taking medicine. At cystoscopy the inside of the bladder is found to be covered with innumerable small cysts concentrated on the trigone and bladder neck. On biopsy, dense lymphocytic infiltrates are found to be present under the mucosa. A urethral dilatation to enlarge the distal urethral ring and meatus can be performed at the time of cystoscopy without increasing the morbidity—dysuria—after the procedure, but there is no evidence that this shortens the course of treatment or prevents further UTIs.

Safe antibacterial prophylaxis is the mainstay of treatment for reflux during childhood and also prevents most UTIs in otherwise susceptible but anatomically and functionally normal girls.

CHILDHOOD ENURESIS

method of
EDMOND T. GONZALES, JR., M.D.
Baylor College of Medicine and Texas Children's Hospital
Houston, Texas

Enuresis is defined as an involuntary loss of urine. Enuresis may occur during the daytime (diurnal enuresis), only at night (nocturnal enuresis), or both day and night (sometimes called mixed enuresis). Enuresis is often further classified as primary, that is, enuresis that has been continuous ever since the child reached the expected age of urinary control, or secondary, that is, enuresis that begins again after a period during which the child was satisfactorily dry. In children who wet only at night, it is also helpful to describe daytime voiding patterns. Some children with nighttime wetting are completely normal during the daytime, whereas other children may have significant daytime voiding dysfunction manifest by frequency and urgency, even if they do not wet. This article addresses the problem of nocturnal enuresis. Symptomatic and troublesome daytime incontinence is not included here in detail.

INCIDENCE OF NOCTURNAL ENURESIS

By the age of 5 years, most children have achieved satisfactory daytime control, but as many as 15% continue to have problems with nocturnal enuresis. The spontaneous resolution of nocturnal enuresis occurs at an incidence of about 15% per year, such that by the age of 14 years, only 1 to 2% of children still have a problem with nocturnal enuresis.

Between 20 and 30% of children who have nocturnal enuresis have secondary enuresis. Once nocturnal enuresis is established, the spontaneous resolution rate appears to be similar for secondary and primary enuresis.

ETIOLOGY OF NOCTURNAL ENURESIS

The cause of nighttime urinary incontinence remains unknown and is somewhat controversial. Enuresis clusters within families, and when either parent has a history of nocturnal enuresis, the incidence of enuresis in the children is more common than in the population at large. When both parents were so affected, the incidence of enuresis in their children can be as high as 75%.

Recent studies have suggested that some children with nocturnal enuresis have abnormally high nighttime urinary volumes due to a blunted secretion of antidiuretic hormone during sleep. This results in rapid bladder filling midway during sleep, leading to the enuretic episode.

Children with a diagnosis of attention-deficit/hyperactivity disorder also seem to be afflicted with an increased incidence of voiding dysfunction. These children, although often affected by nocturnal enuresis, usually also have a significant problem with diurnal enuresis simultaneously and can be quite difficult to treat.

No other single factor has been clearly defined as a cause of nocturnal enuresis alone. Common explanations in the past such as psychologic factors, intrinsic urodynamic abnormalities, allergic reactions, or sleep disorders have not been established to play a primary causative role in nighttime wetting.

The concept of a sleep disorder deserves special mention. Children as a group spend more time in deep sleep than adults; however, children who wet have not been shown to have different sleep patterns than age-matched control subjects who do not wet. Deep sleep, however, may be a factor in the actual episode of wetting in that a full bladder might not be recognized by the sleeping child.

Regardless of the specific cause of nocturnal enuresis, in the overwhelming majority of these children the enuresis resolves spontaneously regardless of treatment. This consistent clinical observation suggests that enuresis can be described as a disorder that results from a maturational lag. Indeed, studies have suggested that children with persisting nocturnal enuresis have a somewhat higher incidence of fine and gross motor abnormalities, speech defects, and reduced spatial and visual motor perception. Whether these changes correlate with an overall delay in the maturation of neurologic development or not, however, continues to be controversial.

EVALUATION OF THE CHILD WITH ENURESIS

The evaluation of a child presenting with urinary incontinence should begin with a specific and thorough history of the current problem. A complete physical examination should always be performed and must include a careful neurologic examination of the lower extremities and perineum as well as inspection of the lower lumbosacral spine for possible vertebral anomalies that would suggest a defect of the lower segments of the spinal cord. A urinalysis and possibly a urine culture should be included in every evaluation. Further diagnostic studies are determined based on the findings of this initial office encounter.

Children with nocturnal enuresis alone (no daytime symptoms, normal physical examination, and normal urinalysis) do not require any additional diagnostic evaluations. In this clinical setting, the incidence of an anatomic abnormality of the urinary tract that would be a cause of the presenting problem is essentially zero. If undue anxiety exists, renal ultrasonography with specific imaging of the bladder is sufficient to reassure the parents or older child.

If there are daytime symptoms associated with the nocturnal wetting, or physical abnormalities are evident, or the urinalysis is infected, then additional studies are warranted. Depending on the age of the child and the history or physical findings obtained, the evaluation may vary. A child younger than 5 years with associated daytime symptoms of urgency, precipitant voiding, and intermittent daytime dampness but with a normal physical examination and a negative urinalysis is unlikely to have any urologic abnormality. Especially in girls, if a significant urologic disorder is present, one expects a history of urinary infection also. In general, in this age group a specific work-up is not obtained in girls who wet but have never had urinary infection. The likelihood of urologic abnormality in boys is likewise quite low. However, boys with infravesical obstructive uropathy may present with voiding dysfunction alone and are less likely to have urinary infection than girls. Therefore, in this population it is prudent to obtain at least a renal ultrasonogram with particular emphasis on the thickness of the bladder wall. In either boys or girls with a history of enuresis and urinary infection, a thorough urologic work-up should be obtained, including at least a renal ultrasonogram and voiding cystourethrogram.

Specific findings that would prompt an imaging evaluation would be continuous urinary incontinence in girls not associated with urgency or symptoms consistent with detrusor instability (this finding suggests an ectopic ureter draining into the distal urethra or vagina), or an obvious neurologic problem by history or physical examination (associated encopresis, lower extremity weakness, lumbosacral anomaly, recognized neurologic disorder). A particularly subtle disorder that can easily be missed on physical examination is female epispadias. This anomaly is characteristically found on examination of the external genitalia and is associated with a bifid clitoris.

TREATMENT OF NOCTURNAL ENURESIS

The treatment of nocturnal enuresis is empirical, because there is little specific information regarding its cause. Treatment can be conveniently divided into pharmacologic approaches and behavioral approaches. It is important to emphasize at this point that there is nothing wrong with no treatment for this disorder. When to treat is often determined by the patient's age as well as the anxiety of the patient or the parents. Traditional measures used to control enuresis, such as significantly limiting fluid intake after dinner or waking the child at random during the night, are not generally thought to be effective means of treatment.

Treatment may also be affected by whether nocturnal enuresis is the only symptom or whether there are associated symptoms of daytime urgency, frequency, and intermittent daytime incontinence. These symptoms suggest an irritable bladder associated with uninhibited contractions. Unless the daytime control can be improved, it is unlikely that satisfactory nighttime control will be achieved. Therefore, in discussing treatment with parents of a child who also has associated daytime symptoms, I generally emphasize the importance of working with the daytime symptoms first and then making an effort to control the nighttime wetting only after we are successful with the daytime disorder. The management of the unstable bladder of childhood is generally initiated with a program of anticholinergic therapy with oxybutynin (Ditropan), hyoscyamine (Levsin), or a similar agent. At times, the initiation of treatment with one of these pharmacologic agents is also beneficial for nighttime control. However, that is not the universal experience, and additional measures to control nighttime wetting are often necessary.

The following description is for the child with nocturnal enuresis alone. Because it is generally conceded that there are no major recognized physical abnormalities associated with nocturnal enuresis, the most important issue regarding the initiation of treatment is age as well as the social impact of the wetting. Because enuresis is exceedingly common even in the 5-year-old child, most physicians do not recommend initiation of treatment until patients are 6 years old or older.

Pharmacologic treatment has been the most common approach to managing nocturnal enuresis. Pharmacologic treatment is not a cure for this disorder; rather, drug therapy only controls the symptoms. When the medication is discontinued, enuresis generally recurs unless the child has reached that age at which he or she would have outgrown the problem anyway. Three drugs are commonly used for control of nocturnal enuresis: desmopressin acetate (DDAVP), imipramine (Tofranil), or one of the anticholinergic agents (oxybutynin or hyoscyamine).

The most common pharmacologic program today involves the use of DDAVP. The use of this agent was prompted by the studies that demonstrated that some children with nocturnal enuresis had higher nighttime urinary volumes with lower specific gravity than an age-matched control group who did not have nocturnal enuresis. Subsequent evaluation of endogenous antidiuretic hormone levels demonstrated a blunted secretory rate in the affected children. The addition of the synthetic analogue DDAVP was subsequently found to be successful in controlling enuresis in a majority of these cases. DDAVP acts on the renal tubule to increase the absorption of filtered water—thereby increasing urinary concentration and decreasing urinary volume. Presumably, by using DDAVP the enuretic child simply does not overfill the bladder during the sleeping hours and therefore has less stimulus for bladder emptying and a reduced rate of nocturnal wetting. The reported rate of success in using DDAVP approximates 60 to 70% of children with nocturnal enuresis. It is currently available only for administration by nasal spray. An oral preparation is currently going through clinical trials but is not yet available for routine administration.

DDAVP has proved to be an effective and safe medication when used as directed. The usual dosage is 2 to 4 sprays at bedtime (10 μg per spray; 40 μg maximal dosage). If used at random during the day, it can cause retention of water with subsequent dilutional hyponatremia, and therefore it is important to emphasize that the drug must be used only in the evening just before going to bed. Side effects otherwise have been minimal and include nasal stuffiness and occasionally headaches. In a child in whom DDAVP is shown to be successful, the drug may become temporarily ineffective if the child develops a significant upper respiratory infection or has seasonal nasal allergies. Presumably, this results in decreased absorption of the administered dose.

Imipramine was the first pharmacologic agent introduced for the treatment of nocturnal enuresis. It is not as successful as DDAVP—reportedly benefiting only 25 to 30% of the children in whom it is used. Tofranil is a complex drug. It is known to have both anticholinergic and alpha-sympathomimetic effects and therefore may directly affect bladder function in the enuretic child. But it is also thought to have a central neurologic effect that may alter sleeping patterns and perhaps change the wetting response for this reason also. The usual dosage is 25 to 50 mg at bedtime (equivalent to about 1 mg per kg per dose).

Imipramine has somewhat more frequent and significant side effects than DDAVP, including increased restlessness and moodiness in the child. Imipramine is also associated with the development of cardiac arrhythmias when taken in excessively high doses. This has resulted in deaths, especially among infant siblings who gain access to the medication. Because imipramine is often used in families with young children, it is important to emphasize to the parents that the medication must be handled responsibly and not be left to the care of the patient. Although still useful in selected cases, imipramine is no longer considered the pharmacologic agent of choice.

The anticholinergic agents commonly used for treatment of dysfunctional voiding and daytime urinary incontinence are the least effective in treating nocturnal enuresis alone. Although these agents can sometimes be beneficial, they are more often used in combination with other approaches to control nighttime wetting when there are also associated daytime voiding abnormalities.

The use of behavioral modification is another approach that may be helpful in controlling nocturnal enuresis. The most successful form of behavioral modification has been the use of one of the alarm units that signals the exact time of wetting. These devices are manufactured as a variety of alarms or vibrating units that are activated by a small sensor worn near the external urethral meatus. The devices are designed to awaken the child during the actual wetting episode. When this is continued on a regular basis, the child can come to recognize during sleep that wetting is about to happen and can either learn to suppress the impending bladder contraction or can be aroused to void in the toilet. The alarm units are usually combined with a program of responsibility reinforcement. This process might include a reward system such as keeping a calendar with stars for each dry night as well as assuming a role in helping to change the bed sheets. When used consistently, the alarm units can be effective in as many as 80% of children.

The problems with this therapeutic approach are many. First, because this is active therapy, the child must exhibit some interest in participating in the program. Many 6-year-old children, I believe, find it difficult to adhere to the schedule and are frightened by the alarm. Second, the child and parents must be patient. The average time to success is 8 to 12 weeks. Third, because of the deep sleep of young children, some fail to be aroused by the device. Fourth, about one third of children who stop wetting with the alarm units have a recurrence within several weeks to months. However, reintroduction of the alarm is usually met with renewed success in short order.

SUMMARY

The timing and approach to management of nocturnal enuresis are obviously variable and affected by the views of the child, parents, and physician. Therapy often involves a combination of different approaches. I usually encourage an initial trial with DDAVP. If this approach is successful, the child obtains immediate relief and has an agent that should restore confidence to allow sleepover activities. The child and parents can then decide whether to use the drug long term or keep it primarily for nights away from home. I personally encourage the latter, because I believe ultimate management is best with behavioral modification. Although requiring a more active role on the part of the patient, this treatment modality does offer the potential for a cure of the problem. Significant daytime frequency and urgency may require the addition of an anticholinergic medication.

URINARY INCONTINENCE

method of
EDWARD J. McGUIRE, M.D.
The University of Texas–Houston
Houston, Texas

Treatment of urinary incontinence depends on a precise diagnosis of the cause of the problem.

LEAKAGE RELATED TO BLADDER DYSFUNCTION

Abnormalities of Bladder Control

True detrusor hyper-reflexia refers to a condition characterized by automaticity of reflex bladder contractility driven by volume. This condition is associated with spinal cord lesions, cerebral diseases, strokes, obstructive uropathy, bladder foreign bodies, and, surprisingly, stress urinary incontinence and genital prolapse. A reflex detrusor contraction elicited by filling the bladder, which typically occurs at a smaller than normal volume, is characteristic of the condition. When patients are aware of the problem, they describe frequent day and night wetting. Some patients may not feel any urgency and may not have any bladder sensation at all. In these cases, which include spinal cord injury and multiple sclerosis, the problem is progressive if untreated.

Diagnosis

The presence of residual urine indicates either a neurogenic or an obstructive condition in most instances. Absence of residual urine generally means it is safe to start empirical therapy, without the imposition of intermittent catheterization. Physical examination may suggest a neurologic condition or demonstrate stress incontinence or genital prolapse. A cystometrogram usually shows a bladder contraction elicited at a smaller than normal volume.

Treatment

Initial therapy is with drugs that delay bladder contractility, including imipramine hydrochloride (Tofranil),* 10 to 25 mg twice daily, and oxybutynin (Ditropan), 2.5 to 5 mg three times daily. Two-drug therapy, e.g., with a tricyclic antidepressant and oxybutynin, is generally more effective than treatment with a single agent. Alpha-blocking agents have also been used to delay reflex bladder contractility in patients with neurogenic conditions. Drug therapy alone is usually not completely satisfactory, and some effort to induce timed voiding, prompted urination, or regular intermittent catheterization is often required to achieve continence. Drug therapy does not usually change subjective ability to anticipate detrusor contractility. Consider, for example, a patient with a spinal cord lesion at a midthoracic level who is wet despite intermittent catheterization. Anticholinergic agents will improve bladder capacity, but inability to anticipate detrusor contractility will persist. A similar problem occurs in neurologically normal patients who are surprised by sudden reflex bladder activity even while receiving anticholinergic agents. Thus, some method of timed voiding or anticipatory voiding is usually required to ensure success.

Definitive Therapy

In women, partial transvaginal vesical denervation is sometimes effective when drugs fail. Ultimately,

---

*Not FDA approved for this indication.

failure of conservative therapy, including drugs and/or intermittent catheterization and timed voiding, can be treated by enlargement of the bladder. There are two basic surgical techniques to achieve a larger bladder. The most commonly employed is an augmentation cystoplasty using small or large bowel, a formidable operative undertaking. Somewhat less morbid, but as yet incompletely evaluated, is a technique called partial detrusor muscle excision wherein part of the detrusor muscle overlying the anterior and lateral walls of the bladder is removed, creating a larger lower pressure reservoir. Complications related to these surgical procedures may be serious.

Other Measures

Pelvic floor exercises and electrical stimulation techniques as well as biofeedback therapy have been used to control hyper-reflexic bladder dysfunction. These methods are generally applied to non-neurogenic dysfunction only. However, electrical stimulation has been used sporadically but with reasonable results in patients with neurogenic vesical dysfunction when the electrical stimulation is applied to the pelvic floor musculature, external urethra, and/or anal sphincter. Stimulation of those structures appears to be associated with indirect and direct inhibition of detrusor contractility.

Idiopathic Abnormalities of Bladder Control

Bladder control abnormalities occur in patients who are ostensibly otherwise normal. Strictly defined as "unstable bladder" is a diagnosis made on the basis of a cystometrogram wherein filling provokes a bladder contractile response that the patient cannot inhibit. As many as 50% of patients with the symptom *urge incontinence* do not show bladder instability on a cystometrogram. In those patients with an abnormal cystometrogram result, a positive response to drugs, behavioral therapy, and timed voiding can be expected. In the other group, when the cystometrogram is normal, there is no pattern to the incontinence that is completely random in character. Wetting is related to neither the bladder volume nor the length of elapsed time since the last voiding. As such, this is a difficult condition to treat effectively. Drugs simply do not work. Anything that can focus the patient's attention on his or her bladder, including timed voiding, voiding diaries, and bladder drills wherein the bladder is emptied at specific times, may help. Other measures including physical therapy, biofeedback, and electrical stimulation may be tried, but the results are uncertain. Patients with normal cystometrograms and motor urge incontinence are generally excluded from clinical trials of these methods because there is no way to prove exactly what is wrong with them. Nevertheless, such patients constitute a relatively large percentage of the incontinent population.

An example of this kind of incontinence occurs in nocturnal enuresis. Patients with this syndrome, when awake, have normal cystometrograms and can control bladder activity perfectly. During sleep, there is a lack of an arousal response, and the bladder contracts when it becomes full. Adult patients with idiopathic instability appear to suffer from an intermittent day and night eneuretic-like syndrome in which cortical appreciation of bladder events is completely lost.

OVERFLOW INCONTINENCE

This is a rare problem that occurs when an overfilled bladder reaches the limits of its viscoelastic distensibility and generates sufficient pressure to overcome urethral resistance, resulting in leakage that is, characteristically, continuous. Diagnosis is by residual urine determination, and the initial treatment is directed at decompression of the bladder by intermittent catheterization until the underlying cause can be identified.

INCONTINENCE AND DEMENTIA

There is no regular relationship between dementia and incontinence. Many patients who are demented are not incontinent, and many patients who are not demented are incontinent. Incontinence occurring in demented patients may be untreatable.

URETHRAL INCONTINENCE

In conditions characterized by a lack of bladder control, the bladder is the expulsive force responsible for leakage. In conditions in which the urethra is at fault, abdominal pressure is the expulsive force inducing leakage. A normal urethra will not leak at any physiologic abdominal pressure, whereas an abnormal urethra will. The severity of the abnormality in urethral function is inversely proportional to the amount of abdominal pressure required to induce leakage. A severely abnormal urethra will leak at low pressure. Such leakage will be associated with minimal physical activity. A urethra that is weakened but still able to resist some degree of abdominal pressure will leak at higher pressures. More vigorous physical activity is necessary in the latter condition to induce leakage. Incontinence related to urethral dysfunction is typically related to activity and is thus termed "stress" incontinence. Although this condition is more common in women than in men, it is produced in a certain percentage of men by a prostatectomy. The history is generally typical, with leakage described as induced by certain activities: coughing, sneezing, lifting, walking, or running. Many patients with stress urinary incontinence related to poor urethral function also have abnormalities of detrusor control. When the urethral problem is dealt with successfully, the abnormalities of detrusor control frequently disappear, but not always. In some instances then, urethral dysfunction appears to be causally related to detrusor dysfunction, but there does not appear to be any way to predict this before

therapy. Physical examination in standing male or female patients with stress incontinence will demonstrate leakage from the urethral meatus driven by a Valsalva maneuver or coughing. Female patients should be examined in both the pelvic examination position and the upright position. Most patients with mild to moderate stress incontinence will not leak in the pelvic examination position, so it is necessary to repeat the examination with the patient standing. Patients with severe degrees of urethral incontinence will leak in the supine pelvic examination position.

In male patients, treatment options are somewhat limited. Most patients suffering sphincteric injury at the time of prostatectomy do not respond to medication. Such patients are candidates for collagen injection therapy, artificial sphincter implantation, or some variety of a male sling procedure. The results of the last are incompletely evaluated. Overall, continence rates with collagen injection or the artificial sphincter range from 40 to 80%, with better results reported after sphincter implantation. In female patients, stress incontinence may be related to urethral hypermobility, in which case a procedure that repositions and replaces the urethra in its normal retropubic position will be satisfactory. Stress incontinence may also result from proximal urethral sphincteric weakness, in which case a suspension procedure will not work. Patients with hypermobility presumably related somehow to impaired pelvic floor muscle activity, or lack of activity, may be treated by pelvic floor muscle exercises, biofeedback, and electrical stimulation. The exact effect of such treatment on the urethra has not been conclusively determined, but many patients are improved by such treatment. Patients with poor urethral function are not well treated by these measures.

Drug Therapy in Female Patients

This is sometimes, but rarely, efficacious. Agents that can be used include imipramine hydrochloride 10 to 25 mg three times daily and alpha-stimulating agents, e.g., phenylpropanolamine as in a sustained-release capsule (Ornade).* Elderly women with urethral dysfunction not related to urethral hypermobility who are severely estrogen deficient may benefit from combined therapy with imipramine hydrochloride,* 10 mg twice daily, and small doses of intravaginal estrogen (Premarin vaginal cream),* one fourth of an applicator every third or fourth day. Such therapy is not effective if the urethra is hypermobile, or in younger women, or in those not severely estrogen deficient.

After a trial of conservative therapy, including biofeedback, pelvic floor exercises, or Kegel's exercises, with or without electrical stimulation, persistent stress urinary incontinence is generally an indication for a surgical procedure. Long-term outcomes after most commonly used surgical procedures are uncertain. The procedures most commonly used by urologists, needle suspension procedures, have been re-

---

*Not FDA approved for this indication.

ported to be associated with relatively poor late outcomes. Better results have been reported in a historical series of retropubic suspensions, but the populations of patients studied are probably different. Better long-term results have been reported with sling procedures.

Injectable Therapy

The Food and Drug Administration recently approved collagen for the treatment of urinary incontinence in men and women. Use in men is restricted to those with normal bladder compliance and intrinsic sphincter dysfunction related to prostatectomy. Results in men are not as good as they are in women. Women with little or no urethral mobility and incontinence related to intrinsic sphincter dysfunction can be satisfactorily treated by injectable agents. Currently, the only approved agent is collagen. About 80% of women so treated, after 2 injections, are markedly improved or dry. Long-term results with collagen beyond 2 years are not available. The material would be expected to be gradually degraded; thus, efficacy on a long-term basis may be a problem.

BLADDER STORAGE ABNORMALITIES

The most important aspect of bladder function is low-pressure urine storage. At capacity, the change in detrusor pressure from that at 0 volume is normally less than 15 cm H_2O. Direct injury, e.g., by chemotherapeutic agents (mitomycin [Mutamycin] and bacille Calmette-Guérin given intravesically and/or cyclophosphamide [Cytoxan] and other agents given parenterally), can induce poor bladder storage, as can radiation therapy. Long-standing untreated obstructive uropathy or chronic catheter drainage can also induce poor compliance (storage). In those instances in which poor storage is the result of obstruction, the process of detrusor muscle hypertrophy may be reversible with treatment. In direct injury, reversal is not usually possible.

Poor storage simply means that bladder pressure rises with volume until intravesical and intraurethral pressures are equal—when leakage occurs. This is like overflow incontinence except that it is pressure related and occurs at moderate, not extreme, volumes. Diagnosis is by a cystometrogram, which determines the bladder pressure response to filling. Patients with poor compliance generally have a history that suggests the bladder might have been injured, directly or indirectly, and leakage is severe.

Poor storage causes incontinence but also puts backpressure on the ureters and causes vesicoureteral reflux. Ultimately, it results in pressure transmission from the bladder to the renal papillae, which induces changes in renal blood flow, cessation of glomerular filtration, and renal failure.

Treatment is directed at reduction in bladder pressure by frequent emptying coupled, if required, with bladder enlargement *or* creation of low-pressure leakage—the price of which is continence.

EPIDIDYMITIS

method of
JOHN N. KRIEGER, M.D.
University of Washington School of Medicine
Seattle, Washington

Epididymitis represents an inflammatory reaction of the epididymis to infection or to local trauma. Epididymitis is a common urologic problem, accounting for more than 600,000 visits to physicians per year in the United States. Acute epididymitis is responsible for more days lost from military service than any other disease and is responsible for 20% of urologic admissions in the military.

CLINICAL PRESENTATION

Painful swelling of the scrotum is the characteristic clinical presentation. In most cases, the pain and swelling are unilateral. The onset may be acute during 1 or 2 days or more gradual. The pain may radiate along the spermatic cord or into the lower abdomen. Symptoms of cystitis or urethritis are common. Dysuria or irritative lower urinary tract symptoms are characteristic. Many men have a urethral discharge, and particular attention should be directed to eliciting a history of genitourinary tract disease or sexual exposure. Some men may have only a nonspecific finding of fever or other signs of infection. This is especially common in hospitalized men who have had urinary tract manipulation, or catheterization, and may be obtunded by medication.

Tender swelling may occur in the posterior aspect of the scrotum. The swelling is usually unilateral and is often accompanied by erythema. Early in the course, the swelling may be localized to one portion of the epididymis. However, the swelling often progresses to involve the ipsilateral testis, producing an epididymo-orchitis. At this point, it is difficult to distinguish the testicle from the epididymis within the inflammatory mass. Scrotal examination reveals the characteristic hydrocele caused by secretion of inflammatory fluid between the layers of the tunica vaginalis. Urethral discharge may be apparent on inspection or stripping of the urethra.

Evaluation for urethritis should be done before the patient voids because micturition may make it difficult or impossible to detect mild urethritis. The nursing staff should be taught to instruct patients with urogenital tract complaints not to void until after the physical examination. This is a common problem when we are asked to consult on management of a patient in the emergency department or in primary care settings.

PATHOGENESIS

Acute epididymitis occurs when uropathogens overcome the host defenses of the male lower genitourinary tract to establish infection of the epididymis. Most cases result from retrograde ascent of organisms through the urethra, prostate, ejaculatory duct, and vas deferens to reach the epididymis. Therefore, infections of the urethra, bladder, or prostate are important risk factors for development of epididymitis. Mechanical factors, such as the flushing action of micturition and ejaculation, should provide some protection against infection. Although the relative significance of such defenses is unclear, extensive clinical experience indicates that structural or functional abnormalities of the lower urinary tract increase the risk for epididymitis.

Prostatic antibacterial factor is an important defense against ascending infections of the male lower genitourinary tract. This zinc-containing polypeptide is secreted by the prostate. Men with chronic bacterial prostatitis have significantly lower levels of zinc in their prostatic fluid than do healthy men, but their serum zinc levels are normal. It is unclear whether reduced zinc concentrations precede the development of prostatic infection or represent a secretory dysfunction resulting from such infections. Prostatic secretions of men with well-documented genitourinary infections contain high concentrations of immunoglobulins. Several studies demonstrated antigen-specific antibody coating of bacteria isolated from men with genitourinary tract infections. The antigen-specific antibody response in prostatic secretions is predominantly secretory IgA and is significantly greater than is the serologic response. Increased concentrations of leukocytes occur in many conditions of the male lower urinary tract, including prostatitis and epididymitis. These humoral and cellular immune responses are important for resolution of tissue-invasive genitourinary infections.

MANAGEMENT OF ACUTE EPIDIDYMITIS

Most cases of acute epididymitis can be classified in one of two categories, nonspecific bacterial epididymitis or sexually transmitted epididymitis. Unusual patients develop epididymitis after genital trauma or with disseminated infections.

Clinical evaluation begins with a history, specifically eliciting recognized risk factors, and a thorough physical examination. Initial laboratory tests include urinalysis, culture, and sensitivity testing for men with presumed nonspecific bacterial epididymitis. Men at risk for sexually transmitted epididymitis should also have a Gram-stained urethral smear, culture for *Neisseria gonorrhoeae,* and testing for *Chlamydia trachomatis.* In the latter group, serologic testing is also recommended for syphilis and for human immunodeficiency virus (HIV) infection.

Nonspecific Bacterial Epididymitis

Infection with coliform or *Pseudomonas* species is the most common cause of epididymitis in men older than 35 years. In most series, gram-negative rods caused more than two thirds of cases of bacterial epididymitis. However, gram-positive cocci are also important pathogens and constituted the most common organisms in other reports.

Patients with bacterial epididymitis often have underlying urologic disease or have a history of genitourinary tract manipulation. After surgery or urethral catheterization, epididymitis may occur weeks or rarely months after the manipulation. Epididymitis constitutes a special risk for men who undergo urinary tract surgery or instrumentation while they are bacteriuric. Acute bacterial prostatitis and chronic bacterial prostatitis are other important predisposing conditions for development of bacterial epididymitis.

Medical management is appropriate for most patients with bacterial epididymitis. Most men with uncomplicated epididymitis are managed as outpatients. Indications for hospitalization include systemic symptoms such as leukocytosis and fever, complications, or associated medical conditions. In these severe cases, parenteral antimicrobial therapy is used until the patient defervesces. Choices for empirical therapy of severe cases include the combination of an aminoglycoside plus a β-lactam agent, or a third-generation cephalosporin. After resolution of the acute systemic infection, therapy is continued with oral agents, guided by the culture and sensitivity results.

For outpatients, empirical treatment is initiated with agents appropriate for both gram-negative rods and gram-positive cocci pending urine culture and sensitivity results. My first choice for management of nonspecific epididymitis in outpatients is the combination of trimethoprim and sulfamethoxazole (Bactrim, Septra), 1 double-strength tablet twice daily for 10 to 14 days. The fluoroquinolones, such as ciprofloxacin (Cipro), ofloxacin (Floxin), and norfloxacin (Noroxin), are alternative medications. If there is evidence of bacterial prostatitis, antimicrobial therapy is continued for 6 to 12 weeks. This initial empirical therapy may be changed, if necessary, after culture results are available.

Nonspecific measures are worthwhile, including bed rest, scrotal elevation, analgesics, and local ice packs. A spermatic cord block with bupivacaine (Marcaine) may be helpful for management of severe pain. I recommend urologic evaluation because structural or functional abnormalities are common among men with nonspecific bacterial epididymitis.

Sexually Transmitted Epididymitis

Sexually transmitted epididymitis is most common in young men. *C. trachomatis* and *N. gonorrhoeae* are the major pathogens. In most series, chlamydiae were identified as the most common cause of epididymitis in younger, sexually active populations. For example, in my institution, *C. trachomatis* infections were documented in 17 (50%) of 34 cases of epididymitis in men younger than 35 years but in only 1 (6%) of 16 cases of epididymitis in men older than 35 years. In the past, these patients were considered to have "idiopathic" nonspecific epididymitis. Sexually transmitted *Escherichia coli* infection also occurs among men who are the insertive partners during anal intercourse.

Patients with chlamydial epididymitis frequently do not complain of urethral discharge. However, 11 (65%) of 17 patients with epididymitis caused by chlamydiae had demonstrable discharge. In most cases, the discharge was scant and watery, characteristic of nongonococcal urethritis. The median interval from the last sexual exposure was 10 days and ranged from 1 to 45 days. Thus, urethral *C. trachomatis* may be carried for long periods before development of overt epididymitis.

In the preantibiotic era, epididymitis occurred in

10 to 30% of men with gonococcal urethritis. However, in more recent series, *N. gonorrhoeae* was identified in 16% of men with epididymitis in military populations and in 21% of men with epididymitis in civilians younger than 35 years. Many patients with epididymitis do not have a history of urethral discharge, and a discharge may be demonstrable in only 50% of such patients. Diagnosis depends on a high index of clinical suspicion, evaluation for presence of urethritis (which may be asymptomatic), appropriate cultures, or antigen detection tests.

Empirical therapy is recommended before culture results are available. Appropriate therapy includes coverage for both *N. gonorrhoeae* and *C. trachomatis* infection. My first choice is the combination of ceftriaxone (Rocephin), 250 mg intramuscularly in a single dose, plus doxycycline (Vibramycin), 100 mg orally two times a day for 10 days. Alternative therapy for epididymitis that is most likely due to enteric organisms or for patients allergic to cephalosporins or tetracycline is ofloxacin, 300 mg orally twice daily for 10 days. Alternatives for coverage of *N. gonorrhoeae* include spectinomycin (Trobicin), 2 grams intramuscularly in a single dose; ciprofloxacin, 500 mg orally in a single dose; or norfloxacin, 800 mg orally in a single dose. Alternatives for coverage of *C. trachomatis* include azithromycin (Zithromax), 1 gram orally as a single dose, or tetracycline hydrochloride, 500 mg orally four times a day for 10 days. Nonspecific measures are helpful, including bed rest, scrotal elevation, analgesics, and local ice packs. A spermatic cord block with bupivacaine may reduce the need for analgesics in men with severe pain.

Patients should be evaluated for other sexually transmitted infections, and treatment of sexual partners is important. Underlying genitourinary tract abnormalities are uncommon in this population. Thus, a complete urologic work-up is indicated rarely for patients with uncomplicated sexually transmitted epididymitis.

Uncommon Causes

Tuberculous epididymitis is the most common manifestation of genital tuberculosis in men, with orchitis and prostatitis less common. The usual symptom is heaviness or swelling. Scrotal swelling with "beadlike" enlargement of the vas deferens is characteristic. Chronic draining scrotal sinuses may occur. The systemic mycoses rarely cause epididymitis; blastomycosis is the most common pathogen and may also cause a draining sinus through the scrotal wall. Men with HIV infection and uncomplicated epididymitis should receive the same treatment as those without HIV infection. However, fungal and mycobacterial causes of epididymitis are more common among patients who are immunocompromised.

In the pediatric population, epididymitis may occur with congenital anatomic abnormalities, such as ectopic ureter or posterior urethral valves.

Epididymitis occasionally occurs after testicular trauma. Many of these men have evidence of genitourinary tract infections with organisms outlined before, but occasional men develop traumatic epididymitis that is not associated with positive cultures or inflammation. I also described an unusual syndrome of noninfectious epididymitis associated with amiodarone (Cordarone) therapy for refractory ventricular arrhythmias.

DIFFERENTIAL DIAGNOSIS

Severe inflammation can lead to an enlarged indurated epididymis that is indistinguishable from the testicle. This can present difficulties in the differential diagnosis of epididymitis from testicular torsion or testicular cancer. The epididymis normally lies posterior to the testis. This demarcation is often preserved in cases of epididymitis. "Reactive" hydrocele formation may render the palpation of intrascrotal structures difficult. Although transillumination frequently identifies hydroceles, color-flow Doppler ultrasonography is my preferred imaging study when the diagnosis is in doubt. Acute epididymitis must be distinguished from testicular torsion at the initial evaluation because uncorrected torsion results in testicular death within 24 hours. Men with swelling and tenderness that persist after completing therapy should be re-evaluated for testicular cancer, tuberculosis, or fungal epididymitis.

COMPLICATIONS

Most patients experience relief of their symptoms within 48 hours. However, swelling and discomfort may persist for weeks or months after eradication of the infecting organism. In some cases, the epididymis remains enlarged or indurated indefinitely. Such men may develop chronic epididymitis, characterized by pain and occasionally by recurrent swelling.

Bacterial epididymitis may be an important focus of organisms causing both local morbidity and bacteremia in men with indwelling transurethral catheters. Genitourinary tract complications of acute epididymitis include testicular infarction, scrotal abscess, pyocele of the scrotum, a chronic draining scrotal sinus, chronic epididymitis, and infertility. Ultrasonography, particularly color-flow Doppler ultrasonography, is useful for the differential diagnosis of complicated cases. Surgery may be necessary for complications of acute epididymal infections but has no role in treatment of tuberculous or fungal epididymitis.

PRIMARY GLOMERULAR DISEASES

method of
W. KLINE BOLTON, M.D.
University of Virginia Health Sciences Center
Charlottesville, Virginia

Primary glomerular diseases are those that affect the glomeruli and are unrelated to a systemic etiology. They are distinguished from secondary glomerular diseases that have an obvious systemic etiology. The latter include systemic lupus erythematosus (SLE), postinfectious glomerulonephritis (GN), systemic vasculitis, amyloidosis, and other systemic diseases. However, in reality, this is a misnomer because all of the primary glomerular diseases recur in transplant recipients, and certain primary glomerular diseases present by chance in allografts transplanted into patients with other causes of end-stage renal disease (ESRD) disappear. It is likely that as a better understanding of the pathogenesis of these disorders is elaborated, fewer will truly be considered primary. Further evidence for the indistinction between these two categories is the notable presence in many of them of vague systemic manifestations such as myalgia or easy fatigability, lack of energy, weakness, cough, or other manifestations that could be considered systemic in nature. In addition, many of the histologic lesions seen on renal biopsy in primary glomerular disorders can be seen with systemic disorders as well. The clinician, in collaboration with the pathologist, is left to assign the designation of primary glomerular disorder versus systemic glomerular disorder. Nonetheless, for purposes of the present discussion, I maintain the traditional classification of those glomerular disorders classically considered primary in nature.

Primary glomerular disorders can be classified into those that are generally nephritic or inflammatory in nature and those that are characterized by an increase in permeability of the glomerular basement membrane (GBM). These "nephritic" versus "nephrotic" syndromes, of course, can overlap.

DIAGNOSIS OF PRIMARY GLOMERULAR DISORDERS

The standard evaluation of the patient with glomerular disease should be the same whether a primary or secondary etiology is considered. (1) Evidence for a systemic disorder should be sought with a thorough history and physical examination as well as appropriate laboratory studies. In this day of cost constraints, broad-spectrum panels of serologic tests are to be discouraged. The clinician should focus on likely causes based on the patient's presentation. In patients with inflammatory nephritic disease, an antineutrophil cytoplasmic antibody (ANCA) assay is essential. In the absence of clinical manifestations of SLE, rheumatoid arthritis, or other rheumatologic disorder, the yield of serologic tests for these clinical entities is cost-ineffective. (2) It should be ascertained whether it is likely that the patient does have a glomerular process. This is best approached by a careful analysis of urinary sediment and renal function studies. In patients with a nephritic syndrome, red blood cells (RBCs) will frequently if not always be dysmorphic in nature, fragmented, and small and show the ravages of passage through damaged GBM on their way to the urinary tract. RBC casts are frequently present but must be sought assiduously in a fresh-spun, first-voided morning urine specimen. It is critical that the urine be properly prepared such that 10 mL of urine is spun at 2000 to 3000 revolutions per minute for 5 to 10 minutes. The supernatant is gently decanted, and the tube is inverted and quickly blotted against a paper towel, leaving only sediment. This sediment can be agitated by flicking the tube bottom and then examined with standard and phase microscopes. The yield is greatly enhanced by use of a vital stain such as Sternheimer-Malbin. The entire slide consisting of one drop of urine should be carefully scanned for evidence of formed elements. (3) The proteinuria should be determined and characterized. A 24-hour urine specimen should be obtained for renal functional studies but most important for a total urinary protein (TUP) determination. The TUP determination should be done by use of a method that detects the entire spectrum of urinary proteins including light chains, Bence Jones proteins, albumin, immunoglobulins, and α_2-macroglobulin. Glomerular diseases are characterized by proteinuria consisting first of albumin, then later of other components of serum. The electrophoretic profile is characteristic for glomerular proteinuria as opposed to tubular and tubulointerstitial proteinuria, which lack a significant component of small-molecular-weight albumin and instead consist of an α_2-macroglobulin peak. The degree of proteinuria is of modest assistance except that tubular proteinuria rarely exceeds 2 grams per 24 hours. Thus, less than this can be either glomerular or tubular; more than 2 grams is usually glomerular in origin. RBCs and RBC casts can be seen in a variety of processes that are not glomerular in origin, such as cortical necrosis, acute tubular necrosis, and acute interstitial nephritis. Thus, whereas their presence is highly suggestive of glomerular diseases, it is not pathognomonic. The presence of white blood cells (WBCs) and WBC casts in the absence of bacteria suggests an inflammatory process in the kidney that may or may not be associated with glomerular disease. Although not invariant, GN with WBC and WBC casts is usually associated with RBCs and RBC casts.

Patients with GN may present clinically with no findings, having been discovered by routine dipstick urinalysis for health or insurance physical examination; may be detected on routine "well visits" to their primary physician; or may complain of features consistent with salt and water retention, such as edema, hypertension, discolored or foul-smelling urine, or other systemic manifestation. A few patients may present with oliguria or anuria in those unusual cases of acute crescentic rapidly progressive GN (AC-RPGN).

In patients who have a nephrotic rather than a nephritic presentation, I use TUP as the sine qua non for the diagnosis. Three grams or more excretion of TUP for 24 hours is considered diagnostic of the nephrotic syndrome. Although the classic definition of this syndrome is hypoalbuminemia, hypercholesterolemia, proteinuria in excess of 3.5 grams per 24 hours, and edema, I have seen many patients who presented with extreme hypoalbuminemia with none of the other presentations, and I have seen patients with 20 grams of proteinuria secondary to amyloidosis with normal cholesterol and albumin levels and no edema. Thus, I use 3 grams per 24 hours TUP as my diagnostic level for nephrotic syndrome.

NEPHRITIC FORMS OF PRIMARY GLOMERULAR DISEASE

This group of primary glomerular disorders presents with either an active urinary sediment with modest proteinuria or with a nephritic-nephrotic profile.

IgA Nephropathy

Diagnosis

IgA nephropathy, Berger's disease or benign recurrent hematuria, is the single most common cause of primary GN in the world today. This is a disease of childhood or young adulthood with a preponderance of males to females. It is more common in individuals of Asian descent, whites, and Native Americans but is less common in African-Americans. Patients generally have chronic, asymptomatic, microscopic hematuria with episodes of gross hematuria that usually occur 1 to 3 days after some type of mucosal infection, such as an upper respiratory infection, gastroenteritis, or cystitis. It can also be associated with physical and emotional stress. The hematuria is usually painless, lasts for a few days, and is self-limited. In the past, it was assumed that this was a totally benign process, but it is now known that at least 20 to 25% of patients have progressive renal dysfunction with heavy proteinuria and require dialytic support. A few patients will develop an RPGN-like course. The prognosis is worse in patients with hypertension, heavy proteinuria unresponsive to prednisone, decreased renal function with increased serum creatinine at presentation, and evidence of chronicity on renal biopsy including glomerulosclerosis and interstitial fibrosis. The presence of crescents also conveys a worse prognosis.

By light microscopy, the renal biopsy specimen shows either minimal changes or mesangial expansion and hypercellularity with increased matrix formation. The immunofluorescence pattern is diagnostic, with strong coarsely granular deposits of IgA and frequently C3 in the mesangium. A few patients may have small deposits of fibrinogen, suggesting that this disease may fall within the spectrum of Henoch-Schönlein purpura. Patients will frequently have elevated serum IgA, and skin biopsy specimens will show IgA deposits. Half of the patients will have circulating immune complexes consisting of IgA. Although the pathogenesis of the disease is unknown, theories include excess formation of IgA-containing immune complexes secondary to mucosal immunity, impaired receptor-mediated clearance of circulating soluble immune complexes, or abnormalities in receptors for IgA-containing complexes within glomeruli. Strong evidence for an abnormality of clearance is provided by the frequent occurrence of IgA nephropathy in patients with hepatic disease, especially cirrhosis.

Treatment

A variety of other diseases may result in a clinical and histologic appearance similar to IgA nephropathy. These include Henoch-Schönlein purpura, a systemic illness associated with joint involvement, gastrointestinal tract involvement, and purpuric rash that is a self-limited form of vasculitis; chronic liver disease of various types, especially including cirrhosis; multiple types of inflammatory bowel disease; dermatitis herpetiformis; IgA gammopathy; and SLE. Spontaneous improvement of the underlying etiologic factor or improvement by therapeutic intervention at the specific cause can result in improvement in the histologic lesion and clinical presentation in these patients.

For idiopathic primary IgA nephropathy, there are no definitively proven therapeutic interventions. A number of different types of treatment, however, have been used with some success. These include treatment with phenytoin (Dilantin), which decreases circulating IgA levels; tetracycline, which decreases hematuria; and alterations in diet to decrease the gluten content as well as gliadin and casein. However, none of these therapeutic interventions has been definitely shown to affect the course of the disease in different trials. A variety of steroids, cytotoxic agents, and cyclosporine have shown limited success. However, long-term treatment with alternate-day prednisone, 15 to 20 mg orally every other day, suggests that this may have some beneficial effect on progression of disease. Studies have suggested that omega-3 fatty acids may also have a beneficial effect and should be administered as 5 grams twice a day. Although the evidence is controversial, a "low-antigen" diet can be attempted in some patients, limiting wheats, breads, and dietary protein. Some clinicians also advocate limitation of alcohol.

My approach is to use pulse methylprednisolone (MP) (Solu-Medrol) therapy for those patients who present with RPGN. In those with more slowly progressive decreasing kidney function, I use high-dose alternate-day long-term prednisone therapy as described in detail later (see RPGN). More recently I have used omega-3 fatty acid supplementation. It is critical that the blood pressure be maintained as close as possible to a mean arterial pressure of 92 mm Hg using first an angiotensin-converting enzyme inhibitor (ACEI) with a 2-gram-per-day low-sodium diet to achieve optimal blood pressure and antiproteinuric effect of the ACEI.

Membranoproliferative Glomerulonephritis

Diagnosis

The diagnosis of membranoproliferative glomerulonephritis (MPGN) is dependent on the histologic finding of hypercellularity in the mesangium with GBM thickening and splitting ultrastructurally. MPGN can be divided into three types on the basis of laboratory and biopsy findings. Type I consists of glomerular deposition of immune complexes in the subendothelial portion of the GBM. In type II MPGN, there are pseudolinear dense deposits along the GBM, Bowman's capsule, and tubular basement membrane, "dense deposit disease." Type III MPGN contains pathologic characteristics of type I and type II with intramembranous deposits. MPGN is a disease of adolescents and young individuals and is slightly more common in whites than in African-Americans. It has a diverse pattern of presentation, with some patients having asymptomatic hematuria and proteinuria for many years that can suddenly develop into acute GN, including RPGN. Yet another quarter of patients can present with nephrotic-range proteinuria, characteristically with an active urinary sediment, as opposed to other types of nephrotic syndrome in which a markedly active urinary sediment is the exception rather than the rule. Patients with MPGN will frequently but not always have a low complement level. The relationship between MPGN and postinfectious GN is unclear because the presence of characteristic "postinfectious humps" is not uncommon in patients with MPGN.

Treatment

Systemic causes of MPGN should be sought and excluded. MPGN is frequently secondary to different causes including infections of various types, hepatitis B and C, and mixed cryoglobulinemia (which is probably hepatitis C). Chronic thrombotic microangiopathy, light chain deposition disease, and various hematologic malignant neoplasms as well as arteriovenous malformations can also be associated with MPGN. Treatment of underlying occult visceral abscess, bacterial endocarditis, or other infection can result in regression or stabilization of the lesion. This includes hepatitis C–associated MPGN when the viremia can be diminished by interferon therapy. Therapy for primary MPGN is controversial, and many different agents have been used including high-dose daily prednisone, alternate-day prednisone, chlorambucil,* cyclophosphamide,* aspirin,* dipyridamole (Persantine),* coumadin (Warfarin),* and other agents. My pattern of treatment has been to use pulse MP followed by alternate-day high-dose steroids in those patients with RPGN or severe inflammatory processes by renal biopsy. As in all forms of glomerular and nonglomerular disease, it is essential that hypertension be controlled, preferably with an ACEI.

Prognosis

MPGN is slowly progressive and inexorably leads to ESRD in approximately 50 to 60% of patients within a decade. The prognosis is worse when the proteinuria is heavier, when tubulointerstitial disease is present, or when marked glomerular fibrosis and scarring or crescents are present. MPGN recurs in the allograft in those patients who receive transplants. Approximately 10% of patients with type I disease will have recurrent disease, with consequent loss of the graft in about 40% of patients; recurrence of dense deposit disease is much more common, approximately 40 to 50% of patients, but with graft loss in about 10%. Thus, the overall graft loss from recurrent disease is approximately equal in the two diseases. There is some suggestion that there is a greater propensity for recurrence and graft loss in living related donors.

Rapidly Progressive Glomerulonephritis

Diagnosis

RPGN is one of the most devastating of the primary glomerular diseases to be seen by the clinician.

*Not FDA approved for this indication.

The syndrome is a group of diseases with acute GN and a decrease in kidney function of 50% or more in a 3-month period or less. Many clinicopathologic entities can present as RPGN, including vasculitis, acute interstitial nephritis, acute tubular necrosis, atheromatous emboli, acute renal vein thrombosis, Henoch-Schönlein purpura, thrombocytopenic purpura, malignant hypertension, and many others. A histologic diagnosis is essential. In addition, the histologic diagnosis must be made as expeditiously as possible because cellular crescents can progress to irreversible fibrous crescents and glomerulosclerosis in as short a period as 2 weeks. RPGN is a *clinical syndrome,* and acute crescentic GN refers to *histologic* findings. Whereas most cases of RPGN are crescentic in nature, a subset of RPGN, especially those with MPGN or IgA nephropathy, can have the same clinical course and generally poor prognosis even in the absence of crescents.

By immunofluorescence and ultrastructural analysis, RPGN can be divided into three groups.

1. RPGN with no immunoglobulin deposit (NID or pauci-immune disease). The immune deposits in the NID variety consist of either no or minimal deposits of IgM and C3. Approximately 70 to 80% will have necrotizing GN and presence of ANCA, suggesting that they are a form of microscopic polyarteritis nodosa. This category of NID GN accounts for around 30 to 50% of RPGN, depending on the geographic region.

2. Immune complex RPGN. In this category, approximately 20 to 25% of patients will have intense deposits of immunoglobulin and C3 in a granular pattern along the GBM and/or mesangium and ultrastructural deposits. Almost all of these can be shown to be secondary to some type of systemic disease, treatment of which effects a beneficial response in many cases.

3. Anti-GBM disease. This category consists of circulating and bound anti-GBM antibodies deposited on kidney and sometimes lung basement membrane. The antigen specificities are the same whether GN, pulmonary hemorrhage, or both are present and can be broadly characterized as Goodpasture's disease. The presence or absence of pulmonary hemorrhage seems to be closely correlated with pulmonary injury such as hydrocarbon exposure, viral infection, or smoking. Approximately 20 to 25% of patients with AC-RPGN have anti-GBM disease, but this can vary by geographic region and can be as low as 5 to 10%. Between 10 and 30% of patients with anti-GBM disease will also have ANCA. The prognosis and response to therapy in double-positive patients appear to be different from those of patients who have anti-GBM disease alone. There is an inverse association between titers of anti-GBM antibodies and ANCAs. Those patients with high ANCA titers tend to have more systemic manifestations and relapses and respond to therapy as if they had vasculitis. This includes the ability to stop hemodialysis support with recovery of sufficient function to maintain the patient

as opposed to those patients who have mostly anti-GBM disease who almost never are able to discontinue dialytic support. Poor prognostic findings in anti-GBM disease including a high degree of crescents, oliguria or anuria, and serum creatinine concentration above 5 to 6 mg per dL are not associated with as poor a prognosis if patients are ANCA-positive as well.

In patients who present with AC-RPGN, it is incumbent on the clinician to obtain anti-GBM and ANCA titers and look for systemic disease. This is especially true in patients with NID who may have microscopic polyarteritis nodosa or Wegener's granulomatosis as the cause of their AC-RPGN.

Treatment

Secondary causes of RPGN should be sought because treatment directed to the underlying disease can be efficacious. This is especially true when an occult infection is present. Appropriate drainage of an infection or antibiotic therapy can result in complete cure, whereas aggressive MP or other cytotoxic agents could be devastating.

In the patient who presents with the clinical picture of decreasing urine output and the clinical syndrome of RPGN, a renal biopsy should be performed within the first 24 hours. Either before the biopsy or immediately thereafter, the patient should be treated with pulse MP 30 mg per kg intravenously every other day for 3 doses up to 3 grams each given during a 20-minute period with hydration and monitoring for blood pressure and arrhythmias. It is essential that the diagnosis be made as expeditiously as possible and therapy be initiated immediately. The overall response to therapy is dependent on how soon therapy is initiated and the degree of fibrosis and scarring present on renal biopsy. In patients with necrotizing GN or presence of ANCA, I also add cyclophosphamide and treat as if this were a form of vasculitis, starting at 2 mg per kg daily and tapering thereafter. The WBC count is monitored to maintain it above 3500 per mm^3 with tapering or cessation of the cyclophosphamide if the WBC count decreases further. The patient is encouraged to drink plenty of fluids to diminish the toxicity associated with hemorrhagic cystitis.

In patients *with vasculitis* who are oliguric or anuric or on dialysis, there is some evidence that plasmapheresis may offer added benefit. Otherwise, plasmapheresis should be limited to patients with anti-GBM disease. Although 14 daily exchanges of 4 liters each is the accepted therapeutic regimen to be followed, there is strong evidence to suggest that the more quickly the diagnosis of anti-GBM disease is made and therapy instituted, the better the prognosis, regardless of the type of therapy. The cost for plasma exchange is significantly greater than pulse MP and/or cyclophosphamide. I routinely treat patients with a tapering dose of oral prednisone consisting of 2 mg per kg every other day for 2 weeks, 1.75 mg per kg every other day for 1 month, 1.5 mg

per kg every other day for 3 months, 1.2 mg per kg every other day for 6 months, and continue this tapering protocol. This dose is adjusted by 75% in patients 60 years and older and is tapered to the next step for complete remission at monthly intervals.

Most patients, including those who are oliguric or anuric or on dialysis, will respond within the first 8 weeks of therapy, with only rare patients responding during the following 2 weeks. If a patient has not responded by 10 weeks, I quickly taper therapy. Using this treatment regimen, I have had few relapses and remissions. If relapse does occur, biopsies are performed and patients are treated as if they have a new-onset GN.

Before the institution of MP pulse therapy and plasma exchange, the death or dialysis rate for AC-RPGN ranged from 80 to 95%. With the advent of rapid diagnosis and treatment, fully three fourths of patients with NID and immune complex disease will be able to show significant improvement and be able to discontinue dialysis. The long-term prognosis is related to the degree of glomerulosclerosis, obsolescence, and interstitial fibrosis. In patients with anti-GBM disease who are diagnosed before the onset of oliguria or the need for dialysis, with less than 50% crescents and a serum creatinine concentration less than 6 mg per dL, the prognosis with conventional therapy including MP or high-dose alternate-day prednisone and/or cyclophosphamide appears to be good. It remains to be shown in prospective randomized controlled trials that plasma exchange in this type of patient adds significantly to conventional therapy with pulse MP. In those patients who have serum creatinine concentrations greater than 6 mg per dL, 50% or more crescents, oliguria or anuria, or dialysis dependence, essentially none will respond unless they are ANCA-positive. If they are ANCA-positive, the response for these patients is much more like that of vasculitis than of anti-GBM disease.

Other Forms of Primary Glomerular Diseases

Because most of the primary glomerular diseases described in the preceding discussion can have vague systemic manifestations at various times during the course of the disease, it is extremely difficult to classify certain diseases as primary versus secondary. It is likely that a number of cases of postinfectious GN of various causes can present and appear to be a primary glomerulopathy. In addition, until the etiology of disease is known, many cases that are likely to be of systemic origin or of known infectious etiology are diagnosed as primary until the underlying disease process is elaborated. Examples of this include malignancy-associated glomerulopathy and MPGN related to hepatitis C viremia. A variety of lesser known entities including C1q and IgM nephropathy have been described and appear to be variants of other more well characterized primary glomerulopathies including minimal change nephrotic syndrome (MCNS) and focal segmental glomerulosclerosis (FSGS). These categories, if they are distinct entities, are much smaller and less well characterized and are best managed as variants of MCNS and FSGS.

NEPHROTIC FORMS OF PRIMARY GLOMERULAR DISEASES

Membranous Glomerulopathy

Diagnosis

Membranous glomerulopathy (MGN) is the most common cause of idiopathic nephrotic syndrome in adults. It accounts for approximately 40% of cases of idiopathic nephrotic syndrome. The presentation of disease can be indolent with long-standing intermittent edema, frothy urine, and few other symptoms. Urinalysis is typically benign, showing oval fat bodies, doubly refractile fat bodies, and fatty casts but little in the way of RBCs, dysmorphic RBCs, or RBC casts. Diagnosis is made by a renal biopsy that reveals classic deposits of IgG, sometimes with C3, in a granular pattern along the GBM. On ultrastructural analysis, there are electron-dense deposits in the GBM initially beginning as a small deposit at the slit pore and increasing in size to involve the width of the basement membrane with formation of strands of normal GBM and domes around these deposits. Three fourths of patients have nephrotic syndrome, with the other quarter having proteinuria less than 3 grams. Approximately 10 to 15% of patients older than 50 years have an occult adenocarcinoma, the prognosis for which is improved by early presentation with proteinuria and discovery rather than development of proteinuria after the diagnosis of malignant disease.

MGN occurs both as an idiopathic variety and as a secondary form. There are many causes of secondary MGN, and if the underlying etiology can be determined and corrected, then treatment is efficacious. One cannot distinguish between primary and secondary MGN on the basis of the renal biopsy. Clues to secondary etiology include deposition of IgM within the membranous deposits and the coexistence of a variety of other systemic diseases or medications. Many medications including heavy metals such as penicillamine and gold can induce this lesion, and also captopril and many other agents. Collagen-vascular diseases such as SLE, infectious agents, hepatitis B and C, syphilis, sickle cell anemia, and thyrotoxicosis have all been associated with the presence of MGN. In view of the significant impact of early diagnosis on malignant disease, I recommend that any patient 50 years and older with the histologic diagnosis of MGN have a careful examination with a chest radiograph, three stool guaiac tests, prostate examination with prostate-specific antigen, and in women thorough pelvic and breast examinations. In some cases, especially if there is any family history or symptoms, sigmoidoscopy would be indicated.

Prognosis

Approximately one fourth of patients will have progressive renal dysfunction, leading to dialysis and ESRD; one fourth will achieve remission; and approximately half will have slow progressive proteinuria for a period of years. Women tend to have a more favorable course, as do younger individuals and those with lesser degrees of proteinuria. As with other glomerular diseases, the presence of hypertension, significant decrease in kidney function or heavy proteinuria, tubulointerstitial disease, and extensive scarring on renal biopsy are poor prognostic signs.

Therapy

Numerous prospective randomized controlled trials have been conducted. These initially appeared to show a beneficial effect of chlorambucil and prednisone, but this consequently has not been confirmed. I recommend general supportive therapy for patients with MGN with normal renal function and minimal edema. In patients with progressive edema or decreased function, I use high-dose alternate-day steroids. The regimen that I use is that described for RPGN, starting with oral alternate-day high-dose prednisone rather than pulse MP. Studies have suggested that the addition of cyclophosphamide* for 6 months may improve prognosis in this group of patients, but the efficacy of this therapeutic regimen remains to be verified. Cyclophosphamide can be associated with hemorrhagic cystitis, gonadal dysfunction in both men and women, and increased risk in the long term for hematopoietic malignancy.

In those patients who develop ESRD related to MGN, the disease can recur in the graft, although this is less likely to occur than with many other types of recurrent nephropathy. It is seldom associated with a decrease in graft function beyond that expected in the general transplant population.

Minimal Change Disease

Diagnosis

MCNS is the cause of approximately 85% of nephrotic syndrome in children and around 20 to 25% in adults. Patients present clinically with the abrupt onset of edema and proteinuria with a relatively benign urinary sediment with little evidence of nephritic abnormalities. Doubly refractile fat bodies, oval fat bodies, and fatty casts may be present. There is frequently a history of atopy in childhood and of various allergies, such as to bee stings and foods, in patients compared with the normal population. Other than general vague symptoms, the presentation of patients other than with edema is nonspecific. In those patients 50 years and older, there is an increased incidence of lymphoma with MCNS. Appropriate treatment of the lymphoma can lead to remission of the process. Reversible MCNS has been described with a variety of nonsteroidal anti-in-

---

*Not FDA approved for this indication.

flammatory drugs and is reversible on discontinuation of the medication.

The diagnosis is made by renal biopsy; as the name implies, findings appear to be normal other than proteinaceous material in Bowman's space and tubules. By electron microscopy, there is swelling and obliteration of the foot process architecture and loss of the negative charge along the basement membrane, thought to play a role in the pathogenesis of the disease. Careful evaluation of the renal biopsy specimen for any evidence of focal sclerosis, tubular atrophy, interstitial fibrosis, or interstitial cellular infiltration should be carried out because FSGS may present in an identical fashion (see later) and has a much different prognosis than MCNS.

Renal function in children and young adults is generally well preserved, but in those 50 years and older, decreased function may be present. The occurrence of acute renal failure has been described with MCNS in elderly patients with severe hypoalbuminemia and massive nephrotic syndrome. The pathogenesis of this syndrome is not clear, but it frequently resolves after a period of dialysis.

Therapy

MCNS is classically immunosuppressive responsive in nature. Renal biopsy is not required for treatment in children because of the high incidence of MCNS in this age group. In children, if a nephritic sediment is present, a renal biopsy *is* indicated, but if a benign sediment is present, then empirical therapy for MCNS is usually instituted. In adults, a biopsy is mandatory, and if MCNS is diagnosed, then treatment with prednisone should be instituted. Although MCNS is spontaneously remitting, therapy with prednisone shortens the time to remission and decreases complications of the nephrotic syndrome including infection and thrombosis with pulmonary embolism.

In children, treatment usually consists of prednisone, 60 mg per m² per day for 6 weeks, followed by 40 mg per m² per day on an alternate-day regimen for an additional 6 weeks, and then discontinuation of treatment. Three fourths of children will respond within 2 weeks, and between 90 and 95% will have achieved remission within 4 weeks. Adults are less responsive than children, but with true MCNS, they should respond as well. I use a regimen of prednisone 1 mg per kg a day for the first month and 0.5 mg per kg a day during the second month, with rapid tapering thereafter. In patients who are unresponsive, I use either azathioprine (Imuran)* 1 to 2 mg per kg for 3 months or cyclophosphamide (Cytoxan) 1 to 2 mg per kg per day for 3 months. Others use chlorambucil (Leukeran)* at a dose of 0.1 to 0.15 mg per kg per day for several months. The other regimen that I have used is the standard alternating high-dose prednisone alone starting with 2 mg per kg and progressing as described before. The advantages of this regimen are few side effects and few relapses. The

disadvantages are a relatively prolonged time, up to 6 months or so, before remission is achieved. It is my habit to treat the first relapse with prednisone alone and for second and consequent relapses to institute immunosuppression along with prednisone.

These various therapeutic regimens have not been compared, but approximately one third of patients will have a good response and remain in remission, one third will have intermittent relapses, and approximately one fourth to one third will have frequent relapses or become steroid dependent.

Steroid-Dependent Patients. In patients who are steroid dependent and develop the side effects of steroid treatment even with alkylating agents, I use cyclosporine (Sandimmune)* at 4 to 5 mg per kg per day for therapy in a pattern used for FSGS. The majority of these patients will undergo remission with cyclosporine therapy, although remission is dependent on continuation of cyclosporine. Cyclosporine nephrotoxicity should be monitored to be certain that more harm is not being done than good. I do not use cyclosporine in patients who are responsive to prednisone or prednisone and alkylating agent.

MCNS has been shown to recur in patients who have developed ESRD and received transplants. It is not entirely clear, however, whether those patients truly had MCNS or FSGS that was initially unrecognized.

Focal Segmental Glomerular Sclerosis

Diagnosis

FSGS accounts for approximately 10 to 15% of cases of idiopathic nephrotic syndrome in adults and is one of the most frequent causes of ESRD in children, although it is not a common disease entity. The presentation is the same as for MCNS, with patients having the onset of edema and frothy urine with examination of the urine being relatively benign. Patients with FSGS may have a few RBCs as part of the normal course of the disease, but RBC casts are not expected. The diagnosis is made by renal biopsy, which shows focal and segmental sclerosis of glomeruli with interstitial fibrosis, tubular atrophy, scarring, and interstitial cellular infiltrates. The FSGS characteristic of this entity may be seen as an end-stage scarring process for any of a variety of different histologic lesions, and this diagnosis is made only in the absence of other underlying pathologic processes. The peak incidence of disease is in the second and third decade, and hypertension is a common feature occurring either after the onset of proteinuria or preceding the onset of proteinuria. In the former case, the prognosis is somewhat better than in the latter. The role of hyperfiltration in the genesis of FSGS is controversial, but there clearly are clinical situations with reduced renal mass in which FSGS appears to develop. These include patients with unilateral kid-

---

*Not FDA approved for this indication.

*Not FDA approved for this indication.

ney, vesicoureteric reflux, hypertensive nephrosclerosis, and oligomeganephronia, all of which may also have a hereditary or congenital abnormality of renal mesenchyme. When other disease processes are present in the renal biopsy specimen, such as proliferative GN or MGN, then the underlying process is said to be primary and the focal sclerosis is considered a scarring process for the underlying process.

Treatment

The response of FSGS to treatment is considerably worse than that of MCNS. It is my opinion that some cases of MCNS can progress to FSGS, but in general, they are distinct disease entities. FSGS is treated with corticosteroids, with approximately one fourth of the patients having remission in response to prednisone and another 20% or so having partial remission. In patients who do have a beneficial effect with prednisone, the prognosis is good. However, in the majority of patients who are unresponsive to prednisone, the prognosis is poor, with most of the patients progressing to ESRD in a period of years. I routinely treat patients with FSGS with a course of prednisone as described before. Signs of poor prognosis are the same as noted previously, i.e., hypertension, increased creatinine, decreased creatinine clearance, and heavy proteinuria as well as histologic evidence of scarring.

In patients who achieve remission with prednisone, relapse off therapy is relatively frequent, especially if prednisone has been tapered quickly. With the slowly tapering high-dose alternate-day prednisone regimen, I have had many fewer relapses than the literature suggests, but there are no prospective randomized controlled trials to direct the clinician in the best therapeutic options. In patients who do not achieve remission in 2 to 3 months, azathioprine* or cyclophosphamide* may be added as described before. Others have used aspirin* and dipyridamole.* This regimen is given as 1 aspirin daily or twice a day with dipyridamole 75 mg three times a day, although the efficacy of this again has not been proved.

In patients who are unresponsive to prednisone and alkylating agents, I have had good success using cyclosporine* therapy as described for MCNS. However, as noted before, it is necessary to maintain the patient with cyclosporine because relapse occurs with discontinuation of therapy. Once again, the clinician must be continuously cognizant of the risk for interstitial fibrosis, scarring, and decreased renal function consequent to cyclosporine rather than to the underlying disease process.

GENERAL APPROACHES TO THERAPY

Edema

Peripheral edema is one of the cardinal signs of glomerulopathy and is much more marked in those patients who have nephrotic syndrome. The first and foremost intervention to use in this situation is sodium reduction because a high-sodium diet not only worsens the edema but makes the patient relatively refractory to diuretic therapy. I usually monitor urinary sodium excretion per 24 hours and aim to maintain the patient between 80 and 100 mEq per day. This equates to an intake of approximately 5 grams of salt per day and is a reasonable diet when patients are taught how to use other seasonings such as garlic, onion, pepper, lemon juice, and lime juice. There are approximately 17 mEq of sodium per gram of sodium chloride and about 42 mEq per gram of sodium.

In patients in whom edema persists, I use furosemide (Lasix) beginning at about 20 to 40 mg per day depending on renal function. I carefully question the patient to be certain there is a brisk diuresis beginning in about 0.5 to 1 hour after oral ingestion, and the patient *has* to be in the vicinity of a restroom during the next few hours! If this is not the case, the diuretic is not working! The dose of diuretic should be increased to the point at which a brisk diuresis ensues, and then this dose can be given two or three times per day. In some patients, it is necessary to give 200 to 300 mg of furosemide at a time. There are some patients who will respond to bumetanide (Bumex) when they do not respond to furosemide. In patients who are unresponsive to 300 to 400 mg of furosemide a day as a single dose, I add a second diuretic, typically either hydrochlorothiazide (HydroDIURIL) or metolazone (Zaroxolyn) 5 to 10 mg per day given 20 minutes before furosemide. Potassium supplements should be used for patients who excrete a large excess of potassium in the urine or who have symptoms of cramping and other problems from hypokalemia.

Patients should be cautioned to keep their legs in a flexed position to increase circulation, to use standard support hose, to exercise by flexing their ankles to increase venous return, and not to sit in a fixed position for prolonged periods.

Hyperlipidemia

Hyperlipidemia is a common complication of patients with glomerulopathy, especially those who have proteinuria. The degree of elevation in lipids parallels that of the increase in urinary protein excretion. Maneuvers that decrease proteinuria will also result in a decrease in serum lipid levels. This type of hyperlipidemia is difficult to treat, and dietary manipulation is of little benefit. Whereas niacin and other methods can be used, including gemfibrizol (Lopid), I routinely use hydroxymethylglutaryl–coenzyme A reductase inhibitors such as pravastatin (Pravachol) or lovastatin (Mevacor). I also encourage patients to exercise on a regular basis and to stop smoking.

Hypertension

Hypertension is perhaps the single most important factor in progression of renal disease and proteinuria.

---

*Not FDA approved for this indication.

I routinely use a mean arterial pressure of 92 mm Hg as the goal for my patients, with slight relaxation of this for patients older than 60 years. Diuretic therapy has usually already been instituted for control of edema. Regardless of whether this is the case, the first line of treatment in patients of this type should be an ACEI such as enalapril (Vasotec) or captopril (Capoten). These and other ACEIs appear to have a specific beneficial effect on preserving renal function as well as decreasing proteinuria, probably by an effect on the negative charge on the basement membrane, by decreasing intraglomerular pressure, and perhaps by other mechanisms. The antiproteinuric effect of ACEI is decreased in patients who do not maintain a low-sodium diet. Other medications include calcium channel blockers, diltiazem (Cardizem) and verapamil (Calan), central antagonists such as clonidine (Catapres), and alpha$_1$-receptor antagonists such as prazosin (Minipress) or doxazosin (Cardura). Other routine blood pressure medications may be used, including beta blockers and peripheral vasodilators, although the latter can be associated with an increase in edema, as can calcium channel blockers.

Diet

The Modification of Diet in Renal Disease study that was recently completed did not show a beneficial effect of a low-protein diet during the period of the trial but did suggest that there might be a beneficial effect during a prolonged time. A low-protein diet can decrease the rate of rise of blood urea nitrogen and thus symptoms, and it results in decreased intravascular volume with decreased protein excretion. Whether specific renal protection occurs, a modest reduction in dietary protein to 0.8 gram per kg per day of good-quality protein should be encouraged but not demanded. Patients should be closely observed to be certain that this does not have a deleterious effect. Some patients are able to tolerate a decrease in protein without difficulty, whereas others find this to be onerous.

ACUTE PYELONEPHRITIS

method of
DOUGLAS W. SODERDAHL, M.D.
Madigan Army Medical Center
Tacoma, Washington

Acute pyelonephritis is an infectious inflammatory disease of the kidney parenchyma and collecting system, which is accompanied by local or systemic signs. *Uncomplicated* infections occur in a urinary tract that is anatomically and functionally correct. *Complicated* infections occur in patients with anatomic or functional abnormalities of the urinary tract or in individuals with underlying defects in natural host defenses.

TABLE 1. **Urinary Pathogens**

Gram-Negative Organisms	Gram-Positive Organisms
Escherichia coli	*Enterococcus faecalis*
85% community acquired	*Staphylococcus saprophyticus*
50% hospital acquired	*Staphylococcus aureus* *
Proteus	
Klebsiella	
Citrobacter *	
Serratia *	
Pseudomonas *	
Providencia *	

*Much higher incidence in nosocomial infections.

EPIDEMIOLOGY

The lifetime risk for the development of urinary tract infection (UTI) is 40 to 50% in women, and although the occurrence of pyelonephritis is low, the risk is real. Nearly 6 million office visits are generated yearly for patients with UTI, and more than 100,000 require hospitalization for pyelonephritis. The majority of acute pyelonephritis is seen in women, with the mean age at diagnosis being 30 years.

ETIOLOGY

Aerobic gram-negative bacteria are the most common agents responsible for pyelonephritis, with *Escherichia coli* being isolated in 85% of community-acquired and 50% of hospital-acquired cases (Table 1). Other less common gram-negative organisms include *Proteus, Klebsiella, Enterobacter, Serratia,* and *Pseudomonas.* These organisms assume a larger role in patients with recurrent infections, stones, urinary tract manipulation, immunocompromised state, or obstruction of the urinary tract.

Gram-positive organisms are rarely seen, with *Staphylococcus aureus* and *Enterococcus* species being the most common uropathogens. Although *Staphylococcus saprophyticus* accounts for 10 to 15% of lower UTI in young women, seldom does it cause pyelonephritis.

ROUTES OF INFECTION

In general, there are three routes by which pyelonephritis can occur: ascending (95%), hematogenous (4%), and lymphatic (rare). The urinary tract can be considered one continuous column of urine extending from the kidneys to the urethra. The perineum may harbor uropathogens, which then ascend in a retrograde manner to the kidney. Women are at increased risk for UTI because bacterial colonization on the external genitalia readily occurs and the urethra is short (4 cm).

Hematogenous spread is generally seen in chronically ill or immunosuppressed patients. The primary source may be infections in virtually any organ system including the skin. Gram-positive pyelonephritis should alert the clinician to consider the possibility of blood-borne infection.

PATHOGENESIS

Colonization of the vaginal mucosa by uropathogens is critical to the development of UTI in women. Cell surface fimbria such as P pili and type 1 pili seen on *E. coli* enable binding to epithelial cells. These fimbriated organisms account for greater than 80% of episodes of pyelonephritis. Patients with certain blood group antigens that aid in bacterial binding have also been shown to have a greater risk for UTI development. In addition, pathogenic bacteria have developed capsular polysaccharides (K antigens) that resist phagocytosis by normal defense mechanisms.

HOST DEFENSES

The body has several protective mechanisms to combat UTI. Intrinsic properties of urine such as high urea content, high osmolarity, and acidic environment are hostile to bacterial growth. Mechanical factors such as frequent and complete bladder emptying also retard the ability of bacteria to cause symptomatic infections. Prostatic secretions in men provide bacteriostatic and bactericidal action. In women, the vaginal introitus and distal urethra are colonized by nonpathogenic bacteria such as diphtheroids, streptococci, and lactobacilli that prevent overgrowth by uropathogens. These natural defenses can be compromised by antibiotic treatment, genital infection, spermicides, and diminished estrogen levels.

SPECIAL SITUATIONS

The incidence of UTI in pregnant patients is 2 to 8%. Of these, 20 to 30% progress to clinical pyelonephritis. Pregnant patients are at increased risk for pyelonephritis owing to decreased ureteral tone and peristalsis and urinary stasis. Aggressive treatment is warranted to eradicate bacteria because pyelonephritis may result in preterm labor, prematurity, and increased perinatal mortality.

Patients with anatomic or functional obstruction from calculi, benign prostatic hyperplasia, neurogenic bladder, or congenital anomalies are also at increased risk as a result of urinary stasis. These abnormalities must be ruled out in patients who fail to respond to conventional treatment.

Pyelonephritis in prepubertal patients poses a unique problem. Anatomic anomalies such as vesicoureteral reflux (VUR) are identified in up to 35% of patients. If these patients are not correctly identified, infection can lead to permanent scarring and loss of renal function. Radiographic evaluation should be obtained after the first documented UTI in all boys and in all white girls younger than 6 years. Because VUR occurs much less frequently in blacks, evaluation might be reserved for infants with a documented infection. Furthermore, all girls with febrile or recurrent infections should be evaluated regardless of age.

Other risk factors including immunocompromised state (e.g., medications, diabetes, human immunodeficiency virus infection), old age, malnutrition, and long-term indwelling urethral catheters must be considered in evaluating and managing patients with UTI.

DIAGNOSIS

The clinical presentation of acute pyelonephritis generally includes an abrupt onset of shaking chills, fever, and flank pain. Significantly, there may not be the anticipated lower urinary tract symptoms of dysuria, frequency, and urgency. Gastrointestinal complaints of nausea, vomiting, and diarrhea are also often present. The patient usually appears ill, with fever (temperature of 38.5 to 40°C) and tachycardia. On physical examination, costovertebral angle tenderness can often be elicited. Laboratory studies may demonstrate significant pyuria (>5 to 10 white blood cells per high-power field), bacteriuria, and polymorphonuclear leukocytosis. Specimens for urine and blood cultures should be obtained before instituting antibiotics. Although 10^5 CFU per mL has been the standard definition of posi-

tive urine culture, levels of 10^2 CFU per mL, properly collected, may indicate significant infection in a symptomatic patient. Blood cultures are positive in approximately 20 to 30% of cases. Tedious bacterial localization methods employing ureteral catheterization and bladder washout techniques are generally not indicated.

Radiologic work-up should be reserved for patients who fail to respond to standard therapy or if there is clinical suspicion that an underlying abnormality may be present in patients with a history of multiple episodes of pyelonephritis, nephrolithiasis, or previous genitourinary surgery. An intravenous pyelogram (IVP) is the initial study of choice. The IVP is most commonly normal; however, radiographic findings associated with pyelonephritis may include a delayed nephrogram phase and increased renal size secondary to obstruction and edema. Ultrasonography and computed tomography are useful in identifying untoward sequelae of pyelonephritis (e.g., renal or perinephric abscess) and may be used if the IVP is nondiagnostic. Radionuclide imaging with gallium Ga 67 citrate– or indium In 111–labeled white cells may localize the infection but fails to distinguish pyelonephritis from renal abscess.

Although the clinical diagnosis of acute pyelonephritis is generally straightforward, differential diagnosis, including nephrolithiasis, pancreatitis, diverticulitis, basilar pneumonia, and pelvic inflammatory disease, may confound even the experienced practitioner.

MANAGEMENT

The goals of successful management of pyelonephritis include (1) eradication of bacteria from the urinary tract, (2) prevention of renal damage, (3) relief of symptoms, and (4) correction of underlying abnormalities, if possible. Supportive measures including antipyretics, analgesics, antiemetics, adequate rest, and hydration are important. However, antibiotic treatment is the cornerstone of therapy, and the route of administration depends on the condition of the patient, the causative organisms, and the presence of complicating factors.

Patients with clinical evidence of pyelonephritis but without sepsis, nausea, or vomiting can be treated with an outpatient regimen (Table 2). Fluoroquinolones are highly effective, have excellent bioavailability, and are recommended first-line agents. Trimethoprim-sulfamethoxazole (Bactrim, Septra) may also be used. However, the 5 to 15% incidence of resistant organisms makes this combination a secondary choice. In female patients, a treatment period of 14 days is usually sufficient. Because prostatic infection so commonly precedes acute pyelonephritis

TABLE 2. **Outpatient Antibiotic Regimens**

Fluoroquinolones

Ciprofloxacin (Cipro) 500 mg PO q 12 h
Enoxacin (Penetrex) 400 mg PO q 12 h
Lomefloxacin (Maxaquin) 400 mg PO q 24 h
Norfloxacin (Noroxin) 400 mg PO q 12 h
Ofloxacin (Floxin) 400 mg PO q 12 h

Trimethoprim-Sulfamethoxazole (Bactrim, Septra)

Trimethoprim 160 mg + sulfamethoxazole 800 mg PO q 12 h

TABLE 3. Parenteral Antibiotic Regimens

Gentamicin 5 mg/kg/24 h ± ampicillin 1 gm q 6 h
Trimethoprim-sulfamethoxazole (Bactrim, Septra) 160 mg of
  trimethoprim + 800 mg of sulfamethoxazole q 12 h
Ceftriaxone (Rocephin) 1–2 mg q 24 h
Ciprofloxacin (Cipro) 200–400 mg q 12 h
Ofloxacin (Floxin) 400 mg q 12 h
Ticarcillin-clavulanate (Timentin) 3.1 gm q 4–6 h*
Imipenem-cilastatin (Primaxin) 250–500 mg q 6–8 h*
Aztreonam (Azactam) 1 gm q 8 h*

*Not a first-line agent.

in men, and because antimicrobials penetrate poorly into the prostatic parenchyma and secretions, 4 weeks of therapy is recommended. The antibiotic regimen may be modified when culture and sensitivity results are available. Repeated urine culture to document resolution is essential.

Patients with severe pyelonephritis generally require hospitalization and treatment with parenteral antibiotics (Table 3). These are administered until the patient is afebrile for 24 hours, after which an appropriate oral regimen is selected according to culture and sensitivity findings. Failure to respond to therapy should prompt further urologic work-up to rule out anatomic or functional abnormalities.

Febrile UTIs in children should be treated as presumed pyelonephritis because clinical diagnostic precision is less reliable in this age group. A short course of parenteral antibiotics followed by an oral regimen is recommended. Pediatric patients at risk for VUR should be maintained with antibiotic prophylaxis (once-a-day dosing) until appropriate urologic work-up can be performed.

Acute pyelonephritis in pregnancy should be treated with hospitalization and parenteral antibiotics, generally a cephalosporin or extended-spectrum penicillin. Owing to concerns regarding fetal cartilage, fluoroquinolones are contraindicated. Likewise, sulfa drugs should not be used in the third trimester because of the possible sequela of kernicterus. Parenteral therapy should be followed by a 2-week course of appropriate oral antibiotics and follow-up culture. Antimicrobial prophylaxis is indicated until delivery in patients with recurrent episodes of pyelonephritis or persistent bacteriuria.

Urine of patients with chronic indwelling urinary catheters always becomes colonized with bacteria. Empirical therapy for this asymptomatic bacteriuria is not indicated lest the growth of pathogenic, multi-drug-resistant organisms be encouraged. However, if systemic findings develop (fever, chills, flank pain, and leukocytosis) in a patient with no other obvious source, prompt treatment with broad-spectrum antibiotics is mandated. Further, an attempt to remove the urinary catheter and provide alternative drainage (spontaneous voiding, clean intermittent catheterization, suprapubic tube) should be attempted if possible.

COMPLICATIONS

If acute pyelonephritis is recognized and treated appropriately, complications are uncommon. Infections associated with obstructive uropathy may be difficult to treat until the abnormality is corrected. Perhaps the most serious complication is the development of septicemia and attendant hypotension, which dramatically increases the risk for mortality.

An unusual complication that is seen most often in diabetic patients is emphysematous pyelonephritis. In this circumstance, gas from the infecting organism (usually from *E. coli*) is released into renal and perirenal tissues. This requires prompt recognition, because it may become a surgical emergency requiring drainage and, in some cases, nephrectomy. In addition, renal and/or perirenal abscess may require open or percutaneous surgical drainage.

Finally, chronic renal scarring from recurrent infections or infections associated with obstruction and/or VUR may occur. Long-term effects of this scarring include loss of renal function, hypertension, and possible renal failure.

PROGNOSIS

Symptoms of pyelonephritis may often improve despite the persistence of the uropathogen. Therefore, it is important to obtain follow-up urine cultures at the end of the treatment period and a repeated urinalysis in 3 to 6 months. Overall, however, the prognosis for complete recovery from an episode of acute pyelonephritis is excellent after prompt treatment in a patient with no complicating factors.

TRAUMA TO THE GENITOURINARY TRACT

method of
PAUL C. PETERS, M.D.
*The University of Texas Southwestern Medical
  School
Dallas, Texas*

Genitourinary injuries are not common and usually are not life-threatening. They may be conveniently divided into (1) those secondary to a blunt external force and (2) those secondary to penetrating trauma, i.e., a bullet or stab wound. A simple approach to management thus evolves. Blunt trauma injuries tax our judgment; operation may be immediate, delayed, or not used at all, depending on the nature of the injury and clinical course of the patient under careful observation and repeated testing. Penetrating injuries demand immediate exploration because of the high incidence of associated injuries. In a series of more than 300 penetrating injuries of the kidney due to low-velocity (<2200 feet per second) missiles, 65% of the patients had associated injuries.

GENERAL PRINCIPLES OF MANAGEMENT FOR THE PATIENT WITH A GENITOURINARY INJURY

Overall inspection is carried out. One looks for bruises over the renal area. Fractured ribs may lacerate a kidney. The rib fracture line may not show until some bone resorption has occurred. Care should be taken to ensure that there is a patent airway, determine the level of consciousness, arrest hemorrhage from bleeding points, ascertain the continuity of the lower urinary tract by passage of a No. 18 French indwelling catheter, and establish access for administration of fluids and blood. A urethral catheter is used to detect concealed hemorrhage from an injured kidney. Abdominal computed tomography (CT) has replaced intravenous pyelography (IVP) to survey the abdomen.

KIDNEY INJURIES (Table 1)

Penetrating renal injuries are usually explored. Time is taken for general evaluation and stabilization, i.e., fluid resuscitation. Renal bleeding may be profuse at first and then stop when the patient's blood pressure falls, giving a false sense of security to the attending physicians, only to recur with a fatal result when blood pressure is restored by fluid resuscitation. Nephrectomy is still occasionally necessary as a lifesaving maneuver; the decision to do surgery is based on the patient's clinical course and nature of the injury as defined by CT, angiography, and other imaging studies as indicated (IVP, chest radiography, conventional radiography, or ultrasonographic studies). CT more precisely defines the extent and location of the renal injury than does IVP and gives additional information about other intraabdominal organs such as liver, spleen, and intestines. A few years ago, contrast studies including IVP were done on people with only a few red blood cells (five or less) in the urine. Ninety-eight percent of these studies were negative for major renal injury.

By selecting those patients for study who have gross hematuria or a history of hematuria with a systolic blood pressure lower than 80 mm Hg at some point since the injury, nearly all the patients with significant renal injury can be determined and a large number of costly negative studies can be avoided. Kennedy and colleagues, in a study at Parkland Memorial Hospital in 1988, showed the dipstick to be reliable in assessing microhematuria in 1485 trauma victims. Blunt trauma victims accounted for 1347 patients (91%) and penetrating trauma for 138 cases (9%). Microhematuria was defined as more than 1 red blood cell per high-power field on microscopic analysis.

Blunt renal injuries tax our judgment most when we have to decide whether to intervene surgically. Once again, I select those patients for imaging studies who have a history of gross hematuria and/or shock. A third factor to consider is the nature of the injury, that is, a fall from 20 feet in height is more likely to cause a significant renal injury than is tripping and falling while walking or running at ground level. Commonsense application in such cases may result in some imaging studies, such as IVP or CT, even when there are no cellular abnormalities in the urine or no history of shock, i.e., pedicle injuries. Another caveat: when IVP is done and one kidney is nonvisualizing, immediate angiography is indicated to define those patients with arterial thrombosis secondary to intimal tear. Such kidneys are occasionally saved by surgical intervention within 8 to 24 hours after injury. When CT is used instead of arteriography, a kidney may show some visualization, although delayed; still later, after injection of the contrast material, the cortex of the kidney may be visualized, the so-called cortical rim sign. Such a patient may have a severe renal arterial injury, and immediate angiography and attempt at reconstructive vascular surgery are indicated. In a 30-year experience at Parkland Memorial Hospital with intimal thrombosis secondary to a renal artery injury, 8 of 30 such kidneys were salvaged.

TABLE 1. **Renal Lesions of Trauma**

Lesion	Frequent Findings	Tests for Diagnosis	Treatment	Complications
Arterial thrombosis	Nonvisualizing kidney at IVP Delayed visualization at CT Cortical rim sign at CT Lack of enhancement with contrast agent	IVP CT Angiography	Surgical revascularization	Postoperative thrombosis, most do not work
Parenchymal tear	Delayed visualization Demonstration of leaking artery by angiography	IVP with selective films if needed	Plug leaking artery with pledget Partial nephrectomy	Postoperative hemorrhage
Collecting system	Extravasation of contrast material	IVP CT Retrograde pyelogram	Stenting or open surgery	Urinoma Continued leak

Abbreviations: CT = computed tomography; IVP = intravenous pyelography.

Polar ruptures of the kidney are usually secondary to blunt trauma. Marked extravasation of urine can usually be seen on imaging studies, especially CT. I prefer to treat polar ruptures by exploration of the kidney, débridement, suture of any bleeding vessels with absorbable suture, and removal of any devascularized fragments. Nephropexy is done to stabilize the kidney if a major partial nephrectomy is done or if there is concern that the kidney might twist on its pedicle. In my experience, if the kidney was left alone and the patient with a polar rupture simply observed, 84% of the patients required surgery later (9 to 10 days). Delayed surgical intervention prolonged the hospital stay 10 to 21 days.

INJURIES TO THE COLLECTING SYSTEM AND URETER

The ureter is well protected in the body, lying anterior to muscles of the back and flank and posterior to the intestine and anterior abdominal wall. The diagnosis is made early in the trauma patient by seeing extravasation of contrast material by IVP or CT with intravenous (IV) contrast enhancement. The diagnosis may be considered later in patients with previous trauma who develop a mass, gastrointestinal disturbance, prerenal azotemia (blood urea nitrogen/creatinine ratio >10:1), or sepsis from infected urinoma. Early treatment may consist of simple insertion of a double-J stent and continued observation. Percutaneous puncture of the kidney may be used to insert an indwelling stent and nephrostomy to divert the urine. Larger openings (rents) greater than 1 cm in the collecting system may not heal promptly as shown by the development of a urinoma, sepsis, or continued extravasation as demonstrated by injected contrast material (IV or retrograde). Surgical intervention is then required. The ureter is divided into thirds for consideration of the various techniques of repair.

Upper Ureter (Upper 10 cm)

Ureteropyelostomy
Ureteroureterostomy

Middle Third (L2–5)

Ureteroureterostomy

Lower Third (L5-Orifice)

Reimplantation into bladder
Transureteroureterostomy

Ileal substitution is done for massive ureteral replacement, i.e., more than 7 cm of ureter, and can be used as a tapered interposition. In pelvic injuries, the ureter may be ligated, a nephrostomy done, and ileal substitution done later with prepared bowel. Again, ureteral closure is done with absorbable suture to prevent stone formation in the urinary tract.

BLADDER INJURIES

Bladder ruptures are classified as extraperitoneal, intraperitoneal, or combined. Intraperitoneal rupture commonly occurs from a blunt external force applied to a full bladder. Extraperitoneal rupture is commonly associated with pelvic fracture, although only about 5% of patients with pelvic fracture have a simultaneous extraperitoneal rupture of the bladder. Diagnosis is made by cystography with emptying films or postdrainage films. Cystography with drainage films is superior to cystoscopy in demonstrating a leak. Treatment is suprapubic cystostomy for 10 days to 2 weeks until the bladder is healed. In some patients, particularly females, an indwelling retention urethral catheter will suffice. Cystography with oblique and postdrainage films is done to ensure complete healing in 10 to 14 days. Bladder rupture is suspected in patients with pelvic injury or those who have sustained a blunt external force to the abdomen by history who, if conscious, complain of severe lower abdominal or suprapubic pain. Like the pain of intestinal ischemia, the pain is not as well localized as is the pain of appendicitis; rebound tenderness is often absent, but pain may be severe. In my opinion, intraperitoneal rupture demands abdominal exploration because of the high incidence of associated injuries.

URETHRAL INJURIES

Urethral injuries are divided into anterior (bulbous and pendulous) and posterior (membranous and prostatic). Anterior urethral injuries are often the "straddle" injuries. A blow or kick to the perineum may also cause anterior urethral rupture. Urethrography will make the diagnosis. With the advent of flexible endoscopic equipment, one can visualize the exact site of injury and consider inserting an indwelling catheter as a stent through the injured area and avoid open surgery in selected cases. Small tears less than 1 cm might be treated this way. For complete transection of the urethra, I still prefer diversion by suprapubic cystostomy using the Lowsley prostate retractor to insert the catheter from below and end-to-end anastomosis of the urethra over a No. 18 Silastic retention catheter used as a stent. Absorbable suture (chromic gut) is used for the anastomosis. The proximal urethra is always fixed to the underlying perineal fascia to prevent excessive movement of the anastomosis. One may inject contrast material through the urethra after 10 to 14 days to see whether it is healed or do voiding cystourethrography (VCUG) through the suprapubic tube.

Posterior urethral transections are uncommon and are usually associated with severe external forces, i.e., crushing injuries of the pelvis. Malgaigne fractures of the pelvis are one of the most common types associated with this infrequent urethral injury. Some are associated with a simple transection of the urethra ranging from simple transection to a massive contusion and complete transection of the urethra with severe injury to the urethral sphincter and, in males, the prostate and adjacent bladder neck. There is occasionally a history of blood at the meatus after injury, and in these cases, it is best to do a urethrogram before passing a catheter. At times, posterior urethral injury can be diagnosed when the bladder shadow is seen by cystography or IVP to be well above the pelvic symphysis. The so-called pie in the sky, the full bladder with a competent internal sphincter, helps to differentiate this urethral injury from extraperitoneal rupture of the bladder, in which condition the bladder shadow, no matter how deformed, reaches the symphysis. Treatment of the injury has been modified by the introduction of stents the day of injury. This is accomplished by introducing a fiberoptic flexible endoscope through the urethral meatus and finding the proximal opening. A wire is then threaded into the bladder; the endoscope is withdrawn; and a catheter, retention type, is passed over the guide wire into the bladder to serve as a stent. If there is associated bladder neck laceration, it will have to be repaired or urinary incontinence will result. The standard surgical approach is still used in many cases. This is to place a suprapubic tube, allow pelvic hemorrhage to resorb and edema to resolve, and then do a combined abdominoperineal approach in 3 to 4 months. Films made at that time will show the length of the definitive stricture. At the time of repair, VCUG is done *at the same time* as the retrograde urethrogram. The patient is asked to expel the piston syringe used to fill the bladder through the suprapubic tube. This allows the sphincter to relax and the urethra to fill to the point where it is strictured off. Work by Defalco and colleagues from Seattle with the fiberoptic approach has shown a lower complication rate of stricture, impotence, and incontinence with use of fiberoptic instruments and immediate realignment. This may supplant the standard approach of immediate cystostomy and delayed repair. A certain number of patients with associated bladder neck lacerations will require open repair of the bladder neck.

GENITAL INJURIES
Penile Injuries

Degloving Injuries

In these cases, the genitalia are caught in machinery (i.e., farm equipment) with resulting avulsion of the skin of the penis and scrotum. The scrotum is used as an immediate pedicle flap. Areas of skin poor in hair bearing are used to finish the closure, if needed. Split-thickness grafts of 0.015 cm thickness are used. Prepuce, if available, is good to use as a donor site.

Penile Amputation

The dismembered part should be thoroughly cleansed and packed on ice until it can be attached by proper vascular techniques. The operation should be performed with use of magnification and 9-0 or 10-0 vascular sutures. An attempt should be made to reconstruct the dorsal arteries and one or two superficial veins. If this is not possible, because of lack of expertise or facilities, the part should be attached by running suture around the circumference of the corpora cavernosa. Even then, one or two

superficial veins can be found and reanastomosed. In spite of denervation, a satisfactory result may be obtained.

Rupture of the Anterior Urethra Confined by Buck's Fascia

Buck's fascia begins at the coronal sulcus and merges imperceptibly with the superficial fascia at the base of the penis. Lesions confined by Buck's fascia will appear as a sleeve of the penis (blood, urine, or pus). The defect in the corpus can usually be palpated and closed with simple interrupted slowly absorbable suture. A urethral catheter is used as a stent for 10 to 14 days. Lesions that rupture through Buck's fascia are more serious and follow the attachments of Colles' fascia in the perineum all the way to the axilla deep to Scarpa's fascia. Early recognition is important. Swelling of the scrotum is seen. Discoloration of the abdomen and flank may be seen later. Drainage deep to Scarpa's fascia, antibiotics, and urinary diversion by suprapubic cystostomy are preferred. Pelvic sonography is indicated to rule out abscesses posterior to the prostate and ischiorectal fossa, which may require drainage, preferably drainage through the perineum.

When the entire perineum is shattered, as by a shotgun blast, the rectum must be carefully inspected; if perforated, it must be closed and an abdominal diverting colostomy done above the site of rectal injury. The urethra and perineum should be débrided and the urine diverted by a suprapubic cystostomy by using a Lowsley prostate retractor that is palpated suprapubically and cut down on. Only obviously dead tissue is discarded, and an attempt is made to end with a central hypospadias, scrotal or perineal, which can be repaired months later. Repetitive débridement may be necessary during the first few weeks of healing.

Testis Injury

Vascular repair may be attempted up to 8 hours after surgery, packing the injured testis in ice in the interim. When the tunica albuginea of the testis is torn, meticulous débridement is done combined with copious irrigation and closure of the tunica albuginea of the testis with chromic gut or Dexon. No drain should be put inside the tunica albuginea. The scrotum may be drained with a dependent Penrose drain.

Vas Injury

A severed vas may be ligated for later repair, or it may be repaired with a direct end-to-end anastomosis by using interrupted 3-0 nylon suture as a stent. The anastomosis can be done with use of magnification and interrupted 8-0 or 9-0 nylon suture. If the scrotum is completely lost, soaks of 0.25% acetic acid may be used over the scrotum. When granulation is present, split-thickness grafts or mobilized flaps of nearby skin are used to cover the testis, usually within 2 to 3 weeks.

PROSTATITIS

method of
ANTHONY J. SCHAEFFER, M.D.
Northwestern University Medical School
Chicago, Illinois

Prostatitis syndrome is one of the most common entities encountered in clinical practice. It is estimated that 50% of adult men experience symptoms of prostatitis at some time in their lives. The symptoms of prostatitis may mimic the symptoms of bladder outlet obstruction from prostatic hyperplasia, which may further confuse the clinician. The differentiation of infectious from noninfectious prostatitis is essential and requires careful attention to details of specimen collection and persistence. New drugs have improved therapy and hold promise for better results in the future.

It is helpful to classify patients into groups commonly encountered: acute bacterial prostatitis, chronic bacterial prostatitis, nonbacterial prostatitis, pelviperineal pain, and granulomatous prostatitis. Table 1 indicates the discriminating variables among these entities.

All patients with bacterial, nonbacterial, or granulomatous prostatitis have evidence of significant inflammation in their expressed prostatic secretions (i.e., 10 or more white blood cells per high-power field [WBC per HPF]), and therefore they cannot be distinguished by the number of inflammatory cells. Patients with bacterial prostatitis, both acute and chronic, are distinguished from those with nonbacterial prostatitis on the basis of microbiologic parameters. For prostate localization studies as described by Meares-Stamey, the patient submits specimens of the first 10 mL of voided urine (VB1), which represents the urethra; the midstream urine (VB2), which represents the bladder; expressed prostatic secretions (EPS) obtained by massaging the prostate; and the first 10 mL of voided urine after prostatic massage (VB3), which represents the contribution of prostatic fluid to the urine. If evaluation shows inflammation in the VB1 (urethritis) or VB2 (cystitis), appropriate antimicrobial therapy is needed to eradicate the infection before attempting evaluation of the prostate. Drugs such as tetracycline and nitrofurantoin should be used because they will eradicate urethral and bladder infection without penetrating the prostatic tissue and thereby reducing the opportunity to document bacterial prostatitis. If the VB1 and VB2 are negative, 10 WBC per HPF in the EPS is diagnostic of prostatitis, and an increase of 10-fold or more in the bacterial count in the prostatic specimens compared with the urethral specimen is diagnostic of bacterial versus nonbacterial prostatitis.

ACUTE BACTERIAL PROSTATITIS

Acute bacterial prostatitis usually presents with dramatic onset of fever, malaise, low back or perineal pain, and myalgia for several days before onset of symptoms of urinary frequency, dysuria, urgency, and varying degrees of bladder outlet obstruction. Palpation of the prostate usually but not always reveals a tender, hard, irregular prostate that is warm to touch. Prostatic massage should be avoided because of the risk of bacteremia, but gentle pressure on the prostate may induce copious amounts of purulent prostatic secretions. Because cystitis usually accompanies acute bacterial prostatitis, the responsible bacterial pathogen can be isolated from bladder urine. *Escherichia coli* and other members of the Enterobacteriaceae family predominate; *Pseudomonas* and *Enterococcus* (*Streptococcus faecalis*) microorganisms are less common.

General Therapy

Most patients are quite toxic and may require admission to the hospital. Supportive measures such as analgesics, antipyretics, hydration, bed rest, and stool softeners should be instituted. If the patient cannot urinate, suprapubic needle aspiration or suprapubic catheter placement is recommended. Urethral catheterization may further exacerbate the prostatic inflammation and lead to complications such as acute epididymitis.

Antimicrobial Therapy

Patients with acute bacterial prostatitis usually respond dramatically to antimicrobial drugs that normally do not achieve therapeutic levels in prostatic fluid. If the patient is septic, I obtain blood cultures and administer gentamicin sulfate or tobramycin sulfate, 3 to 5 mg per kg of body weight per day divided into three intramuscular or intravenous doses, plus

TABLE 1. **Classification of Prostatitis Syndromes**

Syndrome	Cystitis	Pain in the Prostate	Evidence of Inflammation (EPS)	Culture-Positive (EPS)	Culture-Positive (Bladder)	Common Etiologic Bacteria	Rectal Examination (Prostate)
Acute bacterial prostatitis	±	+	+	+	+*	Enterobacteriaceae	Abnormal
Chronic bacterial prostatitis	±	±	+	+	+†	Enterobacteriaceae	Normal
Nonbacterial prostatitis	0	±	+	+	0	?	Normal
Pelviperineal pain	0	±	0	0	0	0	Normal
Granulomatous prostatitis	0	±	+	±	0	*Mycobacterium tuberculosis*, ?	Abnormal

*Acute bacterial prostatitis is nearly always accompanied by bladder infection.
†Characterized by recurrent bacteriuria, at varying intervals up to several months, after antimicrobial therapy is stopped.
Abbreviation: EPS = expressed prostatic secretion.
Modified from Stamey TA: Pathogenesis and Treatment of Urinary Tract Infections. Baltimore, Williams & Wilkins, 1980, p 344.

ampicillin, 1 gram administered intravenously every 6 hours, or an intravenous fluoroquinolone such as ciprofloxacin (Cipro) 400 mg every 12 hours or ofloxacin (Floxin) 400 mg every 12 hours. If the patient can take oral antimicrobial agents, a fluoroquinolone such as ciprofloxacin* 750 mg every 12 hours, ofloxacin 400 mg every 12 hours, norfloxacin (Noroxin) 400 mg every 12 hours, lomefloxacin (Maxaquin)* 400 mg every day, or enoxacin (Penetrex)* 400 mg every 12 hours can be used. Although 2 weeks of therapy is probably adequate, 4 weeks is preferred to ensure that all bacteria are eliminated from the prostate.

Operative Therapy

Surgical intervention is generally not indicated for acute bacterial prostatitis. Prostatic abscess is a rare complication that should be suspected in patients whose symptoms and clinical course do not respond to appropriate antimicrobial therapy. If a large, localized, tender, fluctuant mass is palpated within the prostate, ultrasonography or computed tomography and perineal or transurethral drainage should be performed. If the prostate gland is hard, several months may be required before it returns to normal consistency. Granulomatous prostatitis in the absence of tuberculosis and rare mycotic infection of the prostate is a histologic stage of resolving acute bacterial prostatitis, which is usually detected as a local area of prostatic induration suggestive of carcinoma. Except for exclusion of carcinoma, no special therapy is warranted.

CHRONIC BACTERIAL PROSTATITIS

Chronic bacterial prostatitis is characterized by relatively asymptomatic periods in between episodes of recurrent bacteriuria. The infection is caused by small numbers of bacteria in the prostatic fluid and is difficult to eradicate with most antimicrobial therapy. The most common pathogens are Enterobacteriaceae and species of *Pseudomonas. Enterococcus* (*S. faecalis*) is also a definite cause of chronic bacterial prostatitis. Other gram-positive organisms have been implicated much less frequently and rarely cause recurrent bacteriuria. Mixed infections involving two or more strains or classes of microorganisms are uncommon.

General Therapy

Men with chronic bacterial prostatitis are usually asymptomatic except for symptoms associated with acute cystitis. Hematospermia and painful ejaculation occur infrequently. Prostate examination is nondiagnostic. Appropriate oral antimicrobial therapy usually controls the acute episode of cystitis. Hot sitz baths and antipyretics are also helpful. Septic episodes requiring hospitalization and parenteral therapy occur rarely.

*Not FDA approved for this indication.

Antibacterial Therapy

Cure of bacterial prostatitis appears to correlate best with the level of antimicrobial drug in the prostatic fluid rather than its level in serum or prostatic tissue. Pharmacokinetic studies in men and dogs indicate that few antimicrobials achieve therapeutic levels in prostatic secretions. Trimethoprim and the fluoroquinolones do diffuse into prostatic fluid and have the best documented success in curing chronic bacterial prostatitis due to susceptible pathogens. Long-term therapy (8 to 12 weeks) appears to be more effective than short-term therapy (2 weeks) in achieving bacteriologic cures. The following recommendations are made for treatment of nonazotemic men with documented culture-susceptible pathogens infecting the prostate:

1. Trimethoprim-sulfamethoxazole (TMP-SMZ, Septra or Bactrim), 1 double-strength tablet (160 mg of TMP and 800 mg of SMZ) orally twice daily for 12 weeks or
2. Trimethoprim (Proloprim or Trimpex), 2 tablets (100 mg each) orally twice daily for 12 weeks or
3. Ciprofloxacin, 500 mg every 12 hours for 4 weeks or
4. Enoxacin, 400 mg every 12 hours for 4 weeks or
5. Lomefloxacin, 400 mg every day for 4 weeks or
6. Norfloxacin, 400 mg every 12 hours for 4 weeks or
7. Ofloxacin, 400 mg every 12 hours for 4 weeks

Specific therapy must always be tailored to meet the individual patient's needs and drug tolerance. (See also the manufacturer's official directive in the use of these agents.) Patients not cured by antimicrobial therapy can be kept comfortable and abacteriuric by use of continuous low-dose suppressive daily therapy with an appropriate oral antimicrobial agent such as nitrofurantoin (50-mg capsule) or TMP-SMZ (a single, regular-strength tablet each day). Bacteriuria will usually recur after cessation of therapy.

Operative Therapy

Transurethral resection of the prostate is the only alternative, short of radical prostatectomy, for surgical management of bacterial prostatitis. However, transurethral prostatectomy can be curative only if all foci of infected tissue and calculi are removed. Because most inflammation in chronic prostatitis occurs in the periphery of the gland and all the ducts from the peripheral zone empty into the urethra distal to the verumontanum, radical transurethral resection with removal of all foci of infected stones and tissues is difficult to achieve and carries a high risk of urinary incontinence. Approximately one third of patients with well-documented bacterial prostatitis have been cured by this technique.

NONBACTERIAL PROSTATITIS

Diagnosis and treatment of this disease are controversial. Nonbacterial prostatitis is about eight times more common than bacterial prostatitis. All of the symptoms and signs are similar to those seen with bacterial prostatitis, except that patients with nonbacterial prostatitis never have bacteriuria and the cause of the inflammatory changes in the prostatic secretions is unknown. *Chlamydia trachomatis* is the most controversial organism implicated in chronic prostatitis, but *Ureaplasma urealyticum* has also received attention. Except in rare cases, attempts to implicate other pathogens in bacterial prostatitis have ruled out infection due to fungi, anaerobic bacteria, trichomonads, and viral agents. The clinical significance of evidence for prostate inflammation, particularly in asymptomatic patients, has been questioned. However, recognition that identifiable groups of patients (such as those with infertility) have significantly increased leukocyte counts indicates that nonbacterial prostatitis may be indicative of an underlying disease.

General Therapy

Because the etiology is unknown, treatment is empirical and often unrewarding. Two important conditions should be considered in a differential diagnosis, interstitial cystitis and carcinoma in situ of the bladder. Thus, for selected patients, it may be reasonable to obtain urine specimens for cytology and perform endoscopic evaluation under anesthesia. If *Chlamydia* or *Ureaplasma* species are likely causes of urethritis associated with prostatitis, I recommend a clinical trial with minocycline (Minocin), 100 mg orally twice daily for 10 days. Unless the response is favorable, further treatment is probably not indicated. Empirical administration of other antimicrobial drugs is almost invariably ineffective and engenders considerable expense, anxiety, and dissatisfaction. Instead, efforts should be made to educate the patient with a frank discussion about the unknown and probably noninfectious etiology of the condition and efforts to relieve symptoms. I generally recommend hot sitz baths for symptomatic flare-ups. Many patients obtain symptomatic relief after short courses of anti-inflammatory agents such as ibuprofen (Motrin), 400 to 600 mg orally three or four times daily. Patients with obstructive voiding symptoms may benefit from therapy with an alpha-adrenergic blocker such as terazosin (Hytrin),* 5 mg orally once daily, or doxazosin (Cardura),* 4 mg orally once daily. Irritative voiding symptoms may respond to therapy with anticholinergics, such as propantheline (Pro-Banthine), 15 mg orally four times daily, or oxybutynin chloride (Ditropan), 5 mg orally two or three times daily. Therapeutic prostatic massage and dietary restrictions regarding the use of alcoholic beverages, coffee, and spicy foods are occasionally beneficial.

Antibacterial Therapy

The use of antimicrobial agents is not warranted for patients with nonbacterial prostatitis. Prostatic biopsy is sometimes necessary to differentiate nonbacterial prostatitis from other forms of prostatitis such as granulomatous prostatitis, but surgical therapy is not indicated.

PELVIPERINEAL PAIN (PROSTATODYNIA)

The term prostatodynia has been suggested for men with symptoms that mimic prostatitis, especially "prostatic pain," but who have negative cultures and no evidence of inflammation in the expressed prostatic secretions. Although some of these symptoms may be of prostatic origin, the term is misleading if the patient's assessment of the etiology of his discomfort is inaccurate. Pelviperineal pain is a more accurate description of this symptom complex because the syndrome probably results from varied causes. Musculoskeletal abnormalities are probably responsible for many of the symptoms. Some patients with this syndrome have apparent functional obstruction in the bladder neck and prostatic urethra. These patients may respond favorably to therapy with an alpha-blocking agent such as those listed before, once daily at bedtime. Other patients with apparent tension myalgia of the pelvic floor respond best to treatment with diathermy, muscle relaxants, and physiotherapy, with or without the use of diazepam (Valium),* 5 mg orally three times daily. Some patients have emotional disturbances that benefit from psychiatric consultation.

OTHER FORMS OF PROSTATITIS

Mycobacterium tuberculosis is still occasionally responsible for prostatitis in men who have generalized tuberculosis. The diagnosis can be confirmed by recovery of the organism from prostatic fluid cultures or prostatic tissue biopsy specimens. Therapy is the same as that for active tuberculosis of the urinary tract and should be continued for approximately 24 months. Rarely, systemic mycotic infections, such as coccidioidomycoses, blastomycosis, cryptococcosis, histoplasmosis, and candidiasis, have been associated with granulomatous prostatitis. Therapy is the same as for the systemic disease.

Nonspecific granulomatous prostatitis is seen occasionally. An eosinophilic type is usually seen in men prone to allergies, particularly in asthmatic patients, and is thought to result from a type of vasculitis. The noneosinophilic variety may represent a granulomatous reaction within the prostate presumably due to extravasation of prostatic secretions from the ducts and acini into the stroma. These conditions present clinically as an acute, febrile illness characterized by irritative and obstructive voiding dysfunction. The prostate is often markedly swollen and indurated. Prostatic biopsy is required for diagnosis and to rule out carcinoma. Both varieties usually respond dramatically to therapy with steroids.

---

*Not FDA approved for this indication.

*Not FDA approved for this indication.

BENIGN PROSTATIC HYPERPLASIA

method of
JOHN D. McCONNELL, M.D.
*The University of Texas Southwestern Medical
Center at Dallas*
Dallas, Texas

PATHOPHYSIOLOGY AND EPIDEMIOLOGY

Benign prostatic hyperplasia (BPH) is a noncancerous enlargement of the prostate gland that produces bothersome lower urinary tract symptoms in aging men. The disease process leading to the development of symptoms commonly referred to as prostatism has three components: histologic prostatic hyperplasia, increase in outflow resistance, and the response of the bladder (detrusor) muscle to obstruction. The presence of histologically identifiable BPH increases from 50% at the age of 60 years to 90% by the age of 85 years. BPH is a true hyperplastic process, involving an increase in the number of both epithelial and smooth muscle cells, as well as connective tissue. Growth of the prostate produces an inward transmission of pressure on the urethra, leading to increased resistance to urinary flow. Studies suggest that the prostate in middle-aged men increases approximately 6 mL per decade of age. The elevated detrusor pressure required to maintain urinary flow in the face of prostate growth occurs at the expense of normal bladder storage function, which leads to urinary frequency, urgency, and nocturia, the most bothersome BPH-related complaints.

The correlation between prostate size, the degree of obstruction, and the severity of symptoms is weak. The gland may enlarge without producing urodynamic obstruction or symptoms. Patients may be physiologically obstructed with minimal enlargement. Therefore, the size of the prostate does not predict the need for treatment, although size may limit treatment options. Most important, the symptoms of BPH are not specific. Other causes of bladder outlet obstruction (e.g., urethral stricture and prostate cancer) and primary diseases of the bladder (e.g., neurogenic bladder and bladder cancer) can produce identical symptoms.

The dominant risk factors for the development of BPH are increasing age and the presence of testicular androgens. Epidemiologic and basic scientific knowledge are still insufficient for understanding the etiology of the disease. By the age of 55 years, approximately 25% of men note a decrease in the force of the urinary stream. The odds of moderate to severe lower urinary tract symptoms are 3.5 times higher in men 70 to 79 years of age relative to 40-year-old men. Although the relationship between prostate size and lower urinary tract symptoms is not linear, adjusting for age, men with prostate volumes greater than 50 mL are 3.5 times more likely to have moderate to severe symptoms than those who do not.

Although androgens do not cause BPH, the development of BPH requires the presence of testicular androgens during prostate development and aging. In the prostate, the enzyme 5α-reductase converts testosterone into dihydrotestosterone, a more potent androgen. Two 5α-reductase enzymes have been discovered, each encoded by a separate gene. Type 1 5α-reductase, the predominant enzyme in skin and liver, is poorly inhibited by finasteride (Proscar). Type 2 5α-reductase is the predominant, if not sole, prostatic 5α-reductase, and it is exquisitely sensitive to inhibition by finasteride. Inhibition of type 2 5α-reductase in men with BPH leads to prostatic epithelial cell involution, resulting in prostate shrinkage and symptomatic improvement.

Prostate smooth muscle represents a significant volume of the gland. Active smooth muscle tone in the human prostate is regulated by the adrenergic nervous system, and the alpha$_{1A}$ receptor is the most abundant adrenoreceptor subtype mediating contraction of the organ. Blockade of this receptor in men with BPH leads to prostatic and bladder neck smooth muscle relaxation, resulting in symptom improvement.

Significant complications of BPH include urinary retention, azotemia, recurrent urinary tract infection, and gross hematuria. The likelihood that a patient with a given symptom complex will develop complete urinary retention is in the range of 1% per year. Mortality from BPH is extremely rare, and serious complications are uncommon. However, if symptoms interrupt normal daytime activities or sleep, create anxiety, or reduce perception of general well-being, the quality of life can decline significantly. Because BPH is primarily a quality of life disease, and because significant variations do exist in individual patients' perception of bothersomeness and treatment risks, the patient should play a central role in determining the need for treatment.

DIAGNOSIS

In the initial evaluation of all patients with BPH, a detailed medical history, focusing on the urinary tract, previous surgical procedures, general health issues, and fitness for possible surgical procedures, is necessary to identify other causes of voiding dysfunction and co-morbidities that may complicate treatment. For some patients, a "voiding diary" may help in determining the frequency and nature of complaints. A digital rectal examination and a focused neurologic examination are done to detect prostate or rectal malignancy, to evaluate anal sphincter tone, and to rule out any neurologic problems that may cause the presenting symptoms. A urinalysis should be performed to detect hematuria, pyuria, or bacteriuria, which may indicate nonprostatic disease or complications of BPH. Measurement of the serum creatinine level should be considered, although the incidence of significant azotemia in this population is only 1 to 2%. Measurement of the prostate-specific antigen (PSA) should be considered in patients with lower urinary tract symptoms because prostate cancer can produce lower urinary tract symptoms, and the addition of serum PSA measurement to the digital rectal examination increases the cancer detection rate.

The American Urological Association (AUA) Symptom Index (also called the International Prostate Symptom Score, or IPSS), as a quantitative symptom-scoring questionnaire, should be used in the initial assessment of each patient presenting with symptoms of prostatism. When the AUA system is used, symptoms should be classified as mild (0 to 7), moderate (8 to 19), or severe (20 to 35). This symptom score should be the primary determinant of treatment response or disease progression in the follow-up period. Symptom severity predicts urinary bother but does not predict the probability of BPH complications (e.g., retention or renal insufficiency).

Additional diagnostic tests include measurement of the urinary flow rate and postvoid residual urine, and pressure-flow urodynamic studies. These tests are not necessary before considering treatment options (especially pharmacologic) in every patient. Levels of postvoid residual urine greater than 200 mL may predict a higher risk that watchful waiting will fail but does not predict a poor response to surgery. Pressure-flow urodynamic studies permit a determination of whether symptoms are due to obstruction or poor bladder function and have modest predictive value before surgery. However, baseline urodynamic measurements do not predict the response to medical therapy. Intravenous urography, renal sonography, and cystoscopy are not routinely indicated unless the patient has concomitant hematuria, infection, or renal insufficiency.

TREATMENT

Patients with mild symptoms of BPH (AUA Symptom Index score of ≤7) should be followed in a strategy of watchful waiting. The probabilities of disease progression or development of BPH complications are uncertain. Until research defines these probabilities, patients in watchful waiting should be monitored periodically by reassessment of the symptom level, physical findings, and routine laboratory testing. If the patient's symptoms progress to moderate or severe levels, as defined by the AUA Symptom Index, it is appropriate to discuss the symptoms with the patient to determine whether the condition is bothersome or is interfering with his health and to offer him active treatment options if applicable.

Patients with moderate and severe symptoms (AUA Symptom Index score of ≥8) should be given information on the benefits and harms of watchful waiting, medical therapy (alpha blockers and finasteride), and surgery. Emerging thermal therapy technologies (transurethral needle ablation [TUNA] and transurethral microwave therapy [TUMT]) are appropriate options, if approved by the Food and Drug Administration (FDA) and reimbursed by the patient's health plan. Information should be presented to the patient in an unbiased format that expresses not only the probabilities of benefits and harms, but the range of uncertainty associated with those probabilities. The physician's opinion about optimal treatment should not be the only information communicated to the patient.

If patients initially choose watchful waiting or treatments other than surgery and later experience symptom progression or deterioration, it is appropriate to then discuss surgery as a treatment option. However, failure to respond to medical or thermal therapy is not an absolute indication for surgery. Many patients who fail to benefit from medical therapy, for example, elect to return to a strategy of watchful waiting rather than accept the risks of surgery.

On the other hand, surgery should not be reserved for those men in whom medical or device therapy fails. If the patient has been fully informed, it is appropriate for him to have the option of electing surgery as his initial treatment. The choice of type of surgery (transurethral resection of the prostate [TURP], transurethral incision of the prostate [TUIP], or prostatectomy) is primarily a technical decision; this choice should be based on the surgeon's experience and judgment and should be discussed with the patient. However, TUIP is an underutilized procedure with lower risk that should be strongly considered for patients in whom the estimated resected tissue weight (if done by TURP) would be 30 grams or less.

The types of BPH patients who should be treated surgically are (1) those with refractory urinary retention in whom at least one attempt at catheter removal has failed and (2) those who have recurrent urinary tract infections, recurrent gross hematuria, bladder stones, or renal insufficiency clearly due to BPH. There is little evidence to suggest that treatment options other than surgery benefit patients with any of these BPH complications. Nevertheless, if patients refuse surgery, or if they have sufficient medical co-morbidity to present an unacceptable risk for surgery, alternative therapies may be considered.

Watchful Waiting

Observational follow-up is an appropriate treatment strategy for the majority of patients. Approximately 20% of men have symptomatic improvement over time, and 50% have stable symptoms. However, the probability of BPH complications without active treatment is uncertain. The patient's symptoms and clinical course should be monitored, usually annually. He should be instructed on behavioral techniques to reduce symptoms, such as limiting fluid intake after dinner and avoiding decongestants.

Surgery

Of all treatment options, prostate surgery offers the best chance for symptom improvement, with the average patient enjoying a 75 to 85% reduction in symptoms. However, surgery also has the highest rates of significant complications. This includes operative morbidity (0.1 to 1%, depending on co-morbidities), incontinence (0.1 to 1.0%, depending on the specific procedure), transfusion (3 to 5%), retrograde ejaculation (25 to 90%, depending on the specific procedure), and an 8 to 10% chance of needing repeated surgery within 8 years. In certain studies, impotence after TURP occurred no more frequently than in untreated control groups. TURP is the most commonly used surgical treatment for BPH. TUIP, a procedure of almost equivalent efficacy, is limited by technical factors to patients in whom the estimated resected tissue weight (if done by TURP) would be 30 grams or less. TUIP can be performed in ambulatory settings or during a 1-day hospitalization and has lower rates of mortality, incontinence, and retrograde ejaculation than TURP. Open prostatectomy is typically performed for patients with very large prostates. Laser prostatectomy is slightly less efficacious than TURP but has a lower risk of bleeding complications. Refinements in standard TURP techniques (electrovaporization) achieve similar results.

Surgery need not always be a treatment of last resort; that is, patients need not undergo other treatment for BPH before they can have surgery. However, it is inappropriate to recommend surgery for a symptomatic patient on the grounds that progression is inevitable and that surgical risk only increases with age. BPH progresses slowly and quite variably among patients.

Alpha Blockers

Selective, long-acting alpha blockers such as doxazosin (Cardura) and terazosin (Hytrin) reduce symptoms by 50% in the average patient. There is no evidence to suggest that one alpha blocker is more effective than another. Titration of the dose is necessary. The starting dose of terazosin is 1 mg at bedtime, with weekly stepwise increases to 2, 5, or 10 mg to achieve the desired improvement. The starting dose of doxazosin is 1 mg, morning or evening, with stepwise increases to 2, 4, or 8 mg. With both drugs, postural hypotension should be excluded before initiating therapy. Thereafter, upward dose adjustments can be made on the basis of symptom improvement versus side effects. Patients should be cautioned that the first dose is most likely to produce orthostatic symptoms that may be especially problematic when the patient gets up at night to urinate. If the alpha blocker is discontinued for several days or longer, therapy should be reinstituted using the initial dosing regimen. Even with dose titration, patients should respond within weeks to a few months. Although the 1-year efficacy has been well documented in controlled trials, long-term efficacy is uncertain.

Side effects of alpha-blocker therapy include postural hypotension (2 to 4%), dizziness (9 to 16%), tiredness (7 to 8%), headache (5 to 9%), and nasal congestion (2%). Up to 10% of patients have discontinued therapy in short-term clinical trials because of side effects. The nonselective alpha blocker phenoxybenzamine (Dibenzyline) is not recommended because of a higher incidence of side effects. Prazosin (Minipress) has not been studied in appropriate clinical trials, and its short half-life requires dosing twice daily. There is no evidence that alpha blockers reduce BPH complication rates or the need for future surgery. Alpha blockers do not affect serum PSA levels.

Finasteride (Proscar)

Finasteride significantly lowers intraprostatic dihydrotestosterone levels without decreasing circulating testosterone levels. The average man treated with 5 mg daily has a 20% reduction in prostate size and a 30% reduction in symptoms. Finasteride is not effective unless the patient has significant prostate enlargement (>30 to 40 mL). At least 6 months of therapy is required to assess the response, but patients who respond can expect continuation of the benefit for at least 5 years. Side effects are limited to impotence (3 to 4%), decreased libido (3 to 4%), and a decreased volume of ejaculate (2 to 3%). Breast tenderness and enlargement occur rarely. Only 1 to 5% of patients in clinical trials were discontinued because of side effects.

Studies demonstrate that long-term use of finasteride significantly lowers the probability of BPH-related complications, such as acute urinary retention and the need for surgery. However, the cost-effectiveness of finasteride as a preventive measure requires further study.

Finasteride causes a 40 to 50% decrease in serum PSA levels in men with BPH even in the presence of prostate cancer. Men with elevated PSA levels should undergo complete evaluation to exclude clinically significant prostate cancer before beginning finasteride therapy. Moreover, any sustained increase in PSA levels while the patient is taking finasteride should be carefully evaluated.

Thermal Therapy

Transurethral heating of the prostate can reduce prostatic mass by coagulation necrosis with resulting symptomatic improvement. The FDA has approved two types of thermal therapy. TUMT utilizing a water-cooled catheter antenna produces improvement in urination that is intermediate between that of medical therapy and TURP. TUNA utilizes endoscopically directed needles that heat the prostate with a radio frequency generator. TUNA also produces results that are intermediate in magnitude. Both technologies can be used in an outpatient setting with local anesthesia, although occasional patients require significant sedation or anesthesia. Complications include post-treatment urinary retention and dysuria. The long-term durability and cost-effectiveness of thermal-based BPH therapies are unproved. Re-treatment rates appear to be significant, and insurers have not fully embraced these therapies.

IMPOTENCE

method of
JACOB RAJFER, M.D.
UCLA School of Medicine
Los Angeles, California

Impotence is defined as the inability to attain or maintain an erection sufficient for vaginal penetration and sexual satisfaction. The problem is age dependent, with an estimated incidence of only 1.9% at the age of 40 years, but this increases to approximately 25% by the age of 65 and 67% by the age of 70 years. In fact, about 10 to 15% of all men will have an impotence problem at some time in their life. Although before 1980 it was commonly believed that erectile dysfunction in the majority of men had a psychologic cause, it is now generally accepted that approximately 90% of impotence cases have a physiologic or organic (nonpsychologic) cause.

PHYSIOLOGY

Penile erection is a hemodynamic event that depends on several concurrent physiologic events (Table 1). Basically,

TABLE 1. **Physiology of Penile Erection**

Increase arterial inflow (arterial dilatation)
Increase cavernosal storage (cavernosal muscle relaxation)
Decrease venous outflow (passive veno-occlusion)

stimulation of the cavernosal nerve via central or peripheral stimuli results in (1) cavernosal arteriolar dilatation, (2) relaxation of the smooth muscle within the corpora cavernosa, and (3) corporeal veno-occlusion. The increase in arterial inflow through the paired cavernosal arteries brings the required volume of blood into the corpora to achieve tumescence while the relaxed corporal smooth muscle causes enlargement of the sinusoids of the corpora, thereby providing a space for the increased arterial inflow to pool into. This engorgement of the corpora with blood in effect compresses the subtunical venules, thereby preventing outflow of blood out of the corpora. Therefore, to obtain a normal erection, the man must have these three vascular events occurring in an orderly and sequential manner.

The arterial and cavernosal smooth muscle relaxation that occurs during penile erection is directly induced by stimulation of the nervi erigentes (S2–4), which in the past were assumed to be part of the parasympathetic nervous system; however, these cavernosal nerves are now considered to belong to the nonadrenergic, noncholinergic nerves that use nitric oxide (NO) primarily as the neurotransmitter for smooth muscle relaxation in the penis via the cyclic guanosine monophosphate (cGMP) second-messenger pathway.

CLASSIFICATION

Physiologically, for a man to obtain an erection, he must have an intact penile vascular tree, an intact cavernosal nerve, and a desire to have sex (libido). Therefore, any abnormality in the patient's vascular, neurologic, or hormonal status may result in erectile dysfunction. It is now accepted that one or a combination of these physiologic causes account for approximately 90% of the cases of impotence, and the majority of these can be related to the vascular side. Indeed, failure of the cavernosal smooth muscle to relax totally and hence retain blood completely in the cavernosa is the most common vascular problem identified in men with erectile dysfunction. Although most men with impotence have a psychologic problem regarding their impotence, the psychologic problem is the primary cause of the dysfunction in only about 10% of men.

EVALUATION

Because there are four major causes of erectile dysfunction, (1) psychologic, (2) hormonal, (3) neurologic, and (4) vascular, in the evaluation of a patient with erectile dysfunction, testing is directed at determining whether the cause of the impotence falls into one or a combination of these four categories. Within this testing algorithm, if a patient is found to have intact hormonal, vascular, and neurologic systems, then by exclusion he must have a primary psychologic problem as the cause of his impotence.

During the initial history taking and physical examination, it should be determined whether certain disease states or surgical procedures that are associated with erectile dysfunction may be present. Examples of these are multiple sclerosis, paraplegia, hypertension, atherosclerosis, pelvic surgery, chronic renal failure, and hyperthyroidism. At the physical examination, specific attention is paid to determine whether certain findings associated with impotence are present such as hypogonadism, Peyronie's disease, atherosclerosis, or subtle neurologic deficits. Regardless of the history and physical examination, however, a basic work-up that usually includes a serum testosterone (T) level and a diagnostic intracorporeal injection of a vasoactive substance is performed. Only a serum T level is initially measured in the hormonal evaluation of the patient, and if the serum T level is normal, it is assumed that the patient does not have a hormonal cause of his impotence. The evaluation then proceeds to the other three possible causes of erectile dysfunction, in particular the vascular system. If the serum T level is low, however, serum luteinizing hormone and prolactin levels to help differentiate a central (pituitary) from a testicular cause of the hypogonadism are measured. If the serum T level is high, there can be only two causes of this: hyperthyroidism or an unsuspected incomplete androgen insensitivity. Thyroid function tests help differentiate these two disorders.

To evaluate the vascular system, a diagnostic test injection of a combination of prostaglandin E$_1$, phentolamine,* and papaverine* (triple therapy) is given intracorporeally and the response of the penis is observed. If the patient obtains a good response (tumescence), particularly with manual stimulation, it is concluded that the patient's penile vascular system is either minimally or completely uninvolved as the cause of the erectile dysfunction. A poor response to the injection suggests that there may be a vascular cause of the dysfunction, and if indicated, these patients may undergo further evaluation of their penile vascular system to pinpoint the cause (inflow and/or outflow problem).

The evaluation of the vascular system in men who fail to respond to a vasoactive substance includes a duplex scan of their penile arteries and dynamic infusion cavernosometry (DIC). These tests identify whether the patient has an inflow and/or outflow problem. Once this is determined, therapy may be suggested. In certain individuals whose failure to store blood in their corpora is identified by DIC, a cavernosogram may be obtained to determine whether a venous surgical procedure may be indicated to correct the "leakage." In studies of men with vascular erectile dysfunction, regardless of their age, most are found to have a failure to store or venous leakage problem when DIC or cavernosography or both are performed. Penile-brachial indices are not used today to evaluate the arterial inflow to the penis because of the nonspecificity of the test. Similarly, nocturnal penile tumescence (NPT) testing is rarely performed in the clinical evaluation except in legal cases because of the exorbitant cost of performing precise hospital-based NPT monitoring. Arteriography of the penile vascular tree is usually reserved for patients who may be candidates for an arterial reconstruction procedure.

TREATMENT

The treatment of impotence can be divided into four categories: (1) medical therapy, (2) mechanical devices (external and internal), (3) surgery, and (4) psychologic treatment. Medical therapy for impotence could involve (1) oral (yohimbine), (2) intracorporeal (vasodilators), (3) hormonal (T), and (4) intraurethral (prostaglandin E$_1$) therapy. Mechanical therapy involves (1) external vacuum devices and/or (2) external penile constrictive and/or restrictive devices. Surgery may involve (1) implantation of a penile prosthesis, (2) arterial reconstruction, or (3) ligation or occlusion of the venous drainage from the penis.

No oral drugs, including yohimbine, which suppos-

---

*Not FDA approved for this indication.

edly stimulates alpha receptors in the central nervous tissue, have been shown to have a dramatic positive effect on the erectile mechanism. Currently in clinical trials are oral phosphodiesterase inhibitors that inhibit the breakdown of cGMP and other drugs that act on the NO-cGMP pathway and that may prove efficacious in the future. Bromocriptine (Parlodel) is an oral drug that inhibits prolactin production and is specifically used in the treatment of men with hyperprolactinemia secondary to a pituitary adenoma. These patients are initially identified by a low serum T level tested during the initial evaluation of the impotence, and the adenoma is confirmed by computed tomography or magnetic resonance imaging of the pituitary-hypothalamic area.

Intraurethral prostaglandin E₁ (alprostadil [Muse]) therapy and intracorporeal injection therapy either singly or in combination with either prostaglandin E₁, papaverine,* or phentolamine* rely on the ability of these drugs to cause corporeal and arterial smooth muscle relaxation in the penis. The intracorporeal injection of triple therapy and the intraurethral application of prostaglandin E₁ alone appear to be effective in inducing an erection in about 35 to 80% of the patients tested. For the intraurethral treatment, there is a special applicator to deliver the drug into the urethra via the meatus while a small-gauge needle is used to deliver the vasoactive drugs directly into the corpora. Regardless of their delivery site, all vasoactive drugs can have side effects such as a prolonged response to the medication (priapism) and urethral and/or corporeal discomfort. In addition, hematoma formation and scarring of the penile tissues may occur with the intracorporeal injections. The medications can be used in men taking anticoagulants and with heart disease.

Hormonal therapy to replace T in hypogonadal patients with impotence can be delivered by intramuscular injections or skin patches. The injection of exogenous T occurs every 10 to 14 days, whereas the patches are worn on a daily basis. During therapy, serum T levels are measured to determine the attainment of therapeutic blood levels. Side effects of T therapy may include aggressiveness, acne formation, erythrocytosis, and, in the aged population, elevation of the serum prostate-specific antigen level.

Vacuum erection devices are the primary nonsurgical, nonmedical, noninvasive treatment of men with erectile dysfunction. The devices utilize a vacuum chamber over the penis to obtain a negative pressure around the penis that seems to draw blood into the corporeal tissue. When tumescence occurs, a restrictive ring is placed at the base of the penis to retain the blood and the tumescence. Some men who are able to obtain an erection but cannot maintain it may benefit by using the restrictive device alone (without the vacuum) once the erection is induced normally. The restrictive ring should not be left on the penis more than half an hour at a time. The

vacuum device is not effective in every patient, and even when it is effective it may not be psychologically acceptable by the patient as a form of treatment.

Surgery for impotence, particularly the insertion of a penile prosthesis, should be offered only after the patient refuses nonsurgical therapy, or such therapy fails. There are two types of prostheses: the semirigid and the inflatable devices. The devices, which are made of bioacceptable compounds, are placed into the corporeal tissues and are a permanent and final form of treatment for the dysfunction. Complications of the surgery include pain, infection, erosion, and/or malfunction of the device, and possible shortening of penile length.

Arterial revascularization as performed today is not an effective procedure in restoring potency except in young men with a specific obstruction to the internal pudendal system. These men usually present with a history of a traumatic event to their pelvis, and the obstruction is confirmed by selective pudendal arteriography. The donor vessel is usually the inferior epigastric, and the recipient is usually the dorsal penile artery; a microvascular anastomosis is required. Venous ligation surgery for men with venous leakage is effective in less than 25% of patients long term and, like the arterial revascularization procedure, should rarely be considered as a form of treatment for impotence except in specific instances.

If the aforementioned testing fails to identify a physiologic cause of the impotence and the patient is categorized as having primarily a psychologic problem, there are two avenues of treatment available. One is to have the patient see a psychologist and/or psychiatrist for the appropriate evaluation and treatment; an alternative is to consider the patient for vasoactive drug therapy for a finite length of time as a form of positive biofeedback therapy. Many patients who opt for the latter regimen find that after they realize that they are able to function without fear of failing, their performance and confidence in their sexual abilities are restored.

ACUTE RENAL FAILURE

method of
JIM REICHMAN, M.D., and
MAYER BREZIS, M.D.
Hadassah University Hospital
Jerusalem, Israel

Acute renal failure (ARF) is a clinical entity characterized by an abrupt (hours to days) decline in renal function resulting in the retention of nitrogenous waste products and a perturbation of water, electrolyte, and acid-base balance. It is typically associated with daily increments in serum urea and creatinine levels greater than 10 and 0.5 mg per dL, respectively. ARF is frequently encountered, occurring in approximately 5% of all hospitalized patients and in up to 30% of intensive care unit admissions. Oliguria (urine output < 400 mL per day) is observed in 50% of patients with ARF, with an associated mortality of 50 to

---

*Not FDA approved for this indication.

80%. Nonoliguric ARF portends a better prognosis, with mortality rates of 15 to 40%. Many cases of ARF are iatrogenic, induced by unnecessary procedures or medications. If primary care and hospital physicians are cognizant of the indications and potential nephrotoxicities of each medication and invasive procedure prescribed, the incidence of ARF may be curbed.

The causes of ARF are divided into three categories: prerenal, intrinsic, and postrenal (Table 1). This classification facilitates the diagnostic process and the application of therapeutic modalities. Prerenal ARF is consequent to renal hypoperfusion and denotes a functional impairment without renal parenchymal damage. It is responsible for 55 to 70% of cases of ARF. Renal hypoperfusion is often due to an absolute decrease in blood volume (hemorrhage, diarrhea, vomiting, diuretics) or a relative decrease in effective blood volume (cardiac failure, hypoalbuminemia, cirrhosis). Careful balance of the volume status in these patients may obviate progression to the prerenal state. Renal arterial occlusion (thromboemboli) and systemic vasodilatation (sepsis, anaphylaxis) also impair kidney perfusion. Drug-induced renal vasoconstriction (cyclosporine, norepinephrine) and hypoperfusion (nonsteroidal anti-inflammatory drugs [NSAIDs]) constitute widespread iatrogenic causes of prerenal ARF. These medications, particularly angiotensin-converting enzyme (ACE) inhibitors, are extremely hazardous in the presence of hypoperfusion or high renin output and should be supplanted by alternative drugs in these settings.

Between 25 and 40% of cases of ARF may be ascribed to intrinsic renal damage. Primary glomerular disease and secondary glomerulonephritis (systemic lupus erythematosus [SLE], postinfectious) reduce renal blood flow, and ARF may ensue. Vascular causes of intrinsic ARF (malignant hypertension, vasopressors, contrast material, thromboemboli) are more prevalent in patients with hypertension, coronary artery atherosclerosis, or peripheral vascular disease. Prolonged renal ischemia (as for prerenal ARF), endogenous toxins (myoglobin, hemoglobin, uric acid), and exogenous toxins (aminoglycosides, amphotericin B, contrast material) can all produce acute tubular necrosis, accounting for about 90% of cases of intrinsic ARF. Acute tubulointerstitial nephritis after various infections, malignancies, or drug use may precipitate intrinsic ARF. Patients with chronic renal failure, volume depletion, or oliguria have a predilection for the development of intrinsic ARF, which typically evolves in the setting of combined risk factors and additional insults (contrast material). Recognition of these predisposing conditions before ordering diagnostic tests and administering drugs discourages indiscriminate imaging with radiocontrast material and encourages scrupulous benefit/risk analysis.

Postrenal ARF, constituting 5% of cases of ARF, indicates obstruction of the urethra or bladder neck, bilateral ureteric obstruction, or unilateral ureteric obstruction in patients with one functioning kidney or chronic renal failure. Common causes include ureteral calculi, blood clots, neoplasms, prostatic hypertrophy or malignancy, retroperitoneal fibrosis, or neurogenic bladder. Analgesic-induced papillary necrosis is a cause of postrenal ARF seen in patients with rheumatoid arthritis or chronic lower back pain.

DIAGNOSIS

History

A thorough history is crucial to the diagnosis and stratification of ARF. Weight gain, edema, and a reduction in urine output are early indices of renal insufficiency. Excessive diarrhea, vomiting, bleeding, sweating, or diuretic use accompanied by dizziness implies a prerenal state. Osmotic diuresis should be suspected in brittle or noncompliant diabetic patients. A diagnosis of adrenal insufficiency should be considered in a chronic steroid user whose steroid therapy was abruptly stopped. A careful drug history is essential. Complaints of chest pain and/or shortness of breath may indicate pulmonary emboli, myocardial ischemia, atrial fibrillation, and/or congestive heart failure with subsequent renal hypoperfusion. Alcoholism may implicate cardiomyopathy, cirrhosis, or rhabdomyolysis as the cause of ARF. Weight loss or fever suggests underlying infection or malignancy. Recent procedures such as angioplasty or surgery support a thromboembolic cause. Complaints of hematuria, purpura, hemoptysis, or a malar rash imply a systemic vasculitis. Finally, symptoms of prostatism or nephrolithiasis implicate postrenal failure as the culprit.

A fundamental part of the history is the inquiry into past medical diseases, focusing on hypertension, diabetes, congestive heart failure, atrial fibrillation, cirrhosis, vasculitides, malignancy, prostatism, nephrolithiasis, and chronic renal disorders. Previous measures of renal function help determine the acuteness of the renal insufficiency.

Physical Examination

A detailed physical examination is a vital part of the diagnostic evaluation. Orthostatic hypotension, tachycardia, dry mucous membranes, or poor skin turgor suggests a decrement in effective blood volume. Elevated jugular venous pressure, moist rales, a displaced point of maximal intensity, a third heart sound, a positive hepatojugular reflex, pitting edema, shifting dullness, fluid waves, and Cullen's (bluish discoloration of the umbilicus) or Grey Turner's (blue or green ecchymoses of the flank) sign all reflect a state of ineffective vascular blood volume. Hypotension in tandem with hyper- or hypothermia implies sepsis or adrenal insufficiency. Abdominal bruits indicate renal artery atherosclerosis, whereas flank tenderness denotes nephrolithiasis, renal vein thrombosis, or pyelonephritis. Roth's spots, fever, and a new or changing cardiac murmur support a diagnosis of endocarditis. A malar rash suggests SLE, whereas concomitant fever, neurologic signs, and purpura implicate thrombotic thrombocytopenic purpura. A systemic blanching rash warrants an investigation of all past and recent medication use, with a focus on a potential agent inducing allergic interstitial nephritis. An enlarged prostate associated with dullness on complete bladder percussion reflects postrenal ARF. Uveitis suggests the diagnosis of sarcoidosis.

Laboratory Analysis

Urinalysis. Examination of the sediment and supernatant of an early-morning fresh urine specimen may further elucidate the cause of ARF. Several agents affect supernatant urine color. Bilirubin and melanin induce a dark brown or yellow color. Red urine may result from porphyria, hemoglobinuria, hematuria, or myoglobinuria; using rifampin, phenazopyridine, or phenolphthalein; or eating beets. A blue-green color suggests *Pseudomonas* infection, the use of methylene blue or amitriptyline, or biliverdin. Turbid white implies pyuria, crystalluria, or chyluria. Hematuria may reflect trauma, nephrolithiasis, neoplasm, cystitis, vasculitis, coagulation defects, or menstruation.

Specific gravity (SG; determined by both the mass and

TABLE 1. **Causes of Acute Renal Failure**

Prerenal Failure

Absolute Decrease in Blood Volume

Hemorrhage
Skin losses (burns, sweating)
Gastrointestinal losses (diarrhea, vomiting, surgical gastric drainage)
Renal losses (diuretics, diabetes insipidus, salt-losing nephropathy, osmotic diuresis, adrenal insufficiency)
Burns

Decrease in Effective Blood Volume

Cardiac dysfunction and/or low cardiac output (myocardial infarction, tamponade, valvular disease, arrhythmias, pulmonary embolism, cor pulmonale, positive-pressure mechanical ventilation)
Liver disease with ascites
Hypoalbuminemia
Fluid pooling (pancreatitis, peritonitis)

Peripheral Vasodilatation

Sepsis
Anaphylaxis
Antihypertensive drugs
Anesthesia

Renal Vasoconstriction

Hypercalcemia
Norepinephrine, epinephrine
Cyclosporine
Amphotericin B
Cirrhosis with ascites

Renal Hypoperfusion with Impairment of Renal Autoregulatory Responses

Cyclooxygenase inhibitors, angiotensin-converting enzyme inhibitors

Hyperviscosity Syndrome

Multiple myeloma, macroglobulinemia, polycythemia

Renal Arterial Occlusion

Bilateral thromboembolism, renal artery stenosis, surgery, trauma, angioplasty, dissecting aneurysm, vasculitis

Intrinsic Renal Failure

Glomerular

Primary glomerulonephritis (membranoproliferative)
Secondary glomerulonephritis (hemolytic uremic syndrome, thrombotic thrombocytopenic purpura, disseminated intravascular coagulation, toxemia of pregnancy, after infection, accelerated hypertension, radiation nephritis, scleroderma, systemic lupus erythematosus, Goodpasture's syndrome, Wegener's granulomatosis)

Vascular

Vasculitis, malignant hypertension, renal vein thrombosis, vasopressors, eclampsia, hyperviscosity syndrome, iodinated contrast agents, nonsteroidal anti-inflammatory drugs

Acute Tubular Necrosis

Ischemia (as for prerenal failure)
Toxins (contrast material, aminoglycosides, heavy metals, cyclosporine, amphotericin B, cisplatin, ethylene glycol, acetaminophen intoxication)
Pigments (hemoglobin, myoglobin)
Proteins (in multiple myeloma)
Crystals (uric acid, oxalate, sulfonamides)

Tubulointerstitial Nephritis

Allergic (β-lactams, sulfonamides, trimethoprim, rifampin, cyclooxygenase inhibitors, diuretics, captopril)
Infectious (pyelonephritis, cytomegalovirus infection, human immunodeficiency virus infection, candidiasis, tuberculosis)
Infiltration (lymphoma, leukemia, sarcoidosis)
Radiation

Renal Allograft Rejection

Postrenal Failure

Ureteric

Calculi, blood clot, papillary necrosis, neoplasm, retroperitoneal fibrosis or hemorrhage, fungus balls, ligation, inflammatory aortic aneurysm

Bladder Outflow Obstruction

Prostatic hypertrophy, calculi, blood clot, neurogenic bladder, neoplasm, prostatitis

Urethra

Phimosis, meatal stenosis, stricture, neoplasm, congenital valve the number of solute particles) provides a rough estimation of urine osmolality (determined by the number of osmotically active particles) except in the setting of excess high-density substances (contrast material, protein, or glucose) or low-density substances (urea). Urine that is isosmotic with plasma has an osmolality of 285 mOsm per kg and an SG of 1.010. A high SG (>1.020) reflects the kidney's ability to concentrate urine and implies a prerenal state. An SG of 1.010 is seen in concert with intrinsic ARF and evidence of tubular and concentrating dysfunction.

Urine pH is normally below 7, but this varies with diet, respiration, infection, and systemic acid-base balance. A urine pH greater than 7 suggests a bicarbonate diuresis or the presence of urease-producing bacteria. Acidic urine is associated with uric acid or cystine stones, whereas alkaline urine accompanies struvite stones. Glucose detected by urine dipstick implies hyperglycemia or proximal tubular dysfunction. Bacteria may reduce nitrates to nitrites, yielding a positive nitrite test in approximately 50% of bacteriuric specimens. Urinary ketones may be seen with diabetic ketoacidosis, starvation, volume depletion, and chronic or acute alcohol intoxication.

Normal adults excrete between 40 and 80 mg of protein per day, with the upper limit of normal being 150 mg per day. The urine dipstick detects predominantly albumin. Detection of immune globulins in suspected cases of multiple myeloma, amyloidosis, lymphoma, or macroglobulinemia can be assessed by mixing 2.5 mL of urine with 7.5 mL of 3% sulfosalicylic acid, which precipitates all proteins. Interpretation must also take into account the concentration of urine; a 1+ protein result in a concentrated specimen with an SG of 1.030 may have no significance, whereas the same result combined with an SG of 1.010 may warrant further investigation.

A more accurate assessment of proteinuria is obtained by the spot urine protein/creatinine ratio, which readily yields an accurate estimate of a 24-hour urine collection. Factors causing false-positive dipstick results include gross hematuria, urine pH greater than 8, phenazopyridine, and contamination with an antiseptic. False-positive tests with sulfosalicylic acid may be due to gross hematuria, radiographic contrast agents, β-lactam antibiotics, and sulfonamides. Mildly increased protein excretion, typically less than 1 gram per day, is common in acute tubular necrosis, whereas 1 to 3 grams per day is observed in tubulointerstitial nephritis. Nephrotic range proteinuria, greater than 3.5 grams per day, is compatible with glomerulonephritis and atheroembolic disease.

Urinary sediment is obtained by centrifuging 10 to 15 mL of urine at 2000 to 3000 rpm for 3 to 5 minutes and then decanting the supernatant. Microscopic examination must not be delayed, because erythrocytes and casts degenerate rapidly, especially in alkaline or dilute urine. Moreover, the urine pH may change and bacteria may proliferate with time. The normal range of erythrocytes is 0 to 2 per high-power field. Dysmorphic erythrocytes are often associated with glomerular disease, whereas normal erythrocyte morphology suggests an extraglomerular source. The normal range of leukocytes is 0 to 2 per high-power field. Leukocyturia usually implies cystitis, pyelonephritis, glomerulonephritis, or interstitial nephritis. Pyuria with negative urine cultures (sterile pyuria) denotes partially treated urinary tract infection, tuberculosis, urethritis, prostatitis, interstitial nephritis, calculi, or papillary necrosis. Eosinophiluria (between 1 and 50% of urine leukocytes) is detected in 90% of cases of drug-induced allergic interstitial nephritis when Hansel's stain is used. Wright's stain is less sensitive, detecting approximately 20% of cases. Eosinophiluria is 85% specific for allergic interstitial nephritis, occurring less commonly in atheroembolization, glomerulonephritis, pyelonephritis, cystitis, prostatitis, and ischemic and toxin-induced ARF.

Red blood cell casts suggest glomerulonephritis but may also be seen with pyelonephritis, tubulointerstitial nephritis, trauma, thromboemboli, and malignant hypertension. White blood cell casts imply pyelonephritis, glomerulonephritis, or tubulointerstitial nephritis. Hyaline casts, devoid of cellular elements, do not reflect renal disease and are visualized in concentrated urine after exercise, fever, or diuretic use. Renal tubular epithelial cells indicate tubular damage and are seen in acute tubular necrosis, tubulointerstitial nephritis, and glomerulonephritis. These cells are 1.5 to 3 times the size of a leukocyte and contain a large round nucleus. In nephrotic range proteinuria, degenerating tubular epithelial cells may be manifested as oval fat bodies with a Maltese cross appearance under polarized light. Coarsely granular or waxy casts represent progressive degeneration of cellular elements or aggregated proteins within a cast, denoting tubular injury. Broad casts indicate chronic renal failure, reflecting stasis in the collecting tubules draining diseased nephrons. They may contain cellular elements. Finally, the presence of squamous epithelial cells reflects vaginal contamination, and a new midstream clean-catch specimen should be obtained. The presence of urinary crystals in ARF may facilitate the diagnostic process. Calcium oxalate crystals may indicate excessive exposure to ethylene glycol, methoxyflurane, or high-dose vitamin C. Uric acid crystals may follow tumor lysis, rhabdomyolysis, or the prerenal state.

Blood Tests. Hepatic catabolism of amino acids generates ammonia, which is subsequently converted to urea. Several factors influence the blood urea nitrogen (BUN) level, so it is not a reliable index of the glomerular filtration rate. Conditions that increase the BUN level include gastrointestinal bleeding, a high-protein diet, tissue trauma, glucocorticoids, tetracycline, and reduction of effective circulating blood volume. Factors that decrease the BUN level include malnutrition and liver disease. The serum creatinine level is a more specific measurement of renal function. ARF secondary to atheroemboli, ischemia, or contrast material results in a rapid elevation of the serum creatinine level (24 to 48 hours), with peak levels in contrast nephropathy appearing earlier (3 to 5 days) than in ischemic or atheroembolic disease (7 to 10 days). Aminoglycosides typically induce a rise in the creatinine level during the second week of therapy. Spurious elevations in the serum creatinine level due to the production of noncreatinine chromogens may be seen in ketoacidosis, cephalosporin administration, and methanol or isopropyl alcohol intoxication. Ingesting large amounts of cooked meat containing creatinine may generate a rise in the serum creatinine level. Various drugs (aspirin, cimetidine, trimethoprim, triamterene, spironolactone, amiloride) inhibit tubular creatinine secretion and may increase the serum creatinine level, especially in the presence of renal insufficiency. Decrements in serum creatinine levels appear with cachexia and increasing age due to pathologic and physiologic decreases in muscle mass, respectively. Although the BUN/creatinine ratio is often cited as a useful measure for distinguishing prerenal from intrinsic ARF, urinary indices are more reliable measurements.

A complete blood count and smear may provide evidence of infection (leukocytosis, leukopenia), hematologic malignancy (blasts, plasma cells, anemia), allergic response (eosinophilia), vasculitis (eosinophilia, anemia, schistocytes, thrombocytopenia), or malignant hypertension (anemia, schistocytes). Abnormal liver function tests may reflect hepatic disease or congestive heart failure, whereas a low albumin level may indicate chronic liver or cardiac disease, nephrotic range proteinuria, or malnutrition. Electrolyte disturbances such as hypokalemia may be secondary to diarrhea, vomiting, hyperosmotic diuresis, or drug-induced diuresis, whereas hyponatremia may be consistent with diuresis, adrenal insufficiency, cirrhosis, nephrosis, or congestive heart failure. Hyperkalemia associated with hyperphosphatemia, hyperuricemia, and hypocalcemia after chemotherapy suggests a tumor lysis syndrome. Severe hypercalcemia can induce ARF. Elevated creatine kinase (MM isoenzyme) levels are observed with tumor lysis or rhabdomyolysis. The presence of antinuclear antibody, antineutrophil cytoplasmic antibody, or anti–glomerular basement membrane antibody supports a diagnosis of SLE, Wegener's granulomatosis, or Goodpasture's syndrome, respectively. A low complement level suggests SLE, postinfectious glomerulonephritis, cryoglobulinemia, or membranoproliferative glomerulonephritis. Finally, monitoring blood levels of aminoglycosides and cyclosporine should be routine when these drugs are administered.

Urinary Diagnostic Indices. The most sensitive urinary index applied for distinguishing prerenal from intrinsic ARF is the fractional excretion of sodium (Fe_{Na}), the percentage of filtered sodium that is excreted (Table 2). An Fe_{Na} of less than 1% is seen with avid proximal tubular reabsorption of sodium and is consistent with the prerenal state. Intrinsic renal damage disrupts tubular function, diminishing sodium reabsorption and producing an Fe_{Na} of greater than 1%. The Fe_{Na} in early and late postrenal ARF resembles prerenal and intrinsic ARF, respectively. Conditions of partial tubular preservation (nonoliguric ischemia, aminoglycoside or contrast nephrotoxicity, rhabdomyolysis, hemolysis, sepsis, burns, hepatorenal syndrome, or acute interstitial or glomerulonephritis) may result in a low Fe_{Na}. Furthermore, the Fe_{Na} may occasionally be greater than 1% in the prerenal state (diuretics, adrenal insufficiency, chronic renal failure with salt wasting, bicarbonaturia associated with natriuresis). The Fe_{Na} is a useful diagnostic tool that may reveal the classification of the ARF. It does not pinpoint the cause but complements the history and physical examination. The renal failure index is a measurement similar to the Fe_{Na}, excluding the serum sodium level. Indices of urinary concentrating ability such as urine osmolality, urine SG, and urine/plasma creatinine or urea ratios are less useful measures for differentiating the prerenal, intrinsic, and postrenal ARF states (see Table 2).

Radiology

Ultrasound imaging of the kidney in ARF is warranted to rule out obstruction. Information regarding kidney size, cyst formation, anatomic abnormalies, stones, neoplasms, retroperitoneal masses, and asymmetry is also provided. Reduction in kidney size is typically seen in chronic renal failure, although several chronic diseases may exhibit normal-sized or enlarged kidneys (multiple myeloma, amyloidosis, diabetes, polycystic kidneys, renal vein thrombosis, infiltrative lesions). Ultrasound imaging provides a noninvasive and rapid anatomic assessment of the kidney, and it can be performed at the bedside in an unstable patient. Doppler ultrasonography may be used to assess the patency of the renal vasculature, although angiography is the "gold standard." Angiography carries the added risks of contrast nephropathy, dislodgment of atherosclerotic plaques, and thromboembolic events. Preliminary observations using magnetic resonance imaging suggest that it may become the procedure of choice for evaluating renal vasculature, hence avoiding the hazards of angiography. Computed tomography affords similar visualization as ultrasonography but often requires radiocontrast material.

Biopsy

Indications for renal biopsy in the setting of ARF are controversial. Prerenal and postrenal causes of ARF do not require biopsy, and most causes of intrinsic ARF (acute tubulointerstitial nephritis, contrast material, endogenous and exogenous toxins, ischemia) can be diagnosed without a biopsy. In cases of intrinsic ARF in which the diagnosis has not been ascertained and the suspected disease is amenable to therapy (Goodpasture's syndrome, Wegener's granulomatosis, thrombotic thrombocytopenic purpura), renal biopsy is indicated. Contraindications to kidney biopsy include a solitary or ectopic kidney, horseshoe kidney, uncorrected bleeding disorder, severe uncontrolled hypertension, renal infection, renal neoplasm, or uncooperative patient.

TABLE 2. **Urine Diagnostic Indices**

Diagnostic Index	Prerenal	Intrinsic*	Postrenal†
Fractional excretion of sodium (Fe_{Na}) (%)‡ $\left[\left(\dfrac{\text{Urine Na} \times \text{plasma creatinine}}{\text{Plasma Na} \times \text{urine creatinine}}\right) \times 100\right]$	<1	>1	>1
Renal failure index‡ $\left(\dfrac{\text{Urine Na}}{\text{Urine creatinine/plasma creatinine}}\right)$	<1	>1	>1
Urine sodium (mmol/L)	<10	>20	>20
Urine creatinine/plasma creatinine	>40	<20	<20
Urine urea/plasma urea	>8	<3	—
Urine specific gravity	>1.020	<1.010	—
Urine osmolality (mmol/kg H_2O)	>500	<350	<350

*Many conditions causing intrinsic ARF are associated with renal hypoperfusion, resulting in urine diagnostic indices similar to those observed in prerenal ARF.

†Diagnostic indices in early obstruction can mimic prerenal indices.

‡More sensitive indices.

MANAGEMENT AND COMPLICATIONS

Prevention

Despite significant advances in supportive care, mortality rates in the setting of ARF have not changed in the past 3 decades. Therein lies the importance of preventive therapy. Foremost, physicians are obliged to know the indications, interactions, and adverse side effects of all medications and procedures prescribed. The need to adjust the drug dosage and/or dose interval in patients with reduced creatinine clearance should be routinely assessed (Table 3). There are myriad alternative medications (cephalosporins instead of aminoglycosides) and procedures (ultrasonography instead of computed tomography with contrast material) for the treating physician to utilize. Recognizing the risk factors for ARF (volume depletion, chronic renal failure) and the synergistic effect of combined insults should discourage the use of potentially nephrotoxic agents (NSAIDs, ACE inhibitors) in high-risk patients.

Hydration and salt loading are the mainstay of prophylactic treatment against ischemic and nephrotoxic injury. This protective effect has been demonstrated in recipients of cisplatin, amphotericin, and radiocontrast material, as well as in postoperative patients. There is no convincing evidence that dopamine, loop diuretics, mannitol, or calcium channel blockers prevent ARF in high-risk patients. Moreover, increased risk of ARF has been shown with furosemide and mannitol treatment. Forced diuresis and alkalinization of urine can limit renal injury due to uric acid, methotrexate, and myoglobin toxicity. The early administration of acetylcysteine sodium (Mucomyst) in acetaminophen overdose and the use of dimercaprol in heavy metal intoxication may obviate renal injury.

Supportive Care

ARF is complicated by intravascular volume overload consequent to reduced water and sodium excretion. Careful assessment of the volume status should be obtained by the physical examination and by monitoring fluid input and output and weighing the patient daily. Prerenal ARF due to hemorrhage should be corrected with packed red blood cells or whole blood, and isotonic saline should be administered for replacement of plasma losses (peritonitis, burns). Hypotonic solutions (0.45% saline) are satisfactory repletion for hemodynamically stable patients with urinary or gastrointestinal losses. Cardiac failure complicated by ARF often requires salt and water restriction. Salt and water limitation is also warranted for ARF due to intrinsic renal disease, and careful matching of input and output (urinary, gastrointestinal, insensible, and drainage site losses) is required. Postrenal causes of ARF should be dealt with promptly, conferring with a urologist, nephrologist, and radiologist for the optimal means of relieving the obstruction. Most patients experience diuresis after relief of obstruction, with potential severe

TABLE 3. **Dosage and Interval Adjustments for Commonly Prescribed Drugs**

Drugs Not Requiring Adjustment

Alprazolam	Furosemide	Miconazole
Amiodarone	Gemfibrozil	Minoxidil
Amitriptyline	Glipizide	Nifedipine
Bromocriptine	Griseofulvin	Nitroglycerin
Carbidopa	Haloperidol	Pentobarbital
Cefoperazone	Heparin	Pentoxifylline
Ceftriaxone	Ibuprofen	Phenytoin
Chloramphenicol	Indomethacin	Piroxicam
Clindamycin	Imipramine	Prazosin
Clonazepam	Isosorbide	Propafenone
Clonidine	Isradipine	Propranolol
Diazepam	Itraconazole	Rifampin
Diazoxide	Ketoconazole	Secobarbital
Dicloxacillin	Labetalol	Semisodium valproate
Diltiazem	Levodopa	Steroids
Diphenhydramine	Lidocaine	Streptokinase
Dipyridamole	Lorazepam	Sulindac
Dobutamine	Lovastatin	Theophylline
Esmolol	Metolazone	Verapamil
Flurazepam	Metoprolol	

Dose Interval Adjustment for Commonly Prescribed Drugs

Drug	Dose Interval (h) for	
	GFR 10–50 mL/min	GFR <10 mL/min
Acetazolamide*	12	—
Acyclovir	12	24
Amantadine	48	96
Amikacin	12	24–48
Amphotericin	24	24–36
Cefazolin	12	24–48
Cefotaxime	12	24–48
Cefoxitin	12	24–48
Ceftazidime	12	24–48
Cefuroxime	12	24–48
Cephalexin	6	8–12
Chlorpropamide*	24	—
Ethacrynic acid*	8–12	—
Ethambutol	24–36	48
Digoxin	36	48
Fluconazole	24–48	48–72
Gentamicin	12	24–48
Methyldopa	12	24
Pentamidine	24–36	48
Procainamide	6–12	8–24
Spironolactone*	12–24	—
Sulfamethoxazole	18	24
Tobramycin	12	24–48

*Avoid if glomerular filtration rate (GFR) is <10 mL/min.

Adapted from Bennett WM, Aronoff GR, Golper TA, et al: Drug Prescribing in Renal Failure: Dosing Guidelines for Adults, 2nd ed. Philadelphia, American College of Physicians, 1991.

volume and electrolyte depletion. Refractory volume overload complicated by intractable hypertension or congestive heart failure or pulmonary edema mandates dialysis treatment.

Oliguric ARF portends a worse prognosis than nonoliguric ARF, perhaps reflecting more severe disease. Pharmacologic methods, particularly diuretics, dopamine, and mannitol, are commonly prescribed to augment urine output. Nonetheless, their efficacy in enhancing survival of patients or attenuating renal injury has not been demonstrated. Despite promising early reports, atrial natriuretic peptide is not beneficial in the treatment of oliguric ARF.

Metabolic Acidosis

ARF is frequently complicated by an elevated anion gap metabolic acidosis. The metabolism of dietary protein produces approximately 1 mmol per kg (patient's weight) per day of nonvolatile acids, which is excreted by the kidney. Acidosis may be compounded by other causes of increased endogenous acid production (diabetes, starvation, or alcoholic ketoacidosis). Bicarbonate repletion is required when serum bicarbonate levels fall below 15 mmol per liter. Bicarbonate should be administered cautiously, because it may precipitate metabolic alkalosis, hypokalemia, hypocalcemia, and volume overload. Refractory acidosis is an indication for dialysis.

Hypo- and Hypernatremia

Hyponatremia often accompanies ARF because of the excess retention of water in comparison to sodium. Overzealous ingestion or administration of water (hypotonic fluids) may be a contributing factor. Water restriction is recommended. Hypernatremia, reflecting absolute volume depletion, may complicate the prerenal state. Treatment options include water or hypotonic or isotonic solutions, depending on the severity of the volume loss.

Hypo- and Hyperkalemia

Hyperkalemia due to impaired potassium excretion and concomitant acidosis is common in ARF, characterized by daily increments of 0.5 mmol per liter in oliguric and anuric patients. Hyperkalemia may be exacerbated in patients with ARF associated with rhabdomyolysis, hemolysis, or tumor lysis syndrome. Management of hyperkalemia requires limitation of dietary potassium and elimination of dietary supplements, potassium-sparing diuretics, and ACE inhibitors. Early electrocardiographic abnormalities, typically developing with levels greater than 6 mmol per liter, include peaked T waves, P wave flattening, first- and second-degree heart block, QRS widening, and ST elevation. Potential lethal cardiac arrhythmias include asystole, bradycardia, complete heart block, and ventricular tachycardia or fibrillation. Neurologic manifestations of hyperkalemia include paresthesias, hyporeflexia, weakness, ascending flaccid paralysis, and respiratory failure. Emergency measures, as illustrated in Table 4, should be employed for potassium levels greater than 6.5 to 7.0 mmol per liter or with evidence of cardiac or neurologic abnormalities.

Initial therapy consists of calcium gluconate (10 to 20 mL of a 10% solution infused over 5 to 10 minutes), which rapidly antagonizes the cardiac and neurologic effects of hyperkalemia; the onset of action is 1 to 2 minutes, and transient effects last approximately 15 to 20 minutes. Calcium administered in solutions containing bicarbonate precipitates, so this combination should be avoided. Sodium bicarbonate (1 to 2 ampules or 44.6 to 89.2 mmol intravenously over 5 to 10 minutes) promotes an extracellular-to-intracellular potassium shift, with a rapid onset of action (10 to 20 minutes) and effects lasting from 1 to 2 hours. Furthermore, bicarbonate combats the metabolic acidosis of ARF. Additional doses can be given at 15-minute intervals if symptoms or signs persist. Circulatory overload, hypernatremia, and symptomatic hypocalcemia may complicate bicarbonate treatment. Intravenous glucose (50 mL of 50% dextrose) and insulin (5 to 10 units of Regular Insulin) induce intracellular potassium uptake within 30 to 60 minutes, with effects persisting for several hours. Hypoglycemia may ensue, so periodic glucose measurements should be obtained. Glucose therapy should be omitted in patients with hyperglycemia.

TABLE 4. **Treatment of Hyperkalemia**

Therapy	Mechanism	Onset	Duration	Side Effects
Calcium gluconate 10%, IV, 1 or 2 ampules or 10–20 mL over 5–10 min	Antagonism	1–2 min	15–20 min	Calcium load
Sodium bicarbonate IV, 1 or 2 ampules or 44.6–89.2 mEq over 5–10 min	Redistribution	10–20 min	1–2 h	Sodium and volume load, alkalosis, symptomatic hypocalcemia
Glucose 50% 50 mL and Regular Insulin 5–10 U IV	Redistribution	30–60 min	Hours	Hyperglycemia, hypoglycemia, volume expansion
Albuterol, beta$_2$ agonist, 10–20 mg nebulized or 0.5 mg IV, or salbutamol	Redistribution	30 min	Hours	Arrhythmias
Sodium polystyrene sulfonate (potassium exchange resin) 15–30 gm PO q 2–4 h plus sorbitol 50–100 mL of a 20% solution, or 50 gm rectally plus 200 mL of a 20% dextrose solution	Elimination	1–2 h	4–6 h	Nausea, vomiting, sodium and volume load, calcium and magnesium depletion, intestinal necrosis
Dialysis	Elimination	Hours	Hours	See Table 6

Albuterol (Ventolin)* 10 to 20 mg nebulized or 0.5 mg intravenously, a beta$_2$-adrenergic agonist, effectively redistributes potassium to the intracellular space 30 minutes after administration. The cation exchange resin sodium polystyrene sulfonate (Kayexalate) binds potassium in exchange for sodium (1 mEq of potassium for 1 to 2 mEq of sodium) in the intestinal tract, thereby effectively reducing total body potassium. The onset of action is 1 to 2 hours, and the duration is 4 to 6 hours. Recommended oral doses are 15 to 30 grams, which may be repeated every 2 to 4 hours. Each gram of resin binds 1 mEq of potassium, and 50 grams decreases the serum potassium level by approximately 0.5 to 1 mEq per liter. Because resin is constipating, the osmotic agent sorbitol (50 to 100 mL of a 20% solution) is administered concurrently to hasten gastrointestinal transit time. Adverse side effects include nausea, vomiting, hypernatremia, volume overload, calcium and magnesium depletion, and, rarely, intestinal necrosis. If oral administration is not feasible, retention enemas may be given (50 grams in 200 mL of a 20% dextrose solution). A rectal catheter is inflated to ensure retention of the enema for 30 to 60 minutes. The onset of action is 1 to 2 hours, and enemas can be repeated every 4 to 6 hours. Colonic necrosis and perforation have been rarely reported with the use of resin exchange enemas in humans (animal studies suggest that sorbitol may be the responsible agent; thus, sorbitol solutions are not recommended for use in enema preparations).

Intractable hyperkalemia is an indication for dialysis treatment, preferably hemodialysis, which extracts potassium more rapidly than peritoneal dialysis. Cation exchange resins combined with dietary restriction of potassium provide adequate therapy for asymptomatic moderate hyperkalemia (less than 6.5 mmol per liter). Hypokalemia is a rare occurrence in ARF, complicating nonoliguric cisplatin or amphotericin nephrotoxicity.

Hyperphosphatemia and Hypocalcemia

Hyperphosphatemia consequent to impaired phosphate excretion is frequently observed in ARF. ARF due to rhabdomyolysis, tumor lysis, or acute leukemia may result in severe hyperphosphatemia. Clinical manifestations include ectopic calcifications of soft tissues such as blood vessels, cornea, skin, kidney, and periarticular tissue, particularly when the calcium-phosphorus product exceeds 70 mg per dL. Moreover, the excess phosphate binding of calcium precipitates hypocalcemia. Phosphate lowering involves dietary phosphate restriction (800 to 1000 mg per day) and administering oral phosphate binders such as aluminum-containing antacids (15 to 30 mL or 1 to 3 capsules orally with meals), calcium carbonate (500 to 1000 mg every 8 hours with meals), or calcium acetate. Side effects of short-term use of aluminum-containing antacids are limited to nausea

and constipation, whereas prolonged use may result in osteomalacia, encephalopathy, and anemia. Because calcium carbonate and calcium acetate can elevate serum calcium levels, they should be employed only when the calcium-phosphorus product is less than 70 mg per dL.

Hypocalcemia is a typical finding in ARF, induced by phosphate binding, skeletal resistance to parathyroid hormone, and reduced levels of 1,25-dihydroxyvitamin D. It is often asymptomatic and is alleviated by the concomitant acidosis of ARF, which reduces calcium binding to albumin and augments ionized serum calcium levels. Hypocalcemia may be more pronounced in ARF associated with rhabdomyolysis, pancreatitis, or excessive bicarbonate infusions. Clinical sequelae of hypocalcemia include paresthesias, tetany, Trousseau's and Chvostek's signs, lethargy, confusion, laryngospasm, seizures, prolonged QT interval, cardiac failure, and hypotension. Symptomatic hypocalcemia necessitates immediate treatment with 2 ampules (20 mL) of 10% calcium gluconate over 10 minutes, followed by a continuous infusion of 60 mL of calcium gluconate in 500 mL of 5% dextrose at 0.5 to 2 mg per kg per hour if symptoms persist. Subsequently, oral calcium supplements may be used. Dialysis should be instituted for refractory hyperphosphatemia.

Hyperuricemia and Hypermagnesemia

Elevated uric acid and magnesium levels are common in ARF, rarely warranting treatment. ARF combined with rhabdomyolysis or tumor lysis may dramatically increase uric acid levels. Acute gouty attacks infrequently complicate hyperuricemia in ARF, and colchicine or steroids are sufficient therapy; NSAIDs are prohibited. Clinical manifestations of hypermagnesemia include areflexia; lethargy; weakness; paralysis; respiratory failure; hypotension; bradycardia; prolonged PR, QRS, and QT intervals; complete heart block; and asystole. Magnesium-containing antacids and laxatives should be avoided in patients with ARF. Emergency treatment of symptomatic hypermagnesemia entails infusion of 10 to 20 mL of a 10% calcium gluconate solution over 10 minutes. Intractable hypermagnesemia requires immediate dialysis.

Uremia

Manifestations of uremia include pericardial effusions, pericarditis, anorexia, nausea, vomiting, ileus, lethargy, confusion, stupor, agitation, psychosis, asterixis, myoclonus, hyper-reflexia, restless legs syndrome, focal neurologic deficits, seizures, coma, and bleeding. Symptomatic uremia is an indication for dialysis.

Hematologic Abnormalities

Uremia causes platelet dysfunction and a reduction in platelet survival time, constituting the pre-

---

*Not FDA approved for this indication.

dominant bleeding diathesis observed in ARF. Severe anemia may result, compounded by stress-induced bleeding ulcers in this population of patients. Temporizing measures include intravenous 1-deamino-8-D-arginine vasopressin (desmopressin, DDAVP, 0.3 μg per kg), conjugated estrogens (0.6 mg per kg per day for 5 days), or cryoprecipitate (1 to 2 units per 10 kg per day). The hemostatic effect of DDAVP occurs after 1 hour and persists for 6 hours. Histamine H₂-receptor antagonists or sucralfate is advocated prophylactically to curtail episodes of gastrointestinal hemorrhage, although reductions in overall mortality have not been demonstrated. Uncontrollable bleeding mandates dialysis treatment. Because hemodialysis reduces platelet counts, involves puncturing a major venous blood vessel, and requires heparin administration, peritoneal dialysis may be preferred in this setting.

Cardiovascular Complications

Cardiac failure, pulmonary edema, and hypertension may evolve in ARF because of volume overload. Electrolyte abnormalities may cause refractory arrhythmias in the setting of persistent acidosis. Initial treatment of cardiac failure, pulmonary edema, and hypertension entails fluid and sodium restriction. Antihypertensive medications should be instituted judiciously; ACE inhibitors are generally prohibited. Intractable cardiac failure, pulmonary edema, and hypertension are indications for dialysis. Uremia-induced pericarditis warrants emergent dialysis treatment. Pulmonary embolism is an infrequent complication, despite prolonged immobilization.

Infection

Infection complicates 50 to 90% of cases of ARF, accounting for up to 75% of deaths. The high prevalence of infection is attributed to the combination of impaired host immunity due to uremia and the excessive number of indwelling instruments (urinary, arterial, and venous catheters; endotracheal and dialysis tubes) breaching mucocutaneous barriers. Furthermore, manifestations of infection in ARF are limited, as urea displays antipyretic properties and may impede the body's ability to elevate white blood cell counts. Abdominal signs may be absent in cases of peritonitis. Hence, daily physical evaluations and the removal of all unnecessary indwelling instruments are critical to the early identification and to the forestallment of infectious complications, respectively. The need for dose and/or interval adjustments of antibiotics and antifungal drugs should be routinely assessed.

Nutrition

Malnutrition in ARF is characteristically multifactorial in origin, consequent to diminished intake and enhanced catabolism induced by uremia and the underlying disease state. Nutrient depletion in drainage fluids or dialysate may further aggravate the state of malnutrition. The role of hyperalimentation in ARF is controversial. A consistent benefit has not been demonstrated, and parenteral nutrition may cause serious complications, including infections, electrolyte abnormalities, acid-base disturbances, and increased urea and fluid load. Consequently, adequate oral or nasogastric tube feeding should be implemented if use of the gastrointestinal tract is feasible. Sufficient calories should be provided (minimum of 30 kcal per kg per day), increasing the caloric input according to the increment in catabolism. To minimize the production of nitrogenous waste, ARF patients should be restricted to 0.6 to 0.8 gram per kg per day of protein of high biologic value. Protein ingestion should be increased to 1 to 1.4 grams per kg per day when dialysis is instituted, because dialysis enhances protein catabolism. In addition, significant quantities of protein are lost across peritoneal dialysis membranes.

Dialysis

The optimal timing, frequency, and intensity of dialysis are unclear. Because dialysis does not expedite recovery or alter the prognosis in ARF, its use should probably be limited to absolute indications, as illustrated in Table 5. The primary modes of dialysis are hemodialysis and peritoneal dialysis, with neither method proven superior in the management of ARF. Variations of hemodialysis include ultrafiltration, continuous arteriovenous hemofiltration dialysis (CAVHD), and continuous venovenous hemofiltration dialysis (CVVHD). The advantages and disadvantages of each technique are listed in Table 6.

Hemodialysis

Hemodialysis for ARF is performed by percutaneous cannulation of the subclavian, internal jugular, or femoral vein. Subclavian and internal jugular cannulation provides a cleaner milieu than the femoral approach, so femoral insertion should be limited to short-term dialysis (<48 hours). Moreover, femoral catheters are more uncomfortable for the patient. Major advantages, disadvantages, and complications are depicted in Table 6. Hemodynamically unstable patients are not candidates for hemodialysis. A disadvantage of hemodialysis is the need for heparin administration, adding another risk for bleeding in patients who are already harboring bleeding diatheses.

TABLE 5. **Indications for Dialysis**

Refractory
   Fluid overload
   Acidosis
   Hyperkalemia, hyperphosphatemia, hypermagnesemia
Symptomatic uremia
Some overdoses and intoxications (e.g., methanol)

TABLE 6. **Methods of Dialysis**

Hemodialysis

Advantages: efficiency, intermittent use, easy access for blood sampling and medication administration

Complications and disadvantages: bleeding, infection, pneumothorax, hypotension, hypertension, nausea, vomiting, cramps, headache, hypoxia, arrhythmias, disequilibrium syndrome, venous stenosis, venous thrombosis, heparin administration

CAVHD or CVVHD

Advantages: more physiologic (continuous), better titration of volume and electrolyte status, minimizes cardiovascular instability

Complications and disadvantages: continuous anticoagulation, supervision in intensive care setting, repeated manipulation of a potential infectious access site, slow removal of filtrate, bleeding, infection

Peritoneal Dialysis

Advantages: no complex machinery, minimal anticoagulation, limited cardiovascular and neurologic disturbances

Complications and disadvantages: peritonitis, protein depletion, hyperglycemia, pulmonary compromise, low efficiency

Abbreviations: CAVHD = continuous arteriovenous hemofiltration dialysis; CVVHD = continuous venovenous hemofiltration dialysis.

Ultrafiltration

Ultrafiltration, except for the lack of dialysate, is similar to hemodialysis. It is employed exclusively to extract volume, resulting in fewer hemodynamic changes.

CAVHD and CVVHD

CAVHD and CVVHD entail a more physiologic mode of renal replacement, relying on continuous ultrafiltration. This affords better titration of volume and electrolyte status and reduces the incidence of cardiovascular instability. CAVHD involves cannulation of the femoral artery and vein or insertion of an arteriovenous shunt. The patient's arterial pressure suffices to promote blood flow through the extracorporeal circuit. CVVHD requires insertion of a double-lumen venous catheter and is contingent on a pump for blood flow. Disadvantages of hemofiltration include continuous anticoagulation, constant supervision in an intensive care setting, repeated manipulation of a potentially infectious access site, and the relative slow removal of filtrate.

Peritoneal Dialysis

Access for peritoneal dialysis is achieved by a cannula inserted percutaneously at the bedside or by a minilaparotomy for more permanent usage. Advantages, disadvantages, and complications are delineated in Table 6. Absolute contraindications to peritoneal dialysis include significant peritoneal fibrosis or a pleuroperitoneal leak; relative contraindications include colostomy or nephrostomy, severe catabolism, peritonitis, recent abdominal surgery, extensive abdominal adhesions, or inguinal or abdominal hernia.

OUTCOME

Of those patients recovering from ARF, less than 5% require long-term dialysis or renal transplantation. Approximately 50% of survivors of ARF exhibit subclinical renal functional or anatomic abnormalities. Furthermore, 5% of survivors display progressive deterioration in renal function subsequent to an initial recovery period. It is important to recognize that ARF is often a marker of severe subclinical disease (cardiovascular) and reflects overall prognosis. Despite profound advances in supportive care, mortality rates in ARF have not changed in the past 30 years. The best treatment is preventive care. Education of the patient and awareness of the physician about the factors contributing to ARF formulate the optimal means of combating ARF.

CHRONIC RENAL FAILURE

method of
JOHN T. HARRINGTON, M.D.
Tufts University School of Medicine
Boston, Massachusetts

The changes in management of patients with chronic renal failure (CRF) during the last 50 years border on the miraculous. In the late 1940s, just after the end of World War II, knowledge of renal physiology was in its early adolescence and knowledge of renal pathology was limited to information gleaned from postmortem examination. Percutaneous renal biopsy did not exist, nor did specialized methods of examination of renal tissue (e.g., immunofluorescence microscopy and electron microscopy). In fact, nephrology as a defined subspecialty of internal medicine did not exist in the United States until the early 1970s. The terminology of renal disease was similarly limited, with "Bright's disease" being used as an all-encompassing term for patients with any type of renal disease. Low-protein diets had been popularized by Addis in the 1930s and 1940s, as it was known that some systemic symptoms of advanced renal failure (e.g., nausea, vomiting, and pruritus) could be alleviated by a low-protein diet, but progress in rigorous quantitative evaluation of such a dietary approach (and its potential complications) had to wait nearly 50 years before being carried out (see later). Management of even such a major complication of CRF as hyperkalemia was also in its infancy. The low-salt rice diet, which contained only 7 mEq of sodium per day, was the only (partially) effective treatment of hypertension in the early 1940s until reserpine was introduced in the late 1940s, followed by thiazide diuretics, ganglionic-blocking agents, and α-methyldopa (Aldomet) in the 1950s.

Such a state of limited information continued for another 10 to 20 years. Only in the last 25 years has a firm understanding of renal physiology, renal pathology, and renal pathophysiology culminated in a revolution in the management of CRF. Dialysis for CRF began slowly in the early 1960s, becoming widespread only after federal reimbursement for chronic dialysis became available in 1973. Similarly, renal transplantation has been widely available only in the last 25 years. At the end of 1993, some 60,000 patients in the United States were alive with a functioning kidney transplant. Overall, approximately 250,000 patients with end-stage renal disease (ESRD) are now alive in the United States as a result of such therapy, compared with an estimated 11,000 patients in 1973. Thus, patients with CRF now at least have the safety net of renal replacement therapy. Moreover, some treatments have more recently been shown to slow the once inexorable progression of chronic renal insufficiency, and it seems likely that in the next 5 to 10 years we will be able to truly halt the progression of CRF.

DEFINITION

CRF has been variably defined by investigators and clinicians in the last half century. Theoretically, one could define it by a specified reduction in glomerular filtration rate (GFR), measured either directly (e.g., inulin) or indirectly by creatinine clearance or serum creatinine levels. Alternatively, one could define CRF symptomatically by the presentation of signs and symptoms of renal failure such as nausea, vomiting, and pruritus or by presentation in florid uremia, requiring immediate institution of dialysis.

The normal GFR in adults is approximately 125 to 130 mL per minute. Individuals with a GFR greater than 40 mL per minute have few if any symptoms attributable to renal insufficiency, whereas uremia is virtually always present if the GFR is below 10 mL per minute. In the remainder of this section, I refer to patients with chronic renal disease (e.g., proteinuria) but with normal renal function as being in phase I; asymptomatic patients with a GFR of 40 to 80 mL per minute as being in phase II; symptomatic patients with a GFR between 10 to 40 mL per minute as being in phase III; and patients with a GFR of less than 10 mL per minute as being in phase IV, that is, ESRD requiring urgent dialysis. A full discussion of the measurement of renal function utilizing inulin or iothalamate clearance, serum creatinine levels, creatinine clearance, or the Cockcroft-Gault formula for approximating creatinine clearance can be found elsewhere.* This discussion assumes that the specific cause of CRF has been determined on clinical grounds or as a result of renal biopsy. At a minimum, all patients with evidence of renal disease should have a full history and physical examination, an estimation of renal function (e.g., serum creatinine levels), quantitative measurement of urinary protein excretion, examination of the urinary sediment by the clinician, and renal echography.

CAUSES

The causes of CRF are many, but at the present time in the United States the majority of patients who progress to ESRD can be conveniently classified as having diabetes, primary glomerular disease, hypertensive renal disease, cystic renal disease, or primary urologic disease. For instance, data from the 1996 United States Renal Data System (USRDS) report on morbidity and mortality in dialysis Medicare patients (approximately 93% of all patients treated for ESRD in the United States) reveal that 56,000 patients began chronic dialysis therapy in 1993 (Table 1). Diabetes, hypertension, and glomerular disease accounted for approximately 70% of the reported cases in 1993. Approximately 54% of the ESRD population is male. The predilection of men for ESRD is especially marked for hypertension, glomerulonephritis, obstructive uropathy, malignancy, congenital or hereditary diseases, and ac-

---

*See Levey AS: Measurement of renal function in chronic renal disease. Kidney Int 38:167–184, 1990.

TABLE 1. Causes of End-Stage Renal Disease in the United States in 1993

Primary Diagnosis	Number	Percentage
Diabetes	19,013	34
Hypertension	15,064	27
Glomerulonephritis	5,655	10
Cystic kidney disease	1,397	2
Other urologic disease	2,199	4
Other diseases	3,620	6
Unknown cause	9,652	17
	56,600	100

quired immune deficiency syndrome–related ESRD. Women predominate in diabetes, most collagen-vascular diseases (e.g., lupus), and interstitial nephritis. The incidence of ESRD is four times higher in blacks than in whites because of a higher incidence of diabetes, hypertension, and glomerulonephritis. Native Americans have the higher incidence of ESRD due to diabetes. The United States and Japan have the highest rates of treated ESRD patients per million population. Canada's rate, the next highest, is approximately one half that of the United States, whereas the rate in Western Europe is approximately one third that in the United States.

REVERSIBLE RENAL FAILURE

Several different pathophysiologic mechanisms can cause a sudden deterioration of renal function in patients with previously stable CRF, so-called acute-on-chronic renal failure. The guiding clinical rule in such situations is to assume initially that the loss of function is due to potentially reversible factors rather than to the natural progression of the patient's underlying renal disease. There are several common causes of reversible renal failure (discussed later) and other less common causes, e.g., hypercalcemia.

Renal Hypoperfusion

Renal hypoperfusion from extracellular fluid volume depletion, congestive heart failure (CHF), or impaired renal hemodynamics (collectively termed "prerenal azotemia") is the most common cause of reversible renal failure. Because both NaCl and H_2O depletion and CHF can lead to comparable reductions in renal perfusion (and thus rises in blood urea nitrogen and serum creatinine concentration), obviously the clinician must first determine the volume status of the CRF patient with a sudden loss of renal function. The history (as always) is critical, as is the physical examination. The clinician should particularly search for a decrease in skin turgor and an orthostatic fall in blood pressure. In complex situations, measurement of pulmonary capillary wedge pressure may be required, but catheterization of the central circulation should not be employed routinely, given recent clinical data suggesting that such catheterization carries a significant risk. Patients with chronic renal insufficiency of any magnitude are susceptible to NaCl and H_2O depletion, but, for several reasons, it is more likely to happen in the patient with symptomatic renal failure. First, it unfortunately remains a common practice to reflexly restrict NaCl intake in patients with chronic renal disease. Second, many patients with chronic renal disease are unable to appropriately lower urinary sodium excretion if dietary intake is unduly restricted. Third, uremic nausea and vomiting may preclude normal dietary sodium intake. Finally, the injudicious use of diuretics may lead to sodium depletion. Sodium restriction, in fact, is not indicated in patients with chronic renal disease who are not edematous and who do not have CHF. Moreover, occasional patients, for instance, those with medullary cystic disease, may require as much as 10 to 15 grams of NaCl per day to remain in sodium balance.

Treatment of NaCl and H_2O depletion consists of (1) cessation of diuretic therapy; (2) institution of a normal NaCl diet and an additional 5 to 10 grams of NaCl per day as salt tablets if the patient can eat; and (3) intravenous administration of isotonic NaCl if the patient cannot eat or severe volume depletion exists. The patient must be weighed at least once and preferably twice daily, a nearly impossible task during today's whirlwind hospital stay. The total volume of saline necessary for repletion cannot be predicted by using serum electrolyte levels but must be determined clinically by evaluation of skin turgor, serial orthostatic blood pressure measurements, and if necessary, central venous pressure measurements. Normal saline (0.9%) is usually all that is required to repair volume depletion. If the patient is severely acidotic (p[HCO_3^-] less than 15 mEq per liter), a convenient intravenous solution to use is 0.45 N saline with 50 mEq of $NaHCO_3$ added to each liter.

CHF can also result in a substantial reduction in renal perfusion (and a disproportionate rise in blood urea nitrogen concentration), so evidence for NaCl and H_2O overload must be sought in all patients with acute-on-chronic renal failure, i.e., edema (particularly sacral edema in the hospitalized patient), rales, and chest radiographic findings of fluid overload. These CHF patients must be salt restricted and treated, e.g., with digoxin, diuretics, or angiotensin-converting enzyme (ACE) inhibitors.

In addition to these classic causes of renal hypoperfusion, we now know that ACE inhibitors and nonsteroidal anti-inflammatory drugs (NSAIDs) can abruptly reduce renal perfusion in certain patients, including patients with borderline volume depletion, CHF, renal artery stenosis, or CRF itself. Accordingly, a meticulous drug history must be taken in these patients, especially asking for a history of the use of ACE inhibitors or over-the-counter and prescription NSAIDs. These agents must be withheld if their use is temporally associated with an abrupt decline in renal function.

Prerenal azotemia from any cause can progress to frank acute tubular necrosis (ATN), especially if the patient is exposed to other nephrotoxins simultaneously (see later). Moreover, CRF patients subjected to a major surgical procedure are at special risk of postoperative prerenal azotemia and ATN. These patients frequently require on-line measurement of pulmonary capillary wedge pressures to determine optimal fluid management.

Urinary Tract Obstruction

The frequency and site of urinary tract obstruction depend on the patient's age, sex, and type of intrinsic renal disease. A few decades ago, intravenous pyelography with nephrotomography was the procedure of choice. At present, renal echography is preferred and, as noted earlier, should be done as part of the baseline evaluation in all patients with renal disease. One needs to look for the presence of two kidneys, the presence of cysts, hydronephrosis in one or both kidneys, significant differences in size (>1.5 cm) between the two kidneys, and so forth. Renal echography demonstrates structure, not function, and color-Doppler studies or isotopic renal scans may need to be done to determine the percentage of function of each kidney in certain circumstances. Ordinarily, if there is no a priori suspicion of obstruction and renal echography shows normal- or equal-sized kidneys without hydronephrosis, no further testing is required. If the patient (with a sudden decline in renal function) has only one kidney and even a trace of hydronephrosis, unilateral retrograde pyelography should be performed. Relief of any obstruction present (using either an internal or an external approach) should be carried out as soon as possible. If the patient is uremic, dialysis should be performed before major surgery.

Urinary Tract Infection

Bacterial urinary tract infection is a common occurrence in patients with a variety of renal diseases. However, acute functional deterioration does not occur unless pyelonephritis is clinically present (e.g., chills, fever, flank, pain, dysuria). However, immunosuppressed patients with fungal pyelonephritis and progressive loss of renal function may not appear as septic as their counterparts with bacterial pyelonephritis. Accordingly, urine fungal cultures should be obtained in patients with pyelonephritis not responding to conventional antibacterial agents. The choice of antibiotics and the route of administration depend on the severity of the infection and the degree of renal failure. In a patient with asymptomatic bacteriuria and mild renal failure (phase II), a trimethoprim-sulfamethoxazole agent (Bactrim, Septra) is appropriate. In patients with more advanced renal failure (phase III), most urinary tract infections can be treated with oral ampicillin, 1.0 to 2.0 grams per day for 10 days or with ciprofloxacin (Cipro) in a dose of 250 to 500 mg twice daily. On the other hand, in patients with severely compromised renal function (advanced phase III; phase IV) and acute pyelonephritis, hospitalization is mandatory and parenteral administration of a cephalosporin and/or an aminoglycoside derivative is indicated. Obviously, urine cultures must be obtained before treatment and antibiotics should be chosen on the basis of in vitro sensitivity tests. Urine cultures should also be obtained 48 to 72 hours after the institution of therapy to determine its efficacy. The loading dose of any antibiotic (or any other drug) given to a patient with renal failure is not different from that given to a patient with normal renal function. However, the subsequent dose and frequency of administration must be adjusted on the basis of renal function (see the 1996 edition of the *Medical Letter Handbook of Antimicrobial Therapy*).

Drug-Induced Renal Dysfunction

In addition to renal hypoperfusion due to the use of ACE inhibitors or NSAIDs, a number of drugs can cause ATN in patients with CRF, just as they can in patients without underlying renal disease. Aminoglycosides and contrast agents remain the most common causes of drug-induced ATN. These agents should be used only when absolutely indicated and then in appropriate dosages. In regard to contrast media, there is some slight evidence that nonionic agents may be less nephrotoxic. More importantly, one should use as small a dose as possible, and not carry out back-to-back studies, still an all too frequent cause of superimposed ATN in CRF patients. In patients in whom contrast media must be given, the latest evidence suggests that 0.45 N saline given intravenously at a rate of 100 mL per hour for 12 hours before administration of contrast material can substantially lower the likelihood of contrast medium–associated acute renal failure.

COMPLICATIONS AND TREATMENT

Hypertension

Hypertension is a major problem in patients with CRF. We have known for years that its control is critical in preventing nonrenal complications of hypertension such as strokes and CHF. We have also known that the prevalence and severity of hypertension increase as renal function slowly deteriorates. Important data have accrued strongly suggesting that strict control of the secondary hypertension of CRF can decelerate the progression of CRF. The U.S. Modification of Diet in Renal Disease (MDRD) study, a multicenter trial of the effects of dietary protein restriction and strict blood pressure control, initially screened 1795 patients with renal disease; few diabetic patients were enrolled in this study. Nearly 1500 patients (83%) were classified as hypertensive. Although 90% or so of the hypertensive patients were being treated actively, nearly 50% had blood pressure levels greater than the Fifth Joint National Committee on Detection, Evaluation, and Treatment of High Blood Pressure criteria for hypertension (>140 mm Hg systolic and >90 mm Hg diastolic). The prevalence of hypertension rose from 66% in patients with a modest reduction (83 mL per minute: phase II) in

GFR to 95% in patients with severe renal failure (GFR $\cong$ 12 mL per minute; phase IV). The prevalence of hypertension was slightly higher in men than in women and substantially higher in blacks than in whites. Moreover, the prevalence of hypertension varied directly with increasing body mass (independently of GFR) and with increasing age. Sophisticated statistical analysis demonstrated the importance of five factors ("predictors") in the hypertension of chronic renal failure (in decreasing order of significance): (1) low GFR; (2) high body mass; (3) black race; (4) increasing age; (5) male sex. Interestingly, salt intake was not a determinant of blood pressure status in the MDRD study.

These data from patients in the baseline cohort of the MDRD study regarding the factors related to the genesis of hypertension are especially important given the overall results of the MDRD study (approximately 840 patients were followed for a full 3 years) as well as similar studies from Europe.* In essence, these studies strongly suggest that the strict control of hypertension (to a level of <125/75 mm Hg) leads to significant slowing of the rate of progression of renal failure, at least in patients with a urinary protein excretion rate of greater than 1 gram per day. In the U.S. MDRD study, hypertension was controlled with a variety of antihypertensive agents, so no conclusions can be drawn from that study regarding the relative importance of using, e.g., ACE inhibitors, calcium channel blockers, or beta blockers. However, in many experimental studies of progressive renal failure (e.g., the remnant kidney model), ACE inhibitors have been shown to lower glomerular capillary pressure, decrease proteinuria, and slow the progression to renal failure. More importantly, in humans with diabetic renal disease, strict blood pressure control with captopril (Capoten), initially 25 mg three times per day, has been shown to significantly retard the progression of diabetic nephropathy (in comparison to a control group of patients whose blood pressure was comparably reduced by antihypertensive agents other than ACE inhibitors), as well as to reduce proteinuria.† In addition, similar studies in patients with IgA nephropathy have shown that ACE inhibitors can retard the progression of renal failure in this common glomerular disease. Thus, in patients with renal failure due to IgA nephropathy or to diabetic nephropathy, ACE inhibitors unequivocally should be employed. Side effects of captopril, such as cough and hyperkalemia, need to be kept in mind. Other ACE inhibitors presumably have a similar protective effect, but the major U.S. study thus far investigated only captopril. Whether angiotensin II receptor antagonists will be similarly renoprotective in

---

*See Klahr S, Levey AS, Beck GJ, et al: The effects of dietary protein restriction and blood-pressure control on the progression of chronic renal disease. Modification of Diet in Renal Disease Study Group. N Engl J Med 330:877–884, 1994.

†See Lewis EJ, Hunsicker LG, Bain RP, Rohde RD: The effect of angiotensin-converting-enzyme inhibition on diabetic nephropathy. The Collaborative Study Group. N Engl J Med 329:1456–1462, 1993.

humans is unknown at present. No clinical trials comparing ACE inhibitors and angiotensin II receptor antagonists have been carried out.

Anemia

Despite the recognition by Richard Bright 150 years ago that anemia is frequently associated with chronic renal failure, the cause of this anemia was imperfectly understood until the 1950s. At that time, experimental studies demonstrated two critical facts: (1) erythropoietin stimulates the production of red blood cells in the bone marrow, and (2) the major site (90%) of the production of erythropoietin is the kidney. Despite these studies, the central role of erythropoietin in causing the anemia of renal failure was not conclusively proved until the molecular cloning of the erythropoietin gene in the early 1980s, and the resultant introduction of recombinant human erythropoietin (rHuEpo) into clinical practice in July 1989. Before rHuEpo's widespread use, the anemia of renal failure was ascribed to various combinations of (1) erythropoietin deficiency, (2) bleeding secondary to the platelet defect present in uremia, (3) shortened red blood cell survival, and (4) suppression of red blood cell production by retained uremic toxins.

We now know both that erythropoietin is essential for supporting erythropoiesis and that rHuEpo can correct the anemia of severe renal failure and of ESRD in the vast majority of patients. Nationally, the mean hematocrit in Medicare dialysis patients using rHuEpo rose from 27% in mid-1989 to 31% in late 1994. The source of erythropoietin in normal individuals is most probably a population of peritubular interstitial fibroblasts signaled to produce increased amounts of erythropoietin by tissue hypoxia (caused by the low circulating red blood cell mass). Early studies demonstrated that rHuEpo, administered intravenously three times per week, raised the hematocrit by 1% per week (with 50 units per kg three times per week) to 1.8% per week (with 150 units per kg three times per week). To maintain the hematocrit in the range of 33 to 38%, doses of rHuEpo of between 20 and 100 units per kg per week were required in the majority of patients, with one third requiring larger doses. Interestingly, when the hematocrit is raised to greater than 30% by rHuEpo, there is substantial improvement in platelet function.

In the last 10 years, rHuEpo has been used successfully in thousands of patients in the United States and around the world. The benefits have been profound. The utilization of blood transfusions has dropped dramatically, thereby reducing or eliminating the risks of the blood-borne viral diseases, as well as iron overload. The higher hematocrit has provided both cardiovascular and noncardiovascular benefits. Moreover, the fatigue of CRF in large part has been found to be due to anemia, not uremia. An improvement in sexual function, especially in men, has been noted as well as improved appetite, lessening of depression, better sleep pattern, and an overall increase in the feeling of well-being.

Do problems persist? The answer, not too surprising, given the complexity of clinical medicine and the cost of rHuEpo, is yes. First, the optimal use of rHuEpo remains controversial, including the best ways of determining the cause of a diminished responsiveness to rHuEpo (e.g., iron deficiency), and what is the best route (and dose) of administration of rHuEpo. There has been some shift from the intravenous to the subcutaneous route simply because the latter route allows a one third or so reduction in dose with similar results, obviously leading to substantial cost savings; rHuEpo can also be given intraperitoneally in patients being treated with peritoneal dialysis. The subcutaneous route is particularly an advantage when rHuEpo is being used in patients whose renal failure has not yet reached the end stage. The bioavailability of subcutaneously administered rHuEpo seems higher when it is injected into the thigh. At present, a conventional starting dose (for the subcutaneous route) is 20 to 30 units per kg (1000 to 2000 units per dose) three times per week, aiming for a target hematocrit of 30 to 35%. Once the target hematocrit level is elevated, a lower dose can be used, often given once per week (e.g., 2000 to 4000 units). Whether or not rHuEpo will prolong life in dialysis patients has not yet been proved, although intuitively it seems likely. The proven reduction in left ventricular end-diastolic diameter after rHuEpo treatment suggests that rHuEpo might decrease the long-term cardiovascular mortality rate, but that remains to be demonstrated. Nevertheless, it is fair to say that treatment with rHuEpo has revolutionized the care of chronic dialysis patients.

Azotemic Osteodystrophy

Abnormalities in calcium and phosphorus handling are virtually universal in patients with progressive renal failure. Phosphate is normally excreted by a combination of glomerular filtration and tubular reabsorption. Typically, the serum phosphate level remains normal until the GFR falls to less than 25% of normal. At that time, phosphate retention and hyperphosphatemia ensue. We have known for years that the rise in the serum phosphate level is associated with a fall in the serum calcium level. The resultant hypocalcemia (in combination with other factors) stimulates parathyroid hormone production, causing the secondary hyperparathyroidism of CRF. The increase in parathyroid hormone production, designed to normalize the serum calcium level, causes a loss of bone calcium. Simultaneously, parathyroid hormone suppresses renal tubular phosphate reabsorption, providing a defense against hyperphosphatemia until the GFR falls to less than 25% of normal. Thus, the majority of patients with CRF have secondary hyperparathyroidism, and if it is not appropriately treated, azotemic osteodystrophy can ensue.

Simultaneously with the hyperphosphatemia, hypocalcemia, and secondary hyperparathyroidism is a deficient renal production of the active form of vitamin D (1,25-dihydroxycholecalciferol). The lack of vitamin D in turn decreases gastrointestinal calcium absorption, leads to negative total body calcium balance, and diminishes bone calcium content in nearly all patients with phases III and IV CRF. If the serum creatinine concentration rises to greater than approximately 4 mg per dL, one should prescribe a calcium supplement, usually calcium carbonate (500 mg two or three times daily with meals), both to provide a source of calcium and to bind phosphate in the gut. Exogenous 1,25-dihydroxycholecalciferal (calcitriol [Rocaltrol]) is required in all patients with ESRD and should be used in most patients with CRF (and proven secondary hyperparathyroidism) and a serum creatinine level of greater than 4 mg per dL (phases III and IV); the dose ranges from 0.25 to 0.75 µg per day. Frequent measurements of the serum calcium level are required to prevent (or detect) hypercalcemia from the exogenous active form of vitamin D. The serum phosphorus level can be maintained below 5 mg per dL by dietary phosphate restriction; this is usually accomplished by simply restricting dietary protein intake to 0.6 to 0.8 kg per day and restricting foods rich in phosphate, such as dairy products and cola-colored soft drinks. In the past, aluminum hydroxide was used to prevent the serum phosphate level from rising above 5 mg per dL, but because of problems with hyperaluminemia (and aluminum-induced bone disease), current practice is to use calcium carbonate rather than aluminum hydroxide. However, if the serum calcium level is greater than 11 mg per dL (or the calcium-phosphate product is >60 to 70), aluminum hydroxide should be used initially because of the risk of provoking more serious hypercalcemia and metastatic calcification. Clinical trials are now under way testing the efficacy of poly[allylamine hydrochloride] (RenaGel), a noncalcium, nonaluminum phosphate-binding agent.* In patients whose plasma bicarbonate concentration has fallen to less than 20 mEq per liter, calcium carbonate may also aid in offsetting uremic acidosis, but often sodium bicarbonate (1 to 2 tablets two or three times per day) is required. With dietary restriction of phosphate and the use of calcium carbonate and exogenous vitamin D, secondary hyperparathyroidism can be ameliorated, pruritus may be reduced, and azotemic osteodystrophy can be prevented.

Protein Restriction

As mentioned earlier, dietary protein restriction has been used for at least 50 years to ameliorate some of the symptoms of progressive renal failure. However, rigorous quantitative investigations of the effect of dietary protein restriction on the progression

of CRF have been available only since the late 1980s. The major U.S. study, the MDRD study (referred to earlier) had inconclusive results overall. Nevertheless, the slower decline in renal function that started 4 months after the initiation of a low-protein diet (0.6 gram per kg per day) in patients with moderate renal insufficiency (GFR of 25 to 55 mL per minute; phase II and early phase III) suggested a small benefit of protein restriction. In addition, a subsequent secondary analysis of the MDRD data revealed an approximately 30% reduction in the rate of decline in GFR in patients with more severe CRF (GFR of 13 to 24 mL per minute; advanced phase III).

Despite these (and other) reports, consensus has not been reached on the efficacy of protein restriction in reducing the rate of decline in GFR in patients with CRF. Before a decade or so ago, clinical investigators would have at least considered conducting a "stronger" study, e.g., using more patients and following up the patients for a longer time period. In the 1990s, a meta-analysis is often done instead. And a rigorous meta-analysis of the effect of dietary protein restriction on the progression of renal disease has been carried out.* These mathematical investigators concluded that dietary protein restriction does indeed retard progression to renal failure, in both patients with insulin-dependent diabetic renal disease and those with nondiabetic renal disease. Unfortunately, even this meta-analysis showed only a slowing of the progression to renal failure, not cessation of progression. Finally, although fears of protein-calorie malnutrition due to rigid adherence to a low-protein diet have been raised, most nutritional studies of patients with CRF suggest that a prescribed protein intake of 0.6 gram per kg per day, with approximately 65% in high-biologic-value protein and a caloric intake sufficient to maintain body weight, is safe. In patients with heavy proteinuria (>10 grams per day), the dietary protein intake must be increased to offset the urinary protein loss, which otherwise could lead to malnutrition. Consultation with a knowledgeable clinical dietitian is required to obtain optimal benefit of a low-protein diet (0.6 gram per kg per day). Patients in phase III or IV CRF should also be instructed in a 2-gram potassium diet (for treatment of hyperkalemia, see the article "Acute Renal Failure"). In patients with diabetic renal disease, a low-protein diet should be used in conjunction with intensive control of blood glucose and blood pressure, the latter preferably with an ACE inhibitor.

RENAL REPLACEMENT THERAPY

Like Gaul, renal replacement therapy has three components: peritoneal dialysis (PD), hemodialysis, and renal transplantation. To lay out the pros and cons of each component and thus help patients make

---

*See Chertow GM, Burke SK, Lazarus JM, et al: Poly[allylamine hydrochloride] (RenaGel): A noncalcemic phosphate binder for the treatment of hyperphosphatemia in chronic renal failure. Am J Kidney Dis 29:66–71, 1997.

*See Pedrini MT, Levey AS, Lau J, et al: The effect of dietary protein restriction on the progression of diabetic and nondiabetic renal diseases: A meta-analysis. Ann Intern Med 124:627–632, 1996.

an informed choice of therapy, it is best that every patient with progressive CRF be referred to a nephrologist when the serum creatinine concentration rises to greater than 2.0 to 2.5 mg per dL. Such an early referral also allows timely creation of a native or an artificial arteriovenous fistula.

PD employs the patient's own peritoneum as the semipermeable membrane across which retained uremic toxins diffuse. PD accounted for 15.1% of all dialysis patients at the end of 1993. Several PD options are available, the most common being continuous ambulatory PD (CAPD). The patient usually has four to six 2-liter exchanges daily, the fluid "sitting" in the peritoneal cavity for 4 to 8 hours (dwell time). Recent studies indicate that the prescribed dose of CAPD is inadequate in as many as 25% of patients. Continuous cycling PD (CCPD) uses several exchanges at night via a programmed cycle system, with one long dwell time during the day. Although the fraction of patients using CCPD has increased, CCPD still accounts for only one tenth of CAPD use. Other PD options exist. Both CAPD and CCPD must be performed daily by the patient and thus require patients with a strong desire for self-care. As the PD technique failure rate remains high, approximately 50% at 3 years, patients must often switch to hemodialysis therapy or opt for renal transplantation.

Hemodialysis, the most common form of renal replacement therapy (approximately 60% of all ESRD patients at the end of 1993), employs a dialyzer (the artificial kidney) to remove uremic toxins and excess NaCl and H_2O. Usually employed three times weekly (for 3 to 4 hours per treatment), virtually all hemodialysis patients are cared for in an outpatient, hospital-based unit or a free-standing dialysis unit. Although home hemodialysis encourages independence of the patient, the fraction of patients using home hemodialysis has been falling since the mid-1980s, accounting for only 2.4% of all ESRD patients at the end of 1993. Less complicated dialysis machinery is in development that could, along with economic incentives, stimulate the regrowth of home hemodialysis as we approach the next millennium. The 1-year death rate for dialysis patients decreased from 36% in 1983 to 26% for those beginning dialysis in 1993. Moreover, hemodialysis patients continue to be plagued by a variety of problems including dialysis-associated hypotension and arrhythmias, as well as serious fistula problems (infection and clotting). Not too surprisingly, these patients continue to have high rates of hospitalization, averaging 11 to 12 days in the hospital annually, although overall, there were fewer admissions and an even greater reduction in the number of days in the hospital in 1993 than in the preceding year.

Renal transplant patients accounted for 27.3% of all ESRD Medicare patients at the end of 1993. A total of 10,954 kidneys were transplanted in the United States in 1993. Cadaveric donors constituted the vast majority (74%) of these allografts, but there has been a steady increase in the number of transplantations from living donors. The number of cadaveric transplantations increased steeply in the decades before 1986. Only a small increase occurred between 1986 and 1990, and there was no increase between 1990 and the end of 1993. As a consequence, the number of patients awaiting a kidney transplant has risen from approximately 9000 in 1984 to nearly 31,000 in 1995. Previously transplanted patients now account for 25 to 30% of candidates on the waiting list. In turn this gap between supply and demand has promoted a greater utilization of living emotionally related transplantation (usually from a spouse). Transplantation from a spousal donor results in similar or perhaps in a 10% increase in survival rate (when compared with parent-to-offspring grafts). Thus, living, emotionally related kidney transplantation has the potential to bring the advantages of transplantation to several thousands of patients. The primary care physician should explore this possibility in all patients with progressive CRF even before they begin dialysis.

Recipients of living related donor and cadaveric donor transplants survive longer than do comparable dialysis patients. Trade-offs exist, however, given the necessity for using potent immunosuppresive drugs such as cyclosporine (Sandimmune), azathioprine (Imuran), prednisone, or OKT3 to combat rejection. The 1-year cadaveric graft survival rate now exceeds 85% in many centers nationwide, and 1-year living related donor graft survival now exceeds 90%, a 16 and 7% increase, respectively, when compared with 1984. The average "half-life" for a cadaver kidney is approximately 7 to 8 years and 14 to 15 years for a living related allograft. Cardiac causes account for approximately 28% of all deaths, with infectious diseases and cancer being the next most common causes of death. All these results of the various options of renal replacement therapy have improved dramatically in the past 25 years. Fifty years ago, when the first edition of this book appeared, none existed. (Virtually all the specific data from this last section were taken from the 1996 *Annual Data Report* of the USRDS, which can be accessed on the Internet at http://www.med.umich.edu/usrds/.)

MALIGNANT TUMORS OF THE UROGENITAL TRACT

method of
RICHARD S. FOSTER, M.D.
Indiana University Medical Center
Indianapolis, Indiana

PROSTATE CARCINOMA

Cancer of the prostate is the most common cancer in men. Adenocarcinoma is the predominant histologic type and is the focus of the following discussion. Rarer histologic subtypes may be managed differently.

The autopsy prevalence of adenocarcinoma of the prostate increases with increasing age. The chance of discovering adenocarcinoma at autopsy in men older than 80 years is greater than 50%. Development of adenocarcinoma is dependent on androgens. One of the greatest difficulties in managing patients with adenocarcinoma of the prostate is the unpredictable natural history of the disease. Although such parameters as the grade of the tumor, prostate-specific antigen (PSA) level, and volume of cancer are predictors of clinical course in the aggregate, these factors are incapable of predicting the clinical course in an individual patient. This singular fact has led to great controversy regarding optimal management of patients with localized disease. Similarly, because some adenocarcinomas of the prostate grow quite slowly, a period of 10 to 15 years may be required for the expression of the natural history of the tumor. Therefore, studies of treatments of prostate cancer require 10 to 15 years of follow-up to determine whether or not therapy is effective. These two facts (extended natural history and unpredictable course in an individual patient) are the reason that few adequately powered comparative studies in the treatment of localized cancer of the prostate exist.

Detection

Although the autopsy prevalence of histologic adenocarcinoma of the prostate is high, only about 10% of men are ultimately diagnosed clinically with the disease. About 2 to 3% die from adenocarcinoma of the prostate. Therefore, earlier detection of the 3% of men destined to die from the disease would be ideal to potentially affect the course of the disease. A larger group of men with histologic-only adenocarcinoma of the prostate would then be spared diagnosis of the disease that would likely not affect their survival. Hence, the goal should be to detect aggressive prostate cancer while not detecting it in the larger group of men who have histologic prostate cancer without any clinical sequelae.

Localized cancer of the prostate was traditionally diagnosed by digital rectal examination. This examination remains an important component of diagnosis. Most cancers detected on digital rectal examination are clinically important. PSA is an enzyme that circulates in the serum and is prostate specific. Adenocarcinoma, benign prostatic hyperplasia, prostatitis, and prostate infarction can all lead to elevations of serum PSA levels. Although PSA assay is the best single test for detection of adenocarcinoma of the prostate, a combination of PSA and digital rectal examination provides the best means of diagnosing localized disease. Most studies have suggested that the majority of patients diagnosed by PSA testing have clinically important cancers, although this area is highly controversial. This has led to considerable discussion regarding the usefulness of PSA as a screening test for adenocarcinoma of the prostate. Although advocates exist for and against screening with PSA, it has yet to be shown that PSA-based screening has decreased the mortality from adenocarcinoma of the prostate. Such screening studies are ongoing.

Localized adenocarcinoma of the prostate is generally asymptomatic. If urinary obstruction, urinary symptoms, perineal pain, weight loss, or bone pain ensues, the disease is generally extraprostatic and therefore not amenable to curative therapy.

Diagnosis and Staging

The diagnosis of localized adenocarcinoma of the prostate is generally made by transrectal ultrasonography and biopsy. Transrectal ultrasonography of the prostate was introduced in the 1980s. It was initially thought that characteristics of the ultrasound image of the prostate correlated with the presence of adenocarcinoma. Hypoechoic areas were generally thought to be diagnostic of adenocarcinoma. Subsequent studies have shown that the ultrasound image of the prostate is not a strong predictor of cancer. Transrectal ultrasonography remains useful as a means of verifying correct positioning of the biopsy needle. At the time of biopsy any palpable nodule is biopsied; if the biopsy is being performed for elevation of PSA levels in the absence of a palpable nodule, six distinct sections (three on each side) of the prostate are generally sampled. Men with normal rectal examinations and mildly elevated PSA levels have an approximate 25% chance of having prostate cancer. An abnormal rectal examination in conjunction with an elevated PSA level increases the probability of the diagnosis of adenocarcinoma.

Prostate carcinoma generally spreads to lymph nodes and bone. The higher the PSA level, the greater the likelihood of metastatic disease. Patients with lower PSA levels (<20 ng per mL) undergo digital rectal examination and bone scanning as staging modalities. If the PSA level is higher, computed tomography (CT) of the pelvis may be useful. Nonetheless, the ability to accurately predict localized disease by clinical tests is poor. Occasionally, laparoscopic removal of pelvic nodes is performed in patients at high risk of metastasis. This modality has the potential of sparing a patient with metastatic disease the morbidity of a lower midline incision.

Treatment of Localized Disease

Patients who are thought to have localized disease on the basis of clinical staging have several choices of therapy. This is because the natural history is unpredictable in an individual patient, and good comparative studies of the treatment modalities have not been performed. Because adenocarcinoma of the prostate may take many years to metastasize and lead to death, the life expectancy of the patient is also an important consideration.

Standard Therapies
Watchful Waiting

In some patients, adenocarcinoma of the prostate may take many years to express its natural history.

Instituting no therapy initially and following the patient with periodic rectal examinations and PSA determinations is known as watchful waiting. Watchful waiting is an option for all patients who present with clinically localized adenocarcinoma of the prostate but is generally applied to older patients who are believed to have a shorter life expectancy. Most patients older than 70 to 75 years with localized disease are managed with watchful waiting. However, any patient considered for watchful waiting should be advised of the inability of the physician to predict the natural history of the disease in an individual patient.

Studies from many centers around the world have shown that watchful waiting in properly selected patients leads to only an approximately 10% chance of dying of prostate cancer 10 years from the date of diagnosis. The grade of the tumor and the volume of localized disease are important predictors of the clinical course of a patient on a watchful waiting regimen. Patients should also be advised that if metastasis occurs, curative therapy for metastatic disease is not available. Rather, the patient is given palliative hormonal therapy.

Radical Prostatectomy

Radical prostatectomy involves the removal of the prostate and the seminal vesicles and the subsequent anastomosis of the bladder neck to the urethra. If adenocarcinoma of the prostate is truly confined to the prostate, the procedure is curative. The surgical approach to the prostate may be either perineal or retropubic. In the retropubic approach the lymph nodes are removed before the removal of the prostate. If nodal metastasis is found at the time of exploration, removal of the prostate is aborted, because pelvic nodal metastasis is a strong predictor of systemic metastasis.

Refinements in surgical technique in the 1980s have decreased the morbidity of the procedure. These refinements have led to less blood loss, a shorter time on the operating table, lower rates of incontinence, and preservation of potency in some men. The description of the anatomy of periprostatic nerves responsible for potency has led to a so-called nerve-sparing prostatectomy, which is capable of preserving erectile ability in selected patients.

Radical prostatectomy is generally an option for patients with a life expectancy greater than 10 years who present with clinically localized disease. Well-done studies comparing radical prostatectomy to external beam radiation therapy for the treatment of localized disease do not exist. Therefore, the choice of proceeding with radical prostatectomy is highly contingent on the patient's wishes.

The most important side effects of radical prostatectomy are incontinence and impotence. Roughly 3 to 5% of patients have significant urinary incontinence after radical prostatectomy and may require a subsequent surgical procedure to correct the incontinence. Another 10 to 15% of patients have stress incontinence after radical prostatectomy. Most studies have shown that approximately 80% of patients are perfectly continent after the procedure. If nerve sparing is done in a properly selected patient, the chance of maintaining potency postoperatively is 50 to 70%. The operative mortality of the procedure is less than 1%. After radical prostatectomy, patients are generally followed up with digital rectal examination (to detect local recurrence) and serial PSA testing. A detectable PSA after radical prostatectomy is an indication of disease recurrence.

External Beam Radiation Therapy

Although no adequately powered direct comparative studies of radical prostatectomy and radiation therapy for clinically localized disease have been performed, single institutional series of each treatment suggest that the efficacy of the two treatments is quite similar. External beam radiation therapy is generally administered in fractions during a period of 5 to 6 weeks. Approximately 10% of patients experience radiation proctitis or radiation cystitis that may be permanent. Sexual potency after external beam radiation therapy is preserved in approximately 60%.

After radical prostatectomy, pathologically confined disease and an undetectable PSA are strong predictors of a good prognosis. Such strong predictors do not exist after external beam radiation therapy. However, sanguine predictors after external beam radiation therapy include a PSA level less than 1 ng per mL and a negative postradiation biopsy. Although PSA testing is routine in clinical practice after radiation therapy, postradiation biopsies are not standard practice.

Investigational Therapies

Cryotherapy

Transperineal freezing of the prostate with liquid nitrogen is called cryotherapy. This treatment was used in the 1960s and 1970s and was abandoned. The availability of transrectal ultrasonography to monitor the amount of freezing has led to a resurgence in this therapy. Long-term (10 years) results of cryosurgical treatment of localized disease are not available, and therefore this procedure must be considered investigational.

Radioactive Seed Implantation

Transperineal placement of radioactive seeds of iodine or palladium is known as prostate brachytherapy. Brachytherapy was used with iodine in the 1970s and was abandoned because it was thought to be no more effective than external beam radiation therapy. The availability of transrectal ultrasonography to place the seeds more accurately has lead to a resurrection of this therapy. Although results 5 years after therapy look promising, no long-term results of modern brachytherapy are available. Therefore, this too must be considered investigational.

Treatment of Metastatic Disease

The most common sites of spread of adenocarcinoma of the prostate are lymph nodes and bones. Most patients are diagnosed with metastatic disease on the basis of an increasing or elevated PSA level. Subsequent verification of the site of metastasis is performed by bone scanning or CT. Metastatic disease is generally treated with either observation or hormonal therapy.

Approximately 70 to 80% of patients with metastatic disease experience a clinical remission if systemic androgens are suppressed. Roughly 90% of systemic androgen is produced in the testis, with the other 10% secreted by the adrenal gland. Suppression of systemic androgen production can be accomplished by either bilateral orchiectomy or administration of luteinizing hormone–releasing hormone (LHRH) agonists.* Estrogens were formerly given orally, but cardiovascular side effects led to the abandonment of this therapy. Bilateral orchiectomy or LHRH agonists suppress testicular production of androgens. Adrenal production of androgens can be blocked at the prostate level by administering oral antiandrogens.* Some studies have suggested that the combination of LHRH agonists and an oral antiandrogen is more effective than LHRH agonists alone. The results of a large cooperative group study of orchiectomy with or without oral antiandrogens should be available soon. This study should determine whether or not oral antiandrogens in conjunction with either orchiectomy or LHRH agonists should be considered standard therapy.

Hormonal therapy is palliative therapy. After the initiation of hormonal therapy, progression of disease is again noted in roughly 1.5 to 2 years. No effective therapy exists for this so-called hormone refractory disease. Numerous studies are being performed to improve the quality of life for these patients.

Some patients are discovered to have metastatic disease but are asymptomatic. Observing these patients until they develop symptomatic metastatic disease is entirely reasonable, because the early initiation of hormonal therapy has not been shown to improve survival in all such patients. Therefore, because hormonal therapy is palliative therapy, some physicians advise withholding it until symptomatic metastatic disease presents.

TRANSITIONAL CELL CARCINOMA

With the exception of the penile urethra, transitional cells line the entire urinary tract. If a patient develops transitional cell carcinoma in one part of the urinary tract, he is at greatly increased risk of developing transitional cell carcinoma elsewhere in the urinary tract. This concept is known as "field change." Therefore, patients who are treated for localized transitional cell carcinoma in one portion of the urinary tract need to be subsequently followed

*Not FDA approved for this indication.

up closely for the development of transitional cell carcinoma elsewhere in the urinary tract. Transitional cell carcinoma is characteristically divided into upper tract and lower tract disease. Upper tract signifies disease above the bladder; lower tract disease is cancer of the bladder or prostatic urethra.

Upper Tract Diagnosis

Hematuria is the most common sign of transitional cell carcinoma. The amount of hematuria does not correlate with the amount of abnormality. For this reason all patients presenting with hematuria require evaluation. This evaluation usually includes intravenous pyelography (IVP), cystoscopy, and urinary cytologic examination. Urinary cytologic examination is effective in diagnosing high-grade tumors but is not sensitive for low-grade transitional cell carcinoma. Conversely, cystoscopy can effectively identify low-grade tumors but may not identify high-grade carcinoma in situ. Therefore, the evaluation includes all three tests: IVP, cystoscopy, and cytologic examination. Urinary assays for antigens produced by transitional cell carcinoma have been introduced. If such tests become relatively inexpensive, they will likely be used more commonly in the future for the diagnosis of transitional cell carcinoma.

Upper Tract Disease

Transitional cell carcinoma of the renal pelvis or ureter is called upper tract carcinoma. Common sites of metastasis include lung, lymph nodes, and bone. Therefore, the staging evaluation includes CT of the abdomen and chest. If localized disease is believed to be present, the treatment of upper tract transitional cell carcinoma is surgical. If the patient has a normal contralateral kidney, standard therapy is nephroureterectomy with removal of a cuff of bladder tissue. The rationale for complete nephroureterectomy as opposed to nephrectomy alone is the high likelihood of associated dysplasia and transitional cell carcinoma in situ in the ureter. The likelihood of discovering diffuse changes of the upper tract urothelium on the side of the tumor is dependent on the grade of the tumor. For this reason, well-differentiated ureteral tumors are sometimes treated by segmental ureterectomy with reanastomosis to the bladder. Patients treated in this fashion are selected on the basis of having a low-grade tumor, generally in the distal ureter. Patients with solitary kidneys are treated more conservatively and monitored more closely after therapy. These more conservative therapies include endoscopic fulguration or resection of the primary tumor. The grade of the tumor is a strong predictor of the likelihood of recurrence.

Lower Tract Tumors

Transitional cell carcinoma of the bladder is more common in males. It is associated with smoking. There is evidence that various organic chemicals are also carcinogens. Because of different natural histories, bladder cancer is characteristically divided into superficial and muscle invasive. Superficial bladder cancer is generally of low grade; muscle invasive bladder cancer is characteristically of high grade. Superficial bladder cancer progresses to muscle invasion only about 10% of the time. Superficial bladder cancer is generally a local control problem, whereas invasive bladder cancer has a high propensity for metastasis and subsequent death from metastatic disease.

The diagnosis of superficial bladder cancer is made by transurethral resection of the bladder tumor. If the tumor does not invade into the muscularis propria it is termed superficial. Transurethral resection of superficial bladder tumors is definitive therapy. However, there is a strong tendency for subsequent recurrence in the bladder. This probably relates to the field change phenomenon. Most superficial bladder tumors are of low grade and rarely metastasize. Because of the high tendency for recurrence, periodic cystoscopy after initial transurethral resection is indicated.

Higher grade superficial bladder cancers that invade the lamina propria or carcinoma in situ of the bladder tend to behave more aggressively. Transurethral resection alone may suffice for some tumors invading the lamina propria, but generally these patients are given further therapy. The transurethral instillation of various agents has been shown to prolong the period of time between recurrences of such tumors. In addition, some intravesical agents have proved effective in the eradication of transitional cell carcinoma in situ. Characteristically, these agents are given once a week intravesically for 6 weeks.

The most common intravesical agent in use is bacille Calmette-Guérin (BCG) (Tice BCG, TheraCys). Although the exact mechanism of action is unknown, it is thought that BCG induces an immunologic reaction that leads to eradication of carcinoma in situ in some patients and prevention of subsequent superficial tumors. Whether or not BCG prevents progression to muscle invasive disease is unknown. Additional intravesical agents include thiotepa (Thioplex)*, and mitomycin (Mutamycin).* These intravesical agents are generally well tolerated. BCG is associated with a significant incidence of dysuria and constitutional symptoms. Rarely, systemic tubercular infection ensues and is treated with systemic antitubercular drugs.

The diagnosis of muscle invasive bladder cancer is made by transurethral resection of the tumor. The presence of tumor invading muscularis propria is indicative of a much more aggressive tumor diathesis. These tumors tend to be multifocal within the bladder, and therefore partial cystectomy (removal of only the tumor) is generally not effective. Therefore, standard therapy of muscle invasive bladder cancer involves cystoprostatectomy with subsequent urinary diversion. These diversions include ileal loop diversion, construction of a continent urinary reservoir, and bladder replacement. Ileal loop diversion in-

volves the creation of a urostomy with subsequent wearing of an appliance to collect the urine. This is the most time tested method of urinary diversion. A continent urinary reservoir is an internal reservoir made of bowel that the patient subsequently catheterizes on a periodic basis to empty the reservoir. No external appliance is necessary. Some patients choose to catheterize in lieu of wearing an external appliance. Bladder replacement is the creation of a reservoir that is anastomosed to the urethra in men or women. Patients then void by a Valsalva maneuver and generally have excellent continence during the day. Approximately 15 to 20% of patients experience nighttime incontinence. The choice of urinary diversion after radical cystoprostatectomy is based on the patient's wishes.

Before cystoprostatectomy, staging includes CT of the pelvis, abdomen, and chest. Roughly 50% of patients who are believed to have localized invasive bladder cancer in fact have micrometastatic disease. Therefore, about 50% of patients who undergo radical cystectomy and urinary diversion subsequently develop metastatic disease. More accurate means of clinically staging patients are urgently needed.

External beam radiation therapy for invasive bladder cancer is associated with long-term disease-free recurrence of only about 15 to 20% of cases. Therefore, external beam radiation therapy is not considered standard therapy, at least in the United States. Concurrent administration of chemotherapy during external beam radiation therapy serves as a radiation sensitizer in some patients. So-called bladder-sparing therapy is being investigated. Although short-term results appear reasonable, recurrence of disease in the bladder in the long term has hampered the acceptance of such protocols. Therefore, they must be considered investigational.

Metastatic Disease

The standard treatment of metastatic transitional cell carcinoma usually involves the administration of methotrexate, vinblastine (Velban), and cisplatin (Platinol), with or without doxorubicin (Adriamycin). Combination of these agents has been shown to be more effective than cisplatin alone. Nonetheless, only about 10 to 15% of patients with metastatic disease experience a complete clinical remission, and some of these remissions are not sustained. Therefore, newer agents are being investigated.

TESTIS CANCER

Germ cell carcinoma of the testis is one of the most common cancers in young men. The presentation is characteristically of a painless firm testicular mass. Metastatic disease presents as lung nodules, back pain, or hemoptysis. Initial treatment of such a tumor involves radical inguinal orchiectomy. The inguinal incision is performed to avoid cutting into the tumor and contaminating the scrotum, which drains to an alternative lymphatic area (inguinal nodes).

---

*Not FDA approved for this indication.

Treatment of the patient after inguinal orchiectomy is dependent on the histologic subtype of the tumor and its clinical stage. Clinical staging involves CT of the abdomen and chest in conjunction with determination of serum levels of alpha-fetoprotein and β-human chorionic gonadotropin (β-HCG). Germ cell tumors of the testis are divided into seminomas and nonseminomas. This division is based on the exquisite sensitivity of seminomas to radiation therapy and the relative lack of sensitivity of nonseminomas to radiation therapy.

Seminoma

The treatment of pure seminoma is based on the clinical stage. Patients who have normal CT results for the abdomen and chest have an approximately 20% chance of having pathologic retroperitoneal disease. Because of this and because of the extreme sensitivity of seminomas to radiation therapy, most patients with no evidence of metastatic disease are treated with low-dose radiotherapy to the retroperitoneum. This is generally well tolerated and associated with a high chance for cure. Seminoma patients with low-volume (<5 cm) retroperitoneal disease may also be treated with radiation therapy. Although radiation therapy in this circumstance effectively controls retroperitoneal disease, these patients may need subsequent chemotherapy for distant metastatic disease. Alternatively, such patients can be treated with cisplatin-based systemic chemotherapy. Most patients with seminoma have an extremely good prognosis even in the presence of metastatic disease. Chemotherapy is generally quite effective in seminoma. Only patients with extremely high volumes of metastatic disease or extensive organ involvement have a poorer prognosis.

Nonseminoma

Approximately 70% of nonseminomas have elevations of serum alpha-fetoprotein or β-HCG levels. In fact, elevation of serum alpha-fetoprotein levels is diagnostic of nonseminoma in a patient with a testicular mass. After radical inguinal orchiectomy, CT of the abdomen and chest is performed. If CT reveals no evidence of metastasis and the serum alpha-fetoprotein and β-HCG levels return to normal, the patient is considered to have no evidence of metastatic disease. However, as with seminoma, roughly 30% of nonseminoma patients with a negative staging workup in fact have metastatic disease, most commonly in the retroperitoneum.

This inaccurate clinical staging has led to various treatment regimens for such patients. One option is a retroperitoneal lymph node dissection, with preservation of sympathetic efferent fibers to preserve emission and ejaculation. This procedure serves two purposes: (1) accurate staging and (2) therapy, because removal of metastatic disease is associated with long-term cure in 50 to 70% of patients. Because such a procedure has low morbidity, it is reasonable to offer it to all patients with no evidence of metastatic disease.

Another method of managing these patients is surveillance. Patients are periodically re-evaluated with serum alpha-fetoprotein and β-HCG levels and CT to identify the 30% of patients with metastatic disease. If metastatic disease is discovered, cisplatin-based chemotherapy is given with a good chance of long-term cure. Although no direct comparative studies of retroperitoneal lymph node dissection and surveillance have been performed, it is generally thought that either of these methods of management yields a chance of cure approaching 100%.

Nonseminoma patients who are found to have retroperitoneal metastatic disease at the time of presentation are categorized into two groups. The first group comprises those patients with minimal retroperitoneal disease only. These patients can be treated with either retroperitoneal lymph node dissection or primary chemotherapy. In general, the decision of which therapy to pursue is based on the patient's preference because the ultimate chance of being cured is similar with either modality.

Patients with distant metastatic disease are treated with systemic cisplatin-based chemotherapy. Approximately 70% of such patients experience a complete clinical remission, and many of these are sustained complete remissions. As with seminoma, some patients present with high-volume metastasis or visceral organ involvement. These patients have a poorer prognosis, but many, in fact, are cured. After systemic chemotherapy for metastatic disease, sometimes a partial clinical remission ensues. This is denoted by normalization of serum alpha-fetoprotein and β-HCG levels but persistence of radiographic tumor. These patients characteristically undergo postchemotherapy removal of residual radiographic tumor. Histologically, these tumors are composed of teratoma, necrosis, or active carcinoma. The finding of active carcinoma in such a patient is an indication for further chemotherapy; removal of teratoma is therapeutic.

ADRENAL TUMORS

Malignant tumors of the adrenal gland are relatively rare. With more routine use of CT, more and more benign adrenal adenomas are being discovered. These tumors increase in prevalence as age increases. Adenomas are generally smaller and are nonfunctional compared with adrenal carcinomas.

Most carcinomas of the adrenal gland produce steroids, generally virilizing steroids. However, this is not a universal aspect of adrenal carcinomas. Therefore, even nonfunctional adrenal tumors that are large are generally approached surgically.

The treatment of adrenal carcinoma is surgical. These tumors may be cured even when large, and therefore aggressive surgical resection is important. Staging involves CT of the abdomen and chest. The discovery of metastatic disease precludes surgical resection of the primary tumor. When an adrenal mass is discovered, a search should be made for other tumors, because metastasis to the adrenal gland is not uncommon, especially in carcinoma of the lung.

Pheochromocytomas may arise in the adrenal gland. Most of these tumors are functional and benign, but approximately 10% are malignant. Nonetheless, because these tumors are functional and have deleterious physiologic effects even if benign, they are generally removed surgically in the absence of metastatic disease.

RENAL CELL CARCINOMA

Renal cell carcinoma is the most common malignant tumor of the kidney. However, in the absence of metastatic disease even the rarer cancers of the kidney are generally treated with radical nephrectomy. Renal cell carcinoma typically presents with hematuria. Alternative presentations include flank pain, an abdominal mass, or one of various paraneoplastic syndromes. The most common tumor of the kidney is not a carcinoma; it is a simple renal cyst. Renal cysts increase in prevalence as age increases and with modern imaging can be effectively distinguished from renal cell carcinoma. Renal cysts are typically fluid filled; renal cell carcinoma is typically solid.

Staging

Currently, most renal cell carcinomas are detected by CT. The patient is typically found to have hematuria, is noted to have a mass at IVP, and proceeds to CT for characterization of the mass. CT effectively diagnoses a solid renal mass, and because renal cell carcinoma typically spreads to lymph nodes, liver, and lung, it serves as a staging study. In conjunction with abdominal CT, either chest CT or chest radiography is necessary. Renal cell carcinoma can metastasize to bone, so determination of the serum calcium level and a detailed history about bone pain are also necessary.

Treatment of Localized Disease

Clinically localized renal cell carcinoma is managed by radical nephrectomy. This involves removal of the kidney and adrenal gland, with dissection in a plane outside Gerota's fascia. Characteristically, lymph nodes are removed for accurate staging of the disease. Lymphatic metastasis is generally synonymous with systemic disease. Therefore, obvious nodal metastasis on clinical staging precludes exploration and radical nephrectomy.

Approximately 5 to 10% of patients with renal cell carcinoma present with tumorous involvement of the veins. This generally includes the main renal vein and the vena cava. In the absence of other metastatic disease, aggressive surgical resection is important because many of these patients are cured surgically. The prognosis after radical nephrectomy is dependent on the pathologic stage. Tumors confined to the kidney generally have a good long-term prognosis,

whereas tumors that have invaded adjacent structures fare poorly. Radical nephrectomy is generally associated with low morbidity. Removal of the kidney may be performed by a transabdominal or a flank approach. The surgical approach is usually determined by the individual characteristics of the tumor (e.g., size, position) and the surgeon's preference.

Increasingly, renal cell carcinoma is diagnosed incidentally. By this it is meant that CT has been ordered for some other reason, only to reveal a small solid renal mass. Although radical nephrectomy is curative in such a situation, surgeons are increasingly employing partial nephrectomy (removal of the tumor alone with preservation of remaining kidney parenchyma). It appears that partial nephrectomy is an effective treatment if patients are well selected for the procedure. Nonetheless, patients should be advised that approximately 5% of the time smaller satellite tumors are present in the same kidney harboring the main tumor. Therefore, patients who choose partial nephrectomy should be monitored postoperatively with CT of the kidney for evidence of any local recurrence.

PENILE CANCER

Cancer of the penis is rare in the United States. The most common histologic subtype is squamous cell carcinoma, and the tumor generally originates on the glans penis or prepuce. Although penile cancer in circumcised men is extremely rare, the routine use of circumcision to avoid penile cancer is probably not warranted. It is thought that poor hygiene is associated with an increased chance of developing penile carcinoma.

Diagnosis and Staging

The diagnosis of penile carcinoma is generally made by inspection of the penis. Interestingly, many men present with large, advanced tumors, presumably because of denial. The diagnosis may be made by biopsy of a penile mass. The finding of squamous cell carcinoma engenders a staging work-up consisting of CT of the pelvis and abdomen and chest radiography. The initial site of metastasis is usually the inguinal lymph nodes.

Treatment

Treatment of the initial lesion is generally surgical. Small lesions on the prepuce may be managed by circumcision. Smaller lesions on the glans may be managed by Moh's surgery, laser ablation, or radiotherapy. Larger lesions are usually managed with partial penectomy. If partial penectomy with a 2-cm margin of normal penis results in a small phallus, total penectomy with perineal urethrostomy is usually indicated.

If inguinal metastasis has occurred, bilateral inguinal lymphadenectomy is indicated, because approximately 50% of these patients are cured by removal of such nodes. Approximately 20% of patients with normal inguinal examinations harbor metastatic disease. This has raised the issue of whether or not prophylactic inguinal lymphadenectomy is reasonable. Because of the morbidity associated with inguinal lymphadenectomy, most physicians believe that prophylactic inguinal lymphadenectomy is not warranted. However, certain characteristics of the primary tumor may indicate an increased chance of occult inguinal metastasis. These factors include a higher grade of tumor and invasion of the corporal bodies.

Metastasis beyond the inguinal lymph nodes is generally associated with a poor prognosis. Chemotherapeutic agents employed in this situation have included cisplatin and bleomycin. Rare patients may survive quite some time after the diagnosis of metastatic disease. In most patients, the diagnosis of metastasis is associated with an extremely poor prognosis.

ANTERIOR URETHRAL STRICTURE

method of
GERALD H. JORDAN, M.D.
Eastern Virginia Medical School and Sentara
 Norfolk General Hospital
Norfolk, Virginia

The urethral stricture has long confounded the urologist. The term "urethral stricture" implies a process in the anterior urethra, that portion of the urethra unique to the male (Figure 1). In the 1500s, strictures were thought to be growths, and this philosophy persisted until the 18th century. The treatment of stricture, in many cases, was left to the hands of barbers, executioners, and mountebanks. As late as the latter part of the 1700s, the relationship of urethral stricture to gonorrhea was disputed. In the mid-1800s, the first real understanding of the significance of urethral stricture was made with Thompson's theory that "the question of the diameter of the urethra must be considered as resolving itself into a measure of its capabilities of being distended."

We now know that a urethral stricture is a scar, the natural result of tissue injury or destruction. Scars tend to contract in their lengthwise axis. If the scar happens to be arranged in a circle, then the scar contraction reduces the circumference of the circle. For example, if the normal urethra is No. 30 French, the diameter of that urethra is approximately 10 mm and the area is approximately 75 mm^2. However, if the circumference is decreased by a scar to No. 15 French, the diameter of the urethra becomes 5 mm and the area is approximately 19 mm^2. It is thus easy to appreciate the profound urodynamic significance that urethral strictures can have. A stricture that is No. 15 French would be considered wide caliber by many, and thus the stricture that is No. 6 or 8 French has even more profound effects.

It was not until the early 1900s that the beneficial effects of diversion were relatively well accepted. In 1914, Hamilton Z. Russell described a technique of urethral reconstruction in which the stricture (the scar) was excised. The urethra was then reapproximated. In most cases, only one

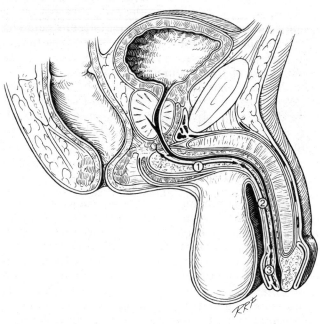

Figure 1. Sagittal section of the male pelvis. The anterior urethra is that portion of the urethra invested with either the corpus spongiosum or the spongy erectile tissue of the glans penis. For the purposes of reconstructive surgery, it can be divided into three sections: (1) the bulbous urethra (that section of the urethra invested by the midline fusion of the ischial cavernosus musculature, (2) the penile or pendulous urethra (that portion of the urethra distal to the investment of the ischial cavernosus musculature), and (3) the fossa navicularis, that portion of the urethra surrounded by the spongy erectile tissue of the glans penis.

wall could be reapproximated, with the remaining wall left to heal by secondary intention. This technique represented the first of the modern approaches to urethral reconstruction for stricture disease.

The classic symptom described by the patient with urethral stricture is diminished force of stream. Many patients, however, endure a diminished stream for years, presuming that their longer stays at the urinal are merely a reflection of what is normal for them. Some young men present with epididymitis as the hailing feature of their urethral stricture. On closer inquiry, these young men then say that it takes them longer than their friends to void. In some cases, the physician can elicit a history of a bloody urethral discharge that follows voiding. This is thought to be due to microtrauma to the urethral epithelium with high-pressure voiding parameters proximal to an extremely narrow caliber stricture. Any young male with unexplained epididymitis should be presumed to have a urethral abnormality until proved otherwise. Epididymitis has been associated with heavy lifting and is thought by some to be due to reflux of urine into the vas deferens. The association of epididymitis with testicular trauma is also well described. However, in the absence of those classic associations, the unexplained epididymitis and the unexplained urinary tract infection must be presumed to be due to anatomic abnormalities.

Another symptom, which is less frequently noted but on inquiry can sometimes be elicited, is diminished volume of ejaculate or perhaps pain with ejaculation. Patients often note that after ejaculation there seems to be remaining ejaculate that drips from the penis. A corollary to this is a history of postvoid residual dribbling. In the patient with a narrow-caliber stricture, the urethra distal to the stricture

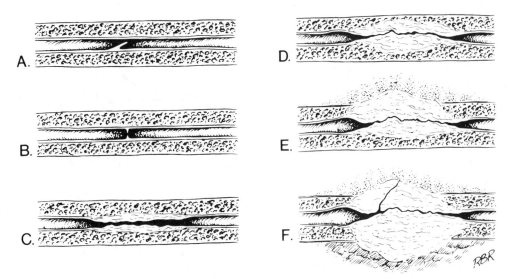

Figure 2. Diagrammatic representation of the categories of anterior urethral stricture disease as proposed by Devine. The categorization of stricture emphasizes the variable involvement of the urethral epithelium and/or corpus spongiosum with the scar. (From Jordan GH: Options for the surgical management of anterior urethral stricture. *In* Webster GD [ed]: Problems in Reconstructive Urology. Philadelphia, JB Lippincott, 1987.)

empties efficiently. However, the urethra proximal to the narrow-caliber area stores urine and/or ejaculate, which then dribbles through the narrowed lumen a few minutes after voiding.

An occasional patient recalls a discrete episode of perineal trauma. At that episode, he may or may not have noticed a bloody urethral discharge. He may or may not notice difficulty with urination immediately after the trauma. However, after that event, and developing in some patients approximately 6 to 8 weeks later, the patient begins to notice a diminished stream.

Although there are many telltale symptoms already described, a number of patients with urethral stricture are discovered purely because they have urinalysis abnormalities that do not clear with antibiotic therapy. In most patients with a stricture, there are white blood cells, evidence of red blood cells, if not red blood cells per se, and not infrequently urethral epithelial cells in the urine. The relationship of urethral stricture to the development of urethral carcinoma is well documented. Given the number of urethral strictures seen, however, urethral carcinoma is quite rare. The hallmark of urethral carcinoma is a patient with a urethral stricture that "just does not act right." In current times, with most strictures secondary to trauma, it is worrisome to see a patient with a urethrocutaneous fistula. Fistulas are usually associated with inflammatory causes of urethral stricture, which in the past implied stricture due to gonococcal urethritis.

The patient suspected of having a urethral stricture should be referred to a urologist. Many times the urologic evaluation is somewhat circumferential to the actual problem because of the vagueness of symptoms and/or findings. If intravenous pyelography is contemplated as the initial study for a patient with voiding symptoms or urinary tract infection, the addition of a voiding film to this study can often be diagnostic. The evaluation per se for urethral stricture includes retrograde urethrography, voiding urethrography, and endoscopy. In addition, a number of centers have used real-time transperineal ultrasonography to assess for urethral stricture. Clinical evaluations are under way to assess the value of intraluminal ultrasonography as an adjunct to the evaluation of anterior urethral stricture disease. By and large, however, the use of ultrasonography—either transperineal or intraluminal—is reserved for *after* the stricture has been documented.

In 1983, Devine suggested a classification of urethral stricture disease such that the results of surgery for urethral stricture disease could be compared in common terms. That classification is shown in Figure 2 and emphasizes that anterior urethral strictures can range from scars confined to the urethral epithelium to extensive scars involving the urethral epithelium, the spongy erectile tissue of the corpus spongiosum, and the adjacent tissues to the corpus spongiosum, and as shown in Figure 2*F*, can be associated with fistula.

The patient with urethral stricture can have problems with recurrent urinary tract infection. This relationship, however, is extremely unpredictable, with some patients having extremely severe urethral strictures from the standpoint of luminal compromise but having had few or no urinary tract infections; whereas another patient with virtually an identical stricture is plagued with almost constant recurrences of urinary tract infection.

TREATMENT

Because the urethral stricture is a scar by definition, all management or cure of urethral stricture is scar revision. The small unsightly scar on a patient's cheek can be revised with a relatively straightforward procedure, but the massively scarred side of the face may require more heroic efforts; the treatment of urethral stricture is absolutely analogous.

Once a stricture has been diagnosed and therapy has been elected, it is my practice to start patients with suppressive antibiotic therapy, and, when not otherwise contraindicated, a synthetic tetracycline in suppressive doses seems to work well. The use of a suppressive antibiotic does seem to offer some protection from recurrences of urinary tract infection, but, more important, the use of that suppressive antibiotic seems to limit patients' symptoms.

The advent of modern tissue transfer techniques has drastically changed the way in which urethral strictures are handled. In years past at many centers, chronic dilatation was almost the only management modality for urethral strictures. Urethral reconstruction was reserved for the exceptional patient. Virtually every university urology program had a

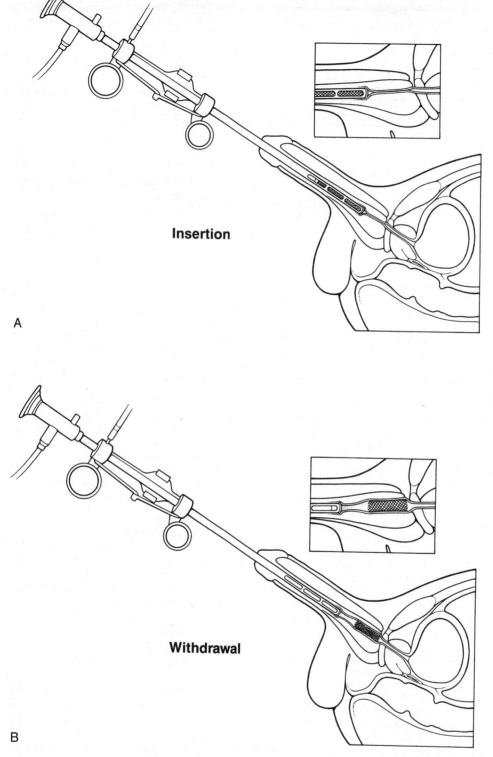

Insertion

A

B

Withdrawal

Figure 3. *A,* Diagrammatic representation of a proximal bulbous urethral stricture. After dilatation of the stricture or internal urethrotomy, the Urolume device is passed through the urethra. *B,* The stent is positioned to span the limits of the stricture and is then deployed. (Courtesy of American Medical Systems, Minnetonka, Minnesota. Medical illustrations by Michael Schenk.)

stricture clinic, and that implied a chronic urethral dilatation clinic. The concept of internal urethrotomy is an old one. However, in 1972, Sachse described the use of internal urethrotomy under direct vision. The change to the technique of internal urethrotomy introduced with his report was that the urologist viewed the incision of the scar, as opposed to the incision's being performed blindly with incision of areas of the urethra that did not require it. Sachse's report turned the management of urethral stricture disease upside down. Chronic dilatation clinics virtually vanished; the art of complex urethral reconstructive surgery, likewise, virtually vanished from many training programs; and, for years, the "gold standard" treatment of urethral stricture was direct visual internal urethrotomy.

It did not take long, however, for many observers to determine that direct visual internal urethrotomy was not the panacea that many thought it would be. Because many of the skills of management of urethral stricture disease (both dilatation and reconstructive surgery) had vanished with the virtual explosion and use of internal urethrotomy, efforts became aimed not at developing new modalities but rather at making direct visual internal urethrotomy "work." These efforts included using varied lengths of time of catheterization after the internal urethrotomy was performed, placing patients on home catheterization or dilatation protocols, using hydrodilatation protocols, and, in many cases, repeatedly applying internal urethrotomy, which in some patients was done in excess of 15 to 20 times.

Fortunately, however, in select centers, there continued to be enthusiasm for surgery for urethral stricture disease. Much of this enthusiasm was aimed at staged procedures. The staged procedures consisted of the marsupialization of the strictured segment for a period (usually 6 months) with a second-stage retubularization. These procedures were somewhat successful but clearly did not offer the success rate that most surgeons demand.

In 1953, Pressman and Greenfield described their experience with reconstruction of the urethra using full-thickness skin grafts. They reported only a small series of patients. However, Devine adopted and improved the technique of full-thickness skin graft urethral reconstruction. In 1976 he described a large series of patients whose strictures were treated with full-thickness skin graft patch urethral reconstruction. After that series, success rates of 80% cure of stricture were noted. That description began a new era of urethral reconstruction. It was an era that used tissue transfer and thus sparked the interest of reconstructive surgeons in devising other modalities of tissue transfer for use with urethral reconstruction. Likewise, the 80% success rate continued to challenge surgeons, and better procedures were sought, developed, and perfected.

The treatment of urethral stricture disease can now be matched directly to the anatomy of the stricture. The information required to know the anatomy of a urethral stricture includes the *length* of the stricture, the *location* of the stricture, the *depth* of the scar (termed "spongiofibrosis"), and the *density* of spongiofibrosis. As mentioned, the combination of retrograde urethrography and voiding urethrography is aimed at determining the length and location of the anterior urethral stricture. The true length of spongiofibrosis, however, remains a different issue. As mentioned previously, ultrasonography has been used in select centers to add information about the anatomy of stricture. Ultrasonography is thought by many to better image the area of spongiofibrosis, and it is known by all who deal with strictures that there can be spongiofibrosis in the face of what appears to

be normally compliant and normal-appearing urethral epithelium.

With accurate knowledge of the anatomy of stricture, treatment can be selected. A major concept that must be understood by all who encounter urethral strictures is deciding whether to *manage* a stricture or *cure* a stricture. It is clear that few strictures are cured by dilatation or internal urethrotomy. There are no current series studying cure rates of stricture using dilatation. Two recent series investigated internal urethrotomy as a curative modality, and those studies showed cure rates of 25 and 33%, respectively. From those studies, it became clear that the strictures that were cured by internal urethrotomy were very short, narrow-caliber strictures of the bulbous urethra associated with virtually no spongiofibrosis. This fact had been presumed by many but was proved by those series.

Options of urethral reconstruction include a host of procedures. Genital full-thickness skin grafts, bladder epithelial grafts, and buccal mucosal grafts are used. With the definition of the genital skin blood supply, many flap techniques for urethral reconstruction have been developed. These techniques truly allow reconstruction of the anterior urethra from the meatus to the apex of the prostate.

As an adjuvant to internal urethrotomy, implantable urethral stents have been developed. The Urolume device has been approved by the Food and Drug Administration. The Urolume is indicated for strictures in the bulbous urethra that are no longer than 3 cm, are at least 1 cm away from the external urethral sphincter, and can have implantation of the stent throughout their length, such that the stent does not extend beyond the middle to distal scrotal urethra (Figure 3). The Urolume has been available in Latin America and Europe for a number of years and seems to have a cure rate of approximately 84%. The Urolume is clearly not a panacea and is being used with a great deal of selectivity in those countries in which it has been available. It was greeted with rampant enthusiasm but is now regarded as appropriate therapy for a select group of patients.

Recent years have been an exciting time for the reconstructive surgeon involved in the treatment of urethral strictures. Depending on the stricture, the surgeon and patient now enjoy, in some cases, as high as a 98.5% cure rate. The vast majority of strictures can be cured and with rates that are 90% or better. The art of anterior urethral reconstruction is returning to training centers, and a disease that could only be managed in the not too distant past is now cured in most cases.

RENAL CALCULI

method of
JOSEPH W. SEGURA, M.D.
Mayo Medical School, Mayo Clinic
Rochester, Minnesota

Renal (and ureteral) calculi are a common reason for emergency department evaluation and are particularly common in the southeastern part of the United States. Part of the reason for this is doubtless dehydration with resultant concentration of urine, but other factors may also be involved. One theory suggests that the soil of this area lacks certain trace elements that are present in other areas, including the Southwest, where the climate is actually hotter but the incidence of stones rather less. Stones occur about 2.5 times more often in men than in women and usually in the third to fifth decades of life. There is a slight but statistically significant predilection for the left kidney over the right.

DIAGNOSTIC EVALUATION

Signs and Symptoms

Stones in the ureteropelvic junction (UPJ) and ureter cause renal colic. Colic is usually severe, unilateral pain that may be felt from the flank, progressing anterolaterally to the lower quadrant and into the testicle or labia. The pain may be intermittent but is characteristic in that there is no position in which the patient feels better. The location of the pain is a general guide to the location of the stone in the ureter, with UPJ stones usually causing flank pain, and stones in the lower ureter often causing pain in the testis and groin. Colic is due to ureteral spasm, and its sudden relief often does not mean that the stone has passed.

When the stone is in the renal pelvis or calyx, the symptoms are usually much less impressive, often being only a vague ache, and there may often be considerable doubt whether the pain is in fact due to the stone.

Patients often have nausea and vomiting and may have a reflex ileus. Stones in the lower ureter often cause urgency and frequency. Gross hematuria is not uncommon, and the patient may have flank tenderness. A low-grade fever may be present, and higher temperatures can be an indication for intervention (see later). Children have symptoms similar to those of adults, but they are often unable to localize the pain and complain more of a stomachache.

Many problems are included in the differential diagnosis. Right ureteral colic has been confused with acute appendicitis; acute diverticulitis may cause questions in left lower quadrant pain; and the symptoms and signs of renal vein thrombosis may be indistinguishable from those due to an upper ureteral stone. The signs and symptoms of cholelithiasis may sometimes be confused with those of right renal stones.

Laboratory Evaluation

Virtually all patients have microhematuria, and many have pyuria. Bacteria may also be seen on urinalysis, and a Gram stain and urine culture should be done for all patients. The urine pH should be noted as well as the presence of any crystals in the urine. Urine osmolality is important but usually not representative under such acute

conditions. Hematologic studies should include the patient's white blood cell count, and a serum creatinine level should be obtained. If the patient is febrile, the possibility of urosepsis should be considered and blood drawn for culture.

Radiologic Evaluation

Because most urinary calculi are radiopaque, a plain film of the abdomen may be sufficient to make the diagnosis, although interpretation of such unprepared films is often difficult. The upper tracts should be assessed in some way, and most urologists prefer to have an intravenous pyelogram (IVP). This enables the physician to determine the site and severity of obstruction and makes the diagnosis in the 20% or so of stones that are radiolucent or poorly calcified. Frequently, there is delayed excretion of contrast medium on the side with the stone. Occasionally, extravasation through a ruptured fornix is noted. Renal ultrasonography is an easy way to detect hydronephrosis, although stones below the UPJ cannot be identified.

There is a trend among many radiologists to use computed tomography instead of the IVP as the radiologic procedure of first resort in the emergency department. Proponents emphasize that stones can be identified whether calcified or not, obstruction detected, and any other abdominal abnormality identified. Although issues of cost must be addressed, this is becoming standard practice in many institutions including our own, despite the fact that most urologists are more comfortable with the IVP.

Retrograde pyelography is ordinarily not indicated for diagnostic purposes on an emergency basis, unless the patient has an allergy to contrast medium and the diagnosis is in doubt for whatever reason.

MANAGEMENT

Factors to Consider

Management of the acute stone event depends on a variety of factors:

1. Stone size
2. Stone location
3. Degree of obstruction
4. Presence or absence of infection
5. Anatomic considerations
6. Severity of symptoms

Stone Size

It should be remembered that 85% of ureteral stones pass spontaneously. The most important indicator of this possibility is the size of the stone. As a rule of thumb, if the stone is smaller than 5.0 mm in diameter, it has about an 85% chance of spontaneous passage; if it is approximately 5.0 mm, about a 50% chance of passage; and if it is larger than 5.0 mm, about a 10% chance of passage. Stones that are smooth and round are more likely to pass than those that are irregular or spiculated. An important predictive point is the patient's history of previous stone passage. Previous passage of large stones may mean that a current stone otherwise unlikely to pass may in fact do so in this particular patient, as long as the stone is on the same side as before. Regrettably, it is not possible to predict exactly *when* a stone will pass, and indeed one of the main reasons to remove passable stones is the patient's exasperation with the uncertainty of the situation.

Stone Location

The intramural ureter is the narrowest point the stone must traverse to pass into the bladder, so that successful passage to this point is not a guarantee of ultimate success. Conversely, stones in the lower ureter are usually small (or else they would not have got this far) and stones in the upper ureter tend to be larger. Also, renal pelvic stones are generally of a size that spontaneous passage cannot be expected.

Degree of Obstruction

Although obstruction with delay in excretion of contrast medium is quite common, it is perhaps more surprising how often obstruction is not present. Markedly delayed function, or indeed nonfunction secondary to obstruction, is often an indication for treatment, although not on an emergency basis, even though the stone is of a size that spontaneous passage might eventually occur. Patients with minimal or no obstruction can be followed up in the hope of spontaneous stone passage.

Infection

Patients who have infected urine with an obstructing stone are candidates for urosepsis. If the urine Gram stain result is positive, if the patient is febrile, or if the patient has a history of frequent urinary tract infections, the possibility of sepsis should be considered. These patients should be given broad-spectrum antibiotics (our preference is ampicillin and gentamicin) and urologic consultation obtained to address the question of bypassing the stone with a stent or placing a percutaneous nephrostomy tube, the choice depending on the clinical situation. One should resist the temptation to remove the ureteral stone at the time of stent placement in case some problem occurs that might prolong the procedure.

Anatomic Considerations

Solitary kidney is the anatomic situation most likely to precipitate treatment, for the obvious reason that anuria could develop at any time. All things being equal, the stone should be removed promptly or at least a double-pigtail stent placed to protect the kidney.

Severity of Symptoms

The pain of renal colic is the most common reason for hospital admission, and spontaneous resolution of pain the most common reason for leaving the hospital without resolution of the stone problem. Multiple such episodes try everyone's patience and may precipitate removal of an otherwise passable stone. Factors such as employment, travel plans, or other issues may have a bearing on stone management.

Surgical Management

Few stones are operated on today. The most common indications for open stone removal are ex-tremely large renal stones, nephrectomy for a nonfunctioning or poorly functioning kidney secondary to stones, certain large ureteral stones, and occasionally ureteral stones that could not be managed by less invasive methods.

Stones are managed by extracorporeal shock wave lithotripsy (SWL), ureteroscopy (URS), or percutaneous nephrolithotomy (PNL). The goal of SWL is to use shock waves to fragment the stone into pieces small enough that spontaneous passage may be expected. The major advantage of SWL is that it is a noninvasive outpatient procedure. Its disadvantages are that more than one procedure is frequently necessary for fragmentation, the passage of fragments is unpredictable and may cause colic, and ancillary procedures such as percutaneous nephrostomy tubes or ureteral stents are often necessary. Although URS can be used anywhere in the ureter, it is particularly effective in the lower ureter. A small ureteroscope is inserted into the lower ureter and the stone evaluated under direct vision. The stone may be either basket extracted or fragmented with a device such as a laser or electrohydraulic probe. The advantages of URS in the ureter are that the single-procedure success rates are quite high (97%) and it is done as an outpatient procedure. It is, however, more invasive than SWL and requires more expertise in the upper ureter. The literature suggests that overall, URS is less expensive in the lower ureter than SWL, although this factor may vary from place to place and time to time.

Stones in the kidney and upper ureter are usually treated with SWL. Because stone-free rates drop and multiple treatment rates rise as the stone increases in size above 2.0 to 2.5 cm, PNL is often employed to remove such large calculi. After a guide wire is placed through the flank into the kidney, a tract is dilated around the wire large enough to insert the nephroscope (about 1.0 cm). The stone is broken up with an ultrasonic probe and the pieces removed. This procedure has high single-procedure success rates, and it can also deal with obstructive uropathies such as UPJ obstruction at the same time. However, it is invasive and requires 2 to 3 days in the hospital.

Medical Evaluation and Management

Some have argued that because stones can be so easily treated, prevention is not as important as it used to be. Although it is true that we no longer are faced with the sequelae of open surgery, stone events still have a price, both in dollars and in morbidity. Most patients with stones are as greatly interested in preventing another such event as their insurance companies are. The average stone patient has a 50% chance of making another stone in a 5-year period if the patient undergoes no evaluation or treatment. Also, there is good evidence that the presence of residual stone particles after SWL causes increased stone formation if the patient has not been medically evaluated or treated.

One may pragmatically divide stone patients into two groups, high- and low-risk patients. Low-risk patients are those who are single-stone formers, without evidence of other stones, with negative family histories. Higher risk patients are those who have multiple stones or a positive family history; have passed stones; or have intestinal disease, hyperparathyroidism, or urinary tract infection, especially when secondary to a bacterium producing urease, uric acid, or cystine stones.

Interest in prevention is highest at the time of the stone event and tapers off afterward. Despite this, metabolic evaluation should wait until the patient has recovered from the acute event and has returned to his or her usual diet and activity. Nevertheless, the basic evaluation that all stone patients should get can be done in the hospital.

All patients should have a plain radiograph of quality adequate to detect other stones; chemistry studies to include the serum calcium level, urine pH, urinalysis, and urine culture; and a stone analysis. The stone history should focus on any dietary excesses, fluid intake, and any surgical procedure known to affect stone formation (e.g., intestinal bypass). Low-risk patients require no further diagnostic evaluation and are ordinarily counseled to increase their fluid intake to produce 2 to 2.5 liters of urine per day. Few patients actually measure this, and as a rule of thumb, they should be told that if their urine is yellow, they are not drinking enough fluid. This simple step in fact reduces the stone recurrence rate in most patients regardless of the cause of their stone disease. The trick is making sure they stay on this program, and the patient's interest should be periodically reinforced by office visits every few months. A plain film of the abdomen about once a year to look for recurrent stones is usually adequate for most low-risk stone formers.

In addition to these steps, higher risk patients should have 24-hour urine studies to include calcium, phosphorus, citrate, oxalate, uric acid, sodium, and creatinine levels. If a qualitative check for cystine is positive, a quantitative measure should be done on the 24-hour specimen. I prefer to do this on the patient's usual diet. There are many diagnostic categories into which stone patients may be placed, and although "idiopathic" is still one of them, it is often possible to select therapy that corrects or treats an underlying abnormality. The following may be thought of as a pragmatic approach for the nonspecialist.

Hypercalciuria

In absorptive hypercalciuria (type 1), the primary defect is increased absorption of calcium from the gut. As there is no specific treatment for the underlying problem, the usual treatment is thiazide diuretics because they reduce urinary calcium levels. Sodium cellulose phosphate is more specific in that it binds calcium in the gut, preventing reabsorption, but it is expensive and poorly tolerated. A second less severe form of hypercalciuria (type 2) that responds to a low-calcium diet alone may be differentiated. Hypercalciuria may also be due to renal leak of calcium at the tubular level. The specific treatment for this is also a thiazide diuretic. On a practical basis, most patients with hypercalciuria are treated with thiazides together with correction of any dietary excess of calcium and measures to increase urine volume.

Normocalciuria

In the absence of other abnormality in the urine or elsewhere, patients with normocalciuria are said to have idiopathic stone disease. The primary treatment is to increase the urine volume to 2 to 2.5 liters per day. When hyperuricosuria is found in patients with calcium stones, treatment is directed toward reducing the urine uric acid levels with allopurinol. More commonly, low urinary citrate levels are identified as the only abnormality, and the rate of stone formation in these patients is often markedly reduced by using oral citrate therapy with potassium citrate. Hyperoxaluria occurs as an inherited disorder causing renal oxalosis. This is often fatal in childhood or the early decades of life. Enteric hyperoxaluria is found in adults and is secondary to increased absorption of oxalate from the gut. This can be due to inflammatory bowel disease and usually happens after intestinal bypass surgery performed for obesity. These groups constitute difficult management problems and should be referred to physicians with a special interest in these entities.

Cystinuria

About 1% of stones are composed of cystine and are found in patients with an autosomal recessive disorder involving the transport of the amino acids cystine, lysine, ornithine, and arginine. Urinary levels of all these amino acids are elevated, but only cystine forms stones owing to its relative insolubility. When the 24-hour concentration of cystine rises above 450 mg per 24 hours, stones begin to form. Therapy is directed to decreasing the concentration of cystine in the urine by increasing the urine volume; increasing the urine pH to enhance solubility; and administering drugs, such as D-penicillamine (Cuprimine) or tiopronin (Thiola), as necessary to decrease cystine excretion. The former drug is less commonly used because it may cause agranulocytosis and nephrotic syndrome. Tiopronin is less toxic and should be used in concert with efforts to raise the pH and increase the urine volume.

Although these measures are theoretically able to dissolve cystine stones, this is usually not possible in practice, and medical management should be used to attempt to prevent new stone formation in cystinuric patients. Small (<1.5 cm) cystine stones occasionally fragment well with SWL, but most require PNL for removal.

Uric Acid Stones

Symptomatic uric acid stones are common (about 10% of stone formers) and often happen in those patients with gout or chronic diarrhea. Patients with certain malignancies and those undergoing cytotoxic chemotherapy may also form uric acid stones. Usually, the 24-hour uric acid levels are normal, and typically the urine is quite acid. Treatment is directed toward raising the pH of the urine above 6.5 to increase the solubility of the uric acid. Agents such as potassium citrate or sodium bicarbonate may be used along with regular measurements of urine pH. The diet should be modified to decrease levels of purine intake from red meat, fish, and poultry and the urine volume maintained at 2 to 2.5 liters per day.

In contrast to cystine stones, it is generally possible to dissolve uric acid stones. Persistent elevations of pH above 7.0 may result in a deposition of calcium over the stone. This is usually obvious on plain radiographs and is an indication that further medical therapy is not warranted. Most such failures are in larger stones, and my preference is to use PNL to remove these calculi.

Struvite Stones

Struvite stones are formed of magnesium-ammonium-phosphate crystals in varied proportions of hydroxyapatite and carbonate apatite. Struvite stones contain varied amounts of calcium and are more or less radiopaque. The sine qua non for struvite stone formation is the presence of urease-producing bacteria in the urine. The most common organisms are *Proteus* species and *Klebsiella* species, but *Pseudomonas,* streptococci, and staphylococci are also weak urea splitters. In the majority of patients, an underlying metabolic and/or an anatomic abnormality predisposing to stone formation may be identified. These patients all have chronic bacteriuria because the bacteria reside inside the stone, and antibiotic therapy is of temporary benefit only.

All the stones must be removed. The highest stone-free rates are achieved with PNL, although acceptable stone-free rates can be achieved with SWL on smaller struvite stones.

The Sexually Transmitted Diseases

CHANCROID

method of
DAVID H. MARTIN, M.D.
Louisiana State University Medical Center
New Orleans, Louisiana

Chancroid, caused by the gram-negative bacillus *Haemophilus ducreyi,* may be the most important cause of genital ulcer disease worldwide. In the United States, the disease had nearly disappeared by the 1970s. However, beginning in the early 1980s, isolated outbreaks began to appear once again. The disease initially occurred primarily among migrant workers and was associated with door-to-door prostitution, but by the mid-1980s, the disease established itself endemically in a number of urban centers such as Dallas, the New York–Philadelphia metroplex, and Miami. Subsequently, the disease appeared in many other cities, especially in the South. In 1988, 5001 cases were reported to the Centers for Disease Control and Prevention (CDC) in Atlanta, Georgia. Epidemiologic research established that the rise in cases during the late 1980s and early 1990s was related to sexual behavior associated with crack cocaine abuse.

Since 1987, the number of reported cases has gradually declined to the point that the disease appears to have disappeared in many locations once again. Only 609 cases were reported to the CDC in 1995. The reasons for the decline in incidence are unclear because there is no evidence that crack cocaine use has diminished significantly. The important lesson learned in the last 10 years is that health care providers in the United States can never completely discount *H. ducreyi* as a cause of genital ulcer disease.

The major public health problem associated with chancroid is that it has been shown to be an important cofactor for the heterosexual transmission of the human immunodeficiency virus (HIV). The number of heterosexual HIV infections attributable to chancroid in the last 10 years is unknown but is likely to have been high.

Classically, chancroid presents as multiple, painful ulcers that have a purulent base and ragged, undermined borders. Because lesions are usually not indurated, they are often referred to in the older literature as "soft chancre." Fifty to 60% of men with chancroid will develop inguinal lymphadenopathy, which is usually unilateral. In a small proportion of cases, the inguinal node mass or bubo becomes fluctuant and may rupture, resulting in a draining abscess. Despite the distinctive features of "classic" chancroid, it is clear that there is considerable overlap among this disease, syphilis, and genital herpes, which makes accurate clinical diagnosis difficult.

For reasons that are not clear, the ratio of male to female chancroid cases ranges from 3:1 to 25:1. In part, this may be because internal lesions in women often go unnoticed, as is the case in primary syphilis. However, the male/female ratio for chancroid cases is higher than that for primary syphilis, suggesting that there may be other reasons for this phenomenon, such as an asymptomatic carrier state in women.

Laboratory confirmation of the diagnosis of chancroid is difficult because *H. ducreyi* has special in vitro growth requirements. Most clinical laboratories cannot successfully cultivate this slow-growing organism. New tests based on DNA amplification technology have been developed, and they appear to be more sensitive than culture. However, it is unclear whether these tests will become available commercially. Therefore, in clinical practice, the diagnosis continues to be one of exclusion. Unfortunately, this approach is not helpful in guiding therapy at the time of the initial encounter with the patient, especially when darkfield microscopy is not available, as is often the case. Therefore, by necessity, treatment is empirical and should be guided by knowledge of the incidence of chancroid in a given area. A useful clue to the presence of the disease is the observation of primary syphilis "treatment failures" resulting from *Treponema pallidum* and *H. ducreyi* co-infection as well as from misdiagnosis of chancroid as syphilis. Another clue is an increased frequency of patients presenting to local acute care facilities for the treatment of painful inguinal buboes. If there is reason to suspect that *H. ducreyi* is present in a given community, then all genital ulcer cases not obviously caused by herpes simplex virus should be treated empirically for both syphilis and chancroid.

TREATMENT

Although increasing resistance to some of the older drugs used to treat this disease has been observed in the last 10 years, there remain a number of drugs both old and new that have good activity against *H. ducreyi*. Ceftriaxone (Rocephin) 250 mg as a single intramuscular dose is effective for both ulcers and buboes. The only drawbacks to this approach are the inconvenience of intramuscular administration and the relatively high cost of the drug.

As with ceftriaxone, there has been no evidence of development of erythromycin resistance among *H. ducreyi* strains worldwide. Erythromycin 500 mg orally four times daily for 7 days is the standard dose. One study has suggested that as little as 500 mg three times a day for 5 days may also be effective.

Sulfonamide resistance among *H. ducreyi* strains has steadily increased worldwide, and more recently, trimethoprim resistance has become a problem in both Thailand and Africa. At one time, a single high dose of trimethoprim-sulfamethoxazole was widely used for chancroid. Whereas increased treatment failure rates were first reported with single-dose therapy, failures have been noted in the Far East and Africa with the multiple-dose regimens as well. Although in vivo and in vitro experience with trimethoprim-sulfamethoxazole in the United States is limited, this drug should probably not be used any longer in view of the availability of effective alternatives.

A number of the newly developed broad-spectrum oral antibiotics have promise in the therapy for chancroid. Among the quinolones available in the United States, ciprofloxacin (Cipro) has been studied most extensively. Studies have shown that a single 500-mg dose is effective, although a failure rate of 26% was reported in HIV-negative Rwandan patients. In the United States, 500 mg twice daily for 3 days is the currently recommended dose. Fleroxacin, a new quinolone not available in the United States, has also been found to cure most cases when it is given as a single dose.

Almost all *H. ducreyi* strains produce β-lactamase and therefore are resistant to amoxicillin alone, but amoxicillin-clavulanate (Augmentin), 500 mg of amoxicillin plus 125 mg of clavulanate three times daily by mouth for 7 days, is effective. Finally, studies in both Africa and the United States have shown that cure rates for the new macrolide azithromycin (Zithromax) given as a single 1-gram oral dose are equal to those for intramuscular ceftriaxone. Azithromycin is available in a 1-gram powdered formulation specifically designed for treating sexually transmitted diseases. This dose form is less expensive than four 250-mg capsules.

Studies from Kenya have suggested that HIV-infected individuals with chancroid are more difficult to treat than are those without HIV infection. Treatment failure rates of 20 to 50% have been reported among these patients after single doses of a number of the drugs discussed, although this experience has not been reproduced in South Africa or in Rwanda. Thus, some experts believe that patients with chancroid who are known to be HIV infected should be treated with one of the multiple-dose regimens. Clearly, HIV-infected patients should be followed up closely for evidence of an appropriate therapeutic response regardless of the therapeutic regimen employed.

Given the difficulty of clinically distinguishing syphilis and chancroid, and because the two diseases may coexist in 10 to 20% of cases, patients suspected of having chancroid who have not had a negative result on darkfield examination should also be treated for primary syphilis unless adequate follow-up can be ensured. An important point to remember is that all recent sexual contacts of patients suspected of having chancroid should be treated as well.

Fluctuant buboes should be drained to prevent rupture. Insertion of an 18-gauge needle into the center of the lesion through normal skin at the margin of inflammation is the simplest approach. However, patients may require one or more repeated aspirations. Incision and drainage is also acceptable as clearly demonstrated by a randomized study comparing this approach with needle aspiration. Large node masses may become fluctuant after treatment with effective antibiotics. This development should not be taken as evidence of treatment failure because the pus aspirated from these lesions is usually sterile.

GONORRHEA

method of
CHARLES B. HICKS, M.D.
Duke University Medical Center
Durham, North Carolina

EPIDEMIOLOGY

Since the mid-1970s, the incidence of gonorrhea in the United States has been steadily declining. *Chlamydia trachomatis* infection is now the most common sexually transmitted disease (STD) reported to the Centers for Disease Control and Prevention (CDC). Nonetheless, gonorrhea remains a serious problem. It is the second most frequently reported infectious disease in the United States; some 700,000 to 800,000 infections are thought to occur annually. Cases are more common among persons younger than 24 years, and the reported incidence of gonorrhea is greater in men than in women, probably because the disease is considerably easier to diagnose in men than in women. There is considerable variability in the incidence of gonorrhea among different ethnic and socioeconomic groups. Factors associated with an increased incidence of gonorrhea include black race, lower socioeconomic status, lesser education, urban residence, illicit drug use, and being unmarried.

As with many bacteria, antimicrobial resistance has become an increasingly difficult problem in the management of infections due to *Neisseria gonorrhoeae*. Beginning with the emergence of penicillinase-producing strains (termed PPNG) in the mid-1970s, *N. gonorrhoeae* has demonstrated a remarkable ability to evolve in response to treatment regimens employing various different antimicrobials. In addition to PPNG, there are now well-documented isolates with resistance to tetracycline, spectinomycin (Trobicin), and recently quinolones. The last strains were first identified in the Far East but have been reported in the United States as well. Since 1986, the CDC has conducted the Gonococcal Isolate Surveillance Project, which regularly monitors the antimicrobial susceptibility of isolates from 25 publicly funded STD clinics representing all areas of the United States. As a result, the emergence of resistance has been quickly identified and appropriate treatment recommendations have been disseminated.

CLINICAL MANIFESTATIONS

The majority of gonococcal infections are confined to the urogenital tract. In men, the urethra is the primary site of disease, with dysuria and a purulent urethral discharge being the most common presenting complaints. Most cases in women involve the endocervix, and in some instances gonorrhea may produce dysuria or a vaginal discharge. Many cases, however, are relatively asymptomatic; in some settings, up to 90% of diagnosed cases may be subclinical. The incubation period for gonorrhea is typically short, averaging 2 to 5 days, but may be more variable in women. Other sites of local infection in men and women include the rectum, the pharynx, and rarely the conjunctivae. More serious gonococcal infections include pelvic inflammatory disease (PID), a term that encompasses endometritis, salpingitis, and peritonitis; and disseminated gonococcal infection (DGI), which may include arthritis, tenosynovitis, dermatitis, and rarely hepatitis, myocarditis, endocarditis, and meningitis.

The diagnosis of gonococcal urethritis in men is generally straightforward, and Gram's stain is often all that is required. The presence of gram-negative diplococci of characteristic morphologic appearance within polymorphonuclear leukocytes is diagnostic of gonorrhea in a smear of urethral exudate material. For suspected infections at other sites (including all infections in women), the sensitivity and specificity of Gram's stain are not adequate for the diagnosis of gonorrhea, and cultures should be done. Treatment decisions in the acute care setting are often made on the basis of the presenting clinical syndrome; diagnostic confirmation is achieved by cultures. Newer diagnostic tests such as amplification methods (polymerase or ligase chain reaction) may be useful in selected settings, but they are much more expensive and are not recommended for routine use.

The diagnosis of gonorrhea is a marker for high-risk sexual behaviors, and other STD pathogens may be acquired at the same time as *N. gonorrhoeae*. A substantial proportion of patients with gonorrhea also harbor the genital tract pathogens (such as *C. trachomatis*) that are responsible for the syndrome nongonococcal urethritis (NGU). Urethritis symptoms may persist if these organisms are not treated simultaneously with the treatment of gonorrhea. Therefore, all patients with gonorrhea must receive antimicrobial regimens that are active against NGU organisms as well. In addition, it is advisable to test for additional STDs in any patient diagnosed with gonorrhea. Serologic tests for syphilis and human immunodeficiency virus infection are recommended whenever possible.

TREATMENT OF ADULTS

Uncomplicated Urogenital, Rectal, or Pharyngeal Infection

Table 1 lists the recommended treatment regimens for uncomplicated gonococcal infection involving the urethra and genital tract as well for rectal gonorrhea. Data on pharyngeal infections are limited; whereas treatment response rates in the pharynx may be somewhat lower, the same regimens are suggested. Although intramuscular ceftriaxone (Rocephin) in a dose of 125 mg is a proven and highly effective treatment, cefixime (Suprax) given as a single 400-mg oral dose is easier to administer and is usually less expensive. Ceftriaxone has the advantage of demonstrated activity against incubating syphilis, but the rarity of syphilis in most areas makes this consideration less important. Quinolones are also effective as

TABLE 1. **Treatment of Uncomplicated Adult Gonococcal Infections***

Preferred Regimens

Cefixime (Suprax), 400 mg orally as a single dose

or

Ceftriaxone (Rocephin), 125 mg intramuscularly as a single dose

Alternative Regimens for Patients Who Cannot Receive β-Lactam Antibiotics

Ciprofloxacin (Cipro),† 500 mg orally as a single dose

or

Ofloxacin (Floxin),† 400 mg orally as a single dose

Alternative Regimen for Patients Who Cannot Receive β-Lactam or Quinolone Antibiotics

Spectinomycin (Trobicin), 2 gm intramuscularly as a single dose

---

*Drugs are listed in order of preference. All regimens must also include therapy for presumptive infection with *Chlamydia trachomatis* and other nongonococcal urethritis pathogens (see Table 2).

†Quinolones are contraindicated in pregnant or nursing women and in children younger than 16 y.

single-dose agents for uncomplicated gonorrhea, but clinically important resistance has been seen in certain geographic areas. Clinicians who use quinolones to treat gonorrhea must be aware of the prevalence of such strains in the area. Quinolones are contraindicated in pregnant women and children because of the potential for damage to articular cartilage. Intramuscular spectinomycin is a useful alternative in some circumstances. In all cases, regimens must also include an antimicrobial that is suitable for the treatment of presumptive infection with NGU pathogens (Table 2).

Pelvic Inflammatory Disease

PID refers to infection of the female upper genital tract, sometimes also involving the peritoneum. A variety of criteria have been proposed for the diagnosis of PID, and most experts believe that it is best to have a low threshold for treatment given the serious sequelae of the disease. PID is almost always a polymicrobial infection in which *N. gonorrhoeae,* when present, is only one of the bacteria responsible. Thus, treatment regimens must be relatively broad spectrum and generally include drugs active against gon-

TABLE 2. **Treatment Regimens for *Chlamydia trachomatis* and the Pathogens of Nongonococcal Urethritis in Patients with Gonorrhea***

Preferred Regimens

Azithromycin (Zithromax), 1 gm orally as a single dose

or

Doxycycline (Vibramycin), 100 mg orally twice/d for 7 d

Alternative Regimens

Ofloxacin (Floxin),† 300 mg orally twice/d for 7 d

or

Erythromycin base, 500 mg orally 4 times/d for 7 d

---

*Drugs are listed in order of preference.

†Quinolones are contraindicated in pregnant or nursing women and in children younger than 16 y.

TABLE 3. **Treatment of Pelvic Inflammatory Disease***

Inpatient Regimens†

Cefoxitin (Mefoxin), 2 gm intravenously q 6 h or cefotetan (Cefotan), 2 gm intravenously q 12 h

plus

Doxycycline, 100 mg intravenously or orally q 12 h

alternatively

Clindamycin (Cleocin), 900 mg intravenously q 8 h

plus

Gentamicin, 2 mg/kg initial dose, followed by 1.5 mg/kg q 8 h, adjusted for renal function

Outpatient Regimens

Cefoxitin, 2 gm intramuscularly, plus probenecid, 1 gm orally, in a single dose

plus

Doxycycline, 100 mg orally twice/d for 14 d, or ofloxacin,‡ 400 mg orally twice/d for 14 d

plus

Clindamycin, 450 mg orally 4 times/d for 14 d or metronidazole (Flagyl), 500 mg orally twice/d for 14 d

---

*Drugs are listed in order of preference.

†Inpatient regimens should be continued for at least 48 h after the patient demonstrates substantial clinical improvement, after which doxycycline 100 mg orally twice daily to complete a total of 14 d of treatment should be given.

‡Quinolones are contraindicated in pregnant or nursing women and in children younger than 16 y.

orrhea and *C. trachomatis*. Patients in whom compliance is suspect or who have severe clinical disease should probably be hospitalized. Women in whom the diagnosis is uncertain (e.g., those who may have an ectopic pregnancy or appendicitis) should also be treated initially as inpatients. Table 3 lists the CDC-recommended treatment regimens for PID.

Disseminated Gonococcal Infection

DGI is an uncommon condition that most often presents as arthritis, tenosynovitis, and/or a papulopustular rash. Patients with DGI should begin therapy in the hospital with regimens active against the gonococcus and *C. trachomatis*. Initial therapy with ceftriaxone, 1 gram intravenously or intramuscularly every 24 hours, plus a single 1-gram dose of oral azithromycin (Zithromax) is recommended. Spectinomycin, 2 grams intravenously every 12 hours, plus azithromycin is suggested for those who cannot be given β-lactam antimicrobials. Parenteral therapy should be continued for 24 to 48 hours after clinical improvement is seen, after which an outpatient regimen of either cefixime (Suprax), 400 mg orally twice daily,* or ciprofloxacin (Cipro), 500 mg orally twice daily, should be given to complete a full week of treatment. Patients with more unusual sites of infection (meningitis, endocarditis) require therapy of longer duration, and consultation with an expert is suggested.

---

*Exceeds dosage recommended by the manufacturer.

TREATMENT OF NEONATES AND CHILDREN

Neonatal Infections

Gonorrhea in neonates is virtually always due to exposure during passage through the birth canal of an infected woman. The most common manifestation of neonatal gonorrhea is gonococcal ophthalmia neonatorum. In the United States, this diagnosis is rare owing to the nearly universal use of ocular prophylaxis in newborns. Recommended treatment is ceftriaxone, 25 to 50 mg per kg intravenously or intramuscularly in a single dose, not to exceed a total dose of 125 mg. Infections at other sites should be treated with single daily doses of ceftriaxone, 25 to 50 mg per kg in consultation with an expert in the field.

Infants born to mothers with gonococcal infection are at high risk for acquiring *N. gonorrhoeae,* and these neonates should be treated whether they are symptomatic or not. The recommended regimen is the same as is recommended for gonococcal ophthalmic infections.

Infections in Children

When gonorrhea is diagnosed in preadolescent children after the neonatal period, the issue of child abuse must be considered, and diagnostic specimens should be obtained in conjunction with the appropriate legal authorities to ensure that the data obtained can be used in legal proceedings if necessary. The recommended treatment of gonorrhea in children is intramuscular ceftriaxone, 25 to 50 mg per kg, up to a maximal dose of 125 mg. For DGI in children, a 7- to 10-day course of intravenous or intramuscular ceftriaxone, 25 to 50 mg per kg per day, is advised. It is not clear how frequently gonococcal infections in children are accompanied by *C. trachomatis* or other NGU pathogens. Most authorities do recommend the routine use of additional antimicrobials in children with gonorrhea but suggest that appropriate diagnostic specimens be obtained with treatment reserved for patients with positive test results.

NONGONOCOCCAL URETHRITIS IN MEN

method of
JACKSON E. FOWLER, Jr., M.D.
University of Mississippi Medical Center
Jackson, Mississippi

Nongonococcal urethritis is the most common sexually transmitted disease syndrome in American men; about 3 million cases occur each year. The disorder is usually manifested by urethral discomfort or dysuria and a purulent or mucoid urethral discharge; it is caused by *Chlamydia trachomatis, Ureaplasma urealyticum,* or *Trichomonas vag-*

inalis in about 40, 20, and 5% of cases, respectively. Studies have suggested that *Mycoplasma genitalium* may also be an important cause of the syndrome. In 35% of affected patients, there is no identifiable microbial agent, and the prevalence of these inflammations appears to be increasing.

The symptoms of *Chlamydia*-positive and *Chlamydia*-negative nongonococcal urethritis are indistinguishable but tend to be less severe than those of gonococcal urethritis. Urethral inflammation is documented by the finding of at least five polymorphonuclear leukocytes per oil immersion field (1000×) in a Gram-stained smear of the discharge or an intraurethral swab specimen. The smear is carefully inspected for the presence of intracellular gram-negative diplococci, which by and large are diagnostic of gonorrhea. If gonorrhea is ruled out, the unstained urethral discharge or a first-voided urine specimen is examined for *T. vaginalis*. This parasite is pear shaped, is slightly smaller than a squamous epithelial cell, and moves with a characteristic twitching motion. Further laboratory studies to determine the causative agent of nongonococcal urethritis do not have an impact on treatment recommendations and are generally not warranted. However, testing for chlamydial infection with an immunoassay or culture of the intraurethral swab specimen may be desirable when the patient is overly concerned about the cause of his illness or the necessity for treatment of his sexual partner. *U. urealyticum* can be isolated by culture, but the organism is not always pathogenic and the significance of a positive culture is generally indeterminate.

TREATMENT

Urethritis produced by *T. vaginalis* is treated with metronidazole (Flagyl), 250 mg by mouth three times daily for 7 days or 2 grams by mouth as a single dose.

Recommended treatments of nongonococcal urethritis that is not due to *T. vaginalis* are shown in Table 1. Doxycycline (Vibramycin), 100 mg orally twice daily for 7 days, is the treatment of choice. Erythromycin stearate, 500 mg by mouth four times daily for 7 days, is recommended if doxycycline therapy is contraindicated or not well tolerated. Azithromycin (Zithromax), 1.0 gram by mouth, is the only single-dose treatment with good activity against *Chlamydia*-positive and *Chlamydia*-negative nongonococcal urethritis and may be the preferable therapy when anticipated compliance with multidose regimens is suspect. However, single-dose azithromycin therapy is substantially more expensive than multidose doxycycline therapy. Ofloxacin (Floxin) is the only fluoroquinolone antibiotic with acceptable activity against *C. trachomatis,* and 300 mg is given twice daily for 7 days. This agent is contraindicated in pregnancy and in children 16 years of age or younger.

Clinical cures are achieved in about 80% of patients with nongonococcal urethritis who are treated with doxycycline, and microbiologic cures are achieved in about 90% with *Chlamydia*-positive infections. Follow-up investigations to assess therapeutic efficacy are not necessary. When there are persistent or recurrent symptoms, objective evidence of urethral inflammation should be documented by microscopic examination of the discharge or an intraurethral swab specimen. Re-treatment with doxycycline for 7 days is appropriate if reinfection or poor compliance is believed to be responsible for the unfavorable outcome. The erythromycin regimen is recommended when the cause of persistent or recurrent symptoms is unclear because *U. urealyticum* may be resistant to doxycycline.

A small proportion of men have persistent but episodic symptoms after the first infection. In these cases, urethroscopy is advisable to rule out a urethral stricture, diverticulum, or condyloma acuminatum, which may simulate nongonococcal urethritis. However, the examination is usually unrevealing. There is no evidence that persistent urethritis of unknown etiology is harmful, but the symptoms may cause substantial concern and anxiety. Self-treatment with a 3- to 5-day course of doxycycline or erythromycin at the onset of symptoms is recommended for the management of these troublesome cases.

OTHER CONSIDERATIONS

The recent sexual contacts of men with nongonococcal urethritis should be identified and treated empirically with doxycycline. This process requires the patient's cooperation and may involve complex social issues. It is most successful if the patient understands the potential risks of an untreated infection in his sexual partner, such as mucopurulent cervicitis or pelvic inflammatory disease, and if the diagnosing physician treats the contact. The clinician must also educate the patient about the importance of protected sex and of a mutually monogamous sexual relationship for prevention of recurrent urethritis and acquisition of such potentially devastating viral diseases as genital herpes and human immunodeficiency virus infection; the physician should never assume that the patient has any knowledge about these issues.

DONOVANOSIS
(Granuloma Inguinale)

method of
MARGARET C. DOUGLASS, M.D.
Henry Ford Hospital
Detroit, Michigan

Donovanosis, a progressive mucocutaneous ulcerative disease of genital, inguinal, or perianal areas, is caused by *Calymmatobacterium granulomatis,* an encapsulated facul-

TABLE 1. **Recommended Treatment Regimens for Nongonococcal Urethritis**

Drug	Dosage
Doxycycline	100 mg q 12 h for 7 d
Erythromycin stearate	500 mg q 6 h for 7 d
Azithromycin	1.0-gm single dose
Ofloxacin	300 mg q 12 h for 7 d

tative intracellular gram-negative bacterium. Endemic in many tropical and subtropical regions, it is relatively rare in the United States, where most cases occur in the South or Southwest. It is a major cause of genital ulceration in southern India, New Guinea, the Caribbean, parts of South America, South Africa, Southeast Asia, and Australian aboriginal regions.

Although it is clearly transmitted sexually, there is controversy regarding whether nonsexual transmission occurs. Infectivity is considered to be low; reported rates of infection in sexual partners vary widely from more than 50% in India to as low as 5 to 15% from studies out of South Africa and Australia.

Clinical disease begins after an incubation period averaging about 3 weeks. A papule or nodule appears at the site of contact. Rapidly progressive ulceration produces beefy red, painless, exuberant, friable ulcers that can be mutilating. Without secondary infection, the base is nonpurulent. In contrast to lymphogranuloma venereum, regional adenopathy is unusual. Subcutaneous inguinal granulomas can mimic buboes.

The genital area is involved in the majority of cases, the inguinal or anal area in about 10 to 25% of cases, and a distal site in less than 5%. The prepuce, coronal sulcus, and frenulum are the most common sites in men. The most common site in women is the labia; vaginal and cervical lesions also occur.

Spontaneous healing, unlikely in established cases, is extremely slow and results in significant fibrosis. Sequelae of chronic infection include strictures, lymphatic obstruction, rectovaginal fistulas, mutilation of external genitalia, and deep local involvement. Systemic disease with bone, liver, or spleen involvement can rarely occur, with possible fatal outcomes.

Complete healing without sequelae can occur with early treatment. Because genital ulcerations facilitate transmission of human immunodeficiency virus (HIV) infection, control of donovanosis in endemic areas is an important public health measure to prevent acquired immune deficiency syndrome.

Reliable culture techniques or serologic tests for donovanosis are not yet available. Diagnosis depends on demonstration of the intracellular organisms (Donovan's bodies) on crushed tissue smear. Donovan's bodies, with their characteristic safety pin appearance, are best seen with Giemsa or various silver stains. The organisms are rarely visualized in formalin-fixed paraffin block specimens, but they can often be found in ultrathin sections from biopsy tissue embedded in plastic.

TREATMENT

Numerous antibiotics have been used for donovanosis, and there is no consensus as to which is the best. Tetracycline 500 mg four times daily, erythromycin 500 mg four times daily, doxycycline (Vibramycin, Monodox) 100 mg twice daily, and trimethoprim 160 mg plus sulfamethoxazole 800 mg (Bactrim DS, Septra DS) twice daily are all considered standard therapies. Treatment should be continued until complete epithelialization has occurred or for a minimum of 2 weeks. Other antibiotics reported to be effective include quinolones and chloramphenicol or streptomycin intramuscularly twice daily to supplement tetracycline in severe cases. Ceftriaxone (Rocephin) 1 gram intramuscularly daily for 7 to 26

days has been reported to be effective when standard therapies have failed and has the advantage of reliable dosage when poor compliance with oral medications is a problem. In all cases, testing should be done for other sexually transmitted diseases including syphilis, gonorrhea, and HIV infection.

LYMPHOGRANULOMA VENEREUM

method of
MARGARET C. DOUGLASS, M.D.
Henry Ford Hospital
Detroit, Michigan

Lymphogranuloma venereum (LGV) is a sexually transmitted disease caused by the LGV serovars of *Chlamydia trachomatis* (L1, L2, or L3). Endemic in Africa, India, Southeast Asia, South America, and the Caribbean, it occurs sporadically elsewhere. In Western countries, the highest frequency of occurrence is in homosexual men, prostitutes, and travelers returning from endemic areas.

Clinical disease has three distinct stages. Three to 30 days after exposure, the primary lesion appears as a small papule or herpetiform ulcer most commonly on the penis, cervix, or posterior vaginal wall. The primary lesion is asymptomatic, heals rapidly without scarring, and often goes unnoticed.

The secondary stage, characterized by regional lymphadenopathy and systemic symptoms, occurs days to weeks after the primary lesion. The lymphadenopathy, unilateral in two thirds of patients, is tender and characterized by initially discrete nodes with overlying erythema. Involvement of multiple nodes and extensive periadenitis result in large inflammatory masses (or buboes). Abscesses developing within buboes can spontaneously rupture, leaving draining sinus tracts. The almost pathognomonic groove sign of LGV occurs when extensive femoral and inguinal adenopathy is separated by the inelastic Poupart (inguinal) ligament.

Inguinal lymphadenopathy is common in men but not in women. Involvement of deep pelvic and lumbar lymph nodes is more common in women and can result in lower abdominal and back pain. Hemorrhagic proctitis or proctocolitis, usually in women or homosexual men as a consequence of anal intercourse, may occur during acute stages of LGV. Presenting with rectal pain, tenesmus, mucopurulent discharge, or bloody diarrhea, it can mimic inflammatory bowel disease. Other possible systemic manifestations of LGV include fever, headache, myalgias, meningitis or meningoencephalitis, pneumonia, and rarely keratoconjunctivitis or polyarthritis.

The late or third stage of disease is most common in women and characterized by perirectal abscesses, fistula formation, and/or stricture or stenosis of the rectum (the anorectogenital syndrome). Chronic lymphatic obstruction can result in elephantiasis of the external genitalia (especially vulva) with ulcerations.

Diagnosis generally depends on a compatible clinical picture and a complement-fixation (CF) titer of 1:64 or greater. Although CF is not specific for LGV serovars, other types of *C. trachomatis* infection (e.g., chlamydial urethritis, cervicitis, or conjunctivitis) rarely have CF titers above 1:16. Microimmunofluorescence is more sensitive in detecting antichlamydial antibodies. Active cases of LGV usually have relatively high levels of IgM (>1:32) and IgG (>1:1200). Lymph node biopsy can support but not confirm the diagnosis. Culture remains impractical for routine use. Amplified DNA probe tests may become the preferred diagnostic method in the future.

TREATMENT

Recommended therapy for LGV is doxycycline (Vibramycin, Monodox) 100 mg orally twice daily, tetracycline 500 mg orally four times daily, or minocycline (Minocin, Dynacin) 100 mg orally twice daily. Erythromycin 500 mg orally four times daily is an alternative. In general, 3 weeks of therapy is recommended. Drainage of fluctuant buboes can prevent rupture and sinus tract formation. Reconstructive surgery may be necessary for late sequelae. Patients with LGV should be checked for human immunodeficiency virus infection as well as for other sexually transmitted diseases. Sexual contacts should be examined for LGV. Although limited data are available regarding therapy for cases of LGV much less for sexual contacts, therapy for asymptomatic contacts for 1 week is recommended.

SYPHILIS

method of
NICHOLAS J. FIUMARA, M.D., M.P.H.
Tufts University School of Medicine–
New England Medical Center
Boston, Massachusetts

Syphilis is an acute and a chronic infectious disease caused by *Treponema pallidum*. Except for congenital syphilis, it is usually acquired by sex and sex play during the infectious period. In acquired syphilis, the disease passes through the primary stage, which is manifested by a chancre (an ulceration at the point of inoculation); a secondary stage, with systemic symptoms, adenopathy, and rash; an early latent stage, which is an asymptomatic period of variable duration with reactive serologic test results; and finally a late stage, which involves the mucocutaneous, osseous, visceral, cardiovascular, and neural systems. Infectious syphilis, however, consists of the primary, secondary, and early latent stages. It is during these three stages that syphilis may be sexually spread. During pregnancy, however, syphilis in all stages is potentially infectious to the developing fetus. Infection by transfusion is rare because of the requirement that all blood for transfusion must have a nonreactive test response, and the spirochete will die within 24 hours under the conditions of blood bank storage. Syphilis, like acquired immune deficiency syndrome, may spread among drug users who share needles.

PRIMARY SYPHILIS

After an incubation period of 9 to 90 days, with an average of 3 weeks, the primary stage appears. It is characterized by the chancre, which emerges at the point of inoculation. Because 90% of all syphilis is sexually transmitted, most chancres appear on the genitals as either single or multiple lesions. Chancres occur after sexual exposure, kissing, and accidental direct inoculation but never after transfusions or in congenital syphilis of the newborn infant. The chancre begins as a papule and soon erodes and becomes ulcerative. It is characteristically painless, indolent, punched out, and clean with a scanty, yellow, serous discharge. The borders of the ulcer are raised, smooth, and sharply defined; the base is finely granular and hard, and the entire lesion is indurated. The neighboring lymph nodes are discretely enlarged, hard, and nonsuppurating. Most chancres of the penis occur on the prepuce, coronal sulcus, glans, or frenulum. Some are intraurethral or are located on the shaft or base of the penis or on the scrotum.

In male homosexuals, anorectal chancres are seen in great frequency. They often occur in the posterior midline of the anal ring and superficially resemble an anal fissure. The patient complains of pain and bleeding on defecation; however, in contrast to an anal fissure, the ulcer is indurated and there is usually bilateral inguinal adenopathy. Chancres of the buttocks are usually asymptomatic. If the patient has had an external hemorrhoid, a chancre may appear at this site as an ulcerated painful lesion. Chancres of the rectum are less common and appear as an ulcerated area that is indurated and looks superficially like a carcinoma. Chancres of the anorectal area appear in less frequency in bisexuals and even less often in female heterosexuals.

In women, the labia are the most common sites, but chancres may appear at the fourchette, urethra, or perineum. The cervix is more frequently involved than the statistics indicate. Some chancres, particularly in women, may be so inconspicuous or so located as to escape notice. Although most appear on the genitals, chancres may be seen anywhere on the body as a result of preliminary sex play.

The diagnosis of primary syphilis is established by the finding of *T. pallidum* on darkfield examination and by the reagin and treponemal blood tests. The blood reagin test may not be reactive if the chancre has been present for less than a week. However, if the rapid plasma reagin (RPR) test is used, it is reactive by the seventh day of the chancre. The Venereal Disease Research Laboratory (VDRL) test may not be reactive in this period and may need to be repeated. The result of the microhemagglutination assay–*T. pallidum* (MHA-TP) test, which is usually performed when the reagin test is reactive, will also be positive. It is even more sensitive than the reagin tests. In 2 to 6 weeks, usually less, the chancre will heal without treatment and the patient progresses to the secondary stage.

SECONDARY SYPHILIS

The secondary stage follows the onset of the chancre by 9 to 90 days with an average of 3 weeks. The chancre is frequently present at the beginning of the secondary stage but is usually healing. The secondary stage appears within 6 months and usually 6 to 8 weeks after infectious exposure. The signs and symptoms of secondary syphilis are protean but may be conveniently grouped within three syndromes.

Early in this stage, the patient complains of an influenza-like or grippelike syndrome consisting of headaches, lacrimation, nasal discharge, sore throat, and generalized arthralgia. There is a slight rise in temperature in addition to a severe loss of weight. There may be secondary anemia, an increase in the white cell count (with an absolute lymphocytosis), and an increase in the erythrocyte sedimentation rate. With these constitutional symptoms, the patient will have enlargement of the lymph nodes. A generalized lymphadenopathy is one of the most common findings of secondary syphilis. The lymph nodes are enlarged but not painful and have a hard, rubbery feel. This adenopathy usually precedes the cutaneous eruption. At about this time, palpation of the abdomen may reveal an enlarged spleen and, less commonly, an enlarged liver as well.

The generalized eruption completes the picture of secondary syphilis. It is often darkfield-positive. Although the eruption of secondary syphilis may mimic a variety of skin diseases, it tends to have certain characteristics that help to identify it as syphilis. The eruption is generalized, painless, and nonpruritic, with the exception of the follicular type. It involves the skin as well as the mucous membranes. On the skin, it tends to follow to some extent the lines of cleavage, especially on the trunk. It has a special predilection for the palms of the hands and soles of the feet. The lesions are discrete and sharply demarcated rather than confluent and have a coppery hue. The color becomes more intensified from the periphery to the center. The eruption of early secondary syphilis is not particularly scaly, with the exception of the hard, indurated papules on the palms and soles. Here the scales tend to be at the periphery rather than at the center (lues cornee). The eruption is bilateral and symmetrical, tending to be more profuse on the upper extremities than on the abdomen and lower extremities. The eruption may be macular, papular, pustular, or more commonly a combination such as maculopapular or papulopustular, but a generalized vesicular or bullous eruption, for all practical purposes, eliminates secondary syphilis. Thus, in any generalized discrete eruption involving the palms and soles, diagnosis of secondary syphilis should be considered until it is proved otherwise. The eruption may last a few weeks to as long as 12 months. This is followed by a period of latency, which—in at least 25% of untreated cases—is interrupted by signs and symptoms of clinical secondary relapse. As stated, of these patients, a little more than one fifth experience one to three additional relapses.

The diagnosis of secondary syphilis is based on the clinical picture of the characteristic rash, the generalized adenopathy, and reactive reagin and treponemal test results. The reagin blood titer is usually higher than that seen in primary syphilis. On occasion, the qualitative RPR or VDRL test result is reported as nonreactive by the laboratory. In such situations, the quantitative reagin will reveal a nonreactive blood test reaction in more concentrated serum, such as undiluted serum 1:1 and 1:2, but as the serum is diluted more and more, such as 1:4 and 1:8 and so forth, a positive reaction is found. This is called the "prozone reaction." Agglutination reactions occur only within fixed limits of antibody and antigen. In the prozone reaction, the patient has a surplus amount of antibody for the amount of antigen used; thus, no agglutination occurs in the more concentrated serum. It is therefore advisable to request that the laboratory perform a quantitative reagin test in a patient with a generalized eruption. The MHA-TP test response is not affected by the prozone reaction, and it will be reactive. Consequently, a reactive MHA-TP test result with a nonreactive qualitative reagin test result alerts the physician to request a quantitative RPR or VDRL test and a treponemal test.

LATENT SYPHILIS

Latent syphilis is a stage of acquired or congenital syphilis that is without signs or symptoms (of early or late

symptomatic syphilis) and characterized by repeatedly reactive reagin and treponemal blood test results and a nonreactive cerebrospinal fluid reagin test result.

Latent syphilis is classified as early latent if the patient has a history of symptoms consistent with primary or secondary syphilis within the past year, a documented nonreactive RPR or VDRL test result within the year, or exposure to a patient with infectious syphilis within the last year. Early latent syphilis is potentially infectious sexually because of the frequency of relapsing secondary syphilis during this period. The diagnosis is established in an asymptomatic patient with no lesions of primary or secondary syphilis who has a repeated positive reagin (RPR) test result and a reactive response to a treponemal test, such as the MHA-TP or fluorescent treponemal antibody absorption test. In the absence of neurologic findings, a lumbar puncture is waived because present-day treatment is curative of asymptomatic neurosyphilis.

RECOMMENDED TREATMENT SCHEDULE FOR SYPHILIS

Early Syphilis: Primary, Secondary, and Early Latent Disease of Less Than 1 Year's Duration

One of the following:

1. Benzathine penicillin G, 2.4 million units intramuscularly weekly for 2 consecutive weeks, a total of 4.8 million units

2. Doxycycline, 100 mg orally two times daily for 15 days

3. Minocycline, 100 mg orally two times daily for 15 days

4. Tetracycline, 500 mg orally four times daily for 15 days

5. Ceftriaxone (Rocephin),* 250 mg intramuscularly daily for 10 days

6. Azithromycin (Zithromax),* 500 mg orally daily for 10 days

The objective of treatment in early syphilis is not only clinical cure—the disappearance of the chancre and rash—but also a serologic cure with the reagin test result reverting to seronegativity. This can be achieved with the recommended schedule in patients suffering their first attack of syphilis. After treatment, the quantitative RPR titer should decline fourfold by the third month, eightfold by the sixth month; all patients with primary syphilis should be nonreactive at 12 months, and those with secondary syphilis in 24 months. Approximately 95% of patients with early latent syphilis less than 1 year in duration should be RPR nonreactive in 2 years, and the remaining 5% within the next 2 years. However, if the patient had previously been infected with syphilis, was treated, and later became reinfected with primary, secondary, or latent syphilis, the reagin titers are slower to decline after treatment; some do not achieve seronegativity as patients with their first infection do.

---

*Not FDA approved for this indication.

The Jarisch-Herxheimer Reaction

After treatment of late primary syphilis, regularly with secondary syphilis, and less often with early latent syphilis, the patient suffers a self-limited episode of chills, fever, headache, and myalgia 2 to 6 hours after an injection of penicillin but not doxycycline or tetracycline; the chancre or rash is exacerbated. It lasts for several hours, and the patient wakes up in the morning refreshed. The Jarisch-Herxheimer reaction was first described by Jarisch in 1895 and by Herxheimer in 1902. It is also seen after treatment of neonatal syphilis. It is believed to be the allergic reaction to the breakdown of the spirochetes. In adults, it can be prevented by the oral administration of steroids before the penicillin injection.

Syphilis of More Than 1 Year's Duration

This category includes latent syphilis of more than 1 year's duration and late (tertiary) stages involving the mucocutaneous, osseous, visceral, and cardiovascular systems but not neurosyphilis.

1. Benzathine penicillin G (Bicillin), 2.4 million units intramuscularly at weekly intervals for not less than 3 weeks

or

2. Doxycycline, 100 mg orally two times daily for 15 days

Patients with a first attack of latent syphilis of 1 to 4 years' duration and treated with the recommended schedules will have a nonreactive RPR test result within 5 years after treatment.

Neurosyphilis

1. Aqueous crystalline penicillin G, 2 to 4 million units intravenously every 4 hours for 14 days
2. Benzathine penicillin G, 2.4 million units intramuscularly daily for 3 weeks
3. Doxycycline, 100 mg orally two times daily for 20 days

Syphilis in Pregnancy

The treatment schedule for syphilis in pregnancy is the same as that recommended for the nonpregnant patient.

Patients Not Allergic to Penicillin

Adequate treatment for the mother requires a minimum of benzathine penicillin G 2.4 million units intramuscularly weekly for 2 consecutive weeks for a total of 4.8 million units. The deciduous teeth are fully formed by the 18th week of pregnancy, and treatment before this time will prevent the formation of the hypoplastic and malformed deciduous teeth. Treatment of the infected mother during the second and third trimester will cure an infected fetus. If the mother is treated with the 2 doses of benzathine penicillin G within 14 days of delivery, the fetus is considered effectively treated and should not develop the early signs of neonatal syphilis, such as the snuffles or rash.

Section 11

Diseases of Allergy

ANAPHYLAXIS AND SERUM SICKNESS

method of
RICHARD D. DeSHAZO, M.D.
University of South Alabama, College of
Medicine
Mobile, Alabama

Anaphylaxis is a potentially life-threatening syndrome resulting from the sudden release of mast cell– and basophil–derived mediators into the circulatory system. The most common cause of anaphylaxis, hypersensitivity reactions to drugs, may occur as often as 1 in every 2700 hospitalized patients and results in 400 to 800 deaths per year from β-lactam antibiotics alone. Insect sting reactions have been estimated to cause about 40 deaths per year in the United States.

PATHOPHYSIOLOGY

Mast cell concentrations in the skin, lungs, and gastrointestinal tract reach 10,000 to 20,000 cells per mm³, with the total mass approximating the size of a human spleen. These cells and their circulating counterparts, the basophils, may be triggered to release the mediators of anaphylaxis by an interaction with one of several mast cell membrane receptors (Figure 1). For instance, certain protein and glycoprotein antigens stimulate the production of IgE antibodies in individuals genetically programmed for this response. These antibodies fix to IgE receptors on the surface of the mast cells and basophils of these individuals. On re-exposure to the antigen, the antigen reacts with antigen-specific IgE, triggering mast cell degranulation and the release of mast cell mediators of anaphylaxis. If the quantity of mediators released is great, anaphylaxis develops.

Complement fragments C3a and C5a, generated in immune complex reactions, may fix to complement receptors on mast cells and trigger mediator release independent of IgE. These reactions and others in which the release of mast cell mediators occurs independent of IgE are anaphylactoid reactions. Anaphylactoid reactions may occur in response to nonsteroidal anti-inflammatory agents, exercise, cold exposure, and iodinated contrast dye, among others (see Figure 1). The mechanisms of anaphylactoid reactions to these agents are unclear.

Mast cell activation is associated with the release of two sets of mediators: preformed granule-associated mediators and the newly formed mediators. The release of preformed mediators explains the rapid onset of symptoms, which usually occur within minutes of exposure to the triggering agent. The production of newly formed mediators appears to explain the protracted symptoms in some individuals.

Mediators of anaphylaxis result in increased vascular permeability with subsequent (1) loss in intravascular volume causing hypotension, (2) smooth muscle contraction associated with the respiratory and gastrointestinal symptoms, and (3) activation of the complement, coagulation, and kinin systems. Trypsin is a mast cell mediator detectable in periperal blood during anaphylaxis. It is useful retrospectively in distinguishing anaphylactic and anaphylactoid reactions from other conditions simulating anaphylaxis and in documenting anaphylaxis in cases of sudden death.

SIGNS AND SYMPTOMS

The signs and symptoms of anaphylaxis are summarized in Table 1 and reflect the wide distribution of mast cells and basophils throughout the body. The majority of deaths from anaphylaxis are associated with respiratory symptoms, primarily asphyxiation from laryngospasm or bronchospasm. A lesser percentage of deaths occurs from cardiovascular symptoms, primarily from refractory shock or states of low cardiac output.

Different individuals have different patterns of anaphylaxis, but urticaria is present in most. The onset of anaphylaxis is often heralded by a brief prodrome of erythema and pruritus of the hands, feet, and genitalia. If not treated immediately, patients may develop more serious symptoms. Although many individuals have combinations of urticaria, angioedema, bronchospasm, and hypotension, isolated symptoms such as hypotension, explosive diarrhea, laryngospasm, or total body erythema may occur in some. The pattern in a given individual is usually recapitulated in recurrent episodes.

Because the symptoms of anaphylaxis are stereotyped, the diagnosis is usually obvious, with few considerations in the differential diagnosis. Acutely, anaphylaxis must be distinguished from vasovagal syncope, in which bradycardia, cool skin, and the absence of urticaria are helpful differential features. Bradycardia does occur in a small percentage of patients with anaphylaxis, however.

NOVEL FORMS OF ANAPHYLAXIS

Several novel forms of anaphylaxis have been reported (Table 2). *Exercise-induced anaphylaxis* is anaphylaxis that occurs with protracted exercise, most often running. A variant form occurs only when exercise is preceded by the ingestion of certain foods, for instance shrimp or celery. Exercise-induced anaphylaxis is not prevented by antihistamine treatment before exercise. If prodromal symptoms occur and exercise continues, syncope may occur. Individuals who are taking *beta blockers* are at risk for unusually severe and protracted anaphylaxis. Treatment with beta-adrenergic blockers is a contraindication to allergy immunotherapy because of the increased risk for severe allergic reactions. Parenteral administration of any drug should be performed with caution in such patients. Up to a third of patients with severe anaphylactic reactions to some drugs have *biphasic anaphylaxis*. In these individuals, a second episode or late phase of anaphylaxis occurs 4 hours or

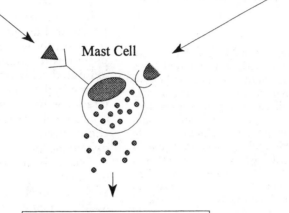

Some Agents Causing Anaphylactic Reactions

Hormones: ACTH, insulin, hydrocortisone
Animal or human proteins: horse serum (snake antivenin, antilymphocyte globulin), seminal fluid, factor VIII, protamine sulfate, monoclonal antibodies
Enzymes: chymotrypsin, chymopapain, streptokinase
Venoms: fire ant, wasp, hornets
Allergen extracts: pollen, mold, dust mite, animal danders
Foods: eggs, milk, shellfish, nuts, chocolate
Drugs: penicillin, cephalosporin, insulin
Ethylene oxide gas on dialysis tubing
Hydatid cyst rupture
Latex

Some Agents Causing Anaphylactoid Reactions

Nonsteroidal anti-inflammatory agents: aspirin, indomethacin, ibuprofen
Diagnostic agents: iodinated contrast media
Opiates
Muscle relaxants: tubocurarine, succinylcholine
Cold
Exercise
Vancomycin
Intravenous immunoglobulin
Polysaccharides: dextran, iron dextran
Idiopathic

Mast Cell

Some Mast Cell Mediators of Anaphylaxis

Preformed
  Histamine
  ECF-A
  NCF-A
  Tryptase
  Chymase
  Peroxidase
  TNF-α

Newly Formed
  Leukotriene C_4, D_4, E_4
  Platelet-activating factor
  Prostaglandin D_2
  Leukotriene B_4
  HETEs
  Interferon-γ
  Adenosine
  Nitric oxide

Pathophysiology of Clinical Symptoms

Increased vascular permeability
Smooth muscle contraction
Platelet activation
Chemotaxis of leukocytes
Activation of complement, kinin and coagulation systems

Figure 1. Mechanisms of mast cell mediator release and anaphylaxis. *Abbreviations:* ACTH = corticotropin; ECF-A = eosinophil chemotactic factor of anaphylaxis; NCF-A = neutrophil chemotactic factor of anaphylaxis; TNF-α = tumor necrosis factor-α; HETE = hydroxyeicosatetraenoic acid.

TABLE 1. **Signs and Symptoms of Anaphylaxis**

Organ System	Signs or Symptom
General	Sense of impending doom, malaise, weakness, disorientation, diaphoresis
Cutaneous	Erythema, urticaria, angioedema, pruritus, warmth
Respiratory	Sneezing, rhinorrhea, nasal congestion, dysphonia, laryngospasm, bronchospasm, asphyxia
Cardiovascular	Tachycardia, hypotension, arrhythmias, faintness, palpitations, myocardial infarction, intraventricular conduction defect
Gastrointestinal	Vomiting, diarrhea, abdominal cramps, tenesmus, diarrhea
Genitourinary	Uterine contractions, bladder urgency
Central nervous system	Syncope, seizure

Modified from Lantner R, Ballow M, deShazo RD: Anaphylaxis and serum sickness. *In* Rakel RE (ed): Conn's Current Therapy. Philadelphia, WB Saunders Co, 1990, pp 673–676.

more after the initial episode. Although this late phase may be attenuated by treatment with corticosteroid therapy during the initial reaction, many authorities believe that the risk for biphasic anaphylaxis warrants hospital admission for observation of all patients with severe anaphylaxis. *Recurrent idiopathic anaphylaxis* is an unusual syndrome in which extensive diagnostic evaluation fails to detect the cause of anaphylaxis and episodes continue. A program of long-term treatment with antihistamines and corticosteroids has been reported to attenuate the frequency and severity of subsequent reactions. *Anaphylaxis in the surgical suite* occurs most commonly on the basis of hypersensitivity to latex or reactions to quaternary ammonium muscle relaxants used during induction of anesthesia. Children with spina bifida who have had recurrent exposure to latex are at special risk for anaphylaxis to latex, which may be present in surgical gloves, connectors for tubing, endotracheal tubes, and other medical material. Medical personnel with a previous history of pruritic hand dermatitis and sneezing or wheezing with latex exposure are also at risk for allergic reactions when exposed to latex gloves or other latex products.

TREATMENT OF ANAPHYLAXIS

The treatment of anaphylaxis centers on the early use of adequate doses of epinephrine and application of the usual and accepted cardiopulmonary resuscitation procedures such as advanced cardiac life support (Figure 2). An airway and appropriate oxygenation should be established. The majority of patients with severe anaphylactic reactions have hypoxemia from

TABLE 2. **Novel Forms of Anaphylaxis**

Exercise-induced anaphylaxis
Food-associated exercise-induced anaphylaxis
Recurrent idiopathic anaphylaxis
Severe anaphylaxis associated with beta-adrenergic blockade
Anaphylaxis in the surgical suite
Biphasic or protracted anaphylaxis

pulmonary ventilation-perfusion mismatches and appear to benefit from oxygen. Intravascular volume should be restored with adequate colloidal solutions, and antihistamines and corticosteroids should be administered liberally to treat and prevent ongoing symptoms. The repeated administration of glucagon* can be lifesaving in patients taking beta blockers, although glucagon may induce nausea and vomiting. Bronchospasm in the presence of hypoxemia may be treated with recurrent or continuous nebulization of beta-adrenergic agents such as albuterol. In the case of persistent hypotension unresponsive to epinephrine or vasopressors, the early initiation of intra-aortic balloon pump therapy has been reported to be lifesaving.

PREVENTION OF ANAPHYLACTIC REACTIONS

Because drug reactions occur more commonly with parenteral administration, drugs should be administered orally when possible. Certain agents, such as parenterally administered β-lactam antibiotics and iodinated contrast agents, are known to be associated with a higher risk for reactions and should be administered with special care. In patients with previous anaphylactoid reactions to contrast dye who require their further use, corticosteroid-antihistamine-ephedrine pretreatment regimens have been shown to block future reactions. Allergies to drugs, food, or biologic agents should be prominently noted on patients' medical charts. Likewise, patients should acquire medical alert bracelets engraved with this information. Several brands of anaphylaxis treatment kits are available for individuals at high risk for anaphylactic reactions, for instance, insect sting reactions or idiopathic anaphylaxis. These include Ana-Kit and EpiPen and EpiPen Jr. auto-injectors. The Ana-Kit allows multiple doses of epinephrine and contains a chewable antihistamine. The EpiPen is spring loaded and does not require the patient to use a syringe for injection. Patients with insect sting anaphylaxis should be referred to an allergist for allergen immunotherapy with insect venom. This technique has been shown to be highly effective in preventing recurrent insect sting anaphylaxis.

SERUM SICKNESS

Serum sickness is a syndrome characterized by combinations of fever, rash, lymphadenopathy, arthralgia, or arthritis that usually occurs 10 to 14 days after exposure to a variety of protein antigens (Table 3). The rash may be either urticaria or cutaneous vasculitis as manifested by palpable purpura. The latter condition occurs on dependent areas such as the lower leg and reflects the leakage of red blood cells into the skin from inflammation in the postcapillary venules. Variants of serum sickness include the syndromes of systemic vasculitis that occur in

---

*Not FDA approved for this indication.

Inject Aqueous Epinephrine 1:1000 (0.01 ml per kg up to 0.5 ml) intramuscularly into the upper arm and massage site. This may be repeated every 5 to 10 minutes while carefully monitoring blood pressure, pulse, respiration, and cardiac rhythm.

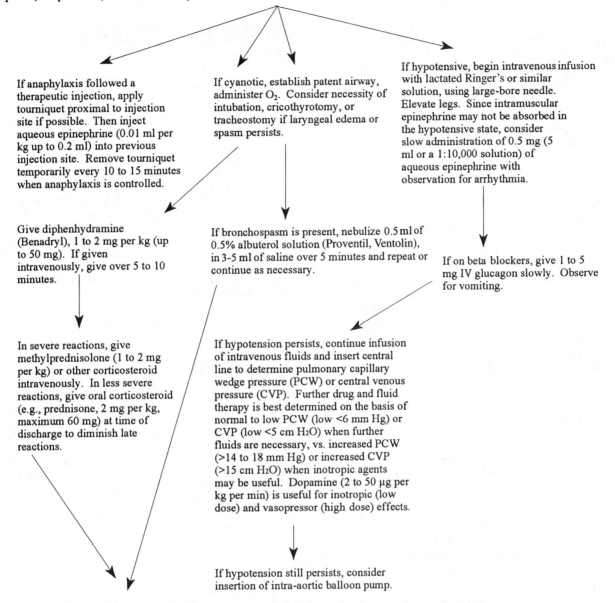

If anaphylaxis followed a therapeutic injection, apply tourniquet proximal to injection site if possible. Then inject aqueous epinephrine (0.01 ml per kg up to 0.2 ml) into previous injection site. Remove tourniquet temporarily every 10 to 15 minutes when anaphylaxis is controlled.

If cyanotic, establish patent airway, administer O₂. Consider necessity of intubation, cricothyrotomy, or tracheostomy if laryngeal edema or spasm persists.

If hypotensive, begin intravenous infusion with lactated Ringer's or similar solution, using large-bore needle. Elevate legs. Since intramuscular epinephrine may not be absorbed in the hypotensive state, consider slow administration of 0.5 mg (5 ml or a 1:10,000 solution) of aqueous epinephrine with observation for arrhythmia.

Give diphenhydramine (Benadryl), 1 to 2 mg per kg (up to 50 mg). If given intravenously, give over 5 to 10 minutes.

If bronchospasm is present, nebulize 0.5 ml of 0.5% albuterol solution (Proventil, Ventolin), in 3-5 ml of saline over 5 minutes and repeat or continue as necessary.

If on beta blockers, give 1 to 5 mg IV glucagon slowly. Observe for vomiting.

In severe reactions, give methylprednisolone (1 to 2 mg per kg) or other corticosteroid intravenously. In less severe reactions, give oral corticosteroid (e.g., prednisone, 2 mg per kg, maximum 60 mg) at time of discharge to diminish late reactions.

If hypotension persists, continue infusion of intravenous fluids and insert central line to determine pulmonary capillary wedge pressure (PCW) or central venous pressure (CVP). Further drug and fluid therapy is best determined on the basis of normal to low PCW (low <6 mm Hg) or CVP (low <5 cm H₂O) when further fluids are necessary, vs. increased PCW (>14 to 18 mm Hg) or increased CVP (>15 cm H₂O) when inotropic agents may be useful. Dopamine (2 to 50 µg per kg per min) is useful for inotropic (low dose) and vasopressor (high dose) effects.

If hypotension still persists, consider insertion of intra-aortic balloon pump.

All patients should be observed for several hours after treatment, because symptoms recur in up to 20% of patients within 8 hours of the resolution of the first episode.

Figure 2. Treatment of anaphylaxis and anaphylactoid reactions. (Modified from Anderson MW, deShazo RD: Anaphylaxis and anaphylactoid reactions. *In* Taylor RB [ed]: Difficult Medical Management. Philadelphia, WB Saunders Co, 1991, pp 25–33.)

association with connective tissue diseases, infection, or tumor. These are often termed "hypersensitivity vasculitis" or "allergic vasculitis" or "Henoch-Schönlein purpura."

Pathogenesis

Experimental serum sickness in the rabbit is a useful model for human serum sickness. When large quantities of antibody and antigen, as soluble immune complexes, fix to receptors in the vascular endothelium of body tissues, the complement system is activated. Complement fragments induce inflammation, which may be limited to the skin or systemic. Serum sickness that occurs after single doses of heterogolous proteins, such as rattlesnake antivenin or diphtheria antitoxin, or after short courses of antibiotics usually resolves spontaneously during a period of weeks. However, if the responsible antigen persists in the circulation, as is the case with DNA in systemic lupus erythematosus, hepatitis B surface antigen in hepatitis B infection, or staphylococcal antigen

TABLE 3. **Representative Antigens Known to Cause Immune Complex Disease in Humans**

Antigens	Syndrome
Therapeutic Agents	
Horse serum products	Serum sickness
Antilymphocyte globulin, snake venom antiserum, streptokinase, monoclonal antibody products	
Drugs	
Cephalosporins, penicillin, amoxicillin, trimethoprim-sulfamethoxazole, fluoxetine, iron-dextran, carbamazepine, and others	
Autologous (Self) Antigens	
DNA	Vasculitis and glomerulonephritis of systemic lupus erythematosus
IgG, IgM	Vasculitis of rheumatoid arthritis and mixed cryoglobulinemia
Tumor antigens	Glomerulonephritis
Colon carcinoma (carcinoembryonic antigen)	
Microbial Antigens	
Hepatitis B	Systemic vasculitis
Plasmodium malariae	
Schistosoma mansoni	Glomerulonephritis
Beta-hemolytic streptococci	
Staphylococcus epidermidis	

Modified from deShazo RD: Immune complex diseases. *In* Bennett JC, Plum F (eds): Cecil Textbook of Medicine, 20th ed. Philadelphia, WB Saunders Co, 1996, pp 1421–1424.

in subacute bacterial endocarditis, syndromes of chronic serum sickness with systemic vasculitis may occur.

Treatment

No controlled treatment trials for serum sickness have been performed. If the agent causing the reaction is being administered or is present at the onset of symptoms, it should be discontinued or removed if possible. For mild cases of serum sickness, symptomatic treatment with antihistamines and/or corticosteroids provides relief. We recommend the use of a long-acting H_1 antihistamine such as hydroxyzine, cetirizine (Zyrtec),* loratadine* (Claritin),* or astemizole (Hismanal)* along with 1 mg per kg of prednisone or equivalent per day divided into 2 doses or more for initial treatment. Improvement usually occurs within 72 hours, whereupon the corticosteroid is tapered over a period of 2 to 3 weeks if symptoms

*Not FDA approved for this indication.

allow. The antihistamine is continued for a longer period and then slowly discontinued.

ASTHMA IN ADOLESCENTS AND ADULTS

method of
SHELDON L. SPECTOR, M.D.
UCLA School of Medicine
Los Angeles, California

There are close to 5000 deaths from asthma in the United States every year. Various guidelines have been developed to improve the quality of care and reduce the mortality rate. There are guidelines from the National Asthma Education Program, guidelines developed by the allergists and immunologists as part of a task force on practice parameters for the diagnosis and treatment of asthma, and even international guidelines. All these guidelines recognize the importance of inflammation, predominantly eosinophilic inflammation, along with reversible airway obstruction.

PATHOPHYSIOLOGY

Throughout the years, pathologists have described mucus plugging, mucosal edema, desquamated eosinophilic inflammation, basement membrane thickening, and smooth muscle and glandular hypertrophy. Bronchial hyper-responsiveness is also characteristic of asthmatics, as quantitated by, e.g., methacholine or histamine inhalation challenge. Various triggers, such as allergens or viral infections, can lead to the hyper-responsive state. In fact, the late phase allergic reaction that follows the early phase reaction after allergen exposure is associated with hyper-responsiveness, and some investigators have postulated that allergic asthma is an ongoing late phase reaction.

An asthmatic subject may manifest physiologic changes, mainly in the large airways, mainly in the small airways, or in both large and small airways.

DIAGNOSIS

History is important; typically the patient mentions chest tightness, wheezing, or shortness of breath. A chronic cough, especially at night, should alert the physician to the diagnosis. These symptoms may occur especially with exercise or allergen exposure, viral respiratory problems, exposure to pollution, or even laughing. Symptoms may occur in association with an occupational exposure or with coexisting illnesses, such as rhinoconjunctivitis, sinusitis, or eczema. A strong family history should alert one to the diagnosis, although its absence does not rule out asthma.

PHYSICAL EXAMINATION

Chest examination may be normal or reveal wheezing with either inspiration or expiration, decreased breath sounds, or signs of hyperventilation. The nose, sinuses, and skin should be examined for associated conditions.

LABORATORY STUDIES

Pulmonary function tests are useful, with spirometry providing more detailed information than peak flow rate.

Spirometry also helps to differentiate obstructive from restrictive airway disease. Pulmonary function tests show increased resistance to airflow and decreased forced expiratory volume. Hyperinflation and ventilation-perfusion abnormalities may be present. Depending on the severity of the asthma, there may be reduced arterial oxygen tension, indicating worsening of asthma or impending respiratory failure. In addition, respiratory alkalosis, pulsus paradoxus, right axis deviation, and right ventricular strain may be present. The positive inhalation challenge to "nonspecific" bronchoconstrictive substances, such as methacholine or histamine, confirms bronchial hyper-responsiveness.

OTHER LABORATORY TESTS

Determination of the total serum IgE is an imperfect determinant of the presence or absence of allergy. However, it can help differentiate, e.g., bronchopulmonary aspergillosis from asthma. Allergen inhalation challenges are rarely used for clinical purposes. A chest radiograph is not useful for the diagnosis of asthma per se but helps to differentiate asthma from other conditions that cause wheezing or possible complications of asthma. If chronic sinusitis is suspected, a sinus radiograph or limited computed tomographic scan might be useful. Eosinophils in the sputum may have diagnostic significance or possibly help to clarify the severity of asthma.

SPECIFIC ALLERGY TESTING

Specific allergy testing helps establish an allergic basis for the patient's symptoms, assists in establishing specific causes for the symptoms, and helps to evaluate the degree of sensitivity. In general, skin tests for immediate hypersensitivity are more sensitive and less costly than in vitro tests, such as the radioallergosorbent test. But the latter may be indicated in patients with dermographism or atopic dermatitis, or for those under the influence of a long-acting antihistamine such as astemizole.

DIFFERENTIAL DIAGNOSIS

Conditions such as chronic bronchitis, vocal cord dysfunction, congestive heart failure, cystic fibrosis, foreign bodies, extrapulmonic obstructive lesions, immunodeficiency resulting in recurrent pneumonia, bronchopulmonary dysplasia, bronchiolitis obliterans, and allergic bronchopulmonary aspergillosis may result in asthmatic symptoms or complicate the course of asthma.

PRECIPITATING OR AGGRAVATING FACTORS

Allergen Triggers

Exposure to high levels of dust mites and cockroaches is associated with a markedly increased risk of developing asthma. Cockroach allergen has been recognized as a major cause of allergic rhinitis and asthma, especially in the urban (especially inner-city) asthmatic population. Trees, grasses, and weed pollens can produce significant exacerbations of asthma at a particular time of year. Molds and fungi are allergens that are known triggers for asthma and rhinitis. *Alternaria* exposure has been associated with known exacerbations of asthma.

Exercise-Induced Asthma

Exercise-induced asthma is probably triggered by cooling of the airways and heat and water loss from the respiratory tract. Warm, humidified air, as well as many pharmacologic agents, can block exercise-induced asthma.

Nocturnal Asthma

Nocturnal asthma represents a distinct entity or (more likely) part of the continuum of persistent asthma. It is associated with physiologic phenomena that occur more commonly or exclusively at night, such as greater hypothermia, decreased pulmonary function, decreased mucociliary clearance, and circadian variations of histamine, epinephrine, and cortisol concentrations.

Nasal Sinus Disease

Sinusitis should be considered in patients with refractory asthma, as well as in asthmatic patients with a persistent cough. Improvement in asthma occurs when sinusitis is properly treated. It should be suspected if nasal polyps are present, as well as certain systemic problems, such as cystic fibrosis.

Gastroesophageal Reflux

Gastroesophageal reflux should be suspected in patients who do not adequately respond to optimal medical therapy or seem to become worse with its initiation. It should also be suspected in patients with primarily nocturnal symptoms. Medical or surgical treatment of gastroesophageal reflux may improve respiratory symptoms.

Aspirin Idiosyncrasy

Many asthmatic patients, perhaps 10 to 15%, have an exacerbation of symptoms with aspirin or nonsteroidal anti-inflammatory agents. These reactions are not IgE mediated and are more common in steroid-dependent asthmatic persons. In addition to vigorous bronchodilator and anti-inflammatory therapy, aspirin desensitization may be a useful therapeutic endeavor.

Other Additives and Preservatives

Sulfites, tartrazine, monosodium glutamate, and other preservatives or additives have been implicated in inducing asthma.

Air Pollution

Air pollution, caused by factors such as sulfur dioxide, nitrogen dioxide, or ozone, is capable of inducing bronchospasm in patients with asthma. One source of air pollution in residential areas, especially in the western states, is household wood-burning devices.

Occupational Asthma

Exposure to fumes, gases, dust, or vapors in an occupational setting can provoke asthma. Symptoms may appear acutely, or hours after exposure. Reactions have been characterized as immunologic, irritant, and pharmacologic. Pre-existing atopy may constitute an increased risk factor for asthma due to occupational agents.

Psychologic Factors and Asthma

Although psychogenic asthma itself probably does not exist, as with any chronic illness, asthma affects psychologic and social aspects of life. Certainly, psychologic factors can make a pre-existing condition worse.

TREATMENT

Goals of Therapy

Although individuals may have specific therapeutic goals, general goals include (1) optimal control of asthma with the use of the least amount of medications possible and minimal side effects, (2) reduction in hospitalization and emergency care visits, (3) prevention of nocturnal symptoms, (4) tolerance to physical activity appropriate for the patient's age, (5) improvement of pulmonary function, (6) minimization of lost time from school, work, or daily activities, (7) improved self-image based on full understanding of the disease, and (8) confidence in the outlined approach to treatment.

Environmental Controls

Environmental control minimizes allergen and irritant exposure. Because house dust mite sensitivity may be a significant risk for the majority of patients, minimizing house dust mite exposure through the use of special pillow and mattress covers would be useful and not too costly. Extensive measures are often limited due to economic and practical considerations. Ideally, one might remove carpets, enclose books in bookcases, and wash sheets, pillowcases, and the rooms themselves, as frequently as possible.

Cockroach allergy is a major cause of inner-city problems. Cockroaches are rarely eliminated without the help of professional exterminators.

Tree, grass, and weed sensitivity may be seasonal. Keeping windows closed helps control pollen contamination, but filtering devices such as high-efficiency particulate air (HEPA) filters and air conditioning can also be helpful. Molds and fungi can occur indoors or outdoors. Although their growth is favored by conditions of high humidity, certain fungal subclasses can grow well in lower, more arid conditions. Although dehumidification, filtration, and air conditioning may be helpful, sometimes more extensive measures are necessary.

Domestic animals, especially dogs and cats, are common causes of allergic reactions. Although most pet owners will not remove these triggers, HEPA filters and removal of the pet from the sleeping area might provide adequate relief. Immunotherapy or allergy injections might also be appropriate for any of these allergic triggers, especially when the owners refuse to remove the pets or control against environmental allergic triggers.

Nonallergic environmental culprits include cigarette smoke, chemical irritants, and strong odors and can be minimized with avoidance and filtering devices. Food allergies, once recognized, can be dealt with through avoidance. Certain allergens, such as peanuts or shrimp, can be quite dangerous; however, they usually play a relatively small role compared with other triggers.

Long-Term Pharmacologic Management

Although a distinction is sometimes made between so-called anti-inflammatory agents and bronchodilators, in reality, certain of these agents, such as theophylline, have both bronchodilator and anti-inflammatory properties. Antileukotrienes (zafirlukast [Accolate]) have recently become available. They are anti-inflammatory in many ways, even though they lack this label officially, and they even have bronchodilator properties.

Agents That Are Mainly Bronchodilators

Beta$_2$-selective agonists are the medications most often employed in the treatment of asthma. They relax smooth muscle and prevent mediator release from mast cells and basophils. The effect of most agents lasts from 4 to 6 hours; however, a 12-hour agent, salmeterol (Serevent), is also available in the United States. Metered-dose inhalers or powder inhalers are preferred for chronic use over oral forms, due to their diminished systemic side effects, such as tremor and anxiety.

Beta agonists are the treatment of choice for the management of acute, severe asthma. There has been concern that overuse of beta agonists has been associated with worsening asthma control and even increased morbidity and mortality. In reality, overuse of beta agonists is a sign of inadequate control with anti-inflammatory and other therapies and should be a clue to the physician and patient that the basic program has to be adjusted.

A tolerance to the beta agonist can also develop with continued use. Tolerance is defined as a decrease in the maximal effect and/or the duration of effect.

Theophylline

Although theophylline is effective in chronic management of asthma, and in some studies is comparable to cromolyn or beta$_2$ agonists, it has been demonstrated to have anti-inflammatory effects as well as bronchodilatory effects. The usual therapeutic levels are 5 to 15 μg/mL. It has a narrow therapeutic range and a significant potential for toxicity, especially due to drug interactions and certain medical conditions such as cardiac decompensation, respiratory failure, hepatic abnormalities, sustained high fever, viral infections, and hypothyroidism. Metabolism of the drug is slowed after administration of cimetidine, oral contraceptives, and antibiotics such as erythromycin, ciprofloxacin, and disulfiram.

Factors such as cigarette smoke, hyperthyroidism, phenytoin or phenobarbital therapy, and the ingestion of certain foods may increase the rate of metabolism.

Anticholinergic Agents

Although anticholinergic bronchodilators are more effective in patients with chronic obstructive pulmonary disease who have partially reversible airflow, they nevertheless may provide benefit to a subgroup of asthmatic patients. Inhaled anticholinergic medications may also be used along with beta agonists to prolong the effect of the latter. They are often an alternative agent when beta agonists have proved to be of minimal benefit or have produced unacceptable side effects.

Primarily Anti-inflammatory Agents

CROMOLYN AND NEDOCROMIL

Cromolyn (Intal) is an effective agent, alone or in conjunction with bronchodilators, in preventing the symptoms of mild to moderate asthma. There is a similar effectiveness when used in a metered-dose inhaler, in a spinhaler, or by nebulization, although individual differences in response may occur. It is a safe compound, and serious side effects are rare. Both cromolyn and nedocromil (Tilade) effectively prevent exercise-induced asthma and both the early and late phase IgE-mediated reaction. In some studies, nedocromil may have been slightly more effective than cromolyn.

CORTICOSTEROID AEROSOLS

Corticosteroid aerosols are one of the most effective agents that can be used in the treatment of asthma, especially in those with moderate to severe disease form. They have become first-line therapy because of their effectiveness in controlling almost every aspect of the inflammatory response. With time, they reduce hyper-responsiveness of the airways.

Beclomethasone, triamcinolone, and flunisolide have been available for many years. Fluticasone has become available in the United States. Its high topical potency might favor its use in the severe asthmatic patient. Adverse reactions to inhaled steroids include thrush, dysphonia, and occasional coughing. There is concern that high doses of these agents can cause osteoporosis in adults and growth retardation in children.

Systemic Corticosteroids

Systemic corticosteroids are useful in the acute management of asthma. When employed early, they prevent relapse and reduce the need for hospitalization. These agents merit special consideration in the fatality-prone asthmatic subject. Because of the potential for significant systemic side effects, the patient should be carefully monitored for suppression of the hypothalamic-pituitary-adrenal axis, bone changes, altered glucose metabolism, hypertension, cataract formation, hypokalemia, and so forth.

Antileukotrienes

This new class of agent, with both bronchodilator and anti-inflammatory–like characteristics, has been tried primarily in patients with mild to moderate asthma but may be particularly useful in certain subgroups of asthmatic subjects, such as those with aspirin idiosyncracy. Zafirlukast, a receptor antago-nist, is the first of the antileukotrienes to be released. It has a convenient, twice-a-day dosing and excellent safety record.

Leukotriene synthesis inhibitors have similar therapeutic potential, and zileuton (Zyflo) is now available.

Ancillary Agents

Although adequate hydration is recommended for patients with asthma, overhydration should be avoided, especially in the elderly and severely ill patient. Fluid overload can lead to pulmonary edema or other adverse circulatory effects.

Guaifenesin and potassium iodide may be worth a trial in some asthmatic patients, although the mechanisms of action are unclear. Steroid-sparing agents, including troleandomycin,* methotrexate,* gold,* intravenous immune globulin therapy,* hydroxychloroquine,* and cyclosporine,* may be effective in some patients with asthma. Certain antihistamines may also serve as bronchodilators. Many investigators have now shown that vigorous treatment of the upper airways provides additional benefit to asthmatic subjects.

Are Generic Products Comparable?

Comparability of inhaled products cannot be assumed. There are potential differences in the response of patients to excipients or other inactive components of these products. Theophylline substitution can also be a potential problem, because one theophylline medication may show diminished efficacy or increased toxicity compared with another, depending on the preparation and on an individual patient's characteristics.

Immunotherapy in the Asthmatic Patient

Allergen immunotherapy should be considered in certain patients as part of a well-planned program that may also include pharmacotherapy and avoidance measures. It plays an anti-inflammatory role and may even decrease the likelihood of the development of asthma in a patient with rhinitis. Although life-threatening reactions during allergen immunotherapy are rare, fatalities can occur. Therefore, careful supervision is required.

Management of an Acute or Severe Attack

Severe acute asthma (status asthmaticus) requires prompt recognition and intervention. More than 4000 deaths result from asthma yearly in the United States.

Oxygen

In the acute asthma exacerbation, ventilation-profusion mismatches occur and the partial pressure of

---

*Not FDA approved for this indication.

oxygen in arterial blood (PaO_2) decreases. Therefore, oxygen administration is indicated. Oxygen is usually given by nasal cannula at 4 to 6 liters per minute, or with a close-fitting mask. Arterial blood gas and pulmonary function monitoring helps decide if the patient is tiring or improving. With increasing obstruction, ventilation is compromised and the partial pressure of carbon dioxide in arterial blood ($PaCO_2$) rises from initially low levels to normal levels. Therefore, a $PaCO_2$ of 40 mm Hg may be a sign of severe asthma.

Intravenous Fluids

The usefulness of hydration is not as clear-cut as was once believed, although one should correct dehydration. Volume overload can be a problem, especially in the elderly patient. An open intravenous line allows administration of other medications, such as theophylline.

Specific Medications

SYMPATHOMIMETICS

Repetitive administration of nebulized $beta_2$-selective agents is usually the initial specific medical treatment of choice. An alternative treatment, more commonly given to children, is subcutaneous injection of 0.3 mL of 1:1000 epinephrine (0.15 to 0.3 mL depending on the child's size). The latter treatment is associated with more cardiac effects.

CORTICOSTEROIDS

Early use of oral or intravenously administered corticosteroids is recommended, because the lag time for the clinical effect is often delayed by several hours. Dose ranges for methylprednisolone are 40 to 125 mg every 4 to 6 hours.

THEOPHYLLINE COMPOUNDS

Intravenous aminophylline may improve diaphragmatic muscle function, thereby benefiting a patient with impending respiratory failure and severe asthma. Although some studies favor its use, others suggest that the addition of methylxanthine does not provide greater bronchodilatation than that achieved by the use of inhaled beta agonists alone and that it only increases side effects. If aminophylline or theophylline is used, it is especially important to monitor blood levels and cardiopulmonary function.

Perhaps theophylline achieves the best results in those individuals who have not been receiving chronic theophylline therapy.

ANTICHOLINERGIC AGENTS

Although anticholinergics such as ipratropium bromide (Atrovent) are of particular benefit in the patient with chronic bronchitis, they can also be used in those with asthma. Other subgroups of responders are certain individuals who do not respond to maximal doses of beta agonists by themselves, and possibly older individuals. Some studies have shown that the combination of the beta agonist with an anticholinergic is superior to either medication alone.

SODIUM BICARBONATE, POTASSIUM CHLORIDE, AND OTHER ELECTROLYTES

Although improved ventilation usually ameliorates acid-base problems with pH values of less than 7.2, intravenous sodium bicarbonate may be indicated to improve the patient's response to other therapy. Many of the agents used in the treatment of asthma can create an electrolyte imbalance, especially potassium loss. Intravenous potassium chloride may be necessary, often with doses at 2 to 3 mEq per kg per day.

Magnesium has been advocated as a beneficial treatment for asthma per se; however, its use is controversial. Magnesium and/or phosphate may also be indicated with reduced serum levels of these salts.

ANTIBIOTICS

Most infections that exacerbate an asthmatic attack are the result of viruses and therefore do not require antibiotic therapy. On the other hand, secondary infections can ensue, with discolored mucus, fever, cough, and either signs of pulmonary involvement or involvement of the paranasal sinuses. Such situations merit the use of an antibiotic.

Need for Hospitalization

The decision to admit a patient can generally be made within the first 1 to 2 hours of treatment. It is based on the observations that a patient is tiring or there is a minimal response to therapy as indicated by flow rates or arterial blood gas measurements. The presence of complications such as cardiac arrhythmias, pneumonia, or pneumothorax might also prompt admission.

If the $PaCO_2$ rises above 50 mm Hg or the PaO_2 falls below 50 mm Hg in the patient who does not have a diagnosis of chronic obstructive pulmonary disease, assisted ventilation may be necessary. Certain fatality-prone asthmatic individuals, e.g., those who have previously required intubation, should also be admitted earlier rather than later.

Fatality-Prone Asthmatic Patients

Risk factors for life-threatening exacerbations of asthma include severe asthma, especially that previously requiring intubation (see previous section) for the control of symptoms, an allergic diathesis, or psychologic factors, so that the patient and physician fail to recognize, or deny, the severity of the patient's asthma. An allergic response to airborne mold (*Alternaria*) has been associated with life-threatening or fatal exacerbations in asthmatic patients.

Psychologic factors such as disregard for asthma symptoms, manipulative use of asthma, poor ongoing care by the patient and family, and significant emotional problems also characterize a high-risk group of asthmatic subjects.

Fatality-prone asthmatic patients require special planning and should have regular follow-up visits for assessment of asthma, along with pulmonary function tests, and possibly referral for specialist care.

Consultation with an Asthma Specialist

Active participation of an asthma specialist in the continuing care of patients with asthma is associated with lower asthma morbidity, including fewer emergency department visits, decreased numbers of hospitalizations, a reduced length of stay in the hospital, a reduced number of days lost from school or work, and a reduction in the global cost of asthma care. Compelling reasons for recommending that a patient consult an asthma specialist include (1) instability of the patient's asthma; (2) the need for identification of possible allergenic or nonallergenic triggers; (3) education of the patient; and (4) clarification of the diagnosis of asthma, if it is in doubt.

It is better to seek consultation early during the treatment program rather than waiting too long. The cooperative interaction between the patient and/or the patient's representative(s), the primary care physician, and the asthma specialist is necessary to maximize the possibility of meeting the goals of asthma therapy.

ASTHMA IN CHILDREN

method of
MARTHA V. WHITE, M.D.
Institute for Asthma and Allergy at Washington Hospital Center
Washington, D.C.

Asthma is one of the most common chronic illnesses of childhood, affecting 5 to 10% of children younger than 20 years. In the United States, asthma and its attendant allergies are the leading cause of time lost from school and work and sick child visits to the physician. Americans spend more than $1 billion each year on asthma, and as many as 50% of asthma patients spend more than 18% of their family income on asthma therapy.

Fortunately, our understanding of the pathophysiology of asthma has improved dramatically in the last 2 decades. We now know that asthma is due to a combination of smooth muscle contraction, excessive secretion of mucus, mucosal edema, and inflammation. Pulmonary autopsy tissue taken from patients who died of asthma reveal epithelial denudement, thickening of the basement membrane, infiltration of the lamina propria by eosinophils and neutrophils, and smooth muscle, goblet cell, and glandular hyperplasia. Airway luminal secretions are excessive and copious and contain increased numbers of eosinophils, neutrophils, mast cells, Creola bodies, Curschmann's spirals, and Charcot-Leyden crystals. These changes were previously thought to occur only in severe asthma, but airway biopsies obtained from patients with mild asthma also demonstrate epithelial denudement, eosinophil and neutrophil infiltration, edema, basement membrane thickening, and mast cell hyperplasia with evidence of degranulation.

Typical asthma attacks consist of an early, short-lived bronchoconstrictive response to an asthma trigger and a late phase reaction (LPR). The LPR consists of inflammatory events occurring 5 to 12 hours after the inciting trigger and is characterized by wheezing that is poorly responsive to bronchodilators. The LPR last hours to days and can render the patient's airways hyper-reactive to additional asthma triggers for prolonged periods. Further exposure to asthma triggers during this hyper-reactive period can initiate an escalating cycle of acute asthma, LPR, and increased hyper-reactivity, which can culminate in a prolonged, recalcitrant asthma attack requiring hospitalization and intravenous corticosteroid administration.

The bulk of evidence suggests that the airway inflammation observed in asthma is caused by mast cell–initiated LPR. Antigen-stimulated mast cells release chemotactic factors, vasoactive factors, and inflammatory leukotrienes and prostaglandins. Mast cells can also induce epithelial cell expression of leukocyte adhesion molecules, such as the vascular cell adhesion molecule, which selectively recruit eosinophils to the site of the allergic reaction. Thus, mast cell–induced up-regulation of adhesion molecule expression may enhance airway inflammation in asthma. Antigen-stimulated mast cells synthesize and release a number of inflammatory cytokines, including interleukin (IL)–3, IL-4, IL-5, IL-8, tumor necrosis factor, and interferon-γ. Activated T cells and macrophages release a similar pattern of cytokines as well as IL-10 and IL-11. The pattern of lymphocyte cytokines produced during the allergic response differs from that of other inflammatory disorders. In most inflammatory diseases studied thus far, IL-2 and interferon-γ, but not IL-4, IL-5 and IL-10, are produced. However, in allergic disorders, IL-4, IL-5, and IL-10 are preferentially produced. These cytokines are important in IgE production as well as eosinophil chemotaxis and survival and thus promote the allergic response. The interleukins and tumor necrosis factor enhance mast cell growth and up-regulate IgE production. Through cytokine production, mast cells may regulate their own function and growth, regulate airway inflammation, and ultimately regulate airway hyper-reactivity.

The degree of airway hyper-reactivity to nonspecific stimuli, such as histamine and methacholine, correlates closely with asthma severity. Furthermore, airway hyper-reactivity increases during the allergy season and during rhinovirus infections. In previous years, bronchodilators, such as theophylline and beta-adrenergic agonists, were used as first-line asthma therapies. Specialists now agree that the primary focus of asthma management should be the reduction and prevention of airway hyper-reactivity and late phase inflammatory reactions. Indeed, guidelines for the management of asthma, which stress the importance of anti-inflammatory medications, have been published through the National Institutes of Health and other world agencies. Consequently, allergen avoidance coupled with inhaled cromolyn sodium (Intal) or inhaled corticosteroids is increasingly being used as a primary form of therapy, and bronchodilators are being employed as second-line symptomatic drugs.

Despite improvements in our understanding of asthma and in delivery systems for asthma medications, the incidence of asthma and of deaths due to asthma is rising. The reason for this is unclear; however, it has been suggested that pollution; passive exposure to tobacco smoke; excessive reliance on symptomatic medications (e.g. bronchodilators) in lieu of lesion-reversing measures (e.g., allergen avoidance, corticosteroid or cromolyn sodium therapy, and immunotherapy) to treat asthma; excessive indoor allergen exposure (e.g., cockroaches, dust mites); and restricted access to long-term follow-up care may be contributing factors. Whatever the reason, asthma must be regarded as a potentially life-threatening disorder. Even in extremely mild cases, disruption of family dynamics, school attendance, and social interactions can be significant. The goals of therapy should be to reduce or eliminate symptoms while normalizing daily activities. This can usually be accomplished with minimal or no side effects. With optimal management, the activities of most children should be unrestricted, allowing a normal lifestyle and reducing the risk of emotional repercussions from asthma.

DIAGNOSIS

Asthma is a disease characterized by episodic wheezing or cough, responsive to defined asthma management protocols, for which other causes have been eliminated. It can present as recurrent cough, especially at night; a cough or wheeze associated with exercise or infections; or frank episodic wheezing, usually with recognizable triggers. The spectrum of severity ranges from a few mild episodes in a lifetime to daily debilitating symptoms. A careful history and a physical examination are the most useful diagnostic aids, and special attention should be given to the timing of symptoms, potential triggers, family history, and exposure to environmental allergens, such as cats, cockroaches and dust mites, and irritants, such as tobacco smoke. A diagnosis of asthma can be confirmed by a postbronchodilator increase of 15% in the forced expiratory volume in 1 second, or 20% in forced expiratory flow ($FEF_{25\%-75\%}$). If spirometry is normal, it may be necessary to perform an exercise challenge to establish the diagnosis. A simple exercise challenge, which can be performed in the office, is supervised running in place or up and down the stairs until the patient feels too tired to continue. Bronchial constriction usually occurs about 10 minutes after the challenge.

Some children normally perform as much as 40% above predicted normal levels for spirometry. These children may have "normal lung functions" during an asthma attack but improve with bronchodilators. Alternatively, if the child has a history of wheezing that cannot be confirmed by physical examination, a diagnosis can be reached by employing a peak flow meter at home and at school, especially during asthma attacks and after bronchodilator use. Children as young as 4 years are capable of performing a peak flow maneuver. For children too young to cooperate, a therapeutic trial with asthma therapy is warranted.

If a more definite diagnosis is required, a methacholine or histamine challenge can be performed to demonstrate airway hyper-reactivity, the hallmark of asthma. An antigen challenge can also be diagnostic of antigen-induced asthma, but it carries the risk of inducing an LPR. These tests are time-consuming, require precision, and are best left to physicians trained in these techniques.

Although it is true that not all that wheezes is asthma, asthma is common, and the other causes of wheezing are rare. The differential diagnosis includes tracheobronchomalacia, cystic fibrosis (particularly in children with nasal polyps or histories of meconium ileus), bronchial stenosis, mass lesions such as lymphomas, foreign bodies (particularly in wheezing of sudden onset), congenital and acquired structural lung disorders such as vascular rings, and many infections such as tuberculosis and infection with *Mycoplasma* or respiratory syncytial virus.

TREATMENT

Environmental Control

Most asthmatic children develop allergies. The development of allergies and the severity of existing allergies depend on the level of exposure to a given allergen. Allergies to foods emerge during infancy, followed somewhat later by allergies to cockroaches, indoor pets, and house dust mites, which are present all year but peak in the winter. Pollen allergies generally develop after three or more seasons of exposure. Children younger than 4 years rarely test positive for pollens.

The diagnosis of allergic triggers can be made by allergy skin testing combined with a temporal pattern of symptoms consistent with the skin test results. Optimization of asthma therapy is difficult without rigorous avoidance of allergic triggers. Exposure to high levels of house dust mites or cockroaches during infancy increases the atopic childs' risk of developing asthma by fourfold in some studies. House dust mite avoidance is accomplished by the use of plastic, allergenproof encasings on all mattresses, box springs, and pillows in the child's bedroom and removal of all venetian blinds and rugs wherever possible. Simplification of the bedroom to eliminate feather bedding, clutter, stuffed furniture, and other dust collectors is also important. Bookshelves should be enclosed or moved to a different room, closet doors closed, and stuffed animals kept to a minimum. Mites in the stuffed animals may be killed by placement in the hot air cycle of the dryer for 10 to 15 minutes. The entire house should be dusted and vacuumed at least weekly, and the bedroom should be cleaned more often. Cockroaches are often carried into the home in paper grocery bags. Mold exposure can be reduced by eliminating potted plants, especially in the bedroom. Persons allergic to outdoor allergens should keep the doors and windows closed during the pollen season (trees in early spring; grass in late spring and early summer; weeds in late summer and early fall; molds in fall). Bathing and dressing for bed after coming indoors for the day eliminate exposure to pollens on clothing and hair.

Animal fur picks up outdoor allergens. Thus, the family pet may be an additional source of pollen exposure. In cases of animal allergy, family pets should be given away. The presence of cats in the house during infancy raises an atopic child's chances of developing asthma by 10-fold. If the family refuses to eliminate the pet, the pet should be kept outside, if possible, and definitely out of the allergic child's bedroom, and the child should be instructed to avoid the animals' saliva.

Passive smoke inhalation is unequivocally deleterious to the pulmonary functions of normal and asthmatic children. In some studies, smoking atopic mothers were four times as likely to have an asthmatic child as nonsmoking atopic mothers. Smoking should not be permitted in the asthmatic child's house.

Immunotherapy

The efficacy of immunotherapy in allergic rhinitis is well documented. Demonstration of the efficacy of immunotherapy in asthma is more difficult because of the etiologic complexities of the disease. However, carefully performed trials of single agents used to treat well-defined allergic asthmatic patients (e.g., cat- or birch pollen–induced asthma) have documented that immunotherapy reduces symptoms and prevents the increases in airway reactivity normally seen during the allergy season. If allergen exposure cannot be completely eliminated, immunotherapy can be helpful in asthmatic patients with known allergic triggers. Although the exact mechanism by which immunotherapy works is unclear, it reduces late asthmatic responses to allergens and, over time, can reduce bronchial reactivity. To be successful, the immunotherapy prescription must contain all relevant allergens, and improvement occurs gradually over 2 or more years. Injections are given once or twice weekly in increasing doses until an optimal dose is achieved. Thereafter, injection intervals are gradually lengthened to monthly.

Severity Assessment

To gauge the success of therapy, it is necessary to determine the maximal lung functions achievable by the patient, often after a therapeutic trial of cromolyn or inhaled corticosteroids plus bronchodilators, as needed. Patients may report fewer symptoms than they are actually experiencing because they have not learned to recognize milder, more chronic pulmonary symptoms of asthma. A daily peak flow graph, filled out thrice daily, is quite helpful, both for the assessment of severity and to help patients recognize asthma symptoms and triggers. Patients soon learn to think of their peak flow meter as their "asthma thermometer." The frequency of bronchodilator use (if used as needed) and nighttime awakenings due to asthma are also good yardsticks for measuring asthma severity.

Cooperative Management

As with diabetes, optimal management of asthma cannot be achieved with crisis care alone. It requires a maintenance program designed to prevent asthma flares and early intervention when flares do occur. Patients and parents should be taught to listen to chest sounds and to monitor peak flow readings, trigger exposure, and symptoms to facilitate physician-patient communication and the early identification of asthma flares. The family and school should be provided with a written medication plan for handling flares based on peak flow readings and response to therapy, including instructions about when to call the physician.

Pharmacologic Management

Pharmacologic products useful in the treatment of asthma can be divided into two groups: (1) anti-inflammatory medications, which heal and prevent airway inflammation that leads to airway hyper-reactivity, and (2) bronchodilators, which relax smooth muscle, thus relieving the acute symptoms of asthma. The anti-inflammatory medications are disease-altering medications that work slowly and do not produce immediate relief of symptoms. Thus a patient's compliance with these products is poor unless their role in asthma management and their expected benefits are clearly outlined for the patient.

Mast Cell Stabilizers

Mast cell stabilizers are probably the safest drugs available for the treatment of asthma. Disodium cromoglycate (Intal) and nedocromil sodium (Tilade) prevent early and late phase allergic reactions. They are not bronchodilators and do not reverse acute symptoms. They work preventively to inhibit inflammation and antigen-induced increases in airway hyper-reactivity. A single dose (2 puffs) inhibits the asthmatic response to exercise or allergen exposure if given 10 to 20 minutes in advance. Maintenance therapy requires 3 or 4 daily doses, and it can take as long as 4 weeks for an effect to be appreciated. Both drugs are provided as unit-dose inhalers. Cromolyn is also provided in a nebulizable form (frequently used in combination with beta agonists). Nedocromil nebulizer solution is in clinical trials. Discontinuation of cromolyn or nedocromil during an asthma attack is counterproductive and not indicated.

Corticosteroids

Corticosteroids are extremely potent antiasthma agents. They reduce inflammation, edema, and mucus secretion and restore beta$_2$-adrenergic responsiveness. Corticosteroids inhibit increases in airway responsiveness and can reverse the baseline airway hyper-responsiveness characteristic of asthma. Several topical formulations delivered by metered-dose inhalers are available (beclomethasone [Vanceril, Beclovent], flunisolide [AeroBid], triamcinolone [Azmacort], and fluticasone [Flovent]). Budesonide (Rhinocort), the first nebulizable corticosteroid, is undergoing clinical trials and is formulated as both a metered-dose inhaler and a solution for nebulization. These potent topical agents are quickly metabolized and rarely cause any of the side effects of oral corticosteroids. In asthmatic patients requiring daily bronchodilator therapy despite cromolyn use, the addition of or substitution with these agents can lead to dramatic clinical improvement. In unstable asthma, best results are obtained after the symptoms are stabilized with oral corticosteroids, followed by maintenance inhaled corticosteroids. From 100 to 200 µg twice daily is the usual dose; however, higher doses may be necessary in more refractory asthma. Nebulized budesonide is used in doses of 250 to 1000 µg per day in one or two divided doses. In the most difficult cases, maintenance oral corticosteroids may be required. Alternate-day dosing is associated with fewer systemic side effects than daily dosing and is the oral regimen of choice.

The key to proper management with oral steroids is to use doses sufficient to cause a dramatic improvement in pulmonary functions and to continue them until pulmonary functions (including FEF$_{25\%-75\%}$) normalize. The patient is then weaned as quickly as possible off oral corticosteroids, and the effect is maintained with inhaled corticosteroids. If a prolonged course of oral corticosteroids is required, the patient may need to be weaned to alternate-day oral corticosteroids before ceasing to take oral steroids completely. Inhaled corticosteroid doses should be increased early during asthma exacerbations. If this fails, a short course of oral steroids should be instituted before the patient's condition deteriorates to the point of requiring emergency intervention.

Pulmonary delivery of any inhaled medication is enhanced by the use of spacer devices (AeroChamber, InspirEase). The AeroChamber may be ordered prefitted with a child's face mask to facilitate delivery of inhaled medications to young children, although nebulization provides superior drug delivery in small children. Inhaled corticosteroids and cromolyn sodium are best given 10 minutes after inhaled beta-adrenergic agonists, because beta agonists cause bronchodilatation and facilitate penetration of subsequent inhaled medications. Gargling or rinsing the mouth with a few sips of water after steroid inhalation is usually sufficient to avoid thrush, the major side effect of inhaled corticosteroids.

Beta-Adrenergic Agonists

Beta agonists are bronchodilators and are effective in treating and preventing early asthmatic responses, but they are less effective in reversing LPRs (Table 1). They are excellent for preventing exercise-induced asthma when given 10 minutes before exercise. Both nonselective (e.g., isoproterenol) and beta$_2$-selective (e.g., metaproterenol, albuterol, terbutaline, bitolterol, and pirbuterol) beta-adrenergic agonists are available. The selective drugs are preferred because they have selective pulmonary effects and fewer cardiac side effects. These preparations are available as metered-dose inhalers, nebulizer solutions, oral preparations, and parenteral preparations.

Delivery by inhalation targets the medication to the lungs and produces fewer systemic effects, such as tremor, nervousness, and palpitations. Nebulizer treatments, often combined with cromolyn or budesonide, are particularly useful in young asthmatic patients and in older children during acute exacerbations of asthma. Ideally, the family should possess a nebulizer for home use and a portable battery-operated unit for travel (which could be rented). There are several lightweight battery-operated models with adapters for plugging into automobile cigarette lighters. In general, the nonportable air compressors have more power than the portable units.

Metered-dose inhalers, preferably used with spacer devices, can be used by older children. The availability of an AeroChamber fitted with a pediatric mask has made the use of metered-dose inhalers possible even in infants, although good studies comparing the two inhalant delivery systems in this age group are lacking. Oral beta$_2$-adrenergic agonists are useful for treating mild asthma, especially in infants, and as adjuncts to inhaled corticosteroids and inhaled beta-adrenergic agonists. In more resistant asthma, the slow-release oral preparations (e.g., albuterol extended, release [Proventil Repetabs]) or long-acting inhaled preparations (salmeterol) are excellent alternatives to theophylline (e.g., Theo-Dur) for nighttime coverage, or to four-times-daily dosing with short-acting beta agonists. Systemic preparations are reserved for office and hospital use, with the exception of epinephrine (EpiPen), used as self-administered emergency treatment for anaphylaxis caused by insect stings, food allergens, or drug reactions.

Theophylline

The use of methylxanthines by asthma specialists has decreased steadily in the last several years, partly because of its side effects and as a result of an improvement in our understanding of the pathogenesis of asthma. It was originally thought that theophylline worked by inhibiting phosphodiesterase; however, other mechanisms, including inhibition of adenosine, are more important. Theophylline, a bronchodilator, is useful in the symptomatic treatment of acute asthma, but it has little effect on the inflammatory component and does not reverse airway hyper-reactivity. It is an effective oral bronchodilator, can be used with twice-daily or once-daily dosing, and is easy to administer; compliance can be ascertained through serum theophylline levels (see Table 1).

Theophylline, at levels slightly above recommended therapeutic levels (5 to 15 μg per mL), is associated with several unpleasant side effects, including a short attention span in predisposed individuals, nausea and vomiting, and behavioral and sleep alterations in some children. Serious theophylline toxicities (e.g., seizure, arrhythmias, death) generally do not occur below 40 μg per mL; however, in rare cases, a seizure can be the first symptom of theophylline toxicity. With the availability of improved delivery systems and toxicity profiles for the beta-adrener-

---

TABLE 1. **Dosing Guidelines for Theophylline, Oral Beta$_2$-Adrenergic Agonists, and Corticosteroids**

Theophylline
Dose to achieve serum concentrations of 5–15 mg/mL

Albuterol	**Prednisolone**
(0.1–0.15 mg/kg q 4–6 h)	Pediapred (5 mg/5 mL)
Ventolin (2 mg/5 mL)	Prelone (15 mg/5 mL)
Proventil (2 mg/5 mL)	
Metaproterenol	**Prednisone**
(0.3–0.5 mg/kg q 4–6 h)	Liquid Pred (5 mg/5 mL)
Alupent (10 mg/5 mL)	

Age (y)

<2	¼–½ tsp tid or qid	5–7.5 mg bid
2–6	½–1 tsp tid or qid	7.5–10 mg bid
6–12	1–1½ tsp tid or qid	10–15 mg bid
>12	1–2 tsp tid or qid	10–20 mg tid

gic agonists, the side effects of theophylline have limited the usefulness of the drug.

Antileukotrienes

The antileukotrienes represent the first new class of antiasthma medications to be licensed in 20 years. These oral medications are effective bronchodilators that also inhibit airway hyper-reactivity. There are three types of antileukotriene drugs; two work by inhibiting the production of leukotrienes C_4, D_4, and E_4 (5-lipoxygenase inhibitors and 5-lipoxygenase–associated protein [FLAP] inhibitors) and the third blocks the binding of leukotriene D_4 to its receptor. Zafirlukast (Accolate), a leukotriene D_4 antagonist, and zileuton (Zyflo), 5α-lipoxygenase inhibitor, have been approved for use in the treatment of chronic asthma in the United States. Leukotriene modifiers are generally well tolerated, although zileuton, but not zafirlukast, causes reversible liver toxicity in about 4% of patients. Their exact place in the pharmacologic armamentarium for asthma is still being established.

Anticholinergics

Anticholinergics act as bronchodilators in most asthmatic patients. Ipratropium bromide (Atrovent), a quaternary isopropyl derivative of atropine, is poorly absorbed and has few of the systemic side effects of atropine, making it the anticholinergic of choice. Although it is not approved by the Food and Drug Administration (FDA) for use in children younger than 12 years, many younger children benefit from its use. It can prolong the effectiveness of concomitantly administered beta-adrenergic agonists and is useful in asthma induced by cold air, irritants, or emotion. Atropine is administered by nebulization, and ipratropium is available as a metered-dose inhaler; both can be used three or four times each day.

Antihistamines

Some data suggest that high-dose nonsedating antihistamines offer statistically, but probably not clinically relevant, benefits in asthma. Previous concerns about the mucus-drying effects of H_1 antihistamines have also proved to be clinically irrelevant. Although antihistamines are probably not much help in asthma, they should not be withheld in children who require them for other reasons, such as allergic rhinitis or eczema.

Antibiotics

The routine use of antibiotics for asthma is not warranted; however, children with frequent asthma attacks often have sinusitis exacerbating their asthma. All asthmatic patients with frequent or difficult asthma, especially those requiring hospitalization, should be evaluated for sinusitis. Chronic sinusitis can be indolent and generally requires 3 to 6 weeks of therapy with appropriate antibiotics. Amoxacillin-clavulanate (Augmentin), cefuroxime axetil (Ceftin), and clarithromycin (Biaxin) are frequently successful. Amoxacillin (Amoxil), erythromycin (E-mycin), cefaclor (Ceclor), and trimethoprim-sulfamethoxazole (Septra, Bactrim) are less effective because of the emergence of drug-resistant strains of bacteria.

Management Strategies

No single asthma management strategy is successful for all patients. Each person has a unique mix of triggers and baseline airway reactivity, necessitating individualization of asthma therapy. However, the following guidelines have been adopted by the National Institutes of Health and apply to most patients.

Occasional mild asthma can be effectively managed with bronchodilators alone. They should be administered by inhalation (2 puffs) because the onset of action is more rapid and side effects are lower by this route. Patients with exacerbations of their asthma symptoms more than twice a week should receive bronchodilators as needed, coupled with daily prophylactic therapy designed to inhibit inflammation and reverse airway hyper-reactivity. Cromolyn is remarkably safe and is an effective prophylactic agent in many children. An adequate trial requires at least 4 weeks of daily administration (2 puffs four times a day). If successful, the patient can be weaned to the lowest daily dose giving normal pulmonary functions and adequate protection from symptoms. Children who respond to disodium cromoglycate will probably also respond to nedocromil, particularly children with cough-variant asthma. In the event of cromolyn failure, inhaled corticosteroids should be instituted. Beclomethasone has been used most extensively in children and has a high topical/systemic ratio. Four puffs twice daily is a reasonable starting dose. If this fails to provide adequate control, a more potent corticosteroid, such as triamcinolone, budesonide, or fluticasone, could be tried. Flunisolide is also an excellent choice, although the taste is prohibitively objectionable to some children. After pulmonary functions have normalized, the dose of inhaled steroids can be reduced to the minimum required to maintain good control. The frequency of bronchodilator use should be monitored as an index of success of prophylactic therapy. Leukotriene modifiers should be added if bronchodilators are required frequently to reverse symptoms. Although the exact role of leukotriene modifiers is still being determined, it may be reasonable to use leukotriene modifiers as first-line anti-inflammatory prophylactic agents.

In cases of moderate to severe asthma with daily debilitating symptoms, the institution of inhaled corticosteroid therapy is often insufficient to achieve adequate control, and a course of oral corticosteroids, administered in divided doses concomitant with inhaled steroids, should be considered. The dose of prednisone required is highly individual, but in general, infants and preschoolers require about 15 to 20 mg per day, whereas school-age children require 30 mg per day. Occasionally, a steroid-dependent asthmatic adolescent may require up to 60 mg per day to effect a remission. The dose should be sufficient to cause a marked improvement in pulmonary functions within a week, and the steroid therapy should be continued until optimal improvement has been achieved. In most patients, complete control can be achieved within 7 to 10 days, but some need longer treatment. The key to success is to use a high enough dose for a sufficient time to maximize lung functions. After control is achieved, the patient should be weaned from the oral steroids as rapidly as is practical and safe.

Education of the Patient

It is often not difficult to achieve good control. However, maintaining control requires the cooperation of a knowledgeable patient or parent who has been taught to recognize triggers and early signs of asthma. Knowledge is a powerful combatant to the fear, confusion, frustration, and desperation experienced by many families attempting to deal with the seemingly unpredictable nature of asthma and its effects on the quality of life and family dynamics.

Patients should be directed to appropriate resources and support groups. Several organizations provide plentiful resources and support for the patient. Allergy and Asthma Network/Mothers of Asthmatics (Fairfax, Virginia; telephone 703-385-4403) publishes a monthly newsletter filled with practical information and numerous educational and practical resources. They also publish a reference list of asthma resources entitled *Team Work*. Local chapters of the American Lung Association sponsor lectures by physicians and paramedics for asthmatic patients and their families, and local Asthma and Allergy Foundation of America chapters sponsor allergy support groups. In addition, the Food Allergy Network publishes helpful information for patients with food allergies, including notices about contamination of commercial foods with possible food allergens.

Patients and their families must be taught to monitor peak flow readings and to record any possible events that may lead to decreases in peak flow. The physician can use this information to help the patient identify triggers and recognize early signs of asthma exacerbations. On the basis of this information, the physician should instruct the patient about avoidance of allergens and other triggers. The patient should also be provided with a written asthma management plan, including a maintenance medication prescription and details of expected medication effects and common side effects. The asthma management plan should detail additional medications that are to be taken when peak flow readings begin to drop or when known triggers, such as an upper respiratory infection, are encountered. It should also give instructions about when to contact the physician. Graded asthma management plans must be individualized, but Figures 1 and 2 can be used as guidelines. Asthmatic patients whose condition deteriorates quickly usually require early intervention with oral

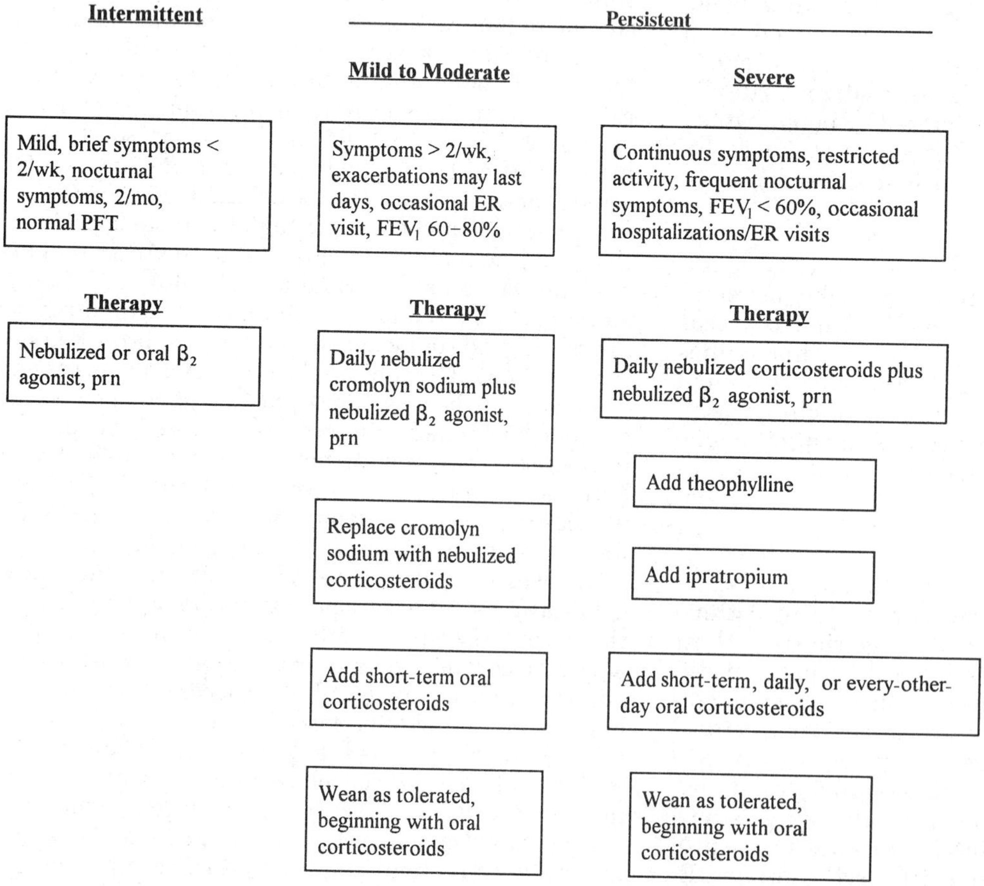

Figure 1. Treatment of asthma in infants and toddlers. *Abbreviations:* PFT = pulmonary function test; FEV_1 = forced expiratory volume in 1 second; ER = emergency room.

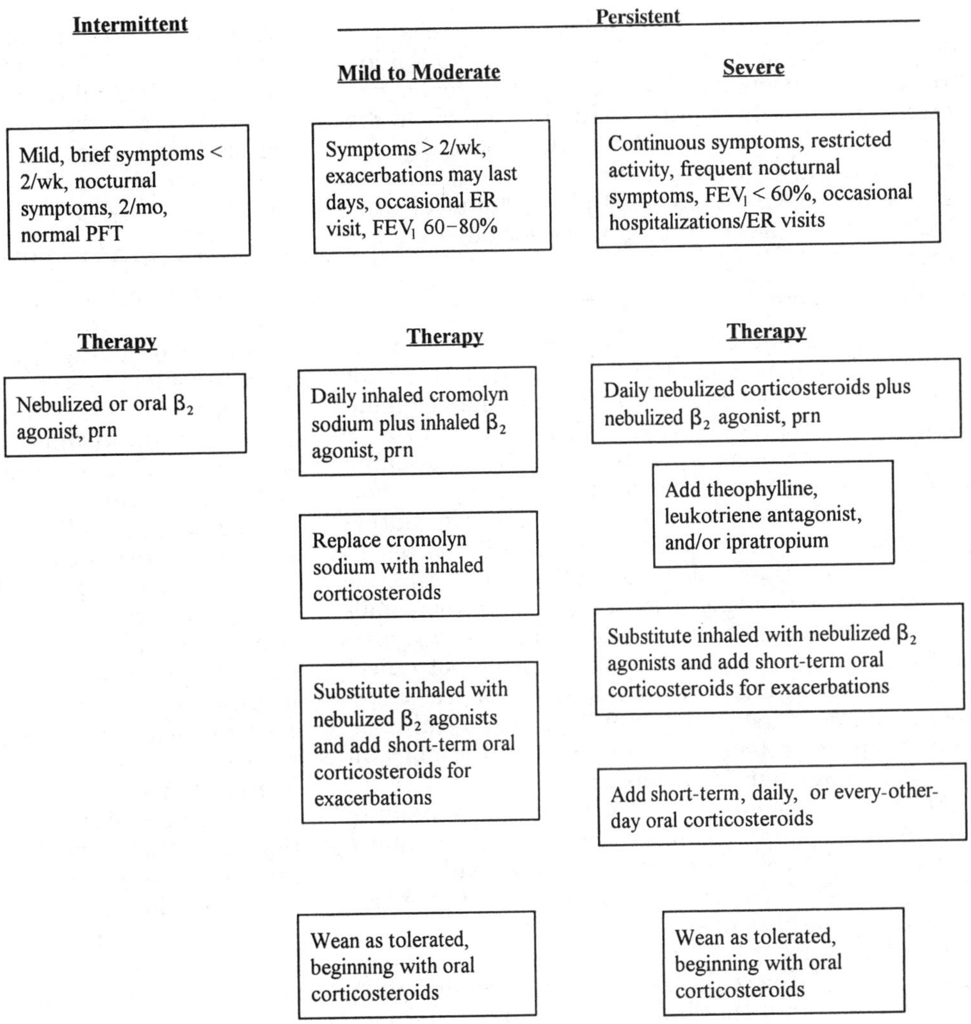

Figure 2. Treatment of asthma in children 4 years old to adolescents. *Abbreviations:* PFT = pulmonary function test; FEV$_1$ = forced expiratory volume in 1 second; ER = emergency room.

corticosteroids to prevent complete deterioration and the need for emergency care.

Emotional Considerations

Parents must be encouraged to expect comparable behavior and, within reason, comparable achievements from their asthmatic and nonasthmatic children. Care must be taken to avoid sibling jealousies over attention given to the asthmatic child. An attitude of achievement and well-being can replace an attitude of defeat if the patient and parent are made to realize that they can control the asthma rather than having the asthma control them. With proper management, most asthmatic children can lead normal lives with normal activities as long as they take their regular medications and premedicate appropriately.

Age Considerations

Relevant asthma triggers and the therapeutic agents available to treat children vary with age.

INFANTS AND TODDLERS

Close monitoring of the asthmatic infant is a challenge, because typical wheezing may be difficult to detect. Parents should pay particular attention to cough and labored breathing, especially labored exhalation that occurs after hard play, nursing, or crying, particularly in association with respiratory infections. Cough and noisy breathing at night should also be monitored. The primary caregiver's observations, recorded in a symptom diary, can be an invaluable aid to the physician.

There are two major types of asthmatic infants: those who wheeze only with infections and frequently improve with age and those who wheeze continuously and experience considerable difficulty. Overlap exists between the two groups, and it is impossible to predict which infant will enter remission.

Response to therapy in infancy is often poor. Milder symptoms can be treated with oral beta-adrenergic agonists; more moderate symptoms may respond to nebulized beta-adrenergic agonists (0.2 to 0.3 mL of 5% solution) diluted in cromolyn (2 mL). In more severe cases in which the combination of beta agonists and cromolyn fail to control symptoms, nebulized budesonide should be given prophylactically in place of cromolyn. Acute severe symptoms unresponsive to beta agonists may necessitate treatment with oral corticosteroids (5 to 7.5 mg of prednisone or prednisolone twice daily). In difficult cases, oral the-ophylline may also be administered if additional bronchodilatation is required (see Figure 1). Pre-scriptions for infants and toddlers should be dis-pensed in duplicate form when indicated so that day care providers can have their own supply. Written asthma management plans complete with medication side effects should also be provided for day care pro-viders.

THREE- TO SIX-YEAR-OLD CHILDREN

Many 3-year-old and most 4-year-old children can perform peak flow maneuvers. This information adds a whole new dimension to the asthma management plan. For instance, in cases with a mild exercise component, the decision about premedicating before moderate exercise can be based on the peak flow reading. Peak flow readings can provide information about airway reactivity, because the differences in peak flow readings before and after bronchodilator use, as well as morning to evening peak flow variabil-ity, seem to correlate positively with airway hyper-reactivity. However, peak flow readings do not reflect small airway disease, which takes the longest to re-solve. Although peak flow readings are a valuable and inexpensive tool, they cannot take the place of complete pulmonary function testing.

Most preschoolers can use metered-dose inhalants delivered through spacer devices. There are many available choices (InspirEase, Inhal-Aid, Aero-Chamber). The InspirEase is compact and provides excellent aerosol delivery to the lungs. Because the bag collapses as the child inhales, it provides excel-lent visual feedback for the child and confirmation for the parent that the child actually inhaled through the mouth. It is important to take a slow deep breath and hold it to maximize aerosol delivery. Most spac-ers contain whistles that blow when the inhalation is too rapid.

Occasional symptoms are best treated with two inhalations of a beta-adrenergic agonist (e.g., albut-erol [Ventolin], metaproterenol [Alupent]). For more persistent symptoms, inhaled cromolyn (2 puffs four times each day) should be administered daily for reversal of airway hyper-reactivity, and bronchodila-tors should be continued as symptomatic medica-tions. As with the younger group, inhaled corticoster-oids are substituted for cromolyn in the event of cromolyn failure, and more severe cases may require a short course of oral steroids (10 to 20 mg twice daily) to achieve control. In difficult cases, cromolyn and inhaled corticosteroids should be used concomi-tantly. Oral beta-adrenergic agonists, ipratropium bromide (Atrovent) 2 puffs four times a day as needed or oral theophylline may be added as additional bron-chodilators. Ipratropium bromide is especially useful if cholinergic mechanisms are involved (e.g., those evoked by emotion or cold weather). This age group is also particularly susceptible to exacerbations with upper respiratory tract infections, and inhaled pro-phylactic medications (cromolyn or corticosteroids) should be increased or instituted at the first sign of

an infection in susceptible patients (see Figure 2). Prescriptions for preschool-age children should be dispensed in duplicate form when indicated, so that day care providers can have their own supply. Writ-ten asthma management plans complete with medi-cation side effects and a peak flow meter should also be given to day care providers.

SIX- TO TWELVE-YEAR-OLD CHILDREN

Children in this age group should take increasing responsibility for their asthma. Younger children should be encouraged to guess their peak flow read-ings and should record the actual values. It has been demonstrated that the regular use of a peak flow meter results in improved perception of airway ob-struction and more accurate early recognition of im-pending exacerbations. As children mature, they should be taught the names of their medications and encouraged to use their peak flow readings to identify their asthma triggers. These children, especially the older ones, can also be given some responsibility (with careful supervision) for keeping their rooms free of clutter and dust and for taking their own medications. A flow-chart on which children can re-cord medications taken, symptoms, and peak flow reading can help to teach self-management skills. Prescriptions for school children should be dispensed in duplicate form so that school nurses can have their own supply. Written asthma management plans complete with medication side effects and a peak flow meter should also be provided for school nurses.

The medications scheme outlined for the 3- to 6-year-old group is also appropriate for this group. If, however, administration of medications at school is undesirable, inhaled corticosteroids should be given instead of cromolyn, because they are frequently more effective than cromolyn if thrice-daily or twice-daily administration is necessary. Inhaled beta-ad-renergic agonists are the bronchodilators of choice, especially if needed for exercise asthma. These agents should always be available for symptom re-versal. If bronchodilators are required several times daily, a long-acting bronchodilator, such as salmet-erol (Serevent) or long-acting albuterol (Proventil Re-petabs), can be used, or theophylline could be pre-scribed. Some specialists prescribe a morning dose of salmeterol given before school to protect against exercise asthma during the school day.

ADOLESCENTS

It is during adolescence that asthma frequently becomes a battleground between parent and patient. All too often, this results in poor asthma control. The need for continual education cannot be overempha-sized. Adolescents must understand that they have control over their disease and that disruption of their lifestyles and the need for additional medications can be reduced if they monitor themselves closely and follow their asthma management plans. It is prefera-ble to allow adolescents to self-medicate at school; however, if school policy does not permit this, dupli-cate prescriptions, asthma management plans complete with medication side effects, and a peak flow meter should be made available to the school nurse.

The agents of choice for reversing inflammation and hyper-reactivity are inhaled corticosteroids, because compliance with four-times-daily dosing of cromolyn is often a problem. Inhaled beta-adrenergic agonists are preferred for symptomatic treatment; however, slow-release albuterol is a good alternative. Ipratropium bromide and oral theophylline are also acceptable choices. Some adolescent girls experience monthly asthma exacerbations immediately before menses. These episodes can be anticipated and should be treated with increased medications as the peak flows dictate.

TREATMENT OF EXACERBATIONS

A 20% fluctuation in peak flow readings is normal. A fall of more than 20%, however, is often a harbinger of an asthma attack and should be the trigger for instituting the backup asthma management plan. Treatment of an asthma exacerbation depends on how quickly the pulmonary functions usually fall. Most children's condition deteriorates slowly over several days or weeks, allowing the physician to take a conservative approach. Others deteriorate rapidly and require hospitalization within 24 to 48 hours. These children must be aggressively managed if hospitalization is to be avoided. In either case, triggers of asthma, such as otitis and sinusitis, or allergen exposure, should be sought and dealt with.

Management of Children Subject to Slow Deterioration

In children subject to slow deterioration, occasional peak flow readings between 70 and 80% of predicted can be treated with an additional dose of an inhaled beta-adrenergic agonist. Nebulized treatments should be used if the response to metered-dose inhalers is poor. Infants with occasional symptoms may also be treated with oral or nebulized beta-adrenergic agonists. However, infants with continual symptoms or children with peak flow readings that stay between 70 and 80% for several days despite four-times-daily bronchodilators should begin taking or increasing their dose of inhaled corticosteroids to reverse the airway hyper-reactivity. Oral beta-adrenergic agonists, ipratropium bromide, or theophylline can be added to give additional symptomatic relief.

If the peak flow readings drop to between 50 and 70% of predicted values or fail to improve on the described regimen, a short course of oral prednisone is probably needed to reverse the attack. The sooner this is instituted, the less is required. I usually prescribe prednisone thrice daily and continue until the peak flows have been normal for 2 days. Prednisone given for 7 days or less can be stopped abruptly. If longer administration is required, the afternoon prednisone dose may be discontinued after improvement has been steady for a few days. Thereafter, prednisone may be slowly discontinued, taking care

not to stop prednisone completely until after the peak flows have normalized. Ideally, these children should have pulmonary function tests done before steroids are discontinued to be sure that the small airways have normalized. The effectiveness of corticosteroids seems to be determined by the incremental dose prescribed. Thus, children taking maintenance oral prednisone may require a higher dose of prednisone during an exacerbation than those not receiving corticosteroids. If peak flows fall below 50% of predicted, the need for hospitalization is likely in the absence of intervention, and oral corticosteroids should be instituted immediately. Precipitating factors, such as sinusitis or otitis, should be sought and treated aggressively.

Management of Children Subject to Rapid Deterioration

Children who require hospitalization within 24 hours of an exacerbation should be managed very aggressively. At the first sign of a likely trigger, such as an upper respiratory tract infection, inhaled corticosteroids should be instituted or increased, and beta-adrenergic agonists should be administered as needed, via nebulization if necessary. If, despite these precautions, peak flow readings drop below 75% of predicted, oral corticosteroids and nebulized beta-adrenergic agonists should be started immediately. Oral beta-adrenergic agonists, ipratropium bromide, or theophylline can be added for additional symptomatic relief. The family should have a supply of prednisone at home, and reliable parents should be given permission to start prednisone on their own if the peak flow readings are down and the patient cannot be seen right away, or if the physician does not return their phone call within a stated period.

For children who do not require hospitalization as often or who tend to deteriorate over 24 to 48 hours, the decision about starting prednisone can be more relaxed. Peak flow readings that are dropping in the morning can be treated with inhaled steroids and nebulized beta-adrenergic agonists. However, it is often wise to begin prednisone if peak flow readings are falling in the late afternoon. It usually takes at least 6 to 8 hours for prednisone to start producing an effect. Because asthma is usually worse in the middle of the night and early morning, the patient's condition can be expected to deteriorate rapidly in the middle of the night, and this is the time when the parents' awareness and the physician's availability are at a low point. Early administration of oral corticosteroids to patients with histories of rapid deterioration can significantly reduce the need for hospitalizations and the cumulative dose of prednisone required.

Exacerbations at School

Occasionally, asthma is worse during the week than on the weekend. The pattern can be confirmed with frequent peak flow readings taken at home and at school. In such cases, antigen exposure at school may be a problem. The best solution is antigen elimination at school. If the offending antigen is the class pet, the solution is simple. Often, the problem is more complex and difficult to correct. In these cases, frequent administration of cromolyn (every 2 hours) while at school may solve the problem. Although administration of cromolyn more often than four times daily is not FDA approved, cromolyn is extremely safe. A lethal dose is unobtainable in animal models, and adverse effects are not seen below several grams (300 mL) per kg per day of inhaled cromolyn sodium.

STATUS ASTHMATICUS

Children presenting with acute severe asthma require both beta$_2$-adrenergic agonists and corticosteroids. Unless the asthma is a component of anaphylaxis, there is little need to use injected epinephrine. Nebulized albuterol, terbutaline, or metaproterenol should be administered every 20 minutes three times (as long as the heart rate remains below 80% of predicted maximum) or until a satisfactory increase in the peak flow reading has been obtained. Methylprednisolone (Solu-Medrol), 2 mg per kg, should be administered intravenously early in the course of treatment. Oxygen therapy is frequently required and when needed can improve the response to beta$_2$-adrenergic agonists.

A sinus radiograph is probably the most useful screening test in status asthmaticus. Radiographic evidence of sinusitis is found in approximately 50% of children hospitalized in status asthmaticus. Often the infection is silent, but proper antibiotic therapy can cause marked improvement in asthma symptoms. Arterial blood gas measurements are also helpful, because the hypoxic lung is poorly responsive to beta$_2$-adrenergic agonists. A chest radiograph is helpful if a pneumothorax or pneumonia is suspected or if other causes for wheezing are sought, and serum theophylline levels should be obtained in patients receiving theophylline.

If hospitalization is necessary, particular attention should be paid to oxygenation, adequate hydration, and expulsion of mucus. Chest percussion should be performed every 4 hours as long as mucus plugging persists. Nebulized beta$_2$-adrenergic agonists and intravenous methylprednisolone are usually required every 4 hours; however, in difficult cases, beta$_2$-adrenergic agonists can be administered more frequently as long as the heart rate remains acceptable. If the patient is receiving cromolyn or theophylline, these agents should be continued. Little added benefit is derived from the addition of these agents during status asthmaticus, and theophylline given acutely can cause numerous unpleasant side effects.

In cases of respiratory failure, the child should be admitted to the intensive care unit for an albuterol drip and possible ventilatory support. The need for either procedure is rare, and both involve risk to the patient. Therefore, if respiratory failure is antici-

pated, it is advisable to refer the child to a physician specifically trained to treat respiratory failure in asthmatic patients.

The adequacy of the discharge plan is as important as the acute treatment. Patients who are not already monitoring peak flow readings should be given a peak flow meter and educated in its use. Unless pulmonary functions have normalized, discharged patients should receive a short course of oral corticosteroids to avert a relapse. Because crisis care alone is inadequate for optimal asthma management, patients not currently receiving long-term follow-up care should receive appropriate referrals. Children not previously evaluated for allergies should also receive appropriate referrals. Following these guidelines can reduce subsequent hospitalizations.

ALLERGIC RHINITIS CAUSED BY INHALANT FACTORS

method of
GAIL G. SHAPIRO, M.D.
Northwest Asthma and Allergy Center
Seattle, Washington

Allergic rhinitis is nasal inflammation resulting from an immune reaction between environmental antigens, known as allergens, and the nasal mucosa. This problem is the most common cause of chronic nasal congestion and may affect as much as 15% of the population. Besides causing discomfort and malaise, allergic rhinitis has been linked to other problems such as sinusitis and middle ear disease.

The pathophysiology of allergic rhinitis relates to the capacity of allergic individuals to produce IgE that specifically recognizes environmental allergens to which they have become sensitized. This IgE coats mast cells and basophils in the nasal mucosa. On re-exposure to allergen, there is an immediate release of preformed mediators from these cells and a later release of newly formed mediators. Hours later there may be a late phase reaction as inflammatory cells such as eosinophils that have been recruited to the airway contribute to mucosal swelling and mucus production, which further augments the inflammatory milieu by producing interleukins and other proinflammatory mediators.

The visible result of this sequence of events is mucosal edema from vasodilatation and vascular leakage, sneezing and itching from neuronal reflex stimulation, and mucus production from stimulation of mucous and serous glands in the mucosa. These changes translate to nasal congestion, pruritus, and rhinorrhea.

DIFFERENTIAL DIAGNOSIS

Although allergic rhinitis is an extremely common cause of chronic rhinitis, other problems should be considered when evaluating the patient with chronic nasal obstruction. Structural anomalies, e.g., severe nasal septal deviation and nasal polyps, distort airway patency. Nasal polyps generally emanate from the sinus cavities into the nasal vault. They occur in nonallergic as well as allergic individuals. Unlike swollen nasal mucosa, which is pink, polyps are grayish, gelatinous projections that droop down from the upper nasal vault and may appear as shiny globules or as large finger-like projections.

Patients may develop hypertrophic, erythematous nasal mucosa secondary to overuse of topical vasoconstrictor nose sprays, a condition known as rhinitis medicamentosa. Similar-appearing mucosa with purulent nasal secretions suggests infectious rhinosinusitis.

Nasal edema with clear, thin secretions may represent vasomotor rhinitis. This condition is seen more often in adults than in children. Typically, sufferers have chronic congestion and rhinorrhea exacerbated by temperature changes, pollution, irritating fumes, and tobacco smoke. These factors probably provoke symptoms on an autonomic rather than an immunologic basis. Some individuals with vasomotor rhinitis complain of copious thin, watery nasal secretions without much congestion.

A condition known as nonallergic eosinophilic rhinitis mimics allergic rhinitis remarkably. Patients complain of congestion and watery rhinorrhea. Their nasal mucosa appears pale and edematous, and secretions are thin and clear. Microscopic examination of the secretions reveals mainly eosinophils. In spite of these findings, results of skin testing to common allergens are negative.

HISTORY

The usual features of allergic rhinitis are nasal congestion, rhinorrhea, sneezing, and nasal itching. Some patients complain of constantly feeling as if they have a cold. Some experience itching of the palate or ear due to common fifth cranial nerve innervation of the nose and ear canal. Youngsters may habitually rub their noses or make strange facial gestures to overcome nasal pruritus. A dark periorbital appearance claims the name "allergic shiners." Allergic rhinitis may be an etiologic factor for chronic or recurrent acute sinusitis as well as for eustachian tube dysfunction and middle ear problems, including infections, effusions, and conductive hearing loss.

Allergic rhinitis may be episodic or continual, depending on the spectrum of allergens affecting the patient. When the predominant ones are pollens, symptoms are confined to pollinating seasons, usually spring and summer. Of course, warmer regions have pollen year-round. In general, trees pollinate in early spring, followed by grasses and then weeds in summer. Ragweed season, the major problem time in the East and Midwest, extends from August until the first frost, usually mid-October.

Usually, people with year-round (perennial) allergic rhinitis have sensitivity to dust, mold, or animal dander and may also react to pollen. Aggravating allergens may exist in the work place or at day care. In taking an environmental history, these factors must be explored.

PHYSICAL EXAMINATION

One should look for previously mentioned clues: nose rubbing, dark circles around the eyes, sneezing, and rhinorrhea. Allergic conjunctivitis may be a concomitant finding that is apparent as injection or edema of the bulbar conjunctiva, sometimes so severe as to produce a gelatinous appearance. The hard palate may show petechiae. These result from negative pressure exerted by the tongue as the patient attempts to scratch the itchy palate, producing unique clucking noises in the process.

The typical appearance of the allergic nasal vault is swollen, pale pink mucosa overlying the turbinates along with thin, colorless secretions. The prototype appearance, however, is frequently replaced by a less classic one. The nasal vault may look normal; the mucosa may be erythematous; secretions may be turbid. These deviations may occur because the patient is asymptomatic at the time of the examination, has an upper respiratory infection, or has a distinctive individual pattern of disease.

DIAGNOSTIC AIDS

The microscopic evaluation of nasal secretions provides valuable information toward making a diagnosis. The patient blows his or her nose into plastic wrap; alternatively, a swab can be used to obtain the specimen. The secretions are wiped onto a glass slide, which is then heat fixed and stained with Hansel's stain. The presence of more than 5 to 10% eosinophils per field suggests allergic rhinitis. However, less common problems such as nonallergic rhinitis with eosinophilia and nasal polyposis (with or without concomitant allergic rhinitis) cannot be discounted. A prevalence of polymorphonuclear cells suggests infectious rhinitis, most likely related to a viral syndrome if acute or to bacterial rhinosinusitis if more long-standing. If there are watery secretions that yield few cells, vasomotor rhinitis is quite likely, although it is also possible that the patient has allergic rhinitis but is currently asymptomatic.

Allergy skin testing plays an important role in distinguishing the several diagnostic possibilities. Extracts of common aeroallergens are applied to the epidermis in such a way as to reproduce the interaction of environmental allergen and mast cell–bound IgE that occurs in the nose. Initial testing is usually carried out with an epicutaneous method, e.g., prick, puncture, or scratch. A drop of an extract of each allergen in question is applied to the skin, and then a needle is used to pierce the skin superficially, enough to bring antigen and mediator-containing cells into contact. Within 15 to 20 minutes, a wheal and flare reaction appears if significant amounts of histamine are released. There is a good correlation between positive epicutaneous skin testing to inhaled allergens and clinical symptoms on exposure. Because this testing is not always adequately sensitive, intradermal skin testing may be needed. A small quantity of allergen is directly injected into the epidermis. Again, a wheal and flare reaction occurring with 15 to 20 minutes of exposure indicates an IgE reaction against the allergen. The correlation of a positive intradermal test and actual symptoms from exposure to a particular allergen is less commanding than that for epicutaneous test reactions.

An alternative diagnostic approach is in vitro measurement of allergen-specific IgE. The patient's serum is incubated with an inert carrier material coated with allergen. Serum IgE to specific allergen reacts with the allergen-carrier complex to form an IgE-allergen-carrier complex that can be radiolabeled and then quantified. The prototype of this is the radioallergosorbent test. In general, such in vitro methods are more costly and less sensitive than skin testing.

The decision to do skin tests or to treat allergic rhinitis empirically depends on the chronicity and severity of the problem. For some situations, brief courses of antihistamines or decongestants provide satisfactory relief and no in-depth evaluation need be done. Sometimes a determination of the total serum IgE may be helpful, giving general information concerning the patient's allergic status. Because this value is elevated in only approximately one half of allergic rhinitis patients, it is helpful when positive but not when negative.

TREATMENT

Avoidance

The common allergens provoking allergic rhinitis are house dust mites, molds, animal protein, and pollens. Insect antigens, especially from cockroaches, are important in certain parts of the United States. Occupational allergens may be important, for example, diisocyanates in industries in which foam rubber is used, wood dust in the lumber industry, and enzymes in the manufacture of household detergents.

The most effective therapy for allergic rhinitis is avoidance of the inciting allergens. In the case of occupational agents or animal exposures, this may represent severe sacrifice. One must weigh the career commitment or emotional attachment against the degree of disease involvement and relief through other modalities.

House dust mites are ubiquitous microscopic creatures that feed off human skin scales. They thrive in climates where the relative humidity is usually greater than 50%. They tend to seep into stuffed furniture, carpet pile, and bedding, where they favor the dark and moist environment. They produce relatively large quantities of fecal material, which is more antigenic than the mites themselves.

Mites do not survive extremes of heat, cold, and dryness. Their proliferation can be minimized by such measures as decreasing ambient humidity, removing carpets, and encasing mattresses, box springs, and pillows in nonporous plasticized covers. Hot-water washing of bedding at a temperature of at least 130°F is helpful, whereas simply drying bedding in a very hot dryer is not as effective. Mites are not well killed by the dryer and are resistant to detergents and bleaches. Treating carpets with chemicals that kill mites (e.g., benzyl benzoate) or that denature their antigen (e.g., tannic acid) can be helpful in situations in which carpet removal is not possible.

Placing stuffed animals and comforters that are not easily washed in the freezer for 12 hours or more has been recommended for dust mite control.

Mold avoidance also involves measures to decrease household humidity. Heating and cooling systems should be checked to eliminate mold reservoirs. A layer of heavy plastic (Visqueen) in the crawl space of a home decreases moisture problems and mold. At times a dehumidifier may be necessary. An application of liquid laundry bleach removes mold growth on window frames and bathroom tiles.

Pollen avoidance is extremely difficult because these allergens are so widespread at certain times of year. Keeping doors and windows closed and using air conditioning effectively filter most pollen from the home. This method is ineffective, however, for people with an outdoors-oriented lifestyle. Similarly, it is impractical in parts of the country where air conditioning is unnecessary for temperature control. High-efficiency filters (electrostatic precipitators, high-efficiency particulate air filters) remove particulate matter including pollens, mold spores, and animal allergens. They, too, are most effective if doors and windows are kept closed. The correlations between their use and control of rhinitis symptoms are unclear.

Although environmental control is theoretically the ideal method for managing allergic rhinitis, it is difficult to institute and to sustain. The impressive improvement one sees in many instances when these preventive measures have been accomplished encourages one to continue with these recommendations. Nevertheless, complicated lifestyles involving such confounding factors as rental homes, dual parental custody of children, and day care settings are important factors that force the use of other approaches.

Pharmacologic Intervention

Antihistamines (Table 1)

Antihistamines are often used as first-line therapy for allergic rhinitis. They competitively inhibit the

TABLE 1. **Classification of Commonly Used Antihistamines**

Class	Generic Name	Trade Name	Suggested Dose for Children (mg/kg/24 h)	Suggested Dose for Adults
Ethanolamine	Diphenhydramine hydrochloride	Benadryl	5.0	25–50 mg qid
	Carbinoxamine maleate	Clistin	0.8*	4–8 mg qid
Ethylenediamine	Tripelennamine hydrochloride	PBZ	5.0	25–50 mg qid
Alkylamine	Chlorpheniramine maleate	Chlor-Trimeton Teldrin	0.35	4 mg qid
	Brompheniramine maleate	Dimetane	0.35	4 mg qid
	Triprolidine hydrochloride	Actidil	0.18	2.5 mg qid
Phenothiazine	Promethazine hydrochloride	Phenergan	0.5	12.5–25 mg qid
	Methdilazine	Tacaryl	0.3	16–23 mg daily (as bid or qid)
Piperazine	Hydroxyzine hydrochloride	Atarax, Vistaril	2.0	10–20 mg qid
Piperidine	Cyproheptadine hydrochloride	Periactin	0.25	4–20 mg daily (4 mg qid)
Miscellaneous	Terfenadine	Seldane	—	60 mg bid
	Astemizole	Hismanal	—	10 mg qd
	Loratadine	Claritin	5–10 mg qd	10 mg qd
	Cetirizine	Zyrtec	5–10 mg qd	10 mg qd
	Fexofenadine	Allegra	—	60 mg bid

*Exceeds dosage recommended by the manufacturer.

allergic mediator histamine at its receptor sites in the airway. Antihistamines block both the vasodilatation and mucous gland hypersecretion consequent to the stimulation of H_1 receptors on blood vessels and sensory nerves, respectively. In terms of symptom relief, antihistamines are most effective for diminishing nasal itch and hypersecretion and are not as helpful in decreasing mucous membrane swelling.

Historically, antihistamines have been classified by chemical structure as falling into one of six categories. Clinicians have become familiar with one or two agents in several groups and have shifted among these as tachyphylaxis or adverse side effects made alternative choices necessary. These so-called first-generation antihistamines are, for the most part, now available to patients over-the-counter. Their value is somewhat dimmed by their propensity to cause drowsiness and anticholinergic effects such as blurred vision, dryness of the mouth and eyes, and urinary retention. These drugs should be used cautiously by older patients, particularly elderly men, and should be strictly avoided in patients with histories of symptomatic prostatic hypertrophy, bladder neck obstruction, and narrow-angle glaucoma. There is concern that these drugs prolong voluntary reaction time, thereby increasing the risk of errors in operating machinery or in driving, even when sedation is not noticed by the patient.

Second-generation antihistamines avoid many of the difficulties associated with the older agents. They have little cholinergic activity and have much less likelihood of causing drowsiness and decreased voluntary reaction time. They are available by prescription and are considerably more expensive than their predecessors. Terfenadine and astemizole are metabolized via the cytochrome P-450 cytochrome system in the liver, and their metabolism can be influenced by other drugs that are metabolized in this way. Elevated levels of these drugs have been associated with prolongation of the QT interval and clinically significant arrhythmia, so that administration of a number of agents is proscribed with these antihistamines. Terfenadine is active within an hour of administration and is effective for about 12 hours. It can be used regularly or on an as-needed basis. Astemizole has a much slower onset of action, often several days, but lasts for days or weeks after the last administration. It is not a good as-needed agent. Loratadine is a 24-hour-duration product that has a rapid onset of action and is not metabolized in the liver. Cetirizine also works for 24 hours and avoids metabolic interaction, but it has an increased incidence of drowsiness compared with the other three second-generation products. The newest member of this family of compounds is fexofenadine, which is a metabolite of terfenadine. It has activity similar to that of the parent compound but is not metabolized in the liver. Two of the second-generation antihistamines, cetirizine and loratadine, are currently available in liquid form for children older than 6 years.

Decongestants

The oral decongestants phenylpropanolamine, phenylephrine, and pseudoephedrine are alpha-adrenergic agents capable of producing nasal mucous membrane vasoconstriction adequate to reduce edema. They work well in conjunction with antihistamines. There are currently a large number of combination products having antihistamine and decongestant in one preparation. Although this increases convenience and compliance, it prevents individualized dosage adjustments. However, because little is currently known about dose-response relationships and the kinetics of most of these preparations, these fixed combinations remain practical and popular.

Topical decongestants are poor choices for treating chronic rhinitis. With repeated use, they tend to cause less sustained decongestion, leading both to overuse and to rebound vasodilatation with increased congestion. This iatrogenic congestion is known as rhinitis medicamentosa.

Cromolyn, long used for asthma therapy, is an alternative to antihistamines as primary therapy for treatment of allergic rhinitis. Nasalcrom is a 4% solution of cromolyn that is used as a nasal spray and seems to act by preventing the release of allergic mediators. The usual dosage is 1 spray per nostril three to six times daily; each spray delivers 5.2 mg of cromolyn. Cromolyn is effective only as a prophylactic agent and for best results must be used regularly rather than after symptoms occur. Adverse effects are uncommon and benign. These include transient sneezing, nasal stinging, and headaches.

Intranasal Corticosteroids (Table 2)

Nasal administration of corticosteroids is an extremely effective therapy for allergic rhinitis. There is growing popularity for using intranasal corticosteroids as first-line therapy, because a number of studies comparing antihistamines and intranasal steroids for allergic rhinitis favor the latter. These drugs appear to diminish histamine release and to decrease the production of allergic mediators. They serve to deter the influx of inflammatory cells such as eosinophils into the mucosa. When used before allergen exposure, they can reduce both immediate and late phase nasal inflammation. They are also helpful soon after therapy is initiated even in situations in which there has not been pretreatment.

Intranasal corticosteroids can control all the manifestations of allergic rhinitis: itch, rhinorrhea, and congestion. They have been shown to decrease bronchial hyper-responsiveness in patients with concomitant asthma. They can be used episodically or for reasonably long periods: weeks and even months. They have been approved for children aged 6 years and older.

The six agents that are currently available vary somewhat in topical potency of the constituent drug, but all are so effective that dose-response comparisons are not likely to show significant differences. They are marketed as once-daily or twice-daily medications. Some are available as aerosols, some as aqueous sprays, and some in both formulations. Although generally well tolerated, they can cause dryness, crusting, and epistaxis. These are counteracted

TABLE 2. **Intranasal Corticosteroids**

Chemical Name	Trade Name	Formulations	Usual Dosage	FDA Approval Age (y)
Beclomethasone	Beconase, Vancenase	a	1 or 2 puffs/side bid	≥6
Budesonide	Rhinocort	a, c	2 puffs/side bid or 4 qd	≥6
Dexamethasone	Dexacort	c	1 or 2 puffs/side bid–tid	≥6
Flunisolide	Nasarel	a	2 puffs/side bid	≥6
Fluticasone	Flonase	a	2 puffs/side qd or 1 puff/side bid	≥12
Triamcinolone	Nasacort	a, c	2 puffs/side bid or 4 puffs/side qd	≥12

Abbreviations: a = aerosol pump; c = chlorinated fluorocarbon propellant.

by decreasing the dosage and using nasal saline before the steroid. There are case reports of nasal septal perforation with intranasal steroid therapy, but these are unusual, and long-term administration is generally well tolerated.

The preparations of intranasal steroid that are available—beclomethasone, dexamethasone, triamcinolone, flunisolide, fluticasone, and budesonide—are described in Table 2. These drugs are sometimes coadministered with antihistamine and/or decongestant for difficult to control rhinitis or rhinoconjunctivitis.

Systemic Corticosteroids

Systemic corticosteroid therapy is rarely needed for allergic rhinitis. In patients who have severe involvement that appears refractory to other therapy, a short course of oral short-acting steroid, e.g., prednisone, is helpful. Long-term use puts the patient at risk of a long list of steroid-induced adverse effects, which may well be more worrisome than the initial rhinitis complaints. Intramuscular steroid injection has produced unsightly keloid formation and subcutaneous fat atrophy, which have been the basis for malpractice suits. Injection of steroids into the turbinates has been associated with blindness due to intra-arterial embolization of the mixture.

Anticholinergic Agents

Intranasal ipratropium (Atrovent) is an atropine-like drug that is useful for decreasing watery secretions that are produced by nasal glands that are sensitive to cholinergic stimulation. Ipratropium in 3 and 6% solutions is available for relief of secretions secondary to upper respiratory infections and nasal allergy. Because the rhinorrhea of allergic rhinitis is relatively easy to treat with antihistamines and nasal steroids, the need for an anticholinergic is unusual. The drug is recommended in a dose of 2 actuations per nostril two or three times per day. It is not absorbed systemically to an appreciable extent and is well tolerated.

Immunotherapy

Immunotherapy, also known as desensitization or hyposensitization, is the injection of allergens to which an individual is immunologically sensitive for the purpose of building tolerance to those allergens. Many studies attest to its usefulness provided that appropriate patients are selected and appropriate allergenic extracts and dosing are used. Immunotherapy is usually reserved for those allergic individuals who continue to have recalcitrant disease after optimal avoidance measures and pharmacologic intervention have been investigated. Frequently, these patients suffer from sensitivity to pollens that are present much of the year, thus reducing the impact of environmental control measures. Patients usually receive injections once or twice weekly for several months and eventually reach a monthly regimen, which is continued for several years. After this, the majority of patients who have had symptomatic benefit will continue to do so because of maintained immunologic tolerance to the specific allergens to which they were immunized.

Before immunotherapy is initiated, a patient's sensitivity to allergens should be confirmed by skin testing. Only clinically significant allergens with such skin test verification should be added to the treatment mixture. Therapy is usually confined to house dust, mite, pollen, and mold allergies. Evidence for efficacy with mold antigens is limited. Standardized cat antigen for immunotherapy has become commercially available.

Benefits of immunotherapy are often achieved in the first year. Most patients receive it for 3 to 5 years. After this time, many of those who have responded seem to retain symptomatic benefit even when immunotherapy is discontinued. Responsiveness is thought to relate to the production of IgE-blocking antibodies, down-regulation of IgE production, and decreased releasability by mediator-containing cells, i.e., mast cells and basophils.

Physicians who administer immunotherapy must be prepared to handle anaphylaxis. Patients are most at risk as they progress to higher antigen doses. Nevertheless, anaphylaxis occurs most commonly immediately after the injection. For this reason patients should remain in the clinic for 20 to 30 minutes after their injection so that they can be observed for possible systemic complications. Quite commonly, patients experience local reactions at the injection site. If a large immediate or late phase local reaction occurs, the dosage should be decreased and then advanced slowly if reactions diminish.

ALLERGIC REACTIONS TO DRUGS

method of
STEPHEN E. WOLVERTON, M.D.
Indiana University School of Medicine
Indianapolis, Indiana

Cutaneous drug reactions (the term is used synonymously in this chapter with "drug allergy") are common, confronting physicians in all fields of medicine. At times these reactions may produce a serious outcome. The subject of cutaneous drug reactions is quite complicated, presenting difficulties for clinicians to master, let alone allowing them to feel reasonably comfortable with managing these patients. The problem is compounded by the fact that a given cutaneous drug reaction may be due to *any* drug the patient is taking, may occur at *any* time in the course of the drug's administration, is potentially caused by *any* route of exposure (oral, parenteral, mucosal), and can be due to medications from *any* potential source (prescription, over-the-counter [OTC], recreational drugs). And if these concerns are not enough, the clinician has no diagnostic test at his or her disposal that is of consistent value in confirming the diagnosis of drug allergy.

In this chapter, I list common errors (pitfalls) and related solutions in the evaluation of patients with cutaneous drug reactions. The lists include common errors that pertain to drug reaction risk assessment, diagnosis, management, and information retrieval. The focus is on drug allergy with cutaneous manifestations, with or without systemic findings as well.

A four-step algorithm is presented in Table 1. Further information on these steps is included in the solutions presented for the various common errors discussed in this chapter. The overall goals in this organizational approach are improved diagnostic precision and minimization of the risks involved with clinical decision-making regarding patients with suspected drug allergy in the form of cutaneous drug reactions.

COMMON ERRORS IN DRUG REACTION RISK ASSESSMENT

Focusing on the Patient's Medication List When First Assessing the Patient

The natural response for most physicians is to first evaluate the patient's medication list for potential "culprits" when a patient presents with a new cutaneous eruption. Given that many patients are taking as many as 5 to 10 medications (prescription and OTC), it is easy to get bogged down surveying the medication list when there is a more streamlined way to approach the key issues.

In contrast, careful categorization of the cutaneous eruption into a specific reaction pattern (e.g., urticaria, morbilliform pattern, erythema multiforme, contact dermatitis) facilitates the clinical decisions for three major reasons. First, the reaction pattern determines the potential risk to the patient if the responsible drug is continued (intentionally or accidentally). High-risk reaction patterns and relatively low risk reaction patterns are detailed in Tables 2 and 3, respectively. Second, the initial characterization of the reaction pattern helps determine the most likely drug cause. Most reviews and chapters on the subject of cutaneous drug reactions present highly divergent lists of common drug causes, depending on the category of drug reaction (reaction pattern). Third, the type of reaction pattern

TABLE 1. Cutaneous Drug Reaction Clinical Diagnosis Algorithm*

Challenge circumstances
  Characterize the reaction pattern
  Evaluate the patient's history of previous drug allergy
  Consider literature experience with the drugs in question
  Give greatest emphasis to drugs started during the past month
Dechallenge
  Observe the response to drug discontinuation if appropriate
  Remember that most cutaneous drug reactions fade in 1–2 wk after drug discontinuation
Rechallenge
  Use intentional rechallenge selectively—primarily with lower risk patterns
  Determine if there has been unintentional (accidental) rechallenge
  Reverse rechallenge (rechallenge all but the drug in question)
Exclusion
  Exclude systemic involvement with high-risk reaction patterns
  Exclude nondrug precipitators of the same reaction pattern

*The greater the number of these four criteria present, the greater the likelihood that a given drug induced the drug reaction.

determines the likelihood that the cutaneous eruption is due to a drug at all.

Labeling the Patient as Having a Drug Allergy, Which Is in Reality a Drug Intolerance

Most clinicians have new patients fill out preprinted history forms, which virtually always have a section in which patients list drug allergies. Many times careful questioning reveals that the "drug allergy" was merely an intolerance or an expected pharmacologic drug effect. Common examples include gastrointestinal intolerance to aspirin, various nonsteroidal anti-inflammatory drugs, and codeine. The problem grows in importance when the patient erroneously claims to be allergic to a member of a large, important drug group such as the β-lactam antibiotics.

The solution is to routinely have the patient carefully describe any previous presumed allergies before formally documenting the drug allergies in the medical record. No doubt there are many times the patient cannot describe the previous rash in sufficient detail to determine the cutaneous reaction pattern. Any suspicion the patient gives that there may have been a previous episode of drug-induced anaphylaxis or severe erythema multiforme (Stevens-Johnson syndrome or toxic epidermal necrolysis) should be taken seriously and recorded in prominent chart locations.

Considering Only the Patient's Skin Findings When There May Be Systemic Findings

The most common cutaneous drug reaction pattern is the morbilliform pattern. Synonyms in common usage include

TABLE 2. Common High-Risk Drug Reaction Patterns

Erythema multiforme minor
Erythema multiforme major (Stevens-Johnson syndrome, toxic epidermal necrolysis)
Vasculitis
Urticaria (possibly with anaphylaxis, anaphylactoid reaction)
Erythroderma (synonymous with exfoliative erythroderma)
Drug hypersensitivity syndrome (see Table 4)

TABLE 3. **Some Examples of Relatively Low Risk Drug Reaction Patterns**

Morbilliform	Fixed drug eruption
Lichenoid (lichen planus–like)	Photosensitivity
Vesiculobullous	Hyperpigmentation
Erythema nodosum	Alopecia

"exanthematous," "maculopapular," and "drug rash." This category of drug reactions is virtually always purely cutaneous, carrying no significant risk of a fatal outcome or significant irreversible morbidity. Exceptions may occur when certain drugs are prescribed (Table 4), in which a drug hypersensitivity syndrome with clinical features reminiscent of infectious mononucleosis can occur. In patients with this hypersensitivity syndrome, the liver is the target organ where reactions may lead to potentially serious complications.

The second most common drug reaction pattern is urticaria, which is far less frequent than the morbilliform pattern. Although the risk of anaphylaxis in patients with drug-induced urticaria is quite low, the potential for this serious complication needs to be considered in every case. Most of the reaction patterns listed in Table 2 gain their high-risk status through the potential for associated systemic features. Exceptions include the burnlike complications from severe erythema multiforme major and rarely from drug-induced blistering diseases such as pemphigus. As a general rule, the clinician should always be aware that the "company" (systemic findings) the cutaneous drug reaction keeps determines the risk from a given reaction pattern.

Overdiagnosing Urticaria or Erythema Multiforme When the Patient Has a Morbilliform Reaction

Morbilliform reactions are characterized by isolated erythematous macules and papules that tend to become confluent during 7 to 10 days. The lesions are somewhat dynamic but do not disappear as new sites become involved. Urticaria, in contrast, typically has lesions present in a given location for less than 24 hours. Erythema multiforme most notably has target lesions, which have at least three concentric rings of contrasting color. The erosive mucous membrane involvement, when present, distinguishes erythema multiforme from other diagnostic contenders.

In my experience, it is common for clinicians to mistake the relatively stable erythema and edema of morbilliform reactions as urticaria. It is also easy to overdiagnose fixed erythematous lesions in morbilliform reactions as targets and fail to note that there are fewer than three zones of color. In both cases, the erroneous diagnosis shifts the patient from a relatively low risk pattern (morbilliform) to a high-risk pattern (urticaria, erythema multiforme) that essentially prohibits drug continuation or rechallenge. The clinician should carefully label the reaction pattern, recalling that somewhat atypical versions of morbilliform reactions are quite common. In most morbilliform reactions,

TABLE 4. **Causes of Drug Hypersensitivity Syndrome**

Anticonvulsants	Other drug causes
Phenytoin (Dilantin)	Dapsone
Phenobarbital	Allopurinol (Zyloprim)
Carbamazepine (Tegretol)	Minocycline (Minocin)

the responsible drug can be continued if it is essential to the patient's overall medical care. Surprisingly often, the cutaneous drug reaction fades away (down-regulates) over 1 to 2 weeks in spite of drug continuation.

COMMON ERRORS IN DRUG REACTION DIAGNOSIS

Considering Only Recently Started Drug Therapy as the Possible Drug Cause

In most cutaneous drug reactions, the responsible drug therapy was started in the preceding 1 to 2 weeks. The great majority of times the causative drug was initially given in the past month. The frustrating reality is that there are many exceptions to these guidelines. There are numerous literature citations of drug allergy in which there was a positive rechallenge involving a drug initially given months or even years before the reaction. The hypersensitivity syndromes due to phenytoin (and related anticonvulsants), dapsone, minocycline, and allopurinol usually present with skin and systemic findings between weeks 3 and 12.

Given the relative imprecision of diagnosing drug allergy, it is reasonable to consider as potential culprits drugs that were recently given for the first time. The key is to avoid limiting one's suspicion to these drugs.

Presuming Laboratory Tests Have a Central Role in Drug Reaction Diagnosis

Unfortunately, no single laboratory test reliably establishes the drug cause or even determines if the clinical scenario was due to any drug. Idiosyncratic reactions can occur on either an immunologic or a metabolic basis; in most cases the exact mechanism is not known. Commonly used tests such as intradermal or scratch testing (assess only type I hypersensitivity and fail to reproduce the drug metabolites often responsible), the radioallergosorbent test (same limitations), and complete blood counts (presence of eosinophils may suggest a drug allergy but provides no guidance toward the responsible drug) all have significant limitations in the vast majority of cases. In general, these tests simply fail to reproduce the biologic circumstances that produced the drug allergy.

Laboratory testing in drug allergy does have two primary purposes. First, laboratory tests may be of value in excluding nondrug precipitators for the same cutaneous reaction pattern. Examples include serologic testing for group A streptococcal infections (urticaria, vasculitis, erythema nodosum) and testing for autoimmune connective tissue diseases with an antinuclear antibody and rheumatoid factor (vasculitis). Second, appropriate tests should be performed to exclude systemic involvement in reaction patterns deemed as high-risk patterns (see Table 2).

Considering Topical Exposures as Possible Causes of Systemic Reaction Patterns

For the most past, systemic drug and related exposures are responsible for common and important reaction patterns such as morbilliform, urticaria, vasculitis, and erythema multiforme. History taking focused on new topical soap, detergent, or fragrance exposures in patients with these reaction patterns is rarely of value. In contrast, topical exposures are virtually always responsible for contact dermatitis. Keeping this inside versus outside exposure dichotomy in mind helps direct the physician's questions to the most likely drug causes in these respective clinical scenarios.

Considering That Skin Biopies Are Essential to the Diagnosis of Cutaneous Drug Reactions

A percutaneous skin biopsy may be of value in determining the reaction pattern but is rarely of value in establishing the drug cause. Patients with a suspected drug cause of vasculitis or erythema multiforme (minor or major) may be clearly placed in the respective diagnostic category, although the diagnostic algorithm listed in Table 1 is necessary to establish the responsible drug. The determination of the reaction pattern risk may therefore be aided by the skin biopsy.

In contrast, a skin biopsy is usually not needed to establish that a morbilliform or urticarial reaction is present in a given patient. Clinical assessment is typically sufficient to establish the presence of these two most common drug reaction patterns. As described previously, the drug reaction diagnostic algorithm is essential to determine the causative drug. It should be noted that the mere presence of eosinophils does not definitively establish that a drug was responsible, although suspicions of drug allergy are increased by the tissue presence of eosinophils. Clearly, the majority of drug reaction patterns are not typified by participation of eosinophils in the aberrant immunologic or metabolic process, making the presence of these cells uncommon in the biopsy specimens of patients with these cutaneous drug reactions.

Failing to Exclude Nondrug Precipitators Before Labeling the Patient as Having a Drug Allergy

I believe that there are numerous occasions in clinical medicine in which a drug is falsely blamed for conditions the "accused" drug did not produce. It is possible to limit the frequency of this scenario by routinely attempting to exclude nondrug causes (such as infections or systemic autoimmune diseases) for the cutaneous reaction pattern present in a given patient. In morbilliform reactions, a history and physical examination alone may be sufficient to exclude the common viral causes of this reaction pattern. A history and the response to specific antiviral therapy may allow the clinician to establish herpes simplex (and not a drug) as the cause of erythema multiforme. In many other scenarios, laboratory testing as described earlier may be required to reliably exclude a nondrug precipitator, thus increasing the likelihood that the drug in question was truly responsible for the new cutaneous reaction.

COMMON ERRORS IN DRUG REACTION MANAGEMENT

Tending to Initiate Wholesale Discontinuation of Medications When Suspecting an Allergic Reaction

It is common for a clinician's first response to a patient with a cutaneous drug reaction to be to initiate widespread drug discontinuation, without regard to the various drugs' duration of administration or the various drugs' reputation for causing the reaction pattern in question. Particularly with lower risk reaction patterns such as morbilliform drug reactions, there are several faulty assumptions that produce this wholesale drug discontinuation. First, there is

the belief that all drugs the patient is taking are equally likely to be responsible for the outcome. Second, there is the assumption that stopping the various drugs does not create a significant new risk. The hazard here is that the drugs in question may be essential for the various diseases being treated. In particular, unnecessary cessation of drugs being prescribed for hypertension, coronary artery disease, dysrhythmias, or seizures (to name a few scenarios) may have potentially disastrous consequences.

The key point here is to compare the inherent risk of the cutaneous drug reaction pattern with the risk of drug discontinuation of any given drug the patient receives. In most cases, there is a chemically unrelated alternative medication that can be given in place of the drug in question after agreement of the physicians involved with the patient's care. Only with the high-risk reaction patterns does the clinician need to be relatively thorough regarding discontinuation of any potential drug cause.

Unilaterally Discontinuing Drugs Without Consulting with Other Physicians Caring for the Patient

A significant percentage of patients have more than one physician prescribing medications for them. Even if there is a primary care physician who is aware of the reasons for the various medications the patient receives, decisions regarding possible drug allergies are often made by consultants such as dermatologists or allergists. It is imperative that any physician who is evaluating a possible medication allergy seek agreement with the prescribing physician before discontinuing *any* medication suspected as the cause.

The reasoning behind this principle is straightforward. Communication between the various physicians involved with the patient's care is not only courteous but also maximizes the quality of care by combining the varied viewpoints, experience, and expertise of the medical team. Such communication should minimize the likelihood of potentially serious medical disease flares through inappropriate cessation of a drug suspected as the cause of a cutaneous drug eruption.

Committing Errors of Overconcern—Erroneously Suspecting a Specific Drug Cause When the Drug in Question is Not Responsible for the Cutaneous Reaction

Whether a drug is falsely blamed for an allergic reaction that is actually a drug intolerance or another chemically unrelated drug was actually the culprit in the allergic drug reaction, the result is the same: a potentially important drug or drug category may be unavailable for future use by the given patient. Furthermore, assigning excessive theoretical risk to morbilliform reactions (in the absence of the drug hypersensitivity syndrome described previously) may have the same net effect—unavailable drugs or drug categories.

Patients who are labeled (whether correctly or incorrectly) allergic to penicillin are conceptually unable to take semisynthetic penicillins (dicloxacillin, cloxacillin), aminopenicillins (ampicillin, amoxicillin), extended-spectrum penicillins (carbenicillin, piperacillin), cephalosporins (cephalexin and many others), monobactams (aztreonam), and other drugs with a β-lactam nucleus in the future. Patients who are labeled allergic to sulfonamides are conceptually unable to take trimethoprim-sulfamethoxazole, sulfasalazine, sulfapyridine, dapsone, diuretics (thiazides, furosemide), or oral hypoglycemic agents (chlorpropamide) that are chemically related to sulfonamides. The risks and ramifications of falsely blaming drugs in either of these drug families are noteworthy. As discussed previously, falsely blaming a drug with subsequent drug discontinuation presents the additional risk of a potentially serious chronic disease flare.

Committing Errors of Underconcern—Failing to Suspect a Specific Drug or Even Failing to Suspect Any Drug as Responsible for a Given Cutaneous Reaction

In contrast to the scenarios of overconcern just described, errors of underconcern also have important implications that relate to potentially serious drug-induced complications instead. A minority of cutaneous drug reactions have the potential for a fatal outcome or significant irreversible morbidity. Clear awareness of the reaction patterns that have such a potential, no matter how rarely these serious outcomes occur, is of tremendous importance. Tables 2 and 3 list reactions that are high risk and relatively low risk. Drug continuation or rechallenge later with any drug suspected of causing one of the high-risk reactions patterns should be undertaken only under exceptional circumstances. In contrast, drugs suspected as causing relatively low risk reaction patterns can be selectively continued or rechallenged later, should the drug in question be essential to the patient's medical care. Morbilliform drug reactions (by far the most common drug reaction pattern) are of relatively low risk unless the patient is taking one of the drugs listed in Table 4, which have been clearly documented to cause a drug hypersensitivity syndrome, thus presenting a much higher risk to the patient.

Failing to Consider a Cross-reaction Between Two Related Drug Groups

The two largest drug families pertinent to drug allergies are the β-lactam antibiotics and the sulfonamide antibiotics (see previous discussion). Although less well documented, other groups such as fluoroquinolones, macrolides, and tetracyclines conceptually have some potential for cross-reaction as well.

The clinician should always consider the possibility of the occurrence of these cross-reactions. The risk of allergy to a cephalosporin in a patient known to be allergic to penicillin is generally quoted at 5 to 20%. If the patient had a prior allergy to penicillin (or to closely related penicillin derivatives) manifesting as a morbilliform reaction, it would be considered acceptable practice to prescribe a cephalosporin, particularly via an oral route. In contrast, prior high-risk reaction patterns such as urticaria, vasculitis, erythema multiforme major, or the drug hypersensitivity syndrome would prohibit the use of a chemically related drug.

COMMON ERRORS IN INFORMATION RETRIEVAL REGARDING DRUG ALLERGIES

Assuming One's Personal Clinical Experience Is Sufficient to Reliably Diagnose the Cause of Cutaneous Drug Reactions

The subject of drug allergy is too complex and unpredictable to fully rely on one's own clinical experience to make these important decisions in most cases. Even researchers or authors in the area of drug allergy do not have adequate experience or insight to make the majority of their clinical decisions without utilizing supplemental published or electronic information. No doubt the principles outlined in this chapter will provide general guidance of tremendous value; however, specific drug tendencies for the various reaction patterns are beyond the scope of this chapter.

Failing to Utilize Established Written and Computerized Database Information on Cutaneous Drug Reactions

Options for pursuing details for specific drug reactions include (but are not limited to) the following: (1) drug compendiums such as the *Physicians' Desk Reference* or *Physicians' GenRx,* (2) *The Medical Letter on Drugs and Therapeutics,* (3) standard dermatology or allergy and immunology textbooks, (4) publications from the Boston Collaborative Drug Surveillance Program, and (5) various on-line services such as Adverse Drug Reaction Reporting System from the American Academy of Dermatology. The reader should be warned that single case reports that are quoted and requoted may be poorly documented and therefore misleading. The clinician should put much greater stock in larger and more rigorous drug reaction studies in the literature.

Putting Too Much Stock in Drug Reaction Tables Derived from Anecdotal Case Reports

Another word of caution is in order. Most major textbooks that have chapters on drug allergy or cutaneous drug reactions present tables with lists of various drug reaction patterns and the drugs reported to commonly cause the various reaction patterns. These lists are not intended to be comprehensive and in addition are usually poorly referenced. The tables should be considered general guides, with other published and electronic references previously discussed serving as more comprehensive resources.

Recently released drugs present problems in drug allergy diagnosis, particularly when referring to standard textbooks and the Boston Collaborative program data. The reader is advised to consult on-line drug reaction databases, drug compendiums, and *The Medical Letter on Drugs and Therapeutics* for information on drug allergy induced by these newer medications.

ALLERGIC REACTIONS TO INSECT STINGS

method of
RICHARD F. LOCKEY, M.D.
*University of South Florida College of Medicine
and James A. Haley Veterans Administration
Hospital*
Tampa, Florida

Stinging insects are responsible for significant morbidity and mortality. Insects of the order Hymenoptera (Greek *hymen,* meaning membrane; *pteron,* meaning wing) account for most instances of insect sting hypersensitivity. Three families are commonly involved: Apidae, which includes the honeybees (genus *Apis*) and bumblebees (genus *Bombus*); Vespidae, which includes the wasps (genus *Polistes*) and yellow jackets and hornets (genera *Vespula, Dolichovespula,* and *Vespa*); and Formicidae, which includes the imported fire ants (genus *Solenopsis*) and harvester ants (genus *Pogonomyrmex*).

The incidence of insect hypersensitivity is estimated at between 0.4 and 4% of persons in the United States and is somewhat higher in people with a history of atopic disease than it is in the general population. There is a 2:1 male/female predominance, and reactions are most common in rural populations and in the younger age group. During the 10-year period between 1950 and 1959, 221 deaths in the United States were attributed to Hymenoptera hypersensitivity, compared with 138 fatalities from venomous snake bites. The incidence of insect-related fatalities is probably higher than reported because some sudden deaths due to insect hypersensitivity are often incorrectly attributed to other causes. One study has detected that high titers of venom-specific IgE are found in the serum of some individuals whose deaths had been attributed to unknown causes. Changes in social patterns as well as physical morbidity often accompany insect allergy. Patients frequently alter lifestyles, work patterns, and leisure activities to avoid future reactions. Some patients become neurotic because of the fear of having a reaction similar to the one they had experienced, particularly if it was a severe systemic reaction.

The incidence of allergic reactions by each insect species varies with its geographic distribution, although hymenop-

teran insects are found throughout the world and in every U.S. state. A 10-year survey of 460 fatalities from all venomous animals, including snakes, in the United States revealed that the stinging insects caused the greatest number of deaths. A different study of 2606 insect sting–hypersensitive persons in the United States found yellow jackets to be incriminated most often, honeybees second, and wasps third.

LARGE LOCAL REACTION

A large local reaction is manifested clinically by an extended area of warmth, tenderness, edema, and erythema emanating from the sting site. For example, a sting on the hand may produce swelling of the hand and entire forearm. Large local reactions do not predispose to systemic reactions, even though the majority of subjects with a large local reaction have a positive skin test and/or in vitro test to hymenopteran extracts. They rarely become infected but are commonly treated as cellulitis in emergency departments and physicians' offices.

SYSTEMIC REACTIONS

Most systemic reactions (anaphylaxis) begin within the first 100 minutes after a sting, and usually within the first 2 to 30 minutes. Some reactions can occur hours after a sting. Generalized urticaria, pruritus, and erythema are the most common clinical manifestations. Angioedema of the lips, periorbital area, tongue, ears, and other cutaneous organs; laryngioedema; asthma; abdominal cramps and diarrhea; or hypotension secondary to vascular collapse (anaphylactic shock) can also occur. Such reactions in their most severe form cause death. It is often possible to identify a specific stinging hymenopteran insect by its nesting characteristics, e.g., wasps build open paper nests under the eaves of homes, in bushes, and in shrubbery around the homes; yellow jackets build their nests in concealed locations, either underground, in wall cavities, or in decaying logs or stumps; and hornets usually build their nests in trees or bushes or on buildings (some hornets build large paper nests and attach them to tree limbs). The honeybee is found throughout the United States in large hives, up to 65,000 per colony. Most honeybee colonies live within manufactured hives and are commercially managed for honey production and pollination. There are at least two species of stinging ants, *Solenopsis* (fire ants) and *Pogonomyrmex* species (harvester ants). *Solenopsis* stings leave a characteristic pustule, which begins as a clear vesicle but becomes cloudy in 24 hours. The pustules are usually umbilicated, surrounded by a large erythematous, slightly painful area. If undisturbed, the pustule remains for 3 to 10 days before rupturing or resolving with subsequent crust formation. Pigmented macules, residual fibrotic nodules, or small scars may form at the site. *Pogonomyrmex* species also sting, and the result is a wheal and flare reaction similar to that from a bee sting.

Sustained anaphylactic reactions may persist for 24 hours or more in spite of appropriate therapy. Rarely, delayed reactions, commonly involving the central nervous system, develop 24 to 96 hours after the sting and may not be associated with a preceding immediate-type reaction. Encephalitis and other neurologic manifestations may rarely occur. Other infrequent and late reactions include serum sickness (mediated by IgE), vasculitis, acute glomerulonephritis with renal failure, and nephrotic syndrome; the exact cause of all of these remains obscure, but they appear to be mediated by immunologic and toxic responses to venom proteins. Localized infections and septicemia can also occur, especially after imported fire ant stings.

Fatalities after insect sting reactions most commonly result from upper and lower airway obstruction, acute vascular collapse, and vascular or hemorrhagic reactions. Deaths most often occur within 1 hour and are more common in older persons, particularly in the presence of underlying disease, such as coronary artery disease or generalized atherosclerosis. Occasional deaths have been reported several days after the sting, associated with sustained or delayed systemic reactions.

DIAGNOSIS

Hymenoptera venoms are used to diagnose and treat bee, wasp, yellow jacket, and hornet allergy, and whole-body extracts to diagnose and treat ant allergy. Ant venoms are not available, and experimental evidence indicates that most of the commercially available whole-body extracts contain the antigens that cause this hypersensitivity state. Skin testing is the most sensitive method of diagnosis, although in vitro techniques (radioallergosorbent test [RAST]) are also reliable methods for determining clinical sensitivity.

TREATMENT

Large Local Reactions

Application of ice packs may be beneficial. Topical steroids are used extensively in clinical practice, but there is little convincing scientific evidence that they are helpful. Antihistamines and analgesics are useful for relieving the pruritus and painful swelling. Systemic corticoids may also be of benefit for large painful reactions. Most local reactions resolve over a few days or a week and do not require treatment, but the sting sites should be kept clean—this is especially true for the imported fire ant sting site—and, if necessary, covered to reduce the chance of secondary infection.

Generalized Systemic Anaphylactic Reactions

Pharmacotherapy

Treatment is the same for any anaphylactic reaction, regardless of cause, epinephrine being the drug of choice (Table 1). Aqueous epinephrine 1:1000, 0.3 to 0.5 mL, subcutaneously or intramuscularly, should be administered immediately (0.01 mL per kg in children, not to exceed 0.3 mL). Epinephrine 1:1000, 0.1 to 0.3 mL, may also be injected directly into the sting site, to delay absorption of venom. Repeated doses for protracted symptoms should be given as necessary or every 15 to 20 minutes. All subjects, but especially those with a history of cardiac disease, should be carefully monitored. Intravenous epinephrine, 1:100,000, given slowly, is indicated for anaphylactic shock not responding to therapy. Parenteral (intravenous or intramuscular) antihistamines, such as diphenhydramine hydrochloride (Benadryl, 5 mg per kg per 24 hours), in divided doses (50 mg, maximal dose 300 mg per 24 hours in children and 400 mg per 24 hours in adults), should be used for persistent urticaria, angioedema, or laryngeal edema in patients who are not responding to epinephrine.

Asthma should be treated with continuous inhalational beta agonists or, when necessary, intravenous

---

TABLE 1. **Treatment of Anaphylaxis**

1. Immediate measures
    a. Give aqueous epinephrine 1:1000, 0.3–0.5 mL (0.01 mL/kg in children, not to exceed 0.3 mL) SC or IM. Repeat as necessary every 15–20 min (twice) to maintain normal blood pressure and control symptoms.
    b. Mix aqueous epinephrine 1:1000, 0.1–0.3 mL in 10 mL of normal saline (1:100,000), give IV over several minutes, and repeat as necessary for anaphylactic shock not responding to therapy. A 1:10,000 dilution may be necessary for IV use.
2. General measures
    a. Place patient in recumbent position. Elevate lower extremities or use the Trendelenburg position.
    b. Establish and maintain an airway (endotracheal tube or cricothyrotomy may be required).
    c. Give oxygen.
    d. Start an IV line with normal saline for fluid replacement and as a route for additional medication. If severe hypotension exists, rapid infusion of volume expanders is necessary (colloid-containing solutions or saline).
    e. Place a venous tourniquet above the reaction site (insect sting or injection) to decrease the systemic absorption of antigen.
3. Specific measures
    a. Aqueous epinephrine 1:1000, 0.1–0.3 mL, at the site of antigen injection will delay absorption of antigen.
    b. Give diphenhydramine hydrochloride (Benadryl, IM or IV, 5 mg/kg/24 h) in divided doses (50 mg) to a maximal dose of 300 mg/24 h in children and 400 mg/24 h in adults.
    c. For asthma, give a beta agonist, albuterol (Ventolin or Proventil), or metaproterenol (Metaprel), 1.25–2.5 mg (0.25–0.5 mL of 5% solution) in 3 mL of saline by in-line nebulized therapy. Repeat as often as necessary.
    d. Aminophylline, 6 mg/kg administered over 20 min IV, followed by a continuous infusion, can be given if the patient still has bronchoconstriction and is not responding to inhaled albuterol.
    Note: Make appropriate adjustments in dosage based on age and other medications being taken, or if the patient is currently using a theophylline preparation.
    e. If hypotension persists, dopamine, 400 mg in 500 mL of D5W, should be given IV at an appropriate rate to maintain normal blood pressure.
    f. Cimetidine (Tagamet), 300 mg, or ranitidine (Zantac), 150 mg IV administered over 5 min, may also be useful.
    g. Glucagon,* 2–5 U given IV over 2 min, may be useful when a beta blocker is complicating anaphylaxis.
    h. A glucocorticosteroid, e.g., methylprednisolone 1–2 mg/kg for 24 h, is usually not helpful in acute anaphylaxis but may be useful in delayed-onset or protracted anaphylaxis.

---

*Not FDA approved for this indication.

aminophylline (6.0 mg per kg) administered over 20 minutes. Intravenous fluid replacement, e.g., saline or colloid-containing solutions, is necessary for persistent hypotension. Pressor agents should be administered if shock persists, and systemic glucocorticosteroids, if given early, may be useful for reversing a protracted anaphylaxis or preventing delayed anaphylaxis. Oxygen therapy and airway patency are essential, and intubation or cricothyrotomy is indicated for severe upper airway edema not responding to therapy. H_2 blockers such as intravenous cimetidine (Tagamet) or ranitidine (Zantac) may be useful for hypotension refractory to usual therapy. Beta blockers potentiate the severity of the anaphylaxis. Glucagon, 2 to 5 units given intravenously over 2 minutes, may be useful when these drugs complicate treatment.

Immunotherapy

Venom immunotherapy for patients who have had systemic reactions may reduce their risk of sting anaphylaxis from 40 to 60% to less than 5%, and if anaphylaxis occurs during maintenance venom therapy, it is almost always less severe than that which occurred before this therapy (Table 2). Immunotherapy is currently not recommended for patients with severe large local reactions, although these are probably of allergic origin. Adult patients who have experienced immediate systemic reactions to the honeybee, yellow jacket, hornet, or wasp should have appropriate venom diagnostic skin tests. Each person should be considered individually as a possible candidate for venom immunotherapy. Physicians and allergist-immunologists trained to care for subjects with severe allergic disease usually treat those who have had any kind of systemic reaction, in particular, those who are most likely to be restung or have altered their lifestyle to avoid being stung. There is some evidence that in adults systemic reactions limited to the skin may not place the person at risk for a more severe systemic reaction or death. More data are needed, and thus these patients are usually treated.

Fatal reactions from stinging insects rarely occur in children and young adults. Most reactions in these age groups are mild (cutaneous symptoms only), and repeated stings result in no reaction or a mild reaction, despite positive skin tests. Venom immunotherapy is not indicated in these patients, although it is recommended for children and young adults with a history of a severe systemic reaction and positive skin or in vitro tests.

Increasing increments of venom or whole-body extracts for ant-induced anaphylaxis are administered in a series of weekly injections until the patient can tolerate a venom dose equivalent to one or more insect stings. Once the maintenance dose is reached and after 1 year of monthly injections, the interval can be increased to every 6 weeks. In most patients, various immunologic parameters are altered; among them are a decrease in venom-specific IgE and an increase in venom-specific IgG or blocking antibody. Treatment occasionally fails, particularly in yellow jacket–hypersensitive individuals and those who do not achieve adequate levels of venom-specific IgG antibodies. The maintenance venom dose for these individuals should be increased to 200 µg from the usual maintenance dose of 100 µg.

Venom immunotherapy can be discontinued when repeated skin tests become negative. Some investigators recommend discontinuance of venom immunotherapy after 5 years, regardless of skin test results, particularly in patients who have had mild to moderate systemic reactions, because the beneficial effects of venom immunotherapy appear to occur after a relatively short course of therapy. Sensitivity, even without treatment, is self-limited in up to 40% of individuals. The converse is true, that is, in individuals with a history of a serious systemic reaction (loss of consciousness and/or severe respiratory distress)

TABLE 2. **Selection of Patients for Venom Immunotherapy**

Sting Reaction	Skin Test and/or RAST	Venom Immunotherapy	Harvester or Fire Ant Whole-Body Extract
In child			
Systemic, non–life-threatening, immediate, generalized urticaria, angioedema, erythema, pruritus	+ or −	No	Yes*
Systemic, life-threatening, possibly cutaneous symptoms but also respiratory symptoms (laryngeal edema or bronchospasm) or cardiovascular symptoms (hypotension, shock)	+	Yes	Yes*
In adult			
Systemic, non–life-threatening or life-threatening	+	Yes	Yes*
	−†	No	No
In child or adult			
Large local (≥2 in in diameter, >24 h duration)	+ or −‡	No	No
Normal (<2 in in diameter, <24 h duration)	+ or −‡	No	No

*Only if the skin test or RAST is positive to ant whole-body extract.

†The patient should be skin retested, with reconstituted extract, in 4–6 wk. If still negative, RAST should be repeated to confirm the negative skin test. The opposite is true for a RAST-negative individual, in whom the skin test should confirm negative RAST results.

‡Patients with large local reactions should not be skin tested.

Modified from Graft DF: Venom immunotherapy: indications, selection of venom, techniques and efficacy. *In* Levine MI, Lockey RF (eds): Monograph on Insect Allergy, 3rd ed. Milwaukee, WI, American Academy of Allergy, Asthma and Immunology. Pittsburgh, Dave Lambert and Associates, 1995, p 97.

TABLE 3. **Measures for Prevention of Hymenoptera Stings and Bites**

What to Do	What Not to Do
Know the stinging insects	Do not use lotions, perfumes, and so forth, which attract insects
Know nesting and foraging behaviors	Do not wear wool, leather, or suede
Remove or destroy nearby nests and hives; have professionals do this	Do not provoke insects or disturb a nest or hive
Wear clean, white, smooth-finish clothes; cover the body as much as possible and practical	Do not go barefoot
Wear white socks and ankle-high shoes	
Keep outdoor living areas clean and free of food refuse and garbage	
Remember that insect repellents are useless for stinging insects	
For biting insects, midges, flies, and mosquitoes, use DEET*-containing repellents on clothes and skin, or apply Avon Skin-So-Soft	

*N,N-Diethyl-3-methylbenzamide. Most insect repellents contain this chemical. It is the only chemical repellent currently approved by the Food and Drug Administration.

From Buckingham RB, Levine MI: Protective measures against insect stings and bites. *In* Levine MI, Lockey RF (eds): Monograph on Insect Allergy, 3rd ed. Milwaukee, WI, American Academy of Allergy, Asthma and Immunology. Pittsburgh, Dave Lambert and Associates, 1995, p 97.

and in whom skin tests remain positive, therapy should be continued for a more prolonged period.

Although venoms have replaced whole-body extract for most Hymenoptera, whole-body extracts are still used for imported fire ant and harvester ant immunotherapy. Patients with systemic reactions to ant stings should be tested with serial dilutions of whole-body extract and started with immunotherapy at a dilution of extract to which they did not react. The dose should be increased to the highest tolerated dose or to 0.5 mL of 1:10 solution, weight to volume. When maintenance therapy is reached, the interval between injections can gradually, over several months, be increased to 6 weeks. Although there is experimental evidence to support the use of whole-body extracts for ant hypersensitivity, "blinded" studies have not been done.

Immunotherapy is not without risk, because patients given this therapy are quite sensitive. Systemic reactions have been reported from such immunotherapy. Therefore, the Hymenoptera extracts should be used only by physicians experienced in immunotherapy or under the guidance of an allergist-immunologist, and only where adequate means for treating systemic reactions are available. Patients should be informed of possible risk and closely observed for at least 20 minutes after each injection.

Patients who have a history of insect hypersensitivity should carry an emergency insect sting kit containing aqueous epinephrine in a prefilled syringe, at least until they reach maintenance doses of immunotherapy. Several are available in the United States, including the EpiPen, Epi E.Z Pen, and Ana-Kit. The two commercially available EpiPens and two Epi E.Z Pens are syringes activated by a pressure mechanism that automatically injects epinephrine, 0.15 or 0.3 mL (0.15 or 0.3 mg); the Ana-Kit includes a self-injecting syringe that contains two 0.3 mL (0.3 mg) doses of epinephrine. Epinephrine, 1.6 to 4.8 mg (10 to 30 inhalations of Medihaler-Epi), can also be used and rapidly achieves plasma levels equal or superior to those of injectable epinephrine. It has the added advantage of being more effective in reversing bronchospasm but could be more difficult to use correctly by the patient in an emergency situation. A Medic Alert bracelet or medallion (Medic Alert Foundation International, 2323 Colorado Avenue, Turlock, CA 95382) should be worn by persons who may be exposed to stings and have had insect-induced anaphylaxis. They should also be instructed on how to avoid being stung (Table 3). Scented hair oils, perfumes, and dark and floral-patterned clothing should be avoided. Patients should wear shoes and avoid insect-populated areas.

Diseases of the Skin

ACNE VULGARIS AND ROSACEA

method of
GUY F. WEBSTER, M.D., PH.D.
Jefferson Medical College
Philadelphia, Pennsylvania

ACNE VULGARIS

Acne vulgaris is a common and variable disease that afflicts nearly all adolescents and adults at some time in their lives. Although not medically dangerous, the cutaneous scars, as well as the emotional ones, can last a lifetime. Studies exist documenting numerous psychologic problems stemming from acne, even to the point of causing decreased employability in adulthood. Fortunately, acne is eminently treatable.

Pathogenesis

A sensible approach to therapy cannot exist without some understanding of the disease's pathogenesis. Acne is truly multifactorial, involving abnormal keratinization, hormonal function, and immune hypersensitivity, and each defect provides a potential target for therapy.

Acne is limited to the pilosebaceous follicles of the head and upper trunk. The primary lesion is the comedo, an impaction and distention of the follicle with improperly desquamated keratinocytes and sebum. The stimulus for comedogenesis is unknown. At puberty, when androgens stimulate sebum production, comedones become engorged and enlarge to the point of visibility. Subsequently, some individuals begin to show signs of inflammation as well. Inflammatory acne is the result of the host response to the follicular inhabitant *Propionibacterium acnes,* which is a member of the normal flora and is a harmless commensal, largely incapable of tissue invasion. The level of anti–*P. acnes* immunity is proportional to the severity of acne inflammation and appears to be causal. The response has many characteristics of hypersensitivity, rather than a necessary immune defense against a pathogen.

Treatment

The first step in the treatment of any disease is to determine the severity of the problem. In diseases such as diabetes and hypertension, severity can be measured and response to treatment followed with quantifiable markers. This is only partially the case in acne. Severity is often overestimated by the patient and minimized by the doctor. Teenagers in particular are stigmatized by fairly trivial acne: in their eyes, severe acne can mean ruination. Thus, simple pimple counts are only partially useful; it is of little benefit to clear 95 of 100 lesions if the patient is left with several large nodules. Grading schemes that rely solely on lesion counts are of greater use in clinical studies than in clinical practice. I prefer to focus on the most severe lesions present, because adequate treatment for them covers all lesser pimples. For the purposes of clinical practice, acne classification can be condensed to just a few categories: purely comedonal (i.e., noninflammatory acne), mild pustular, scarring papular, and nodular.

Patients (and their parents) usually need to have a few common misconceptions dealt with before treatment begins. The misconceptions share the feature of blaming the patient for the disease and are to be avoided. Above all, patients (and parents) need to realize that cleanliness has nothing to do with acne. The black tip of a comedo is oxidized sebum, not dirt, and cannot be removed by scrubbing. Vigorous washing may actually make things worse! Second, parental admonitions notwithstanding, diet has never been shown to affect acne. Finally, stress reduction does not play a big role in controlling the disease.

Comedonal Acne

Noninflammatory acne is the mildest form of disease but can be the hardest to treat. Comedones are usually firmly ensconced in the follicle and, untreated, cannot be expressed without some risk of scarring. Topical tretinoin (Retin-A) (retinoic acid) cream is the standard against which all other anticomedonal agents are compared. Applied once or twice daily, it inhibits comedo formation and clears even severe comedonal acne in a few months. The only significant drawback is the irritation that is common with the preparation. Typically, irritation is greatest after a few weeks, and it usually does not require intervention. If desired, a moisturizing lotion may be prescribed. Because their skin is inherently irritable, patients with atopic diseases may not tolerate topical tretinoin even with moisturization.

Two newer drugs are also useful for noninflammatory acne. Adapalene (Differin) is a naphthoic acid derivative that binds to nuclear retinoid receptors. It is effective for comedonal acne and also has a measure of anti-inflammatory activity. It appears to be equivalent to topical tretinoin, but with somewhat less irritation. Azelaic acid (Azelex) is a dicarboxylic acid that has both antibacterial and comedolytic effects. Topical application is effective in reducing comedones, and it is the least irritating of the preparations. The side effect of hypopigmentation may be desirable in some patients.

Inflammatory Acne

TOPICAL THERAPY

Mild papulopustular acne rarely results in scarring and typically is responsive to aggressive twice-daily topical therapy. Usually, two drugs are prescribed, an antibacterial and a comedolytic (discussed in the preceding paragraph). Benzoyl peroxide at 2.5, 4, 5, 8, or 10% is an extraordinarily effective anti–P. acnes drug. Its major disadvantage is irritation, which can be minimized by using lower concentrations in a cream vehicle. Topical erythromycin and clindamycin (Cleocin T) are available as alcoholic solutions, lotions, creams, and gels, all of which are about equally effective. Acne that does not respond to erythromycin is usually also resistant to clindamycin. A combination of erythromycin and benzoyl peroxide in gel form is often found to be superior to topical antibiotic alone. Azelaic acid 20% cream is also an effective alternative to topical macrolide preparations.

During the past 2 decades, several reports have documented the acquisition of antibiotic resistance by P. acnes during acne therapy, most commonly with topical clindamycin and erythromycin. Extracutaneous infections with resistant organisms resulting from acne therapy have not been reported. Relatively resistant P. acnes strains are more commonly seen in acne that is refractory to therapy, but not always. When resistance is suspected, culture and susceptibility testing is not needed, because therapeutic failure in acne should automatically prompt a change in medication. The addition of benzoyl peroxide to the topical regimen is the easiest way to eliminate resistant organisms.

ORAL THERAPY

Acne that is resistant to topical treatment or that manifests as scarring or nodular lesions typically requires oral antibiotics to improve. Many of the antibiotics useful in acne also have an anti-inflammatory activity in the disease, which is nearly as important as the anti–P. acnes effect. Many physicians prefer to begin using tetracycline or erythromycin at 1 gram per day in divided dosage. I find this drug to be often insufficient and usually begin with doxycycline (Vibramycin) or minocycline (Minocin) at 100 to 200 mg per day. Most patients are significantly improved after 4 to 6 weeks. Patients are instructed to take the medication with food, a maneuver that minimizes stomach complaints and maximizes compliance at the cost of a slight decrease in absorption. Patients should be warned that they may sunburn more easily. Oral antibiotic therapy may be continued for months or years with little concern, given the decades-long track record of these drugs in acne.

If, for some reason, minocycline or doxycycline cannot be used, reasonable alternatives include trimethoprim-sulfamethoxazole (Bactrim, Septra), clarithromycin (Biaxin), azithromycin (Zithromax), and ciprofloxacin (Cipro). In general, cephalosporins and penicillins are not very effective in acne therapy. The increased cost of some of these newer drugs may make using isotretinoin (Accutane) an attractive option if long-term treatment is needed.

Because all acne begins with follicular impaction, it is appropriate to add a topical comedolytic such as tretinoin, azelaic acid, or adapalene to oral antibiotics, and most patients greatly benefit from it. Even with combination therapy, the physician should expect at least 4 to 6 weeks to pass before seeing maximal improvement.

Isotretinoin. Isotretinoin revolutionized the therapy of severe acne about 20 years ago. For the first time, a short course of medication was able to control severe acne and change the course of disease even after the drug was discontinued. Isotretinoin is a synthetic retinoid that inhibits sebaceous gland differentiation, corrects the keratinization defect in the follicle, and also has a measure of anti-inflammatory activity. Its major indication is severe nodular acne, but it is commonly used for significant acne that is resistant to oral antibiotics as well.

Side effects of isotretinoin are mostly dose related and are not always trivial. Most patients complain of dry skin, lips, and eyes. In dry seasons, it is common to see epistaxis and flares of atopic dermatitis due to the drug. About one third of patients show an elevation in triglyceride levels during the first month of therapy. Usually, dietary modification or dosage reduction keeps the triglyceride level from rising too high. Thinning of hair occurs infrequently but can be particularly distressing. Hair usually regrows after the drug is discontinued. Patients with severely inflamed lesions may have a severe flare of disease accompanied by systemic complaints similar to those seen in serum sickness. Administration of prednisone, 20 to 40 mg per day, at the initiation of isotretinoin therapy is sensible in selected severe cases. Rarely, patients complain of myalgias while taking isotretinoin and show significant elevations of creatinine kinase and transaminase levels. Because creatinine kinase measurement is rarely ordered, hepatitis is often incorrectly diagnosed. Restriction of exercise and reduction of dosage usually correct the problem. Depression is another rare, but documented, adverse effect of isotretinoin. Dosage reduction or discontinuation usually is required.

Isotretinion is listed as a drug capable of causing pseudotumor cerebri, although tenuously, because most patients with pseudotumor related to isotretinoin use were also treated concurrently with a tetracycline, a well-established cause of the problem. It is therefore contraindicated to co-administer the two medications. Patients with a history of pseudotumor from another medication have safely taken isotretinoin without recurrence of disease.

The most feared side effect of isotretinoin is its

teratogenicity. A majority of fetuses developing during isotretinoin therapy are severely malformed. Two means of birth control are required for all fertile women taking the drug and should be continued for one or two menstrual periods after therapy is stopped. It is now clear that after a course of isotretinoin, fertility and development are normal. There are no known deleterious effects on the fertility of male patients.

Some laboratory monitoring is required during treatment. A lipid panel, Sequential Multiple Analyzer (SMA 12/60), complete blood count, and pregnancy test are sufficient pretreatment tests. At 1 month, tests are repeated, and if the results are normal, only the pregnancy test need be repeated each month. The correct dosage of isotretinoin is a matter of some controversy, and clearly, there is a point at which greater efficacy is outweighed by increased side effects. I prefer to use 0.75 to 1 mg per kg per day. Lower dosages often require longer than the standard 4 or 5 months of treatment and have a higher long-term failure rate.

Hormonal Therapy. It is clear that virilized women have a higher incidence of acne, but it is mistaken to assume that any woman with acne has a hormonal derangement. In fact, the majority of hyperandrogenic women do not have significant acne. Treatment-resistant acne, especially in a woman with irregular menses, should be investigated with at least measurements of total and free testosterone as well as dehydroepiandrosterone sulfate. If these substances are elevated, two approaches may be taken, suppression with either low-dose oral corticosteroid or oral contraceptives. Currently, Triphasil is the only contraceptive approved for acne therapy.

Acne and Pregnancy

No drugs can be unequivocally guaranteed to be safe in pregnancy, but several have come into general use in this situation. Erythromycin, topical or oral, is usually held to be safe, although it is often poorly tolerated in patients whose lower esophageal sphincter is already relaxed. Benzoyl peroxide rapidly decomposes into benzoic acid and hydrogen peroxide and is probably safe for use during pregnancy.

ROSACEA

Rosacea is largely limited to the fair-skinned, easily blushing patient. Early disease may simply be a more persistent blush on the cheeks or a fixed telangiectasia. Inflammatory papules that resemble acne, but lack a comedo, arise in some and often become granulomatous. Sebaceous hyperplasia is common and reaches its zenith on the nose, where a nobby, swollen overgrowth known as rhinophyma may develop. (The actor W. C. Fields was such a case.) About 50% of rosacea patients have significant ocular involvement, which may range from mild conjunctivitis to styes, hordeola, and even corneal damage.

Diet clearly plays a role in rosacea, but food never gave anyone the disease. Anything that increases blood flow to the face makes rosacea worse. Spicy food, hot food, and alcohol are most commonly identified as triggers, but it is hard to document that abstinence will ultimately make a difference for the patient.

Rosacea may be treated topically using metronidazole (MetroGel). Available as a cream or gel, this preparation helps in mild to moderate inflammatory disease. The physician should allow about 6 weeks of therapy before switching to a stronger drug.

Topical steroids are often used to treat rosacea, a practice that should be discouraged. Although initially responsive to weak compounds, the rosacea quickly exhibits tachyphylaxis, requiring stronger and stronger preparations that both damage facial skin and eventually potentiate the rosacea.

Oral antibiotics are often the best therapy for severe rosacea and are most effective in ocular rosacea. Tetracyclines work best, but erythromycin may occasionally be useful. I generally prescribe doxycycline 100 mg twice daily for 1 or 2 months, and then taper the dosage to daily or alternate-day dosing. Because the drug probably acts more as an anti-inflammatory than an antibiotic, these low dosages are not as homeopathic as they might seem.

HAIR DISORDERS

method of
WILMA F. BERGFELD, M.D.
Cleveland Clinic Foundation
Cleveland, Ohio

The diagnosis of hair disorders is complex and necessitates an evaluation of the clinical presentation, history, physical examination, and appropriate laboratory tests. The patient with hair loss commonly presents with several different complaints that are helpful in the diagnosis. Such complaints as "My hair is falling out by the roots," "My hair does not seem to grow," "The texture of my hair has changed," "My hair breaks off," and "My scalp hair is thinning" reflect several disorders (Table 1):

Alterations of hair growth cycles
Failure to regenerate hair
Decreased rate of growth
Fragile hair
Inflammatory skin disease
Permanent alopecia
Cutaneous neoplasms (see Table 1)

Understanding normal hair growth patterns is essential for correct interpretation of the hair loss events. Important facts are as follows: scalp hair grows in an asynchronous pattern, with approximately 80% of hair follicles in an anagen phase (active) and 10 to 20% in a telogen phase (resting). Any alteration of hair growth cycling manifests clinically as increased shedding of scalp hair, representing either a telogen or a dystrophic anagen hair fiber. Other variations are induced by age, sex, and season (Table 2).

Diagnostic office techniques include visual examination of all the hair-bearing skin sites as well as of the nails.

TABLE 1. **Classification of Alopecia**

Nonscarring

Alterations in hair growth cycles
Telogen effluvium
   Androgenic alopecia
Anagen effluvium
   Alopecia areata
   Drugs
Alterations in hair shaft (trichodystrophies)
   Inherited
   Acquired
      Trichorrhexis nodosa
      Trichotillomania

Scarring or Inflammatory

Lupus erythematosus
Lichen planus
Scleroderma
Infectious

The specific techniques are hair pulls, hair clipping, hair plucks, light microscopy examination of hair fibers and scalp scales, bacterial and fungal cultures, and biopsies (Table 3).

ALTERATIONS OF THE HAIR GROWTH CYCLE

The complaint "My hair is coming out by the roots" represents an alteration in the cyclic growth pattern of scalp hair and may manifest as a telogen or anagen shed. The mechanism appears to reside in the severity of insult to the growing germinal center of the anagen hair follicle. A severe insult, interrupting keratinization and changing of the anagen hair follicle to a resting or dying hair follicle, produces a telogen follicle. This results in a telogen shed and reduced hair diameter.

Telogen Shed (Effluvium)

Normally, telogen (resting) follicles represent approximately 20% of the total volume of scalp hair. Any premature interruption of the anagen phase induces more telogen hair follicles. Ultimately, this results in increased shedding of excessive telogen hair. This change is experienced 6 weeks to 4 months after the initial cause. The diagnosis of telogen effluvium can be made by excessive hair loss, telogen hair as demonstrated with hair pull, hair clipping, hair pluck

TABLE 2. **Normal Scalp Hair Growth Patterns**

Average total number of scalp hairs is 100,000 hairs.
Fastest growth is between 15 and 30 y.
Slow growth occurs in the elderly.
Average rate of growth is 0.35 mm/d.
Hair grows faster in summer than in winter.
Active growth period is 2–5 y before replacement.
Average daily loss is 25–100 hairs/d.
Female hair grows faster than male hair.
Fiber diameters and shapes vary in different races
   and nationalities.

TABLE 3. **Examinations for Hair Disorders**

Pattern of hair loss
Length and diameter of hair fiber
Hair pull, clipping, pluck
Light microscopy examination of hair
Scalp skin condition
Scrapings of scales and hair for potassium hydroxide
   testing and culture
Biopsy

with light microscopy examination of the hair fiber, and a biopsy.

The etiology of telogen effluvium is generally elucidated by history, with special concentration on events that have preceded the shed by 6 weeks to 4 months.

In general, simple cases of telogen effluvium are self-limited, and no treatment is necessary. However, chronic or persistent telogen shed heralds androgen alopecia or other metabolic or disease states. In addition, severe weight reduction diet and certain drugs are also causative agents (Table 4). If telogen shedding persists, a more intense medical evaluation is needed.

Anagen Shed (Effluvium)

The anagen shedding is the result of a major insult to the growth center, general bulb, of the growing anagen hair follicle. The arrest of keratinization produces a progressively narrowing hair shaft that is fragile and fractures easily on its exit from the scalp's skin. This type of shedding generally occurs 1 to 2 weeks after the insult. Typical causes are chemotherapeutic agents, antimetabolites, alkylating agents, and cytotoxic agents (Table 5).

ALOPECIA AREATA, AN AUTOIMMUNE DISEASE

Alopecia areata is considered an autoimmune disease that affects 1 to 2% of the population. It commonly manifests as an oval patch, singular or multiple, and with occasional confluent patches. It is an inflammatory, nonscarring alopecia. Twenty percent of cases of alopecia areata proceed to alopecia totalis, affecting the whole scalp, and 1% to alopecia universalis, or total body hair loss. Alopecia areata is asso-

TABLE 4. **Causes of Telogen Effluvium**

Childbirth (post partum)
Androgenic alopecia
Febrile illness (postfebrile)
Surgical shock, anesthesia
Drugs
Alopecia areata
Endocrinopathies
Nutritional and metabolic deficiencies
Chronic infection
Collagen-vascular disease
Chronic disease
Hereditary, androgenic alopecia

TABLE 5. **Causes of Anagen Effluvium**

Anticoagulants	Alkylating agents
Antimetabolites	Alopecia areata
Cytotoxic agents	

ciated with atopy, Hashimoto's thyroiditis, and other autoimmune diseases. Minor nail dystrophies are common. The primary diagnosis is based on the hair pull and light microscopy examination of hair fibers that identify dystrophic anagen hair fibers, and biopsy of involved areas.

Treatment depends on the extent of the disease and age of the patient. For mild to moderate patchy disease, topical corticosteroids are the preferred treatment. For more extensive or recalcitrant disease, triamcinolone acetonide (Kenalog suspension, 10 mg per mL) can be injected into the involved sites with a 30-gauge needle, delivering tiny injections of 0.1 mL to each small site. The total amount should not exceed 10 to 15 mg of triamcinolone per visit every 6 to 8 weeks.

Other options for marked to severe disease are topical minoxidil (Rogaine), anthralen (Drithocreme), and topical contact sensitizers such as diphenylcyclopropenone (DPCP). The expected result of sensitization therapy is approximately 40% cosmetically acceptable regrowth of hair. DPCP is difficult to obtain in the United States, being more readily available in Europe and Canada. Other treatment options include psoralen (methoxsalen [Oxsoralen]) plus ultraviolet A radiation (PUVA) and systemic corticosteroids. The use of systemic corticosteroids is controversial because of the prolonged duration of therapy and the potential side effects, i.e., cataracts, osteopenia, osteoporosis, and growth retardation.

Patients with alopecia areata need a source of disease-specific information and support therapy, such as the National Alopecia Areata Foundation (710 Sea Street, No. 11, San Rafael, CA 94901-3853).

ANDROGENIC ALOPECIA

Androgenic alopecia, an autosomal dominant disorder, is the most common alopecia in humans, with a prevalence of 23 to 87%. In both sexes, it presents with a central scalp alopecia and is associated with clinical signs of sexual development (puberty) and androgen excess. Central alopecia is more severe in males than females, manifesting as several distinct areas of partial or complete alopecia. In the female, there is a more diffuse thinning rather than complete baldness. Androgenic alopecia can be heralded by a chronic telogen effluvium and failure to regenerate terminal hair.

Female androgenic alopecia often appears in women with strong family histories of baldness or a personal history of hirsutism, acne, abnormal menses, or other signs of androgen excess. Sudden onset of the signs of androgen excess should prompt the search for a neoplasm. Genetically predisposed women may present with androgenic alopecia in youth (puberty) or in perimenopausal or postmenopausal times. Young women have a higher incidence of acquired adrenal hyperplasia, polycystic ovaries, or both. In general, menopausal women have lower levels of hormones, especially estrogen and testosterone. Androgen excess screening should include measurements of total testosterone and dehydroepiandrosterone sulfate as well as other laboratory tests, such as a complete blood count, Sequential Multiple Analyzer (SMA 12/60), ferritin measurement, thyroid screening, and antinuclear factor measurement (Table 6).

In men, the treatment of androgenic alopecia consists of creative hairstyles, hair pieces, hair transplantation, and scalp reduction. Medical therapies include topical minoxidil twice a day and selected antiandrogens. Finasteride (Proscar)* has been studied and appears to be a therapeutic option.

Women have similar treatment options, but in addition to antiandrogens, estrogen replacement therapy can be used. These agents include estrogen-dominant oral contraceptives (Demulen 1/50)* or conjugated estrogen (Premarin),* 0.625 mg, given daily or in conjunction with a progesterone such as medroxyprogesterone (Provera).* The Provera dose may range from 2.5 to 10 mg, depending on the dosing schedule. Spironolactone (Aldactone)* in doses of 50 to 200 mg has been used as an antiandrogen successfully. If adrenal suppression is needed for androgen excess, dexamethasone,* in doses of 0.125 to 0.25 mg at bedtime, may be used for 4 months or longer.

HAIR SHAFT ABNORMALITIES

Hair shaft abnormalities (trichodystrophies) may be inherited or acquired. Inherited abnormalities may indicate a systemic disorder and may be associated with mental retardation, short stature, hypogonadism, and other metabolic disorders. Examples of trichodystrophy are pili torti (corkscrew hairs), Menkes' (kinky-hair) syndrome, trichorrhexis nodosa in argininosuccinicaciduria, trichoschisis (transverse fractures to the hair), and trichothiodystrophy (sulfur-depleted hair).

Acquired physical and chemical damage to the hair

---

*This is not listed in the manufacturer's product information and is not FDA approved.

TABLE 6. **Screening Tests for Women with Probable Androgenic Alopecia**

Complete blood count
Sequential Multiple Analyzer (SMA 12/60)
Ferritin
Thyroid screen (thyroxine, thyroid-stimulating hormone, microsomal antibody)
Antinuclear antibody
Androgen excess screen (dehydroepiandrosterone sulfate, total testosterone)

may be caused by sunlight, hair care techniques, and chemical processes. Bleaching, "perming," straightening, coloring, and curling may result in fragile hair that is easily broken with normal handling. Usually, this entity manifests as a complaint of failure to grow and is associated with short hair and normal scalp hair density. Treatment consists of gentle handling and normal shampooing with the use of conditioners or volumizers. If the cause is not repeated, the hair normally regrows within 1 year.

Trichorrhexis Nodosa

Trichorrhexis nodosa is the most common trichodystrophy that can be either inherited or acquired. The inherited form can be associated with aminoaciduria. The more common acquired form is the result of physical and chemical trauma. The history includes the use of straighteners, hot combing, permanent waves, and coloring procedures. Characteristically, the hair breaks off suddenly and becomes strikingly short in the affected areas. Diagnosis is made by hair clipping and microscopic identification of nodes or fractured nodes ("broomstick deformity"). Treatment consists of discontinuation of hair care procedures except for normal shampooing and the use of conditioners or volumizers.

Traction Alopecia

Hair loss caused by traction results from physical damage to the hair shaft, alterations in the growth cycle, and scalp inflammation. Diagnosis is made by hair pluck, hair clipping, and scalp biopsy. Dystrophic anagen, multiple-catagen hair follicles, and a variety of traumatic changes to the hair can be noted.

If traction is repetitive and long-term, scarring, permanent alopecia may result. Practices such as tight braiding, wearing a ponytail, using elastic hair bands, and rollers, and extremely repetitive teasing of the hair are responsible for most cases and should be discontinued.

Trichotillomania

Trichotillomania is a traction alopecia related to an underlying psychologic, compulsive disorder. It is commonly seen in young and old women. In general, the condition is produced by repetitively pulling, tugging, plucking, or clipping. The hair loss manifests in a bizarre pattern. Individuals presenting with incomplete hair loss and a short stubble of hair on the scalp, eyebrows, lashes, or other hairy areas should be suspected of having trichotillomania. Light microscopy examination of clipped hair demonstrates fractures of the terminal ends. Scalp biopsy is often diagnostic. Therapy requires psychologic counseling. The use of anticonvulsants and antidepressants can be helpful. Such drugs include clomipramine (Anafranil), fluoxetine HCl (Prozac), and sertraline HCl (Zoloft).*

---

*Not FDA approved for this indication.

NONINFECTIOUS INFLAMMATORY SCALP DISORDERS

Noninfectious inflammatory scalp disorders are divided into scarring and nonscarring disorders. The causes of scarring alopecia include chronic lupus erythematosus, lichen planopilaris (lichen planus follicularis), and morphea (localized scleroderma). The most important nonscarring inflammatory alopecia is alopecia areata. The evaluation of all chronic patchy inflammatory and noninflammatory alopecias comprises potassium hydroxide testing, fungal cultures, scalp biopsy, and optional serologic testing, depending on history.

Lupus Erythematosus

Cutaneous lupus erythematosus may present with or without associated systemic disease. In the scalp, it manifests as erythematous, indurated alopecic patches or patchy noninflammatory alopecia similar to alopecia areata. The inflammatory type results in skin atrophy, hypopigmentation or hyperpigmentation, and permanent loss of hair. Diagnosis is made from clinical history, skin biopsy for light microscopy examination and direct immunofluorescence testing, and laboratory testing for lupus erythematosus, such as antinuclear antibody profile.

Therapy consists of the use of topical and intralesional corticosteroids. Potent topical corticosteroids such as fluocinonide (Lidex) may be applied at bedtime. Cutaneous atrophy and striae are the most common side effects, resulting from overuse of potent topical steroids. Intralesional triamcinolone acetonide (Kenalog), 2.5 to 10 mg per mL, may be injected every 6 to 8 weeks as needed. Side effects of intralesional triamcinolone have already been discussed. Topical corticosteroids and antimalarial agents may be helpful in refractory cases. On occasion, oral corticosteroids are given. Quiescent, "burnt-out" lesions are best treated with hair transplantation or scalp reduction.

Lichen Planopilaris

Lichen planopilaris represents a patchy inflammatory and scarring alopecia, often manifesting as follicular hyperkeratosis and erythema. It occurs primarily in adults and may be difficult to differentiate from cutaneous lupus erythematosus. Searching for associated skin lesions of lichen planus, skin biopsy for light microscopy, and immunofluorescence studies may differentiate the two disorders.

Treatment of lichen planopilaris involves the use of corticosteroids. Guidelines for the use of topical corticosteroids are essentially the same as those in chronic cutaneous lupus erythematosus. Individual lesions in lichen planopilaris are often quite small and widespread, so intralesional corticosteroids are often impractical. Oral corticosteroids (prednisone) are often effective. The initial dose of 1 mg per kg per day is tapered as signs of inflammation respond.

Oral corticosteroid therapy may be long-term, therefore requiring monitoring of side effects. Topical antiinflammatory agents, antiseborrheic shampoos, and keratolytic agents can be helpful. Chronic scarred, burnt-out areas are best treated with surgical intervention, such has hair transplantation or scalp reduction.

Morphea (Localized Scleroderma)

Morphea, or localized scleroderma, is a relatively uncommon scarring alopecia. The clinical and histologic features usually permit easy diagnosis; therefore, a biopsy is recommended. Treatment regimens are usually unsuccessful but include topical and intralesional corticosteroids as well as antimalarial agents. Quiescent, burnt-out lesions are best treated with hair transplantation or scalp reduction.

INFECTIOUS DISORDERS

Tinea Capitis

Tinea capitis may manifest as an intensely inflamed, boggy, alopecic patch or a patchy, noninflammatory alopecia accompanied by only mild scaling. Tinea capitis is common, especially in children, and a high index of suspicion must be maintained in all presentations of alopecia.

Tinea is caused by fungi of the genera *Trichophyton* and *Microsporum*. Diagnosis of fungal infections requires fungal culture or demonstration of the organism by means of a potassium hydroxide test. A helpful technique is to rub a moistened gauze pad over the affected scalp; in noninflammatory cases, vigorous rubbing gives a better yield. The short, broken fragments of hair that adhere to the gauze are ideal for potassium hydroxide examination.

The treatment of choice is oral griseofulvin (Gris-PEG). The dosage depends on the practical size of the oral preparation prescribed (ultra-microsize griseofulvin is better absorbed). To be absorbed, griseofulvin must be given with a fatty meal. For children, the dose can be mixed with ice cream. The only common side effect is headache, which generally resolves with a temporary reduction in dosage. Local cleansing with selenium sulfide lotion (Selsun) and application of topical antifungals in conjunction with oral griseofulvin may be helpful. Intensely inflamed lesions may require a short course of systemic corticosteroids, such as prednisone (1 mg per kg per day), in addition to griseofulvin. Secondary bacterial infection responds to oral antibiotic therapy. Newer oral antifungals, such as ketoconazole (Nizoral), itraconazole (Sporanox),* and terbinafine (Lamisil),* may be helpful.

Syphilis

The incidence of secondary syphilis has risen in the last several years, especially among youth. Secondary syphilis often manifests as papulosquamous lesions on the trunk, with or without similar lesions on the palms and soles. Hair loss associated with secondary syphilis may have a characteristic moth-eaten appearance or may mimic alopecia areata. Especially in urban areas, a high index of suspicion should be maintained. Diagnosis is best made with serologic testing for syphilis; however, darkfield examination of skin scrapings and skin biopsies can be helpful. Treatment of uncomplicated syphilis may be given according to current Centers for Disease Control and Prevention guidelines. Complicated cases are best treated in conjunction with a specialist in infectious disease.

NEOPLASTIC DISORDERS

A variety of benign and malignant tumors may interrupt hair growth or destroy hair follicles. The patient may have only an alopecic patch or may have a palpable tumor. The diagnosis rests on a skin biopsy. Common neoplasms of the scalp are epidermoid and pilar cysts, melanocytic nevi, organoid nevi, seborrheic keratosis, warts, basal cell carcinoma, and metastatic disease from the breast, lung, and kidney.

CANCER OF THE SKIN

method of
PHILIP L. BAILIN, M.D.
Cleveland Clinic Foundation
Cleveland, Ohio

Nonmelanoma skin cancer is the most common cancer affecting humankind. It is estimated that approximately 1 million new skin cancers will occur in the United States in 1998. There are two major types of nonmelanoma skin cancer, basal cell carcinoma (BCC), which accounts for approximately 80%, and squamous cell carcinoma (SCC), which accounts for 15% or more. The two types share a number of etiologic factors, the most prominent of which are genetic predisposition (light skin, eyes, hair color; inability to tan easily) and excessive long-term cumulative exposure to ultraviolet A or B radiation. Other etiologic factors are remote exposure to ionizing radiation, arsenical compounds, and coal tar derivatives and long-term immunosuppression. Burn scars and chronic ulcerations may develop foci of SCC, and infection with certain serotypes of human papillomavirus may predispose to SCC. BCCs have an extremely low metastatic potential (<0.01%) but may be locally aggressive. SCCs arising in sun-damaged skin have a low metastatic rate (<5%), whereas those arising in ulcerations or on mucous membranes may have a considerably higher metastatic potential.

Therapeutic options for these cutaneous malignancies are multiple and fortunately offer high cure rates for primary tumors in most cases. For primary BCC, the overall cure rate is approximately 95%, and for primary SCC, the cure rate is in the 80% range. Certain clinical or histologic features have been demonstrated to be associated with reduced cure rates. Among these are large size (>2 cm), location in the midfacial triangle or around the ears, infil-

---

*Not FDA approved for this indication.

trative histologic subtypes (e.g., morpheaform BCC), and recurrence after any of the standard recognized therapies. For this group of "high-risk" tumors, the cure rate drops to the 50 to 60% range with conventional therapy.

The first step of any therapeutic program for these tumors must be biopsy for histologic confirmation. Although an excisional biopsy may be performed, it is usually more prudent to initially obtain a tissue sample with a shave or punch biopsy. Either of these methods provides a specimen for diagnosis (and subtyping) but leaves the lesion to be treated subsequently by any one of several potential modalities, the appropriate choice of which depends on the specific lesion, the particular patient, and the physician's preferences and skills.

SURGICAL THERAPIES

Electrodesiccation and Curettage

Electrodesiccation and curettage rely on the relative difference in palpable texture between tumor tissue and normal dermis. The palpable or visible borders of the tumor are marked, and the area is infiltrated with local anesthetic. The lesion is then scraped with a surgical curet, which removes the softer gelatinous tumor tissue. When normal dermal tissue is encountered, it is palpably firmer and grittier, and often the surgeon can actually hear a rough scraping sound. The base is then lightly electrocoagulated. This sequence is normally repeated three times (each time with a successively smaller curet) to complete the procedure.

Because this technique offers no histologic margin control, it is best used for low-risk tumors. It should be avoided for infiltrating histologic types, midfacial lesions, or recurrent lesions. If the surgeon encounters subcutaneous adipose tissue as curettage is carried out, the procedure should be abandoned and another modality chosen, because the tactile difference between normal and malignant tissue is no longer valid.

Healing of the coagulated wound base proceeds by second intention during a period of several weeks. This technique frequently leaves a depigmented irregular scar, so cosmesis is often less than optimal.

Surgical Excision

Standard elliptical excision is a common therapeutic choice for BCC and SCC. Its main benefits are that it provides a complete specimen for pathologic examination (including traditional margin control) and that it results in a sutured wound that usually gives acceptable cosmetic results in any area. However, the surgeon must preoperatively decide on the surgical margin to be taken. This is a problem with poorly defined lesions or lesions that reside on irregular tissue planes. There is little tactile feedback as the surgeon cuts, so infiltrating lesions are likely to be incompletely removed. Also, if the lesion is large, a local flap or skin graft may be required for closure. If this type of closure is done and the pathology report subsequently identifies residual tumor, the reconstruction may have to be sacrificed.

Mohs' Micrographic Surgery

The technique of Mohs' micrographic surgery is based on the sequential excision of thin layers of tissue starting with the clinically evident tumor. Debulking of any gross tumor mass may be accomplished first with scalpel or curet. As the layer is removed, it is divided into pieces, each of which will fit onto a standard glass microscopic slide. The edges of each piece are color coded with dyes, and a map is drawn illustrating the orientation and location of the tissue specimen on the patient. The specimens are then processed in a specialized laboratory as horizontal frozen sections. This technique enables the complete base and peripheral margin of the excisional specimen to be examined microscopically. If any tumor is identified at the margins, the surgeon may return to the operative field to remove another layer from the specific area of involvement while sparing the areas that are tumor free. Thus, the technique provides total margin control with maximal tissue conservation.

Mohs' surgery is time and resource intensive. It is therefore reserved for high-risk skin cancers—which may be defined as recurrent tumors, tumors of the midfacial triangle or periauricular area, infiltrating histologic subtypes, lesions with clinically indistinct margins, and tumors more than 2.0 cm in diameter. Cure rates with Mohs' surgery approach 98% for primary BCC and 90% for primary SCC. For recurrent tumors (which have only a 50 to 60% cure rate with conventional methods), Mohs' surgery yields an 85 to 90% cure rate.

NONSURGICAL THERAPIES

Cryotherapy

Compared with surrounding normal tissues, nonmelanoma skin cancers are quite sensitive to cryogenic injury. Liquid nitrogen is a low-cost, readily available cryogen that can be conveniently stored in an office setting and easily delivered to the patient's skin in a highly controlled manner. Studies have confirmed that tumor cells are consistently damaged irreversibly and lethally when exposed to a double freeze-thaw cycle, in which the target tissue is twice frozen to a temperature of at least $-20°C$. Such a level of freezing can be monitored by special thermocouple electrodes placed in the skin beneath the tumor, or with clinical indicators, such as the progression of the ice front peripheral to the tumor or the fixation of the target skin to underlying structures such as cartilage or bone.

Cryotherapy causes local edema and necrosis that usually heal with a soft but hypopigmented scar. It is indicated in patients who are poor surgical candidates. It is not effective on the scalp (too vascular for adequate freezing) or on the lower extremities (commonly, delayed healing). No pathologic specimen results from the procedure, so the completeness of removal cannot be documented. Therefore, an ample margin must be clinically selected both peripherally and in depth.

Radiation Therapy

Although ionizing radiation is a well-recognized cause of skin cancer, it also remains a most effective therapeutic option in certain circumstances. Patients who are elderly, debilitated, or not surgical candidates for various reasons may be treated with either orthovoltage or electron beam. If the total dose (4500 to 6000 R) is fractionated over several weeks, the tumor may be adequately treated without the acute side effects commonly associated with radiation therapy. Late secondary changes in the skin (atrophy, telangiectasia, discoloration, malignant transformation) may still occur after 15 to 20 years, so most physicians do not utilize this modality in patients younger than 60 years.

Chemotherapy and Immunotherapy

Although topical chemotherapy with 5-fluorouracil (5-FU) is effective for premalignant lesions such as actinic keratosis and Bowen's disease, it is not reliable for the treatment of skin cancer. The agent does not penetrate deeply enough into the skin to ensure destruction of aggregates of cells within the dermis or along adnexal epithelium. There has been some enthusiasm regarding the efficacy of 5-FU intradermal implants, but these are still investigational.

Immunotherapy with intralesional interferon alfa* has been reported to be effective in small solid or nodular variants of basal cell carcinoma. It is given several times weekly for courses of varied lengths. This agent is associated with minor flulike side effects. However, it has been disappointing for larger tumors and tumors with an infiltrative pattern.

Laser Therapy

Carbon dioxide laser vaporization has been shown to be effective on superficial BCC and has been used with good results on SCC in situ. This modality is particularly recommended for patients who are taking anticoagulants or have pacemakers that are incompatible with electrocoagulation. Likewise, the carbon dioxide laser may be used as a form of scalpel to perform excisional or Mohs' surgery in such compromised patients.

Photodynamic therapy involves the administration of a potent photosensitizing agent either intravenously or topically over the area of the tumor. The malignant cells take up the chemical and retain it, but it is cleared from the normal tissue. After the clearance period, the tumor area is irradiated with high-intensity laser light, which activates the photosensitizer and causes tumor cell death. This therapy is still investigational for cutaneous malignancy but has been proved to be of great value for tumors

of indistinct margins and in patients who are not candidates for conventional therapy.

CUTANEOUS T CELL LYMPHOMA

method of
BIJAN SAFAI, M.D., D.Sc.
New York Medical College
Valhalla, New York

Cutaneous T cell lymphomas (CTCLs) are primarily lymphomas of the skin that encompass a heterogeneous group of skin disorders (Table 1). The T in these disorders is the T lymphocyte (T cell). They are, however, wildly disparate in clinical presentation, course of disease, and prognosis. The choices and indications for treatment and the response rates are quite different. The appropriate medical management and the choice of therapeutic modalities should, therefore, be based on the clinical presentation and the natural course of the disease in various subgroups. Practicing physicians are encouraged to utilize the clinical and laboratory findings to properly classify the disorder in a given patient and be able to choose the most appropriate and effective therapeutic modalities.

This brief article is intended to familiarize reader with basic information about this group of lymphomas and to provide a summary of the currently utilized therapeutic modalities.

CLINICAL PRESENTATION

Mycosis Fungoides. The classic form of CTCLs was initially described by Alibert in 1806 in a patient who had a desquamating eruption that evolved into "mushroom-like" tumors. Alibert chose the name mycosis fungoides to describe the condition. Mycosis fungoides manifests initially as erythematous scaly patches on the skin that later become more infiltrated and form raised plaques. In the late stages of the disease, large nodules and tumors appear that may break down and manifest with large ulcerated fungating masses. Secondary infections are quite common. In the tumor stage, the disease may manifest as involvement of lymph nodes or other internal organs. It is noteworthy that the patch stage of the disease may last for many years. With proper treatment, this stage may not progress to the plaque and tumor stage.

Parapsoriasis (Pre–Mycosis Fungoides). Before the patch stage of CTCL, some patients may present with a skin eruption that lacks the clinical and histologic criteria

TABLE 1. **Clinical Subtypes of Cutaneous T Cell Lymphoma**

Mycosis fungoides
Parapsoriasis en plaque
Tumor d'emblée
Exfoliative erythroderma
Poikiloderma atrophicans vasculare
Follicular mucinosis
Pagetoid reticulosis
Granulomatous mycosis fungoides
Sézary's syndrome
Adult T cell leukemia-lymphoma
Lymphomatoid papulosis

*Not FDA approved for this indication.

denoting mycosis fungoides. This stage is variably called parapsoriasis or pre–mycosis fungoides. The literature contains descriptions of patients with parapsoriasis or pre–mycosis fungoides who have lived 30 to 50 years without progressing to classic mycosis fungoides. A definitive diagnosis of mycosis fungoides in such cases is quite difficult.

Tumor D'emblée. Mycosis fungoides d'emblée was first described by Vidal and Brocq in 1885. It manifests as sudden (d'emblée) development of skin tumors without the patch and plaque stages. This form of the disease has a worse prognosis.

Exfoliative Erythroderma. Desquamation and generalized erythrodermas are the presenting manifestations in exfoliative erythroderma. Patients do not show the classic progressive stages from patch to plaque and to tumors. The prognosis of this type of T cell lymphoma is much better, and patients usually live long. The clinician should note the similarity in clinical presentation between this form and the more severe form of CTCL, Sézary's syndrome. The differential diagnosis of this subtype includes atopic dermatitis, psoriasis, contact dermatitis, and drug eruption.

Poikiloderma Atrophicans Vasculare. Although poikiloderma atrophicans vasculare is characterized by hypopigmentation, hyperpigmentation, telangiectasia, and atrophy, pruritus may also be a prominent symptom. Ulceration may occur on the dry, atrophic skin. Poikilodermatous skin lesions may be seen as part of the clinical presentation of other medical illnesses, such as dermatomyositis, lupus erythematosus, acrodermatitis chronica atrophicans, xeroderma pigmentosa, poikiloderma congenitale, dyskeratosis congenita, and arsenicum.

Follicular Mucinosis (Alopecia Mucinosa). Follicular mucinosis manifests as grouped follicular papules devoid of hair and with or without signs of inflammation. The disease may regress spontaneously but may be followed by remissions and exacerbations and subsequent development of plaques and tumors of mycosis fungoides.

Pagetoid Reticulosis (Woringer-Kolopp Disease). Pagetoid reticulosis manifests as solitary patches that resemble patch stage of mycosis fungoides both clinically and histologically. The course of the disease is, however, more chronic and indolent.

Granulomatous Mycosis Fungoides. The granulomatous form of mycosis fungoides is characterized by papular and nodular lesions resembling the tumor stage that resolve into a poikilodermatous presentation. This condition is associated with long survival.

Sézary's Syndrome. Initially described by Sézary and Bouvrain in 1838, this syndrome manifests with generalized erythroderma, enlarged lymph nodes, pruritus, thickening of the palms and soles with fissures, loss of hair, nail dystrophy, ectropion, edema of the skin, and infiltrated lesions on the face (leonine face). Presence of large abnormal mononuclear cells with cerebriform (folded) nuclei is one of the hallmarks of this condition; these cells are present in skin lesions of patients with Sézary's syndrome and mycosis fungoides and have proved to be of the helper T cell subset of lymphocytes. On the basis of the presence of these cells in the skin and peripheral blood, mycosis fungoides and Sézary's syndrome are considered to be part of a broader spectrum of CTCLs. Thus, it is believed that Sézary's syndrome is the leukemic form of mycosis fungoides. Patients with Sézary's syndrome have a shorter survival and a worse prognosis than those with other forms of CTCL.

Adult T Cell Leukemia-Lymphoma (ATL). This form of CTCL was first described in Japan in 1977. It has a different geographic distribution from that of mycosis fungoides; it is limited to clusters in southern Japan, the West Indies, and the southern part of the United States. The course of the disease is acute, with skin lesions appearing in patch, plaque, or tumor stages separately or one after the other and with rapid progression and shorter survival. Other features are circulating abnormal lymphocytes and hypercalcemia. The ATL cells are reported to be TAC-positive in most cases. In rare cases of ATL, the abnormal T cells in skin and peripheral blood have been reported to be of the suppressor T subset rather than the helper T subset, that are usually seen in mycosis fungoides and Sézary's syndrome. It has been demonstrated that ATL is one of the clinical manifestations of infection with the human T cell lymphotropic virus type I. More than two thirds of patients with ATL have skin involvement in the form of patches, plaques, and/or nodules; generalized erythroderma; and poikiloderma.

Lymphomatoid Papulosis. Characterized by recurrent self-healing papules and nodules, lymphomatoid papulosis histologically shows features of a malignant lymphoma but clinically follows a benign course. Ten to 20% of cases, however, are reported to progress to aggressive lymphoma. The cells of this disease are Ki1-positive. The cell involved in lymphomatoid papulosis has been shown to be a T cell, and therefore, this entity is also classified as one of the CTCLs.

EXTRACUTANEOUS INVOLVEMENT

In patients with CTCL, occurrence of extracutaneous disease is uncommon except in late or terminal stages of the disease. Several autopsy reports, however, suggest that extracutaneous involvement is common. These reports support the clinical and laboratory findings noted during the late stages of the disease. However, in the early stages, internal involvement is quite rare.

Enlarged lymph nodes are usually seen in the tumor stage of mycosis fungoides and early in the course of Sézary's syndrome. Postmortem data demonstrate lymph node involvement occurs in 60%, spleen in 50%, and liver and lung in 40% of patients. Bone marrow involvement in mycosis fungoides is rare; 2% of all patients and 5% of erythrodermic patients have positive bone marrow biopsies. Bone marrow is commonly reported to be involved in Sézary's syndrome. Skeletal involvement is rarely reported in CTCL, but if it does occur, osteolytic lesions, osteoblastic lesions, and diffuse osteoporosis may be seen. Involvement of the oral cavity is also rare and usually occurs during dissemination of the disease. The most commonly reported intraoral site is the tongue; the lesions are usually indurated and ulcerated nodules.

STAGING CLASSIFICATION

Staging classification has been shown to be helpful in the management of most human cancers, including lymphomas and leukemias. With CTCL, however, staging classification seems to be less effective for management, mostly because of the heterogeneous presentation. At least five different staging classifications have been suggested. The clinical staging classification is based on the TNM nomenclature, in which T represents the skin stage, N represents the peripheral lymph nodes, and M represents visceral organ involvement. Another variable is B, which represents peripheral blood involvement. However, because it is not clear whether peripheral blood is an independent prognostic variable unrelated to node and/or visceral involvement,

TABLE 2. **TNM Classification for Cutaneous T Cell Lymphoma**

Skin (T)

T0	Clinically and/or histologically suspicious lesions
T1	Limited plaques, papules, or eczematous patches covering less than 10% of skin surface
T2	Limited plaques, papules, or eczematous patches covering 10% or more of skin surface
T3	Tumors (one or more)
T4	Generalized erythroderma

Lymph Nodes (N)

N0	No clinically abnormal peripheral lymph nodes; pathologic findings not CTCL
N1	Clinically abnormal peripheral lymph nodes; pathologic findings not CTCL
N2	No clinically abnormal peripheral lymph nodes; pathologic findings positive for CTCL
N3	Clinically abnormal peripheral lymph nodes; pathologic findings positive for CTCL

Peripheral Blood (B)

B0	Atypical circulating cells not present (less than 5%)
B1	Atypical circulating cells not present (5% or more)

Visceral Organs (M)

M0	No visceral organ involvement
M1	Visceral involvement (must have pathologic confirmation)

Modified from Bunn PA, Lamberg SI: Report of the Committee on Staging and Classification of Cutaneous T-Cell Lymphomas. Cancer Treat Rep 63:725–728, 1979.

the B has not been incorporated into the staging classification for this disorder (Tables 2 and 3). Staging systems based only on skin involvement and lymph nodes have been recommended for general use, because the information needed is readily available, requiring only thorough physical examination of the patient (Table 4).

DIAGNOSTIC PROCEDURES

To confirm the diagnosis of CTCL and identify the subtype as well as the stage of the disease, the following procedures should be performed. The information yielded enables the physician to select appropriate treatment modalities for a given patient.

Clinical Examination. The physical examination should include a total skin examination and lymph node palpation. From these clinical findings, one can easily identify the subtype as well as the stage of the disease.

TABLE 3. **Staging Classification for Cutaneous T Cell Lymphoma**

Stage	Skin	Lymph Nodes	Visceral Involvement
IA	T1	N0	M0
IB	T2	N0	M0
IIA	T1,T2	N1	M0
IIB	T3	N0,N1	M0
III	T4	N0,N1	M0
IVA	T1–T4	N2,N3	M0
IVB	T1–T4	N0–N3	M1

Modified from Lamberg SI, Bunn PA Jr: Cutaneous T-cell lymphomas. Summary of the Mycosis Fungoides Cooperative Group–National Cancer Institute Workshop. Arch Dermatol 115:1103–1105, 1979. Copyright 1979, American Medical Association.

TABLE 4. **Clinical Staging Classification for Cutaneous T Cell Lymphoma**

Clinical Stage	T Category (Skin)	No. of Clinically Enlarged Nodal Sites
1	T0–T1	0–1
2	T0–T1	2–8
	or	
	T2	0–1
3	T2	2–8
	or	
	T3	0–8
4	T4	0–8

Modified from Lamberg SI, Green SB, Byar DP, et al: Clinical staging for cutaneous T-cell lymphoma. Ann Intern Med 100:187–192, 1984.

Histopathologic Examination. The diagnosis of CTCL is based on a combination of clinical and histopathologic findings. In most cases, multiple skin biopsies are preferred, because they increase the chance of detecting the characteristic histopathologic findings. In the patient with Sézary's syndrome or erythrodermic mycosis fungoides, the histopathologic diagnosis of the skin lesions may not be as easy and helpful as it is in the patient with mycosis fungoides. One of the essential features in the histologic diagnosis is the presence in the epidermis of atypical lymphocytes with large hyperchromatic, convoluted nuclei and scanty cytoplasm, which are known as mycosis fungoides cells.

In early stages of mycosis fungoides (parapsoriasis and pre–mycosis fungoides), it is usually difficult to establish a histopathologic diagnosis. If clinical suspicion of mycosis fungoides cannot be corroborated, close regular follow-up with repeated biopsies is warranted.

In the plaque stage of mycosis fungoides, the epidermis usually shows acanthosis and elongation of the rete ridges. Mycosis fungoides cells are seen in the epidermis or dermis. Epidermotropism and Pautrier's microabscesses are prominent, and the dermis shows a patchy bandlike infiltrate of lymphocytes and histiocytes and occasional eosinophils and plasma cells.

In the tumor stage, the epidermis may show ulceration secondary to an extensive infiltrate, consisting mainly of mycosis fungoides cells, that occupies much of the dermis and penetrates into the subcutis.

In Sézary's syndrome, Pautrier's microabscesses are rarely present in the epidermis. The upper dermis shows a dense infiltrate of lymphoctyes, histiocytes, and Sézary cells (see next section). The latter cells are indistinguishable from the mycosis fungoides cells seen in the plaque stage of mycosis fungoides.

Peripheral Blood Smear. Examination of a peripheral blood smear enables detection of the presence of circulating Sézary cells, which are large mononuclear cells with folded and cerebriform nuclei. The presence of more than 15% Sézary cells in peripheral blood is a minimal requirement for the diagnosis of Sézary's syndrome, although this is not uniformly agreed on by all experts. In the case of mycosis fungoides, circulating Sézary cells are found only in rare instances and in low percentage.

In a few case reports, small Sézary cells are observed that are not identifiable by light microscopy. For this reason, electron microscopic examination has been performed and found to be useful. With the leukemic form of CTCL, the higher the number of atypical cells, the worse is the prognosis.

Immunologic Studies. These assays are usually not helpful in confirming the diagnosis of CTCL or its subtype. Most patients have normal immune reactivity even in the late stages of the disease.

Nuclear Contour Index. Quantitative determination of the nuclear hyperconvolution of mycosis fungoides cells using morphometry (nuclear contour index) reveals that the atypical lymphocytes in mycosis fungoides have greater nuclear indentation and higher nuclear contour index values than those seen in benign skin diseases. The nuclear contour index is obtained by examining electron micrographs, measuring the length of the nuclear membrane of a suspected cell, and then dividing this value by the square root of the cross-sectional area.

Cytophotometry (DNA Histogram Study). In more than 65% of patients with suspected mycosis fungoides in whom light microscopy studies were not definitive, DNA histograms of lymphoid cells are abnormal. It is believed that with this technique, one might predict which patients would subsequently develop typical histologic changes of CTCL.

Cytogenetic Studies. Various studies for CTCL have shown a wide range of heteroploidy. No specific pattern of chromosomal abnormalities is seen. In one report, chromosome abnormalities were frequently detectable before morphologic changes became apparent. In addition, cytogenetic findings supported the impression that CTCL is a disease in which various clinical manifestations represent a chronologic sequence, with the cytogenetic findings paralleling the clinical symptoms. In other words, patients with minimal chromosomal changes had the best survival, and those with more extensive chromosome abnormalities had more advanced stages of disease. Those patients who developed clonal abnormalities had a poorer prognosis and a shorter survival.

Computer-Assisted Studies. Two new computerized techniques, laser flow microfluorimetry (studying DNA content and structure) and automated image analysis (studying chromatin dispersion), promise additional refinement in detecting aneuploid cell populations in the blood of patients suspected of having CTCL.

T Cell Receptor Gene Rearrangement. Lymphocytes express antigen recognition molecules, that is, immunoglobulin (Ig) in B cells and T cell receptors (TCRs) in T cells. Genes for Ig and TCRs have certain homologies, including similar nucleotide segments and rearrangements to become functionally active during early B or T cell development. Therefore, analysis of the Ig and TCR alpha and beta chain gene rearrangements has become useful for determining the lineage and clonality of lymphoid neoplasms. A third gene that rearranges in T cells, designated the T cell gamma gene, also exhibits sequence similarity with Ig gene segments and undergoes rearrangement in both suppressor/cytotoxic and helper T cells. Using methods to detect T cell receptor gene rearrangements for beta and gamma chain in 30 patients with ATL and 17 patients with non-ATL T cell neoplasms, Matsuoka and colleagues reported T beta gene rearrangement in all 47 cases; T gamma gene rearrangement was seen in all but one ATL patient. Other studies have used these advances to obtain strong evidence that some CTCL precursors, variants, or early lesions are neoplastic in nature. Wood and associates reported a case of pagetoid reticulosis in which the atypical cells were deficient in multiple T cell antigens. Rearranged bands of beta and gamma T cell receptor genes were noted in DNA from lesional skin. The rearranged bands did not represent inherited DNA polymorphism, because DNA extracted from peripheral blood that was concurrently obtained lacked these bands. This lack also indicated that the clonal population identified in the skin was not circulating in the blood. These findings suggest the biologic potential to evolve into a more aggressive form of the disease.

Computed Tomography. Computed tomography is not considered clinically useful in the early plaque phase of CTCL. During the nodal phase, computed tomography is useful for determining lymph node involvement.

Lymphangiogram. Lymph node involvement in CTCL is an important determinant of extracutaneous involvement. Although the lymphangiogram is rarely used today, it can demonstrate the extent of lymph node involvement in this disease.

TREATMENT

Once a diagnosis of CTCL has been established, the extent of involvement should be assessed. Regardless of the extent of the disease, symptomatic care is warranted. Liberal use of emollients and moisturizers to treat the dry, scaly, pruritic eruption is suggested. Topical steroids and oral antihistamines may be helpful and should be added to the regimen. If skin infections are seen, topical systemic antibiotics or both are recommended.

For patients with stage IA disease, options for treatment vary from periodic examination with no treatment, except for lubrication and occasional use of topical steroids and ultraviolet B (UVB) exposure, to continuous topical treatment with corticosteroid. However, if progression is noted or if the disease manifests beyond this early stage, topical chemotherapy, the combination of PUVA (psoralen plus ultraviolet A), or electron beam therapy should be considered.

Topical Chemotherapy

Mechlorethamine hydrochloride (nitrogen mustard, HN_2)* has been used as a topical cutaneous medication for mycosis fungoides since the 1950s. It is a proven regimen for control of early stage CTCL, with 94% complete remission in stage IA and 59% in stage IB. The exact mechanism of action is not known. A 10-mg vial of nitrogen mustard is dissolved in water (120 mL or more); the solution is then applied daily to the entire skin surface, including all uninvolved areas. Limitations of this treatment modality include relapses occurring steadily over the years, a high rate of hypersensitivity reactions, the need for continuous daily application, lack of effectiveness in the tumor stage of the disease, and high cost. Long-term use of nitrogen mustard could cause severe aggressive squamous cell carcinomas.

Another modality is the topical use of carmustine (BCNU), an alkylating agent with the ability to inhibit DNA repair. In one report, complete remission was achieved in 84% of stage IA and 52% of stage IB patients with mycosis fungoides.

---

*Not FDA approved for this indication.

Psoralen Plus Ultraviolet A

In the presence of UVA (longwave ultraviolet light of wavelengths 320 to 400 nm), methoxsalen (psoralen), a photosensitizing furocoumarin compound with an action spectrum centered at 340 to 360 nm, produces photoadducts with thymine in the DNA of mammalian cells. This effect has been shown to inhibit DNA synthesis in human epidermal cells as well as fibroblasts. Use of PUVA in CTCL has demonstrated clinical clearing, especially in early-stage lesions.

Limitations of this modality include many relapses if PUVA is not maintained continuously or even during the maintenance period. In addition, the risk and the degree of carcinogenicity of PUVA therapy remain to be resolved.

Radiotherapy

More than 30 years ago, conventional x-ray therapy was the most effective palliative treatment for CTCL. Since the 1950s, however, electron beam therapy has been utilized. In contrast to x-rays, electrons with appropriate energies penetrate only the upper dermis. Thus, the skin alone can be treated without systemic effects.

Any of the several multiple-field techniques for delivering electron beam therapy are acceptable, including four-, six-, or rotational-field techniques; the choice of technique depends on the equipment and expertise available at each institution. One protocol involving once-weekly radiation for 6 consecutive weeks resulted in disappearance of skin lesions and median duration of remission of more than 1.5 years. Another study showed a 24% 5-year disease-free survival.

Limitations of electron beam therapy include its expense and availability. In addition, uniform exposure of the entire skin surface is technically, dosimetrically, and physically difficult. Adverse local cutaneous effects include alopecia, atrophy of skin, damage to sweat glands, radiodermatitis, and edema of the skin.

Systemic Chemotherapy

Because PUVA, electron beam therapy, and topical chemotherapeutic agents penetrate only the epidermis and upper dermis, systemic chemotherapy is necessary to treat any visceral or lymph node involvement by CTCL. Single agents, including systemic mechlorethamine, methotrexate, high-dose methotrexate with L-leucovorin rescue, bleomycin,* doxorubicin (Adriamycin)* and VP-16,* produced complete but short-term remissions. However, single agents have not been shown to cure any patients with internal CTCL. Combination chemotherapy used in CTCL includes the following regimens: (1) mechlorethamine, vincristine, prednisone, and procarbazine,*

(2) bleomycin and methotrexate, (3) cyclophosphamide, doxorubicin, vincristine, and prednisone, and (4) chlorambucil and prednisone. The number of patients treated with any one regimen is small, and as yet there are no convincing data that any one regimen is better than the others. Moreover, some investigators believe that combination chemotherapy may actually reduce survival.

Cyclosporine

A profound immunosuppressive agent, cyclosporine (Sandimmune)* blocks antigen-specific T cell proliferation, possibly by decreasing expression of interleukin-1 (IL-1) and IL-2 receptors on T cells, thus down-regulating their activation. Cyclosporine has been utilized in selected refractory cases of CTCL, with a temporary response at the expense of profound immunosuppression and renal toxicity.

Purine Nucleotide Analogues

Purine nucleotide analogues have shown promising results in patients with advanced CTCL. Fludarabine (Fludara),* cladribine (Leustatin),* and pentostatin (Nipent)* have all yielded a response rate of 30 to 40%. Toxicity includes bone marrow and immune suppression as well as neurologic dysfunction.

Retinoids

Retinoids, including etretinate and isotretinoin, have demonstrated antiproliferative and antineoplastic activity. In a study involving patients with extensive mycosis fungoides, retinoid therapy achieved a 44% objective clinical response rate. Doses of 1.5 to 2.0 mg per kg per day of retinoid were used, and lymph node remissions were reported. A later study using combined systemic chemotherapy (cyclophosphamide, bleomycin, and prednisolone) with oral retinoids in 20 patients with progressive tumor-stage disease showed no further disease progression with treatment. In addition, long-term retinoid therapy may prolong remission after systemic chemotherapy is terminated. Retinoids have also been used in combination with interferon.

Combined Therapeutic Modalities

Combined therapy employing electron beam irradiation with systemic chemotherapy (single agents such as mechlorethamine, or combinations) has shown some promising results. One study reported good results with a protocol of total body electron beam therapy, followed by six monthly cycles of chemotherapy (doxorubicin once monthly and cyclophosphamide daily for 14 days). In 50 patients with stages I or II mycosis fungoides, such treatment achieved complete clinical remission with a follow-up period of up to 75 months in some cases. Despite

---

*Not FDA approved for this indication.

*Not FDA approved for this indication.

the good response, all patients continued to show karyotypic abnormalities in circulating lymphocytes.

Leukapheresis

Leukapheresis involves passage of anticoagulated whole blood from a catheter placed in one antecubital vein through a continuously operating centrifuge and back into the body. As the blood components separate, the lymphocyte-enriched buffy coat is selectively removed, thus reducing the circulating "leukemic" T cells. It is believed that this procedure causes disequilibrium of T cells between the soft tissues and the intravascular compartment, with subsequent migration of cells from the skin to the blood.

Photopheresis

In photopheresis, extracorporeal anticoagulated whole blood is subjected to PUVA photochemotherapy. One study showed that the combination of UVA and methoxsalen caused an 88% loss of viability of target lymphocytes, whereas the drug alone was inactive; 27 of the 37 patients in this study who had otherwise resistant CTCL responded to the treatment.

Antibodies

Polyclonal anti–T cell globulin administered intravenously has been shown to bind to essentially all normal blood mononuclear cells as well as the malignant cells of CTCL. With the advent of monoclonal antibodies, this form of therapy with more specific and selective antibodies against CTCL cells may prove to be extremely rewarding. Antithymocyte globulin (Atgam)* and IL-2 antibodies are currently undergoing trial.

Interferon

The largest series of patients with CTCL treated with interferon* showed a 50% response rate. Whether interferon works because of its antiviral, antiproliferative, or immunomodulatory properties remains unanswered. Further documentation of this work is obviously needed. Interferon alfa-2a (Roferon-A) and alfa-2b (Intron A) have been used with dosages as high as 12 million units three times weekly. Toxicity is dose dependent and includes fevers, chills, myalgia, malaise, anorexia, and even bone marrow suppression. Median time to optimal response is reported to be 4 to 6 months, which is quite long, and treatment has to be continued in responding patients for years. Interferon has been used in combination with photopheresis, PUVA, and retinoids. Even complete responses are reported with the combination therapy.

---

*Not FDA approved for this indication.

Interleukin-2 Fusion Toxin (DAB389IL2)

A chimeric protein, IL-2 fusion toxin contains diphtheria toxin and IL-2 gene. It targets those cells bearing IL-2 receptors and releases the toxin fragment intracellularly after internalization of the ligand-receptor complex. It is reported that 30 to 40% of those patients whose T cells have IL-2 receptors have responded to this approach. Obviously, more detailed trials are needed before the final results can be determined.

Thymopentin

A pentapeptide similar to thymopoietin, thymopentin has been used in some cases of Sézary's syndrome with up to 60% response rates. Further studies are under way.

Autologous Bone Marrow Transplantation

In the treatment of CTCL, autologous bone marrow transplantation may prove to be helpful.

SELECTION OF APPROPRIATE TREATMENT FOR A GIVEN SUBTYPE OF CTCL

For early-stage disease, a nonaggressive approach should be taken. First, emollients, gentle skin care, topical antipruritics, and moderate exposure to sunlight should be used, as this regimen tends to produce substantial improvement. High-potency topical steroids (class 1 to 3) along with antineoplastic treatment should be avoided at this time. UVB seems to work by reducing the number of proliferated epidermal Langerhans' cells as well as the thymus-like cytokines. For disease of plaque stage, more aggressive topical treatments should be used, consisting of aqueous topical nitrogen mustard, topical carmustine (BCNU), and PUVA. Some authorities suggest that extracorporeal photopheresis is needed at this point.

In the tumor phase, more aggressive systemic therapy is necessary. Total body electron beam therapy, chemotherapeutic regimens, and the experimental treatments discussed earlier have been used. Other potential therapies are autologous bone marrow transplantation, adenosine analogues, pentostatin, fludarabine phosphate, antithymocyte globulin, and δ-aminolevulinic acid photodynamic therapy.

Alopecia mucinosa (follicular mucinosa) is treated with diaminodiphenylsulfone. Poikiloderma atrophicans vasculare should be treated aggressively to prevent progression to mycosis fungoides plaque and tumor stages. It has been treated with topical mechlorethamine, three times a week, but one case study reported the development of melanoma and dysplastic nevi after such treatment. Generalized erythroderma (exfoliative dermatitis) is secondary to underlying benign or malignant causes, which can be treated by determining the true cause. PUVA and photopheresis have been used with success for this disease. Pagetoid reticulosis (Woringer-Kolopp disease) is optimally treated by low-dose radiotherapy or topical nitrogen mustard; however, controversy exists as to whether or not this is a benign disease that can be treated with intralesional steroids. Granulomatous mycosis fungoides tends to be resistant to current treatments.

Lymphomatoid papulosis has been treated successfully with low-dose methotrexate, at 5 to 25 mg orally, which decreases the risk of transformation into a malignant process. It is also treated with PUVA but has been shown to have a high rate of relapse on discontinuance of treatment. Interferon alfa-2a has also been tried, although it also was shown to have a high rate of relapse. (Hexadecylphosphocholine) is an experimental topical treatment that has been shown to be effective.

Mycosis fungoides d'emblée needs more aggressive treatment than earlier stages. The recommended treatment is a combination of topical and systemic therapy. One study obtained good results with a combination protocol of total skin electron beam irradiation (30 Gy), followed by six monthly cycles of systemic chemotherapy with either mechlorethamine or cyclophosphamide with vincristine, procarbazine, and prednisone. Topical immunotherapy, with mechlorethamine hydrochloride as the immunogen, was also shown to create prolonged remission. In primary CD30 cutaneous T cell lymphoma, the prognosis is excellent, with more than 90% of patients so treated alive and disease free after 5 years. This stage of disease has been successfully treated with methotrexate at doses of 25 mg or less given every 1 to 4 weeks.

Treatment of Sézary's syndrome consists of photochemotherapy in addition to a cytotoxic drug. The most common cytotoxic drug used is low-dose chlorambucil. Systemic corticosteroids are also used. In ATL the first-line treatment is with total body irradiation at 100 to 150 Gy. This form of the disease has been treated successfully with a combination chemotherapy called the RCM (response-oriented cyclic multidrug) protocol.

PAPULOSQUAMOUS DISEASES

method of
MICHAEL ZANOLLI, M.D.
Vanderbilt University Medical Center
Nashville, Tennessee

The papulosquamous diseases are a varied group of cutaneous disorders with a common morphologic feature, papules or plaques with overlying scale. There are important distinguishing features for each disorder, such as initial presentation and involvement of mucous membranes. The diseases vary in their histopathology, and a skin biopsy may facilitate the diagnosis if the characteristic clinical features are not all present at the time of evaluation. Dermatophyte-type fungal infection of the skin and chronic

TABLE 1. **Papulosquamous Diseases**
(A Partial but Essential List)

Tinea corporis*	Chronic cutaneous lupus*
Psoriasis	Pityriasis rubra pilaris
Lichen planus	Pityriasis lichenoides
Pityriasis rosea	Parapsoriasis
Secondary syphilis	Cutaneous T cell lymphoma
Seborrheic dermatitis	

*Not discussed in this article.

cutaneous lupus erythematosus are also to be considered in the differential diagnosis of papulosquamous diseases; but those disorders and their treatment are presented elsewhere in this text. A partial but essential list of papulosquamous disorders is shown in Table 1.

PSORIASIS VULGARIS

Psoriasis is an inflammatory disease of the skin that affects approximately 2 to 3% of the population in North America. The mean age at onset is between 20 and 30 years, and the course is usually chronic, with intermittent remissions and exacerbations. Persons of any age may be affected, from young children to elderly patients. In patients with psoriasis, involved areas of skin demonstrate an increased cellular mitotic rate, rapid proliferation of epidermal cells with resultant scaling, abnormal differentiation of keratinocytes, and increased vascular proliferation within the plaques. The pathogenesis and etiology have not been completely elucidated, but the identification of an increased frequency of HLA-Cw6 and HLA-B17 in affected families indicates the need for continued investigation and special attention to a dysregulation or inappropriate stimulation of immune-mediated inflammation.

Clinical Types

There are distinct clinical variants of psoriasis vulgaris: plaque, guttate, erythrodermic, and pustular. Plaque-type psoriasis is the most common form. The clinical presentation of plaque-type psoriasis is characterized by variably sized, well-demarcated erythematous plaques with an overlying thick, adherent silvery-white scale most commonly located on the extensor surfaces of the elbows and knees. The scalp, umbilicus, and intergluteal cleft are also common sites of involvement. Bilateral symmetrical involvement of the extremities is a consistent feature of psoriasis.

Guttate psoriasis is characterized by smaller papules, 1 to 2 cm in diameter, with an acute eruptive onset. The trunk is the predominant site of involvement. Psoriatic erythroderma manifests as generalized intense erythema and prominent shedding of scales. Pustular psoriasis has three subsets—generalized, localized, and hand and foot—that share the feature of sterile pustules ranging from 2 to 3 mm in diameter within the affected areas or regions of the body.

Areas of involvement other than the skin include the nails, which may demonstrate pits of the nail plate as well as onychodystrophy in 30 to 50% of patients with psoriasis. The joints may also be affected with an inflammatory process, and up to 45% of patients with psoriasis have joint complaints of arthralgias or stiffness. True psoriatic arthritis with synovitis and/or joint destruction is less common, occurring in 7 to 15% of patients. Psoriatic arthritis manifests most commonly as a peripheral asymmetrical oligoarthritis involving the hands and feet. Larger joints such as the knees and hips may also be affected. Depending on genetically determined factors, the arthritis associated with psoriasis may also take the form of a spondyloarthritis or a rheumatoid factor–negative symmetrical polyarthritis.

Treatment

The approach to the treatment of psoriasis encompasses the physical characteristics and the psychologic impact. Consequently, the provider of care must assess the extent to which the disease alters the daily activities of the patient and take this assessment into account when counseling the patient about the disease process and available treatments. Another major consideration is the balance between the risks and benefits of a proposed treatment. It must be remembered that the tendency to express the disease is an inherited trait, most likely from multiple genes, and treatment does not remove this tendency but merely modifies the expression of the disease. The goal of the health care provider is to bring the psoriasis into remission or an inactive state, which may mean leaving residual lesions on selected areas of the body rather than proceeding to more aggressive treatment. Whenever factors that are known to provoke the activity of psoriasis are present, such as streptococcal infection, alcohol excess, certain drugs, or excessive stress, they should be addressed appropriately.

The treatments for psoriasis are divided into three main categories: topical, ultraviolet light, and systemic. These may be used as monotherapy or in combination, depending on the severity of the disease, the potential risks for side effects, and the overall health of the patient. An underlying and basic principle in any treatment regimen for psoriasis is daily lubrication and moisturizing of the skin.

Topical Therapy

Topical corticosteroids are the most common form of therapy for psoriasis in the United States. The potency of the particular compound used depends on the location and severity of the psoriasis. In general, thicker plaques on the trunk or extremities require application of the superpotent class (class I) of corticosteroids such as augmented betamethasone (Diprolene) or clobetasol (Temovate) for a 2-week period, followed by the use of these drugs 2 days per week to help maintain the response achieved. An alterna-tive is to use a less potent class of topical corticosteroids after the initial 2-week induction period.

Parts of the body that are more susceptible to the skin atrophy associated with the use of corticosteroids are the face, groin, axilla, and genital areas. In these locations, the use of superpotent topical corticosteroids should be avoided, and a less potent class of compound should be used.

Tar preparations are still of value in the treatment of psoriasis, especially when used for the treatment of mild scalp psoriasis in the form of shampoos and on limited plaque-type psoriasis of the skin. Patients are sometimes reluctant to accept tar treatments because of the odor and staining properties of these compounds. The use of crude coal tar in an emollient base is still an essential part of the Goeckerman therapy for resistant psoriasis when used in combination with ultraviolet B (UVB) light.

Anthralin compounds (Drithocreme, Micanol) have never been used to the same extent in the United States as they are in Europe—especially the United Kingdom. This chemical is known to have beneficial effects on psoriasis, and it is especially useful for the treatment of well-marginated, thick plaques. Patients must be educated as to the proper use of the medication to avoid skin irritation and possible burning. The other major consideration with anthralin therapy is its staining properties, which result from oxidation of the anthralin molecule. Micanol, the most recent formulation of anthralin, encapsulates the anthralin molecule in a liposome without decreasing its efficacy, and has less associated irritation and staining than previous formulations.

Another alternative in the treatment of mild to moderate plaque-type psoriasis has been the development of vitamin D_3 analogues for topical use. Calcipotriene (Dovonex) has been shown to be as effective as medium- to high-potency topical steroids in the treatment of psoriasis. One of the additional benefits is that there does not appear to be any associated atrophy with long-term use. The main side effect, which occurs in approximately 10% of patients, is mild irritation of the skin at the site of its use. This is especially prominent on the face and in body folds. The total amount of this product to be applied to the skin is limited to 100 grams per week in patients with normal renal function, to avoid possible calcium metabolism alterations and hypercalcemia.

Topical retinoid therapy for psoriasis had previously been too irritating or was ineffective as a treatment option. A newly developed topical retinoid, tazarotene (Tazorac), has been shown to be useful and effective for limited body surface involvement. This new compound has the additional benefit of being applied only once a day, but the total body surface area to be treated must be less than 20%. Irritation can still occur but is usually manageable by the patient.

Phototherapy

UVB is one of the primary treatments of moderate to severe psoriasis and is effective therapy for 70 to

80% of patients with plaque-type psoriasis. The use of erythemogenic doses of UVB at least three to five times a week has a more beneficial effect than less aggressive treatment regimens. Therapeutic UVB light is best delivered under the supervision of a trained dermatologist.

The use of photochemotherapy, in the form of psoralens plus ultraviolet A (PUVA) treatments, is one of the major advancements in the therapy for psoriasis in the past 25 years. This treatment modality is quite effective in treating psoriasis, with 85 to 90% of patients having an excellent response. PUVA treatment also requires that the supervising physician be proficient in its delivery and familiar with the potential side effects of the treatment program. The oral dose of the oil emulsion form of methoxsalen is 0.5 to 0.6 mg per kg and must be given 1 to 1.5 hours before the delivery of the UVA. The dose of UVA depends on the skin type of the patient, which is measured by the patient's inherent response to ultraviolet light and ability to tan.

The most significant side effects to be considered with the use of PUVA and UVB therapy are the potential for severe phototoxic reactions resulting in blistering of the skin, ocular damage unless appropriate precautions are taken for protection, and the long-term risk of promoting cutaneous malignancies, including melanoma. Textbooks are available on the subject of phototherapy for psoriasis and the application of these treatment modalities in other cutaneous diseases.

Systemic Medications

Systemic antibiotic therapy is used to treat recognized infections in patients with exacerbations of psoriasis, but it is often overlooked as a treatment for the overall disease state. Infections are known to exacerbate the condition, and antibiotic use should be considered a management option in selected patients.

Methotrexate is one of the more effective agents utilized for severe, extensive, or debilitating psoriasis and psoriatic arthritis. This medication can be delivered orally or given parenterally through a subcutaneous or intramuscular route. The use of methotrexate should be reserved for cases that are resistant to the less toxic and potentially less dangerous forms of therapy described previously. If there is normal renal function in an otherwise healthy adult, the usual dose is 15 mg per week in a divided dose taken 1 day a week. Once there is an adequate response, which may take 4 to 6 weeks, the dose may be reduced to a maintenance level of 7.5 to 10 mg per week. Laboratory monitoring on a monthly basis for acute effects on the hematopoietic system and for signs of long-term effects on the liver, such as fibrosis and cirrhosis, is essential. Monitoring of the state of the liver is especially important, because patients with psoriasis appear to have a higher incidence of hepatic abnormalities than patients with rheumatoid arthritis. The single best test for the accurate evaluation of the state of the liver continues to be liver biopsy to determine whether any histologic changes have taken place. It is recommended that patients without risk factors for methotrexate use have a liver biopsy after receiving 1.5 grams of the medication. Longitudinal laboratory evaluation, including a complete blood count with platelet count and liver enzyme measurements, should be done every 2 to 4 weeks during the first 2 months of therapy and then every 4 to 8 weeks during maintenance therapy.

Systemic retinoid therapy is an important consideration for treating pustular psoriasis or when specific locations, such as the hands and feet, are involved. The retinoid most commonly used for the treatment of psoriasis is etretinate (Tegison). The efficacy of etretinate is most pronounced with the generalized form of pustular psoriasis, for which it can be used as a monotherapy. Utilization of retinoids for severe, resistant plaque-type psoriasis can be combined with other treatment modalities, such as PUVA and UVB. When retinoids are combined with either form of phototherapy, the total dose and number of treatments necessary to reach a complete response are reduced. The usual dose of etretinate, whether used alone or in combination therapy, is between 0.5 and 1.0 mg per kg per day. Once the desired response is attained, the retinoid dose can be tapered over weeks and then discontinued, depending on the clinical setting.

The side effects of the systemic retinoids are myriad, with the primary consideration being the potent teratogenic properties of this class of compounds. It is imperative that precautions be taken to prevent pregnancy during therapy with retinoids. The half-life for etretinate is 100 to 120 days, making it a drug to be avoided for any woman with childbearing potential. In reported cases, there were measurable blood levels of etretinate or metabolites in the serum up to 2 years after discontinuation of therapy due to storage in and slow release from the adipose tissue. Obviously, caution and education of patients must be undertaken when this drug is used, and the physician should be familiar and comfortable with all the precautions and long-term follow-up needed for its safe and effective use. Acitretin, the acid metabolite of etretinate, has been approved by the Food and Drug Administration for use in psoriasis. This drug must also be used with caution, but its half-life is much shorter at 15 days, and it is not stored in the adipose tissue. Concomitant use of alcohol can cause conversion of acitretin back to etretinate, which is to be avoided.

Among the possible immune-suppressing agents that have been used to treat psoriasis, cyclosporine* has received the most attention. Only the most severe cases of psoriasis should even be considered for treatment with this agent, because of the possible side effects associated with its use, such as hypertension and nephrotoxicity. However, in some cases, cyclosporine can be considered for short-term use, with long-term maintenance to be accomplished with

---

*Not FDA approved for this indication.

a less hazardous form of therapy, such as PUVA. The usual dose of cyclosporine for the treatment of psoriasis is 3 to 5 mg per kg per day initially, which should be adjusted to a lower dose for maintenance, depending on the response to therapy.

LICHEN PLANUS

Lichen planus is an inflammatory disease of unknown cause that affects less than 1% of the population. It is characterized by small, polygonal, flat-topped, smooth papules that are erythematous to violaceous. The sites of predilection are the flexor surfaces of the forearms and wrists as well as the neck, thighs, and shins. These papules are characteristically intensely pruritic. The scalp may be involved, progressing to a scarring alopecia in some cases.

Lichen planus also involves the mucous membranes in about 66% of cases. Classically, it manifests as a reticulated white patch with fine lines, called Wickham's striae. The buccal mucosa is the most commonly involved site, but the disease may occur in any area of the oral or genital mucosa.

Drug-induced lichen planus can be associated with a number of different medications, including angiotensin-converting enzyme inhibitors, antimalarials, thiazide diuretics, and the antibiotics streptomycin and tetracycline (Table 2). It is essential that any diagnosis of a lichen planus type of skin change be accompanied by a history of previous drug use and discontinuation of any drugs associated with the development of a lichen planus–type reaction.

Treatment

Therapy for lichen planus must take into consideration that approximately 66% of patients undergo spontaneous remission within 1 year.

The initial therapeutic modality most commonly used for lichen planus is topical corticosteroids. Class I or II topical corticosteroids are required to cause regression of active lesions (Table 3). Intralesional corticosteroids, such as triamcinolone, at a strength of 5 to 10 mg per mL, are effective treatment for lesions on the trunk or extremities. For extensive or generalized disease, a 2- to 4-week course of oral prednisone, beginning at 40 mg per day and followed by a tapering of the dose, can be instituted to control the eruption. Intramuscular corticosteroids may also be of use in the active stage of the disease.

Antihistamines such as hydroxyzine may be help-

TABLE 2. Selected Drugs Associated with Induction of a Lichen Planus–Like Eruption

Captopril	Chloroquine	Penicillamine
Enalapril	Quinidine	Thiazides
Gold	Tetracyclines	Chlorpropamide
Phenothiazines	Streptomycin	Tolazamide
Quinacrine		

TABLE 3. Ranking of Some Commonly Used Topical Steroids by Potency

Brand Name	Generic Name
Group I (Super Potency)	
Temovate cream 0.05%	Clobetasol propionate
Temovate ointment 0.05%	Clobetasol propionate
Diprolene cream 0.05%	Betamethasone dipropionate
Diprolene ointment 0.05%	Betamethasone dipropionate
Psorcon ointment 0.05%	Diflorasone diacetate
Ultravate ointment 0.05%	Halobetasol propionate
Group II (High Potency)	
Cyclocort ointment 0.1%	Amcinonide
Elocon ointment 0.1%	Mometasone furoate
Florone ointment 0.05%	Diflorasone diacetate
Halog cream 0.1%	Halcinonide
Lidex cream 0.05%	Fluocinonide
Lidex gel 0.05%	Fluocinonide
Lidex ointment 0.05%	Fluocinonide
Topicort cream 0.25%	Desoximetasone
Topicort ointment 0.25%	Desoximetasone
Group III (High Potency)	
Aristocort cream (HP) 0.5%	Triamcinolone acetonide
Diprosone cream 0.05%	Betamethasone dipropionate
Elocon ointment 0.1%	Mometasone furoate
Florone cream 0.05%	Diflorasone diacetate
Maxiflor cream 0.05%	Diflorasone diacetate
Uticort ointment 0.025%	Betamethasone benzoate
Valisone ointment 0.1%	Betamethasone valerate
Group IV (Medium Potency)	
Cutivate cream 0.05%	Fluticasone propionate
Elocon cream 0.1%	Mometasone furoate
Halog ointment 0.025%	Halcinonide
Kenalog cream 0.1%	Triamcinolone acetonide
Synalar cream 0.2%	Fluocinolone acetonide
Synalar ointment 0.025%	Fluocinolone acetonide
Westcort ointment 0.2%	Hydrocortisone valerate
Group V (Medium Potency)	
Aclovate ointment 0.05%	Alclometasone dipropionate
Diprosone lotion 0.05%	Betamethasone dipropionate
Kenalog lotion 0.1%	Triamcinolone acetonide
Locoid cream 0.1%	Hydrocortisone butyrate
Synalar cream 0.025%	Fluocinolone acetonide
Uticort cream 0.025%	Betamethasone benzoate
Valisone cream 0.1%	Betamethasone valerate
Westcort cream 0.2%	Hydrocortisone valerate
Group VI (Medium Potency)	
Aristocort cream 0.1%	Triamcinolone acetonide
Locorten cream 0.03%	Flumethasone pivalate
Synalar solution 0.05%	Fluocinolone acetonide
Synalar cream 0.01%	Fluocinolone acetonide
Tridesilon cream 0.05%	Desonide
Valisone lotion 0.05%	Betamethasone valerate
*Group VII (Low Potency)**	
Nutracort cream 1%	Hydrocortisone
Hytone cream 1%	Hydrocortisone

*Includes other preparations containing dexamethasone, flumetasone, prednisolone, and methylprednisolone.

From Arndt KA, LeBoit PE, Robinson JK, Wintroub BU (eds): Cutaneous Medicine and Surgery: An Integrated Program in Dermatology, Vol 1. Philadelphia, WB Saunders Co, 1996, p 162, as modified from Flowers FP: Topical corticosteroid use in a dermatologic practice: An algorithm for appropriate use. University of Florida Continuing Education Proceedings, November 1987, pp 4–9.

ful in ameliorating the intense pruritus that many patients experience. PUVA (see earlier discussion of psoriasis treatments) has also been reported to be efficacious in the treatment of generalized symptomatic lichen planus. Involvement of the oral or genital mucosa can be treated with topical corticosteroids, but medium- or low-potency agents should be used in these regions.

PITYRIASIS ROSEA

Pityriasis rosea has a characteristic clinical presentation. Classically, patients have a prodrome of mild nausea, anorexia, low-grade fever, and occasionally, mild arthralgias. Within 2 days to 3 weeks, the initial plaque—called the herald patch—may appear in 50% of patients. The herald patch is characterized as the largest of the skin lesions, with a salmon color, oval shape, and peripheral collarette of scale. It may occur anywhere on the skin but is most commonly found on the trunk. This is followed by smaller salmon-colored oval plaques with collarettes of scale, most commonly on the abdomen and trunk in a "fir-tree" distribution; these lesions are mildly pruritic in up to 75% of patients. The total duration of the eruption ranges from 4 to 16 weeks. Rare cases may take a more protracted course, lasting up to 6 months.

Treatment

Often, because pityriasis rosea is self-limited, the only therapy necessary is reassurance and education of the patient. Emollients and/or medium-potency topical corticosteroids may be helpful in ameliorating any mild symptoms that may be present. If the patient is experiencing significant pruritus or extensive involvement, 5 to 10 erythemogenic doses of UVB therapy can improve the symptoms considerably and shorten the overall duration of the disease.

SECONDARY SYPHILIS

The clinical presentation of syphilis is classified into primary, secondary, and tertiary stages. Secondary syphilis must be considered in the differential diagnosis of any of the papulosquamous disorders. The lesions are circular erythematous papules or plaques, often indurated, with an overlying light scale or shallow erosion. The scale may present as a ring on the outer edge of the papule. These lesions can occur on the trunk, abdomen, and extremities. Involvement of the palms and soles is characteristic of syphilis, as is the presence of mucous patches on the oral mucosa, which occur in only a minority of cases. Lymphadenopathy is also commonly present, and the patient should be examined for the presence of epitrochlear node enlargement.

Treatment

Several therapeutic regimens are listed by the Centers for Disease Control and Prevention (CDC) to treat secondary syphilis. If the patient has had syphilis for more than 1 year or for an indeterminate period, the recommendation is benzathine penicillin, 2.4 million units intramuscularly each week for 3 consecutive weeks. The alternatives are doxycycline

(Vibramycin) 100 mg twice a day for 4 weeks, and tetracycline, 500 mg four times a day for 4 weeks. The course is different for patients known to have syphilis for less than 1 year, patients with neurosyphilis, pregnant patients, and neonates. The reader is advised to refer to the latest CDC guidelines regarding the treatment of syphilis.

SEBORRHEIC DERMATITIS

Seborrheic dermatitis is a common cutaneous disease with a characteristic appearance. The yeast *Malassezia furfur* is known to be present in increased numbers in active lesions, and their eradication causes the disease expression to subside.

Clinically, seborrheic dermatitis may manifest in infancy as thick, greasy, yellow to white scales and crusts on a mildly erythematous base. Characteristically, the scalp is involved as well as the intertriginous regions. The face, neck, chest, groin, and intergluteal area may also be involved in extensive disease affecting infants. In adolescents and adults, the disease manifests as pink to erythematous plaques with thin, white, greasy scales. Classic sites of distribution are the scalp, eyebrows, nasolabial folds, postauricular regions, external auditory canals, and central chest.

Treatment

Mild seborrheic dermatitis responds to treatment with antifungal medications that have activity against yeast. The use of ketoconazole (Nizoral) in the form of shampoo or cream usually obtains a satisfactory response within 2 to 3 weeks. The initial response may be accelerated with concomitant class V or VI topical corticosteroids, and their use should then be tapered to avoid epidermal atrophy in the central facial area.

Intermittent biweekly use of shampoos inhibiting the growth of the *M. furfur* yeast, such as those containing ketoconazole, selenium sulfide, and zinc pyrithione, is usually enough to maintain good results in mild cases.

PITYRIASIS RUBRA PILARIS

Pityriasis rubra pilaris is a rare cutaneous disease that may be either inherited or acquired. Initially, the lesions are hyperkeratotic follicular papules with underlying orange erythema. Classically, these first occur on the scalp and face and eventually progress to involve the trunk and legs. Characteristically, within large plaques or orange erythema, there are small "islands" of normal skin. The palms and soles develop thick hyperkeratosis. At this later stage, the initial hyperkeratotic follicular papules are less conspicuous in areas of diffuse erythema but tend to remain perceptible on the dorsal digits, providing insight into the diagnosis.

The acquired type of pityriasis rubra pilaris in adults has a fluctuating course, with an 80% chance of spontaneous resolution within 3 years. The childhood presentation of the familial type of pityriasis rubra pilaris does not remit, but the clinical features are partially responsive to therapy.

Treatment

Both topical and oral medications have been used in the treatment of pityriasis rubra pilaris. Lubricating lotions containing keratolytic agents, such as salicylic acid, lactic acid, and urea, in low concentrations may aid in controlling the symptoms of dry scaling skin, but these agents do not promote regression of the disease. Oral vitamin A* at a dosage of 1×10^6 IU† per day for 2 weeks has been demonstrated to be helpful, but this treatment regimen would need to be given under close supervision owing to the toxicity of vitamin A at this dose.

The availability of systemic retinoids, such as isotretinoim (Accutane) and etretinate, has essentially replaced the need for high-dose vitamin A. A high dosage of either of the retinoids, at 1 to 2 mg per kg† per day for 2 to 3 months, has demonstrated beneficial effects by decreasing the duration of disease activity and shortening the expected course of the disease. Methotrexate, in low doses of 2.5 to 5 mg every 2 to 3 days, has also been shown to help alleviate the symptoms of skin disease. With any of these systemic treatments, there are potentially serious side effects. These agents are best given by physicians who are familiar with the side effects as well as with the type of monitoring required by patients receiving such therapy.

PITYRIASIS LICHENOIDES (ACUTA AND CHRONICA)

Pityriasis lichenoides can be separated into a self-limited variant—pityriasis lichenoides acuta (Mucha-Habermann disease)—and a more persistent variant, pityriasis lichenoides chronica. Pityriasis lichenoides acuta manifests as a generalized eruption of pink to light brown papules with overlying thin scales usually smaller than 1 cm. This disease characteristically displays individual lesions in various stages of activity, from early erythematous papules to older lesions with a central scale crust, which may leave a residual scar.

Pityriasis lichenoides chronica manifests as recurrent crops of pink to erythematous papules with thin overlying scales. Crusting or scarring is not a consistent component of the clinical presentation, and the individual plaques tend to measure up to 2 cm, larger than in the acute form.

Histopathologic changes are characteristic of this disorder and are helpful in accurately confirming the clinical suspicion. Both forms usually occur on the trunk and proximal extremities.

Treatment

Pityriasis lichenoides acuta may be treated with an oral antibiotic such as erythromycin or tetracycline in combination with topical corticosteroids. Many cases respond to exposure to natural sunlight, most likely from the effects of UVB. Therapeutic UVB is useful for both the acute and chronic forms; however, a maintenance schedule is usually needed for severe cases, because early recurrence is common if the treatment schedule is discontinued after the initial response is seen. However, the best results for both acute and chronic forms when treated with ultraviolet light are obtained with PUVA. Methotrexate, in low doses of 5 to 7.5 mg per week, has also been reported to be effective in recalcitrant cases.

PARAPSORIASIS

The term parapsoriasis encompasses two types of parapsoriasis—large plaque and small plaque. This category of cutaneous disease is not related to psoriasis vulgaris through any common pathophysiologic mechanism and has a completely separate histopathology. Large plaque parapsoriasis is characterized by well-demarcated, erythematous to light brown plaques with a surface described as "cigarette-paper wrinkling" that is due to epidermal atrophy. Plaque size may range from 5 cm to greater than 10 cm. The sites of predilection are the lower trunk, buttocks, and thighs, or a bathing trunk distribution. The breasts are also commonly involved in women. It is estimated that large plaque parapsoriasis may progress to cutaneous T cell lymphoma in 5 to 10% of patients. At present, there is no means of accurately predicting which patients are at risk. Therefore, patients with this histologic diagnosis are treated as if they have the potential for developing cutaneous T cell lymphoma.

Small plaque parapsoriasis manifests as round erythematous plaques with fine scales less than 5 cm in diameter. The plaques are usually well demarcated. The most common sites of involvement are the trunk and proximal extremities. Small plaque parapsoriasis does not appear to have the same malignant potential as the large plaque variety.

Clinicopathologic correlation of biopsies from multiple sites is usually needed to arrive at an accurate diagnosis.

Treatment

A range of treatment modalities for parapsoriasis is available, depending on the extent of the disease. Medium- to high-potency topical corticosteroids applied twice daily may cause temporary regression of localized plaques, which recur after discontinuation of treatment. Ultraviolet radiation with either UVB or PUVA is the treatment of choice to obtain long-term remission. Maintenance therapy after induction of a remission is necessary for this disease and should continue for at least 6 months after regression

---

*Not FDA approved for this indication.
†Exceeds dosage recommended by the manufacturer.

of the lesions. The highest rates of remission are accomplished with PUVA therapy. Topical nitrogen mustard is also efficacious but is necessary only for the large plaque variant.

Small plaque parapsoriasis generally does not require therapy of the same aggressiveness. Both topical corticosteroids and phototherapy have been used. With either type of parapsoriasis, the patient should be examined at 6- to 12-month intervals for evaluation of recurrence or progression of the disease. Repeated biopsies may be necessary to adequately follow the clinical course.

CUTANEOUS T CELL LYMPHOMA

Cutaneous T cell lymphoma (CTCL), or mycosis fungoides, is a malignant neoplasm of a clonal population T cells that originates in the skin. The diagnosis requires histologic identification of the malignant lymphocytes. The light microscopic characteristics of the lymphocytes, in addition to a gene rearrangement of the T cell receptor molecule, confirm the diagnosis.

There are four main clinical presentations:

1. Patch-stage CTCL is characterized by well-demarcated erythematous macules with overlying fine scale, most commonly on unexposed areas.
2. Plaque stage may progress from the patch stage or may arise spontaneously. It consists of well-demarcated, erythematous to violaceous plaques with thick overlying scale that can occur on any area of the skin.
3. Tumor stage is characterized by erythematous to violaceous nodules that most commonly arise on the face and in the body folds. These nodules may ulcerate and become secondarily infected.
4. Erythroderma stage, or Sézary's syndrome, can arise as progression from pre-existing disease or de novo. There is diffuse, intense erythema with overlying white scale and concomitant fever, chills, and, often, disturbances in temperature regulation. A markedly thickened epithelium of the hands and feet known as tylosis may accompany this form of disease.

Treatment

Patch and plaque stages of CTCL may be treated with several different modalities alone or in combination. They include topical nitrogen mustard, PUVA, total skin electron beam radiotherapy, and single-drug chemotherapy in extensive disease. Selection of the therapeutic modality most beneficial for the individual patient depends on the extent and stage of disease at the time of diagnosis. See also the preceding article on CTCL.

AUTOIMMUNE CONNECTIVE TISSUE DISORDERS

method of
RICHARD D. SONTHEIMER, M.D.
University of Texas Southwestern Medical Center
Dallas, Texas

LUPUS ERYTHEMATOSUS

The cutaneous manifestations of lupus erythematosus (LE) can be divided into those that are histopathologically specific for LE (LE-specific skin disease) and those that are not (LE-nonspecific skin disease). Space allows only a discussion of LE-specific skin disease here. The three categories of LE-specific skin disease are acute cutaneous LE (ACLE), subacute cutaneous LE (SCLE), and chronic cutaneous LE (CCLE).

ACLE in its localized form is more commonly recognized as the butterfly rash of systemic LE (SLE), whereas the most common and widely recognized form of CCLE is classic discoid LE (DLE). Because ACLE is often accompanied by active SLE, patients with this form of cutaneous LE often require systemic immunosuppressive therapy with drugs such as prednisone, azathioprine (Imuran),* and/or cyclophosphamide (Cytoxan),* and such therapy is usually adequate to quell their cutaneous inflammation. Sunscreens, topical corticosteroids, and aminoquinoline antimalarials such as hydroxychloroquine (Plaquenil) can have a steroid-sparing effect in ACLE.

SCLE is usually associated with lesser degrees of systemic illness, whereas CCLE, especially the classic DLE lesions, often occurs as an isolated clinical entity. SCLE and CCLE lesions often respond in a similar manner to the topical and systemic modalities discussed here.

Education of the Patient

Most patients with SCLE and DLE lesions are photosensitive, with many reacting to both short-wavelength (ultraviolet B [UVB]) and long-wavelength (ultraviolet A [UVA]) light. Such patients should use a commonsense approach to avoiding unnecessary sun exposure. This would obviously preclude sunbathing in natural or artificial (tanning booth) settings; exposure to sunlight at high altitudes; exposure to sunlight around highly reflective surfaces such as snow, sand, and water; and exposure to unshielded sources of artificial ultraviolet light, including standard fluorescent lighting. Whenever possible, they should wear broad-brimmed hats and tightly woven, long-sleeved shirts or blouses. Especially designed clothing is available for these purposes (Solumbra Ultra Sun Protective Clothing, Frogwear Sun Protective Clothing). In addition, such

---

*Not FDA approved for this indication.

patients should be instructed on the proper and regular use of water-resistant, broad-spectrum sunscreening agents.

All patients receiving a diagnosis of any form of LE are often initially quite fearful of the very worst possible outcome from SLE. To allay undue fears, cutaneous LE patients should be counseled appropriately about prognosis concerning their particular variety of LE. For example, patients presenting with isolated DLE skin lesions on only the head and neck (localized DLE) have less than a 5% chance of ever developing a life-threatening form of SLE. In addition, it would appear that only about 10% of patients presenting with SCLE lesions subsequently develop severe manifestations of SLE.

Local Therapy

Sunscreens

Patients should select products having a sun protection factor of at least 15 for adequate UVB protection. Ingredients such as avobenzone (Parsol 1789) and micronized titanium dioxide greatly enhance a product's ability to provide UVA protection. Sunscreens should be applied at least 30 minutes before sun exposure, and they should be reapplied after bathing or swimming, because many are quite water soluble, even when advertised to be water-resistant or water-repellent. Repeated application of sunscreens every 2 hours while in a hot, sweaty environment is also advisable.

Topical Corticosteroids

Topical corticosteroids are helpful at least partially in many patients with SCLE and DLE lesions. The superpotent class I fluorinated steroid creams and ointments (e.g., clobetasol propionate [Temovate] and betamethasone dipropionate [Diprolene]) are the most likely to be beneficial. These preparations should be used carefully on the face and intertriginous areas, because they have the capacity in themselves to produce cutaneous erythema, telangiectasia, and atrophy (2-week cycles of alternating use and nonuse can minimize this risk). Some physicians prefer the use of medium-strength topical steroids such as triamcinolone acetonide, 0.025 to 0.1% creams and ointments, when treating sensitive areas such as the face. Occlusive therapy with corticosteroid-impregnated tape (e.g., flurandrenolide) or plastic wrap (Saran) can potentiate the beneficial effects of topical corticosteroids but also carry a higher risk of local side effects. Class I or class II topical steroid solutions and gels are best employed for treating the scalp.

Intralesional Corticosteroids

Intralesional application of corticosteroids is indicated for particularly hyperkeratotic lesions or lesions that are unresponsive to topical corticosteroids. Triamcinolone acetonide (Kenalog) suspension, diluted to 2.5 to 5.0 mg per mL with either 1% lidocaine (Xylocaine) or normal saline, can be used. Intralesional corticosteroids themselves can produce cutaneous and subcutaneous atrophy (deep injections into the subcutaneous tissue enhance this risk). A 30-gauge needle is preferred because it produces only mild discomfort on penetration, especially when injected perpendicularly to the skin. The active borders of lesions should be thoroughly infiltrated.

Surgical and cosmetic intervention in cutaneous LE carries finite risks. Cutaneous LE is characterized by a tendency for nonspecific mechanical trauma to the skin, including surgical incision or laser ablation, to exacerbate the disease (Koebner's phenomenon). Injection of atrophic lesions with collagen or other similar materials should also be avoided. DLE lesions often produce permanent scarring alopecia, cosmetically disturbing dermal atrophy, and pigmentary changes. A patient often obtains great psychologic benefit from the use of a wig or corrective camouflage cosmetics designed to minimize the dystrophic appearance of dyschromic facial lesions. Covermark and Dermablend are examples of such therapeutic cosmetics.

Intralesional Antimalarials

Intralesional chloroquine hydrochloride (Aralen)* has been reported anecdotally to be of benefit for refractory cutaneous LE lesions; however, I have little personal experience with this modality.

Systemic Therapy

Unfortunately, the local measures just described often do not contain the activity of SCLE or DLE skin lesions. In such cases, the use of systemic therapy with one or more antimalarial agents should first be considered. The patient and physician, however, must be convinced that the potential benefits of systemic therapy outweigh the risks.

Antimalarials

One or a combination of the aminoquinoline antimalarials can be effective in approximately 75% of cutaneous LE patients who have failed to benefit from the local measures described previously. The risks of retinal toxicity should be discussed with the patient, and a pretreatment ophthalmologic examination should be carried out. (It is now recognized that the risk of antimalarial retinopathy is extremely rare if recommended daily dose maximums of these agents are not exceeded—hydroxychloroquine, 6.5 mg per kg per day; chloroquine,* 4 mg per kg per day.) Patients should have follow-up ophthalmologic evaluations every 6 to 12 months while receiving this therapy.

Hydroxychloroquine sulfate, 400 mg per day by mouth, should be given for the first 6 to 8 weeks of treatment to reach equilibrium blood levels. Once an adequate clinical response has been achieved, the daily dose should be decreased to a maintenance dose

---

*Not FDA approved for this indication.

of 200 mg per day for at least a year to minimize chances of recurrence; some authorities recommend even longer periods of inductive treatment. If no response is seen after 8 to 12 weeks, quinacrine hydrochloride, 100 mg per day (currently available in the United States only through compounding pharmacies such as Panorama Pharmacy, 1-800-247-9767), can be added to the hydroxychloroquine without enhancing the risk of retinopathy (quinacrine does not cause retinopathy). If after 4 to 6 weeks, adequate clinical control has not been achieved, consideration should be given to replacing the hydroxychloroquine with chloroquine diphosphate,* 250 mg per day (hydroxychloroquine and chloroquine should not be used together because of enhanced risk for retinal toxicity). In Europe, chloroquine is generally held to be more efficacious in cutaneous LE than hydroxychloroquine, perhaps owing to the earlier therapeutic responses that might be seen as a result of the shorter period required to reach equilibrium blood levels with chloroquine.

A number of side effects other than retinal toxicity are associated with the use of antimalarials. In general, quinacrine is associated with a higher incidence of side effects, such as headache, gastrointestinal intolerance, pruritus, lichenoid drug eruptions, and mucosal or cutaneous pigmentary disturbance, than is either hydroxychloroquine or chloroquine. Quinacrine commonly produces a yellow discoloration of the entire skin in fair-skinned individuals, which is completely reversible on discontinuation of the drug. Quinacrine can produce significant hemolysis in patients with glucose-6-phosphate dehydrogenase (G6PD) deficiency. Each of the aminoquinoline antimalarials can rarely produce bone marrow suppression. Toxic psychosis, grand mal seizures, neuromyopathy, and cardiac arrhythmias were observed with the use of high doses of these drugs in the past; however, these reactions are quite uncommon with the lower daily dose regimens that are used today.

When hydroxychloroquine and chloroquine are used, complete blood counts as well as liver and renal function tests are recommended before therapy, at 4 to 6 weeks after beginning therapy, and every 4 to 6 months thereafter; screens for hematologic toxicity are recommended more often when using quinacrine. Some authorities advocate confirming that patients are not deficient in G6PD activity before starting antimalarial therapy to reduce the risk of acute hemolysis—this is more important with the use of quinacrine. Patients who have overt or subclinical porphyria cutanea tarda are at especially high risk for developing acute hepatotoxicity when treated with therapeutic doses of antimalarials for cutaneous LE. It is also advocated to check urine β-human chorionic gonadotropin initially in women with childbearing potential, although evidence indicates that the pregnancy risk with the currently recommended dosage regimens of antimalarials appears to be minimal.

Non-immunosuppressive Options for Antimalarial-Refractory Disease

Some otherwise refractory cases (SCLE more than DLE) respond to diaminodiphenylsulfone (dapsone).* An initial daily dose of 25 mg by mouth twice daily can be tried. The dose can be increased up to 200 to 300 mg per day if necessary. Significant dose-related hemolysis and/or methemoglobinemia can result from the use of dapsone, especially in individuals deficient in G6PD activity. (Complete blood counts and liver function tests should be monitored regularly while a patient is taking dapsone, and the physician should be familiar with this drug before using it.) Thalidomide works especially well in antimalarial-refractory cutaneous LE; however, because of its teratogenicity and neurotoxicity, it is available in the United States only through a Food and Drug Administration compassionate use investigational new drug approval. Other drugs that can be of value to selected cases of refractory cutaneous LE are isotretinoin (Accutane),* etretinate (Tegison),* gold (auranofin, Myochrysine),* and clofazimine (Lamprene)*; however, each of these agents is associated with significant side effects. Vitamin E, phenytoin (Dilantin),* and sulfasalazine* have also been reported to be of value in uncontrolled trials.

Systemic Corticosteroids

Every effort should be made to avoid the use of systemic corticosteroids in patients with LE limited to the skin. However, occasionally a patient is encountered who has especially severe and symptomatic skin disease. In such a patient, moderate daily doses of oral corticosteroids (prednisone, 20 to 40 mg per day, given as a single morning dose) can be used as supplemental therapy during the loading phase of antimalarial therapy. Every effort should be made to reduce the dose of corticosteroids at the earliest possible time, because of the many complications of long-term corticosteroid therapy in LE patients, especially avascular bone necrosis. When the disease activity is controlled, the daily dosage should be reduced by 5- to 10-mg decrements until activity flares again or until a daily dosage of 20 mg per day is achieved. The daily dose should then be lowered by 2.5-mg decrements (some prefer to use 1-mg dose decrements once the dose falls below 10 mg per day). If the disease flares while the dose is being decreased, the prednisone should be raised to the last dose at which no clinical or laboratory activity was evident.

Alternate-day corticosteroid therapy has not been successful in suppressing disease activity in the majority of patients with cutaneous LE or SLE. However, some patients can be switched from daily to alternate-day therapy after their disease has come under control. The following protocol can be useful for making the switch from daily to alternate-day therapy. If x represents the daily dose, then the pa-

---

*Not FDA approved for this indication.

*Not FDA approved for this indication.

tient should be started on a 2x dose on the "on" day and a ¾x dose on the "off" day. One week later, the off day dose should be decreased to ½x. After another week, the off day dose should be ¼x. One week after that, the off day dose should be discontinued altogether. This protocol is more successful than others in preventing disease flares during the switch from daily to alternate-day therapy. Many patients with SLE, however, do not tolerate an alternate-day schedule, often having mini-flares on the off day.

Prednisolone rather than prednisone should be used in patients who have significant underlying liver disease, because prednisone requires hydroxylation in the liver to become biologically active. Any amount of prednisone given as a single oral dose in the morning has less adrenal-suppressing activity than the same amount given in divided doses throughout the day. However, any amount of this drug, taken in divided doses, has a greater LE-suppressing activity than does the same amount of drug given as a single morning dose.

Other Immunosuppressives

Azathioprine,* 1.5 to 2.0 mg per kg per day by mouth, can play a steroid-sparing role in the severely affected patient with cutaneous LE. Methotrexate,* 7.5 to 25 mg by mouth one day per week, is also gaining popularity in this regard. The physician should become thoroughly familiar with the proper use of these drugs, including side effects and drug interactions, before using them (space does not allow for a complete discussion of this subject here). Anti-CD4 monoclonal antibody therapy has also been reported to be of value in refractory cutaneous LE.

DERMATOMYOSITIS

Highly characteristic inflammatory skin changes accompany the pattern of proximal skeletal muscle inflammation and weakness that is the hallmark of the juvenile and adult forms of classic dermatomyositis (DM). It is not unusual for the skin manifestations of classic DM to precede the muscle manifestations by 6 months. In approximately 10% of all patients with DM, skin inflammation occurs as an isolated clinical finding for periods of 2 years or longer (amyopathic DM or dermatomyositis sine myositis). It is now well documented that adult-onset classic DM (and perhaps amyopathic DM as well) can be a sign of evolving occult malignancy, especially ovarian carcinoma in women. All patients with classic and amyopathic DM should be carefully evaluated for associated internal malignancy. Women should receive state-of-the-art screening for ovarian carcinoma, including transvaginal ultrasonography and blood CA 125 levels in addition to a Pap smear and bimanual pelvic examination.

Education of the Patient

Because cutaneous DM involvement in many patients is photosensitive, the same measures concerning ultraviolet light avoidance and photoprotection described for patients with cutaneous LE should be followed by patients with DM.

Patients should be re-evaluated for internal malignancy every 6 to 12 months after diagnosis for at least the first 2 years of their illness. They should be told to report immediately any clinical changes that develop for 2 years after the diagnosis of DM, so that the physician can determine whether such symptoms might reflect an evolving internal malignancy.

Patients with amyopathic DM should be told to report any evidence of muscle weakness or other symptoms of systemic DM involvement (e.g., pulmonary or cardiovascular symptoms). Asymptomatic DM patients should be re-evaluated for the development of muscle weakness on a regular basis (muscle examinations, creatine kinase and aldolase blood levels).

Local Therapy

Local therapy should include the regular use of sunscreens as described for LE patients. The skin manifestations of DM are characteristically extremely pruritic, and at times patients can experience disability from intense itching alone. Substantive emollients (e.g., Eucerin, Aquaphor, plain Vaseline) should be employed liberally, especially after bathing, and nonsensitizing topical antipruritics should be provided (e.g., Sarna Anti-Itch, Prax, Lubriderm with 0.25% menthol and 0.50% phenol). The use of potent topical corticosteroids as described for LE patients can provide some relief from inflammation and pruritus; however, systemic therapy is usually required in all but the most mildly affected patients.

Systemic Therapy

Potent sedating antihistamines such as doxepin (Sinequan),* 10 to 25 mg at bedtime, and nonsedating antihistamines such as loratadine (Claritin), 10 mg every morning, and cetirizine (Zyrtec), 5 to 10 mg every morning, can provide some relief. For those not requiring a nonsedating antihistamine during the day, hydroxyzine (Atarax, Vistaril), 25 to 50 mg by mouth four times a day, is a less costly alternative.

Single-agent or combination antimalarial therapy used in the protocol described previously for cutaneous LE can occasionally provide relief of the cutaneous manifestations of DM; however, these drugs as a rule are much more effective for cutaneous LE. Dapsone has been suggested to be of value in cutaneous DM in the dosage ranges given for cutaneous LE. In my experience, dapsone is most helpful for patients with the more limited forms of cutaneous DM.

---

*Not FDA approved for this indication.

*Not FDA approved for this indication.

Prednisone, 60 to 80 mg per day, has classically been the drug of choice for patients having both the cutaneous and the muscle manifestations of DM. The cost/benefit ratio of systemic corticosteroids in the management of patients having only the cutaneous manifestations of DM must be carefully considered. For those patients with classic DM not responding to prednisone alone after 2 months of therapy, azathioprine* and methotrexate* in the regimens described for LE patients are often used. These drugs can also be of benefit to the severely affected patient with only cutaneous manifestations of DM.

High-dose intravenous gamma globulin, chlorambucil (Leukeran),* and cyclosporine (Sandimmune)* are used for the most severely affected patients who have shown no response to previously discussed agents.

SCLERODERMA

Cutaneous involvement is the defining clinical aspect of both the localized (morphea, linear scleroderma) and systemic (limited cutaneous systemic sclerosis [SSc], diffuse cutaneous SSc) forms of scleroderma. The key clinical distinction between the localized and systemic forms of scleroderma is the presence or absence of acral involvement—Raynaud's phenomenon, periungual nail fold telangiectasia, ischemic digital infarcts or ulcers, stellate digital scars, and sclerodactyly. These acral changes are hallmarks of SSc, whereas they are notably absent in morphea and linear scleroderma.

The cutaneous changes of scleroderma evolve through three stages. The early inflammatory, edematous stage is replaced by a fibrotic stage that eventually evolves into an atrophic stage. Most treatment modalities for this disorder have a better chance of working if they are begun during the initial inflammatory, edematous stage.

Education of the Patient

Patients with Raynaud's phenomenon should avoid cold exposure as much as possible and should be educated about the use of layered clothing and electrically warmed gloves and mittens. Such individuals should also be actively encouraged to stop smoking. The use of vasoconstricting medications, including ergotamine, beta blockers, and sympathomimetic amines such as pseudoephedrine in over-the-counter decongestant and allergy preparations and ephedrine in nutritional supplements, should be avoided. Stress management techniques such as temperature biofeedback can mitigate an important trigger factor for Raynaud's attacks. The use of vibrational tools should be curtailed. Patients with SSc should be advised to avoid environmental stimuli such as silica or polyvinyl chloride exposure, which are known to precipitate or exacerbate this illness.

Because patients are always frightened by any diagnosis of scleroderma, the physician should address the issue of prognosis at the outset. Patients presenting with morphea and linear scleroderma rarely ever develop life-threatening manifestations of SSc. The limited cutaneous form of SSc is compatible with decades of survival. Patients presenting with early forms of diffuse cutaneous SSc should be encouraged to participate in properly designed controlled clinical trials of new therapeutic modalities whenever possible.

Local Therapy

Sclerodermatous skin is typically dry and pruritic. Thus, the same moisturization and antipruritic measures described previously for DM patients should be recommended to patients with scleroderma. Broad-spectrum topical antibiotics such as mupirocin (Bactroban) can be of value in the finger ulcerations that are associated with severe Raynaud's phenomenon. Semiocclusive hydrocolloid dressings such as Duo-Derm used in conjunction with topical antibiotics can promote ulcer healing. It has also been reported anecdotally that topical vasodilators such as nitroglycerine ointment, when applied to the intact skin surrounding digital ulcers, can promote healing.

Systemic Therapy

Digital ulcers that become acutely painful are often secondarily infected and can benefit from systemic antibiotics directed at staphylococci.

Calcium channel blockers such as nifedipine have become the mainstay for treating Raynaud's phenomenon. Sustained-release forms of nifedipine, such as Procardia XL,* are preferred because of ease of dosing and lower risk of side effects. The initial dose of Procardia XL is 30 mg per day; this can be increased to 60 to 90 mg per day as needed. Other calcium channel blockers, including amlodipine, diltiazem,* felodipine,* isradipine,* and nicardipine,* have also been used in patients with Raynaud's phenomenon but do not appear to have clear advantages over nifedipine. Some physicians also recommend the use of peripheral alpha-adrenergic receptor blockers such as prazosin,* terazosin,* and doxazosin.* Platelet-directed therapy such as the combination of aspirin,* 81 to 325 mg per day, and dipyridamole (Persantine),* 50 to 100 mg three or four times daily, or pentoxifylline (Trental),* 400 mg three times daily, is also used by some. Anticoagulant therapy, including subcutaneous injection of low-molecular-weight heparin three times per week, has also been recommended for severe Raynaud's phenomenon. Drugs that have been used for severe Raynaud's phenomenon and are not currently available in the United States are intravenous and oral prostaglandins and prostaglandin analogues, including iloprost and cicaprost as well as the serotonin antagonist ketanserin.

*Not FDA approved for this indication.

*Not FDA approved for this indication.

Other investigational approaches are intravenous calcitonin gene–related peptide and relaxin.

Treatment of sclerodermatous involvement of the skin and internal organs is extremely difficult. A number of systemic non-immunosuppressive agents have been reported anecdotally to be of benefit for scleroderma—antibiotics, aminoquinoline antimalarials, colchicine,* phenytoin sodium,* potassium aminobenzoate (Potaba), dimethyl sulfoxide (DMSO),* sulfasalazine (Azulfidine),* plasmapheresis, and interferon gamma.* However, there is currently little good evidence to support the routine use of any of these agents. In addition, a number of immunosuppressive drugs, including prednisone, azathioprine,* chlorambucil,* cyclosporine,* and antithymocyte globulin,* have also been used; however, there is little evidence from controlled clinical trials to support the use of any of these agents in scleroderma. My personal experience suggests that prednisone and antimalarials can provide some symptomatic relief during the early inflammatory, edematous phase of the disease.

There is now a wide clinical experience to suggest that long-term therapy with D-penicillamine can be of value for the cutaneous and systemic manifestations of morphea and localized scleroderma and SSc. The problem is that therapeutic doses of D-penicillamine* (750 to 1000 mg per day) are associated with a high rate of side effects, including bone marrow suppression and renal toxicity.

Ultraviolet light therapy in the form of photopheresis has been quite controversial in the treatment of scleroderma. The consensus currently is that this modality, although quite safe, does not provide enough benefit to justify its enormous cost. Uncontrolled trials in Europe have suggested that both topical bath and conventional oral 8-methoxsalen photochemotherapy may have benefit in morphea or localized scleroderma.

Surgical Therapy

Cervical sympathectomy and digital microsurgical sympathectomy have been used for severe Raynaud's phenomenon. Although these procedures can provide some initial relief, symptoms often recur with time.

*Not FDA approved for this indication.

CUTANEOUS VASCULITIS

method of
JOSEPH L. JORIZZO, M.D.
Bowman Gray School of Medicine of Wake Forest University
Winston-Salem, North Carolina

Vasculitis is a much-abused clinicopathologic concept. Lack of both a common terminology and a common system of classification of vasculitis among medical specialties and

TABLE 1. **Classification of Necrotizing Vasculitides by Gilliam and Fink, Presented at Medical Grand Rounds on September 9, 1976, at University of Texas Southwestern Medical Center**

Leukocytoclastic vasculitis (hypersensitivity angiitis or allergic vasculitis)
  A. Schönlein-Henoch purpura
  B. Hypocomplementemic vasculitis
  C. Essential mixed cryoglobulinemia
  D. Other disease-related dermal vasculitides
Rheumatic vasculitis
  A. Systemic lupus erythematosus
  B. Rheumatoid vasculitis
  C. Scleroderma
  D. Dermatomyositis
  E. Acute rheumatic fever
Granulomatous vasculitis
  A. Churg-Strauss allergic granulomatous angiitis
  B. Wegener's granulomatosis
  C. Limited Wegener's granulomatosis
Polyarteritis nodosa
  A. Classic type
  B. Limited type (skin and muscle)
  C. Hepatitis B antigen–associated vasculitis
  D. Vasculitis in drug addicts
  E. Vasculitis after serous otitis media
Giant cell arteritis
  A. Temporal arteritis
  B. Polymyalgia rheumatica
  C. Takayasu's disease

Modified from Jorizzo JL: Classification of vasculitis. J Invest Dermatol *100*:106S–110S, 1993.

even within specialties such as dermatology has created an environment of confusion, miscommunication, and missed investigative opportunity. The most elegant basic investigative techniques are misapplied if the population of patients studied is misclassified and not comparable. A number of systems of classification of vasculitis have been published, none of which has achieved universal acceptance. The classification developed at my institution is included (Tables 1 through 3). The gross clinicopathologic characteristics of vasculitides, at least as they manifest cutaneously, can be determined from careful inspection of the skin. Categorization into small-vessel vasculitis or larger vessel vasculitis is often easily accomplished clinically but should be confirmed histopathologically by the microscopic demonstration of leukocytoclastic vasculitis.

TABLE 2. **1900 American College of Rheumatology Criteria for Hypersensitivity Vasculitis (Traditional Format*)**

Age at disease onset > 16 y
Medication at disease onset
Palpable purpura
Maculopapular rash
Biopsy, including arteriole and venule, with histologic changes showing granulocytes in a perivascular or extravascular location

*At least three of the five criteria must be present. The presence of three of five criteria is associated with a specificity of 83.9% and a sensitivity of 71.0%.
From Jorizzo JL: Classification of vasculitis. J Invest Dermatol *100*:106S–110S, 1993.

TABLE 3. **Proposed Working Classification of Vasculitis**

I. Small-vessel necrotizing vasculitis
  A. Necrotizing venulitis
  B. Schönlein-Henoch purpura
  C. Essential mixed cryoglobulinemia
  D. Waldenstrom's hypergammaglobulinemic purpura
  E. Associated with collagen-vascular disease
  F. Urticarial vasculitis
  G. Erythema elevatum diutinum
  H. Rheumatoid nodules
  I. Reactive leprosy
  J. Septic vasculitis
II. Larger vessel necrotizing vasculitis
  A. Polyarteritis nodosa
    1. Benign cutaneous form
    2. Systemic form
  B. Granulomatous vasculitis
    1. Wegener's granulomatosis
    2. Allergic granulomatosis
    3. Lymphomatoid granulomatosis
  C. Giant cell arteritis
    1. Temporal arteritis
    2. Takayasu's disease
  D. Larger vessel vasculitis with collagen-vascular disease
  E. Nodular vasculitis

From Jorizzo JL: Classification of vasculitis. J Invest Dermatol *100*:106S–110S, 1993.

SMALL-VESSEL VASCULITIS

Small-vessel necrotizing vasculitis would be the preferred designation for leukocytoclastic vasculitis of postcapillary venules. These small-vessel vasculitides may affect the skin without systemic illness or may be classic cutaneous manifestations of systemic disease. The typical cutaneous lesions consist of palpable purpuric lesions on the lower extremities. When encountering a patient with these findings, the clinician would do best to adopt the following evaluation approach. First, it would always be appropriate to confirm the clinical diagnosis histopathologically. Such patients are generally managed by a health care team, and clinicopathologic correlation ensures a better acceptance of the diagnosis, in light of my introductory comments. The next step is to determine the extent of the disease. Because there is evidence that small-vessel necrotizing vasculitis is a classic circulating immune complex disease in the skin, one could accomplish this by answering the question, "Where else could the immune complexes deposit?" The third step is to exclude underlying disease. It is important to realize that 50% of patients in most clinical series do not have detectable underlying disease. The attempt to exclude underlying disease, however, can be accomplished by answering the question, "What is the antigen in the immune complexes?" General categories are drug effects, infections, and a miscellaneous group of diseases considered to be associated with immune complexes. This group includes malignancies, especially myelodysplastic disorders; connective tissue vascular diseases such as systemic lupus erythematosus, rheumatoid arthritis, and juvenile dermatomyositis; diseases such as inflammatory bowel disease and chronic hepatitis; and less common diseases such as Behçet's disease.

In regard to the step of evaluating for systemic disease by answering the question, "Where would immune complexes deposit?": Patients often have general features of serum sickness–like illness, including myalgias, arthralgias, and fever. They may develop (1) proteinuria or hematuria owing to a deposition of complexes in the kidney glomeruli; (2) central or peripheral, diffuse or focal neurologic findings; (3) nonerosive polyarthritis due to synovial involvement; (4) abdominal pain or gastrointestinal bleeding due to gastrointestinal tract involvement (pathologically, the gastrointestinal lesions are almost identical to those in the skin, with palpable purpura presenting in various sites of the bowel); or (5) plural effusions, pleurisy, and pericarditis. Other less common manifestations result from deposition of immune complexes in other internal sites.

LARGER VESSEL VASCULITIS

Diagnosis of larger vessel vasculitis in the skin also requires clinicopathologic correlation. Clinical lesions typically include multiple peripheral gangrene at sites such as digits. Lesions usually have a wedge shape to the infarction, suggesting occlusion of a proximal small or medium-sized muscular artery with "downstream infarction." Another clinical presentation consists of necrosis of lesions in a livedo reticularis pattern; this again is due to occlusion of a small or medium-sized connecting vessel, such as the vessels connecting the superficial and deep plexus in skin. Clinicians must be aware that other occlusive states can result in identical clinical findings, such as occlusion of arteries of similar size by emboli; from hyperviscosity states, such as would occur with antiphospholipid antibodies; or from intense vasospasm, such as would occur with Buerger's disease or ergot intoxication.

Histologic confirmation of vasculitis affecting larger vessels requires incisional biopsy of deep tissue. The microscopic appearance of the specimen is characterized by a panarteritis with leukocytoclasia and aneurysmal dilatation of vessel walls, such as would be seen in polyarteritis nodosa. Findings of granulomatous vasculitis such as would be seen in Wegener's granulomatosis or in Churg-Strauss syndrome have been well described. Larger vessel vasculitis can also occur in patients with systemic lupus erythematosus, rheumatoid arthritis, and juvenile dermatomyositis. A thorough evaluation for internal involvement and for etiology is similar to that done for patients with small-vessel necrotizing vasculitis and is warranted for all patients.

TREATMENT

General Measures

It is important to realize that the simple presence of palpable purpura with histologic confirmation of small-vessel necrotizing vasculitis does not automatically dictate aggressive systemic therapy. Perhaps the only cutaneous indication for systemic therapy would be extensive cutaneous necrosis. No treatment is an option for patients with simple palpable purpura. Close monitoring for internal organ involvement and a search for etiology as discussed previously are always warranted. It is possible that reversal of an underlying precipitant such as a drug, treatment of an infection, or treatment of an autoimmune disorder might result in prompt resolution of the reactive vasculitis. Bed rest or support stockings can be crucial in promoting healing of lesions on dependent sites, such as the lower extremities. Gradient support stockings, as opposed to simple support stockings, are required. Potent topical corticosteroids may result in more rapid clearing of cutaneous lesions, but their long-term use can induce cutaneous atrophy, and they would not be useful for ulcerated or deeper lesions. Adjunctive therapy with agents such as nonsteroidal anti-inflammatory drugs (NSAIDs) can be quite useful in controlling the non-specific systemic serum sickness–like aspects of the illness, such as myalgias, arthralgias, and low-grade fever, but it is important to rule out infection and other causes of these manifestations first rather than to simply suppress the signs and symptoms. Patients with small-vessel necrotizing vasculitis who have significant internal involvement and all patients with more serious larger vessel vasculitis require systemic therapy.

Corticosteroids

Systemic corticosteroids are still the treatment of choice for severe vasculitic syndromes, particularly for patients with small-vessel necrotizing vasculitis who have rapidly progressive internal manifestations such as renal, neurologic, or cardiopulmonary disease and for patients with larger vessel vasculitis. Systemic corticosteroids are important adjuncts to therapy for larger vessel vasculitis. The mortality from syndromes such as polyarteritis nodosa and Wegner's granulomatosis has been altered more by the aggressive, appropriate use of systemic immunosuppressive therapy with agents such as cyclophosphamide than by oral corticosteroids alone.

It is important to realize that there have been no prospective double-blind placebo-controlled studies to show the efficacy of systemic corticosteroids in any form of vasculitis. Because of the potential for high-dose systemic corticosteroids to induce adverse reactions, physicians must be well informed about the risks of this therapy and the care of its complications. It is also important to realize that too rapid a taper of systemic corticosteroids in systemic circulating immune complex diseases can be associated with severe adverse consequences due to rebound. This is particularly a problem with low-dose, short-taper treatments, such as would occur with "dose pack" regimens.

If systemic corticosteroid treatment is strongly indicated, therapy should be initiated, usually at 1 mg per kg per day, in a single oral morning dose (prednisone 60 to 80 mg per day). Split-dose therapy carries a proportional increase in clinical response and in side effects, so that it offers no advantage over a higher single daily dose regimen. Alternate-day therapy is effective in diseases such as dermatomyositis and bullous pemphigoid but appears to be less advantageous in circulating immune complex diseases such as necrotizing vasculitis syndromes. Systemic daily corticosteroid therapy should be tapered to zero over several weeks to months while all affected organ systems are monitored closely, by clinical and laboratory examinations, for rebound. Pulse therapy with massive doses of methylprednisolone (Solu-Medrol), given at 1 gram per day intravenously for 3 to 5 days, has been used in patients with life-threatening vasculitis in an attempt to gain rapid control of the disease process. There is debate about this approach and whether the long-term disease management is benefited as much as it is by lower maintenance corticosteroid requirements. Initial reports described a risk of cardiac arrhythmias due to sudden electrolyte shifts, but this may be controlled by slower infusion of the pulse dose.

Methotrexate

Weekly low-dose pulse methotrexate* in "rheumatologic" doses of 5 to 15 mg accompanied by 1 mg per day of folic acid supplementation can be a safer alternative to high-dose systemic corticosteroid therapy for patients with milder vasculitis. This drug can also be used as an important corticosteroid-sparing drug for patients who identify themselves as requiring unacceptably high doses of systemic prednisone. Close monitoring by using established protocols such as those published by the American Academy of Dermatology for psoriasis or by the American College of Rheumatology should be followed, including regular hematologic and liver function test monitoring. Although there is some controversy about the role of liver biopsy and monitoring for liver disease, it does seem clear that routine liver function testing alone cannot predict liver fibrosis in these patients. Therefore, if patients require long-term therapy and the cumulative dose of methotrexate exceeds 2 grams, liver biopsy should be considered. Methotrexate has advantages over several other immunosuppressive drugs in its relatively rapid onset of action and in its negligible contribution to increasing the risk of internal malignancy. Obviously, aggressive pregnancy prevention is required in patients with childbearing potential because of the possible risks to the fetus.

Azathioprine

Patients who require large doses of prednisone may benefit from the addition of azathioprine (Imuran),* to the regimen as a single oral dose of 100 to 200 mg per day (use not listed by the manufacturer). Evidence of benefit can be delayed for as long as 4 to 6 weeks. Close monitoring for the possibility of hematologic toxicity is required. Long-term risks of azathioprine therapy are being reviewed particularly by rheumatologists, who seem to be finding a lower risk of internal malignancy due to reduced immune surveillance than was observed in the renal transplant population.

Cyclophosphamide

Cyclophosphamide (Cytoxan)* has been shown by a group at the National Institutes of Health to be

---

*Not FDA approved for this indication.

the treatment of choice for larger vessel vasculitis syndromes such as Wegener's granulomatosis and polyarteritis nodosa. The dosage schedule was usually like that for azathioprine; however, a newer pulse regimen has been described in which patients often receive doses of 1 gram by intravenous infusion once a month for an adult, which is tapered to every 3 months with improvement. This pulse approach may be associated with lower toxicity.

Side effects with cyclophosphamide are similar to those with azathioprine, with the added significant toxicity for cyclophosphamide of hemorrhagic cystitis. Careful attention to adequate hydration is required to prevent this complication.

Miscellaneous Therapies

Other systemic therapies and approaches have been used. Patients with small-vessel vasculitis that is difficult to manage, but is not severe enough to require therapy with systemic corticosteroids or immunosuppressive agents, may be treated with milder agents. Some of these agents may also play a role in treating larger vessel vasculitis, such as benign cutaneous polyarteritis nodosa. In addition, several new approaches have been used in patients with resistant systemic disease in the setting of small-vessel necrotizing vasculitis or with larger vessel vasculitis.

Antihistamines have been advocated, because local histamine release in tissue might trigger deposition of circular immune complexes by producing gaps in postcapillary venules in patients with small-vessel vasculitis. In my view, these drugs are seldom effective in treating vasculitis.

NSAIDs have been used to treat vasculitis, because products of acid metabolism may play a role in producing the gaps just described and because platelet aggregation is inhibited by these agents. It appears that although NSAIDs may be used in controlling serum sickness–like features of the illness, they are seldom beneficial in treating the vasculitis. Systemic antibiotics are postulated to have an effect on neutrophil chemotaxis, and they have been used by some clinicians to treat vasculitis. In my opinion, these are not terribly effective in this setting. Antimalarial agents such as hydroxychloroquine (Plaquenil)* have been used in the treatment of various forms of vasculitis. They are generally safely used if patients are closely monitored for signs of ocular, hematologic, and other toxicity. Results, in my opinion, have not been particularly beneficial.

Colchicine,* in doses of 0.6 mg two or three times daily, was thought to be of some benefit in treating mild cases of small-vessel vasculitis, although one double-blind prospective controlled study failed to show statistically significant benefit. Anecdotally, however, I have combined colchicine and dapsone therapies with some synergistic benefit. The mechanism of action in other neutrophilic dermatoses is believed to be inhibition of neutrophil migration. Side effects such as diarrhea and nausea respond to lowering of the dose. Hematologic status requires that monitoring for neutropenia be done in elderly patients.

Dapsone* has been reported to be an effective treatment of various forms of small-vessel vasculitis, particularly erythema elevatum diutinum (a chronic plaque form of small-vessel vasculitis). Oral doses of 50 to 200 mg per day may be used, but hematologic monitoring must be aggressive owing to the risk of methemoglobinemia and hemolysis. Baseline glucose-6-phosphate dehydrogenase activity is worth assessing because of the risk of life-threatening hematologic consequences in patients deficient in this enzyme. Plasmapheresis has been described as a mode of clearing circulating immune complexes in conditions such as vasculitis. A number of exchanges are required, and they must be performed in a hospital setting. Although this therapy might be useful as a lifesaver in patients with acute flares of disease, it is not clear that there is long-term benefit to this approach.

High-dose immune globulin G* has been reported to be quite beneficial in patients with severe vasculitis. This therapy appears to be well tolerated, but the high cost greatly limits its benefit.

Other immunosuppressive approaches, such as with chlorambucil (Leukeran)* or cyclosporine (Sandimmune),* can be life-threatening in selected patients. These drugs can have considerable toxicity, and great experience in their use would be required to prescribe these drugs. Other selected agents such as the antileprosy drug clofazimine (Lamprene) and thalidomide, which can be used with single-case investigational new drug approval through the Food and Drug Administration, have been reported to be beneficial in selected vasculitic syndromes such as the pustular vasculitis of Behçet's disease.

---

*Not FDA approved for this indication.

DISEASES OF THE NAILS

method of
HOWARD P. BADEN, M.D.
Cutaneous Biology Research Center
Massachusetts General Hospital and Harvard
Medical School
Boston, Massachusetts

The nail plate protects the end of the finger but also aids in fine movement of the fingers. Disorders of the nail most commonly result from trauma, infection, or dermatologic disease. Less commonly, they may be a manifestation of systemic disease or medications.

ANATOMY OF THE NAIL

The nail plate grows out from the matrix, which is the living layer that lies under the proximal nail fold and

---

*Not FDA approved for this indication.

extends out on some digits, where it appears as a white half-moon called the lunula. The hardness of the plate results from its compact proteinaceous structure. The cuticle grows out on the plate and forms a seal between the fold and the plate. The sides of the plate are bounded by the lateral nail fold, but no cuticle is present. The plate is firmly attached to the bed, and separation of these layers occurs at the hyponychium, which appears white owing to the presence of air.

The most proximal region of the matrix gives rise to the epithelium of the nail bed, which allows the plate to grow over the bed without becoming detached. The dermal papillae run in parallel rows in a longitudinal direction; for this reason, injury to vessels may cause splinter hemorrhages. There is no fat between the nail bed and bone, which explains why blunt trauma to the nail is so painful and results in hemorrhage. Fingernails grow continuously at about 0.1 mm per day, whereas toenails grow about 50% more slowly.

ONYCHOLYSIS

Onycholysis is a common nail problem that occurs more frequently in women than men. It often involves more than one finger. The white color represents separation of the plate from the bed and results from scattering of light by air under the plate. In most patients, onycholysis is an idiopathic disorder. However, it may be seen in psoriasis and fungal infections; in the latter, it is most commonly associated with subungual hyperkeratosis. In the idiopathic type, practically no scale is present. Bacteria may grow as saprophytes. *Pseudomonas* is a common bacterium, causing a greenish discoloration of the plate. Similarly, *Candida* species may be isolated; rarely, *Candida albicans* is found. Specific treatment with ketoconazole, topical or systemic, does not affect the onycholysis, although the yeast infection may be eradicated.

The course of onycholysis is unpredictable, but spontaneous healing may occur. Cutting the nails short does seem to reduce the extent of involvement and the time to healing. In the absence of any known cause or effective treatment, the most practical solution is to use nail polish to hide the cosmetic defect. Patients should be warned not to clean too vigorously under the nail, because this practice may cause a subungual abcess, usually from *Staphylococcus aureus.* If an abscess occurs, a 4-mm hole should be made in the plate with a circular punch to establish drainage, a culture obtained, and appropriate antibiotic treatment initiated.

INFECTIONS OF THE NAIL
Paronychia

Acute paronychia commonly follows injury to the nail fold and manifests as redness, swelling, and tenderness. Pus is generally present and can be released by elevating or lancing the fold with a blade, unless it is already draining. A specimen for culture should be obtained and the patient started with an antibiotic that is appropriate for *S. aureus,* which is

the most common pathogen. If *C. albicans* is found, it should be treated with ketoconazole (Nizoral), 200 mg per day. The nail should be soaked in warm water four times a day for 15 minutes to encourage drainage of pus, should be covered with a nonocclusive gauze dressing between treatments, and should be protected from the environment.

Chronic paronychia may follow an acute episode and is particularly common in individuals whose hands are frequently immersed in water. The nail fold is red, edematous, and separated from the plate, resulting in the formation of a space above the plate that allows entrance of foreign materials. Acute flares may occur periodically. A variety of bacteria may be cultured as well as *C. albicans,* but the condition behaves like an irritant reaction, not an infection. Treatment of this condition with systemic or topical antibiotics and antiyeast drugs rarely leads to resolution. The most effective treatment is protecting the hands from excessive wetting and irritants, which is best accomplished with cotton gloves worn inside loose-fitting plastic gloves. Topical corticosteroids of high potency may be tried to reduce inflammation, but one must watch for evidence of infection. In resistant cases, excision of the unattached nail fold eliminates the dead spaces and results in healing.

Tinea Unguium

Fungal infection of the nails most commonly starts in the toenails, principally the nails of the large toes. The most common organisms are the dermatophytes. Subungual hyperkeratosis at the distal or lateral margins of the plate is the earliest change, and fragmentation of the nail plate is a later finding. The infection eventually involves all the toenails and may spread to the fingernails. Because treatment involves months of systemic drug therapy, it is important to confirm the diagnosis by microscopic examination of scales as well as culture. To obtain material for mycologic examination, the nail not attached to the bed should be cut off, and the scales close to the point of attachment of the plate to the bed collected. If suspicion of infection is high and examination of scales shows no organism, paraffin sections of the nail should be cut and stained with periodic acid–Schiff.

Cure of tinea of the fingernails and toenails is now possible using either itraconazole (Sporanox), 100 mg twice daily, or terbinafine (Lamisil), 250 mg per day. Fingernails require 6 weeks of treatment, and toenails 3 months. The cure rate runs at about 70%. When infection extends to under the nail fold, the time of treatment should be longer, at least until several millimeters of normal nail have grown out. Itraconazole has a more consistent activity against *C. albicans* and should be used when there is mixed infection. Itraconazole may cause serious arrhythmias when taken with cisapride (Propulsid). Drug interactions are less likely with terbinafine. Intermittent or pulse therapy with both drugs at double the usual dosage for 1 week a month has been reported to be effective; this treatment does not have approval of the Food and Drug Administration (FDA). I am aware of an unusually high incidence of drug eruptions with itraconazole at the higher dose and believe it is best to stick to the approved regimen for either drug until more data are available.

Warts

Warts commonly affect the fingernails, involving the folds and hyponychium. They can at times be extensive, particularly in the proximal nail fold, and cause pressure on the matrix, leading to a distorted nail plate. Warts do have a reasonably high rate of spontaneous resolution, so treatment should be conservative, particularly for lesions present for a short period. In patients with a few and small lesions, fulguration and cryosurgery are the methods of choice. For extensive lesions, it is advisable to avoid surgical procedures; the best approach is to instruct the patient to paint the lesions with a thoroughly combined mixture of equal parts of 85% lactic acid and flexible collodion and to cover the lesions with waterproof tape for 8 hours. The tape is removed and the treated areas are abraded with an emery board while wet. This process is repeated nightly until the warts are gone.

Injection of warts with bleomycin (Blenoxane),* at 0.1 to 0.5 unit per mL or 5-fluorouracil,* at 1 to 2%, can be used, but pain can be a problem and recurrences are not unusual. Persistent warts, particularly those resistant to therapy, should undergo biopsy to exclude the diagnosis of virally induced squamous cell carcinoma.

Herpes Simplex

Primary and recurrent herpes simplex of the ends of the fingers is common in health professionals as a result of exposure to saliva, which contains the virus in 2 to 5% of normal adults. It is important not to confuse these lesions with bacterial infection, so as to avoid surgical incision. The indications for use of acyclovir are the same as in treatment of herpes infections in other areas of the body—acyclovir (Zovirax), 200 mg five times a day for 5 days.

Candidiasis

Infection of the nail plate with *C. albicans* occurs as a primary event in the mucocutaneous candidiasis syndrome. *C. albicans* may also be isolated in chronic paronychia and onycholysis, in which it is a secondary invader. Oral ketoconazole or itraconazale is effective in the management of primary candidiasis but is not helpful in secondary infections in paronychia or onycholysis. The length of treatment depends on a number of factors, particularly whether the patient is immunocompetent.

---

*Not FDA approved for this indication.

NAIL DISORDERS FROM TRAUMA

Chipping and horizontal and vertical splitting of the nails can result from excessive exposure of the nail to water, and occasionally from nail cosmetics. This problem is aggravated by using the nails as tools and by incorrect grooming. The nails should be cut when wet and then smoothed with an emery board when they are dry by filing in one direction and avoiding a back-and-forth movement. The nail hardener Nailtique is widely used for chipping and splitting, and many patients believe it helps. Patients who take the time to use it become more careful with their nails, which may in part explain its popularity. I have observed one case of contact dermatitis of the nail bed due to Nailtique. Nail wrapping, when done by an experienced manicurist, can be effective for individuals with exceptionally fragile nails.

Trauma to the nail fold through "playing" with it, biting, or excessive manicuring results in defects in the plate that manifest as variously shaped grooves. Repeated trauma may cause permanent injury to the matrix and persistent grooves. The best treatment is avoidance of the injury. A number of cuticle lubricants help the cuticle retain water and remain soft.

Blunt trauma to the nail can result in a hematoma that may take several days to become apparent if the injury occurs under the nail fold. Unless there is extreme pain, it is best to avoid treatment. Nail drills are designed for making a hole to relieve the pressure, but a hole may be burned in the nail plate if a paper clip heated in an open flame is used.

Onychogryphosis is a nail dystrophy of the large toes resulting from trauma, usually from poorly fitting shoes. The nail is extremely thick and curved. Clipping and filing the nail constitute the most conservative treatment, but when the condition becomes too painful, the nail should be removed and the matrix permanently destroyed or removed.

Ingrown Nail

Failure to cut toenails straight across and wearing tight shoes may result in growing of the nail plate into the lateral fold. In the early stage, the symptoms are pain, redness, and swelling. When the fold is pierced, symptoms and physical findings are magnified, and granulation tissue becomes apparent. Treatment of the early stage involves packing cotton in the nail groove and under the free edge of the nail. If the changes have progressed beyond the stage at which this is possible, clipping off the offending piece of plate and soaking will give immediate relief. When the acute process has subsided, the edge of the nail plate should be removed and the exposed matrix cauterized with phenol to permanently prevent regrowth of the offending edge of the nail plate.

In pincer nails, there is marked horizontal curvature of the nail, which pinches the skin at the free end of the plate, resulting in pain. Although trauma is blamed, this is not always the case. Ingrown nail can result, and the treatment is the same as for that condition.

CUTANEOUS DISEASES AFFECTING THE NAIL

The most common skin disease affecting the nail is psoriasis. It characteristically causes pits or depressions of the nail plate surface. This results from focal involvement of the proximal end of the matrix, causing faulty keratinization. Other changes are a rough surface, onycholysis, subungual hyperkeratosis, and total disintegration of the plate. These changes may be indistinguishable from those caused by a fungal infection of the nails.

Lichen planus also commonly affects the nails. The earliest change is a red to violaceous papule of the fold or bed. When the matrix is involved, roughness of the surface, pits, longitudinal grooves, and splits may appear. With severe involvement, there is destruction of the matrix with loss of nail, and one may observe focal attachment of the fold to the plate, called pterygium.

Pitting and roughness of the nail plate surface may be seen in alopecia areata and an idiopathic disorder called twenty-nail dystrophy, in which all of the nails are involved.

These disorders can be diagnosed by biopsy of the matrix, which should be done when lichen planus is suspected because of its tendency to cause scarring and disfigurement of the nail unit.

Various types of dermatoses (e.g., contact dermatitis, atopic dermatitis) that affect the hands may involve the nail folds and extend to the matrix. Such involvement results in dystrophy of the nails, with horizontal grooves predominating.

Treatment of these nail disorders is problematic, because it is difficult for topical agents applied to the nail folds to reach the involved matrix. Except in some patients with lichen planus, the changes are reversible; with time, new nails will grow out. The newer class I topical corticosteroids, when applied at night to the nail apparatus under a plastic film, can have a beneficial therapeutic effect, but the nail fold skin should be watched for signs of atrophy. Corticosteroids (3 to 5 mg per mL of triamcinolone acetonide [Aristocort]) can be injected under the fold close to the nail; however, this should not be done routinely because of the pain and the risk of infection. It has been advocated in patients with lichen planus whose disease appears to be progressing to scarring, and in this situation it may be indicated. In the dermatoses, topical corticosteroids are helpful for the skin changes, but the nail plates take some time to grow out normally.

SYSTEMIC DISEASES AFFECTING THE NAIL

Color changes may be the nail abnormalities most commonly observed with a systemic disease or as a result of its treatment. Splinter hemorrhages under the nail plate can be seen in normal individuals but are characteristic in subacute bacterial endocarditis and scurvy. Because these are such treatable condi-

tions, they must be considered in the differential diagnosis. Periungual telangiectasia and redness are constant features of collagen-vascular disease. Other changes that may be observed are redness of the lunula, loss of the pulp of the digit, and nail plate dystrophy.

Acquired clubbing of the nail manifests as exaggeration of the horizontal and longitudinal curvature of the nail. The angle formed by the dorsum of the nail plate and the surface of the digit proximal to the nail in clubbing is greater than 180 degrees (Lovibond's angle). It can be seen in association with bronchopulmonary disease or cyanotic cardiovascular disease. It has also been observed with intrathoracic neoplasms, colitis, and cirrhosis.

Reports of pigmentation associated with drug therapy have been increasing, and a careful drug history should be taken. Many chemotherapeutics can cause pigmentation. Both the plate and bed may be involved. Phototoxic reactions to drugs, the tetracyclines being the most common, manifest as painful redness of the plate followed by onycholysis. Ultraviolet A light is the responsible wavelength; it can penetrate the plate and may be focused on the bed.

TUMORS

The most common tumor of the nail unit is a mucous (myxoid) cyst, which manifests as a painless translucent nodule usually on the proximal nail fold. It is commonly connected to the joint space and contains highly viscous material. It frequently causes grooves in the nail plate through pressure on the matrix. It is treated by freezing with liquid nitrogen but is more reliably eradicated by marsupialization. The most common malignant lesion of the nail unit is a squamous cell carcinoma of the nail bed, which may be the result of a wart with oncogenic potential. It is most effectively treated by microscopically controlled surgery (Mohs'). Pigmented bands of the nail plate are most commonly caused by a nevus in the matrix, but the presence of a malignant melanoma is a serious risk. Spread of pigment to the surrounding soft tissue (Hutchinson's sign) is strongly suggestive of malignant melanoma. Treatment of melanoma of the nail is partial or complete amputation of the digit.

KELOIDS

method of
A. PAUL KELLY, M.D.
Martin Luther King, Jr. / Charles R. Drew
  Medical Center
Los Angeles, California

Keloids are hard benign cutaneous growths of various sizes and shapes that result from an excessive tissue response to skin trauma. Humans are the only animal that forms keloids, and the etiology is unknown. African-Americans have a much higher incidence than whites do; however, once keloids develop, the recurrence rate is the same in both races. The onset of keloids is greatest in the 15- to 19-year age group, whereas they seldom develop in senior citizens. There is no significant sexual difference in keloid formation. More than 40% of the patients have a family history of similar lesions.

Keloids and hypertrophic scars are often confused clinically, although they are different. Keloid scar tissue progressively invades surrounding normal tissue, whereas hypertrophic scars remain confined to the area of the tissue damaged by the initial injury. Hypertrophic scars enlarge by pushing out the margins of the scar rather than by invasion of normal tissue as seen in keloids.

Keloids may occur at sites of ear piercing, surgical scars, burns, vaccinations, severe acne, chronic inflammation, tattoos, and other forms of skin trauma, although some, especially midchest keloids, seem to develop spontaneously. The most common sites of keloid formation are the earlobes, neck, abdomen, chest, and upper back. They rarely occur on the nose, eyelids, hands, or scalp. Pruritus is the most common symptom, occurring in 50 to 60% of the patients. Less frequent are burning, tenderness, and pain. Yet, most patients seek therapy for cosmetic reasons.

TREATMENT

The first rule of keloid therapy is prevention. Nonessential cosmetic surgery should be withheld from known keloid formers (those with only earlobe lesions should not be considered in this category). All surgical wounds should be closed with minimal tension, incisions should not cross joint spaces, deltoid incisions should be avoided, incisions should follow skin creases whenever possible, and sutures should not be buried.

Keloid therapy may be divided into four categories: (1) topical modalities; (2) physical modalities; (3) pharmacologic agents; and (4) surgical.

Topical Modalities

Topical corticosteroids*
Topical retinoids*

Physical Modalities

Cryotherapy*
Radiation therapy*
Laser therapy*
Pressure therapy*
Silicone gel sheets*
Ligatures*

Pharmacologic Agents

Intralesional steroids*
Interferon alfa-2b (Intron A)*
Interferon gamma (Actimmune)*
β-Aminopropionitrile (BAPN)†
Colchicine*

---

*Not FDA approved for this indication.
†Not available in the United States.

Surgery

Primary closure*
Secondary closure*
Flaps*
Grafts*

Treatment Preferences

There is, however, one factor that influences the success of all therapies: the patient's compliance, especially if office visit appointments are not kept.

There is no single therapeutic modality that is best for all keloids. The type of therapy used is determined by location, size, and depth of the lesion; age of the patient; the patient's compliance; and past responses to treatment.

My treatment of choice for most earlobe keloids as well as for those in locations other than the midchest is the combined liquid nitrogen, intralesional steroid, and surgical approach with postoperative silicone gel and pressure. After briefly freezing (longer than 25 seconds may result in hypopigmentation, especially in dark-skinned individuals, which lasts 18 months or longer) the keloid with liquid nitrogen to produce tissue edema and slight local anesthesia, triamcinolone acetonide (Kenalog-40) should be injected into the papillary dermis (where most collagenase activity takes place) of the keloid with a Luer-Lok syringe and a 27-gauge needle. The action of triamcinolone is thought to be due to inhibition of tissue alpha globulins that block collagenase from breaking down collagen. The patients should be warned that they may get hypopigmentation at the injected sites, which may last 6 months or longer. The keloids should be injected every 2 to 3 weeks, and the injections are continued as long as the keloid is getting softer and smaller. Once regression ceases, the keloid should be excised after using a mixture of equal parts 2% lidocaine with epinephrine and triamcinolone 40 mg for local anesthesia. Small lesions can be closed primarily, but for larger lesions, part of the overlying epidermis can be used as an autograft to facilitate postoperative closure. Some authors claim less recurrence if the lesion is allowed to heal secondarily. If primary closure is used, the physician should not bury any sutures because this seems to stimulate increased keloid recurrence. Also, primary closure sutures should be left in place for 10 to 14 days, because earlier removal may result in wound dehiscence. A week after the sutures have been removed or the second-intention postoperative site has epithelialized, triamcinolone injections should be resumed in the postoperative site every 2 to 3 weeks for four times.

For earlobe keloids, postoperative pressure earrings with silicone sheeting on the clips should be worn for 3 to 4 months. For keloids on the trunk and extremities, the sticky silicone gel sheets should be

---

*Not FDA approved for this indication.

used with some type of pressure-gradient elastic garment (Jobst) 12 to 20 hours a day.

Topical tretinoin (Retin-A)* applied daily is sometimes effective in causing mild regression and alleviating the symptoms of keloids. It seems to be more effective when used with a class I or II topical corticosteroid.

Cryotherapy as the sole therapeutic modality has been reported to be successful in treating keloids and preventing recurrences. However, the long freeze time required produces a fair amount of morbidity and will cause those with darker skin to have marked hypopigmentation at the treated sites for 18 months or longer.

Adjuvant radiation therapy should be initiated within the first 48 hours after surgical excision; 250 to 300 cGy should be administered on 4 successive days, for a total of 1000 to 1200 cGy.

Laser therapy is sometimes successful in treating keloids, especially the neodymium:yttrium-aluminum-garnet (Nd:YAG) or the carbon dioxide laser. However, adjuvant therapy is necessary to prevent recurrences.

Pressure is an excellent adjuvant therapy or may be used alone. Pressure of 20 to 30 mm Hg, 24 hours a day for 2 to 4 months after surgery, is required to prevent recurrence.

Silicone gel sheets or silicone sheeting helps prevent keloids when it is used 12 to 20 hours a day for 3 to 4 months after keloid removal. The sticky gel sheets must be cleaned daily and changed every 2 to 3 weeks, whereas the sheeting will last for the duration of the keloid. The younger the patient and the shorter the duration of the keloid, the better the therapeutic response to silicone. Although silicone may be effective, its mechanism of action is unknown.

Ligatures may be used for pedunculated keloids when surgery is contraindicated or refused by the patient. A 4-0 nonabsorbable suture is tied around the base of the keloid and a new one applied every 2 to 3 weeks. The suture gradually cuts into and strangles the keloid. Some patients claim the lesions are sore for the first 24 to 48 hours after the ligature is applied.

Interferon alfa and interferon gamma have been successful in the hands of a few investigators. Interferon injections are not successful in causing existing keloids to regress completely and preventing their recurrence. However, when interferon alfa-2b is used immediately postoperatively at approximately 1 million units per cm of the wound length and 1 week later at the same dose, recurrences seem to be completely prevented or markedly delayed.

Other pharmacologic agents that have had limited success are β-aminopropionitrile, antihistamines, and colchicine.* One tablet of colchicine should be taken 3 times a day for 3 to 4 months. It should be initiated at the time of suture removal because earlier use may retard wound healing.

---

*Not FDA approved for this indication.

The myriad of solo therapies and combination therapeutic approaches indicate that at present, no ideal treatment is available for keloids. New and different modalities are being tested, but because keloids have no animal model, therapeutic investigations are somewhat hampered. As of yet, the keloid gene has not been identified; however, once it is discovered, gene therapy may be effective in preventing keloid formation.

WARTS

method of
KARL R. BEUTNER, M.D., PH.D.
Solano Dermatology Associates and University of California, San Francisco
San Francisco, California

Warts are the most common clinical manifestation of infection with human papillomavirus (HPV). There are at least 100 genotypes of HPV, which have been further classified on the basis of the infection at different anatomic sites. In the immunocompetent host, when HPV infection is clinically noted, it is seen in the form of warts. The development of squamous cell carcinoma in warts is extremely rare in immunocompetent patients but is a frequent complication in immunosuppressed patients, particularly in sun-exposed skin. Warts can be classified on the basis of anatomic location or morphologic type. The two major morphologic types of common warts are verrucae vulgaris and flat warts. Verrucae vulgaris are keratotic papules. Warts are confined entirely to the epidermis. Wart thickness is determined by the thickness of the infected epidermis. Flat warts are slightly raised, flat-topped, papular lesions that are rarely more than a few millimeters in diameter. Warts can also be classified anatomically; the major classifications are periungual, plantar, and facial. Warts can be found on any cutaneous surface.

The differential diagnosis of verrucae vulgaris, or common warts, includes molluscum contagiosum, Gottron's papules of dermatomyositis, acrochordon, perforating granuloma annulare, acrokeratosis verruciformis, lichen nitidus, lichen planus, seborrheic keratosis, actinic keratosis, and squamous cell carcinoma. The differential diagnosis of a flat wart would include freckles, lichen planus, or appendigeal tumors. The differential diagnosis of plantar warts includes clavus (corn), acquired digital fibrokeratoma, calus, and foreign body. The diagnosis of warts is established predominantly by physical examination, but it can be histologically confirmed.

Warts appear to be most common in children. Patients with atopic dermatitis show a predilection to cutaneous infections, including viral warts. Individuals who do wet work or have hyperhidrosis have warts more frequently, which are also more extensive and difficult to treat. If the environmental conditions can be modified, treatment can be facilitated. In addition, warts that occur in areas that are shaved, such as the face of men and legs of women, tend to be spread by this hair removal process. Extensive cutaneous warts appear to be a complication of chronic immunosuppression. Warts on sun-exposed skin of immunosuppressed patients frequently become squamous cell carcinoma. What appears to be an inflamed wart in immunosuppressed patients may turn out to be a squamous cell carcinoma. About one half to two thirds of warts will resolve in immunocompetent patients within 1 to 2 years.

The reason to treat warts, in addition to their cosmetic appearance, includes that depending on their location, warts can be painful, are susceptible to trauma, can present mechanical problems, and are a source of infection to others.

Currently available treatments include surgery, cryosurgery, scissors excision, curettage, blunt dissection, electrosurgery, laser surgery, and infrared coagulation; trichloroacetic acid, dichloroacetic acid, and the keratolytic salicylic acid; and contact sensitization with dinitrochlorobenzene, diphencyprone, or squaric acid. The selection of treatment, in part, is dictated by the anatomic location of the warts, the number of warts, the previous treatment, the patient's preference, and the clinician's experience.

CRYOTHERAPY

Cryotherapy is most often performed with liquid nitrogen applied by the spray technique, with a large loosely wound piece of cotton on a wooden stick, or with a cryoprobe. Cryotherapy cannot be done effectively with a small, tightly wound cotton-tipped applicator, which simply cannot hold an adequate amount of liquid nitrogen to effectively freeze a wart.

Cryotherapy is moderately painful and highly dependent on the operator's experience. The extent of the freeze is determined by the thickness of the wart and the anatomic location. Inadequate freezing results in poor efficacy; excessive freezing results in greater pain, scarring, and, in rare instances, damage to nerves and nail beds. Clinicians should not undertake cryotherapy without proper training and/or supervision.

SURGERY

The surgical approach requires achieving local anesthesia. This is most commonly obtained with an injection of lidocaine. Once anesthesia is obtained, surgery should be painless with only mild pain in the postoperative period. Surgical approaches that can be used are scissors excision, curettage, blunt dissection, electrodesiccation, laser vaporization, or coagulation with an infrared coagulator. The blunt dissection is most commonly achieved with plantar warts. With the surgical approach, scarring may be more common, particularly on the hands and feet.

CAUSTIC AGENTS

Dichloroacetic acid has been used for sequential treatment of warts, particularly in the plantar areas. Availability of this treatment approach varies considerably.

KERATOLYTICS

Keratolytics, predominantly in the form of various salicylic acid preparations, have been a mainstay of home treatment of warts for decades. Unlike trichloroacetic acid or dichloroacetic acid, salicylic acid is not caustic. It appears to work by drawing water into the wart and allowing it to be easily pared away. The solid dosage form is 40% salicylic acid plasters. The liquid forms consist of various concentrations of salicylic acid in either acrylic or flexible collodion. Salicylic acid plasters for the treatment of plantar warts should be applied to the wart and a small area of surrounding tissue and held in place by a cloth type of adhesive tape. The plaster can be left on for 2 to 3 days. After removal, the area should be pared with a scalpel blade or with coarse sandpaper or a pumice stone. This process is continued until the wart is gone as indicated by the return of normal dermatoglyphics. This approach should never produce bleeding and should not result in pain. If either of these occurs, the patient should be instructed to stop therapy.

The liquid keratolytics are applied most commonly after the patient soaks the area in warm to hot water. The area is lightly dried, and the keratolytic is applied as film. This is repeated daily until the wart resolves.

MISCELLANEOUS TREATMENTS

A variety of treatments, such as topical 5-fluorouracil cream (Efudex),* tretinoin (Retin-A),* and tretinoin creams, have sometimes been used. The scientific basis for the use of these drugs is not clear.

CONTACT SENSITIZER

The current theory is that patients who are infected with HPV and do not develop warts, or patients who develop warts that resolve spontaneously, do so because the body makes an adequate immune response. The theory of immunotherapy for warts is the elicitation of low-grade delayed-type hypersensitivity reaction in the vicinity of the wart. This local immune response results in recruitment not just of cells specific to the contact sensitizer but of cells that are able to recognize a wide variety of epitopes. By stimulating this response, the hope is to accelerate the host's immunologic recognition of the wart infection. Common contact sensitizers that have been employed for this include dinitrochlorobenzene and squaric acid. Unfortunately, there are no standardized preparations or protocols available for these agents.

TREATMENT BY ANATOMIC SITE

Whereas a variety of factors influence the treatment of warts, anatomic site may be the major determinant.

---

*Not FDA approved for this indication.

Warts on the Face

Two major types of warts are seen on the face most commonly. The major therapeutic challenge of the face is the removal of the warts without significant scarring in the form of hypopigmented or hyperpigmented macules. Although there is little proof of its efficacy, topical tretinoin is frequently used for multiple flat warts on the face. Alternative treatment would include light electrocautery or cryotherapy. With cryotherapy or other surgical approaches to multiple warts, people with olive-skinned complexion or darker should be cautioned that they may have significant hyperpigmented or hypopigmented macules. For filiform warts on the face, particularly in men who shave, light cryotherapy is effective. These warts often have a base of less than 1 mm and when frozen properly will rarely result in significant scarring.

Warts on the Hands

Care should be taken with ablative and surgical modalities on warts on the proximal nail fold. Overaggressive treatment in this area can result in damage to the nail matrix and transient or permanent nail dystrophies. The current mainstay of treatment of warts on the hands is cryotherapy. The second line of therapy would be a surgical approach, but again cautioning patients about scarring.

Overaggressive surgical treatment on the hands can result in damage to the nerves that run along the lateral aspect of the digits.

Plantar Warts

Keratolytics in the form of salicylic acid plasters are ideal for the feet. Deep plantar warts sometimes can be anesthetized and bluntly dissected with little or no bleeding and good wound healing. The problem is that other ablative modalities result in pain; having a sore hand is one thing, but having a surgical site or wound on the foot can result in much more disability than the same procedure performed on the hand. For this reason, the use of a keratolytic is the preferred method. Salicylic acid plasters, when used properly, will alleviate this wart-related pain by softening the area and not producing additional therapeutically induced pain.

CONCLUSION

In the treatment of warts, patients should have reasonable expectations of therapies, and this would include induction of a wart-free period. Patients should be told prospectively that recurrences do happen. A treatment no worse than the disease is also desired. Patients should also be warned that ablative modalities in active wart infection can sometimes result in koebnerization of the warts or an increase in the number and size of warts. Sometimes in this case, the central area where the wart had originally been treated is clear and is surrounded by a rim of wart tissue referred to as a "doughnut" wart. Although warts are clearly transmitted from person to person, there is no clear interventional method available to prevent transmission to household or other social contacts.

CONDYLOMATA ACUMINATA

method of
LIBBY EDWARDS, M.D.
Carolinas Medical Center
Charlotte, North Carolina

Genital warts are benign tumors produced by a form of the human papillomavirus (HPV) that is usually sexually transmitted. Visible warts occur in about 1% of adults between the ages of 18 and 45 years. However, sensitive testing by the polymerase chain reaction technique shows evidence of HPV in up to 40% of sexually active people even when the skin appears normal.

Genital warts have varying appearances. Warts may be filiform with acuminate, keratotic tips. They may be lobular, resembling raspberries. Occasionally, genital warts are pedunculated and attached by a narrow stalk. At other times, genital warts are flat. In addition, genital warts tend to be grouped, and they may be skin colored, pink, or brown. When they occur on moist skin, the surface is often white. Warts that are flat or hyperpigmented are more likely than warts of other morphologic appearances to exhibit histologic dysplasia and carcinogenic HPV types.

Treatment

The management of warts requires sensitive and informative education so that patients can both resolve personal issues and become prepared for the often lengthy treatment process. First, patients should understand that there are currently no specific, effective antiviral agents for HPV. Therefore, eradication of warts is often difficult. Because the virus cannot be selectively destroyed, most wart therapies function by destroying the skin harboring the virus. This is generally painful, slow, and/or expensive. Second, warts can live in a latent form in the skin, so that recurrences soon after therapy are usual. Even after apparently effective treatment, warts sometimes recur months or years later, especially during illness or immunosuppression. Third, because of this latency, the apparent incubation period from exposure to the appearance of clinical warts can vary enormously, from weeks to years. This as well as the nearly ubiquitous nature of subclinical HPV makes contact tracing difficult or impossible. Because this is usually a sexually transmitted disease, warts can be passed from one partner to another. Therefore, avoidance of intercourse is the only sure way to prevent spreading genital warts.

TABLE 1. **Comparison of Current Therapies**

Medication	Elimination Rate (%)	Recurrence Rates (%)	Advantages	Disadvantages
Podophyllin	22–80	30–60		Slow, sometimes erosive
Podofilox	45–88	35–60	Home use	Slow, somewhat irritating
Trichloroacetic acid, dichloroacetic acid	<80	30–60		Slow, irritating
Imiquimod	40–77	13	Home use	Slow, mildly irritating
Interferon	36–62	21–25	No erosions, no irritation	Slow, expensive, requires multiple injections
Cryotherapy	69–79	45	Faster than chemotherapy	Painful, occasional dyspigmentation
Excision	100	12	Fast	Painful, scarring
Hyfrecation	100	9	Fast	Painful, scarring
Laser	100	9–72	Fast	Painful, expensive

However, condoms can help minimize transmission, and those patients with a stable relationship have already exposed their partner. Also, the length of time required to eliminate clinical warts is so long as to make abstinence impractical for most people. Finally, elimination of the visible wart does not signify elimination of the virus, so that a (smaller) risk of transmission remains after therapy. However, patients need to understand that genital warts are usually a nuisance only and most often do not cause significant symptoms or produce important medical disease. Still, the presence of a sexually transmitted disease, especially a chronic one, often produces significant damage to self-esteem and to intimate relationships. Some HPV types are also carcinogenic, producing dysplasia within the warts of the external genitalia and, more important, predisposing the patient to invasive squamous cell carcinoma. This transformation occurs primarily on the areas where squamous epithelium and glandular epithelium meet, such as the cervix and anus.

A second important aspect of management of condylomata acuminata is an evaluation for vaginal and cervical involvement and, if perianal warts are present, for rectal disease. For most women with genital warts, yearly Pap smears are adequate for the early detection of cervical dysplasia. Anoscopy for those patients with perianal disease is generally sufficient to evaluate for the presence of warts within the anal canal. However, patients with flat warts, and particularly those with pigmented flat warts, should be assessed especially carefully because this morphologic form is most often associated with those HPV types known to carry a higher risk for dysplasia and squamous cell carcinoma. A small skin biopsy of one of these warts can be performed, and if it shows changes of dysplasia, the patient (if female) or the female partner can be regarded as high risk for squamous cell carcinoma of the cervix. Any significantly abnormal Pap smears should be evaluated more fully with colposcopy. Patients with external warts showing dysplasia on a biopsy specimen but having normal cervical Pap smears should have Pap smears performed twice yearly.

Finally, the wart tumor should be eliminated when possible (Table 1). This is usually performed by chemical, physical, or surgical destruction. A comparison of the effectiveness of these methods is difficult, because various studies are not comparable. Different end points, different numbers of applications of medication, and different follow-up periods produce widely varying results.

Podophyllin at a concentration of 20% in benzoin is a time-honored therapy that slowly eliminates many warts when it is applied once every 1 to 2 weeks in the office. This therapy has been largely replaced by the home application of podofilox (Condylox), a much milder, purified form of podophyllin. Podofilox is applied by the patient to the warts twice a day for 3 consecutive days each week until visible warts are eliminated. Other chemical modalities often used in an office setting include trichloroacetic acid and dichloroacetic acid preparations. These medications are most useful for flat warts. Trichloroacetic acid (Tri-Chlor) and dichloroacetic acid (Bichloracetic Acid) are reapplied as soon as erosions from the previous application have healed, usually every 2 to 4 weeks.

Fluorouracil cream 1% (Fluoroplex)* is a medication that is indicated for the removal of actinic keratoses, but it has been shown to be effective for the treatment of genital warts. It is applied once or twice daily to the warts until a brisk inflammatory response eliminates the visible wart. Erosion, exudation, and pain are usual. Unlike the other therapies, this medication is sometimes used in the vagina for internal warts. An applicatorful is inserted into the vagina once a week. This therapy is limited by the erosive vaginitis that can occur and by its teratogenic potential in a sexually active population that is generally of childbearing potential.

The application of liquid nitrogen is effective for

---

*Not FDA approved for this indication.

the treatment of genital warts. This destructive therapy is faster than the application of chemicals, but it is generally more painful. Temporary white or dark areas on the skin can occur after healing, especially on the penile shaft.

The most common surgical therapies include hyfrecation (an electric needle), laser therapy, and snipping exophytic warts. The advantages include the elimination of all visible wart during one office visit, but the primary disadvantage is pain. Even these therapies are often followed by recurrence, because latent wart virus can be detected in normal, surrounding skin.

A recent addition to the armamentarium of wart therapies is imiquimod 5% cream (Aldara), a topical interferon inducer. This agent does not remove warts by destruction of skin; rather, it provokes an immune response. Patients apply this medication to warts overnight three times a week, with the most common side effect being mild to moderate local irritation. Another new therapy is intralesional fluorouracil in a collagen matrix.* Although effective, three injections into each wart for weeks are required, and the medication produces significant ulcerations in many patients.

Recurrence is common with all of these therapies. The usual course of genital warts is recurrence and re-treatment until warts finally disappear when the virus is eliminated by the patient's immune response or the virus becomes latent.

---

*Not available in the United States.

MELANOCYTIC NEVI (MOLES)

method of
WILLIAM A. CARO, M.D.
Northwestern University Medical School
Chicago, Illinois

The melanocytic nevus (mole) represents the most common tumor of humans, and the average individual has 25 to 50 such lesions located anywhere on the skin surface. Nevi are treated by surgical removal, and the important decision will be which lesions require treatment.

The most important reason for removing nevi is the prevention of malignant melanoma. A small percentage of certain nevi have the capacity to transform into malignant melanoma, and because of this possibility, all removed nevi should be examined microscopically. Nevi are also removed because of frequent irritation or because the patient finds them cosmetically undesirable.

In addition to removal of nevi for cosmetic reasons, the decision whether to remove a nevus depends on a number of factors including (1) type of nevus, (2) clinical behavior of the lesion, (3) location, and (4) age of the patient.

TYPES OF NEVI

Intradermal Nevus

On microscopic examination, this nevus has nests of nevus cells confined to the dermis. The lesions are round to oval and are elevated with a dome-shaped, polypoid, or verrucoid configuration. They may be pedunculated or sessile, and the margins are sharply outlined from the normal surrounding skin. Color ranges from dark brown to flesh colored, and pigmentation is usually uniform. Many such lesions contain hairs. Intradermal nevi ordinarily do not transform into malignant melanoma and require no treatment unless they undergo change or are subject to irritation.

Junction and Compound Nevi

The junction nevus has nests of nevus cells at the dermoepidermal junction, and compound nevi have nests both at the dermoepidermal junction and within the dermis. Junction nevi are flush with the skin surface (macular) and range from tan to deep brown with uniform pigmentation. Compound nevi are elevated but may have a macular pigmentary component. Malignant melanomas that arise from nevi develop from junction or compound nevi, although this change is infrequent. Removal of ordinary junction and compound nevi is usually unnecessary.

Dysplastic (Atypical) Nevus

Dysplastic nevi differ from ordinary intradermal, junction, and compound nevi in both clinical and microscopic appearances. Such lesions may have a higher incidence of malignant transformation, especially in individuals with multiple dysplastic nevi. Individuals with multiple dysplastic nevi, with a family history of similar multiple lesions, and with another member of the family having had a malignant melanoma are at particular risk for the development of malignant melanoma.

Dysplastic nevi differ from ordinary nevi in having irregular borders, often not sharply defined; variation in pigmentation with different shades of tan and brown and often some red; and larger size, often greater than 5 mm. Dysplastic nevi are usually junctional or compound, and microscopically they are characterized by atypical melanocytic cells at the dermoepidermal junction. The degree of microscopic atypia frequently cannot be predicted by the clinical appearance, and nevi suggestive of being dysplastic should be excised.

Blue Nevus

This is a lesion composed of pigmented melanocytes deeper within the dermis. Although it is benign, the normal deep blue to black color of the lesion allows confusion with malignant melanoma. Surgical excision and microscopic examination resolve the problem.

Spindle and Epithelioid Cell Nevus (Spitz Nevus)

These lesions occur primarily in childhood but are also seen in young adults and less commonly in older individuals. The lesions are usually solitary and favor the face, trunk, and extremities. They are dome shaped and usually erythematous to orange rather than pigmented. They have a minimal malignant potential, but the histopathologic picture, although distinctive, may have features suggesting malignant melanoma. In certain lesions, microscopic differentiation from malignant melanoma may be difficult. Radical treatment is not indicated, and simple excision suffices when treatment is desired.

Congenital Pigmented Nevus

Although most nevi arise sometime after birth and are termed acquired nevi, the congenital pigmented nevus is present at birth. Such lesions may symmetrically involve large areas of the body, such as the trunk, chest, or upper back (bathing trunk or garment nevi), and often have coarse hairs. Surface configuration and degree of pigmentation vary. Because malignant melanoma may often arise from an area of such a giant congenital nevus, complete surgical excision is indicated. Such excision is usually performed in stages with skin grafting. Small congenital nevi have but a minimal tendency for malignant transformation, and opinions differ as to whether all such small lesions should be excised.

CLINICAL BEHAVIOR OF LESIONS

Nevi that undergo change without a ready explanation should be removed. Enlargement of a previously quiescent lesion signals the need for treatment, as does pigmentary change occurring in individual lesions. These pigmentary changes include darkening, development of irregular pigmentation, and diffusion of pigment from the lesions into the surrounding skin. These changes must be distinguished from changes affecting all nevi, such as the darkening that occurs during pregnancy. This darkening is physiologic in nature, and the affected lesions usually require no treatment. The development of pigmented satellite lesions also dictates the need for removal, although the development of a depigmented halo about an ordinary nevus signals an early stage of regression and usually does not require treatment. Other changes necessitating removal include unexplained inflammation; the development of symptoms such as itching, pain, or tenderness; and bleeding and ulceration.

LOCATION

Lesions located in areas subjected to repeated trauma should be removed. There has been debate on the handling of nevi on the palms, soles, and genitalia. Clinicians in the past had advocated removing all such lesions because most are junction nevi, but because approximately 10 to 15% of the population has such lesions, with only rare transformation into malignant melanoma, removal of all these lesions is neither practical nor necessary. Such lesions should be observed and removed only if they are subjected to repeated trauma or if they begin to change. Lesions appearing de novo beneath the fingernails or toenails usually represent active junction nevi and should be excised.

AGE OF PATIENT

Most nevi in children are junctional or compound but do not require removal unless behaving suspiciously. In older people, macular hyperpigmented spots may develop over exposed areas, and these represent lentigines with epidermal hyperpigmentation but no nevus cells. These lesions should be removed or examined by biopsy if their appearance is atypical. An older patient will uncommonly develop a larger, irregularly pigmented, macular to slightly rough lesion over a sun-exposed area, especially the face. This lesion, lentigo maligna or melanotic freckle of Hutchinson, frequently evolves into malignant melanoma and should be removed.

TREATMENT

The treatment of nevi is surgical removal with microscopic examination. Small, elevated lesions may be safely removed by tangential excision parallel to the skin surface and light cautery or electrodesiccation to achieve hemostasis. This technique leaves an excellent cosmetic result, but on occasion there may be some repigmentation, a harmless development. This technique is not used for deeper lesions or where the nature of the lesion is not obvious clinically.

Nevi are also treated by surgical excision and suturing, and the resulting linear scar may or may not be noticeable, depending on local factors. This technique is always used when the clinical diagnosis is in doubt. A lesion clinically suspected to be malignant melanoma should be completely excised but without an attempt to extend the margin of excision. If benign histologically, the lesion will have been conservatively and appropriately treated; if it is malignant, a further carefully planned surgical excision will be required.

Nevi should not be destroyed by techniques such as cautery, fulguration, or electrodesiccation. Such procedures prevent the obtaining of biopsy material and often leave a less desirable cosmetic result because of the amount of tissue destruction.

CUTANEOUS MELANOMA

method of
ARTHUR J. SOBER, M.D., and
RICHARD G. B. LANGLEY, M.D.
*Harvard University Medical School and
    Massachusetts General Hospital
Boston, Massachusetts*

Cutaneous melanoma is an increasingly frequent and potentially lethal malignancy of melanocytes. Approximately 50% of melanomas arise within pre-existing nevi, including common melanocytic nevi, dysplastic nevi, and congenital nevi. Melanoma may also arise from the malignant transformation of melanocytes in normal skin.

INCIDENCE

The incidence of cutaneous melanoma is increasing more sharply than that of any other malignancy in men and is second only to lung cancer in women. In the United States, the incidence of melanoma has been increasing 4% each year during the period 1973 to 1991. The current lifetime risk for an American's developing melanoma has been estimated to be 1 in 87 and may increase to 1 in 75 by the year 2000.

DIAGNOSIS

Early diagnosis with prompt surgical excision is the most important principle in cutaneous melanoma management. At present, approximately 50% of melanomas are self-diagnosed by the patient; 25% are diagnosed by physicians, and the remaining by a spouse or another individual. A cardinal feature of a skin lesion that proves to be a melanoma is a change observed during a period of months. A change in a pre-existing nevus or a new pigmented lesion appearing in an adult or the development of any symptoms (itching) or signs (enlargement, asymmetry, darkening, bleeding, ulceration) should prompt referral for assessment of a pigmented lesion. The most common change noted initially in early melanoma is increased size and color change. Proposed criteria for clinical recognition of a melanoma are summarized by the ABCD acronym: A, asymmetry; B, border irregularity; C, color variegation; D, diameter greater than 6 mm. Small superficial spreading and nodular melanomas may lack some or all of these clinical criteria.

BIOPSY

A biopsy should be performed on any pigmented lesion in which the diagnosis of melanoma is suspected. If the lesion is small, a complete excision with narrow margins is recommended. An incisional biopsy or punch biopsy may be performed when the lesion is large and complete excision cannot be easily done. A biopsy of the lesion should remove the most raised area, if it is raised, and remove the darkest area, if it is flat. Incisional biopsies do not increase the risk for metastasis or affect the prognosis. Shave biopsies should not be performed, because the lesion can be transected, precluding accurate determination of tumor thickness if a diagnosis of melanoma is made.

CLASSIFICATION

Four clinical and pathologic subtypes of melanoma have been identified.

Superficial Spreading Melanoma

Superficial spreading melanoma (SSM) is the most common type of melanoma occurring in whites and represents 70% of all melanomas. SSMs occur most commonly on the legs of women and the upper back of men. SSMs have a long radial growth phase, often several years before the development of invasive melanoma. It may initially present as an area of darkening within a pre-existing nevus with gradual expansion and variegated changes in color; brown, black, blue, gray, pink, and white hues are found. SSMs are initially flat surfaced (although they may be minimally raised at the edge) with loss of fine skin markings. The borders of SSM may be irregular with notching or scalloping. The vertical growth phase is usually heralded by the development of nodules within the plaque.

Nodular Melanoma

This is the second most common form of melanoma representing approximately 15 to 30% of all tumors. In contrast to SSM, these more frequently arise in uninvolved skin and have an invasive or vertical growth phase from the onset. Nodular melanomas may not fulfill the ABCD criteria, often being a symmetrical papule or nodule and blue-black in color or amelanotic.

Lentigo Maligna Melanoma

Lentigo maligna melanoma (LMM) constitutes approximately 4 to 15% of all melanomas and invariably occurs on chronically sun-exposed skin, particularly on the head

and neck area of an older patient. LMM has a long radial growth phase and can be present for long periods in its precursor form, lentigo maligna, before invasion occurs. LMM arises from lentigo maligna, which some consider a form of melanoma in situ. The exact risk for progression of lentigo maligna to LMM is unknown but has been estimated at 5 to 30%.

Acral Lentiginous Melanoma

Acral lentiginous melanoma represents approximately 5 to 10% of all melanomas. These have a site predilection to palms, soles, and subungal or mucosal areas. In contrast to the other forms of melanoma, these occur more commonly in darker pigmented patients (Asians, blacks, and dark-skinned whites). In the nail, they may occur as a pigmented band with darkening of the proximal nail fold known as Hutchinson's sign.

RISK FACTORS

Epidemiologic and genetic studies have identified certain risk factors for melanoma. It is important to identify individuals at increased risk of developing melanoma for effective screening and educational efforts.

Phenotypic Features

Phenotypic features associated with an elevated risk for melanoma include light skin pigmentation, ease of developing sunburn, blond or red hair color, blue or gray eyes, and freckles. Individuals with these phenotypic features who have intermittent and intense exposure to sunlight appear to be at a particularly elevated risk for developing melanoma. Severe sunburn in children and adolescents is associated with at least a twofold increase in melanoma.

Dysplastic Nevi (Clinically Atypical Nevi)

Dysplastic nevi (clinically atypical nevi) are a type of acquired melanocytic lesion that have atypical features including irregular border, color variegation, and size greater than 6 mm. Dysplastic nevi may be sporadic or familial. Patients with familial dysplastic nevi inherit this in an autosomal dominant mode and appear to have an elevated risk for developing melanoma. Familial-associated melanoma syndrome in patients with clinically atypical nevi and a family history of melanoma, in at least two first-degree relatives, have a lifetime risk for developing melanoma that approaches 100%. Studies have localized a tumor suppressor gene, $p16^{INK4}$ on chromosome 9p21, and identified this as a candidate gene for familial cutaneous melanoma, noting mutations in up to 50% of these families. This gene may also be involved in sporadic melanoma.

PROGNOSTIC FACTORS

Certain clinical and histologic prognostic factors have been identified in cutaneous melanoma.

Clinical Factors

Sex. Female sex confers a better prognosis.
Age. Older patients have a poorer prognosis.
Anatomic Location. Extremity melanomas have a better outcome than truncal or scalp melanomas.

TABLE 1. **Three-Stage System for Melanoma**

Stage I	Five-Year Survival Rate (%)
Thickness (mm)	
≤0.75	96
0.76–1.49	87
1.50–2.49	75
2.50–3.99	66
≥4.00	47
Stage II	
Nodal metastasis	36
Stage III	
Distant metastasis	5

Histologic Factors

Thickness. The vertical thickness of the primary tumor as measured by Breslow is the most important histologic factor in determining prognosis of melanoma; increasing thickness of melanoma portends a progressively worse prognosis (Table 1). with increasing thickness, there is a greater chance of metastasis. Whereas only a quarter of intermediate-thickness melanomas (1.5 to 4 mm) have nodal metastases, more than 60% of melanomas of 4 mm or greater thickness have nodal metastasis.

Nodes Involved. The number of nodal metastases is also a prognostic indicator. With only one node involved, the prognosis is comparatively better than when more than two nodes are involved.

Ulceration. The presence of ulceration confers a poorer outcome.

Mitoses. The greater the number of mitoses, the poorer the prognosis.

Other. Tumor-infiltrating lymphocytes are believed to be a favorable prognostic feature, whereas regression is believed to portend a poorer prognosis.

MANAGEMENT

Excision

Complete excision of the primary tumor is the most important aspect in the clinical management of melanoma. Considerable controversy surrounds the choice of resection margins in melanoma. Current clinical management guidelines from the Melanoma Center at the Massachusetts General Hospital are outlined in Table 2. For in situ melanomas, a 0.5-cm margin is recommended on the basis of current National Institutes of Health consensus guidelines. A World Health Organization prospective randomized study comparing 1- and 3-cm margins has, for melanomas less than 1.0 mm thick, confirmed the efficacy and safety of 1.0-cm margins. The Intergroup Melanoma Study demonstrated in a prospective randomized trial for melanomas of intermediate thickness (1.0 to 4 mm) that there was no significant difference in survival or local recurrence when 2- and 4-cm margins were compared. For melanomas greater than 4 mm in thickness, there are no established guidelines, although many surgeons prefer margins of 2 to 3 cm. If the melanoma is in proximity to a vital organ or when wider margins entail a more complicated procedure, smaller margins are often used.

Elective Lymph Node Dissection

The value of performing elective lymph node dissection remains an ongoing controversy in surgical oncology. Retrospective studies suggest that there is a benefit in the 5-year survival rate in the range of 10 to 30%, although controlled prospective studies are pending and existing studies have not established any significant difference to date. A new technique that is gaining increasing acceptance is the sentinel node biopsy procedure. In this procedure, a blue dye is injected around the site of the primary melanoma. This dye drains to the first node (the sentinel node). This sentinel node is then identified intraoperatively and examined pathologically. If this node is negative, it is assumed that the remainder of the nodes are negative and no further surgery is recommended. If the node is positive, a lymphadenectomy is performed. Skip metastasis to nonsentinel nodes is believed to occur in less than 2% of the patients. A refinement of this technique involves the use of a radioactive tracer, technectium Tc 99m, with gamma probe localization to identify the sentinel node, facilitating minimally invasive surgery.

Adjuvant Therapy

Until recently, there has been no standard therapy for patients with resected melanoma who are at high risk for recurrence (adjuvant therapy). Studies have shown a benefit to the use of high-dose interferon alfa in patients with resectable node-positive melanoma. The Eastern Cooperative Oncology Group EST 1684 trial has demonstrated improvement in median relapse-free survival and 5-year survival of interferon alfa–treated node-positive resected patients

TABLE 2. **Management of Patients with Stage I and II Melanoma**

Treatment for Lesion Size of			
≤0.75 mm	0.76–1.49 mm	1.50–4.00 mm	>4.00 mm
1-cm excision margin	1- to 2-cm excision margin	2-cm excision margin ± Sentinel node studies ± Adjuvant therapy for node-positive melanomas*	2- to 3-cm excision margin ± Adjuvant therapy

*See text for discussion.

TABLE 3. **Melanoma Follow-up Schedule at Massachusetts General Hospital Melanoma Center***

Lesion Thickness (mm)	Frequency of Follow-up (mo)	Duration of Follow-up (y)
≤0.75	6	1–2, then annually
0.76–1.49	6	5, then annually
≥1.5	3	2
	6	Next 3 y, then annually

*Ten-year follow-up for all melanoma patients. Those with dysplastic nevi require more frequent follow-up and follow-up for life.

compared with control subjects. At the Massachusetts General Hospital Melanoma Center, adjuvant therapy with interferon is discussed with patients who are node-positive and had complete resection or with certain high-risk primary melanomas. Ongoing trials with interferon in combination or comparison with other adjuvant agents (i.e., melanoma vaccines) and other adjuvant therapies, where appropriate, may also be discussed.

Systemic Therapy

The treatment of metastatic melanoma remains disappointing despite extensive trials with chemotherapy, immunotherapy with interleukin-2 alone, interleukin-2 in combination with tumor-infiltrating lymphocytes or natural killer cells, monoclonal antibodies, melanoma vaccines, and combination chemoimmunotherapy. At present, there is no standard effective regimen for metastatic melanoma, although future and ongoing trials hold promise.

Follow-up

The follow-up of a patient diagnosed with melanoma is tailored to the risk for recurrence or the risk for development of a second primary. This follow-up schedule is outlined in Table 3.

PREMALIGNANT LESIONS

method of
THOMAS G. HILL, M.D.
*Skin Cancer and Cosmetic Surgery of Georgia
Decatur, Georgia*

With the dramatic rise in melanoma and nonmelanoma skin cancer comes an increased need for earlier recognition and appropriate management of precancerous skin lesions. In recent years, melanoma has become the third leading cancer killer in the United States. In addition, the frequency of squamous cell carcinoma (SCC) and basal cell carcinoma (BCC) has increased significantly, producing ever more disfigurement and deformity. Rare precancerous conditions are not discussed. A small punch biopsy of any suspicious lesion, however, is always a reasonable diagnostic choice.

Examination of skin biopsy material by a dermatopathologist, rather than a general pathologist, is more likely to yield a correct diagnosis. The physician should remain aware that the biopsy specimen is only a small portion of the average lesion and may well not include the area of worst disease. If the diagnosis is in doubt, multiple 2-mm biopsies may be used to sample various areas of a suspicious lesion. Therapy is based on the worst area sampled.

Most precancerous and cancerous tumors occur in fair-skinned individuals and are directly related to cumulative sun exposure. Prevention of actinic damage is easily accomplished by use of a sunscreen with a sun protection factor (SPF) of 15 or higher, use of a 30 SPF sunscreen for intense exposure, and avoidance of sun during the middle of the day.

TUMORS THAT MAY LEAD TO SQUAMOUS CELL CARCINOMA

Actinic Keratosis

Actinic keratosis (AK) is the most common precancerous skin lesion. AKs are ill-defined, usually mildly inflamed, scaly lesions that are often palpable because of their keratotic nature. They are found on exposed sites, are not infrequently hyperpigmented, and may itch (Table 1).

Appropriate treatments of AKs include cryosurgery, shave excision, electrodesiccation, spot dermabrasion with refrigerant anesthesia, or surgical excision for resistant lesions. Treatment of these lesions is important because 1 to 3% will eventuate in SCC. Cryosurgery is usually the best choice if the physician is skilled in the modality. Cryosurgery is generally effective, does not scar if it is properly done, and is cost-effective. Permanent hypopigmentation may result from this technique, particularly on the lower extremity.

TABLE 1. **Tumor Associations with Precancerous Lesions**

Tumor	Precancerous Lesion
Squamous cell carcinoma	Actinic keratosis
	Leukoplakia
	Oral florid papillomatosis
	Cutaneous horn
	Bowenoid papulosis
	Bowen's disease
	Arsenical keratoses
	Erythroplasia of Queyrat
Basal cell carcinoma	Nevus sebaceus
	Syringocystadenoma papilliferum
	Fibroepithelioma of Pinkus
Malignant melanoma	Lentigo maligna
	Giant hairy nevus
	B-K mole syndrome
	Large congenital nevus
Dermatofibrosarcoma protuberans	Dermatofibroma
Mycosis fungoides	Parapsoriasis en plaques
Breast, genital, or anorectal carcinoma	Paget's disease

Use of 5-fluorouracil (5-FU, Efudex) is controversial. Advocates of 5-FU tout the low expense and nonsurgical nature of this therapy. Unfortunately, if it is applied properly to the entire exposed area daily for 4 to 6 weeks, most patients experience severe reactive inflammation, which often leads to actual ulceration. This may occur even when topical corticosteroids are used to blunt the inflammatory response. The worst objection to 5-FU therapy is that it is only a temporary solution. Patients must be re-treated every year or two with attendant erythema, discomfort, and photophobia because 5-FU therapy is not curative.

Full-face dermabrasion in patients with severe actinic damage and extensive AKs has been shown to decrease the subsequent number of SCCs and BCCs that will develop in later life.

Leukoplakia

Leukoplakia means "white plaques" and generally refers to the same pathologic process as that operating in AK but on mucous membranes. A small biopsy of any unusual lesion is always indicated because invasive SCC arising in a mucous membrane may be associated with up to a 30% metastasis rate. Isolated lesions of leukoplakia usually respond to simple cryosurgery, but excision may be necessary, particularly in extensive lesions. Vermilionectomy with mucous membrane advancement skin flap may be necessary in the most severe presentations.

Bowenoid Papulosis

Flat, wartlike lesions may occur on the genitalia and are caused by several subtypes of human papillomavirus. These lesions are similar to dysplasia of the cervix caused by the same viral subtypes. In both sexes, they may eventuate in SCC, which may invade locally or metastasize. Simple excision is the safest management option, but cryosurgery, electrodesiccation, and shave excision can also be effective. Topical podophyllin is not appropriate for this condition.

Unusual Precancerous Conditions

Oral florid papillomatosis is a rare presentation of leukoplakia as large numbers of tiny intraoral papillomas. Tobacco exposure is thought to be causative. However, these lesions are less likely to experience malignant degeneration.

Cutaneous horns are horny excrescences that usually have SCC or a wart at the base. Warts are more common before age 40 years; SCC is more common after age 60 years. Biopsy is appropriate, followed by therapy indicated by the pathologic process.

Bowen's Disease

Bowen's disease (BD) is actually an SCC developed in situ. BD lesions often appear eczematous, are well demarcated, and are persistent in the same location.

Surgical excision is the preferred therapy, because the in situ malignant lesion often extends down into hair follicles and skin appendages (such as sweat glands).

Erythroplasia of Queyrat is BD of the penis. Tissue-conserving Mohs' surgery is the treatment of choice.

Arsenical keratoses are florid and usually thicker AKs in persons exposed to arsenic. Most arsenic exposure occurred in the Southeast with potassium triarsenate used to treat the cotton pest, boll weevil.

Keratoacanthoma

Keratoacanthoma (KA) is a tumor that was taken much too lightly by many physicians until multiple case reports of "metastasizing KA" began to appear in the literature 2 decades ago. Because the metastasizing KA often resulted in death, the safest approach to the KA is to surgically excise it as a low-grade SCC. Injection of KAs with triamcinolone, 5-FU,* and bleomycin has been advocated, as have curettage and electrodesiccation. None of these modalities approaches the certainty of cure that excisional surgery offers.

TUMORS THAT MAY PRODUCE BASAL CELL CANCER

The precursor lesion for the majority of BCCs has not been identified. Nevus sebaceus of Jadassohn, syringocystadenoma papilliferum, and fibroepithelioma of Pinkus are rare lesions that may occasionally degenerate into BCC.

LESIONS THAT MAY PRODUCE MALIGNANT MELANOMA

Because the actual risk for malignant melanoma in America has increased more than 1800% in the past 50 years, early recognition and appropriate management of precursor lesions have assumed increased importance. Projections based on this trend forecast further increases in malignant melanoma for the next 10 to 20 years, resulting in even more deaths from the disease. Education of patients and awareness of physicians are complementary and equally important as we face this trend.

Lentigo Maligna

Lentigo maligna (LM) lesions are irregular pigmented lesions usually on exposed sites in the elderly. LM is essentially in situ malignant melanoma with a slightly lower tendency to metastasize early. Pathologic examination of these lesions by step-section technique may reveal one or more foci of invasive malignant melanoma, necessitating further tissue removal. Conservative excision is the preferred treatment of LM.

---

*Not FDA approved for this indication.

Atypical Mole Syndrome

Atypical mole syndrome (AMS) is characterized by the presence of large numbers of unusual-looking nevi, many of which are larger than usual. AMS patients may also have many nevi below the waist and may have several precancerous (dysplastic) lesions. These patients are much more likely to develop one or more malignant melanomas during a lifetime.

ABCDs of nevi refer to asymmetry, irregular borders, blue or black color, and larger diameter. Underlying mild inflammation can often be a valuable indicator of changing nevi as well. Narrow excision of suspicious lesions is appropriate with additional tissue removal if indicated or dermatopathologic examination. Lifetime periodic examination of AMS patients and sunscreen protection and sun avoidance are appropriate.

B-K Mole Syndrome

This unusual familial condition features multiple peculiar nevi in patients with a strong family history of malignant melanoma. Patients with B-K have been studied photographically, and the transition from "B-K moles" to malignant melanoma has been documented many times. This is clearly different from the usual malignant melanoma patient who has no precursor lesion in 60 to 70% of cases. The lifetime malignant melanoma risk in B-K patients approaches 100%.

Large Congenital Nevi

Large congenital nevi, defined as greater than 20 cm in size and present within the first year of life, present an approximate 10% risk for malignant melanoma. Risk is generally proportionate to size. Surgical removal, if practical, is recommended by either staged excision or excision with skin grafting, because malignant melanoma developing in large congenital nevi has a greater than usual metastatic potential.

SKIN LESIONS RARELY ASSOCIATED WITH MALIGNANT NEOPLASIA

Dermatofibroma

Dermatofibroma (DF) is a firm and often hyperpigmented nodule in the skin, usually on extremities. Changing DFs occasionally degenerate into a locally aggressive malignancy, dermatofibrosarcoma protuberans. Changing DFs should be excised.

Parapsoriasis en Plaques

This rare disease is characterized by indurated psoriasiform plaques with varying distribution. Multiple skin biopsies for a span of years are often required to establish the diagnosis. This condition tends to evolve into cutaneous T cell lymphoma.

These patients should be referred to a specialty center for management.

Miscellaneous Conditions

Neurofibromatosis, pachyonychia congenita, dyskeratosis congenita, and epidermodysplasia verruciformis are rare, familial conditions with a known tendency to malignant degeneration. Affected persons should be followed up clinically with surgical intervention if necessary.

BACTERIAL INFECTIONS OF THE SKIN
method of
JAMES E. RASMUSSEN, M.D.
University of Michigan Medical Center
Ann Arbor, Michigan

IMPETIGO

Impetigo is the most common bacterial infection of the skin. It can occur at almost any age from the neonatal period through the geriatric population. Although impetigo is a minor problem that can be treated easily with topical medications in most situations, it can be the source of serious bacterial and nonbacterial complications in some patients.

The classic clinical varieties have traditionally been separated into bullous and nonbullous (crusted) on the basis of morphologic and bacterial distinctions. In recent years, it has become apparent that both bullous and nonbullous forms have a predominantly staphylococcal etiology. Patients of any age can develop impetigo, although it is much more common in the first 5 to 10 years of life. Factors that increase the prevalence of the disease and its severity include young age, increased temperature and humidity (tropical and subtropical climates), local skin trauma, and exposure to other infected patients and other skin diseases that feature damage to the epidermal barrier (e.g., varicella, herpes, atopic dermatitis). Because of its contagious component, epidemics are much more commonly found under conditions of increased population density.

Impetigo is particularly common during the summer months when increased temperature and humidity favor insect bites, increased local skin exposure, and scratching. The initial lesion is a small pustule that is often not even noticed. Those lesions that are infected with coagulase-positive *Staphylococcus aureus,* which produces an exfoliative toxin, quickly develop flaccid blisters in the outer portion of the epidermis. In some patients, this results in clinically obvious, clear, thin-walled vesicles and bullae. In many patients, the lesions rupture rapidly, spreading peripherally and leaving only a small rim of crust and blister, which with casual inspection may mimic ringworm. Bullous impetigo is much more common in the warm, moist areas of the body, particularly favoring the axilla and diaper areas. It is a particular problem during the neonatal period when the umbilical stump offers a site of easy colonization. Blisters can be particularly widespread during the first few years of life, particularly in the neonatal period.

In most patients, however, the initial lesion develops a serous, yellow-brown exudate that dries into the "golden crusts" of impetigo. Almost all serous exudate, whether from scratching or trauma, will dry into a similarly colored lesion. Crusted impetigo usually carries a heavy mixed flora of both staphylococci and streptococci, although streptococcus predominates in about 10 to 15% of patients. These lesions seem to be much slower in onset than bullous impetigo, which favors a more explosive development. Crusted lesions of impetigo are often present for weeks to months before the patient seeks medical attention. Crusted impetigo is much more often associated with local symptoms of tenderness and regional symptoms of lymphadenopathy and lymphangitis, which are also a cause for medical concern. Crusted lesions of impetigo are much more common on exposed areas of the body, such as the hands, feet, and legs, and areas particularly prone to trauma, such as the knees and elbows.

Predisposing factors for both bullous and nonbullous impetigo are commonly present. This includes the history of insect bite, minor trauma, a recurrent cold sore on the lips, a resolving crusted phase of varicella, and chronic skin diseases such as atopic eczema.

The diagnosis is usually based on clinical parameters and a typical history without systemic signs and symptoms. It is not usually necessary to do Gram's stain and/or a culture because coagulase-positive penicillinase-producing *S. aureus* is usually the predominant organism in both bullous and nonbullous lesions. Therapy should be directed toward the staphylococcal component of the disease.

Therapy can be directed topically and/or systemically. If lesions are few and if the patient has no other risk factors, topical antibiotics such as mupirocin (Bactroban) have been shown to be as effective as a systemic antibiotic. Patients with more widespread lesions, those who fail to respond to local therapy, or those with risk factors should be treated with adequate doses of systemic antibiotics. Although it is logical to assume that the antibiotics should be directed toward the coagulase-positive penicillinase-producing staphylococci, it has been shown in numerous studies that even in the face of cultural resistance to one or more of these antibiotics, clinical response is usually prompt in most settings. I favor the use of erythromycins, cephalosporins, or semisynthetic penicillins. It is rarely necessary to use more exotic and expensive antibiotics.

Although it probably makes parents feel good to increase local hygiene, soap and water, topical antibacterial soaps, and scrubbing rarely do much of anything, in my opinion. Disinfection of towels and bedding is probably appropriate, particularly in a setting where there are multiple children in the household.

The therapy for impetigo probably depends as much on local bacteriology and customs as it does on anything else. It is important to know whether a large percentage of staphylococcal strains in your community are resistant to erythromycin, cephalosporins, or other antibiotics, although, as I previously mentioned, this does not usually have a great effect on therapy. It seems logical to assume that it would do so, however. Additional and follow-up laboratory evaluation also depends on community situations because in areas where I practice, nephritogenic streptococci are uncommon. It is usually not necessary to do urinalysis before and after.

Other systemic complications from impetigo are uncommon. Cellulitis may occur occasionally but usually responds well to systemic antibiotic therapy. Septicemia is also a distinctly uncommon complication. Staphylococcal scalded skin syndrome can begin with impetigo, and this obviously needs systemic therapy.

FOLLICULITIS, FURUNCULOSIS, AND CARBUNCULOSIS

Folliculitis is a term applying to a wide spectrum of diseases that begin with an infection of the hair follicle. Those that remain localized and produce only a small pustule are called folliculitis. With deeper penetration and rupture outside of the hair follicle, a tender nodule is produced that is referred to as a furuncle. When these become massive in size, and particularly when they are located on the back of the neck, they are called a carbuncle. Obviously, size, symptoms, complications, and therapy relate to the size and number of the lesions.

Simple folliculitis is a common problem and usually occurs in the more humid, covered areas of the body. It is particularly common under diapers, under tight-fitting clothing such as underwear, and in those employed in jobs that feature exposure to heat and grease. It tends to be a recurrent problem, perhaps because of re-exposure but also because of the problem of chronic nasal carriage. The risk factors are the same as for impetigo, although local trauma does not seem to play as major a role. Soaking in a contaminated whirlpool can produce a gram-negative infection ("hot tub buns," hot tub folliculitis).

Clinically, lesions range in size from small follicular pustules, to the large tender nodules of a boil (furuncle), to the large mass on the back of the neck (carbuncle). Lesions of folliculitis are more likely to produce itching; as the furuncle and carbuncle become apparent, local pain and systemic symptoms of fever and lymphadenopathy are more common. It is common to see a pattern of recurrent folliculitis and furunculosis. All varieties of this disease can feature either an indolent or an explosive course. The natural progression is from an erythematous papule to a nodule to a large mass. Most larger lesions eventually develop a pustule or a pointing core that may drain copious amounts of yellow material and result in a large scar. Folliculitis and furunculosis tend to favor the larger, softer areas of the body such as the thighs, buttocks, abdomen, and axillary area. Carbuncles are found primarily at the back of the neck, primarily because of the number of follicles and other anatomic considerations.

The diagnosis is usually based on the clinical appearance. Not all small pustules are infected by staphylococci. In fact, many diseases that feature pustules are not directly infected. A typical example is acne. Gram's stains and cultures are not usually necessary unless that patient has failed to respond to therapy or the disease is recurrent.

For patients with localized folliculitis or a few lesions of furunculosis, local treatment with topical antibiotics may be appropriate and effective. Some of the topical antibiotics used for the treatment of acne (clindamycin phosphate [Cleocin T], topical erythromycins) as well as mupirocin and local antibacterial soaps are effective both in treatment and for reducing the risk for the development of further lesions. Patients with multiple or tender nodules of furunculosis or carbunculosis should be treated with doses of systemic antibiotics that are effective against coagulase-positive *S. aureus*. Large fluctuant nodules should be incised and drained, but no lesion should be incised before it is ready. This is a traumatic, painful procedure that produces significant scarring.

If the disease is recurrent, the course of therapy should extend for a period of months rather than the 5 to 10 days typically suggested. In addition, patients with recurrent disease should have their nares treated with a topical antibiotic such as mupirocin for a few days.

CELLULITIS

Cellulitis is the least common of bacterial skin infections. It usually occurs in the setting of some local skin trauma and, for purposes of therapy and prognosis, can be divided into types that are associated with sepsis and those that are not.

Damage to the skin is the most common local risk factor. Insect bites, abrasions, surgical wounds, and chronic lymphedema are important factors in the etiology and spread of this disease. In addition, immunosuppressed patients are particularly prone to the development of cellulitis. Finally, some may have a particularly aggressive form of cellulitis, which has received a considerable amount of adverse publicity in the lay press ("flesh-eating bacteria," necrotizing fasciitis). Although cellulitis can occur in any locale, it is common on the face (where it is termed erysipelas) and on the extremities, particularly where local edema is a problem. Cellulitis accompanied by substantial pain should alert the clinician to the possibility of necrotizing fasciitis, which is a true medical and surgical emergency.

Cellulitis presents clinically as a relatively rapidly expanding, tender, red, slightly firm area of skin. Systemic signs and symptoms can be severe but most of the time are minor or not apparent. There may be an associated ascending lymphangitis, particularly if the lesion is located on the extremity. Most lesions of cellulitis occur around a local site of skin trauma, although those on the face (erysipelas) usually occur in what appears to be intact skin. It is important for the clinician to be aware that not everything that is red and warm represents cellulitis. Localized reactions to insect bites, urticaria, thermal burns, and other skin conditions can feature inflammation without cellulitis. These distinctions are usually made on clinical grounds.

A diagnosis of cellulitis is usually dependent on the history and the physical examination. Culture of the leading edge of the lesion by tissue aspiration, skin biopsies, and blood cultures are usually not appropriate unless the patient is immunosuppressed or is significantly ill. Most cellulitis is caused by streptococci, but there are some situations when staphylococci are primarily involved. In immunosuppressed patients, however, it is imperative that culture be obtained by appropriate methods. These patients sometimes have infection with unusual bacteria and fungi.

Treatment depends on the patient's condition and underlying risk factors. Asymptomatic patients (the majority of patients with erysipelas and localized cellulitis) can usually be treated with oral antibiotics. Hospitalization and the intravenous administration of antibiotics are not usually required in this situation, although they are commonly used. Patients with fever or other signs and symptoms of septicemia should be admitted to the hospital for appropriate cultures and intravenous administration of antibiotics. Cephalosporins and penicillinase-resistant penicillins are usually the drugs of choice. Patients with recurrent cellulitis should be vigorously examined for local entry sites, such as tinea pedis or chronic open sores. In these patients, long-term antibiotics, with treatment duration measured in weeks and months instead of days, are usually appropriate. The clinical lesions of cellulitis usually defervesce within 2 to 6 days except in areas of local edema, when resolution may take weeks.

Complications are uncommon unless the cellulitis is accompanied by sepsis.

VIRAL DISEASES OF THE SKIN

method of
STEPHEN K. TYRING, M.D., Ph.D.
University of Texas Medical Branch
Galveston, Texas

Whereas many families of viruses produce lesions of the skin, the clinical manifestations of three of these families are usually limited to the skin and mucous membranes. These virus families include most herpesviruses as well as papillomaviruses and poxviruses. Twenty-six antiviral drugs have received Food and Drug Administration (FDA) approval thus far, and many are used in therapy for viral diseases of the skin and mucous membranes. However, treatment of most viral lesions of the skin is mainly symptomatic.

HERPESVIRUSES

When the word "herpes" is used, one often thinks of genital herpes or cold sores. It is true that both conditions are due to infection with the herpes simplex virus (HSV), but the human herpesvirus (HHV) family actually comprises eight members, seven of which are closely associated with human disease. In fact, the herpesviruses are so common that almost everyone in the United States has been infected and affected by them. These seven herpesviruses are (1) HSV-1, most often associated with cold sores; (2) HSV-2, most often associated with genital herpes; (3) varicella-zoster virus (VZV), the cause of both chickenpox and shingles; (4) Epstein-Barr virus, the cause of infectious mononucleosis; (5) cytomegalovirus, which is associated with certain birth defects and is a frequent cause of eye disease, including blindness, in patients with acquired immune deficiency syndrome (AIDS); (6) herpesvirus 6, the cause of roseola, a usually mild childhood disease; and (7) HHV-8, which has been closely associated with Kaposi's sarcoma both in patients seropositive for the human immunodeficiency virus and in patients with classic Kaposi's sarcoma. Although presence of HHV-8 DNA as well as antibodies to HHV-8 correlates closely with the presence of Kaposi's sarcoma and with the risk of developing Kaposi's sarcoma, HHV-8 has not yet been proved definitively as the cause of this tumor. The following discussion focuses on the HSV and VZV.

Herpes Simplex Viruses

In general, HSV-1 and HSV-2 are found at different sites in the body, with HSV-1 responsible for at least 90% of cold sores and HSV-2 causing at least 90% of recurrent genital herpes. The remaining cases of cold sores and genital herpes are associated with HSV-2 and HSV-1, respectively. The initial infection with either type of HSV can be the most disabling, with widespread blistering of the body site associated with severe discomfort and a healing time of 3 to 4 weeks (without therapy). Often, however, a person's first symptomatic episode is not a true primary infection because the virus may already have been in the body for an extended time. Recurrences are usually less severe but still bothersome, and lesions usually heal in less than 2 weeks without therapy. The majority of persons who are infected with either HSV-1 or HSV-2 have no symptoms, although the virus can hide in the person's body, specifically in one or more nerves. Although not everyone who has a primary (initial) outbreak of herpes will have a recurrence, the average number of recurrences in the year after primary genital infection with HSV-2 is four episodes. In contrast, the number of recurrences in the

year after primary genital infection with HSV-1 is only one episode. Antibodies to HSV-1 and HSV-2 can be found in millions of adults who deny ever having had an outbreak of cold sores or genital herpes.

Clinical manifestations of HSV infection usually progress from a prodrome of burning and tingling to erythema, then blisters, then ulcers, then crusts, and finally healing. What triggers an outbreak of herpes is not always clear, but it often follows some type of emotional or physical stress, which can be intense sunlight exposure for cold sores or menstruation for genital herpes or for herpes labialis in women. However, the triggering event is often not known. In persons whose immune systems are impaired, such as with cancer, with AIDS, or in organ transplant patients, episodes of HSV infection can be chronic in that one recurrence does not completely heal before the next recurrence starts.

Whereas HSV infection in otherwise healthy persons can be uncomfortable, the effects are usually temporary. In contrast, genital herpes in a pregnant woman can result in birth defects or even death of the infant. In the past, HSV-2 was thought to be responsible for cervical cancer. However, another virus, the human papillomavirus (HPV), is now believed to be primarily responsible for this cancer, although HSV-2 may still act as a "helper virus."

HSV infection is not restricted to the mouth and genitalia; both HSV-1 and HSV-2 can affect any site on the body. Herpetic infection of the eyes can be severe, resulting in impaired vision or even blindness if it is not treated. Although it is a rare occurrence, HSV can also infect the brain, producing herpes encephalitis, a potentially fatal condition. In addition, HSV-1 has been associated with Bell's palsy. The majority of cases of herpesvirus infections are transmitted by asymptomatic viral shedding. Although this route of transmission was suspected for a number of years, studies have demonstrated that HSV-2 can be frequently cultured from the anogenital areas of women with histories of recurrent genital herpes even in the absence of any signs or symptoms of recurrence.

Treatment

The time of healing of herpetic lesions can be markedly shortened by antiviral therapy, and in fact, some episodes can be totally prevented if therapy is initiated early enough during the prodromal phase or if daily suppressive therapy is given to those individuals who have frequent recurrences. Whereas a number of antiherpes drugs are available, such as idoxuridine (Herplex, Stoxil), trifluridine (Viroptic), and vidarabine (Vira-A), the first safe, systemic, and effective antiherpes drug was acyclovir (Zovirax), which is available as a cream, a capsule, and an intravenous preparation (Table 1). Both oral and intravenous forms of acyclovir are highly effective, but neither acyclovir nor any other drug has been demonstrated to rid the body of HSV. Acyclovir is safe, rarely producing any side effects. It is activated by thymidine kinase produced by the virus and there-

TABLE 1. **Treatment of Herpesvirus Infections**

Herpes Simplex Viruses			Varicella-Zoster Virus	
		Acyclovir* NORMAL HOSTS		
Treatment			Treatment	
Initial Episode 200 mg PO 5 times/d × 10 d (or 400 mg PO tid), or 5 mg/kg IV q 8 h × 5–10 d, or 5% ointment topically qid × 7 d†	*Recurrent Episode* 200 mg PO 5 times/d ×5 d (or 400 mg PO tid)	Suppression 400 mg PO bid	*Primary Varicella: Children* 20 mg/kg PO qid × 5 d (maximal dose, 800 mg PO qid)	*Herpes Zoster* 800 mg PO 5 times/d × 7–10 d
			Primary Varicella: Adults 800 mg PO 5 times/d × 7–10 d	
		IMMUNOCOMPROMISED PATIENTS		
200–400 mg PO 5 times/d × 7 (recurrence) or 10 (initial) d, or 5 mg/kg IV q 8 h × 7–10 d,‡ or 5% ointment topically qid × 7 d†		≥400 mg PO bid	10 mg/kg IV q 8 h × 7–10 d§	10 mg/kg IV q 8 h × 7–10 d
		Famciclovir NORMAL HOSTS		
Treatment			Treatment *Herpes Zoster*	
Initial Episode 250 mg PO tid × 10 d	*Recurrent Episode* 125 mg PO bid × 5 d	Suppression 250 mg PO bid	500 mg PO tid × 7 d	
		Valacyclovir NORMAL HOSTS		
Treatment			Treatment *Herpes Zoster*	
Initial Episode 1 gm PO bid × 10 d	*Recurrent Episode* 500 mg PO bid × 5 d	Suppression 500 mg PO qd	1 gm PO tid × 7 d	

*Doses of acyclovir are for adults with normal renal function unless otherwise noted.
†Less effective than the oral or the intravenous routes; topical therapy should be used only for minor outbreaks.
‡A dose of 250 mg/m² of body surface area should be given to children younger than 12 y.
§A dose of 500 mg/m² of body surface area should be given to children younger than 12 y.

fore works only where it is needed, i.e., in cells infected by HSV. In addition to the fact that it is a treatment and not a cure, the primary drawbacks to the use of acyclovir are its low bioavailability and the need for frequent dosing. Five 200-mg capsules a day are recommended to treat a recurrence, although many patients find that one 400-mg tablet three times daily (tid) is more convenient and equally effective. One 400-mg tablet twice daily (bid) is recommended for prophylaxis in recurrence-prone individuals.

Two new treatments for herpes simplex have recently become available, famciclovir (Famvir) and valacyclovir (Valtrex). These drugs have higher bioavailability than does acyclovir and require infrequent dosing. For the treatment of recurrent genital herpes, famciclovir is taken 125 mg orally bid for 5 days (see Table 1). Therapy for first-episode genital herpes with famciclovir uses 250 mg orally tid for 10 days. Suppression of recurrent genital herpes requires famciclovir 250 mg orally bid.

Valacyclovir is taken 500 mg orally bid for 5 days to treat an episode of recurrent genital herpes. First-episode genital herpes can be effectively treated with valacyclovir 1 gram orally bid for 10 days. Vala-cyclovir 500 mg orally once daily can effectively suppress recurrent genital herpes in most patients. Vaccines for prophylaxis and treatment of HSV as well as other antiherpes drugs are currently under investigation.

Varicella-Zoster Virus

VZV is a unique herpesvirus in that it causes two different diseases, chickenpox and shingles (also known as herpes zoster). Chickenpox is highly contagious and can be spread by airborne droplets, sneezing, or coughing. In children, chickenpox is usually not a severe disease and resolves in 2 to 3 weeks in otherwise healthy persons. In some adults and in children with impaired immunity, however, chickenpox can be a serious and potentially fatal disease. Whereas symptomatic treatment is usually sufficient in most children, chickenpox in persons with cancer, AIDS, and other immunodeficient states requires antiviral therapy (e.g., acyclovir).

When the skin lesions of chickenpox heal, the virus remains latent in a cranial nerve ganglion or in the dorsal root of a spinal nerve and can later reappear to produce a completely different disease, shingles (herpes zoster). Shingles affects approximately 20% of persons at some time in their lives. It is more common in persons older than 50 years, but it can be seen in persons of any age, and it is not uncommon in younger individuals with impaired immunity. The skin lesions of shingles appear first as erythema, then vesicles, and then pustules, which finally progress to crusts that fall off after 3 to 4 weeks. These skin lesions follow the distribution of a single nerve and are therefore seen only on one side of the body, often the trunk, but sometimes on the arm, leg, or face. If the nerves that supply the eye are affected, partial or total loss of vision can result if shingles is not treated.

Although shingles is caused by the same virus, it is much less contagious than chickenpox. A person who has never had chickenpox can develop this disease after direct contact with the skin lesions of a person with shingles. Shingles, however, cannot be passed from one person to another, because it develops only from a reactivation of latent VZV in the nervous system of a person who has had chickenpox.

Treatment

Acyclovir is FDA approved for the treatment of chickenpox and herpes zoster, but antiviral therapy is not always indicated in otherwise healthy persons with these conditions. When acyclovir is used for therapy of VZV infections, however, the dosage must be significantly higher than that for treatment of HSV infections. Specifically, acyclovir, 800 mg orally five times per day for 7 to 10 days, is necessary for treatment of herpes zoster or of chickenpox in adults. If the patient is severely immunocompromised or otherwise requires intravenous therapy, the recommended dosage is 10 mg of acyclovir per kg of body weight tid. Acyclovir cream has no proven efficacy in treatment of VZV infections. Systemic acyclovir is clearly indicated for VZV infections in immunocompromised patients, for chickenpox in adults, and for shingles in patients older than 50 years. It is important to treat VZV infections as early in the course as possible because starting acyclovir after the third day of development of vesicles has questionable benefits.

Both famciclovir and valacyclovir are approved for the treatment of shingles. With dosing three times daily, both agents are more convenient than is acyclovir: famciclovir 500 mg orally tid or valacyclovir 1 gram orally tid (each for 7 days).

Because disseminated zoster is rare, the usual reason for treating shingles is to shorten the duration of postherpetic neuralgia (PHN). Acyclovir is of only modest benefit in decreasing PHN. Prednisone was widely used for decreasing PHN before the availability of acyclovir but is associated with more side effects. Two studies compared the efficacies of acyclovir or prednisone (or prednisolone) with those of the drugs in combination. Both studies demonstrated that this combination produced no greater benefits regarding PHN than did acyclovir monotherapy, but one investigation demonstrated that acyclovir plus prednisone yielded added benefits for certain quality of life parameters. Although PHN is more easily prevented than treated, therapy can be undertaken with analgesics, antidepressants (e.g., amitriptyline [Elavil]*), substance P inhibitors (capsaicin [Zostrix]), and nerve blocks. A VZV vaccine widely used in Japan and Europe became available in the United States for prophylaxis of chickenpox in 1995.

HUMAN PAPILLOMAVIRUSES

More than 80 HPV types have been identified. Members of the HPV family have not been successfully grown in tissue culture, but HPV types can be distinguished by DNA hybridization. Some HPV types are common, whereas others are extremely rare. One or more of approximately 18 different papillomaviruses can be found in epidermodysplasia verruciformis, which is a rare condition, but most of these HPV types are not found in other clinical settings. A limited number of HPV types are associated with a high rate of malignant conversion to squamous cell carcinoma when infected skin is exposed to ultraviolet light (e.g., sunlight). More common HPV infections can be divided into anogenital and nonanogenital types.

Anogenital HPV Infections

These HPV types can be classified as having low malignant potential (e.g., HPV-6 and HPV-11), intermediate malignant potential (e.g., HPV-31, HPV-33, and HPV-35), and high malignant potential (e.g., HPV-16 and HPV-18). Types 6 and 11 are responsible for venereal warts, condylomata acuminata, which is considered the most common viral sexually transmitted disease. These warts can present as verrucous, flat, or pedunculated papules on the skin and mucous membranes. In addition to being a cosmetic problem, they can produce large cauliflower-like lesions that are painful and malodorous, bleed easily, and can block the passage of body fluids. Not only can genital warts make sexual intercourse difficult, they can actually grow so large during pregnancy that they can interfere with vaginal delivery.

Treatment

Initial therapy for genital warts is usually symptomatic, involving chemotherapeutic and cytodestructive techniques. Chemotherapeutic agents include dichloroacetic acid, trichloroacetic acid, 5-fluorouracil cream, and podofilox (podophyllotoxin, Condylox). The last-named agent is the active ingredient in the crude resin podophyllin, which was widely used in the past but has toxic potential, contains mutagens, and lacks reproducible clinical results. The reproducible clinical activity and low toxicity of podofilox have made it the chemotherapeutic agent of choice for many physicians.

Cytodestructive treatment of genital warts in-

---

*Not FDA approved for this indication.

cludes cryotherapy using such agents as liquid nitrogen. Surgical therapies include simple excision, laser surgery, and electrosurgery.

Until recently, the only antiviral drugs approved for treatment of genital warts were interferon alfa-2b (Intron A) and interferon alfa-n3 (Alferon N), which have been demonstrated to eliminate more than 70% of genital warts when they are used intralesionally or subcutaneously (locally). A mild flulike syndrome is often seen after the first injection of interferon, but almost all patients develop tolerance to side effects by the second or third in a series of injections. Although the recurrence rate of genital warts after clearing with interferon is usually less than that after nonantiviral therapy, the clinical response with interferon therapy is often slower than with other therapies. Therefore, interferon has not become a popular treatment for genital warts owing to (1) the fact that it must be given by injection, (2) the potential for systemic side effects, and (3) its expense. In large lesions, interferon may not be effective as monotherapy.

Interferon is most efficacious in combination with nonantiviral therapy. For example, with smaller genital warts, the patient can self-administer topical podofilox twice daily for 3 days, stop therapy for 4 days, and then repeat the cycle as necessary. During the same period, the patient can simultaneously receive local subcutaneous interferon therapy two or three times per week. Alternatively, large or numerous genital warts can be surgically removed and the area treated with local subcutaneous interferon to reduce the recurrence rate. Either combination should result in a rapid response due to the nonantiviral therapy and a low recurrence rate due to the interferon treatment.

More convenient and potentially more effective antiviral therapies should be available by prescription in the near future. Imiquimod (Aldara) is an inducer of endogenous interferon as well as a spectrum of immune-enhancing cytokines. It is applied topically by the patient as a 5% cream (three times per week) to the genital warts. It was proved to be highly effective in otherwise healthy patients and is associated with a low recurrence rate. Systemic side effects are rare; local inflammation is usually mild to moderate and well tolerated by almost all patients. Imiquimod was approved by the FDA in March 1997 for treatment of external anogenital warts.

A second antiviral agent under investigation for genital warts is cidofovir, which inhibits viral DNA polymerase. Cidofovir has been effective as a 3% topical gel in clearing warts in AIDS patients. Although it produces local inflammation, it has not been associated with systemic side effects. Cidofovir has not yet been evaluated in otherwise healthy persons with condylomata acuminata.

Nonanogenital HPV Infections

The most common HPV-related lesions outside of the anogenital area include plantar warts (HPV-1), verruca vulgaris (common warts, HPV-2), and flat warts (HPV-3). Aside from their appearance and their potential for infectivity, most warts are asymptomatic except when located on weight-bearing surfaces. Plantar warts can make standing or walking uncomfortable.

Treatment

Neither interferon nor any other antiviral drug is approved for treatment of nongenital warts, although a few case reports suggest that interferon may have some efficacy against these warts. Standard therapy for nongenital warts includes salicylic or lactic acid, keratolytic compounds, cantharidin, liquid nitrogen, electrosurgery, and sometimes even laser surgery. Cimetidine appeared effective in one study but was no better than placebo in another investigation.

POXVIRUSES

The only poxvirus infection commonly seen today is molluscum contagiosum, in which 4- to 6-mm smooth papules with a central umbilication can present as a (usually) non–sexually transmitted disease on any part of the body in children and as a (usually) sexually transmitted disease on the genitalia of adults. A much more aggressive presentation of molluscum contagiosum has become more frequent recently because of the prevalence of AIDS. Molluscum lesions can cover much of the body surface in AIDS patients. Less common diseases due to poxviruses include orf and milker's nodules, which are occasionally seen on the hands of persons who work with sheep and cattle. Both diseases may be due to the same virus, which produces nodules, tender plaques, or abscesses but no systemic symptoms.

Treatment

Therapy for molluscum contagiosum in non-immunocompromised patients is usually simple and can involve such procedures as expressing the molluscum body from an incised papule or use of liquid nitrogen with or without curettage. Because AIDS patients often have many thousands of molluscum papules, the success of such simple destructive therapies for them is limited. Interferon alfa* therapy is effective in eradicating molluscum contagiosum in non-immunocompromised patients but has limited usefulness in AIDS patients. Self-administered topical application of podofilox, however, is fairly effective even in AIDS patients. When podofilox is combined with systemic interferon, the clinical effects are often additive to synergistic. A much more convenient and effective therapy, however, for molluscum contagiosum in AIDS patients is topical use of cidofovir gel, which is currently undergoing clinical studies for this indication.

No specific antiviral therapy exists for orf or milker's nodules, but none is needed because both conditions spontaneously resolve in 3 to 4 weeks.

---

*Not FDA approved for this indication.

PARASITIC DISEASES OF THE SKIN

method of
W. P. DANIEL SU, M.D.

Mayo Clinic and Mayo Foundation and Mayo Medical School
Rochester, Minnesota

MYIASIS

With increased travel to tropical countries, physicians should be familiar with myiasis. Myiasis may be produced by the invasion of human tissue by Diptera larvae. Eggs or larvae are deposited in the skin, mucous membranes, or open wounds, and larvae burrow into the skin and subcutaneous tissue, causing inflammation. Various fly larvae can cause myiasis, which occurs most commonly in immigrants or travelers from tropical climates such as South and Central America and tropical Africa.

The human botfly *Dermatobia hominis* is a common cause of furuncular myiasis. Diagnosis is made by finding larvae in the opening of erythematous nodules or ulcerations.

Treatment

Treatment involves physical removal of the larvae and wound care. If the larvae cannot be removed readily with forceps, the larval opening to the skin should be covered with petrolatum (Vaseline), which causes the larvae to migrate externally seeking air. Chloroform or ether can also be used if the larvae can be reached with forceps. After the larvae are removed, the wound is irrigated and treated with antibiotic dressings. The patient should be observed for about 2 weeks, and any newly hatched larvae in the wound should be removed. Physical removal of the larvae and prevention of secondary bacterial infection usually result in complete resolution of myiasis.

SCABIES

Scabies is a disease that affects all age groups and socioeconomic classes. The scabies mite *Sarcoptes scabiei* is spread by close contact and may be found among family members, playmates, and other close contacts. The female mite burrows into the stratum corneum and deposits her eggs. Larvae emerge in 3 to 5 days and mature in about 2 weeks. The mite may continue to live in the stratum corneum for as long as 2 months. Mites are dependent on their hosts for survival, but they have been found to survive for as many as 3 days on clothing, bedding, or furniture without a host.

Initially, the infestation may be asymptomatic for as long as 1 month. Sensitization and pruritus then develop in response to the scabies mite or to its scybala (feces); pruritus is generally worse at night. Cutaneous lesions include papules, excoriations, and burrows. Vesicles are seen more often in children and infants. Burrows are identified as short (<1 mm), white, linear lesions that are often on an erythematous papular base. A black speck at the end of the burrow indicates the mite. Lesions characteristically involve the interdigital spaces, volar surface of the wrists, elbows, axillary folds, areolae, buttocks, umbilicus, and genitals. Lesions on the head and neck are rare in adults but may be seen in infants.

Typically, 6 to 12 adult mites are present in a patient with scabies. Norwegian, or crusted, scabies, in which several hundred mites are present, represents a rare florid form of the disease. It is more common in immunocompromised patients, such as those with acquired immune deficiency syndrome (AIDS), and in people who are institutionalized. These patients have generalized crusted eczematous lesions that may involve the face and fingernails.

Scabies can be diagnosed by examination of skin shavings. A No. 15 scalpel blade is used to scrape the stratum corneum from a typical burrow onto a glass slide. This scraping is best done in a fresh lesion that has not been excoriated. Often, multiple lesions need to be scraped. A drop of oil and a coverslip are put on the slide, which is then examined with a 10× objective. The presence of a mature mite, eggs, or scybala establishes the diagnosis of scabies.

Treatment

The treatment of scabies is simple and effective. Because the initial phase is asymptomatic, family members and close contacts should also be treated, even if they do not have clinical evidence of infestation. Bed sheets and clothing should be laundered because the most common cause of treatment failure is reinfection. Treatment kills the scabies mite but does not remove the mite or scybala from the stratum corneum. Thus, continued pruritus can be expected for 2 to 4 weeks, until the dead mites are shed with the stratum corneum. The pruritus can be treated with topical steroids or antipruritic medication.

Treatment with lindane (γ-benzene hexachloride [Kwell]) 1% lotion has been the mainstay of therapy for scabies and has a cure rate of 95 to 98%. The lotion should be applied from the neck down (taking care to include the web spaces and intertriginous areas), left on the skin overnight, and washed off with soap and water the next morning. The face and scalp should also be treated in children and in adults with Norwegian scabies. It is advisable for the patient to be treated again in 5 to 7 days. Although the safety and efficacy of lindane have been established by its use worldwide, there are reports that it has a neurotoxic effect. However, these cases are rare and involve patients who were overtreated. Nonetheless, lindane is not advised for treatment of pregnant women, nursing mothers, or infants.

Precipitated sulfur 6% in petrolatum is the treatment of choice for infants and pregnant women or nursing mothers. It should be applied daily for 3 consecutive days without being removed. The patient should not bathe during the treatment. The entire body should be treated in infants because the head and neck are often involved.

Crotamiton (Eurax) 10% cream is an antiscabietic medication that has antipruritic effects. However, it has poor ovicidal activity and, thus, a lower success rate. It must be applied daily for 3 to 5 consecutive days without removal.

Patients with scabies may become secondarily infected. The secondary impetiginization and residual pruritus should also be treated. Infection may be treated with topical antibiotic ointments or appropriate oral antibiotic medications that have anti-staphylococcal and antistreptococcal activity. The pruritus may be treated with antihistamines given orally and with corticosteroids applied topically. Complete resolution of the pruritus may require 2 to 4 weeks.

Permethrin (Elimite) 5% cream is a newer antiscabietic medication that is as effective as lindane. Permethrin can be used with a single application. It is applied, left on overnight, and washed off with soap and water the next morning. Because permethrin is not associated with any neurotoxic effect, it is useful for treating infants who are older than 2 months. The head should also be treated. I prefer permethrin rather than lindane in children. Permethrin has not been approved by the Food and Drug Administration for use in pregnant patients, but it is a better choice than lindane if the treatment is necessary in these patients. For other adults and older children, one must keep in mind that lindane lotion is usually effective, safe when used as directed, and considerably less expensive than permethrin cream.

PEDICULOSIS

The insects of the Anoplura order can cause the infestation called pediculosis in humans. The three organisms of dermatologic importance are *Phthirus pubis* (pubic louse or crab louse), *Pediculus humanus corporis* (body louse), and *Pediculus humanus capitis* (head louse). The diagnosis is made by finding the lice or nits by examination with a $10 \times$ hand lens. The eggs (nits) of the pubic and head lice are attached to the hair shafts, whereas those of the body lice are laid in the clothing. The nits remain viable for as long as 1 month. After they hatch, they develop into adults in 2 to 3 weeks. Adult lice live for as long as 1 month on the host but die within a few days without feeding. All of these organisms are transmitted by physical contact; therefore, people who have had close contact with the patient should be evaluated and treated. Clothing and bedding should be professionally laundered or laundered in hot water and dried in the hot cycle of the clothes dryer. Pruritus is common in all forms of pediculosis and is often the presenting symptom. It resolves in days to weeks with treatment.

Head lice are found on the scalp, behind the ears, and on the posterior aspect of the neck. Infestation is common among school-age children. Often, a lack of good hygiene is not a factor. Nits, or eggs, appear as whitish nodules tightly adherent to the hair shaft. When the hair is combed, a characteristic metallic sound is made as the comb strikes the nits. Nits are laid at the base of the hair shaft. Because the hair grows at a rate of 1 cm per month, the length of infestation can be estimated by the distance of the nit from the scalp. Adult lice may be seen moving in the scalp.

Treatment

Single treatment with permethrin 1% (Nix) has a 98% cure rate. This medication is formulated in a cream-rinse base and should be applied to the hair and scalp for 10 minutes after shampooing and then rinsed out. Adverse reactions are rare. Pyrethrins (RID) and lindane 1% shampoo can also be used in a similar fashion but should be reapplied after 7 days because they have poor ovicidal activity. After a single treatment with RID, as many as 25 to 30% of the residual ova may hatch. Residual egg casings (nits) can be removed with a fine-toothed comb or fine forceps. Combs and brushes should be soaked in hot water or a pediculicidal shampoo.

Pubic lice may affect pubic, body, and axillary hair; the eyelashes; and the posterior aspect of the scalp. Anogenital pruritus is often the presenting symptom. Nits can be seen attached to hairs, and slow-moving lice can be identified as 1- to 2-mm crawling insects clinging to the hairs or attached to the skin. Pubic lice are often sexually transmitted but can be transferred from infected towels or bedding. Lindane 1% cream is the treatment of choice for pubic lice; it is applied to the affected areas for 10 minutes and washed off with soap and water. Treatment should be repeated in 7 days. Permethrin 5% cream can be used in a similar fashion. Scalp, beard, and axillary hair and the eyelashes should also be inspected. Eyelash involvement can be treated by removing the nits with fine forceps, by applying petrolatum to the eyelashes three to five times daily for 1 week, or by applying physostigmine (Eserine)* 0.25% ophthalmic ointment three to five times daily for 3 days.

Body lice are most common among people who live under poor conditions, for example, street people and refugees from war or natural disasters. *P. humanus corporis* is the vector for several human diseases, including typhus (*Rickettsia prowazekii*), louse-borne relapsing fever (*Borrelia recurrentis*), and trench fever (*Rochalimaea quintana*). The lice and eggs are found in the seams of clothing. Adult lice feed on covered areas of the skin, such as the waistline, neckline, and trunk, and produce papular, erythematous, macular, and urticarial lesions. Pruritus and secondary infection are common. Treatment requires improving the patient's environment. Clothing should be placed in a plastic bag for incineration or laundered with hot water and dried in a hot clothes dryer for at least half an hour. Nonwashable personal items should be dry-cleaned or sealed in a plastic bag for

---

*Not FDA approved for this indication.

10 days. The pruritus can be treated with topical corticosteroids.

CREEPING ERUPTION (LARVA MIGRANS)

The nematode larvae of *Ancylostoma braziliense*, dog and cat hookworm, is the most common organism causing cutaneous larva migrans, which is characterized by twisting, winding linear skin lesions produced by burrowing larvae. Infection occurs when humans come in contact with soil infected by contaminated dog or cat feces. Outdoor workers and children walking barefoot or playing in the sand are infected in endemic areas, commonly tropical regions. The larvae penetrate the epidermis. This infection produces erythematous papules and, 1 to 2 days later, pruritic, slowly progressive, serpiginous burrows, which commonly involve the feet, interdigital toe webs, knees, buttocks, and hands.

Treatment

Because humans are an unnatural host, the disease is often self-limited and resolves in 1 to 3 months. A patient with few lesions can be treated with electrocautery or cryotherapy. Care must be taken to treat the leading edge of the burrow, where the larvae are located. Patients with many lesions can be treated with thiabendazole (Mintezol) (500 mg per 5-mL suspension) applied to the burrows three times daily until the lesions resolve. For patients with numerous lesions, thiabendazole (25 mg per kg per day) may be given orally for 2 consecutive days. Side effects include dizziness, anorexia, nausea, vomiting, and diarrhea. A single 400-mg dose of albendazole (Albenza) given orally has also been shown to be effective.

STRONGYLOIDIASIS (LARVA CURRENS)

Strongyloides stercoralis (the dwarf threadworm) has a worldwide distribution. It is found in soil, in humans, and in at least 1% of dogs in the eastern United States.

Immunodeficiency states, as in recipients of organ transplants, in patients receiving corticosteroids, and occasionally in patients with AIDS, can result in hyperinfection syndrome and its high mortality. These patients, when infected with *Strongyloides*, are also more susceptible to bacterial infections and recurrent sepsis. The larva migrates with the bacteria either adherent to its surface or within its lumen.

Chronic urticaria, abdominal cramping, and diarrhea are classic symptoms of strongyloidiasis. Recurrent dyspnea and wheezing are common. Some patients may be asymptomatic, and fatigue or malabsorption may be the only clues to the diagnosis.

The cutaneous lesions of strongyloidiasis are produced by the moving larvae on the skin, which migrate rapidly, thus the term "larva currens." Larva currens occurs mostly on the trunk and perianal skin. It is a linear or papular migrating (10 cm per hour) urticarial pruritic rash with crops on the abdomen, groin, buttocks, thighs, back, and chest.

In disseminated disease, larvae can be found in most organs. In an immunocompromised host, one must be alert to the presence of a periumbilical petechial or purpuric rash. The parasite is readily found in biopsy specimens of these skin and extracutaneous lesions.

Treatment

Thiabendazole has been used to treat strongyloidiasis. The recommended dosage in uncomplicated cases has been 25 mg per kg twice daily for 2 days taken after meals and repeated after 1 week. For immunocompromised patients, continuous treatment for 5 to 15 days may be necessary.

The treatment preferred by the World Health Organization is albendazole, 400 mg daily for 3 days for adults and children older than 2 years. Albendazole is teratogenic and has not been approved for use by the Food and Drug Administration.

Toxic symptoms are frequent. Thiabendazole may cause vomiting, dizziness, headache, delirium, pruritus, and malodorous urine. It may also cause hyperglycemia, hypotension, liver dysfunction, and hypersensitivity reactions.

Concomitant administration of theophylline may result in severe vomiting associated with higher blood levels of the drug. Mebendazole (Vermox),* has been used (1.5 grams daily for 14 days).† It has few unpleasant side effects and has been given safely in massive doses, but its effect in resistant cases is uncertain.

---

*Not FDA approved for this indication.
†Exceeds dosage recommended by the manufacturer.

FUNGAL DISEASES OF THE SKIN

method of
EDGAR B. SMITH, M.D.
University of Texas Medical Branch
Galveston, Texas

The superficial fungal infections, dermatophytosis, candidiasis, and tinea versicolor, are common and frequently lead to both self-treatment with over-the-counter agents and visits to physicians. All of these conditions are due to organisms that invade the outermost layer of the epidermis, the stratum corneum, and produce varying degrees of inflammation in the underlying cutaneous structures. Although these infections often have typical clinical features, they may be simulated by other inflammatory skin diseases. Therefore, mycologic confirmation with potassium hydroxide preparation or culture, or both, should always be sought to ensure most effective management. This principle is even more important now that effective but expensive agents are available for treatment of infections of the nails.

DERMATOPHYTOSIS

The dermatophytes are a class of fungi that live in the stratum corneum of humans or animals and in soil. Although there are many species, most infections in the United States are due to five species: *Trichophyton rubrum, Trichophyton tonsurans, Trichophyton mentagrophytes, Microsporum canis,* and *Epidermophyton floccosum.* Clinical manifestations of the infection vary somewhat with the causative organism but more with the site of infection and the host inflammatory response.

Dermatophytosis of the scalp, tinea capitis, is the most common fungal infection of children and is most commonly due to *T. tonsurans.* This organism invades the hair shaft and produces spores within the hair (endothrix infection). It does not produce fluorescence on Wood's light examination. Clinical findings can vary from slight scaling suggestive of seborrheic dermatitis to classic ringworm with scalping patches or plaques with broken hairs to kerion formation with marked edema and the presence of exudate. It is common to find infection in other family members, and examination and treatment of all in the household are recommended. In Europe and in some cities of the United States, the most common cause of scalp infections is *M. canis,* which normally infects dogs and cats. This organism is more likely to produce classic scalp ringworm and does cause fluorescence of hairs on Wood's light examination. Dermatophytosis of the scalp should be treated with oral ultramicronized griseofulvin (Gris-PEG, Fulvicin, Grisactin), 10 to 15 mg per kg per day in either a single dose or divided doses for 6 to 8 weeks. Patients who cannot tolerate griseofulvin or fail to respond should be treated with oral ketoconazole (Nizoral), 200 mg per day for the same length of time. Topical therapy is not effective, but frequent washing with povidone-iodine (Betadine), selenium sulfide (Selsun, Exsel), or ketoconazole shampoos reduces the spread of infectious spores.

Dermatophytosis of nonhairy skin, or tinea corporis, is characterized by scaling patches or plaques with sharp margins. Infections due to *M. canis* frequently result in multiple lesions and tend to be more inflammatory. Chronic infections, which can be extensive, are most commonly due to *T. rubrum.* Tinea cruris (infection of the inguinal folds) occurs frequently in athletes or those who work outdoors in hot, humid climates and is commonly due to *T. rubrum* or *E. floccosum.* Tinea cruris and solitary lesions respond well to topical treatment with any of the imidazoles (clotrimazole [Mycelex], miconazole [Micatin, Monistat], econazole [Spectazole], ketoconazole, oxiconazole [Oxistat], sulconazole [Exelderm]), the allylamines (naftifine [Naftin], terbinafine [Lamisil]), or ciclopirox olamine (Loprox). Oral griseofulvin, ultramicronized, 500 mg two times a day for 4 to 6 weeks, is the treatment of choice for extensive infec-

tions or those due to multiple inoculations. Griseofulvin-resistant infections due to *T. rubrum* are a growing problem, and oral ketoconazole, 200 to 400 mg per day, should be given. Infections resistant to both griseofulvin and ketoconazole have responded to topical naftifine or terbinafine; the new oral agents itraconazole (Sporanox), 200 mg twice daily for 1 week, and terbinafine, 250 mg daily for 1 month, have been reported to be effective, although these drugs have not yet been approved by the Food and Drug Administration (FDA) for this indication.

The most common dermatophyte infections in adults are those of the feet and nails. There are three variants of tinea pedis: the interdigital type, with scaling and itching of the webs between the toes; the inflammatory type, with vesicles involving the toes or the instep (most commonly due to *T. mentagrophytes*); and the plantar hyperkeratotic variety (like the interdigital type, usually due to *T. rubrum*), with slight redness and itching but marked thickening and scaling of the skin of the sole. Dermatophytes do not commonly cause infections of the hands, but when they do, they produce chronic disease of the palmar skin and are usually unilateral. The common toe web infections and the inflammatory form usually respond well to topical treatment for 4 to 6 weeks with the imidazole, allylamine, or ciclopirox creams mentioned earlier. Recurrences are common and require either intermittent therapy or prophylactic use of an antifungal powder (tolnaftate [Tinactin] or undecylenic acid [Desenex]). Chronic infections should be treated with either oral griseofulvin or ketoconazole. The topical allylamines naftifine and terbinafine are often effective in the more resistant infections, and the new oral agents itraconazole and terbinafine, although not yet FDA approved for infections of the feet, are effective in the same dose schedules as for tinea corporis.

Dermatophytosis of the nails (onychomycosis, or tinea unguium) is common (especially toenail infections) and often responds poorly to treatment. The most common form is distal subungual onychomycosis, which is usually due to *T. rubrum* and is characterized by separation of the nail from the nail bed, subungual scaling and thickening, and white to brown discoloration of the nail. Infections of the fingernails respond reasonably well (60 to 70%) to oral ultramicronized griseofulvin, 500 mg two times a day for 6 to 8 months, but the cure rate for toenails is poor even with up to 24 months of therapy and avulsion of the nails. Frequent clipping and filing of the infected nail, with application of a topical allylamine (naftifine or terbinafine) twice daily after bathing or after brief soaking in warm water, will sometimes result in a cure. However, the recent approval of itraconazole and terbinafine for nail infections due to dermatophytes now allows much more effective therapy. Itraconazole should be given either 200 mg daily for 3 months or as the equally effective but more economical pulse dose schedule, 200 mg twice daily for the first week of the month for 3 months. The section of the package insert regarding drug interactions should be consulted and patients specifically warned to avoid terfenadine (Seldane), astemizole (Hismanal), and cisapride (Propulsid). Terbinafine is given at a dose of 250 mg daily for 3 months. Published studies suggest that fluconazole (Diflucan) may also be effective, but optimal dosing schedules have not been determined. The less frequent superficial white onychomycosis due to *T. mentagrophytes* is exhibited as white spots on the dorsum of the nail plate. The condition responds well to any of the topical antifungal agents. Proximal subungual onychomycosis, with whitish discoloration of the proximal nail, occurs most frequently in persons who have human immunodeficiency virus disease or who are otherwise immunosuppressed, and the condition usually clears with correction of the immune problem and use of oral griseofulvin.

CANDIDIASIS

Cutaneous candidiasis is usually due to *Candida albicans*, a yeast normally found in the gastrointestinal tract. The most common forms of infection involve the inguinal folds, perineum, and perianal and vaginal areas and are characterized by redness, superficial erosion, and itching or pain in the skinfolds. Typically, satellite papules, pustules, or scaling macules occur around the borders of the larger patches. Other skinfolds can be involved. Although candidiasis is a common cause of disease of the inguinal folds in healthy athletes and those whose work produces excessive sweating, predisposing factors such as obesity, diabetes, immunosuppression, oral contraceptives, and treatment with antibiotics or systemic steroids are frequently noted in the patient's history. Cutaneous candidiasis usually responds well to topical treatment with any of the imidazoles, or with nystatin (Mycostatin) or ciclopirox olamine creams, applied twice daily for 2 weeks. Allylamines are almost as effective as the imidazoles. Extensive or refractory disease should be treated with oral ketoconazole, 200 mg per day, or the newer triazoles (itraconazole or fluconazole). Predisposing causes should be corrected, if possible.

TINEA VERSICOLOR

Tinea versicolor is due to the lipophilic yeast *Malassezia furfur*, which is normally found in small quantities of the skin. Overgrowth of this organism produces discrete and confluent, slightly scaly patches or plaques on the upper trunk and proximal part of the arms. It occurs most frequently in young adults and is much more common in the summer and in hot, humid climates. As the name suggests, the involved skin can be slightly hyperpigmented or, more commonly, hypopigmented. The treatment of choice is selenium sulfide, 2.5% suspension, applied with water to the scalp, neck, upper trunk, and extremities for 10 minutes daily for 1 week. Patients should be warned that the pigmentary changes will persist for weeks to months. Topical antifungal creams are effective, but the extensive skin involvement makes their cost prohibitive. Alternative treatments include the use of ketoconazole shampoo in the same way or, in extensive or resistant cases, oral ketoconazole, 400 mg in a single dose, or 200 mg per day for 10 days.

DISEASES OF THE MOUTH

method of
ROY S. ROGERS, III, M.D.
*Mayo Medical School and Mayo Clinic and
 Mayo Foundation
Rochester, Minnesota*

Disorders of the mouth may be caused by many different factors, most frequently congenital, nutritional, immunologic, traumatic, infectious, or neoplastic. The resulting condition may be limited to the mouth or may be part of a systemic disease. To correctly assess the scope of the problem, careful examination of the oral cavity and of the skin should be supported by a general medical evaluation. The treatment may be local, systemic, or a combination of both and may require cooperation of several specialties, such as dermatology, dentistry, primary care, internal medicine, and others.

LIPS

Cleft Lip and Cleft Palate. This congenital anomaly occurs in approximately 1 in 1000 births and is the result of failure of the facial processes to fuse during the seventh week in utero. Combinations of cleft lip and cleft palate occur more frequently than isolated clefts. The upper lip is more often affected than the lower lip, and unilateral lip clefts are much more common than bilateral ones. Surgical repair of cleft lips should take place at 1 to 2 months of age to facilitate eating and drinking. Closure of a cleft palate is usually delayed until age 18 months to allow undisturbed growth of the maxilla, but this time is still early enough to aid development of speech. Surgery of cleft lips allows excellent cosmetic and functional results, but the remaining functional problems associated with cleft palate may leave some patients with psychologic problems.

Congenital Lip Pits and Fistulas. These congenital malformations of the lips may occur as isolated defects or in combination with oral clefts. They are mostly found in the lower lip where they present as unilateral or bilateral depressions on the vermilion surface. The pits are harmless and may be excised for aesthetic reasons.

Melanin Pigmentation of Lips. Multiple freckles on the lips, especially the mucosal surface of the lower lip, are found in Peutz-Jeghers syndrome. This hereditary disorder consists of melanotic spots of the face, mouth, and sometimes hands and feet together with intestinal polyps. The syndrome may be present from birth but usually appears in infancy. The facial pigmentation fades in life, but the oral pigmentation persists. The multiple brownish or almost black patches are round or irregular in shape, measure 1 to 5 mm in diameter, and are irregularly distributed throughout the mouth. The intestinal polyps may give rise to recurrent abdominal pain and minor intestinal obstruction. Their potential for malignant transformation is small. Observation of the oral pigmentation may lead to the diagnosis of Peutz-Jeghers syndrome.

Labial Melanotic Macules. Single or few brown macules may appear on the vermilion of the lips in young adults. The labial melanotic macule is histologically a benign lentigo. No treatment is necessary. The lesion may be removed for cosmetic purposes but may resolve spontaneously.

Fordyce Granules. These ectopic sebaceous glands are a developmental anomaly that can be found on the mucosal surface of the lips and the buccal mucosa. The grouped or clustered yellowish spots are benign and require no treatment.

Mucus Retention Phenomenon. This common lesion involves accessory salivary glands and their ducts. It occurs most frequently in the lower lip but can also affect other parts of the mouth. Caused by traumatic severance of a salivary duct, an expanding collection of material develops within the tissues. Clinically, a superficial lesion appears as a raised, bluish cyst up to 10 mm in diameter; a deeper lesion presents as lip swelling. After formation within a few days, the lesions may persist at a stable size for months. Some lesions regress and enlarge periodically and, unless treated, will persist. Treatment consists of excision of both the lesion and its contributory salivary gland.

Hemangioma. This benign vascular malformation may be congenital or may arise later in life. Clinically, a localized hemangioma presents as a red or blue, blood-filled lesion that blanches when pressure is exerted. If it is superficially located or is large, it may produce an elevated lesion. Removal is indicated if the lesion is cosmetically disfiguring and because it carries a certain risk of bleeding.

Angioedema. Angioedema is an immediate-type allergic reaction that can occur as part of an allergic reaction after a bee sting or drug administration. Rarely, angioedema presents as an inherited disorder characterized by the deficiency of a complement enzyme, C1 esterase inhibitor. Both forms present clinically as diffuse swelling of the lips and the adjacent parts of the face, the region around the eyes, and sometimes the hands and feet. If the swelling affects the pharynx, a life-threatening emergency may develop. Angioedema develops rapidly and usually resolves in 24 to 36 hours. In severe, life-threatening conditions, injection of 0.5 to 1 mL of epinephrine 1:1000 intravenously or subcutaneously is recommended. Systemic antihistamines and cold compresses may be used in less severe cases.

Contact Cheilitis. Contact cheilitis is a delayed-type allergic reaction to a variety of substances. The most frequent causative agent is cinnamaldehyde, which may be contained in dentrifrices, mouth-washes, lipsticks, cosmetics, foods, and other substances. The patients usually complain of soreness, burning, or dryness of the lips. Clinically, contact cheilitis manifests as erythema, swelling, and scaling of one or both lips. Other oral tissues may also be involved, mainly the gingivae and tongue. Identification and elimination of the offending allergen are the cornerstone of therapy but may be difficult to achieve without patch testing. Cool compresses, topical fluorinated corticosteroids, and protective salves are helpful in reducing the inflammation.

Bullous Erythema Multiforme. This acute, self-limited dermatosis ranges from a mild disease to a severe condition that may endanger the patient's sight or life. The condition may be idiopathic or the result of infection or drug administration. Recurrent herpes simplex virus infections are the most common cause of recurrent erythema multiforme. Typical clinical findings are blister formation and extensive hemorrhagic crusts. There may be erosions and sloughing of the oral epithelium. The oral involvement may be associated with fever and skin and ocular involvement. Acute attacks last 3 to 6 weeks and may recur periodically. In severe cases, large doses of systemic corticosteroids may be necessary to treat the condition. In less severe cases, cold compresses, topical corticosteroid salves, and protective salves are helpful.

Angular Cheilitis. Painful fissures may develop at the corners of the mouth (perlèche). Angular cheilitis may be associated with vitamin deficiency, neonatal thrush, or *Candida* infection in elderly patients. In the elderly, the reduction of vertical dimension of the jaws creates deep folds where saliva can produce intertrigo. Local treatment with nystatin (Mycostatin) cream or ointment and drying to prevent maceration are helpful. The oral source of the infection must also be treated, and any systemic factors should be corrected, otherwise relapse will occur.

Recurrent Herpes Simplex. The most common infectious disease of the lips is the recurrent herpes simplex virus infection. After the primary infection, the virus persists in the trigeminal ganglion, and recurrences are possible throughout the rest of an infected person's life. Recurrences start as a pricking or burning sensation followed by formation of multiple small vesicles, which rupture and form shallow ulcers. During the vesicular stage, the lesions are infectious. The ulcers are covered by fibrinous crusts and heal within 2 weeks. Owing to the self-limited nature of the disease, the treatment is symptomatic. Topical medications such as witch hazel or 70% alcohol applied after unroofing of the vesicles have been helpful. Systemic acyclovir (Zovirax) 200 mg five times daily for 5 days may be useful in severe cases if it is administered early in the course of the infection.

Verruca Vulgaris. Caused by the human papillomavirus, oral warts can be found in association with warts of the skin. Clinically, single or multiple, small, white, cauliflower-like growths may be found on the lips or commissures. Treatment consists of excision or destruction of the lesion by electrosurgery or similar methods. The lesions are of minor significance but may pose a cosmetic problem.

Leukoplakia. The clinical term "leukoplakia" denotes an asymptomatic white patch that cannot be wiped off and cannot be identified as any other disease process. A relationship to tobacco use and alcohol abuse or to chronic mechanical injury exists. The histologic findings range from hyperkeratotic and thickened epithelium to early infiltrating carcinoma. Because a certain risk of malignant transformation exists and because early squamous cell carcinomas may present as white patches, the lesion should be examined histologically. After biopsy, the lesion may regress if the proximate causes are corrected.

Actinic Cheilitis. This condition frequently affects the lower lip after many years of exposure to sunlight. It starts as dryness and fine scaling, later followed by thickening of the epithelium and development of gray-white plaques. Vertical fissuring and crusting may appear. Later, warty nodules may form, which may evolve into a squamous cell carcinoma. Photoprotection with sun-blocking lipsticks should be emphasized. Suspicious lesions should be studied histologically. Extensive actinic cheilitis can be treated by carbon dioxide laser ablation.

Squamous Cell Carcinoma. This is the most common oral malignancy and accounts for more than 90% of all oral cancers. The vermilion border of the lower lip is frequently involved owing to its exposure to sunlight and its susceptibility to actinic damage. It affects middle-aged and elderly men. Clinically, an early lesion appears as an innocuous-looking white patch or thickening. In later stages, it forms an indurated, warty, or ulcerated growth. Therapy consists of surgical removal. The prognosis is good, because the tumors are usually well differentiated and slow to metastasize.

TONGUE

Median Rhomboid Glossitis. Traditionally said to represent a development defect of the tuberculum impar, this condition rarely occurs until the third or fourth decade of life. It is characterized by an irregularly shaped, smooth red patch on the mid-dorsum of the tongue; it is usually slightly depressed. Median rhomboid glossitis may well represent a chronic hyperplastic candidiasis. If the lesion does not respond to anticandidal therapy, a biopsy may be indicated to exclude carcinoma.

Fissured Tongue. The fissured or grooved tongue is a developmental defect. It is seen in Down, Sjögren's, and Melkersson-Rosenthal syndromes, but it occurs most often as an isolated defect that increases in prevalence with advancing age. No treatment is necessary. If halitosis is a problem, vigorous cleansing of the fissures with a soft-bristled toothbrush is indicated.

Furred Tongue. This condition is commonly seen with upper respiratory tract infections, fevers, soft diet, and smoking. It is due to failure of normal desquamation or hypertrophy of the filiform papillae

or both. Brushing the tongue with a soft-bristled toothbrush and a dentifrice is satisfactory in most instances for treatment.

Black Hairy Tongue. Elongation of the filiform papillae of the tongue presents clinically as a hairlike overgrowth. Its brownish black pigmentation is attributed to proliferation of pigment-producing bacteria that inhabit the tongue. Although the cause is unknown, heavy smoking, antibiotics, and the use of mouthwashes have been implicated. Treatment includes brushing of the tongue with a soft toothbrush and using a dilute (1%) hydrogen peroxide mouthwash. Tobacco and other oral irritants should be avoided. Extremely elongated papillae may be snipped with scissors.

Benign Migratory Glossitis (Geographic Tongue). As its name implies, this harmless condition is characterized by migratory, white annular lesions with atrophic centers. It is most commonly encountered among pediatric patients in whom the prevalence may be as high as 15%. In general, the cause is obscure, although it may be associated occasionally with psoriasis or Reiter's disease. Geographic tongue is often asymptomatic, although a burning discomfort may occur. This is generally mild and self-limited. A mild hydrogen peroxide mouth rinse and bland diet may help.

Glossodynia (Burning Tongue). This is one of the most vexing problems of oral medicine. It often afflicts middle-aged and elderly women. Patients complain about painful burning, stinging, or itching sensations of the tongue or other oral mucous membranes. The "true" glossodynias have no morphologic aberrations or show only mild fortuitous changes (furred, geographic, or fissured tongue). "Secondary" glossodynias have abnormal morphologic features or symptoms (hypogeusia, dysgeusia). In many cases of burning tongue or burning mouth, psychogenic factors are relevant, most commonly emotional conflict, depression, and cancerophobia. The differential diagnosis includes pernicious anemia and various vitamin deficiencies, zinc deficiency, xerostomia, diabetes mellitus, recent antibiotic therapy, gastric reflux, allergic contact stomatitis, denture sore mouth, and other causes, including hormonal changes. Before glossodynia is ascribed to depression or psychogenic factors, a careful evaluation for organic causes, including contact stomatitis, should be undertaken.

Smooth Tongue. Generalized, marked redness and smoothness of the tongue due to atrophy of the filiform papillae are classically associated with nutritional deficiencies such as iron deficiency anemia, sideropenic dysphagia (Plummer-Vinson syndrome), malabsorption states (sprue), pellagra, and pernicious anemia. The condition may be painful, and angular cheilitis may be associated with it. Treatment is directed at correction of the underlying disease.

Macroglossia. A variety of conditions may lead to an enlarged tongue. It may be seen as a developmental defect and in Down syndrome. Tumors such as hemangiomas, neurofibromas, and thyroglossal duct cysts may cause an enlarged tongue. Infectious processes such as actinomycosis, tuberculosis, and syphilis and metabolic processes such as hypothyroidism, amyloidosis, and multiple myeloma are other causes of an enlarged tongue.

White Patches on Tongue. White patches on the tongue may be observed in association with different diseases, including lichen planus, candidiasis, acquired immune deficiency syndrome (AIDS), and squamous cell carcinoma.

Herpetic Geometric Glossitis. This infection with the herpes simplex virus occurs in immunosuppressed hosts. Patients present with painful linear fissures on the central tongue dorsum. These take on a geometric pattern. These lesions respond to systemic acyclovir but may recur and require re-treatment.

Oral Hairy Leukoplakia. A frequent prodromal sign of AIDS is the presence of a hairy-type leukoplakia on the lateral margins of the tongue. Diagnosis of this lesion is important, because in patients with hairy leukoplakia, the risk of developing full-blown AIDS is approximately 75%. Clinically, the unilateral or bilateral lesions are symptom free but have a whitish, corrugated, hairlike surface that cannot be wiped off. A biopsy may be helpful, but further AIDS-specific tests are necessary to establish the diagnosis. A similar picture can occur in immunosuppressed transplant recipients.

Squamous Cell Carcinoma of Tongue. Intraoral carcinoma frequently affects the tongue (40% of all cases). Typically, men older than 60 years are affected, and patients frequently have a history of tobacco or alcohol abuse. Most tumors are on the lateral border of the anterior two thirds of the tongue. An early carcinoma may present as an inconspicuous, painless, white or red patch or small nodule. In later stages, the lesion usually forms a thickened, indurated painful ulcer. Treatment consists of surgical removal of the tumors and of palpable regional lymph nodes. The prognosis is greatly influenced by the stage of the disease and is poor in advanced lesions with regional lymph node metastasis.

BUCCAL MUCOSA, FLOOR OF MOUTH, AND PALATE

White Mucosal Lesions

Leukedema. This opalescent, translucent appearance of the buccal mucosa is a variant of normal. The milky white color disappears on stretching of the buccal mucosa. It is more common in Americans of African descent.

Candidiasis. *Candida albicans* produces infections mainly in infants, debilitated or immunosuppressed patients, and patients taking oral antibiotics or corticosteroids for prolonged periods. The lesions can present as white, curdlike plaques; hyperplastic indurated plaques; atrophic inflamed plaques; or a leukoplakic area. The white, cheesy patches can be wiped off, leaving an eroded, bleeding surface. The

diagnosis is confirmed by microscopic examination of scrapings or by culture. Treatment is directed at correcting the underlying condition in conjunction with local therapy. The use of antifungal agents such as nystatin locally applied as solution or oral clotrimazole troches (Mycelex troches) often suffices. In resistant palatal infections of denture wearers, anticandidal creams such as clotrimazole (Lotrimin, Mycelex), econazole (Spectazole), and others may be applied under the denture plate. Systemic treatment with oral antiyeast antibiotics such as fluconazole (Diflucan) 100 mg daily for 2 weeks is occasionally indicated.

Nicotine Stomatitis. In nicotine stomatitis, the palatal mucosa is thickened and gray-white in color, with multiple small red dots that represent the orifices of minor salivary glands. The lesions usually regress slowly on cessation of smoking and are not considered premalignant. Atypical or persistent lesions should be studied histologically.

Oral Burns. Any caustic agent may injure the oral epithelium, leaving a sloughing, white membrane. An oral burn can be observed after placement of an aspirin tablet in the oral vestibule to relieve toothache. Healing of the lesion is usually uneventful, and treatment is symptomatic.

Leukokeratoses. Leukokeratoses are benign white plaques, usually caused by chronic trauma such as cheek biting, sucking of the buccal mucosa, ill-fitting dentures, or malpositioned teeth with sharp edges. Benignity is recognized by the distribution of the lesions and not by their morphologic appearance and is best confirmed by biopsy if any doubt exists. Avoidance of tobacco, scrupulous oral hygiene, correction of dental abnormalities, and removal of irritating factors are followed by improvement. As with all leukoplakic lesions, induration, irregular thickening, ulceration, or erythroplasia should alert the clinician to the need for additional tissue samples to exclude malignancy.

Leukoplakia. Leukoplakia is a clinical term for a white patch on the oral mucosa that cannot be wiped off and cannot be identified as any other disease process. The white appearance of the mucosa is the result of hyperkeratosis of the oral epithelium. Leukoplakia is a relatively common oral lesion. Although any oral site may be involved, lesions of the buccal mucosa and the mandibular mucosa are the most common. The cause appears to be multifactorial, including abuse of tobacco, local irritation, and local trauma. If the cause is eliminated, the lesion frequently regresses. If a lesion does not respond to specific therapy, it should be studied histologically to exclude early squamous cell carcinoma.

Papilloma. Papillomas (warts) of the oral cavity, caused by the human papillomavirus, are most frequently seen on the soft palate, tongue, and lips. The typical appearance is warty and keratotic. Excisional biopsy is diagnostic and therapeutic.

Verrucous Carcinoma. Warty nodules occur in the buccal or sulcular mucosa or the floor of the mouth. This lesion is often induced by the use of smokeless tobacco. The wart virus may play a permissive role in its development. Verrucous carcinomas are locally destructive but rarely metastasize. Surgical excision is the treatment of choice, but radiation therapy should be avoided.

Squamous Cell Carcinoma. The second most common site for oral carcinoma is the floor of the mouth, whereas the buccal mucosa and the palate are less frequently affected. The typical patient is an elderly man. The most important cause is heavy tobacco use, including smokeless (chewing) tobacco. Heavy alcohol use seems to have a synergistic effect. Early lesions often present as innocuous-appearing areas of leukoplakia or erythroplakia; more advanced lesions usually present as indurated ulcers. Treatment consists of wide excision or radiotherapy. Early carcinomas (stages I and II) have a good to fair prognosis; advanced lesions (stages III and IV) have a poor prognosis.

Lichen Planus. Oral lichen planus usually presents as bilateral, lacelike keratosis of the buccal mucosa, forming a striated or netlike pattern. Other oral areas, such as the gingivae, tongue, or palate, may also be involved. Lesions on the dorsal surface of the tongue appear profusely opaque. The oral lesions are often associated with lesions of the skin, which most commonly occur on the flexor aspects of the wrist and lower legs bilaterally. To confirm the diagnosis of oral lichen planus, routine histopathologic and immunofluorescence studies of nonulcerated lesions may be helpful. Lichen planus does not require treatment unless the patient complains of painful symptoms. Painful lesions may be treated with topical or intralesional corticosteroids. In more severe cases, oral prednisone in daily doses of 40 to 60 mg may be given for 14 days and then tapered over 2 weeks, although this form of therapy is only palliative.

Red and Pigmented Lesions

Erythroplakia. These red patches are often dysplastic and many are malignant. All erythroplakic areas must be studied histologically. Local excision is preferred.

Denture Stomatitis. Poor oral hygiene in denture wearers can lead to inflammation of the soft tissues beneath the denture and secondary candidiasis. Most often the maxilla is affected, with a red and painful mucosa. Treatment consists of thorough daily cleaning of the denture and removal of the denture at night. If secondary candidiasis is present, nystatin tablets, clotrimazole troches, or oral fluconazole 100 mg daily for 7 days may be prescribed. Construction of a new denture is occasionally necessary.

Amalgam Tattoo. This is an exogenous pigmentation, produced when silver amalgam filling material becomes implanted in soft tissue during dental restoration procedures. The tattoo is blue-black and asymptomatic. Its nature may be confirmed by a radiograph, revealing radiopaque metallic particles. If it is confirmed radiographically, further treatment is unnecessary; otherwise, excisional biopsy may be

indicated. The differential diagnosis includes pigmented nevus and malignant melanoma.

Pigmented Nevus. Benign pigmented nevi of all types may occur in the oral cavity. These include lentigines and junctional, compound, and blue nevi. Except for the blue nevus, these lesions are generally brown-black. They may be raised or flat and are relatively unchanging. All pigmented lesions should be excised to exclude the possibility of melanoma. A radiograph may be obtained to exclude amalgam tattoo.

Oral Kaposi's Sarcoma. This is encountered in about 15% of patients with AIDS. These lesions may be the first clinical manifestation of AIDS. Oral Kaposi's sarcoma represents a malignant neoplasm of capillaries. It is most frequently located on the palate, where reddish brown or red to blue nodules are noted. The lesion may be treated by surgery, radiation, or intralesional chemotherapy.

Malignant Melanoma. Primary malignant melanoma of the oral mucosa is rare. Most of the oral lesions arise on the maxillary mucosa. Clinically, the melanoma may present as a nodular, superficial spreading, or lentiginous lesion. Oral melanomas require wide surgical excision. The prognosis depends on the stage of the malignancy but in general is poor for oral melanomas.

Erosive, Ulcerative, and Vesiculobullous Lesions

Recurrent Aphthous Stomatitis (Canker Sores). This condition is characterized by recurrent, painful shallow ulcerations that may occur on any area of the oral mucosa except the anterior hard palate and the attached gingivae. The cause is multifactorial. Some patients have "correctable causes" such as ulcerative colitis; Crohn's disease; gluten-sensitive enteropathy; deficiency of vitamin B_{12}, folic acid, or iron; or estrogen-sensitive aphthosis. However, the cause remains obscure in most patients. Recurrent aphthous stomatitis occurs mainly in teenagers and young adults, being more common in women than in men. The shallow ulcerations may be single or multiple and can range from less than 2 mm to more than 10 mm in size. They have a yellowish gray pseudomembranous base and are surrounded by an erythematous halo. Fever and lymphadenopathy may be associated. The lesions are self-limited and resolve in 7 to 14 days but recur often, ranging from quarterly to almost continuously. Treatment of recurrent aphthous stomatitis is symptomatic and consists of avoidance of spicy, acidic, and salty foods as well as sharp, hard foods. A mixture of diphenhydramine (Benadryl elixir) and Kaopectate in equal parts used as a mouth rinse six times a day may be helpful. Also, 3 mL of 2% viscous lidocaine (Xylocaine) held in the mouth for 3 minutes before meals provides relief of pain. The identification of associated diseases or deficiencies and correction of these problems may lead to a remission.

Recurrent Intraoral Herpes Simplex Stomati-

tis. This viral infection is the result of reactivation of the herpes simplex virus. It is found much less frequently than herpes simplex infection of the lips. Intraorally, it predominantly involves the hard palate and attached gingivae. The condition is self-limited and requires only symptomatic treatment. Healing usually occurs within 7 to 10 days.

Herpangina. Herpangina is an infection of the posterior oral cavity and pharynx by coxsackievirus. It usually affects children and young adults. Small vesicles are seen on the soft palate and uvula and symmetrically on the tonsillar pillars. They quickly rupture, leaving small, painful ulcerations. Fever, lymphadenopathy, headache, and malaise along with oral and abdominal pain are associated. The distinctive clinical findings confirm the diagnosis. Treatment is symptomatic, and healing occurs rapidly.

Pemphigus Vulgaris. Oral lesions may be the presenting manifestation of 50% of patients with pemphigus vulgaris. It is an autoimmune disease that presents as oral blisters of varying sizes. These slough, leaving painful ulcerations with a whitish pseudomembranous base. The most frequently involved sites are the buccal mucosa, palate, and gingivae. Patients are usually in their fifth or sixth decade. An early diagnosis of pemphigus vulgaris will facilitate early treatment and may prevent extensive lesions in this potentially fatal disease.

Cicatricial Pemphigoid. At least 85% of patients with cicatricial pemphigoid have oral lesions. They may present with desquamative gingival lesions or with mucosal lesions that become erosions. Other mucosal surfaces may be involved, such as ocular, nasal, laryngeal, or esophageal mucosa or genital and perianal tissues, as well as skin. As with oral pemphigus, early diagnosis is important. Topical and systemic corticosteroids may be required. Many patients respond to dapsone or sulfapyridine. These nonsteroidal anti-inflammatory agents are particularly useful in immunobullous diseases.

Bullous Pemphigoid. Approximately one third of patients with bullous pemphigoid develop oral lesions. These blisters are less friable than those in pemphigus vulgaris, but as with all oral blisters, they break easily to become erosions or ulcerations. Treatment of bullous and cicatricial pemphigoid, as of pemphigus vulgaris, consists of systemic corticosteroids and, occasionally, immunosuppressive drugs.

GINGIVAL AND PERIODONTAL MEMBRANES

Eruption Cyst. Eruption of the deciduous or, less frequently, the permanent dentition may cause single or multiple bluish red swellings of the mucosa that covers the erupting tooth. Treatment is rarely necessary, because the tooth will erupt through the lesion. Alternatively, it may be treated by surgically exposing the affected tooth. The eruption of the deciduous dentition in young children may produce considerable discomfort, and topical anesthetic ointment such as 5% lidocaine may be necessary to relieve it. Analgesics may also be used for pain control.

Pericoronitis. This is an inflammatory reaction that develops around erupting third molar (wisdom) teeth. Occasionally, if these inflamed areas become infected, they produce pain and swelling. Submandibular lymphadenopathy may be associated with severe pericoronitis. For treatment of the infection, penicillin or erythromycin is indicated, 1 gram per day for a week. To prevent recurrence of the condition, removal of the offending tooth is often necessary.

Localized and Generalized Enlargement of Gingival Tissue. Localized enlargement of the gingivae may be inflammatory in nature, resulting from a periodontal abscess, or it may be hyperplastic owing to local irritating factors forming a reparative granuloma (epulis). Plaque and calculus deposits are the most common irritants. However, faulty dental restorations may also be responsible. As many as 20 to 40% of the patients treated with phenytoin (Dilantin) or cyclosporine (Sandimmune) develop a generalized enlargement of the gingivae. If the gingival overgrowth poses aesthetic problems, interferes with mastication, or prevents adequate oral hygiene, the tissue must be surgically removed. After surgical treatment, excellent oral hygiene and the construction of a positive-pressure mouthguard may reduce the regrowth of the tissue.

Leukemic Infiltrates. Leukemic infiltrates into the gingival tissue may be responsible for diffuse enlargement. The overgrown tissue appears pale and bleeds easily. Because of the risk of severe hemorrhage, surgery is contraindicated. Gentle cleaning of the teeth helps reduce irritation from dental deposits. If hemorrhage occurs, topical hemostatic agents (Gelfoam) and a periodontal dressing are applied.

Acute Necrotizing Ulcerative Gingivitis (Trench Mouth, Vincent's Infection). This destructive infection of the gingiva predominantly affects young adults. It is often caused by a synergistic infection with *Fusobacterium fusiforme* and *Borrelia vincentii*. Stress, fatigue, and heavy smoking are predisposing factors. Although the condition is rare, it is frequently found in AIDS patients. The lesions are usually localized to the interdental papillae, but in severe instances, lesions may also involve the buccal mucosa and pharynx. Clinically, the lesions appear as craters or punched-out areas with a yellowish necrotic surface. There may be considerable discomfort, and analgesics may be necessary to control the pain. In severe infections, with fever and adenopathy, antibiotic treatment (penicillin, erythromycin, or metronidazole) is indicated. Pronounced improvement is usually noted 4 to 5 days after antibiotic treatment has been initiated. After the acute phase has passed, cleaning of the teeth and oral hygiene measures (brushing, flossing) must be started and maintained, otherwise the infection will recur. Surgery occasionally is necessary to recontour the craters in the interdental gingiva. Mild infection may be treated by warm hydrogen peroxide mouth rinses and improvement in oral hygiene.

Gingivitis and Periodontitis. These are the most common inflammatory diseases that involve the supporting structures of the teeth. Gingivitis consists of inflammation of the gingival margin and is caused by accumulation of plaque and calculus at the junction of the gingiva and the tooth surface. The affected tissue appears red and swollen and bleeds easily. Treatment consists of thorough removal of all plaque and calculous deposits and meticulous oral hygiene with brushing and flossing. In periodontitis, the inflammatory process also involves the periodontal ligament and alveolar bone. Periodontitis is characterized by separation of the gingivae from the teeth; it may cause extensive bone resorption and, if untreated, may lead to tooth loss. The term for separation of the gingivae from the teeth is "periodontal pockets." In advanced disease, when pockets are more than 4 mm deep, surgical correction is necessary. Postsurgically, a high standard of oral hygiene should be maintained, or the periodontitis is likely to recur.

Chronic Desquamative Gingivitis. Diffuse erythematous sloughing of the marginal gingiva is most often seen in postmenopausal women but is occasionally encountered in other patients. It may be the clinical manifestation of several different disorders, including bullous or cicatricial pemphigoid, lichen planus, contact stomatitis, or pemphigus vulgaris. A biopsy should be performed to establish an accurate diagnosis. Treatment is directed at the primary condition. Besides scrupulous oral hygiene, topical or systemic corticosteroids may help suppress the inflammatory reaction.

TEETH AND JAWS

Congenital Absence of Teeth. Complete absence of teeth (anodontia) is rare, whereas absence of several teeth (oligodontia) is more common. Most likely to be missing are the third molars and, less commonly, the maxillary lateral incisors and second premolars. If missing teeth are diagnosed at an early age by dental radiography, the spaces that would have been occupied by the teeth can be maintained by orthodontic appliances until a permanent bridge can be constructed or the spaces closed orthodontically.

Enamel Hypoplasia. Enamel hypoplasia may result from excess fluoride in drinking water (fluorosis) or from disease states during childhood (chickenpox, measles).

Developmental Anomalies. Developmental anomalies of the enamel (amelogenesis imperfecta) or dentin (dentinogenesis imperfecta) are rare disorders that make the teeth more susceptible to dental caries. These teeth may require extensive restorative procedures.

Anomalies of Dental Pigmentation. A tooth may be discolored as a result of trauma that causes hemorrhage in the pulp chamber. Necrotic pulp tissue should be removed and replaced by a root canal filling. Administration of tetracycline to a pregnant woman during the last trimester of pregnancy or to the child during the formative stage of the teeth may produce a yellow to gray discoloration of the child's teeth. Minocycline can cause tooth discoloration in children or adults.

Premature Loss of Teeth. This may be attributable to trauma, caries, histiocytosis X, or genetic disorders such as hypophosphatasia, cyclic or chronic neutropenia, or Papillon-Lefèvre syndrome.

Malposition and Malocclusion of Teeth. Malposition and malocclusion of teeth may present aesthetic and functional problems. Discrepancies in occlusion require orthodontic treatment. If severe problems of prognathism, retrognathism, or open bite occur, surgical correction is necessary to restore proper occlusion and cosmetic appearance.

Dental Caries. Dental caries is a chronic destruction of the tooth caused by microorganisms, in particular *Streptococcus mutans*. It is characterized by progressive demineralization of the calcified components of the tooth and the destruction of its organic components; this leads to cavity formation. Although the disease affects all age groups, it is most prevalent in young persons up to the age of 20 years. Administration of topical or systemic fluoride is an effective measure to prevent tooth decay. Once a carious lesion has developed in a tooth, the infected tooth substance must be removed and replaced by a filling or artificial crown. If left untreated, the process will continue and eventually lead to pulpitis or periapical abscess formation.

Pulpitis. Pulpitis is an acute or chronic inflammation of the pulp tissue of a tooth. Most frequently, it is caused by caries; less frequently, by trauma to the tooth. In acute pulpitis, the patient experiences severe pain that may be difficult to control with analgesics. For treatment, the diseased pulp tissue must be removed and a medicated dressing placed in the pulp chamber. Later, the tooth may require a root canal filling. Teeth with extensive carious destruction may have to be extracted. If left untreated, the inflamed pulp tissue may degenerate and a periapical abscess may eventually develop. This also requires endodontic treatment (root canal filling) or tooth removal. Additional antibiotic therapy may be necessary to control the infectious process. If the abscess is left untreated, facial cellulitis and fascial plane infections may develop.

Osteomyelitis. Osteomyelitis is an inflammatory process of the bone that primarily involves the marrow and secondarily affects the bony trabeculae and cortex. Most commonly, it is caused by an odontogenic infection such as an infected postextraction alveolus or a periapical lesion. The mandible is more commonly involved. Clinically, acute osteomyelitis is manifested by severe pain, elevated temperature, regional lymphadenopathy, and leukocytosis. The teeth may become loose, and eating may become painful. If the mandible is affected, paresthesia or anesthesia is sometimes experienced. When, in addition, periostitis develops, the skin or oral mucosa may be red and swollen. Bacterial culture and sensitivity tests are needed to determine the proper antibiotic agent for treatment.

Odontogenic Tumors. These develop from odontogenic epithelium or mesenchyme that persists in the jaws after the teeth have developed. Surgical removal of the tumor is the treatment of choice.

Ameloblastoma. Ameloblastoma is the most common significant odontogenic tumor and accounts for approximately 1% of all oral tumors. It usually affects individuals in the third to fifth decades and is most often located in the mandible. The tumor is benign and slow growing and, with increasing size, may lead to facial deformity and loosening of the teeth in the affected area. It may develop into a large multilocular cystic lesion and destroy a large portion of the jaw. This can easily be detected on dental radiographs. Ameloblastomas are the most aggressive benign odontogenic tumors, and large lesions may require extensive resections.

Odontoma. Odontoma is the most common odontogenic tumor. It is benign and considered a hamartomatous lesion that consists of enamel and dentin. Most odontomas are small lesions and do not exceed the size of a tooth. They are usually symptomless, being discovered only on routine radiographic examination, where they appear as an area of opacity. Surgical removal will confirm the clinical diagnosis.

Malignant Odontogenic Tumors. Malignant odontogenic tumors are rare, but odontogenic carcinomas and odontogenic sarcomas have been described. Both tumors are characterized by aggressive local behavior, may lead to extensive bone destruction, and may invade adjacent tissues. Pain and swelling are prominent features. Surgical treatment is necessary.

Odontogenic Cysts. These cysts arise from odontogenic epithelium and are of developmental origin or result from inflammation. On dental radiographs, they appear as well-circumscribed radiolucent areas. The lesions are slowly enlarging but if left untreated can be quite destructive. In most instances, an odontogenic cyst can be treated by removing the cyst lining and the associated tooth, if one is present.

Odontogenic Keratocysts. Odontogenic keratocysts are cysts that have a keratinized lining. Thorough removal of the lining is necessary, because these cysts frequently recur, and a few may undergo malignant transformation.

SALIVARY GLANDS AND REGIONAL LYMPH NODES

Sialolithiasis. Obstruction of the duct of a salivary gland by calcified stones is not uncommon. If the stone is small and close to the orifice, it can often be removed with a fine probe. If the stone is large and inaccessible, surgical removal of the entire gland is indicated.

Sialadenitis. This is an inflammatory reaction involving the major salivary glands, which may become swollen and painful. The usual cause is obstruction of the major duct by a mucous or bacterial plug. Systemic antibiotics should be administered and fluid intake increased. The gland usually returns to normal in 1 to 2 weeks. However, if the symptoms persist, surgical removal of the gland may be necessary.

Xerostomia. Dry mouth is a relatively common complaint of patients older than 50 years. Drug therapy, often in the form of antidepressants, anticholinergics, and antihypertensives, may be responsible for xerostomia. Patients should always be questioned about any medications they are taking. In patients who have received radiation to the head and neck, xerostomia may develop as the result of atrophy of the salivary glands. Sjögren's syndrome and Mikulicz's disease must also be excluded. Xerostomia is difficult to treat because there is no consistently effective way to increase salivary flow once a gland has atrophied. Artificial saliva (Xero-Lube, Salivart) can be used to relieve dryness of the oral mucosa. Stimulation of salivary glands can be provided by oral pilocarpine therapy (Salagen) or sugar-free sialagogues (gum, candies). If the problem is drug induced, a change of medication should be considered. Patients with xerostomia are prone to dental caries and candidal infections. Fluoride mouth rinses are helpful in reducing dental decay, and nystatin oral suspension is beneficial in oral candidiasis.

Lymph Node Enlargement. Lymph node enlargement should always be viewed with suspicion. Nodal involvement in the submental or submandibular area may be caused by dental infection. A thorough oral examination should be performed to rule out any malignancy. Oral squamous cell carcinoma, for example, may present with metastasis to regional lymph nodes.

STASIS ULCERS

method of
JESS R. YOUNG, M.D.
Cleveland Clinic
Cleveland, Ohio

Venous stasis ulcerations continue to be a common problem. More than a half-million Americans have, or have had, stasis ulcers. It is a serious social economic problem, with an estimated loss of 2 million workdays annually in the United States.

ETIOLOGY

The basic underlying mechanism in chronic venous insufficiency is venous hypertension. This hypertension is created either by obstruction of the outflow or by reflux from incompetent valves. Obstruction is most often due to venous thrombosis but may result from congenital abnormalities or from extraluminal compression with tumors or cysts. Incompetent valves can be secondary to scarring or destruction with thrombi. They can also be caused by the floppy, incompetent valves seen in primary valvular insufficiency. As a result of this venous hypertension, excessive fluid and red blood cells are lost to the extracellular spaces, fibrosis occurs, and there is poor nutrition of the surrounding tissue. The stasis ulcer itself is often associated with an incompetent perforating vein leading into the area of the ulcer.

CLINICAL FEATURES

Edema is often the first sign of venous insufficiency. It will first be noted at the end of the day, disappearing overnight, but slowly becoming more persistent if untreated. The next evidence of venous insufficiency is usually pigmentation. The excessive venous pressure causes rupture of tiny venules and capillaries with subsequent extravasation of hemoglobin into the tissues.

In some patients, stasis dermatitis will develop with erythema, weeping, scaling, and pruritus. Patients with stasis dermatitis will occasionally develop a generalized eczematous eruption as a sensitization or autoallergic (id) reaction.

A few patients will develop an indurated, erythematous, tender, subcutaneous cellulitis on the medial aspect of the leg just proximal to the medial malleolus. This sterile, indurated cellulitis may spread up and down the calf on the medial side and occasionally may involve the posterior and lateral aspects of the lower leg. This condition has also been termed "liposclerosis." It is often mistaken for thrombophlebitis or bacterial cellulitis.

Stasis ulcerations usually occur in the vicinity of the malleoli, especially the medial malleolus. Less commonly, they may occur on the posterior and lateral aspect of the calf. Brown pigmentation is usually present in the surrounding skin. The leg is often edematous. The base of the ulcer is usually moist with extensive granulation tissue and is often secondarily infected. The ulcer may vary greatly in size, at times extending around the whole circumference of the calf. Pain is not a prominent feature of stasis ulcers. If pain is present, it is usually relieved by elevation of the limb.

TREATMENT

Many different treatments of stasis ulcers, both medical and surgical, have been proposed. The multitude of approaches emphasizes the fact that no one outstanding method exists for treating these ulcers. The choice of treatment is somewhat dependent on the size of the ulcer, the presence and extent of stasis dermatitis, the presence of arterial insufficiency, and the severity of secondary infection.

Acute Dermatitis

If weeping acute dermatitis accompanies the stasis ulcer, the leg is best treated by bed rest and wet compresses. Compresses should be changed every 2 to 3 hours. The wet dressings should not be enclosed in a plastic covering because this will result in maceration of tissues and will prevent the evaporation necessary to promote healing. One of the following solutions is suggested for compresses: (1) aluminum acetate (Burow's solution) 0.5%, (2) isotonic saline solution 0.9%, or (3) acetic acid solution 1%. Between compresses, a drying anti-inflammatory topical steroid or steroid-antibiotic ointment or cream may help clear the dermatitis. If there is evidence of secondary infection with cellulitis or bacteremia, a culture should be done and appropriate antibiotic therapy initiated.

Subacute Dermatitis

When the acute phase of the dermatitis has subsided and the patient becomes more ambulatory, recurrence of edema must be prevented. If this is not done, acute dermatitis may promptly recur. A wet-to-dry compression dressing program can be instituted (Table 1). Either isotonic saline solution 0.9% or boric acid solution 3% can be used, and the dressing is changed at least twice daily. The dressing is held in place by a lightweight compression liner stocking with 8 to 10 mm Hg compression. During the day when the patient is active, this compression liner stocking is covered by a heavy support stocking with 30 to 40 mm Hg compression. The dressing is changed at bedtime, and the light liner stocking alone is worn over the dressing during sleep.

For patients who are unable to manage the compression dressing program, the use of a modified Unna paste boot is often effective. The boot consists of flesh-colored rolled bandages impregnated with a paste of zinc oxide, calamine, glycerin, and gelatin. Directions for applying the paste boot are well illustrated on the package. It is usually changed at weekly intervals unless excessive drainage necessitates changing more frequently. If excessive discomfort occurs at home, the patient should be instructed to cut off the dressing and to return to the physician's office for further evaluation.

Chronic Stasis Cellulitis

No bacterial infection is present in chronic stasis cellulitis, and the inflammation does not respond to antibiotics. Best results are achieved by rest and elevation of the leg with local application of heat to

TABLE 1. **Wet-to-Dry Compression Dressings**

Soak the legs and feet in lukewarm water with Dreft or Ivory Snow for 5 to 10 min and dry well, especially between toes.

Apply a moisturizing cream such as Nivea, Lanolor, or Lubriderm to the legs and feet, but not between the toes.

Moisten a 4 × 3 in gauze pad with the prescribed solution, either 0.9% saline or 3% boric acid. Place it directly over the ulcer. Place a dry 4 × 3 in gauze pad over that.

Apply a clean compression liner stocking (8–10 mm Hg compression) over the dressing.

Apply a heavy (30–40 mm Hg compression) elastic stocking over the liner stocking.

Change this dressing every 8 to 12 h as instructed.

When the dressing is applied, it is wet. When it is later removed, it should be dry and stuck to the wound. Ideally, it should be pulled off dry to débride the wound. If this causes excessive pain, moisten the dressing before removing.

When the dressing is changed at bedtime, do not apply the heavy elastic stocking over the liner stocking.

the inflamed area. Warm, wet dressings are probably more effective than dry heat. The healing process may be expedited at times by giving nonsteroidal anti-inflammatory agents. After 1 to 3 weeks, the patient can usually tolerate an elastic stocking and resume normal activities. In a few patients, cellulitis appears to resist all forms of treatment. If no improvement has been noticed after 8 to 12 weeks of treatment, excision of the indurated subcutaneous area and skin grafting should be considered. The patient must continue to wear a heavy elastic stocking after the operation.

Stasis Ulcers

The general principles of management of a stasis ulcer are the same as those outlined for chronic stasis dermatitis (see Table 1).

If there is considerable secondary infection, an Unna boot or an occlusive dressing should not be applied. Bed rest and compresses, as described previously, are recommended until the infection subsides. Topical antibiotic ointments may be used between the compresses. If cellulitis, lymphangitis, or septicemia is present, systemic antibiotic therapy is indicated. The choice of antibiotics should be dictated by the culture and sensitivity reports.

Topical enzymes and dextran polymer beads (Debrisan or DuoDerm beads) can be used to débride leg ulcers and to try to develop a healthy granulation tissue. I have not been impressed that these agents offer any advantages over the more conservative measures outlined previously.

Occlusive or semiocclusive dressings have been developed that do more than cover the wound and keep it clean. Some examples are DuoDerm, Op-Site, Tegaderm Bioclusive, and Vigilon. There can be excessive accumulation of fluid under some of these dressings, especially Op-Site. Infection and cellulitis can be exacerbated if these dressings are used on an infected ulcer. They are best used when all infection is cleared, good granulation tissue is present, and re-epithelialization is sought. Some clinical trials have indicated that ulcer healing is equally effective with the regular compression dressings (see Table 1).

Large ulcers, small ulcers that have failed to respond to these conservative measures, or persistently recurring ulcers should be referred for split-thickness skin grafting.

Generalized Eczematization

In patients with stasis ulcerations, a generalized eczematous eruption may develop as a sensitization or id reaction. This can often be controlled by topical corticosteroids and oral antihistamines such as cyproheptadine (Periactin), 4 mg four times daily, or diphenhydramine (Benadryl), 50 mg four times daily. In patients with severe autoeczematization, systemic corticosteroids, orally or intravenously, may be necessary.

TABLE 2. **Stocking Wear and Care**

Put the stockings on in the morning before getting out of bed.
Take the stockings off at night. Do not sleep in them.
Hand wash the stockings in a mild soap or detergent and rinse well. Roll them in a towel to remove excess moisture, then lay them flat to dry.
Rubber gloves, such as Playtex or Sigvaris, can be used when putting on the stockings. The grooves in the palms and fingers of the gloves help to grip the stockings when putting them on.
Never roll or fold the stocking down when it is pulled up too high. Pull it down again. This will cause a wrinkle, but then pinch the wrinkle and snap it. The wrinkle should disappear.
Stockings will last approximately 4 to 6 mo before they lose their elasticity. Therefore, they should be replaced at about that time.

Chronic Venous Insufficiency

After the stasis ulcerations have healed, the treatment of chronic venous insufficiency is not finished. The patient must be impressed with the fact that he or she has a lifelong problem and that continuous supportive measures will be necessary to prevent future complications.

Elastic bandages and proprietary light compression elastic stockings are usually not satisfactory for most of the patients. Patients with mild to moderate venous insufficiency will usually do well with an off-the-shelf elastic stocking such as Jobst, Camp, Sigvaris, Bauer & Black, Juzo, and Medi stockings. A compression of 30 to 40 mm Hg is generally desired. Patients with large legs, those with irregularly contoured legs, and those with recurrent ulcerations in spite of regular elastic stockings should obtain individually measured, custom-made, pressure-gradient stockings such as the Jobst custom-made stocking. Unless the patient has impressive thigh edema, a below-knee stocking usually suffices. If thigh edema is a problem, a waist-high leotard elastic support is usually easier to wear and more effective than a thigh-high elastic stocking.

Elastic stockings should be put on before arising and should be removed just before retiring. Proper care should be given the stockings (Table 2). It is usually necessary to purchase new stockings every 4 to 6 months because the stockings stretch with wear. A lubricating cream or lotion should be applied at bedtime to keep the skin of the legs from becoming excessively dry. Exercise of the legs should be encouraged, but the patient should be instructed to avoid prolonged standing or sitting with the legs hanging down.

PRESSURE ULCERS
method of
G. ALLEN HOLLOWAY, JR., M.D.
Maricopa Medical Center
Phoenix, Arizona

Pressure ulcers are an unfortunately common problem and are usually painful, aesthetically unpleasant, and frequently difficult to heal. They occur because of excessive external pressure, particularly over bone prominences, which causes ischemia and necrosis of underlying tissues. Although pressure appears to be the primary causative factor, friction, shear, and moisture are often contributive as are the age and general state of health of the patient. It is in the elderly patient, frequently with multiple medical problems and a poor state of nutrition, that they are most likely to occur. With the increase in the aging population, greater numbers of people are at risk and an increasing proportion of our health care dollars will be spent in their prevention or treatment. Avoidance of the problem by prevention is much preferable to the necessity for treatment. Recognition of the at-risk patient and potential ulcerations at early stages is critical to success. The Agency for Health Care Policy and Research (AHCPR) initially published a set of guidelines for pressure ulcer prevention that have become a de facto standard.* A second set of guidelines addressing the treatment of established ulcers have also become widely adopted.† These well-researched and well-prepared documents should be available and referred to by every health care provider charged with caring for this problem.

PREVENTION

Most pressure ulcers can be prevented. However, this requires vigilant care in recognizing risk factors and settings that put the patient at risk. Assessment tools have been developed to identify the at-risk patient and to provide a level of severity for clinical documentation. A staging system has also been developed to permit consistent evaluation and documentation of existing lesions. Both systems are discussed in the AHCPR 1992 guidelines and should be adopted and used in some form in all clinical situations where pressure ulcers are encountered and treated.

Prolonged pressure, immobility, malnutrition, and moisture are the predominant factors leading to breakdown, which usually starts invisibly in the subcutaneous tissues. The skin, which is the tissue most resistant to the pressure-induced ischemia, is last affected so that there is often significant underlying necrosis by the time the skin ulcerates. Pressure ulcers can occur anywhere tissue sustains prolonged pressure, so when unexplained ulcerations occur in unexpected areas, e.g., lateral foot, calf, knee, or arm, one needs to consider and look for a source of pressure such as a bed rail, wheelchair footrest, or other such item. Once identified, the pressure must be relieved by either appropriate cushioning or positioning of the patient. Heels are particularly vulnerable to prolonged pressure and must be meticulously watched and protected. The commonly seen foam and sheepskin booties are virtually useless, and some form of heel suspension, be it a splint, foam "moonboot," or support under the calf, is a must. Foam mattresses should be at least 4 inches thick for patients at bed rest in addition to turning, and many types of seat cushions other than foam are available for patients at risk for ischial ulcers when sitting. Turning patients at regular intervals, the duration of which should be determined by the individual patient's risk, is still the mainstay of prevention and should be diligently pursued. For patients at higher risk and in special situations, such as intensive care units, low-air-loss beds and assorted types of mattress overlays are available that provide a greater degree of pressure relief.

TREATMENT

General

Conditions contributing to inadequate healing, including vascular disease, systemic disease or infection, and limited mobility, must be improved when possible. Nutritional deficiency can severely retard healing and must be addressed, and caloric supplementation by enteral or parenteral routes is frequently necessary. Dietetic consultation is important and should be obtained where available. Most patients should receive oral daily multivitamins when possible or, if not, parenteral supplementation.

Antibiotics, oral or parenteral, are not indicated unless there is specific evidence of cellulitis or systemic infection involving soft tissue or bone. If systemic infection is suspected, a source must be sought and appropriate cultures done. Swab cultures of wounds are generally not indicated because all chronic wounds are contaminated and bacteria found in this type of culture are often not those causing the infection. Biopsy cultures at débridement are preferable, but culturing of expressed pus may prove helpful.

Local Wound Care

Local care can be divided into two phases: debris removal and healing. Larger amounts of necrotic debris are usually best removed surgically. Wound edges that are undermined must generally be trimmed and the wound "saucerized" for optimal healing. Significant tracking must be carefully probed for and opened or excised when found because tracks that remain are impossible to rid of bacteria and are often the source of recurrent infection. Bone that is obviously infected must be surgically débrided or resected. Smaller quantities of debris can often be removed by autolytic débridement. The traditional wet-to-dry gauze dressings should be avoided because desiccation kills healthy cells. I prefer moist-to-moist dressings, which do not dry out the underlying cells but are effective in removing debris and allowing the formation of new granulation tissue. Enzymatic débridement has proved to be of limited value in my hands. Use of antiseptic solutions such as povidone-iodine, Dakin's (hypochlorite) solution, hydrogen peroxide, and acetic acid is to be avoided because all have been shown to be toxic to new cells. There is also no evidence that any greater effect is achieved by the removal of contaminating bacteria other than by rinsing with water.

When reasonable débridement has been achieved, healing should begin and dressings should be se-

---

*Pressure Ulcers in Adults: Prediction and Prevention. Clinical Practice Guideline, Number 3. Rockville, MD, Agency for Health Care Policy and Research, Public Health Service, U.S. Department of Health and Human Services, 1992. AHCPR publication 92-0047.

†Treatment of Pressure Ulcers. Clinical Practice Guideline, Number 15. Rockville, MD, Agency for Health Care Policy and Research, Public Health Service, U.S. Department of Health and Human Services, 1995. AHCPR publication 95-0652.

lected to support this. Healing is accomplished by the patient, with the role of the provider being to achieve the optimal environment for this to occur. Moist saline gauze is a useful "filler" and can be lightly packed into the wound to fill vacant space. Dressings do not need to be sterile, especially in the nonhospital setting, and packs of clean gauze pads are much more cost-effective unless required otherwise by health care intermediaries. Other fillers including gels and newer products are also available. These may be covered with occlusive dressings such as petrolatum gauze, films, or hydrocolloids to prevent drying out and can be changed as infrequently as every 3 to 5 days, allowing lesser nursing care requirements as well as improved comfort of the patient.

Pressure Relief

Relief of pressure is the key to both prevention and healing of pressure ulcers. Critical to this is the provision of good nursing care and turning the patient as often as is necessary to prevent further injury or to allow healing. Ideally, the goal is to eliminate all pressure to the involved area, but this is usually not possible. Frequency of turning should not be less than every 2 hours, but elderly, debilitated, and malnourished patients should be turned more frequently whenever possible. Four-inch-thick foam mattresses provide comfort and some degree of pressure relief and may be adequate to allow healing in many cases. However, air- or water-filled mattresses give improved pressure relief and in the patient at greater risk are usually cost-effective. For the highest risk patients, low-air-loss mattress overlays or beds or fluidized bead beds provide the best pressure relief and their higher cost may well be justified, especially in patients with larger or multiple ulcers when positioning is difficult and other methods have failed. However, even these high-technology systems usually do not give adequate heel protection and additional measures as presented before are indicated and necessary.

Other Treatments

Patients with stage III or IV pressure ulcers may present a more difficult problem and may not be able to be healed by positioning and wound care alone. This is especially true in patients lacking protective sensation or who have had previous skin breakdown. These patients may well benefit by additional plastic surgical procedures, which include skin grafts, rotation flaps, myocutaneous flaps, and free flap grafts. It is important to work with a plastic surgeon who deals with this type of problem and who can provide good advice as to when these procedures should be considered and in which patients. Optimal wound therapy is followed by surgical excision of the ulcer and involved tissue and placement of the indicated flap or graft. The patient is usually maintained on a low-air-loss or fluidized bead bed for 2 to 3 weeks

after the procedure before gradually beginning graduated pressure to the treated area. Because the underlying lack of protective sensation and mobility limitation are still present in most of these patients, recurrence is unfortunately common even in the well motivated.

New treatment modalities continue to be developed. Electrical stimulation, cytokine growth factors, dermal substitutes, and vacuum-assisted wound closure, to name a few, are currently being evaluated, but results to confirm their efficacy and safety are not yet available.

ATOPIC DERMATITIS

method of
HARRY LEO ROTH, M.D.
*University of California, San Francisco
San Francisco, California*

Atopic dermatitis is a chronic, familial, relapsing, pruritic dermatitis characterized by early age at onset and associated with allergic rhinitis and asthma. The exact pathophysiologic mechanism is not determined, but there are multifactorial causes attributed to different authors since the term "atopic dermatitis" was coined by Hill and Sulzberger some 70 years ago (Table 1).

Because this is a multifactorial condition, all of the factors cited must be evaluated and addressed in the treatment plan.

Because "eczema" and "dermatitis" are generic terms, it became apparent that a better definition of the condition called atopic dermatitis was needed. Hanifin and Rajka collaborated and made the list shown in Table 2, of major and minor criteria for the diagnosis of atopic dermatitis.

The differential diagnosis should include seborrheic dermatitis, psoriasis, drug eruption, contact dermatitis, fungus infection, and, in more severe extensive cases, lymphoma, mycosis fungoides, and exfoliative erythroderma. Fungus cultures and skin biopsies may be necessary to aid in the diagnosis.

TREATMENT

The most important part of the therapy starts at the first visit when the physician explains the nature of the condition to the patient or the family of the patient. The expectation of a cure must be dispelled, and the need for "control of symptoms and appearance" must be emphasized. A plan must be

TABLE 1. **Pathophysiologic Factors of Atopic Dermatitis**

Psyche	Physiologic alterations
Acute viral infection	Increased itch response
Xerosis	Heredity
Contactants	Aeroallergens
Sweat retention	Antigen-antibody reaction
Bacterial infection	Viral infection
Alterations in cytokine production	Elevation of phosphodiesterase values

TABLE 2. **Major and Minor Criteria for Diagnosis of Atopic Dermatitis**

Must Have Three or More Major Characteristics

Pruritus

Typical morphology and distribution—a bilateral symmetrical dermatitis usually involving the flexures of the arms, legs, and neck

Chronic or chronically relapsing dermatitis

Personal or family history of atopy (asthma, allergic rhinitis, eczema)

Must Have Three or More Minor Characteristics

Xerosis

Ichthyosis (palmar hyperlinearity, keratosis pilaris)

Immediate (type 1) skin test reactivity

Early age at onset

Tendency toward cutaneous skin infections (especially *Staphylococcus aureus* infection and herpes simplex), impaired cell-mediated immunity

Tendency toward chronic hand and foot dermatitis

Nipple eczema

Cheilitis

Recurrent conjunctivitis

Dennie-Morgan infraorbital line

Keratoconus

Periorbital darkening

Facial pallor centrally with peripheral facial erythema

Pityriasis alba

Anterior neck folds

Itch when sweating

Intolerance to wool and lipid solvents

Perifollicular accentuation

Food intolerance

Course influenced by environment or emotional factors

White dermatographism, delayed blanch

From Hanifin JM, Rajka G: Diagnostic features of atopic dermatitis. Acta Derm Venereol *60*(Suppl 92):44–47, 1980.

made and the patient must be told that he or she will be a partner in the nursing management of this chronic condition, which usually has a good prognosis.

Compliance is the key to success of therapy, and an effort should be made to ensure that topical therapy is applied on a regular basis. Do not allow patients to apply medication "when it itches"; rather, explain that prevention of inflammation will lead to decreased pruritus and comfort. The proper technique of applying medication should be shown to patients by the physician or physician's assistant. I suggest that small droplets of cream or ointment be dotted on the trunk or extremity and the flat of the hand used to make sweeping strokes downward with the hair growth. This spreads the medication on evenly and minimizes provoking a bout of itching with excess rubbing. The amount of medication applied is important. It takes about 15 to 25 grams of cream to cover an adult body per day. Most patients apply too little medication because of a fear of using topical steroids based on improper information. It often takes 450 grams (1 pound) of cream to cover an adult's body per month. A prescription and adequate number of refills should be given to ensure continuity of medication until the next appointment.

Because atopic individuals have increased aware-

ness of pruritus, and the pruritus response is exaggerated, the immediate skin environment should be controlled as much as possible. High temperatures and high humidity should be avoided to prevent sweat retention. The use of a room air conditioner may be needed. Low humidity should be clearly avoided because dryness of the skin, especially in wintertime, produces increased pruritus. Leaving pots of water in the bedroom and allowing them to evaporate is a simple device; buying a room humidifier that keeps the room humidity at about 70% is more reliable. The wearing of woolens should be avoided as well as rough-textured, tight and binding, or heavy clothing that could be sweat producing. Nylon clothing may lead to increased sweat retention. Avoid "stay pressed" cotton and polyester blends that contain formaldehyde resins, which may cause irritation or contact allergy; 100% cotton is the ideal fabric. Empirically, avoid house dust, tobacco smoke, external pollens, and animal dander in the immediate environment.

Trigger factors known to produce itching should be avoided and include the following common factors: (1) aeroallergens as determined by history or scratch testing; (2) contactants that are irritants or true contact allergens; (3) dryness of the skin; (4) stress, which is treated with stress reduction and behavior modification; (5) foods that are known allergens, usually in infancy; (6) prevention of active *Staphylococcus aureus* infection, herpes simplex virus infection, and cutaneous fungus infection.

The choice of topical therapy is based on the anti-inflammatory properties of the medication, the base, and the economic confines of treating a chronic disease. The most common topical steroids used are 0.1% triamcinolone acetonide (Aristocort) and 1% hydrocortisone. I prefer the ointment over the cream because of more moisturizing and less exposure to preservatives and emulsifiers, but patients occasionally will not tolerate the occlusive effect of ointment. It is applied twice daily as described before. It is good practice to have the patient bring the containers of medications to the office and be sure that they are using adequate amounts of the correct medication. Reinforce the nursing program on each follow-up visit. As the patient improves, decrease the class of the steroid to a level that will control the erythema and pruritus. Always encourage a hydration program. In cases in which more anti-inflammatory effect is needed, I use 2.5% hydrocortisone (Hytone), 0.05% desonide (DesOwen), 0.05% aclometasone dipropionate (Aclovate), and for short times, 0.2% hydrocortisone valerate (Westcort) on the face. For more severe involved areas on the trunk, 0.005% fluticasone propionate (Cutivate), 0.1% mometasone furoate (Elocon), 0.1% halcinonide (Halog), 0.05% betamethasone dipropionate (Diprosone), 0.05% fluocinonide acetonide (Lidex), 0.05% betamethasone dipropionate in augmented base (Diprolene AF), 0.25% desoximetasone (Topicort), and 0.05% diflorasone diacetate (Psorcon) are used. The use of class I topical steroids such as 0.05% halobetasol propionate (Ultravate) or 0.05% clobetasol propionate (Temovate) should be confined to small areas and not used for more than 2 weeks. When using the more potent topical steroids, one can often get an adequate therapeutic effect by using them once a day and applying moisturizers on the alternate application. Always monitor the patient for signs of striae, bruising, telangiectasia, and atrophy.

One of my favorite prescriptions that uses less steroid is mixing 2 ounces of 0.05% fluocinonide acetonide or 0.1% amcinonide (Cyclocort) cream with 6 ounces of Complex 15 lotion to make 8 ounces. This is easy to apply to the body and is more economical. For antipruritic effect, one can substitute Doak Tar lotion for the Complex 15 lotion. Alternative nonsteroidal topical therapy is cold tap-water compresses using Burow's solution, or more simply, dilute acetic acid made by mixing 1 tablespoon white household vinegar to 1 quart of ice water. Crushed ice put in a Ziplock bag and held against the skin, Aveeno Anti-Itch cream or lotion, Sarna lotion, PrameGel, and Estar gel are helpful.

Atopic dermatitis of the scalp can be treated with a tar shampoo such as T/Gel or DHS Tar. When this is not adequate, the addition of 1% hydrocortisone (Texacort scalp lotion), 0.1% halcinonide (Halog solution), 0.05% fluocinonide acetonide (Lidex solution), 0.05% betamethasone dipropionate (Diprolene lotion), or 0.05% clobetasol propionate (Temovate solution) after the shampoo may be used for short-term therapy.

Systemic therapy should include antibiosis for clinical folliculitis, impetiginization, and markedly excoriated skin. I use erythromycin 250 mg four times a day and dicloxacillin 250 to 500 mg four times a day for 7 to 10 days. I find that chronic therapy leads to the development of resistant strains of *Staphylococcus*. In selected cases of poor response, cultures and bacterial sensitivity studies should be done and appropriate antibiosis instituted. Systemic oral steroids in the form of prednisone usually given in doses of 10 to 60 mg per day are miraculous, but the side effects are well known and there is rebound when the patient stops the drug. Patients usually stop topical therapy when they feel well, which contributes to the rebound. I use systemic therapy only when the patient presents with a generalized flare of the disease, usually after being without medication or secondary to a generalized infection. Although controversial, I prefer to ration such steroid therapy in the form of intramuscular triamcinolone acetonide (Kenalog-40), 40 to 60 mg. I try to keep these injections limited to a maximum of 2-month intervals. Besides use of antihistamines for the often accompanying allergic rhinitis, antihistamines are used for their antipruritic effect, and I take advantage of the long half-life and soporific effect of hydroxyzine (Atarax) 10 to 100 mg taken 3 hours before sleep. Doxepin (Sinequan)* in doses of 25 to 150 mg is also prescribed as a single bedtime dose taken 3 hours before bedtime.

*Not FDA approved for this indication.

Cetirizine (Zyrtec), the metabolite of hydroxyzine, in doses of 5 to 10 mg every 12 to 24 hours has been effective.

The use of ultraviolet A or B or in combination can be helpful if redness, dryness, and burning can be avoided. I give suberythema doses of ultraviolet B twice weekly, usually after the patient takes a bath with coal tar (Zetar emulsion), 1 ounce per tub. Ultraviolet A can be given with methoxsalen (Oxsoralen-Ultra) 10-mg capsules, 0.6 mg per kg, taken 1 or 2 hours before therapy. Depending on skin type, therapy is limited to a maximum of 15 joules per treatment, with 15 or 20 treatments given.

Newer experimental drugs that are being evaluated are thymopoietin, a synthetic five-carbon thymus-stimulating hormone; cyclosporine; and interferon gamma.

ERYTHEMA MULTIFORME

method of
MARCIA G. TONNESEN, M.D.
State University of New York School of Medicine
Stony Brook, New York

Veterans Affairs Medical Center
Northport, New York

Erythema multiforme (EM) is an acute, self-limited inflammatory disorder of the skin and mucous membranes. Traditionally, EM has been considered to be a disease spectrum that included EM minor, EM major, Stevens-Johnson syndrome (SJS), and toxic epidermal necrolysis (TEN). Therefore, these entities are addressed in this article. Currently, however, the definition and nosology of EM are undergoing evolution as diagnostic criteria are refined and subsets in the EM spectrum are identified as distinct disease entities. Recent evidence supports a clear distinction between EM, with acrally distributed skin lesions and an etiologic link to herpes simplex virus (HSV) infection, and SJS, with centrally to widely distributed skin lesions, mucous membrane involvement, and an etiologic link primarily to drug reactions.

ERYTHEMA MULTIFORME

EM is a relatively mild, frequently recurrent, cutaneous illness characterized by the sudden onset of a symmetrical erythematous eruption with a primarily acral distribution. Mucosal involvement, when present, is usually limited to the oral cavity. Skin lesions begin as fixed erythematous macules, develop into edematous papules, and may become bullous. At least some of the lesions evolve to form characteristic target lesions. Individual lesions occasionally burn or itch, appear in successive crops, and resolve within 2 to 4 weeks. The majority of cases of recurrent EM are associated with HSV infection and typically occur 7 to 10 days after the appearance of a recurrent HSV lesion (oral, genital, or other location). Subclinical episodes of herpes can also precede EM. Herpes-associated EM is currently believed to result from an HSV-specific host immune response in the skin.

STEVENS-JOHNSON SYNDROME

SJS is a severe mucocutaneous illness characterized by an extensive blistering eruption with a primarily truncal distribution and mucosal erosions, typically involving the mouth and conjunctivae. A prodrome with constitutional symptoms typically heralds the onset of the eruption. Skin lesions begin as erythematous or purpuric macules, frequently develop central vesiculation, and may progress to widespread bullae formation with epidermal necrosis. Epidermal detachment may involve up to 10% body surface area. Painful mucosal erosions may result in characteristic hemorrhagic crusted lips, a foul-smelling mouth, decreased oral intake, and difficulty with micturition. Ocular involvement may produce red sore eyes with photophobia, conjunctival erosions and inflammation with residual scarring, and lacrimal abnormalities. Permanent visual impairment may occur. Disease duration is 4 to 6 weeks. Recurrences are infrequent. SJS is now recognized as strongly related to drugs and linked to some infections, particularly *Mycoplasma pneumoniae,* but never to herpesvirus infection.

TOXIC EPIDERMAL NECROLYSIS

TEN is characterized by widespread sheetlike necrosis and sloughing of the epidermis, involving greater than 30% of the body surface. (Epidermal detachment between 10 and 30% of body surface area is now classified as overlap SJS-TEN.) After a 1- to 3-day prodrome of fever and flulike symptoms, the cutaneous eruption begins as a burning or painful erythema, often distributed symmetrically on the face and upper body. It then rapidly extends to involve significant or total body surface area within hours to 2 to 3 days. Involvement of multiple mucosal surfaces is present in nearly all patients. The order of frequency is oropharynx (which in severe cases may extend to involve the larynx and tracheobronchial tree), eyes, genitalia, anus. TEN can be considered a manifestation of "acute skin failure" with abnormal barrier function resulting in fluid and electrolyte loss, protein loss, increased susceptibility to infection, impaired thermoregulation, altered immune status, and increased energy expenditure. Morbidity is significant, and the mortality rate is often 30% or greater. The leading cause of death is sepsis. Drugs are now considered by many to be the only documented cause of TEN. The major offenders include anticonvulsants, sulfonamides, other antibiotics, allopurinol, and nonsteroidal anti-inflammatory agents, although many other drugs have been implicated. Although the mechanism is unknown, a specific defect in the detoxification of reactive drug metabolites and a resultant lymphocytotoxic reaction may be pathogenic factors in epidermal necrosis.

THERAPEUTIC APPROACH

Optimal therapeutic intervention is hindered by the fact that specific pathogenic mechanisms of tissue injury have not yet been completely defined. In addition, few controlled studies have been performed to evaluate the effectiveness of therapeutic interventions. Elimination of any identified or presumed precipitating factors is of prime importance. Successful therapy should combine symptomatic and supportive measures with observation for and treatment of associated complications, depending on the clinical characteristics and severity of the episode. Typically, EM is mild and self-limited and requires only symptomatic care. However, because of the degree and extent of epidermal and mucosal involvement that occurs in SJS and TEN, careful monitoring is critical, hospitalization is often required, and supportive care is usually necessary.

Elimination of Etiologic Factors

Any suspected or unnecessary drug should be withdrawn and avoided in the future. *M. pneumoniae* and other infections, if diagnosed, should be appropriately treated. In recurrent herpes-associated EM, a course of acyclovir (Zovirax),* 200 mg orally five times daily for 5 days, should be initiated at the first symptom of HSV infection.

Symptomatic Measures

For pruritic or painful skin lesions, systemic antihistamines or analgesics may provide symptomatic relief.

Skin Care

For crusted erosive skin lesions, mild drying, débridement, and cleansing as well as a soothing antipruritic effect can be achieved with open wet-to-damp compresses of tepid water applied for 20 minutes three or four times per day or with frequent bathing in lukewarm to cool water for 20 minutes two or three times per day. Lesions should be observed for signs of secondary infection, cultures performed when indicated, and treatment initiated with the appropriate systemic antibiotic. Topical acyclovir and topical corticosteroids have not been shown to be of benefit.

Mouth Care

When extensive painful mouth lesions are present, good oral hygiene is critical to minimize infection and discomfort. Hydrogen peroxide (1.5%) mouthwash every 2 hours provides gentle débridement. Topical anesthetics such as dyclonine (Dyclone), viscous lidocaine, or a 1:1 mixture of Kaopectate and elixir of diphenhydramine used as a mouthwash often provide relief from painful erosions. A liquid or soft diet, usually better tolerated, contributes to the maintenance of hydration and nutrition.

Eye Care

Because of the potential for long-term sequelae resulting in visual loss, careful monitoring of eye involvement is mandatory, and early consultation with and continuing care by an ophthalmologist are strongly recommended. Suggested therapeutic measures might include irrigation and compresses to cleanse the eye, lysis of adhesions, and instillation of topical antibiotics when indicated.

---

*Not FDA approved for this indication.

Supportive Care

Because of the extensive epidermal and mucosal necrosis and detachment that can occur in SJS and TEN, careful monitoring is critical, hospitalization is often required, and intravenous fluid therapy and nasogastric or parenteral feeding may be necessary to maintain hydration and nutrition.

Preventive Measures

Because of the common etiologic association between recurrent HSV infections and EM, measures that attempt to prevent recurrences of HSV may lessen the frequency of subsequent episodes of EM. Avoidance of sun exposure through the use of sunscreens (sun protection factor of 15 or higher), sunsticks (sunscreen-containing lip balm [Chap Stick]), and protective clothing and by minimizing sun exposure from 10 AM to 3 PM (the peak period for ultraviolet B) may reduce ultraviolet light–induced HSV recurrences. Attempts should be made to minimize stress, a well-known precipitating factor of HSV. Topical antiviral preparations have not been clearly shown to prevent or abort recurrent HSV infections. Prophylactic administration of acyclovir has resulted in abolition of recurrent HSV infections and of ensuing episodes of EM. Therefore, in patients with frequently recurring, debilitating, and documented herpes-associated EM, the treatment of choice is daily oral acyclovir for a period of 6 months or longer. The recommended starting dose is 400 mg orally twice daily, with tapering of the dose after the disease is brought under control. Because of the known occurrence of acyclovir resistance and the unknown long-term side effects of chronic acyclovir therapy, the drug should be stopped periodically and the need for its continuance reassessed. In drug-associated SJS or TEN, withdrawal and future avoidance of the implicated drug are mandatory.

Reduction of Morbidity and Mortality

The indication for the use of systemic glucocorticosteroids in EM, SJS, and TEN is highly controversial, because no controlled studies have been conducted to document efficacy. However, because SJS and TEN can progress to widespread epidermal necrosis with a mortality rate as high as 30%, early use of systemic steroids in the progressive phase of the disease process in an attempt to decrease the extent of tissue damage is advocated by some. In contrast, systemic steroid use is condemned by others because some retrospective reports have suggested that patients treated with systemic steroids have an increased incidence of morbidity, prolonged hospitalization times, and mortality. Therefore, if systemic steroids are used, once disease progression ceases and the wound healing process begins, or if no response is noted within 2 to 3 days, treatment should be abruptly discontinued to minimize risk of associated complications.

If extensive, advanced tissue necrosis occurs or is already evident (approaching 20% of total body surface area involvement), immediate transfer of the patient to a burn unit under the care of a surgical burn specialist is strongly advocated. Therapeutic burn unit recommendations consist of (1) measures to guard against iatrogenic infection, including withdrawal from systemic steroids, limitation of antibiotic use to specific culture-proven infections, avoidance of indwelling lines and catheters whenever possible, daily cultures of skin and of blood and urine, and aggressive treatment of sepsis if it occurs; (2) supportive care consisting of use of an air-fluidized bed, respiratory and physical therapy, intravenous fluid therapy, tube feedings, adequate pain relief, and continuing care by an ophthalmologist; (3) avoidance of all unnecessary medications, particularly those that are known etiologic factors of SJS-TEN, such as sulfonamides (including sulfa-containing eye preparations, diuretics, and topical dressings); and (4) skin care with emphasis on early gentle débridement followed by application of a dressing to protect the denuded dermis from desiccation and to facilitate rapid re-epithelialization. Reduced mortality and faster healing result from the use of synthetic dressings, biologic dressings, silver nitrate dressings, allografts, or porcine xenografts.

Education of the Patient

For EM, patients should be reassured regarding the usual benign, self-limited course and educated regarding the frequent association with recurrent HSV infections. For SJS and TEN, patients should be advised that the course is self-limited but potentially severe and educated regarding the frequent association with certain drugs.

BULLOUS SKIN DISEASES
method of
ROBERT E. JORDON, M.D.
University of Texas–Houston Medical School
Houston, Texas

The bullous skin diseases continue to challenge physicians both diagnostically and therapeutically. On the basis of intensive investigative efforts, it is now clear that a large number of these blistering diseases have an autoimmune or immunologic pathogenesis. Early immunologic studies of bullous diseases, such as pemphigus, bullous pemphigoid, and dermatitis herpetiformis, are also credited with ushering in the modern era of immunodermatology. Not only have these investigative efforts shed light on the pathogenesis of these diseases, but such studies have allowed us to better classify all blistering skin diseases. In addition, better therapeutic regimens have evolved. In this article, I discuss the major clinical findings, appropriate diagnostic studies, and therapeutic approaches for patients with autoimmune bullous skin diseases. Table 1 lists the major members (and variants) of the autoimmune bullous disease group.

GENERAL PRINCIPLES OF DIAGNOSIS AND THERAPY

Patients with suspected autoimmune bullous diseases should have appropriate diagnostic tests performed as early as possible. Such diagnostic evaluation would include routine histopathology, direct immunofluorescence (IF) studies, and when appropriate, indirect (serum) IF studies. For routine histopathologic examination, biopsy of a fresh small early blister should be done. For direct IF, a fresh early small blister is chosen for patients with pemphigus; skin adjacent to an intact blister (perilesional skin) or erosion is appropriate for all of the other autoimmune blistering skin diseases. A correct diagnosis can usually be established by employing these two diagnostic tests. Indirect IF is useful in assessing the levels of autoantibodies in the serum of these patients and in the diagnosis of patients with epidermolysis bullosa acquisita.

Because most of the autoimmune bullous diseases are induced by specific immunopathologic mechanisms, drugs used in the treatment of these diseases should be anti-inflammatory or immunosuppressive or both. These medications should be instituted as soon as the appropriate diagnosis has been determined and in doses sufficient to suppress new blister formation. Combinations of medications may be used for long-term management.

PEMPHIGUS

Pemphigus constitutes a group of blistering skin diseases considered universally fatal before the availability of corticosteroid drugs. Diseases in this group include pemphigus vulgaris, pemphigus vegetans, pemphigus foliaceus, pemphigus erythematosus, drug-induced pemphigus, and paraneoplastic pemphigus.

Pemphigus vulgaris, the most common form of the disease, often begins with erosions and ulcerations of the oral mucosa. Within 2 to 4 weeks, this is most often followed by flaccid, weeping bullous lesions of the skin, usually on the trunk and scalp. These flaccid blisters rupture easily and extend peripherally, producing large denuded areas. Lesions may arise on seemingly normal skin or on erythematous bases. Common sites include the scalp, face, back, and chest, although the disease when generalized may involve any cutaneous or mucous membrane surface. The usual age at onset is in the fourth and fifth decades of life, although all groups, including children and the elderly, may develop this disease. Pemphigus vegetans, a rare variant of pemphigus vulgaris, is characterized by vegetative weeping lesions, most commonly in the axillae and groin. Pemphigus affects all races and ethnic groups, although it is more common in peoples of Jewish or Mediterranean origin.

Although less common than pemphigus vulgaris, pemphigus foliaceus represents a superficial, less severe form of the disease. Cutaneous manifestations include slowly spreading eczematoid lesions, crusts, scales, and shallow erosions. Oral lesions are extremely rare. The scalp, face, upper chest, and back are commonly involved sites, although the disease may progress to involve the entire body, presenting as a generalized exfoliative erythroderma. Sun exposure appears to aggravate this condition. All age groups may be affected, again including the elderly and children. Variants of this superficial form of pemphigus include Brazilian pemphigus foliaceus or "fogo selvagem," endemic to South Central Brazil, and pemphigus erythematosus, a localized form of pemphigus foliaceus that mimics lupus erythematosus (LE) including a malar rash. All forms of pemphigus are characterized histopathologically by intraepidermal bulla formation and acantholysis (loss of cohesion of individual epidermal cells). In pemphigus vulgaris, blister formation occurs deep within the epidermis so that the basal cells form the floor of the blister cavity. Pemphigus foliaceus, a more superficial form, is characterized by blister formation occurring in or near the granular layer in the upper epidermis. Large numbers of eosinophils may be present in the inflammatory reaction.

Both forms of pemphigus are characterized immunopathologically by the presence of autoantibodies that react with keratinocyte cell surface antigens. Thus, these autoantibodies react precisely at the sites of the primary histopathologic lesions and partially explain the process of acantholysis. Some of these antibodies have been shown to activate components of the complement system. Antigens have now been identified for both forms of pemphigus and include adhesion proteins of the epidermis. The main keratinocyte antigen reactive with pemphigus vulgaris autoantibodies appears to be desmoglein III; in pemphigus foliaceus, it is desmoglein I. These are both components of the desmosomes, or the attachment plates, of individual keratinocytes and belong to the cadherin family of adhesion proteins. By direct

IF staining, IgG and complement deposits are also seen on the surface of the keratinocytes in areas of disease activity. These deposits may be seen in both oral and cutaneous lesions, and these are now considered hallmark diagnostic findings for the diagnosis of pemphigus.

The mainstay of therapy for all forms of pemphigus continues to be systemic corticosteroids. Pemphigus vulgaris still poses the greatest threat to the patient, especially during acute episodes or widespread disease. At this stage of the disease process, no other form of therapy has replaced high doses of corticosteroids. The initial dose should be sufficiently high (100 to 150 mg* of prednisone per day) to completely suppress new blister formation. If the disease is confined to the oral cavity, 80 mg of prednisone per day should be sufficient. I usually have patients take prednisone as a once-a-day dose, usually in the morning to minimize side effects. Most patients with pemphigus foliaceus will respond to lower prednisone doses, 60 to 80 mg daily, depending on the disease severity. With cessation of new blister formation (usually 2 to 4 weeks), the prednisone dose may be lowered to 40 to 60 mg per day. Further reductions, however, should be more gradual. At 60 mg per day, I usually try to convert the patient slowly to alternate-day steroid therapy. This may be accomplished by reducing the prednisone dose on alternate days at approximately 2- to 3-week intervals. If I can successfully taper patients to an alternate-day therapeutic regimen and maintain remission, I do not add additional drugs such as immunosuppressives. If I encounter difficulty in converting to alternate-day steroids, immunosuppressive agents, including azathioprine,† cyclophosphamide,† and methotrexate,† may be employed, especially in patients with pemphigus vulgaris. My favorite approach is to use azathioprine, because fewer side effects are usually encountered. With any form of immunosuppressive therapy, careful monitoring of the blood elements and liver enzymes must be maintained. Plasmapheresis, to lower circulating autoantibodies, may also be employed at this stage if further control is needed. I normally advise calcium supplementation for all patients who need long-term corticosteroid therapy. Gold therapy† has also been used and found to be successful in selected pemphigus patients. In addition, I have found hydroxychloroquine† to be a marvelous steroid-sparing agent in patients with pemphigus foliaceus. This drug can be started along with prednisone in doses of 200 mg twice daily. As with any antimalarial, periodic eye examinations to rule out retinitis are required.

Drug-induced pemphigus usually takes the form of pemphigus foliaceus. The two most commonly associated drugs are D-penicillamine (Cuprimine) and captopril (Capoten). Cessation of the offending medication usually results in the disappearance of the skin lesions. Paraneoplastic pemphigus, the newest member of the group, is almost always associated with an underlying lymphoma or lymphocytic leukemia. Because of the underlying neoplastic process, the prognosis of this form of pemphigus is poor.

PEMPHIGOID

Four disease processes constitute this group. These include bullous pemphigoid, herpes (pemphigoid) gestationis, cicatricial pemphigoid, and localized scarring pemphigoid (Brunsting-Perry). The major disease in this group, bullous pemphigoid, is an autoimmune subepidermal blistering disease that primarily affects elderly patients. This disease process has long been confused with other blistering diseases of the skin and was not officially recognized as a separate distinct disease until the specific IF findings were reported. The major clinical feature of bullous pemphigoid is the presence of large, tense bullae arising on normal-appearing skin or erythematous bases. The inner aspects of the thighs, the flexural surfaces of the forearms, the groin, the axillae, and the lower abdomen are common sites of involvement. Oral lesions occur in less than one third of patients and, unlike in pemphigus vulgaris, are rarely the initial manifestation. The disease is usually self-limited, and the patient's health usually remains good. The mortality is low, although because of the age of many of these patients, death from unrelated causes may intervene before the disease has run its course. On histopathologic examination, bullous pemphigoid shows subepidermal bulla formation with primarily an infiltrate of eosinophils and lymphocytes. By direct IF, these patients have IgG deposits and C3 deposits at the basement membrane zone. Perilesional skin is the site of choice for biopsies submitted for direct IF assay in patients with bullous pemphigoid. In addition, circulating autoantibodies (IgG type), again directed toward the basement membrane zone, are present in the serum of these patients. The antigenic sites, reactive with bullous pemphigoid autoantibodies, reside on the polar tips of basal keratinocytes associated with hemidesmosomes. Both routine histopathology and direct IF studies should be employed for correct diagnosis of this condition.

The therapy for bullous pemphigoid is similar to that for diseases of the pemphigus group, except that lower doses of corticosteroids and immunosuppressives will often suppress blister formation in this disease. Starting doses of prednisone 80 to 100 mg per day will usually bring about clinical remission. Immunosuppressive agents, particularly azathioprine, are extremely useful in maintenance therapy and in combination with alternate-day corticosteroids. Careful monitoring of blood elements and chemistries must be maintained if immunosuppressives are used. Because of the age of most bullous pemphigoid patients, a constant vigil for underlying medical problems and infection must also be maintained. High-dose tetracyclines* (1 to 2 grams per

---

*Exceeds dosage recommended by the manufacturer.
†Not FDA approved for this indication.

*Not FDA approved for this indication.

day) have also been employed in this disease process and have been found useful in selected patients.

Herpes gestationis is a relatively rare, highly pruritic blistering skin disease of pregnancy and the immediate postpartum period. Estimates suggest an incidence of herpes gestationis to be one case per 10,000 to 50,000 deliveries. The disease is misnamed, because there is no relationship to herpesvirus infection. The disease usually appears in the fifth or sixth month of pregnancy, but earlier onsets in the first trimester have been documented. Several cases have occurred in the immediate postpartum period. It is a self-limited disease, but with subsequent pregnancies, blistering may occur earlier and be more intensive. Estrogen- and progesterone-containing medications have been reported to reinitiate the disease process and should be avoided. Like bullous pemphigoid, large tense blisters, in addition to vesicular lesions, are common in this disease. Common sites of involvement include the abdomen, the extremities, the umbilicus, and the trunk. The histopathologic appearance of this disease is subepidermal blister formation, with eosinophils being the major cell infiltrate. Direct IF studies reveal C3 deposits at the basement membrane zone, usually in the absence of IgG, in a pattern similar to bullous pemphigoid. These patients also have autoantibodies in their serum that are difficult to detect by routine indirect IF staining. In vitro C3 staining techniques, however, reveal an IgG complement-fixing autoantibody reactive with the basement membrane zone. The antigen in this disease is located on the polar tips of basal keratinocytes. It appears to be a component of the hemidesmosomes found on basal cells.

Treatment of herpes gestationis is less than satisfactory. If skin lesions are limited, topical corticosteroid preparations may be used. Most patients, however, have more extensive involvement with concomitant severe pruritus. Prednisone 20 to 40 mg daily usually provides adequate control. The dosage should be regulated to provide the patient symptomatic relief rather than complete control. Therapy must be continued into the postpartum period, because flaring of the disease usually occurs after delivery and with the resumption of normal menses. In most instances, the disease disappears approximately 6 months after delivery. If the disease persists in the postpartum period, immunosuppressives such as azathioprine may be added to corticosteroid therapy. The disease may also recur during subsequent pregnancies.

Cicatricial pemphigoid is a rare, chronic subepidermal blistering disease that primarily involves the mucous membranes. This condition is characterized clinically by its chronicity and for lesions to produce scarring. Most common sites are the oral and ocular membranes, but the nasal mucosa, pharynx, larynx, esophagus, genitalia, anus, and skin may be affected. Although clinically cicatricial pemphigoid bears little resemblance to bullous pemphigoid, investigative studies suggest that the two diseases (at least some forms) may be related. Cicatricial pemphigoid is also histopathologically characterized by subepidermal bulla formation. Direct IF studies reveal deposits of IgG and C3 at the basement membrane zone in perilesional tissue. Fibrin deposits are common and almost universally present in ocular conjunctival specimens. These deposits are also present in the lamina lucida region of the basement membrane zone as they are in bullous pemphigoid. One set of patients appears to have autoantibodies reactive with the 180-kilodalton protein associated with bullous pemphigoid and herpes gestationis. Another set of patients appears to have autoantibodies reactive with laminin 5 or epilegrin, which is located deeper in the lamina lucida. The diagnosis is established by clinical findings and appropriate direct IF studies. A variant of cicatricial pemphigoid, localized pemphigoid of the Brunsting-Perry type, involves primarily the skin of the head and neck area. IF findings in this disease process are similar.

Treatment of this disorder is less than satisfactory. The mainstay of treatment is systemic corticosteroids and immunosuppressives such as azathioprine.* Dapsone* has been useful in selected patients primarily with oral disease. However, I have found this drug to be ineffective in patients who have ocular manifestations. Topical steroids are of little value, although local injections into or adjacent to lesions are sometimes helpful. In treating patients with this condition, starting doses of prednisone are 60 to 80 mg given as a once-a-day dose. Once the disease process has been controlled, the patient should be switched to alternate-day corticosteroid therapy. Immunosuppressives, such as azathioprine, may be added if switching to alternate-day prednisone therapy proves difficult.

DERMATITIS HERPETIFORMIS

Dermatitis herpetiformis is a chronic subepidermal blistering dermatosis characterized by pruritic grouped vesicles. The extensor surfaces of the body, including the shoulders, buttocks, elbows, and knees, are common areas of involvement. The major symptom is intense burning pruritus that may be incapacitating. The disease usually begins in the third and fourth decades of life, and once it makes its appearance, it is generally lifelong. On histopathologic examination, these patients reveal subepidermal blister formation with collections of neutrophils (microabcesses) within the tips of the dermal papillae at the dermal-epidermal junction.

Dermatitis herpetiformis is a genetic disease with a high prevalence of HLA-B8 and HLA-DR3. The disease is characterized immunologically by the presence of IgA deposits by direct IF within the tips of the dermal papillae, a finding that is now considered the best diagnostic test for this disease process. The etiology of the disease, however, remains unknown.

The mainstay of therapy for dermatitis herpetiformis is dapsone, a drug that is thought to interfere

---

*Not FDA approved for this indication.

with neutrophil function. The dose varies among patients, although most respond to 25 to 50 mg daily. The response is dramatic, and the patient's symptoms usually subside within 24 to 48 hours. Because dermatitis herpetiformis is a lifelong disease, patients may be required to take dapsone for the rest of their life. Careful monitoring of blood work for side effects is therefore crucial. Adherence to a gluten-free diet is helpful in most patients and will allow some reduction in drug dosage. Recent evidence suggests that adherence to a gluten-free diet also diminishes the development of lymphoma in these patients. As an alternative to dapsone, sulfapyridine, 2 to 4 grams daily in divided doses, is thought to be as effective as dapsone. The drug is difficult to obtain, however, and may not be available in all areas. If sulfapyridine is used, fluid intake must be maintained at a high level to avoid crystallization of the drug in the urinary tract. In patients who are sensitive to both dapsone and sulfapyridine, colchicine* in usual therapeutic doses has also been found to be effective.

LINEAR IMMUNOGLOBULIN A BULLOUS DERMATOSES

Two blistering diseases are included in this group, linear IgA bullous dermatosis of adults and chronic bullous disease of childhood.

Linear IgA bullous dermatosis is a subepidermal blistering disease characterized by tense blisters of varying size and more erythema than is seen in dermatitis herpetiformis. The disease process may be confused with dermatitis herpetiformis, but one does not see the high frequency of HLA antigens HLA-B8 and HLA-DR3, nor do these patients have granular IgA deposits in the tips of the dermal papillae. Instead, these patients have linear IgA deposits at the basement membrane zone as seen by direct IF, usually in the basal lamina. On histopathologic examination, these patients show subepidermal bullae and may have papillary microabscesses of neutrophils as seen in dermatitis herpetiformis. As in patients with dermatitis herpetiformis, many of these patients respond to sulfones* and sulfapyridine. Dosage for these patients is similar to that in dermatitis herpetiformis.

Chronic bullous disease of childhood is a subepidermal blistering disease that affects preschool-aged children. Most pediatric dermatologists think that this is a common blistering disease of childhood but that many cases may be mild. The disease is characterized clinically by tense bullae of varying size, with a predilection for the flexural areas and the groin. Lesions may be generalized with grouping; annular configurations are common. The disease course is punctuated by periodic remissions with decreasing exacerbations. The disease usually does not persist into the teens or adult life, a feature that separates this disease process from other blistering diseases, including linear IgA bullous disease of the adult. Chronic bullous disease of childhood is characterized histopathologically by subepidermal blister formation, and most commonly, neutrophils are present in the inflammatory infiltrate. Direct IF, which is most useful diagnostically, shows linear IgA and, often, C3 deposits at the basement membrane zone. Patients with this disease process are quite responsive to sulfones and sulfapyridine. Extremely small doses of dapsone,* for example, often control this disease process.

EPIDERMOLYSIS BULLOSA ACQUISITA

Epidermolysis bullosa acquisita is a rare subepidermal blistering disease associated with milia formation and scarring. Unlike the hereditary forms of epidermolysis bullosa, this form is acquired and has an autoimmune etiology. Sites commonly affected include the extensor surfaces of joints, the dorsal surfaces of the hands and feet, and areas subjected to trauma. The disease is usually chronic, lasting for many years, and unfortunately is recalcitrant to most therapeutic modalities. Epidermolysis bullosa acquisita is characterized histopathologically by subepidermal bullae formation with an inflammatory infiltrate that is variable. Neutrophils are often seen in the inflammatory infiltrate; at times, no inflammatory infiltrate is present. Direct IF examination of perilesional skin demonstrates linear IgG and often C3 deposits at the basement membrane zone similar to bullous pemphigoid. Likewise, these patients have autoantibodies in their serum (IgG type) that react with the basement membrane zone. It has now been shown that these autoantibodies react with antigens located beneath the lamina densa of the basement membrane zone thought to be type VII collagen. As mentioned earlier, this disease process is most difficult to treat. Some patients respond to dapsone and/or sulfapyridine. Others do not. Prednisone and immunosuppressives have been used in some patients with limited success. Plasmapheresis, and more recently photophoresis, have been tried in a few patients and may offer some hope to these patients.

BULLOUS LUPUS ERYTHEMATOSUS

Bullous lesions of LE represent a rare yet more frequently recognized manifestation of this disease process. Bullous lesions are more commonly seen in patients with systemic LE and are often found as clusters of tense blisters. Bullous lesions of LE tend to be more common in black persons and tend to appear in crops of blisters in a fashion similar to dermatitis herpetiformis. Bullous LE is characterized histopathologically by subepidermal blister formation and a rich neutrophilic infiltrate that appears to be identical to the papillary microabscesses seen in dermatitis herpetiformis. Direct IF examination, however, is typical for LE, that is, granular IgG and

---

*Not FDA approved for this indication.

*Not FDA approved for this indication.

IgM deposits rather than IgA at the dermal-epidermal junction. This form of LE must be differentiated from other autoimmune blistering diseases such as bullous pemphigoid, epidermolysis bullosa acquisita, and erythema multiforme, and patients who present with this form of LE must have a work-up for a possible flare of systemic LE. The treatment of choice for the bullous lesions is dapsone* 25 to 100 mg daily. Most patients respond dramatically to this therapy. However, patients who present with bullous lesions of LE may be undergoing a severe flare of systemic LE. Such flares, if involving other organ systems, must be assessed and treated appropriately.

---

*Not FDA approved for this indication.

CONTACT DERMATITIS

method of
JOHN E. WOLF, Jr., M.D.
Baylor College of Medicine
Houston, Texas

The skin is, among many other things, a barrier—an interface between a person's internal and external environments. It is generally an effective barrier but is thus exposed to many noxious agents, both physical and chemical. These agents may cause contact dermatitis, an inflammation of the skin first described by Pliny the Younger in the first century AD.

There are two general types of contact dermatitis—irritant and allergic—and these, in turn, like any other form of dermatitis (eczema), may be acute, subacute, or chronic. The management of contact dermatitis must account for these variations and must be prefaced by careful description and accurate diagnosis.

Irritant contact dermatitis results from exposure of the skin to inherently injurious chemicals or toxins and does not require allergic sensitization. Examples include dermatitis caused by detergents, household or industrial cleansers, or the sting of the Portuguese man-of-war *Physalia physalis*. On the other hand, allergic contact dermatitis follows exposure to a substance capable of sensitizing the skin; subsequent re-exposure may elicit a contact dermatitis. The classic illustration is *Rhus* contact dermatitis (poison ivy).

AVOIDANCE AND PHYSICAL PROTECTION

With either form of contact dermatitis, a critical component of proper management is identification of the inciting agent followed by careful avoidance of that substance. In the case of irritant contact dermatitis, this information is generally obtained by a probing history of the patient, sometimes combined with a careful examination of the home or work place. Evaluation of allergic contact dermatitis may also include open or closed patch testing.

Once an inciting or provocative agent has been identified, the patient must make every effort to avoid further contact with that substance, which may be difficult. A bricklayer with a contact allergy to chromates may be unable to avoid contact with chromate-containing cement. Seemingly ubiquitous substances such as nickel may also be difficult to avoid. Short of outright avoidance, the use of protective clothing such as gloves, boots, masks, and long-sleeved shirts may help. Barrier creams, especially in an industrial setting, may also be useful.

TREATMENT

Acute Contact Dermatitis

Acute contact dermatitis, irritant or allergic, is usually a weeping, oozing, exudative process, which is often accompanied by vesicles or bullae and is sometimes complicated by secondary bacterial infection. The application of cool or tepid soaks or compresses may be both soothing and drying; tap water or Burow's solution (Domeboro) may be used. Colloidal oatmeal (Aveeno) baths may also be comforting. Itching is often intense and may be controlled by antihistamines such as diphenhydramine (Benadryl) or hydroxyzine (Atarax) or one of the newer, less sedating antihistamines such as cetirizine (Zyrtec), loratadine (Claritin), astemizole (Hismanal), and fexofenadine (Allegra). Astemizole has been associated with rare cases of serious cardiovascular adverse events.

Most cases of acute contact dermatitis require the use of topical and/or systemic corticosteroids for effective management. Systemic steroids, used for the more severe cases, may be administered either orally (as prednisone, 40 to 60 mg daily for 7 to 14 days) or intramuscularly (as triamcinolone acetonide [Kenalog] or betamethasone acetate [Celestone]). Oral steroids are generally tapered during a 1- to 2-week period, whereas intramuscular preparations may persist for 1 week (betamethasone) to 3 weeks (triamcinolone). The well-known contraindications for the use of systemic corticosteroids must, of course, be considered when deciding whether to use them in the treatment of acute contact dermatitis.

For an acute contact dermatitis, topical corticosteroids are most often prescribed in the form of a lotion, cream, or solution. Solutions are particularly useful for hair-bearing areas or for sites such as the ears or interdigital spaces, whereas lotions may be spread easily over larger areas of affected skin; creams may be ideal for hands, feet, or smaller patches of contact dermatitis. In any format, topical corticosteroid preparations may be mild (hydrocortisone), moderate (hydrocortisone valerate [Westcort], desonide [Tridesilon], hydrocortisone butyrate [Locoid]), potent (desoximetasone [Topicort], fluocinonide [Lidex], amcinonide [Cyclocort]), or superpotent (augmented betamethasone dipropionate [Diprolene], diflorasone diacetate [Psorcon], halobetasol propionate [Ultravate], clobetasol propionate [Temovate]) formulations. Milder preparations should be used on the face, breasts, groin, and axillae. With the potent or superpotent preparations, local (atrophy, telangiectasia, striae) or even systemic (adrenal axis suppression) side effects are potential problems. The superpotent steroids must be used with special caution.

Chronic Contact Dermatitis

In the chronic form, allergic or irritant contact dermatitis generally produces thickening, lichenification, and fissuring, often intermixed with acute or subacute manifestations of the eczematous process. As with acute contact dermatitis, secondary infection may be a problem and necessitate the use of topical antibiotics such as mupirocin (Bactroban) or systemic antibiotics such as penicillin, erythromycin, tetracycline, or cephalosporins. The dry, cracked, thickened skin of chronic contact dermatitis is generally treated with the application of moisturizing or emollient lotions, creams, and ointments, rather than with the baths, soaks, and compresses that are most helpful in acute forms of the disorder. Likewise, when topical corticosteroid preparations are used, creams or ointments are generally favored over the less emollient lotions and solutions. Because a chronic disease process predicts a prolonged therapeutic course, the physician must be especially vigilant when using the more potent topical corticosteroid preparations. Certainly the same caveat applies to systemic corticosteroids, which should be used carefully and infrequently to control severe flare-ups of chronic contact dermatitis. Pruritus is, indeed, a problem here, as with the acute process, and oral antihistamines may provide at least temporary relief.

PATCH TESTING

The complete evaluation of patients when a diagnosis of contact dermatitis is suspected will generally include patch testing. The birth date of modern patch testing may be traced to a presentation of Jadassohn in 1895. Whereas patch testing does require training and experience, especially in the interpretation or "reading" of tests, its use has been greatly facilitated by the development of a new standardized system (allergen patch test, TRUE Test) in which materials are already incorporated in easy to apply test strips. Only when a causative agent is identified can contact dermatitis be optimally managed.

SKIN DISEASES OF PREGNANCY

method of
KIM B. YANCEY, M.D.
National Cancer Institute, National Institutes of Health
Bethesda, Maryland

Skin changes during gestation include normal physiologic manifestations of pregnancy itself, exacerbations of existing skin disorders, coincidentally acquired skin diseases, and specific dermatoses of pregnancy. The last vary widely in their incidence and potential severity and often require specialized care to ensure their correct diagnosis and management.

HERPES GESTATIONIS

Diagnosis

Herpes gestationis (HG) is a rare, nonviral, vesiculobullous and/or urticarial skin disease of pregnancy and the puerperium. HG has no relationship to an existing or prior viral infection. Instead, its designation refers to the characteristically grouped (i.e., herpetiform) distribution of lesions in patients with this disorder. HG may present during any trimester of pregnancy or begin within 24 to 72 hours of delivery. Interestingly, severe exacerbations of HG often occur immediately after delivery, and it is crucial to evaluate all patients carefully at that time (including individuals whose earlier disease was controlled by treatment or relatively inactive). HG usually resolves within several weeks of delivery, although temporary flares of disease may develop when patients resume menses or are exposed to oral contraceptives. In addition, HG tends to recur in subsequent pregnancies and often presents earlier during gestation in such cases.

Patients with HG typically present with lesions on their abdomen and extremities; interestingly, the umbilicus is often involved. In severe cases, lesions may also affect the palms, soles, chest, and back; mucous membrane involvement is rare. HG is a polymorphic skin disease (i.e., lesions may demonstrate a variety of different morphologies). Classically, lesions consist of erythematous, urticarial papules and plaques that enlarge peripherally and are often rimmed by vesicles and blisters. Lesions are typically pruritic and often interfere with these patients' ability to sleep or perform routine activities comfortably. Infants born to affected mothers also occasionally demonstrate skin lesions of this same character. However, such lesions are usually limited in extent, are transient, last only a few weeks, and require minimal supportive care.

Biopsies of lesional skin from patients with HG demonstrate teardrop-shaped subepidermal blisters and an eosinophil-rich leukocytic infiltrate along the epidermal basement membrane and within the upper dermis. Although characteristic, these findings do not specifically distinguish HG from other subepidermal blistering or inflammatory skin diseases. This distinction is typically provided by direct immunofluorescence microscopy studies that reveal continuous deposits of C3, the third component of complement, in the epidermal basement membrane of these patients' normal-appearing perilesional skin. These C3 deposits, the immunopathologic hallmark of HG, signify the existence of complement-fixing IgG anti–basement membrane autoantibodies in these patients. These autoantibodies are directed against specific proteins in skin that normally function to promote the adhesion of epidermis to epidermal basement membrane. Current experimental evidence indicates that HG is an autoantibody-mediated disease in which subepidermal blisters develop as a consequence of complement activation, mast cell degranulation, and granulocyte accumulation. Although the cause of autoantibody formation in these patients is unknown, HG's relationship to pregnancy and other endocrinologic stimuli (e.g., oral contraceptives) suggests that the pathophysiologic mechanism of this disease is hormonally modulated.

Immunopathologic studies have shown that in addition to C3, approximately 40 to 50% of patients with HG have deposits of IgG (or other immunoglobulins) in situ in their epidermal basement membranes as well as circulating IgG anti–basement membrane autoantibodies. Such studies illustrate the importance of studying these patients' skin for evidence of cutaneous deposits of C3 in epidermal basement membrane rather than testing their serum for evidence of circulating autoantibodies that are demonstrable in a minority of patients. Because these patients' autoantibodies are of the IgG isotype, they are able to cross the placenta, enter the fetal circulation, deposit in fetal skin, and cause skin lesions. Whereas some studies have suggested that HG is associated with an increased risk of fetal morbidity and mortality, this notion is currently somewhat controversial. At present, there is general agreement that these pregnancies have an increased risk of prematurity and that these patients and their offspring require specialized care.

Treatment

The goal of therapy in patients with HG is to prevent new lesions, relieve intense pruritus, and care for sites of blisters and erosions. Decisions about treatment should be directly based on the character, extent, and severity of each patient's disease. In mild cases of HG, vigorous use of potent topical corticosteroids such as 0.05% fluocinonide (Lidex) or 0.1% triamcinolone acetonide (Kenalog) four to six times each day* may control the eruption and relieve symptoms. However, at some point in the course of their disease, most patients with HG require treatment with moderate doses of systemic corticosteroids administered daily. Doses of 20 to 60 mg of prednisone each morning usually relieve pruritus and halt lesion formation within several days. Dividing doses of daily corticosteroids into morning and evening doses (i.e., given every 12 hours) has been used to hasten improvement in patients with severe disease. Once the eruption and pruritus have been controlled, daily doses of prednisone should be tapered by approximately 5 mg every 1 to 2 weeks until lesions develop or symptoms recur. For patients with a postpartum flare of disease, daily prednisone should be restarted (or increased) at a dose of 20 to 40 mg each morning; postpartum patients unable to tolerate oral medications should be treated with an equivalent daily morning dose of hydrocortisone given intravenously. Severe postpartum flares of disease may require as much as 60 mg of daily morning prednisone (used in combination with other systemic immunosuppressives in rare cases). In managing this disease, the

*Exceeds dosage recommended by the manufacturer.

minimally effective dose of corticosteroids should be employed to control the eruption. Moreover, a modest amount of disease activity (e.g., several new vesicles or urticarial plaques developing every 2 to 3 days) is acceptable and should not warrant more aggressive therapy. Patients using corticosteroids after delivery should be counseled about appropriate nursing practices. If systemic corticosteroids are used during pregnancy, physicians should be alert to possible reversible adrenal insufficiency in newborns. Notably, studies have indicated that there is no significant difference in the incidence of uncomplicated live births in HG patients treated with systemic corticosteroids versus those managed with more conservative forms of therapy. For weeping or eroded lesions, open wet dressings of saline or tap water for 10 minutes three to four times each day should promote drying and débridement. Individual blisters should be allowed to remain intact to promote wound protection and re-epithelialization; large uncomfortable blisters can be drained by aspiration. Skin lesions should be examined carefully for evidence of bacterial infection, which should be cultured and treated appropriately. As noted earlier, lesions in newborns are usually transient, require only local care, and resolve as maternal autoantibodies are cleared from these infants' circulation.

PRURITIC URTICARIAL PAPULES AND PLAQUES OF PREGNANCY

Diagnosis

Pruritic urticarial papules and plaques of pregnancy (PUPPP) is a distinctive pruritic eruption that typically presents during the third trimester of gestation in primigravidas. Although the exact incidence of PUPPP is unknown, it is generally regarded to be the most common specific dermatosis of pregnancy. Lesions in patients with PUPPP almost always begin on the abdomen and typically present in periumbilical striae distensae. Other common sites of involvement include the buttocks and proximal extremities; facial involvement is rare. Although pruritus in patients with PUPPP is characteristically severe, excoriations are uncommon. PUPPP usually responds to treatment or resolves soon after delivery; it does not tend to flare post partum, recur in subsequent pregnancies, or develop in patients later exposed to oral contraceptives. PUPPP is not associated with an increased risk of fetal morbidity or fetal and maternal mortality. Lesions in infants born of mothers with PUPPP are uncommon. Several studies have demonstrated that patients with PUPPP have an increased average maternal weight gain, newborn birth weight, and incidence of twinning—findings suggesting that abdominal distention (or a reaction to it) may play a role in the development of PUPPP.

Lesions in PUPPP consist of small, erythematous, urticarial papules that usually coalesce into large urticarial plaques. Although uncommon, vesicles may be seen in some patients. In severe cases, large portions of the body may be involved. Biopsies of lesional skin from patients with PUPPP show a superficial or mid-dermal perivascular mononuclear cell infiltrate, dermal edema, and occasional eosinophils. Although not diagnostic, these findings are consistent. In contrast to HG, there is no evidence of specific immunoreactants in these patients' epidermal basement membranes or evidence of specific autoantibodies in their circulation. Because there is no specific laboratory test for PUPPP, the diagnosis of this disorder is largely based on its characteristic clinical presentation.

Treatment

PUPPP is best treated by the application of potent topical corticosteroids (i.e., 0.05% fluocinonide or 0.1% triamcinolone acetonide) four to six times each day.* This treatment usually relieves pruritus and halts lesion formation. Less potent topical corticosteroids as well as less frequent treatment schedules should be employed after the eruption is controlled. In patients who are improving, therapy should be gradually tapered rather than abruptly stopped. Patients with severe disease may require treatment with 20 to 40 mg of daily prednisone each morning. This treatment usually promptly controls the eruption as well as the associated pruritus. Prednisone can be tapered fairly quickly in patients with PUPPP, typically by 5 mg at 2- to 3-day intervals. Topical corticosteroids represent the mainstay of treatment for this disease. In general, oral antihistamines are less effective in relieving pruritus than is aggressive use of potent topical corticosteroids.

PRURIGO GRAVIDARUM

Diagnosis

Prurigo gravidarum (PG; also known as recurrent cholestasis of pregnancy) is a hepatic condition that usually occurs late in pregnancy and demonstrates cutaneous manifestations of pruritus and (in severe cases) jaundice. The initial manifestation of PG is pruritus, which may be either localized or generalized in distribution; secondary excoriations may be observed. In general, pruritus exceeds the onset of jaundice by 2 to 4 weeks. PG tends to remit soon after delivery but typically recurs in subsequent pregnancies. It may also recur in susceptible individuals after their exposure to oral contraceptives. Although the exact cause of this disorder is unknown, PG is believed to be hormonally induced in susceptible individuals. Underlying hepatic impairment in these patients is often supported by elevated determinations of liver function tests. Some reports have suggested that there is an increased incidence of prematurity, stillbirth, and postpartum hemorrhage in patients with PG. The incidence of such adverse events is highest in patients with both pruritus and

jaundice. The diagnosis of this disorder is based on clinical and laboratory findings as well as a personal and/or family history of pruritus during pregnancy.

Treatment

Therapy in patients with PG is entirely symptomatic. Emollients, topical antipruritics, topical corticosteroids, and in selected cases antihistamines with or without cholestyramine (Questran)* may be beneficial. Some have suggested that patients with PG (because of potential fat malabsorption) receive supplemental vitamin K immediately before delivery to avert complications of hemorrhage.

IMPETIGO HERPETIFORMIS

Diagnosis

Impetigo herpetiformis (IH) is the nosologic designation for a form of pustular psoriasis whose onset is triggered by pregnancy. Although rare, this disease may be life-threatening. It is often accompanied by significant constitutional symptoms such as fever, chills, nausea, vomiting, and diarrhea. Moreover, in severe cases, it may be complicated by hypoalbuminemia, hypocalcemia, and tetany. IH typically begins as a series of grouped erythematous plaques that are rimmed by small sterile pustules. Lesions predominate in flexural areas, expand peripherally, and show new pustules forming at their leading edge. IH may progress to involve substantial portions of the body surface. In advanced cases, involvement of mucous membranes and nail beds also occurs. Biopsies of lesional skin from patients with IH demonstrate alterations that are identical to those seen in pustular psoriasis.

Treatment

Systemic corticosteroids are the mainstay of treatment for these patients. Prednisone in daily doses as high as 60 mg each morning are often required to control the eruption. Prednisone should be tapered slowly to avoid flares of disease. All patients should be closely monitored for evidence of hypoalbuminemia, hypocalcemia, fluid loss, or infection. Patients with IH require specialized care and careful monitoring by dermatologists, obstetricians, and pediatricians.

---

*Not FDA approved for this indication.

PRURITUS ANI AND VULVAE
method of
MARILYNNE McKAY, M.D.
Emory University School of Medicine
Atlanta, Georgia

Acute-onset perineal itching is most often due to one of the following: *Candida* infection, irritant and contact

---

*Exceeds dosage recommended by the manufacturer.

dermatitis, urinary tract infection, hemorrhoids, pinworms, and condylomata. Fecal contamination of the anus can be extremely irritating, as can overcleansing; contact dermatitis may develop after application of medications such as neomycin, benzocaine, or those containing preservatives such as ethylenediamine. Cleanliness, the use of bland emollients, and treatment of infection or infestation will generally resolve perineal itching that has been present for a few days to a few weeks.

Diagnostic tests for acute itching should specifically rule out infection, and examination of the female patient should include a vaginal smear for *Candida, Trichomonas,* and bacterial vaginosis (*Gardnerella*). Even though bacterial vaginosis is not typically itchy, the characteristic odor often induces patients to overcleanse or douche with irritating solutions. Recurrent candidiasis is common; culture specimens for *Candida* should be taken from the vagina, and anal culture should be considered in both sexes. Risk factors for *Candida* infection include antibiotics for sinusitis, urinary tract infections, or acne; steroids or other immunosuppressants; human immunodeficiency virus infection; and estrogen therapy (oral contraceptives, estrogen replacement). Itching due to estrogen deficiency may be important in perimenopausal women, because dry mucosal epithelium is easily irritated. Systemic disorders that may be associated with itching include diabetes, uremia, and hepatitis.

Chronic perineal itching is more difficult to evaluate than itching of recent onset, because the likelihood of discovering an underlying cause is significantly diminished when itching has persisted for months. With chronic pruritus, repeated episodes of itching and scratching cause local thickening of the skin called lichen simplex chronicus (LSC). LSC is identified by a leathery scaly texture with accentuation of normal skin lines. Irritable nerve endings in LSC lesions trigger an "itch-scratch-itch" cycle that typically continues long after the initial insult has resolved. LSC is secondary to rubbing and scratching, and this chronic skin change must be treated separately from the usual primary causes of acute perineal itching. Lichen sclerosus is an entirely different condition that may itch or burn; this dermatosis typically presents with thin, pale, friable skin around the anus and/or vulva.

If there are visible skin changes, a biopsy should be considered to differentiate LSC from other genital dermatoses such as psoriasis, lichen planus, or lichen sclerosus as well as to rule out malignant neoplasms such as intraepithelial neoplasia (carcinoma in situ) or extramammary Paget's disease. A 3- to 4-mm punch biopsy specimen should be taken from the thickest areas of any lesions (plaques, scarring, thickening). Acetowhitening (application of vinegar or 3 to 5% acetic acid for 1 to 2 minutes) can be used to highlight thickened areas if there is a history of genital warts (human papillomavirus [HPV]). If HPV infection is found on the vulva, colposcopy of the vagina and cervix is recommended; if on the anus, proctoscopy. Biopsy of multifocal lesions, typical of HPV-associated intraepithelial neoplasia, should be done.

THERAPY

As mentioned before, the etiology of acute-onset perineal itching is most likely to be discovered by diagnostic testing. Therapy for infections should reduce itching within a few days, but *Candida* may be especially recalcitrant. Women with a tendency for recurrent candidiasis may need to use vaginal creams such as clotrimazole (Gyne-Lotrimin) or terconazole (Terazol) once a week for several months. An effective *Candida* suppression regimen is oral fluconazole (Diflucan), 150 to 200 mg weekly for 2 months, tapering to biweekly for 2 months, then monthly. For relatively mild itching, 1% hydrocortisone cream is effective, especially when it is mixed with pramoxine, a mild anesthetic (Pramosone, Zone-A).

Proper cleansing is the single most important factor in management of perineal itching. After each bowel movement or possible soiling, the patient should cleanse gently with Tucks pads, Balneol or Cetaphil lotion, or a mild soap (Neutrogena, Purpose) followed by cool-water rinses. Plain white unscented toilet tissue is recommended, but Tucks cloth pads are probably better. The patient should be advised to pat the skin gently, because rubbing can be irritating. Tight or occlusive garments should be avoided; this includes plastic-backed panty shields, which can contribute to maceration—perfumes in these products can be irritating as well. Cotton underwear and the avoidance of fabric softeners are often helpful.

There is debate over whether spicy or caffeine-containing foods contribute to pruritus ani; probably the best course is to advise the patient to adopt a bland diet at first and then add back one or two items a week to see whether symptoms are exacerbated. Some patients already realize that certain foods worsen their problem. Food allergens are another possible factor, and an elimination trial of milk, tomatoes, corn, and nuts should be considered.

Older patients who complain of burning or stinging rather than itching (and who usually have minimal skin change as a result) may actually suffer from a cutaneous dysesthesia. Low-dose tricylic antidepressants such as amitriptyline (Elavil)* or nortriptyline (Pamelor)* are especially effective. Begin with 10 to 20 mg at bedtime and increase by 10 mg weekly to a dose of 30 to 50 mg per day. It may take 4 to 6 weeks to reach an adequate therapeutic dose. Once improvement has been maintained for a month or two, the dosage can gradually be tapered.

For LSC, the mainstay is topical steroid therapy. Caution is always advised in using fluorinated topical steroid preparations in intertriginous areas; side effects include skin thinning, striae formation, and rebound erythema and burning. On the other hand, nonfluorinated class VII preparations such as hydrocortisone are unlikely to be effective in severe thickened LSC. Short-term application of a high-potency class I steroid ointment such as betamethasone dipropionate 0.05% (Diprolene) or clobetasol propionate 0.05% (Temovate) can be extremely effective; I prescribe twice-daily applications for 3 to 4 weeks, then once daily for 3 to 4 weeks. Evaluation of the patient at 6 to 8 weeks almost always reveals significant improvement, sometimes for the first time in years. At this point, the potency and/or frequency of application should be decreased, using only the

*Not FDA approved for this indication.

strength necessary to control symptoms. Triamcinolone acetonide 0.1% (Kenalog, Aristocort) may be used as a short-term stepdown to maintenance therapy with 1% hydrocortisone. Fluorinated steroids are recommended for use only on LSC or severe lichen sclerosus; they are contraindicated for erythema and burning, both of which can be worsened by their use. Overuse of potent topical steroids on vulvar skin will cause steroid rebound dermatitis with burning and erythema; perianal skin is more likely to develop thinning and telangiectasia.

It often takes 3 or 4 weeks for a topical steroid to begin to affect well-established LSC, and itching typically flares from time to time during the healing process. The patient must be told that this does not mean that the medication is not working, especially if symptom-free intervals indicate that treatment is progressing satisfactorily. The patient's anxiety is often a significant factor in episodic itching, and reassurance is an important part of therapy.

URTICARIA

method of
CHARLES D. KENNARD, M.D.
Wilford Hall Medical Center
Lackland AFB, Texas

Urticaria, which is recognized by wheals in the dermis, is a common affliction with a lifetime incidence of 15 to 20%. Angioedema is a similar condition, with acute edema involving the dermis and subcutaneous tissues, often of the perioral or genital regions or upper aerodigestive mucosa. Identification and avoidance of causative agents that directly or indirectly precipitate the whealing eruption constitute the most direct and effective therapy. This therapeutic approach is most applicable in cases of acute urticaria. Unfortunately, in most cases of long-standing urticaria, it is not possible to determine the triggering factors. Nevertheless, the treatment of urticaria may be guided by an understanding of the various pathophysiologic mechanisms involved even when clearly identifiable causes have not been identified. In this manner, trials of various medications, guided by the clinical response within the limits of acceptable side effects, may be necessary to find the optimal therapy.

EVALUATION: ACUTE URTICARIA

Urticaria is recognized by the appearance of variably pruritic wheals. The individual lesions persist for up to 24 hours, and crops of wheals may recur sporadically. Urticaria usually resolves spontaneously within a few months. Cases that resolve within 6 to 12 weeks have been called acute urticaria; cases lasting longer are considered chronic. Food and medication exposures are the most common causes of acute urticaria. The patient is often suspicious of a possible offending agent, and the history alone may be sufficient to suggest the culprit. Elimination and addition diets may be useful in the evaluation of some cases. However, a period of 2 to 3 days between additions or deletions of a dietary item must be observed to differentiate true sensitivity from the normal variations in disease activity. Intracutaneous skin testing can rule out IgE-dependent

food sensitivity, such as is seen with nuts, fish, and eggs. Other urticaria-inducing foods include shellfish and strawberries. Substances in food, such as salicylates, tartrazine, and benzoic acid derivatives (*p*-aminobenzoic acid [PABA]), can cause urticaria. Cross-reaction to *Candida* and food yeasts may be manifested as urticaria; such patients may be helped by anticandidal therapy and a diet low in yeast.

A detailed medication history should be obtained. Penicillin is the medication most commonly causing urticaria, which it does through IgE-dependent mechanisms. Radiocontrast media, opiates, and other medications can produce urticaria by directly causing mast cell degranulation without IgE mediation. Aspirin, perhaps through interactions with the arachidonic acid metabolic pathways and inhibition of prostaglandin synthesis, can produce urticaria and/or angioedema. In some patients, aspirin-induced urticaria is seen in association with nasal polyps and asthma, often with a familial pattern.

Contact urticaria is, in my opinion, an unusual form of urticaria. The most frequent source of contact urticaria is probably latex. Patients with an IgE-mediated hypersensitivity to latex are often medical workers or patients with frequent contact with catheters or other latex-containing medical equipment. Reactions may be severe, with rapid anaphylaxis and collapse. Thus, testing for such possible latex allergic responses must be performed in controlled settings with appropriate supportive equipment and trained personnel immediately available.

Hereditary angioedema is an autosomal dominant trait having a deficiency of serum inhibitor of the activated first component of complement. It is manifested by acute isolated *painful*, rather than pruritic, edema. Angioedema can potentially cause fatal upper airway obstruction, precipitated by trauma or other stress. A frequently noted presentation is laryngeal edema after dental procedures. The biochemical marker is usually a lack of C1 esterase inhibitor, although functional deficiency of the inhibitor with normal levels of the inhibitor by immunoassay is seen in 15% of cases. Evaluation should include assay of C4 levels, which are chronically low, C1 inhibitor immunoassay, and possibly a functional assay if the immunoassay levels are normal.

EVALUATION: CHRONIC URTICARIA

In an uncertain proportion of patients, initially episodic urticaria progresses to a continuous, chronic form of the disorder. This chronic urticaria remits in about 50% of cases within 1 year, but 20% of patients continue to have urticaria for more than 20 years. Diagnostic testing is relevant to this subgroup with chronic urticaria. Efficacious and cost-effective evaluations require an individualized approach to the patient's clinical condition and often to the patient's emotional need to know a cause of the urticaria.

Unfortunately, the etiology of chronic urticaria is determined in less than 25% of cases. Again, the medical history may be most helpful: patients may have an opinion about the triggering of the urticaria, or they may have sinusitis, arthralgias, urinary symptoms, or constitutional symptoms pointing to an underlying etiology. Such symptoms may direct the physical examination to the indicated areas, with laboratory examinations as indicated from the findings. A "shotgun" approach to laboratory studies rarely uncovers an infection or connective tissue disease as the cause of urticaria that was not suggested by the history or physical examination. However, some studies have indicated that occult sinus infections may be a treatable cause of urticaria. Thus, a useful screening protocol of laboratory examinations for patients with chronic urticaria may be those confirmatory tests for conditions specifically suggested by the patient's history or physical examination, with a sinus radiograph series for all other patients.

For extreme cases, when the initial evaluation is negative and symptoms have persisted for several months, more in-depth laboratory testing could include the erythrocyte sedimentation rate to screen for inflammatory or occult neoplastic processes. A complete blood count with differential might show an elevated white blood cell count as an indication of an infection, with eosinophilia possibly implicating a helminthic disease, atopy, or drug eruption. Hepatitis B and infectious mononucleosis may both be associated with urticaria and have abnormal serum transaminase levels and abnormal liver function values. Abnormal renal function tests and urinalysis may indicate nephritis or urinary tract infection. Antinuclear antibodies, rheumatoid factor, serum complement (C3 and C4), and/or cryoglobulins may point to autoimmune disease or cold-induced urticaria. Cold-induced urticaria may also be detected by simple testing with an ice cube applied to the forearm. Cholinergic urticaria can be diagnosed when extremely small urticarial papules appear on a large background flare after a provocative challenge of perspiration-inducing exercise. Pressure urticaria and other forms of physical urticarias may be confirmed through appropriate stimulatory challenges. Stool guaiac testing and chest radiograph may reveal occult malignancies that rarely present through urticaria. Urticarial vasculitis, an uncommon whealing eruption, is characterized by individual lesions that persist for greater than the 24 hours of duration specified in the diagnosis of other urticarial disorders. Urticarial vasculitis is often associated with hepatitis B or C, mononucleosis, and autoimmune disorders.

THERAPEUTIC APPROACH

Acute Urticaria

Because the cause of acute urticaria is most likely to be an ingested food or medication, avoidance of the offending substance may be all that is required for relief. Symptoms of whealing and pruritus are usually controllable with oral antihistamines of the H_1 class. Hydroxyzine (Atarax), 10 to 50 mg three or four times daily, is my choice for urticaria because it appears to have less "hangover" from bedtime doses, and tolerance to side effects often develops early in treatment. Diphenhydramine (Benadryl), 25 to 100 mg three or four times daily, is effective but is often overly sedating for daytime use. Cyproheptadine (Periactin), 4 mg four times daily, is especially useful for cold-induced urticaria. Chlorpheniramine (Chlor-Trimeton), 8 to 12 mg twice daily, or triprolidine (Actidil), 2.5 mg four times daily, may produce less drowsiness, but central nervous system (CNS) stimulation or irritability is seen in some patients; sustained-release forms are available. To lessen these side effects, newer, nonsedating antihistamines have been produced; see the discussion in the section on chronic urticaria. When these methods are ineffective, oral prednisone, 40 mg each morning tapering over 10 to 14 days, should give relief.

In the case of hereditary angioedema, long-term prophylaxis can be achieved with oral androgens. Stanozolol (Winstrol),* 2 mg three times daily, and then reduction of dose to the lowest possible is effective. Short-term prophylaxis in a previously untreated patient can be achieved with 2 units of fresh-frozen plasma.

Severe urticaria or angioedema that is accompanied by signs of compromised respiration or the potential for circulatory collapse may require subcutaneous injection of epinephrine, 0.3 to 0.5 mL of 1:1000. Supplemental oxygen should be given in accordance with the patient's clinical picture, and pulse oximetry readings and intravenous access should be established in such cases and intubation and tracheostomy should be immediately available. Intravenous diphenhydramine, 50 to 100 mg, may be a useful supplement. In cases of severe reactions, systemic corticosteroids and hospitalization for observation and airway management are indicated.

Chronic Urticaria

Unfortunately, the vast majority of chronic urticaria cases do not have an easily identifiable cause, but the end result is the same: histamine that has been released from mast cells interacts with the H_1 receptor on dermal vasculature, producing edema. Thus, antihistamines are the therapeutic cornerstone in chronic urticaria. Other general, nonspecific treatment should include the avoidance of possible triggering factors such as opiates, aspirin, heat, exercise, and alcohol if these factors are present.

Side effects are common in traditional H_1 antihistamine therapy; sedation occurs regularly with all classes of traditional H_1 antihistamines. The sedation at bedtime may provide relief from the exacerbation of pruritus that plagues many patients as they attempt to fall asleep. Tachyphylaxis to this hypnotic effect may develop with continued use. Additional side effects that may be seen with this class of medication include dizziness, incoordination, blurred vision, diplopia, and paradoxical symptoms of CNS stimulation, particularly in young children and elderly people. Seizure activity may be induced in patients with focal lesions in the CNS. Anticholinergic effects such as dryness of mucous membranes, urinary retention, palpitations, agitation, and increased intraocular pressure may be seen. Phenothiazine class antihistamines can produce a cholestatic jaundice. Because traditional H_1 antihistamines can induce hepatic microsomal enzymes, medications such as warfarin (Coumadin), griseofulvin (Gris-PEG), and phenytoin (Dilantin) that are metabolized by this route may have decreased effectiveness.

A new generation of antihistamines has been developed that do not significantly cross the blood-brain barrier, have little anticholinergic activity, and are nonsedating. Most of these second-generation antihistamines have a prolonged half-life, permitting once-daily dosing. For these reasons, nonsedating an-

---

*Not FDA approved for this indication.

tihistamines are the treatment of choice for chronic, idiopathic urticaria. Fexofenadine (Allegra), 60 mg twice daily or 120 mg once a day, astemizole (Hismanal), 10 mg once daily, loratadine (Claritin), 10 mg daily, and cetirizine (Zyrtec), 10 mg daily, are all effective with little or no sedation. With cetirizine, the incidence of sedation is slightly higher than in placebo. Astemizole may produce increased appetite with or without weight gain. Astemizole and loratadine should be taken on an empty stomach. Astemizole can cause torsades de pointes, a potentially fatal ventricular arrhythmia, when it is taken in overdosage. This can also occur when it is taken concomitantly with medications that would compromise its hepatic metabolism by the cytochrome P-450 enzyme system or in the face of medical conditions limiting the liver's metabolic capacity or predisposing to a prolonged electrocardiographic QT interval.

ALTERNATIVE THERAPIES

For some patients who do not respond to H_1 antihistamines alone, the addition of an H_2 antagonist such as cimetidine (Tagamet),* 400 mg four times daily, may aid in the control of symptoms. Beta agonists such as terbutaline (Brethine),* 2.5 mg orally three times daily, and other agents that raise mast cell intracellular cyclic AMP levels may have a small effect on controlling chronic urticaria in some patients, but they cannot be relied on as first-line medications for this disorder. The calcium channel blocker nifedipine (Procardia),* 10 mg up to three times daily, can rarely improve the control of chronic, idiopathic urticaria when added to a regimen of traditional or nonsedating H_1 and H_2 antihistamines. Tricyclic antidepressants are potent antagonists of H_1 histamine receptors. Doxepin is 700 times more potent on a molar basis than diphenhydramine as an in vitro H_1 blocker, and doxepin (Sinequan),* 10 mg three times daily, can be more effective than diphenhydramine in controlling symptoms. Doxepin has been formulated in a topical form (Zonalon cream), but unless urticarial symptoms are restricted to a specific area of skin, it would offer no benefit in the treatment of chronic urticaria. Systemic corticosteroids may give temporary respite from an overwhelming bout with chronic urticaria. However, the severe side effects associated with the prolonged use of corticosteroids, such as adrenal suppression and exacerbation of hypertension and diabetes, prevent their regular or sustained use in chronic urticaria. Oral cyclosporine (Sandimmune),* 6 mg per kg per day, can produce rapid resolution of severe, chronic urticaria and angioedema. Cost and systemic immune suppression limit its use. Studies have shown evidence for a circulating histamine-releasing factor, perhaps an IgG autoantibody to IgE, and patients with severe, chronic idiopathic urticaria can have significant improvement for up to 2 months by a week-long course of plasmapheresis.

---

*Not FDA approved for this indication.

PIGMENTARY DISORDERS

method of
NORMAN LEVINE, M.D.
University of Arizona College of Medicine
Tucson, Arizona

Skin pigmentation is the body's best defense against ultraviolet (UV) light radiation and is an important cultural and social characteristic. Almost all of what gives the skin its characteristic hue is from melanin, a complex protein produced in epidermal melanocytes. Disorders of pigmentation occur when there is an abnormal number of melanocytes, when an inappropriate amount of melanin is synthesized, or when the pigment is deposited in anomalous sites.

HYPERPIGMENTARY DISORDERS
Melasma

Clinical Findings

Melasma is a reticulated hyperpigmentation of the face, neck, and forearms that occurs most commonly in women taking oral contraceptives or in those who are pregnant ("the mask of pregnancy"). Men and nonpregnant women may also be affected. Hormonal and genetic factors are operative, but the exact cause of this malady is unknown. Sunlight exacerbates the condition.

Treatment

If the extra pigment is located primarily in the epidermis, the patches are tan. These lesions respond well to bleaching agents. Pigment that is situated deeper in the dermis is blue or gray and does not lighten well, even after prolonged treatment. A combination of hydroquinone cream (Viquin Forte) applied twice daily and tretinoin cream 0.025% (Retin-A) applied at night for 4 to 6 months can produce substantial lightening. The combination can cause irritation when it is first used. This can be minimized by using the tretinoin cream every other night for the first 2 to 3 weeks and then increasing the frequency of application to a nightly treatment program. Azelaic acid 20% cream (Azelex) applied twice daily with or without tretinoin 0.025% cream for 6 months may also bleach the patches.

Physical means of removing the excess pigment may be helpful in those with fair skin and mainly epidermal melanin deposition. Mid-depth trichloroacetic acid or glycolic acid chemical peels or laser resurfacing will lighten the skin, but recurrences are common.

It is critical that assiduous sun avoidance be followed during therapy. Some hydroquinone products such as Viquin Forte and Solaquin Forte contain sunscreens. All patients with melasma should also use additional sunscreen agents during and after treatment (Table 1). The product should have a sun protection factor of at least 15. Water-resistant products are preferred in those who exercise outdoors or who sweat heavily.

TABLE 1. **Sunscreens**

Brand Name	Sunscreen Type	Characteristics
Ti-Screen Natural	Physical blocker	Chemical free; difficult to rub in completely
Oil of Olay Daily UV Protectant	Chemical sunscreen	Emollient base
PreSun Active Gel	Chemical sunscreen	Greaseless vehicle; waterproof
Coppertone Sport	Chemical sunscreen	Waterproof; less runoff in eyes
Durascreen 30	Combination chemical and physical sunscreen	Wide range of ultraviolet protection

Solar Lentigo

Clinical Findings

Solar lentigines present in most whites older than 60 years. They are largely confined to sites of chronic sun exposure and presumably arise as a protective mechanism against UV light injury. The lesions are stellate brown macules that occur mostly on the dorsa of the hands, on the face, and over the shoulders.

Treatment

Because solar lentigines have no malignant potential, treatment is for cosmetic purposes only. Bleaching creams containing hydroquinone or azelaic acid work slowly and incompletely in most cases. The addition of tretinoin cream may improve the results somewhat. Light liquid nitrogen cryotherapy or destruction by electrodesiccation and curettage is effective for localized lesions; there is a risk for post-therapy hypopigmentation, particularly with cryotherapy. Mid-depth trichloroacetic acid or glycolic acid chemical peels can eradicate multiple lesions in a single sitting. The neodymium:yttrium-aluminum-garnet laser, the Q-switched ruby laser, and the resurfacing carbon dioxide laser are effective at removing lentigines, but the treatments are costly.

Drug-Induced Hyperpigmentation

Clinical Findings

Several medications can produce abnormal skin or nail pigmentation because of either deposition of the drug or its metabolite in the skin or drug-induced increased melanin production by melanocytes (Table 2). Several medications such as 5-fluorouracil, gold, and amiodarone (Cordarone) produce preferential darkening in sun-exposed sites. Other medications such as zidovudine (AZT), bleomycin (Blenoxane), and cyclophosphamide (Cytoxan) cause pigmented bands in the nails. Minocycline (Minocin) is used in acne and may produce brown-gray discoloration in old acne scars. The color change seen with medication reactions ranges from tan to slate gray to blue-black.

Treatment

In most instances, the dyspigmentation that appears with drugs slowly fades after the drug is discontinued. Certain medications such as gold and topical hydroquinone are responsible for color changes that are irreversible. The use of sunscreens is encouraged in patients with drug-induced hyperpigmentation to minimize additional pigment production from the sun.

Postinflammatory Hyperpigmentation

Clinical Findings

After an epidermal injury such as occurs with a superficial burn, melanin either is carried into or falls into the dermis where it is engulfed by macrophages. This pigment may remain indefinitely and cause clinical macular hyperpigmentation. If the melanin is close to the surface, the lesions are tan or brown. As the pigment is deposited deeper in the dermis, the skin becomes gray or blue-gray.

Treatment

If the pigment is superficial, the areas can be lightened somewhat with the regimens noted before for melasma. This will not work well in deep dermal melanosis. Laser therapy is ineffective in most cases. Sunscreens are helpful for minimizing increased tanning in sites that are already dark.

HYPOPIGMENTARY DISORDERS

Vitiligo

Clinical Findings

Vitiligo is a common condition of uncertain etiology characterized by loss of skin pigment. The characteristic lesion is a milk white macule or patch. The hair

TABLE 2. **Medication-Induced Pigmentary Abnormalities**

Medication	Clinical Characteristics
Busulfan (Myleran)	Generalized increased skin color resembling Addison's disease
Doxorubicin (Adriamycin)	Pigmented nail bands and palmar creases
5-Fluorouracil (fluorouracil)	Increased pigment in sun-exposed sites
Minocycline (Minocin)	Gray pigment in old scars and/or on the legs, or a generalized muddy color
Hydroxychloroquine (Plaquenil)	Brown or gray discoloration of the shins, trunk
Gold (Myochrysine)	Permanent blue-gray color in sun-exposed areas
Estrogen (Premarin)	Melasma
Amiodarone (Cordarone)	Gray discoloration in sun-exposed sites
Zidovudine (AZT, Retrovir)	Nail pigmentation; diffuse Addison's-like pigmentation
Levodopa (Sinemet)	Diffuse hyperpigmentation

in the affected sites may also be white. The lesions often have a remarkably symmetrical distribution. There is also a variety in which the depigmentation occurs in a segmental pattern.

Treatment

Treatment can be tailored to suit the extent of the disease, the location of the depigmented patches, the degree of psychosocial disruption that the condition causes, and the amount of time that the patient has to treat this chronic problem. For limited lesions, a trial of high-potency topical corticosteroids such as clobetasol (Temovate) applied twice daily for at least 3 months is indicated. For facial lesions, less potent corticosteroids such as fluocinonide (Lidex) 0.05% cream are safer but still can produce cutaneous atrophy and steroid-induced rosacea if used for a prolonged period.

The most effective therapy for widespread vitiligo is photochemotherapy (psoralen plus ultraviolet A [PUVA]). It is not indicated for children younger than 10 years or for those with lesions predominantly over the hands, elbows, and knees; these sites rarely repigment with any treatment. Methoxsalen (Oxsoralen) may be applied in a 0.1% concentration in Cetaphil lotion 30 minutes before exposure to a carefully monitored, slowly increasing dose of ultraviolet A (UVA) radiation. Oral methoxsalen is easier to administer and has somewhat less phototoxicity associated with it. Nausea and fatigue occur with this modality, however. A dose of 0.6 mg per kg is administered 90 minutes before UVA exposure. Treatments are given two or three times per week, never on successive days. A minimum of 50 treatments is usually needed to get repigmentation.

For dark-skinned patients with depigmentation involving greater than 50% of the body, bleaching of the uninvolved skin may cause the skin tones to be uniform by transforming the whole integument into a white color. Monobenzyl ether of hydroquinone (Benoquin) 20% cream applied twice daily for 3 to 6 months to the normal skin can cause permanent loss of pigment. Before embarking on this treatment, the patient must understand that he or she will never have normal skin color again. This medication is difficult to obtain in the United States.

Vitiliginous skin contains no protective melanin. Thus, the patient is highly susceptible to sunburning and the chronic effects of sun exposure, such as actinic keratoses and skin cancer. Daily sunscreen use and protective clothing will aid in retarding the development of sun-damaged skin.

One should not underestimate the extent of the psychologic devastation that may accompany the progression of vitiligo. Support and reassurance can be therapeutic. Referral to a trained cosmetologist who can teach the patient the proper use of cover-up cosmetics is helpful. Self-tanning products containing dihydroxyacetone such as Self Tanning Lotion by Almay or Sunless Tanning Lotion by Vaseline Intensive Care can also help to cover the white spots.

Idiopathic Guttate Hypomelanosis

Clinical Findings

Idiopathic guttate hypomelanosis is an extremely common condition in which patients develop asymptomatic confetti-like white macules on the extremities. The spots are rarely larger than 1 cm in diameter and have no tendency to involute spontaneously. Thus, during many years, one can acquire hundreds of hypopigmented macules. The cause of this condition is unknown but may in some way be related to sun exposure.

Treatment

Careful destruction with trichloroacetic acid (25%) can occasionally cause isolated lesions to repigment. For the individual with hundreds of lesions, a full-extremity trichloroacetic acid chemical peel may result in a more uniform pigmentation. This is particularly true for the person with concomitant sun-damaged skin who has generalized cutaneous mottling.

Pityriasis Alba

Clinical Findings

Pityriasis alba is a common form of hypomelanosis that occurs mainly in children and young adults with atopic dermatitis. The lesions begin as poorly defined pink, scaly papules that evolve into hypopigmented plaques with a fine, powdery scale. The lesions are found on the face and upper trunk. This is probably an example of postinflammatory hypopigmentation after a flare of eczema.

Treatment

Mild or moderate-strength topical corticosteroids such as desonide (DesOwen) cream or triamcinolone (Kenalog) 0.1% cream applied twice daily help to reduce any residual inflammation and thus to delimit the process. Emollient creams will mask the scale and improve the appearance and texture of the skin. Judicious sun exposure will stimulate the epidermal melanocytes to produce more melanin and will darken the affected sites.

SUNBURN

method of
JOHN H. EPSTEIN, M.D.
*University of California, San Francisco
San Francisco, California*

Adverse reactions to the sun have been occurring with increasing frequency, in no small part owing to the general public's desire to develop a "good suntan." The most common of these is the phototoxic event, the sunburn reaction. It is caused by the ultraviolet rays (UVR) that compose 3 to 5% of the solar radiation that arrives at the earth's surface. In the early 1930s, the UVR was divided into three spectra because of apparent different photobiologic properties: ultraviolet C (UVC), 200 to 280 nm; ultraviolet B (UVB), 280 to 320 nm; and ultraviolet A (UVA) 320 to 400 nm. UVC rays from the sun do not penetrate to the earth's surface because of absorption by ozone in the stratosphere. This stratospheric ozone also absorbs about half of the incident UVB rays and none of the UVA rays. Essentially no rays shorter than 290 nm reach the earth's surface from the sun. However, photodamage of the skin can occur from UVC rays emitted by artificial sources such as germicidal lamps. Window glass absorbs UVB and UVC radiation but transmits UVA rays.

The sunburn reaction is characterized clinically by erythema with or without edema (depending on the amount of exposure) that starts a few hours after exposure, usually reaches a peak at 12 to 24 hours, and starts to subside by 72 hours with the onset of hyperpigmentation followed by desquamation of the dead cells. The erythematous skin is warm, painful, and tender. The desquamation phase may be pruritic. The intensity of the reaction may vary from from a mild erythema to blister formation, that is, from a first-degree to a superficial second-degree type of thermal burn. The severity of the reaction varies with the amount of UVR exposure and the susceptibility of the individual. People with light skin, hair, and eyes who do not tan well sunburn much more readily and severely than dark-complected people who tan well. However, everybody can sunburn with enough exposure to UVR.

Although the sunburn response is clinically defined by the erythema resulting from vasodilatation, it is a much more complicated process. Biologically it consists of immediate DNA damage in the epidermis with inhibition of DNA, RNA, and protein synthesis and mitosis formation that occurs shortly after exposure. DNA repair then occurs, and the cells in which the damage cannot be repaired die, forming the apoptotic sunburn cells that will eventually slough (peeling). By 24 hours, new cell formation occurs with increased DNA, RNA, and protein synthesis and mitosis formation that reaches a peak at 48 hours as a rule but may persist a week or more. New pigment formation in the melanocytes and pigment migration into the malpighian cells subsequently occur. However, if one receives enough UVR to produce new pigment, one has received enough UVR to cause damage. Labilization of lysosomal membranes with release of lysosomal enzymes and prostaglandin formation and release are part of the sunburn response as well. DNA and connective tissue damage also occurs in the dermis. This whole photobiologic response, not just the erythema, should be considered the sunburn reaction.

The rays primarily responsible for the sunburn reaction are those in the UVB spectrum. However, UVA radiation has been shown to significantly augment the acute damaging effects of UVB rays. UVA rays can also produce erythema and new pigment formation (tanning) by themselves. The amount of UVA radiation required to produce erythema is 1000 times that required for UVB to produce an erythema in human skin. Suberythemogenic amounts of both UVB and UVA can damage the skin. Indirect exposure to UVR also occurs from skylight and reflected radiation. White surfaces such as snow and white sand can reflect 80% of the incident ultraviolet radiation. In general, water is not a good reflector of ultraviolet radiation; as a result, one can have a severe sunburn develop on a cloudy day. In addition, the greater the elevation, the greater the ultraviolet exposure. It has been calculated that the UVB exposure increases by 4% for every 1000 feet above sea level.

PREVENTION AND TREATMENT

The best treatment for any adverse reaction is prevention. Although the intensity of UVA rays remains relatively constant throughout the daylight hours, UVB radiation is concentrated during the central portion of the day. Therefore, avoidance of sun exposure between 10 AM and 3 or 4 PM (depending on latitude) will eliminate exposure to 60% of the UVB rays. Wearing a hat with a wide brim can protect the head and neck against 70% of the incident UVR. Clothes with long sleeves and long pants can provide 100% protection. Lightweight sun-protective clothing that is comfortable to wear on hot summer days is available.

Sunscreens, which contain substances that absorb and/or reflect UVR, are useful for protecting unclothed skin. Their efficacy against UVB penetration is defined by the sun protection factor (SPF). The SPF represents the amount of UVB radiation required to produce a minimal erythema, that is, the minimal erythema dose (MED) through the sunscreen divided by the MED without the sunscreen:

$$SPF = \frac{MED \text{ with sunscreen}}{MED \text{ without sunscreen}}$$

A sunscreen with an SPF of 15 will prevent 94% of the UVB rays from reaching the skin. However, 6% will penetrate. Thus, applying the sunscreen two times will not provide an SPF of 30. A sunscreen with an SPF of 30 will prevent about 96% or 97% UVB penetration. In general, all people should use a sunscreen with at least an SPF of 15 when they are going to be in the sun. Although reapplication of the sunscreen will not increase the SPF value, it is useful to reapply every 2 hours or so to ensure that it is still in place and functioning. Many sunscreens also contain good UVA absorbers.

Once the acute exposure and reaction have occurred, the amount of therapy necessary depends on the degree of injury. A mild erythematous response rarely requires any specific treatment. Moderate reactions can be treated with cold, wet dressing (cold water is as effective as any of the special compresses), soothing lukewarm baths using oatmeal or cornstarch and baking soda, and aspirin 300 to 600 mg (5 to 10 grains) every 4 hours as needed for pain and pruritus. Widespread skin involvement may cause weakness, chills, and malaise, requiring bed rest and, at times, hospitalization. Severe involvement with or without systemic symptoms justifies short-term corticosteroid therapy. An initial dosage schedule of 10 mg of prednisone three times a day for 2 to 3 days may reduce the amount of inflammation present. The dosage should then be rapidly reduced (5 mg per day during the next few days). Nonsteroidal anti-inflammatory medications may supply some relief for the inflammation and discomfort.

Section 13

The Nervous System

BRAIN ABSCESS

method of
MORTON N. SWARTZ, M.D.
Massachusetts General Hospital
Boston, Massachusetts

Brain abscess is a purulent collection within the brain parenchyma, most commonly in the cerebrum, occasionally in the cerebellum, and rarely in the brain stem or medulla. The incidence is approximately 1 per 10,000 hospital admissions. Brain abscesses occur more commonly in adults than in young children.

PATHOGENESIS

Predisposing initiating infections or specific clinical settings may provide the clinical clue suggesting brain abscess in the diagnosis of a cerebral syndrome that might suggest some other process (e.g., tumor, stroke). There are five principal settings in which brain abscesses develop (Table 1). Brain abscess associated with a contiguous site of infection (e.g., otogenic, rhinogenic abscesses) probably develops as a result of direct extension from adjacent osteomyelitis (and epidural infection) or from retrograde thrombophlebitis of diploic or emissary veins. Otogenic brain abscesses occur more commonly in the temporal lobe but also in the cerebellum, particularly in children. Rhinogenic brain abscesses tend to be in the frontal lobes.

Brain abscesses secondary to hematogenous spread occur more frequently in the distribution of the middle cerebral artery and at the gray–white matter border. Since the advent of computed tomography (CT), multiple abscesses have been reported in more than 10% of patients (particularly those with hematogenous dissemination) with brain abscess.

Brain abscess is almost never a consequence of bacterial meningitis. When the conditions do occur together, meningitis has usually followed leakage or rupture of a preexisting abscess into a cerebral ventricle. The rare exception is abscess due to *Citrobacter diversus* complicating neonatal meningitis due to the same microorganism.

After introduction of pathogenic microorganisms into the brain, ingress of polymorphonuclear leukocytes, increased vascular permeability, and edema ensue. This stage of poorly demarcated presuppurative inflammation, lasting some days before frank suppuration and liquefaction necrosis, is often referred to as the stage of "bacterial cerebritis."

MICROBIAL ETIOLOGY

About 50% of the bacteria isolated from brain abscesses are anaerobes, and the other 50% are facultative, mainly streptococcal species and members of the Enterobacteriaceae (Table 2). About 40% of brain abscesses are due to two or more bacterial species, often mixtures of anaerobes and facultative bacteria. *Nocardia, Eikenella, Actinobacillus, Haemophilus aphrophilus,* and *Listeria monocytogenes* are bacterial species occasionally involved in brain abscess.

Various fungi such as *Aspergillus, Mucor, Candida, Pseudallescheria boydii,* and *Cladophialophora bantiana* (formerly *Cladosporium trichoides*) are occasionally the cause of brain abscess, typically in immunocompromised patients. Protozoa *(Toxoplasma gondii, Entamoeba histolytica, Acanthamoeba)* and helminthic diseases (cysticercosis, paragonimiasis, echinococcosis, schistosomiasis) may be the cause of lesions resembling brain abscess in appropriate epidemiologic settings.

In immunocompromised hosts, a variety of uncommon pathogens must be included among possible causes. In patients with defects in cell-mediated immunity, these would particularly include *T. gondii, Nocardia asteroides, Cryptococcus neoformans, L. monocytogenes, Salmonella,* and mycobacteria. Defects in neutrophils predispose to infections with Enterobacteriaceae, *Pseudomonas, Staphylococcus aureus,* and fungi as well as the usual pathogens in brain abscess. In patients with acquired immune deficiency syndrome (AIDS), focal central nervous system (CNS) lesions are caused by a variety of processes that occur more frequently in this setting than does brain abscess due to

TABLE 1. **Predisposing Factors for Brain Abscess**

Predisposing infections (40–50%)*
Otogenic
Otitis media (usually chronic) and mastoiditis—25% of all brain abscesses
Rhinogenic
Frontal, ethmoidal, or sphenoidal sinusitis
Pleuropulmonary
Lung abscess, bronchiectasis (including cystic fibrosis), empyema
Odontogenic
Dental infections (~2% of brain abscesses)
Other contiguous sites
Face and scalp infections; osteomyelitis of skull
Right-to-left cardiovascular shunts (5–10%)
Cyanotic congenital heart disease
Pulmonary arteriovenous malformations
Trauma
Penetrating head trauma—e.g., gunshot wounds, pencil points
Neurosurgical trauma—craniotomy infections, head tongs
Hematogenous spread from definable distant foci (~10%)
Intra-abdominal infections, pelvic infections, skin infections
Acute bacterial endocarditis (usually due to *Staphylococcus aureus*)—these are uncommon, usually multiple, small, and secondary to embolic events
Cryptogenic (15–20%)
None of the above predisposing factors are present; probably the result of transient occult bacteremia or a small right-to-left shunt (e.g., patent foramen ovale)

*Percentage of all brain abscesses.

TABLE 2. **Organisms Causing Brain Abscess**

Organism	Frequency of Isolation (% of Cases)
Anaerobes	45–50
Peptococcus, Peptostreptococcus, other "anaerobic streptococci"	10–15
Bacteroides, Prevotella, and Fusobacterium species	20–25
Actinomyces, Propionibacterium species	5
Eubacterium, Veillonella, Clostridium species	5
Aerobes and facultative organisms	50–55
Streptococci (including Streptococcus milleri group)	20
Enterobacteriaceae and Pseudomonas aeruginosa	10–15
Staphylococcus aureus	5–10
Haemophilus species	2
Nocardia species	1
Other (Eikenella, Actinobacillus, Listeria, fungi)	10

the common bacterial causes in the non-immunosuppressed population (Table 3). In patients with AIDS, such brain abscesses must be differentiated by clinical features and CT or magnetic resonance imaging (MRI) from other causes of brain lesions that also occur in that setting. These other causes are primarily (1) progressive multifocal leukoencephalopathy (involving white matter, predominantly in parieto-occipital area and cerebellum; nonenhancing hypodense lesions at CT; hypodense signal abnormalities on T1-weighted MRI scans; and hyperintense lesions without mass effect on T2-weighted scans); and (2) primary CNS B cell lymphoma (at CT, lesions are often hyperdense, with surrounding edema, variable contrast enhancement, and a mass effect resembling that of brain abscess).

CLINICAL FEATURES

In most patients with brain abscess, particularly those of hematogenous origin, symptoms have been present for

TABLE 3. **Cause of Brain Abscess in Patients with AIDS and in Other Immunosuppressed States**

Common cause
  Toxoplasma gondii: most common cause of mass lesion in AIDS patients (occurs in 4–8% in United States; commonly, multiple lesions in cerebral hemispheres and basal ganglia on CT and MRI with ring enhancement, surrounding edema, mass effect; almost invariably serum IgG antibodies present
Less common causes
  Bacterial brain abscesses due to *Salmonella, Nocardia, Streptococcus pneumoniae, Listeria*
  Cryptococcus neoformans (cryptococcoma)
  Fungi—*Aspergillus, Mucor, Candida*
  Mycobacterium tuberculosis (tuberculoma)
  Mycobacterium avium-intracellulare
  Acanthamoeba

Abbreviations: AIDS = acquired immune deficiency syndrome; CT = computed tomography; MRI = magnetic resonance imaging.

less than 2 weeks before diagnosis. Headache, localized or generalized, is present in 80%; nausea and vomiting in 60%; and fever (temperature of ≥100°F) in only 50%. In some, the course is more indolent, mimicking a brain tumor. The state of consciousness is altered to various degrees in about 50%. Seizures and stiff neck each occur in about 30% of patients with brain abscess. Papilledema occurs in about 50% of patients, but only relatively late in the course.

Focal neurologic deficits are detected in about 50% of patients, and the nature of the deficits depends on the location of the abscess. Temporal lobe abscess is associated with ipsilateral frontotemporal headache, anomic aphasia (difficulty naming objects) if in the dominant hemisphere, a superior homonymous quadrantanopia, and only minimal contralateral motor or sensory defects. The initial symptom of cerebellar abscess is often suboccipital or postauricular headache, followed by the development of coarse nystagmus, vomiting, ataxia of the ipsilateral arm and leg, and weakness of the conjugate gaze to the side of the abscess. Signs of increased intracranial pressure are often more prominent with cerebellar than cerebral abscesses. The features of frontal lobe abscess include headache; inattention; drowsiness and depressed cognition; contralateral hemiparesis; and unilateral motor seizures. Parietal lobe abscesses produce cortical sensory deficits and sensory extinction, homonymous hemianopia or visual inattention, and mild hemiparesis.

LABORATORY FINDINGS

A peripheral leukocytosis (cell count of ≥10,000 per mm³) is present in two thirds of patients with brain abscess, but its absence does not rule out the diagnosis. Blood cultures may be positive in some patients with hematogenous brain abscess. Lumbar puncture is dangerous in the presence of elevated intracranial pressure and may lead to herniation. Imaging studies are indicated as the initial diagnostic procedure. Occasionally, stiff neck or focal cerebral signs may be prominent and lead to performance of a lumbar puncture in a patient in whom a brain abscess was not initially suspected. In such a case the cerebrospinal fluid findings may be a mild lymphocytic pleocytosis (10 to 300 lymphocytes per mm³), a normal glucose level, and a mildly elevated protein level. It is important to recognize that a cerebral abscess may leak (or rupture) into a ventricle, producing a polymorphonuclear pleocytosis and secondary bacterial meningitis, a grave complication.

IMAGING STUDIES

Imaging studies (CT, MRI) are invaluable in diagnosing brain abscess, defining the features of the lesion (solitary, multiple, multilocular), and indicating their location. At CT the characteristic appearance of an abscess includes a hypodense center, peripheral rim enhancement, and a variable surrounding area of edema. With contrast medium, a relatively uniform ring of enhancement (sometimes thinner along the medial margin) is present. Similarly, MRI with contrast medium (gadolinium) shows a ring-enhancing mass with surrounding vasogenic edema. MRI is the more sensitive radiologic procedure for demonstrating an abscess.

Bacterial cerebritis is the earliest stage of brain abscess, and one that is difficult to recognize specifically with either CT or MRI. With CT without contrast medium, the involved area appears as a vague hypodense area. MRI is more sensitive to early edematous changes (area of high signal intensity on T2-weighted images). Early cerebritis shows little or no contrast enhancement with CT or MRI. In a later stage of cerebritis, there is development of a thin, often incomplete and ill-defined, rim of enhancement. With delayed CT, the rim may fill out and contrast material diffuse into the hypodense center in cerebritis (but not in abscess).

MANAGEMENT OF PATIENTS WITH SUSPECTED BRAIN ABSCESS

Contrast-enhanced CT or MRI is indicated for the evaluation of patients with headache, altered consciousness, and focal cerebral deficits, particularly in the presence of any of the predisposing factors (see Table 1) for brain abscess. Lumbar puncture is deferred until a CNS mass lesion has been excluded. If the clinical course has been rapid or if meningitis is a possibility because of stiff neck, blood cultures are promptly obtained and empirical antimicrobial therapy is instituted before CT or MRI.

Involvement of a neurosurgeon is essential at the outset in the management of a suspected brain abscess. The presence of a predisposing ear infection (mastoiditis, chronic otitis media) or sinusitis warrants otolaryngologic consultation, but the initial attention must be directed toward treatment of the brain abscess. Empirical antimicrobial therapy is begun promptly in patients whose clinical findings and MRI or CT features are consistent with brain abscess, even if immediate neurosurgical intervention is required. Several initial antimicrobial regimens have been employed in adults directed against the most frequent aerobic and anaerobic pathogens. In one, penicillin G (4 million units intravenously every 4 hours), or ampicillin (2 grams intravenously every 4 hours), is combined with metronidazole (Flagyl) (15 mg per kg as a loading dose, followed by 7.5 mg per kg every 6 hours, intravenously). In another (which I favor), cefotaxime (Claforan) (2 grams intravenously every 4 to 6 hours) is added to the regimen of penicillin G (or ampicillin) plus metronidazole. In another regimen, cefotaxime replaces penicillin G and is used in combination with metronidazole. In the past, chloramphenicol was used for coverage of anaerobes, but it has largely been replaced by metronidazole.

Because no combination of two, or even three, antimicrobials will cover the entire spectrum of organisms involved in brain abscess, specific delineation of the infecting agent should be sought by blood cultures and by stereotactic aspiration of the lesion. Less common organisms detected by such methods and requiring different antibiotic therapy include *S. aureus* (nafcillin, 9 to 12 grams intravenously daily; or vancomycin, 2 grams intravenously daily) and *Pseudomonas aeruginosa* (ceftazidime [Fortaz], 6 to 8 grams intravenously daily*).

Surgery is needed for microbiologic diagnosis and drainage in most patients. Stereotactic CT-guided aspiration is generally the procedure of choice. Excision

is usually indicated for treatment of large posterior fossa abscesses, abscesses associated with foreign bodies, and fungal abscesses (due to the difficulty of treatment with available antimicrobials).

The stage of bacterial cerebritis should be recognized and can be cured with the use of antibiotics alone, but it requires both initial CT or MRI diagnosis and careful documentation of resolution by imaging. Between 1975 and 1985, 67 cases of "brain abscess" (many representing late cerebritis) treated only medically were reported in the literature, the great majority successfully. Aspiration during the cerebritis stage may be dangerous because of possible hemorrhage.

DURATION OF THERAPY

The duration of therapy is based on several factors: (1) whether cerebritis or abscess is present, (2) the nature of the infecting organism, (3) the clinical response, (4) the resolution of changes on CT or MRI, and (5) whether aspiration or excision is performed. For cerebritis, 4 weeks of parenteral antimicrobial therapy is reasonable. For an abscess that has been aspirated and treated with appropriate antimicrobials in a patient who is clinically and radiographically improving, a 6-week course of parenteral treatment is recommended. In patients in whom contraindications to surgery exist, a 6- to 8-week course of parenteral therapy with close clinical and CT (every 1 to 2 weeks) monitoring is appropriate. The duration of therapy is not based on complete resolution of all CT or MRI abnormalities, because after a cure, residual enhancement may persist for up to 2 to 6 months or longer. If *Nocardia,* a difficult to treat organism, is the cause, prolonged intravenous (followed by oral) therapy with trimethoprim-sulfamethoxazole (TMP-SMZ) (Bactrim, Septra) is necessary (for a total course of 6 to 12 months if surgical excision has been performed; 12 months or longer if excision is not performed and the patient is immunosuppressed). Addition initially of a second drug (third-generation cephalosporin, imipenem, or amikacin) to TMP-SMZ may be considered for a known *Nocardia* brain abscess until a clinical response is evident.

PATIENTS WITH AIDS

The management of adults with AIDS and consistent contrast-enhancing CNS lesions is directed initially, empirically, at the most frequent cause of such lesions in this setting, i.e., cerebral toxoplasmosis. Combination therapy with pyrimethamine (Daraprim) (a loading dose of 200 mg the first day followed by 50 to 75 mg orally daily) plus sulfadiazine (1.0 to 1.5 grams orally every 6 hours) is employed in adults. Folinic acid (leucovorin [Wellcovorin], 10 to 20 mg daily orally) is added to reduce pyrimethamine-induced myelotoxicity. If sulfadiazine cannot be used, clindamycin (Cleocin) (600 mg orally every 6 hours, or 600 mg up to 1200 mg intravenously every 6 hours) is an alternative. Because the MRI or CT

---

*Exceeds dosage recommended by the manufacturer.

appearance of toxoplasmosis cannot be distinguished accurately from that of other conditions (bacterial or fungal abscesses, lymphoma, metastatic malignancies), failure to respond clinically and by neuroimaging within 7 to 14 days of treatment is an indication for aspiration or biopsy. A negative *Toxoplasma* serologic IgG test prompts early biopsy.

In immunosuppressed patients other than those with AIDS, early biopsy is usually indicated because of the spectrum of possible causes (see Table 3).

CORTICOSTEROID THERAPY

Corticosteroids are used intravenously only to reduce cerebral edema and a mass effect in patients with increasing neurologic deficit and a depressed level of consciousness due to increased intracranial pressure. Disadvantages in their use include decreased antibiotic entry into the CNS, delayed healing, and reduction of the degree of contrast enhancement at CT (obscuring the initial diagnosis or confusing interpretation of follow-up scans).

OUTCOME

The introduction of the newer neuroimaging techniques (CT, MRI) and the use of image-directed stereotactic aspiration have had a major impact on the outcome of brain abscess. Current diagnostic and therapeutic approaches have reduced mortality in the antibiotic era from 40% to 0 to 24%.

ALZHEIMER'S DISEASE

method of
LEON J. THAL, M.D.
University of California, San Diego, School of Medicine
La Jolla, California

Alzheimer's disease (AD) is the most important dementing illness because of its high prevalence. In the United States, 5 to 10% of the population older than 65 years is afflicted with AD. In 1990, there were approximately 4 million individuals with AD, and this number is expected to reach 14 million by the year 2050. AD is the fourth leading cause of death for adults, resulting in more than 100,000 deaths annually. Current costs to the nation are estimated at $90 billion per year.

Although there are many causes of the dementia syndrome, AD, including cases of dementia with Lewy bodies, makes up approximately 65% of all cases (Table 1). About 50% of patients have classic AD, and neuropathologic examination demonstrates senile plaques, neurofibrillary tangles, and vascular amyloid. Another 15% present with an Alzheimer-like dementia that may be accompanied by fluctuations in consciousness, frequent hallucinations, and extrapyramidal symptoms (EPS). At autopsy, these patients are found to have abundant plaques, few tangles, and cortical Lewy bodies. These two entities are difficult to separate clinically. Other common causes of dementia include mixed dementia, in which both the changes of AD

TABLE 1. Common Causes of Dementia

Disease	Approximate Percentage
Alzheimer's disease (AD)	50
Dementia associated with Lewy bodies	15
Mixed dementia (AD and vascular)	10
Vascular dementia	5
Other degenerative conditions including frontotemporal dementia	5
Treatable dementia (infections, tumor, alcohol, hydrocephalus, epilepsy)	5
Reversible dementias (drugs, depression, metabolic)	5
Miscellaneous disorders	5
	100

and vascular disease are present (10%), pure cerebrovascular dementia (5%), and other neurodegenerative disorders such as the frontotemporal dementias including Pick's disease (5%). In another 5% of cases, treatable dementias may result from subdural hematoma, hydrocephalus, seizures, chronic infections, some tumors, and alcohol abuse. About 5% of dementias may be reversible, including those due to drug toxicity, depression, and unsuspected metabolic disturbances such as hepatic dysfunction, hyponatremia, disorders of calcium metabolism, vitamin B_{12} deficiency, and thyroid disease. A variety of miscellaneous disorders account for the remaining cases.

Every patient presenting with a dementia syndrome should undergo a complete evaluation for potentially reversible or treatable conditions (Table 2). A detailed history is needed from a collateral source including the approximate onset, duration, and course of the illness. A history of cognitive fluctuations, delusions, and hallucinations should also be sought. Physical examination with particular attention to vision and hearing is essential. Mental status testing should include evaluation of recent memory, remote memory, orientation, language, calculations, abstractions, judgment, and visuospatial relations. This can be accomplished by a simple office examination, which may be sup-

TABLE 2. Evaluation of the Patient with the Dementia Syndrome

By the examiner
  History from collateral source
  Physical examination, vision, hearing
  Mental status testing
  Neurologic examination
Testing
  Blood for CBC; metabolic screen; thyroid test; vitamin B_{12} level; serologic examination; HIV (if indicated)
  Chest radiograph
  ECG
  Brain imaging: CT, MRI
  EEG (if indicated)
  LP (if indicated)
  Psychometric testing (if indicated)
  In uncertain cases, may consider
    Apolipoprotein E genotyping
    CSF tau and A_β1–42

Abbreviations: CBC = complete blood count; HIV = human immunodeficiency virus; ECG = electrocardiogram; CT = computed tomography; MRI = magnetic resonance imaging; EEG = electroencephalogram; LP = lumbar puncture.

plemented with a standardized cognitive screening test such as the Mini-Mental State Examination (MMSE). A physical neurologic examination is performed with particular attention to the presence or absence of focal motor or sensory findings; gait disturbances; and EPS such as masked facies, bradykinesia, tremor, or rigidity. Blood tests for common metabolic disorders that may produce the dementia syndrome should include thyroid function and a serum vitamin B_{12} level. Human immunodeficiency virus testing should be performed if risk factors are present. A brain-imaging procedure should be performed at least once in all individuals with the dementia syndrome to identify structural and potentially treatable causes of dementia in particular, tumors, hydrocephalus, and strokes. An electroencephalogram is not required but may be helpful in instances of suspected seizures or if the diagnosis of depression presenting as dementia is a consideration. Lumbar puncture is not routinely recommended but should be performed when significant systemic illness or cancer is present and central nervous system infection, hydrocephalus, or other unusual dementias are suspected. In addition, cerebrospinal fluid levels of the proteins tau and A_β 1–42, which occur in the lesions of AD, may be useful in increasing the accuracy of the antemortem diagnosis of AD. Psychometric testing is not essential but may be helpful in diagnosing early dementia when the bedside or office mental status testing fails to reveal significant cognitive deficits in spite of a suggestive history; in separating dementia from depression; and in determining or predicting an individual's ability to work, drive, and live independently.

In most cases, AD presents in a stereotyped fashion and leads to death in 10 to 12 years. Memory loss, recent greater than remote, is the most common initial complaint (Table 3). On average, patients decline by 3 to 4 points per year on the MMSE; however, variability is common, and the standard deviation of this change (3 to 4 points) is large. Language disturbance usually develops during the first several years of disease, characterized by decreased spontaneous output and difficulty with naming objects and later by comprehension deficits. Visuospatial impairment can readily be demonstrated in most AD patients. Early in the course of the illness, many AD patients are unable to draw a clock and set the hands correctly. Behavioral disturbances are common, peak in the middle stages of the disease, and include depression, delusions, wandering, agitation, insomnia, hallucinations, and disinhibition. Although abnormal neurologic findings are generally absent, primitive reflexes, extrapyramidal features, myoclonus, and seizures may occur as the disease progresses. The presence of EPS early in the course of the disease strongly suggests the diagnosis of dementia associated with Lewy bodies. Institutionalization, most often necessary in the later stages of the disease, may be precipitated by incontinence, agitation, wandering, insomnia, and physical disability.

Although the etiology of AD has not been firmly estab-

lished, numerous risk factors have been identified, the most important of which is age (Table 4). The prevalence of the illness rises rapidly with age, doubling every 5 years after the age of 65 years, reaching 28 to 47% for the population older than the age of 85 years. A family history of multiple affected first-degree relatives increases the risk fourfold. Recently, the E_4 allelic variant of apolipoprotein E, a cholesterol-carrying protein, has been associated with AD. The apolipoprotein E status and genetics account for about 50% of the attributable risk for AD. Other weaker risk factors include female sex, low educational levels, antecedent head trauma, and myocardial infarction.

The genetics of early-onset AD have been revolutionized during the past decade and provide clues to the etiology of the disease. A small number of families have been found to have genetic defects, generally single-base-pair substitutions. There are three chromosomal loci involved: on chromosome 21 in or near the gene coding for amyloid precursor protein; on chromosome 14 in a gene called presenilin 1; and on chromosome 1 in a gene called presenilin 2 (Table 5). Although these three genetic loci result in early-onset AD in rare families, the presence of the gene coding for the apolipoprotein E_4 allele is a major risk factor for the development of AD after the age of 50 years and is associated with both a higher overall risk and an earlier age at onset. Controversy currently exists about whether or not screening for the apolipoprotein E_4 allele can enhance sensitivity and specificity for the diagnosis of AD. A consensus conference has recommended that apolipoprotein E genotyping not be used to predict the future risk of AD in symptom-free individuals and said that its utility for increasing the accuracy of diagnosis in patients presenting with the dementia syndrome is not clear. Further population-based clinicopathologic data are needed to determine the clinical utility of apolipoprotein E genotyping in dementia.

TREATMENT

There are no truly satisfactory therapies for AD. Treatment should begin with a comprehensive evaluation that includes education of the family and manipulation of the environment before pharmacologic therapies are considered. It often requires several

TABLE 3. Common Clinical Features of Alzheimer's Disease

Memory loss
Language disturbance
Visuospatial disturbances
Behavioral changes including depression,
    agitation, delusions, hallucinations
Absence of focal neurologic findings

TABLE 4. Risk Factors for Alzheimer's Disease

Major	Minor
Age	Female sex
Apolipoprotein E genotype	Low level of education
Genetics	Head injury
Positive family history	Myocardial infarction
Familial AD	

TABLE 5. Genetics of Alzheimer's Disease

Chromosome	Gene	Age at Onset (y)	Percentage with AD
21	APP	30s–50s	<1
14	Presenilin 1	40s–60s	<1
1	Presenilin 2	40s–60s	<1
19	Apolipoprotein E_4	Late onset	40–60

Abbreviation: APP = amyloid precursor protein.

TABLE 6. **Noncognitive Pharmacologic Treatment**

Depression	Delusions
Fluoxetine (Prozac)	Risperidone
Paroxetine (Paxil)	Haloperidol
Sertraline (Zoloft)	Thioridazine
Venlafaxine (Effexor)	Insomnia
Nortriptyline (Pamelor)	Warm milk
Anxiety	Trazodone
Lorazepam (Ativan)	Diphenhydramine (Benadryl)
Alprazolam (Xanax)	Zolpidem (Ambien)
Buspirone (BuSpar)	Short-acting benzodiazepine
Agitation	
Trazodone (Desyrel)	
Haloperidol (Haldol)	
Risperidone (Risperdal)	
Thioridazine (Mellaril)	

visits before the diagnosis is accepted and a plan of action can be initiated.

Noncognitive Pharmacologic Treatment

Behavioral symptoms, including depression, anxiety, agitation, delusions, and insomnia, occur frequently in patients with AD (Table 6). There are no absolute rules for treating these symptoms. Because inappropriate pharmacologic intervention can produce more harm than good, careful evaluation of the patient's medical condition and the severity of symptoms is of paramount importance before deciding on treatment. Not all symptoms require treatment. For example, although as many as one third to one half of AD patients have delusions, in many instances they are mild and do not require treatment. General principles of geriatric psychopharmacology must be emphasized. Once a decision to use pharmacologic intervention is made, a specific target symptom should be identified. The degree of symptom reduction anticipated by the physician, caregiver, or both should be noted. Treatment should be initiated at the lowest possible dose. The patient should be monitored frequently, and after the symptom has been controlled, judicious dose lowering or withdrawal should be considered. Intermittent dosing may be useful for reducing side effects, especially when treating anxiety or agitation. Pharmacologic intervention may result in significant side effects, including sedation, disinhibition, depression, falls, incontinence, parkinsonism, tardive dyskinesia, and akathisia.

Approximately 15 to 20% of AD patients experience depression at some point during the course of their illness. If the depression requires therapy, fluoxetine (Prozac) 10 to 20 mg per day, paroxetine (Paxil) 20 to 40 mg per day, and sertraline (Zoloft) 50 to 100 mg per day are available as selective serotonin reuptake inhibitors (SSRIs). Venlafaxine (Effexor) 50 to 100 mg per day is an inhibitor of both serotonin and norepinephrine reuptake that may be useful in some refractory cases. Nortriptyline (Pamelor), a classic tricyclic antidepressant, may also be effective in doses of 25 to 100 mg daily. The SSRIs are generally preferred to tricyclic agents not only because of their greater efficacy, but also because they induce fewer side effects, such as orthostasis, dry mouth, or cardiac problems. However, weight must be monitored because weight loss may occur in 10 to 15% of patients taking SSRIs.

Anxiety may accompany AD, especially in its early stages. It can be relieved by small doses of lorazepam (Ativan) 0.5 mg per dose, alprazolam (Xanax) 0.25 mg per dose, or buspirone (BuSpar) 5 mg per dose, as needed.

Agitation occurs frequently in AD and is often cited as an important factor for institutionalization. Precipitating factors for agitation should be sought, such as physical discomfort, excessive sensory stimulation, or improper environment. Mild outbursts can sometimes be handled behaviorally by distracting patients or allowing them to wander in an enclosed space. If agitation is sufficiently troublesome and without obvious remedial cause, it may require treatment. There is no consensus regarding the class of agents best suited for the treatment of agitation. Few studies have compared neuroleptics with benzodiazepines or other sedatives. Recent empirical evidence suggests that trazodone (Desyrel), with starting doses of 25 to 50 mg at bedtime and increments to 200 mg per day, may be as effective in controlling agitation as neuroleptics. Neuroleptic treatment can control agitation and reduce disability. Haloperidol (Haldol) may be used in doses ranging from 0.25 to 2 or 3 mg per day. Unfortunately, many AD patients develop EPS with haloperidol. Neuroleptics should generally be avoided in individuals suspected of having Lewy bodies associated with dementia because of the propensity to develop severe EPS. Clozapine (Clozaril) is generally not used because of the need for blood testing to guard against the development of agranulocytosis. Risperidone (Risperdal) in doses of 0.5 to 2 mg per day may control agitation in some AD patients with less risk of inducing EPS. Thioridazine (Mellaril) 10 to 30 mg per day in divided doses may control agitation without inducing EPS, but doses greater than 70 to 80 mg per day should not be used because there is a high risk of confusion secondary to anticholinergic side effects.

Delusions should be treated only when significantly disturbing to the patient or caregiver or when they clearly have an impact on the quality of life. Risperidone, haloperidol, and thioridazine are frequently the first-line drugs.

Insomnia is best managed by environmental manipulation. Keeping the patient awake during the day and reducing the amount of nighttime fluids frequently helps. Adequate exposure to daytime bright light may help to reset the body's natural circadian rhythm and re-establish an improved sleep-wake cycle. The use of warm milk at bedtime should be tried first. If this fails, a nighttime dose of trazodone 25 to 100 mg or diphenhydramine (Benadryl) 25 to 50 mg might suffice. These agents are recommended because there is relatively little tolerance to their sedating effect. Alternatively, zolpidem

TABLE 7. **Cognition-Enhancing Agents**

Ergoloid mesylates (Hydergine)
Tacrine (Cognex)
Donepezil (Aricept)

(Ambien) 5 mg or short-acting benzodiazepines can be used. Benzodiazepines should be used only intermittently to prevent the development of tolerance.

Cognition-Enhancing Agents
(Table 7)

In the past, the only agent available for the treatment of memory impairment in the elderly was ergoloid mesylates (Hydergine), a metabolism-enhancing mixture of three ergot alkaloids. Although extensively tested in elderly individuals with cognitive impairment, the exact mode of action of this agent remains unknown. About 5% of patients treated with doses of 3 to 9 mg seem to improve regarding subjective cognitive dysfunction, depressed mood, and composite global scores. However, studies using objective psychometric testing have generally failed to document improvement in AD patients. The side effects of the ergoloid mesylate agent are minimal; rarely, it may cause headache. Mildly impaired patients not wishing treatment with other agents may be treated with up to 9 mg per day in three equally divided doses. If improvement is not observed after 2 to 3 months, the drug should be discontinued.

In the 1970s, multiple laboratory investigators described a marked decrease in levels of cortical choline acetyltransferase, the synthetic enzyme for acetylcholine, in patients with AD. Decreases in the levels of this enzyme were correlated with the degree of cognitive impairment on mental status testing. During the past 15 years, numerous cholinesterase inhibitors have been developed aimed at enhancing cholinergic transmission. Three large multicenter trials involving more than 2000 AD patients led to the approval of tacrine (Cognex) for the treatment of AD in 1993. In these trials, tacrine produced a small degree of improvement in patients with AD, equivalent to the amount of decline an average AD patient would undergo during a period of approximately 6 months. However, only 15 to 20% of AD patients exposed to tacrine had a large enough therapeutic effect to be observable by the family and clinician without the use of psychometric testing. In controlled clinical trials, 40 to 50% of tacrine-treated patients develop reversible elevations in serum transaminase levels. In addition, approximately one third develop significant digestive system complaints consisting of nausea, vomiting, or diarrhea. Transaminase monitoring must be carried out every other week for at least the first 15 weeks after the initiation of tacrine treatment, after which the monitoring frequency may be decreased. In clinical practice, dose escalation is generally carried out more slowly than in controlled clinical trials, and the frequency of transaminase

elevations and side effects is likely to be lower. Treatment is generally initiated with 40 mg daily in four divided doses then increased to 80 mg daily in four divided doses. Further increments are best carried out by increasing the dose 20 to 40 mg per month to a maximal tolerated dose or 160 mg daily. Because of the small clinical effect (generally 1 to 3 points on the MMSE), the side effect profile, and the need for laboratory monitoring, many patients and clinicians are reluctant to use tacrine. A second cholinesterase inhibitor, donepezil (Aricept), was released in early 1997. It appears to have the same effectiveness as tacrine, is relatively free of hepatotoxicity, and produces a lower incidence of gastrointestinal distress. In addition, it may be dosed once daily at 5 or 10 mg. Numerous other cholinesterase inhibitors are currently in clinical trials and are likely to reach the marketplace within the next several years.

Experimental Treatment
(Table 8)

Numerous compounds are currently in clinical trials for AD. Agents designed to improve cognition include cholinesterase inhibitors, muscarinic agonists, nootropic agents, and agents designed to alter noncholinergic transmission and/or receptors. Some are now being tested for their ability to slow the rate of decline or delay the onset of AD including anti-inflammatory agents, antioxidants, and hormones such as estrogens. Many of these trials are based on observational studies that suggest that the use of these agents is associated with a reduced risk of developing AD. Recently, both the antioxidant α-tocopherol (vitamin E), at a dosage of 1000 IU twice daily, and selegiline, a monoamine oxidase B inhibitor, at a dosage of 5 mg twice daily, were demonstrated to result in approximately a 6-month delay in the time to reach important milestones in AD, including loss of basic activities of daily living, progression to severe dementia, institutionalization, and

TABLE 8. **Experimental Treatment of Alzheimer's Disease**

To improve cognition
  Cholinesterase inhibitors
  Muscarinic agonists
  Nootropic agents
Agents or classes of compounds to alter noncholinergic transmitters and/or receptors, slow decline, or delay onset
Acetyl-L-carnitine
MAO-β inhibitors*
Hormones, especially estrogens*
Calcium channel blockers*
Anti-inflammatory agents*
Antioxidants, especially vitamin E
Trophic factors, especially NGF
Agents that reduce apolipoprotein E_4 levels
Drugs to prevent deposition or enhance removal of amyloid

*Not FDA approved for this indication.
Abbreviations: NGF = nerve growth factor; MAO = monoamine oxidase.

death. Trials of compounds that alter apolipoprotein E_4 status and/or amyloid deposition have not yet been carried out.

Therapeutic Role of the Physician

In the care of the AD patient, the physician often serves as the primary family adviser. The nature of the illness, the expected course, and anticipated problems need to be discussed with the caregivers, and issues related to finances, legal planning, wills, placement, and withholding of treatment need to be addressed. Complex problems related to driving, the use of appliances, wandering, inappropriate sexual behavior, and impact on the family need to be managed. The physician must be an adviser as well as a source of helpful referrals. Knowledge about local facilities such as day care centers, Alzheimer support groups, and sources of information for family members can be as useful in managing the patient as is the writing of prescriptions. *The 36 Hour Day* by Nancy Mace and Peter Rabins should be recommended reading for caregivers. Contact with a local Alzheimer's Association support group should be encouraged. Contact with the National Alzheimer's Association (312–335–8700) should be made. The availability of centers that specialize in the care of AD patients and also carry out controlled clinical trials should be made known to the patient and family. Knowledge of home health service agencies, skilled nursing facilities capable of handling AD patients, social workers, and legal advisers is a necessary part of the physician's armamentarium.

PRIMARY INTRACEREBRAL HEMORRHAGE

method of
RALPH G. GREENLEE, JR., M.D.
University of Texas Southwestern Medical Center
Dallas, Texas

In recent years effective antihypertensive therapy has reduced the incidence of intracerebral hemorrhage (ICH) to 10% of strokes. Although ICH is more lethal than ischemic stroke, early recognition, thorough etiologic evaluation, and assiduous clinical management can significantly modify the individual patient's mortality. It is often not appreciated that functional recovery from ICH is often better than that from a comparable initial deficit due to ischemic infarction. This is because the parenchymatous hematoma expands as an ovoid mass, with the initial neurologic deficit due primarily to compression of neural structures rather than ischemic death of those structures. The initial deficit usually develops during 30 to 60 minutes. Much of the ensuing neurologic deterioration is as a result of increased intracranial pressure (ICP) and focal edema around the hematoma. Thus, the goal of therapy for ICH is to minimize the size of the hemorrhage by appropriate antihypertensive therapy and to minimize increased ICP.

The hematoma itself eventually resolves to leave a slitlike cavity lined by a glial scar.

Certain stroke syndromes are relevant to the recognition and clinical management of ICH. They are predicated on the presence or absence of hypertension and on an infratentorial or supratentorial location of the hemorrhage. Thus, a clinical history of coexisting hypertension and the location of intraparenchymal blood at computed tomography (CT) provide the basic framework for further diagnostic evaluation and management of ICH.

HYPERTENSIVE INTRACEREBRAL HEMORRHAGE

Up to 80% of hemorrhagic strokes are associated with a clinical history of chronic hypertension. The ictus usually, but not always, occurs when the patient is active. Hypertensive hemorrhages usually originate from the same small penetrating vessels that are affected by hypertensive microvascular disease. Thus, hematoma formation is almost always localized to one of four anatomic regions: (1) putamen and caudate regions adjacent to the internal capsule (50% of cases), (2) thalamus (22% of cases), (3) pons (10% of cases), and (4) cerebellar hemispheres (20% of cases). Each of the four locations produces a relatively distinct clinical stroke syndrome, as illustrated in Table 1. Hypertension as a cause for hematoma located solely in the cerebral cortex or deep white matter is rare.

The clinical deficit resulting from hypertensive ICH reaches its maximal extent rapidly but can continue to worsen if blood pressure remains uncontrolled. Clinical worsening after the initial ictus and the blood pressure has been controlled is usually due to edema, ventricular obstruction, or both. Increased ICP is suggested by nausea, vomiting, and a decreased level of alertness. The development of coma in ICH usually implies a poor prognosis for functional survival. Supratentorial hemorrhages can result in transtentorial herniation, and frequent clinical re-examination of the patient is necessary. Once hypertension has been controlled, progressive clot enlargement as verified by CT should raise suspicion for a coagulopathy or underlying vascular malformation.

NONHYPERTENSIVE INTRACEREBRAL HEMORRHAGE

ICH without an associated history of hypertension has a less predictable anatomic distribution but is more likely to involve the cerebral cortex or deep white matter. A wide variety of underlying pathologic conditions can produce these hemorrhages. Diagnostic consideration should be given to the possibility of an aneurysm or arteriovenous malformation (AVM) in these settings. Prolonged bleeding times due to systemic causes or the use of anticoagulants must be excluded. Amphetamine and cocaine substance abuse and even excessive use of a nasal spray with sympathomimetic agents can lead to ICH. Amyloid angiopathy is a condition seen usually in elderly patients with dementia and often results in recurrent cortical hemorrhages.

The clinical presentation of nonhypertensive ICH depends on the anatomic location of the hemorrhage. The hematoma in nonhypertensive ICH has a greater tendency to continue to expand. This is a useful as a differential point in those patients who present with mild to moderate hypertension and progressing neurologic deficit.

TABLE 1. **Some Clinical Signs Usually Associated with Hypertensive Intracerebral Hemorrhage Depending on Location**

Location	Motor and/or Sensory	Pupils	Eye Deviation
Putamen	Contralateral hemiparesis; hemianesthesia	Normal	Contralateral conjugate gaze
Thalamus	Contralateral hemiparesis; hemianesthesia	Small	Conjugate downward deviation
Cerebellum	Ipsilateral facial weakness; ipsilateral truncal ataxia; ipsilateral limb ataxia	Small	Ipsilateral conjugate gaze paresis; sixth nerve paresis
Pons	Quadriparesis	Pinpoint	Ipsilateral horizontal gaze paresis, ocular bobbing

LABORATORY EVALUATION OF INTRACEREBRAL HEMORRHAGE

Clinical laboratory evaluation in all forms of ICH should be directed toward the differential diagnosis outlined in Table 2. CT should be performed as soon as the diagnosis of ICH is suspected. Hemorrhages as small as 1 cm in diameter can be localized by CT, although small pontine hemorrhages can be missed because of volume averaging or bone artifact. CT localization is extremely useful in terms of guiding further evaluation and management of ICH of any cause. Evidence for associated vascular malformations including aneurysms, AVMs, and venous angiomas should be sought by CT, especially if the hematoma is immediately subcortical or if there is dissection of blood into the subarachnoid space. Frontopolar hematomas are often associated with anterior cerebral artery aneurysms. If the clinical history arouses suspicion of tumor, follow-up contrast-enhanced CT revealing ring enhancement around the hemorrhage provides evidence for hemorrhage into a pre-existing tumor cavity. CT performed 10 to 14 days after the clinical ictus can be confusing, as blood can appear isodense and may go unnoticed as such. Magnetic resonance imaging is superior to CT in identifying late-stage hematomas, posterior fossa lesions, and AVMs. Whenever the cause of ICH is not obvious, cerebral angiography should be performed in patients deemed appropriate surgical candidates.

Lumbar puncture (LP) after an ICH is unnecessary for diagnosis, carries the risk of precipitating herniation or ventricular rupture, and should be avoided. It may be indicated only in those rare cases in which an associated intracranial infection is a possibility.

Many formulas for prognosis in ICH have been developed. Most include the size and location of the hematoma, level of consciousness, and age of the patient. The level of consciousness at the onset of ICH is perhaps the most useful, as most patients presenting in coma have a poor prognosis. This can be important in directing further diagnostic and therapeutic management strategies. Noncoma-tose patients with hematomas less than 3 cm in diameter often make an excellent functional recovery despite an initially severe neurologic deficit.

MANAGEMENT

Guidelines for the management of ICH are similar to those of ischemic stroke and include the establishment of adequate ventilatory support, vascular access (including arterial line placement when indicated), maintenance of adequate cardiac output, and correction of serum glucose and electrolyte disturbances. Initially, patients should have fluid restriction to daily maintenance levels. CT should be performed as soon as possible to distinguish a hemorrhage from an ischemic stroke.

An elevation in blood pressure is a normal response to stroke of any cause. Treatment of malignant hypertension is indicated to minimize the risk of increasing clot size and the development of intracranial edema. However, excessive reduction of blood pressure to normotensive levels or below can prove more harmful than beneficial as autoregulatory function of cerebral vasculature in ICH is often impaired and results in ischemic infarction of the tissue surrounding the hematoma. As a guideline, blood pressure above 180/110 mm Hg should be treated initially. It is suggested that blood pressure be lowered by no more than 25% in the immediate 1 to 2 hours or to a diastolic pressure of 100 to 110 mm Hg. Further reduction to more normotensive levels can be achieved more slowly during the ensuing 2 to 3 days. Antihypertensive agents can be given orally or intravenously. With significant elevations in blood pressure, intravenously administered agents are preferred because they allow more instantaneous and predictable titration of blood pressure (Table 3). Ni-

TABLE 2. **Some Common Causes of Nonhypertensive Intracerebral Hemorrhage**

Iatrogenic (oral anticoagulants)
Amyloid angiography
Vascular anomalies (AVM and aneurysm)
Anticoagulant therapy
Sympathomimetic drugs
Inflammatory or autoimmune arteritis
Thrombocytopenia
Coagulopathy associated with hematogenous tumors
Bleeding into tumor
Sagittal sinus thrombosis

TABLE 3. **Intravenous Antihypertensive Agents**

Sodium nitroprusside (Nipride) (50 mg in 250 mL D5W): Initial dose as 0.5 µg/kg/min; titration not to exceed 10 µg/kg/min

Nitroglycerin (Tridil): Initial dose of 10 µg/min; titration not to exceed 200 µg/min

Labetalol (Trandate): Initial dose of 10 mg; then 20–80 mg every 10 min, not to exceed 300 mg total dose; alternatively, an infusion of 2 mg/min may be used in sustained malignant hypertension

troprusside and nitroglycerin are potent systemic vasodilators and can elevate ICP. Labetalol (Normodyne) thus has theoretical advantages over nitroprusside. Patients already on a regimen of calcium channel blocking agents or angiotensin-converting enzyme inhibitors can be treated urgently with their intravenous equivalents, but experience with these agents has not been well documented in ICH. The use of sublingual agents is discouraged because of the risk of poorly controllable hypotension.

Clinical signs of increased ICP may be due to rebleeding, cerebral edema, hydrocephalus with cerebrospinal fluid outflow obstruction, or combinations of these factors. Repeated CT should be used to discern the interplay of these issues. In the setting of clinical deterioration with impending brain herniation, mannitol (20%) may be given in a dose of 1 gram per kg intravenously as an initial bolus, followed by 20 to 25 grams every 6 hours to keep serum osmolality at approximately 310 mOsm per liter. Dexamethasone (Decadron) is of unproven value in ICH but can be given as an initial 12-mg intravenous bolus followed by 4 to 6 mg every 4 to 6 hours for 48 to 72 hours to reduce vasogenic edema surrounding the intracerebral clot. Intubation with forced hyperventilation to PCO_2 of 25 mm Hg has an immediate effect of reducing ICP by reducing cerebral blood volume. Raised ICP secondary to CSF obstruction should be treated urgently with ventriculostomy.

Seizures can occur in ICH, and phenytoin (Dilantin) given prophylactically is suggested, especially in cortical and lobar hemorrhages. The loading dose is 15 to 20 mg per kg. If phenytoin is given intravenously, it should be mixed in an isotonic solution and administered no faster than 50 mg per minute. Daily maintenance doses vary from 4 to 8 mg per kg to achieve a plasma level of 10 to 20 μg per mL. Fosphenytoin (Cerebyx) offers a convenient alternative to phenytoin as a loading agent as it can be administered more rapidly. The loading dose of 15 to 20 mg of phenytoin per kg can be given at a rate of 150 mg of phenytoin per minute.

Surgical intervention in the management of hypertensive ICH remains controversial, and with the exception of cerebellar hemorrhage, definitive indications do not exist. Surgical removal of hematomas located in lobar sites has been successfully employed in the face of progressive obtundation and impending herniation. However, cerebellar hemorrhages, even if secondary to hypertension, are a special situation in which urgent surgical evacuation of the hematoma can be lifesaving. Patients with cerebellar hematomas less than 2 cm and no evidence of brain stem compression, hydrocephalus, or depressed sensorium can be managed medically, if under close observation. Patients with cerebellar hematomas 3 cm or larger should be immediately assessed for surgical evacuation, especially if there is a depressed level of consciousness, as there can be good functional recovery after hematoma evacuation despite presentation in stupor or coma. ICH associated with amyloid angiopathy can usually be managed medically, but if surgi-

cal intervention is deemed necessary, the need for meticulous hemostasis cannot be overstated.

The general approach to management of nonhypertensive ICH does not differ from that of hypertensive ICH, but a search for the cause becomes more imperative (see Table 2). Patients taking oral anticoagulants can be presumed to have suffered a hemorrhagic intracerebral complication unless other potential causes are evident. Anticoagulants should be discontinued and administration of vitamin K and/or fresh-frozen plasma initiated to restore hemostatic function. Hemorrhage associated with amphetamine or cocaine can be associated with an immune-mediated arteritis, and corticosteroids may be added pending diagnostic angiography to confirm arteritis. When an aneurysm or AVM is the cause of ICH, the timing of surgical intervention depends on the clinical status of the patient and the discretion of the attending neurosurgeon. Surgery to treat AVMs can usually be delayed to later in the clinical course as the risk for early rebleeding is less than that associated with aneurysmal hemorrhage.

ISCHEMIC CEREBROVASCULAR DISEASE

method of
FRANK M. YATSU, M.D.
University of Texas–Houston Medical School
Houston, Texas

Unprecedented claims for the first unequivocal success in treatment of ischemic strokes was reported in 1995. This accomplishment with the use of the thrombolytic agent tissue plasminogen activator (t-PA) (Activase) in a randomized, prospective, double-blind study has fired the interest of stroke investigators and clinicians in treating acute ischemic strokes and also in identifying factors that may predispose to the dreaded complication of intracerebral hemorrhage. Clearly, the use of t-PA is a double-edged sword, but because the prospects of reversing neurologic deficits with ischemic strokes treated early are substantial, a more detailed discussion of this new therapy is provided under the section on therapies. Simultaneous efforts to minimize complications of "reperfusion" and to salvage ischemically vulnerable neurons with "neuroprotective agents" are advancing in parallel to more refined treatment guidelines. These exciting potentials for adjunctive therapies are also discussed in the section on therapies, as are efforts to optimize impaired hemorheologic factors.

Although the dramatic benefits from t-PA have revolutionized the conceptual thinking about stroke therapy, the unfortunate reality is that the majority of patients seen with ischemic strokes do not qualify for t-PA because of exclusionary criteria. For this reason, this chapter reviews the important epidemiologic factors related to ischemic strokes and their differential diagnosis, diagnostic workup, and therapeutic options for each, both acutely and for preventive measures. Up to a quarter of acute ischemic strokes may be so devastating as to be lethal, and no aggressive management strategies are warranted in such cases.

EPIDEMIOLOGY

Stroke is a generic term referring to the acute or subacute onset of neurologic deficits that can be explained by either vascular occlusion (the focus of this chapter) or vascular rupture. Despite their declining incidence, strokes remain the major neurologic disorder in America and are the third major cause of death and disability. The annual costs, both direct and indirect, of strokes in the United States are considerably more than $20 billion annually. The risk factors for atherosclerosis, the primary cause of strokes, are similar to those for coronary artery disease and include hypertension, cigarette smoking, diabetes mellitus, elevated lipid levels, excess alcohol intake, and perhaps obesity, a sedentary life, and stress. Intervention in patients with these risk factors must be undertaken to reduce stroke incidences. Although elevated cholesterol levels had for some time been thought not to be an important factor causing atherosclerotic strokes, increasing evidence shows a strong relationship. In fact, recent studies on cholesterol lowering using the 3-hydroxy-3-methylglutaryl coenzyme A reductase inhibitors, such as pravastatin (Pravachol), in patients with moderately elevated serum cholesterol levels, principally in the form of low-density lipoprotein, showed a reduction in coronary artery disease end points but also in the incidence of strokes.

STROKE CLASSIFICATION

A number of classifications exist for strokes, but a practical one is to divide them initially into the two major types: (1) ischemic strokes and (2) hemorrhagic strokes, as determined by neuroimaging studies of the brain (Table 1). Each category is divided into subcategories. The importance of the classification is in providing a reference point for the differential diagnosis of strokes. It remains axiomatic in medicine that unless an entity is thought of, it will not be diagnosed.

A detailed discussion of the differential diagnosis of ischemic strokes is beyond the scope of this article, but the history, examination, and initial screening laboratory studies, including neuroimaging and noninvasive vascular studies, should provide clues to the most likely cause of the stroke syndrome. For example, patients younger than 50 years would have a higher risk of cardioembolic strokes and of the miscellaneous causes noted in Table 1 such as the antiphospholipid syndrome, both suggested by screening tests.

COMMON STROKE SYNDROMES, THEIR TREATMENT, AND USE OF TISSUE PLASMINOGEN ACTIVATOR

Transient Ischemic Attacks

The term "transient ischemic attack" (TIA) is a fixture in medical nomenclature, but it does not precisely explain the pathophysiologic events in all patients presenting with temporary neurologic deficits such as the common symptoms hemiparesis, aphasia, and slurred speech. TIAs refer to these symptoms lasting typically for a matter of minutes to perhaps hours. Although the majority of such transient symptoms in elderly patients are likely due to extracranial atherosclerotic disease, or even cardiogenic emboli, the differential diagnoses in Table 1 should be considered, particularly in younger patients. For example,

TABLE 1. **Stroke Classification**

I. Ischemic strokes
  A. Atherothrombotic brain infarction (ABI) or thrombotic strokes (ABI is a continuum, from TIAs to progressing and completed strokes)
  B. Cardioembolic stroke
    1. Arrhythmias: atrial fibrillation but also sick sinus syndrome
    2. Valvular abnormalities, e.g., mitral valve prolapse; prosthetic valves; bacterial endocarditis; nonbacterial thrombotic endocarditis due to occult cancer; mitral annulus calcification; subaortic stenosis
    3. Cardiomyopathies: after myocardial infarction and cardiomyopathies
    4. Anatomic or neoplastic, e.g., patent foramen ovale, atrial myxoma
  C. Lacunar syndromes (These refer to small cystic areas of brain infarction corresponding to arteriole occlusion frequently due to long-standing hypertension and have typical symptoms)
  D. Miscellaneous causes
    1. Arterial abnormalities other than atherosclerosis, e.g., the arteritides, migraine, dissection, moyamoya syndrome, fibromuscular dysplasia
    2. Venous (cortical) diseases with thrombosis: hypercoagulable states and postpartum women; use of both anticoagulation and thrombolytic agents should be considered
    3. Erythrocytes: polycythemia vera and sickle cell anemia
    4. Platelets: thrombocytosis, especially for counts $>10^6/mm^3$
    5. Serum proteins, e.g., antiphospholipid antibodies (lupus anticoagulant, anticardiolipin antibodies), protein C and S and antithrombin III deficiencies, macroglobulins, homocyst(e)inemia
II. Hemorrhagic strokes
  A. Subarachnoid hemorrhages
  B. Intracerebral hemorrhages

Abbreviation: TIA = transient ischemic attack.

transient symptoms may occur from metabolic disorders involving hepatic, renal, or calcium metabolism, as well as seizures with or without brain mass lesions. All of these latter considerations are not common, but the setting of the patient provides clues for these unusual causes. For example, in a patient with known migraine who during an attack develops focal neurologic signs such as hemiparesis or unilateral blurring of vision, the cause is most likely vasospasm. The concern with extracranial stenosis causing TIAs is that they are a harbinger for subsequent fixed strokes.

Surgical Treatment of Transient Ischemic Attacks

For the largest group of patients with TIAs with significant extracranial occlusive disease, the best treatment of stenosis greater than 70% is carotid endarterectomy by experienced surgeons. Three randomized prospective studies from North America and Europe published in 1991 attest to the effectiveness of this approach. For stenoses between 30 and 69%, studies are continuing to enroll patients to determine whether surgery or the best medical therapy, such as antiplatelet agents (e.g., aspirin), is superior. It is likely on the basis of extrapolating available data that the conclusions will be that neither form of treatment is superior; however, certain patients, such as those with a contralateral occluded carotid artery or those with increased risk factors, such as hypertension or diabetes, may benefit from surgery.

A related issue is performing carotid endarterectomy on subjects with asymptomatic carotid bifurcation stenosis of greater than 70%. A prospective randomized study in the United States showed a slight reduction in stroke occurrence in those receiving surgery, but this hotly debated issue suggests that physicians considering surgery should seek consensus within their practice group. As criteria are refined in this group of patients, likely those in the greatest danger of strokes and therefore likely to benefit will be patients with the previously noted risk factors or contralateral carotid artery occlusion.

Medical Treatment of Transient Ischemic Attacks

In patients who do not qualify for surgery as noted previously and who have TIAs due to extracranial occlusive disease, antiplatelet agents such as aspirin reduce stroke occurrence. Authorities on this subject disagree on the proper dosing of aspirin, but one 350-mg aspirin tablet per day is a reasonable starting dose. If symptoms continue, the dose can be increased. The use of four 325-mg aspirin tablets is associated with an increased incidence of gastrointestinal symptoms. Although this is debated, some authorities recommend adding dipyridamole (Persantine), 75 mg three times daily, to aspirin, and others recommend adding pentoxifylline (Trental),* 400 mg three times daily, to aspirin to optimize hemorheologic characteristics and minimize strokes.

For aspirin failures, that is, if TIAs continue or increase in frequency, so-called crescendo TIAs, carotid endarterectomy should be considered in surgical candidates.

Treatment of Completed Strokes

Completed strokes are by far the most common ischemic stroke encountered, and the degree of disability determines acute and chronic therapeutic approaches. Acutely, for moderately severe strokes, patients are optimally managed in an intensive care or stroke care unit for monitoring of cardiac and pulmonary status, because many of these patients have other medical problems, particularly cardiopulmonary disease. If viable recovery is reasonable, decisions to be aggressive with the use of intracranial pressure monitoring and the use of dehydrating agents, such as mannitol, require consultation with intensivists experienced in these problems. Furthermore, consideration must be given to other neurologic complications such as seizures and to medically related issues, including bladder, bowel, renal, hepatic, skin, joint, psychiatric, and other considerations. Complications from fluid and electrolyte imbalances must, of course, be watched for assiduously. Physio-

TABLE 2. **Thrombolysis (Tissue Plasminogen Activator) in Acute Ischemic Strokes**

Acute ischemic stroke
↓
Duration: ≤3 h from onset
↓
CT of brain: no hemorrhage or clear infarction
↓
Laboratory studies: Hct, platelets, PT and PTT
↓
If above negative or normal, use IV t-PA therapy
↓
Dosing of t-PA: 0.9 mg/kg; 10% in 1 min, remaining t-PA in 60 min
↓
Hourly neurologic examinations × 6, then every 2 h for first 24 h
↓
Repeat CT and blood studies at day 2

Abbreviations: CT = computed tomography; Hct = hematocrit; PT = prothrombin time; PTT = partial thromboplastin time; t-PA = tissue plasminogen activator.
Data from The National Institute of Neurological Disorders and Stroke rt-PA Stroke Study Group: Tissue plasminogen activator for acute ischemic stroke. N Engl J Med 333:1581–1587, 1995.

therapy and occupational therapy should be started as soon as possible to maximize recovery and minimize complications such as contractures. Depression is a frequent complication of strokes, because of both the reality of the disability and the occurrence of a "chemical imbalance" in the brain that causes endogenous depression. Antidepressants can be effective, particularly selective serotonin reuptake inhibitors.

For patients with moderate deficits that are not life-threatening, considerations for the prevention of stroke recurrence relate to whether the cause is cardiogenic or atherothrombotic disease. With a cardiogenic cause, such as atrial fibrillation, patients younger than 75 years should optimally have anticoagulation with an International Normalized Ratio of between 2.0 and 3.0. However, patients should not have anticoagulation in the acute period, and computed tomography (CT) of the brain should not show hemorrhage. For those older than 75 years, aspirin may be as beneficial because of the greater degree of hemorrhagic complications with anticoagulation in these patients. In patients with atherothrombotic strokes with moderate deficits, acute therapeutic considerations include efforts acutely to improve circulation to the ischemic "penumbra" or shadow where decreased blood flow threatens to cause infarction.

Treatment of Completed Strokes with Tissue Plasminogen Activator* and Adjunctive Therapies

For patients who qualify for t-PA therapy intravenously, the physician must abide by the criteria published in the December 1995 issue of the *New England Journal of Medicine,* as shown in Table 2, and subsequently approved by the Food and Drug Admin-

*Not FDA approved for this indication.

*Not FDA approved for this indication.

istration as an accepted guideline for ischemic stroke therapy.

Clinicians interested in using t-PA should consult experienced individuals who have used the drug. Experience and caution are perhaps the most important attributes to have when using t-PA, because violations of the protocol may have disastrous consequences, particularly intracerebral hemorrhage. For example, it is crucial to appreciate subtle changes of brain infarction such as effacement of brain sulci or signal attenuation at CT as exclusionary criteria.

The use of other thrombolytic agents such as streptokinase or urokinase is either not successful or is of unproven effectiveness. Whether direct intrathrombal injection of thrombolytic agents through an arterial catheter is successful is yet unproved; this form of therapy may prove to be the best approach for clot dissolution, but the time delay, a critical element in determining success, may be a limiting factor for its success. Adding heparin after completion of thrombolytic therapy, as is done with cardiac cases, is not yet agreed on because the danger of hemorrhage is increased.

As noted previously, no definitive acute ischemic stroke therapy other than t-PA is available, and therefore efforts to optimize recovery remain uncertain but worth considering until proved effective or otherwise. Currently available treatment strategies focus on efforts to (1) minimize hypercoagulability, (2) offer neuroprotective therapies, and (3) improve hemorheologic characteristics to allow greater perfusion of ischemic areas. For the first goal, aspirin, unless contraindicated, is warranted because platelet hyperaggregability is present. For the second goal, a number of agents are being studied, but none has been proved definitively beneficial, with perhaps the exception of nimodipine to prevent calcium entry into neurons, provided hypotension is avoided. Finally, for the third goal, the use of agents such as pentoxifylline* to reduce viscosity is worth considering, although proven benefits are short term. A number of clinical studies are addressing each of these areas of therapy of acute ischemic strokes, and their results are awaited with great expectation.

For subacute and chronic considerations for patients with moderate strokes due to atherothrombosis, minimizing the risk factors discussed previously is critical. Accomplishing this task successfully requires the direct involvement and participation of the patient's caring physician. Whether chronic anticoagulation or aspirin will reduce stroke recurrence in these at-risk patients will be elucidated in a large, ongoing prospective study in the United States.

Diagnostic Studies for Ischemic Strokes

In addition to CT and magnetic resonance imaging of the brain to help elucidate the cause and character of the stroke syndrome, other studies help with both

diagnosis and management. These include the previously noted noninvasive tests for carotid stenosis, such as the duplex scanner, and transcranial Doppler study for intracerebral arterial abnormality, which may also provide information on whether emboli are being showered to the brain by identifying events termed high-intensity transient signals. Magnetic resonance angiography (MRA) is becoming more successful in identifying arterial and venous abnormalities, both extra- and intracranially, such as dissection, moyamoya syndrome, arteritis, venous sinus thrombosis, and, of course, atherosclerotic lesions. MRA is especially successful when two- and three-dimensional time-of-flight techniques are used to minimize the signals from turbulence, which may give false-positive images for stenosis.

Single photon emission computed tomography (SPECT) is helpful in identifying the pattern of cerebral blood flow in ischemic stroke patients. SPECT is particularly useful in selecting patients with TIAs or minimal persisting neurologic deficits who are good risks for carotid endarterectomy; this is determined by assessing cerebrovascular reserve demonstrated by an increase in cerebral blood flow in response to acetazolamide (Diamox), which provokes vasodilatation. A lack of vascular reserve would increase the risk for hemorrhage or brain infarction. In the future, functional magnetic resonance imaging should provide similar information.

When indicated, transthoracic and transesophageal echocardiography should be used to identify potential causes of cardiogenic or aortogenic emboli. Only these studies can identify with certainty patent foramen ovale and mitral valve prolapse with redundancy or valve thickening, which are prone to cause thromboembolism.

REHABILITATION OF THE STROKE PATIENT

method of
ELLIOT J. ROTH, M.D.
*Northwestern University Medical School and
Rehabilitation Institute of Chicago
Chicago, Illinois*

BACKGROUND

In addition to being the third most common cause of death in the United States, stroke is the leading cause of severe disability. The consequences of stroke can range from minimal and minor to extensive and severe. Rehabilitation efforts are instituted to reduce the impact of the stroke and its consequences on the patient's functioning. In this way, rehabilitation attempts to enhance quality of life. The goals of rehabilitation, as outlined by Roth, are to (1) prevent, recognize, and manage co-morbid medical illnesses and secondary intercurrent medical complications; (2) provide training in skills to maximize functional independence; (3) facilitate optimal psychosocial coping and adaptation by the patient and family; (4) promote

---

*Not FDA approved for this indication.

reintegration into family, home, work, leisure, and community activities, and also resumption of prior life roles; and (5) enhance the quality of life for stroke survivors.

Although training to improve the ability to perform activities of daily living (ADLs) constitutes a major portion of the rehabilitation effort, other interventions are also important. A partial list of these other activities includes teaching the patient and family about stroke, its consequences, preventive techniques, and strategies to prevent secondary problems; psychologic support and counseling for the patient and family; facilitation of a smooth transition to the postdischarge environment through training, planning, and recruiting community resources; and medical management of actual and potential comorbidities.

To understand the real and potential impact of stroke and rehabilitation on the patient's functioning, it is helpful to understand the Model of Disablement according to the World Health Organization. In this classification system, *pathologic* problems are the changes in the brain caused by the stroke; *impairment* describes the specific neurologic deficits that result from the pathologic dysfunction; *disability* is the impact of these problems on a person's ability to perform ADLs; and *handicap* or *societal limitation* refers to changes in the ability of the individual to perform activities in a social context. Traditional rehabilitation efforts are not thought of as affecting pathologic problems, and the impact of rehabilitation efforts on impairment are thought to be minimal (if any); it is the focus of most rehabilitation interventions to reduce the disability and, to a somewhat lesser extent, the handicap or societal limitations.

Variations exist across strokes and across individuals with stroke in the specific types, patterns, combinations, and severity levels of neurologic deficits, and in the extent to which neurologic recovery reduces the level or extent of each impairment type. Although any of a number of clinical manifestations may occur after stroke, the most common impairment is loss of voluntary motor control, with hemiparesis or hemiplegia. Other neurologic deficits may occur in the areas of consciousness and alertness, cognition (problems in attention; concentration; orientation; memory; and executive functions such as judgment, abstract reasoning, and problem solving), motor planning (apraxias), language (aphasias), behavior (impulsivity), mood (e.g., depression, anxiety), visual fields (hemianopia), visuospatial perception (e.g., unilateral hemineglect, agnosias), cranial nerve function (e.g., facial palsy, extraocular muscle palsy), speech production (dysarthria), swallowing (dysphagia), muscle tone and motor control (spasticity, rigidity, synergy patterns), balance (ataxia), motor coordination, sensation, bladder and bowel continence, endurance, and tolerance (e.g., fatigue, deconditioning). Although it is difficult to determine with accuracy the frequency with which patients with stroke experience impairments, it is estimated that more than 50% have some form of neurologic deficit.

It is important to note that reduction of impairment through spontaneous natural recovery of neurologic functioning is common after stroke. Most patients with stroke experience some degree of improvement in one or more of the neurologic deficits that stroke causes. The amount of impairment reduction that occurs after stroke is variable, but one way to evaluate the effect of poststroke natural recovery is to compare the frequencies of each of the neurologic deficits between the early and late poststroke stages. For example, the prevalence of hemiparesis has been reported to decline from nearly 75% during the initial presentation to about 33% at 1-year follow-up, aphasia from 33

to 20%, and dysarthria from about 50 to about 15%. Most (but not all) improvement in physical functioning occurs within the first 3 to 6 months.

When it exists, natural recovery occurs in a relatively stereotyped predictable pattern in most (but not all) patients. For example, in about 75% of patients with stroke-induced spastic hemiparesis, motor recovery tends to evolve through a series of stages from complete flaccid hemiplegia to increasing tone and spasticity, emergence of synergy patterns in extremity movement, and finally gradually increasing isolated voluntary movement of the muscles in the weak extremity. Common patterns are also seen by which language, perception, cognition, and other neurologic functions improve.

The mechanisms by which natural recovery of neurologic functioning occurs after stroke are of substantial interest to both clinicians and investigators. The first group of mechanisms, accounting for early (within the first 3 to 6 months) poststroke recovery, is through the resolution of local harmful factors, such as reduction of cerebral edema, reabsorption of local toxins, improvement of local circulation, and recovery of partially damaged ischemic neurons. The second proposed group of mechanisms, which can occur early or late, is neuroplasticity, or the ability of the brain to modify its structural and functional organization in response to injury. Although a variety of forms of plasticity have been proposed, the two most plausible include collateral sprouting of new neuronal synaptic connections and unmasking of previously latent functional neuronal pathways. Both these mechanisms may be stimulated by injury or by environmental influences such as those that occur during rehabilitation interventions, although these interactions are controversial.

Impairment reduction is not the only type of recovery that occurs after stroke. The major focus of poststroke rehabilitation is on the improvement in the disability level. Although an individual's ability to perform daily functional tasks is thought to be largely dependent on, and often limited by, the type, severity, and pattern of neurologic deficit, it is important to note that disability is related to impairment in subtle and complex ways. Several factors other than the neurologic deficit are often relevant in the ultimate determination of the functional outcome. Some of these other factors that might influence disability level include the motivation level; ability to learn; type and amount of rehabilitation and training; level of emotional and social support; coping and adaptation ability; and number, severity, and impact of co-morbid medical conditions.

Estimates of the frequencies of the various types and severity levels of disabilities after stroke vary, but studies suggest that about 67% of stroke patients are unable to feed, dress, groom, or toilet themselves independently, and that 75% are unable to walk independently in the acute phase after stroke onset. It is important to note that extensive clinical observation and many formal reports have indicated that the figures reflecting the frequencies of various disability types tend to improve over time. For example, dependence on others at 6 months after stroke declines to about 33% for feeding and dressing skills, to about 10% for grooming, to about 20% for toileting, and to about 15% for walking.

Although the extent to which rehabilitation has contributed to this rather consistent finding of disability reduction has been questioned, several clinical trials and considerable clinical experience have supported the concept that rehabilitation improves functional performance levels over and above the amount that might be expected by natural neurologic recovery alone.

MEDICAL CO-MORBIDITIES

Not all the factors that affect the stroke patient's ability to function are direct physical consequences of the stroke. Among the more important impediments to successful rehabilitation and functional independence are the pre-existing medical conditions and the secondary intercurrent medical complications that are common among stroke survivors. The institution of preventive techniques to reduce the incidence and impact of these co-morbid medical conditions is likely to help to enhance functional performance.

One of these complications, venous thromboembolic phenomena, has an estimated frequency of 25 to 75% for deep venous thrombosis and about 10% for pulmonary embolism. Various pharmacologic measures (especially standard and low-molecular-weight heparin) have been found to be beneficial in preventing these events. Physical measures have not been found to be as effective in preventing these problems, but investigation into their efficacy continues. Pneumonias occur in about 33% of stroke patients, largely due to the high frequency with which dysphagia and aspiration accompanies stroke. Evaluation of swallowing function, establishment of alternative feeding routes when needed, and institution of swallowing therapy are useful measures. Initiation of a feeding regimen, whether it is oral, nonoral enteral, or parenteral, helps to reduce the likelihood of malnutrition, which appears to be a fairly common complication of stroke. Bladder and bowel dysfunction can usually be managed with regulation of fluid and diet, medications, and implementation of a timed scheduled toileting program. Although pressure sores are fairly common in stroke patients, these can be prevented with proper positioning techniques. Falls, which are also common in stroke survivors, can be prevented through functional training, supervision, and environmental modifications.

Probably one of the most common complications of stroke is shoulder dysfunction, which can consist of pain, subluxation, or both, occurring in about 70 to 80% of stroke survivors. Although reflex sympathetic dystrophy syndrome (shoulder-hand syndrome) occurs with some frequency, the more common problem causing shoulder dysfunction is the set of musculoskeletal conditions that arise from local factors, such as tendinitis, bursitis, spasticity (which by itself can cause pain or subluxation in some patients), and altered muscle-tendon mechanics; these altered mechanics may result from the weakness and spasticity from the stroke, or from inappropriate positioning or handling of the patient after the stroke. Proper positioning, training in proper transfer and movement techniques, range-of-motion exercise, splinting, and medications help to prevent and treat these common problems.

REHABILITATION DURING THE INITIAL PHASE

Consideration of rehabilitation as an integral part of *all* medical management, instead of as a distinctly separate phase of care, facilitates the inclusion by stroke care professionals of rehabilitation intervention in the early poststroke stage. This is important, because it has been suggested by both clinical experience and a few clinical studies that stroke patients' outcomes can be enhanced by the implementation of rehabilitation practices as soon as it is medically feasible after stabilization, ideally within the first day or two after the onset of stroke. Many of the problems that impede rehabilitation efforts in the later stages derive from the deconditioning that occurs early after the stroke, resulting from the stroke itself, from co-morbid medical conditions, or from the institution of prolonged forced bed rest during treatment of the acute stroke. This is a preventable problem.

Stroke patients should be encouraged to regain as much mobility and independence as possible as early as possible to prevent certain complications (such as venous thromboembolism, pneumonias, pressure sores, soft tissue and joint contractures, constipation, and depression) and to provide opportunities to practice skills that will be important later. Specific early poststroke interventions might include aggressive range-of-motion stretching exercises and frequent position changes, placement of the patient in the upright position to improve orthostatic tolerance, psychologic counseling, education of the patient and family, training and encouragment of independence in the performance of personal care skills, mobility and ambulation training, and bladder and bowel management. Early evaluation of swallowing function enables clinicians to initiate some form of feeding, either through the normal route or by an alternative means, and to begin training in swallowing techniques. Provision of appropriate nutrition and hydration can help to prevent infection, fluid and electrolyte problems, and the fatigue that often accompanies stroke. Early identification of depression facilitates appropriate treatment, which may help to improve motivation and thereby favorably influence the outcome. The ultimate goal of these interventions is to facilitate an easy transition to the formal rehabilitation program or the next poststroke stage, and in that way to improve long-term functional and psychosocial outcomes.

LEVELS OF REHABILITATION CARE

A variety of levels and types of rehabilitation and postacute services now exist, allowing professionals to select from a "menu" of choices of settings to enable them to more directly meet the stroke patient's specific needs at the time. Because these needs evolve, an ideal complete *system* of care provides not only the services at each of the several levels along the continuum of care, but also a systematic method of assessment, follow-up, and transfer between levels. Full integration of the system requires communication and collaboration among all elements of the system to facilitate the easy and smooth transfer of patients, flow of information, and sharing of expertise across the various levels of care.

Comprehensive acute inpatient stroke rehabilitation is the traditional interdisciplinary team-facilitated physician-directed program of care conducted in a coordinated fashion on an inpatient unit. This level of care is most appropriate for patients who require and can tolerate 3 hours or more of therapy per day, and who require both 24-hour-a-day nursing care and at least daily physician supervision.

Subacute inpatient rehabilitation, on the other hand, is appropriate for patients who require or can tolerate a less intensive therapy schedule, but who still need a comprehensive and coordinated therapy program for functional training. One to 3 hours of therapy each day is typical. Most commonly conducted in skilled nursing facility environments, the level of intensity of nursing and medical needs is usually less in subacute inpatient rehabilitation than it is in intensive rehabilitation, although around-the-clock nursing care is available and periodic physician supervision is required.

Relatively new in the continuum of postacute care for stroke survivors is "day rehabilitation," a comprehensive coordinated program of outpatient therapy services designed to enhance functional status. For patients who do not require an inpatient stay, but who can benefit from all the therapy services provided during acute inpatient rehabilitation, day rehabilitation fulfills their needs in what is often a more comfortable environment (outpatient facility) and cost-efficient manner.

Two other levels of postacute care are commonly used for stroke survivors. Traditional outpatient therapy is appropriate for stroke patients who require single therapy services to meet specific focused objectives on an outpatient basis, but not necessarily in as coordinated or comprehensive or extensive a fashion as the group who benefits from day rehabilitation. Other patients derive substantial benefit from home therapy services, because the home is the environment that is most familiar to the patient and family, and therapy in the home allows the patient and family to learn specific functional tasks in the setting in which those skills will be applied most frequently.

All the main principles of rehabilitation, including those directed toward improving function, preventing complications, facilitating psychosocial adaptation, promoting community reintegration, and enhancing the quality of life, can be applied in any setting. Factors that may be useful to the clinician in the determination of the ideal setting and level of rehabilitation for an individual patient include the rehabilitation potential (based on the patient's cognitive functioning, ability to learn, motivation, prior and present level of functioning, degree of medical stability, physical endurance to participate actively in the therapeutic exercise program, and likelihood of achieving functional gains during rehabilitation), level of available social and financial resources, medical and nursing needs, and availability of appropriate resources in the community.

REHABILITATION PRINCIPLES

The variety of stroke presentations and recovery patterns, and the diversity with which stroke patients present and respond to their disabilities, make it necessary to individualize the rehabilitation management program for each patient. However, several common themes and a few general principles of rehabilitation that are applicable to a variety of problems in a number of situations can be enumerated.

Probably the most important distinguishing feature of rehabilitation is its reliance on a team approach to care. The multiplicity and complexity of problems with which the stroke patient presents demand that evaluation and treatment of stroke patients be comprehensive and holistic. Therefore, the adoption of a coordinated approach that calls for the care to be provided by an interdisciplinary team of experienced rehabilitation professionals working collaboratively seems the most rational method. It is critical that the activities be coordinated and not fragmented or duplicative, and it is helpful when skills developed in one specific functional area are used to facilitate the achievement of favorable outcomes in other specific areas. A rehabilitation team conference helps to facilitate communication, monitoring of the patient's progress, and treatment planning.

Because the central focus of rehabilitation includes the facilitation of learning and adaptation, a rehabilitation setting can be thought of as a "school" as much as it is a hospital or health care environment. For patients to reacquire skills or learn ways to compensate for new deficits in a logical coherent manner, it is necessary to apply principles of learning theory to the conduct of the rehabilitation program. This means that skills training is performed using graded levels of task difficulty. The opportunities for repetition of skill performance and for supervision are emphasized, as are the provision of immediate feedback and guidance from professionals to the patient on task performance, and the creation of an environment that fosters "protected practice." In this way, the rehabilitation program encourages and facilitates progress.

Another important feature of rehabilitation is its goal-directed nature. The focus of the treatment is on specific functional and behavioral goals that specifically address the patient's particular needs. The goals, and therefore the rehabilitation activities, must be practical, realistic, and mutually agreed on by the patient, family, and treatment team.

REHABILITATION INTERVENTIONS

Although environmental influences such as rehabilitation interventions may have some limited effect on reducing the frequency and severity of stroke-induced impairments, the effectiveness of such so-called remediational interventions on stroke-related neurologic deficits such as weakness is controversial. The major focus of rehabilitation efforts is on reducing the type and level of disability experienced by the patient, primarily through training in what have been called "compensatory" activities. The goal of compensatory training is to improve the ability of the patient to carry out a functional task in the presence of the neurologic impairment. Specific therapeutic interventions that are used to enhance functional performance include skills training, demonstration, provision of opportunity for practice, provision of feedback on skill performance, therapeutic exercises (passive, strengthening, endurance, functional), physical modalities, prescription of adaptive equipment, education, behavioral techniques, and supportive counseling. Medications and surgical techniques can also be used.

The most common (but not the only) focus of the stroke rehabilitation program is the functional loss caused by motor deficits resulting from the stroke. The degree of weakness is usually less pronounced in the lower extremity than in the upper extremity, and the therapy interventions are usually more successful in restoring mobility and ambulation than in improving the level of independence for upper limb self-care activities. Therapeutic exercise programs consist of positioning, passive and active range-of-motion exercises to prevent contracture and reduce tone, progressive resistance exercises to improve strength, and fitness training. Functional training in the performance of personal care skills, mobility activities, and instrumental ADLs form the main focus of most rehabilitation efforts. An example of compensatory skills training is teaching the patient one-handed techniques for feeding, dressing, bathing, and toileting. Another example is helping the patient to learn to walk independently with a spastic hemiplegic lower extremity. Instrumental ADL training occurs by practicing skills in a home or community setting, such as practice in housekeeping, laundering, or shopping. The emphasis of all the functional training is on specific *practical* skills that will be needed by the patient in the home or community environment after discharge.

A number of neuromuscular facilitation exercise approaches have been developed to improve motor control, symmetry, and balance in stroke patients, but no single approach has been documented as superior for the treatment of stroke-related deficits. The most common clinical practice is to incorporate elements of the various methods. Several newer techniques have been under development in the treatment of stroke-related deficits. Biofeedback, a technologic method used to provide external signals to the patient to increase awareness of his or her level of motor control, has had variably successful results in selected patients, as has the use of neuromuscular electrical stimulation. "Forced use" treatment, in which the patient is restricted from using the more functional limb to force the use of the hemiplegic limb, has also been found to be variably successful in selected patients. Treatment of spasticity, which can complicate stroke, includes proper positioning, therapeutic exercise, medications, casting, orthotic use, motor point or peripheral nerve injections of blocking agents, and surgical releases.

Although weakness and motor control problems are the most prominent deficits that result from stroke, they are not the only problems that stroke patients experience. For some patients, visuospatial perceptual deficits, including unilateral hemispatial neglect, right-left disorientation, and the various agnosias, have the greatest adverse impact on functioning of all the various impairment types. Treatment methods include increasing the patient's own awareness of deficits, providing visuospatial cues to compensate for perceptual losses, prism glasses, and computer-assisted training.

Aphasia, which occurs in about one third of stroke survivors, can be a severely disabling problem for certain stroke patients. Treatment of aphasia focuses on determining and utilizing the most effective means by which the patient can communicate, which might take place in individual supervised practice or group speech therapy and could include encouragement of verbalizations, conversational coaching, oral reading, melodic intonation therapy (which relies on available "musical" neural pathways to facilitate communication), teaching of compensatory strategies, encouragement of the use of gestures and sign language, and augmentative communication devices.

Depression and other emotional problems occur in a significant proportion of stroke survivors and have been found to both inhibit rehabilitation efforts and limit functional outcomes. These problems may be endogenous, resulting directly on an organic basis from the stroke itself, or reactive, in relation to the recent disability and dependence, or both. Treatment approaches for depression are varied and consist of peer and professional counseling through psychotherapy and/or the supportive rehabilitation environment, and medications. For some patients, the reduction of impairment and disability alone that occurs during the recovery phase helps to resolve the depression. For certain patients, treatment of the depression, by psychotherapy or by medication, helps to improve functional outcomes.

Even in the absence of serious depression, attention to psychosocial issues is critical because the motivation level and coping ability play extremely important roles in the participation of the patient in the treatment program and in the ultimate achievement of favorable outcomes.

An important aspect of rehabilitation is its attention to the quality of life and community issues that extend beyond traditional medical interventions. In this capacity, the rehabilitation treatment team works with the stroke survivor to address the return to as many community activities as possible in which the patient was previously involved; some of these include sexuality, spirituality, driving a vehicle, employment, education, and recreation.

One of the distinguishing characteristics of rehabilitation is its emphasis on family involvement; families are considered members of the rehabilitation team. In addition to didactic education and counseling, helping to prepare family members for their roles in planning and providing for the future care of the patient is a critical element of the rehabilitation process. Examples of components of a family education program include stroke and its consequences;

medications, their uses and side effects; medical complications, their prevention and recognition; safety training and injury prevention; swallowing training; maintenance of nutrition and hydration; methods of management of bladder catheters, feeding tubes, and respiratory equipment; training in the performance of specific functional skills for which the patient needs assistance (e.g., transfers, toileting, dressing); and a home exercise program.

Adaptive equipment can be used to help the patient achieve certain specific goals, usually to facilitate the achievement of maximal functional independence. Examples of adaptive devices that enable the patient to perform personal care activities independently include "built-up" eating utensils; grooming and bathing aids; dressing devices; and toilet, tub, and shower equipment. Resting hand splints help to maintain the hand and wrist in an ideal position for function and to prevent contracture.

Providing assistive devices for walking, such as canes or walkers, means the difference between walking and wheelchair use for many patients. Providing transfer aids and well-fitted wheelchairs may mean the difference between bed rest and assuming the upright position. Factors to consider when selecting and fitting a wheelchair for a patient include body size and habitus, posture and the ability to maintain the upright position independently, and an optimal method for locomotion (e.g., one-arm-drive manual, electric power operated). Advances in wheelchair design have greatly enhanced the ability of the rehabilitation professional to customize the wheelchair to meet the patient's specific needs. Ankle-foot orthoses are often used to improve the position of the foot in standing and walking, as a means of facilitating an optimal gait pattern. This improves the appearance, comfort, endurance, and quality of performance of gait. Technologic advances have facilitated the development of specially adapted and electronically operated devices to facilitate communication (for those with speech or language dysfunction) and environmental control (for those with motor dysfunction). One of the critical concepts with regard to all these equipment types—whether "high-tech" or "low-tech"—is the importance of training the patient and/or family in the proper use of these devices.

PERSPECTIVE

Rehabilitation is as much a philosophy or approach to care as it is a set of specific clinical activities to perform. This means that rehabilitation principles can be applied at any level or any location of care, and at virtually any time during the poststroke course of care. It also means that activities that extend beyond the traditional therapeutic exercise program are considered rehabilitation interventions; some of these activities include psychologic counseling education of the patient and family, and discharge planning. The recent Post-Stroke Rehabilitation Clinical Practice Guideline published by the U.S. Agency for Health Care Policy and Research outlined

several important principles of stroke rehabilitation. These universal principles confirm and support those that have been enumerated in this discussion.

It is important that the approach to care be holistic and carried out by an interdisciplinary team of professionals that establishes realistic and mutually agreed on goals and provides treatment in accordance with a carefully developed rehabilitation management plan designed to meet patients' specific needs. A critical but often overlooked set of interventions are the methods to prevent recurrent stroke, venous thromboembolism, pneumonia, contracture, and pressure sores, and also those measures that address functional health issues, such as bowel, bladder, skin, and nutrition problems. Initiating the rehabilitation training early by mobilizing the patient and encouraging the resumption of self-care activities as soon as possible is also important. The main emphasis of most stroke rehabilitation programs is to provide compensatory training for sensorimotor deficits, and to evaluate and manage communicative and cognitive-perceptual disorders. This can be done in a variety of levels, types, and settings of rehabilitation. The involvement of the patient and family in the process is essential, as is reliance on principles derived from learning theory. Addressing psychologic problems and facilitating a smooth transition to the community by appropriate discharge planning, family teaching, and securing community resources may facilitate the achievement of favorable long-term outcomes.

SEIZURES AND EPILEPSIES IN ADOLESCENTS AND ADULTS

method of
ANTONIO V. DELGADO-ESCUETA, M.D.
*UCLA and West Los Angeles VA Medical Center
Los Angeles, California*

A team approach is vital to the successful management of epilepsy. The social stigma of epilepsy and its dire consequences to the emotional state and quality of life of the patient can sometimes be worse than the seizures themselves. Thus, the primary care physician in charge should manage and coordinate the efforts of specialists, including neurologic, pharmacologic, psychologic, psychiatric, and social service professionals, and should foster understanding among the patient's family, employers, and school personnel.

The team approach should (1) verify that seizures are epileptic in nature; (2) define seizure types and the epilepsy syndrome; (3) prove the likely cause of epileptic seizures and stop trigger factors; (4) establish an early treatment plan with appropriate antiepileptic drugs; (5) monitor seizure control, recognize adverse effects on the patient's quality of life, and plan future discontinuation of antiepileptic drugs when complete suppression of seizures is achieved; and (6) evaluate for possible surgical treatment, if seizures are resistant to antiepileptic drugs.

The term "epilepsy" is derived from a Greek word meaning a condition of being overcome or seized. The term is used to describe the brain's innate ability to produce paroxysmal depolarization shifts within neurons and recurrent electroencephalographic discharges such as focal spikes or diffuse bilateral 1.5- to 6-Hz spike-and-wave complexes. Clinically, a person's consciousness and senses may be abruptly suspended, and motor, sensory, or behavioral symptoms result.

An individual seizure is distinguished from epilepsy per se, with the latter term being reserved for three or more recurrent seizures. Epileptic seizures should be distinguished from nonepileptic convulsive seizures produced by cerebral ischemia or hypoxia, hypoglycemia, convulsive drugs such as cocaine, and withdrawal from alcohol, barbiturates, and benzodiazepines. Pseudoepileptic behavior produced by conversion hysteria must not be mistaken for epilepsy.

VERIFY THAT SEIZURES ARE EPILEPTIC

When a patient loses consciousness episodically, epilepsy should be differentiated from syncope, pseudoepileptic seizures, drop attacks, and drug-induced or withdrawal seizures. Although closed-circuit television videotaping with biotelemetry of the electroencephalogram (CCTV-EEG) and Holter monitoring of the electrocardiogram have shown important clinical differences among these conditions, the history and setting are frequently the most important determinants of the diagnosis.

Twenty percent of patients believed to have epilepsy actually experience nonepileptic seizures. Four common causes of nonepileptic seizures are hyperventilation, hysteria, alcohol withdrawal, and cocaine use. The provoking factor for hyperventilation is sometimes difficult to discover. Rapid shallow breathing is present, and the patient feels lightheaded, with trembling limbs and often trembling of the whole body. Excessive loss of carbon dioxide produces paresthesias in the hands, face, and feet; carpopedal spasms may develop. Sometimes, somnambulism from non–rapid eye movement parasomnias and narcolepsy are mistaken for epilepsy.

Syncope

Syncope occurs in as many as 25 to 30% of young, healthy adults. Postural tone and consciousness are suddenly lost, and the patient falls. Most frequently, syncope is due to a temporary decrease in cerebral blood flow resulting from a fall in systemic arterial pressure, and/or a decrease in cardiac output resulting from cardiac arrhythmias, sick sinus syndrome, complete heart block, or vasovagal syncope. The clinical picture of pallor, flaccidity, upward deviation of the eyes, and loss of consciousness in simple syncope is paralleled by the appearance of 2- to 4-Hz high-amplitude slow waves on the electroencephalogram (EEG). The persistence of cerebral anoxia for more than 15 seconds is reflected by tonic spasms and one or two generalized jerks (convulsive syncope). The EEG becomes slow and low voltage but promptly returns to normal after consciousness is regained. Less commonly, syncope can be produced by hypoglycemia or hypoxia, characterized by gradual loss and recovery of consciousness.

Aortic valvular stenosis, hypersensitive stretch receptors in the carotid sinus, micturition, explosive vigorous coughing, pain, and orthostatic hypotension can all produce syncope.

Pseudoepileptic Psychogenic Seizures

An audience is usually present during hysterical or psychogenic seizures. Consciousness is preserved, amnesia is absent or patchy, and movements that simulate epileptic convulsions do not have tonic-clonic phases or in-phase clonic movements of the upper extremities. Movements are out of phase, chaotic, and bizarre without stereotype. Side-to-side head movements are observed in one third of patients and forward pelvic thrusting in almost half of those experiencing psychogenic seizures. The duration is usually longer than the average 70 seconds of a tonic-clonic convulsion. The attack ends abruptly with the patient alert and showing no postictal tiredness, sleep, or Todd's paralysis. A prior psychiatric history is usually present; psychogenic seizures are seldom the sole symptom and sign.

Both psychogenic seizures and epileptic seizures can exist together in the same patient. The EEG and prolactin levels are especially useful in differentiating the two events. A main indication for CCTV-EEG intensive monitoring is the differentiation of pseudoepileptic from epileptic seizures. The EEG, during and immediately after epileptic seizures, is most always abnormal. Between epileptic seizures, the EEG is abnormal in 40 to 60% of patients. The EEG is normal between, during, and after hysterical attacks. Serum prolactin levels increase within 20 minutes of a tonic-clonic convulsion or complex partial seizure but do not change with pseudoepileptic hysterical seizures.

Drop Attacks

Episodic ischemia of the brain stem, which may occur in elderly patients with insufficient blood flow throughout the vertebrobasilar system, is usually of atherosclerotic origin. Transient ischemic attacks affecting the brain stem can cause episodic loss of tone with falls. Consciousness is usually preserved and no convulsions are present. EEGs between episodes are normal.

Drug-Induced or Withdrawal Seizures

A history of psychiatric problems, post-traumatic seizures, and convulsions induced by abstinence is not uncommon in chronic alcoholism. Seizures can be induced by alcohol, but withdrawal seizures are more common. Tonic-clonic seizures appear 24 to 48 hours (up to 7 days) after alcohol withdrawal. Confusion, delusions, and visual, tactile, and auditory hallucinations (alcoholic hallucinosis) accompany agitation and can progress to delirium tremens lasting up to 5 days. Hypoglycemia can complicate the picture. Subdural or epidural hematoma must be excluded. Smoking of crack or cocaine paste can produce tonic-clonic convulsions that appear at the height of or immediately after the high. In severe cocaine toxicity, respiratory depression, cardiac arrhythmias, a hypermetabolic state, and status epilepticus can occur. Alcohol withdrawal convulsions, delirium tremens, and cocaine convulsions are medical emergencies and can be effectively treated with benzodiazepines. Ventricular dysrhythmias in cocaine toxicity can be treated with intravenous propranolol (0.5 to 1 mg).

DEFINE SEIZURE TYPES AND EPILEPSY SYNDROME (Table 1)

In the United States, at least 150,000 new cases of epilepsy are diagnosed each year and about 1,416,000 epilepsy patients are receiving antiepileptic drugs. The age-adjusted prevalence of epilepsy is 6.25 per 1000. Incidence

TABLE 1. **International Classification of Epileptic Seizures and Epilepsies**

Seizures	Epilepsies
I. Partial (focal, local) seizures	I. Localization-related epilepsies
A. Simple partial seizures (consciousness not impaired)	1. Idiopathic (age related)
1. With motor symptoms	Benign childhood epilepsy with centrotemporal spikes
2. With somatosensory or special sensory symptoms	Benign childhood epilepsy with occipital paroxysms
3. With autonomic symptoms	2. Symptomatic
4. With psychic symptoms	a. Epilepsies involving the limbic system
B. Complex partial seizures (with impairment of consciousness)	b. Epilepsies not involving the limbic system
1. Beginning as simple partial seizures and progressing to impairment of consciousness	Frontal
a. With no other features	Temporal
b. With features as in I.A.1 to I.A.4	Central
c. With automatisms	Parietal
2. With impairment of consciousness at onset	Occipital
a. With no other features	II. Generalized epilepsies
b. With features as in I.A.1 to I.A.4	1. Idiopathic (age related)
c. With automatisms	Benign neonatal familial convulsions
C. Partial seizures evolving to secondarily generalized seizures	Benign neonatal convulsions
1. Simple partial seizures evolving to generalized seizures	West's syndrome (idiopathic cases)
2. Complex partial seizures evolving to generalized seizures	Epilepsy with myoclonic-astatic seizures (idiopathic and familial cases of Lennox-Gastaut-Dravet syndrome)
3. Simple partial seizures evolving to complex partial seizures to generalized seizures	Childhood absence epilepsy (pyknoepilepsy)
II. Generalized seizures (convulsive or nonconvulsive)	Epilepsy with (myo)clonic absences
A. Absence seizures	Juvenile absence epilepsy
1. Absence seizures	Benign juvenile myoclonic epilepsy (impulsive petit mal)
2. Atypical absence seizures	Epilepsy with generalized tonic-clonic seizures on awakening
B. Myoclonic seizures	2. Symptomatic
C. Clonic seizures	a. Nonspecific cause (age related)
D. Tonic seizures	Neonatal seizures
E. Tonic-clonic seizures	Early myoclonic encephalopathy
F. Atonic seizures (astatic seizures)	West's syndrome (infantile spasms, Blitz-Nick-Salaam-Krampfe)
III. Unclassified epileptic seizures	Lennox-Gastaut-Dravet syndrome
Includes all seizures that cannot be classified because of inadequate or incomplete data and some that defy classification in hitherto described categories (this includes some neonatal seizures, e.g., rhythmic eye movements, chewing, and swimming movements)	b. Specific cause
	Progressive myoclonus epilepsies, e.g.,
	Lafora's disease
	Unverricht's disease
	Unverricht-Lundborg-Hartung disease
	Kufs' disease
	Zeman's disease
	3. Epilepsies undetermined whether focal or generalized
	4. Special syndromes

From Proposal for revised clinical and electroencephalographic classification of epileptic seizures. From the Commission on Classification and Terminology of the International League Against Epilepsy. Epilepsia 22:489–501, 1981. © The International League Against Epilepsy.

rates are highest in the very young (newborns and infants, especially), drop to a relatively constant rate between 10 and 70 years of age, and increase again thereafter. Acquired epilepsies characterized by partial and secondary tonic-clonic seizures are the most common forms. They occur frequently in the first 5 years of life, somewhat less often in persons 5 to 10 years of age, and more often in those older than 20 years. The incidence of genetic epilepsies with grand mal tonic-clonic convulsions peaks during adolescence and early adulthood. Juvenile myoclonic epilepsy (JME) is a disease of adolescence. Absence epilepsies are usually childhood disorders and rarely occur in patients younger than 3 years or older than 20 years.

The type of seizure must be identified (see Table 1), and then the epilepsy syndrome and cause are determined. Are seizures the manifestations of a genetic form of epilepsy or of a structural lesion? Genetic epilepsies often manifest as generalized seizures and rarely as focal seizures. Epilepsies symptomatic of structural disease often manifest as focal seizures and secondarily as generalized convulsions.

It is essential to obtain from the patient and relatives a detailed case history and description of the first and subsequent attacks. Are the seizures partial or generalized? Is the epilepsy syndrome idiopathic or symptomatic? In partial epilepsies, the first seizure and its aura can give clues about its site of origin. Changes in character in subsequent attacks may suggest progression of a structural lesion or reflect the effects of antiepileptic drugs. The EEG is indispensable when epilepsy is suggested. It should be obtained with the patient awake and asleep, and with photic stimulation and hyperventilation. Hyperventilation often provokes pyknoleptic absences in childhood absence epilepsy. In complex partial seizures, nasopharyngeal, nasoethmoid, or sphenoid electrodes may be necessary.

IDENTIFY UNDERLYING CAUSES

Brain magnetic resonance imaging (MRI) or computed tomography (CT) or both are recommended in all adults with symptomatic partial seizures. Positron emission tomography with fluorodeoxyglucose is recommended in surgical candidates. MRI T1- and T2-weighted axial and coronal planes can image neuronal migration disorders, such as cortical dysplasia and hamartomas; clarify the picture of cavernous hemangioma detected earlier by CT as calcifications; and detect low-grade glioma undiagnosed by CT. MRI can demonstrate atrophy of the hippocampus by volume measurements of the hippocampus. Coronal planes can show hippocampal atrophy and gliosis. Routine MRI may not be necessary in benign epilepsy syndromes, such as JME, juvenile or childhood absence epilepsy, or rolandic epilepsy.

Postictal hemiparesis (Todd's paralysis) and postictal dysphasia point to a focal cerebral lesion. Provoking factors such as sleep deprivation, alcohol, and sleep or awakening states must be identified. Clusters of seizures before or during menses (catamenial seizures) are often present. When seizures start in childhood, adolescence, and young adulthood, the birth history is of value. Headaches and visual hemisensory or hemimotor complaints suggest a focal lesion. Seizures associated with fever and meningeal signs suggest meningitis or encephalitis and warrant a lumbar puncture.

The age at the onset of seizures can suggest the cause of epilepsy. Seizures that start in childhood and adolescence commonly have a genetic origin or are related to birth injuries or cerebral cortical dysplasias and hamartomas. Seizures beginning in the second and third decades of life are associated with postnatal head trauma, central nervous system infections, cerebral cortical dysplasias, arteriovenous malformations, and aneurysms. Seizures in the fourth and fifth decades of life are usually due to cerebral neoplasms, trauma, or cerebrovascular disease. During the sixth decade and beyond, cerebrovascular disease, neoplasms, and degenerative diseases cause seizures.

ESTABLISH AN EARLY TREATMENT PLAN

When to Start Treatment

Figure 1 is an algorithm for the approach to antiepileptic drug treatment of epilepsies. Antiepileptic therapy is obligatory for generalized or partial epilepsies. Uncontrolled convulsions and prolonged complex partial status epilepticus can cause selective cell damage in the cerebral cortex, hippocampus, amygdala, and cerebellum. Physical injuries, skull and limb fractures, rare spinal cord transections, and rare sudden death provide even more compelling arguments for treatment of tonic-clonic convulsions.

Antiepileptic treatment is seldom indicated, however, after a single tonic-clonic seizure. Most of these patients have no risk factors for epilepsy and have normal neurologic and EEG examinations. Approximately 25% of these patients do develop epilepsy. A strong family history, an aura, absence or complex partial (focal) onset, abnormal neurologic examination, and epileptiform EEG patterns require immediate investigation and treatment. Treatment may be postponed if a single tonic-clonic seizure is related to sleep deprivation (>36 hours), stress, extreme fatigue, drug or alcohol withdrawal, or use of cocaine.

Starting with Monotherapy

The aim of treatment is to control seizures without drug toxicity. Treatment should begin with one antiepileptic, preferably the drug of choice. Using one drug makes the management of toxicity easier, improves the patient's compliance, avoids drug interactions, and makes it easier to monitor and control idiosyncratic side effects. A single drug can improve control in 40% of patients previously receiving polytherapy. Single-drug treatment of partial, complex partial, and secondary tonic-clonic seizures with phenytoin (Dilantin), carbamazepine (Tegretol), or primidone (Mysoline) results in satisfactory long-term seizure control in 60% of patients and complete eradication of seizures in 40 to 60%. Frequent seizures, especially acute symptomatic seizures associated with an acute medical or neurologic illness, require an oral loading dose of 15 mg of phenytoin per kg. Otherwise, gradual institution of drug therapy is usually adequate.

The trough plasma level should be measured at steady state. If seizures persist at steady state, the dosage should be raised until seizures stop or toxic

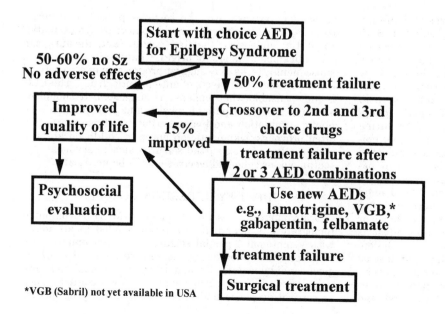

Figure 1. Approach to medical treatment of the epilepsies. *Abbreviations*: AED = antiepileptic drug; Sz = seizure; VGB = vigabatrin.

*VGB (Sabril) not yet available in USA

side effects develop. For some drugs such as primidone and carbamazepine, peak plasma levels may correlate with dose-dependent side effects. Dosage should produce therapeutic results at trough levels and without toxicity at peak levels. If seizures persist despite therapeutic or toxic drug levels, a second drug of choice is added. When trough levels of the second drug reach high therapeutic ranges, the first drug is gradually withdrawn (cross-over). If seizures persist, a third drug of choice is added and the second withdrawn as previously described. Cross-over must be carefully planned to avoid seizure breakthrough or unanticipated side effects. If single entry drugs fail, the drugs may be given in combination.

Shifting to Monotherapy from Polytherapy

Often patients return to monotherapy because of continuing seizures despite polypharmacy. Because 34% of patients receiving two drugs and 44% of patients receiving three or more antiepileptic drugs report adverse drug reactions, single-drug therapy is desirable.

Cross-over from polypharmacy to monotherapy starts with the gradual introduction of a first drug of choice. When therapeutic plasma levels of that drug are reached, the dosages of the other drugs can gradually be reduced. As drugs are withdrawn, plasma levels of the first drug of choice commonly rise. Nonessential drugs and those with interactions and undesirable side effects are withdrawn first. Withdrawal usually occurs over a 1- to 3-month period, with monitoring of plasma drug levels. An 8-hour outpatient CCTV-EEG monitoring session can be helpful.

DRUGS OF CHOICE

Table 2 shows the common epilepsy syndromes with the first- and second-choice antiepileptic drug treatments.

Primary Generalized Genetic Epilepsies

About 40% of adults and children with epilepsy suffer from genetic epilepsies with primary generalized seizures. Generalized seizures are present when epileptogenic discharges involve both cerebral hemispheres from the onset. Early loss of consciousness is the rule. Generalized seizures may involve only loss of consciousness (absence) or convulsive movements (tonic-clonic, myoclonic, tonic, or clonic). Early childhood myoclonic, myoclonic-astatic, absence, benign juvenile myoclonic, and tonic-clonic or clonic-tonic-clonic grand mal epilepsies can be best recognized by their onset in childhood and adolescence. Almost all are genetically transmitted. Structural lesions are rare. The EEG shows bilaterally symmetrical and synchronous 2.5- to 3.5-Hz or 3.5- to 6-Hz spike- or polyspike-wave complexes.

The first drug of choice for primary generalized convulsive epilepsies such as pure grand mal,

TABLE 2. Common Epilepsy Syndromes with Choice Antiepileptic Drugs

Syndrome	First Choice	Second Choice
Idiopathic		
Absence only	ETHS	VPA
Absence plus grand mal	VPA	LTG
		ETHS + PHT or ETHS + CBZ
Juvenile myoclonic epilepsy	VPA	LTG
Benign childhood epilepsy, e.g., rolandic epilepsy	CBZ	VPA
Symptomatic		
Lennox-Gastaut-Dravet	VGB* alone or with CBZ	VPA + CBZ
Temporal lobe epilepsy	CBZ or PHT	LTG
Frontal lobe epilepsy	CBZ or PHT or VPA	LTG

*Not available in the United States but being considered by FDA.
Abbreviations: ETHS = ethosuximide (Zarontin); VPA = valproate (Depakote); VGB = vigabatrin (Sabril); CBZ = carbamazepine (Tegretol); LTG = lamotrigine (Lamictal); PHT = phenytoin (Dilantin); CNZ = clonazepam.

juvenile myoclonic, photosensitive, and combined absence–grand mal epilepsies is sodium valproate (Depakote). Valproate suppresses about 80 to 90% of grand mal tonic-clonic, 80 to 95% of myoclonic, and as much as 90% of absence attacks. If valproate does not stop myoclonic seizures, clonazepam (Klonopin) or lamotrigine (Lamictal) can be used. When valproate fails to stop grand mal attacks, lamotrigine, phenytoin, carbamazepine, or primidone should be tried, but these drugs can aggravate absences. Isolated absence attacks are still best treated with ethosuximide (Zarontin). Vigabatrin (Sabril)* alone or combined with carbamazepine is now the first choice for the drop attacks of myoclonic-astatic epilepsy or Lennox-Gastaut-Dravet syndrome. Valproate plus carbamazepine is a second choice drug combination in Lennox-Gastaut-Dravet syndrome. Lamotrigine is the third choice drug. Clonazepam or valproate combined with carbamazepine or lamotrigine combined with carbamazepine can also be tried. As a last resort, felbamate can be used. *If felbamate is used, the patient should sign a consent form.*

Before valproate monotherapy is initiated, a complete blood count, platelet count, bleeding time, and liver function tests should be done. The patient should be warned of possible signs of serious hepatic dysfunction such as loss of appetite, nausea, vomiting, abdominal pain, lethargy, easy bruising, or malaise. A complete blood count and hepatic function tests should be performed again and valproate plasma levels measured after 10 days. Serial complete blood counts, hepatic function tests, and careful clinical monitoring should be carried out every month for the first 6 months. Elevation of serum transaminase levels is usually transient and dose related. In

*Not available in the United States.

sporadic cases, it may mean serious and even fatal hepatic dysfunction; 1.5 patients per 10,000 receiving polytherapy including valproate and 2.7 patients per 100,000 receiving monotherapy have experienced fatal hepatic failure. In these cases, valproate therapy has been continued for less than 6 months. With rare exceptions, all patients in the United States who experienced valproate liver failure had unusual congenital syndromes, mental retardation, or organic brain diseases. Hepatic failure seems to be idiosyncratic and age related, with children younger than 2 years being the group at primary risk (1 in 7000 during monotherapy and 1 in 500 during polytherapy). The frequency of hepatic failure declines with age and is extremely rare with monotherapy (11 in 37,000). Rarely, valproate has also produced thrombocytopenia, increased platelet aggregation, and hypofibrinogenemia. Hyperammonemia has also been reported.

The dose of valproate is gradually increased from one 250-mg capsule daily to achieve trough plasma levels of 60 to 80 µg/mL (usually 250 mg three times daily). The final dosage may be 500 mg three times daily. Valproic acid is quickly absorbed and eliminated and controls attacks at lower dosages (15 to 18 mg per kg) when used alone. Nausea and vomiting appear when the dose is increased too quickly. Gastric irritation may be reduced by taking the capsules after meals. Weight gain, hair loss, and tremors are common side effects.

Ethosuximide controls 60% of childhood absence epilepsy that is not associated with tonic-clonic seizures. It is quickly absorbed (0.5 to 4 hours), and steady state is reached in 1 week. It has an average half-life of 24 to 30 hours in children, longer in adults. Dose-dependent side effects include nausea, vomiting, anorexia, dyspepsia, night terrors, motor unrest, agitation, and paranoid psychoses. Rash and thrombocytopenia may suggest uncommon idiosyncratic side effects, such as aplastic anemia and agranulocytosis.

Clonazepam can be useful as a third treatment option for atonic drop and myoclonic and absence seizures. Peak plasma concentrations occur in 1 to 4 hours. The half-life is 20 to 50 hours. Doses start with 0.5 mg daily increased every 3 to 5 days until seizures are controlled or sedation prohibits further dosage increments. Ataxia and irritability can result.

Symptomatic Partial Epilepsies

Symptomatic partial epilepsies account for 60% of adult and about 40% of childhood epilepsies. Symptomatic partial epilepsies have a localized origin. Neurologic signs may be present, and onset can occur at any age. Between seizures, the EEG can show localized epileptiform spikes. During the onset of seizures (ictus), the EEG shows epileptogenic discharges related to the lesion. During seizures, the most common EEG pattern consists of localized, rhythmic, low-voltage 16- to 30-Hz rapid potentials that can propagate and spread.

Partial seizures arise from an anatomic or functional system limited to part of one or both cerebral hemispheres. Localization and the preferred routes of spread determine clinical features. Partial seizures are divided into three major subgroups: simple, complex, and secondarily generalized seizures. In simple partial seizures, consciousness is never lost. In complex partial seizures, consciousness is impaired. Synonyms include psychomotor seizures, fugus epileptique, and Damner attacken. Simple or complex partial seizures can develop into secondary tonic-clonic seizures. Complex partial seizures should be differentiated from absence seizures because the choice of drug for each of these disorders differs. Most absence seizures last 10 seconds or less. Psychomotor seizures last an average of 3 minutes, and most are not longer than 5 minutes. An aura precedes 44% of complex partial seizures. Full consciousness returns slowly. Absence seizures have no aura, and full consciousness returns abruptly. Automatisms in complex partial seizures are more complex than automatisms of absence. Walking or running, perseverative bilateral arm or leg motions such as kicking and defensive flailing, and bimanual, bipedal movements can appear at the onset of psychomotor attacks. Such complex motor movements have not been reported in absence seizures. Between seizures (interictus), local spikes or spike-wave formations appear in the EEG. If a circumscribed lesion is present, the term "focal epilepsy" is most appropriate. If the site and side of seizure onset vary (which is often the case in benign childhood syndromes), the term "localization related" is more appropriate.

Acquired generalized epilepsies manifest generalized seizures, but focal or diffuse cerebral abnormality may be recognized by the presence of abnormal neurologic signs, background EEG changes, and brain images. Organic brain disease can also manifest as generalized tonic seizures, myoclonic jerks, infantile spasms, or atonic attacks, as in West's syndrome of infancy, symptomatic Lennox-Gastaut-Dravet syndrome, and the progressive myoclonus epilepsies. Temporal lobe and frontal lobe epilepsies are the most common forms of acquired epilepsies and account for almost half of all epilepsies in children and adults.

Carbamazepine, phenytoin, and valproate are the first-tier drugs for partial and secondarily generalized epilepsies. These three drugs are equally successful in monotherapy of new-onset partial epilepsies. Phenobarbital and primidone are less well tolerated. Primidone commonly causes ataxia, vertigo, nausea, and drowsiness. Phenobarbital, carbamazepine, phenytoin, primidone, and valproate have no significant differences in efficacy. The choice among these five drugs is determined by their toxicity.

Drowsiness, dizziness, nystagmus, blurred vision, diplopia, and nausea are pronounced at the onset of carbamazepine therapy and at peak plasma levels (Table 3). These side effects can be prevented by starting at lower doses and gradually increasing therapy. Carbamazepine is absorbed slowly, reaching

TABLE 3. **Commonly Used and New Antiepileptic Drugs**

Drug	Usual Daily Doses*	Time Required to Reach Steady State (d)	Therapeutic Range (mg/mL)†	Elimination Half-Life (h)‡	Protein Binding (%)	Toxicity
Commonly Used Drugs						
Valproic acid (Depakote)	1000–3000 mg (divided)	1–2	40–150	6–15	80–95	Nausea, vomiting, somnolence
Ethosuximide (Zarontin)	1000 mg (divided)	7–10	50–100	20–60	0	Nausea, fatigue, GI upset, psychoses
Clonazepam (Klonopin)	10.5 mg (divided)		0.005–0.070	20–40	45	Sedation, ataxia, impaired cognition
Carbamazepine (Tegretol)	1000–1600 mg (divided)	3–6	4–12	18.7 (11–22)	66–89	Dizziness, diplopia, ataxia, blurred vision
Phenytoin (Dilantin)	300–400 mg	7–28	10–20	22 (highly variable)	90	Nystagmus, ataxia, somnolence, GI discomfort
Primidone (Mysoline)	750 mg (divided)	1–5	4–12	15.6	20–25	Sedation, nausea, dizziness, ataxia
Phenobarbital (Luminal)	120 mg (divided)	10–30	15–40	96	40–60	Sedation, dizziness; hyperactivity in children
New Antiepileptic Drugs						
Gabapentin (Neurontin)	900–1800 mg (divided) and 1800–2400 mg (divided)	1–2	1–2	5–7	5–9	Somnolence (20%), dizziness (18%), ataxia (13%), fatigue (10%), headaches, diplopia
Lamotrigine (Lamictal)	75 to 500 mg	7–10	1–10	29 (14–60)	55	Headaches (30%), nausea (18%), dizziness (38%), diplopia (28%), rash, ataxia (20%)
Felbamate (Felbatol)	15–60 mg/kg or 2400–3600 mg	7–28	20–80	12–24	25–35	Headaches (25–40%), nausea (35%), decreased appetite (10–20%), insomnia (20%), weight loss, hepatic failure, bone marrow suppression

*This is an eventual dose; a lower dose is necessary when initiating therapy.
†Therapeutic levels may change with multiple drugs.
‡Half-life may also change with multiple drugs; half-lives are given for adult dosages. Steady state is reached in four half-lives.
Abbreviation: GI = gastrointestinal.

peak plasma levels in 2 to 8 hours (24 hours). Leukopenia occurs in 10%. Idiosyncratic side effects include rash, icterus, anemia, and edema. Bone marrow depression has been reported rarely. An incidence of 0.5 case per 100,000 treatment years with carbamazepine or 2 cases per 75,000 patients has been reported for aplastic anemia. Hypersensitivity reactions with rashes, exfoliative dermatitis, Stevens-Johnson syndrome, and systemic lupus erythematosus rarely occur.

Ataxia and nystagmus are dose dependent with phenytoin, but sedation is usually not a problem. Dysmorphic effects, including coarsening of facial features, gum hypertrophy, and hirsutism, appear with chronic use in children, adolescents, and women. Cerebellar degeneration can appear after chronic therapy. Stevens-Johnson syndrome occurs in 1 of 20,000 persons. A lupus-like syndrome, pseudolymphoma, exfoliative dermatitis, and a fatal hepatic necrosis can also occur. Exanthema, fever, hepatitis, and lymphadenopathy indicate withdrawal of the drug. Peak plasma levels appear in 2 to 8 hours; phenytoin has a half-life of 24 hours. Up to 96% is bound to plasma proteins. Phenytoin should not be administered intramuscularly because it precipitates. Toxic neurologic side effects related to peak plasma levels indicate a reduction of dosage. Despite these limitations, 50 years of experience has proved that most adults can safely use phenytoin for effective seizure control.

Disulfiram (Antabuse), chloramphenicol, sulfamethizole, and phenylbutazone all inhibit the metabolism of phenytoin, increasing the risk of intoxication. Phenytoin accelerates the metabolism of warfarin and dicoumarol. This effect causes a risk of bleeding if phenytoin is withdrawn. Phenytoin lowers serum folate levels, occasionally producing macrocytic anemia. It also interferes with vitamin D metabolism, producing osteopenia. Antagonism with vitamin K can be important during pregnancy. Supplemental vitamin K should be administered to the pregnant woman and to the neonate to prevent hemorrhagic disease of the newborn.

Sedation, cognitive impairment, and sometimes impotence are the major drawbacks of phenobarbital. Transient sedation is prominent during the initiation of treatment. Most patients develop tolerance within a few weeks. Blood phenobarbital levels of 30 mg per mL or higher usually produce drowsiness. Some patients complain of tiredness with low levels. Hyperactivity, agitation, or sleeplessness can appear as paradoxical reactions, especially in children and elderly patients. Systemic toxicity is uncommon.

Primidone may produce listlessness and difficulty in rousing from sleep during the first few months of use. Sixty percent of patients discontinue primidone therapy by the end of the first year. Partial and complex partial seizures are poorly controlled. The initial dose should be low and the dosage increased cautiously. After 1 year, primidone has minimal sedative side effects when used as the sole drug. Patients who continue to use the drug successfully for 1 year continue to do so for the next 5 years. It can be considered an acceptable alternative drug. When primidone is used in combination with phenytoin, increased biotransformation to phenobarbital can lead to side effects similar to those reported for phenobarbital. Systemic side effects have been rare. Primidone's efficacy may be separate from that of its metabolites. When drugs must be used in combination, primidone can be used effectively with phenytoin or carbamazepine.

New Antiepileptic Drugs

The new antiepileptic agents lamotrigine, gabapentin, and felbamate are broad spectrum, should be considered third-tier agents, and are presently recommended as add-on antiepileptic drugs.

Two monotherapy trials in Europe showed that *lamotrigine* (Lamictal), at doses of at least 300 to 500 mg daily, is as effective as phenytoin or carbamazepine in reducing partial, complex partial, and secondarily generalized seizures as a single entry agent. It is also effective in reducing atonic drop seizures of Lennox-Gastaut-Dravet syndrome. Sodium valproate inhibits the metabolism of lamotrigine, doubling the elimination half-life from 29 to 60 hours. Enzyme-inducing antiepileptic drugs such as phenytoin, carbamazepine, and phenobarbital reduce the half-life of lamotrigine about 50%. Rashes, including Stevens-Johnson syndrome, a lupus-like syndrome, and toxic epidermal necrolysis, are reasons for discontinuing lamotrigine in 6 to 10%. A gradual ascension of dose from 50 mg daily for 2 weeks and then 100 mg daily for 2 weeks is scheduled until 300 to 500 mg daily is reached.

Gabapentin (Neurontin) has an advantage over other antiepileptic agents in that it is not metabolized, is not protein bound, and does not produce significant pharmacokinetic changes in other antiepileptic agents. The sole elimination pathway is renal excretion. Gabapentin (at least 1200 to 1800 mg to as much as 3000 to 4000 mg daily) reduces the frequency of partial, complex partial, and secondarily generalized seizures as an add-on agent and is ideal for elderly patients.

Felbamate (Felbatol) is particularly potent and has wide clinical spectrum. Felbamate (maximal dose of 45 mg per kg per day or 3600 mg per day) is particularly effective in reducing atonic seizures, generalized tonic-clonic seizures, and total seizure frequency in the Lennox-Gastaut-Dravet syndrome. Felbamate is also effective as a single entry drug or as adjunctive therapy in partial seizures. When felbamate is administered with phenytoin, phenytoin concentrations increase. With felbamate administered at 1800 to 2400 mg per day, the phenytoin dose should be reduced by 20%; at 3600 mg of felbamate per day, the phenytoin dose should be reduced by 40%. At 3600 mg of felbamate per day, the mean carbamazepine levels decrease 30%, whereas the carbamazepine epoxide levels increase 60%. Felbamate increases steady-state plasma valproic acid concentrations by as much as 50% with 2400 mg of felbamate per day. Mean felbamate trough concentrations increase with valproate and drop slightly with carbamazepine or phenytoin therapy. Because felbamate therapy is limited by hepatic toxicity in 1 per 6000 and bone marrow suppression in 1 per 10,000, a signed consent form should be obtained.

Metabolism of Antiepileptic Drugs

To predict the time of drug actions, toxic effects, and drug interactions, the practicing physician should be familiar with the absorption, distribution, protein binding, elimination characteristics, and half-lives of each of the antiepileptic drugs (see Table 3). Absorption varies from one drug to another and among patients. Peak plasma concentrations appear most often at 4 to 24 hours. Carbamazepine, primidone, and phenobarbital dosages must be increased slowly, because peak plasma levels may rise quickly. Phenytoin and phenobarbital increase the metabolism of carbamazepine, reducing its half-life from 20 to 10 hours. This may result in early-morning seizures in spite of drug intoxication in the evening.

Body distribution and full antiepileptic effects are dependent on plasma protein binding. Only the free or non–protein-bound fraction crosses the blood-brain barrier. Carbamazepine forms an active metabolite, 10,11-epoxycarbamazepine, which may be responsible for some of its clinical action and untoward side effects. Primidone forms two active metabolites: phenylethylmalonamide and phenobarbital. No antiepileptic action of the metabolites of phenytoin has been shown.

The half-life of a drug determines the steady state, as well as the number of doses needed per day (see Table 3).

All antiepileptic drugs are eliminated by first-order kinetics; that is, a direct relationship exists between dosage and plasma levels. The exception is phenytoin, which saturates liver enzyme capacity at high levels. Metabolism is dependent on plasma levels, so that at the high end of the therapeutic range, the dosage should be adjusted by small amounts (25 mg).

Various conditions modify metabolism or protein binding. Adults older than 65 years metabolize drugs more quickly. The dose may be kept unchanged, however, because the unbound protein fraction is larger. Serious kidney failure increases the free fraction of phenytoin. The absolute plasma concentration is unchanged, however. Liver dysfunction can also change protein binding and impair metabolism. During serious medical illnesses and pregnancy, it is wise to follow plasma levels often. The blood levels in newborn infants of treated mothers are similar to the levels in the mother. Antiepileptic drugs pass into breast milk, but the concentration is significantly lower than that in the mother's plasma.

Antiepileptic Drugs During Pregnancy

All five main antiepileptic drugs (carbamazepine, phenytoin, valproate, primidone, phenobarbital) are potential teratogens when ingested during pregnancy. Major anomalies such as spina bifida rarely occur after valproate monotherapy (1.5%) or carbamazepine (0.9%) exposure of the fetus in utero. Urogenital and congenital heart abnormalities are reported with any of the five drugs. Oral-palate cleft is increased 3-fold to 10-fold after phenytoin or carbamazepine exposure in utero. Minor craniofacial and limb anomalies, especially epicanthal folds and distal phalangeal hypoplasia, can occur in offspring after the use of any of the five drugs during pregnancy. Fortunately, most pregnancies (90 to 95%) in which there is antiepileptic drug exposure still result in normal offspring. Birth defects in general, however, are two to three times more common in pregnancies exposed to antiepileptic drugs than in those unexposed to antiepileptic drugs. A positive family history of birth defects should serve as a warning. If an antiepileptic drug is absolutely necessary, monotherapy with the smallest effective dose should be used. Plasma levels of antiepileptic drugs must be monitored monthly. Vitamins, including folic acid (15 mg per day) and vitamin K, are important supplements. Serum and amniotic fluid alpha-fetoprotein and acetylcholinesterase levels detect 78% of open spina bifida but not closed lesions. Ultrasound imaging detects 96% of open and closed spina bifida. The newborn should receive 1 mg of vitamin K (phytonadione) immediately after birth, and clotting factors should be monitored closely.

Status Epilepticus

Status epilepticus occurs when seizures persist for 30 minutes or when a series of convulsions continues without recovery of consciousness. This is a medical emergency and requires immediate treatment to prevent brain damage or death. There is no single ideal drug for the treatment of status epilepticus. A step-by-step protocol is given in Table 4. If the patient continues to convulse after 60 minutes, general anesthesia with a barbiturate (usually pentobarbital) should be initiated.

FOLLOW-UP AND MONITORING OF SEIZURE CONTROL AND QUALITY OF LIFE

Follow-up is guided by an understanding of the prognosis and psychosocial complications of epilepsy. The prognosis depends to a great extent on the age at onset. An excellent outcome is seen in idiopathic generalized epilepsies of childhood and adolescence. Generalized seizures caused by progressive brain disease have a poor prognosis. Partial epilepsies with psychomotor symptoms can be difficult to treat and may require surgery. Nocturnal tonic-clonic seizures have a good prognosis.

Sixty to 79% of patients with absence seizures become free from seizures with ethosuximide or valproic acid therapy. Ninety percent of patients with pure grand mal or primarily generalized tonic-clonic seizures become free from seizures with valproic acid, carbamazepine, or phenytoin therapy. Ninety-five percent of patients with juvenile myoclonic epilepsy are completely free from seizures when receiving valproic acid.

Many economic, social, and educational conditions influence the course of epilepsy. Patients are commonly asked to leave school or give up a job. They are considered to be high accident risks. The epilepsy victim is even thought to have a special tendency to criminality. No evidence supports any of these assumptions, however.

Persons with epilepsy are often handicapped by depression or cognitive and behavioral problems associated with epilepsy or antiepileptic drugs. Emotional immaturity and personality disorders may develop because of defective rearing, overprotection, and rejection. The physician should act as an advocate for the patient and should develop a support system that includes family, school, and vocational personnel. A multidisciplinary team is needed.

The practicing physician often has to cope with these issues alone. The clinician must be an educator. The patient should have a calendar for recording seizures and a list of drugs and dosages. The patient should expect follow-up visits at least every 3 months for the first year and every 6 months subsequently. Patients must understand the necessity of follow-up examinations, complete blood counts, and liver function tests. In a seizure-free condition, patients should have no mental or psychiatric abnormalities and can have a normal life expectancy. Death can be caused by suicide, status epilepticus, accidents, or brain tumor.

Plan Withdrawal of Antiepileptic Drug Treatment When Treatment Is Successful

Almost all genetic epilepsies with primary generalized seizures have an excellent prognosis. Sixty to 95% are stopped by drug treatment. Genetic partial epilepsies, such as rolandic epilepsy, are usually controlled by monotherapy, and clinical features usually disappear by the age of 16 years. The prognosis and recurrence of seizures after withdrawal of an antiepileptic drug, therefore, depend on the specific epilepsy syndrome. A high frequency of seizures, abnormal mental function during inadequate control of seizures, repeated tonic-clonic status as observed in Lennox-Gastaut-Dravet syndrome, severe myoclonic epilepsy of infancy, and the progressive myoclonus

TABLE 4. **Management of Tonic-Clonic Status Epilepticus**

Step	Time from Initial Observation and Treatment (min)	Procedure
1	0	Assess cardiorespiratory function. If unsure of diagnosis, observe one tonic-clonic seizure and verify the persistence of unconsciousness after the seizure. Insert oral airway and administer oxygen if necessary.
		Insert an indwelling IV catheter. Draw venous blood for stat levels of anticonvulsants, glucose, electrolytes, and urea. Draw arterial blood for stat pH PO_2, HCO_3. Monitor respiration, blood pressure, and ECG. If possible, monitor EEG.
2	5	Start IV infusion through indwelling venous catheter of normal saline containing vitamin B complex. Give a bolus injection of 50 mL of 50% glucose.

Three options are available as the first drug regimen:

Step	Time from Initial Observation and Treatment (min)	Procedure
		Option 1, IV bolus of lorazepam (Ativan)
3	10–30	Give 0.1 mg/kg lorazepam as IV bolus at 4 mg over 2 min. Repeat the same dose in 15 min if control is not achieved.
		Option 2, diazepam (Valium)-fosphenytoin (Cerebyx) combination
3	10–30	Infuse diazepam IV no faster than 2 mg/min until seizures stop, or to total of 20 mg (do not dilute). Also start IV drip of 750 mg of fosphenytoin prodrug (75 mg/mL) concentrate in tetraglycol and TRIS at 40–50 mg/min. Rate of infusion should be watched carefully and no faster than 150 mg/mL.
		Option 3, IV phenobarbital
3	10–30	Give IV infusion of phenobarbital at 100 mg/min until seizures stop or a total dose of 10 mg/kg is administered. If seizures continue, continue infusing phenobarbital at 50 mg/min until a total dose of 20 mg/kg is reached.

If first-option drugs do not control seizures, EEG monitoring and endotracheal intubation are recommended during the remaining steps.

Step	Time from Initial Observation and Treatment (min)	Procedure
4	30–50	If seizures reoccur or persist, IV fosphenytoin can be given if lorazepam is used as the first option. If diazepam-fosphenytoin is used as the first option, lorazepam can be tried as the second drug. If phenobarbital is used as the first option, fosphenytoin or lorazepam can be administered as the second regimen. Fosphenytoin may be increased to 30 mg/kg or to a level of 30 mg/mL.
5	60–80	If seizures continue, general anesthesia can be instituted with:

(1) IV pentobarbital loading dose of 15 mg/kg over 1 h followed by monitor and infusion of 1–2 mg/kg/h until seizures stop or EEG burst suppressions occur.

or

(2) Thiopentone given at 2 mg/min in normal saline by a microdrip set for 30–60 min. Reduce dose to 0.5 mg/min when controlled. Dose can be increased to anesthetic levels if necessary to achieve control. EEG monitoring to ascertain a burst-suppression pattern and seizure control is required. Alternatively, other anesthetizing barbiturates can be used.

or

(3) Halothane and neuromuscular junction blockade administered by an anesthesiologist. Once control is achieved, EEG monitoring is recommended continuously or as frequently as is technically possible in the obtunded patient, to ensure that electrographic status has not recurred.

Abbreviations: ECG = electrocardiogram; EEG = electroencephalogram; TRIS = tris(hydroxymethyl)aminomethane.

encephalopathies are all associated with poor prognosis. In contrast, 80% of patients whose seizures are completely controlled during the first year of treatment remain free from seizures in the subsequent 3 years. Children older than 5 years with generalized seizures, such as absence seizures, who have normal neurologic examinations and normal IQ and whose seizures have been controlled for 2 to 4 years have a 75% chance of remaining seizure free after withdrawal of antiepileptic drugs. The exception is the juvenile myoclonic epilepsy of Janz and awakening clonic-tonic-clonic seizures, in which electroclinical traits persist for life. Withdrawal of antiepileptic drugs is not indicated in these patients.

Antiepileptic drugs can be withdrawn gradually after 2 years of complete control in cases of rolandic epilepsy and pure childhood absence seizures, and after 4 years of complete control in cases of simple partial epilepsy, complex partial epilepsy, absence associated with tonic-clonic seizures, and grand mal tonic-clonic seizures.

A minimal 5-year follow-up is recommended after withdrawal of therapy. EEGs and clinical visits should be scheduled at 6 months and 1 year. CCTV-EEG monitoring can also be used to confirm the absence of epileptic seizures.

Because symptomatic partial seizures are often due to atrophic nonprogressive structural changes, they stand a good chance of control and even cure. Seizures from tumors, vascular malformation, and cerebral infarctions are unlikely to be cured. Control of attacks should be the goal. Partial seizures occurring early in life and in newborns have a favorable prognosis. Early treatment in adults also produces a favorable prognosis as long as an underlying progressive structural disease is not present.

EVALUATION FOR POSSIBLE SURGICAL TREATMENT WHEN PATIENT IS DRUG RESISTANT

Of all patients with refractory seizures, approximately 10% can benefit from anterior temporal lobectomy, amygdalohippocampectomy, or cortectomy if the epileptogenic zones are adequately identified.

Refractory complex partial seizures can be due to noncompliance, inadequate drug dosage, improper choice of drugs, or the presence of precipitating or aggravating factors such as a stressful home or work place, alcohol, sleep deprivation, and menses. Structural lesions such as an arteriovenous malformation or occult neoplasm must be identified.

If none of these factors are operative and the patient's complex partial seizures or secondary tonic-clonic seizures have been present for at least 3 or 4 years, show no signs of remission, and are of such severity and frequency as to interfere seriously with life, surgical treatment should be considered. Evaluation for surgery should be carried out without undue risk to life and without producing serious neurologic deficits. Excellent motivation and compliance are essential.

The evaluation process for surgical treatment is aimed at differentiating temporal from extratemporal epilepsy. Surgical resection of epileptogenic zones has varied percentages of success in eliminating seizures completely or eradicating 95% of epileptic attacks (Table 5).

After epileptogenic zones are localized by specialized techniques, it is determined whether they can be removed without impairing speech or memory. If the focus is within the anterior temporal lobe, the seizure may be arising primarily from medial (hippocampus or amygdala or both) or lateral structures. If seizures are extratemporal, they may originate from the frontal, parietal, or occipital lobes. An essential and indispensable test for speech and recent memory is the modified Wada test. It is routinely performed in all patients being evaluated for surgery. Sodium amylobarbitone is injected into one internal carotid artery, and tests for speech and memory are conducted during contralateral hemiplegia and the presence of ipsilateral hemispheric, high-amplitude, 1.5- to 3-Hz slowing on the EEG. Hemispheric lateralization of speech or memory is established by appropriate testing.

The decision to perform selective amygdalohippo-campectomy if there is medial temporal epilepsy or anterior temporal lobectomy if there is combined medial and lateral temporal epilepsy is based on two conditions: (1) that focal or regional seizures originate in one hippocampus or anterior temporal lobe, and (2) that there is no evidence of memory impairment originating in the contralateral temporal lobe. When seizures originate from the lateral temporal or extratemporal cortex, it is especially important to outline the precise site and extent of the seizure focus by chronic stereoelectroencephalography, subdural or epidural electrode recordings, and intraoperative electrocorticography. Intraoperative evoked potentials mapping the primary motor cortex and, if necessary, eloquent areas of the hemisphere dominant for language, usually precede cortical resections.

EPILEPSY IN INFANTS AND CHILDREN

method of
BARRY R. THARP, M.D.
Baylor College of Medicine
Houston, Texas

THE FIRST SEIZURE

A child's initial seizure may be due to an acute illness, such as a metabolic or infectious disorder; may be idiopathic but self-limited; or may be the beginning of epilepsy. If a specific acute cause is not found, a decision must be made about initiating chronic antiepileptic drug (AED) treatment. If there is no history of a prior neurologic illness and the child is neurologically normal and has a normal electroencephalogram (EEG), the risk of a subsequent seizure is approximately 26%. If the seizure appears to be the consequence of a static encephalopathy such as cerebral palsy and the EEG is abnormal, the recurrence risk may be as high as 60%. In the former situation no treatment is indicated. In the latter case, treatment is not required but should be considered, particularly if the seizure was partial (focal), the EEG shows a focal abnormality, or there is a history suggesting prior minor seizures.

SEIZURE TYPE AND EPILEPTIC SYNDROME

As part of the initial work-up the physician should attempt to determine the specific type of seizure the child experienced and, if possible, the seizure syndrome category into which the child falls (Tables 1 and 2). A syndrome as defined by the International League Against Epilepsy is "an epileptic disorder characterized by a cluster of signs and symptoms customarily occurring together. These include such items as type of seizure, etiology, anatomy, precipitating factors, age of onset, severity, chronicity, diurnal and circadian cycles and sometimes prognosis." A syndrome diagnosis allows one to more accurately define the epileptic disorder and may provide a long-term prognosis and the risk for subsequent seizures of a different type. The identification of a syndrome is easier if the child has already had seizures for some time or the EEG shows a pattern typical for a particular syndrome, e.g., an absence syndrome with a spike at 3 cycles per second and slow wave discharges (Table 3). Several epileptic syndromes have now been shown to be due to a specific gene mutation,

TABLE 5. **Results of Tailored Surgical Resection of Epileptogenic Zones**

Epilepsy Type	Complete Elimination or 95% Eradication of Seizures (%)
Temporal lobe epilepsy	
Medial	95
Lateral	80
Combined medial-lateral	85
Combined temporal and frontal	80
Frontal lobe epilepsy	
Medial	80
Dorsolateral	
Nondominant hemisphere	70
Dominant hemisphere	40
Parietal lobe epilepsy	80

TABLE 1. Classification of Epileptic Seizures

1. Focal (partial, localization related)
  1.1 Simple partial (consciousness not impaired)
    1.1.1 With motor signs
    1.1.2 With sensory symptoms
    1.1.3 With autonomic symptoms or signs
    1.1.4 With psychic symptoms (disturbance of higher cortical function)
  1.2 Complex partial (consciousness usually impaired)
    1.2.1 Simple partial seizures followed by impairment of consciousness
    1.2.2 With impairment of consciousness at onset
  1.3 Partial seizures evolving to secondarily generalized
    1.3.1 Simple partial seizures evolving to generalized seizures
    1.3.2 Complex partial seizures evolving to generalized seizures
    1.3.3 Simple partial seizures evolving to complex partial evolving to generalized seizures

2. Generalized seizures
  2.1 Nonconvulsive generalized
    2.1.1 Absence seizure
    2.1.2 Atypical absence seizure
  2.2 Convulsive generalized
    2.2.1 Myoclonic
    2.2.2 Clonic
    2.2.3 Tonic
    2.2.4 Tonic-clonic
    2.2.5 Atonic (drop attack)

3. Unclassified

Adapted from Proposal for revised clinical and electroencephalographic classification of epileptic seizures. Epilepsia 22:489–501, 1981.

and the abnormal protein encoded by the mutated gene has been identified.

BASIC PRINCIPLES OF ANTIEPILEPTIC DRUG THERAPY

Monotherapy is the goal of treatment. It is characterized by better compliance, fewer side effects, lesser teratogenicity, lower cost, and, in most instances, better seizure control than polytherapy. Drug interactions are avoided, and pharmacokinetics are simplified. The half-life and, therefore, dosage intervals are usually longer and compliance is enhanced. Seizure frequency may actually decrease as the number of drugs is reduced.

Polypharmacy may be necessary in children with more than one seizure type and those refractory to monotherapy. One usually combines AEDs that have different pharmacologic actions. Phenytoin (Dilantin) and carbamazepine (Tegretol) are therefore usually not given together. The synergistic interaction of two AEDs may be associated with improved seizure control. Children with refractory generalized nonconvulsive seizures (petit mal), for example, occasionally require a combination of divalproex sodium (Depakote) and ethosuximide (Zarontin) or lamotrigine (Lamictal).

The AED chosen for initial therapy should be one that has relatively low toxicity and few side effects, is highly effective for a particular seizure type or syndrome, has a long half-life that will afford rela-

TABLE 2. Classification of Epileptic Syndromes and Drugs Used to Treat Them

Syndrome	Antiepileptic Drug
Idiopathic epilepsies	
Localization related (partial, focal)	CBZ, PB, VPA, LTG,† PHT, GBP,† VGB,‡ PRM, CRZ
Generalized epilepsies	
Absence seizures	ESM, VPA, LTG,† CNZ
Generalized tonic-clonic	CBZ, VPA, PHT, PB
Juvenile myoclonic	VPA, PHT, LTG†
Myoclonic absence	VPA, ESM, LTG,† CNZ
Symptomatic	
Localization related	CBZ, PB, VPA, LTG,† PHT, GBP,† VGB,‡ PRM, CRZ
With generalized seizures	
Infantile spasms	ACTH, prednisone, VGB,‡ VPA (?), CNZ (?)
Lennox-Gastaut syndrome	VPA,* LTG,† CNZ, CRZ

* Not FDA approved for this indication.
† Not FDA approved for children.
‡ Not available in the United States.
Abbreviations: PHT = phenytoin (Dilantin); CBZ = carbamazepine (Tegretol); CRZ = clorazepate (Tranxene); CNZ = clonazepam (Klonopin); ESM = ethosuximide (Zarontin); GBP = gabapentin (Neurontin); LTG = lamotrigine (Lamictal); PB = phenobarbital; PRM = primidone (Mysoline); VGB = vigabatrin; VPA = valproate (divalproex sodium); ACTH = corticotropin.

tively smooth serum levels and good compliance, is cost-effective, and, in younger children and infants, can be administered as an oral suspension. Table 4 lists the common AEDs used in pediatrics. A drug with a long half-life, e.g., ethosuximide, phenytoin, and phenobarbital, may be administered once a day.

Elimination kinetics should also be considered when choosing the initial AED. Linear or first-order kinetics (a constant fractional amount of the drug eliminated per unit of time independent of the concentration of the drug in the serum) is preferable to nonlinear or dose-dependent, saturable or concentration-dependent kinetics (as the level of the drug increases the elimination declines as the elimination mechanisms become saturated). Divalproex sodium and phenytoin are in the latter category.

INITIATION OF THERAPY

The kinetics of a drug determines the initial dose and the interval between dosage increments. With linear kinetics, one is better able to anticipate serum levels after each dosage increase, whereas drugs with nonlinear kinetics may require closer monitoring of levels. Phenytoin has linear kinetics until the serum level approaches the therapeutic range, when nonlin-

TABLE 3. Absence Syndromes

Childhood absence epilepsy
Juvenile absence epilepsy
Juvenile myoclonus epilepsy
Epilepsy with myoclonic absences
Lennox-Gastaut syndrome
Myoclonic astatic epilepsy

TABLE 4. Drug Therapy for Seizures

Drug	Dosage		Blood Level	Side Effects	Laboratory
	Starting	Maintenance			
Carbamazepine (Tegretol)	5–10 mg/kg/d	10–40 mg/kg/d	5–12 µg/mL	Diplopia, drowsiness, dizziness, headache, rash, behavioral changes, occasionally increased seizures and/or new seizures (drop attacks), low serum sodium (rare), leukopenia and aplastic anemia (rare), hepatotoxicity (rare), level increased by erythromycin	CBC after initial 4–6 wk, then prn; if initial WBC low (particularly ANC) repeat as needed
Clonazepam (Klonopin)	0.03 mg/kg/d	0.2 mg/kg/d	Not used	Behavioral changes, drowsiness, swallowing dysfunction causing increased secretions	If clinically indicated (e.g., bruising, unexplained fevers)
Clorazepate (Tranxene)	0.3 mg/kg/d	0.4–3 mg/kg/d	Not used	Sedation, ataxia, swallowing dysfunction with increased drooling, behavioral changes	Not required
Divalproex sodium (Depakote) Valproate (Depakene)	15 mg/kg/d	60–80 mg/kg/d	50–150 µg/mL	Drowsiness, behavioral changes, nausea, anorexia, weight gain, alopecia, tremor, thrombocytopenia, easy bruising, leukopenia, hepatic necrosis (rare), pancreatitis (rare)	Hepatic function tests every 1–2 mo during the first 6 mo of therapy (optional), amylase if abdominal pain, CBC and plts at high doses
Ethosuximide (Zarontin)	5–10 mg/kg/d	20–30 mg/kg/d	40–100 µg/mL (may increase to 150)	Drowsiness, rash, behavioral changes, headaches, hiccoughs, nausea, vomiting, aplastic anemia (rare), lupus-like syndrome (rare), Stevens–Johnson syndrome (rare)	CBC and plts after first 1–2 mo, prn thereafter
Felbamate (Felbatol)	15 mg/kg/d	45–60 mg/kg/d	50–100 µg/mL	Headache, insomnia, vomiting, anorexia, aplastic anemia (common), hepatic failure (common), not recommended except in refractory epilepsy	CBC and plts every 2 wk, hepatic function tests every month
Gabapentin (Neurontin)*	10 mg/kg/d	40–80 mg/kg/d	Not established (probably 7–12 µg/mL)	Sedation, behavioral changes, ataxia, nausea, weight gain, headache, increased seizures	CBC and plts every 3 mo for first 6 mo, chemical panel prn (routine monitoring may not be necessary)
Lamotrigine (Lamictal)*	Monotherapy 1 mg/kg/d; Add to VPA 0.5 mg/kg/d; Add to inducer (PB, CBZ, PHT) 2 mg/kg/d	10–12 mg/kg/d; 2–5 mg/kg/d; 15–20 mg/kg/d	Not established	Rash, behavioral changes, sedation, headache, nausea, occasionally seizures worsen, tremor	CBC and plts every 3 mo for first 6 mo, chemical panel prn (routine monitoring may not be necessary)
Phenytoin (Dilantin)	4–8 mg/kg/d	4–8 mg/kg/d (older children, adolescents 300 mg/d)	10–20 µg/mL	Rash, dizziness, behavioral changes, gingival hyperplasia, hirsutism, coarse facies, lupus syndrome (rare), hepatic toxicity (rare), Stevens–Johnson syndrome (rare)	Routine laboratory tests not recommended
Fosphenytoin (Cerebyx)	Status epilepticus 20 mg PE/kg (infusion rate < 150 mg/min)				
Phenobarbital	3–4 mg/kg/d	4–6 mg/kg/d	10–40 µg/mL	Behavioral changes, hyperactivity, sedation, rash, Stevens–Johnson syndrome (rare)	Routine laboratory tests not recommended
Primidone (Mysoline)	1–2 mg/kg/d	10–20 mg/kg/d	5–12 µg/mL (phenobarbital level 1.2 × higher)	See phenobarbital; also dizziness, nausea and vomiting, particularly at initiation of therapy	Routine laboratory tests not recommended

*Not FDA approved for children.
Abbreviations: VPA = valproate; PB = phenobarbital; CBZ = carbamazepine; PHT = phenytoin; CBC = complete blood count; plts = platelet count; WBC = white blood cell count; ANC = absolute neutrophil count.

ear kinetics take over. At this point, extremely small increases in dose result in large increases of the serum level and potential toxicity. At high serum levels, the half-life is significantly longer. A minimal increase in daily dosage is required to attain the desired level, and in some instances an increase made every other day may suffice.

Most AEDs should be started at about 10 to 25% of the planned maintenance dose. AEDs with a long half-life can be started at close to the maintenance dose. If seizures are frequent, the dose can be increased at intervals approximating 5 half-lives. This allows the serum level to plateau between each dosage increment. The dose should be increased until seizures stop (regardless of the serum level), there are unremitting side effects, or levels reach a supratherapeutic range without a significant impact on the seizure frequency. If side effects appear and are tolerable, the dosage should be held at that level for up to 2 weeks to determine whether the symptoms are transient. If side effects disappear and seizures continue, the dosage increases can continue at a slower rate. If the initial seizure frequency is low, the AED dose should be increased to the lower end of the therapeutic range and stabilized until a satisfactory observation period passes. If seizures continue, further slow increments can be made.

It may be necessary to give patients larger than standard doses of an AED to reach therapeutic levels. Although low levels may be caused by poor compliance, they may be secondary to hypermetabolism of the AED, i.e., the clearance is higher because of increased hepatic metabolism. If levels are not increasing as anticipated and noncompliance is unlikely, the child should be given a loading dose under medical observation and levels measured for the next 24 hours. If the levels remain low, high daily doses are indicated.

As a child grows, the clearance of the AED decreases and approaches adult rates in the late first decade and adolescence. Serum levels remain stable for many years even though the per-kilogram dose declines, and frequent measurement of the serum levels is not necessary. If a child is placed on another long-term therapy, for example, for asthma, it may be necessary to measure the AED level after the dosage of the new drug has been stabilized. It is helpful to have a baseline level once seizure control has been attained to compare with levels obtained during periods of seizure recurrence.

Serum levels should be used as guides to therapy only. Each individual has his or her own optimal therapeutic level, which may be outside the usual range. I often increase carbamazepine levels to the midteens and divalproex levels to 150 to 180 μg per mL. In the latter case, dose-related hematologic (low platelet counts) and neurologic (tremor and behavioral changes) side effects may occur.

When seizures are resistant to the initial AED, a second is added. If the initial drug had been partially effective, it should be continued until reasonable levels of the new AED are achieved and then tapered. If the initial AED was ineffective, it can be tapered as the dose of the second drug is increased. The pharmacokinetics of the second drug may be altered by the first, and serum levels may have to be monitored to determine when the second drug is in the low therapeutic range.

Ideally, daily AED doses should be repeated at intervals slightly shorter than the half-life to avoid excessive swings in the serum levels. The longer the half-life, the less frequent the dosing. Patients taking AEDs in a single daily dose have the advantage of "makeup" dosing, i.e., if a dose is missed one day, a double dose can be taken the next day. Makeup dosing of AEDs with short half-lives might lead to high levels and accompanying side effects a few hours after medication is taken. Compliance is improved when medications are taken on schedule and prompted by an association with a routine activity of daily living, e.g., morning hygiene or lunch.

DISCONTINUANCE OF ANTIEPILEPTIC DRUGS

The current practice is to discontinue anticonvulsants 1 to 2 years after the last seizure. The overall risk of recurrence is approximately 30%. The risk is higher if the EEG done at the time of discontinuance is abnormal; the child was older than 12 years at the onset of seizures or has a particular epileptic syndrome, e.g., juvenile myoclonic epilepsy; or the neurologic examination is abnormal. The recurrence risk after 2 seizure-free years is under 15% if the child is young, has a normal EEG, is neurologically and intellectually normal, and has a negative family history of seizures.

The drugs should be withdrawn slowly one at a time. The rate of tapering is not relevant, but abrupt discontinuance is not recommended. We usually taper each drug over several weeks, using a somewhat longer withdrawal period with AEDs that have long half-lives.

LABORATORY MONITORING

I usually obtain a complete blood count, platelet count, and blood chemistry tests as baseline and to screen the child for occult disease before initiating a new AED. Routine follow-up laboratory testing is not recommended in the otherwise healthy individual.

STATUS EPILEPTICUS

Seizures that continue for 30 minutes or recurrent seizures without return of consciousness constitute status epilepticus. The physician must make a decision on a case-by-case basis about the urgency of the situation and whether intravenous, rectal, or oral therapy suffices. Initial treatment consists of supporting vital functions and stopping the seizures as quickly as possible. The benzodiazepines (BZDs) (lorazepam [Ativan], diazepam [Valium], and midazolam [Versed]), phenobarbital, and phenytoin are the standard treatments. Fosphenytoin (Cerebyx) will soon replace phenytoin for parenteral administration because it lacks the unfavorable side effects of phenytoin, i.e., pain at the injection site, venous occlusion, cardiac toxicity necessitating extremely slow intravenous administration, poor absorption after intramuscular injection, and poor solubility in intravenous glucose-containing solutions. It is administered as phenytoin sodium equivalents (PE), i.e., the same dose as used for phenytoin. Fosphenytoin should not be administered faster than 150 mg PE per minute. Most physicians initiate therapy with one of the BZDs and follow with a longer acting AED, e.g., phenytoin. The BZD dose may be repeated once if the initial dose is ineffective, but further injections are usually not effective and lead to respiratory depression and the need for intubation. Phenobarbital given after a BZD increases the risk of respiratory depression.

An injectable form of valproate sodium (Depacon) has recently been released. It can be use for continuance of maintenance therapy in a child unable to take oral medication or in treating some forms of status epilepticus.

NEONATAL SEIZURES

Ideally, seizures should be confirmed by a simultaneous EEG, as many abnormal movements in neonates are not epileptic. If an emergency EEG is not available, treatment should be initiated for behaviors that have a high correlation with epileptic EEG patterns, including focal and multifocal clonus, focal tonus involving the limbs or eyes, and, occasionally, myoclonus. Other less clearly epileptic behaviors should be treated on a case-by-case basis and attempts made to obtain an EEG after therapy is initiated.

After an AED is administered intravenously, the clinical manifestations of seizures often cease and the electrical seizures continue unabated. Only the EEG can confirm the persistence of these subclinical seizures.

Hypoglycemia should be treated promptly with 25% intravenous glucose, hypocalcemia with 100 to 200 mg of intravenous 5% calcium gluconate per kg, and hypomagnesemia with 0.2 to 0.4 mEq of 50% magnesium sulfate per kg per 24 hours intravenously.

The standard intravenous AEDs are phenobarbital (20 to 30 mg per kg) and fosphenytoin (20 mg PE per kg). The rate of administration has not been established for neonates but should probably not exceed 3 to 5 mg per kg per minute. Intravenous BZDs are useful initially but are less effective as long-term therapy.

If the electrical and clinical seizures stop, the AED should be discontinued 1 to 2 weeks after the last seizure.

FEBRILE SEIZURES

Two to 5% of all children experience at least one febrile seizure between the ages of 6 months and 5 years. In most cases chronic therapy is not initiated. If the seizures recur frequently or are unusually prolonged or associated with prolonged apnea, or if the family prefers therapy, the physician has two choices: (1) long-term phenobarbital (maintaining serum levels above 15 μg per mL) or (2) rectal diazepam (0.33 mg per kg) every 8 hours until the fever subsides. Chronic phenobarbital therapy often produces hyperactivity, a personality change, or, less commonly, sedation necessitating discontinuance of the drug.

RECTAL THERAPY

Rectal BZDs are an effective and relatively safe emergency treatment, particularly in patients who live at some distance from a medical facility, those requiring emergency therapy while traveling, and those whose seizures occur in clusters. Diazepam (0.3 to 0.5 mg per kg) is the most commonly used rectal AED. In the United States, the parenteral solution is the only preparation currently available for rectal use. Respiratory depression may occur at high doses; therefore, the individual administering the medication should be trained in cardiopulmonary resuscitation. I have also found it useful to give a test dose under the physician's observation to determine its effect on mentation and respiration.

Many AEDs can be given rectally for short periods, e.g., postoperatively, if the patient is unconscious, if a parenteral form of their chronic AED is not available, or during illnesses when oral intake is limited. The currently available oral suspensions of clonazepam (Klonopin) (0.1 mg per kg), valproate (maintenance dose diluted with an equal volume of water), and carbamazepine (maintenance dose diluted with an equal volume of water) may be used for short periods. Carbamazepine has a significant cathartic effect. Secobarbital (Seconal),* 5 mg of the parenteral solution per kg, also produces adequate anticonvulsant levels 30 to 90 minutes after instillation.

INFANTILE SPASMS

Infantile bilateral flexion and extension spasms typically appear between 4 and 12 months of age, occur in clusters, and are usually accompanied by a slowing of development and a characteristic EEG pattern (hypsarrhythmia). Infants are divided into three groups. The *symptomatic* group is associated with various static encephalopathies including perinatal hypoxia-ischemia; infections; congenital brain malformations and chromosomal disorders; the neurocutaneous syndromes, particularly tuberous sclerosis; and inherited metabolic disorders. In *cryptogenic* cases, an encephalopathy is suspected but none is identified; in *idiopathic* cases, development is normal before the onset of the spasms. More than 85% of children have significant long-term neurologic sequelae. The prognosis is worse in children with symptomatic spasms.

---

*Not FDA approved for this indication.

The treatment of choice is intramuscular corticotropin (ACTH) in doses of 20 to 30 units of ACTH (Acthar Gel) daily for 2 weeks. If spasms continue, the dose is increased to 30 to 40 units for 4 weeks. If there is no response, the ACTH is tapered over 1 to 2 weeks and prednisone therapy, 2 mg per kg, is begun and continued for 4 weeks. If spasms stop, the treatment is tapered and the child is reassessed at 2 and 4 weeks. In some infants, intramuscular injections are impracticable or refused by the family. In these instances prednisone therapy is initiated. Side effects include irritability and insomnia, cushingoid changes, and hypertension. Elective immunizations should be postponed during steroid therapy.

Divalproex, clonazepam, and, in Europe, vigabatrin (Sabril) have also been used to treat spasms, but controlled studies comparing their efficacy to that of steroids are needed.

THE KETOGENIC DIET

There has been a resurgence of interest in the ketogenic diet because of concerns over the toxicity of AEDs. The diet consists of three to four parts fat to one part protein and carbohydrate. The high fat content and relative absence of carbohydrate produce a persistent ketosis, which appears to have a direct anticonvulsant effect. The diet is not curative but suppresses seizures in approximately 50% of patients, particularly those between 7 and 10 years of age. The diet is continued for at least 2 years and should be supervised by a well-trained dietitian.

ATTENTION-DEFICIT/HYPERACTIVITY DISORDER

method of
BENNETT A. SHAYWITZ, M.D.
Yale University School of Medicine
New Haven, Connecticut

Attention-deficit/hyperactivity disorder (ADHD) is now recognized as the most common neurobehavioral disorder of childhood, affecting children across the full span of development, from preschool to school age and continuing into adult life. Investigators have reported a wide array of prevalence estimates: early studies using teachers' ratings indicated prevalence rates between 10 and 20%; later studies indicated prevalence rates of 3% up to 15%. More recent reports indicate prevalence rates between 2 and 11%. ADHD now constitutes perhaps 50% of referrals to child neurologists, neuropsychologists, behavioral pediatricians, and child psychiatrists; furthermore, on the basis of studies examining the prevalence of stimulant medication usage in children, it appears that the disorder is being diagnosed more frequently now than a decade ago.

The diagnosis of ADHD is established on the basis of a history of symptoms representing the cardinal constructs of ADHD—inattention, impulsivity, and, at times, hyperactivity. How to quantitate these symptoms and then how many symptoms are necessary for diagnosis remain an issue in ongoing research. However, at the present time, *Diagnostic and Statistical Manual of Mental Disorders*, fourth edition (DSM-IV) criteria, diagnostic criteria developed by consensus agreement of a panel of experts, form the basis of the most widely recognized diagnostic schema. These symptoms can be assessed systematically and quantified to some degree by using symptom rating scales for teachers and for parents.

In addition to specific symptoms of the disorder, certain overall trends or characteristics are evident. Symptoms diagnostic of ADHD manifest a developmental trend; that is, until 3 years of age activity levels increase but then continue a downward trend, so that by adolescence gross motor hyperactivity is generally no longer present. However, attentional deficits persist. Awareness of this developmental pattern is particularly important because it is at times mistakenly assumed that inasmuch as the child is no longer hyperactive, he or she is free from problems and no longer in need of, for example, special education services.

Not only do the symptoms of ADHD vary over time, they also exhibit situational variability. The variability not only extends to different settings and situations but also refers to the lack of predictability of the child's behavior that is often seen from minute to minute or day to day, even in similar situations. Current DSM-IV criteria require that the symptoms of ADHD be present in two or more settings, for example at home and in school.

MANAGEMENT

Management of ADHD represents a complex and intricate balance of a variety of treatment strategies encompassing educational, cognitive-behavioral and pharmacologic interventions, what has been termed a multimodality approach. Establishing the diagnosis, using DSM-IV criteria, is the initial focus of management, and once this has been accomplished, the diagnosis and its implications must then be interpreted to the child, his or her parents, and critical school personnel. Management of ADHD encompasses two general domains: (1) nonpharmacologic (educational and cognitive-behavioral and other psychologic and psychiatric approaches); and (2) pharmacologic therapies. Educational management of children with ADHD not only must recogize the frequently associated learning disability but in addition must recognize and deal effectively with academic issues related to the inattention and impulsivity. Such approaches have been reviewed previously and include minimizing distracting stimuli by preferential seating in carrels or in a self-contained classroom; providing a one-on-one tutorial by increasing teacher availability through the use of aides or in a resource room; ensuring structure and predictable routines; monitoring and, if necessary, modifying nonacademic structured times such as in the lunchroom, recess, or physical education; teaching organizational and work-study skills, such as organizing materials and time. Cognitive-behavioral therapy (CBT), a term representing a host of cognitive components and behavioral strategies including operant techniques (positive and negative reinforcement) and parent counseling, has come to represent a widely employed alternative to pharmacotherapy. Unfortunately, both short- and long-term gains with CBT have been quite limited, and a number of investigators have questioned whether CBT combined with pharmacotherapy offers any advantages to pharmacotherapy alone. However, formidable methodologic difficulties plague such studies and may obscure the effects of combined CBT and pharmacotherapy. Several reports suggest that CBT may, in fact, be a useful adjunct to pharmacotherapy. Individual psychotherapy may be a helpful component of therapy in some children who have serious psychiatric problems or are unable to cope with their disability. Although the exclusive use of psychotherapy is rarely recommended in ADHD, it is often employed as part of multimodality therapy—individual and group psychotherapy for the child and for the parents.

Medication is the most widely used modality in the management of ADHD. Stimulants represent the treatment of choice, not only because so much is known about their actions and side effects, but because until recently few effective alternatives have been available. More recently, a number of other classes of compounds have been used successfully in ADHD. These include antidepressants* (tricyclic agents such as imipramine [Tofranil] and desipramine [Norpramin]; bupropion [Wellbutrin]; fluoxetine [Prozac]), anticonvulsants (carbamazepine [Tegretol]*), and miscellaneous drugs (guanfacine [Tenex],* clonidine [Catapres]*). Except for the tricyclic agents, experience with their use is relatively limited. They were reviewed by Spencer and colleagues in 1996.†

Historically, a stimulant, D-amphetamine, was the first agent found to be effective in the treatment of hyperactivity, and since that initial report abundant evidence from many investigative groups supports the belief that stimulants (amphetamine, methylphenidate [MPH] [Ritalin], pemoline [Cylert]) are effective in reducing activity levels and improving attention in 60 to 70% of children with ADHD. In contrast to the plethora of studies documenting the salutary effects of stimulants on attention and activity in children with ADHD, their effects on cognitive function remain controversial. Despite some early studies suggesting a positive effect of stimulants on learning or academic achievement, the consensus indicates that stimulants should not be expected to improve reading or learning and achievement. Despite the half-century of experience with stimulants in children, the effects of these agents on aggressive kinds of behaviors is still not clear. Aggressive behavior, as determined by 5-minute-long observations during relatively short-term amphetamine administration, is, indeed, reduced. As reviewed by Pelham and Murphy,‡ it is likely that combined pharmaco-

therapy and behavioral therapy is more effective than either alone in children with both conduct disorder (and/or oppositional disorder) and ADHD.

To a great extent, the decision to initiate pharmacotherapy is based on a number of diverse and difficult to define general factors such as the physician's clinical judgment; her or his understanding of the child, the family, and the school environment; and knowledge of educational practices within the community. However, two specific considerations are educational placement and focus on target symptoms.

Educational Placement

Educational placement represents perhaps the most critical factor in the success of pharmacotherapy, because stimulant therapy will almost certainly be ineffective unless the child's educational placement is satisfactory. Thus, it is vital for the physician to do everything to ensure that the school system has properly evaluated the child and that the most appropriate school placement has been effected.

Focus on Target Symptoms

Before prescribing medication the physician must determine which particular symptoms are the targets of the treatment and decide at which times these symptoms are most troublesome. Contrary to popular notions, hyperactivity alone is seldom a sufficient reason for initiation of pharmacotherapy. In fact, hyperactivity tends to abate with increasing age, no matter what treatment is employed.

In general, stimulants are more effective for amelioration of attentional difficulties in school than for improvement of the child's behavior or performance at home. In part, this dichotomy between satisfactory improvement at school with relatively less improvement at home correlates with the biologic availability of the stimulant. It also reflects the fact that those characteristics of attentional deficit that are most amenable to the effects of stimulants, for example, being able to follow a complicated set of directions amid the distractions caused by 25 other children, are put to the test in school. It is rare for the child to be placed in a similiar stressful situation at home.

Not surprisingly, prediction of clinical response to stimulants does not appear to depend on either an abnormal neurologic examination or an abnormal electroencephalogram. Some investigators have suggested that such a prediction can be reliably determined using double-blind, placebo-controlled methodology to assess the child's performance on specific tests conducted in a laboratory setting. Although such procedures may be advantageous in particular situations, they are generally not necessary, and most experienced clinicians consider the administration of medication in the child's real-life setting the only valid therapeutic trial. Parenthetically, it should be noted that a positive response to stimulants may be observed in nonhyperactive children, and thus

---

*Not FDA approved for this indication.

†See Spencer T, Biederman J, Wilens T, et al: Pharmacotherapy of attention-deficit hyperactivity disorders across the life cycle. J Am Acad Child Adolesc Psychiatry 35:409–432, 1996.

‡See Pelham WE, Murphy HA: Attention deficit and conduct disorders. In Hersen M (ed): Pharmacological and Behavioral Treatment: An Integrative Approach. New York, John Wiley & Sons, 1986, pp 108–148.

improvement in symptoms with therapy should not be construed as implying that the diagnosis of ADHD was, indeed, correct.

Children with ADHD are characteristically extremely sensitive to alterations in their environment and need more time to adjust to new situations. Thus, we recommend initiation of pharmacotherapy only if the child has had an opportunity to adjust to any environmental alteration. This means that in most cases medication should not be initiated simultaneously with the child's beginning a new school year or with his or her entrance into a classroom setting that has just been changed. Such a practice not only allows the physician to determine the child's baseline functioning without medication, but more important, gives the child an opportunity to adjust to the new environment before beginning stimulant therapy. However, if past experience suggests that pharmacotherapy has made such a difference in the child's behavior that entry into a new class without medication would probably result in the child being viewed in a negative fashion by the new teachers, it would seem most reasonable to consider beginning medication before entry into the new environment. In practice, such a situation is most likely to arise when the child enters, for example, a middle or a junior high school setting and must contend with the additional stresses of a new setting, departmentalized programs, and older peers.

Administration and Dosage

Both the pharmacokinetics and the behavioral effects of MPH are indistinguishable whether it is given with breakfast or 30 minutes before breakfast. A reasonable approach is to begin with an initial dosage of 0.3 mg per kg given in the morning immediately before the child leaves for school. Thus, by the time the child reaches school, MPH should be absorbed, and peak levels should be attained within 2 to 3 hours. The school should be encouraged to place the child in academic subjects during these morning hours so that the effects of the drug on attentional processes are maximal when the child needs the most help. Thus, by lunchtime, and in afternoon classes (ideally, nonacademic subjects), the medication effect will be waning but the need for the drug not as great. Clinical response is monitored by obtaining weekly feedback from the parents and, most important, from the school. This may be accomplished most efficiently by weekly rating scales filled out by the child's primary academic teacher(s). If the child is not responding satisfactorily after 2 weeks of treatment, the MPH dosage should be increased to 0.6 to 0.8 mg per kg. If there is no response after 2 weeks at this dose, the physician should consider switching to another medication and possibly reassessing the patient.

Determining the most effective dose of medication is further complicated because an optimal dosage for one target symptom may not be optimal for a different symptom. Thus, Sprague and Sleator have suggested that although high doses of MPH (1.0 mg per kg) may produce improvement in global measures of activity, scores on memory tasks and performance on attentional tests may be poorer at a high dose compared with a low dose (0.3 mg per kg). However, other investigators have found that within a range of 0.3 to 0.8 mg per kg, performance on both behavioral and cognitive tasks improves in a dose-related fashion. Swanson and colleagues suggested that depending on the cognitive task, the relationship of dose to performance may follow either a quadratic (U-shaped) function or a linear function.

At least one study documents what many clinicians know only too well: poor compliance in taking stimulant medications may be a significant problem in children with ADHD. Poor compliance in taking medications may explain some of the variability and conflicting results of various studies of the effects of stimulants.

On many occasions the child will do well in the morning at the 0.3 mg per kg dose but the effects appear to wear off by early afternoon. In this situation, it is reasonable to add another 0.3 mg per kg dose in the morning (for a total morning dose of 0.6 mg per kg). If afternoon function is still problematic, a second 0.3 mg per kg dose may be given 3 hours later. Experience has shown that "piggybacking" a second dose in this manner before the initial dose has worn off eliminates the problems seen with decreasing availability of the medication. Another option would be to employ a stimulant with a longer duration of action, such as amphetamine, or pemoline. However, although D-amphetamine has an apparent biologic half-life of 6.6 hours for tablets and 8.4 hours for the sustained-release preparation, the behavioral effects last no longer than 4 hours with either form. The dose of amphetamine (Dexedrine) is calculated as approximately two thirds of the MPH dose, milligram per milligram. Still another possibility is to consider the use of the sustained-release preparation of MPH (SR-20). Pemoline also provides a longer duration of action. Although not as widely used as MPH and amphetamine, the improvement rate in ADHD after pemoline therapy is similar to that observed with the other stimulants. Furthermore, its action may continue even after treatment is stopped. It is supplied in capsules of 18.75, 37.5, and 75 mg. The dosage varies between 0.5 and 3.0 mg per kg, with a starting dose of 18.75 mg per day and a dosage range between 37.5 and 112.5 mg per day. However, pemoline may adversely affect liver function, and periodic monitoring of liver function tests is required when the drug is used. This necessity for frequent blood sampling has limited the clinical usefulness of the agent.

Another important issue that must be considered is whether medication should be administered daily, or just on school days, with drug holidays when the child is away from school. Administration solely during school offers the advantage of limiting potential toxicity while maximizing the effect of MPH when it is most needed, i.e., during the school day. I usually prescribe MPH each school day but omit the drug on weekends, school holidays, during the summer, and for the first 4 to 6 weeks of the new school year. Discontinuing MPH at the end of one school year enables evaluation of how the child will do without medications and offers a regular opportunity to discontinue medications permanently. Thus, if it appears that the patient is doing well without medication during the initial portion of the new school year, I do not resume pharmacotherapy. However, careful follow-up is critical because as the school year continues and academic pressures increase, initial sanguine assumptions about the lack of a need for medication may prove to be overly optimistic.

Clearly, such a procedure may need to be modified in particular situations. Thus, on occasions when a particular child's impulsivity and activity are preventing optimal peer and family interaction, I have continued MPH therapy on weekends. Furthermore, if the child's response to medication has been so dramatic that starting a new school year without medication would be detrimental to his or her best interests, consideration should be given to initiating treatment as soon as school begins.

Side Effects

Insomnia or sleep disturbances and decreased appetite represent the most frequently observed side effects of stimulants, with weight loss, irritability, and abdominal pains almost as common. These and a host of other less frequent side effects (e.g., headaches, nausea, dizziness, dry mouth, constipation) usually disappear as the child becomes tolerant to the medication, or resolve if the dosage is reduced. Cardiovascular function in ADHD children receiving oral stimulants is reassuringly normal. Whether MPH affects growth remains an important question. This problem may be minimized if the drug is discontinued for a time to allow catch-up growth to occur. In practice this suggests that if the medication could be omitted for long periods (e.g., summer vacations, holidays, weekends) the total yearly dose would be reduced and presumably the detrimental effects on stature lessened.

GILLES DE LA TOURETTE SYNDROME

method of
JOSEPH JANKOVIC, M.D.
Baylor College of Medicine
Houston, Texas

Gilles de la Tourette syndrome (TS) is a chronic, childhood-onset neurologic disorder manifested by motor and vocal tics and often accompanied by neurobehavioral problems such as obsessive-compulsive disorder (OCD), attention-deficit/hyperactivity disorder (ADHD), and lack of impulse control. Once considered a rare psychiatric curiosity, TS is now recognized as a relatively common neurologic

and behavioral disorder. Because the clinical criteria are not well defined, the prevalence rates have been estimated to vary between 0.1 and 1%.

The cause of TS is yet unknown, but the disorder appears to be inherited in nearly all patients. The clinical expression of this genetic defect may be different in various family members. The clinical heterogeneity, marked fluctuation severity, and bizarre nature of some of the symptoms are some of the reasons why the disorder is often not recognized or is misdiagnosed. Educational efforts directed to physicians, educators, and the general public have increased the awareness about TS. Many patients, however, still remain undiagnosed, or their symptoms are wrongly attributed to "habits," "allergies," "hyperactivity," "nervousness," and many other conditions.

Tics, the clinical hallmark of TS, consist of relatively brief and intermittent movements (motor tics) or sounds (phonic tics). Currently accepted criteria require both types of tics to be present for the diagnosis of TS. Motor tics are usually abrupt in onset and rapid (clonic tics), but they may be slower, causing a briefly sustained abnormal posture (dystonic tics) or an isometric contraction (tonic tics). *Simple motor tics* involve only one group of muscles, causing a brief, jerklike movement or a single, meaningless sound. Examples of simple clonic motor tics include blinking, nose twitching, and head jerking; simple dystonic tics include blepharospasm, oculogyric movements, bruxism, sustained mouth opening, torticollis, and shoulder rotation; and tensing of abdominal or limb muscles is an example of a tonic tic. *Complex motor tics* consist of coordinated, sequenced movements resembling normal motor acts or gestures that are inappropriately intense and timed. They may be seemingly nonpurposeful, such as head shaking or trunk bending, or they may seem purposeful, such as touching, throwing, hitting, jumping, and kicking. Additional examples of complex motor tics include gesturing "the finger" (copropraxia) or imitating gestures (echopraxia). *Simple phonic tics* typically consist of sniffing, throat clearing, grunting, squeaking, screaming, coughing, blowing, and sucking sounds. *Complex phonic tics* include linguistically meaningful utterances and verbalizations, such as shouting of obscenities or profanities (coprolalia); repetition of someone else's words or phrases (echolalia); and repetition of one's own utterances, particularly the last syllable, word, or phrase in a sentence (palilalia).

Most motor and phonic tics are preceded by premonitory feelings or sensations, such as "a burning feeling" in the eye before an eye blink, "a tension or a crick in the neck" relieved by stretching of the neck or jerking of the head, a "feeling of tightness or constriction" relieved by arm or leg extension, "nasal stuffiness" before a sniff, "dry or sore throat" before throat clearing or grunting, and "itching" before a rotatory movement of the scapula. The sensations or feelings that often precede motor tics usually occur out of a background of relative normalcy and are clearly involuntary, even though the movements (motor tics) or noises (phonic tics) that occur in response to these premonitory symptoms may be regarded as semivoluntary or involuntary. Many patients report that they have to repeat a particular movement to relieve the uncomfortable urge and until "it feels good." The "just right" feeling has been associated with compulsive behavior, and as such the involuntary movement may be regarded as a compulsive tic. Some complex motor tics may be difficult to differentiate from compulsions, but compulsions are often preceded by or associated with a feeling of anxiety or panic, as well as an irresistible urge to perform the movement or sound because of a fear that if it is not promptly or properly executed something "bad" will happen.

In addition to motor and phonic tics, patients with TS often exhibit a variety of behavioral symptoms, particularly ADHD and OCD. These co-morbid conditions often interfere with learning, academic and work performance, social adjustment, and psychosocial development. A common link between the motor and behavioral manifestations of TS is a loss of impulse control. Indeed, many of the behavioral problems, such as uncontrollable temper outbursts, seen in patients with TS can be attributed to poor impulse control. Some TS patients exhibit inappropriate sexual aggressiveness, and antisocial, oppositional, violent, and self-injurious behavior. Conduct disorders and problems with discipline at home and in school are among the most frequently discussed topics during an office visit.

Although the pathogenetic mechanisms of TS are still unknown, the weight of evidence supports organic rather than psychogenic origin. Sleep studies have provided additional evidence that tics are truly involuntary, in that tics are often present in all stages of sleep. Quantitative magnetic resonance imaging studies have found subtle, but possibly important, reductions in the volume of caudate nuclei in patients with TS. In contrast, the corpus callosum has been found to be larger in children with TS than in normal control subjects. Positron emission tomography (PET) has shown variable rates of glucose utilization in basal ganglia of patients compared with control subjects, but fluorodopa uptake and the density of dopamine receptors, as determined by PET studies, have demonstrated no significant abnormalities. An alteration in the amounts of central neurotransmitters has been suggested, chiefly because of relatively consistent responses to modulation of the dopaminergic system. Dopamine antagonists and depletors generally have ameliorating effects on tics, whereas drugs that enhance central dopaminergic activity exacerbate tics. Other biochemical abnormalities in postmortem brains include low serotonin levels, low glutamate levels in the globus pallidus internum, and low cyclic AMP levels in the cortex.

The most intriguing hypothesis, supported by increased ^{3}H-mazindol binding in postmortem brains and by increased binding of the dopamine transporter ligand 2β-carboxymethoxy-3β-4(^{123}I)iodophenyl trepane demonstrated by single photon emission computed tomography, suggests that TS represents a developmental disorder resulting in dopaminergic hyperinnervation of the ventral striatum. This portion of the basal ganglia is anatomically and functionally linked to the limbic system. The link between the basal ganglia and the limbic system may explain the frequent association of tics and complex behavioral problems. A disturbance in sex hormone levels and activity and certain excitatory neurotransmitters that normally influence the development of these structures may be ultimately expressed as TS. This hypothesis may explain the remarkable sex difference in TS, with males outnumbering females by 3 to 1, the exacerbation of symptoms at the time of puberty and during the estrogenic phase of the menstrual cycle, the characteristic occurrence of sexually related complex motor and phonic tics, and a variety of behavioral manifestations with sexual content. According to this hypothesis, the gene defect in TS results in an abnormal production of gonadal steroid hormones and increased trophic influence exerted by the excitatory amino acids causing disordered development and increased innervation of the striatum and the limbic system. Further studies are needed to test this hypothesis.

Finding a genetic marker, and ultimately the gene, has been the highest priority in TS research during the past decade. Unfortunately, despite a concentrated effort by many investigators, the TS gene has thus far eluded this intensive search. Assuming that genetic heterogeneity is not an important factor in TS, more than 95% of the genome has already been excluded. Linkage disequilibrium has been demonstrated between the D4 receptor locus (on chromosome 11) and TS. Current concepts of the genetics of TS support a sex-influenced autosomal dominant mode of inheritance with a nearly complete penetrance for males and 56% penetrance for females when only tics are considered and 70% when OCD is included. Common bilineal transmission may lead to frequent homozygosity and the high density of TS observed in some families. Furthermore, because this type of transmission violates the standard principle of one-trait–one-locus it may hinder linkage studies and may explain why a gene marker has not yet been identified for TS despite intense collaborative research effort. Twin studies, showing 89% concordance for TS and 100% concordance for either TS or chronic motor tics, provide strong support for the genetic etiology of TS.

DIAGNOSIS

Without a specific biologic marker, the diagnosis depends on a careful evaluation of the patient's symptoms and signs by an experienced clinician. To aid in the diagnosis of TS, the Tourette Syndrome Classification Study Group (TSCSG) formulated the following criteria for definite TS: (1) both multiple motor and one or more phonic tics have to be present at some time during the illness, although not necessarily concurrently; (2) tics must occur many times a day, nearly every day, or intermittently throughout a period of more than 1 year; (3) the anatomic location, number, frequency, type, complexity, or severity of tics must change over time; (4) the onset must be before the age of 21 years; (5) involuntary movements and noises must not be explained by other medical conditions; and (6) motor and/or phonic tics must be witnessed by a reliable examiner directly at some point during the illness or be recorded by videotape or cinematography. Probable TS type 1 meets all the criteria except 3 and/or 4, and probable TS type 2 meets all the criteria except 1; it includes either a single motor tic with phonic tics or multiple motor tics with possible phonic tics. In contrast to the criteria outlined by the *Diagnostic and Statistical Manual of Mental Disorders*, fourth edition (DSM-IV), the TSCSG criteria do not include a statement about "impairment." There is considerable controversy about the DSM-IV criteria, which require that "marked distress or significant impairment in social, occupational or other important areas of functioning" be present.

TREATMENT

The first step in the management of TS is proper education of the patient, parents and other family members, teachers, and other individuals who interact with the patient about the nature of the disorder. School principals, teachers, and students can be helpful in implementing the therapeutic strategies. In addition, the parents and the physician should work as partners in advocating the best possible school environment for the child. This may include preferential seating; assignment sheets; shorter writing assignments; one-on-one tutoring; extra break periods and a refuge area to "allow" the release of tics; waiving time limitations on tests; and other measures designed to relieve stress. National and local support groups can provide additional information and can serve as a valuable resource for the patient and the family.*

Not all patients require pharmacologic therapy; counseling may be sufficient for those with mild symptoms. Medications, however, may be considered when symptoms begin to interfere with peer relationships, social interactions, academic or job performance, or activities of daily living. Because of the broad range of neurologic and behavioral manifestation and varied severity, therapy of TS must be individualized and tailored specifically to the needs of the patient. The most troublesome symptoms should be targeted first. Medications should be instituted at low doses and titrated gradually to the lowest, but effective, dosage and tapered during nonstressful periods (e.g., summer vacations). Another important principle of therapy in TS is to give each medication and dosage regimen an adequate trial. This approach avoids needless changes made in response to variations in symptoms during the natural course of the disease.

Tics

The goal of treatment should not be to completely eliminate all the tics, but to achieve a tolerable suppression. Of the pharmacologic agents used for tic suppression, the dopamine-receptor–blocking drugs (neuroleptics) are clearly most effective (Table 1). Although haloperidol (Haldol) has frequently been recommended in the past and pimozide (Orap) is the only neuroleptic actually approved by the Food and Drug Administration for the treatment of TS, I prefer fluphenazine (Prolixin) as the first-line anti-tic pharmacotherapy. If fluphenazine fails to adequately control tics, I substitute pimozide. Both fluphenazine and pimozide are started at 1 mg at bedtime and increased by 1 mg every 5 to 7 days. If these drugs fail to adequately control tics, I then try haloperidol, risperidone (Risperdal), thioridazine (Mellaril), trifluoperazine (Stelazine), molindone (Moban), or thiothixene (Navane). Risperidone, a neuroleptic with both dopamine- and serotonin-blocking properties, has been shown to be effective in reducing tic frequency and intensity in some patients. It is not clear whether some of the new atypical neuroleptics, such as olanzapine (Zyprexa), will be effective in the treatment of tics and other manifestations of TS. Tetrabenazine, a monoamine-depleting and dopamine-receptor–blocking drug, is a powerful anti-tic drug, but regrettably it is not readily available in the United States.

The side effects associated with neuroleptics, such as sedation, depression, weight gain, and school phobia, seem to be somewhat less frequent with flu-

TABLE 1. Pharmacology of Tourette's Syndrome

Drugs	Initial Dosage (mg/d)	Clinical Effect
Dopamine receptor blockers		Tics
Fluphenazine	1	+ + +
Pimozide	2	+ + +
Haloperidol	0.5	+ + +
Risperidol	0.5	+ +
Thiothixene	1	+ +
Trifluoperazine	1	+ +
Molindone	5	+ +
Dopamine depleters		Tics
Tetrabenazine	25	+ +
CNS stimulants		ADHD
Methylphenidate	5	+ + +
Pemoline	18.75	+ +
Dextroamphetamine	5	+ +
Noradrenergic drugs		Impulse control and/or ADHD
Clonidine	0.1	+ +
Guanfacine	1.0	+ +
Serotonergic drugs		OCD
Fluoxetine	20	+ + +
Clomipramine	25	+ + +
Sertraline	50	+ + +
Paroxetine	20	+ + +
Fluvoxamine	50	+ + +
Venlafaxine	25	+ + +

Abbreviations: CNS = central nervous system; ADHD = attention-deficit/hyperactivity disorder; OCD = obsessive-compulsive disorder.

phenazine than with haloperidol and the other neuroleptics. The most feared side effects of chronic neuroleptic therapy include tardive dyskinesia and hepatotoxicity. In addition, pimozide may prolong the QT interval, and therefore patients treated with the drug must have an electrocardiogram (ECG) before starting therapy. I obtain another ECG about 3 months later and once a year thereafter. Tardive dyskinesia, usually manifested by stereotypic involuntary movements, is only rarely persistent in children. Tardive dystonia, a variant of tardive dyskinesia most frequently encountered in young adults, however, may persist and occasionally progresses to a generalized and disabling dystonic disorder. Other movement disorders associated with neuroleptics include bradykinesia, akathisia, and acute dystonic reactions. Therefore, careful monitoring of the patients is absolutely essential, and whenever possible the dosage should be reduced or even discontinued during periods of remission or during vacations. Tetrabenazine has a major advantage over other neuroleptics in that it does not appear to cause tardive dyskinesia.

Of the non-neuroleptic drugs, clonazepam (Klonopin)* is sometimes useful, particularly in patients with clonic tics. Motor tics can be ameliorated by local injections of botulinum toxin.† By preventing the release of acetylcholine from the nerve terminal, the toxin causes focal chemodenervation, and the

---

*Tourette Syndrome Association, 42–40 Bell Boulevard, Bayside, NY 11361–2857.

*Not FDA approved for this indication.
†Not yet approved for use in the United States.

resulting weakness may be partly responsible for its beneficial effects. Another mechanism by which botulinum toxin improves tics is its effect on the local premonitory sensations. Presumably by lessening the "tension" in the muscles, botulinum toxin prevents the urge to perform a tic. In addition to ameliorating motor tics, botulinum toxin injections have been useful in the treatment of phonic tics, including severe coprolalia. In addition to pharmacologic therapy, behavioral and muscle relaxation techniques, such as stress management and biofeedback, may play an important ancillary role.

Behavioral Symptoms

Attention-Deficit/Hyperactivity Disorder

Behavioral modification, school and classroom adjustments, and other techniques described previously may be useful in some selected patients for the management of behavioral problems associated with TS, but in my experience these approaches are rarely effective and at best play an ancillary role. Such behavioral strategies, however, may provide important emotional support for the patient and the family members and may be helpful in raising self-esteem and improving motivation.

When these measures are insufficient to maintain good academic performance and to allow a satisfactory adaptation, pharmacologic therapy may need to be employed. I use clonidine (Catapres),* a presynaptic alpha$_2$-adrenergic agonist used as an antihypertensive because it decreases plasma norepinephrine levels, in mild cases of ADHD and impulse control problems. Although initially thought to be effective in controlling tics, clonidine has been shown to be ineffective as an anti-tic agent. However, the drug is quite useful in controlling a variety of TS-related behavioral symptoms, particularly ADHD and problems with impulse control. The usual starting dose is 0.1 mg at bedtime, and the dosage is gradually increased up to 0.5 mg per day in three divided doses. The drug is also available as a transdermal patch (TTS-1, TTS-2, TTS-3, corresponding to 0.1, 0.2 and 0.3 mg) that should be changed once a week, using a different skin location. Side effects include sedation, lightheadedness, headache, dry mouth, and insomnia. Although the patch can cause local irritation, it seems to cause fewer side effects than oral clonidine. Another drug increasingly used in the treatment of ADHD and impulse control problems is guanfacine (Tenex),* available as 1- or 2-mg tablets. Pharmacologically similar to clonidine, guanfacine may be effective in patients in whom clonidine failed to control the behavioral symptoms. Guanfacine may have some advantages over clonidine in that it has a longer half-life, it appears to be less sedating, and it produces less hypotension. It also seems to be more selective for the alpha$_2$-noradrenergic receptor. Although both clonidine and guanfacine appear to be effective in the treatment of attention deficits with and without hyperactivity, they appear to be particularly useful in the management of oppositional, argumentative, impulsive, and aggressive behavior. Although less effective than methylphenidate (Ritalin), the drugs have an advantage over methylphenidate in that they do not increase tics. The most frequently encountered side effects of the two drugs include sedation, dry mouth, itchy eyes, postural hypotension, and headaches. The beneficial effects may not be appreciated for several weeks after the initiation of therapy, and the symptoms may markedly intensify if the medications are withdrawn abruptly. We have found deprenyl or selegiline (Eldepryl),* a monoamine oxidase B inhibitor, to be effective in controlling the symptoms of ADHD without exacerbating tics. It is not clear how deprenyl improves symptoms of ADHD, but the drug is known to metabolize into amphetamines. Other drugs frequently used in relatively mild cases of ADHD include imipramine (Tofranil),* nortriptyline (Pamelor),* and desipramine (Norpramin).* Because of potential cardiotoxicity, ECG or cardiologic evaluation may be needed before the initiation of desipramine therapy, and follow-up ECGs should be obtained every 3 to 6 months.

A central stimulant, methylphenidate, although clearly effective in the treatment of ADHD, may exacerbate or precipitate tics in 25% of patients. If, however, the symptoms of ADHD are troublesome and interfere with a patient's functioning, it is reasonable to use this, or other central nervous system stimulants such as pemoline (Cylert) or dextroamphetamine (Dexedrine) and titrate the dosage to the lowest effective level (see Table 1). The initial dose for methylphenidate is 5 mg in the morning, and the dose can be gradually increased to 20 to 30 mg per day. Besides the possible development of tolerance, other potential side effects of these stimulant drugs include nervousness, insomnia, anorexia, and headaches. The dopamine-receptor–blocking drugs can be combined with the central nervous system stimulants if the latter produce unacceptable exacerbation of tics.

Obsessive-Compulsive Disorder

Although imipramine and desipramine have been reported to be useful in the treatment of OCD, the most effective drugs are the selective serotonin reuptake inhibitors (SSRIs). These include fluoxetine (Prozac), fluvoxamine (Luvox), clomipramine (Anafranil), paroxetine (Paxil),* sertraline (Zoloft),* and venlafaxine (Effexor).* No comparative study has been performed of the various agents in patients with TS and OCD, but clomipramine, fluvoxamine, and fluoxetine seem to be particularly effective. The initial dosage of clomipramine is 25 mg at bedtime, and the dosage can be gradually increased up to 250 mg per day, using 25-, 50-, or 75-mg capsules after meals or at bedtime. Fluoxetine and paroxetine should be

---

*Not FDA approved for this indication.

*Not FDA approved for this indication.

started at 20 mg after breakfast, and the dosage can be increased up to 80 mg per day. In contrast to clomipramine and fluvoxamine, the other SSRIs should be started as a morning, after breakfast dose. In addition to the SSRIs, anxiolytics, such as alprazolam and clonazepam, have been used with modest success. Likewise, monoamine oxidase inhibitors, trazodone, and buspirone have limited efficacy in the treatment of OCD. In patients with extremely severe and disabling OCD, in whom optimal pharmacologic therapy has failed, psychosurgery, either limbic leucotomy or cingulotomy, may be considered as a last resort. Although stereotactic infrathalamic lesions can improve OCD and even tics, such procedures can be complicated by severe disturbances in speech, swallowing, and gait.

HEADACHE

method of
SEYMOUR DIAMOND, M.D.
Diamond Headache Clinic
Chicago, Illinois

Headache is among the most frequent complaints. It is estimated that 45 million Americans experience headaches of significant morbidity in any one year. The majority of headache patients remain undiagnosed, primarily owing to either the patient's not informing the physician of the headache complaints or the physician's lack of understanding and attention to the complaint.

To facilitate an understanding of the various headache disorders, a simple classification may provide the physician with a basic tool for treating the headache patient (Table 1). Most headache patients are suffering from tension-type (muscle contraction) headaches, either episodic or chronic. Of those seeking care by their physicians, 8 to 10% are suffering from some form of vascular headache. Only 2% of these patients are suffering from headaches with an organic basis. The proportion of patients seeking help at specialized headache or pain clinics varies; most have vascular headaches. I have modified the complex classification of the International Headache Society, published in 1988,

TABLE 1. Classification of Headache

Vascular	Tension Type (Muscle Contraction)	Traction and Inflammatory
Migraine	Episodic or chronic	Mass lesions
With aura (classic)	Anxiety	Diseases of the eye, ear, nose, throat, teeth
Without aura (common)	Depression	
	Post-traumatic	
Complicated		Cranial neuralgias
Ophthalmoplegic		Allergy
Hemiplegic		Infection
Basilar artery		Arteritis
Cluster		Temporomandibular joint dysfunction
Facial		
Toxic		Cervical osteoarthritis
Hypertension		Chronic myositis

TABLE 2. Headache History Form

How many types of headache?
Initial onset of headache?
Location of pain?
Frequency of headache attacks?
Severity of pain? Qualities of pain (throbbing, aching, tightness)?
Any exertional aspects to headache?
Duration of headache attack?
Any warning symptoms of headache (aura or vague premonitory symptoms)?
Any sleep disturbance (with or without presence of headache)?
Any family history of headache?
Any relationship to menses (if applicable)?
Any seasonal relationship to headaches?
How would you describe your personality or emotional status?
Any previous testing for headaches?
Any previous medications for headaches? What was the response?
Any current medications for headaches?
Any current medications for other medical illnesses?
What is previous medical, surgical, and (if applicable) obstetric history?
Any allergies to medications or foods?
Any relationship to alcohol?
Are you a smoker?
How much caffeine do you consume daily?

to facilitate understanding by the practicing physician (see Table 1).

A detailed and relevant history geared to the headache patient is the most important factor in making correct diagnoses (Table 2). By careful questioning and directing of the inquiry, a specific headache profile evolves that makes the diagnosis in many instances, for the majority of patients with headache have negative neurologic and physical examination findings. The essentials of a headache history should be set down in a short, concise manner so that a pattern evolves and the clinicians will be able to identify the kinds of headache that are present.

Although the history is by all means the most important factor in diagnosis of the headache patient, additional evaluation may be required. Table 3 lists the suggested studies for headache evaluation.

TABLE 3. Headache Work-up

General: History and physical examination
If focal disease, mass lesions, or hydrocephalus is suspected: CT or MRI
If arterial disease is suspected: Angiograms
If aneurysm is suspected: Magnetic resonance angiography
If infection is suspected: Lumbar puncture (immediately)
If giant cell arteritis is suspected:
  Erythrocyte sedimentation rate (by the Westergren method)
  Temporal artery biopsy, antinuclear antibody

Occasionally Indicated in Special Situations

For chronic facial pain: Radiographs of the temporomandibular joints
If disease of cervical spine is suspected:
  Cervical spine radiographs
  EMG—for signs of radiculopathy or spinal cord compression
  Myelography, rarely
If idiopathic headache without any clinical findings:
  CT, MRI, spectroscopy, or PET

Abbreviations: CT = computed tomography; MRI = magnetic resonance imaging; EMG = electromyography; PET = positron emission tomography.

VASCULAR HEADACHES

Migraine Headaches

The term "migraine" is a French word based on the Greek *hemikrania*, which means "half-a-head." Migraine is typically a periodic headache that usually occurs unilaterally but may become generalized. The frequency of migraine varies from one or two per year to as many as two attacks per week. For most patients, the migraine attack lasts 4 to 24 hours, a few continuing more than 24 hours. Migraine is often described as a "sick" headache owing to the various associated symptoms, including nausea, vomiting, photophobia, phonophobia, lightheadedness, scalp tenderness, blurred vision, and cold extremities.

Migraine can be subdivided into two categories: migraine with aura (classic) and migraine without aura (common or nonclassic). This division is based on the occurrence of a warning in migraine with aura, which approximately 20 to 30% of migraine patients report. The most frequently occurring warnings or prodromes are visual in nature and are listed in Table 4. In addition to the visual manifestations of the aura, the patient with migraine with aura may experience a "slow march" of paresthesias throughout the body. The patient may also notice a strange odor surrounding the body before the migraine attack. Patients without aura do not describe these specific prodromes. However, these patients may note various premonitions presenting 2 to 72 hours before the onset of the acute attack. These premonitions are generalized and include a feeling of well-being, depression, fatigue, a surge of energy, hunger, anorexia, irritability, anxiety, talkativeness, and restlessness. For those patients with complicated migraine, characterized by persistent neurologic symptoms, referral to a headache clinic or neurologic specialist is indicated. The initial onset of migraine usually occurs in the second or third decade of life. It may occur during childhood, and some patients may not experience their first attack until the fourth or fifth decade. Migraine frequency and intensity usually diminish with advancing age. Approximately 60% of migraine sufferers are females, and 70% of these report a relationship between the migraine attacks and menses. By the end of the first trimester of pregnancy, migraine usually disappears. Most of these patients note a disappearance of their migraine attacks after menopause.

Most migraine patients report a family history of similar headaches. During the headache history, the interviewer should determine whether there is a familial history of migraine by establishing the diagnosis. In 1993, one study genetically "linked" a region of DNA on human chromosome 19 to the clinical diagnosis of familial migraine. A variety of studies have been conducted on the personality profile of the migraine patient. In my clinical experience, I have noted that these patients are often compulsive, neat, rigid, and perfectionistic and often build an environment too great to handle.

Therapy

Migraine treatment should be divided into four categories: nonpharmacologic measures; abortive therapy; pain relief (symptomatic) measures; and prophylactic therapy. Both physician and patient should be aware that making the appropriate selections can be a painstaking process that may require frequent office visits and many thoughtful, interactive discussions. It is also important for patients to be apprised of the fact that migraine headache is a disorder whose symptoms may wax and wane throughout the course of a lifetime. Therapeutic selections chosen within the framework of one set of circumstances or one stage of life may be ineffective and/or inappropriate in the framework of another. Thus, whereas pharmacologic therapy can greatly reduce pain and suffering, it is not likely to render the patient completely headache free, given the complex variables involved.

NONPHARMACOLOGIC MEASURES

Reduction of the various migraine triggers should be the initial stage of migraine therapy. The physical triggers include weather changes, altitude changes, bright lights, hormones, oversleeping, excessive fatigue, and missing a meal. Psychic provocateurs include stress, depression, anxiety, fear, and repressed hostility. Studies have been inconclusive on the effect of diet on migraine, but in my clinical experience, I have noted many patients relating their acute attacks to specific foods. All the patients at the Diamond Headache Clinic receive a diet that limits foods containing vasoactive substances, such as tyramine, which may precipitate an acute migraine attack (Table 5). Instructing patients about the various triggers and encouraging avoidance or elimination of these provocateurs may greatly benefit them in reducing the frequency and severity of the attacks.

Stress reduction, relaxation training, and biofeedback may be excellent adjunctive therapy in those patients for whom psychologic factors act as triggers. I have found biofeedback particularly helpful in children and young adults.

ABORTIVE THERAPY

Sumatriptan Succinate (Imitrex). The most recent addition to the armamentarium of acute migraine therapies is the drug sumatriptan. As a serotonin receptor agonist that inhibits release of 5-hydroxytryptamine, norepinephrine, acetylcholine, and substance P, sumatriptan is highly effective in

TABLE 4. **Visual Prodromes of Migraine with Aura**

Positive	Teichopsia or fortification spectra Zigzags Flashing lights and colors
Negative	Scotomata Hemianopsia
Metamorphopsia	Illusions of distorted size, shape, and location of fixed objects

TABLE 5. **Headache Diet**

Each day eat 3 meals with a snack at night or 6 small meals spread throughout the day.

All food, especially high-protein foods, should be prepared and eaten fresh. Do not eat leftovers held for more than 1 d.

The foods listed in the "caution" column have smaller amounts of tyramine or other vasoactive compounds. Avoid these foods if you are taking an MAOI. (Caffeinated beverages may be used in allowed amounts.)

Each person may have different sensitivities to a certain level of tyramine or other vasoactive compounds in foods. If you are taking an MAOI, use restricted foods in limited amounts.

Beverages

Allowed	*Use with Caution*	*Avoid*
Decaffeinated coffee	Limit caffeinated beverages to no more than 2 servings per day	All alcoholic beverages not specified in caution column
Fruit juices	Limit alcoholic beverages to one serving: wine, vodka, or scotch	
Club soda and sparkling water		
Caffeine-free carbonated beverages		

Meat, Fish, Poultry, Eggs

Allowed	*Use with Caution*	*Avoid*
Freshly purchased and prepared meats	Bacon	Products that are
Fish and poultry	Sausage	Aged
Eggs	Hot dogs	Dried
Tuna fish, tuna salad (with allowed ingredients)	Corned beef	Fermented
	Ham	Smoked
	Any luncheon meats with nitrites added (may not be high in tyramine)	Pickled
		Pepperoni
	Meat with tenderizer added	Salami
	Caviar	Liverwurst
		Nonfresh meat or liver
		Pickled herring

Dairy

Allowed	*Use with Caution*	*Avoid*
Milk	Parmesan or romano as a garnish (2 tsp) or minor ingredient	Aged cheese
Processed cheese	Yogurt	
	Buttermilk	
	Sour cream	

Breads, Cereals, Pasta

Allowed	*Use with Caution*	*Avoid*
Commercially prepared yeast products	Homemade yeast breads and coffee cake	Any with restricted ingredients
Products leavened with baking powder	Sourdough breads	
All hot and dry cereals		
All pasta		

Vegetables

Allowed	*Use with Caution*	*Avoid*
Any vegetables not on avoidance list	Raw onion	Fava or broad beans
		Sauerkraut
		Fermented soy products such as miso and pickles

Fruits

Allowed	*Use with Caution*
All fruits not on restricted list	Limit intake to one-half cup per day from each group: citrus; avocados; bananas; figs; raisins; papaya; passion fruit; red plums

Nuts and Seeds

Avoid
All nuts: peanuts, peanut butter, pumpkin seeds, sesame seeds, walnuts, pecans, and others

Soups

Allowed	*Use with Caution*
Soups made from allowed ingredients	Canned soups with
Homemade broths	Yeast
	Meat extracts
	MSG

Desserts and Sweets

Allowed	*Use with Caution*	*Avoid*
Any made with allowed foods and ingredients	Chocolate-based products	Mincemeat pie

Table continued on following page

TABLE 5. **Headache Diet** *Continued*

Ingredients Listed on Food Labels

Allowed	*Avoid*
Any not listed in the restricted section	MSG* (in large amounts)
	Nitrites* (found in processed meats)
	Yeast, yeast extracts, brewer's yeast
	Meat extracts
	Meat tenderizers (papain, bromelin)
	Seasoned salts (containing MSG)
	Soy sauce
	Teriyaki sauce

Fats, Oils, and Miscellaneous

Allowed	*Use with Caution*	*Avoid*
All cooking oils and fats	Fermented vinegars (wine, apple, others)	Mixed dishes made with restricted ingredients: macaroni and cheese, beef stroganoff, cheese blintzes, Asian foods, pizza
White vinegar		
Commercial salad dressing with allowed ingredients in small amounts		Frozen dinners: read labels to check for restricted ingredients
All spices not listed in restricted ingredients		

*MSG and nitrites do not have the same effect as tyramine-containing foods but can cause headache in many people.
Abbreviations: MAOI = monoamine oxidase inhibitor; MSG = monosodium glutamate.

blocking inflammation and producing vasoconstriction in dilated cranial arteries, and it has become the agent of choice in the abortive treatment of migraine. Unlike the ergot preparations, sumatriptan has, in many cases, demonstrated efficacy even in the advanced stages of a migraine attack. A 20-mg dose of nasal spray is now available.

The drug is available for oral or parenteral administration and has been shown to provide relief in approximately 80% of migraineurs. If the first dose offers at least partial relief, a second dose may be repeated after an hour, or anytime within the next 24 hours in those patients who experience a recurrence of migraine symptoms. At the Diamond Headache Clinic, a specific protocol is followed for titrating the oral dose during successive headaches. This protocol is described in Table 6. Regardless of whether the oral or injectable form is used, a 5-day hiatus is observed between treatment days.

Sumatriptan is generally well tolerated. Minor and transient side effects, such as flushing, throat discomfort, neck and chest tightness or pain, tingling,

TABLE 6. **Selected Abortive Therapies in the Treatment of Migraine**

Medication	Route	Dosage
Sumatriptan succinate (Imitrex)	SC	6 mg; may repeat after 1 h; up to 12 mg/24 h. Maintain 5-d hiatus between treatment days.
Sumatriptan succinate	PO	Start with 25 mg; may repeat same dose in 2 h; up to 50 mg tabs/24 h. If ineffective, next headache start with 50 mg; may repeat same dose in 2 h; up to 100 mg/24 h. If ineffective, next headache start with 75 mg; may repeat same dose in 2 h; up to 125 mg/24 h. If ineffective, next headache start with 100 mg; may repeat same dose in 2 h; up to 150 mg/24 h. Maintain 5-d hiatus between treatment days.
Ergotamine tartrate (Ergostat, Ergomar)	SL	2 mg under tongue at earliest sign of headache; may repeat q 30 min up to 6 mg/d, 10 mg/wk. Maintain 5-d hiatus between treatment days.
Ergotamine tartrate with caffeine (Cafergot, Wigraine)	PO	1 mg at earliest sign of headache; may repeat 1 mg q 30 min up to 6 mg/d, 10 mg/wk. Maintain 5-d hiatus between treatment days.
Ergotamine tartrate with caffeine (Cafergot)	PR	One suppository at earliest sign of headache; may repeat at 60 min up to 2/d, 5/wk; may begin with ½ suppository followed by ½ within next hour. Maintain 5-d hiatus between treatment days.
Dihydroergotamine (D.H.E. 45)	IV, IM, SC	Individualize dose to patient, usually in the range of 0.5 to 1.5 mg. IV, IM usually administered in hospital or office; SC useful in home; often coadministered with metoclopramide or other antiemetic.
Isometheptene mucate with dichloralphenazone and acetaminophen (Midrin)	PO	2 capsules stat, then 1 q h up to 5 capsules/24 h, or 2 stat, then repeat 2 capsules in 1 h, then stop.
Aspirin	PO	900 mg at onset.
Naproxen sodium (Naprosyn)	PO	825 mg at onset; repeat 275–550 mg q 30–60 min; up to 1375 mg/d.
Flurbiprofen (Ansaid)	PO	50–100 mg at onset; repeat q 6 h.
Etodolac (Lodine)	PO	300 mg tid.
Mefenamic acid (Ponstel)	PO	500 mg at onset.
Diclofenac sodium (Voltaren)	PO	50–75 mg bid to qid.

nausea, and local irritation at the site of injection (if the autoinjectable form is used), typically resolve quickly. Sumatriptan is contraindicated in patients with basilar or hemiplegic migraine, ischemic heart disease, or Prinzmetal's angina and cannot be used concomitantly with ergot-containing preparations.

Ergotamine and Derivatives. Until sumatriptan arrived on the scene, ergotamine had been a first-line choice in the abortive treatment of migraine headaches for many years. Still commonly prescribed, ergotamine is an alpha-adrenergic blocking agent with a direct stimulating effect on the smooth muscle of peripheral and cranial blood vessels, and it produces depression of central vasomotor centers. The compound also has the properties of serotonin antagonism.

Regardless of the route of administration (orally, sublingually, rectally, or nasally), ergotamine has proved effective in no more than 50% of patients with migraine. Because absorption of ergotamine and related drugs is variable, the route of administration chosen for use should be dependent on what is most acceptable to the individual patient. Sublingual preparations should be considered if the oral route is too slow or is not well tolerated. Rectal suppositories* are the best absorbed of the nonparenteral preparations and are especially helpful for those patients who experience nausea during an attack. However, they would not be the preparation of choice for those patients who find them awkward to use or who experience associated diarrhea. Doses should be increased to a single effective dose administered as early as possible in subsequent attacks. Patients experiencing migraine with aura should be instructed to use the drug during their prodromal phase, although some headache experts question initiating therapy at this stage. To prevent rebound headache, a 5-day hiatus must be maintained between treatment days.

Side effects of ergotamine administration include nausea, vomiting, diarrhea, cramping, dizziness, transient paresthesias, stroke, hypertension, myocardial ischemia or infarction, and peripheral vasospasm. Ergotamine preparations are generally contraindicated in elderly patients and/or in patients with peripheral vascular disease, thrombophlebitis, severe hypertension, coronary ischemia, angina, renal or hepatic disease, or recent infection. Excessive consumption of the ergots may lead to symptoms of vasoconstriction and ultimately to ergotism.

One of the ergot derivatives, D.H.E. 45 (dihydroergotamine), whose efficacy in aborting migraines seems to be associated with its central serotonergic effects, has been found to be highly effective in its intramuscular form and even more effective intravenously. Side effects, which include nausea, flushing, leg cramps, numbness or burning around the injection site, diarrhea, and chest or throat tightness, tend to be of short duration. A nasal form of this agent is available.

Isometheptene Mucate (Midrin). The use of a combination medication containing isometheptene (a sympathomimetic amine that acts by constricting dilated cranial and cerebral arterioles), combined with dichloralphenazone (a mild sedative), and acetaminophen (an analgesic) may be indicated in certain patients who cannot use ergotamine or its derivatives. This medication is most helpful for aborting mild to moderately severe migraines when it is taken at the earliest stages of an attack, and it produces few if any side effects. It is contraindicated in patients with uncontrolled hypertension and/or severe cases of renal or hepatic disease, hypertension, or organic heart disease and in those patients who are receiving monoamine oxidase inhibitor (MAOI) therapy.

Nonsteroidal Anti-inflammatory Agents. For patients with mild to moderately severe migraine attacks, the nonsteroidal anti-inflammatory drugs (NSAIDs) are often an excellent first choice for abortive treatment. A possible explanation for their effectiveness involves their ability to inhibit prostaglandin synthesis and thus prevent neurogenically mediated inflammation in the trigeminovascular system. They may also interfere with serotonin neurotransmission and modulate vasoconstriction. In mild cases, aspirin may be effective. Side effects of short-term NSAID therapy are generally minor and may include nausea, abdominal distress, dyspepsia, diarrhea, dizziness, and tinnitus. Because of their capacity to induce gastrointestinal bleeding, however, these drugs should be avoided in patients with peptic ulcer disease. They are also contraindicated in patients with kidney or renal dysfunction.

Status Migraine

A migraine attack that lasts several days or weeks is referred to as status migraine. When other abortives have failed, and there are no contraindications for use, the treatment of choice for status migraine is intravenous dihydroergotamine and/or corticosteroid therapy. Repetitive intravenous D.H.E. 45, generally administered with metoclopramide (Reglan)* or another antiemetic, breaks the headache cycle sufficiently long enough to facilitate the patient's transition to a more targeted prophylactic approach. Long-acting dexamethasone or other steroid preparations may be used independently or in conjunction with D.H.E. 45 administration for the same purpose. General precautions for the administration of glucocorticoids should be observed, and treatment should be limited to less than one per month.

PROPHYLACTIC THERAPY

Prophylactic therapy (Table 7) should be considered in those patients experiencing two or more migraine attacks per month. This form of therapy is also indicated for patients whose attacks are severe enough to greatly affect their quality of life and ability to function, for whom abortive therapies have been unsuccessful, or for whom abortive therapies are contraindicated.

Several prophylactic trials are reasonable as long

---

*Not available in the United States.

*Not FDA approved for this indication.

Table 7. **Selected Prophylactic Therapies in the Treatment of Migraine**

Medication	Route	Dose
Propranolol (Inderal)	PO	60–160 mg/d
Propranolol long-acting	PO	60–160 mg/d in once-daily dose
Timolol (Blocadren)	PO	10–20 mg/d
Nadolol (Corgard)	PO	20–120 mg/d
Metoprolol (Lopressor)	PO	100–200 mg/d
Atenolol (Tenormin)	PO	25–100 mg/d
Methysergide (Sansert)	PO	2 mg tid
Divalproex sodium (Depakote)	PO	250–200 mg/d
Verapamil (Calan)	PO	120–480 mg/d
Nimodipine (Nimotop)	PO	30 mg tid to qid
Nicardipine (Cardene)	PO	20–30 mg bid to tid
Flunarizine (Sibelium)	PO	10 mg/d
Protriptyline (Vivactil)	PO	5–30 mg/d
Desipramine (Norpramin)	PO	25–150 mg/d
Amitriptyline (Elavil)	PO	10–150 mg/d
Doxepin (Sinequan)	PO	10–150 mg/d
Nortriptyline (Pamelor)	PO	10–150 mg/d
Imipramine (Tofranil)	PO	10–150 mg/d
Fluoxetine (Prozac)	PO	10–80 mg/d
Sertraline (Zoloft)	PO	50–200 mg/d
Paroxetine (Paxil)	PO	20–60 mg/d*
Phenelzine (Nardil)	PO	15–60 mg/d
Trazodone (Desyrel)	PO	50–300 mg/d
Bupropion (Wellbutrin)	PO	200–300 mg/d
Venlafaxine (Effexor)	PO	37.5–75 mg bid
Aspirin	PO	81 mg qd
Ketoprofen (Orudis)	PO	50–75 mg bid to tid
Naproxen (Naprosyn)	PO	250–750 mg qd
Naproxen sodium (Anaprox)	PO	250–750 mg qd
Fenoprofen calcium (Nalfon)	PO	600 mg tid
Flurbiprofen (Ansaid)	PO	50–100 mg bid
Indomethacin (Indocin)	PO	25–50 mg tid
Piroxicam (Feldene)	PO	20 mg q AM
Nabumetone (Relafen)	PO	500–750 mg bid
Diclofenac sodium (Voltaren)	PO	50 mg qd to bid
Clonidine (Catapres)	PO	0.1 mg tid
Cyproheptadine (Periactin)	PO	Up to 4–8 mg qid; begin with 4–8 mg q PM; increase to maximum if needed

*Exceeds dosage recommended by the manufacturer.

as the provider is sufficiently comfortable and familiar with *both* the diagnosis *and* subsequent selections. With significant potential for reducing frequency, duration, and intensity of attacks, these therapies can be instrumental in the functional restoration of patients with chronic migraine.

Once administration has begun, trials should be long enough (if sufficiently tolerated) to ensure that therapeutic levels have been achieved, yet short enough to avoid prolonged courses of nonproductive therapies. A time frame for trials of approximately 4 to 6 weeks is reasonable but may differ according to the medicine chosen and the individual response time of the patient. Beyond this period, if patients do not report improvement, evaluation for a different prophylactic choice may be warranted. Four agents have been approved by the Food and Drug Administration for the indication of migraine prophylaxis: methysergide, propranolol, timolol, and divalproex sodium.

Propranolol (Inderal). Propranolol, a nonselective beta-adrenergic receptor blocking agent, is considered to be the drug of choice in migraine prophy-laxis. The capacity of this drug to produce a blockade of beta-adrenergic receptors that results in inhibition of arterial dilatation and its ability to induce blockade of catecholamine-induced platelet aggregation are among the mechanisms of action that may account for its effectiveness.

Propranolol is especially beneficial for migraineurs with concomitant hypertension, angina pectoris, or thyrotoxicosis. At the Diamond Headache Clinic, I prefer the long-acting form of propranolol (Inderal LA), which allows one daily dosage and enhances the patient's compliance. The most common side effects include fatigue, gastrointestinal disturbances, insomnia, nightmares, hypotension, cold extremities, decreased resting heart rate, and sexual dysfunction. The drug is contraindicated in patients with asthma, chronic obstructive lung disease, congestive heart failure, or atrioventricular conduction disturbances and in patients receiving treatment with insulin, oral hypoglycemic drugs, or MAOIs. Abrupt withdrawal in patients with coronary heart disease may exacerbate coronary ischemia and lead to unstable angina or myocardial infarction.

Other Beta Blockers. If propranolol is contraindicated, treatment with another beta blocker may be considered. Both timolol (Blocadren) and nadolol (Corgard)* have demonstrated successful prophylaxis in many patients. For asthmatics or those with bronchial disorders, a cardioselective beta blocker, such as metoprolol (Lopressor)* or atenolol (Tenormin),* may be substituted.

Divalproex Sodium (Depakote). The effectiveness of this anticonvulsant agent in preventing migraine may be due to its capacity to increase synaptic levels of γ-aminobutyric acid. It can be considered first-line therapy for patients with coexisting seizures, mania, or anxiety. I have found that blood levels do not correlate with clinical efficacy. Its side effect profile includes nausea, gastrointestinal distress, sedation, tremor, blood dyscrasias, coagulation abnormalities, pancreatitis, and hepatotoxicity. Baseline complete blood count and liver function tests should be obtained before therapy and at frequent intervals thereafter, especially during the first 6 months of treatment. Double-blind studies have confirmed its efficacy. In a retrospective study of long-term therapy with this drug conducted at my clinic, divalproex sodium demonstrated efficacy in the treatment of headache, with gains maintained for at least 63 months. Also, this agent can be considered safe for prolonged treatment.

Calcium Channel Blockers. The effectiveness of calcium channel blockers in migraine prophylaxis appears to be related to their ability to block the influx of calcium ions across the cell membrane of vascular smooth muscle and thereby inhibit arterial vasospasm as well as to block platelet serotonin release and aggregation. Their effects on cerebral blood flow, neurotransmission, and neuroreceptor blockade may also enhance their efficacy. As with other agents that depend on down-regulation of serotonin receptors, their full effects may not be realized for 2 to 4 weeks after initiation of treatment.

Verapamil (Isoptin, Calan)* is a papaverine-derived calcium entry blocker with antiplatelet effects. The drug is orally active and has long-term effects that promote its usefulness as a migraine preventive. Constipation is among the most common side effects of therapy, but as with any of the calcium blockers, flushing, lightheadedness, hypotension, rash, and nausea may also occur.

Nimodipine (Nimotop)* has the highest marked selectivity for cerebral vasculature but has also been associated with more behavioral changes, sedation, and other central nervous system effects than other calcium blockers. Muscle pains have also been reported.

In some parts of the world, flunarizine (Sibelium)*† is used for migraine prevention. Nicardipine (Cardene)* has also demonstrated some prophylactic benefits. Two other calcium channel blockers, nifedipine (Procardia)* and diltiazem (Cardizem),* have not been shown to be particularly useful for this purpose.

Patients using calcium channel blockers should be monitored carefully for adverse symptoms related to postural hypotension. This is especially important in patients who are concurrently taking other antihypertensive agents including beta blockers. Because of their negative inotropic effects, calcium blockers should be used with caution in patients with concomitant congestive heart failure. Abrupt withdrawal of these agents should be avoided because of their potential to induce chest pain, rebound angina, or exacerbation of symptoms.

Antidepressants. The antimigraine effect of the antidepressant agents is believed to be relatively independent of their antidepressant effect, although the exact relationship remains uncertain. Tricyclic antidepressants* (TCAs) are known to block the reabsorption of serotonin and, to a lesser degree, norepinephrine at nerve endings. They also exhibit anticholinergic and antihistaminic activity that may contribute to their efficacy. With chronic TCA administration, the initial reabsorption effects are followed by slower, adaptive changes at the serotonin and norepinephrine receptor levels. The net effect is a reregulation of abnormal receptors and consequent stabilization of the neurotransmitter relationship. Clinically, this down-regulation results in relief of symptoms and may explain the 2- to 3-week lag time that generally occurs between initiation of treatment and the appearance of therapeutic effects.

TCAs are not considered to be a first-line migraine preventive but may be useful in some patients, particularly those with coexisting migraine and tension-type headache. Amitriptyline (Elavil), one of the oldest antidepressants used in migraine therapy, along with doxepin (Sinequan), nortriptyline (Pamelor), and imipramine (Tofranil), tends to be more sedating than protriptyline (Vivactil) or desipramine (Norpramin). These agents may also cause constipation, dry mouth, weight gain, blurred vision, tachycardia, orthostatic hypotension, sexual dysfunction, and urinary retention and are not recommended in patients with narrow-angle glaucoma, prostatic hypertrophy, or cardiac conduction disturbances.

Some of the newer antidepressants including the selective serotonin reuptake inhibitors* and others appear to operate more specifically at serotonin receptors and have a different side effect profile. As with the TCAs, however, a lag time of 2 to 3 weeks may occur before therapeutic effects are evident. Among the selective serotonin reuptake inhibitors, fluoxetine (Prozac), sertraline (Zoloft), and paroxetine (Paxil) have been beneficial, although nausea, insomnia, agitation, weight loss, and sexual dysfunction may be associated with their use. Among the other antidepressants, bupropion (Wellbutrin)* and trazodone (Desyrel)* have demonstrated some efficacy in migraine prophylaxis. Bupropion, however, has been known to produce agitation, anxiety, insom-

---

*Not FDA approved for this indication.
†Orphan drug.

*Not FDA approved for this indication.

nia, and seizures and is therefore contraindicated for use in patients with a history of seizures or in those who are prone to electrolyte disturbances (e.g., patients with bulimia). Trazodone has been associated with priapism and should be avoided in male migraineurs.

One of the MAOIs, phenelzine (Nardil),* has been found to help in the preventive treatment of migraine. It is not a first-line antidepressant agent but may be considered for use in refractory cases. Monoamine oxidase (MAO) is the enzyme system responsible for the metabolic decomposition of biogenic amines throughout the body. Inhibition of MAO results in an increase in the concentration of endogenous epinephrine, norepinephrine, and serotonin in storage sites throughout the nervous system. Drugs that inhibit MAO activity have a wide range of clinical effects and must be monitored with extreme caution because of their potential interaction with several foods and drugs.

Adverse effects reported with MAOIs include dizziness, insomnia, hypomania, orthostatic hypotension, dry mouth, blurred vision, urinary retention, impotence, peripheral edema, and weight gain. Patients should be warned to avoid alcoholic beverages, tyramine-containing foods, and sympathomimetic drugs. When the body's MAO is inhibited, ingestion of large amounts of tyramine may result in a hypertensive crisis of sufficient severity to cause myocardial infarction or cerebrovascular accident. Owing to the residual MAOI effects, a 2-week "washout" period is necessary before tyramine-containing foods or interactive drugs may be ingested.

Clonidine (Catapres).* Clonidine is a centrally acting alpha-adrenergic agonist whose efficacy in migraine prophylaxis is not comparable to the beta blockers. Clonidine has been found to be particularly helpful, however, in those patients who experience food-related attacks. Its mechanism of action may be related to its ability to block vasomotor reflexes and subsequently decrease vascular reactivity. It is also effective in those patients withdrawing from opiates. Side effects associated with clonidine include drowsiness, dry mouth, constipation, disturbances of ejaculation, orthostatic hypertension, and depression.

Cyproheptadine (Periactin).* Cyproheptadine has been used successfully in the treatment of childhood migraine. Its antiserotonin and antihistamine effects have suggested its use for treatment of migraine in adults, although results in this category have been marginal. Sedation and excessive weight gain also limit its usefulness.

Methysergide (Sansert). Closely related to the naturally occurring ergot alkaloids, methysergide is a semisynthetic lysergic acid derivative that lacks intrinsic vasoconstrictive properties. Its effectiveness in migraine prevention may be related to several mechanisms of action including (1) peripheral serotonin antagonist effects on vascular receptors, (2) inhibition of serotonin release from platelets, and (3) central serotonin agonist effects.

Although methysergide is one of the most effective agents for migraine prophylaxis, it is generally reserved for use in patients with frequent, severe, disabling migraines that do not respond to less toxic agents. Adverse effects include nausea, vomiting, abdominal pain, ataxia, insomnia, drowsiness, leg cramps, paresthesias, edema, weight gain, hair loss, and hypotension. Long-term use of methysergide has been associated with retroperitoneal fibrosis, pleuropulmonary fibrosis, and fibrotic thickening of the cardiac valves. Therefore, patients receiving methysergide therapy should be evaluated at regular intervals, should not be kept on therapy for more than 4 to 6 months consecutively, and should be given a 4- to 6-week drug hiatus between treatment periods. The drug is contraindicated in patients with a history of collagen diseases or fibrotic disorders as well as peripheral vascular disease, coronary artery disease, severe hypertension, and thrombophlebitis.

NSAIDs. The NSAIDs have a unique place in the treatment of migraine in that their anti-inflammatory and analgesic properties make them appropriate choices for abortive, symptomatic, and prophylactic therapy. As platelet antagonists with the potential to affect abnormalities of platelet aggregation, and thus levels of serotonin, NSAIDs are of particular interest in the preventive treatment of those who suffer from chronic migraine. Data collected from the U.S. Physicians' Health Study raise the possibility that regular use of aspirin or other platelet-active drugs in this category might reduce the recurrence of migraine by approximately 20%. Among the agents available, those listed in Table 7 have all been shown to be of benefit for prophylactic purposes.

Gastrointestinal toxicity is the adverse side effect seen most often within this category of drugs. The risk of gastrointestinal toxicity escalates with increased dose (thus, the lowest possible dose should be used), chronic use, alcohol ingestion, and smoking and in patients with a history of peptic ulcer disease. Patients should be monitored for gastrointestinal bleeding and for evidence of liver and/or kidney disease, both of which have been associated with chronic NSAID use.

Menstrual Migraine

Some 60 to 70% of female migraineurs will note a relationship between their menstrual cycle and the incidence of their migraine attacks, with severe headaches occurring immediately before, during, or after their period and/or ovulation. Approximately 60% of female migraineurs will also note a remission in their headaches after the first trimester of pregnancy. Almost 70% of these patients will experience a decrease or complete remission after menopause.

Oral contraceptives have been observed to increase the frequency, severity, and duration of attacks and should thus be avoided in migraine patients. Similarly, estrogen replacement therapy should be avoided or limited in postmenopausal patients because of the potential to exacerbate or restart mi-

---

*Not FDA approved for this indication.

TABLE 8. **Selected Prophylactic Therapies in the Treatment of Menstrual Migraine**

Medication	Route	Dose*
Aspirin	PO	81 mg qd
Ketoprofen	PO	50–75 mg bid to tid
Naproxen	PO	250–750 mg qd
Naproxen sodium	PO	250–750 mg qd
Fenoprofen calcium	PO	600 mg tid
Flurbiprofen	PO	50–100 mg bid
Indomethacin	PO	25–50 mg tid
Piroxicam	PO	20 mg q AM
Nabumetone	PO	500–750 mg bid
Diclofenac sodium	PO	50 mg qd to bid
Propranolol	PO	40 mg bid
Metoprolol	PO	50 mg/d
Methylergonovine maleate	PO	0.2 mg bid
Phenobarbital ⎫ Ergotamine tartrate ⎬ Bellergal-S Bellafoline alkaloids ⎭	PO	40 mg ⎫ 0.6 mg ⎬ 1 tablet bid 0.2 mg ⎭
Methysergide	PO	2 mg tid
Estradiol, transdermal patch	TD	0.05 mg continuous delivery system for twice-weekly application; to be used at onset of period and continued through flow
Danazol	PO	200 mg bid to tid; to be taken on a daily basis (i.e., not to be limited to perimenstrual use)

*Except where otherwise indicated, any of the therapies are to be started 3 days before the onset of the period and continued through flow.

graine attacks. If patients still choose to begin or continue estrogen replacement, they should be prescribed a daily uninterrupted regimen of the lowest dose of hormone available.

The perimenstrual use of certain agents may be helpful in preventing menstrual migraine, including the NSAIDs; methylergonovine maleate (Methergine); methysergide; a combination product containing phenobarbital, ergotamine tartrate, and Bellafoline; and standard migraine prophylactic agents. The selected agents (Table 8) should be started 3 days before the onset of menstruation (based on the patient's closest estimation) and be continued through the menstrual flow. Brief courses of corticosteroids or tranquilizers may also be of benefit, as may low-dose danazol. The use of transdermal estrogen patches* can offer some preventive relief if applied at the onset of menses.

Cyclical Migraine

Certain patients with migraine experience a "clustering" of their attacks followed by a relatively long period of remission. Intermittent use of prophylactic agents such as beta blockers, calcium channel blockers, NSAIDs, and methysergide can be used to treat this cyclical type of migraine. Lithium carbonate* has also been used successfully in patients with this migraine pattern.

SYMPTOMATIC THERAPY

Although the patients may have used abortive agents appropriately, the symptoms associated with migraine may persist. Narcotic analgesics may be used to control the pain of infrequent attacks but

*Not FDA approved for this indication.

should be avoided in patients who experience chronic migraine. If not contraindicated, the NSAIDs are an excellent alternative (Table 9). Among those NSAIDs that have been used successfully for this purpose, ketorolac (Toradol) is available for intramuscular administration and, as such, can be used effectively in emergency department or outpatient settings. Transnasal administration of butorphanol (Stadol), a potent mixed agonist-antagonist synthetically derived opioid analgesic, has also been shown to provide effective pain relief. Although drowsiness or dizziness may occur, this dosage form may offer an advantage to those patients whose nausea and vomiting prohibit the use of oral medications.

Because gastric stasis often accompanies migraine attacks, the effectiveness of analgesic medications may be enhanced by the addition of a drug, such as metoclopramide, that increases peristalsis and promotes gastric emptying. The drug should be avoided in adolescents, however, and used sparingly in adults because of its potential to produce dysarthria.

Butorphanol is a synthetic kappa agonist and mu antagonist opioid analgesic that is available for parenteral administration. It is not a controlled substance. Its lipophilic nature promotes a quick absorption by the transnasal route. Because the nasal mucosa is highly vascular, it is conducive for rapid uptake and absorption of butorphanol and similar agents. The authors of one investigation believed that transnasal butorphanol was comparable or superior to placebo and methadone in relieving the acute pain of migraine. The advantages to using this agent by the transnasal route are the increased rate of onset of action and the decrease in the risks associated with parenteral administration. Because of pos-

TABLE 9. **Selected Symptomatic Therapies in the Treatment of Migraine**

Medication	Route	Dose
Aspirin	PO	500 mg bid
Ketoprofen	PO	12.5–25 mg bid
Naproxen sodium	PO	275–550 mg bid
Ibuprofen	PO	200–400 mg q 4 h
Ketorolac	PO	10 mg qid
Ketorolac	IM	60 mg bid
Butorphanol nasal spray (Stadol NS)	NS	1 mg in one nostril; if pain persists, an additional 1 mg dose may be used within 60–90 min; the 2-dose sequence may be repeated q 3–4 h
Lidocaine 4%	NS	2 drops in affected nostril, may repeat hourly, up to 3 doses in 24 h
Metoclopramide	PO	10–20 mg at onset; may repeat q 6–8 h
Metoclopramide	IM	10–20 mg at onset; may repeat q 6–8 h
Metoclopramide	IV	10 mg at onset; may repeat in 6 h
Chlorpromazine HCl	PO	25–50 mg; may be repeated at 6-h intervals
Chlorpromazine HCl	PR	100 mg; may be repeated at 6-h intervals
Chlorpromazine HCl	IM	25–50 mg; may be repeated at 6-h intervals
Chlorpromazine HCl	IV	0.1 mg/kg slow IV push; may be repeated at 6-h intervals
Prochlorperazine	PO	25–50 mg; may be repeated at 6-h intervals
Prochlorperazine	PR	25 mg; may be repeated at 6-h intervals
Prochlorperazine	IM	10 mg; may be repeated at 6-h intervals

sible dependence problems, it should not be used on a daily basis. At the Diamond Headache Clinic, a 3- to 4-day interval between use is mandatory.

When nausea and vomiting are present, suppository forms of both analgesic and antiemetic drugs can be administered. Prochlorperazine (Compazine) and chlorpromazine (Thorazine) are among the most commonly prescribed antiemetic drugs for adjunctive migraine therapy and, as previously mentioned, have actually shown efficacy as migraine abortives in emergency department settings owing to their dopaminergic and adrenergic effects. However, given the likelihood that some patients who are chronically exposed to neuroleptics will develop the potentially irreversible extrapyramidal reactions associated with tardive dyskinesia, it is prudent to limit their use and advise patients of this risk before beginning treatment.

Cluster Headaches

Another form of vascular headaches, cluster headache, is characterized by its occurrence in series. These series usually last 1 to 3 months, occurring on a daily basis from once to several times per day. The series are self-limiting and usually disappear abruptly, and the patient may be headache free for months to years. The sex distribution in cluster headaches is in contrast to that in migraine, with a male predominance of 5:1. Although the onset of cluster headaches may be at any age, these headaches typically begin in the third and fourth decades of life. A seasonal relationship has also been noted, with an increase in the occurrence of the series in spring and autumn.

The pain of an acute cluster headache is extremely severe and is characterized by its short duration, from a few minutes to a few hours. These headaches rarely last more than 4 hours. However, patients may complain of several attacks in one day, often awakening them at the same time each night. Acute cluster attacks are always unilateral and are usually around the eye. During a series, the site is usually consistent. The headaches may change sides with the next series. Associated symptoms include tearing, facial flushing, conjunctival injection, sweating, nasal congestion, rhinorrhea, and partial Horner's syndrome. Patients with cluster headaches describe the pain as burning, boring, constant, and knifelike. The severity of the acute headaches has driven some sufferers to consider suicide. Some unfortunate patients experience chronic cluster headaches, which are characterized by no remission; management of these may be quite difficult.

Abortive Therapy

Owing to the brief duration of the acute attacks, abortive therapy must be immediate. The options for this form of therapy are listed in Table 10. Sumatriptan has recently been approved for the indication of cluster abortive therapy. Previously, the drugs of choice for abortive therapy were the ergotamine derivatives, which should be used at the first signs of the headache. The use of oxygen therapy has also been recommended for acute cluster headaches. Oxygen should be administered by mask at 8 to 10 liters per minute for 10 minutes. This type of therapy may be inconvenient for many cluster sufferers.

The use of 4% lidocaine (Xylocaine) solution applied to the sphenopalatine fossa by nasal drips has reportedly been beneficial in abortive therapy for cluster headaches. Also, 10% cocaine hydrochloride in a saline solution has been used successfully when administered in the same way as the lidocaine. Owing to the short duration of these headaches, analgesics may not be required unless the headache has not responded to recommended therapy.

TABLE 10. **Abortive Therapy for Cluster Headache**

Medication	Dosage
Sumatriptan (Imitrex)	
Subcutaneous	6 mg; may repeat after 1 h; up to 12 mg/24 h
Oral	25 mg, may repeat dose in 2 h, up to 50 mg/24 h. May increase to 50 mg dose with next attack, up to 100 mg/24 h. May increase to 75 mg dose with next attack, up to 125 mg/24 h. May increase to 100 mg dose with next attack, up to 150 mg/24 h.
Ergotamine tartrate with caffeine	
Oral (Cafergot; Wigraine)	2 tablets at onset, may repeat 1 tablet q 0.5 h, up to 6/d, 10/wk
Rectal (Cafergot)	1 suppository at onset, may repeat in 1 h, up to 2/d, 5/wk
Sublingual (Ergomar)	1 tablet at onset, may repeat 1 tablet q 0.5 h, up to 3/d, 5/wk
Dihydroergotamine	
Parenteral: D.H.E. 45	1 mg IM at onset, may repeat in 1 h, up to 3 mg/d, 5 mg/wk
Oxygen (by mask)	8–10 L/min for 10 min
Sumatriptan (Imitrex)	
Subcutaneous	6 mg s at onset of headache; may repeat 1 mg in 1 h; up to 12 mg/d
Oral	25 mg at onset; may repeat same dose in 2 h; up to 50 mg/d
Lidocaine 4% solution (Xylocaine)	1 mL (15–16 drops) to affected nostril, repeat in 5 min, prn, up to 4 times/d; if nasal congestion is present, use Neo-Synephrine 0.5% nasal solution 3 to 5 min before instilling lidocaine
Cocaine HCl 10% solution	2 drops into affected nostril or both nostrils, 4 times/d, prn

Prophylactic Therapy

The treatment of choice in cluster headache is prophylactic therapy to decrease the frequency of the attacks and rapidly resolve the series (Table 11). In cluster prophylactic therapy, the agent of choice is methysergide. Because of the self-limiting nature of cluster headaches, the complications of prolonged methysergide therapy do not pose a problem. Methysergide is prescribed at 2 mg three times daily.

Corticosteroids.* Corticosteroids may be added to this regimen. The rationale for this therapy is not clear. It has been attributed to the multiple effects of corticosteroids on inflammation. Again, the self-limiting nature of cluster headaches sustains the short-term use of the corticosteroids. Methylprednisolone (Medrol), 16 mg, in an alternate-day dose pack

---

*Not FDA approved for this indication.

TABLE 11. **Prophylactic Therapy for Cluster Headache**

Medication	Dosage
Methysergide (Sansert)	2 mg tid
Corticosteroids	
Methylprednisolone (Medrol)	16 mg qod
Prednisone	30 mg/d
Triamcinolone (Aristocort)	4 mg/qid
Verapamil (Isoptin, Calan, Verelan)	240–480 mg/d
Lithium carbonate (Eskalith; Lithobid)	300 mg tid/d
Histamine desensitization	Total of 21 treatments of histamine phosphate in 250 mL of normal saline; first treatment, 2.75 mg of histamine phosphate; treatments 2–21, 5.5 mg of histamine phosphate
Cluster Headache Variants	
Indomethacin (Indocin)	25–50 mg tid

has been used successfully in combination with methysergide. Prednisone 30 mg daily in divided doses or triamcinolone (Aristocort) 4 mg four times daily may also be considered. The corticosteroids should be discontinued gradually.

Verapamil.* The calcium channel blocker verapamil has demonstrated efficacy in the prophylaxis of episodic and chronic cluster headaches. Verapamil may be used concomitantly with the corticosteroids. The usual dose is 240 to 480 mg daily in divided doses.

Lithium Carbonate (Eskalith, Lithobid).* The effective action of lithium carbonate in treating episodic or chronic cluster headache is unknown. It has been suggested that lithium alters electrical conductivity in the central nervous system and affects sodium, calcium, and magnesium metabolism. Lithium also inhibits the action of the antidiuretic hormone and reduces rapid eye movement sleep. Its ordinary half-life is 24 hours, it is completely absorbed in 6 to 8 hours, and it is excreted by the kidneys.

The usual dose of lithium carbonate is 900 mg per day in divided doses. To prevent toxicity, tests of serum lithium levels should be performed on a monthly basis; the level should not exceed 2.0 mEq per liter. Side effects are usually mild and transient and include polydipsia, polyuria, fatigue, and tremor. Persistent nausea and vomiting, blurred vision, and fasciculations may occur, and seizures may ensue with lithium toxicity. If this happens, the drug should be discontinued immediately and fluid and electrolyte replacement initiated.

Histamine Desensitization*

For cluster headache patients refractory to standard prophylactic agents, histamine desensitization therapy may be considered. First described by Bayard T. Horton during the 1930s, histamine desensitization has been confirmed as a safe and effective

---

*Not FDA approved for this indication.

therapeutic modality. This type of therapy is most effectively administered in an inpatient setting. At the Diamond Headache Clinic, I have successfully used this therapy for more than 20 years. Therefore, I attempted to confirm its efficacy in recidivist chronic cluster headache patients. The study was performed on both a retrospective and a prospective basis and involved 150 patients who had previously received intravenous histamine therapy. Therapy involved 21 intravenous treatments of histamine phosphate mixed with 250 mL of normal saline, with initial dose of histamine at 2.75 mg and all subsequent mixtures with histamine 5.5 mg. Adjustments in the rate of infusion were based on the patient's tolerance. Patients received two treatments within 24 hours, unless the patient could tolerate three treatments within 24 hours.

After 4 weeks of follow-up, 30% reported no headache, and 34% had a reduction in the frequency of attacks. A total of 64% reported more than 50% reduction in the frequency ($P < .05$). Headache frequency increased or remained unchanged in 12%. In 64%, histamine desensitization therapy was effective in preventing or reducing the frequency of attacks to more than 50%. Duration was improved in 39% and severity in 77%. Associated symptoms improved in 45%. I concluded that intravenous histamine therapy is an effective treatment of intractable chronic cluster headaches.

Surgery for Cluster Headaches

The treatment of cluster headaches is invariably medical. However, for some patients with intractable cluster headaches, surgical intervention may be considered. Surgical procedures that have been used in the treatment of cluster headache include resection of the greater superficial petrosal nerve, section of the nervus intermedius, and ablation of the sphenopalatine ganglion. Other procedures such as percutaneous radiofrequency gangliorhizolysis, a partial trigeminal root section, and glycerol injections of the trigeminal cistern have been suggested. The results of these procedures are equivocal. It should be stressed that surgical intervention should be considered only after other methods of treatment have been exhausted and the patient is desperate.

Cluster Headache Variant

Some patients present with a syndrome similar to that of cluster headaches but with some atypical symptoms. Cluster headache variant syndrome consists of three types of pain that can occur in any combination. The patient may experience (1) atypical cluster headaches (of atypical location, duration, and frequency), which may occur several times per day; (2) multiple jabs (sharp, variable pains lasting only a few seconds), which occur several times per day and are often related to exertion or head movement; and (3) background vascular headaches (chronic, continuous, usually sharply localized, and often unilat-

eral) of variable severity, which usually are throbbing or become throbbing during exertion.

Treatment

Indomethacin (Indocin) is the agent of choice in treating cluster headache variant. The favorable response to indomethacin, in doses of 25 to 50 mg three times daily, is a diagnostic feature of this syndrome. Chronic paroxysmal hemicrania is a subtype of this syndrome, and it is also relieved by indomethacin. For patients unresponsive to indomethacin, a TCA or the addition of lithium carbonate to the regimen may be considered.

TENSION-TYPE (MUSCLE CONTRACTION) HEADACHES

Tension-type headaches occur episodically or are chronic in nature. Typically, they are a steady, nonpulsatile ache. Patients describe the pain as a "tightness" occurring bilaterally or at the occiput, a bandlike sensation about the head (similar to a tight hat), viselike, a weight, pressure, drawing, and soreness. The headache is often accompanied by pain and tightness in the neck. On palpation, the physician may find several tender areas or nodules, which are sharply localized.

Episodic tension-type headaches are usually related to some type of emotional distress or fatigue. Patients with episodic tension-type headaches rarely seek medical attention for their problem and usually rely on over-the-counter analgesics for pain relief. Patients with chronic tension-type headaches report a daily, continuous headache. These patients also have a multitude of emotional, psychic, and somatic complaints. Chronic tension-type headaches may occur at any age but are usually seen after the third decade. Although both sexes are affected, women appear to predominate, possibly because they are more likely to seek treatment. Depression is the most frequently cited cause of chronic tension-type headaches. The presence of a sleep disturbance, such as early or frequent awakening, will confirm this diagnosis.

Prophylactic Therapy

Because of the continuous pattern of chronic tension-type headaches, the use of habituating agents, such as narcotics, tranquilizers, and barbiturates, is not recommended. Prophylactic therapy is the treatment of choice to prevent a dependence problem.

Antidepressants. Antidepressants are the agents of choice in the prophylaxis of chronic tension-type headaches. As stated previously, their role is increasingly being recognized.

TCAs* are known to interfere with the uptake of the neurotransfer amines into the synaptic stores, resulting in the increased availability of epinephrine, norepinephrine, and similar amines, which may pro-

---

*Not FDA approved for this indication.

TABLE 12. **Effects of Antidepressants**

Drug	Serotonin Inhibition	Norepinephrine Inhibition	Dopamine Inhibition	Sedative Effects	Anticholinergic Effects
Amitriptyline	Moderate	Weak	Inactive	Strong	Strong
Doxepin	Moderate	Moderate	Inactive	Strong	Strong
Nortriptyline	Weak	Fairly potent	Inactive	Mild	Moderate
Imipramine	Fairly potent	Moderate	Inactive	Moderate	Strong
Trimipramine	Weak	Weak	Inactive	Moderate	Moderate
Protriptyline	Weak	Fairly potent	Inactive	None	Strong
Desipramine	Weak	Potent	Inactive	Mild	Moderate
Maprotiline	Weak	Moderate	Inactive	Moderate	Moderate
Venlafaxine	Potent	Potent	Weak	Mild	Mild
Trazodone	Fairly potent	Weak	Inactive	Strong	Mild
Fluoxetine	Potent	Weak	Inactive	None	Mild to none
Bupropion HCl	Weak	Weak	Weak	None	None
Sertraline HCl	Potent	Weak	Weak	None	None
Paroxetine HCl	Potent	Weak	Weak	None	None

mote their pharmacologic activity. The presence of a sleep disturbance will be instrumental in the selection of the TCA (Table 12). Amitriptyline (Elavil) and doxepin (Sinequan), in large bedtime doses, are often effective for patients with early or frequent awakening. In the absence of a sleep disturbance, nortriptyline (Aventyl), 25 mg at bedtime, or protriptyline, 5 to 10 mg three times daily, may be indicated. Protriptyline is the least sedating of the TCAs, and the majority of a day's dose should be given in the morning. Imipramine, 25 to 150 mg daily, or trimipramine (Surmontil), 75 to 200 mg daily, may also be considered.

Newer antidepressants are now available, such as trazodone.* Trazodone, in doses of 75 to 300 mg daily, has a low profile for cardiovascular and anticholinergic effects; drowsiness is the most commonly reported side effect. Persistent priapism has been reported with trazodone therapy. Fluoxetine (Prozac),* a bicyclic antidepressant, has been the subject of much publicity. Its action is slower than that of TCAs, but it is less likely to produce the frequent adverse effects associated with the TCAs. Fluoxetine in headache prophylaxis is usually prescribed in doses of 20 mg four times daily. One of the newest antidepressants, bupropion HCl,* is not related to the TCAs. For headache therapy, it is usually prescribed in doses of 100 mg two or three times daily. At the Diamond Headache Clinic, I reported the results of a retrospective study on the efficacy and safety of venlafaxine (Effexor).* Similar to other antidepressants, the effectiveness of venlafaxine on chronic headache is linked to its immediate effects on the neurotransmitters. Its specific actions include inhibition of both norepinephrine and serotonin uptake and weak inhibition of dopamine reuptake. Thirty-six of 97 patients using venlafaxine 75 mg twice daily noted improvement in their headaches, and any reported side effects were mild and transient. I concluded that this antidepressant could be effectively and safely used in the treatment of chronic tension-type headaches.

For patients refractory to other forms of antidepressants, the MAOIs* may be considered. The MAOIs are generally considered second-line concomitant therapy and have possible food interactions. Phenelzine 15 mg three times daily is the MAOI of choice in headache therapy. Previously, the concomitant use of an MAOI with a TCA was strictly avoided because of reported cases of morbidity. However, most of these cases were due to concomitant use of imipramine with the MAOIs. Concomitant therapy should be initiated cautiously, preferably in an inpatient setting. Reports have noted that amitriptyline has been effective in the treatment of the reaction caused by eating tyramine-containing foods while receiving MAOI therapy. A 5- to 14-day washout period is required before starting treatment with fluoxetine or bupropion after discontinuation of MAOI treatment.

Abortive Therapy

For episodic tension-type headaches, simple over-the-counter analgesics usually suffice. As stated previously, the patient with chronic tension-type headaches is prone to dependency problems because of the continuous pattern of pain. All analgesics containing narcotic, barbiturates, or tranquilizers should be strictly avoided in the patients. Over-the-counter analgesics containing caffeine may also be excessively consumed, and the patient may experience a caffeine withdrawal headache when the medication is missed.

COEXISTING MIGRAINE AND TENSION-TYPE HEADACHES (MIXED HEADACHE SYNDROME)

Most patients presenting at a specialized headache clinic are suffering the coexisting migraine and tension-type headaches. These patients present with periodic severe migraine attacks as well as a daily continuous milder tension-type headache. Manage-

---

*Not FDA approved for this indication.

*Not FDA approved for this indication.

ment of these complex patients is difficult. The dual nature of this headache syndrome may require specific agents for the migraine as well as the tension-type headaches. Initiation of a copharmacy approach to these patients should be undertaken only in an inpatient setting. The antidepressants are especially beneficial to patients with coexisting migraine and tension-type headaches.

Because of the frequency and severity of the pain, these patients are especially prone to developing rebound headaches with ergotamine preparations as well as analgesics. Successful treatment can be achieved only if the dependency problem has been resolved. Inpatient therapy, with a multidisciplinary approach, can be effective in treating the patient with coexisting migraine and tension-type headaches. The criteria for admission of headache patients to a specialized inpatient unit are provided in Table 13. These patients require continuity of care, because they have often consulted a multitude of physicians. They have also been treated with most conventional therapies. Referral for psychologic or psychiatric consultation may be indicated, and the use of both pharmacologic and behavioral therapies should be considered.

HEADACHE IN CHILDHOOD

As stated previously, headaches may occur at any age. The onset of migraines is often noted during childhood and adolescence. A thorough history and physical examination are essential, as well as an inventory of emotional and psychologic factors that may be contributing to the child's headache.

TABLE 13. **Criteria for Admission to Inpatient Headache Unit**

Prolonged, unrelenting headache, with associated symptoms such as nausea and vomiting, which, if allowed to continue, would pose a further threat to the patient's welfare.
Status migraine.
Dependence on analgesics, caffeine, narcotics, barbiturates, or tranquilizers. Withdrawal from these agents must be undertaken in an inpatient setting.
Habituation to ergots; ergots taken on a daily basis, when stopped, will cause a rebound headache.
Pain accompanied by serious adverse reactions or complications from therapy; continued use of such therapy aggravates pain.
Pain in the presence of significant medical disease; appropriate treatment of headache symptoms aggravates or induces further illness.
Chronic cluster headaches unresponsive to treatment.
Treatment that requires copharmacy with drugs that may cause a drug interaction and necessitates careful observation within a hospital milieu. For example, concomitant therapy using monoamine oxidase inhibitors and beta blockers.
Patients with probable organic cause of their headaches, requiring the appropriate consultations and perhaps neurosurgical intervention.
Headache in the presence of ergot or analgesic toxicity.
Severe headache in the presence of severe psychiatric disease.
Severe headache necessitating frequent parenteral medication.

Treatment

In the abortive treatment of childhood headaches, the use of habituating analgesics must be strictly avoided. The drug of choice for pediatric migraine is cyproheptadine,* 4 to 8 mg, at bedtime. Propranolol,* 10 mg daily, has also been effective for some young patients. Children with headache are especially responsive to biofeedback training; this has been attributed to their willingness to learn new techniques. Also, children have not developed the chronic pain pattern often seen in adult headache sufferers.

POST-TRAUMATIC HEADACHE

The severity of the injury is not especially parallel to the degree or severity of the ensuing headache. Many patients incur severe trauma to the head without experiencing a subsequent headache. Other patients, within a few days of minor head trauma, complain of severe headaches. There is often a delayed onset of symptoms, which may persist for many years.

To rule out a possible organic cause for the headaches, diagnostic examinations must be considered, including computed tomography of the head and/or the cervical spine and MRI. Referral to the appropriate specialist, such as an orthopedic surgeon or a neurosurgeon, may be indicated.

Treatment

Treatment is, of course, dependent on the diagnosis. Some patients experience an initial onset or an exacerbation of migraine headaches and should be treated accordingly. The antidepressants are especially useful in the post-traumatic headache syndrome, possibly because of their action in pain control. The use of muscle relaxants, such as cyclobenzaprine (Flexeril),* 10 mg three times daily, may be indicated if neck pain is associated with the headache. Physical therapy, including massage and deep heat, may also be effective. The prognosis of this syndrome varies. In my clinical experience, I have not observed the relief of symptoms contingent on the outcome of pending litigation.

TRACTION AND INFLAMMATORY HEADACHES

The term traction and inflammatory headaches refers to headaches resulting from inflammation, traction and displacement, and distortion of the pain sources of the head, such as the cranial vessels. A traction headache can have a variety of organic causes, such as hematomas, aneurysm, abscesses, brain tumors, nonspecific brain edema, or lumbar puncture. Diseases of the eye (such as glaucoma), ears, and sinuses trigger inflammatory headaches.

---

*Not FDA approved for this indication.

Treatment

The management of these headaches is directly related to their cause. For example, a patient with a subdural hematoma or brain tumor should be referred for neurosurgical consultation. Appropriate antibiotic therapy should be instituted for the patient with headache due to abscess. Most patients with headaches due to organic disease do not seek treatment at a specialized headache clinic. The physician should be cognizant of the importance of immediate and appropriate diagnostic evaluation for patients with recent onset of headache or for those whose headache pattern has changed. Some organic headache syndromes, such as trigeminal neuralgia and temporal arteritis, can be treated medically.

Trigeminal Neuralgia (Tic Douloureux)

Some forms of facial pain are believed to be related to the cranial nerves, excluding major neuralgias, such as the trigeminal and glossopharyngeal. Trigeminal neuralgia is characterized by episodic, recurrent unilateral pain that rarely occurs before the age of 50 years. The pain is of high intensity, and the description of trigger zones typifies this syndrome. In trigeminal neuralgia, the patient avoids touching, washing, or shaving the face, biting or chewing, or any maneuver that could stimulate the pain site. These trigger zones are usually on the face, in particular above the nares and mouth. Many patients with trigeminal neuralgia lose weight because they avoid stimulating the oral cavity.

The distribution of the pain usually affects the second or third division of the fifth cranial nerve. Patients describe the pain as a unilateral sharp jab, short and momentary, and compare it to electric shocks. It typically lasts less than 20 to 30 seconds. Episodes of pain are followed by pain-free periods. The sex distribution of trigeminal neuralgia is 2:1, female to male.

Some patients will present with a postinfectious neuralgia, usually due to herpes zoster that has localized in a facial area. Postherpetic neuralgia usually presents in the elderly, and the pain is especially intense and prolonged. Its severity and duration are often associated with depression and habituation to analgesics.

Treatment

The treatment of choice in trigeminal neuralgia is anticonvulsant therapy (Table 14). Anticonvulsants reduce the sensitivity of the trigger zones and provide pain relief, often dramatically, within 4 to 24 hours. The first-line drug is usually carbamazepine (Tegretol) with initial doses of 200 mg per day, which may be increased to 800 to 1200 mg daily, in divided doses. If the medication is well tolerated and the pain is relieved, therapy may continue for several months. The medication is titrated according to the severity of the pain. Phenytoin (Dilantin),* up to 400

TABLE 14. Medical Therapy for Trigeminal Neuralgia

Medication	Dose (mg/d)	Precautions
Carbamazepine (Tegretol)	200–1200	Monitor for blood disorders
Phenytoin (Dilantin)	200–400	Central nervous system, hematopoietic, oral symptoms
Chlorphenesin (Maolate)	800–2400	Drowsiness
Baclofen (Lioresal)	30–60	Drowsiness, weakness, nausea, vomiting

mg per day in divided doses, may be added to the carbamazepine regimen if the patient is unresponsive. If this two-drug combination therapy produces no response, chlorphenesin (Maolate),* 800 to 2400 mg per day, or baclofen (Lioresal),* in maximal doses of 60 mg daily, may be added. Because many patients with trigeminal neuralgia are elderly, the incidence of toxicity is increased. Complete blood counts should be performed periodically to effectively monitor the patient receiving anticonvulsants.

If the patient remains refractory to the three-drug regimen, neurosurgical intervention may be considered. Surgical procedures for trigeminal neuralgia include radiofrequency rhizotomy, glycerol injection into the trigeminal cistern, and microvascular compression of the trigeminal root (Jannetta's procedure). Again, all medical alternatives should be tried before considering surgical therapy for this disorder.

To prevent the sequelae of postherpetic neuralgia, the TCAs should be started in proximity to the initiation of acyclovir (Zovirax)* therapy. The residual pain may be decreased with this combination therapy and preclude the use of habituating analgesics.

Temporal Arteritis

Headache is the most common presenting complaint of the patient with temporal arteritis. This disorder is caused by an inflammatory process to the cranial arteries. The physician should be alert to any patient older than 50 years, with the initial onset of headache, who was previously asymptomatic. The female/male ratio is 2:1. Associated symptoms include night sweats, weight loss, aching of joints, low-grade fever, and jaw claudication. The site of the headache is usually localized to the affected scalp vessels, and pain on chewing is a characteristic symptom of this disorder. On examination, the area around the temporal artery is tender and the skin may appear red. These physical signs vary according to the arteries involved.

Treatment

Early diagnosis is critical because 50% or more of untreated cases result in irreversible blindness. The diagnosis can be confirmed by an erythrocyte sedi-

*Not FDA approved for this indication.

*Not FDA approved for this indication.

mentation rate obtained by the Westergren method. If this is elevated above 40 mm per hour, a temporal artery biopsy should be performed. Therapy with corticosteroids can be initiated while awaiting the results of the biopsy to avoid delayed treatment. Prednisone, 40 to 60 mg daily, is the drug of choice in temporal arteritis. A low maintenance dose of 10 to 20 mg daily may be required for a prolonged period.

EPISODIC VERTIGO

method of
ROBERT W. BALOH, M.D.
UCLA School of Medicine
Los Angeles, California

Treatment of vertigo can be divided into three general categories: specific, symptomatic, and rehabilitative. Specific therapies are directed at the underlying cause of vertigo and have the potential for eliminating vertigo. Symptomatic therapy is used to control troublesome symptoms during the acute stage and may also be used when a specific treatment does not exist. Rehabilitation is appropriate when damage to the vestibular system is expected to persist; this type of treatment is used to reduce symptoms of dizziness, gait imbalance, and oscillopsia.

SPECIFIC THERAPY FOR VERTIGO SYNDROMES

Motion Sickness

Unaccustomed exposure to prolonged motion can cause marked autonomic symptoms in susceptible persons. Typically, these symptoms include perspiration, nausea, vomiting, increased salivation, yawning, and malaise. The syndrome is worsened when there is a conflict between visual cues and vestibular cues about self-motion. For example, reading or sitting in an enclosed space while in motion in a boat or car gives the visual system the miscue that the environment is stationary, while the vestibular system receives strong self-motion cues. This mismatch can be reduced by viewing the environment—the horizon from aboard ship, or the road while driving—so that self-motion can be accurately perceived. For susceptible persons, use of a vestibular suppressant with moderate sedating action (Table 1) helps prevent the development of symptoms by diminishing the sensation of motion detected by the inner ear.

Benign Positional Vertigo

Patients with benign positional vertigo develop brief episodes of vertigo after a position change—typically, when turning over in bed, getting in and out of bed, lifting the head after bending over, or extending the neck to look up (top-shelf vertigo). The syndrome usually results from free-floating otoconial debris within the posterior semicircular canal, which causes gravity-dependent movement of the cupula. It can follow any form of damage to the inner ear (e.g., trauma, infection, surgery) but most commonly occurs spontaneously, particularly in older people. The physical examination is usually normal. However, rapidly moving the patient from the sitting to the head-hanging position (the Dix-Hallpike test) induces a torsional, vertical nystagmus when the affected ear is down (upper pole of the eye beats toward the ground). The nystagmus appears after a brief latency, lasts for less than 1 minute, and fatigues with repeated positioning. A positioning maneuver is used to move the debris along the posterior canal and out its opening into the utricle, effectively curing the syndrome (Figure 1). The maneuver can be reapplied several times in succession until the positional nystagmus disappears. Patients are cautioned to keep the head elevated at least 45 degrees above the horizontal for 48 hours after the procedure to prevent the debris from reentering the posterior semicircular canal.

Acute Prolonged Vestibulopathy

An acute episode of severe vertigo with nystagmus, nausea, and vomiting that gradually resolves over days to weeks can result from any lesion that causes an acute imbalance in the peripheral or central vestibular pathways. Infection involving the vestibular nerve and inner ear is the most common cause. Findings and specific therapies for several syndromes are listed in Table 2. Symptomatic treatment is usually necessary to control acute vertigo and nausea as the work-up progresses, and vestibular rehabilitation is often needed to speed recovery. The brain has a remarkable ability to compensate for an acute vestibular imbalance, particularly after peripheral vestibular lesions.

Relapsing Vestibulopathy

Recurrent attacks of vertigo result when there is a sudden temporary and largely reversible impairment of resting neural activity of one labyrinth or its central connections, with subsequent recovery to normal or near-normal function. Common syndromes resulting in recurrent episodes of vertigo are listed in Table 3. Key factors in the differential diagnosis include the duration of typical vertigo attacks (minutes versus hours) and the presence or absence of hearing loss and abnormalities at electronystagmography. Symptomatic therapy can be used during acute, severe attacks of vertigo but is less effective when used daily because of the long-term, chronic nature of these conditions. Treatment aimed at relieving the underlying disorder is critical.

Chronic Vestibulopathy

Processes that cause slow loss of vestibular function, or that involve both labyrinths simultaneously,

TABLE 1. **Antivertiginous, Antiemetic Drugs**

Drug	Dosage	Action		Major Side Effects	Precautions
		Sedative	*Antiemetic*		
Antihistamines					
Meclizine (Antivert, Bonine)	Oral: 25 mg qd–qid	±	+	None	Asthma, glaucoma, prostate enlargement
Dimenhydrinate (Dramamine)	Oral: 50 mg q 4–6 h	+	+	None	Same as above
Promethazine (Phenergan)	Oral: 25 mg q 6 h Suppository: 50 mg q 12 h IM: 25 mg q 4–6 h	+ +	+	Extrapyramidal reactions*	Same as above plus history of seizures
Benzamide					
Metoclopramide (Reglan)	Oral: 5–10 mg q 6 h IM or IV: 10 mg q 4–6 h	+	+ + +	Extrapyramidal reactions*	Liver or kidney disease, bowel obstruction, pheochromocytoma
Phenothiazine					
Prochlorperazine (Compazine)	Oral: 5–10 mg q 6 h Suppository: 25 mg q 12 h IM: 5–10 mg q 6 h	+	+ + +	Extrapyramidal reactions*	Known hypersensitivity
Benzodiazepines					
Diazepam (Valium)	Oral: 2, 5, 10 mg bid–qid IM: 5–10 mg q 4–6 h IV: 5–10 mg (slow) q 4 h	+ + +	+	Respiratory depression, drug dependency	Glaucoma
Butyrophenone					
Droperidol (Inapsine)	IM or IV: 2.5–5 mg q 12 h	+ + +	+ +	Extrapyramidal reactions*	Known hypersensitivity, liver or kidney disease

*Tardive dyskinesia, dystonia, akathisia, oculogyric crisis, parkinsonism.

do not usually result in attacks of severe vertigo. Such syndromes may give rise to recurrent, transient sensations of mild vertigo, nonspecific dizziness, or progressive gait imbalance. Associated symptoms and signs are necessary for diagnosis in these cases. For example, slowly growing tumors of the eighth nerve or cerebellopontine angle (acoustic neuroma) rarely produce vertigo. They usually manifest as unilateral tinnitus and hearing loss and can cause facial weakness or central signs; magnetic resonance imaging and brain stem auditory evoked response testing are diagnostic, and surgical consultation is indicated. Exposure to ototoxic drugs (particularly aminoglycosides) can result in bilateral vestibular damage, which causes gait imbalance and oscillopsia. Therapy includes discontinuation of the drug and the use of a vestibular rehabilitation program.

SYMPTOMATIC THERAPY OF VERTIGO

Normally, the vestibular nuclei receive a balanced, tonic input from the vestibular receptors in the inner ears. Any asymmetry in this tonic firing rate causes vertigo. Antivertiginous drugs are believed to act by suppressing the firing rate of primary afferent neurons and by reducing transmission of impulses from primary to secondary vestibular neurons, thereby decreasing the imbalance resulting from a vestibular lesion. Antiemetic drugs work by suppressing the brain emetic centers or input to these centers, including signals from the vestibular nuclei. Commonly used drugs and their dosages are listed in Table 1. The effectiveness of these drugs has been determined empirically, and it is often difficult to predict which drug or combination of drugs will be most effective in any given patient.

A single drug or drug combination should be chosen on the basis of the known effects of each drug and the severity and time course of the patient's symptoms. Acute, severe vertigo with nystagmus is an extremely distressing symptom, and sedation is useful during the early phase of treatment, e.g., with diazepam (Valium) or droperidol (Inapsine). Side effects can be serious, and parenteral treatment should be reserved for settings in which emergency resusci-

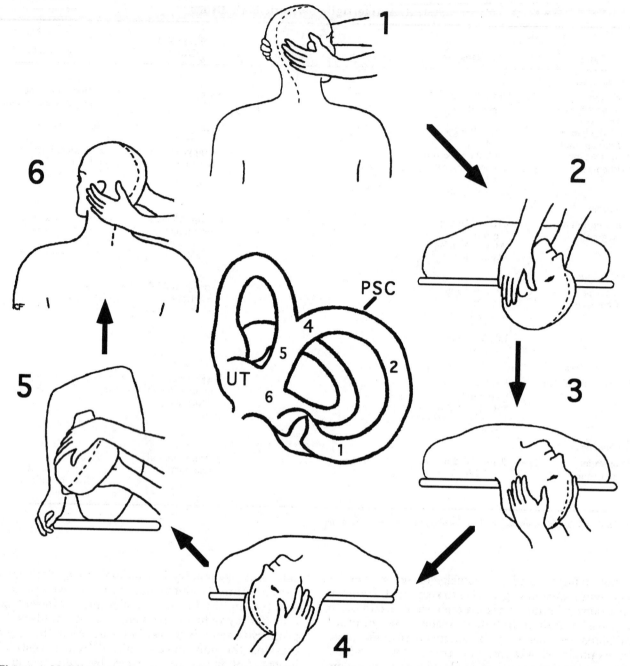

Figure 1. Modified Epley maneuver for treating benign positional vertigo affecting the right ear. (1) The patient is seated upright, with the head facing the operator, who is standing on the patient's right. The patient should grasp the forearm of the operator with both hands for stability. (2) The patient is then rapidly moved into the supine position, allowing the head to extend just beyond the end of the examining table, with the right ear downward. This position is maintained until the nystagmus ceases. (3) The operator moves to the head of the table, repositioning the hands as shown. (4) The head is quickly rotated toward the left, stopping with the right ear upward. This position is maintained for 30 seconds. (5) The patient rolls onto the left side, while the examiner rapidly rotates the head leftward until the nose is directed toward the floor. This position is then held for 30 seconds. (6) The patient is rapidly lifted into the sitting position, now facing left. The entire sequence should be repeated until no nystagmus can be elicited. For treating the left ear, begin with the patient's head to the left and move to the left ear down position.

tation equipment is available. When nausea and vomiting are prominent, a potent antiemetic such as prochlorperazine (Compazine) or metoclopramide (Reglan)* can be combined with an antivertiginous medication. Severe, infrequent vertigo spells associ-

ated with nausea can be managed on an outpatient basis with promethazine (Phenergan) taken orally or as a suppository at the onset of symptoms.

Chronic, frequently recurrent vertigo is a different therapeutic problem, because the patient must attempt to carry on normal activities, and sedation is undesirable. Milder antivertiginous medications,

---

*Not FDA approved for this indication.

TABLE 2. **Diagnosis and Management of Common Causes of Acute Peripheral Vestibulopathy**

Syndrome	Vertigo History	Examination	Treatment
Viral neurolabyrinthitis	Develops over hours; resolves over days; prior flulike illness	Nystagmus, vomiting, ± high-frequency hearing loss	Consider steroids (Medrol Dosepak); vestibular rehabilitation
Bacterial labyrinthitis	Abrupt onset; history of ear infection, or headache and fever	Profound hearing loss, nystagmus, otitis media or meningitis	Antibiotics based on culture results; surgical débridement; vestibular rehabilitation
Stroke	Abrupt onset; age >50 y, prior history of vascular disease, other neurologic symptoms	Signs of brain stem or cerebellar infarct, nystagmus, unilateral hearing loss, changes on magnetic resonance imaging	Supportive measures; vestibular rehabilitation
Trauma or labyrinthine concussion	Abrupt onset following head trauma, plus other neurologic symptoms	Nystagmus, hearing impairment, hemotympanum, ± facial weakness, temporal bone fracture on computed tomography	Surgical consult for seventh nerve injury; vestibular rehabilitation

such as meclizine (Antivert), 25 mg every four hours,* can be used for less severe vertigo. These drugs are generally not indicated for long-term, daily use, because they tend to interfere with the normal process of compensation to vestibular disorders. Diazepam can be used episodically, but its prolonged use on a daily basis results in chemical dependency. Rehabilitation therapy or a specific treatment aimed at the underlying condition is a better choice of therapy for persistent symptoms of dizziness.

*Exceeds dosage recommended by the manufacturer.

TABLE 3. **Diagnosis and Management of Common Causes of Relapsing Vestibulopathy**

Syndrome	Vertigo Duration and History	Examination	Treatment
Autoimmune inner ear disease	Hours duration; rapidly progressing bilateral hearing loss	Hearing loss, ± inflammatory process in eye, joints, other organs ± elevated ESR	Steroids: prednisone, 100 mg qd; Solu-Medrol, 1 g qd
Meniere's syndrome	Hours duration; aural fullness, tinnitus, hearing loss	Low-frequency hearing loss during attacks, ENG abnormal	1-g sodium diet; diuretics; surgery if vertigo is uncontrolled
Migraine-associated vertigo	Minutes to hours duration; prior history of aura or unilateral throbbing headache	Normal, ± ENG abnormalities	Migraine prophylaxis: acetazolamide (Diamox),* 250 mg bid; propranolol LA, 80–160 mg qd; imipramine, 50–100 mg qd
Syphilitic labyrinthitis	Similar to that in Meniere's disease; history of sexually transmitted disease or congenital infection	Bilateral progressive hearing loss, ENG abnormalities, signs of congenital syphilis	Penicillin and steroids: benzathine penicillin,* 2.4 million U IM q wk × 6 wk; prednisone, 60 mg qod × 3 mo
Vertebrobasilar insufficiency or transient ischemic attacks	Minutes duration; abrupt onset, age >50 y, prior history of vascular disease, other neurologic symptoms	Normal between attacks; nystagmus, ataxia, other neurologic signs during attacks	Antiplatelet therapy: aspirin, 325 mg qd; ticlopidine (Ticlid), 250 mg bid

*Not FDA approved for this indication.
Abbreviations: ENG = electronystagmography; ESR = erythrocyte sedimentation rate.

VESTIBULAR REHABILITATION

When the vestibular system has been permanently damaged, the initial state of imbalance at the level of the brain stem nuclei results in acute vertigo. Gradually, the patient adapts to this imbalance through a process of compensation, which requires intact vision and depth perception, normal proprioception in the neck and limbs, and intact sensation in the lower extremities. Central pathways are also integral to compensation, and damage to these areas results in a less effective recovery.

Clinicians have long been aware that vestibular compensation occurs more rapidly and is more complete if the patient begins exercising as soon as possible after a vestibular lesion. Controlled studies in primates have supported this general clinical observation. Baboons whose hind limbs were restrained by plaster casts after a unilateral vestibular lesion showed markedly delayed recovery of balance compared with lesioned animals that had been allowed normal motor exploration. Visual experience is also necessary; lesioned animals kept in light compensated faster than those kept in darkness. Compensation is accelerated by stimulant drugs and slowed by sedation. For these reasons, vestibular exercise programs should be instituted as soon as possible after an injury to the vestibular system has been identified, and the use of sedating drugs and vestibular suppressants should be limited to the acute stage.

In addition to vertigo, vestibular lesions interfere with reflexes controlling eye movement during active head motion and with postural righting reflexes. This interference can result in symptoms of oscillopsia caused by head movements and a tendency to veer or fall to the side when walking. These symptoms, and the associated dizziness, can be improved by active exercises designed to speed compensation. Vestibular exercises should begin as soon as the acute stage of nausea and vomiting has ended and the underlying disease process is subsiding. Many of the exercises result in dizziness. This sensation is a necessary stimulus for compensation; antivertiginous medications should be avoided during this period to maximize the beneficial effect. Exercises should be done at least twice daily for several minutes but may be done as often as the patient can tolerate.

While nystagmus is present, the patient should attempt to focus the eyes and to move and hold them in the direction that provokes the most dizziness. Once the nystagmus diminishes to the point that a target can be "held" visually in all directions, the patient should begin eye-head coordination exercises. A useful exercise involves staring at a visual target while oscillating the head either from side to side or up and down. The speed of the head movements can be gradually increased, as long as the target can be kept in good focus. Target changes, in which the patient uses combined eye and head movements to "jump" quickly back and forth between two widely separated visual targets, are also useful. Blinking during these fast head turns can help reduce symptoms of dizziness or visual blurring.

The patient should attempt to stand and walk while nystagmus is still present. It may be necessary to walk in contact with a wall, or using an assistant, in the early stages. Slow, supported turns should be made initially. As improvement occurs, head movements should be added while the patient is standing and walking—at first slow, side-to-side or up-and-down movements, then fast head turns in all directions. Learning to combine fast head turns with brief eye closure or blinks during walking turns can increase stability and decrease dizziness.

Compensation requires from 2 to 6 months. Dizziness that persists beyond this time indicates either the presence of an ongoing, recurrent vestibular illness or poor compensation. The patient's history should be reviewed, and any vestibular suppressants should be discontinued. Evidence of central involvement or impairment of vision, proprioception, or sensation should be evaluated. If all areas are normal, no evidence of active disease is present, and no medications are in use, a program of habituation to dizziness should be instituted. All movements that provoke dizziness should be identified, and they should then be repeated as often as possible to maximize the symptom. This approach will gradually result in habituation to the provoking stimulus.

MENIERE'S DISEASE

method of
C. GARY JACKSON, M.D.
The Otology Group
Nashville, Tennessee

Meniere's disease is a capricious disorder of the inner ear. The disease is episodic, with spells punctuated by periodic remission. Its cause is unknown. An overaccumulation of inner ear endolymph is thought to dilate the membranous labyrinth. The resulting overpressure produces the disorder's characteristic symptom complex.

Meniere's disease is a specific entity, the diagnosis of which is clinical. This diagnosis must be accurate and consistent with this form of balance disorder. Characteristically, an attack of Meniere's disease is heralded by the onset of ear pressure or fullness followed by loud, roaring tinnitus and a downward fluctuation in hearing. The events precede an acute attack of true whirling vertigo by minutes to days or weeks. The true vertigo typically lasts minutes to hours, the whole attack encompassing 2 to 5 hours. Hearing returns to normal after the attack, and tinnitus and pressure abate. The disease is exacerbated by barometric pressure changes, hormonal fluctuations, stress, tension, anxiety, and cigarette abuse.

This disorder is typically unilateral, but in 15 to 40% of cases, it is bilateral. The auditory symptoms are poorly addressed by therapy, and although bothersome, they do not threaten lifestyle. It is the vertigo that is the Meniere's disease sufferer's most disabling symptom and to which most therapy is directed.

DIAGNOSIS

The general physical and otoneurologic examination is usually unremarkable in Meniere's disease. Pure tone and speech audiometry is often characteristic, exhibiting diminution of low-tone hearing. The symptoms of this disorder are neurologic, and therefore, a long list of diagnostic possibilities must be excluded before this diagnosis is derived. Magnetic resonance imaging with gadolinium is necessary to evaluate the neuraxis for neoplasm, especially acoustic neuroma.

TREATMENT OPTIONS

The therapy for Meniere's disease is medical or surgical. Treatment is steeped in controversy owing to the inconclusiveness surrounding the etiology. The erratic natural history of the disorder confounds statistical validation of treatment options. The goal of treatment is to eliminate the disabling symptom of vertigo. A subobjective, rarely achievable in the long term, is relief from the inexorable progression of the sensorineural hearing loss.

Medical Therapy

Medical therapy is aimed at (1) reducing the inner ear fluid overpressure (endolymphatic hydrops) and (2) controlling vertigo.

Treatment of Endolymphatic Hydrops

A sodium-restricted diet forms the basis of dietary management of Meniere's disease. Salt intake is restricted to 1500 mg per day. Organized education is critical to successful compliance. Alcohol and caffeine may be provocative and are recommended to be used in moderation. Nicotine should be excluded. Once dietary compliance is established, variances from the diet usually provoke symptoms.

Body fluid management is augmented by diuretic therapy. Thiazides in combination with potassium-sparing agents are popular (Dyazide, Maxzide). Electrolytes require intelligent surveillance.

Dietary compliance and diuretic therapy alone are often adequate for control of Meniere's disease.

Symptomatic Vestibular Suppression

Vestibular suppressants are used in conjunction with dietary and diuretic therapy when the latter inadequately control active vertigo.

Diazepam (Valium)* is the single most effective outpatient vestibular suppressant. It is thought to diminish resting activity of vestibular nuclei neurons as well as to affect cerebellovestibular inhibitory transmissions. Individual responses to this agent are quite variable. Idiosyncratic reactions may be more objectionable than the symptoms for which it is prescribed. Dosages must be individualized and range from 1 to 5 mg orally every 8 hours. Individual treatment courses should be short, and the drug should be discontinued when clinical benefit is realized.

The excitatory neurotransmitter of the vestibular system is thought to be acetylcholine. Anticholinergics diminish neuron excitability in the vestibular

nuclei and, in combination with diazepam, are useful in therapy for Meniere's disease. Glycopyrrolate (Robinul), 2 mg orally twice daily, can be used. Similar agents suffice (e.g., propantheline [Pro-Banthine], atropine). Dry mouth, blurred vision, and bladder outlet symptoms may be objectionable.

The antihistamines, including meclizine (Antivert), are not useful in Meniere's disease. Antidopaminergic agents act on the medullary chemoreceptor trigger zone and vomiting center and are useful intravenously in managing the *acute* episode (droperidol [Inapsine]). Vasodilators are no longer recommended.

The majority of cases of Meniere's disease (75 to 80%) can be controlled by medical therapy. Dietary therapy and diuretic therapy are regarded as long-term treatment. Labyrinthine sedation is short-term, symptomatic therapy that is reinstituted for symptom flare-ups, *not* for quiescent punctations in the episodic course of this disorder. An adequate trial of medical management should last approximately 6 weeks. After 6 weeks of treatment failure, the patient can be judged to have medically refractory Meniere's disease, and candidacy for more invasive formats explored.

Streptomycin Therapy

Streptomycin* is an ototoxin that selectively destroys first the balance and then, in higher dosages, the hearing apparatus. Chemical ablation of the vestibular apparatus can thus be achieved while hearing is preserved.

First described in 1956, streptomycin therapy is reserved for medically refractory cases of bilateral Meniere's disease. Throughout the course of therapy, hearing and balance are monitored by audiology and electronystagmography (ENG) or caloric response, respectively. Protocols involve treatment to vestibular ablation or by titration to response. Treatment to ablation is associated with permanent disequilibrium and oscillopsia. The titration method is, therefore, preferred.

Streptomycin sulfate, 1 gram twice daily, is given intramuscularly for 5 days (10 grams), and the monitoring baseline studies are repeated. Therapy is continued in 5-gram intervals until symptoms cease, oscillopsia occurs, hearing level falls, or balance function on ENG becomes reduced, at which point titration ends. Average doses range from 20 to 30 grams. The effect is cumulative; more drug can be given later as indicated. Unexplained improvement in hearing or stabilization occurs in approximately a third of cases.

Intratympanic Injections

The intratympanic injection of steroids* or aminoglycosides,* which are thought to access the labyrinth via transport across the round and oval windows, has become popular. An array of protocols exist that highlight the transtympanic injection of compounds into the middle ear space on an outpatient

---

*Not FDA approved for this indication.

*Not FDA approved for this indication.

basis, in small amounts, and in repeated doses until vertigo spells are relieved. Deafness is possible in 10% of patients, and significant hearing loss in another 25%. The relief from vertigo is quite good in 85% of patients, but new data suggest that the effect is short term (2 to 5 years). Research in this area is ongoing.

Surgical Therapy

Surgery for Meniere's disease is reserved for those who have medically refractory disease and are incapacitated by their vertigo (20%). If the patient's hearing is serviceable (50 decibels, 80% speech discrimination), an operation to conserve hearing is offered. If hearing is poor, a "destructive" procedure may be suggested. The success of cochlear implantation, as well as the significant incidence of bilateral Meniere's disease, proposes destructive surgery reluctantly. Surgery for Meniere's disease remains controversial.

Labyrinthectomy

Removing the balance contents of the inner ear is a destructive procedure in which hearing is also sacrificed. The procedure is generally reserved for unilateral Meniere's disease in its late stages, when hearing is essentially gone. Although a transcanal approach is feasible, removal of the semicircular canals with the utricle and saccule via mastoidectomy is preferred. The extent of postoperative dizziness depends on the patient's preoperative residual vestibular function. Complete postoperative compensation is augmented by vestibular rehabilitation. Success is achieved in 9 of 10 patients. Risks are low, and outcome is excellent.

Endolymphatic System Surgery

A conservation procedure in which hearing is preserved, endolymphatic system surgery (ELSS) is commonly referred to as shunt surgery. It is the only option that, at least on theoretical grounds, addresses the issue of hearing as well as balance in Meniere's disease.

The endolymphatic sac is an appendage of the membranous labyrinth that is contentiously believed to be a pressure regulator of, or an absorption site for, endolymph. Theoretically, the sac can be exposed to "shunt" fluid or to restore the function of this anatomy to eliminate endolymphatic hydrops.

Even though ELSS is minor, its application remains controversial. My practice has abandoned this procedure save in exceptional circumstances. The procedure is generally regarded as a first step that is successful in the short term. Initial success is *significantly* downgraded after 3 to 5 years. The procedure is low risk and appealing to some. The risk to hearing loss is 5%.

Vestibular Nerve Section

Selective vestibular nerve section (VNS), while preserving hearing, is the only surgical modality that, *in the long term*, offers freedom from vertigo at rates

(90 to 95%) exceeding those seen in the untreated natural history of Meniere's disease (75 to 80%). VNS is a complicated, intracranial operation performed via a middle cranial fossa (MFVNS) or suboccipital exposure (SOVNS) route while hearing is monitored.

In MFVNS, the skull is entered via a temporal craniotomy. The temporal lobe is retracted, and the contents of the internal auditory canal are microsurgically exposed. In SOVNS, the skull is entered via the suboccipital route. Gentle cerebellar retraction exposes the VII/VIII nerve complex for selective VNS. The risk to hearing is 5% or less. The risk of craniotomy notwithstanding, headache can be a problem in some 20% of patients after SOVNS.

VIRAL MENINGITIS AND ENCEPHALITIS

method of
J. RICHARD BARINGER, M.D.
University of Utah School of Medicine
Salt Lake City, Utah

The distinction between viral meningitis and encephalitis is important in assigning an etiology for the condition but also in considering appropriate treatment. Acute meningitis induced by viruses commonly has a relatively abrupt onset characterized by fever, headache, vomiting, and photophobia, with or without stiffness of the neck. It may be accompanied by a variety of other symptoms, including malaise, muscle aches, and rash. Meningitis and encephalitis are distinguished from each other by the signs in the latter pointing to involvement of the parenchyma of the brain. One must immediately suspect that the brain parenchyma is involved in the patient who has symptoms of meningeal involvement but who, in addition, has difficulty with memory, confusion, hallucinations, dysphasia, seizures, or focal motor or sensory deficits. In patients with only meningitis, involvement of the parenchyma due to a concomitant vasculitis can produce signs of parenchymal damage, but this is usually a late rather than an initial sign in the course of the disease.

CLINICAL AND DIAGNOSTIC FEATURES

The presence of signs and symptoms pointing to meningitis and/or encephalitis mandates an examination of the cerebrospinal fluid (CSF). The CSF formula may be similar in virally induced meningitides and encephalitides, consisting of a usually lymphocytic pleocytosis attended by a modest elevation of CSF protein values and normal glucose values, the exception being the occasionally lowered glucose values that have been described in mumps meningitis. The CSF pressure may be normal or elevated in either condition.

The presence of symptoms or signs pointing to involvement of the brain parenchyma mandates the use of computed tomography (CT) or magnetic resonance imaging (MRI) to determine whether a pattern consistent with herpes simplex virus (HSV) involvement might be present or to demonstrate other pathologic conditions. Because of the greater sensitivity and resolution that can be obtained with MRI than with CT, it is preferable that MRI with contrast enhancement be utilized in such cases. Electroencephalography may be of additional aid in pointing to the possibility of parenchymal involvement of the brain and occasionally in providing a pattern consistent with HSV encephalitis.

DIFFERENTIAL DIAGNOSIS

It is vital to consider alternative diagnoses in patients who present with signs of meningeal involvement with or without signs or symptoms of parenchymal involvement of the brain, and in whom the CSF formula consists of a lymphocytic pleocytosis. The concept that this constellation of symptoms and findings equates with "viral meningitis" has led to numerous diagnostic misfortunes. The syndrome is more properly designated aseptic meningitis, one cause of which is viral infection. A host of other disease entities may demonstrate this constellation of findings but have other causes, mandating entirely different approaches. A variety of bacterial diseases may mimic the clinical and CSF findings that are more commonly seen in virally induced meningitis. Often, patients presenting with signs and symptoms of meningitis may have received prior antibiotic treatment directed at presumed sinus, otic, or other upper respiratory tract disease, and the treatment has been sufficient to blunt the usual pyogenic meningeal response to bacterial organisms and rendered the CSF cultures negative. In such cases, cultures and Gram stains of the CSF may be unrevealing, and screening for bacterial antigens may provide the only clue to the underlying etiology.

Parameningeal foci of infection, such as epidural or subdural empyemas or intraparenchymal abscesses caused by bacteria, may manifest as acute meningitic or encephalitic processes, with CSF formulas consisting of mild lymphocytic pleocytosis with minimal elevations of CSF protein. A history of antecedent mastoid or sinus disease, or pyogenic infection elsewhere in the body, may provide clues to the presence of a parameningeal focus. Often, careful imaging with contrast-enhanced MRI may be necessary to demonstrate these processes involving relatively silent areas of the brain.

Bacterial endocarditis can occasionally announce its presence through involvement of the central nervous system. It manifests often with focal signs or symptoms, but sometimes simply with confusional states attended by mild abnormalities in the CSF resulting from hematogenous septic infarcts in the brain.

Finally, a number of bacterial organisms can produce the picture of a meningitis, with or without involvement of brain parenchyma, in which the CSF formula consists of a predominantly mononuclear or lymphocytic pleocytosis. *Brucella*, *Mycobacterium tuberculosis*, and *Listeria monocytogenes* may cause meningeal infection, resulting in a CSF formula that suggests aseptic meningitis. Although tuberculosis classically produces a great elevation of CSF protein values and a conspicuous lowering of the CSF glucose values, neither finding is uniform. *L. monocytogenes* should be considered if the patient has signs of meningeal involvement with a CSF pleocytosis but also has signs pointing to involvement of the brain stem. Syphilis as a cause of meningitis is seen uncommonly enough to be forgotten, with potentially tragic consequences. In certain geographic regions of the country, notably the Northeast coast and the upper Midwest states, *Borrelia burgdorferi*, the cause of Lyme disease, must now be considered as a cause of the aseptic meningitis syndrome, particularly in

people who have been out of doors in tick-infested regions, and especially in those with a history of rash, arthritis, carditis with conduction defects, or a cranial neuropathy.

Although fungal infections more commonly cause subacute meningitis, the course of such an infection can be relatively acute, and the CSF formula is characterized by a mononuclear and/or lymphocytic pleocytosis consistent with an aseptic meningitis syndrome. Often, the CSF protein values are elevated, and the glucose values are sometimes depressed. The diagnosis rests on suspicion of this etiology in any patient who is immunosuppressed, but it must be kept in mind that non-immunosuppressed patients can acquire cryptococcal or other fungal meningitides. Patients who live or who traveled in the southwestern United States, where *Coccidioides* is prevalent, particularly those who may have been digging in soil in these areas, must be regarded as possibly having *Coccidioides*-induced meningitis.

Another condition that can occasionally manifest as acute aseptic meningitis with lymphocytic predominance is involvement of the meninges by sarcoidosis or carcinoma. Modest elevations of the protein and depression of glucose values characterize the CSF in both of these conditions. In carcinomatous meningitis, the CSF glucose values are often extremely low. Although CSF cytology is often positive in patients with carcinomatous meningitis, repeated sampling of the CSF may be required to establish the diagnosis. In sarcoidosis, the diagnosis often rests on the demonstration of typical involvement by sarcoid of other organs, including lung and liver, the presence of cranial neuropathy, or the demonstration by MRI of a typical involvement of the basal meninges, optic chiasm, and hypothalamus. Finally, one must be alert to the occasional patient who is sensitive to one of a variety of drugs or therapeutic agents that produce a CSF pleocytosis with the picture of meningitis through an idiosyncratic reaction. Such reactions can be seen rarely with nonsteroidal anti-inflammatory drugs, cimetidine, trimethoprim-sulfamethoxazole, carbamazepine, or ciprofloxacin, or with administration of OKT3 antibody.

Viral Meningitis and Encephalitis

Echovirus and coxsackievirus are common causes of acute meningitis, and although they may predominate in summer and early fall, they can be seen at any time of the year. These infections may be attended by rash, and myalgia is often a prominent component of the illness. Recovery from these infections is usually prompt and uncomplicated, but a significant proportion of the patients suffer rather prolonged and debilitating headache. The diagnosis can be based on the recovery of virus from the stool and occasionally from the CSF, the demonstration of viral genomes by polymerase chain reaction (PCR) analysis of the stool or CSF, or the subsequent development of neutralizing antibodies. There is no specific treatment for these conditions. HSV-2 occasionally causes meningitis in adults, usually in the wake of an acute genital HSV infection; the process is usually self-limited and may even be subclinical. Treatment with intravenous acyclovir may be considered in symptomatic individuals.

Viral encephalitides are seen in community epidemics in various parts of the United States, often in association with mosquito vectors. These RNA viruses, formerly designated arboviruses, produce varying degrees of parenchymal involvement. The involvement of the nervous system by eastern equine encephalitis virus usually produces the most severe neurologic involvement and sequelae, whereas western equine encephalitis virus and St. Louis encephalitis virus produce lesser degrees of parenchymal involvement. No specific treatment is available for involvement of the nervous system by these viruses.

Rabies involvement of the nervous system is seen only occasionally in the United States, but it must be considered in any patient with an acute encephalitis characterized classically by the development of hydrophobia and laryngeal spasms. The disease must be considered when there is any history of exposure to possibly infected dogs, skunks, or bats. It must be seriously considered in individuals who have traveled to a part of the world where rabies in dogs is prevalent, such as the Middle East, Africa, or the Indian subcontinent. Prompt washing of the animal bite, administration of rabies immune globulin, and vaccination of exposed individuals with human diploid cell vaccine offer the best hope for avoidance of the disease. No treatment has been demonstrated to be effective once symptoms of nervous system involvement are evident.

Herpes Simplex Encephalitis

The most common sporadic encephalitis in the United States is caused by HSV. In children and adults, this is almost always due to the type 1 or oral strain of the virus, whereas in newborns either HSV-1 or HSV-2 can be the etiologic agent. In adults and children, the encephalitic process may begin with headache and fever or may be initiated by a seizure with the subsequent development of focal signs of dysphasia or hemiparesis. Few, if any, clinical signs serve to distinguish encephalitis caused by HSV from encephalitis caused by other viruses or, for that matter, from a variety of other conditions involving the nervous system, such as those described previously. Vascular disease, in my experience, remains one of the often confusing conditions that can mimic the picture of HSV encephalitis. A history of the sudden development of olfactory or gustatory hallucinations, or prominent memory loss, should immediately enhance one's suspicion of the possibility of herpetic involvement of the nervous system. However, the rapid evolution of confusion and coma in such patients commonly obscures these symptoms. Patients presenting with a history and signs compatible with herpes encephalitis should be treated promptly with acyclovir (Zovirax), in a dose of 10 mg per kg intravenously every 8 hours (30 mg per kg per day), while confirmatory tests are in progress.

The two tests that are most helpful in confirming the diagnosis of herpes encephalitis are contrast-enhanced MRI of the brain and PCR analysis of the CSF for HSV-1 genomes. MRI is frequently abnormal within the first day or two of the development of herpes encephalitis. It characteristically shows involvement of the medial temporal, insular, and subfrontal regions of the brain with areas of diffuse high signal intensity on T2-weighted images. Later in the course, contrast enhancement of the cortical ribbon in these areas can be demonstrated. A small, seemingly independent lesion in the cingulate cortex is often an additional helpful diagnostic tip-off in patients with herpes simplex encephalitis. It should be noted that the MRI findings are often positive in the first few days of the development of herpes encephalitis, when CT either is negative or shows only equivocal evidence of involvement of medial temporal lobe structures. Thus, a negative CT result early in the illness should not be used to rule out herpes encephalitis.

Analysis of the CSF is of great help in making the diagnosis of herpes encephalitis. The general CSF formula of a lymphocytic or mixed pleocytosis with a mild elevation of protein value and a normal or very slightly depressed glucose level does not serve to distinguish herpes encephalitis from other encephalitic conditions. The presence or absence of red blood cells in the CSF should not be relied on in considering the diagnosis. The application of PCR analysis for HSV genomes to CSF samples has provided a reasonably rapid and highly specific way of demonstrating the presence of HSV DNA in the CSF. This test is often positive on the initial spinal tap and is almost invariably positive on days 2 through 12 after the development of symptoms, becoming negative in many cases after that time. Because occasional cases have been described in which the CSF PCR analysis for HSV is negative on the first or second day of the development of the illness, the PCR analysis should be repeated in 24 to 48 hours in questionable cases with an initially negative result.

Electroencephalography may be helpful in suggesting the diagnosis of herpes encephalitis, especially if the electroencephalogram (EEG) reveals high-voltage periodic activity in the regions of the temporal lobe. The electroencephalographic changes may be quite nonspecific, however. It is extremely rare for cases of herpes encephalitis to be accompanied by a normal EEG. An abnormal EEG is thus of value in enhancing suspicion of the disease; if the EEG is normal, the probability of herpes encephalitis is low.

Brain biopsy was formerly employed to establish the diagnosis of herpes encephalitis, but it is unnecessary if MRI and CSF PCR findings are confirmatory; its use is now confined to cases in which these findings are inconclusive. Biopsy tissue should be cultured for bacterial and fungal pathogens as well as viruses, and the tissue subjected to PCR analysis for viral genomes.

TREATMENT

The general management of patients with viral encephalitis or for encephalitis due to HSV consists of supportive treatment, usually in an intensive care unit. Seizures, if present, should be treated with phenytoin (Dilantin) or carbamazepine (Tegretol) in appropriate doses. The management of increased intracranial pressure is sometimes difficult in these patients. The raised intracranial pressure is caused by a combination of cytotoxic edema and vasogenic edema. Cytotoxic edema results from damage to neurons and other cells, with consequent intracellular swelling and edema. Vasogenic edema is produced by alteration in the blood-brain barrier with leakage of fluids from the vascular compartment into the intercellular compartment of the brain.

The treatment of vasogenic edema is most effectively accomplished by the administration of steroids. Dexamethasone is used in divided daily doses of 10 to 40 mg, depending on the seriousness of the increased intracranial pressure and the extent of shift of midline structures. The theoretical impairment of viral clearance from the administration of anti-inflammatory steroids is outweighed by their frequent salutary effect on reversing the component of vasogenic edema that is often present in these patients.

The treatment of cytotoxic edema is often much less effective. Patients should be maintained in a head-up posture in bed, and the administration of hyposmolar fluids should be carefully avoided. Although the treatment of brain edema mandates restriction of fluid intake, particularly the intake of hyposmolar fluids, this restriction must be carefully balanced against the necessity to maintain adequate fluid volume for renal perfusion and to compensate for fluid losses due to fever. An additional consideration is the tendency for patients receiving acyclovir for herpes encephalitis to develop crystalluria with renal failure, which can be obviated to some extent by adequate administration of intravenous fluids. The use of mannitol to decrease brain edema can be considered in situations in which the preceding measures are insufficient. It should be remembered, however, that mannitol is used to create an osmotic gradient between the intravascular and brain interstitial compartments. It thus works most effectively where an intact blood-brain barrier prevents the leakage of mannitol out of the vascular compartment. To the extent that the blood-brain barrier is disrupted in patients with viral encephalitis, mannitol may leak into the parenchyma in areas of damage and may be ineffective or may even cause a reversal of the desired osmotic gradient. Hyperventilation may be utilized to maintain a lowered PCO_2, which may be helpful in temporarily reducing cerebral edema.

The general care of patients with viral encephalitis of any cause deserves attention. Patients must be carefully positioned so as to avoid vomiting and consequent aspiration if the airway is not protected by intubation. Careful attention should be paid to turning and skin care to avoid the development of decubitus ulcers. Turning together with careful tracheal aspiration should be employed to prevent the development of atelectasis and/or hypostatic pneumonia, and radiographs of the chest should be obtained periodically to monitor the pulmonary status. Heparin should be administered subcutaneously, and intermittent compression stockings should be applied to mitigate the possibility of leg vein thrombosis and subsequent pulmonary embolism. Finally, patients who are in stupor or coma for prolonged periods should receive physical therapy to prevent limb contractures, which may significantly interfere with eventual return to function.

Treatment of Herpes Encephalitis

Acyclovir is administered intravenously in the treatment of herpes encephalitis in a dose of 10 mg per kg of body weight every 8 hours. The drug is preferentially phosphorylated to its active form by virally encoded thymidine kinase. Furthermore, the active drug more effectively inhibits virally encoded DNA polymerase than cellular DNA polymerases. This feature contributes to a favorable therapeutic ratio. Because the drug is excreted by the kidneys, the dose may need to be reduced in patients with renal failure. Hydration must be adequate to prevent crystalluria. A drug-induced encephalopathy may complicate treatment, especially in patients with compromised renal function. Despite these problems, acyclovir is usually well tolerated. One should not hesitate to initiate acyclovir therapy in patients suspected of having herpes encephalitis while confirmatory tests are in progress. It is advised that the drug be given intravenously for 10 days in confirmed cases of herpes encephalitis. Because there is a low but definite rate of recurrence of herpes encephalitis after completion of the 10-day course, many authorities consider that the minimal course of intravenous treatment should be 14 days.

REYE'S SYNDROME

method of
ALAN R. SEAY, M.D.
*University of Colorado School of Medicine and
The Children's Hospital
Denver, Colorado*

Reye's syndrome is an acute metabolic encephalopathy associated with hypoglycemia, hepatocellular injury, and hepatic dysfunction that affects children primarily between the ages of 5 and 18 years, although infants and adults may also be affected. The association between acute encephalopathy and fatty degeneration of the liver was recognized as early as 1929 by Brain, Hunter, and Turnbull, but the full significance of this association was not appreciated and described until the reports of Johnson and associates from North Carolina and Reye and colleagues from Australia in 1963.

The disease has a biphasic course, commencing with a viral respiratory or gastrointestinal illness, with infections by influenza B virus or varicella-zoster virus among the most common precipitants. As the patient is recovering from the prodromal illness, the second phase begins, with vomiting and progressive encephalopathy (Table 1). Diagnostic laboratory changes include threefold or greater increase in serum transaminase levels, prolonged prothrom-

TABLE 1. **Clinical Stages of Reye's Syndrome**

Stage	Signs and Symptoms
I	Lethargy
	Vomiting
	Appropriate responses to verbal stimuli
II	Delirium, confusion
	Combative
	Reactive, dilated pupils
	Responsive to pain
III	Coma
	Decortication
	Hyperventilation
IV	Coma
	Decerebration
	Disconjugate eye movements
	Abnormal or absent oculovestibular reflexes
	Sluggish pupillary light reflexes
	Cheyne-Stokes respirations
V	Coma
	Flaccidity
	No response to pain
	Absent brain stem reflexes
	Fixed pupils
	Absent spontaneous respirations

bin time, and elevated blood ammonia concentration. Approximately 40% of patients have hypoglycemia, and metabolic acidosis with compensatory respiratory alkalosis is typical. Cerebrospinal fluid pressure is elevated, but other cerebrospinal fluid studies are normal. Although electroencephalopathy shows nonspecific diffuse, generalized slowing, it is of limited usefulness in the initial diagnosis of Reye's syndrome. Similarly, neuroimaging tests demonstrate nonspecific changes consistent with cerebral edema and increased intracranial pressure. Liver biopsy is of diagnostic help in demonstrating accumulation of microvesicular fat, depletion of hepatic glycogen, and swollen mitochondria with disrupted cristae.

The fundamental cause of Reye's syndrome is not known, but the clinical features and biochemical derangements are indicative of a generalized disturbance of mitochondrial function. A strong epidemiologic link between salicylate intake and Reye's syndrome has been observed during the past 10 years, although the exact nature of this relationship is not fully understood. Coinciding with the decrease in salicylate use for childhood febrile illnesses in the United States from 1980 to 1989, there was a dramatic reduction in the number of children between 5 and 10 years old reported with Reye's syndrome.

Table 2 lists disorders that can demonstrate clinical features similar to those of Reye's syndrome and that should be considered in the differential diagnosis.

TREATMENT

Treatment goals are to correct existing metabolic derangements, prevent and treat secondary systemic and metabolic complications, and reduce increased intracranial pressure. These goals are achieved by providing intensive monitoring and supportive care. The aggressiveness of therapy is based on the stage of the patient's illness (Table 3).

Stage I

The patient should be hospitalized, and oral intake discontinued. Intravenous, hypertonic dextrose solution (10 to 15%) with maintenance electrolytes is infused at 1600 mL per m^2 per 24 hours. Vitamin K_1 (phytonadione [AquaMEPHYTON]) is given intramuscularly at a dose of 5 mg or intravenously at a

TABLE 2. **Differential Diagnosis of Reye's Syndrome**

Toxins and ingestions
  Salicylates
  Acetaminophen
  Valproic acid
  Amiodarone
  Aflatoxin
  Hypoglycin
  Margosa oil
  Insecticides
Inborn metabolic disorders
  Medium chain acetyl-CoA dehydrogenase deficiency
  Carnitine deficiency
  Organic acidurias
  Carbamoyl phosphate synthetase deficiency
  Mitochondrial cytopathies

TABLE 3. **Treatment of Reye's Syndrome**

Stage	Treatment
I	D10W + electrolytes (1600 mL/m²/24 h)
	Vitamin K₁ (5 mg IM or 1 mg IV)
II	Same as stage I *plus*
	Admit to intensive care unit
	Cooling blanket
	Pentobarbital sedation
III	Same as stage II *plus*
	Intracranial pressure monitor
	Intubation
	Hyperventilation
	Mannitol therapy
IV and V	Same as stage III *plus*
	Consider pentobarbital coma

dose of 1 mg. This dose is repeated every 24 hours if initial coagulation tests are abnormal and is continued until results of coagulation tests approach normal. Serum electrolytes and glucose concentration should be monitored every 6 to 8 hours.

Stage II

The patient who progresses to stage II disease should be monitored and treated in an intensive care unit. The head of the bed is elevated 30 degrees, and the patient is stimulated as little as possible. Monitoring of vital signs and neurologic function is carried out at least hourly. A cooling blanket and antipyretics are used to control fever. For severe agitation, 1 to 2 mg of pentobarbital (Nembutal) per kg may be given intravenously every 1 to 2 hours. Nasogastric and urinary catheter tubes are inserted to accurately monitor fluid and electrolyte imbalance. Hypertonic glucose solution (15 to 20%) with maintenance electrolytes is infused at a rate of 1200 to 1600 mL per m^2 per 24 hours. The serum concentration of glucose is kept at about 200 mg per dL, and the urine output is maintained at about 1 mL per kg per hour. Serum osmolality and serum concentrations of glucose, electrolytes, ammonia, calcium, and lactate are measured every 2 to 4 hours. Arterial blood gas measurements are done every 4 hours or more frequently as indicated.

Stage III

The same measures used for stage II disease are employed for stage III. In addition, an intracranial monitoring device is placed to monitor and aggressively treat raised intracranial pressure. The patient is paralyzed with pancuronium bromide (Pavulon), 0.1 to 0.2 mg per kg* intravenously, and then is intubated. Arterial and venous catheters are placed to monitor cardiovascular function. With use of a mechanical ventilator, the $Paco_2$ is kept at 25 mm Hg. Intravenous boluses of 20% mannitol, 0.5 gram per kg per dose, are given when intracranial pressure

*Exceeds dosage recommended by the manufacturer.

TABLE 4. **Metabolic and Systemic Complications of Reye's Syndrome and Their Treatment**

Complications	Treatment	Comments
Hypoglycemia	*Acute:* 50% glucose, 1 mL/kg as IV bolus *Maintenance and prevention:* Use electrolyte solution that contains 10–15% dextrose for stage I and II disease and 20% for stage III to V disease	
Hypocalcemia	*Acute:* 10% calcium gluconate, 1 mL/kg (+9 mg elemental calcium/kg) as IV bolus *Maintenance:* Include 30–50 mg of elemental calcium/kg/24 h in electrolyte solution	Progressive fall in serum calcium value suggests pancreatitis.
Hypophosphatemia	In electrolyte solution, replace potassium chloride with potassium phosphate	Potassium phosphate cannot be used in electrolyte solutions that contain calcium.
Thrombocytopenia	Platelet transfusion	
Bleeding diathesis	Vitamin K₁, 1 mg IV or 5 mg IM q 24 h or Fresh-frozen plasma, 10–20 mL/kg/24 h	
Hypotension	5% albumin or plasmanate, 10–15 mL/kg IV over 0.5 h to maintain central venous pressure between 6 and 15 cm H₂O Vasopressors Calcium chloride	Give calcium chloride if hypotension is resistant to volume expanders and vasopressor or if there is a history of phenothiazine intake.
Pancreatitis	Treatment directed at metabolic complications and shock	Suggested by hypotension, fluctuating glucose levels, and progressive hypocalcemia.
Renal failure	Hemodialysis or peritoneal dialysis	
Seizures	*Acute:* 50% glucose, 1 mL/kg as IV bolus, then phenytoin loading dose, 20 mg/kg as IV bolus *Maintenance:* Phenytoin, 5 mg/kg/24 h	Exclude fluid, electrolyte, or glucose abnormalities. Administer phenytoin through a peripheral venous catheter.

exceeds 20 mm Hg and are repeated as often as necessary to keep intracranial pressure less than 20 mm Hg and to keep serum osmolality at about 310 mOsm per liter. Adjustments are made in $PaCO_2$ and mannitol infusions and general supportive measures are carried out as necessary to maintain a cerebral perfusion pressure of 50 mm Hg or greater, to protect the brain from ischemic injury.

Stages IV and V

All measures described previously are used for the patient in stage IV or V disease. If intracranial pressure does not respond to measures described previously, a reduction may be achieved by use of high-dose pentobarbital therapy. An intravenous bolus of pentobarbital, 5 mg per kg, is given, followed by an infusion of 1 to 3 mg per kg every 1 to 4 hours. Continuous electroencephalographic monitoring is required, and the pentobarbital dose is adjusted to produce a burst-suppression pattern and to maintain a pentobarbital blood level at 30 to 40 μg per mL. After intracranial pressure has been kept below 20 mm Hg for 24 to 48 hours, the pentobarbital is tapered over 24 to 36 hours. Pentobarbital coma can be complicated by bradycardia, hypotension, and cardiovascular collapse. High-dose pentobarbital therapy is reserved for severely affected patients in whom other measures to lower intracranial pressure have failed.

Complications

Metabolic and systemic complications that can develop in Reye's syndrome are listed in Table 4. Rapid detection and treatment of these disorders are important to ensure a good outcome for the patient. Although high concentrations of ammonia can be reduced by exchange transfusions, sodium benzoate therapy, or other measures, it is not certain what long-term benefits these treatments have in Reye's syndrome.

Seizures occur frequently in patients with Reye's syndrome. When they occur, reversible metabolic derangements should be sought and corrected. Anticonvulsant therapy is initiated with an intravenous loading dose of phenytoin (Dilantin), 20 mg per kg. This is followed by intravenous doses of phenytoin, 5 mg per kg per 24 hours, to maintain serum concentrations between 10 and 20 μg per mL.

OUTCOME

Although the case-fatality rate in Reye's syndrome has declined during the past several years, it remains at about 25%. Approximate case-fatality rates for patients based on stage of illness are stage I, 5%; stage II, 10%; stage III, 25%; stage IV, 45%; and stage V, 60%. Permanent sequelae include mild cognitive dysfunction, seizures, and retardation. These sequelae are most likely to occur in patients who reach stages III to V, those with extremely high ammonia levels, and those younger than 1 year.

MULTIPLE SCLEROSIS

method of
DONALD H. SILBERBERG, M.D.
University of Pennsylvania Medical Center
Philadelphia, Pennsylvania

PERSPECTIVE

Multiple sclerosis (MS) is a disorder of unknown etiology, defined by its clinical characteristics and by typical scattered areas of brain, optic nerve, and spinal cord demyelination. Clinical diagnosis requires evidence on neurologic examination of two or more central nervous system (CNS) white matter lesions, preferably with at least a month's interval between symptoms in a patient of the appropriate age, in whom evidence is lacking of any other explanation for the signs and symptoms. Common symptoms include transient tingling paresthesias of the hands or feet, unilateral loss of vision, weakness or incoordination, and voiding dysfunction.

Despite the fact that its cause is still mysterious, treatments have been developed that seem to alter the course of MS. Agents that reduce the number of relapses, such as recombinant interferon beta (interferon beta-1a [IFN-β-1a; Avonex]; interferon beta-1b [IFN-β-1b; Betaseron]) and copolymer 1 (Copaxone), have been approved by the Food and Drug Administration and are being considered for approval in many other countries. A variety of other agents are the subject of many clinical trials worldwide.

Before considering specific options, a few observations may help to provide a perspective useful in understanding approaches to treatment:

Although MS is a common cause of disability among young individuals, its behavior is unpredictable in a particular person; it does not necessarily disable, nor does it appreciably shorten the life span in most. The history of attempts to treat MS is replete with examples of claims made on the basis of anecdotal experience or uncontrolled trials. The extraordinary variability and unpredictability of MS coupled with the characteristic spontaneous improvement (remission) after a relapse make it impossible to judge therapeutic efficacy except in the setting of a randomized, double-blind (masked), controlled clinical trial.

Both the initial cause of MS and the mechanisms by which MS may continue to damage the CNS remain unknown.

Some of the therapeutic approaches that are currently available seem to modify the clinical expression of MS over the short term. None, however, fully interrupt the disease process. The search for evidence of the longer term effects of these agents on clinical disability is the subject of current studies.

The management of individuals with MS may include therapies designed to modify the course of the disease but almost always includes other components such as psychologic support, the use of medications intended for purely symptomatic treatment, physical therapy, and occupational therapy.

DIAGNOSIS

The implications of the diagnosis of multiple sclerosis are profound. The prospect of possible future disability, financial hardship, and disruption of personal and family life descend on an individual when MS is even mentioned as a possibility. The physician must therefore be clear in his or her own mind about the relative certainty of the diagnosis and must be careful not to overstate the position when presenting it to the patient.

A case in point is the young patient who appears for a second opinion after months of testing and often treatment, usually occasioned only by vague sensory symptoms, or fatigue. She does not seem to have MS, but she has become both disabled by and attached to the diagnosis of MS and does not want to hear of alternative explanations such as anxiety or depression. This situation can often be avoided by accepting the fact that it is both legitimate and appropriate to defer suggesting a diagnosis when there is still a degree of uncertainty.

MS is defined by its clinical characteristics coupled with its histopathologic appearance. Multiple areas of inflammation and demyelination in the myelinated tracts (white matter) of the brain, optic nerve, and spinal cord impair conduction of the nerve impulse. Depending on their location, affected individuals commonly develop such problems as unilateral impairment of vision, disordered sensation, incoordination, weakness, difficulty controlling urination, or cognitive dysfunction.

The clinical diagnosis requires evidence on neurologic examination that indicates two or more sites of CNS white matter abnormality, with at least a month's interval between symptoms. A critical requirement is the lack of evidence for any other possible explanation for the signs and symptoms. It is particularly important to look for evidence of alternatives such as acute disseminated lupus erythematosus in young women or a herniated intervertebral disk in the face of spinal cord dysfunction. The need to exclude other disorders leads to consideration of the role of imaging and cerebrospinal fluid (CSF) examination in diagnosis and management.

Imaging

Magnetic resonance imaging (MRI) is the most sensitive way in which to identify one or more white matter abnormalities and simultaneously search for evidence of alternative explanations for dysfunction. Gadolinium (gadopentetate dimeglumine [Magnevist]) enhancement, indicating blood-brain barrier leakage, provides evidence of current or very recent disease activity. In an individual with a monophasic disorder such as optic neuropathy occurring for the first time, the presence of four or more separate areas of abnormality makes it somewhat more likely that MS will develop in the future (see the section "Monophasic Demyelination"). Although some locations, such as the periventricular white matter and the corpus callosum, are more typically affected by MS, MRI findings must be considered as almost totally nonspecific, despite the sensitivity of the technique. Signal alterations like those of MS also occur in many other disorders.

When MRI is unavailable, computed tomography is an efficient way in which to exclude confounding diagnoses, although it is much less sensitive for visualizing the brain abnormalities of MS per se.

Cerebrospinal Fluid

CSF examination may help to increase confidence in the diagnosis, both by excluding other disorders (e.g., neurosyphilis) and by providing supportive, although nonspecific, data. Within a year after an initial symptom, about 85% of individuals with MS develop CSF oligoclonal bands.

These are discrete separate peaks visualized in the gamma-globulin region by electrophoresis. However both oligoclonal bands and an increased rate of IgG synthesis within the CNS also occur in a variety of chronic infections and in neurosarcoidosis. Measurement of CSF myelin basic protein may be used to reflect current disease activity as reflected by release of the protein but has no diagnostic specificity.

NATURAL HISTORY

At any given time MS affects approximately 0.1% of the population in the United States, Canada, Europe, Australia, and New Zealand. More women than men develop MS; the lifetime risk among northern Europeans approaches 1 in 500. It is rare in sub-Saharan Africa and less common in Japan and among other Asian populations than among whites. The observed variations in population prevalence and studies of multiplex families and twins have led to evidence for both a genetically determined capacity to develop MS and an environmental trigger, probably an infectious agent. The role of infections has been reinforced by studies showing that individuals with established MS are more likely to experience a relapse after respiratory or other incidental infections.

MS usually produces its first clinical symptoms in those between the ages of 15 and 55 years. Although the first symptoms may occur beyond these extremes, the average age at onset is 33 years. Most patients (90%) recover clinically to some extent from individual bouts of demyelination, producing the classic *relapsing-remitting* course of the early disease. The timing of new relapses is totally unpredictable for an individual, but relapses occur at average intervals of about 16 months. Within approximately 15 years of onset, about 50% of patients develop what is now known as a *secondary progressive* course. This may signify an accumulation of residual deficits from individual bouts, with less capacity to recover from each subsequent episode. Fortunately, about 30% of individuals experience a *benign course*, avoiding any troublesome disability for many years.

An unfortunate subset of about 10% develop a *primary chronic progressive* course from the outset. These individuals never experience a significant remission, although many stop progressing for variable, sometimes long, periods. The MRI characteristics of this group are somewhat different from those of relapsing-remitting patients, pointing to the possibility that they in fact have a different disorder, but this is by no means certain.

Monophasic Demyelination

Individuals who have experienced one episode such as optic neuropathy or partial transverse myelopathy present special challenges. Overall, about 50% experience a second clinical episode within 10 years, indicating that they have definite MS, assuming that other causes have been excluded on both occasions. If it is a woman, or if four or more areas of abnormality compatible with MS are seen by MRI, or if there are CSF gamma-globulin abnormalities at the time of the first episode, the odds rise to 60 or 65%.

What explains the 35 to 40% who do not develop a second clinical episode? There are at least three possibilities:

1. Some patients have experienced an episode of acute disseminated encephalomyelitis, the CNS inflammation and demyelination that can sometimes follow an infection or immunization. By definition, acute disseminated encephalomyelitis is a monophasic disorder. The clinical, MRI, and CSF findings are often identical to those of an MS relapse, and the histopathologic findings are virtually indistinguishable.

2. Perhaps some who develop the "MS process" are able to limit it to the initial bout.

3. Some subsequently develop additional areas of abnormality visualized by MRI but in CNS areas that are not clinically eloquent, and thus these patients remain asymptomatic. These individuals do not have, and may never develop, clinically definite MS.

This conundrum is an important part of the reason for avoiding the diagnosis of MS until it is clinically definite. However, it is possible that the time immediately after a first episode may be the most advantageous point at which to start therapeutic agents designed to stop or slow the MS process. The clinical trial of IFN-β-1a currently under way among monosymptomatic patients is exploring this possibility.

TREATMENT (MANAGEMENT) CATEGORIES

Three broad categories include most of the available approaches to management. These are

Psychologic support
Disease course modification
Symptom relief

Psychologic Support

In the absence of a curative treatment, efforts to help the person with MS and the family deal emotionally with uncertainty about future disability, current symptoms and disability, and work-related issues are often the treating physician's most significant contribution.

Many approaches can contribute to helping: the supportive psychotherapy provided by an understanding physician, nurse, or other professional; the opportunities to learn and share in support groups; specific counseling by a psychiatrist, psychologist, marriage counselor, or other appropriate individual; participation in clinical trials; physical and occupational therapy; cognitive therapy; antidepressants and other psychotropic medications—some or all have a role at some time for most individuals with MS.

Disease Course Modification

Controlled clinical trials have led to the acceptance of five agents in an effort to either

Hasten recovery from a relapse: adrenal corticosteroids
Reduce the severity and frequency of future exacerbations, and perhaps prevent progression to disability: IFN-β-1a, IFN-β-1b, and copolymer 1
Slow progression: methotrexate (Table 1)

The premise for the use of each is that MS is an immunologically mediated disease. However, the evidence for this remains indirect: (1) the tissue re-

TABLE 1. **Treatments to Modify the Course of Multiple Sclerosis**

Clinical Classification	Treatments Assessed in Controlled Trials
Relapsing-remitting Acute relapse	Corticosteroids, e.g., prednisone; methylprednisolone (Medrol)
Prevent relapses	Interferon beta-1a (Avonex) Interferon beta-1b (Betaseron) Copolymer 1 (Copaxone)
Primary or secondary progressive	Methotrexate (Rheumatrex)

sponse has features of an immunopathologic process; the CNS lesions contain most of the cells that would be needed for a variety of immune responses, exhibiting perivenular mononuclear cell infiltration and an absence of any overt histopathologic evidence of an infection; (2) one finds frequent elevation of CSF gamma-globulin levels and a common oligoclonal pattern in the gamma-globulin region on CSF electrophoresis, apparently synthesized by plasma cells in areas of demyelination; and (3) several of the genetic loci associated with MS occur in the region of the genetic locus of the major histocompatibility complex that regulates immune responses.

Evidence that the pathogenesis of MS entails an immunologic process specific to the disease awaits future research. Meanwhile, virtually all available agents that have been used as immunosuppressants or immunomodulators for other disorders have been or are being tried in MS.

The currently approved agents used in an effort to modify the course of MS are considered in relation to their indications.

Acute Relapse (Exacerbation, Bout)

It is now well established that intercurrent infections, viral or bacterial, are associated with many relapses. The infection may occur 2 or 3 weeks previously, or concomitantly. For this reason, the first priority in managing a patient experiencing an acute worsening of pre-existing symptoms, or new symptoms, is to detect and treat any existing infection. Cystitis, for example, may be asymptomatic, particularly if bladder or urethral sensation is impaired, and yet may precipitate a relapse. Often the associated neurologic symptoms improve within several days of treatment, making it unnecessary to consider the use of corticosteroids.

Conversely, in a patient whose neurologic functioning is temperature sensitive, fever associated with infection may cause a pseudorelapse, or pseudobout. Other causes of body temperature elevation may also lead to profound, but transient, degradation of function, particularly in the patient who has had a recent relapse. Sun exposure, a very warm ambient temperature, exercise, or a hot bath or shower is often responsible for this, and patients should be so counseled. Fortunately, no permanent problems result,

but a rise in body temperature can cause increased weakness, loss of vision, or other symptoms lasting several hours after restoration of normal core temperature. Swimming in a cool pool is a useful way to exercise without overheating. Also, cooling jackets are available for the same purpose.

Corticosteroids

The advent of adrenocorticotropic hormone (ACTH) and synthetic glucocorticosteroids in the early 1950s ushered in the modern history of the treatment of MS. The uncontrolled observations that patients seemed to recover from acute relapses more quickly when treated with ACTH led to widespread use, and then to many therapeutic trials, controlled and uncontrolled. These supported the original observation that treatment often yielded faster recovery, but no controlled trial has shown long-term reduction in disability.

Of cortisol's many properties, those most relevant to MS appear to be the anti-inflammatory and anti-edema effects. Both reduction in edema and transient restoration of the blood-brain barrier are readily demonstrable by MRI. Cortisol's ability to energize some individuals may give the appearance of neurologic improvement even though underlying function has not changed.

The use of the oral glucocorticoids prednisone, prednisolone, dexamethasone, and betamethasone, and more recently the use of high-dose intravenous methylprednisolone (IVMP), have largely supplanted ACTH treatment. Before considering which, if any, to use in an attempt to reduce the impact of an acute exacerbation, it is important to remember that all are capable of producing serious side effects, ranging from psychosis to peptic ulcer, even in the short term.

Oral prednisone, from 20 to 60 mg per day for 1 to 3 weeks, is prescribed by many neurologists for acute exacerbations, even though the efficacy of this treatment has not been shown in a controlled trial. The questionable efficacy of this dosage range seems clear from a large treatment trial of patients with acute optic neuritis, comparing oral prednisone with an oral placebo, and with IVMP, 1 gram daily for 3 days. The readily quantifiable visual impairment produced by optic neuritis provides an easy and reproducible measure compared with measurement of motor or other dysfunctions. Optic neuritis patients fared as well with placebo as with prednisone at each time point in follow-up. Patients treated with IVMP recovered vision more quickly but had no better function after 6 months than did the prednisone or placebo group. Despite this evidence, many experienced clinicians prescribe oral prednisone for more moderate exacerbations, with the hope that some benefit follows without the greater risk of the much larger dose intravenous therapy.

Uncontrolled trials of high-dose oral prednisone, 200 mg per day, paved the way for the introduction of high-dose IVMP for acute relapses. The available evidence is that high-dose IVMP shortens the time to improvement, but produces no longer term benefit. The demonstration of even this limited efficacy has led to the widespread use of IVMP for the treatment of acute exacerbations.

IVMP treatment regimens that have been used in controlled trials range from 500 mg daily for 5 days to 15 mg per kg per day for 3 days with or without a following period of oral prednisone therapy. It is appropriate to limit this treatment to individuals who are otherwise well, for relapses that produce threatening disability over the course of at least several days. This allows the significant number of attacks that resolve promptly on their own to do so. One should make it clear to the patient that the treatment goal is entirely to try to shorten the duration of the attack, and the potential risks should be carefully spelled out. With the understanding that the study to determine the optimal dose and duration has yet to be done, one can prescribe 15 mg per kg per day for 4 days, or fewer days if improvement is prompt, and follow with oral prednisone. Prednisone is often started at 60 mg daily, then tapered and discontinued over the course of a week.

Salt restriction helps to prevent edema, and the use of an H_2 blocker such as ranitidine (Zantac) is a reasonable precaution. Many patients require a short-acting hypnotic such as zolpidem tartrate (Ambien) for sleep. If an affective disorder or psychosis emerges during treatment, it is safest to administer an appropriate psychotropic drug before the next course of corticosteroids.

Long experience makes it clear that longer term use of corticosteroids on a daily or every-other-day basis does little other than to induce adrenal suppression, Cushing's syndrome, osteoporosis, and the other well-known side effects. However, a trial is under way to determine if monthly treatment with IVMP alters the development of disability.

Prevention of Relapses and Disability

IFN-β-1b

Interferons were discovered in the course of the search for naturally occurring substances that protect cells from viral infection. Interferons represent a large, heterogeneous family of glycoproteins that have multiple antiviral and immunomodulatory properties, many of which are still being discovered. IFN-β-1b (Betaseron) is a nonglycosylated recombinant molecule, produced in *Escherichia coli*, that substitutes serine for cysteine at one site. A randomized trial led to the finding that in ambulatory, relapsing-remitting patients subcutaneous injection of IFN-β-1b, 8 million IU (250 μg) every other day, produced a 33% decrease in the number of relapses over the course of 2 years. It also seemed to reduce the severity of attacks. Subsequent experience suggests that a modest reduction of disability also occurs with continued use.

IFN-β-1b administration produces a marked reduction in the number of gadolinium-enhancing lesions seen by MRI. The hope is that reducing the aspect of disease activity that expresses itself as a relapse, and is associated with leakage of the blood-brain barrier, will achieve a reduction in actual progression to demyelination and neurologic dysfunction. Although studies to date suggest that this is occurring, it will take much longer follow-up of treated patients to make an accurate determination. This applies to IFN-β-1a and to copolymer 1 as well. The major indications for the use of each of these agents is therefore to reduce the number and severity of relapses in individuals with relapsing-remitting MS (see later).

ADVERSE EFFECTS

After each injection of IFN-β-1b, about 30% of patients develop transient viremia-like symptoms that last for 24 to 36 hours. These muscle aches, and sometimes slight body temperature elevation, are usually relieved by acetaminophen (Tylenol) and decrease or stop occurring after several months of treatment. If these effects are severe, the physician may choose to start with a lower dose, e.g., 4 million IU for the first several weeks. The second most troublesome problem is a reaction at the sites of the subcutaneous injections: local skin erythema, induration, pain, and occasionally necrosis. To reduce this, the injection site must be rotated on a regular schedule. All patients should be monitored for the possible development of anemia, leukopenia, or elevation of serum transaminase levels. Blood studies are usually obtained at 3-month intervals for the first year and then semiannually. A small proportion of those receiving IFN-β-1b develop psychiatric depression or have an exacerbation of pre-existing depression. The physician must inquire about mood and be prepared to treat or seek consultation if depression becomes apparent.

An additional concern is that many patients (reportedly 38% after 3 years of treatment) develop neutralizing antibody to IFN-β-1b, and this is associated with decreased clinical efficacy. At the present time, Berlex Laboratories offers testing in patients who the physician believes are failing to respond clinically. The detection of neutralizing antibodies can be used to support the discontinuation of treatment in an individual who seems unresponsive.

IFN-β-1a

IFN-β-1a (Avonex), which has an amino acid sequence identical to that of naturally occurring IFN-β, is a glycosylated recombinant product of a mammalian cell line. In a controlled trial, the treated participants received weekly intramuscular injections of 6.6 million IU (33 μg). The trial was designed to study the time to onset of progression of disability. Treatment resulted in less disability progression compared with placebo. IFN-β-1a also reduced the annual relapse rate by 32% and reduced the number and volume of gadolinium-enhancing lesions.

ADVERSE EFFECTS

The flulike symptoms described previously occur with the same frequency after weekly intramuscular injections of IFN-β-1a. Because the injected amount is smaller, and intramuscular, no skin irritation occurs at the injection site. Analyses to date show that 22% of treated individuals develop neutralizing antibody activity at 2 years. The relationship of antibody activity to clinical efficacy has not yet been determined.

Indications for the Use of IFN-β

The primary reason for prescribing either IFN-β-1a or IFN-β-1b is to reduce the number and severity of relapses in individuals with relapsing-remitting MS who are still ambulatory and who have experienced frequent relapses. The expectations for either preparation are framed by the results of a single controlled trial in each instance. The more recent IFN-β-1a trial was designed to determine primarily if disease progression was slowed as well; a relatively modest effect was found. Although no effect on disability was found with the initial 2-year trial of IFN-β-1b, postmarketing studies show that it too seems to retard disability progression somewhat.

Copolymer 1

Copolymer 1 (Copaxone) is a mixture of synthetic polypeptides that was developed to partially resemble myelin basic protein, one of the major components of myelin. Two controlled trials in relapsing-remitting patients showed both a reduction in the number of attacks and less disability among treated individuals at the end of 2 years. The larger, more recent study showed a 29% reduction in the number of relapses per year. A similar study among patients, most of whom had secondary progressive MS, showed a trend toward efficacy that did not reach statistical significance.

ADVERSE EFFECTS

Copolymer 1 is administered as a daily subcutaneous injection of 20 mg. Mild discomfort occurs at the injection site in most patients. The only other adverse effects in the most recent trial were brief episodes of anxiety, flushing, chest tightness, and cardiac palpitations that occurred in 15% of those receiving the drug. Although some patients developed antibodies to copolymer 1 during the study, these did not correlate with clinical response.

Indications for the Use of Copolymer 1

As with the preparations of IFN-β, the primary reason for prescribing copolymer 1 is to reduce the number and severity of relapses in individuals with relapsing-remitting MS who are still ambulatory and who have experienced frequent relapses. It too seems to retard disability progression somewhat.

Treatment Decisions

Thus, the clinician and patient are faced with several decisions concerning these agents, IFN-β-1a,
IFN-β-1b, and copolymer 1 (Table 2). The first is whether to start treatment at all with an agent that must be injected subcutaneously or intramuscularly for an indefinite period. The treatment effects are modest but seem far better than anything available in the past. For an individual patient the inherent variability of MS makes it virtually impossible to determine efficacy, and the patient must understand at the outset that the purpose in treating is to reduce the number of new relapses and prevent disability, but not to reduce existing disability.

Once the decision is made to start therapy with one of these agents, the next difficult decision is which one to choose.

IFN-β-1a has the advantage of requiring injection only once a week, but many patients are uncomfortable self-administering an intramuscular injection. Its use avoids injection site irritation, but flulike side effects occur in many. The trial design demonstrated a favorable effect in preventing progression of disability, but the time available for the evaluation of IFN-β-1a has been the shortest of these three agents.

IFN-β-1b is familiar to most U.S. neurologists by virtue of its earlier introduction. Most patients can self-administer the subcutaneous injection but must do so every other day, and many must deal with injection site reactions. Flulike symptoms occur. Post-trial data show some effect in reducing the progression of disability.

Copolymer 1 also reduces the relapse rate by about one third and is associated with a reduction in the progression of disability. It requires a daily injection, but by the subcutaneous route, and does not produce any lasting local or systemic reactions.

Thus, at this time, there is no clear and convincing basis for recommending one agent over another. The decision must be reached by the patient and physician together, taking into account each of the different features.

The next decision is how long to treat, or when to stop. There is no evidence that the administration of any of these agents offers a therapeutic effect beyond the time that it is being used. As a result, the decision to stop treatment is usually prompted by intolerable side effects or apparent therapeutic failure, perhaps buttressed by demonstration of neutralizing antibody titer in the case of IFN-β-1b.

TABLE 2. **Therapy to Prevent Relapses and Disability in Multiple Sclerosis**

Drug	Dose	Route	Origin
Interferon beta-1a (Avonex)	33 μg 1/wk	IM	Cultured cell line
Interferon beta-1b (Betaseron)	250 μg every other day	SC	Recombinant *Escherichia coli*
Copolymer 1 (Copaxone)	20 mg daily	SC	Chemical synthesis

PRIMARY OR SECONDARY PROGRESSION

Attempts to stop or slow the development of disability among those with progressive MS have been extraordinarily frustrating. Several immunosuppressant drugs have been used extensively, particularly azathioprine (Imuran) and cyclophosphamide (Cytoxan). However, no convincing evidence from controlled, masked studies supports the use of either for this purpose. A well-controlled trial of cyclosporine (Sandimmune) showed a modest effect, but this was less impressive than its toxicity. Many studies of these and other drugs are under way. At this time, the agent that has been shown to have the most favorable benefit/risk ratio, albeit with a modest effect of slowing progression, is low-dose methotrexate (Rheumatrex).

Methotrexate

Methotrexate inhibits both humoral and cell-mediated immunity by its activity as a dihydrofolate reductase inhibitor. Low doses have been effective and relatively nontoxic in treating psoriasis and rheumatoid arthritis. In a 2-year randomized, placebo-controlled, double-blind study of patients with chronic progressive MS, most of whom had secondary progressive disease, 7.5 mg of oral low-dose methotrexate per week was associated with less loss of upper extremity function and less progression as seen by MRI. No significant adverse reactions occurred. It thus seems to be a viable choice for patients with progressive MS, with the reservation that to date the treatment effect demonstrated is small.

Symptom Relief

Virtually every symptom or disability that an individual with MS may develop can be addressed constructively (Table 3). The willingness and ability of the clinician to manage symptom relief are critical, because curative treatments do not yet exist. The wide range of potential problems makes it obvious that the patient often benefits from a multidisciplinary approach, with the neurologist serving as the focal clinician. A full description of the management of some of the categories of problems encountered by individuals with MS would require an article equivalent in length to this one. What follows is an outline of possibilities that can serve as a stimulus to further reading and to selection of appropriate consultants and caregivers when needed.

Mobility

The main factors that contribute to a loss of mobility, or loss of dexterity of the hands, are weakness, spasticity, impaired position sense, and incoordination due to impairment of cerebellar function. Useful approaches include the following.

A controlled study demonstrated that a supervised, vigorous training program increased muscle strength

TABLE 3. **Symptom Relief in Multiple Sclerosis**

Symptom	Treatment
Mobility	Physical therapy
	Occupational therapy
	Orthotics
	Nerve blocks
Fatigue	Amantadine (Symmetrel)
Voiding dysfunction	
Difficulty storing	Oxybutynin (Ditropan)
Nocturia	Imipramine (Tofranil)
Difficulty emptying	Self-catheterization
Bowel dysfunction	Fluid, bulk
	Training
	Stool softeners
	Suppositories, and so forth
Sexual dysfunction	Counseling
	Lubricants; urologic treatments
Psychiatric disturbances	Counseling
	Antidepressants, other psychotropics
Pain	
Meningeal	Corticosteroids, when otherwise indicated
Root entry zone	Carbamazepine (Tegretol)
Dysesthesias	Amitryptiline (Elavil)
Flexor-extensor spasms	Baclofen (Lioresal)
Paroxysmal movements	Carbamazepine

and endurance and improved patients' sense of well-being, compared with inactivity. Skilled physical therapy and the patient's willingness to exercise represent the most important way to try to maximize strength. As described previously, it is sometimes important to avoid overheating during exercise; the patient must establish the limits. The use of appropriately prescribed orthotic devices often means the difference between walking and not walking. Gait training can often help the patient to circumvent limitations in a safe manner.

Spasticity may take the form of difficulty in muscle relaxation that impairs walking, and/or spontaneous flexor or extensor spasms. Because the tightness produced by spasticity often enables an individual to walk despite weakness, pharmacologic treatment of spasticity must be prescribed carefully. The mainstay of treatment is baclofen (Lioresal), which seems to inhibit presynaptic excitatory transmission. It is a safe drug; its main side effect is drowsiness, although that is an advantage when used at bedtime to prevent nocturnal flexor spasms. The hypnotic effect decreases with repeated use. One starts with the lowest dose that may be effective, e.g., 5 mg per day, and advances gradually to as much as 200 mg per day,* divided as a four-times-a-day schedule. The average person benefits from 40 to 80 mg per day. Although it is often used as an adjunct, diazepam (Valium) is less effective than baclofen and also causes drowsiness, and its longer metabolic (not therapeutic) half-life may lead to rising blood levels with time.

Dantrolene (Dantrium) represents a second-line al-

---

*Exceeds dosage recommended by the manufacturer.

ternative, added to or replacing baclofen if needed. It acts primarily to decrease muscle contractility peripherally, although it may also induce drowsiness. It has the disadvantage of occasionally being hepatotoxic. Again, one starts with a low dose, 25 mg per day, advancing if needed to as much as 400 mg per day, on a four-times-a-day schedule. A second alternative, tizanidine (Zanaflex), has reached the U.S. market. It is an alpha$_2$-adrenergic blocker that presumably reduces spasticity by increasing presynaptic inhibition of motor neurons.

Spasticity so severe that it no longer responds to oral drugs may be managed by placement of a baclofen programmable pump to deliver a continuous infusion into the lumbar subarachnoid space. A next measure to consider is the use of botulinum toxin type A (Botox) injections to achieve temporary nerve block by blocking calcium-mediated acetylcholine release at the neuromuscular junction. If this is successful, injections must be repeated every 2 to 4 months. If needed to prevent decubitus ulcers or facilitate hygiene, longer lasting nerve blocks can be achieved with alcohol or dilute phenol.

Two ways to deal with impaired proprioception are (1) helping the patient to understand that vision can be used to compensate for impaired position sense, i.e., looking at the walking surface and avoiding walking in total darkness, and (2) suggesting gait aids such as a cane, Canadian crutch, or walker, which provide a more stable base.

Cerebellar ataxia, producing tremulous movements or dysmetria, can be disabling even when strength, muscle tonus, and proprioception are intact. Unfortunately there is no ready solution. Drugs such as carbamazepine (Tegretol), clonazepam (Klonopin), propranolol (Inderal), and isoniazid help only a small proportion of patients. Stereotactic thalamotomy may provide relief but may also cause hemiparesis and or dysphasia. Occupational therapy can sometimes improve function, primarily by teaching the patient how to circumvent or avoid the most tremulous movements.

Fatigue

Chronic fatigue is one of the most common symptoms that trouble MS patients. Sleep deprivation and temperature elevation must be excluded as causes. Amantadine (Symmetrel) 100 to 300 mg per day sometimes provides relief, with virtually no risk. If 300 mg per day does not help, neither will a higher dose.

Voiding Dysfunction

Voiding dysfunction presents as either failure to empty the bladder or difficulty in storing urine, or a combination of both. Failure to empty may represent a major health hazard, potentially leading to cystitis, hydroureter and hydronephrosis, renal calculi, and pyelonephritis. Effective management strategies have been developed, but the choice of an approach must be determined by a correct understanding of the underlying pathophysiology. Unfortunately, this cannot be determined by the history alone, because any of the categories of dysfunction may produce frequency and urgency, incontinence, or nocturia.

The minimal evaluation is urinanalysis to exclude infection or a renal disorder. Ideally, urodynamic testing should be done to provide detailed information. If more complete testing is not readily available, measurement of the pre- and postvoid residual urine by catheterization or ultrasonography helps to determine appropriate therapy. If the residual is less than 100 mL, the first step is to advise avoidance of caffeine. Next, partial relief of urgency may be obtained with an anticholinergic such as oxybutynin (Ditropan) 2.5 mg twice daily to 5 mg three times daily. Nocturia may be relieved by restricting fluids after supper, and if an anticholinergic is inadequate, by imipramine (Tofranil) 10 to 25 mg at bedtime, or desmopressin nasal spray (DDAVP) 0.1 to 0.2 mL at bedtime. With the latter, serum sodium levels should be monitored weekly for several weeks and then every 3 months.

Failure to empty is best treated by intermittent self-catheterization four times daily. Many other treatment options can be considered. If progression to bladder contracture or other problems suggest the need for an indwelling catheter, urology consultation should be obtained beforehand.

Bowel Dysfunction

Measures to address the common problem of constipation in MS include

Maintenance of adequate fluid intake
Bulk foods, e.g., bran
Exercise
Elimination of unnecessary anticholinergic medications
Establishment of a regular schedule of defecation
Stool softeners
Suppositories
Fleet Enema
Manual extraction

Many individuals defecate only two or three times per week, which is acceptable. However, patients must understand the implications of the development of bowel obstruction, should their constipation become more severe and unmanageable, and the need to ask for help.

Sexual Dysfunction

The causes of the varieties of female and male sexual dysfunction that occur in MS are as complex as they are difficult for many patients to describe. The physician usually must, and should, ask questions to elicit the relevant history. The approaches to treatment include counseling, the use of vaginal lubricants in women, the use of yohimbine, topical (urethral) or injected agents, and penile prostheses for erectile dysfunction in men. Specialist consultation is often invaluable in addressing these issues.

Cognitive Dysfunction

Cognitive dysfunction is more common in the more severely physically disabled individual with MS, but it can develop before other clinical signs are prominent. Neuropsychologic testing helps to quantify impairment and to determine to what extent depression may contribute. Management involves recognition, discussion of any imposed limitation, help in identifying alternative ways in which to handle tasks, and often referral to a psychiatrist or psychologist to help deal with the emotional impact of the loss of such critical functions.

Psychiatric Disturbances

Anxiety is often the initial response to the diagnosis of MS. Depression is common after subsequent relapses or progression. A sleep disorder may develop, adding to fatigue. Other psychiatric disorders occur with the same frequency as in the general population. When cognitive dysfunction coexists, accurate diagnosis may be more difficult. However, all these problems are amenable to treatment, whether by the supportive measures outlined previously (see "Psychologic Support"), more formal psychologic counseling, or psychotropic medications. Although the measures taken are identical to those used for any individual with the same psychiatric problem, the pharmacotherapist should keep in mind that MS lesions may alter the patient's response to psychoactive drugs. This may require somewhat more frequent monitoring and willingness to change drugs than would be needed in the absence of a CNS disorder.

Emotional lability, the occurrence of unwarranted laughing or crying, is a special problem that can occur as the result of bilateral impairment of the cerebral corticospinal and associated tracts from any cause. Although it is not the result of depression, it is often helped by amitriptyline (Elavil), 25 to 50 mg or more, at bedtime.

Pain

The several varieties of pain that may occur in the course of MS are all treatable:

Meningeal pain results from inflammation or edema near the meningeal surface, such as the characteristic pain on eye movement associated with optic neuritis. It subsides as the inflammation decreases over the course of several days to 3 or 4 weeks. Treatment with corticosteroids hastens recovery from the discomfort as well as the return of function.

Inflammation and demyelination of the root entry zone can cause lancinating pain; when this occurs at the origin of the trigeminal nerve, the lancinating pain may be indistinguishable from the idiopathic trigeminal neuralgia that more often occurs in older individuals. The most effective treatment for this or lancinating pain in the distribution of any other nerve root is usually carbamazepine, 200 to 1200 mg daily in divided doses. Alternative therapies include phenytoin (Dilantin), amitriptyline, baclofen, and misoprostol (Cytotec). Rarely, alcohol injections or surgical treatment is needed.

Painful, spontaneous dysesthesias may last months. These probably result from altered conduction within the spinothalamic tracts. Amitriptyline, 50 to 250 mg per day, often helps. Carbamazepine may be added or used alone.

Flexor and extensor spasms may be quite painful; reducing the spasms by avoiding unnecessary cutaneous stimuli and by using baclofen is effective.

Joint, back, and muscle pain can result from the stresses imposed by gait alterations or postural imbalance, and by contractures that develop if a paretic extremity is not put through its full range of motion at least twice daily. Prevention by physical therapy is the best management; treatment involves a wide range of physical therapy measures, the use of analgesics and anti-inflammatory agents, and sometimes injection of corticosteroids into a joint or tendon area.

Paroxysmal Movement Disorders

Tonic spasms (brief, sometimes painful spontaneous dystonic movements of a hand, or hand and arm) result primarily from cervical spinal cord lesions. These are almost always self-limited, occurring for weeks to months. Hemifacial spasm (paroxysmal, unilateral, spontaneous contraction of the facial muscles) is also usually self-limited. Both problems respond well to carbamazepine, usually to 200 to 600 mg per day. Phenytoin is the second-line drug of choice.

FUTURE DEVELOPMENTS

At the time of this writing, more than 125 randomized clinical trials of at least 20 different agents are in various stages of completion, around the world. Additional approaches are just moving from the laboratory to pilot studies in patients. In addition to the aim of preventing relapses and stopping or slowing progression, strategies are being pursued to try to improve the repair processes that follow the acute lesion. Finally, trials are under way to develop the optimal timing and dosage schedules for existing therapies. It is therapeutic to share with those who have MS the promise of these future developments.

MYASTHENIA GRAVIS

method of
STANLEY H. APPEL, M.D.
Baylor College of Medicine
Houston, Texas

Myasthenia gravis (MG) is an autoimmune disorder of the neuromuscular junction characterized by weakness and fatigability of skeletal muscles. The incidence of MG has been estimated at less than 1 in 100,000 with a prevalence of 10 to 15 per 100,000, but because MG is probably underdiagnosed the prevalence rate may be much higher. Most commonly, the disease has a peak incidence in younger women in their second to third decades and in older men in their sixth to seventh decades.

CLINICAL SYMPTOMS AND SIGNS

The weakness in MG is quite variable with respect to the muscle groups involved and the rate of progression. The extraocular and eyelid muscles can be affected early, giving rise to double vision and ptosis. The disease gradually becomes more generalized, involving the limb muscles, especially proximal musculature such as the deltoid and iliopsoas. The pattern of involvement also compromises the triceps muscles and the finger extensors and flexors. Weakness tends to fluctuate during the day and from day to day, with improvement after a period of rest and increases in severity as the day progresses or with increased exertion. Bulbar muscle weakness especially of the pharyngeal muscles results in swallowing difficulty, regurgitation of liquids, and aspiration of food and secretions. Pharyngeal muscle weakness can result in nasal speech, and jaw muscle fatigue can lead to impairment in chewing. Weakness of the respiratory muscles can lead to difficulty in breathing, and to a respiratory myasthenic crisis. Exacerbations can be provoked by infections, stress, and emotional disturbances, altered hormonal states such as hyperthyroidism or hypothyroidism, various medications such as antiarrhythmics (e.g., quinidine and procainamide), aminoglycoside antibiotics, diuretics (by inducing hypokalemia), the magnesium salts (Maalox, milk of magnesia), and beta-blocking agents.

PATHOPHYSIOLOGY

The major physiologic changes in MG are at the neuromuscular junction and are primarily the result of acetylcholine receptor (AChR) antibodies' decreasing the number of AChRs on the muscle postsynaptic membrane. As a consequence, the postsynaptic muscle membrane is markedly simplified, the space between the motor nerve terminal and the muscle membrane is widened, and the concentration of AChRs in the postsynaptic muscle membrane is reduced. These changes lower the safety margin of conduction of information from nerve to muscle, such that the acetylcholine normally released from the nerve has a reduced likelihood of giving rise to a muscle action potential. The failure of transmission is due to widening of the synaptic cleft as well as to the decreased AChR concentration and is accentuated when repetitive activity lowers the number of acetylcholine "packets" released from the motor terminal.

AChR antibodies can be detected in the serum of more than 80% of MG patients. The serum concentration of these antibodies may not correlate well with the degree of weakness, nor predict the severity of disease in individual patients. In a small percentage of patients, AChR antibodies may be absent with bungarotoxin immunoprecipitation assays, but detectable with assays of AChR turnover in tissue culture. Improvement in the clinical state after treatment is commonly associated with a reduced titer of such antibodies, but only over the long term.

The factors that trigger the autoimmune response giving rise to AChR antibodies are incompletely understood. Seventy percent of patients have thymic hyperplasia with germinal centers, and 15% of patients with MG have a thymoma or may develop thymoma during the course of the illness. Thymomas are usually benign and well differentiated. Removal of the hyperplastic or neoplastic thymus by surgery results in improvement of the MG, but the exact mechanism of this improvement is not clear. A number of other autoimmune disorders have been associated with MG, including lupus erythematosus, rheumatoid arthritis, thyroid diseases, and autoimmune anemias.

DIAGNOSTIC PROCEDURES

Of greatest importance in diagnosing MG are the clinical history and physical examination. Pharmacologic tests may be of value because inhibiting the enzyme acetylcholinesterase (AChE), which catalyzes the breakdown of acetylcholine, can improve symptoms. Edrophonium chloride (Tensilon), a short-acting AChE inhibitor, can be injected intravenously to a total dose of 10 mg. A muscle group that fatigues on examination such as eyelid levators, deltoid, or iliopsoas should be tested. Initially, 2 mg is injected and the muscle strength is monitored after 1 minute. In the absence of any improvement, subsequent injections of 3 and 5 mg are given, with monitoring of changes in strength over the next several minutes. Beneficial effects may last at least 5 to 10 minutes. Caution is urged, because patients may be extremely sensitive to small amounts of edrophonium chloride, and respiratory crisis can occur, although it is uncommon in MG patients not receiving AChE inhibitors. An Ambu bag should be available when the test is done to breathe for the patient if necessary. In elderly patients, cardiovascular problems such as bradycardia or complete heart block have been reported. A false-positive edrophonium test with briefly improved strength may be seen in patients with amyotrophic lateral sclerosis, as well as occasionally in patients with brain stem lesions with compromise of cranial nerves. Patients who do not respond to edrophonium chloride may require intramuscular neostigmine (Prostigmin) 0.5 mg or pyridostigmine (Mestinon) 60 mg orally as a diagnostic test, but responses to these medications over several days are usually of less specific diagnostic value.

Electromyography (EMG) is usually of considerable diagnostic value. In approximately 80% of patients with generalized MG, a decreasing response of greater than 15% is noted after stimulation at 3 Hz. The facial and proximal limb musculature is more likely to exhibit a positive decreasing response than distal limb musculature. In patients with pure ocular MG, the sensitivity of repetitive nerve stimulation is less than 50%. Single-fiber EMG is extremely sensitive to the impaired neuromuscular transmission of MG, especially in the facial musculature. However, such tests are usually less specific, and other disorders must be excluded.

Eighty percent of patients with acquired autoimmune MG have serum antibodies against the AChR. Less than 50% of patients with ocular MG have similar AChR antibodies. The presence of an elevated concentration of AChR antibody in a patient with clinical features is in accord with the diagnosis of MG, although false-positive tests can be seen uncommonly in other autoimmune disorders without clinical myasthenia. The absence of AChR antibodies does not exclude MG. The presence of elevated titers of striational antibodies should raise concern about possible thymoma. Computed tomography of the anterior mediastinum is necessary to rule out possible thymoma as well as to provide evidence of thymic hyperplasia.

TREATMENT

There is no single ideal treatment for MG because no large, double-blind, controlled trials have been carried out for any therapeutic regimen in MG. The treatment plan for each patient needs to be individualized and constantly reassessed to optimize therapeutic benefits. Treatment can be divided into (1) symptomatic therapy (AChE inhibitors) and (2) attempts to influence the natural history with thymectomy and immunosuppression with corticosteroids, azathioprine, and/or cyclosporine, as well as plasmapheresis and intravenous immunoglobulin.

Anticholinesterase Agents

AChE inhibitors do not modify the natural history of disease but can improve muscle strength. These agents are effective because they prolong the availability of acetylcholine and enhance neuromuscular transmission despite the widened synaptic cleft and the decreased density of AChRs on the muscle surface membrane. The most widely used AChE inhibitor is pyridostigmine bromide. The usual initial dose is 60 mg every 4 to 6 hours during the day. The pharmacologic action of the drug begins within 30 minutes, peaks at 2 hours, and declines during the subsequent 2 hours. Dosing intervals should be determined by both the duration and the extent of benefit achieved. If weakness occurs 3 hours after the dose, the interval between doses can be shortened and the actual dose increased. It is rarely necessary to exceed 120 mg every 3 hours.

It is important to appreciate the variable response of different muscles and the necessity to adjust the dosage to provide optimal response in the muscles that are weakest. At all times safeguarding respiration should be the primary concern. Even when a dose results in improved strength in the extremities, if it causes labored breathing, then the dosage needs to be adjusted downward. Patients with swallowing difficulty should have their doses timed to coincide with optimal strength for chewing and swallowing during meals. If the patient has difficulty with weakness on awakening in the morning, sustained-released pyridostigmine (Mestinon Timespan 180 mg) may be prescribed at bedtime to improve strength in the early morning so that the patient can swallow the usual 60-mg tablet at that time. Because of the variable absorption of the sustained-release preparation, it should not be used for daytime treatment. The most common side effect of AChE inhibitors is diarrhea, which can be treated with loperamide hydrochloride (Imodium) or diphenoxylate hydrochloride with atropine sulfate (Lomotil). In addition, taking food with the medication can minimize side effects. AChE inhibitors can increase bronchial secretions and may precipitate episodes of bronchospasm in patients with asthma; caution is advised. Bradycardia appearing after parenteral administration of edrophonium chloride is sufficiently short-lived not to require therapy. However, it can be treated with 0.6 to 1.2 mg of intravenous atropine sulfate.

The benefit of AChE inhibitors is often limited, and their effectiveness is usually greatest earlier in the course of the disease. In an attempt to eliminate all weakness, patients may be overdosed and develop signs of a cholinergic crisis exacerbating weakness, impairing respiration, and severely altering central nervous system function. These side effects can be avoided if one keeps in mind that AChE inhibitors provide only symptomatic therapy and that more definitive treatment is usually required to alter the fundamental course of the disease.

Other AChE inhibitors, used less frequently, include neostigmine bromide, which is administered orally in 15-mg tablets every 4 to 6 hours. Ephedrine may also enhance neuromuscular transmission and increase acetylcholine release from presynaptic cholinergic terminals. The combination of ephedrine and AChE inhibitors may be synergistic. The dose of ephedrine* is 25 mg two or three times a day.

Thymectomy

Thymic hyperplasia with germinal centers is present in 70% of cases and thymomas are present in 10 to 15%. Thymomas are usually benign and spread locally rather than metastasize. These tumors should be removed to prevent local spread as well as to benefit MG. I recommend thymectomy for most patients with MG before the age of 60 years. The optimal benefit for thymectomy is reported to occur in young women early in the course of the disease, although in my experience, improvement occurs in both men and women even much later in their disease. In patients older than 60 years, little thymus tissue may be present, and the benefit of thymectomy is much less. In the past, transcervical approaches have been recommended because of decreased morbidity, but the inadequate removal of the thymic tissue makes this a less beneficial approach. A sternum-splitting transthoracic approach with full exploration of the anterior mediastinum provides maximal benefit for patients. With a skilled surgical team, there is minimal morbidity with transthoracic surgical thymectomy. Optimal preparation of the patients with either plasma exchange or immunosuppression may be required in patients with significant weakness. Skilled postoperative management in an intensive care unit is critical to achieve the best outcome. Extubation can be accomplished within hours after surgery, and attention to pulmonary function is imperative, with deep-breathing exercises and intermittent positive-pressure breathing to avoid atelectasis and infection. Judicious use of pain medication permits the patient to rapidly improve respiratory function.

The requirement for AChE inhibitor medication may be markedly altered after thymectomy, and patients may become exquisitely sensitive to such medi-

---

*Not FDA approved for this indication.

cation. I usually withhold AChE inhibitor medication for at least 24 hours after surgery. If the patient's breathing deteriorates after extubation, intramuscular AChE inhibitors such as pyridostigmine intramuscularly or intravenously (2 mg intramuscularly or 0.7 mg intravenously = 60 mg orally) can be administered every 4 hours as a substitute for oral pyridostigmine tablets. In addition, if the patient was receiving corticosteroid therapy before surgery, intravenous methylprednisolone should be given during the course of the surgery and continued postoperatively. Some experts have successfully avoided postoperative complications of thymectomy by treating patients with plasma exchange and corticosteroids for 4 to 6 weeks before surgery.

After thymectomy, patients may experience an immediate benefit lasting several days. However, patients are more likely to experience a more lasting benefit beginning several months to several years after surgery. Occasionally in patients with disease that does not respond to other regimens, repeated transthoracic surgery may be required to re-explore anterior mediastinum, searching for residual thymic tissue. Although repeated thymectomy is not commonly carried out, it may provide a significant benefit to a patient who had responded well initially and then several years later had recurrence of MG weakness. Removal of the thymus in infants or children does not have deleterious effects on development of immune system function.

Immunosuppression

Corticosteroids

The absence of placebo-controlled, double-blind clinical trials is most evident in the different empirical regimens of corticosteroids employed by different experts in MG. All such experts agree that corticosteroids can result in significant improvement of myasthenic weakness ranging from diplopia and ptosis to severe respiratory compromise. Despite the different approaches, a number of common principles have evolved: (1) Corticosteroids should be used early in the course of the disease. (2) When therapy is initiated, high-dose corticosteroids give a more immediate benefit than low-dose therapy in patients with myasthenic weakness. (3) In older patients with diplopia and ptosis, corticosteroids may be far more effective than AChE inhibitors. (4) Relatively rapid exacerbation of weakness can occur early in the course of high-dose corticosteroid therapy; the major therapeutic aim should be to safeguard respiration. (5) The greatest limitation to chronic corticosteroid therapy is the presence of adverse side effects including diabetes, ulcers, hypertension, increased fluid retention, increased appetite and weight gain, cataracts, bone demineralization and osteoporosis, and aseptic necrosis of bone. Recurrent infections may also result from immunosuppression. (6) Reducing corticosteroid doses too quickly may exacerbate myasthenic weakness. It is better to reduce the medication dose slowly

and obviate the necessity of returning to high-dose regimens. (7) Once benefit with corticosteroids is achieved, every-other-day therapy is quite effective and may reduce the likelihood of side effects.

When therapy with corticosteroids is initiated, the presence of underlying disorders that would exacerbate side effects needs to be evaluated. For example, in the presence of diabetes, ulcers, hypertension, osteoporosis, or chronic infection, the potential complications of corticosteroids may contraindicate their use. In all instances when chronic corticosteroid treatment is planned, careful and continuous medical follow-up must be available to minimize potential side effects.

In general I follow two regimens, one for patients with significant generalized weakness that requires hospitalization, and the other for patients with mild MG given on an outpatient basis. Patients with significant limb weakness, oropharyngeal weakness, or respiratory insufficiency, in the absence of contraindications for corticosteroids, are started with high-dose intravenous methylprednisolone (Solu-Medrol)* therapy at 1000 mg per day for 5 days with careful monitoring of blood glucose, salts, blood pressure, and vital capacity. Calcium at 1.5 grams per day, in the form of calcium lactate or calcium gluconate, and H_2 antagonists are also administered. The major concern is a steroid-induced exacerbation of respiratory muscle weakness during the first 4 to 5 days of therapy. In the presence of deteriorating respiratory function, the patient should be moved to the intensive care unit and plans made to assist respiration. Corticosteroid therapy can be continued, and plasma exchange or intravenous immune globulin (IGIV) may be of value. After successful completion of therapy, the patient is discharged and prescribed 80 mg of prednisone* per day for 7 days followed by 60 mg of prednisone per day for 2 weeks. Patients who have improved symptomatically can be switched to 60 mg alternating with 20 mg every other day for 2 weeks, 60 mg alternating with 10 mg every other day for 2 weeks, and then 60 mg per day every other day. Thereafter, the prednisone dose is lowered by 10 mg per day every 4 weeks, with side effects carefully monitored. Severe exacerbation of weakness, whether during the initial intravenous steroid phase or subsequently, prompts me to hospitalize the patient and consider alternative therapies such as plasmapheresis or intravenous globulins. As long as respiration is safeguarded within the hospital setting and preferably in an intensive care unit, I have noted no untoward effects of this regimen, and the majority of patients show significant improvement in a period as early as 4 days or as late as 6 months.

MG patients with mild weakness can have their treatment initiated in an outpatient setting with a daily dose of 60 mg of prednisone per day for approximately 2 weeks. When improvement occurs, the dose is then changed to 60 mg alternating with 20 mg for 2 weeks, then to 60 mg alternating with 10 mg for 2

---

*Not FDA approved for this indication.

weeks, followed by 60 mg every other day. Doses are gradually decreased over many months by 10 mg per month to the lowest dose that can sustain clinical improvement, usually 15 to 20 mg every other day. A gradual decrease of the steroid dose must be dictated by the patient's individual response, balancing the benefit in the myasthenic weakness with untoward side effects.

Although I do not routinely use a regimen of incrementing-dose prednisone, other experts have found it an effective way to treat the disease and at the same time avoid the early respiratory side effects. Prednisone is begun at 20 mg per day with increments of 10 mg per day each week until the patient achieves clinical benefit or reaches a level of 60 mg per day. After definite improvement has been achieved for at least 1 to 2 weeks, an alternate-day dose that is slightly less than twice the daily dose is employed. This dose is continued until maximal improvement is achieved, and then the prednisone is reduced slowly to the minimal needed dose.

In nearly all patients, corticosteroid therapy needs to be continued for at least several years, unless side effects preclude such a regimen. The maintenance dose of corticosteroid needs to be individualized for each patient, and minimal doses need to be established.

Other Immunosuppressive Drugs

Azathioprine (Imuran)* can provide improvement in MG, but the delay in clinical efficacy may be at least 6 months. Azathioprine may be most effective when used in combination with prednisone in patients refractory to prednisone therapy alone. The usual dose is 2 to 3 mg per kg per day, starting with an initial dose of 50 mg per day and increasing by 50 mg per day every 3 days to a total of 150 to 200 mg per day for adult patients. Complete blood counts and liver function tests should be checked every 2 weeks during the first month and monthly for 6 months and every 3 to 6 months thereafter. If the white blood cell count decreases to approximately 3000 per mm³, the dose should be temporarily reduced and then gradually increased after the white blood cell count rises above 3500 cells per mm³. Treatment should also be discontinued if serum transaminase concentrations exceed twice the upper limit of normal, and the drug can be restarted at lower doses when such liver function tests have returned to normal. White blood cell counts can be increased with corticosteroid therapy. Patients receiving azathioprine and prednisone must be monitored with lymphocyte counts as an alternative. Counts below 1000 per mm³ are comparable to the 3000 per mm³ whole white blood cell counts in the absence of corticosteroids. An acute idiosyncratic reaction with flulike symptoms or myalgia may necessitate stopping azathioprine. Gastrointestinal irritation can be minimized by giving divided doses after meals. Because of potential mutagenic side effects, females of childbearing age should avoid the medica-

tion. The use of azathioprine may also be limited by its expense.

Cyclosporine (Sandimmune)* has been reported to benefit patients with MG. Treatment can begin at 5 mg per kg per day in two divided doses taken 12 hours apart. Serum concentrations at trough levels can be monitored monthly. The major side effects of concern are nephrotoxicity and hypertension. If serum creatinine concentrations as well as blood urea nitrogen increase to more than 150% of pretreatment values, the dosage of cyclosporine should be reduced. Regardless of side effects, the dose should be gradually reduced to the least amount maintaining improvement. In general, the high cost of cyclosporine, as well as its potential toxicities including hepatotoxicity, limits its usefulness in MG.

Cyclophosphamide (Cytoxan)* can be useful in patients with MG refractory to other immunosuppressant drugs. It can be used intravenously at 400 mg per day in divided doses for 5 days as well as orally at 150 to 200 mg per day. Frequent toxic side effects including alopecia, leukopenia, anorexia, and cystitis, as well as the increased risk of delayed malignancy, limit its usefulness on a chronic basis.

Plasmapheresis (Plasma Exchange)

Plasma exchange removes circulating factors including antibodies from the serum of myasthenic patients and can achieve short-term benefits under appropriate circumstances. Patients with sudden worsening of myasthenic weakness for any reason, including recent institution of corticosteroid therapy; patients with the need to improve strength before surgery; and patients refractory to corticosteroid therapy or in whom corticosteroid side effects become unacceptable may experience temporary but definite benefit with plasma exchange. Our protocol is to remove 2 liters of plasma three times a week for a total of six exchanges in 2 weeks. Improvement may last for weeks or months. During the course of plasma exchange we administer prednisone orally at 30 mg per day as well as 100 mg of cyclophosphamide each evening after the exchange. After the six exchanges, the prednisone dose is changed to 50 mg alternating with 10 mg every other day, and the dose of cyclophosphamide (100 mg per day) is continued for 1 month and then stopped. The prednisone dose is then gradually lowered until a minimal beneficial dose is achieved. In our experience, the combination of these immunosuppressive drug regimens together with plasmapheresis has resulted in prolonged benefit. Repeated exchanges have been required less than once a year using this regimen. Adverse reactions have been relatively minimal but do include hypotension, thromboembolism, and transitory cardiac arrhythmias. Of greater concern are the potential complications of shunts placed to maintain vascular access, such as pain, infection, bacterial endocarditis, and thrombophlebitis. Another concern is that plas-

---

*Not FDA approved for this indication.

*Not FDA approved for this indication.

mapheresis is expensive and therefore not always an available option.

Intravenous Immune Globulin

Most patients with MG who receive high-dose IGIV* note within several days a benefit that can last for a number of weeks. The benefit may be substantial in an individual patient, but it is quite variable from patient to patient. In the presence of infection or other medical contraindications to plasmapheresis, IGIV may be quite helpful. In addition, it may provide short-term benefit in any patient with sudden worsening of myasthenic weakness. The usual dose is 400 mg per kg per day for 5 successive days given intravenously. Side effects include chills, headache, and fever. Renal failure can occur in patients with impaired renal function. In addition, if the patient has selective IgA deficiency, an anaphylactic reaction to the IgA may occur. An additional concern is the transmission of hepatitis C by IGIV. Human immunodeficiency virus is not known to be transmitted by IGIV. The major disadvantages of IGIV are its high expense and the variable response in different patients.

TREATMENT PLAN

Treatment of Associated Diseases

Exacerbation of myasthenic weakness requires immediate attention. Infection of any sort can exacerbate weakness and may precipitate oropharyngeal or respiratory dysfunction. Hypothyroidism and hyperthyroidism may aggravate myasthenic weakness and must be treated vigorously. Various neuromuscular blocking agents such as D-tubocurarine compromise neuromuscular transmission and worsen myasthenic weakness. Antibiotics including aminoglycosides, antiarrhythmics, and beta-adrenergic blocking drugs also can aggravate myasthenic weakness.

An annual influenza immunization is recommended, because any infection can aggravate myasthenic weakness. However, vaccination may occasionally also worsen MG. Immunization against pneumococcus is also recommended, preferably before initiating immunosuppressive regimens, because the latter may impair effectiveness of such vaccinations.

Ocular Myasthenia Gravis

In patients in whom weakness is limited to the extraocular muscles and eyelids, AChE inhibitor medication should be started first. If the response to AChE inhibitors is inadequate, corticosteroids are usually the most effective immunosuppressive agents. The development of cataracts is one of the major side effects to be monitored. Thymectomy, plasmapheresis, and IGIV are usually far less effective in ocular myasthenia and should be considered only if corticosteroid therapy is ineffective or contraindicated.

*Not FDA approved for this indication.

Neonatal Myasthenia Gravis

Approximately 15% of infants born to MG mothers may develop weak sucking and crying and impaired swallowing and respiration at birth or within the first several weeks postnatally. Neither the titer of AChR antibodies nor the mother's clinical status can predict which infants will be affected. The infants' symptoms can last from several weeks to several months, with no recurrence of the MG later in life. Because all children of myasthenic mothers should be assessed for neonatal MG, the pregnant myasthenic woman should deliver in an institution with special expertise in MG, and both obstetrician and pediatrician should be alerted to this possible condition. The diagnosis in the infant can be confirmed by an edrophonium test and therapy administered consisting of AChE inhibitors such as pyridostigmine (4 to 10 mg) orally or by nasal gastric tube every 4 hours as needed. Intravenous neostigmine (0.05 to 0.1 mg) every 4 hours may be given if needed. In neonates with respiratory weakness, plasma exchange may be required.

During pregnancy, the clinical state of myasthenic women is unpredictable. Symptoms and signs may improve, worsen, or remain unchanged. Side effects of many drugs used in MG may contraindicate their use in pregnant women with MG. AChE inhibitors enhance uterine contractions, and immunosuppressant cytotoxic drugs should be avoided because of their potential mutagenic effects. Regional anesthesia is to be preferred for delivery; cesarean section is not warranted by the MG but only by obstetric indications. Barbiturates rather than magnesium sulfate should be used to manage preeclampsia if it occurs.

Despite the presence of AChR antibodies in mother and newborn infant, breast-feeding does not exacerbate myasthenic weakness in the infant. Decreased fetal movement in utero suggests a diagnosis of intrauterine myasthenia and may warrant plasma exchange or IGIV therapy to prevent the development of arthrogryposis multiplex congenita.

Generalized Myasthenia Onset in Patients Younger than 60 Years

Patients should be started with AChE inhibitors as initial symptomatic therapy. Transthoracic surgical thymectomy is recommended for most patients. In patients presenting with steady progression of limb weakness before bulbar and respiratory involvement or with respiratory or swallowing muscle weakness, corticosteroids and/or plasma exchange may be needed to reduce the postoperative risk of pulmonary dysfunction. After thymectomy, if disabling weakness continues, immunosuppression with prednisone is advocated.

Generalized Myasthenia Gravis Onset in Patients Older than 60 Years

Treatment is begun with AChE inhibitors as with younger patients. Thymectomy is not considered the first option. Instead, corticosteroid therapy is initiated, and plasma exchange and IGIV as follow-up therapies are considered. With this regimen, other immunosuppressive drugs such as azathioprine or cyclosporine have not been required. However, other experts start azathioprine therapy at the same time as high-dose prednisone to provide a corticosteroid-sparing effect.

Seronegative Myasthenia Gravis

Approximately 10 to 15% of patients with autoimmune acquired MG do not have detectable AChR antibodies by serum immunoprecipitation assays. These patients are more likely to be younger, to be males without thymoma and with less frequent thymic hyperplasia, and to have an atrophic, an involuted, or a normal thymus. The history and physical examination as well as the response to AChE inhibitors and decreasing response on the EMG are the same as with seropositive MG patients. Treatment of patients with seronegative autoimmune MG is the same as that for seropositive patients. The absence of AChR antibodies does not imply an unsatisfactory response to thymectomy, immunosuppression, plasma exchange, or IGIV.

Penicillamine-Induced Myasthenia Gravis

The use of D-penicillamine (Cuprimine, Depen) for rheumatoid arthritis, Wilson's disease, or cystinuria has resulted in myasthenic weakness in some patients. Weakness is usually mild and confined to the ocular muscles. Edrophonium chloride tests as well as EMG and an elevated serum AChR antibody are usually positive for MG. The mechanism of D-penicillamine–induced MG is likely to be an enhanced immunologic reaction against the AChR. Stopping the D-penicillamine therapy as well as using AChE inhibitors should ameliorate the condition, but if symptoms persist, the patient should be treated as for autoimmune MG.

Myasthenic Crisis

The most critical complication in MG is the myasthenic crisis, which is characterized by significant weakness in breathing and in swallowing. Myasthenic crisis may occur as a consequence of infection or surgery, or after marked exacerbation of the disease, possibly in the presence of rapid tapering of immunosuppressive drugs.

Several decades ago, before the introduction of immunosuppression, large dosages of AChE inhibitors were employed, and respiratory failure from overdose was a frequent clinical problem. With the present regimens, respiratory failure from excess AChE inhibition (cholinergic crisis) is a far less common occurrence.

Impaired respiration from any cause requires emergency intervention. The patient should be admitted to the hospital immediately. Decreasing vital capacity below 50% of normal, or below 2 liters, should prompt the patient's transfer to an intensive care unit experienced in the management of respiratory insufficiency. The edrophonium test is contraindicated in an effort to distinguish myasthenic from cholinergic crisis. Edrophonium can strengthen limb muscles at the same time as it is weakening respiratory function. The critical issue is to safeguard respiration. This can be best accomplished by decreasing all AChE inhibitors and using ventilation. Prompt intubation and ventilatory support, as well as careful monitoring of the patient's fluid, electrolyte balance, and nutrition, are mandatory.

Special attention must be given to the possible presence of any infection, because fever as well as infection may worsen myasthenic weakness and make recovery from pneumonia difficult. Furthermore, in the presence of immunosuppressive drugs, patients are vulnerable to infection and need to be treated early and vigorously. At the slightest indication of infection, even in the absence of evidence of respiratory failure, material for cultures should be obtained and empirical therapy begun. Too often aminoglycoside antibiotics are withheld because of their adverse effects on myasthenic weakness. However, if necessary, these drugs can be used, especially in an intensive care unit setting where the patient is already receiving ventilatory support.

Ventilation and respiratory assistance must be provided when the vital capacity falls below 1 liter or 25% of normal. This corresponds to an inspiratory force of more than -20 cm H_2O, a tidal volume of 4 to 5 mL per kg of body weight, and a forced vital capacity of less than 15 mL per kg of body weight. Intubation should be carried out by an expert in ventilatory management with a low-pressure, high-compliance, cuffed endotracheal tube. A volume-controlled respirator set to provide tidal volumes of at least 10 mL per kg of ideal body weight and an automatic sighing every 10 to 15 minutes is preferred. The pressure of the tube cuff should be checked frequently and the tube position verified. Inspired gas must be humidified to at least 80% at 37°C to prevent drying of the tracheal bronchial tree. In addition, frequent aseptic aspiration can be undertaken to remove tracheal secretions.

If the patient cannot be weaned from the ventilator, because of continuing complaints of fatigue and shortness of breath, I have successfully carried out plasmapheresis or IGIV therapy. In the presence of infection in the intensive care unit, corticosteroids may be contraindicated. In my experience with patients in myasthenic crisis secondary to infection, decreasing corticosteroid therapy and eliminating AChE inhibitors together with initiating appropriate antibiotic coverage and IGIV therapy result in the best outcome.

With the availability of immunosuppressive drugs and increasing expertise in ventilatory management, myasthenic crisis has become a less common problem. The outlook for patients with MG has improved dramatically, and more than 90% can lead to meaningful, productive lives. There is no single best way to treat an individual MG patient, but the enhancement of neuromuscular transmission and the varied immunosuppressive regimens can reverse pathophysiologic processes in a meaningful way and lead to dramatic improvement in the quality of patients' lives.

Congenital Myasthenic Syndromes

Congenital MG must be considered in all childhood- or adult-onset seronegative MG, especially patients with a positive family history. However, many patients with myasthenic syndrome have an autosomal recessive inheritance, and the family history may be negative. These inherited myasthenic syndromes are due to genetically mediated abnormalities of presynaptic and/or postsynaptic structures impairing the safety of neuromuscular transmission. They are not mediated by AChR antibodies. Symptoms may occur at birth, in childhood, or later in adult life. In different syndromes, clinical weakness ranging from diplopia and ptosis to more generalized weakness has been described. For rational therapy, precise diagnosis and knowledge of the site of defect are required. In familial infantile myasthenia, in which the resynthesis or vesicular packaging of acetylcholine is impaired, AChE inhibitors are of great value. However, patients with deficiency of end-plate AChE may not benefit. Patients with inherited AChR deficiency may benefit from AChE inhibitors. However, if such deficiency is accompanied by a prolonged open time of the AChR channel, therapy with AChE inhibitors over time can lead to myopathy.

TRIGEMINAL NEURALGIA

method of
KIM J. BURCHIEL, M.D.
Oregon Health Sciences University
Portland, Oregon

CLINICAL PRESENTATION

Trigeminal neuralgia (tic douloureux) is typically described as fleeting, lancinating pain lasting seconds to minutes that occurs in the sensory distribution of the trigeminal nerve. The pain commonly strikes the third (mandibular) division of the nerve along the jaw or lower teeth or tongue; less commonly it affects second (maxillary) and first (ophthalmic) divisions. Frequently, more than one distribution is affected, and the pain seemingly radiates from one division to the other. The pain is almost always unilateral, although very rarely, bilateral trigeminal neuralgia can be seen. The typical pains are always paroxysmal, often described as "electrical" in quality by patients.

There is usually a perioral trigger zone in the second or third division. Triggering stimuli often include talking, eating, oral hygiene activities such as toothbrushing, and wind or cold temperatures on the face. Light tactile, nonnoxious stimulation of the trigger zone produces the typical neuralgic pains commonly seen. Frequently, the pain oc-

curs spontaneously either from environmental stimuli or without apparent trigger. Because of the triggerability of the pain, patients often do not groom the affected side of the face during acute episodes and may not eat or even swallow oral secretions.

The disorder is often characterized by pain-free intervals, which can last from months to even years. After a pain-free interval, the pain returns exactly as before the hiatus. Neurologic examination in the typical case reveals no deficit. Sensory loss, even minimal, in the area of the pain or of the trigger zone suggests structural pathology or severe compression of the nerve in the posterior fossa.

This disorder primarily affects older patients (60 years and older), but individuals from their teens to older than 90 years can be affected. There is a slight predominance of females to males with the disorder, and the pain is slightly more common on the right side of the face.

Atypical trigeminal neuralgia combines features of typical idiopathic trigeminal neuralgia, i.e., brief, lancinating, unilateral electrical pains, with a constant background pain that is usually described as either aching or burning. These pains are likewise unilateral, and facial sensory loss is more common.

Secondary trigeminal neuralgia represents approximately 2% of cases of trigeminal neuralgia, and atypical pain is more common. There is always a sensory loss, and patients are found to have tumors or vascular lesions that cause compression of the nerve. The age range is usually lower than that for typical idiopathic trigeminal neuralgia, and male and female incidences are about equal.

Symptomatic trigeminal neuralgia occurs in association with multiple sclerosis and may manifest as either typical or atypical pains. Approximately 1% of patients with multiple sclerosis develop trigeminal neuralgia, which in rare cases is the presenting complaint. Thirty to 35 years is the average age at presentation for symptomatic trigeminal neuralgia.

Post-traumatic trigeminal neuralgia occurs approximately 5 to 10% of the time after facial trauma or oral surgery. It is reported to be seen in between 1 and 5% of patients after removal of impacted teeth. The painful episodes are sharp and episodic and are often triggered, like the pain of typical trigeminal neuralgia. Superimposed is a background of dull, throbbing, or burning pain like that of atypical trigeminal neuralgia. These post-traumatic pain problems may represent either trigeminal "neuroma" or deafferentation pain, i.e., pain after *loss* of nervous system input. This diagnosis overlaps substantially with atypical facial pain.

Atypical facial pain may be included with a number of disorders that come under the rubric pain of psychologic origin in the head and face. There is no known physical cause or pathophysiologic mechanism for this type of pain. Once other causes of the pain are ruled out, such as sinus disease and migrainous neuralgia, the diagnosis of atypical facial pain should be considered. Usually, there is also proof of contributing psychologic factors, and the characteristics of this group of patients overlap those in the American Psychiatric Association definition of psychogenic pain disorder. The pain is usually described as diffuse or nonanatomic in the orofacial region. There is a steady, often burning or aching quality. Atypical facial pain may mimic other syndromes. There is often obvious psychopathology, including delusions, hallucinations, and multiple physical complaints. There may also be conversion or pseudoneurotic symptoms and signs. Psychologic evaluation reveals signs of somatization, depression, and illness behaviors. Patients typically exhibit excessive treatment- or medication-seeking behavior. Neurologic examination is almost invariably normal, although there may be poorly localized tenderness and vague, nonreproducible sensory loss.

DIAGNOSIS

The diagnosis of typical trigeminal neuralgia is usually not difficult if it is considered. Again, a patient with unilateral, fleeting, lancinating, electric shock–like facial pains in the trigeminal sensory distribution generally has trigeminal neuralgia. The pains are alleviated by carbamazepine (Tegretol), which in itself is a diagnostic test, because no other orofacial pain responds to this anticonvulsant. The diagnosis of the overlap syndrome, atypical trigeminal neuralgia, may be more problematic, but again, fleeting pains are the hallmark of the disorder. Patients with constant pain only (atypical facial pain) should be treated nonsurgically and not without thorough diagnostic evaluation, in most cases including psychologic evaluation.

Although the diagnosis of trigeminal neuralgia is generally made from clinical criteria, computed tomography or magnetic resonance imaging of the head should be performed to rule out the uncommon instance of intracranial pathology. The latter may be preferable because of its superior imaging of the posterior fossa and of demyelinating disease.

ETIOLOGY

The underlying cause of trigeminal neuralgia is still debated. In typical trigeminal neuralgia, considerable evidence suggests that cross-compression of the nerve at its entry into the pons by an artery or vein may be the inciting event. Demyelination may occur at this point of cross-compression. Some autopsy results in patients with trigeminal neuralgia and multiple sclerosis indicate that demyelination within the descending tract of the trigeminal nerve or within the nerve itself can be correlated with the disorder. As mentioned previously, other structural lesions, such as tumors, aneurysms, and arteriovenous malformations, rarely can cross-compress the nerve and produce quite typical pain.

TREATMENT

Medical Management

The medical treatment of typical idiopathic trigeminal neuralgia is usually quite rewarding. Carbamazepine is started in doses of 100 mg twice daily and then increased by 200 mg per day every 2 to 3 days, until a final daily dose in the range of 800 to 1000 mg is reached.

Before this medication is started, a baseline white blood cell (WBC) count is obtained, because not uncommonly, mild leukopenia can occur during medical treatment. Rarely, a non–dose-dependent and idiosyncratic bone marrow suppression (aplastic anemia) can occur early in treatment, which must be watched for diligently. The WBC count is typically repeated a week after therapy is begun, approximately 3 to 4 weeks later, and then every several months while the patient is taking the drug. Most typical cases of trigeminal neuralgia respond to carbamazepine to some extent. In fact, as mentioned previously, this

response is a powerful and reliable diagnostic confirmation of trigeminal neuralgia.

Limitations of carbamazepine treatment are hypersensitivity reactions that preclude use of the drug and, at higher doses, symptoms of drowsiness, mental dullness, subjective dizziness, and ataxia. These latter, common symptoms can be quite troublesome in elderly patients.

A newer agent, gabapentin (Neurontin)* may be as effective as carbamazepine. Gabapentin seems to be better tolerated, although it also can produce drowsiness, dizziness, and mental dullness at higher doses. It is typically begun at 300 mg per day and the dose is increased by 300 mg every 2 to 3 days until relief is achieved. Some patients can tolerate as much as 2400 mg per day, but most experience side effects at 1500 to 1800 mg per day. Alternatively, baclofen (Lioresal)* may be substituted with good effect. This drug is started at 5 mg twice daily and then increased by 5 to 10 mg every 2 to 3 days to a maximal dose of 80 mg per day. Baclofen is not usually helpful in patients who are otherwise able to take carbamazepine or gabapentin but who continue to have neuralgic pains at high doses and are intolerant of the side effects. The anticonvulsant phenytoin can also be used but is rarely of additional benefit when the other drugs have failed.

In general, about 70% of patients respond at least initially to medical management. However, as time goes on, the drugs become ineffective in many patients, and the pain "breaks through" the pharmacologic therapy. In fact, for most patients followed up carefully for many years, medical management eventually fails.

Surgical Management

The surgical approach to trigeminal neuralgia is likewise highly effective. The procedures can generally be considered in two groups, percutaneous procedures and microvascular decompression. Dozens of other operations have been developed in the past 5 or 6 decades, but these two surgical approaches seem to hold most of the surgical attention and promise at present.

Percutaneous procedures are generally performed on an outpatient basis or with, at most, a brief stay in the hospital. In general, the risks of the procedures are minimal, and for this reason, they are generally thought to be more appropriate for the elderly (older than 65 years) or debilitated patient. The risk of death from these operations is close to zero, and morbidity is usually minimal or acceptable.

Currently, three main percutaneous procedures are performed: percutaneous radiofrequency trigeminal gangliolysis (PRTG), percutaneous retrogasserian glycerol rhizotomy (PRGR), and percutaneous balloon microcompression (PBM). In all these procedures, with the patient under local or brief general anesthesia, a needle or trocar is inserted from a point

---

*Not FDA approved for this indication.

on the cheek just lateral to the corner of the mouth, and then, under fluoroscopic guidance, the needle is introduced into the ipsilateral foramen ovale. The position of the needle is fluoroscopically verified in the lateral position, and then the gangliolysis is performed.

The PRTG procedure uses radiofrequency (RF) heating of the tip of an electrode to produce a thermal lesion in the ganglion, with the production of appropriate facial numbness in the area of pain or the trigger zone as the end point. RF lesions are produced using brief general anesthesia with a short-acting intravenous anesthetic.

The PRGR procedure is likewise performed using a spinal needle, until cerebrospinal fluid (CSF) from the trigeminal cistern is encountered. With the patient in the sitting position, a trigeminal cisternogram is obtained using radiopaque, water-soluble contrast material. After the contrast dye is removed, anhydrous glycerol (approximately 0.3 mL) is instilled into the cistern. The patient remains in the seated position with the neck flexed slightly forward for 2 hours to obtain the maximal neurolytic effect.

The PBM procedure uses a trocar placed into the region of the trigeminal ganglion, whereupon a balloon catheter is inserted into this region and is inflated for 2 minutes. The PRGR and PBM procedures do not routinely produce facial numbness, which therefore is not used as an end point. Sporadically, considerable numbness can be produced by the glycerol procedure, although it is reportedly rare with the balloon compression technique.

The alternative procedure, which is more commonly applied to younger (less than 65 years) and healthy patients with typical or atypical trigeminal neuralgia, is the microvascular decompression procedure. With the patient under general anesthesia, a small incision is made behind the ear. A 2.5- to 3-cm craniectomy is performed, the dura is opened, and the cerebellum is microsurgically retracted, revealing the trigeminal nerve. Typically, an artery or other vascular cross-compression of the nerve is identified at the pontine entry area of the nerve; the vascular structure is padded away from the nerve with polytetrafluoroethylene (Teflon) felt. This operation has a low but nonzero mortality rate, between 0.1 and 0.5% in most series. It does not ordinarily produce numbness, but complications involving hearing loss, dizziness, cerebellar syndrome, CSF leaks, meningitis, and diplopia have been seen in a few patients. Serious morbidity probably averages between 1 and 5%.

Results of Surgical Therapy

The best way to compare the outcome of pain-relieving procedures such as these is to look at the point at which 50% of patients can be statistically expected to experience return of pain. Initial efficacy for these surgical procedures is quite good. Most series report that more than 90% of patients are pain free after any of the procedures previously described. If the pain recurs, a percutaneous procedure can be repeated, and by that means, almost all patients can be successfully treated. If microvascular decompression initially fails to relieve the pain, a percutaneous procedure can be performed after an appropriate recovery interval and is also highly likely to result in a pain-free state.

For the PRGR procedure, the expected pain-free interval is approximately 1.5 to 2 years, and similar results have been seen with the PBM technique. The PRTG procedure produces about twice the pain-free interval, or about 3 to 4 years; for microvascular decompression, the pain relief can be expected to last an average of 15 years.

OPTIC NEURITIS

method of
NEIL R. MILLER, M.D.
Wilmer Eye Institute
Baltimore, Maryland

The term "optic neuritis" describes a set of clinical signs and symptoms that are assumed to be produced by inflammation of the optic nerve.

CLINICAL MANIFESTATIONS

Optic neuritis usually occurs in patients between 15 and 45 years of age, with women being affected about four times as often as men. Most patients present with blurred vision in one eye preceded or accompanied by pain. The pain may be sharp or dull, and it is often exacerbated by movement of the affected eye.

Visual acuity in an eye with optic neuritis varies considerably, from a minimal decrease in central vision to no perception of light in about 4% of patients. Color vision is almost always impaired, even when central vision is normal or nearly so. Almost all patients with optic neuritis have a defect in the central visual field of the affected eye that occasionally may extend into the peripheral visual field. True central scotomas are rare, however, with many patients having arcuate, altitudinal, and even hemianopic defects in the central field.

Patients with unilateral optic neuritis always have a relative afferent pupillary defect (Marcus Gunn pupil) on the affected side, as do many patients with asymmetric bilateral optic neuritis. However, some patients with bilateral optic neuritis have no evidence of a relative afferent pupillary defect despite clinically asymmetric bilateral optic neuritis, indicating that the actual damage to both optic nerves is more symmetrical than the clinical picture would suggest.

The optic disk in an eye with optic neuritis may appear swollen, normal, or pale. If the disk is swollen, the optic neuritis is called papillitis or anterior optic neuritis, and it is assumed that the inflammation is occurring within the intraocular portion of the optic nerve. If the disk is normal in appearance, the disorder is called retrobulbar optic neuritis or, simply, retrobulbar neuritis. Retrobulbar neuritis occurs about twice as often as papillitis; however, whether the optic disk appears swollen or normal has no visual or systemic prognostic significance in a patient with optic neuritis. Optic atrophy in a patient with acute optic neuritis indicates previous damage to the optic nerve, because it takes at least 4 to 6 weeks to develop optic pallor after an acute optic neuropathy.

NATURAL HISTORY

The characteristic course of optic neuritis is one of maximal visual loss during about 2 weeks, followed by some recovery in the subsequent 2 to 12 months. Recovery is complete in many patients, but others complain that visual function is not as good as it was before the attack, even when visual acuity returns to 20/20 or better in the previously affected eye. Such patients usually have evidence of persistent optic nerve dysfunction that can be demonstrated by clinical, electrophysiologic, or psychophysical testing.

DIAGNOSIS

Most patients who experience an attack of isolated optic neuritis eventually develop multiple sclerosis (MS), and it is thus believed that the majority of cases of optic neuritis are caused by demyelination. Indeed, the risk that MS will occur after an attack of isolated optic neuritis ranges from 25 to 75% within the first 5 years. The major risk factor is abnormal magnetic resonance imaging (MRI) features at the time of the attack of acute optic neuritis. Patients in whom MRI shows multiple periventricular white matter lesions at the time of an attack of apparently isolated optic neuritis have a much higher risk of developing MS than do patients with normal MRI features at the time of the optic neuritis attack. Other risk factors for the development of MS after an attack of optic neuritis are a previous attack of optic neuritis in the other eye, previous transient neurologic dysfunction, and a family history of MS.

Optic neuritis may occur as the initial manifestation of, or in the setting of, systemic inflammatory disorders other than MS, such as various viral exanthema, syphilis, sarcoidosis, systemic lupus erythematosus, and Lyme disease (Table 1). A special form of optic neuritis, called neuroretinitis, can also occur in any of these inflammatory disorders as well as with cat-scratch disease caused by *Bartonella henselae*. Neuroretinitis is characterized by optic disk swelling associated with formation of a "star figure" composed of lipid exudate in the macula.

Pathologic processes other than inflammation may cause an acute optic neuropathy that mimics optic neuritis (Table 2). These include compression, ischemia, infiltration, and toxic processes. In addition, Leber's hereditary optic neuropathy may manifest as initially unilateral visual loss that mimics optic neuritis, although affected patients never complain of ocular or orbital pain, and the other eye is always affected sooner or later.

TABLE 1. **Causes of Optic Neuritis**

Most Common	Less Common	Least Common
Multiple sclerosis	Idiopathic Postviral	Granulomatous inflammation, especially syphilis or sarcoidosis
		Collagen-vascular (autoimmune) disorders
		Infectious mononucleosis
		Adjacent inflammation of paranasal sinuses or orbit

TABLE 2. **Differential Diagnosis of Optic Neuritis**

Other optic neuropathies
  Compressive
    Orbital
    Intracanalicular
    Intracranial
  Ischemic
  Toxic
  Nutritional (deficiency)
  Infiltrative
  Hereditary (particularly Leber's disease)
  Glaucoma
  Drusen of the optic disk
Intraocular disease
  Retinal disease
  Retinal vascular disease
  Diseases of the ocular media
    Corneal disease
    Cataract
Nonorganic visual loss
  Conversion reaction
  Malingering

Because the diagnosis of optic neuritis is based entirely on clinical grounds, the responsibilities of the physician for a patient with presumed optic neuritis are (1) to eliminate the possibility of a process that is causing an optic neuropathy that is mimicking optic neuritis and (2) if no such lesion is present, to determine whether there is an underlying and potentially treatable cause for the optic neuritis. The minimal evaluation of such a patient includes a complete systemic and neurologic history. If there is no history suggesting an underlying inflammatory disorder such as syphilis, sarcoidosis, systemic lupus erythematosus, or Lyme disease, it probably is not necessary to obtain serologic studies. If the history is unreliable or is suggestive of a systemic inflammatory disease, however, the physician may wish to obtain some or all of the following evaluations, depending on the setting: a complete blood count, erythrocyte sedimentation rate, serum tests for syphilis, assay for antinuclear antibodies, assay for angiotensin-converting enzyme, Lyme titers, assay for human immunodeficiency virus, and a chest radiograph. Patients with presumed optic neuritis that is painless, patients with bilateral presumed optic neuritis, and patients whose vision does not improve spontaneously or with treatment (see later) should undergo a blood test for the mitochondrial DNA mutations that are associated with Leber's hereditary optic neuropathy. Patients with neuroretinitis should be questioned about exposure to kittens, and they should undergo an assay for *B. henselae* titers.

There are two schools of thought regarding neuroimaging in patients with presumed optic neuritis. Many experts believe that one need not obtain any neuroimaging studies in a "typical" case of optic neuritis and that neuroimaging should be performed only if the clinical presentation is atypical for optic neuritis (i.e., subacute, slowly progressive, painless) or if vision does not begin to improve spontaneously or with treatment (see later) within 3 to 6 weeks. Others, myself included, prefer to perform MRI of the orbits and optic chiasmal region in patients with presumed retrobulbar neuritis, not only to make certain that there is no evidence of a mass compressing the intracranial portion of the affected optic nerve but also to determine the patient's risk of development of MS. Given the significant amount of information obtained from MRI, there would seem to be little or no justification for performing computed tomography or any other type of neuroimaging in a patient with acute optic neuritis.

Patients with optic neuritis whose history, physical findings, or both suggest the diagnosis of MS should undergo a complete neurologic examination. Other tests that may be considered in such patients are testing of evoked potentials (visual, brain stem, somatosensory) and a lumbar puncture with cerebrospinal fluid analysis for protein, glucose, cells, and IgG content as well as for oligoclonal bands and myelin basic protein.

TREATMENT

Patients with isolated demyelinating optic neuritis recover spontaneously within weeks to months without treatment. The results of the Optic Neuritis Treatment Trial, sponsored by the National Institutes of Health, indicate that a 3-day course of intravenous methylprednisolone (Solu-Medrol), given in four divided doses of 250 mg every 6 hours, followed by a 10-day course of oral prednisone in a single dose of 1 mg per kg per day, and begun within the first 8 days after onset of visual loss, results in a more rapid improvement in all parameters of vision (e.g., visual acuity, contrast sensitivity, color vision, visual field), in about 2 to 3 weeks, than does either low-dose oral prednisone alone or no treatment; however, neither high-dose methylprednisolone nor low-dose prednisone improves ultimate visual outcome compared with no treatment. In addition, oral prednisone alone, in the dose just described, is associated with a higher incidence of both recurrent optic neuritis in the previously affected eye and optic neuritis in the other eye than is seen with no treatment and with high-dose methylprednisolone followed by low-dose oral prednisone.

There is some evidence that high-dose intravenous methylprednisolone followed by low-dose oral prednisone reduces the risk of MS in the first 2 years after an attack of optic neuritis in patients with abnormal MRI features at the time of the optic neuritis. I therefore recommend that high-dose intravenous methylprednisolone followed by a short course of oral prednisone be considered in any patient with acute optic neuritis when a more rapid improvement in vision compared with the natural history of the condition is required or when MRI performed at the time of the attack shows abnormal features consistent with demyelination.

Although I cannot explain the apparent adverse effects of low-dose oral corticosteroids in patients with acute optic neuritis, I do not recommend their use for such patients. There is no evidence that other anti-inflammatory agents have any effect on the extent or speed of recovery of visual acuity, color vision, contrast sensitivity, or visual field in patients with acute demyelinating or idiopathic optic neuritis. Systemic corticosteroids may be extremely valuable in treating the rare cases of optic neuritis associated with certain systemic inflammatory disorders, such as sarcoidosis and systemic lupus erythematosus. The early use of steroids in patients with these conditions may avert profound, irreversible visual

loss. Similarly, patients with optic neuritis caused by syphilis, Lyme disease, or cat-scratch disease may benefit, both visually and systemically, from early and aggressive use of systemic antibiotics.

GLAUCOMA

method of
RONALD L. GROSS, M.D.
Cullen Eye Institute
Houston, Texas

Glaucoma is a leading cause of irreversible blindness in the world. In the United States alone, 600,000 people have been blinded by glaucoma. It is the leading cause of irreversible blindness among African-Americans, and it numbers among the three most common causes overall. In the United States, 1.5 million people are affected by glaucoma, and another 1.0 million may have the disease but are not yet diagnosed.

Increasing age is a major risk factor for glaucoma, which affects 4% of the population older than 65 years, and nearly 15% of the population older than 80 years. African-Americans are affected 10 times more commonly than are whites; and in African-Americans, glaucoma has an earlier onset and more aggressive course. Immediate family members of affected patients have a 10- to 15-fold higher risk of developing glaucoma than the general population. Patients with myopia, diabetes, and systemic hypertension are also more likely to be affected by glaucoma.

Glaucoma refers to several conditions characterized by typical visual field loss due to optic nerve damage. Elevated intraocular pressure is the most important risk factor. The progressive damage to the optic nerve can be slowed or halted by an adequate reduction in intraocular pressure. In most cases, the elevated pressure is due to obstruction of the outflow of aqueous humor. This fluid is produced in the posterior chamber and normally passes between the iris and the lens through the pupil into the anterior chamber of the eye, exiting through the trabecular meshwork into the episcleral venous circulation. An obstruction to outflow increases aqueous humor volume, raising the intraocular pressure and damaging individual axons of the optic nerve in a typical manner. Visual field testing evaluates the function of the optic nerve, which exhibits characteristic abnormalities in glaucoma. Although intraocular pressure plays an important role in glaucoma, the site of damage is the optic nerve. Its appearance and function are key factors in diagnosis and treatment. Other local or systemic factors that affect the optic nerve, such as systemic hypotension, may exacerbate the condition.

GLAUCOMA SUSPECTS

Patients with elevated intraocular pressure without change in optic nerve appearance or visual field abnormality are glaucoma suspects. Only 10 to 20% of these patients will develop glaucoma, but they are at increased risk compared with the general population.

PRIMARY OPEN-ANGLE GLAUCOMA

The most common form of glaucoma, affecting nearly two thirds of patients, is primary open-angle glaucoma (POAG). The disease is bilateral but may be asymmetrical. It is caused by increased resistance to aqueous humor outflow through the trabecular meshwork that results in a mild to moderate elevation of intraocular pressure. It is a chronic disease, and because intraocular pressures are not elevated markedly, it is often asymptomatic. There is no pain or redness of the eye. The visual field loss tends to be peripheral and slowly progressive, so the patient may have no visual complaint. When central vision is affected, the disease is far progressed and more difficult to control.

POAG is insidious, so early diagnosis is the most important factor in preventing visual loss. Patients older than 35 years should be evaluated every 3 years. Older adults, African-Americans, individuals with a family history of glaucoma, and persons with other ocular or systemic problems (e.g., ocular trauma, myopia, diabetes, systemic hypertension) are at an increased risk and should be evaluated more frequently.

Glaucoma screening consists of four components: (1) medical and family history, (2) visual acuity testing, (3) examination of the optic nerve, and (4) measurement of intraocular pressure.

Examination of the optic nerve is greatly enhanced by pupillary dilatation. The optic nerve is composed of the retinal ganglion cell axons. The surface of a normal optic nerve is normally flat or slightly elevated, with a small, central, pale, depressed physiologic cup. This cup is surrounded by neural rim tissue that is normally orange-red. The appearance of the normal optic nerve and its cup varies among individuals. It is important to document the appearance of the optic nerve so that any change can be recognized. In glaucoma, early damage to nerve fibers at the inferior and superior poles of the disk result in a vertical elongation of the optic cup, with narrowing of the neural rim and pallor of the optic nerve. The vessels of the optic disk tend to be displaced nasally.

Glaucoma should be suspected if cupping represents greater than one third of the surface of the disk, extends to the rim of the disk, or results in an optic cup that is larger vertically than horizontally; if there is asymmetry between the optic disks of the patient's eyes; if a flame-shaped hemorrhage is present in the nerve fiber layer near the border of the optic disk; or if there is a definite change in the appearance of the optic disk from that of a previous evaluation.

Intraocular pressure measurement is also important in screening for glaucoma. The best way to measure intraocular pressure is tonometry. This method requires topical anesthetic but is painless and accurate. A pressure above 22 mm Hg is suggestive of glaucoma and warrants further evaluation. Intraocular pressure fluctuates in all patients, more so in those with glaucoma. Therefore, patients with damage may not have elevated pressures at any one time of measurement. Conversely, glaucomatous damage is not always present in patients with elevated intraocular pressures.

Treatment

Treatment consists of reducing intraocular pressure. Medical therapy is instituted initially, using the minimal concentration, frequency, and number of medications to control the disease and minimize side effects. Although administered topically, these drugs may cause systemic effects.

Medications

Antiglaucoma medications are as follows.

Beta Blockers. Beta blockers decrease intraocular pressure by reducing the secretion of aqueous humor. The potential side effects of ocular drops are the same as for systemic use of these agents and include exacerbation of reactive airway disease, bradycardia, systemic hypotension, decreased libido, and altered mentation. These agents should not be used in patients with heart block or heart failure, asthma, or obstructive lung disease.

Sympathomimetic Agents. Sympathomimetic drugs, such as epinephrine (Epifrin) and dipivefrin (Propine), 0.1% increase aqueous humor outflow. Their potential side effects include systemic hypertension, headache, cardiac palpitations, and arrhythmias. Alpha-adrenergic agonists also decrease aqueous humor production. Systemic effects may include dry mouth and somnolence. The most common problem is development of a topical allergic response.

Miotics. Parasympathomimetic agents such as pilocarpine (Pilocar) improve aqueous humor outflow through the trabecular meshwork. Often, these agents have ocular side effects due to the ciliary body spasm and pupillary miosis. Systemic cholinergic effects are rare. Cholinesterase inhibitors, such as echothiophate iodide (Phospholine Iodide), are topical agents that can inhibit systemic cholinesterase. Patients taking these drugs should not receive agents such as succinylcholine during general anesthesia.

Carbonic Anhydrase Inhibitors. Carbonic anhydrase inhibitors reduce intraocular pressure by depressing aqueous humor production. For long-term use, the topically applied form is preferred because of its greater safety. The long-term use of oral carbonic anhydrase inhibitors is controversial, as they can cause urinary frequency, anorexia, nausea, depression, malaise, peripheral neuropathy, kidney stones, and, rarely, aplastic anemia. Taken orally, they may lower serum potassium concentrations and so should be used with caution in patients taking non–potassium-sparing diuretics or digoxin. Carbonic anhydrase inhibitors are sulfonamides and so are contraindicated in patients allergic or sensitive to these medications.

Prostaglandins. The newest class of antiglaucoma agents that increase aqueous humor outflow, prostaglandins appear to have few systemic effects, with the primary concern being a progressive, irreversible increase in iris pigmentation in some patients.

Topical Application and Treatment Duration

To reduce the systemic absorption of all topical ophthalmic drops, nasal lacrimal duct compression or simple eyelid closure should be performed for 3 to 5 minutes after instillation of each drop.

Treatment is advanced for POAG until intraocular pressure has been reduced significantly in comparison with the level at which damage occurred. If this target level is reached, the patient is followed up closely with evaluation of the optic nerve and visual field evaluations to be sure that no further progression has occurred.

Other Modalities

If medical therapy is unsuccessful in adequately lowering intraocular pressure, surgical methods are considered. Argon laser surgery can be used to treat the trabecular meshwork to increase aqueous humor outflow. It is successful in approximately 80% of patients with POAG, with 50% of these 80% showing a treatment effect for up to 5 years. Several other surgical procedures are also designed to provide alternative aqueous humor outflow or reduce its production.

PRIMARY ANGLE-CLOSURE GLAUCOMA

Primary angle-closure glaucoma (PACG) is an ocular emergency. The onset is acute with severe symptoms. Patients at risk are those with "narrow angles," usually in an eye that is hyperopic, resulting in close apposition of the lens and iris. When an attack occurs, flow between the lens and iris is stopped. Aqueous humor continues to be secreted, forcing the iris anteriorly, covering the trabecular meshwork, and preventing outflow. Within a very short time, intraocular pressure can rise to a dangerous level.

The acute attack may be precipitated by physical or emotional stress or by dilatation of the pupil in response to dim lighting or the use of eye drops. The predisposition to angle closure is uncommon (1% of the population), and the majority of patients at risk never have an attack. Physicians should not hesitate to dilate pupils to facilitate examination of the posterior segment of the eye. Antihistamines and other medications with autonomic effects may dilate the pupil slightly, which could precipitate an attack in a predisposed patient. When such agents are used in their recommended dosage, however, this effect is rare.

Unlike patients with POAG, a patient with PACG exhibits severe symptoms, including ocular pain and redness, blurred vision, rainbow-colored halos around lights, headaches, and, frequently, nausea and vomiting. Usually only one eye is affected. On examination, that eye is red, the pupil is mid-dilated, the cornea is cloudy, and on tactile tension the eye is quite firm.

Treatment

If an acute attack of PACG is suspected, the patient should be immediately referred to an ophthalmologist; in the meantime or if referral is not possible, treatment should be instituted. It should include a topical beta blocker, 1 drop every 30 minutes, and pilocarpine 2%, 1 drop every 15 minutes for 1 hour; also, acetazolamide (Diamox), 500 mg, if not contraindicated. Osmotic diuretics, such as nitroglycerin or isosorbide (IsMO) orally or mannitol intravenously, 1 to 1.5 grams per kg of body weight, can be given if necessary.

Medical therapy is usually effective in lowering intraocular pressure and stopping the attack. Later, a laser peripheral iridotomy is performed to make an opening in the iris, which allows aqueous humor flow to the trabecular meshwork and prevents future attacks. In some patients, all effects of the attack cannot be reversed, and long-term therapy is required.

PRIMARY DEVELOPMENTAL GLAUCOMA

Primary developmental glaucoma is a rare condition in which glaucoma is caused by abnormal development of the anterior segment, including the outflow channels. In 75% of affected patients, the condition is bilateral. Patients with developmental glaucoma usually present within the first year of life, initially with excessive tearing. In addition, the infant with developmental glaucoma may have enlarged eyes as a result of the increased intraocular pressure in eyes that are immature and relatively elastic. Photophobia or light sensitivity is a common symptom, as is frequent blinking or blepharospasm. The treatment of developmental glaucoma is primarily surgical. Developmental glaucoma must also be considered as one cause of a cloudy cornea at birth.

SECONDARY GLAUCOMAS

One of the most common forms of secondary glaucoma is steroid-induced glaucoma. It occurs when corticosteroid eye drops or, rarely, systemic or inhaled corticosteroids are used for up to several weeks. In 15% of normal patients and 95% of patients with POAG, intraocular pressure may increase by 15 mm Hg after treatment with long-term topical corticosteroids. Once this effect is identified, discontinuation of the steroid with treatment of the glaucoma will usually control the intraocular pressure. However, it may take weeks to months. There is no concentration or type of corticosteroid that will avoid the pressure rise. Other ocular complications can also result from steroid use, including cataract formation and exacerbation of viral infections. Therefore, great care should be exercised when prescribing these drops.

Secondary glaucoma may also be caused by ocular trauma, retinal vein occlusion, intraocular inflammation, intraocular tumors, diabetes, and cardiovascular disease. Any patient suspected of having secondary glaucoma should be referred to an ophthalmologist for evaluation as soon as possible.

ACUTE PERIPHERAL FACIAL PARALYSIS
(Bell's Palsy)

method of
GORDON B. HUGHES, M.D.
The Cleveland Clinic Foundation
Cleveland, Ohio

Acute facial palsy can result from many causes, including tumor, trauma, infection, and stroke. When there is no obvious acquired cause and the patient is otherwise healthy, the most common cause (approximately 20 new cases per 100,000 population per year) is "idiopathic" Bell's palsy. Abundant experimental and clinical evidence now indicates that the primary cause of idiopathic Bell's palsy is herpesvirus. Of the herpesvirus family, herpes simplex virus almost always is the cause, although herpes zoster auricularis (Ramsay Hunt syndrome) without shingles (zoster sine herpete) can mimic herpes simplex Bell's palsy.

Symptoms of Bell's palsy include general malaise, facial pain, dry eye, dysacusis, dysgeusia, and facial hypesthesia; other cranial nerves can also be involved. Whether there is a prodrome or not, acute disease implies that the palsy progresses over days, with the first day of visible weakness defined as day 1, and maximal nerve injury occurring by day 14. Thus, Bell's palsy is acute, unilateral weakness or paralysis of the face due to peripheral facial nerve dysfunction with no readily identifiable cause and with some degree of recovery within 6 months.

Physical examination excludes lesions that can mimic Bell's palsy. The clinician should document in the chart that (1) all facial nerve branches are involved diffusely, (2) the otoscopic examination is normal, (3) there are no skin blebs or blisters (herpes zoster), and (4) there is no ipsilateral parotid gland mass. These points distinguish Bell's palsy from overt infection, tumor, trauma, and stroke. In contrast, Bell's palsy does not cause segmental palsy (one branch or division), slowly progressive palsy, facial twitching, or delayed recovery beyond 6 months (this last has been reported but is extremely rare). Such clinical presentations must be thoroughly evaluated for a neoplasm or other lesion.

Other than audiometric, human immunodeficiency virus, and Lyme testing in appropriate cases, Bell's palsy does not require any further diagnostic work-up. However, I prefer to perform gadolinium-enhanced magnetic resonance imaging (MRI) of the ipsilateral temporal bone and adjacent soft tissues if the face is completely paralyzed, to reassure the patient further and to support the presumptive clinical diagnosis. On MRI examination, herpetic inflammation of the facial nerve, usually near the geniculate ganglion, should not be misdiagnosed as facial neuroma; it resolves over weeks or months.

TREATMENT

To prevent exposure keratitis in Bell's palsy, eye care is of paramount importance in all but extremely mild cases and may require months of care until recovery is adequate. The patient should wear some kind of eyeglasses when outside. I prescribe sterile ophthalmic lubricant solution during the day, sterile ophthalmic lubricant ointment at night, and a moisture chamber over the eye at night. One convenient, inexpensive chamber can be created by applying a small square of clear plastic wrap to the face with gentle hair-setting tape. To avoid scratching the globe, tape should not be placed directly on the eyelid. In the most severe cases, an eyelid weight to facilitate passive closure can be temporarily placed in a short outpatient procedure using local anesthesia, then removed when paralysis resolves. Tarsorrhaphy is not recommended.

The American Academy of Otolaryngology–Head and Neck Surgery recommends that recovery be measured and reported according to the House-Brackmann grading system, as shown in Table 1. Grade I is normal function; grade VI is paralysis; grades II to V are intermediate. "Estimated function" refers to the subjective impression of global facial movement. "Measurement" refers to objective voluntary movement of the mouth and eye, evaluated as follows: a centimeter scale divided into four equal parts is used. On the involved side, maximal voluntary lateral movement of the corner of the mouth and elevation of the eyebrow are each measured on a scale of 0 to 4. The resultant sum is 0 to 8, with 0 being paralyzed, 2 to 7 intermediate, and 8 normal. Thus, facial nerve grading combines subjective estimate and objective measurement.

With no treatment other than eye care, 84% of patients have normal or near-normal recovery (grade I or II), often within 3 weeks. Maximal recovery occurs by 9 months in all patients. Medical and surgical treatment attempts to improve recovery in the 16% of patients with more severe disease. In my practice, treatment consists of prednisone and famciclovir (Famvir)* in all cases and surgical nerve decompression in rare, highly selected cases.

---

*This use of famciclovir is not listed in the manufacturer's official directive.

TABLE 1. **House-Brackmann Facial Nerve Grading System**

Grade	Description	Measurement*	Function (%)	Estimated Function* (%)
I	Normal	8/8	100	100
II	Slight	7/8	76–99	80
III	Moderate	5/8–6/8	51–75	60
IV	Moderately severe	3/8–4/8	26–50	40
V	Severe	1/8–2/8	1–25	20
VI	Total	0/8	0	0

*See text for explanation.
From Hughes GB: Acute peripheral facial nerve paralysis. *In* Britton BH (ed): Common Problems in Otology. St. Louis, Mosby–Year Book, 1991, pp 229–246.

In the acute stage of Bell's palsy (first 14 days), I prescribe prednisone, 1 mg per kg per day orally in two divided doses (usually 30 to 40 mg twice daily in an adult), and famciclovir, 500 mg orally three times daily for a total of 10 days or until the acute stage has passed, if there is no medical contraindication. Prednisone then is tapered and stopped, and famciclovir is stopped. Famciclovir is not approved for use in infants. In a prospective, controlled study of Bell's palsy, Adour and colleagues determined that final recovery was better with prednisone and acyclovir (Zovirax)* (a similar antiviral agent) than with prednisone and placebo ($P < .05$).

Highly motivated patients who are first seen after 2 weeks of palsy can be treated similarly but more briefly, although treatment efficacy is questionable after the acute phase has passed.

Surgical decompression of the labyrinthine and perigeniculate regions of the facial nerve remains controversial; simple decompression of the mastoid portion is not helpful. Some published data suggest that middle cranial fossa decompression performed within 14 days of onset can help certain highly selected patients, compared both with the natural history of disease and with prednisone therapy (results have not been compared yet with those of prednisone-famciclovir therapy) (Bruce J. Gantz, personal communication). These highly selected candidates for surgery have no voluntary movement on clinical examination, no voluntary motor unit potentials on electromyography, and less than 10% compound muscle action potential on electroneurography (evoked electromyography). Decompression must be performed by the middle cranial fossa approach and within 14 days of onset. Compared with spontaneous recovery, approximately 50% of patients undergoing decompression have better results, and 50% have similar results.

Although reports from several treatment centers are still preliminary, surgery appears to play a small but important role in the total management of Bell's palsy. Family practitioners, internists, and neurologists, however, should be reassured that eye care and medical management without surgery are appropriate and helpful for the vast majority of patients with Bell's palsy.

---

*Not FDA approved for this indication.

PARKINSONISM

method of
STANLEY FAHN, M.D.
*The Neurological Institute of New York,
Columbia-Presbyterian Medical Center
New York, New York*

Parkinsonism is a symptom complex comprising any combination of six cardinal features: (1) rest tremor; (2) akinesia or bradykinesia; (3) rigidity; (4) loss of postural reflexes; (5) flexed posture; and (6) the freezing phenomenon. At least two of these six cardinal features, with at least one of them being either item 1 or 2, must be present for a diagnosis of definite parkinsonism. There are many causes of parkinsonism (Table 1), which can be conveniently divided into four categories: primary (idiopathic); secondary (symptomatic) (i.e., a known cause, such as neuroleptic drugs); parkinsonism-plus syndromes (symptoms of parkinsonism mingled with other neurologic abnormalities, including such disorders as progressive supranuclear palsy, multiple system atrophy, cortical-basal ganglionic degeneration); and other hereditary degenerative diseases (e.g., juvenile Huntington's disease, Wilson's disease).

Parkinson's disease (PD) (primary parkinsonism) is the most common form of parkinsonism encountered by neurologists and primary care physicians. Because PD is treatable, it is emphasized in this chapter. PD begins insidiously and steadily worsens, as do most of the other parkinsonian syndromes. The diagnosis of PD has prognostic and therapeutic significance because it almost always responds to at least a moderate degree to levodopa therapy, whereas the parkinsonism-plus disorders do not. With time, the clinical distinctions of the parkinsonism-plus disorders become more apparent with the development of other neurologic findings, such as cerebellar ataxia, loss of downward ocular movements, and autonomic dysfunction (e.g., postural hypotension, loss of bladder control, and impotence). There are no practical diagnostic laboratory tests for PD, and the diagnosis rests on clinical features or excluding some of the other causes of parkinsonism based on laboratory tests (Table 2). A response to levodopa is most helpful in the differential diagnosis. The cause of PD is unknown, but it is widely believed that multifactorial genetic and environmental factors are responsible. More than 10% of patients have a positive family history of the disorder, and a mutation in the gene for alpha-synuclein has been discovered in a few families.

Although PD can develop at any age, it is most common in older adults, with a peak age at onset of about 60 years.

TABLE 1. **Classification of Most Cases of Parkinsonism**

I. Primary (idiopathic)
Parkinson's disease
II. Secondary (symptomatic)
A. Drugs
1. Dopamine-receptor blockers
2. Dopamine storage depletors
B. Postencephalitic
C. Toxins—Mn, carbon monoxide, MPTP, cyanide
D. Vascular
III. Parkinsonism-plus syndromes
A. Progressive supranuclear palsy
B. Multiple system atrophy
1. Striatonigral degeneration
2. Shy-Drager syndrome
3. Olivopontocerebellar degeneration
C. Cortical-basal ganglionic degeneration
D. Dementia syndromes
1. Alzheimer's disease
2. Normal pressure hydrocephalus
3. Diffuse Lewy body disease
IV. Heredodegenerative diseases
1. Wilson's disease
2. Juvenile Huntington's disease
3. Hallervorden-Spatz disease

Abbreviation: MPTP = 1-methyl-4-phenyl-1,2,5,6-tetrahydropyridine.

TABLE 2. **Helpful Diagnostic Criteria for Parkinsonism**

Syndrome	History	Examination	Laboratory
Parkinson's disease	Often begins with tremor and unilaterally	Lacks (1) ataxia, (2) early dementia, (3) early balance difficulty Good response to levodopa	—
Drug induced parkinsonism	Neuroleptics	Resembles PD	—
Postencephalitic parkinsonism	Encephalitis	Oculogyric crises	—
Mn intoxication	Mn exposure	Cock walk	—
Carbon monoxide intoxication	Coma from carbon monoxide	Can have dystonia	MRI: pallidal atrophy
MPTP induced parkinsonism	Drug abuser	Resembles PD	—
Vascular parkinsonism	Strokes	Usually no tremor	MRI: lacunae
Brain tumor	Headache	Pyramidal tract papilledema	MRI: tumor
Head trauma	Trauma within weeks of onset	Resembles PD	—
Progressive supranuclear palsy	Early unsteadiness; no response to levodopa	Supranuclear gaze defect; nuchal dystonia; facial dystonia; little tremor	MRI: atrophy of midbrain
Striatonigral degeneration	Loss of response to levodopa	Little tremor	—
Shy-Drager syndrome	Syncope; loss of bladder function; male impotence	Postural hypotension	No rise of plasma NE level on standing
Olivopontocerebellar degeneration	Early unsteadiness	Ataxia	MRI: cerebellar atrophy
Cortical-basal ganglionic degeneration	Stiffness	Unilateral rigidity; apraxia; myoclonus	—
Alzheimer's disease	Dementia; hallucination with levodopa	Memory loss	MRI: cortical atrophy; ventricular dilatation
Normal pressure hydrocephalus	Urinary incontinence; possible dementia	Grasp reflex of feet; unable to crawl	MRI: huge ventricles
Wilson's disease	Juvenile onset	K-F rings	Low ceruloplasmin level
Huntington's disease	Juvenile onset; family history	Dementia; personality change	MRI: caudate atrophy; gene test
Hallervorden-Spatz disease	Usually juvenile onset	Dystonia often present	MRI: iron in globus pallidus

Abbreviations: PD = Parkinson's disease; MRI = magnetic resonance imaging; NE = norepinephrine; K-F = Kayser-Fleischer; MPTP = 1-methyl-4-phenyl-1,2,5,6-tetrahydropyridine.

The likelihood of developing it increases with age, with a lifetime risk of 2%. Almost all symptoms and signs are related to progressive loss of dopamine-containing neurons in the substantia nigra, with an associated reduction in dopamine concentration in the caudate nucleus and putamen. The discovery of this biochemical correlation led to the most important advance in therapy 30 years ago: replacing dopamine with its precursor, levodopa. Unfortunately, after several years of use, levodopa often produces unpleasant complications, and then the clinician needs to spend considerable effort in controlling these problems, frequently utilizing a combination of anti-PD drugs and sometimes neurosurgery. Thus, a strategy is often used whereby levodopa is usually not initiated when the diagnosis is first made, but only when the symptoms are becoming troublesome to the patient. Treatment is aimed at controlling symptoms, for no drug or surgical approach has unequivocally been shown to prevent further progression of the disease. However, concepts of neuroprotection in PD have emerged, based on a popular hypothesis that the dopamine-containing neurons succumb to oxidative stress initiated by the metabolism of dopamine by monoamine oxidase types A and B (MAOA and MAOB) to form hydrogen peroxide and free radicals.

PRINCIPLES OF THERAPY

The strategy of treating patients with PD depends on the phase of the disease, which is always progressive, and on specific clinical features requiring special attention. The following principles serve as guidelines.

Keep the patient functioning independently as long as possible. Because of the inability to stop the progression of the disease, the long-term goal of the physician is to keep the patient functioning independently for as long as possible. Although levodopa is the most effective drug, 80% of patients develop complications of disabling response fluctuations and dyskinesias after 6 years of levodopa therapy, and younger patients (younger than 60 years) are particularly prone to these problems. Some physicians therefore use dopamine agonists, rather than levodopa, when beginning therapy, in an attempt to delay the onset of these problems.

Individualize therapy. The treatment of PD needs to be individualized, i.e., each patient presents with a unique set of symptoms, signs, responses to medications, and a host of social, occupational, and emotional problems that need to be addressed. Practical guides are the severity of the patient's symptoms, the degree of functional impairment, the expected benefits and risks of available therapeutic agents, and the age of the patient. Younger patients are more likely to develop motor fluctuations and dyskinesias;

older patients are more likely to develop confusion, sleep-wake alterations, and psychosis.

If therapies are established as protective, such as drugs or surgery, they should be given priority. If any drug could slow the progression of the disease process, it should be incorporated early.

Patients should be encouraged to remain active and mobile. PD leads to decreased motivation and increased passivity. An active exercise program, even early in the disease, can often avoid this. Furthermore, such a program involves patients in their own care, allows muscle stretching and full range of joint mobility, and enhances a better mental attitude toward fighting the disease.

TREATMENT OF EARLY PARKINSON'S DISEASE

The earliest stage of PD is when the symptoms are noticed and the diagnosis is made but the symptoms are not yet troublesome. Although there is debate as to whether or not levodopa is responsible for the development of response fluctuations and other complications that occur, there is general agreement that in the early stage of PD when the symptoms are noticed but not troublesome, symptomatic treatment is not necessary.

Selegiline (Eldepryl) is a relatively selective inhibitor of the enzyme MAOB. Unlike MAOA inhibitors, which can induce a hypertensive crisis if the patient ingests tyramine-containing foods (the "cheese effect"), selegiline is free of this risk if the dose is not increased beyond 10 mg per day. Selegiline has mild symptomatic benefit and is metabolized to methamphetamine and amphetamine. When given early in the course of the disease, selegiline can extend the duration of the need of levodopa by an average of 9 months. There is controversy about whether selegiline has some neuroprotective action in addition to its mild symptomatic one, and some physicians use this drug in this early phase, although long-term follow-up indicates that discontinuing selegiline brings back the same degree of parkinsonian severity as in a control group of nontreated patients. The dose of selegiline should not exceed 5 mg twice daily, and because of its long half-life, many physicians believe that a much smaller dose could be equally effective, although this has not been tested. If insomnia develops, 5 mg in the morning, avoiding later doses, can usually correct this. Male impotence is less common than insomnia. When selegiline is used in the presence of levodopa, it potentiates this drug and lower doses of levodopa can usually be used. Selegiline does not prevent the development of levodopa-induced complications of fluctuations and dyskinesias.

My own preference is to use tranylcypromine (Parnate),* an inhibitor of both MAOA and MAOB, rather than selegiline, which inhibits only MAOB. As measured by cerebrospinal fluid concentration of the metabolite of dopamine, selegiline partially inhibits dopamine oxidation, reducing hydrogen peroxide formation by only 20%. Therefore, inhibiting both MAOA and MAOB would likely more completely inhibit oxidation of dopamine and reduce hydrogen peroxide formation. This requires the patient to be placed on an MAO inhibitor (MAOI) diet, avoiding the ingestion of large amounts of tyramine that would cause the cheese effect. When tyramine cannot be deaminated in the gut, it causes release of norepinephrine from sympathetic nerve terminals, thereby raising blood pressure and potentially creating a hypertensive crisis. The dose of tranylcypromine is 10 mg thrice daily. Insomnia and male impotence are fairly common adverse effects that would require shifting the times of the dosings or reducing or discontinuing the drug. A side benefit is the lifting of any existing depression. Levodopa cannot be given in the presence of an inhibitor of MAOA because the combination produces a volatile blood pressure. Meperidine (Demerol) and the antidepressants, tricyclics and selective serotonin reuptake inhibitors, are to be avoided with any MAOI, including both selegiline and tranylcypromine, because of the potential for psychiatric and autonomic reactions that could be fatal.

I also recommend to my patients that they take high doses of the antioxidants ascorbic acid (vitamin C)* and tocopherol (vitamin E),* solely based on the oxidant stress hypothesis of the pathogenesis of PD. A controlled clinical trial has shown that tocopherol by itself is ineffective in slowing down the progression of PD. But a combination of ascorbic acid and tocopherol potentiates the antioxidant efficacy of both. I have been using this combination in early PD patients since 1979 and have not found any harmful effects. The doses I gradually reach in four divided doses are 3000 mg per day of ascorbic acid and 3200 units per day of d-α-tocopherol. There is evidence that the natural form of tocopherol (d isomer) achieves higher blood levels than the synthetic racemic (dl-α) form.

TREATMENT OF MILD PARKINSON'S DISEASE

Mild PD is that stage when symptoms and signs begin to interfere with daily activities. In clinical practice, a global judgment for initiating symptomatic drug therapy is usually made in discussions between the patient and the treating physician.

If the delay in initiating symptomatic treatment was so prolonged that the symptoms threaten the patient's occupation or endanger the patient because of falling, one needs to begin levodopa therapy. The advantages of using levodopa in preference to a dopamine agonist when the symptoms are this pronounced are that a therapeutic response is virtually guaranteed, and nearly all patients with PD respond to levodopa relatively quickly. In contrast, only a minority of patients with severe symptoms benefit sufficiently from a dopamine agonist given alone, and it takes more time (months) to build up the dose to

---

*Not FDA approved for this indication.

*Not FDA approved for this indication.

adequate levels to discover this. If levodopa is to be used, tranylcypromine therapy must be discontinued 2 weeks earlier. If selegiline is the MAOI used, therapy with this drug can be continued. Antioxidant vitamins, if used, can also be continued.

If the symptoms are not severe enough to require levodopa, a dopa-sparing strategy should be used in young patients. Delaying the initiation of levodopa delays the time that complications such as fluctuations occur, so a dopa-sparing strategy seems particularly important for patients younger than 61 years because they have a high likelihood of developing such complications from chronic levodopa therapy. The choices are dopamine agonists, amantadine, and anticholinergics. Therapy with the MAOI and antioxidant vitamins can be continued in the presence of any of these drugs.

For patients older than 70 years, levodopa therapy should be used. Not only is there less need for a dopa-sparing strategy in these elderly patients, but they are more susceptible to cognitive and behavioral difficulties from other antiparkinsonian drugs; levodopa has a better benefit/risk profile against these types of complications than do the others.

Dopamine agonists are usually more effective than either amantadine or anticholinergics. The agonists currently available are the ergots* pergolide (Permax) and bromocriptine (Parlodel). The nonergots pramipexole and ropinirole may soon be marketed. Ergots can rarely induce red, inflamed skin (St. Anthony's fire), which is reversible on discontinuation of the drug. Each of the dopamine agonists easily induces orthostatic hypotension, particularly when the drug is first introduced. After that period, this complication is much less common. Therefore, it is best to start with a tiny dose (bromocriptine 1.25 mg at bedtime; pergolide 0.05 mg at bedtime) for the first 3 days and then switch from bedtime to daytime dosing for the remainder of the first week. The daily dose can be increased gradually (bromocriptine 1.25 mg per day every week; pergolide 0.125 mg per day weekly), building the dosage up to a four-times-a-day dosing schedule until benefit or a dose of about 40 mg per day (bromocriptine) or 4 mg per day (pergolide) is reached. I use the lowest dose that provides adequate benefit.

I prefer starting with pergolide, because in my experience it appears to be more powerful than bromocriptine. Also, bromocriptine appears to have greater psychotoxicity. If pergolide does not offer sufficient benefit, one can consider trying bromocriptine therapy and then adding amantadine or an anticholinergic (see later). If none of these agents are helpful or tolerated, the patient moves into the next stage of illness, the stage in which levodopa is required. Nausea and vomiting are other potential side effects that would limit the usefulness of the dopamine agonists. These symptoms are usually avoided by increasing the dose slowly. In countries where the peripherally acting dopamine antagonist domperidone is available

(e.g., in Canada and in Europe), this drug blocks these gastrointestinal side effects. The usual dose is 10 to 20 mg thrice daily. Even if a dopamine agonist is effective, most patients require the addition of levodopa within a year or two after its introduction.

When the new dopamine agonists pramipexole and ropinirole become available, it will take some time to compare their effectiveness with that of pergolide to know the comparative advantages of the different agents.

Amantadine (Symmetrel) is a mild indirect dopaminergic, acting by augmenting dopamine release from storage sites and possibly blocking reuptake of dopamine into the presynaptic terminals. It also appears to have some anticholinergic properties. In the mild stage of PD it is effective in about two thirds of patients. A major advantage is that substantial benefit, if it occurs, is seen in a couple of days. Unfortunately, its benefit in more advanced PD is sometimes short-lived, with patients reporting a falloff effect after several months of treatment in the absence of concomitant levodopa therapy. The falloff appears to be caused by a depletion of already-reduced dopamine stores so that the effect of amantadine is exhausted. A common adverse effect is livedo reticularis (a reddish mottling of skin) around the knees; occasional adverse effects are ankle edema and visual hallucinosis. Sometimes when the drug therapy is discontinued, there can be a gradual worsening of parkinsonian signs, indicating that the drug has been helpful. The usual dosage is 100 mg twice daily, but sometimes a higher dose (up to 400 mg per day*) may be required. Amantadine can be useful, not only in the early phases of symptomatic therapy, thereby forestalling the introduction of levodopa or reducing the required dosage of levodopa, but also in the advanced stage of the disease as an adjunctive drug to levodopa and the dopamine agonists. Amantadine is excreted mostly unchanged in the urine, so the dose needs to be reduced in patients with renal impairment. The half-life is long, about 28 hours, so twice-daily dosing is adequate.

Anticholinergic drugs are less effective antiparkinsonian agents than the dopamine agonists. The anticholinergics are estimated to improve parkinsonism by about 20%. Many clinicians find that if tremor is not relieved by an agonist or levodopa, the addition of an anticholinergic drug is often effective. Sometimes, the anticholinergic can lessen tremor severity even in the absence of levodopa therapy, so clinicians can use such an agent as monotherapy for tremor. If not helpful, then continuing to use the drug while a dopamine agonist or levodopa is added can be helpful. Later, if tremor is relieved by the dopaminergic agent, one can try to discontinue the anticholinergic. Commonly used anticholinergics are trihexyphenidyl (Artane) and benztropine mesylate (Cogentin), but there are many others. To minimize adverse effects, one should start with low doses (trihexyphenidyl 1 mg twice daily; benztropine 0.5 mg twice daily) and

---

*Not FDA approved for this indication.

*Exceeds dosage recommended by the manufacturer.

increase gradually to 2 mg three times daily for trihexyphenidyl and 1 mg three times daily for benztropine.

Peripheral anticholinergic effects include blurred vision (treated with pilocarpine eye drops or if glaucoma is present), dry mouth, and urinary retention. Central side effects are predominantly forgetfulness and decreased short-term memory. Occasionally hallucinations and psychosis can occur, particularly in elderly patients. I avoid these powerful anticholinergics in patients older than 70 years. If tremor persists in this age range despite the presence of levodopa or dopamine agonists, I use drugs with a weaker anticholinergic effect, such as diphenhydramine (Benadryl),* orphenadrine (Norflex),* cyclobenzaprine (Flexeril),* and amitriptyline (Elavil).* Diphenhydramine and amitriptyline can cause drowsiness; therefore, they can also be used as hypnotics. For tremor control, one needs to increase the dose gradually until at least 50 mg three times daily is reached for diphenhydramine and orphenadrine; 20 mg three times daily for cyclobenzaprine; and 25 mg three times daily for amitriptyline.

TREATMENT OF MODERATE PARKINSON'S DISEASE

Moderate-stage PD is when the disability is beyond the scope of efficacy of dopamine agonists, amantadine, anticholinergics, and selegiline; treatment with levodopa is necessary to control symptoms. The rule of thumb is to use the lowest dosage that brings about adequate symptom reversal, not the highest dosage that the patient can tolerate, in an attempt to avoid response fluctuations and dyskinesias. Levodopa is combined with carbidopa (Sinemet and generics), a peripheral decarboxylase inhibitor that prevents the formation of dopamine peripherally, thereby usually avoiding the otherwise common peripheral adverse effects of nausea, anorexia, and vomiting. Many patients require at least 50 to 75 mg of carbidopa per day to have adequate inhibition of peripheral dopa decarboxylase. If the dose of levodopa is less than 300 mg per day, then one should use the 25/100-mg tablets of carbidopa/levodopa and not the 10/100-mg tablets. In some patients, even 75 mg per day of carbidopa is inadequate, and nausea, anorexia, or vomiting still occur. In such patients, one needs to use higher doses of carbidopa; carbidopa tablets (Lodosyn) can be obtained by special request from Sinemet's manufacturer (DuPont Pharma).

Carbidopa/levodopa is marketed in both standard-release (Sinemet and generics) and sustained-release (Sinemet CR) tablets, which provides a longer plasma half-life and lower peak plasma levels of levodopa compared with standard Sinemet. Unfortunately, Sinemet CR has not been shown to avoid the development of response fluctuations. A prebedtime dose of Sinemet CR may allow the patient some mobility during the night. Disadvantages are the lack of a rapid response with each dose and a delayed response that can be excessive, resulting in sustained severe dyskinesias that cannot be controlled except by sedating the patient. Moreover, the response to individual doses of Sinemet CR is less predictable than that to standard Sinemet. It is complicated to use both standard Sinemet and Sinemet CR to smooth out fluctuations, but this is often necessary. Finally, one should keep in mind that not all of the carbidopa/levodopa in Sinemet CR is absorbed. A dose of Sinemet CR is equal to about two thirds to three quarters of an identical dose of standard Sinemet.

I prefer Sinemet CR as a first-line drug in patients older than 70 years to slow the rate of absorption and lessen the peak plasma level of levodopa, making it less likely that the patient develops peak dose drowsiness or confusion. For younger patients, in whom cognitive adverse effects are less likely to occur, I use standard carbidopa/levodopa when levodopa is necessary. I want to observe the response so that I can better monitor the effectiveness of the drug.

Sinemet CR is available in two strengths, a carbidopa/levodopa 50/200-mg tablet that is scored and can be broken in half, and a 25/100-mg unscored tablet. Crushing either tablet destroys the slow-release property because the matrix is no longer intact. When Sinemet CR is added to the therapy of a patient taking a dopamine agonist, a dose of 25/100 mg three times daily (built up gradually by 25/100 mg per day weekly) often suffices. When it is used alone, it often is necessary to use these dosages after meals to reduce initial nausea and vomiting; the dose can later be increased to 50/200 mg three or four times daily. If greater relief is required, a dopamine agonist should then be added.

Standard carbidopa/levodopa is available in 10/100-, 25/100-, and 25/250-mg tablets. Because of the desire to have at least 75 mg per day of carbidopa, one should start with the 25/100-mg tablets when the drug is introduced. An increase by 25/100 mg per day per week until three-times-daily dosing is achieved is often adequate. Not every symptom of PD responds equally well. Bradykinesia and rigidity respond best, whereas tremor can be more resistant. If a response is seen, but with symptoms later returning or worsening, increasing to 50/200 mg three times daily is a reasonable goal before adding a dopamine agonist. If agonists are already being taken and there is still an inadequate response, the dosage of levodopa should be increased gradually, switching to the 25/250-mg tablets as necessary. A dose of 25/250 mg four times daily may be required. A reasonably high dose before concluding that levodopa is ineffective is 2000 mg of levodopa per day.

A patient's response to levodopa is an important piece of information to help differentiate PD from parkinsonism-plus syndromes. If the response is nil or minor, it is most likely that the disorder is not PD. However, an adequate response does not ensure the diagnosis of PD, because some patients in the early

---

*Not FDA approved for this indication.

stages of multiple system atrophy or progressive supranuclear palsy may improve; later in these diseases, when dopamine receptors are lost, the response is lost. The only effective drugs in such a situation are the anticholinergics and amantadine, even though only mildly so.

TREATMENT OF ADVANCED PARKINSON'S DISEASE

Advanced PD is that stage of the disease when (1) there is sufficient disability to interfere with independence despite levodopa therapy, (2) there is sufficient loss of postural reflexes, (3) the freezing phenomenon has developed to make walking difficult, (4) there is pronounced flexed posture, or (5) complications (fluctuations, dyskinesias, psychosis) from levodopa have developed so that they are the focus of treatment. Because only the last group is somewhat amenable to therapy, the discussion concentrates on methods to overcome these complications.

There is usually a pattern of progressively worsening motor complications in patients who are taking chronic levodopa therapy. Response fluctuations usually begin as mild wearing-off (end-of-dose failure), which is when an adequate dosage of levodopa does not last at least 4 hours. Typically, in the first couple of years of treatment, there is a long-duration response so that the timing of doses of levodopa is not important. Over time, a short-duration response occurs, and patients develop the wearing-off phenomenon. The "offs" tend to be mild at first but over time become deeper with more severe parkinsonism; simultaneously, the duration of the "on" response becomes shorter. Eventually, many patients develop sudden "offs" in which the deep state of parkinsonism develops over minutes rather than tens of minutes, and the "offs" are less predictable in terms of timing with the dosings of levodopa. Many patients who develop response fluctuations also develop abnormal involuntary movements, i.e., dyskinesias.

Fluctuations

The wearing-off phenomenon, when mild, may be ameliorated with the addition of selegiline (introduced as 2.5 mg daily, and increasing to 5 mg twice daily, as necessary). Selegiline potentiates the action of levodopa, and its introduction can induce confusion and psychosis, particularly in the elderly patient, and dyskinesias. A lower dose of levodopa may be necessary. Sinemet CR can also be effective in patients with mild wearing-off, and one can gradually switch from standard carbidopa-levodopa to Sinemet CR, beginning with the last dose of the day and working forward each day. Because it takes more than 1 hour for slow-release medication to become effective, most patients also require supplemental standard carbidopa/levodopa to obtain an adequate response. One can attempt to use standard carbidopa/levodopa alone, giving the doses closer together, but ultimately most patients develop progressively

shorter durations of effectiveness from these doses, so patients could require as many as 6 doses or more per day. Then eventually, dose failures often develop. Dopamine agonists, which have a longer biologic half-life than does levodopa, can also be used in combination with standard Sinemet or Sinemet CR. These drugs seem to be the most effective agents when used in combination with levodopa to reduce the severity of the "off" states, and I tend to employ pergolide for this purpose. The addition of dopamine agonists can increase dyskinesias, however; in this situation the levodopa dosage needs to be reduced. If the fluctuations cannot be brought under control with these approaches, liquefying the carbidopa/levodopa and having the patient sip doses repeatedly throughout the day is often useful. Carbidopa/levodopa can be dissolved in ascorbate solution (2000 mg per 1000 mL of tap water) or in a carbonated beverage, both of which provide the acidity to dissolve and preserve the levodopa. A fresh supply of liquefied carbidopa/levodopa should be prepared daily by adding the total daily amount to 1000 mL of the acidic solution and having the patient consume this volume in small calculated amounts at frequent times throughout the day. The liquid formulation can more quickly resolve "off" states and also allow small dose adjustments that are not possible with tablets.

Peripheral catechol O-methyltransferase inhibitors (COMTI) have been found useful for treating wearing-off. COMT is the enzyme that catalyzes the conversion of dopa and dopamine to their methylated derivatives, so COMTIs extend the duration of levodopa's effect. Two COMTIs are being investigated, tolcapone and entacapone, and they should be marketed in the near future. Tolcapone, with a longer half-life, is taken three times daily, whereas entacapone is taken simultaneously with each dose of carbidopa/levodopa. Diarrhea and hepatic enzyme changes are sometimes adverse effects of tolcapone.

Sudden, random "offs" are more difficult to treat. The first approach is to use a dopamine agonist as the major therapeutic agent and reduce the amount of levodopa as much as possible to serve as a supplementary drug. If this fails, the patient needs to try liquefied carbidopa/levodopa, taking frequent, small doses throughout the day.

Dose failures are episodes when the patient fails to respond to each dose of levodopa, and delayed "ons" are increased durations before levodopa takes effect with a given dose. Both these situations seem to be related to poor gastric emptying, and they can be overcome by dissolving levodopa in liquid before it is ingested. For this problem, individual doses of carbidopa/levodopa can be liquefied when they are needed. The dose dissolves readily in carbonated water. Cisapride (Propulsid),* which is a prokinetic agent that increases gastrointestinal motility, may reduce the number of dose failures. A dose of 10 mg three times daily, up to 20 mg four times a day, may be beneficial in overcoming dose failures, may

---

*Not FDA approved for this indication.

shorten the time of response to a dose, and even help overcome constipation, which is common in PD.

Response varies in relation to meals because levodopa is absorbed only from the small intestine. Absorption is thus dependent on the passage of levodopa intact through the stomach to enter the small intestine. There are at least three variations of levodopa responsiveness in regard to meals. First, taking levodopa after or during a full meal results in a delayed and weaker response to levodopa than taking levodopa about 20 minutes before the meal. Second, patients who had normally taken levodopa with or after a meal find that if they take it before a meal, the response is much greater and they might develop peak-dose dyskinesia. If either of these two variations is present, it can be corrected by accommodating the timing of dosages of levodopa according to the pathophysiology of the particular problem. The third variation relates to high-protein meals. Competition with other amino acids in the diet can interfere with transport of levodopa across the intestinal mucosa and across the blood-brain barrier. Only seldom does this competition with other amino acids pose a major problem for patients, and most accommodate to protein in their diet. In those individuals in whom protein in a meal interferes with their response to levodopa, it is necessary to plan a meal strategy. Having nonprotein meals at breakfast and lunch, and making up for this lack by having higher protein meals at dinner, is usually effective. The patient then has the "offs" at night when he or she can best afford to be "off."

The freezing phenomenon is often listed as a type of fluctuation because the patient transiently has difficulty initiating or continuing a movement. The most common motor activity affected is walking. Start hesitation, target hesitation, turning hesitation, startle (fearfulness) hesitation, and sudden transient freezing are the most common forms of freezing, as if the feet are glued to the floor. Of major importance is the need to distinguish between "off freezing" and "on freezing." Off freezing is best explained as a feature of PD, and its treatment is to keep the patient from getting to the point of off freezing. On freezing remains an enigma, and this problem tends to be aggravated by increasing the dosage of levodopa. It may lessen by reducing the dosage of levodopa but usually resists treatment. Patients have developed "tricks" to help overcome freezing, such as stepping over an inverted cane.

Dyskinesias

Levodopa-induced dyskinesias are involuntary movements that occur in two major forms—chorea and dystonia. Choreic movements are irregular, purposeless, nonrhythmic, abrupt, rapid, unsustained movements that seem to flow from one body part to another. Dystonic movements are more sustained contractions. Choreic movements occur sooner and are more common than dystonia, but with continuing treatment, individual patients can develop more dys-

tonic dyskinesias and less chorea. Many patients probably have a combination of chorea and dystonia. Dystonia is a more serious problem than chorea because it is usually more disabling.

Peak-dose dyskinesias occur shortly after the time when the plasma concentration of levodopa is at its peak and the brain level is too high. Reducing the individual dose can resolve this problem. The patient may need to take more frequent doses at this lower amount because reducing the amount of an individual dose also reduces the duration of benefit. Another approach is to substitute higher doses of a dopamine agonist while lowering the dose of carbidopa/levodopa. Dopamine agonists are less likely to cause dyskinesias and therefore can usually be used in this situation quite safely. If lowering the dose of levodopa results in more severe "off" states, the agonists become more important. Sinemet CR is not helpful because there is the danger of increased dyskinesias at the end of the day as the blood levels become sustained from frequent dosing. Once dyskinesias appear with Sinemet CR, they last for a considerable time because of the slow decay in the plasma levels. In some patients, peak-dose chorea and dystonia occur at subtherapeutic doses of levodopa, and lowering the dosage renders a patient even more parkinsonian. There is little choice but to use smaller and more frequent doses, coupled with dopamine agonists and other antiparkinsonian drugs, such as amantadine. Such patients are candidates for stereotaxic pallidotomy (see later).

Diphasic dyskinesias occur at the beginning and end of a dose, not at the peak plasma and brain levels of levodopa. They tend to particularly affect the legs with a mixture of chorea and dystonia. Because the mechanism is unclear, treatment of diphasic dyskinesias is difficult. I use pergolide as the major pharmacologic agent with supplementary levodopa.

"Off dystonia" and "off painful cramps" could be listed as both dyskinesias and fluctuations, because these dystonias occur when the patient is "off." Dystonic spasms can either be a sign of levodopa overdosage, as in peak-dose dyskinesias, or occur when the plasma level of levodopa is low, such as in early morning before the first dose of levodopa. "Off" dystonia can occur anytime the patient is "off." Preventing "offs" is the best way to control them. I use pergolide as the major pharmacologic agent with supplementary levodopa. Baclofen (Lioresal)* has also been reported to benefit some patients. Bedtime Sinemet CR may be useful to prevent early morning dystonia, but some patients need to set the alarm early to take a dose of carbidopa/levodopa and then fall back to sleep and awaken at their usual time.

Nonmotor Complications

Mental changes of psychosis, confusion, agitation, hallucinations, paranoid delusions, and excessive

---

*Not FDA approved for this indication.

sleeping are probably related to activation of dopamine receptors in nonstriatal regions, particularly the cortical and limbic structures. Elderly patients and patients with concomitant dementia are extremely sensitive to small doses of levodopa, but all patients with PD, regardless of age, can develop psychosis if they take excess amounts of levodopa as a means to overcome "off" periods. Psychosis and hallucinations can often be eliminated by reducing the dosages of antiparkinsonian drugs. All antiparkinson drugs have the potential to induce psychosis, so the less efficacious drugs should be withdrawn first. Accordingly, selegiline, amantadine, anticholinergics, and dopamine agonists should be withdrawn in that order. If psychosis persists, a gradual reduction of levodopa can be tried, but a return of parkinsonism may be the price. Instead, psychosis can often be controlled by using clozapine (Clozaril), an atypical antipsychotic agent because it rarely causes drug-induced parkinsonism or antagonizes the antiparkinsonian effect of levodopa. Unfortunately, clozapine induces agranulocytosis in approximately 1 to 2% of patients. Patients must have their blood counts monitored weekly for this potential complication and then discontinue the drug if leukopenia develops. Other adverse effects include drowsiness (bedtime dosing is therefore recommended) and seizures with high doses. If clozapine is not tolerated, one can try relatively weak antipsychotics, such as molindone (Moban), pimozide (Orap), or risperidone (Risperdal). Olanzapine (Zyprexa), a new antipsychotic, needs to be evaluated in PD patients. If antipsychotics produce an increase of parkinsonism, it is preferable to lower the dosage of carbidopa/levodopa to avoid the psychosis, rather than maintain the antipsychotic at that high dosage. An intact mental function is more important than an intact motor function.

It is not safe to discontinue levodopa suddenly, for such action can induce the neuroleptic malignant syndrome.

An altered sleep-wake cycle of drowsiness during the daytime, particularly after a dose of levodopa, and insomnia at night are fairly common in elderly persons and often accompany confusion. If a patient becomes drowsy after each dose of medication, this is a sign of overdosage; reducing the dosage can correct this problem. Sometimes, substituting Sinemet CR for standard Sinemet may help because this provides a slower rise in plasma and brain levels of levodopa. If the patient is generally drowsy during the daytime and remains awake at night, this makes it difficult for those caring for the patient to look after him or her effectively. It is important to get the patient to follow a sleep-wake schedule that fits with the rest of the household. To correct the problem it may be necessary to use a combination of approaches. Efforts must be made to stimulate the patient physically and mentally during the daytime and force him or her to remain awake, otherwise the patient would not be able to sleep at night. At night the patient should then be drowsy enough to be able to sleep. If this fails, it may be necessary to use stimulants in the morning and sedatives at night to reverse the altered state. This should be done in addition to prodding the patient to remain awake during the day. Drugs such as methylphenidate (Ritalin) and amphetamine are usually well tolerated by patients with PD. A 10-mg dose of either of these two drugs, repeated once if necessary, may be helpful. To encourage sleep at night, a hypnotic may be necessary. It should be noted that strong sedatives, such as barbiturates, are poorly tolerated by patients with PD. Milder hypnotics, such as benzodiazepines, are usually taken without difficulty. Short-acting benzodiazepines would be preferable, but if the patient awakens too early, a longer acting one may need to be used.

Orthostatic hypotension from levodopa is aggravated by other drugs taken by the patient, such as tricyclic antidepressants. These other drugs should be discontinued. If orthostatic hypotension remains, it can sometimes be managed by the use of support stockings, NaCl, and fludrocortisone (Florinef),* but often the dosage of levodopa needs to be reduced.

Constipation is common in PD. It may be further aggravated by anticholinergics. The role of levodopa is uncertain. This drug does not ordinarily relieve the problem, and some patients believe it makes it worse. For those who have bloating due to suppression of peristalsis when they are "off," keeping them "on" with levodopa is beneficial. Besides changing dietary habits by increasing intake of fiber and dried fruits, the drug cisapride* may help by enhancing colonic transit.

TREATMENT OF DEPRESSION

Depression is a common nonmotor symptom in PD, probably related to the reduction of all brain monoamines in this disease. Depression must be treated, not only for its own sake, but because its presence interferes with a good response to antiparkinsonian drugs. It often responds to tricyclic antidepressants, such as amitriptyline (Elavil), nortriptyline (Pamelor), and protriptyline (Vivactil). Because of its anticholinergic and soporific effects, amitriptyline can be useful for these properties as well as for its antidepressant effect. Protriptyline, on the other hand, has no anticholinergic effect and can be useful when this property is not needed. Selective serotonin reuptake inhibitors, such as fluoxetine (Prozac), sertraline (Zoloft), and paroxetine (Paxil), are also effective agents for treating depression in PD but may aggravate parkinsonism if antiparkinsonian drugs are not being used concurrently. The newer agents nefazodone (Serzone) and venlafaxine (Effexor) with a combination of serotonin and norepinephrine reuptake inhibition are also effective. Electroconvulsive therapy can be effective in patients with severe, intractable depression, and it can transiently improve the motor symptoms as well.

---

*Not FDA approved for this indication.

SURGICAL THERAPY FOR PARKINSON'S DISEASE

Neurosurgical therapy for PD reached its peak in the 1960s and declined after the introduction of levodopa. There is now a renaissance with new surgical techniques and brain targets available. In the 1960s the most common operation was a thalamotomy. Today, there are also pallidotomy, deep brain stimulation, and fetal tissue implantation.

Thalamotomy and Thalamic Stimulation for Tremor

In the 1950s and 1960s, before the introduction of levodopa therapy, stereotactic thalamotomy was a common therapeutic approach for patients with PD. Thalamotomy is most efficacious for tremor, with successful relief in as many as 90% of patients. It is much less effective against bradykinesia, which is usually more disabling. Therefore, after the introduction of levodopa therapy, its use was greatly diminished, except for intractable tremor. The target for treating tremor is the ventral intermediate nucleus of the thalamus, which is in the lateral tier of nuclei. A recently developed alternative to this lesioning is to implant a stimulating electrode into this nucleus to deliver high-frequency chronic stimulation, which is just as effective in relieving tremor. Turning the stimulator off results in a return of tremor. There is a risk of dysarthria with a thalamotomy, and this risk increases to 15 to 25% with bilateral lesions. Stimulation is less of a risk and can be applied to both sides of the brain with less risk of serious complications, but the stimulator is costly, and it can take weeks before the settings of current, frequency, and voltage are determined by trial and error for the optimal settings.

Pallidotomy and Pallidal Stimulation for Dyskinesias

The globus pallidus was a target for lesioning for parkinsonism in the 1950s but was largely abandoned in favor of the ventral intermediate nucleus as the preferred target to control tremor. However, a Swedish neurosurgeon continued to explore the pallidum, searching for a site in this nucleus for a superior result against other parkinsonian features. The ventroposterior part of the internal segment of the globus pallidus (GPi) was discovered to be the best target for reducing parkinsonian symptoms. However, ventroposterior pallidotomies were largely ignored until it was discovered that this target can also eliminate levodopa-induced dyskinesias, as well as provide a modest reduction of tremor and bradykinesia. This operation has now gained acceptance in overcoming contralateral dyskinesias. The duration of benefit remains uncertain, but ideally placed lesions have controlled dyskinesias for at least 2 years. Ipsilateral dyskinesias may also be transiently reduced. Contralateral reduction of tremor, rigidity,

and bradykinesia is also seen, but the extent of the benefit is more variable than that for dyskinesias. If the lesion is not made in a perfect location, the benefits of surgery can be lost in a number of months. Microelectrode recordings to locate the perfect target within the GPi appear to be the preferable method. With the control of dyskinesias, patients are able to take higher doses of levodopa, providing benefit in reducing the number and severity of the "off" phenomena, as well as dyskinesias. Parkinsonism is otherwise not improved more than what is achieved with levodopa therapy, and surgical complications of dysarthria have been observed with bilateral pallidotomies. The freezing phenomenon is not relieved by this procedure and may even be made worse. Because the optic tract runs near the target site, a potential complication is impairment of the contralateral visual field. However, stimulating the target or recording via microelectrodes identifies if the electrode is in the optic tract, so the surgeon can avoid producing a lesion in this region. Implanting stimulating electrodes in the ventroposterior GPi is now being tested, showing a similar response to that of creating a lesion in this target. It may allow bilateral procedures with fewer adverse effects.

Subthalamic Nucleus Stimulation

The subthalamic nucleus (STN), which sends excitatory efferents to the GPi, is overly active in PD. In animal models of PD, lesioning the STN results in a marked reduction of the parkinsonian signs. Because surgical lesions of the STN run the risk of the patient's developing hemiballismus, electrical stimulation of the STN in patients with PD is being tested instead. So far the results have been promising, showing that the procedure provides relief of contralateral bradykinesia and other signs of parkinsonism. STN stimulation, however, can also induce contralateral chorea and ballismus, so careful adjustment of the current, voltage, and frequency is required. The degree of benefit is about the same as that from levodopa therapy but would theoretically avoid the problems of fluctuations and mental side effects often encountered with levodopa therapy. Too few cases have been reported to know the full range of adverse effects, the degree of benefit, and the duration of benefit.

Embryonic Dopaminergic Mesencephalic Tissue Implants

Transplantation of embryonic mesencephalic dopamine cells into the striatum of patients with PD is being investigated. The first successful ones were implanted unilaterally, and a report of a 6-year follow-up reveals the implants continue to be effective. Moreover, the report revealed increasing improvement over time. Fluorodopa uptake into the striatum, as shown by positron emission tomography, is dramatically increased, reversing the loss of uptake that normally occurs in patients with PD. Tests are now under way to determine the results of bilateral transplants. A single autopsy of one patient who had a successful transplantation 18 months after the transplantation showed that the embryonic dopamine neurons survive, grow nerve processes, innervate, and make synaptic contact with the host's striatal tissue. So far, those patients who have shown improvement have not relapsed, and indeed, many patients have been able to reduce their dosage of levodopa and some have even discontinued medication. It is likely that such fetal dopamine cell transplants may be supported and nourished by the fetal glial tissue that accompanies it. Whether the PD pathologic process present in the host's brain will eventually attack and destroy these grafted neurons is not known. There are many questions to be answered, including the amount of tissue required, the best targets for the implants, the nature of the cellular tissue (i.e., cell suspension or solid tissue), the type of symptoms that can be helped, the degree of improvement, the duration of improvement, the type of complications and their rate, the preferable age of the host, and the impact of the duration of the disease. Many of these factors are under investigation. Although this technique seems promising, it should be considered investigational. The concern in using human embryonic tissue raised by some and the limited supply of this tissue have led to investigations with embryonic porcine cells. Also, attempts are being made to develop a permanently viable dopaminergic cell line that could be a future source of tissue for implants.

PERIPHERAL NEUROPATHY

method of
PETER JAMES DYCK, M.D.

Mayo Clinic
Rochester, Minnesota

Among diseases affecting the nervous system, those affecting peripheral nerves are some of the most common. There may be as many as 100 or more causes of peripheral nerve disease, including such common varieties as mechanical nerve laceration, contusion, repetitive compression and entrapment (e.g., spinal stenosis, intervertebral disk and carpal and cubital tunnel syndromes), malnutrition, alcoholism, infection (leprosy, human immunodeficiency virus [HIV] infection, and borreliosis), immune disorders (e.g., acute and chronic inflammatory demyelinating neuropathies, necrotizing vasculitis, and inflammatory ganglionopathies), metabolic disease (e.g., diabetes mellitus [DM], uremia, porphyria, hepatic disease, and amyloidosis), tumors, cancer, lymphoproliferative disorders, and genetic abnormalities. Two decades ago, there were almost no treatments for peripheral neuropathy. Today, some neuropathies are preventable and many others can be treated, sometimes with amazing benefit. Here I provide the greatest coverage to disorders for which there is specific treatment.

Generally, specific therapy is needed for a given variety of peripheral neuropathy. Neuropathy from malnutrition, vitamin B_{12} deficiency, or thyroxine deficiency is treated by providing the deficient ingredient—food, vitamin B_{12}, or thyroxine. Leprosy is treated by providing specific antimicrobial therapy. Other neuropathies are treated by withholding the injurious medicinal or toxic agent and sometimes by giving a medication that removes the injurious agent from the body, e.g., a chelating agent in heavy metal neuropathies. In immune-mediated neuropathies, treatments often are less specific but nevertheless may be quite effective. It may be that there are therapies to improve neuropathy regardless of the cause of the injury. Such a general beneficial effect, however, remains to be proved. Certain neurite outgrowth factors, antioxidants, and anticytokines might have such a generalized beneficial effect, but proof is needed.

DIFFERENTIAL DIAGNOSIS

Therapy depends on accurate diagnosis of the specific variety of neuropathy to be treated. In general, three approaches may be used to diagnose the cause of a given patient's neuropathy; they are the gestalt approach, the shotgun approach, and the 10-step approach. In the gestalt approach, one diagnoses the variety of neuropathy from the pattern of anatomic involvement, the class and proximal to distal level of neuron involvement, course of disease, and other clinical features. In the shotgun approach, after establishing that neuropathy is present, one orders all available tests that might identify the specific cause of neuropathy to find the one that shows an abnormality and presumably explains the neuropathy. In the 10-step approach, one systematically characterizes a patient's neuropathy into one of 16 specific anatomic-pathologic patterns of involvement; next, the correctness of the anatomic-pathologic pattern is confirmed by electrophysiologic, quantitative sensory, quantitative autonomic, or other tests; and then each variety, in a shorter list of possibilities, is ruled in or out by further testing. The third approach is preferred over the first two because it is cost-effective and most likely to give the correct diagnosis.

MECHANICAL INJURIES OF NERVE

Laceration, contusion, stretch, single or repetitive compression, and entrapment of nerve are among the most common of nerve diseases. Certain medical conditions, for example, DM, inherited tendency to pressure palsy, pregnancy, hypothyroidism, and acromegaly, predispose a patient to repetitive or compression nerve injury. Certain habits of living or occupations (e.g., repetitive flexion and extension of wrists) may be associated with nerve injury. Radiculopathy from cervical or lumbosacral disks, vertebral stenosis, entrapment or repetitive injury neuropathy (carpal tunnel and cubital tunnel), and peroneal neuropathies are common.

In assessing focal nerve injuries, the physician should identify the nerve and site and then assess for underlying predisposition and cause. A primary objective should be to prevent further injury by avoidance of repeated injury and use of protective splints or pads. A patient's work requirements or recreational activities may need to be changed. Surgical relief of compression, reconnection of severed nerves, or insertion of a graft may be needed. Specialized textbooks should be consulted for further information.

TYPES AND CAUSES OF NEUROPATHY

Malnutrition, Vitamin Deficiency, and Alcoholism

Worldwide, neuropathy related to malnutrition, vitamin deficiency, or alcoholism is common, but in Western countries, it tends to be restricted to segments of society (homeless, lactating mothers, or elderly patients) who do not eat regularly or do not eat a balanced diet, are alcoholic, or have systemic disease (e.g., cancer, malabsorption, or specific metabolic diseases). Typically, these patients develop a chronic symmetrical sensorimotor polyneuropathy. The pattern of clinical involvement depends on whether small or large fibers are preferentially affected. If large fibers are affected, the patient tends to exhibit sensory ataxia. If intermediate and small fibers are affected, the patient may report prickling, lancinating and burning pain, and autonomic disturbances.

Prevention

The causes and prevention of epidemic hunger, poor nutrition, and alcoholism are generally beyond the remedy of individual physicians. In Western countries, homelessness, mental illness, alcoholism, and other chronic diseases are often involved.

Diabetic Neuropathy

DM is made up of at least three disorders: insulin-dependent DM, non–insulin-dependent DM, and secondary DM. Varieties of neuropathies occurring in DM are distal symmetrical polyneuropathy, sensorimotor lumbosacral plexus neuropathy, truncal radiculopathy, upper limb mononeuropathies, cranial neuropathies (especially cranial nerve III—extraocular muscle weakness with pupillomotor sparing), autonomia, and hypoglycemic polyneuropathy. Present evidence suggests that the symmetrical polyneuropathies are related to metabolic derangement and microvessel dysfunction. The focal and asymmetrical neuropathies probably relate to immune and vascular mechanisms.

Diabetic Polyneuropathy. There is good evidence that the frequency of clinically evident distal symmetrical polyneuropathy and abnormality of nerve conduction are partially preventable by rigorous glycemic control. Such control is possible with frequent plasma glucose monitoring and frequent insulin injection by pump or by multiple single doses of insulin. Pancreas transplantation induces euglycemia but is at this time restricted to patients with severe diabetic complications. It appears that the progression of polyneuropathy can be stopped with euglycemia.

Whether reversal of distal symmetrical polyneuropathy is possible has not yet been established. A variety of agents (in addition to glycemic control) are being investigated: aldose reductase inhibitors, antioxidants (e.g., α-lipoic acid), methylguanidine, nerve growth factors, and fatty acids (e.g., linolenic acid).

Diabetic Lumbosacral Plexus Neuropathies. Also called proximal diabetic neuropathy, femoral neuropathy, diabetic amyotrophy, and Bruns-Garland syndrome, diabetic lumbosacral plexus neuropathy tends to occur in non–insulin-dependent DM and in old age. There is increasing evidence that inflammation of nerve blood vessels and ischemia are involved in nerve fiber degeneration. At this time, no controlled clinical trials of immunotherapy have been completed.

Upper Limb Mononeuropathies. Hand weakness and atrophy in DM are usually attributable to carpal tunnel syndrome or cubital tunnel syndrome and only infrequently to brachial plexus neuropathy, cervical radiculopathy, or manifestation of severe diabetic neuropathy.

Oculomotor Neuropathy. The characteristic feature of oculomotor neuropathy is extraocular muscle weakness with pupillomotor sparing. This is usually a self-limited disease, usually improving in days, weeks, or months. Specific treatment has not been found.

Autonomia. It is not uncommon to have mild asymptomatic autonomic alterations in diabetic polyneuropathy. Generally, specific treatment is not available or needed. Other diabetic patients may develop severe visceral dysautonomia with such symptoms as postural hypotension, gastric atony with satiety, nausea and vomiting, cramping abdominal pain, night diarrhea, and sexual erectile dysfunction.

Other Metabolic Neuropathies

Uremic Polyneuropathy. Uremic polyneuropathy is a consequence of end-stage kidney disease caused by DM, glomerulonephritis, pyelonephritis, amyloidosis, polycystic kidneys, or other kidney disease. The complication of polyneuropathy is more apt to occur in patients treated with hemodialysis than with peritoneal dialysis. Successful renal transplantation is usually associated with gradual improvement of uremic neuropathy.

Porphyric Neuropathy. A variety of inherited disorders involving the heme molecule may be associated with peripheral neuropathy. Usually, the disorder is provoked by ingestion of certain chemicals, e.g., barbiturates and sulfone drugs. In acute intermittent porphyria, delirium is associated with a generalized paralytic neuropathy that may be life-threatening. Identification of persons with the metabolic disorder and avoidance of precipitating agents are most important. When general paralysis develops, the patient must be admitted to an intensive care unit. Mechanical support and fluid balance will need to be given.

Hepatic Neuropathy. Several varieties of neuropathy have been described in association with hepatocellular failure. Specific treatment other than liver transplantation is not available.

Amyloidosis. The protein molecule involved in amyloid fibril formation is the basis for classification of amyloidosis. The proteins implicated are monoclonal light chains (in primary amyloidosis), transthyretin, gelsolin, and apolipoprotein A-I (in inherited amyloidosis) and protein A (in secondary amyloidosis). A variety of immune therapies have been tried for primary amyloidosis, but the results have been disappointing. For some patients with inherited amyloidosis, liver transplantation may offer a worthwhile treatment. Because of the great expense of liver transplantation and shortage of available livers, it would appear prudent to limit the procedure to relatively young persons with early tissue involvement rather than end-stage disease.

Acromegaly. Acromegaly may be associated with a hypertrophic neuropathy.

Infections

Worldwide, infection is one of the major causes of peripheral nerve disease. Leprosy, herpes zoster, and borreliosis (Lyme disease) are common debilitating disorders for which treatment is now available. Altered immunity plays an important role in the expression of these neuropathies. Treatment of these disorders is discussed elsewhere.

Acute Immune Polyradiculoneuropathies, Guillain-Barré Syndrome

There appear to be several variants of Guillain-Barré syndrome (GBS): a demyelinating disorder in which the brunt of the immune attack is on Schwann cells or myelin (acute inflammatory demyelinating polyradiculoneuropathy); another in which the attack is on motor axons; and another in which the attack is on sensory and motor axons. There probably are two closely related syndromes, the Miller-Fisher syndrome (extraocular paralysis and ataxia) and pandysautonomia. The following discussion is based on therapeutic trials in GBS.

Treatment

In previous times, treatment was restricted to recognition that the disorder was GBS, provision of cardiorespiratory support, avoidance and treatment of infection, maintenance of fluid and food intake, avoidance and prevention of bed sores, and symptomatic treatment of anxiety. Today, these therapeutic measures remain important, but the emphasis is on early recognition of the patients who will develop generalized paralysis, with the view to providing plasma exchange (PE) or immune globulin infusion (IGIV),* in hopes that total paralysis can be avoided or shortened. Both PE, usually given once a day for 5 consecutive days and removing approximately 75

to 85% of circulating plasma proteins on each of these days, and IGIV, 0.4 gram per kg of body weight once or twice a week, reportedly reduce the duration of severe weakness or paralysis. The value of corticosteroids in modulating the course of GBS remains controversial. Sometimes a coexisting infection should be treated with appropriate antibiotic medication.

Generally, the diagnosis is based on recognition of the temporal relation to a preceding upper respiratory infection; the development, over hours, days, or a week or two, of a polyradiculoneuropathy causing muscle weakness of both distal and proximal segments of limbs and of trunk; characteristic electrophysiologic findings; and increased cerebrospinal fluid protein without cells. How the physician should proceed after he or she thinks that the patient may have GBS depends on the expertise of the physician, the stage of the disease, and the availability and nearness of treatment options. If neurologic involvement is mild to moderate, the neurologic impairment is not worsening rapidly, the patient has competent family members who can effect rapid transfer to hospital, and there is a full-service medical facility nearby, it may be reasonable to follow the patient medically as an outpatient.

Whether the patient is at home or in the hospital, the neurologic status must be carefully monitored as frequently as necessary. Simple functional tests, such as ability to walk on toes, and heels and to arise from a kneeled position, first on one side then on the other, are rapid and useful. Helpful for this purpose is to examine a standard group of muscles for strength, muscle stretch reflexes of upper and lower limbs, and sensation at standard sites. The Neuropathy Impairment Score (NIS) provides a standard score from such an examination (Table 1; see later discussion). As soon as it is judged that the patient is in danger of generalized or respiratory paralysis, he or she should be admitted to an intensive care facility, and tracheotomy may need to be performed.

Concurrently, or preferably before this stage, PE or IGIV should be given. Once it has been decided that PE will be used, an exchange is given daily for 5 days, and then twice weekly (distributed approximately equally over time) for another 3 weeks. If IGIV is to be used, an intravenous infusion of 0.4 gram per kg of body weight is given twice per week for the first week, and then once weekly for another 3 weeks. There are situations in which PE or IGIV may not be useful. The patient who comes under a physician's care after a week or more of severe paralysis with established generalized denervation on needle electromyography may not profit from these therapies. Some patients improve only to worsen again. In such cases, additional PE or IGIV therapy should probably be given.

Maintenance of an airway, adequate suctioning, mechanical respiration, prevention of lung stasis or aspiration, treatment of pneumonia, maintenance of adequate hydration and electrolyte balance, and avoidance and treatment of infection can be done only in adequate facilities with good and caring nurs-

---

*Not FDA approved for this indication.

TABLE 1. **Neuropathy Impairment Score***

			Right	Left	Sum
Cranial Nerves	1	3rd nerve			
	2	6th nerve			
	3	Facial weakness			
	4	Palate weakness			
	5	Tongue weakness			
Muscle Weakness†	6	Respiratory			
	7	Neck flexion			
	8	Shoulder abduction (deltoid)			
	9	Elbow flexion (biceps brachii)			
	10	Brachioradialis			
	11	Elbow extension (triceps brachii)			
	12	Wrist flexion			
	13	Wrist extension			
	14	Finger flexion			
	15	Finger spread (interossei)			
	16	Thumb abduction (thenar)			
	17	Hip flexion (iliopsoas)			
	18	Hip extension (gluteus max.)			
	19	Knee flexion (biceps femoires)			
	20	Knee extension (quadriceps)			
	21	Ankle dorsiflexors (tibialis ant. +)			
	22	Ankle plantar flexors (gastroc sol.)			
	23	Toe extensors			
	24	Toe flexors			
Reflexes‡	25	Biceps brachii			
	26	Triceps brachii			
	27	Brachioradialis			
	28	Quadriceps femoris			
	29	Triceps surae/gastroc soleus			
Sensation§ I. Finger: (terminal phalanx)	30	Touch-pressure			
	31	Pin-prick			
	32	Vibration			
	33	JP			
G. Toe: (terminal phalanx)	34	Touch-pressure			
	35	Pin-prick			
	36	Vibration			
	37	JP			
Total _____					

*The objective is to provide a single score of neuropathic deficit and subset scores for abnormalities abstracted from a neurologic examination in which all of the assessments are made. The examiner scores deficits according to what he or she considers to be normal, considering the test, the anatomic site, and the patient's age, sex, height, weight, and physical fitness.

†To score muscle weakness: normal = 0; 25% weak = 1; 50% weak = 2; 75% weak = 3; paralyzed = 4. Increments of scoring between 3 and 4 are just able to move limb against gravity = 3.25; just able to move limb when gravity is eliminated = 3.5; flicker of muscle without movement = 3.75. Patients 75 y or younger should be able to walk on their toes and heels; inability to rise from a kneeled position is not scored as abnormal after age 60 y.

‡To score reflexes and sensation: normal = 0; decreased = 1; absent = 2. For patients 50–69 y old, decreased ankle reflexes are scored as 0, and absence of ankle reflexes is scored as 1. In patients 70 y or older, absence of ankle reflexes is scored as 0.

§Touch-pressure, pinprick, and vibration (V. Mueller, Chicago, tuning fork, length 25 cm, made from ½ × ¼ in stock; 156 Hz with counterweights) are assessed on the dorsal surfaces of the terminal phalanx of the index (I.) finger and the great (G.) toe. Joint motion is tested by moving the terminal phalanx of the index finger and the great toe.

Modified from Dyck PJ, Sherman WR, Hallcher LM, et al: Human diabetic endoneurial sorbitol, fructose, and myo-inositol related to sural nerve morphometry. Ann Neurol 8:590–596, 1980; and data from (revised): Dyck PJ, Kratz KM, Lehman KA, et al: The Rochester Diabetic Neuropathy Study: Design, criteria for types of neuropathy, selection bias, and reproducibility of neuropathic tests. Neurology 41:799–807, 1991; and Dyck PJ, Litchy WJ, Lehman KA, et al: Variables influencing neuropathic endpoints: The Rochester Diabetic Neuropathy Study of Healthy Subjects. Neurology 45:1115–1121, 1995.

ing personnel. Personal accounts of patients who have lived through paralytic attacks emphasize the need for explanation, reassurance, and kindness, as well as continuous and gentle care. Frequent passive movement of uncomfortable limbs, gentle massage, and skin care are required.

There is a suggestion that longer and more intensive treatment may be needed for the axonal varieties of GBS.

Chronic Inflammatory Demyelinating Polyradiculoneuropathy

Chronic inflammatory demyelinating polyradiculoneuropathy (CIDP) shares many features with acute inflammatory demyelinating polyneuropathy (GBS)—polyradiculoneuropathy due to an inflammatory demyelinating process; a cytoalbuminologic dissociation; low nerve conduction velocity, dispersion, or conduction block; and an immune basis—but departs from it in having a different course, outlook, and treatment. CIDP usually begins insidiously, worsens slowly or in steps, and tends to wax and wane. There also appears to be a lower frequency of respiratory paralysis. In an early series of 53 patients followed up for an average of 7.5 years, a small percentage of mostly untreated patients with CIDP had died, a small percentage had recovered, and the remainder had smoldering disease.

Specific Treatment

In controlled clinical trials, three modalities of treatment were shown to be efficacious—prednisone, PE, and IGIV. Other immune-modulating therapies may also be efficacious but have not been adequately studied. Generally, a course of PE or IGIV has a much greater and more rapid beneficial effect than prednisone. Prednisone use, especially for long times and high dosages, is commonly associated with serious complications (e.g., hyperglycemic, hyperosmolar coma, psychosis, cataract of the lens, altered physical appearance, infection, osteoporosis). By contrast, PE or IGIV treatment is generally well tolerated. There are two types of complications with PE. Acute and relatively mild complications include lightheadedness, fever, and rash. Occasional patients may experience anaphylaxis. With prolonged intermittent use, iron deficiency anemia may occur. Complications that may occur with IGIV are lightheadedness, nausea, rash, and low-grade fever. Of more concern is the possibility of anaphylaxis (extremely infrequent) or transmission of a viral infection, such as hepatitis or HIV infection.

The diagnosis and treatment of CIDP should probably be supervised by physicians with expertise in neuromuscular disease. Before deciding on treatment, the physician should answer these questions: Does the patient have CIDP? Is it severe enough to justify expensive treatment? Is the disease improving? Do the potential benefits of the putative treatment outweigh the risks? Does the chronicity of the disease preclude a likely good outcome?

Assuming that the answers to these questions are answered in favor of treatment, I usually begin with PE or IGIV treatment. I set up a surveillance plan to monitor the severity of neuropathic symptoms and impairments and then decide on the treatment schedule and dosing to be given for the ensuing 6 weeks or 3 months. The intent is to titrate the treatment dosage to the response at regular intervals, e.g., every 6 weeks, 3 months, or 6 months. Symptoms may be quantitated by using the Neuropathy Symptoms and Change (NSC) score, which tallies the number of symptoms, their severity, and their change from the preceding surveillance time. Neuropathic impairment is judged by using the NIS; summated compound muscle action potentials (CMAPs) of ulnar, median, peroneal, and tibial nerves; sensory nerve action potentials of ulnar and sural nerves (or subsets of these); and vibration detection threshold of the great toes using the CASE IV system and the 4, 2, and 1 stepping algorithm. The NIS is shown in Table 1. It provides a standard composite score of neuropathy impairment and grades weakness as a percentage decrease from normal to paralysis.

Next, one should decide whether PE or IGIV will be used. The two treatments are approximately equivalent in efficacy, cost, and risk. Venous access is less of a problem with IGIV. What schedule should one begin with? It depends on the course and severity of the disease and should be individualized. A typical patient with moderately severe disease might be given 0.4 gram per kg of body weight of IGIV once a week for 4 weeks, then 0.2 gram per kg for a further 4 weeks. The infusions can be given in an outpatient setting or even in the home by a specialized nursing service equipped to deal with anaphylactic reactions.

Within 1 week of the last treatment, the patient is re-evaluated by using NSC, NIS, nerve conduction, and quantitative sensory tests. One seeks evidence that the patient has responded unequivocally to treatment. If improvement has not occurred, the diagnosis may be in error, the modality of treatment is not efficacious, or the dosage schedule is not sufficient. If the patient has CIDP, one expects unequivocal improvement with optimal treatment using PE, IGIV, or both. Assuming that improvement occurred from the first treatment period, one decides after the evaluation what treatment should be given for the next interval (no treatment, or increased or decreased treatment).

With the approach of titrating dosage and frequency of treatment to response, it is sometimes possible to maintain an essentially normal status with a low dosage given infrequently. Some patients who fail to respond to PE or IGIV occasionally respond to oral prednisone given in dosages of 80 to 15 mg on alternate days, with the dosage being decreased exponentially over 6 to 9 months. Prednisone in smaller dosages, e.g., 45 and 10 mg on alternate days, or azathioprine (Imuran),* e.g., 2 or 2.5 mg per kg, may be used to try to decrease the dosage or

---

*Not FDA approved for this indication.

frequency of PE or IGIV treatment. If prednisone is used, it is necessary to set up surveillance to prevent or recognize hyperglycemic hyperosmolar coma, infection, osteoporosis, and the other complications already mentioned. If azathioprine is used, periodic surveillance of the leukocyte count and assessment for hepatotoxicity are needed.

Polyneuropathy Associated with Monoclonal Gammopathy of Undetermined Significance

There is a chronic polyradiculoneuropathy associated with IgG, IgA, or IgM monoclonal protein of undetermined significance (monoclonal gammopathy of undetermined significance [MGUS]). The finding of a monoclonal protein may raise the question of an associated lymphoma, amyloidosis, and other lymphoproliferative diseases, although most commonly it is unassociated with these disorders. Generally, the course of MGUS polyneuropathy is slowly progressive. PE, compared with sham PE, has been shown to be efficacious for MGUS polyneuropathy. Responsiveness, however, was shown to be almost entirely attributable to responsiveness in the IgG and IgA MGUS neuropathy groups. The approach and dosages are like those described previously for CIDP. Commonly, prednisone and melphalan* (Alkeran) are used for the latter condition, but proof that it helps neuropathy has still not been shown.

Primary Amyloidosis Neuropathy

At present, efficacious treatment for primary amyloidosis neuropathy has not been demonstrated.

Inflammatory Polyganglionopathy, Sensorimotor Neuropathy, and Multiple Mononeuropathy Sometimes Associated with Sjögren's Syndrome

The disorders are immune neuropathies that especially affect spinal ganglia and sensory nerves and are sometimes associated with dry eyes and mouth owing to inflammation of lacrimal and salivary glands and with serologic abnormalities. Sometimes the involvement of lacrimal and salivary glands is minimal. Serologic abnormalities are present only in a small percentage of cases. Although immune-modulating therapy is used, there is as yet no convincing evidence that it is efficacious.

Necrotizing Vasculitis

Disorders with necrotizing vasculitis typically affecting large arterioles or small arteries (polyarteritis nodosum, rheumatoid arthritis with necrotizing vasculitis, Wegener's granulomatosis, Churg-Strauss syndrome, and hypersensitivity angiitis) characteristically induce a disorder with involvement of first one nerve, then another nerve (multiple mononeuropathy). Often, affected patients have systemic disease (fever and malaise), multiple tissue involvement, and serologic abnormality (elevated antinuclear antibody, rheumatoid factor, estradiol nuclear antibody, or antineutrophil cytoplasmic antibody). Usually, tissue diagnosis is desirable. In overwhelming disease, methylprednisolone (Solu-Medrol), given intravenously in dosages of 1000 mg for 2 or 3 days, may be needed. In less fulminant cases, prednisone in dosages of 80 mg per day for perhaps a week, followed by rapid reduction to a dosage level sufficient to inhibit systemic features, serologic abnormalities, and new tissue complication, is used.

Inflammation of small nerve vessels without (or with little) systemic involvement is typical of nonsystemic vasculitic neuropathy. It also induces a multiple mononeuropathy. Sometimes, low dosages (10 to 15 mg per day) of prednisone may stop new nerve lesions from developing.

Sarcoid Neuropathy

Although sarcoidosis often affects cranial nerves, it occasionally induces a peripheral polyneuropathy. A history or association of cranial neuropathy, uveitis, rash, and systemic symptoms such as fever and elevated angiotensin-converting enzyme should bring this diagnosis to mind. The tissue reaction is a noncaseating granuloma with KPI-positive histocytes and giant cells especially affecting the perineurium. Polyneuropathy is only infrequently caused by sarcoidosis. Although cranial polyneuropathy appears to respond to prednisone, peripheral polyneuropathy does not respond as readily.

SYMPTOMATIC TREATMENT IN NEUROPATHY

Muscle Weakness

The approach to treatment must vary with the distribution and severity of weakness, the anticipated course of disease, the needs of the patient, and the availability of help from family and physical medicine and rehabilitation. Paralysis of bulbar and respiratory muscles due to peripheral neuropathy generally requires immediate tracheotomy and assisted mechanical respiration. Tube feeding may also need to be instituted. Acute generalized axial and limb weakness usually requires total nursing care, including frequent turning and positioning and care of tissues to relieve discomfort and to prevent bedsores, cushioning of nerves vulnerable to compression, and to prevent contracture. Which orthotic devices should be used and when are beyond the scope of this discussion. Generally, for all paralytic diseases, it is advisable to use active physical fitness exercises and to maintain full range of movement of joints. Direct electrical stimulation of muscles is not considered by most experts to be useful.

---

*Not FDA approved for this indication.

Neuropathic Pain

Pain attributable to peripheral neuropathy is of several kinds and is recognized as being neuropathic from the character, distribution, association with other sensory symptoms, association with clinical findings of neuropathy, and lack of evidence of another cause of pain. The descriptions of pain include sharp needle-like pricks or jabs, pulses or surges, superficial burning, and deep aching. The distribution of the pain depends on which neural structures are affected. In symmetrical distal lower limb sensorimotor polyneuropathy, the pain is in the toes, feet, or distal legs. In lumbosacral plexus neuropathy, it is in the buttock, groin, and anterior thigh. In brachial plexus neuropathy, the pain is in the posterior and lateral shoulder and into the upper arm. Associated sensory symptoms are "asleep" or prickling numbness of the part, a tightly wrapped or constricted feeling of the part, a retained sock or cotton ball feeling on the sole of the foot, and other similar symptoms. Associated clinical findings are muscle weakness, sensory loss, and autonomic disturbance in the region of painfulness.

Symptomatic treatment of pain should not be continued without a determined effort to identify its underlying cause and the responsible variety of neuropathy. It is especially important to identify remediable causes of neuropathy—infections, toxic conditions, malnutrition, deficiency, immune factors, neoplasia, compression, and so on. Assuming this has been achieved, what can be done about symptomatic relief of pain?

The physician should begin by understanding the factors involved in the pain experience. The possible implications of a disease process, lack of adequate sleep, and anxiety and depression may be important in facilitating a patient's pain. Explanation of the medical problem and assurance that support is available may help. Good footwear and avoidance of some types of activity may lessen pain. Cool soaks of the feet followed by petroleum jelly salve or lotion to maintain hydration of the skin may be soothing and prevent callus, which when compressed in walking may be painful. The feet should be inspected daily for callus, infection, and ulcer. I also pay attention to the activities of daily living, emphasizing the need to engage in life so as not to ruminate on the medical problem. I strongly encourage a physical fitness program to maintain muscle bulk, range of motion of joints, and cardiovascular reserve, and generally to help the patient feel better.

Pharmacologic approaches may be helpful but should be only a part of the overall program. There are no medications that will relieve all the discomfort of neuropathic pain without creating excessive drowsiness or addiction. The goal, therefore, should be to ameliorate the pain to enable the patient to cope and live with it. It is necessary, therefore, for the physician to try to establish the time of day or night when the pain comes and have the patient use medications for this time. If the pain is mild and not troublesome, analgesics may not be needed. For mild discomfort that begins toward the end of the working day, is troublesome in the evening hours, and interferes with falling asleep, use of an analgesic or sedative (e.g., plain or enteric-coated acetylsalicylic acid, 60 mg; acetaminophen, 325 mg, or 650 mg of extended-release preparation) may prove to be useful. For more severe and chronic pain, the two groups of drugs most commonly used are the tricyclic antidepressants and the anticonvulsants. Readers should consult other articles in this book and specialized textbooks on the management of chronic pain.

Autonomic Disturbance

Gastroparesis, gastrointestinal dysfunction, diarrhea, sphincter disturbances, postural hypotension, impotence in the male, and sudomotor increase or decrease are extremely troublesome manifestations of autonomic neuropathy. The reader should see articles in this book and specialized reviews for the management of these disorders.

ACUTE HEAD INJURIES IN ADULTS

method of
DONALD W. MARION, M.D.
University of Pittsburgh Medical Center
Pittsburgh, Pennsylvania

Traumatic brain injury remains a common cause of death and disability in the United States. Approximately 180 to 220 persons per 100,000 per year suffer a head injury, and 14 to 30 persons per 100,000 die each year as a result. Ten percent of these victims have severe injuries that render them comatose, 20% have moderate neurologic deficits but are still conscious, and 70% have mild injuries. Most victims of head injury are between the ages of 15 and 24 years, and men are two to three times more likely to suffer a head injury than women. A positive blood alcohol level is detected in 50 to 60% of head-injured patients. The most common causes of traumatic brain injury are motor vehicle accidents, falls, and assaults. In the country as a whole, motor vehicle accidents account for the majority of head injuries, but in large urban areas, assaults and gunshot wounds are a more common cause. In the elderly, falls may be a more common cause than motor vehicle accidents.

PATHOPHYSIOLOGY OF HEAD INJURIES

Neurologic outcome after traumatic brain injury is a result of injuries to the brain that occur at the time of the trauma (primary brain injury) and by delayed neurochemical and metabolic changes that occur during the first few hours and days after the injury (secondary brain injury). Primary injuries to the skull and brain are a result of impact, translational, and rotational forces applied to the head. The types of skull and brain injuries that occur depend on the type of force applied. For example, direct impact to the head, such as a blow to the head with a rigid object, is far more likely than a motor vehicle accident to result in a skull fracture and intracranial hematoma. High-speed motor vehicle accidents cause severe rotational forces to the head, diffuse brain injuries, and brain swelling, and less commonly, intracranial hematomas. Primary injuries include skull fractures, subdural and epidural hematomas, contusions, and diffuse axonal injuries.

Secondary injury occurs during the first few hours and days after the trauma. Several pathophysiologic abnormalities exacerbate brain tissue injury and lead to brain swelling. Early after the injury, cerebral blood flow is typically less than half of normal values, the blood-brain barrier is disrupted, and cerebrovascular autoregulatory mechanisms responsible for modulating normal cerebral blood flow are disrupted. In some cases, these changes may exist for several days after the injury. The abrupt decrease in cerebral blood flow and the inability of the cerebrovasculature to maintain an adequate blood supply to damaged areas of the brain result in ischemia. Focal and, in some cases, global cerebral ischemia leads to the release of high levels of excitotoxic amino acids, lactate, and oxygen free radicals. Disruption of the blood-brain barrier and other factors result in an intense inflammatory response around contusions and underlying subdural hematomas. All of these conditions increase brain tissue injury, swelling, and ischemia.

The challenge for the contemporary neurotraumatologist is to intervene early after traumatic brain injury to prevent as much secondary injury as possible. On the basis of our current understanding of the pathophysiologic abnormalities associated with secondary brain injury, the treatment of these patients should focus on enhancing cerebral blood flow, avoiding therapies that can exacerbate ischemia, and identifying and applying therapies that effectively reduce the production of oxygen free radicals and suppress the inflammatory response.

TREATMENT

Mild Head Injuries

The majority of patients with head injuries have only a brief period of loss of consciousness, followed by several minutes of amnesia for the event. In more severe cases, retrograde amnesia for several minutes may occur. On evaluation, victims may be neurologically normal or somewhat confused or disoriented. An estimated 2 million people per year suffer head injuries, but only 400,000 require hospitalization. The challenge is to identify those patients who are at risk for the development of intracranial mass lesions or brain swelling and delayed neurologic deterioration. Risk factors include mechanism of injury, age, predisposing medical conditions (e.g., use of an-

ticoagulants), duration of loss of consciousness, and duration of pre- or post-traumatic amnesia (Table 1). If any of these risk factors exist, the patient should be taken to an emergency department and undergo a thorough evaluation, in most cases including computed tomography (CT) of the head. The patient should be observed with serial neurologic examinations for a minimum of 1 hour. Neurologic assessment should include cranial nerve, motor, and sensory function, as well as the more subtle neuropsychologic and cognitive functioning. If any abnormality persists, the patient should be admitted for observation for 24 hours and closely monitored for neurologic deterioration. In most cases, those patients with post-traumatic lesions identified by CT should also be hospitalized and have an additional CT examination within 12 to 24 hours to rule out enlargement of intracranial mass lesions. When discharged from the hospital or the emergency department, the patient and family members should be carefully informed, both verbally and with written instructions, about the symptoms and signs of delayed brain injury and whom to contact if these symptoms occur. The significance of increasing headaches, lethargy, nausea or vomiting, or new onset of focal neurologic deficits should be emphasized.

Moderate to Severe Head Injuries
Prehospital Management

The first priority in the initial evaluation of the patient with moderate to severe head injury is to restore and/or maintain normal oxygenation and blood pressure. Most severely head injured patients who are rendered comatose benefit from early endotracheal intubation and controlled ventilation. Portable pulse oximetry should be used to verify arterial oxygen saturations of greater than 96%, and supplemental oxygen should be provided to achieve this level. A ventilatory rate of 10 to 12 breaths per minute (arterial P_{CO_2} of 35 to 40 mm Hg) is recommended. In larger patients, higher ventilatory rates may be required to provide adequate minute ventilation. Patients who suffer neurologic deterioration while being observed are at high risk for the development of intracranial mass lesions and may also benefit from higher ventilatory rates until the mass lesion is removed. Hypotension is aggressively treated by placement of several large-bore intravenous catheters and administration of isotonic crystalloid or colloid solutions as necessary to restore a mean blood pressure of 90 to 100 mm Hg.

After the airway is secured, normal oxygenation is ensured, and the blood pressure is stabilized, a rapid assessment of injuries is conducted. A rigid cervical spine collar is applied, and the patient is placed on a back board. Any points of active bleeding are tamponaded with external dressings. The neurologic status is assessed in terms of the Glasgow Coma Scale score (Table 2). Any asymmetry in motor functioning or eye opening is noted, and pupil size and reactivity to light are documented.

TABLE 1. **Risk Factors for Delayed Neurologic Deterioration After Head Injury**

Mechanism
   High-speed motor vehicle accident
   Fall of more than 8 ft
   Injury that causes significant damage to other areas
     of the body
Age greater than 65 y
Medical conditions
   Long-term anticoagulation therapy
   Presence of cerebrovascular malformation
Duration of loss of consciousness more than 5 min
Pre- or post-traumatic amnesia for longer than 10 min

TABLE 2. **Glasgow Coma Scale Scoring***

Measure	Score
Eye Opening	
Spontaneously	4
To verbal command	3
To painful stimuli	2
None	1
Verbal Response	
Oriented and converses	5
Disoriented and converses	4
Inappropriate words	3
Incomprehensible sounds	2
No audible sounds	1
Motor Response	
Follows verbal commands	6
To painful stimuli	
Purposeful localization	5
Withdraws from stimulus	4
Flexor posturing	3
Extensor posturing	2
No response	1

*Total score equals eye opening + verbal response + motor response; scores range from 3 to 15.

At this point, the patient is rapidly transported to a trauma center capable of definitive neurosurgical intervention. For transport times longer than 15 to 20 minutes, serial neurologic assessments should be documented every 10 to 15 minutes. Early contact by telephone or radio should be made with the trauma center, and medications given to the patient coordinated through the neurosurgeons and other health care providers at the trauma center.

Emergency Department Management

Transfer of the severely head injured patient to a trauma center certified by the American College of Surgeons or state trauma certification systems is highly recommended. Such trauma centers typically have a trauma surgeon in house 24 hours a day and a neurosurgeon available within 10 minutes of notification. The patient is initially evaluated according to the guidelines of the Advanced Trauma Life Support protocol of the American College of Surgeons. The primary survey is conducted to identify all life-threatening injuries and to assess the level of consciousness of the patient. Life-threatening chest or abdominal injuries are immediately identified and treated. Cervical spine radiographs are obtained to rule out cervical spine instability. A diagnostic peritoneal lavage or diagnostic abdominal ultrasound scanning is done to rule out significant intra-abdominal hemorrhage. The patient is taken to the CT suite and has CT of the head to identify any surgical intracranial mass lesions. If abdominal ultrasound scanning or diagnostic peritoneal lavage has not been performed, most comatose head-injured victims also have CT of the abdomen and, if thoracic hemorrhage is suspected, CT of the chest.

If the blood pressure is difficult to control, or the diagnostic peritoneal lavage is positive, the patient may be taken immediately to surgery without CT of the head. In these cases, an intraoperative air ventriculogram can be obtained to detect large intracranial mass lesions.

Once CT of the head is done, whether or not a craniotomy is indicated is determined by the size and location of intracranial hematomas or hemorrhagic contusions. Approximately 20% of comatose head-injured patients have one or more hemorrhagic contusions, and 20% have an acute subdural hematoma. In most cases, lesions larger than 25 to 30 mL, particularly those within or adjacent to the temporal lobes, should be evacuated. In addition to the size and location of the mass lesion, the decision to operate is based on the patient's neurologic status, change in the neurologic status, presence or absence of pupil abnormalities, and age. For example, an 80-year-old patient who is admitted with a fixed and dilated pupil and a Glasgow Coma Scale score of 3 or 4 is not likely to have a functional recovery, even though he or she may have a large subdural hematoma that can be evacuated. In such cases, the decision is often made not to intervene surgically.

Intensive Care Management

Once all life-threatening and surgical issues are resolved, the patient with severe to moderate head injury is transferred to an intensive care unit staffed by nurses familiar with the management of patients with head injuries. An intracranial pressure monitor is placed for continuous intracranial pressure monitoring in all patients who are unable to follow commands and have post-traumatic intracranial abnormalities at CT. I prefer a ventriculostomy catheter placed into the right lateral ventricle and fluid-coupled to a transducer; this device permits intermittent cerebrospinal fluid drainage as a potential treatment for raised intracranial pressure.

Every attempt is made to normalize the patient's physiologic and hemodynamic parameters. The mean arterial blood pressure is kept at 100 ± 10 mm Hg. The central venous pressure is kept at 6 to 15 cm H_2O, the arterial Pco_2 at 35 ± 2 mm Hg, and the arterial Po_2 higher than 98 mm Hg. In addition, the core body temperature is maintained at 37 ± 5°C. The head is kept in the midline, and compression of the soft tissues of the neck is avoided. For the first 24 hours after injury, I keep the head of the bed flat to enhance cerebral perfusion. Cerebral perfusion pressure (mean arterial pressure minus intracranial pressure) is maintained above 70 mm Hg with the use of vasopressor agents if necessary. A 20-gauge Silastic catheter is inserted into the internal jugular vein with its tip in the jugular bulb, usually on the right, and frequent assessments of the arterial jugular venous oxygen content difference are obtained. Our goal is to maintain these values at less than 7 vol%. The hemoglobin is maintained at 10 to 12 mg per dL, sodium and potassium values are normalized, partial thromboplastin time and prothrombin time are normalized, and any other hematologic or electrolyte abnormalities are corrected.

The presence or absence of cervical spine instability must also be determined early after injury. Good-quality lateral, anteroposterior, and open-mouth odontoid radiographs of the cervical spine, when properly interpreted, will identify more than 99% of unstable cervical spine injuries. The lateral view must include the C7–T1 interspace. The most common reasons for missed cervical spine injuries are inadequate radiographs or improper interpretation of the radiographs. In patients who are alert and awake and have neck pain, flexion and extension films are recommended.

Phenytoin (Dilantin) is administered to all patients who have post-traumatic parenchymal injuries, such as contusions, subdural hematomas, and diffuse brain swelling. Therapy is discontinued after 7 days unless the patient has delayed post-traumatic seizures, in which case the therapy is continued for 6 months to 1 year. An H_2 blocker is given to lower the risk of stress ulcers. Sequential pneumatic compression devices are applied to the lower extremities. Nutritional supplementation, preferably enteral, is begun within 48 to 72 hours after the injury, and the goal is to reach 2000 to 2500 kcal per day.

Management of Elevated Intracranial Pressure

Brain swelling occurs after most severe traumatic brain injuries. A primary goal of the critical care of severely head injured patients is to prevent elevated intracranial pressure. Normal intracranial pressure is less than 12 to 15 mm Hg. Most studies find a significant increase in mortality and morbidity when intracranial pressure exceeds 20 mm Hg for prolonged periods.

I use a stepwise approach to the management of elevated intracranial pressure (Table 3). Therapies are added only when the previous one fails to reduce intracranial pressure. If there is an abrupt increase

TABLE 3. **Stepwise Approach to Management of Elevated Intracranial Pressure**

---

1. All physiologic and hemodynamic parameters normalized
   - Pco_2 35 ± 2 mm Hg
   - Po_2 > 98 mm Hg
   - Mean arterial pressure 100 ± 10 mm Hg
   - Central venous pressure 6–15 cm H_2O
   - Core temperature 37 ± 5°C
2. Systemic neuromuscular paralysis (vecuronium or pancuronium)
3. Narcotic sedation (morphine or fentanyl)
4. Intermittent CSF drainage
5. Mannitol (25–50 gm q 3–4 h)
   - Not used if serum osmolality exceeds 315 mOsm
   - Urine output replaced milliliter per milliliter with isotonic saline solution
6. Furosemide (40 mg q 4 h)
   - Not used if serum osmolality exceeds 315 mOsm
7. Pentobarbital to achieve electroencephalographic burst suppression
8. Moderate hypothermia (32–33°C for 24 h)

Abbreviation: CSF = cerebrospinal fluid.

in intracranial pressure after the pressure had previously been well controlled, CT of the head is performed immediately. In addition, follow-up CT of the head is routinely performed within 12 to 24 hours after the patient is admitted, particularly for those patients in whom small contusions, subdural, or epidural hematomas were documented at the initial CT. Approximately 20 to 30% of such lesions are found to be larger at follow-up CT.

When intracranial pressure remains below 20 mm Hg for 24 to 48 hours without treatment, the ventricular catheter is removed. Shortly thereafter, most patients can be weaned from mechanical ventilation. Patients who remain comatose for longer than 5 to 10 days usually benefit from the placement of a tracheostomy and feeding jejunostomy tube for long-term care. During the second week after injury, physiatry personnel should be involved with care on a day-to-day basis to coordinate a routine of bedside physical therapy and occupational therapy. Long-term anticoagulation therapy should be considered for patients who have little or no spontaneous extremity movement.

Complications

The most common complications that occur early after severe traumatic brain injury are infectious, pulmonary, and gastroenterologic. Pneumonia occurs in 30 to 50% of intubated head-injured patients in the intensive care unit. These infections are usually treated with broad-spectrum antibiotics until the organism and antibiotic sensitivities are identified, at which point antibiotic coverage is adjusted. Atelectasis and pneumothorax are also common complications. The most common gastroenterologic complication is paralytic ileus and gastrointestinal hemorrhage from stress ulcers. I start all severely head injured patients on H_2 blockers on admission to the intensive care unit. Other less common complications are pituitary insufficiency as a result of damage to the hypothalamus, pituitary stalk, or pituitary gland. Within 4 to 5 days after admission, the comatose head-injured patient should have a screening endocrine battery, including cortisol, prolactin, growth hormone, and thyroid function studies.

Longer term complications include post-traumatic hydrocephalus, heterotopic ossification, decubitus ulcers, malnutrition, and spastic contractures. Many of these complications are prevented or limited with aggressive daily physical therapy routines. The risk of deep venous thrombosis or pulmonary embolism is lowered with the use of anticoagulant therapy.

PROGNOSIS

Mild Head Injuries

Most patients who suffer mild head injuries have a complete recovery by 3 months after injury. However, some studies have found that as many as two thirds of mildly head injured patients may have significant neurobehavioral deficits, memory problems, and headaches until then. A few studies have found that two thirds of mildly head injured patients remain unemployed after 3 months. Patients with mild traumatic brain injury are particularly at risk for postconcussive syndrome, which manifests as headaches, dizziness, and reduced energy levels. As many as 47% of victims of mild head injury complain of headaches 3 months after injury.

Severe Traumatic Brain Injury

The prognosis for patients with severe traumatic brain injury has changed a great deal in the last 10 to 15 years. In 1985, mortality rates for patients who suffered closed head injury were 36 to 40%, and the rate of functional recovery was 20 to 30% at 1 year after the injury. Several more recent studies have found a mortality rate of approximately 20% and good recovery rates of 35 to 45% at 1 year after injury. This improved outcome is attributed to the focus on enhancing cerebral perfusion and avoiding therapies that may exacerbate early cerebral ischemia. A prospective randomized trial of the use of therapeutic moderate hypothermia has demonstrated even further improvement in outcomes for those patients who are treated with cooling to 32 to 33°C for 24 hours early after injury.

ACUTE HEAD INJURIES IN CHILDREN

method of
ANDREA E. HERBERT, M.D.
University of Florida College of Medicine
Gainesville, Florida

Trauma is the leading cause of mortality among children, accounting for more than half of all deaths in patients aged 1 to 14 years. Head injury is the most common cause of traumatic death in the United States. For those patients who do survive, the morbidity of head injury may be devastating developmentally and psychologically as well as financially. Therefore, physicians must have a clear understanding of the evaluation and treatment of pediatric head injury. The following discussion describes guidelines for the management of pediatric head injury practiced at the University of Florida, and several important concepts are reviewed.

EVALUATION

The first concept in attending children with head injuries is that neurologic deterioration or improvement is a continuum, so no single physical examination can accurately determine the need for therapeutic intervention or predict the outcome. Caring for children with head injuries requires frequent and sometimes virtually continuous neurologic assessment. This goal necessitates an accurate and rapid evaluation of the patient's neurologic status at any time. To this end, the Glasgow Coma Scale (GCS) (Table 1) was developed to aid physicians in the rapid assessment of trauma patients. This scale is the most commonly used quantitative clinical assessment system for defining points along the neurologic continuum. The GCS guides therapeutic decisions of physicians and provides highly accurate

TABLE 1. Glasgow Coma Scale*

Measure	Score
Verbal Response	
None	1
Incomprehensible sounds	2
Inappropriate words	3
Confused	4
Oriented	5
Eye Opening	
None	1
To pain	2
To speech	3
Spontaneously	4
Motor Response	
None	1
Abnormal extensor	2
Abnormal flexion	3
Withdraws	4
Localizes	5
Obeys	6

*Maximal score = 15; minimal score = 3.

outcome determination. Employing the assessment of three variables—eye opening, best verbal response, and best motor response—this point system can be used in patients of all ages. Without relying on detailed neurologic examination, the GCS gives an excellent idea of the level of neurologic function in the head-injured patient and also gives a good estimate of the prognosis. Because infants and toddlers may be unable to communicate or follow the commands needed for the GCS, the Children's Coma Scale (Table 2) was developed for patients younger than 3 years.

The second concept is that children have a better prognosis than adult patients with the same severity of apparent injury. This fact demands an aggressive approach to the care of the head-injured child. Clinical outcome in pediatric head injury is a result of the primary traumatic event and certain secondary events occurring as complications of that primary event. As physicians, we have only a preventive control over the primary event. Certain injuries are not compatible with survival, and no amount of intervention can retrieve a patient from inevitable demise in these situations. Treatment must be initiated as early as possible by

TABLE 2. Children's Coma Scale*

Measure	Score
Ocular Response	
Fixed pupil and EOM paralyzed	1
Fixed pupils or EOM impaired	2
EOM intact, reactive pupils	3
Pursuit	4
Verbal Response	
Apneic	1
Spontaneous respirations	2
Cries	3
Motor Response	
Flaccid	1
Hypertonic	2
Withdraws from painful stimuli	3
Flexes and extends	4

*Maximal score = 11; minimal score = 3.
Abbreviation: EOM = extraocular muscles.

trained personnel at the accident scene. The aggressive multidisciplinary approach to the treatment of head injuries, both at the accident scene and in the emergency department, is directed toward minimizing the secondary insults on an already injured brain. Fortunately, most head injuries, especially in children, are compatible with survival, so that if the secondary events are prevented and treated, a positive outcome can be expected in a high percentage of cases.

The third concept of managing head injury in children involves the fact that the volume of the intracranial contents is fixed (except in very small children). Any mass occurring intracranially must be accommodated by the normal contents of the intracranial cavity; otherwise, the intracranial pressure (ICP) will increase. If the process is general and results in edema of the brain, a general rise in ICP occurs. With focal edema or blood accumulation, various herniation syndromes can ensue after the normal compensatory mechanisms have been exhausted.

The final concept is that children suffer different kinds of head injuries from those seen in adults. This fact is related both to the anatomic differences between the child's and adult's brains and skulls and because of etiologic differences in head injury in children. Several properties unique to the infant's skull are important in the pathophysiology of infant head injury. The skull is thin and the sutures are not fused, making the brain susceptible to deformational forces. Furthermore, the base of the skull is smoother than that in older children and adults, resulting in a lower incidence of basilar contusions and contrecoup injuries.

Radiographic examination is essential in the evaluation of mild and severe head injury (Table 3). At the University of Florida, we routinely perform computed tomography (CT) in children with a loss of consciousness or an altered level of consciousness. The head CT should be performed without use of a contrast agent to determine the presence of acute blood. Bone windows from the head CT reveal skull fractures and suture diastasis. Skull radiographs are also useful in the evaluation of skull fractures. A lateral cervical spine film, performed as part of head CT, is useful in the evaluation of cervical fractures.

TYPES OF INJURY

Head injury in infants is most commonly secondary to falls and abuse. In older children, head injuries are frequently related to falls and sports injuries and are often minor. The most serious injuries are usually due to acute deceleration forces during motor vehicle accidents.

Head injury related to birth trauma is less common now

TABLE 3. **Radiographic Assessment of Minor Head Injury**

Type	When
None	Minor head injury
	Good social structure
Skull radiographs	Deformity
	Point tenderness
	Scalp hematomas
Long-bone radiographs	Head injury of questionable etiology
Head CT	Persistent complaints

Abbreviation: CT = computed tomography.
Modified from Mickle JP: Acute head injuries in children. *In* Rakel RE (ed): Conn's Current Therapy 1990. Philadelphia, WB Saunders Co, 1990, pp 863–865.

TABLE 4. **Hospital Admission Criteria in Mild to Moderate Pediatric Head Injury**

Loss of consciousness	Skull fracture
Seizures	Focal neurologic deficit
Persistent vomiting	Severe headache
Prolonged memory deficit	Possibility of child abuse

than in the past. Birth trauma injuries result from slow deformational forces and are characterized by tears in the falx and tentorium and by draining venous sinuses. Skull fracture, usually a greenstick fracture, occasionally occurs with a forceps delivery. These fractures may require elevation for cosmetic reasons. The cephalhematoma that is seen in the newborn after vaginal delivery is secondary to the subperiosteal accumulation of blood. Such hematomas usually resorb spontaneously, although they may become calcified and form a bony protrusion.

The distinction between minor and major head injury is an important one. A minor head injury is one in which there is no loss of consciousness and the neurologic examination is normal. Most of these cases can be managed on an outpatient basis as long as good parental supervision is available (Table 4). Minor head injury can have delayed sequelae detrimental to the patient, necessitating careful initial evaluation as well as adequate follow-up. Serious head injury is classified as loss of consciousness associated with neurologic deficit. Severe head injury is also defined as a GCS score of less than 8. A neurosurgeon should be involved in all cases of serious pediatric head injury.

"Shaken baby syndrome" is a constellation of findings, the most grave and potentially fatal of which is neurologic injury. Infants are anatomically susceptible to this type of head injury because of a relatively large head, poor control of neck muscles, and smooth cranial base. If the infant is held by the shoulders and shaken, a typical brain injury results. Findings consistent with this brain injury are subarachnoid hemorrhage, subdural hematoma, cerebral contusion, and retinal hemorrhage. Diffuse cerebral swelling is often present and may be refractory to medical management. Any child who has minimal external signs of trauma with neurologic damage should be suspected of having been abused. In these cases, radiographs of long bones and the chest should be obtained to look for old fractures.

Several secondary insults occur in children with severe head injury: shock, anoxia or hypoxia, hydrocephalus, seizures, infection, increased ICP, and intracranial lesions, including epidural, subdural, subarachnoid, parenchymal, and intraventricular hemorrhages and diffuse axonal injury.

Epidural hematomas are a relatively uncommon complication of head injury. Traditional treatment consists of surgical evacuation of the epidural clot. Risk factors for acute deterioration include a skull fracture over a major vessel and/or diagnosis less than 6 hours after the trauma. The classic presentation of an epidural hematoma is a postconcussive lucid interval, pupillary dilatation, and motor deficit. Subdural hematomas are the most common intracranial lesions seen in children younger than 2 years and are also treated by surgical drainage. Subarachnoid hemorrhage is often associated with diffuse axonal injury or diffuse brain swelling. Diffuse axonal injury is common in children and is often the cause of delayed neurologic deterioration.

Skull fractures are common injuries in children. Infants can lose a significant amount of their blood volume from a skull fracture, and for this reason we admit young children with skull fractures for observation and serial hematocrit determinations. A depressed skull fracture is elevated surgically if it (1) is open, (2) is depressed at least full thickness of the skull, or (3) causes significant cosmetic defect. The depressed or diastatic skull fracture can be associated with a dural tear. Children with a dural tear must be followed up closely, because they are at risk for developing a growing skull fracture, an uncommon problem clinically manifesting as a palpable nontender swelling in the area of a previous linear skull fracture; such a fracture is repaired surgically. Basilar skull fractures are also seen in severe head injury and usually extend through the floor of the frontal fossa or the temporal bone. Affected patients must be evaluated for facial and vestibulocochlear nerve injury and cerebrospinal fluid (CSF) leak. Serial physical examinations, audiologic examinations, and repeated head CT are mandatory for monitoring these patients.

TREATMENT

Initial treatment of severe pediatric head injury consists of immediate resuscitation using advanced cardiac life support guidelines (Table 5). Children fare better than adults with the same severity of head injury, thereby demanding an aggressive approach to the pediatric head-injured patient. If the head CT does not reveal a potential surgically correctable lesion, the severely head injured patient must be admitted to the intensive care unit and monitored for increased ICP. A coordinated team approach involving pediatricians, intensivists, and neurosurgeons provides the most thorough care of the child (Tables 6 and 7). Mortality is significantly increased in children with severe head injuries with coexisting systemic hypotension or hypoxia.

Intracranial hypertension is a major concern of clinicians treating trauma patients, owing to the potential for ischemia. ICP monitoring is an invasive method used to measure intracranial hypertension. Any child with a GCS score of 7 or less is monitored with an ICP monitor. An ICP monitor measures ICP and cerebral perfusion pressure (CPP), the current parameter used to assess cerebral blood flow. CPP is the ICP subtracted from the mean arterial pressure (CPP = MAP − ICP); a normal CPP is higher than 70 mm Hg. The advantages of ICP monitors are early detection of intracranial mass lesions, limitation of

TABLE 6. Medical Treatment of the Child with Serious Head Injury

What	How
Phenytoin (Dilantin)	15 mg/kg loading dose; 5 mg/kg/d maintenance
Phenobarbital	Same as phenytoin
Diazepam (Valium)	1–5 mg IV to stop seizure
Antibiotics	IV; broad-spectrum agent in contaminated wounds
Mannitol*	0.25–1 gm/kg IV for rapid decompression prn
Diuretics	1 mg/kg IV furosemide (Lasix) prn
Pentobarbital	15 mg/kg IV loading dose; titrate as needed to control intracranial pressure

*Can push serum osmolarity as high as 310 mOsm.

Modified from Mickle JP: Acute head injuries in children. *In* Rakel RE (ed): Conn's Current Therapy 1990. Philadelphia, WB Saunders Co, 1990, pp 863–865.

indiscriminate use of ICP management therapies, reduction of ICP via CSF drainage, and assistance in prognosis.

Elevation of ICP to greater than 20 to 25 mm Hg or a decrease in CPP to less than 70 mm Hg is an ominous sign of neurologic deterioration in head-injured patients and requires immediate intervention. This is accomplished by utilizing the stepwise decision-making therapeutic regimen outlined in Table 8. Aggressive hyperventilation (PO_2 less than 25 mm Hg) has previously been the cornerstone in management of traumatically brain injured patients because it rapidly reduces ICP. Hyperventilation should be used for only brief periods when there is acute neurologic deterioration or for longer periods when increased ICP is resistant to sedation, CSF drainage, induced paralysis, and diuretics. Head position is maintained at 30 degrees to decrease cerebral venous pressure and improve elevated ICP.

Mannitol is an effective osmotic diuretic for lowering ICP after severe head injury. The use of mannitol should be restricted to intracranial hypertension that does not respond to sedation, CSF drainage, or hyperventilation. Also, mannitol may be used in patients with signs of impending herniation or pro-

TABLE 5. Sequence of Events in the Care of the Child with Serious Head Injury

Event	How
1. Evaluate	General physical examination
	Examination of central nervous system
2. Resuscitate	Secure airway, intubate
	Treat shock
	Stabilize
3. Triage	Continue resuscitation
	To operating room
	To intensive care unit

From Mickle JP: Acute head injuries in children. *In* Rakel RE (ed): Conn's Current Therapy 1990. Philadelphia, WB Saunders Co, 1990, pp 863–865.

TABLE 7. Intensive Care Unit Monitoring of the Child with Serious Head Injury

1. Monitoring of vital signs: serial central nervous system examination (Glasgow Coma Scale)
2. Input/output
3. Central venous pressure
4. Arterial blood gases
5. Serum electrolytes
6. Hemogram
7. Intracranial pressure monitor
8. Multimodality somatosensory evoked potentials and brain stem auditory potentials
9. Serial CT

Modified from Mickle JP: Acute head injuries in children. *In* Rakel RE (ed): Conn's Current Therapy 1990. Philadelphia, WB Saunders Co, 1990, pp 863–865.

TABLE 8. **Stepwise Events in the Control of Increased Intracranial Pressure***

1. Head elevated to 30 degrees
2. Sedation and/or paralysis
3. Keep normothermic
4. Diuresis: loop diuretics vs. mannitol
5. Cerebrospinal fluid drainage
6. Hyperventilate briefly for acute neurologic deterioration, P_{CO_2} 30–35 mm Hg
7. Pentobarbital coma
8. Surgical decompression

*Higher than 20 mm Hg.
Modified from Mickle JP: Acute head injuries in children. *In* Rakel RE (ed): Conn's Current Therapy 1990. Philadelphia, WB Saunders Co, 1990, pp 863–865.

gressive neurologic deterioration. These patients must be followed up with frequent serum osmolarity measurements, and mannitol must be discontinued if osmolarity exceeds 310 mOsm, to prevent renal failure. Euvolemia must be maintained with adequate fluid replacement during mannitol administration. There is a risk of mannitol accumulation in the brain, which is why bolus administration rather than continuous infusion is recommended.

Barbiturates are sometimes effective in controlling elevated ICP that is refractory to preceding measures. Pentobarbital coma (high-dose pentobarbital) has been shown to decrease mortality in the setting of uncontrolled ICP. The use of barbiturates for prophylactic treatment of elevated ICP is not recommended. The major side effects of such use are cardiac depression and hypotension, often requiring pressors to support CPP.

Antiseizure medications are recommended for the prophylaxis of early post-traumatic seizures (PTSs) (occurring within 7 days of injury) in patients at high risk for seizures after head injury. Current studies do not support the use of antiepileptic drugs for preventing late PTSs. Patients at high risk for PTSs include those who have intracranial lesions, those in whom the GCS score is less than 10, and those who have seizures within 24 hours of injury.

Multimodality somatosensory evoked potentials and brain stem auditory evoked potentials are helpful in detecting early signs of deterioration in a seemingly stable comatose child. They are also useful in predicting outcome in the comatose child. A poor outcome can be reliably predicted by the combined use of somatosensory and auditory evoked potentials. A good outcome can also be predicted, but with a 10% rate of false optimism.

In conclusion, the management of head injury requires a multispecialty team approach. Head CT should be performed when neurologic status is declining or for any unexplained rise in ICP. This will facilitate detection of surgical lesions. ICP monitoring should be continued as long as the child is comatose or not improving. Routinely, we replace ICP monitors after 1 week to prevent infection. Recognizing and treating hypotension rapidly in head-injured

children are essential in preventing cerebral ischemia and improving the patient's outcome.

BRAIN TUMORS

method of
N. SCOTT LITOFSKY, M.D., and
LAWRENCE D. RECHT, M.D.
University of Massachusetts Medical Center
Worcester, Massachusetts

Brain tumors represent a heterogeneous group of neoplasms that have different presentations, prognoses, and treatments. Defining a single approach to these lesions can therefore be difficult. To facilitate decision-making, we have noted that management issues for all brain tumor patients generally are classifiable into one of three possible categories: (1) symptoms arising from tumor or treatment effects on normal brain, (2) issues concerning correct diagnosis of the lesion, and (3) specific therapeutics of the particular brain tumors. The management of brain tumor symptoms spans the patient's entire clinical course; management decisions here are for the most part histology independent, depending more on tumor location, the presence of mass effect, the patient's age, and the particular symptoms encountered. Decisions concerning making the proper diagnosis—specifically, when to operate and how much tumor to remove—are also for the most part histology independent, being affected mainly by such issues as location and the patient's age. Only the specific therapy of brain tumor is crucially dependent on tumor histology.

We have found that dealing with brain tumors is much easier if treatment issues are first classified and dealt with. Such an approach facilitates management by non–neuro-oncologists, because most treatment decisions are related to symptoms and are therefore largely histology independent. Furthermore, it emphasizes the importance of attending to symptoms, the effective treatment of which can markedly improve quality (and sometimes quantity) of life.

SYMPTOMATIC ISSUES

Seizures

Seizures are an important cause of morbidity in the brain tumor patient. In approximately 40% of patients with gliomas, seizure is the earliest manifestation of the disease, and 55% have had at least one spell by the time the tumor is diagnosed. Seizure frequency and pattern may vary as tumor size and pathology change. Status epilepticus is a common occurrence and may be a presenting symptom. In addition to the morbidities commonly associated with idiopathic epilepsy, seizures in tumor patients are particularly dangerous because of their propensity to increase intracranial pressure (ICP) in a patient with impaired compliance; this can result in sudden death due to cerebral herniation.

Although surgical resection can provide effective relief in patients with persistent refractory seizures secondary to infiltrative tumors in the temporal or frontal lobes, pharmacologic therapy remains the mainstay of treatment. Pharmacotherapy is unique for brain tumor patients in a number of aspects:

1. Brain tumor patients are frequently receiving other medications that may interact with anticonvulsants. For example, patients taking phenytoin (Dilantin) frequently require higher doses of drug when they are also taking dexamethasone; conversely, when steroids are tapered, serum phenytoin levels may rise to toxic levels.

2. Brain tumor patients frequently receive cranial radiotherapy, which may predispose to Stevens-Johnson syndrome and erythema multiforme reactions; this is especially common with phenytoin.

3. Patients frequently have other neurologic impairments that can make anticonvulsant side effects more distressing. For example, brain tumor patients are particularly prone to develop shoulder-hand syndrome and diffuse arthralgias that can be discomforting enough to warrant withdrawal of the medication.

Despite these complications, phenytoin is generally the first-line drug. If breakthrough seizures develop or allergic reactions occur, carbamazepine (Tegretol), phenobarbital, or valproate (Depakote) can be substituted. In lower grade neoplasms, tumor resections can be performed specifically to relieve epilepsy when medical management is ineffective. Patients with brain tumors are prone to develop seizures after intravenous contrast medium for computed tomography (CT). This tendency can be minimized by preprocedural administration of 5 to 10 mg of diazepam intravenously.

Mass Effect

Patients commonly present with symptoms related to mass effect from the tumor. These symptoms can be subdivided into symptoms of elevated ICP and those of focal neurologic deficits.

Brain tumors raise ICP either by the local effects of tumor mass coupled with vasogenic edema or by producing obstruction of cerebrospinal fluid (CSF) pathways leading to the development of hydrocephalus. Elevated ICP may therefore manifest itself in a variety of ways. Headache results from distortion of the dural membranes and intracranial blood vessels. The headache is typically described as holocranial and occurs on arising, because recumbency at night decreases venous drainage of the brain, and mild hypoventilation as the patient is sleeping causes cerebral vasodilatation. Patients may also experience vomiting, which is a result of pressure on the area postrema. Nausea may not be present, and the vomiting occurs most often in the morning (along with a headache) and is frequently projectile. Chronically elevated ICP may also produce progressive cognitive abnormalities with resultant changes in personality and behavior or, alternatively, progressive diminution in the level of consciousness.

Medical and mechanical therapies are available that can treat both mechanisms responsible for elevated ICP. For patients with brain masses and symptoms or signs of elevated ICP, the head of the bed should be elevated at least 30 degrees to increase cerebral venous drainage and reduce intracranial volume. In addition, limiting fluid intake to 1.5 liters per day may help reduce the amount of edema fluid produced.

Analgesics may make the patient more comfortable. However, patients with large intracranial masses who hypoventilate even mildly may rapidly decompensate because of their limited cerebral compliance; therefore, sedation, with its attendant hypoventilation, should be avoided. Codeine is thus preferable to other narcotic analgesics, because it is less sedating. Antiemetics are also helpful to reduce vomiting and improve the patient's comfort. Trimethobenzamide (Tigan), at a dose of 250 mg every 6 hours orally or 200 mg every 6 hours rectally, is preferable to prochlorperazine (Compazine) or promethazine (Phenergan). Phenothiazine agents, although good antiemetics, can reduce the seizure threshold, an effect that should be avoided.

The most serious effect of elevated ICP is cerebral herniation. Management of this neurologic emergency includes hyperventilation by the patient and the administration of osmotic diuretics and steroids. Hyperventilation requires intubation, and its effect rapidly attenuates; however, lowering P_{CO_2} immediately causes cerebral vasoconstriction and decreased intravascular blood volume, effectively reducing ICP and potentially reversing the herniation syndrome. P_{CO_2} should not be lowered to below 25 mm Hg, which may cause cerebral ischemia. Osmotic diuretics such as mannitol are also useful; their onset of action is slower than hyperventilation. An initial dose of 1 gram per kg, followed by 0.25 gram per kg every 4 to 6 hours, reduces the extracellular brain water volume and can control elevated ICP for several days. An initial dose of furosemide (Lasix) at 1 mg per kg can also hasten the response through its vasodilative effect on the peripheral vasculature.

Glucocorticoids such as dexamethasone (Decadron) and methylprednisolone (Medrol) stabilize cell membranes and reduce vasogenic edema. Because their onset of action requires at least 30 to 60 minutes, they should be used only in conjunction with other modalities if the situation is an emergency. They are particularly useful, however, in the chronic management of elevated ICP. Dexamethasone is most commonly utilized. The initial dose is 10 mg, followed by 4 mg every 6 hours. It may be given either orally or intravenously, the latter route being necessary in urgent cases when the patient is unable to take oral medication.

Mechanical therapy can also be provided by placement of a ventriculostomy. This surgical procedure can be performed relatively quickly by a neurosurgeon to divert CSF. Such intervention may rapidly reduce ICP and reverse a herniation syndrome, making it the treatment of choice for the deteriorating patient with hydrocephalus. The ventricular catheter can be removed once the CSF pathway is opened by reduction of edema, or by surgical decompression of tumor bulk. If continued CSF diversion is required after these maneuvers, placement of a permanent ventriculoperitoneal shunt may be necessary.

Patients may develop focal neurologic deficits from mass effect as well. These symptoms and signs include hemiparesis from frontal, parietal, or thalamic masses; aphasia from dominant temporal lobe masses; hearing loss from vestibular schwannomas; visual loss from parasellar masses (such as pituitary adenomas, optic nerve and hypothalamic gliomas, and dorsum sella meningiomas); and hypothalamic-pituitary insufficiency from sellar and suprasellar masses.

Treatment for these symptomatic issues is similar to that described for elevated ICP. Dexamethasone is effective in reducing neural compression by decreasing edema and may significantly improve the symptoms. Often, however, surgical decompression of the affected structure by removal of the offending mass is required for improvement. If the symptoms are related to endocrine insufficiency, replacement therapy is the most effective method of improving the clinical condition. In the specific instance of visual loss from a sellar or suprasellar mass with an elevated prolactin level (usually a pituitary prolactinoma), treatment with bromocriptine (Parlodel) may rapidly shrink the tumor and improve vision.

Immediate and Long-term Symptoms Related to Treatment

Over the years, the treatment of patients with brain tumors has become more intensive, resulting in better response and survival rates. These more aggressive therapies are also associated with morbidities that must be distinguished from tumor progression.

Although operative mortality has decreased significantly, medical and neurologic morbidities of neurosurgical procedures remain problematic. Postoperative infections, including subdural empyema and meningitis, can be significantly reduced by the administration of prophylactic antibiotics. Abscesses are particularly difficult to differentiate from tumor both radiographically and clinically. Fever and high leukocyte count may suggest infection, but they are not invariably present in patients who are taking steroids. Abscess should therefore be a consideration in any patient developing signs of neurologic deterioration postoperatively, especially if imaging studies reveal an enlarging concentric ring lesion.

Shunt malfunctions can also produce symptoms and signs mimicking tumor recurrence; correction will reverse symptoms and afford effective palliation. Therefore, a high index of suspicion for malfunction is required in tumor patients with shunts, and appropriate imaging studies must be performed before clinical worsening is attributed to tumor progression.

Radiation and chemotherapy, although mainstays of neuro-oncologic treatment, may also result in early and delayed neurologic side effects that may either mimic tumor recurrence or impair quality of life. External beam irradiation may result in symptomatic worsening either during its administration or as a delayed effect occurring from weeks to months after its completion. The early reactions are related to cerebral edema and usually respond to steroid administration. The delayed effects are more serious and usually represent a form of cerebral radionecrosis. This latter development is often indistinguishable, in conventional imaging studies and clinical manifestations, from tumor recurrence and represents a difficult diagnostic and therapeutic problem. We have found thallium 201, single photon emission computed tomography particularly useful in helping differentiate necrosis from recurrence; if decreased uptake in the area of imaging abnormality is noted, necrosis is the more likely diagnosis. Often, however, biopsy is the only way to make the diagnosis. Surgical excision is sometimes required for symptomatic relief. No medical treatments are very effective, although reports of improvement after therapeutic anticoagulation are promising.

A number of more subtle long-term complications also arise in irradiated patients. Endocrine deficiency is a common occurrence. This generally results from the effects of irradiation (and possibly chemotherapy) on the hypothalamus and pituitary. A decrease in gonadotropin hormones is most common, and patients frequently develop either amenorrhea or impotence. Thyroid dysfunction is also a common occurrence, and patients should be periodically screened for this problem.

A more vexing long-term complication of treatment is a deterioration in cognitive capabilities. Both very young and very old patients are particularly vulnerable to this development. Furthermore, the effects occur more frequently with higher total and fractionated doses of radiation and are probably aggravated by the addition of chemotherapy. The underlying pathologic process probably represents a leukoencephalopathy that is reflected by increased white matter abnormalities seen by magnetic resonance imaging (MRI). A gradual deterioration in cognitive abilities coupled with other signs of white matter dysfunction, especially gait dysfunction, characterize the disorder. Unfortunately, no effective treatments exist for this problem.

Deep Venous Thrombosis and Pulmonary Embolism

Deep venous thrombosis (DVT) and pulmonary embolism (PE) occur frequently in the brain tumor patient and present a difficult management problem. Immobilization of the patient and release of tissue thromboplastin from the brain tumor make peripheral venous thrombosis especially common in brain tumor patients, with incidence figures as high as 33%. Thrombosis can occur at any time of the disease, although it is more likely to develop in the first 6 weeks after craniotomy.

Patients with brain tumors who develop leg swelling or pain should be screened for DVT with impedance plethysmography. Patients who develop sudden shortness of breath or an encephalopathy of uncertain etiology should be evaluated for PE with radionuclide lung scanning. In those in whom DVT or PE is documented, treatment is indicated.

The optimal therapy remains uncertain because of the risk of anticoagulating a patient with a brain tumor who has recently undergone craniotomy. Placement of a Greenfield filter or other type of vena caval interruption procedure has been advocated as a safer alternative to anticoagulation in the immediate postoperative period (i.e., within 4 weeks). However, the documented long-term morbidities of this procedure make it a less desirable choice for other patients, especially because anticoagulation is relatively safe with an extremely low incidence of intracranial hemorrhage.

Although steroids are liberally used in patients with malignant brain tumors, they are not without serious long-term complications. Myopathy, glucose intolerance, osteoporosis, avascular necrosis of the hips, and mental status changes can all result from their use. Unfortunately, these problems often develop in a patient who needs the symptomatic benefit that steroids can provide. In these situations, oral glycerol (Osmoglyn), a potent osmotic diuretic that can achieve the same benefits as mannitol, can be substituted. Although the medication may be quite unpalatable for many patients, most tolerate it when it is mixed with orange juice. Frequently, its addition allows a reduction in or even discontinuation of glucocorticoid dosage.

DIAGNOSTIC ISSUES

Sometimes a definitive diagnosis of a brain lesion can be made on the basis of imaging and clinical criteria alone, such as when a cancer patient develops multiple enhancing lesions in the setting of progressive systemic disease. Often, however, establishing a definitive diagnosis is essential for planning specific therapy. Because tissue is required for a definitive diagnosis, a surgical procedure can be designed to make a tissue diagnosis as well as to decompress the lesion and improve symptoms. In some instances, however, diagnosis should be made by biopsy only, without specific therapeutic benefit to the patient.

Obviously, an adequate diagnostic work-up must be done before an appropriate surgical procedure can be performed. Patients between 20 and 40 years of age with parenchymal lesions are at risk for human immunodeficiency virus (HIV)–related central nervous system (CNS) masses. If the patient is HIV-positive, stereotactic biopsy can establish whether the lesion is related to an opportunistic infection or to CNS lymphoma. Conversely, patients older than 40 years are more likely to have metastatic lesions. Therefore, screening tests consisting of a rectal examination with stool guaiac, urinalysis, skin and breast examinations, complete blood count, and chest

radiograph may suggest a primary focus. If a primary lesion is identified, resection of a single parenchymal metastatic lesion will result in an improved prognosis. For multiple lesions, empirical radiotherapy is usual if a primary lesion is identified, and stereotactic biopsy can confirm the pathology if no primary lesion is found.

Most patients with newly diagnosed mass lesions do undergo some type of surgical procedure for either diagnostic or therapeutic purposes. Open craniotomy is necessary if therapeutic decompression (and acquisition of pathologic material) is desired. In most instances, this operation requires administration of general anesthesia. In some masses, such as meningiomas and metastatic neoplasms, there are well-defined planes between the tumor and the brain; these lesions can often be grossly totally removed. Other lesions, such as anaplastic astrocytoma and glioblastoma multiforme (GBM), send macroscopic or microscopic infiltrating fingers of tumor out from their tumor bulk; they can never be completely resected, but they can be significantly decompressed to reduce mass effect. If craniotomy is judged not to be indicated, stereotactic biopsy is the preferable means of acquiring tissue for diagnostic purposes. This procedure can be performed with local anesthetic using CT or MRI guidance with minimal risk.

The choice of which surgical approach to use depends on a number of factors, including neuroimaging appearance, whether symptoms of mass effect are present, and the patient's age. Extra-axial lesions are well suited for surgical excision, because they can often be totally removed. Lesions that are exerting significant mass effect on imaging studies are also suitable for surgical decompression if they do not involve eloquent cortical or subcortical structures. Stereotactic approaches are usually not appropriate for hemorrhagic lesions, which are probably better handled by craniotomy. On the other hand, lesions involving the deep nuclear structures of the thalamus, basal ganglia, and brain stem are usually not amenable to surgical decompression, even if they have significant mass effect. If multiple lesions are present, stereotactic biopsy is likewise preferred.

The patient's age is an important determinant of surgical approach. For many childhood tumors, the patient has a more favorable prognosis with more radical excision of the mass. Therefore, if the lesion is in a surgically accessible location, craniotomy for resection is preferable. On the other hand, very elderly patients may not tolerate craniotomy well. Unless the lesion has significant mass effect, stereotactic biopsy is indicated in such cases.

SPECIFIC THERAPEUTIC ISSUES

A tumor's histology becomes particularly important when one is considering specific therapies such as radiation, chemotherapy, and immune and endocrine therapies that are administered specifically to eradicate tumor or control its growth. Even in this particular area of treatment, however, other factors must be taken into account. For example, in the decision whether to administer radiation therapy, the patient's age must be taken into account, because of the high incidence of deleterious effects that occur in very young and very old patients.

The following brief survey orients the physician to some of the more common brain tumors encountered. Because these are relatively rare events for which many clinical investigations are ongoing, we advise that whenever possible, patients should be evaluated in settings where multidisciplinary (i.e., neurosurgery, radiation therapy, oncology) input is available.

Brain Metastasis

In patients older than 40 years, brain metastasis is the most common cause of brain tumor. Lung and breast cancers are the most frequent primary tumors; although most brain metastases develop late in the clinical course, when systemic cancer is obvious, they may also be evident at time of presentation and not uncommonly may herald the diagnosis. For this reason, newly diagnosed brain tumor patients should have at least a chest radiograph (CT of the chest in patients with a smoking history), mammogram, and urinalysis, and CT of the abdomen if there is a suspicion of an intra-abdominal or retroperitoneal lesion, before neurosurgical intervention.

The prognosis of patients with intracranial metastasis from systemic cancer is poor, with median survivals being less than 6 months. However, certain patients, especially those with no evidence of systemic disease at the time of neurologic presentation, may do much better.

From a therapeutic standpoint, brain metastases are approached differently depending on whether they are single or multiple. MRI most accurately determines the number of intracranial lesions. In patients with two or more lesions, whole-brain radiation therapy, generally consisting of 10 fractions of 300 cGy per fraction, is the treatment of choice. Because of the long-term neurologic side effects of this high-fractionation scheme, it has been our practice to administer an equivalent total dosage using only 200 cGy per dose in patients who are deemed to be capable of longer term survival. In addition, if one larger lesion, especially in the posterior fossa, is causing significant neurologic deficits unresponsive to dexamethasone, surgical decompression may rapidly improve symptoms.

Management of a single intracranial metastatic lesion depends on its location and the patient's symptoms. If the patient has a lesion in noneloquent brain or has significant symptoms of mass effect, surgical resection followed by radiation therapy provides the best long-term care. On the other hand, if the patient has minimal neurologic signs and the lesion is in or adjacent to eloquent brain, radiation therapy alone eliminates possible neurologic deficits related to surgery. Because of the many studies documenting better outcomes in surgically treated patients, it has been our approach to consider all patients with single

lesions, stable or inactive systemic disease, and reasonable performance status for surgical resection unless a contraindication exists.

High-Grade Gliomas

High-grade or malignant gliomas are the most commonly encountered primary brain tumors. They affect mostly middle-aged adults, although they can occur at any age. The most malignant tumor of this group is the GBM, characterized pathologically by the presence of endothelial proliferation and tissue necrosis. Anaplastic astrocytomas are distinguished from glioblastomas by the absence of necrosis. A number of factors affect prognosis; the patient's age (younger is most favorable), the presence of necrosis on pathologic section (unfavorable), and postoperative performance status are the most commonly associated factors.

Unfortunately, these tumors are incurable, and treatment is geared toward maximal palliation. Debulking of as much tumor as deemed safe, combined with postoperative external beam radiation therapy to maximal brain tolerance (approximately 60 Gy), is associated with median time to tumor progression in patients with GBM of less than a year. Increasing the radiation dosage has minimal added effect and increases toxicity, as do newer radiation therapy modalities such as stereotactic radiosurgery. The addition of chemotherapy, administered either as a single agent or in combination, modestly increases survival, mainly by increasing the number of longer term survivors. Patients with anaplastic astrocytomas have slightly better prognoses, and 5-year survivals, although uncommon, do occur.

Although chemotherapy is generally associated with at best a modest efficacy, reports indicate that a particular subtype of malignant glioma, the aggressive oligodendroglioma, may be particularly chemosensitive to a combination of procarbazine (Matulane), CCNU (lomustine [CeeNu]), and vincristine (Oncovin). A number of other experimental chemotherapies and immune therapies are currently being evaluated, but none so far has proved superior to the standard conventional approach of surgery, external beam irradiation, and single-agent chemotherapy.

Low-Grade Gliomas

Although gliomas represent a continuum of tumor types, it has been clinically useful to separate them into higher (i.e., malignant) and lower grades; however, it is important to remember that although clinically less aggressive, the low-grade tumors also are often incurable and represent low-grade malignancies rather than benign tumors. The most common tumor type is the diffuse fibrillary astrocytoma; oligodendroglioma and mixed tumor types are other important tumor types.

These tumors tend to occur at younger ages, usually between 20 and 50 years. They tend to arise in the cerebral hemispheres and manifest as a seizure or seizures. They pose a particularly difficult clinical problem when they produce an isolated seizure in an otherwise young, healthy patient whose imaging studies reveal an unenhancing supratentorial lesion without mass effect, because it is unclear whether early intervention results in improved outcome for the patient.

Unfortunately, although at the outset these tumors frequently behave indolently, at some point (usually within 7 to 8 years), they begin to behave more like their malignant counterparts. It is not clear whether early irradiation postpones this event or prolongs survival, although a number of retrospective series suggest this. It has been our practice to approach each case individually and make clinical decisions based on the potential for complete resection, the patient's age (the older the patient, the sooner the tumor will become more aggressive, so we tend not to postpone treatment), and the preference of the patient and physician.

Central Nervous System Lymphomas

Primary CNS lymphomas were once considered rare, but their incidence is increasing, especially in the acquired immune deficiency syndrome (AIDS) population but also in the elderly. These tumors are identical in histology to non-Hodgkin's lymphomas that occur systemically. They tend to be multifocal and occur in deep periventricular locations; however, it is impossible to distinguish these tumors from GBM preoperatively.

Owing to their oncolytic actions versus lymphomas, the administration of glucocorticoids may result in a complete disappearance of the lesion; when this occurs, it strongly suggests lymphoma as a diagnosis. On the other hand, because such therapy obscures the ability to make the diagnosis, it is recommended that at least a biopsy specimen be obtained if possible before the long-term administration of steroids in patients in whom lymphoma is suspected.

Stereotactic biopsy is indicated to make the diagnosis; retrospective data indicate that more extensive surgery may be associated with a poorer outcome. Radiotherapy affords long-term palliation, but the median survival of these patients is still only slightly longer than a year. A number of reports demonstrate that CNS lymphomas are sensitive to chemotherapy; effective regimens include high-dose methotrexate and more intensive therapies. We thus routinely administer chemotherapy preirradiation to newly diagnosed, non–immunosuppressed patients with CNS lymphoma.

In patients with AIDS and CNS lymphoma, irradiation offers effective palliation; although survival is not appreciably increased, the pattern of disease is changed, and patients generally succumb to other complications of their disease. Chemotherapy has not proved particularly effective in this cohort of patients, although ongoing studies continue.

Meningiomas

Meningiomas are extraparenchymal tumors that arise from leptomeningeal tissue and produce symptoms by compressing contiguous neural structures. They are benign in the sense that they can be cured if totally removed; if total removal is not possible, however, further tumor growth can occur, which can produce further neurologic deficits or death. Thus, the goal of surgery is total resection of the tumor and its dural attachment without damage to surrounding neural and vascular structures. This may not be possible if the tumor has invaded the skull base or is attached to neural or vascular structures the excision of which would cause unacceptable neurologic morbidity. In these instances, the goal of surgery should be to remove as much of the tumor bulk as possible.

If a complete resection can be performed, no further therapy is necessary. When only partial removals are accomplished, radiation therapy focused on the residual component of tumor can be just as effective in preventing recurrence as complete excision in the long term. Using a focused form of radiation minimizes the complications of radiation therapy on normal brain. No truly effective chemotherapeutic agent has been identified for adjuvant therapy. RU486 (mifepristone), the "morning after" birth control pill, has been shown to have some efficacy in some cases, but further study is necessary before this agent or others become part of the standard care.

Not all meningiomas require therapy. In many patients, lesions are discovered incidentally during evaluation of unrelated symptoms. In these cases, close follow-up with serial imaging every 6 months to a year can establish a growth pattern of the lesion. Surgical removal is indicated when progressive growth is documented or symptoms or signs develop.

Medulloblastomas

Medulloblastomas are primitive neuroectodermal tumors that arise most commonly in the cerebellum. They represent the most common malignant brain tumor of childhood. They affect mainly young children or adolescents; occurrence after 20 years of age is much less frequent. Until the early 1970s, less than one third of patients with medulloblastomas survived 5 years after treatment. Owing to several factors, including earlier diagnosis, safer anesthesia, advances in surgical techniques, improved postoperative care, and more effective use of radiotherapy, 5-year disease-free survival rates approaching 50% are now common.

Generally, patients can be characterized as those with average risk (no disseminated disease, no marked hydrocephalus, total or near-total resection, and age greater than 4 years), and those with poor risk (some combination of disseminated disease, hydrocephalus or tumor infiltration of the brain stem, a less than total resection, or age younger than 4 years). Medulloblastomas, unlike most other brain tumors, have a high likelihood of disseminating to other CNS sites early in the course of illness, and more than 30% of patients have either CSF cytologic or imaging evidence of leptomeningeal disease at diagnosis (which can be asymptomatic). Therefore, every newly diagnosed patient should have MRI of the spine, lumbar puncture for cytology, and bone marrow examination as part of the staging work-up.

Because many patients with medulloblastoma develop tumor outside the primary tumor site after local radiotherapy, the entire neuraxis is usually irradiated to improve long-term disease control. Conventionally, 36 cGy is given to brain and spine and an additional 20 cGy is administered to the local disease site. Children with poor-risk indicators may benefit from chemotherapy; other children do not. The optimal chemotherapy regimens for both initial and recurrent disease are currently being studied in prospective trials.

The Locomotor System

RHEUMATOID ARTHRITIS

method of
JOHN T. SHARP, M.D.
Tifton Medical Clinic
Tifton, Georgia

The course of rheumatoid arthritis (RA) is highly varied, and unfortunately clinical and laboratory features that correlate well with the future outcome in studies on groups of patients are of limited value in predicting disease progression in individual patients. A small percentage of patients have rapidly progressive disease from the onset with the development of major systemic manifestations, a rapid onset of disability, and early death. Other patients have a remitting course and mild disease that is easily managed during exacerbations and develop minimal disability, even many years after disease onset. The large majority of patients have relentlessly progressive disease that over time leads to erosion of juxta-articular bone, dissolution of cartilage, contracture of muscles and supporting soft tissues, joint deformities, major functional impairment, and some shortening of life expectancy.

Controlled therapeutic trials in RA, begun in the late 1940s, have become standard requirements for the introduction of new drugs and provide basic information on the short-term benefits and risks of new agents. As a result, we can state with confidence that several of the drugs available slow the rate of joint damage, but no agent currently available will completely halt disease progression in all patients, and not one is a cure. Furthermore, no truly long-term trials have ever been conducted, the longest being about 2 years, and most trials are 1 year or less. One year is a small fraction of the duration of disease in the average patient who has onset before the age of 50 years and has only a modest reduction in life expectancy.

The physician who wishes to take charge of the medical care of patients with RA must be familiar with the expected course of RA, the variability of the progression rate, and the usefulness of clinical and laboratory process measures and must have a clear set of treatment objectives. Periodic use of appropriate outcome measures is essential to assess the effectiveness of long-term treatment.

Pain relief is often the patient's primary reason for consulting a physician and must often be the physician's main short-term objective. At the same time, he or she must educate the patient in terms of the expected course of the disease and set the goal of treatment to control inflammation to achieve long-term pain control and prevent progressive joint damage. The physician must keep clearly in mind that the persistence of signs of joint inflammation accurately predicts future joint damage, whereas pain does not, an observation that has been repeatedly confirmed.

Modes of treatment available include physical and occupational therapy, several classes of drugs, and reconstructive surgery for patients with serious deformities. The principles of maintaining good muscle strength, a full range of motion, and joint protection and continuing a general exercise program to maintain whole-body condition should be explained to the patient on the first or second visit and as early as possible in the course of the disease. Many physicians will want to carry out this instruction themselves. Patients with more severe problems and persistent symptoms usually benefit greatly from a few visits to a physical therapist trained in managing patients with rheumatoid arthritis, and follow-up visits several times a year may be indicated.

A large number of drugs belonging to one of several classes are available for RA (Table 1). Only a small minority of patients with extremely mild disease or those with remitting disease who have short and nondestructive exacerbations do well for prolonged periods with a nonsteroidal anti-inflammatory drug (NSAID) without other treatment. The majority of patients require disease-controlling antirheumatic therapy (DCART) in addition to an NSAID to prevent or slow joint damage. Some may benefit from low-dose, intermittent corticosteroid therapy for short periods, but prolonged use of steroids is to be avoided. Instituting treatment early in the disease to antedate serious joint damage is an important goal. Even treatment that is effective in slowing or stopping bone and cartilage destruction will not lead to healing after cartilage is destroyed or large erosions have developed. Early disease in this context refers to that period before joint destruction occurs and cannot be defined in specific units of time. Some patients do not develop significant erosions or cartilage loss for months or years, but the majority of patients with continually active disease have some evidence of joint damage in 4 to 24 months, and a small number of patients may develop small erosions in a few weeks. Joint contractures and deformities due to soft tissue changes can also occur

TABLE 1. **Drugs Available to Treat Rheumatoid Arthritis**

Representative nonsteroidal anti-inflammatory drugs
    Etodolac (Lodine)*
    Nabumetone (Relafen)*
    Ibuprofen (Motrin)
    Fenoprofen (Nalfon)
    Meclofenamate (Meclomen)
    Diclofenac (Voltaren)
    Naproxen (Naprosyn)
    Piroxicam (Feldene)
Drugs used to control disease
    Sulfasalazine (Azulfidine)
    Hydroxychloroquine (Plaquenil)
    Minocycline (Dynacin, Minocin)
    Gold salts (Myochrysine, Solganal)
    Methotrexate (Rheumatrex)
    Azathioprine (Imuran)
    Cyclosporine (Sandimmune)

---

*Drugs thought to have the least gastrointestinal toxicity.

rapidly. Because the course of the disease in the early stages is even more unpredictable than later, the recommended treatment will vary depending on the duration of symptoms and the physical findings at the time the patient is first seen.

TREATMENT SCHEMES ARE TAILORED FOR DIFFERENT TYPES OF PRESENTATIONS

Arthralgia Without Joint Swelling

A patient who presents with mild or moderate joint pain of only a few days' duration and has no definite swelling on examination and a normal or only mildly elevated erythrocyte sedimentation rate (ESR) and/or C-reactive protein (CRP) can be treated initially with an NSAID alone for a short time while the physician observes the patient to determine whether the diagnosis will become more certain. Many such patients who are suspected of being in the earliest stages of RA have complete remission of symptoms without resolution of the diagnostic problem. In fact the majority of patients considered to have "possible" RA under an older arthritis classification system, in which this patient fits, have a remission and remain free of arthritis for 5 years or longer. Many never develop further manifestations of arthritis.

The choice of which NSAID to use depends in large measure on whether the patient is in the older age group and more prone to the gastrointestinal side effects of these drugs and whether the patient has a history of peptic ulcer disease, gastroesophageal reflux symptoms, or gastritis. Nabumetone has few or no adverse gastrointestinal effects but unfortunately is less effective in controlling arthritis symptoms than other NSAIDs. Acetaminophen does not induce gastritis or flare in ulcer disease but has little or no anti-inflammatory effect. Etodolac appears to have less gastrointestinal toxicity than many of the other NSAIDs, but the risk of bleeding or perforation of an ulcer is not eliminated. All patients given an NSAID should be advised of the risk of developing gastritis and ulcer disease and their complications. Simultaneous administration of misoprostol (Cytotec) or an H_2-blocking agent reduces the frequency of serious complications but does not eliminate them. Because the risk of death from the gastrointestinal side effects of NSAIDs is greatest in individuals older than 65 years, patients in this age group, as well as those with a prior history of peptic ulcer, should routinely be given medication for ulcer prophylaxis.

Persistent Swelling in Multiple Joints

Because treatment designed to slow or stop joint damage should not be long delayed in patients with active inflammation, careful and frequent observation of patients with early symptoms to detect the onset of joint swelling is necessary. Assuming that diagnostic studies have ruled out other causes of polyarthritis, when unequivocal joint swelling develops in several joints, particularly when multiple small joints are involved, a DCART along with an NSAID is prescribed. The treatment is the same for the patient who has unequivocal swelling in multiple joints when first seen.

In the initial stages of the disease, sulfasalazine (Azulfidine)* is recommended beginning with a dose of 500 mg twice daily to establish the patient's tolerance and increasing to 1 gram twice daily in 7 to 14 days if the blood count and urinalysis remain normal and no evidence of allergy develops. A further increase to 1 gram three times daily is considered after another 2 to 6 weeks if improvement is limited or negligible. Many patients do well on sulfasalazine along with an NSAID, and in some patients all signs of active synovitis disappear. If the patient remains symptom free without physical findings in the joints for 6 months or longer, the risk of stopping medication is discussed with the patient and a slow reduction in dose of sulfasalazine may be started. If the patient has been in complete remission for a year or longer and the dose has been reduced to 1 gram per day or less for several months, medication can be stopped with careful follow-up to detect exacerbation early if it occurs.

Steroid Use Should Be Very Limited

At any time during the course of the disease, if a single joint or small number of joints exhibit signs of severe inflammation and are the dominant symptom, after the physician rules out septic arthritis, intra-articular injection of a slow-acting steroid often provides relief that persists until a slower acting DCART becomes effective. Sterile gloves, needles, and syringes and single-dose vials of medication that are never reentered are used to avoid any risk of introducing an infection into a susceptible joint. After careful preparation of the skin and subcutaneous site, 40 to 80 mg† of triamcinolone hexacetonide mixed with 0.5 to 1 mL of lidocaine 2% is injected into the knee, shoulder, or ankle, and 20 to 30 mg† is injected into an elbow or wrist. The dose for finger joints is 5 to 8 mg.† Because there usually is a definite systemic effect of the intra-articular injection, only one large joint is injected at one time in most instances. Severe deterioration of joints that were repeatedly injected was seen when intra-articular steroid treatment was first introduced and excessive enthusiasm led to frequent, repeated injections. Consequently, it is recommended that intra-articular injection not be given in any one joint more often than two or three times per year. For this reason, the main value of joint injection is to help a patient manage an exacerbation while introducing other effective therapy that has a lag before suppressing inflammation. Care must be taken when a joint is injected to avoid introducing medication directly into a tendon, because this causes deterioration in the tendon, which may rupture at a later time.

---

*Not FDA approved for this indication.
*Exceeds dosage recommended by the manufacturer.

Patients who have severe symptoms and those who respond slowly may be given a short course of systemic steroids in an attempt to gain quicker control of the inflammatory process. When used in this way, prednisone is given in a single morning dose of 10 to 20 mg daily for 5 to 7 days, followed by 20 mg every second day, with dose reduction every 7 to 14 days. The patient is informed that steroids are expected to be withdrawn after 2 to 8 weeks.

Alternative DCART medication used as first treatment may be hydroxychloroquine (Plaquenil), 200 mg twice daily for 2 months and then once daily, or minocycline, 100 mg twice daily. General experience, confirmed by meta-analysis, indicates that hydroxychloroquine is not as effective as sulfasalazine. Minocycline (Minocin)* has not had broad enough usage to be ranked among the DCARTs, but controlled trials suggest that it has a limited effect or is effective in only a minority of patients. Personal experience suggests it should be ranked low among the DCARTs. Tenidap has been reported to substantially reduce the progression of joint damage in RA, but the drug has not yet been released, and exactly where it will fit in the treatment plan for the usual patient with RA is yet to be determined. If its toxicity profile, which is still being investigated, is found to be low, then it may be an appropriate drug for early treatment.

Poor Response to Initial Treatment

If the patient has little or no improvement and swelling persists in multiple joints after a 2- to 4-month trial of sulfasalazine* or alternative DCART, or if a steroid is required to control symptoms and there is difficulty in withdrawing it, the patient is advised that gold or methotrexate treatment is more likely to control the disease process. After thorough explanation of the toxic effects of these medications, treatment is changed to either intramuscular gold or oral methotrexate, whichever is elected. The majority of patients elect methotrexate because it is taken by mouth and has fewer early side effects. It also has a shorter lag period before effectiveness is apparent. Some elect gold because of the risk of serious liver disease with long-term use of methotrexate, and patients who are unwilling to give up alcoholic beverages or who already have some form of liver disease should not be given methotrexate. The initial dose of methotrexate is 7.5 mg *once each week*. Weekly dosing should be emphasized to the patient because so few medications are given at this interval; the patient may not hear instructions unless special attention is given to getting this point across. It must be stressed that the mistaken use of methotrexate daily in this dose can lead to disastrous toxicity. If the patient does not have definite and marked improvement after 4 weeks, the dose is increased stepwise to 15 mg per week at intervals of every 2 to 4 weeks. Infrequently, the dose is increased to 20 mg weekly,

*Not FDA approved for this indication.

usually only in large, nonobese patients. Initially, a complete blood count is obtained weekly to monitor bone marrow toxicity. After 1 month, the blood is checked at 2- to 4-week intervals, except for the first week after the dose is increased. The majority of patients improve symptomatically when given methotrexate. Most have prompter improvement in symptoms than decrease in signs of inflammation. If no improvement has occurred after 6 to 10 weeks of methotrexate therapy at 15 mg per week, treatment failure is probable, and if there is no benefit in 12 to 16 weeks, there is little hope that continuing treatment will induce a response.

Intramuscular gold may be given as a water-soluble compound, Myochrysine, or as a suspension in oil, Solganal. The water-soluble compound is preferable unless the patient develops nitritoid reactions, manifested by flushing and tachycardia. Before injections are started, a careful history is taken to rule out gold allergy, which is most often manifest as a rash at sites of contact with gold-containing jewelry. Even patients with a negative allergy history are given a test dose of 5 mg intramuscularly. If the patient remains free of rash for 5 days, weekly injections of 50 mg of Myochrysine or Solganal are begun. A complete blood count with platelet count and differential and a urinalysis are obtained before each injection, and the patient is questioned about rash, itching, mouth ulcers, cough, dyspnea, and diarrhea as long as gold is given. Some patients notice a decrease in morning stiffness and joint pain in the first 4 to 6 weeks, but most patients will not have clear evidence of benefit until treatment has been continued for 2 to 3 months. Injections are continued at weekly intervals until 8 to 10 weeks after all signs and symptoms of inflammation have disappeared or until the total cumulative dose of gold compound is 1 to 1.5 grams. If no improvement has occurred after 5 to 6 months, the likelihood of a later response is remote. In those patients who have remission of all signs of inflammation, the injection interval is reduced to every 2 weeks for 6 months and then if the patient continues to do well to every 3 weeks. If the patient remains in complete remission for 18 months or longer, discontinuation of injections is considered and discussed with the patient, but there are no helpful data to guide the physician in advising the patient as to the likelihood of exacerbation. There is no scientific basis for giving gold injections at intervals longer than every 4 weeks.

Poor Response to Methotrexate or Gold

There is no clear answer to the question of how to advise patients who have had an unsatisfactory response to gold or methotrexate. If only one of the two drug therapies has failed and there are no contraindications, the patient may be given a course of the alternative drug. However, because at this point the patient will have had continual joint inflammation for several months, there is real concern that irreversible joint damage has already begun or is imminent. At this point, a trial of combinations of DCARTs is recommended by some experts. Other possibilities are treatment with azathioprine (Imuran) or cyclosporine (Sandimmune).* Larger doses of steroids provide some symptomatic relief for most patients, but such a course is almost always associated with serious side effects and is not recommended.

Only one combination has proved effective in a carefully controlled trial. Combining methotrexate, hydroxychloroquine, and sulfasalazine resulted in greater responses than treatment with methotrexate alone or the combination of sulfasalazine* and hydroxychloroquine. Experience with this drug combination is still limited, so the physician who offers this treatment regimen to an RA patient should proceed with extreme caution and thorough monitoring for possible side effects, although this combination was well tolerated in the reported trial.

In spite of the enthusiasm expressed by some rheumatologists for combinations of DCARTs, controlled trials of combinations are few and all but the combination just discussed previously have been disappointing. No better results were seen in patients treated simultaneously with methotrexate and gold than with either agent alone. Combining penicillamine and hydroxychloroquine gave results worse than those with a single treatment. Azathioprine and methotrexate given together did not improve responses over treatment with methotrexate alone. Anecdotal reports of greater improvement with other combinations are impossible to evaluate because of serious bias in selecting patients, the lack of a constant study design, the frequent use of variable doses of steroids, and the lack of meaningful comparisons. Whether combining two drugs known to be partially effective will result in an improved response in the patient in whom a single agent has failed to produce a satisfactory result cannot be answered in more detail at this time. In the meantime, the practicing physician should recommend proven treatment whenever possible and must recommend unproven treatment with great caution, making it quite clear to the patient that he or she is embarking on unproven, experimental therapy with potentially serious side effects. Cyclosporine given in a dose of 5 mg per kg or greater is frequently associated with significant loss of renal function in treatment intervals as short as 6 to 12 months. In one study, a reduction of the dose of cyclosporine to 2.5 mg per kg resulted in a smaller loss of renal function with what was judged to be an acceptable decrease in therapeutic benefit. However, in view of the long duration of treatment required in RA, even a small decrease in renal function, if progressive, may carry too great a risk of renal failure to be acceptable.

Azathioprine has been used extensively in Europe and Canada, but in my experience it is not as effective as gold and methotrexate and is used only in patients in whom other treatments have failed or in those with milder forms of rheumatoid vasculitis. Cyclophosphamide (Cytoxan)* was tried in RA in the 1960s, but long-term use was associated with increased incidence of tumors and is contraindicated except in those patients who have vasculitis with visceral, life-threatening involvement.

OSTEOPOROSIS IS A COMMON OCCURRENCE IN RHEUMATOID ARTHRITIS

Because RA is more common in women, osteoporosis is common in RA patients. Reduced physical activity and the common use of steroids increase the likelihood of developing symptomatic bone disease, and there is some evidence that the systemic effects of generalized inflammation induce earlier and perhaps more severe osteoporosis. All patients with RA should be instructed in exercises and prescribed calcium and vitamin D supplementation to lessen bone loss and delay the onset of pathologic fractures with special emphasis for those on steroids. Patients in whom steroid therapy is started should be given cyclical etidronate (Didronel),* calcitonin injections (Calcimar), or estrogen replacement therapy for postmenopausal women to counteract the steroid bone-wasting effect. Alendronate (Fosamax)* and pamidronate (Aredia)* are being tested to determine their effectiveness in counteracting the bone loss induced by corticosteroids. Because the new bisphosphonates are more effective than etidronate in reducing osteoclast activity and have less effect on osteoblasts, if trials prove them to be effective and free of serious side effects, they will be the preferred prophylactic agents in most cases. Estrogens have been reported to reduce the extent of osteoporosis in glucocorticoid-treated postmenopausal patients and are an important option for the patient who does not have a family history of breast cancer. A progestin should be used with estrogen in each patient who still has her uterus.

OBESITY SHOULD BE AVOIDED, AND PATIENTS SHOULD MAINTAIN GOOD GENERAL CONDITIONING

Measures recommended to maintain good general health include a diet designed to avoid both obesity and excessive weight loss. There is some evidence that a diet rich in saturated fats may increase the symptoms of active synovitis and large amounts of polyunsaturated fats may reduce symptoms. The quantity of fat required to produce this limited relief is outside the usual intake, making fish oil and other unsaturated fat products of little practical significance for the ordinary patient. A general exercise program is prescribed to help the patient reduce pain and maintain a sense of well-being. Exercise specifically tailored to the individual patient's joint involvement helps maintain joint function and delays or

---

*Not FDA approved for this indication.

*Exceeds dosage recommended by the manufacturer.

prevents joint deformities. Joint use should be non-stressful when possible. Exercise for weight-bearing joints should not include jogging, running, long-distance walking, or other activities that include repetitive high impact. Power use of the upper extremities should be replaced by range-of-motion exercises. Exercising against water resistance in a heated swimming pool, when available, is optimal but not essential. Dipping the hands in hot wax is often quite soothing and in addition requires exercising the fingers to remove the wax coat that forms. Care must be taken to carefully control the temperature of the wax to prevent burns, and wax should never be used over an open flame because of the risk of fire.

SURGICAL MEASURES ARE HELPFUL IN REHABILITATING THE PATIENT WITH SOME TYPES OF DEFORMITIES

Patients who have long-standing disease without complete control of inflammation eventually develop irreversible damage and deformities with functional limitation. Some surgical procedures may provide relief of pain and improved function. In the feet, resection of the metatarsal heads and realignment of the toe proximal interphalangeal (PIP) joints often provide dramatic relief of foot pain and restoration of pain-free weight bearing. Sometimes a prosthesis can be used to replace the metatarsophalangeal (MTP) joint of the big toe in combination with resection of the other MTP joints. Surgical arthrodesis of the MTP joints in my experience has not been successful and should be avoided.

Total joint replacement for hip and knee involvement is usually successful if bone stock is not severely osteoporotic from long-term disuse and steroid therapy. Wrist and shoulder joint replacement procedures are frequently successful in the hands of experienced orthopedists but are infrequently performed by the general orthopedist. Total joint replacement for elbows and ankles has not been regularly successful and needs further refinement. Patients who have had joint prostheses implanted will be more susceptible to septic arthritis for the rest of their lives, and this susceptibility is increased by the use of steroids and immunosuppressive drugs. All endoscopies and dental and surgical procedures on these patients should be done with antibiotic prophylaxis.

Cervical spine involvement is common in RA and may lead to serious spinal cord damage in patients with disease of several years' duration. All patients undergoing surgery, general anesthesia with intubation, bronchoscopy, or gastroesophagoscopy should have lateral cervical spine films taken before the procedure with the neck in the flexed and extended positions to rule out C1–2 instability. Patients who develop symptoms of intermittent cord compression from C1–2 displacement have a good chance of improvement with surgical fusion, but success is not universal. The asymptomatic patient who has 8 mm or more of displacement of C1 on C2 is a candidate for elective cervical fusion. In formulating advice for this patient, the physician must weigh the risks of the surgery, the prolonged restricted mobility in the postoperative period, and the frequent failure of fusion against the risk of sudden, unheralded spinal cord injury with irreversible effects.

OUTCOME MEASURES ARE USED TO JUDGE THE EFFECTIVENESS OF TREATMENT

Measuring the effectiveness of therapy for RA is a serious challenge for all who undertake treatment of these patients. The problem requires selecting the appropriate methods to assess inflammation in the active stages of the arthritis and to measure joint damage in persisting disease. Evaluating the results of these measurements requires some knowledge of the expected course of the disease. If responses were dichotomous, namely, treatment either induced a complete remission or had no effect, then assessing response to treatment would be quite simple. Unfortunately, we do not have agents that accomplish this goal regularly or frequently. The physician instead commonly observes some improvement occurring slowly over a few weeks and is left to wonder whether the modest improvement is a response to treatment or a spontaneous change in disease, the "brownian movement" of disease expression. Regularly spaced, repeated observation of several key features of the disease permits the physician to visualize changes in disease activity over time and provides a reasonable basis for continuing or changing treatment. A visual analogue scale is useful in assessing pain. The modified health assessment questionnaire is simple and quickly filled out and provides basic data on daily functions. Physical examination should record the swollen joints, and an ESR or CRP provides an index of inflammatory activity. These observations should be made at 4- to 6-week intervals when treatment is first started or treatment is changed because of a flare or poor response to prior treatment. If the patient is doing well with limited evidence of disease activity, recording these objective indices of disease activity two or three times a year for 1 or more years provides invaluable baseline data if the patient has a later flare. In prolonged remissions, recording this information once yearly and sometimes even less frequently may be adequate. A detailed record of joint deformities every 4 to 12 months is important in long-term follow-up. Yearly radiographs of the hands and feet during periods of active disease and for 1 or 2 years after apparent remission occurs provide a permanent record and the best information on the progression of joint damage. Comparison of joint films over the course of the disease gives a clear indication of the effectiveness of treatment when interpreted along with observations on joint swelling and a plot of the ESR or CRP. In interpreting films, a simple count of the number of metacarpophalangeal, PIP, intercarpal, and MTP joints that show erosions and/or joint space narrowing gives an index of the severity of the disease that correlates well with more detailed scoring methods that are used in controlled trials. A count of the joints that have developed new erosions or have become narrowed when comparing films done at intervals gives an indication of whether treatment is controlling joint damage, but the physician should keep in mind that there is a lag phase before treatment becomes effective with most agents, so that new erosions in the first 4 to 8 months of treatment may not represent treatment failure if other evidence of response is present, such as complete resolution of joint swelling and normalization or marked drop in ESR or CRP.

ADVERSE DRUG REACTIONS ARE COMMON

Adverse reactions to drugs occur all too often with the agents used in the treatment of RA, and patients must be thoroughly informed of these risks before beginning any medication regimen and constantly monitored as long as therapy with these drugs is continued. As mentioned earlier, gastritis and peptic ulcer disease are common side effects with all the NSAIDs with the possible exception of nabumetone. Diarrhea is fairly common with meclofenamate (Meclomen) and diclofenac (Voltaren) and less common with other NSAIDs. Some patients receiving prolonged treatment develop an enteropathy with extensive small bowel inflammation. Toxic hepatitis is an infrequent but serious complication that may occur with any of the NSAIDs, and a liver chemistry profile is recommended in the first 6 to 8 weeks after starting treatment and two to four times a year while treatment is continued. Bronchospasm is frequently aggravated or induced in patients who have asthma, and some patients develop nasal polyps. Interstitial nephritis is an uncommon but potentially serious NSAID reaction because continued treatment will likely lead to renal failure. Most cases are nonprogressive and perhaps reversible when caught early and NSAID ingestion is stopped. It is not clear whether switching to another NSAID is safe in this situation.

Gold injections are associated with frequent side effects. Monitoring for gold toxicity is important for reducing the risk of prolonging serious reactions. A complete blood count, including a platelet count and differential, and a urinalysis are performed and the results carefully reviewed before each injection. The patient is queried about symptoms related to skin, pulmonary, and gastrointestinal reactions. Rashes are common, occurring in approximately 15% of patients. Lesions vary from trivial, small, itching, keratotic plaques to life-threatening and sometimes fatal toxic epidermatolysis and exfoliative dermatitis. Any generalized rash requires stopping medication, and if the rash continues to spread or vesicular or bullous lesions develop, steroid therapy is needed. Toxic epidermatolysis is best treated in a burn unit with measures to reduce serum loss and to prevent infection.

Bone marrow toxicity is the most frequent life-threatening adverse reaction to gold injections, occurring in about 1% of patients. Thrombocytopenia and agranulocytosis are usually reversible in a few weeks so that most patients survive if the reaction is caught early and if treatment is effective in controlling bleeding and infection. Aplastic anemia occurs rarely and responds irregularly to treatment with cytotoxic drugs and bone marrow transplantation.

Renal toxicity is manifest by proteinuria, which may persist for a prolonged period after stopping gold injections but eventually clears without apparent residuals. Progressive renal damage leading to kidney failure is apparently quite rare. Pulmonary toxicity is an infrequent complication that presents as interstitial lung disease and may rapidly lead to pulmonary failure. Most patients respond to steroid therapy and survive with the use of respiratory support during the exudative and inflammatory phase of the reaction. In some patients gold induces an enteropathy. Diarrhea can be severe, with 15 or more bowel movements per day that can persist for months. Weight loss can be extensive in these patients. Toxic hepatitis was thought to be common in the early days of use of this agent, but when the viral cause of hepatitis was discovered, it was apparent that most of these cases were due to improper needle and syringe technique. An occasional case of toxic hepatitis is still seen in patients receiving gold, but most of these patients are also taking an NSAID, and determining which is the cause has not been possible. Neuritis is a rare reaction to gold therapy.

Methotrexate has fewer side effects than gold therapy in the early stages of treatment but is not free of significant reactions. Rashes are uncommon. Bone marrow suppression is dose related and forms the basis for increasing the dose stepwise when initiating treatment. Patients who are receiving antifolates, e.g., anticonvulsants, should be started with small doses, and the dose should be raised more slowly in these patients. Some physicians routinely give folic acid while administering methotrexate, but the evidence is not clear that folic acid does more than increase the dose of methotrexate required to achieve optimal clinical benefit. In therapeutic mishaps when an excessive dose of methotrexate is mistakenly taken, citrovorum factor (leucovorin calcium [Wellcovorin]) limits serious toxicity if given within the first 12 to 24 hours after methotrexate.

Interstitial lung disease occurs regularly in patients taking methotrexate, perhaps as often as 1 to 2%. Fatal reactions have been reported, and prompt diagnosis with institution of respiratory support and steroid therapy is important in rescuing these patients. Gastrointestinal reactions to methotrexate include nausea, vomiting, abdominal pain, and diarrhea, which can frequently be avoided by giving the medication parenterally.

Cirrhosis of the liver occurs in patients who receive long-term therapy with methotrexate and is serious because it is not reversible and is associated with a high mortality. Alcohol intake increases the risk of developing cirrhosis and should be avoided by all patients. Patients who are not willing to forgo alcohol should not be treated with this drug. The risk of cirrhosis is related to the total or cumulative dose. It is not thought that ingestion of less than 1500 mg of methotrexate is associated with a significant risk, which for the average patient means that the first 100 to 150 weeks of treatment are unlikely to cause cirrhosis. In one survey the reported incidence of cirrhosis was 1 in 1600 patients at 5 years of treatment, but went up much more rapidly in the second 5 years. It is thought that the polyglutamates of folic acid that are a regular product of methotrexate metabolism and are stored in the liver with an extremely long half-life may be responsible for the liver fibrosis. Study has begun on methotrexate congeners that are more completely metabolized in the hope that they will retain therapeutic effect and cirrhosis will be avoided.

Patients taking methotrexate should have a weekly complete blood count for 2 to 4 weeks when the drug is first started and after each upward adjustment in dose. If the patient has tolerated a constant dose for several weeks, monthly blood counts are usually adequate for monitoring the bone marrow effects. Liver chemistry profiles are checked monthly when the drug is first started. If these remain normal for 3 to 4 months the liver chemistry profiles are checked every 3 to 4 months for the first 5 years of treatment and thereafter every 1 to 2 months. Some experts advise a liver biopsy after 5 years because liver chemistry profiles are not sensitive in detecting the early stages of cirrhosis. The drug must be stopped if liver chemistry profiles are abnormal for 2 months or longer and if a biopsy shows early signs of cirrhosis.

Sulfasalazine* is generally well tolerated. Rash and bone marrow suppression are the most frequent reactions. The rash is frequently urticarial, but any type of drug eruption may occur. Leukopenia and thrombocytopenia are the most common bone marrow reactions and are reported to occur in 1 to 2% of patients. The effects on blood usually are not abrupt, so a complete blood count 2 weeks after initiating therapy and monthly thereafter usually detects counts that are slowly declining before severe reactions occur. Interstitial nephritis is an occasional reaction, and rarely toxic hepatitis has been reported.

Hydroxychloroquine can cause macular degeneration, and its use must be monitored by an ophthalmologist. Ocular reactions are thought to be partly dose related, so prolonged use of doses greater than 400 mg daily are not recommended, and 200 mg is preferred. Rash, gastrointestinal symptoms, and occasionally depression of leukocyte and platelet counts are other side effects of hydroxychloroquine.

Minocycline* may cause a rash, and some patients develop nausea. Penicillamine has a large number of side effects. Penicillamine may induce rash, leukopenia, thrombocytopenia, myopathy, myasthenia, proteinuria and nephrotic syndrome, and other connective tissue disease–like reactions. Because of these

*Not FDA approved for this indication.

side effects, together with its low efficacy, penicillamine is rarely recommended. Azathioprine causes bone marrow suppression in a dose-related fashion, and patients taking the drug must be carefully monitored because the effective dose is close to the toxic level. In addition, evidence has raised the possibility that lymphomas may be more frequent in subjects who have taken azathioprine for a prolonged period. Cyclosporine* has serious renal toxicity as discussed previously, and hepatotoxicity has been seen in some transplant patients.

FUTURE TREATMENT

In the last decade, much has been learned about the mechanism of synovial inflammation in RA, and this has resulted in the development of new and novel drugs that are now being tested for therapeutic benefit and safety. The most promising of these block the inflammatory effects of interleukin-1 and tumor necrosis factor-α. In addition, monoclonal antibodies to the CD4$^+$ lymphocyte antigen have the ability to modulate the synovial lymphocyte infiltration. None of these agents are close to being sufficiently well tested to be released. Although none of the new agents being tested may prove to be appropriate for general use, it is clear that the development of new therapeutic agents is now more firmly derived from a rational, scientific base, so the outlook for more effective treatment in the future is brighter than ever.

*Not FDA approved for this indication.

JUVENILE RHEUMATOID ARTHRITIS

method of
ROBERT W. WARREN, M.D., PH.D., M.P.H.
Baylor College of Medicine
Houston, Texas

Juvenile rheumatoid arthritis (JRA) is a chronic disease of joints and other tissues that affects approximately 250,000 children in the United States. JRA is subdivided into three major subgroups, based on the clinical course in the first 6 months of illness. These subgroups are (1) systemic, characterized by spiking fevers, evanescent rash, and other extra-articular disease; (2) pauciarticular, with four or fewer affected joints; and (3) polyarticular, with five or more affected joints. Only a small minority of JRA patients have an illness like adult rheumatoid arthritis (RA); unlike adults with RA, the majority of children who are treated appropriately recover from JRA without significant disability. The mortality rate in the United States is less than 1%.

JRA must be differentiated from arthritis of other causes. Indeed, more likely causes of childhood arthritis include trauma and infectious and postinfectious etiologies. Whereas these processes usually resolve over days to weeks, the arthritis of JRA persists in at least one joint for a minimum of 6 weeks. The formal diagnosis of JRA also requires age at onset younger than 16 years and exclusion of other inflammatory joint diseases. There are no diagnostic laboratory tests; antinuclear antibody (ANA) and rheumatoid factor assist in subclassification of JRA, but not its diagnosis.

GENERAL MANAGEMENT

There is no specific cure for JRA. No medication safely and totally quells the inflammation of JRA. Continuing or recurrent inflammation produces secondary phenomena, including joint destruction, soft tissue contractures, and growth abnormalities, with accompanying psychologic trauma.

MEDICAL FOLLOW-UP

Excellent home- and community-based care is critical for the child with JRA, but every child with active JRA should also be evaluated periodically by a health care team that specializes in the care of children with arthritis. The frequency of such visits depends on the diagnosis and the problems of specific patients but should be no less frequent than annually. A systemic JRA flare or acutely increased joint symptoms in any JRA patient should command immediate medical attention.

EDUCATION AND COUNSELING OF FAMILY AND PATIENT

The family's understanding and commitment to the care of the child with JRA is the most critical element in management. Common family concerns are physical deformity and the possible dangers of physical therapy and aspirin therapy. The physician's role in education of the patient and family should be supplemented by literature on diseases and medication, family support groups (such as those sponsored by the parent-run American Juvenile Arthritis Organization), and professional assistance by rheumatology nurses, social workers, and child psychologists.

Family anxieties and concerns are normal. On the other hand, the JRA-provoked psychosocial dysfunction in the patient and family may far outstrip and outlast active or even residual joint disease. The need for psychosocial intervention must be periodically assessed.

MEDICATIONS

Nonsteroidal Anti-inflammatory Drugs

Nonsteroidal anti-inflammatory drugs (NSAIDs) remain first-line medical therapy for all forms of JRA. Responses to NSAID therapy generally occur within weeks. Despite the fact that no one NSAID has proved to be more efficacious than the others, there are differences in chemical structure and unpredictable differences in a patient's response; thus, changing to another NSAID is reasonable in therapeutic failures. On the other hand, the rare child with aspirin allergies should not be given any other NSAID. Although anecdotally successful, the simultaneous use of two NSAIDs has not been carefully studied in JRA, nor is the practice approved by the Food and Drug Administration, because of the risk of significant additive side effects.

Used for decades for children with JRA, aspirin is inexpensive and efficacious; no other NSAID is clearly superior. Compliance with aspirin therapy is much easier to measure than that with other drugs, although more difficult to obtain because of the frequency of administration and parental worries about aspirin's efficacy and about Reye's syndrome. Aspirin is often begun in doses as low as 80 mg per kg per day to decrease the chance of toxicity, but 90 to 100 mg per kg per day (to a maximum of 4 grams per day) divided three or four times daily is usually required for a therapeutic serum salicylate level of 20 to 30 mg per dL. Illnesses affecting gastrointestinal absorption, low serum albumin levels, other medications, and aspirin coating can influence the obtained level. Levels should be reached 7 to 10 days after the initiation or any change of therapy, including the institution or withdrawal of other drugs, or with the advent of any signs of salicylate toxicity (e.g., tinnitus, hyperpnea).

A number of prescription salicylate derivative drugs are marketed, including choline magnesium trisalicylate (Trilisate), which is approved for use in children. Potential advantages include twice-daily dosing, a liquid form (500 mg per 5 mL), less gastrointestinal intolerance, and the lack of an effect on platelet function. Disadvantages include higher cost and the lack of a chewable, small children's tablet. Dose ranges are identical to those of aspirin.

Many other NSAIDs are used by pediatric rheumatologists in the care of children with JRA, although only tolmetin (Tolectin) and naproxen (Naprosyn) are currently approved for use in children from 2 to 14 years of age. Tolmetin is available in 200-mg tablets and 400-mg capsules, and therapy should be initiated at 20 mg per kg per day divided into 3 doses and increased to 30 mg per kg per day (maximum 1.6 grams per day) if well tolerated. Tolmetin bioavailability is decreased by food and milk. Naproxen is available in 250-, 375-, and 500-mg tablets as well as a suspension of 125 mg per 5 mL. Naproxen may be given on a twice-daily schedule, with doses of approximately 15 mg per kg per day (maximum 1 gram per day). Other commonly used NSAIDS include ibuprofen (Motrin), 40 mg per kg per day in three or four divided doses (maximum 2.4 grams per day); diclofenac (Voltaren), 2 to 3 mg per kg per day in two divided doses; and indomethacin (Indocin),* 1.5 to 3 mg per kg per day, in two to four divided doses depending on form (maximum 150 mg daily). Indomethacin is often considered the most potent NSAID, but its usefulness is sometimes limited by dosing schedules and side effects, particularly those affecting the central nervous system. Physicians

---

*Not FDA approved for this indication.

should be aware that the lower dose, over-the-counter versions of naproxen, ibuprofen, and other NSAIDS may be more appropriate and less expensive.

Potential adverse effects of NSAID therapy include gastrointestinal symptoms, such as vomiting, abdominal pain, gastritis, ulcer disease, and constipation. Parents should report complaints of abdominal pain, vomiting, and hematochezia. Although children seem less likely to develop these problems than adults, they are not exempt and should thus take NSAIDs with meals or snacks. Buffered products offer little additional protection. Antacids, sucralfate (Carafate), and H$_2$ blockers such as ranitidine (Zantac) are used with variable effect, and misoprostol (Cytotec) is occasionally used. A hemoglobin level or hematocrit and red blood cell indices should be obtained at least every 4 months to assess occult blood loss. Mild liver function abnormalities sometimes occur in children taking NSAIDs; rarely, children develop significant hepatitis or even liver failure, which is generally rapidly reversible. Liver function studies should be obtained within 1 month of beginning or changing therapy and thereafter, if values are normal, as indicated by careful physical examination. Liver function should be more closely monitored and NSAID therapy decreased if serum transaminase values consistently exceed twice normal. Therapy should be temporarily discontinued with significant transaminase elevation and then restarted at a lower dose after recovery. NSAIDs, and particularly salicylates, should be temporarily discontinued when there is a presumed increased risk for Reye's syndrome (e.g., after exposure to influenza or chickenpox).

Renal effects of NSAIDs include hematuria and decreased creatinine clearance. Urinalysis should be performed every 3 to 4 months, and blood urea nitrogen and serum creatinine levels every 6 months. Some nephrologists recommend that creatinine clearance be checked yearly. Finally, significant central nervous system effects (e.g., hallucinations) are rare adverse effects of aspirin and other NSAIDs that necessitate discontinuance of the drug.

Other Agents

In most patients, NSAIDs alone will not control the polyarticular arthritis of systemic or polyarticular JRA, as judged by clinical examination and evidence of progressive, erosive joint disease by diagnostic imaging. Therapy with other medications is then indicated, and NSAIDs are often continued. Given the natural history of polyarticular JRA, many subspecialists begin aggressive second-line medication early in the treatment program in the hope of preventing permanent joint changes.

For such children, the medication of choice is usually methotrexate,* typically in an oral dose of approximately 10 mg per m^2, once weekly. If this dose is ineffective, higher doses are sometimes used, and the medication may be given intramuscularly, subcutaneously, or intravenously as appropriate. Although methotrexate is generally well tolerated, parents are often reticent about the use of a chemotherapeutic drug; indeed, although the risks of secondary malignancy and decreased fertility are apparently quite small, they merit discussion. Teenagers should be particularly counseled about the risks of pregnancy, given the reported teratogenic effects of methotrexate, and birth control advised, as appropriate. Teenagers taking methotrexate should also be warned about the increased risk of liver damage with alcohol ingestion. Patients taking methotrexate should be monitored for liver and bone marrow toxicity with blood counts and chemistry profiles at least every 1 to 2 months. Renal function should also be studied periodically. Treatment with folic acid daily (0.5 to 1.0 mg orally) or folinic acid weekly the day after methotrexate administration (1.25 to 5 mg orally) may help limit side effects of methotrexate. Sulfasalazine* is also an appropriate second-line agent, particularly for patients with aggressive spondyloarthropathy, although it is generally considered not as potent as methotrexate. Dosage is 40 to 50 mg per kg per day in two divided doses, reaching the maximal dose with increments over 1 to 2 months with close monitoring for bone marrow toxicity, in particular. The coated preparation (Azulfidine EN-tabs) may be better tolerated in terms of nausea. As with methotrexate, laboratory monitoring is essential.

Children who do not respond well to methotrexate and NSAID therapy are sometimes treated with steroids (see later), but experimental combination therapy is also sometimes used by pediatric rheumatologists. Methotrexate therapy is typically continued and used with hydroxychloroquine (Plaquenil), sulfasalazine, cyclosporine (Sandimmune), or other agents. Azathioprine (Imuran) may also be used. Other experimental therapies include cyclophosphamide and intravenous immunoglobulin infusions. The efficacy of biologic agents for JRA is unknown, but preliminary studies suggesting the efficacy of agents such as anti–tumor necrosis factor in RA are encouraging. Of note, although approved for use in children, intramuscular gold is now only rarely used to treat children with JRA, because of a poorer benefit/risk ratio compared with methotrexate. Oral gold preparations are ineffective in children. Similarly, penicillamine is now an unusual therapy for children with JRA.

Corticosteroids

Systemic steroids are rarely used in the treatment of JRA. Intravenous steroids are indicated in the therapy of acutely ill children with systemic JRA and polyarticular JRA patients, who require hospitalization. Methylprednisolone (Solu-Medrol) may then be given intravenously, 0.25 to 0.5 mg per kg every 6 hours. Methylprednisolone may also be given in crises as pulse intravenous therapy, generally 30 mg

---

*Not FDA approved for this indication.

*Not FDA approved for this indication.

per kg per dose, to a maximum of 1 gram. In addition, systemic oral steroids are occasionally needed to control chronic symptoms in systemic JRA, such as severe anemia and rheumatoid lung disease. They may also rarely be necessary to control extremely active, severe polyarticular arthritis that is unresponsive to other medications. In these circumstances, oral prednisone is given daily or preferably every other day, in as low a dose as possible for therapeutic effect. Systemic steroids have no place in the therapy of pauciarticular JRA, except for severe uveitis. Possible benefits of systemic steroids must always be balanced against the well-described major short- and long-term risks, and these should be discussed in detail with the family.

Intra-articular steroid injections of triamcinolone hexacetonide (Aristospan) are now often used in the therapy of JRA. Intra-articular steroid injections have a role in pauciarticular JRA, as well as in flares of single and few joints in polyarticular disease. The recommended dosage is 5 to 40 mg of triamcinolone (depending on the age of the child and on the particular joint), which can be mixed with preservative-free lidocaine; this should be injected no more than twice a year per joint. Activity of the joint should be limited for 1 to 3 days after the injection. Although most patients respond well, there are potential problems associated with intra-articular injections. These include minimal or brief overall response, postinjection arthritis flare, and the psychologic trauma of intra-articular injection. Risks of bleeding, damage to joint cartilage, and infection should be minimal. Some systemic absorption of the drug may occur, and therefore brief adrenal suppression is theoretically possible. Secondary poor bone growth and weakness of surrounding structures near the injected joints have not been confirmed.

Topical steroids are used in the eye for treatment of uveitis (discussed later).

PHYSICAL AND OCCUPATIONAL THERAPY

Physical therapy and occupational therapy are essential elements in the treatment of JRA. The goals of therapy are to maintain and improve the range of motion, strength, and function. Specific guidelines and components for physical therapy for JRA include the following:

1. A home-, school-, and community-based exercise program should be planned and supervised by a licensed physical and/or occupational therapist. Normal activities that accomplish the desired joint motions should be strongly encouraged. Swimming and bicycle and tricycle riding are excellent activities for the child with JRA.

2. Splinting is used for many purposes in JRA, including reducing pain, protecting joints, improving contracture and muscle strength, and increasing function. Night splinting is a highly successful and standard technique for reducing peripheral joint con-

tractures, particularly at the wrist and knees. On the other hand, daytime use of immobilizing splints should at most be only a temporizing measure while other therapies are being instituted. Dynamic splints, which hold joint position and yet encourage specific joint motions against resistance to increase strength, are sometimes used in JRA patients. Shoe inserts and other orthotic devices such as metatarsal bars and pads, as well as comfortable, well-supported shoes, reduce pain. Serial casting is a technique occasionally used to reduce joint contractures unresponsive to physical therapy and splinting.

3. Localized therapy, and sometimes mild pain relievers such as acetaminophen, can be extremely useful in decreasing joint stiffness and discomfort. Warm baths, local application of moist heat, and frequent changes of position can combat joint stiffness. "Icing" a joint can temporarily decrease discomfort and is used as an adjunct in serial casting.

SURGERY

Orthopedists should see children with severe leg length discrepancy, cervical spine disease, and subluxed and/or extremely restricted joint movement or severe pain. However, surgery is not a cure for JRA; in fact, synovectomy may worsen the disease. On the other hand, surgery can be extraordinarily valuable as a reconstructive modality. Unilateral epiphyseal stapling can improve leg length discrepancy in the growing child with asymmetrical pauciarticular arthritis. Specific operations to be considered in the child with severe deforming polyarticular arthritis include soft tissue releases, metatarsal head resection, pin traction for joint subluxation, and cervical spine stabilization. Selective joint replacement may be considered for the older adolescent and young adult patient.

PREVENTION AND TREATMENT OF EYE DISEASE

JRA is a major cause of blindness in children. Chronic, occult iridocyclitis is most common in ANA-positive pauciarticular JRA, and less common in systemic and polyarticular JRA. The risk for eye disease does not correlate with the activity of arthritis. Eye pain and photophobia are uncommon complaints, and ophthalmoscopic examination rarely suggests uveitis until significant eye damage has occurred. Thus, slit-lamp examination must be done as frequently as every 6 weeks in the young, female, ANA-positive, new pauciarticular JRA patient; in the older patient with systemic or polyarticular JRA, the examination should be performed at least annually. The consulting ophthalmologist should direct any needed therapy for iritis, which generally includes topical steroids and a mydriatic agent.

ANKYLOSING SPONDYLITIS AND OTHER SPONDYLOARTHROPATHIES

method of
FRANK C. ARNETT, M.D.

The University of Texas–Houston Health Science
*   Center*
Houston, Texas

DEFINITIONS AND ETIOPATHOLOGIC CONSIDERATIONS

Ankylosing spondylitis (AS) is a member of a family of chronic systemic inflammatory diseases termed the "spondyloarthropathies" (SpAs) (Table 1). These disorders are characterized by an inflammatory process affecting spinal joints (sacroiliitis, spondylitis) and/or peripheral joints (arthritis), as well as axial and peripheral bony sites (entheses) where tendons and ligaments are attached (enthesitis). A variety of extra-articular inflammatory manifestations may also occur. Although this family includes several distinct clinical entities (AS; reactive arthritis, or Reiter's syndrome; psoriatic arthritis; and enteropathic arthritis), the rationale for grouping them together is based on their sharing many clinical, radiographic, and epidemiologic features, as well as a genetic association with the major histocompatibility complex class I allele HLA-B27. Moreover, many patients demonstrate overlapping clinical features of several of these disorders (undifferentiated SpA), making specific disease classification impossible. Finally, evolving research findings suggest that similar pathophysiologic mechanisms may underlie all these diseases.

Reactive arthritis may serve as the paradigm for the other spondyloarthopathies, because it is known to be triggered by certain specific microorganisms infecting the gut or genitourinary tract. Although these microorganisms cannot be cultured from joint fluid or tissue, there is now incontrovertible evidence that that these bacteria are present in affected peripheral joint tissues, where they may persist for many years. Living but metabolically inactive *Chlamydia trachomatis* microorganisms have been demonstrated in synovial macrophages and fibroblasts by electron microscopy and by polymerase chain reaction. Bacterial antigens of the enteric bacterial causes of reactive arthritis (*Shigella, Salmonella,* and *Yersinia*) have also been demonstrated in joint tissues; however, living organisms have not been convincingly demonstrated. A bacterial cause of primary AS is also suspected but not yet proved, and, similarly, a bacterial cause of psoriatic arthritis and enter-opathic arthritis. The role of HLA-B27 is still unknown; however, it appears likely to promote bacterial persistence and/or dissemination. Transgenic rats and mice expressing the human HLA-B27 gene develop the clinical disease features of human SpAs; however, normal gut bacterial flora is also essential because animals raised in the germ-free state remain well. These discoveries have led to consideration of antimicrobial therapeutic approaches in patients with SpAs (see later).

EPIDEMIOLOGY, CLINICAL FEATURES, AND COURSES

Primary AS affects 0.1 to 0.2% of the white population and is less common in black persons. In fact, the prevalence of AS parallels the frequency of HLA-B27 in various populations and develops in approximately 2% of HLA-B27– positive individuals overall. The disease risk is 10-fold higher, however, in HLA-B27–positive relatives of patients with AS. Men are affected more often than are women (3:1). First symptoms typically occur in young adults or teenagers.

As usually begins insidiously with "inflammatory back symptoms" (Table 2). With time, pain and stiffness, accompanied by decreased spinal mobility, may progress into the thoracic and cervical regions leading to complete bony fusion (bamboo spine) and a kyphotic posture. The spectrum of disease severity, however, is broad. Patients in whom there is an early age of disease onset, hip involvement, and failure to respond to medications have a worse long-term prognosis. The majority of patients, however, remain functional and continue to work despite chronic pain and physical limitations. Death from AS is infrequent but may occur in those sustaining spinal fractures, especially cervical, or developing systemic complications such as cardiac involvement or amyloidosis (see Table 2).

Reactive arthritis (Reiter's syndrome) is a peripheral arthritis and enthesitis syndrome, often accompanied by mucocutaneous lesions, which develops 2 to 6 weeks after certain gastrointestinal or venereal infections (see Table 2). The inciting event is often asymptomatic or not remembered. Its prevalence varies among populations and locales, being dependent on both the frequencies of HLA-B27 and the endemic infectious agents that cause the disease. Males predominate in the sexually transmitted form (10:1), but the sex ratio is equal in the postenteritis form. Approximately 20% of HLA-B27–positive individuals develop reactive arthritis after exposure to the arthritogenic enteric pathogens. The disease is self-limited in the majority of patients, lasting 4 to 12 months, but residual joint complaints are common, and relapses may occur. Morbidity most often results from chronic arthritis and enthesitis of the feet, refractory uveitis, complicating spondylitis in 10 to 12%, and rarely aortitis or amyloidosis.

Psoriatic arthritis develops in 5 to 7% of the 1 to 2% of the white population with cutaneous psoriasis. Males and females are affected equally. Genetic susceptibility is strong. HLA-B27 appears to predispose only to spinal involvement. The pattern of arthritis is variable but distinctive (see Table 2), and it pursues a chronic, slowly progressive course that is less likely to lead to disability than rheumatoid arthritis.

Enteropathic arthritis occurring in patients with ulcerative colitis or Crohn's disease is uncommon and takes two forms. A peripheral nondeforming, oligoarticular, asymmetrical arthritis appears in 15 to 20% of patients and parallels the inflammatory activity of the bowel disease (see Table 2). This clinical picture shows no association

---

TABLE 1. **Spondyloarthropathies**

Predominant spinal arthritis and enthesitis
    AS (primary)
    AS secondary to ulcerative colitis or Crohn's disease
    AS secondary to psoriasis
Predominant peripheral arthritis and enthesitis
    Reactive arthritis after venereal infections (*Chlamydia* or
        Ureaplasma)
    Reactive arthritis after bacterial gastroenteritis (*Shigella,*
        Salmonella, Yersinia, or *Campylobacter*)
    Juvenile-onset SpA
    Psoriatic arthritis
    Arthritis secondary to ulcerative colitis and Crohn's disease
    Undifferentiated SpAs

Abbreviations: AS = ankylosing spondylitis; SpA = spondyloarthropathy.

TABLE 2. **Features of Spondyloarthropathies**

Clinical Features

Primary and Secondary AS

Sacroiliitis and spinal arthritis and enthesitis: alternating buttock pain, low back pain, and/or stiffness worsened by inactivity and improved by more than 3 mo of exercise

Pain symptoms and loss of spinal mobility gradually ascend to involve lumbar, thoracic, and cervical spinal segments resulting in ankylosis and typical "stooped forward" kyphotic deformity

Peripheral joint pain and/or stiffness, especially of hips, shoulders, or knees, in approximately one third of patients

Episodes of monocular iritis (25%); aortic valve regurgitation and/or atrioventricular heart block (5%); apical pulmonary fibrosis (occasionally cavitary) (1%); amyloidosis (1%); cauda equina syndrome (rare)

Overt ulcerative colitis or Crohn's disease or psoriasis in secondary forms of AS; occult bowel inflammatory lesions in primary AS

Family history of AS, reactive arthritis, psoriasis, or inflammatory bowel disease (also in others listed later)

Reactive Arthritis (Reiter's Syndrome)

Asymmetrical oligoarthritis, especially of lower limb joints

Dactylitis, i.e., "sausaging" of toes or fingers

Enthesitis, especially of plantar or Achilles tendon insertions (heel pain)

Conjunctivitis (or iritis in 20%)

Urethritis (sterile or venereally acquired) or cervicitis or prostatitis

Mucocutaneous lesions: keratoderma blennorrhagicum, circinate balanitis, painless oral ulcers, onychodystrophy

Antecedent venereal or diarrheal illness within 6 wk (occult bowel inflammation in latter group)

Psoriatic Arthritis

Cutaneous psoriasis and nail pitting and/or onychodystrophy

Asymmetrical oligoarthritis or symmetrical polyarthritis

Distal interphalangeal joints often involved

Dactylitis

Laboratory Features

Seronegative: negative tests for rheumatoid factor and antinuclear antibodies

HLA-B27–positive: 90% of primary AS, 50% of secondary AS, 75% of reactive arthritis, and less frequent in psoriatic arthritis

Radiographic: sclerosis and erosions and bony fusion of sacroiliac joints (sacroiliitis); bony fusion of apophyseal joints; ossification of spinal ligaments (syndesmophytes); peripheral joints and entheses show periostitis, bony erosions, cartilage loss, and bony fusion

with HLA-B27. Sacroiliitis or spondylitis, indistinguishable from primary AS and unrelated to the peripheral arthropathy, develops in 10% of patients with inflammatory bowel diseases. HLA-B27 is found in 33 to 50% of such patients. Colectomy for ulcerative colitis eliminates the peripheral arthritis but has no effect on the spondylitis.

DIAGNOSIS

Diagnosis of each of the SpAs is based primarily on clinical and radiographic grounds. The most specific finding for AS is radiographic sacroiliitis. Plain radiographs may be negative early in disease, and computed tomography and magnetic resonance imaging are more sensitive (but expensive) in demonstrating inflammatory changes in these joints. Blood typing for HLA-B27 is rarely indicated, although in preradiographic AS it may prove a useful

adjunct in supporting (or not) a high likelihood of disease (being expected to be positive in more than 90% of cases but in only 8% of the normal white population).

In reactive arthritis, attempts should be made to identify the precipitating infection, especially *C. trachomatis,* by using culture or molecular probes in patients with urethritis or cervicitis. In postenteric reactive arthritis, stool cultures are usually negative after arthritis appears, unless the patient still has bowel symptoms. Serologic tests for the enteric pathogens are not reliable.

Other laboratory tests are nonspecific. Acute phase reactants, such as the erythocyte sedimentation rate and C-reactive protein, are elevated in the majority of patients, as are serum levels of IgA. Tests for rheumatoid factor and antinuclear antibodies are negative.

MANAGEMENT

The goals of therapy are to (1) reduce pain and stiffness, (2) maintain good posture and joint range of motion, and (3) modify the course of disease, if possible. Nonsteroidal anti-inflammatory drugs (NSAIDs) remain the agents of first choice for improving the symptoms of pain and stiffness (Table 3) and allowing the institution of a sound physical therapy program (Table 4). Salicylates usually are not effective in any of the SpAs. Similarly, propionic acid derivatives tend to be less effective than indoleacetic acid–based drugs; however, there is a great deal of individual variability of patients in response and tolerability. Several agents may need to be tried in sequence before the most effective one is found. Phenylbutazone was once a commonly used and effective NSAID for the SpAs; however, its use has been largely abandoned because of rare but life-threatening hematologic side effects.

Long-acting or second-line drugs, especially certain antibiotics, are being increasingly used. The rationale for antibiotic therapy is based on epidemiologic and experimental evidence that the ongoing inflammatory response in these diseases is driven by bacterial infection. Several clinical trials have demonstrated the clinical efficacy of such an approach,

TABLE 3. **Principles of Nonsteroidal Anti-inflammatory Drug Therapy for Spondyloarthropathy**

Educate patient about benefits and potential risks of NSAIDs.

Choose nonsalicylate NSAID: indomethacin (Indocin), tolmetin (Tolectin), sulindac (Clinoril), piroxicam (Feldene), diclofenac (Voltaren), oxaprozin (Daypro), etodolac (Lodine); proprionic acid derivatives and other NSAIDs usually less effective, e.g., ibuprofen (Motrin, Advil, Nuprin), ketoprofen (Orudis, Oruvail), flurbiprofen (Ansaid), naproxen (Naprosyn), nabumetone (Relafen).

Prescribe full-dose NSAID.

Do not use combinations of NSAIDs.

Use timed-release forms (when available) to prevent night pain.

Allow 2- to 3-wk trial of NSAID.

Try another agent if current one gives suboptimal response.

Add cytoprotective agent for GI intolerance or history of peptic ulcer.

Abbreviations: NSAID = nonsteroidal anti-inflammatory drug; GI = gastrointestinal.

TABLE 4. **Education and Physical Therapy for Spondyloarthropathy**

Education*
  Natural history of disease
  Purpose and goal of each modality of treatment
  Promotion of appropriate work and leisure habits and positions for posture, sitting, sleeping, and so forth
Physical therapy
  Prevention of spinal and peripheral joint contracture
  Maintenance of full range of joint motions
  Specific regular exercises to include extension of spine; deep breathing exercises (maintain chest expansion); range of motion of neck, shoulders, hips, knees
  Most appropriate recreational activities (e.g., swimming, weight training)
  Use of heat or cold to relieve pain and relax muscles
Physician's reassessment and reinforcement of program over time

*Useful information for patients is available from the Arthritis Foundation (USA), Spondylitis Association of America, Arthritis Society of Canada, National Ankylosing Spondylitis Society (NASS) (United Kingdom), and the Arthritis and Rheumatism Council (ARC) (United Kingdom).

as well as the lowering of acute phase reactants, thus demonstrating the potential for disease modification. The greatest experience has been with sulfasalazine (Azulfidine)* (2 to 3 grams daily), which has been proved to be more efficacious than placebo in primary AS, reactive arthritis, and psoriatic arthritis. This drug also has a long history of use in the inflammatory bowel diseases. The sulfapyridine moiety rather than the salicylate appears to be the effective ingredient. More recently, clinical trials have demonstrated that in patients with reactive arthritis, early and aggressive tetracycline or erythromycin treatment of new venereal infections prevents relapse, and one study has shown that a 3-month course of a tetracycline shortens the duration of postchlamydial but not postenteric reactive arthritis. Early antibiotic treatment of bacterial gastroenteritis does not appear to prevent the subsequent development of reactive arthritis, and limited numbers of trials of fluoroquinolone antibiotics in chronic reactive arthritis have, thus far, shown disappointing results (Table 5).

Methotrexate (Rheumatrex)* in oral doses of 7.5 to 15 mg weekly may also be helpful in treating refrac-

*Not FDA approved for this indication.

TABLE 5. **Antibiotics for Treatment of Spondyloarthropathies**

Sulfasalazine (Azulfidine)* 0.5–1.5 gm twice daily
  Early and/or progressive AS
  Postenteric reactive arthritis
  Severe psoriatic arthritis
  Enteropathic arthritis—peripheral and axial forms
  ? Prevention of recurrent iritis
Tetracyclines (doxycycline or minocycline) 100 mg twice daily
  Venereally acquired (Chlamydia) reactive arthritis (3 mo)
  Reinfection with Chlamydia in patient with previous reactive arthritis (1 mo) (also treat sexual partner)
Fluoroquinolones (ciprofloxacin, Floxin)*
  ? Acute or chronic postenteric reactive arthritis

*Not FDA approved for this indication.

tory cases of SpA, especially psoriatic arthritis. Similarly, azathioprine (Imuran)* at oral doses of 100 to 200 mg daily may be beneficial. Gold therapy (Myochrysine, Solganal, Ridaura)* and hydroxychloroquine (Plaquenil)* do not appear to be effective in these diseases.

Repository corticosteroid injections (Aristospan, Depo-Medrol, Celestone) may prove effective for refractory peripheral joint arthritis, sacroiliitis, or enthesitis, although injections of the Achilles tendon should be avoided because of the potential for inducing tendon rupture. Brief courses of low-dose daily corticosteroids (prednisone ≤10 mg daily) may be beneficial in some patients, but their chronic use is discouraged. Analgesics and muscle relaxants may be useful adjuncts to the other therapies, but addictive drugs should be avoided.

COMPLICATIONS

Iritis

Ocular symptoms, especially pain, redness, photophobia, or blurred vision, warrant immediate referral to an opthalmologist to confirm the diagnosis and begin therapy, usually with topical corticosteroids and mydriatics. Refractory cases may require systemic corticosteroid therapy. Some evidence suggests that sulfasalazine* therapy of the arthritis reduces the incidence of iritis.

Cardiac Disease

There is no known medical treatment of aortic valvulitis or heart block. Most patients with these complications ultimately require surgical valvular replacement or pacemaker implantation, respectively.

Amyloidosis

Secondary amyloidosis usually presents as proteinuria and should be confirmed by rectal or subcutaneous fat pad biopsy rather than renal biopsy, from which internal bleeding may occur. There is no definitive treatment for this complication, although low-dose colchicine* 0.6 mg twice daily is worthy of trial.

Suspected Spinal Fracture

A high index of suspicion for fracture is warranted in all AS patients, even after seemingly trivial trauma. Plain radiographs are often unreliable in detecting fractures, and computed tomography or magnetic resonance imaging of the suspected area may be necessary. If a fracture is present, an experienced trauma surgeon or neurosurgeon should be consulted immediately.

Total Hip Replacement

Prosthetic hip replacements may be necessary in AS patients, even at a young age, and most have a

*Not FDA approved for this indication.

good outcome. AS predisposes to an increased risk of heterotopic ossification, and postoperative radiation may be necessary if signs begin to appear.

TEMPOROMANDIBULAR DISORDERS

method of
JOSÉ DOS SANTOS, JR., D.D.S., M.S.
University of Texas Health Science Center at San Antonio, School of Dentistry
San Antonio, Texas

In the presence of some form of temporomandibular disorder (TMD), the clinician must be aware that he or she will be assessing a case that may embody a wide range of variables involving the diagnosis, prognosis, and treatment of the masticatory system.

As significant segments of the population are affected by this problem, TMD is a subject of concern in the dental profession. This disorder is not entirely comprehended, particularly the mechanisms that may subject the patient to acute or chronic pain. Therefore, the term TMD refers to a group of symptoms affiliated with acute or chronic functional and structural diseases of the masticatory apparatus.

Elements that can induce the beginning of, an increase in, or a solution of TMDs are numerous and distinct. Such elements may encompass actual pathologic changes within the joints; systemic conditions altering muscle function, connective tissue biology, nerve transmission, or blood flow; the patient's psychologic attitudes; and the emergence of occlusal prematurities and interferences.

EVALUATION OF THE PATIENT

During the diagnostic evaluation of the patient's TMD, the clinician must initially keep in mind the functional status of the masticatory system. If some functional disorder is suspected, it is important to attempt to detect symptoms such as those discussed in the following sections.

Pain

A good reason to consider pain a primary symptom for diagnosis, especially in patients with TMDs, is the probability of making a differential diagnosis of other entities that may require evaluation and treatment by other medical specialists (for example, a neurologist). These entities include migraine, trigeminal neuralgia, angiomas, brain tumors, multiple sclerosis, reflex sympathetic dystrophy (causalgia), glossopharyngeal neuralgia, systemic lupus erythematosus, and headaches.

Mechanisms of Referred Pain. Typically, acute pain may be felt at the primary site of the noxious stimulation. In some instances, pain may be felt in an anatomic region distant from the primary area of injury. This phenomenon is called referred or secondary pain. This phenomenon has been thought to occur through cumulative mechanisms influencing other neural divisions; however, the theory of excitation of the central nervous system may be the best explanation of this category of pain. According to this theory, a volley of painful sensory impulses reaching the central nervous system may stimulate nearby and inactive internuncial neurons, producing a consequent reaction.

Deafferentation and Chronic Pain. Physiologic, neurochemical, and morphologic changes in somatosensory pathways may result from the transmission of pain from peripheral structures to the central nervous system. These phenomena may produce partial or total loss of sensory supply to and from a particular region of the body, or deafferentation. Although not fully explained, deafferentation may underlie the development of chronic orofacial pain, because this phenomenon induces sensory alterations that may cause changes in the somatosensory pathways of the trigeminal nerve. Some theories about chronic pain consider that alterations in these pathways may produce localized organic changes in the structures of the central nervous system. This process may be initiated by trauma, compression, degeneration, and so forth, in orofacial regions, which may lead to painful conditions such as trigeminal neuralgia, atypical facial neuralgia, and other forms of disorders involving the craniomandibular structures.

Craniomandibular Pain in Peripheral Structures. Common peripheral clinical features of pain are dental and periodontal symptoms. Direct noxious stimulation or irritation of some peripheral structures may also lead to symptoms of facial pain of cutaneous, mucosal, and periosteal origin, for example, (1) trauma to the skin covering the face (e.g., contusion, laceration, burning) or infection (abscesses and cellulitis); (2) infective lesions of the mucous membrane covering the oral cavity, nose, sinuses (e.g., sinusitis, nasal infections); and (3) fractures or osteomyelitis affecting the periosteum covering the craniomandibular skeleton.

Craniomandibular Pain Originating from Muscles. Pain may be caused by hyperactivity of a muscle, leading to fatigue. It has been shown that psychologic or physical stress may lead to increased activity of jaw muscles. Although many causes can be identified (for example, muscle contracture; dyskinesia; dystonia; fibromyalgia; myositis), the two most encountered sources of muscle pain that may have special meaning in craniomandibular disorders are muscle splinting and muscle spasm, or trismus.

Craniomandibular Pain of Temporomandibular Joint Origin. Pain experienced in the region of the temporomandibular joint (TMJ) occurs mainly when the articular surfaces are destroyed by extensive degenerative disease or when there is production of abnormal mechanical tension in the fibrous capsule of the joint (due to some form of acute malocclusion consequent to inflammation of the capsule or posterior attachment). The arthralgia can be described as a dull, depressing, not well localized discomfort of variable intensities.

Craniomandibular Pain of Vascular Origin. This type of discomfort occurs far more commonly than has been customarily detected by either medical or dental professionals. It is elicited by chemical or mechanical irritation of the plexiform system of unmyelinated nerve fibers that are embedded in the adventitial sheaths of the blood vessels supplying the craniofacial tissues (mainly branches of the supraorbital, facial, and superficial temporal arteries). Such irritation may occur in patients with vascular diseases, e.g., arteriosclerosis or temporal arteritis, that are well recognized by competent physicians. Much more often it results from episodic immoderate dilatation of blood vessels, as in migraine. That is, when mechanically distorted, these blood vessels noxiously stimulate sensory receptors and afferent fibers within the vascular and perivascular tissues. Vascular pains have an obnoxious pounding feature and are habitually followed by a feeling of nausea and autonomic effects such as lacrimation and photophobia. The pain is considerably dispersed and totally deceptive as far as neurologic parameters of localization are concerned, because the vascular arborization (where the pain is felt) crosses other neurologic limits.

Craniomandibular Pain of Neurologic Origin. Pains felt in the face and masticatory structures that arise from some sort of neurologic disturbance have similar characteristics. The pain is brilliant, arousing, and burning. The pains are promptly localized by the patient, taking as reference the neuroanatomic distribution of the nerves. The stimulus-response association is invariably nonproportional, and sometimes the response is much more intense than the stimulus. In general, the most significant neuropathies encountered in clinics are (1) neuromas, which are a disorganized mass of nervous tissue; (2) scar tissue, which is formed after a surgical or accidental nerve amputation; (3) inflammation of sensory fibers, for instance, neuritis; (4) herpes zoster, which is a neuritic involvement of the ganglion, sensory root, or medullary tract of a nerve by the chickenpox virus and; (5) trigeminal neuralgia, an idiopathic neuralgia that includes changes in the fibers of the ganglion and dorsal root.

Referred Craniomandibular Pain. Pain may be referred to craniomandibular structures from different structures. Such pain includes the following:

1. Pain from mucosal tissues of the nose and paranasal sinuses, where afferent extensions from the sensory receptor system converge synaptically with neurons in the spinal nucleus of the trigeminal nerve.

2. Pain from a group of maxillary and mandibular teeth, where regions of the face innervated by the mandibular and maxillary branch of the fifth nerve may be dispersively painful. Some masticatory muscles may also display some form of dysfunction capable of referring sparse pain to teeth and orofacial structures. Sometimes, due to its magnitude, this kind of pain can easily be mistaken for trigeminal neuralgia; for this reason it is known as atypical facial neuralgia.

3. Pain of myogenic origin involving the masticatory and cervical muscles, where trigger mechanisms (located in the body of a given muscle) may produce discomfort radiating to the craniofacial structures. This category of pain is common in the presence of muscle tension headaches, which complicate the craniomandibular symptoms.

Familiarity with various biologic mechanisms and concepts pertaining to head and neck musculature is essential for diagnosis and treatment of many functional disturbances associated with the masticatory system. In particular, from an occlusion standpoint, the clinician should be aware of the complex role played by the musculature in physiologic interactions between various components (e.g., teeth, muscles, joints). In addition, there may be intervening muscle actions from conscious and unconscious emotional sources.

4. Pain related to temporomandibular arthropathies. Inherent pain and dysfunction as result of these arthropathies may produce secondary myalgia and muscle spasm so that the area of complaint in the craniomandibular structures may be considerably larger than the site of origin. The patient's problem may consist of the chief complaint, or the condition may remain subacute and not be discovered until palpation or provocation tests are performed. Pain is elicited at rest, on movement, or both.

Painful stimulation of the joint structures typically leads to induced predominant contraction of flexor muscles. Free nerve endings, which are common in joint capsules, may be activated by vigorous twisting or stretching of the capsule (which may occur during extreme bruxing movements).

5. Pain of vascular origin. In this case it is also common to have the combination of secondary central excitatory effects plus vascular pain. The vascular component of masticatory and neck muscle pain is the most influential and has been considered the main source of myalgia. Areas of reference on the head and face together with complex symptoms of masticatory pain and dysfunction may often develop as a result of secondary pain induced by vascular problems.

Craniomandibular Pain of Psychologic Origin. Pain of psychologic origin proves the involvement of the psyche and the soma. The term "pain experience" has been suggested as an alternative to "pain," because it includes the individual's integration of all effects of noxious stimuli (for example, reactions to a pain threat, physical sensations, and physiologic reactions). Some psychosocial factors, such as beliefs attributed to pain, the age of the individual, and ethnic background, seem to contribute to the pain response.

Joint Sounds and Incoordination

Masticatory muscle asynchrony and alteration in TMJ structures may be responsible for incoordination of mandibular motions and sounds. To illustrate, it is possible to detect that the incoordination of some movements may be caused by the presence of gross occlusal interferences. Other correlated findings are the occurrence of inadequate molar support; the presence of excessive slide in centric; the type of occlusion that produces instability of dental arches; the possible presence of massive hidden occlusal interferences; and so forth.

Limitation of Movements

TMJ disturbances may include chronic and acute traumatic arthritis; rheumatoid arthritis; progressive degeneration of the joints (osteoarthritis); and congenital alterations. All these entities are capable of limiting and modifying the pattern of mandibular motion.

Occlusal Relationships

Aspects of the functional analysis of occlusion are related to possible influences that some distorted interocclusal relationships may contribute to the instability of the masticatory system. Naturally, the absence of teeth, the degree of mobility, the presence of atypical facets of wear, tooth sensitivity, crown fractures, root fractures, trauma from occlusion, and other findings are all prominent factors to be taken into consideration in the preparation of therapy for TMDs.

Parafunctional Habits

The role of occlusion as a trigger for the onset of parafunctional habits has not been clearly defined; however, more important is not to disregard the deleterious effects of these habits at the level of dentition.

Another neurologic pathway mechanism produces another type of parafunctional habit. It is represented by forceful clenching of the jaws. Although this parafunctional process does not produce active reduction of tooth structures, it may cause painful masticatory muscle dysfunction. There are also some speculations about free gingiva retraction and localized periodontal bone loss as related to cervical lesions of the teeth (abfraction). These noncarious cervical lesions may be the result of excessive forces exerted on the occlusal surfaces of the teeth, producing tension stresses on the cervix of the crowns with possible consequent fracture and dislocation of the enamel rods.

TREATMENT PLANNING

The most rational approach to treatment planning is to use one's best judgment based on clinical evaluation to achieve a preliminary diagnosis and to establish an essentially conservative treatment plan. Depending on the patient's response to the initial phase of treatment, more definitive diagnosis can then be made, bringing with it a more reliable prognosis. Thus, in the patient's interest, the initial therapy should be based on management of symptoms using conservative methods, such as behavior modification through counseling and diet restriction; mild non-narcotic analgesics (nonsteroidal anti-inflammatory drugs); mental relaxation and meditation (biofeedback); psychologic consultation; physiotherapy; masticatory muscle exercises; transcutaneous neural stimulation; or institution of bite splint therapy (this last approach, in some cases, may act more as a diagnostic tool than treatment appliance).

Sometimes the personality of the patient plays a significant role in all processes. Perfectionist individuals are not so easily convinced of some facts, but they are the most cooperative in finding solutions for their predicaments. Consultation with other health professionals to provide a combination of other forms of therapy may produce good dividends in clinical practice.

Conservative management of the patient's symptoms may involve the following therapies.

Drugs

Although the most widespread use of pharmacologic agents is for the control of chronic pain afflicting the orofacial regions, this does not mean that there are no indications for their use in acute cases. Many important aspects of the clinical case must be identified before medication is prescribed, including indications and contraindications for the drug, side effects, complications, and so forth.

Injections

The infiltration of anesthetics, steroids, sclerosing agents,* and hyaluronidase (Wydase)* solutions into affected areas may produce significant relief of pain. However, there are some limitations, such as anatomic difficulties, need for advanced training of the therapist, or the presence of intense pain. The strategy for such treatment is the interruption of the vicious circle of pain, allowing a temporary absence of pain, to provide conditions for the recovery of the masticatory system. In general, the injections are

*Not FDA approved for this indication.

applied at the level of the masticatory musculature (intra- and extramuscular) and into the TMJs.

Physical Agents

The clinician may also use some physical agents for TMD treatment. There are a great variety of procedures as well as indications. Such procedures may be used as adjuncts for relief of symptoms and may be combined.

Therapy with both cold and heat alleviates pain through a counterirritant effect, acting directly on the peripheral innervation of the masticatory system, especially at the level of free nerve endings.

Exercises

Exercises are considered relevant for the functional recuperation of the masticatory system, even when complications involving cervical structures are considered. Therapeutic exercises use the motive action of masticatory muscles, promoting mandibular movement in such a way that the patient becomes the main agent during the treatment. Some clinicians consider therapeutic exercises necessary for the resolution of residual subclinical stages, and even for the prevention of future cases of dysfunction.

Electrostimulation

The most accepted electrostimulation technique is referred to as transcutaneous electrical nerve stimulation and in dentistry is applied at the level of peripheral nociceptive receptors. This modality has been considered by clinicians as an effective way to control skeletal masticatory muscle and neurogenic pains on a temporary basis.

Biofeedback

Every living being possesses a complex or simple internal organic mechanism that provides a constant biofeedback loop to regulate biologic functions. With instrumentation, external biofeedback approaches add an extra motivation to these mechanisms to promote homeostasis of selected physiologic functions. Electromyographic biofeedback may be an effective way to help to control masticatory muscle tension.

Intraoral Appliances

Occlusal bite plane splints are a notable landmark in the symptomatic treatment of TMDs. Although there is no defined explanation for their therapeutic actions, they have proved to be effective for many patients. Substantial reductions in symptoms of masticatory muscles and TMJs have been observed. There are many designs of these appliances, but considering the reversible aspect of the therapy, the stabilization type of appliance, with a flat surface for occlusal contact and anterior guidances, is considered the best choice.

Some patients will probably have to use an intraoral appliance for a long time, or for the rest of their lives. If the appliance is not designed to change the alignment of the dentition, this should not be an unbearable burden. Fortunately, some patients never complain about this long-term use.

Summary of Reversible Therapy

The reversible character of the initial therapy is correlated with the amount of information gathered in the process of reaching the final diagnosis and prognosis. In a more advanced stage of the treatment process, one can use irreversible types of therapy, namely occlusal adjustment, oral reconstruction, orthodontics, orthognathic surgery, and so forth.

Modalities of treatment for TMDs are various, and almost invariably a combination of procedures constitutes a successful basis of therapy. We must not forget the cyclical nature of the disorders afflicting the masticatory system, because this cyclical nature may be misleading when checking the results of any sort of treatment. Because of the cyclical characteristic of TMDs, many patients may erroneously believe that they have an inherent ability to overcome any kind of disorder afflicting the masticatory system. In some instances, the resolving or recuperative power of the system during acute episodes accounts for the probability that in some ethnic groups a large number of patients with TMD never seek professional help.

Occlusal Evaluation

Some therapeutic approaches for TMDs may consist of the evaluation of the patient's occlusion and methods to treat it. However, questions concerning the type of treatment needed to manage a TMD at the level of the dentition are difficult to answer. It is important to understand that the dental practitioner, like any health professional, should just try to manage dysfunctional conditions first, to be able to equilibrate the occlusion. It is almost impossible to predict any defined cure for problems only at the level of the dentition, because in the majority of cases there is no definite solution to some dysfunctional problems, especially in chronic conditions. A continuous conservative approach is sometimes the best we can do. Trying to modify the patient's occlusion may produce more added problems than benefits, especially when the patient becomes conscious of his or her bite.

Some chronic symptoms are not totally related to the dentition. Chronicity is sometimes the result of a lack of physical and emotional ability to cope with pain. Physical and emotional stress may lead to masticatory muscle hyperfunction, causing the aggravation and continuation of masticatory dysfunction. In some cases, it is wise to have professional consultations with other specialists to define the cognitive aspects of pain to develop behavioral strategies. The list of psychologic and behavioral factors is quite long, and these factors have a strong tendency to interact. It is important to remember that the patient's cooperation in this management process is of extreme importance.

There is some belief that malocclusion may be a precipitating factor for TMDs. However, the term malocclusion just implies the comparison of some person's occlusion to a parameter of alignment of the dental arches. Therefore, any deviation from this parameter does not imply tendency to a dysfunctional problem. If the patient has an occlusion that functions properly and is free of symptoms, it may be considered normal for that individual and there is no reason for great concern about alignment of the teeth.

Restorations in the patient's mouth may result in some slight imperfections; however, they probably would not generate an enormous set of problems, because these slight imperfections may be acting in the normal range for that person. Some occlusal schemes are mostly guided by the canines (canine-protected occlusion), and because of this almost no interference to eccentric movements is usually present. Therefore, the morphology of the occlusal surfaces might have little influence on these movements. However, to improve the stability and function of the masticatory apparatus, provisions for occlusal adjustment might be able to deliver more predictable self-perpetuating results to the system.

In cases of aggressive parafunctional habits, some clinicians are concerned with possible occlusion overclosure. It is not easy to define overclosure clearly, especially concerning the loss of the vertical dimension of occlusion, in these cases. Sometimes, interarch deviations are the result of a distorted tridimensional position of the mandible. Images of the TMJs may disclose that the patient's condyles are not evenly seated on the glenoid fossae. This condition might be due to temporary incoordination of masticatory muscles. Judicious use of a stabilization-type of bite splint (an orthotic appliance), followed by continuous recall of the patient and adjustment of the bite splint, may help to correct muscle incoordination, producing satisfactory results.

Patients may really have painful episodes, not just in their imagination. However, the exact contributing cause or causes for the distress are almost impossible to determine. It is important to realize that the occlusion, although sometimes representing an important contributing factor, is not solely responsible for the patient's suffering.

In some extreme conditions, patients may have a very low level of tolerance to small imperfections of their dentition, and some of them may even perceive prematurities smaller than 20 μm. However, the masticatory system of most individuals has the ability to overcome and to adapt to such small imperfections. Naturally, the dental practitioner cannot see or adjust such microscopic defects. This is why it so important for the clinician to be aware of these extreme conditions when planning rehabilitation procedures to avoid adding more problems for a person with a propensity to dysfunction.

Occlusal Adjustment

Occlusal adjustment refers to the equilibration of the natural dentition through the use of different approaches. There are many techniques for occlusal adjustment. All are equally good when they comply with the occlusal philosophic concepts on which they are based. Although many procedures may be attempted to accomplish an occlusal adjustment (from simple spot grinding to complex orthognathic surgery), it is important to note that the great majority of occlusal adjustment procedures are carried out using selective grinding or prosthetic rehabilitations. The most widespread technique for occlusal adjustment employs a selective grinding technique, according to the concept of freedom in centric.

If an intervention at the level of dentition is planned suggesting the application of the freedom-in-centric concept for selective grinding, it is necessary to understand that this concept is based on the principles of an "ideal" occlusion, in which after completion of the adjustment procedures (1) there will be no need for neuromuscular adaptation of the masticatory system; (2) the vertical dimension of occlusion in maximal intercuspation and centric relation might be the same when all interferences for closing in centric are eliminated; (3) masticatory forces might be directed axially on a flat platform on the depth of the occlusal fossae, which will allow a certain degree of freedom for centric and eccentric movements of the jaw; (4) there might always be freedom for condyle movements; and (5) the clinical application of this concept might promote occlusal stability.

BURSITIS, TENDINITIS, MYOFASCIAL PAIN, AND FIBROMYALGIA

method of
ROBERT M. BENNETT, M.D.
Oregon Health Sciences University
Portland, Oregon

Nonarticular musculoskeletal pain is the leading cause of pain and disability in the United States. This should not be surprising as muscle is the largest organ in the body, accounting for 40% of body weight. There are 696 muscles in the human body, and most have attachments to two bones, with the tendon passing over the intervening joint.

The smooth functioning of the musculotendinous unit is aided by the encasement of some muscles by tendon sheaths and the interposition of bursae between bony prominences and muscle bellies or tendons. The majority of patients who present to their physician with a complaint of rheumatic pain have a disorder of the musculotendinous unit rather than a true arthritis. Common syndromes involving bursae, tendons, and muscles are given in Tables 1 through 3. Some patients have a history of persistent widespread musculoskeletal pain, often in association with profound fatigue and many other somatic symptoms; this is called the fibromyalgia syndrome. Fibromyalgia may be the final result of inadequately managed regional pain states. The diagnosis of nonarticular musculoskeletal pain is often challenging to contemporary physicians as it depends on a careful clinical examination rather than imaging and blood tests.

GENERAL PRINCIPLES OF MANAGEMENT

Most patients presenting with bursitis, tendinitis, or myofascial pain have a predisposing cause for the initiation of the problem. In many cases, perpetuation of the problem is due to repetitive activities that irritate the involved structures. The most difficult part of treatment is to identify precisely and eliminate these aggravating factors. Biomechanical dysfunction may be an important contributory factor (e.g., scoliosis or unequal leg length). In some patients, there is an underlying systemic disease, such as rheumatoid arthritis, gout, or Reiter's disease. In patients with septic bursitis or septic tenosynovitis, there is usually a history of a penetrating injury. When a site of infection is not apparent, one should search for a focus of blood-borne sepsis, such as staphylococcal skin lesions, gram-negative sepsis from urogenital instrumentation, or gonococcemia from pelvic inflammation.

Several points are important in the overall management of these conditions:

1. Explain to the patient why he or she has the condition, and explain the expected results of therapy. This should include the time course for recovery and possible complications of treatment.

2. Provide information on the avoidance of aggravating factors.

3. If the patient is in a work situation that is aggravating or perpetuating the condition, prescribe

TABLE 1. **Commonly Involved Bursae**

Site	Symptom	Finding
Subdeltoid	Shoulder pain	Tender subcutaneous swelling
Olecranon	Elbow pain	Tender subcutaneous swelling
Trochanteric	Lateral hip pain	Tenderness over greater trochanter
Ischial (weaver's bottom)	Pain on sitting	Tenderness with pressure over ischium
Prepatellar (housemaid's knee)	Painful knee	Subcutaneous swelling over patella
Infrapatellar (clergyman's knee)	Painful knee	Subcutaneous swelling below patella
Anserine	Painful knee	Tenderness over medial aspect of knee
Iliopectineal	Painful groin	Tenderness over inguinal triangle
Achilles (pump bump)	Painful heel	Subcutaneous swelling at back of Achilles tendon
Calcaneal	Painful heel	Tenderness on pressure over calcaneum

TABLE 2. **Commonly Involved Tendons**

Site	Symptom	Finding
Supraspinatus	Shoulder pain	Painful arc
Bicipital	Shoulder pain	Local tenderness anteriorly
Infraspinatus	Shoulder pain	Pain on internal rotation
Extensor pollicis brevis and abductor pollicis longus (de Quervain's tenosynovitis)	Wrist pain	Pain on ulnar deviation of wrist
Lateral epicondyle muscle attachments	Elbow pain	Tenderness just below lateral epicondyle
Patellar tendon	Knee pain	Local tenderness
Finger flexors	Trigger finger	"Catching" on extension of finger
Tibialis posterior	Ankle pain	Local pain under medial malleolus
Peroneal tendons	Ankle pain	Local pain under lateral malleolus

appropriate time off from work for recovery and counsel on modification of the job description.

4. Provide biomechanical rest when appropriate, e.g., splinting, slings, or instruction in the use of a cane.

5. Provide pain relief.

6. Provide anti-inflammatory treatment when appropriate.

7. Prescribe a long-term plan of stretching and muscle-strengthening exercise to minimize recurrence of the problem.

BURSITIS

When inflammation of a bursa is superficial, such as of the shoulder, knee, elbow, or Achilles tendon, the diagnosis is usually obvious (see Table 1). Deep bursae, such as those around the hip joint and the ischial tuberosity, do not present with obvious swelling; a diagnosis must be inferred from local tenderness and exacerbation of pain by activation of the associated muscles. In difficult cases, the temporary elimination of pain after the local instillation of an anesthetic is a useful diagnostic tool. Bursitis seldom shows up on plain radiographs, and expensive imaging studies are not routinely advocated. If possible, one should aspirate the bursa because the finding of synovial fluid helps confirm the diagnosis of bursitis.

TABLE 3. **Commonly Involved Sites of Myofascial Pain**

Location of Trigger Point	Symptom
Trapezius (most commonly upper portion)	Shoulder and neck pain, often headache
Sternomastoid (often multiple trigger points)	Atypical facial pain, headache
Masseter	Temporomandibular pain syndrome
Suboccipital	Headache—occipital, retro-orbital, forehead
Levator scapulae	Stiff neck
Gluteus medius (upper portion)	Pain in low back and buttock
Muscles inserting into greater trochanter	Lateral hip and thigh pain
Tensor fasciae latae	Lateral thigh pain
Muscles inserting into upper border of patella	Knee pain

If the fluid is not clear (as is the case in most instances of "irritated" bursitis), it should be sent for culture and examined for the presence of crystals.

Noninfective bursitis is treated as follows. The involved areas should be rested (e.g., the provision of a sling for subdeltoid bursitis or instruction in the use of a cane in the contralateral hand for trochanteric bursitis). The quickest and usually most complete relief is obtained by an appropriately placed corticosteroid injection. After the bursa is aspirated, a mixture of 1% procaine (about 3 mL) containing 1 to 2 mL of a long-acting corticosteroid preparation, such as triamcinolone hexacetonide (Aristospan Intralesional [into the bursa, not the joint]), prednisolone tebutate (Hydeltra-TBA), betamethasone acetate (Celestone Soluspan), methylprednisolone acetate (Depo-Medrol), or dexamethasone acetate (Decadron-LA), can be instilled. Prompt amelioration of discomfort within about 5 minutes of giving this injection (due to the effect of the local anesthetic) gives some reassurance that the injection has been accurately placed and the diagnosis is correct. In some cases, the injection of a long-acting corticosteroid preparation, which is usually microcrystalline, provokes an acute inflammatory response akin to gout. This is almost always averted if the patient is prescribed concomitant nonsteroidal anti-inflammatory drugs (NSAIDs) (e.g., indomethacin [Indocin SR], 75 mg twice daily), ibuprofen (Motrin or Rufen, 800 mg three times daily), ketoprofen (Orudis, 75 mg twice daily), naproxen (Naprosyn, 500 mg twice daily), or nabumetone (Relafen, 500 mg twice daily). Therapy with NSAIDs should be continued for approximately 1 week after all symptoms have subsided and the patient has embarked on a program of gentle return to normal activity. If aggravating factors have been eliminated, the patient seldom needs repeated injections. A recurrence of the bursitis within 7 days of injection should arouse concern regarding possible septic bursitis, and a reaspiration should be performed. Septic bursitis is usually caused by *Staphylococcus aureus*, which is often penicillin resistant. The physician should always consider the possibility of the patient's having undiagnosed diabetes, being an intravenous drug abuser, or being immunocompromised with human immunodeficiency virus infection. It is important to note that septic bursitis is *not* treated with local antibiotics. In many patients, systemic treatment with oral dicloxacillin (Dynapen, 500 mg four times a day for 10 days) is an effective regimen. Patients who have a serious underlying illness should be treated more vigorously with intravenous antibiotics, such as oxacillin (Prostaphlin), 2 grams four times a day for 7 days, followed by oral dicloxacillin. In patients who are allergic to β-lactams, the appropriate antibiotic is dictated by the culture report. At the initiation of therapy, it is most important that the bursal contents be drained through a 16- to 18-gauge needle. This drainage often has to be repeated two or three times over the course of the first week of treatment. In those rare cases in which reaccumulation of infected bursal fluid is recurrent, despite appropriate antibiotics, the possibility of open surgical drainage needs to be discussed with an orthopedic surgeon.

TENDINITIS

Tendons may tear or be partially ruptured but are never truly inflamed. The term "tendinitis" refers to an inflammation of the peritendinous tissues or synovial sheaths (tenosynovitis). Awareness of this distinction is not purely academic because the injection of corticosteroids into a tendon, particularly if repeated, may lead to its subsequent rupture. Most instances of tendinitis result from overuse or unaccustomed activity; hence rest or splinting (or both) is an important ingredient in successful treatment. In most instances, tendinitis is an acute or subacute response to repetitive irritation (see Table 2). An accurately placed injection of corticosteroids provides the quickest symptomatic relief. The simultaneous injection of a local anesthetic provides immediate confirmation that the correct anatomy has been injected. A knowledge of the relevant anatomy is essential to the success of such injections. Tendons are not injected; rather the small space between the exterior surface of the tendon and the peritendinous sheath is infiltrated with the mixture of corticosteroids and local anesthetic. To avoid snagging the tendon, it is important that the bevel of the needle be face downward and parallel to the long axis of the tendon. After injection, use of the tendon should be minimized for about 1 week. Local corticosteroids should not be used in patients with Achilles tendinitis because of its propensity to rupture. In competitive athletes, peritendinous injections should be avoided in relation to the infrapatellar tendon and the supraspinatus muscle, for similar reasons. Unresolved tendinitis, which becomes chronic, eventually leads to weakening and sometimes disruption of the tendon (e.g., a ruptured rotator cuff). Both biomechanical causes (e.g., excessive repetitive wrist action in de Quervain's tenosynovitis) and anatomic causes (e.g., an acromioclavicular osteophyte irritating the supraspinatus tendon) should be sought and eliminated in chronic cases of tendinitis. Physical therapy plays an important role in the rehabilitation of subacute and chronic tendinitis. Two phenomena need to be reversed, namely impaired blood supply and progressive shortening. The use of therapeutic ultrasound techniques both improves tendon perfusion and enhances tendon extensibility. This should be combined with an initial program of isometric exercises followed by isotonic stretching exercises. Finally, the patient should engage in progressive eccentric muscle contractions (i.e., muscle contraction while the muscle-tendon elongates); this is especially effective in restoring tendon length and at the same time promotes the orderly alignment of newly formed collagen bundles.

MYOFASCIAL PAIN

Minor muscle tears consequent to injury, unaccustomed activity, or repetitive use may cause a painful irritative focus in a muscle, commonly referred to as a "trigger point." In my experience, this is the most common cause of nonarticular rheumatic pain; it presents as a regional musculoskeletal pain syndrome (see Table 3). Many patients who have myofascial pain are initially misdiagnosed as having bursitis, tendinitis, a radiculopathy, or a nerve entrapment syndrome. Trigger points are not visualized on routine imaging studies. Thus, these patients may have significant dysfunction that cannot be substantiated by routine tests, and they may be erroneously labeled as malingering or having a "functional syndrome." Many patients with a primary arthritis or tendinitis and/or bursitis develop biomechanical imbalance, which leads to a secondary myofascial pain syndrome. Failure to recognize the evolution of such a myofascial pain syndrome results in apparent treatment failures. The finding of a single or several trigger points should suggest the diagnosis of a myofascial pain syndrome. The characteristics of a trigger point are as follows:

1. Symptoms of regional musculoskeletal pain
2. Local pain on pressure of the trigger point, often with centrifugal referral
3. Pain on stretching the involved muscle
4. Pain on contraction of the involved muscle
5. Functional shortening of the involved muscle
6. Increased consistency of muscle on palpation of the trigger point area
7. Temporary relief of pain by the precise injection of 1 to 3 mL of 1% procaine hydrochloride into the trigger point area

The essential prerequisites of myofascial therapy are as follows:

1. Identification and elimination of aggravating factors
2. The accurate injection of the myofascial trigger points as detailed subsequently
3. Passive stretching of the involved muscle after the local anesthetic has taken effect, often aided by spraying the overlying skin with a vapocoolant spray before passive stretching

In most patients, this treatment regimen needs to be repeated for a period of several weeks and occasionally several months. Recalcitrant cases are usually due to failure to eliminate an aggravating factor, imprecise injection of the trigger point, or failure to inject satellite trigger points. Trigger points are usually injected with 3 to 5 mL of 1% procaine. Whether the addition of a small amount of local corticosteroid (e.g., 0.25 mL of Hydeltra-T.B.A.) provides increased benefit has not been carefully studied. There is certainly no rationale for injecting concentrated corticosteroids into a myofascial trigger point; furthermore, insoluble corticosteroid preparations may leak back into subcutaneous tissues and cause an unsightly area of skin atrophy.

The technique for performing trigger point injection is as follows. After the skin is cleaned, a 24- to 26-gauge needle is inserted only as far as the deep dermis. The needle is then slowly advanced into the area of the trigger point, and the patient is instructed to tell the physician when an acute increase of pain is noted. There are two reliable signs that a trigger point has been entered: (1) the patient's experience of a sudden pain, often with a centrifugal pattern of referral, and (2) a feeling of increased resistance to the progression of the needle tip. In superficial muscles, a transient twitch response of the muscle may be observed. Approximately 0.5 mL of fluid is injected and the needle is then reinserted (without its leaving the original skin puncture) into an adjacent area of muscle. This "peppering" procedure is repeated until no more pain is experienced. For the average-sized trigger point, the total amount injected is between 1 and 5 mL. The beneficial effects from such an injection typically occur after a lag period of 2 to 5 days. Patients should be informed that they may experience an immediate relief of the pain from the effects of the local anesthetic, but there may be a temporary increase in pain for a few days. There are often several trigger points responsible for myofascial pain syndrome; hence more than one trigger point may need to be injected at the same time. Because large volumes of local anesthetic (more than 15 mL) may cause dizziness, tinnitus, muscle fasciculations, bradycardia, hypertension, and rarely convulsions or cardiorespiratory arrest, the number of injections should be limited. Repeated visits for the injection of satellite trigger points are scheduled at 1- to 6-week intervals. Anaphylaxis is a rare complication from all local anesthetics, and physicians doing these procedures should have a ready availability of airway oxygen, 1:1000 epinephrine, and intravenous diazepam (Valium). Injections in the upper back and other locations close to the thorax may result in a pneumothorax if the needle penetrates the pleura or lung. An awareness of this potential problem and the entering of trigger points at an oblique angle to the surface of the chest wall minimize the likelihood of this complication. The efficacy of trigger point injections is often enhanced by performing "myofascial spray and stretch" immediately after the injections. Spray and stretch consists of an application of a vapocoolant spray, such as dichlorodifluoromethane-trichloromonofluoromethane (Fluori-Methane) over the muscle with simultaneous passive stretching. The cool spray is used as a distraction technique based on the gate theory of pain; actual cooling of the muscle should be avoided. A fine stream of the spray is aimed toward the skin directly overlying the muscle with the active trigger point. A few sweeps of the spray are passed over the trigger point and the zone of reference. This is followed by a progressively increasing passive stretch of the muscle.

FIBROMYALGIA

During the past decade, there has been an increasing realization that many patients presenting with widespread musculoskeletal pain can best be classified as having the fibromyalgia syndrome. Simplistically, fibromyalgia can be thought of as widespread myofascial pain, in that such patients have multiple myofascial tender points. There is now good evidence that such patients have an abnormality in their central processing of both pain sensations (hyperalgesia) and nonpain sensations (allodynia). The American College of Rheumatology has defined the fibromyalgia syndrome in terms of widespread musculoskeletal pain (defined as pain in three or more quadrants of the body plus axial pain) and the presence of 11 or more of 18 specifically designated tender points. In reality, most fibromyalgia patients present with a syndrome of complicated somatic distress that is thought to be both a manifestation of a "pain centralization state" (neuroplasticity) and the psychologic distress engendered by chronic pain (Table 4). There is no cure for this disorder, and most patients can be expected to be symptomatic for many years with a reduced quality of life and varied levels of psychosocial dysfunction. However, engagement in a productive lifestyle and minimization of dysfunction can often be achieved by paying attention to four major areas: pain, exercise, sleep, and psyche.

Pain

The use of NSAIDs in these patients is usually disappointing; it is unusual for fibromyalgia patients to experience more than a 20% relief of their pain, but many consider this to be worthwhile. Narcotics (propoxyphene, codeine, oxycodone) may provide a

TABLE 4. **Clinical Features of Fibromyalgia**

Nearly Always Present	Often Present
Total body pain	Recurrent headaches
Multiple tender points on examination	Irritable bowel syndrome
Severe fatigue	Atypical paresthesias
Nonrestorative sleep (alpha-delta sleep)	Cold sensitivity (often Raynaud's phenomenon)
Postexertional increase in muscle pain	Restless leg syndrome
Reduced functional ability	Aerobic deconditioning

worthwhile short-term relief of pain, but tolerance quickly develops in most patients, and their prescription needs to be restricted in a controlled manner. Tramadol (Ultram), a recently introduced analgesic, seems to provide partial, but significant, pain attenuation in many fibromyalgia patients—it is currently undergoing controlled trials. The severity of pain and the location of "hot spots" typically vary from month to month, and the judicious use of myofascial trigger point injections and spray and stretch (see the section on myofascial pain) is worthwhile in selected patients but should be viewed as an aid to active participation in a regular stretching and aerobic exercise program. Evaluation by an occupational and physical therapist often provides worthwhile advice on improved ergonomics, biomechanical imbalance, and the formulation of a regular stretching program. Hands-on physical therapy with heat modalities is reserved for major flares of pain, as there is no evidence that long-term therapy alters the course of the disorder. The same comments can be made for acupuncture, transcutaneous electrical stimulation, and various massage techniques.

Exercise

A gentle program of stretching and aerobic exercise is essential to counteract the tendency for deconditioning that leads to progressive dysfunction in fibromyalgia patients. Before stretching, muscles should be warmed either actively by gentle exercise or passively by a heating pad, warm bath, or hot tub. Stretching aids in the release of the often tightened muscle bands and when properly performed provides pain relief. The amount of the stretch is important. Stretching to the point of resistance and then holding the stretch allow the Golgi tendon apparatus to signal the muscle fibers to relax. Stretching to the point of increased pain precipitates a contraction of additional fibers and has a deleterious effect. The stretch should be gentle and sustained for 60 seconds. Often patients must work up to this amount of time and start with 10 to 15 seconds *on* and then 10 to 15 seconds *off*. There is good evidence that fibromyalgia patients benefit from increased aerobic conditioning, but many are reluctant to exercise because of increased pain and fatigue. However, most patients can be motivated to increase their level of fitness if they are provided realistic guidelines for exercise and have regular follow-up. Exercise prescription should emphasize nonimpact loading exercise such as walking, the use of stationary exercycles, and water therapy. The eventual aim is to exercise three or four times a week at 60 to 70% of the maximal heart rate for 20 to 30 minutes. Most patients cannot start out at this level but need to establish a regular pattern of exercise. I have found that an acceptable initiation for most patients is to start with two or three daily exercise sessions of only 3 to 5 minutes each. The duration should then be increased until they are doing three 10-minute sessions, then two 15-minute

sessions, and finally one 20- to 30-minute session performed three times per week.

Sleep

All fibromyalgia patients complain of fragmented nonrefreshing sleep. A treatable cause of the sleep disturbance should always be sought. For instance, a small number of patients have sleep apnea and benefit from continuous positive airway pressure therapy. Other patients have nocturnal myoclonus associated with a restless leg syndrome and may often be helped by the prescription of clonazepam (Klonopin),* 0.1 mg at bedtime, or carbidopa-levodopa (Sinemet),* 10/100 at bedtime. In the majority of patients, the sleep disturbance seems to be rooted in psychologic distress or due to pain itself. For instance, a regional myofascial pain syndrome consequent to a whiplash injury may cause a persistent sleep disruption, which eventually leads to the appearance of widespread musculoskeletal pain consistent with the fibromyalgia syndrome; this transition from regional pain to widespread pain typically occurs over a period of 6 to 18 months. In some patients, trochanteric bursitis or subacromial bursitis and/or tendinitis causes a sleep disruption every time the patient turns over onto that side, and appropriate treatment of the bursitis (see the previous section) may lead to a more restorative sleep pattern. In many fibromyalgia patients, the sleep disturbance may be helped by the judicious prescription of a low-dose tricyclic antidepressant (TCA).* The doses required to promote restorative sleep in fibromyalgia are not in the range required to treat depression. There seems to be no logical way of knowing which TCA to prescribe. The ideal medication would produce restorative sleep with a feeling of being refreshed on awakening with no side effects. In reality, some patients are excessively sensitive to TCAs and have a severe sense of "morning hangover"; this may be helped by switching from one of the more sedative agents to a more stimulant TCA. Other patients find TCAs unacceptable owing to anticholinergic side effects, such as tachycardia, dry mouth, and constipation. Most TCAs cause some weight gain, but in certain patients this may amount to 20% of their initial body weight and is thus unacceptable. I often initiate TCA therapy with a trial of four medications taken for 6 days each with a 1-day washout between. Patients can be advised to start medication on a Friday evening to minimize the inconvenience of a possible hangover the next morning. If the patient has not taken a TCA before, the following drugs and dosages can typically be used: amitriptyline (Elavil, Endep),* 10 mg at bedtime; doxepin (Sinequan, Adapin),* 10 mg at bedtime; nortriptyline (Pamelor, Aventyl),* 10 mg at bedtime; trazodone (Desyrel),* 25 mg at bedtime; and cyclobenzaprine (Flexeril), 10 mg at bedtime—cyclobenzaprine has a TCA structure and is also a muscle relaxant. Unless the patient

---

*Not FDA approved for this indication.

has a concomitant major depressive illness, I do not routinely advocate selective serotonin reuptake inhibitors (SSRIs) such as fluoxetine (Prozac),* because they may exacerbate insomnia and cause agitation. When SSRIs are used in patients with concomitant major depression, I usually prescribe a low-dose TCA, such as trazodone, 50 mg at bedtime. Some fibromyalgia patients are intolerant of TCAs due to a persistent daytime hangover effect. In such cases, I use zolpidem (Ambien), 10 mg at bedtime, with instructions not to use it more than three times a week.

Psyche

Patients with chronic pain often develop secondary psychologic disturbances, such as depression, anger, fear, withdrawal, and anxiety. Sometimes these secondary reactions become the major problem; however, it is a common mistake to attribute *all* the patient's symptoms to an aberrant psyche. The prompt diagnosis and treatment of these secondary features are essential to effective overall management of fibromyalgia patients. Some patients develop a reduced functional ability and have difficulty being competitively employed. In such cases, the treating physician needs to act as an advocate in sanctioning a reduced or modified load at work and at home. The overall philosophy of treating fibromyalgia patients, however, is to provide them with realistic expectations of what can be done to help and to de-emphasize the role of medications. Frequent visits to physical therapists, masseurs, and chiropractors or a dependence on repeated myofascial trigger point injections should be discouraged. Unless the patient has an obvious psychiatric illness, referral to psychiatrists is usually nonproductive. Psychologic counseling, particularly the use of techniques such as cognitive restructuring and biofeedback, may benefit some patients who are having difficulties coping with the realities of living with their pain and associated problems.

*Not FDA approved for this indication.

OSTEOARTHRITIS

method of
DAVID H. NEUSTADT, M.D.
University of Louisville School of Medicine
Louisville, Kentucky

Osteoarthritis (OA) (degenerative joint disease, osteoarthrosis) is by far the most commonly encountered rheumatic disorder and the major cause of disability and reduced activity in persons older than 50 years. Radiographic evidence of OA is found in up to 85% of people older than 65 years. Autopsies indicate evidence of OA in weight-bearing joints of almost all persons by the age of 45 years. In spite of the evidence of pathologic changes of OA found in skeletons of the Java and Neanderthal men and dinosaurs, OA was confused with rheumatoid arthritis (RA) until the turn of the present century. It is characterized pathologically by involvement of cartilage, varying from fissures and microfibrillations in early disease to virtual destruction in advanced disease. Weight-bearing or shearing forces are transmitted to the subchondral bone, leading to sclerosis and cyst formation. Osteophytes develop at the margins of joints, and new cartilage proliferates over these bony spurs. An inflammatory component occurs in most patients with symptomatic OA. The traditional belief that OA is simply a wear and tear condition associated with advancing years is no longer tenable. This mistaken belief is considered the major reason for the slow progress of cartilage research and investigation into the etiology and pathogenesis of OA. During the past decade, much new knowledge on cartilage, including metabolic changes, genetic mutations, metalloproteinases, and inflammatory mediators, has fostered considerable excitement and interest in new approaches for the prevention and treatment of OA.

Although the cause of OA is unknown, contributing factors include heredity, trauma, overweight, overuse of joints, and aging. OA may be classified into primary (idiopathic) and secondary forms. Secondary OA results from trauma or repetitive overuse of a specific joint; an inflammatory form of arthritis such as RA, repeated attacks of gout, or septic arthritis; developmental problems such as congenital dysplasia of a hip or slipped capital femoral epiphysis; or metabolic and miscellaneous causes including hemophiliac arthropathy, ochronosis (alkaptonuria), and osteonecrosis. Thus, OA may be considered a (final) common pathway resulting from a host of many different problems. Joints commonly affected in OA include the large weight-bearing and frequently used joints, such as the hips and knees, spine, distal interphalangeal (DIP) joints (Heberden's nodes), and trapeziometacarpal (thumb base) and first metatarsophalangeal joint (bunion). Joints usually spared in OA include the metacarpals, the wrists, the shoulders, and the ankles (except in ballet dancers).

The onset of OA is insidious, and the course is slowly progressive. Clinical features include variable pain and stiffness, manifested by limited motion; bony enlargement with or without tenderness; synovitis of the knees; and functional impairment (with varus or valgus deformities) when advanced involvement of the knees or hips develops. There are no specific laboratory abnormalities or (disease) markers of the disease, except in ochronosis. Radiographs and other imaging procedures demonstrate evidence of OA, manifested chiefly by a narrowed joint space, osteophyte formation, and secondary subchondral sclerosis. There may be a lack of correlation between symptoms and underlying structural findings (thus the dictum "We don't treat x-rays"). Special subsets of OA and significant associated conditions include inflammatory (cystic erosive) OA, crystal pyrophosphate dihydrate disease (chondrocalcinosis), and diffuse idiopathic skeletal hyperostosis.

MANAGEMENT

The optimal management program for OA should be individualized to the specific problems and clinical syndromes presented by each patient (Table 1).

General Considerations

Realistic reassurance that the patient does not have a serious potentially crippling disease such as

TABLE 1. **Comprehensive Management Program for Osteoarthritis**

Education of the patient and family
Coping measures
Measures to reduce joint loading
Physical therapy; occupational therapy assistive devices
Pharmacotherapy
Intra-articular and lavage therapy
Arthroscopy and surgery

RA and provision of adequate understanding of what to expect are of paramount importance for successful management. Education of the patient is the basic foundation of the treatment program. The updated OA booklet provided by the National Arthritis Foundation is a useful supplement to education. There is increasing interest in involving spouses and other family members in coping skills training. Understanding the patient's problem permits reasonable delegation of responsibilities for chores and engaging in combined social activities. Patients and spouses who are better informed about the disease and its outlook are generally better able to manage and cope with the illness. Cognitive-behavioral techniques help patients confront the variability of symptoms and the effects of rest, exercise, and emotional aspects.

Prophylactic Measures

Reducing the impact of the load and shearing force on an osteoarthritic joint may not only diminish symptoms, but also retard progression of the disease. Explaining the biomechanical factors helps the patient understand the need for rest and protection of the affected joints. Weight reduction by dietetic means is strongly encouraged for the overweight patient. Protective and preventive measures for knee involvement include avoiding weight-bearing knee bending, stair climbing, jogging, and prolonged walking. Knee bending during weight bearing can be avoided by using a high stool or chair, elevated toilet seat, knee supports, and assistive walking devices (Table 2).

Physical and Occupational Therapy

The most important aspect is specific instructions for balanced rest and exercise (preferably at home). Exercises should be mainly isometric (nonmovement) such as quadriceps strengthening, stretching, and range-of-motion exercises.

TABLE 2. **Measures to Protect Knees**

Avoid knee bending when weight bearing
Avoid steps
Use high chair or high stool
Use elevated toilet seat
Use cane or crutches for prolonged walking
Do quadriceps muscle-strengthening exercises

Instructions should be given in joint protection with measures to conserve energy and on the use of any needed assistive aids, such as canes, crutches, splints, back supports and braces, cervical supporting collars, and proper shoes with any needed orthotics.

Heat modalities should be prescribed in the form of moist hot packs, soaks, a Bed Buddy (microwave collar), and a warm pool for water aerobic exercises. These measures ameliorate discomfort, as well as facilitate the exercise program. Diathermy, shortwave, and ultrasound methods are relatively expensive and time-consuming. Available evidence suggests that these forms of treatment provide no additional benefit in terms of pain relief or improved function. The use of a hot tub or Jacuzzi, especially after exercise or work, may be of palliative benefit.

Job and recreational activities must be assessed and modified if necessary to avoid overuse of affected joints. Sexual counseling may be needed in some patients with severe knee, hip, or back involvement.

PHARMACOTHERAPY

The basic program of education and reassurance of the patient, joint rest and protection, and physical measures may control symptoms in some patients with early or mild OA. Many patients, however, require drug therapy. Although no available drugs predictably reverse or halt the inexorable progression of the disease, the drugs do reduce pain and inflammation.

Analgesics

Some patients with OA have minimal inflammation and can be managed with analgesics alone. Analgesic agents currently available include acetaminophen (Tylenol), propoxyphene (Darvon), and tramadol (Ultram). Effective dosages of acetaminophen are 1.0 to 1.3 grams administered three or four times daily. Adverse effects are rare, but caution must be exercised in patients with pre-existing renal or liver conditions. Propoxyphene is effective, especially in combination with acetaminophen (Darvocet-N 100), and may be given in a dosage of 1 tablet at 4- to 6-hour intervals to supplement the acetaminophen, as needed for pain. Side effects are usually minimal, with the patient occasionally intolerant because of nausea and lightheadedness. Tramadol can be given in 50-mg tablets up to three or four times daily for pain relief. It is generally well tolerated, with nausea, vomiting, and dizziness the most common adverse effects.

Anti-inflammatory Agents

A report has compared acetaminophen, 4 grams daily, with ibuprofen, 1200 or 2400 mg daily, in OA of the knee. The clinical results demonstrated no difference in efficacy among the three treatment groups. Critical analysis of this "comparative" study, however, discloses a rather short duration of the treatment trial (4 weeks) and a relatively low anti-inflammatory dosage (2400 mg) of ibuprofen. Nevertheless, in my experience and that of others, pain in some OA patients is not adequately controlled with pure analgesics, whereas aspirin and nonsteroidal anti-inflammatory drugs (NSAIDs) may provide significant clinical improvement. Nonacetylated salicylates are widely used in OA. Compounds currently available include salsalate (Disalcid), choline magnesium trisalicylate (Trilisate), and magnesium salicylate. These agents are weak prostaglandin (cyclooxygenase) inhibitors, thus avoiding the anticlotting effect and potential adverse effect on the gastrointestinal tract and kidney. Side effects are relatively infrequent and minor with nonacetylated salicylates when administered in a dosage of 1 to 1.5 grams twice daily. Salicylism with ototoxicity is a rare occurrence. If simple analgesics and salsalate fail to provide adequate relief, one of the many currently available NSAIDs may be selected for a therapeutic trial. The chief limiting factor in the use of NSAIDs is the possible induced gastric pathologic changes and disturbed renal function. Cost and compliance must also be considered. Many of the NSAIDs are now available in dosage forms that can be given once or twice daily, which helps overcome the compliance problem. Currently available NSAIDs are all similar in their proposed mechanism of action but vary considerably in their pharmocokinetics, dosage, clinical response, and side effects. The variability of the effects of different NSAIDs in patients is significant and unpredictable. All NSAIDs are metabolized in the liver, but two available compounds, sulindac (Clinoril) and nabumetone (Relafen), are prodrugs and are not converted to active drugs until after absorption. The prodrug effect may partially spare the gastrointestinal tract and also produces less suppression of renal prostaglandins. Etodolac (Lodine) reportedly has fewer gastric complications, and endoscopy does not demonstrate the typical gastric erosions found in the gastric mucosa of the majority of patients taking NSAIDs. Concomitant prophylactic use of misoprostol (Cytotec) has been recommended to protect gastric mucosa in patients with a previous history of peptic ulcer or gastrointestinal bleeding. Unfortunately, misoprostol causes cramps and diarrhea in a relatively high percentage of patients. The question of potential deleterious effect on cartilage versus "chondroprotective" properties by various NSAIDs is under study but remains unsettled. It has been discovered that prostaglandin synthesis in humans is catalyzed by two forms of cyclooxygenase, cyclooxygenase-1 (COX-1) and cyclooxygenase-2 (COX-2).

COX-1 is constitutively expressed and is considered responsible for suppression of physiologic functions such as gastric mucosal protection. In contrast, COX-2 is not constitutively expressed but is induced by mediators and is responsible for inflammation without any significant effect on the gastric mucosa and kidney. The development of agents that selectively inhibit the COX-2 pathway without any gastro-intestinal or renal effect would be an extremely important advance in avoiding the serious adverse events. Clinical investigation of two different COX-2–inhibiting compounds is in progress. A preliminary analysis has shown effectiveness with no effect on platelet function and no significant gastrointestinal side effects. This is an extremely promising area of research and may represent an important advance in the drug therapy of OA.

CYSTIC EROSIVE OSTEOARTHRITIS

Cystic erosive OA, the genetically determined clinical syndrome manifested by the lumpy-bumpy nodes of the DIP joints (Heberden's nodes) and proximal interphalangeal joints (Bouchard's nodes), rarely causes significant pain, except during the early developing stage. It is important to strongly reassure the patient that this is not a serious crippling disease, emphasizing the distinction of the knobby nodes from the swelling (synovitis) of RA. However, if the thumb base joint (trapeziometacarpal) is involved, abduction splinting and/or local injection may be necessary for relief. Occasionally, when OA of the fingers is symptomatic, warm soaks; the application of an analgesic balm, such as triethanolamine, after the warm soaks; and the wearing of spandex gloves during the night are sometimes useful. When a digital node is inflamed, local instillation of a few drops of a corticosteroid suspension often provides prompt relief. If symptoms persist, a cautious trial with one of the topical analgesic pepper plant creams (capsaicin) such as Zostrix or Dolorac may be worthwhile. Capsaicin is an inhibitor of substance P, the neuropeptide pain mediator. The topical cream is safe, and a local burning or transient stinging sensation is the only troublesome adverse effect.

INTRA-ARTICULAR CORTICOSTEROIDS

After many years of controversy concerning intra-articular corticosteroid therapy in OA, there is now consensus that the procedure is of considerable value when administered skillfully and when indicated. Although early on it is still preferable to attempt to control symptoms by simple measures with oral therapy, rather than by local injection, when faced with relatively acute conditions such as synovitis of the knee or inflamed Heberden's node, quick and sometimes lasting relief can be obtained with intrasynovial steroid instillation. This form of treatment must always be considered an adjunct to a conventional management program.

A large painful knee effusion is the strongest indication for arthrocentesis, followed by a local corticosteroid injection. The potential deleterious effect of instability's developing in the knee can be avoided by giving injections at infrequent intervals and prescribing a strict (postinjection) rest regimen. Instructions are given to refrain from all weight-bearing activity for 3 days, except getting up for meals and going to the bathroom. The patient is advised to reduce "loading" of the injected knee by using a cane or crutches with a three-point gait during all weight bearing for 2 to 3 weeks. This routine delays escape of the steroid suspension from the joint cavity and promotes a longer duration of response to the injection. I have observed numerous patients with OA of the knee associated with large painful recurrent synovitis who had been given three to five or more local injections with only transient benefit. When a strict postinjection rest program was imposed, these patients obtained substantial improvement in the duration of the effect and some achieved indefinite "cures." The remote risk of introducing infection from the procedure is minimized by adhering to a meticulous aseptic technique.

Another important indication for arthrocentesis and intra-articular steroid therapy is OA associated with crystal synovitis due to calcium pyrophosphate dihydrate, so-called pseudogout. Diagnosis is confirmed by radiographic findings of chondrocalcinosis and polarized microscopic identification of the specific crystals. Treatment, including aspiration and administration of intra-articular steroids, is usually successful in controlling the acute synovitis.

JOINT LAVAGE AND ARTHROSCOPY

Clinical improvement in the symptoms and signs of OA of the knee has been reported after two-needle tidal irrigation and closed joint lavage. Lavage of the arthritic knee may also be performed with arthroscopic visualization. A double-blind evaluation including a sham lavage group is currently ongoing.

Arthroscopy permits detailed inspection of the joint cavity. Associated abnormality such as ligamentous and meniscal tears can be observed in conjunction with osteoarthritis. Calcified loose bodies can be removed, and débridement can be carried out. The procedure may "buy time" for a patient not yet ready or willing to consider joint replacement. The success rate is variable. Studies using the office small-gauge or needle arthroscope (1.6 mm in diameter) are currently under way.

INVESTIGATIONAL FORMS OF THERAPY (DISEASE-MODIFYING DRUGS)

The purpose of the investigational disease-modifying drugs is to play a role in either enhancing the biosynthesis of cartilage matrix or preventing enzymatic degradation and inhibiting catabolic cytokine activity in an attempt to induce cartilage repair and restore joint homeostasis.

The use of the descriptive term "disease-modifying drugs," well established in RA, is relatively new to the OA field. The International League of Associations for Rheumatology recommended that the designation be limited to agents that "prevent, retard progression of, or reverse morphologic changes" to qualify an agent as a disease modifying drug. Although several agents meet the criteria in animal models of OA, no available therapeutic agent predictably alters the underlying pathogenesis of OA. However, research has been carried out with certain novel noteworthy approaches.

Several intramuscular preparations, Arteparon,* an extract of bovine lung and trachea cartilage, and Rumalon,* an extract of bovine bone marrow and cartilage, have shown some evidence of favorably modifying OA in animal models of OA and in uncontrolled studies in human subjects in Europe. Both compounds showed stimulation of cartilage synthesis and inhibition of protease enzymes, but unfortunately bleeding associated with the heparinoid structure of the agents and reports of anaphylaxis have led to their removal from the overseas market. Sodium pentosan sulfate, Cartrofen, another heparinoid agent, an extract of beech hemicellulose, inhibits lysosomal and metalloproteinase enzymes and increases the production of hyaluronic acid. It lacks an antigenic protein, thus avoiding the potential problem of anaphylaxis, and a calcium form has the advantage of oral absorption but has not yet been studied in patients with OA. Confirming evidence of a true disease-modifying effect will require a randomized controlled long-term study in humans.

Tetracycline and its congeners (doxycycline, minocycline) have shown evidence of inhibiting enzymatic degradation of cartilage, including that by stromelysin, collagenase, and gelatinase, in canine, guinea pig, and rabbit models of OA. A proposed long-term clinical trial in human subjects is now in progress.

Tenidap (Enable),† a new anti-inflammatory agent with additional inhibiting properties of interleukin-1 and interleukin-6, now undergoing investigation in a large multicenter trial, may have a significant disease-modifying effect.

Hydroxychloroquine (Plaquenil) and chloroquine have been administered successfully in RA and systemic lupus erythematosus for many years. More recently, anecdotal and retrospective uncontrolled studies have reported the efficacy of hydroxychloroquine in retarding the progression of inflammatory (cystic) erosive OA. It has been suggested that the beneficial action of hydroxychloroquine is due to its inhibitory effects on lysosomal (enzyme) activities. In addition, hydroxychloroquine has demonstrated inhibition of the secretion of interleukin-1. Experience thus far indicates that this agent is promising in inflammatory OA, and a prospective placebo-controlled study would be a worthwhile contribution.

Other so-called novel therapeutic approaches under study without conclusive significant data include insulin-like growth factors, transforming growth factor-β, and glucosamine, a proteoglycan component and a growth factor for cartilage.

Superoxide dismutase (orgotein),‡ a protein extract of bovine liver, removes superoxide and hydroxyl radicals, which are considered involved in the patho-

---

*Not available in the United States.
†Investigational drug in the United States.
‡Not FDA approved for this indication.

genesis of joint damage in OA. In a multicenter placebo-controlled intra-articular study of superoxide dismutase in OA of the knee, statistically significant clinical improvement did not occur. It has been suggested that superoxide dismutase may have a specific beneficial effect on cartilage, but no conclusive evidence has been demonstrated.

Evidence has shown that nitric oxide a highly reactive free radical, plays a significant role in the pathogenesis of inflammatory arthritis and inhibits proteoglycan synthesis. Inhibitors of nitric oxide synthase reduce swelling and other evidence of inflammation in animal models of arthritis.

NEW APPROACHES

A variety of new experimental approaches for the treatment of OA are currently under development.

Hyaluronate (Hyaluronic Acid)

Hyaluronate, a glycosaminoglycan, responsible for the viscosity and lubrication of normal synovial fluid, has been studied as a substance capable of restoring the properties of synovial fluid and cartilage and reducing pain and stiffness in the osteoarthritic knee.

Several preparations, Orthovisc, hylan (Synvisc), and Hyalgan, are available in Canada and Europe, and Hyalgan and Synvisc were approved in 1997 by the FDA Arthritis Advisory Committee, clearing the way for the clinical use of this new form of intraarticular therapy. This mode of therapy is called viscosupplementation, because clinical improvement is thought to be due to supplementing the viscous properties of altered synovial fluid. It may also have a beneficial protective effect on the chondrocyte. Adverse effects are limited to rare transient local reactions. For enhanced efficacy, because of a relatively short half-life of hyaluronate, three or four injections are administered at 5- to 7-day intervals.

Electromagnetic Field Therapy

Pulsed electromagnetic field therapy has a long history of use, chiefly for treatment of delayed nonunion fractures. Relatively preliminary studies in knee OA suggest that this form of therapy may be useful; however, data are inadequate to critically assess the effects. Further study of a larger number of patients is required for confirmation of the value of this form of treatment.

Chondrocyte Transplantation

Chondrocyte transplantation was initially developed and carried out in Sweden for localized cartilage damage resulting from trauma in rather young subjects. A subsequent report described relatively successful treatment of 23 patients with chondral defects of the knee given autologous chondrocyte transplantation, combined with periosteal grafting.

Preliminary additional uncontrolled clinical trials to determine efficacy have described no significant adverse effects. However, the expectation that the procedure will "cure" OA lesions remains an unmet possibility for the future. Regeneration of articular cartilage is a complex process and will require longterm evaluation of the function of the new cartilage and prospective controlled clinical studies to confirm the value of the procedure.

Gene Therapy

Gene therapy is an exciting new technology that holds promise for the future but requires considerable further investigation and refinement. Techniques to introduce gene transfer in conjunction with autologous cultured chondrocytes are being explored.

SURGERY

When appropriate medical (nonoperative) management fails to adequately control pain, and associated (functional) disability significantly interferes with lifestyle, surgical procedures should be considered.

Available procedures include osteotomy for joint malalignment (varus knee deformities); débridement, especially for specific lesions such as calcified loose bodies or meniscal tears; and arthrodesis (fusion) for unstable joints, when joint replacement is not indicated or declined. Arthrodesis may be the optimal procedure in young, overweight, active patients with severe OA involving a single knee. Partial or total arthroplasty, especially total knee and hip replacement, may be carried out in patients in whom medical management fails to adequately control symptoms. An estimated 120,000 total hip replacements, most of which are for OA, are performed each year in the United States.

POLYMYALGIA RHEUMATICA AND GIANT CELL ARTERITIS

method of
LOUIS A. HEALEY, M.D.
University of Washington School of Medicine
Seattle, Washington

Polymyalgia rheumatica and giant cell arteritis are in some way related but exactly how is not known. Both affect older patients and both occur much more often in whites. The two syndromes are often seen in the same patient, although not always at the same time. They appear to be separate syndromes rather than two manifestations of a single underlying giant cell arteritis. Polymyalgia rheumatica may be persistent or recurrent, whereas temporal arteritis is almost always a single episode; documented recurrences are rare.

TREATMENT

Polymyalgia rheumatica is the more common of the two syndromes; it is characterized by pain in the neck, shoulders, or hips that persists for at least 1 month. Morning stiffness is especially pronounced and provides a helpful clue to the diagnosis. Arthroscopy and biopsy have demonstrated that the pain and stiffness are caused by a nondestructive inflammation of synovial tissues in and about the shoulder and hip. The erythrocyte sedimentation rate is often elevated, and symptoms respond dramatically to prednisone and so invariably that if the response is not seen within a week the diagnosis should be doubted. Aspirin and other anti-inflammatory drugs are less effective than prednisone. The usual dose is 10 or 20 mg a day, which is tapered to a maintenance dose of 5 to 7.5 mg per day after the clinical response. Methotrexate* is effective for the rare patient who requires a higher dose of prednisone.

The subsequent disease course is unpredictable. Some patients, perhaps two thirds, can discontinue prednisone therapy after 2 years, but others need to continue to take the medication for much longer to prevent the pain and stiffness from returning. Despite prolonged treatment, these patients remain free from symptoms on 5 mg per day and develop no joint destruction or steroid side effect. In patients who stop the prednisone therapy, recurrence is frequent, appearing in about 30%, any time from months to years later. The recurrence may be similar to the initial episode of polymyalgia rheumatica, or the synovitis may involve wrists and metacarpophalangeal joints and look like seronegative rheumatoid arthritis, but again, responding to low-dose prednisone and without joint destruction.

Polymyalgia rheumatica and temporal arteritis often appear coincidentally or within months of one another, but at times, the interval between their appearance may be as long as 10 years. Many patients apparently have only polymyalgia; they respond well to low-dose prednisone and never develop clinical evidence of arteritis. The frequency of concurrence varies in different populations, but in North America it is approximately 15%. Thus, temporal artery biopsy and high-dose steroid treatment are not recommended for every patient with polymyalgia. If patients have no clinical symptoms to suggest cranial arteritis, then polymyalgia rheumatica is treated with low-dose prednisone, but the patients are informed that there is a 15% chance of developing arteritis. They should be instructed in the significance of headache, diplopia, blurred vision, and jaw claudication and should be told to alert their physician if these symptoms appear. It is useful to give these patients a list of such symptoms as shown in Table 1.

Giant cell arteritis responds to prednisone, but because of the risk of blindness it is necessary to treat

TABLE 1. **Symptoms Suggestive of Temporal Arteritis**

Temporal or occipital headache
Transient blindness or blurring of vision
Transient double vision
Pain in the jaw when chewing or talking

with at least 50 mg of prednisone per day. This high dose should be maintained for 1 month even though symptoms such as headache respond rapidly. This schedule suppresses the inflammation so that late recurrences of arteritis with vision loss are rare (less than 1%). The steroid dose is tapered after a clinical response. The erythrocyte sedimentation rate, which is initially a good indicator of inflammation and a useful clue to the diagnosis of arteritis, is not a good guide to continuing therapy, as it does not accurately reflect the activity of the arteritis in the subsequent course. Attempting to maintain a normal erythrocyte sedimentation rate almost invariably results in steroid toxicity of osteoporosis. Temporal arteritis is usually a single episode with complete recovery even though a late recurrence of polymyalgia rheumatica is possible.

OSTEOMYELITIS

method of
LAYNE O. GENTRY, M.D.
St. Luke's Episcopal Hospital and Baylor College of Medicine
Houston, Texas

Treatment of osteomyelitis has evolved dramatically since the introduction of antibiotics in the 1940s. The current standard therapy for osteomyelitis is a lengthy parenteral regimen of a broad-spectrum cephalosporin or a penicillinase-resistant penicillin combined with an aminoglycoside. Extended regimens of parenteral antibiotics, however, are associated with toxicity, long hospital stays, high costs, and inconvenience to the patient. Therapeutic options have expanded to include effective oral agents and the use of local antibacterial treatment. The cornerstones of effective management remain early diagnosis and aggressive treatment, including thorough débridement and the institution of sensitivity-specific antibiotics.

PATHOPHYSIOLOGY

Bone infections are classified by the system of Waldvogel and colleagues as either hematogenous or osteomyelitis secondary to a contiguous focus of infection (either with or without vascular insufficiency). Hematogenous osteomyelitis is seen primarily in infants and children. Typically, invasive gram-positive cocci, such as *Staphylococcus aureus*, spread by the bloodstream to the metaphyses of long bones in children. A single pathogenic organism is almost always recovered from the bone. Hematogenous osteomyelitis in adults, although rare, often involves the vertebrae, which are vascularized and thus susceptible to hematogenous seeding associated with intravenous catheters and intravenous drug abuse.

---

*Not FDA approved for this indication.

Osteomyelitis in adults almost always derives from a contiguous focus of infection. Organisms may be inoculated directly into the bone after an open fracture, a penetrating wound, or a surgical procedure, or they may extend from an adjacent soft tissue infection. In contrast to hematogenous osteomyelitis, contiguous or direct inoculation infection is often polymicrobial. Although *S. aureus* remains the most commonly isolated pathogen, other gram-positive and gram-negative organisms are frequently seen. In osteomyelitis due to direct inoculation, *Pseudomonas aeruginosa* and coagulase-negative staphylococci are frequently the cause.

In the subgroup of contiguous focus disease with vascular insufficiency, most patients have diabetes mellitus. Infection, usually involving the small bones of the feet, may be initiated by minor trauma of the foot. Often, culture of infected bone yields multiple organisms, with the most common being coagulase-positive and coagulase-negative staphylococci, enterococci, *Streptococcus* species, gram-negative bacilli, and anaerobes. Accompanying peripheral neuropathy may mask the presence of pain in diabetic patients. Furthermore, fever and systemic toxicity are not usually present. Impaired circulation to the infected site may necessitate amputation.

Hematogenous osteomyelitis and contiguous focus osteomyelitis have been further classified as acute or chronic disease. In acute disease, signs and symptoms have been present for less than 3 months, and in chronic disease, signs and symptoms have been present for more than 3 months. Acute osteomyelitis, often diagnosed in children with bacteremia, may respond favorably to a short-term regimen of parenteral antibiotics followed by oral therapy. Patients may present with a suppurative infection accompanied by edema, vascular congestion, and small vessel thrombosis. Chronic osteomyelitis is usually diagnosed in adults after trauma or major orthopedic surgery and may require a lengthy regimen of parenteral antibiotics. The hallmarks of chronic disease are a nidus of infected dead bone or scar tissue, an ischemic area of soft tissue, and a refractory clinical course.

In contrast to the system proposed by Waldvogel and colleagues, Cierny and Mader have developed an alternative classification system. Their universal staging system defines the clinical stage of osteomyelitis based on the combination of four anatomic types of bone infections and three physiologic host conditions.

DIAGNOSIS

Laboratory Studies

For patients in whom osteomyelitis is suspected, laboratory data may be suggestive of or inconclusive for infection. Unfortunately, no laboratory test specifically indicates the diagnosis of osteomyelitis; however, laboratory results are important in assessing the patient's health status and predicting the response to treatment. Usual laboratory tests include a complete blood cell count with differential, an erythrocyte sedimentation rate (ESR), urinalysis, and serum chemistry tests. The white blood cell count is usually elevated only in early stages of the disease and is often normal in patients with chronic osteomyelitis. The ESR is commonly elevated before therapy and may return to normal levels with successful therapy. The return of the ESR to normal levels during therapy is a favorable prognostic sign. The ESR, however, is less reliable in immunocompromised patients, in patients with sickle cell anemia, and in newborns.

Imaging Studies

In the early stages of osteomyelitis, findings on conventional radiographs may be normal. Changes to the bone may not be detectable on radiographs for 10 to 14 days after injury and infection. The earliest changes are deep soft tissue swelling, which may be difficult to detect, followed by periosteal elevation and radiolucent areas of bone destruction. In contiguous focus and chronic osteomyelitis, radiographic changes are subtle and often nonspecific.

Radionuclide scans allow an earlier diagnosis of osteomyelitis. Scintigraphy with technetium Tc 99m methylene diphosphonate offers excellent sensitivity, especially within the first 2 weeks (Table 1). In fact, ^{99m}Tc scans may be positive 2 to 3 days after infection. Sensitivity, however, is lower in newborns and in patients with sickle cell anemia. Unfortunately, the specificity of ^{99m}Tc scans is low. False-positive results may occur in patients with tumors or infarction or in patients with bone injury involving the periosteum. Furthermore, distinguishing osteomyelitis from cellulitis, septic arthritis, or areas of noninfected inflammatory processes may be difficult. An additional disadvantage is that bone scans remain positive for 6 weeks to 6 months after therapy because of bone metabolism and remodeling. Nevertheless, ^{99m}Tc scanning combined with a detailed evaluation of patients and careful radiography constitutes an effective diagnostic strategy for many cases of chronic osteomyelitis.

Gallium Ga 67 citrate scans have been used to diagnose osteomyelitis. Because gallium citrate binds to proteins involved in inflammation and infection, excessive purulent material and active phagocytosis at the site of infection are necessary to produce a positive scan. Advanced infections may be more reliably detected with this method because of increased numbers of white blood cells. Disadvantages with gallium citrate scans include higher doses of radiation, poor resolution in small bones, and a waiting period of 48 to 72 hours after injection before imaging can be performed.

Indium 111–labeled leukocyte scanning, in which a patient's own white blood cells are labeled in vitro and reinjected, and imaging is performed 24 to 48 hours later, is less useful in evaluating osteomyelitis. False-positive results may occur in patients with infarction, rheumatoid arthritis, healing fractures, noninfected prostheses, and metastatic cancer. This technique may be more useful in complicated cases or as an adjunct for detecting infections associated with orthopedic prostheses.

Computed tomography is useful in selected patients. It is helpful in evaluating bones such as the spine that are difficult to view. Magnetic resonance imaging (MRI) is

TABLE 1. **Comparison of Radiographic and Radionuclide Techniques in Osteomyelitis**

Procedure	Sensitivity	Specificity	Cost
Radiographic			
Radiography	Good*	Poor	Inexpensive
CT	Good	Good	Expensive
MRI	Excellent	Excellent	Very expensive
Radionuclide scans			
Technetium 99m	Excellent	Poor	Moderate
Gallium 67	Moderate	Poor	Expensive
Indium 111	Moderate	Moderate	Expensive

*Sensitivity is poor before 2 wk.
Abbreviations: CT = computed tomography; MRI = magnetic resonance imaging.

highly sensitive in detecting and assessing the extent of infection of the musculoskeletal system. In addition to its sensitivity in detecting infection early, MRI has excellent specificity, especially in distinguishing bone tumor or infarction from osteomyelitis. MRI is the technique of choice for detecting and assessing the extent of infection in the spine and is a favored technique for staging the extent of infection in long cortical bones before definitive open débridement. The expense of MRI, however, precludes its use on a routine basis. A limited MRI technique with specialized views and minimal use of gadolinium contrast material has been used to control costs.

Two experimental imaging techniques have been used to diagnose osteomyelitis: the ^{99m}Tc-hexamethylpropylene-amineoxime–labeled leukocyte scan and a ^{99m}Tc-labeled antigranulocyte antibody. Limited studies indicate that the sensitivity, specificity, and diagnostic accuracy of both modalities compare favorably with those of the ^{99m}Tc bone scan.

Bacteriologic Culture

The "gold standard" for diagnosis of osteomyelitis is aerobic and anaerobic culture of a biopsy specimen obtained under direct vision during surgery. Alternatively, at our center, culture of multiple specimens obtained by needle biopsy with a bone biopsy needle under ultrasonic or radiographic guidance has been a reliable, cost-effective method of diagnosing osteomyelitis. Specimens for culture should be obtained before starting antibiotic therapy. Swab cultures of sinus tracts are not usually accurate because organisms that colonize the sinus tract may not be present in bone. Blood cultures may be positive in patients with hematogenous osteomyelitis but are rarely positive in patients with chronic osteomyelitis.

MANAGEMENT

Treatment of chronic osteomyelitis requires complete surgical débridement of necrotic, avascular, infected bone and soft tissue and a prolonged regimen of antibiotic therapy. The most effective strategy for optimal care of the patient with osteomyelitis is the institution of appropriate antimicrobial therapy (Table 2) based on culture and sensitivity results after complete surgical débridement and after microbiologic confirmation of the diagnosis by biopsy. The most frequent underlying factor in failure of therapy in patients with chronic osteomyelitis is inadequate débridement.

In children with acute hematogenous osteomyelitis, antibiotic therapy alone may be sufficient. If the child responds initially, a regimen of combined intravenous and oral antibiotics may be used. Intravenous therapy should be administered for 1 to 2 weeks, followed by oral therapy for 2 to 3 additional weeks. Although oral quinolones are effective in treating osteomyelitis, they should not be used in children because of the potential for cartilage damage. Most children respond favorably to antimicrobial therapy; however, if the response is slow, antibiotic therapy should be continued and the need for surgery addressed. In adults with acute hematogenous osteomyelitis, surgical débridement is often required.

For adult staphylococcal osteomyelitis, a β-lactamase–resistant penicillin is an appropriate initial choice for methicillin-susceptible strains. A combination regimen of a semisynthetic penicillin and rifampin (Rifadin) has been used successfully to treat methicillin-sensitive S. aureus. Vancomycin (Vancocin) should be used in patients with a methicillin-resistant S. aureus or a coagulase-negative staphylococcal infection. Again, rifampin may be added to increase antistaphylococcal activity. After 4 weeks of parenteral therapy, patients may be switched to an

TABLE 2. **Antimicrobial Therapy for Osteomyelitis in Adults**

Organism	Drug	Regimen
Methicillin sensitive	Nafcillin (Unipen)	2 gm IV q 6 h
Staphylococcus aureus	Oxacillin (Prostaphlin)	2 gm IV q 6 h
	Cefazolin (Kefzol, Ancef)	2 gm IV q 8 h
Methicillin resistant	Vancomycin (Vancocin)*	1 gm IV q 12 h
S. aureus and other staphylococci		
Streptococcus species	Ampicillin (Omnipen, Principen)	2 gm IV q 6 h
Enterococcus species	Ampicillin + gentamicin (Garamycin)†	2 gm IV q 6 h
		1 mg/kg q 8 h
Enterobacteriaceae	Ciprofloxacin (Cipro)	750 mg PO q 12 h
	Ticarcillin-clavulanate (Timentin)	3.1 gm IV q 6 h
	Imipenem-cilastatin (Primaxin)	0.5 gm IV q 6 h
Pseudomonas aeruginosa	Ceftazidime (Fortaz, Tazidime)	2 gm IV q 12 h
	Ceftriaxone (Rocephin)	2 gm IV q 24 h
	Ciprofloxacin (Cipro)	750 mg PO q 12 h
	Semisynthetic penicillin‡	
	Piperacillin (Pipracil)	3 gm IV q 6 h
	Ticarcillin (Ticar)	3 gm IV q 6 h
	with	
	Aminoglycoside‡	
	Amikacin (Amikin)	15 mg/kg/d
	Gentamicin (Garamycin)	5 mg/kg/d
Anaerobes	Clindamycin (Cleocin)	0.9 gm IV q 8 h
	Metronidazole (Flagyl)	0.5 gm IV q 8 h

*Studies show that adding rifampin (Rifadin) may increase efficacy.
†Use the combination for the first 2 wk, followed by ampicillin alone.
‡Use a semisynthetic penicillin in combination with an aminoglycoside.

oral agent. In patients treated with oral agents, close outpatient follow-up and compliance are essential. Although some studies have shown that oral therapy with ciprofloxacin (Cipro) is effective in treating staphylococcal osteomyelitis, reports of variable efficacy and of resistance in some strains of *S. aureus* and *Staphylococcus epidermidis* indicate that oral ciprofloxacin should not be used as monotherapy for treating staphylococcal osteomyelitis. The oral regimen of ofloxacin (Floxin) and rifampin has been effective in patients with *Staphylococcus*-infected implants; however, in the United States ofloxacin is not approved by the Food and Drug Administration for osteomyelitis. At our center, most strains of *S. aureus* isolated from cortical (nonsternal) bone are methicillin susceptible; however, more than 70% of coagulase-negative staphylococci are methicillin resistant.

Most cases of osteomyelitis caused by *Streptococcus* species are treated with ampicillin. *Enterococcus faecalis*, however, is an increasingly troublesome pathogen in acute infections, especially those associated with infected prostheses. Fortunately, *E. faecalis* is an unusual cause of osteomyelitis of long bones without prostheses. Standard recommended therapy for enterococcal infections is gentamicin (Garamycin) plus ampicillin (Omnipen) for 2 weeks, followed by ampicillin alone for 2 more weeks. Because of the potentially serious nature of an associated bacteremia in acute infections, aggressive therapy is necessary until acute symptoms resolve and blood cultures become negative.

For bone infections caused by ciprofloxacin-sensitive Enterobacteriaceae, oral therapy with ciprofloxacin is an effective and inexpensive choice. In addition to the economic savings of reducing the hospital stay and pharmacy and supply costs, oral therapy reduces the complications and inconvenience associated with prolonged intravenous infusion of antibiotics. For patients with diabetes mellitus, aggressive therapy is warranted because infections in these patients are often caused by multiple pathogens, including both gram-positive and gram-negative aerobes and anaerobes. Antibiotic therapy in patients with diabetes should be based on culture and sensitivity results. A typical regimen may include a broad-spectrum cephalosporin or a quinolone combined with metronidazole (Flagyl) or a regimen of clindamycin (Cleocin) and ticarcillin-clavulanate (Timentin).

Pseudomonas infections of the bone may be treated with the third-generation cephalosporin ceftazidime (Fortaz). The extended-spectrum penicillins may act synergistically with the aminoglycosides against more resistant strains of *Pseudomonas*; however, evidence of efficacy in osteomyelitis is not definitive, and toxicity associated with a 28-day regimen of intravenous aminoglycosides is a serious concern. Because the quinolones have been associated with the development of resistance in *P. aeruginosa*, progress must be monitored carefully if ciprofloxacin is used as monotherapy in pseudomonal osteomyelitis.

Antibiotic-impregnated polymethylmethacrylate (PMMA) beads have been used for local treatment of bone infections; however, they have not been approved for use in the United States. PMMA beads deliver a high concentration of antibiotic to the localized area of infection without causing high serum concentrations, which are associated with nephrotoxic, ototoxic, and allergic complications. Local concentrations of antibiotic may be 5 to 10 times higher than those associated with intravenous administration. In addition, PMMA beads, which are usually removed after 2 to 4 weeks, may be useful in temporarily filling dead space in large wounds. The most effective antibiotics used in PMMA beads have been the aminoglycosides. Although they offer an effective means of sterilizing local areas of infection, PMMA beads should be used in conjunction with systemic antibiotics, not as an alternative to conventional therapy.

COMMON SPORTS INJURIES

method of
ALLAN V. ABBOTT, M.D.
University of Southern California School of Medicine
Los Angeles, California

Sports injuries can result from both acute trauma and chronic (overuse) injury. Acute trauma can cause disruption of ligamentous, musculotendinous, or bone structures. If the acute trauma causes no pain and only microscopic damage but is repeated again and again, an overuse syndrome can develop. Overuse injuries with both inflammation and pain are commonly seen by primary care physicians.

The RICE-DIETS (Table 1) mnemonic summarizes the management of most sports injuries.

MOST COMMON INJURIES

The most common injuries to athletes are relatively minor. Contusions or bruises are characterized by inflammation, edema, erythema, hemorrhage, and pain at the site of an acute blow or trauma. Abrasions to the skin may be simple or may overlay more serious injuries. Abrasions should be promptly and thoroughly cleaned to remove dirt and foreign particles, and covered with antibiotic ointment and a sterile dry bandage. Lacerations should be cleaned and closed as appropriate with adhesive strips or sutures. Tenosynovitis is inflammation of the synovium surrounding a tendon and usually results from overuse or a direct blow. The tendon swells, causing pain with motion and sometimes pain at rest. Treatment should be directed to reduce inflammation, swelling, and stiffness of the involved joint. A stretching and strengthening program should follow.

SPRAINS AND STRAINS

Sprains are damaged ligaments, and strains are damaged muscles and/or tendons (Table 2). Most

TABLE 1. **RICE-DIETS Management of Sports Injuries**

Rest minimizes additional injury. The length of rest needed depends on the injury; as little as 1 or 2 d for minor contusions to 8–10 wk for a second- or third-degree sprain.

Ice decreases inflammation and minimizes edema, pain, and muscle spasm. Ice should be applied (never directly to the skin) for 20- to 30-min periods every 1 to 2 h during the first 48 h.

Compression further reduces microhemorrhage and decreases pain and swelling. A cold elastic wrap over a foam or felt pad is effective. An air splint is sometimes preferred but makes ice application difficult.

Elevation to above the level of the heart improves drainage of serous fluids and decreases venous pooling. Elevation adds to the benefits of ice and compression.

Drugs including nonsteroidal anti-inflammatory drugs (such as ibuprofen [Motrin] 200–800 mg q 6–8 h, or naproxen [Naprosyn] 250–500 mg q 12 h) or aspirin (325–650 mg q 6 h) can reduce both pain and inflammation. Drugs that decrease inflammation should be considered especially during the first 3–5 d after injury.

Incision and drainage and injection can be important for large and fluctuant hematomas. Injections of steroids and local anesthetics should be reserved for acute exacerbations of chronic bursitis or tenosynovitis.

Exercise Therapy or rehabilitation begins after acute inflammation improves, often as soon as 2–3 d after acute injury. Progressive range-of-motion exercises and hot and cold applications should be followed by progressive resistance exercises.

Surgery is reserved for certain injuries such as unstable fractures and third-degree sprains and strains.

sprains and strains resulting from sports injuries are to the knee, ankle or foot, wrist or hand, and shoulder.

KNEE INJURIES

Knee sprains are managed with the RICE-DIETS regimen. Second- and third-degree strains are of particular concern, and acutely injured knees should be re-examined in 24 hours. *Tears of the anterior cruciate ligament* (ACL) sometimes result when the knee is locked and the athlete is struck from the front. An ACL injury is suggested if there is immediate pain and if hemarthrosis with moderately severe swelling develops within a few hours after the injury. Radiographs rule out fractures. Mild ACL injuries can be treated with functional rehabilitation. In more severe ACL injuries, the drawer test with the knee in 15 to 20 degrees of flexion (Lachman's test) is abnormal. Rapid consultation and arthroscopy provide precise diagnosis and treatment. *Posterior cruciate ligament tears* are less common and may result from severe hyperextension injuries, or a blow or fall to the front of a flexed knee. The knee may not swell, and the popliteal fossa is tender. The posterior drawer test may be positive if the posterior capsule is also torn. Surgical consultation is indicated.

Collateral ligament sprains usually result from a blow to the side of the knee with the foot planted. Collateral ligament injuries are more common medially. Swelling and tenderness are seen over the ligament. Ligament integrity should be tested by using varus and valgus stress on the knee. First-degree and many second-degree collateral ligament strains can be treated with functional knee rehabilitation. Opening of the joint on stress, which can be confirmed by radiography, suggests a second- or third-degree sprain, and surgery is indicated.

Meniscus tears frequently occur as the result of blows to the knee or from sudden twisting movements. These tears can cause the knee to pop, click, lock, or "give way." The typical joint-line pain and swelling depend on the severity and type of tear. Radiographs rule out fractures. Symptomatic treatment and knee rehabilitation may be adequate for minor meniscus injuries; however, if the symptoms persist, arthroscopy is indicated for both diagnosis and repair.

Patellofemoral pain syndrome is a common knee problem resulting from overuse. It is commonly seen in runners, especially in young women, and is often related to abnormal tracking of the patella. The patient describes a soreness or aching under the patella aggravated by activities such as walking, climbing or descending stairs, or squatting, or after sitting for long periods. The knee may also occasionally give way or have pain or crepitation on movement of the patella under pressure. There may be tenderness to patellar compression or to pressure over the medial facet. Radiographs are usually not helpful. The RICE-DIETS regimen is helpful with emphasis on knee rehabilitation including progressive quadriceps-strengthening exercises. The correction of biomechanical foot abnormalities with orthotics may be helpful.

TABLE 2. **Description of Sprains and Strains**

First-degree: Minimal stretching or tear of fibers with no decrease in range of motion and minimal functional disability.

Second-degree: Rupture of up to 80% of tissue fibers. Pain and edema are more marked and range of motion is limited. Pain and swelling improve within 2–3 wk, and the athlete may convert a second-degree to a third-degree injury by returning to full exercise too soon. Complete healing requires 8–10 wk.

Third-degree: Complete rupture of the ligament or musculotendinous unit. There is complete loss of function of that unit, usually with severe pain, ecchymosis, and swelling. A chip or avulsion fracture may be present on radiographs. Surgical repair may be required, and at least 8 wk of complete protection is needed.

ANKLE AND FOOT INJURIES

Ankle sprains are the most common ankle injuries, usually resulting from inversion and injury to the lateral ankle ligaments. Swelling, ecchymosis, and tenderness are evident over the injured ligaments. In first-degree sprains, the RICE treatment is sufficient. If weight bearing is painful, or if the anterior drawer test is abnormal compared with the opposite ankle (or >3 mm motion), the talofibular and possibly the calcaneofibular ligaments may be torn. Radiographs are indicated to rule out fractures. Early mobilization and the use of functional bracing have been shown to be effective treatment for all grades of ankle sprains. After 24 to 48 hours of RICE, the patient can begin partial or full weight bearing while wearing an inflatable inversion-eversion splint (Air-Cast) that allows some dorsiflexion and plantar flexion for 6 to 8 weeks. If there is gross ankle instability or if pain and inflammation persist, orthopedic consultation may be appropriate.

Plantar fasciitis is the most common cause of heel pain resulting from running. As the result of overuse, pain and tenderness occur at the base of the heel where the plantar fascia inserts into the calcaneous. Predisposing factors include running on hard flat surfaces, pes planus, overpronation, and tight calf muscles. The patient has pain with the first steps in the morning or at the beginning of a workout, and the pain decreases during exercise. Radiographs are not usually helpful and may reveal a bone spur that is unrelated to the diagnosis or management. This condition often responds to correction of overpronation or other imbalance of the foot with orthotics or special shoes. The RICE regimen is appropriate with rehabilitation exercises emphasizing calf muscle stretching and foot muscle strengthening. Many persistent cases of plantar fasciitis respond to treatment with a posterior splint that holds the ankle and foot in mild dorsiflexion during sleeping hours.

WRIST AND HAND INJURIES

Most *wrist sprains* can be managed cautiously with splints, re-examination, and rehabilitation. A *scaphoid (navicular) fracture* is easily missed on initial radiographs and can result from a fall on an outstretched hand. There is pain on gripping and tenderness in the anatomic snuffbox. These fractures are often inappropriately treated as sprains with subsequent fracture nonunion. If a scaphoid fracture is suspected, a thumb spica cast should be applied until the radiograph is repeated in 10 to 14 days when the fracture will be more evident.

Ulnar collateral ligament injury to the thumb (gamekeeper's thumb) may result from forced abduction of the thumb in baseball, football, falls, and so forth. The athlete complains of pain and swelling over the ligament, and weakness of pinch. Radiographs rule out fracture or avulsion fracture, and ligament stressing rules out third-degree tears that may require surgical repair. Most first- and second-degree sprains can be treated with a thumb spica cast or splint for 5 to 6 weeks. *Finger sprains* are immobilized with splints or "buddy" taping to the adjacent finger. *Finger dislocations* can be managed similarly if there is no fracture, the relocation was simple, and the examination and function are normal; otherwise orthopedic consultation is appropriate.

TENNIS ELBOW

The term "tennis elbow" has been used for years to describe pain at or near the origin of the extensor carpi radialis brevis, at or near the lateral epicondyle. It occurs most commonly in white, middle-aged men, and nearly always in the dominant hand. Tennis, hammering, or any forceful activity with gripping and lateral wrist movement can lead to tennis elbow, especially in "weekend" athletes. There is pain with gripping objects with the involved hand, especially with the wrist extended. Morning stiffness and achiness throughout the day are common symptoms. On physical examination, tenderness over and just distal to the lateral epicondyle and pain on extension of the pronated wrist are usually diagnostic. The RICE regimen is effective, and emphasis should be placed on education of the patient and prevention through attention to conditioning. Tennis players should address the technique and style of swing, especially during the backhand stroke. Tennis elbow bands that wrap around the forearm, placing pressure over the epicondyle and forearm, are helpful for some patients. A nonsteroidal anti-inflammatory drug may be helpful during the first few weeks.

SHOULDER INJURIES

Shoulder dislocations (third-degree injuries) are most frequently anterior. Often as the result of forced external rotation and abduction to the shoulder, the athlete complains of severe pain and resists moving the shoulder. Radiographs reveal anterior displacement and are important to rule out fracture. Prompt reduction and maintenance in a sling for 3 to 4 weeks are appropriate for first-time dislocations. Recurrent dislocations may not require immobilization. Rehabilitation is important to restore balanced shoulder strength and to reduce the likelihood of recurrence.

Second-degree shoulder injuries are easily misdiagnosed, and an athlete with a second-degree injury who returns to competition too early could easily convert the injury to a third-degree one. While a second-degree injury is healing, the athlete can return to some other type of training that will allow some overall conditioning during rehabilitation of the shoulder. The complex anatomy and function of the shoulder require a thorough examination. Symmetry is noted, and motor strength, sensory function, pulses, deep tendon reflexes, and active and passive range of motion are tested. Strains to the deltoid, rotator muscles, or biceps tendon can result from a number of severe, sudden, or repeated shoulder motions in sports. The rotator cuff, consisting of the supraspinatus, infraspinatus, teres minor, and sub-scapularis muscles, can receive small tears and repeated minor trauma leading to inflammation, scarring, and soft tissue impingement in the subacromial space. Larger tears can result from falls or sudden jerks to the arm. The examination reveals crepitus, clicking, and some weakness or pain on abduction of the shoulder. Atrophy of the deltoid or of the supraspinatus may be apparent in the suprascapular fossa. Treatment is with the RICE-DIETS regimen, with emphasis on early progressive resistance exercises within the limits of pain.

Acromioclavicular (AC) injuries can result from a fall on an outstretched arm or a direct blow to the shoulder. The severity of injury is often indicated by the amount of deformity and the tenderness of the AC joint. A second-degree injury with negative radiographs is treated with immobilization in a sling and swathe for 2 to 3 weeks, then with progressive strengthening exercises. Third-degree disruption of the AC ligament is usually obvious on examination and radiographs. However, with an intact coracoclavicular ligament, plain radiographs may be normal, and the diagnosis is confirmed by bilateral upright stress radiographs (with 5 to 10 pounds held in each hand), revealing subluxation of the distal clavicle from the acromion. Third-degree separation is treated with immobilization or surgery and requires orthopedic consultation.

Sternoclavicular injuries result from various blows to the shoulder injuring the sternoclavicular ligaments. Treatment consists of the RICE-DIETS regimen with a sling and swathe or figure-eight wrap for 1 week for first-degree injury and 4 to 6 weeks for second-degree sprains. Complete disruption or third-degree injury should be handled by orthopedic consultation.

Impingement syndrome is a painful decrease in shoulder motion resulting from repeated overhead motion as in throwing sports, swimming, or tennis. There is overuse injury to the general area of the supraspinatus and biceps tendons as they pass under the acromion. Impingement causes a "painful arc" as the athlete moves the shoulder between 70 and 120 degrees of abduction. The impingement sign is positive when internal rotation with the arm in 90-degree forward flexion causes pain. There is usually tenderness to palpation anteriorly over the supraspinatus tendon, long head of the biceps, and/or subacromial bursa. Radiographs are usually unremarkable. Initial treatment consists of rest from the offending activity, ice, and anti-inflammatory drugs. Rehabilitation is essential and consists of stretching of the rotator cuff muscles and progressive resistance exercises. Finally, prevention of recurrence requires proper training and educating the athlete to improve the technique of the offending throw, stroke, or serve.

Section 15

Obstetrics and Gynecology

ANTEPARTUM CARE

method of
VAL A. CATANZARITE, M.D., PH.D.
*Mary Birch Hospital for Women/Sharp
Memorial Hospital
San Diego, California*

The role of prenatal care has shifted dramatically during the past several decades as the technology for predicting, detecting, and treating abnormalities of pregnancy and the fetus has evolved. Thirty years ago, pregnancy care involved the patient, her family, and her physician. Now, unseen participants range from the patient's attorney, to talk show hosts and writers of "medical miracle" articles for newsstand tabloids, to health maintenance organization stockholders. Today's health care environment presents ever changing opportunities, obstacles, and challenges, but as always, excellent care rests on the relationship among physician, patient, and family.

Prenatal care optimally begins with a preconception visit during which potential risks to the pregnancy may be discussed, baseline laboratory tests obtained, and prenatal care planned. During this visit, expectations for the pregnancy can be explored and a realistic view reinforced. Exposures to potential teratogens—including alcohol—should be evaluated before conception and folate supplementation initiated. The couple will need to recognize that pregnancy often requires lifestyle changes. The prospective mother may need to limit activity and travel, particularly in the third trimester. Couples need to plan for adequate time off after delivery. There are many excellent books regarding pregnancy, and reading in advance of pregnancy may be helpful, especially for first-time parents.

Notwithstanding the busy schedule of the obstetrics practice, I try to start these visits in an office, not an examination room, and end by giving out my business card and encouraging the couple to call back with questions.

PRECONCEPTION OR FIRST PRENATAL VISIT

History

Obstetric and Gynecologic History

The reproductive health history includes maternal age, gravidity, parity, and outcomes of all prior pregnancies. Obstetric history tends to repeat itself! Obtaining records for prior complications may yield important information relevant to the current pregnancy. Particular attention must be paid to abnormal fetal outcomes, such as miscarriage, intrauterine death, and large-for-gestational-age or small-for-gestational-age infants, and to symptoms and circum-

stances preceding premature births. About one third of women who deliver prematurely in their first pregnancy will do so again. Preeclampsia developing remote from term, or with "atypical" features, has a 30 to 50% recurrence risk.

Currently, in the United States, the rate of cesarean section is between 20 and 25%. Most women who have had a prior, low-transverse cesarean section are candidates for a trial of labor during subsequent pregnancies.

The gynecologic history is also important. Surgeries, particularly cone biopsy and myomectomy, may have implications for pregnancy management. Past and current birth control methods and plans for postpartum contraception can be explored. For the patient who is seen while planning a pregnancy, use of a menstrual calendar can be initiated.

The history should specifically include sexually transmitted diseases. Syphilis, gonorrhea, and chlamydial infection can have adverse effects and are easy to detect and treat, particularly before pregnancy. The patient who has a history of herpes often needs reassurance that except if she has active genital lesions in labor, her delivery route will not be affected. The patient with a history of pelvic inflammatory disease should be made aware of the risk for ectopic pregnancy, and sonography should be planned early to confirm an intrauterine gestational sac.

Acquired Immune Deficiency Syndrome

The specter of acquired immune deficiency syndrome looms large in the thinking of many reproductive-aged women. The American College of Obstetricians and Gynecologists has recommended that all women be offered screening for human immunodeficiency virus (HIV). In certain areas of the country, HIV seropositivity is found in up to 3% of newborn infants. Fortunately, with antenatal diagnosis of HIV infection and zidovudine chemoprophylaxis, the rate of vertical transmission from mother to newborn drops from 27% to about 8%. The *preconception* diagnosis for prospective mother or father may result in reconsideration of the decision for pregnancy.

Medical Conditions

The past medical history is an essential component of the preconception or first prenatal visit. Allergies to drugs or medications are noted. Particularly for health care workers, latex allergy is increasingly common and demands awareness of both patient and physician. A "checklist" patient information form,

TABLE 1. **Human Teratogens Commonly Used by Women in Reproductive Years**

Carbamazepine (Tegretol)	Tetracycline
Ethanol	Trimethadione
Isotretinoin (Accutane)	Valproic acid (Depakene)
Lithium	Warfarin (Coumadin)
Phenytoin (Dilantin)	

specifically listing such conditions as hypertension, cardiac problems, tuberculosis, pneumonia, asthma, kidney disease or kidney infections, bladder infections, gastrointestinal diseases, hepatitis, endocrine disorders, anemia, and neurologic or neuromuscular complaints, can be completed by the patient before the office visit to streamline the history-taking process. Prior surgeries, major injuries, and transfusions are also included.

Medications

Relatively few drugs or medications are known teratogens (Table 1), but it is not unusual for patients to use over-the-counter drugs on a routine basis. The patient who is taking a potential teratogen can often be switched to a different drug. I encourage patients to discontinue all nonprescription drugs except for acetaminophen during the preconception period and during the early pregnancy.

Alcohol

Heavy alcohol consumption is surprisingly common in women of childbearing age. Full-blown fetal alcohol syndrome, with symmetrical growth retardation, craniofacial and central nervous system abnormalities, and, in some cases, cardiac and musculoskeletal abnormalities, occurs in 30 to 50% of offspring of women who drink 2 ounces of absolute alcohol (four or five mixed drinks) per day. Alcohol effects are present in more than 10% of infants born to women drinking even 1 ounce of absolute alcohol daily. The recommendation is for pregnant women to abstain from alcohol; however, no fetal risk has been proved with a single episode of binge-drinking, even during embryogenesis.

Cigarette Smoking

Cigarette smoking causes preterm delivery and fetal growth disturbances. Also, children exposed to secondhand smoke have an increased rate of respiratory disease. All pregnant women, and their husbands, should be advised to quit. Nicotine patches may be helpful in smoking cessation and may be used in pregnancy.

Drug Abuse

The use of "street drugs" is a source of continued concern to the obstetrician. Although the rate of intravenous drug use in most areas of the country is relatively low, potent methamphetamine preparations ("crystal," "ice," "crank") and highly refined cocaine ("crack") are readily available and commonly abused. These can cause growth retardation and preterm delivery as well as placental abruption. In addition, cocaine is increasingly seen as a cause of serious neonatal complications and neurodevelopmental problems in childhood.

Family History and Pedigree

Significant health problems among first- and second-degree relatives may have an impact on pregnancy planning. A genetics screening questionnaire is used by many obstetricians but does not replace the family history by interview. Particular attention should be paid to stillbirths or anomalous children and to familial patterns of birth defects, neuromuscular disorders, or mental retardation. The ethnic background of the parents is important. Blacks in the United States have a 10% rate of carriage of sickle cell trait or hemoglobin C trait. Hemoglobin E, heterozygous or homozygous, is common in patients of Southeast Asian origin. α-Thalassemia and β-thalassemia are seen in individuals of Asian, African, and southern European (Greek and Italian) ancestry. Detection of hemoglobin variants or thalassemias may warrant genetic counseling and prenatal diagnostic testing. Tay-Sachs disease, uniformly lethal to the neonate, is an autosomal recessive condition with a carrier rate of about 1 in 30 among people of Jewish ancestry, 1 in 10 to 20 among French Canadians and Cajuns, and 1 in 150 in the general population. Carrier testing is recommended if either partner is in an at-risk group. Cystic fibrosis is a relatively common autosomal recessive condition among northern Europeans. Carrier testing for many cystic fibrosis mutations is available, but routine carrier screening is not yet recommended.

Detailed genetic counseling is indicated for women older than 35 years at delivery, patients with family history of inheritable disorders or birth defects, patients with teratogen exposures, and consanguineous couples.

Social History

The living circumstances, employment, exercise habits, and lifestyle of a couple may need to be modified as pregnancy progresses. Some women expect to be able to continue 12- to 16-hour work days through pregnancy; others assume that they need to quit work as soon as they become pregnant. The medical and obstetric history often allows prediction of activity limitations, and this is helpful before conception.

Domestic violence is common in all social classes and reportedly increases in frequency during pregnancy. Some cases are apparent, but the diagnosis can be elusive. Both physician and staff must be attuned to the possibility and be unafraid to ask specific, open-ended questions about past or present physical abuse.

Physical Examination

Vital signs, including blood pressure, pulse, and respirations, as well as the general appearance of the patient are noted.

Head, Eyes, Ears, Nose, and Throat Examination

Dental disease is common. The patient should continue regular dental care, and her dentist can be reassured that procedures under local anesthesia, including fillings and extractions, can be safely undertaken during pregnancy. I encourage patients to have their dentists call with inquiries regarding safety of pain medications and choices of antibiotics.

The thyroid is slightly enlarged in size during normal pregnancy and may have a somewhat "mushy" feel.

Breasts

Breasts enlarge in size during pregnancy and become tender. With the glandular proliferation, the texture of the breasts may become difficult to evaluate. However, any firm masses should be evaluated for the possibility of malignancy; breast cancer is among the most common cancers seen during pregnancy.

Respiratory System

The respiratory rate and depth of breathing increase during pregnancy. The lungs should remain clear.

Cardiovascular System

A soft (1–2/6) systolic ejection murmur in the pulmonic area reflects the increased cardiac output of pregnancy. An S_3 may also be heard in the normal patient. An S_4 or any diastolic or loud systolic murmur of grade 3 or higher should be further investigated.

Abdominal Examination

Abnormal physical findings in the upper abdomen, such as hepatosplenomegaly, are uncommonly encountered during pregnancy. These may be obscured in late pregnancy by the growing uterus and fetus.

The uterus rises out of the pelvis at approximately 14 weeks' gestation but may be palpable abdominally in the slim patient as early as 12 weeks or so. From about 18 to 38 weeks, the size of the uterus, measured in centimeters from the pubic symphysis to the top of the fundus, should be within about 2 cm of the gestational age in weeks.

Pelvic Examination

During even early pregnancy, the vaginal walls and cervix soften and take on a bluish or "cyanotic" appearance (Chadwick's sign).

The uterine size is not appreciably increased until 6 to 8 weeks' gestation; Hegar's sign, softening of the isthmic portion of the uterus (the part between the cervix and the fundus), is usually appreciated at 6 to 8 weeks.

Clinical sizing by an experienced examiner during the first trimester is a fairly accurate means of confirming menstrual dates in gestational age assessment. The uterine diameter, in centimeters, matches the gestational age within about 2 weeks from 6 to 12 weeks. Beyond the 12- to 14-week range, however, clinical uterine sizing becomes less accurate.

Evaluation of the adnexa is obscured by the growing uterus after 10 to 12 weeks. The corpus luteum may be palpable at 4 to 10 weeks as a slightly tender, 4- or 5-cm adnexal mass. Any adnexal mass larger than 5 cm should be evaluated by sonography.

In addition to uterine sizing, evaluation of pelvic architecture is part of the initial examination. The "obstetric conjugate"—the distance from the underside of the pubic symphysis to the sacral promontory—is normally 11 cm or more. The bi-ischial diameter in most patients exceeds 8.5 cm. The angle of the pubic arch, the convergence of the pelvic side walls and of the sacrum, and the prominence of the ischial spines allow a determination of pelvic type (gynecoid, anthropoid, android, or platypelloid) and, in rare cases, reveal an abnormality or deformity that precludes a trial of vaginal delivery.

Laboratory Evaluation

Routine laboratory tests performed at the preconception or first prenatal visit are summarized in Table 2. A complete blood count includes a hematocrit and red blood cell indices. In cases of anemia, the red blood cell indices may suggest a cause. A microcytic anemia is seen in thalassemias as well as in iron deficiency states. The lower limit of normal for platelet count during pregnancy is 150,000 per mm³. Any count below 100,000 per mm³ deserves further investigation.

Determination of the blood type, Rh antigen, and antibody screen (indirect Coombs' test) is important for three reasons. First, the Rh-negative patient whose spouse is Rh-positive is at risk to become sensitized during the pregnancy or at the time of

TABLE 2. **Laboratory Tests During Pregnancy**

First Visit

Blood type, Rh, antibody screen
Complete blood count
Urinalysis and culture if indicated
Rubella titer
Venereal Disease Research Laboratory or rapid
    plasma reagin test
Hepatitis B surface antigen
Pap smear
Gonococcus and chlamydial cultures
Human immunodeficiency virus antibody
Glucola 50-gm screen*
Hemoglobin electrophoresis*
Hepatitis C antibody*
Tay-Sachs screening*

Subsequent Testing

15–19 wk: Serum marker screening ("expanded alpha-
             fetoprotein screening")
26–28 wk: Glucola 50-gm screen (low-risk patients)
             Glucose tolerance test (high-risk patients)
36–38 wk: Group B streptococcus culture

*In at-risk patients.

delivery. Rh_0 D immune globulin prophylaxis is indicated after any significant bleeding episode, at 26 weeks, and after delivery if the infant is Rh-positive. Second, the presence of irregular antibodies may place the fetus at risk for erythroblastosis fetalis, or hemolytic disease of the newborn, and require further evaluation and/or treatment of the fetus during the latter half of gestation. Finally, obstetrics is a "bloody business." The patient whose antibody screen is negative can be safely transfused, with type-specific, non-crossmatched blood in the event of hemorrhage.

Urinalysis (and culture, if indicated) is performed at the first prenatal visit. Asymptomatic bacteriuria occurs in 5 to 10% of pregnant (and nonpregnant) women; however, during pregnancy, the rate of progression from asymptomatic bacteriuria to pyelonephritis is much higher than in the nonpregnant state, and eradication of asymptomatic bacteriuria is recommended. The presence of abnormalities on urinalysis, such as proteinuria or red blood cell casts, suggests the possibility of chronic renal disease.

The rubella titer is determined at the first visit. For the patient who is being seen before pregnancy and who does not plan pregnancy for the next 6 months, rubella vaccination can be given. Otherwise, the nonimmune patient can be vaccinated after delivery.

Hepatitis B screening is also done. A positive hepatitis B surface antigen test result may indicate acute or chronic infection. Newborn disease can be prevented by passive and active immunization. Hepatitis C testing is considered in patients with a history of transfusion or of drug or alcohol abuse. About 2% of pregnant women carry hepatitis C antibody. These patients need surveillance for chronic disease. Breast-feeding is generally discouraged, because hepatitis C can be transmitted at delivery or via breast milk.

Toxoplasmosis screening is offered to selected patients with cats or who report ingestion of raw or undercooked meats.

Syphilis is again increasing in prevalence during pregnancy; congenital syphilis can be prevented by prompt treatment. A positive screening test result (rapid plasma reagin or Venereal Disease Research Laboratory test) should trigger a fluorescent treponemal antibody absorption test and further evaluation.

Papanicolaou's (Pap) smear, gonococcus culture, and *Chlamydia* culture are routinely performed during pregnancy by most obstetricians. The abnormal Pap smear is evaluated as in the nonpregnant state. Gonorrhea is best treated with intramuscular ceftriaxone. Chlamydial carriage is treated with a tetracycline in the nonpregnant patient but with azithromycin (Zithromax) or erythromycin during pregnancy. Of course, the patient's sexual contacts must also be treated.

MULTIDISCIPLINARY CARE AND TEAM APPROACH

A hallmark of modern obstetric practice is a team approach to care of the patient. Evaluations by a

TABLE 3. **Indications for Referral for Maternal-Fetal Medicine Consultation and/or Care**

Medical Conditions

Hypertension requiring medications
Diabetes
Cardiac disease except mitral valve prolapse
Severe asthma
Renal impairment or chronic proteinuria
Collagen-vascular disease
Anticardiolipin antibody
Hereditary anemias (e.g., sickle cell)
Symptomatic hyperthyroidism
Neuromuscular disorders (e.g., myasthenia gravis)
Morbid obesity

Obstetric Factors

Maternal age >35 y or <15 y
Uterine anomaly
History of cervical incompetence, diethystilbestrol exposure, or
    extensive cone biopsy
Prior history of
    Very premature delivery
    Preterm severe preeclampsia
    Unexplained stillbirth
Isoimmunization
Monochorionic twins
Higher order multiple gestation (≥triplets)

nutritionist, social worker, and/or health educator are often helpful in initial assessment and/or ongoing pregnancy care. A crucial question for the obstetric care provider is whether the patient is best served by referral for consultation with specialists in other fields of medicine or for evaluation or global care with a maternal-fetal medicine subspecialist. It is common practice for health insurers and managed care organizations to try to hold down referrals. It is the role of the obstetrician to be the patient's advocate, and one of the most difficult ethical challenges is to provide excellent care despite financial pressures of managed care organizations. Some of the conditions that warrant referral are summarized in Table 3.

OBSTETRIC SONOGRAPHY

As is discussed later, I recommend a high-resolution sonogram to all pregnant women at 16 to 20 weeks' gestation. Additional ultrasound scans may be indicated; some of the reasons are given in Table 4.

Ectopic Pregnancy

In normal pregnancy, a gestational sac is seen with vaginal ultrasound examination at 5.5 weeks, and it is seen in more than 90% of patients in whom the quantitative human chorionic gonadotropin (hCG) level exceeds 2000 mIU per liter. The gestational sac is seen with abdominal scanning at about 6 weeks' gestation or when the quantitative β-hCG level exceeds 6000 mIU per liter. An extrauterine gestational sac or even an extrauterine embryo is occasionally seen with ultrasound examination. However, the primary importance of sonography is to demonstrate

TABLE 4. **Indications for Sonography**

Ectopic pregnancy
Adnexal masses
Pregnancy dating
Diagnosis of fetal anomalies
Multiple gestation
Size-dates discrepancy
Third-trimester bleeding
Suspected malpresentation
Guidance for invasive procedures (chorionic villus
  sampling, amniocentesis, percutaneous umbilical
  blood sampling)
Assessment of fetal health (biophysical profile scoring,
  Doppler velocimetry)

an intrauterine pregnancy. Then, the risk of ectopic pregnancy is reduced to about 1 in 10,000 (the rate of coexistent ectopic and intrauterine pregnancies).

Adnexal Masses

Ultrasound examination is recommended whenever an adnexal mass of 5 cm or larger is palpated during pregnancy. Depending on the size and on the appearance of the mass at ultrasonography, surgical removal of the mass may be indicated.

Pregnancy Dating

Accurate dating of the pregnancy is critical in planning prenatal care. Obstetric dogma has been that in women with regular menstrual cycles, conception occurs about 14 days before the date of the first *missed* menstrual period. Therefore, for patients with 28-day cycles, the due date is assumed to be 40 weeks from the last period. There are surprisingly few data to support this time-honored method of calculation! If a patient knows her conception date, the due date can be reliably calculated by adding 38 weeks. In the patient with a regular menses, a known last period, and a concordant first-trimester physical examination, calculation of a *tentative* due date from the menstrual history is appropriate. However, an overwhelming body of evidence demonstrates that pregnancy dating is best confirmed by sonography. When sonography is performed between 7 and 12 weeks, the gestational age, as inferred from the crown-rump length of the embryo, is accurate within 7 days. Between 13 and 22 weeks, the gestational age inferred from measurements of biparietal diameter, femur length, and abdominal circumference is accurate within 10 days. Between 22 and 26 weeks, the gestational age is accurate within approximately 2 weeks. A single scan performed after about 26 weeks' gestation has an error range of ±3 weeks and, therefore, is not particularly useful in judging gestational age. The reason for this is that with ultrasonography, there is much more variation in fetal size at a given gestational age during the third trimester than in the first or second trimester.

Some patients present late in pregnancy, without any solid criteria for dating. In these cases, either clinical or ultrasound dating can be used, but the unreliability of either method must be recognized in obstetric decision-making.

Growth Abnormalities

Ultrasound examination can also be used to evaluate patients with size-date discrepancy. A variety of formulas and tables for estimation of fetal weight by use of ultrasonography have been developed and, in general, are accurate within 15% of the actual weight.

In the patient with size less than dates, sonography can show intrauterine growth retardation (IUGR) or oligohydramnios. If the fetal weight estimate is less than the 10th percentile for confirmed gestational age, the diagnosis of IUGR is strongly suspected.

Symmetrical IUGR may be due to fetal chromosomal defects and congenital infections or may represent an end-stage effect of asymmetrical IUGR. Symmetrical IUGR requires careful, individual assessment.

Asymmetrical IUGR is usually due to maternal or uteroplacental factors. Management includes serial assessments of growth and amniotic fluid volume as well as twice-weekly nonstress tests if the gestational age is 26 weeks or more.

Oligohydramnios (amniotic fluid index of ≤5 cm) is another cause for size less than dates. Causes include ruptured membranes, fetal urinary tract abnormalities, and decreased fetal urine output due to uteroplacental insufficiency.

In the patient with size greater than dates, common sonographic findings include macrosomia (estimated fetal weight >90th percentile for dates), polyhydramnios, and large fibroids.

The finding of fetal macrosomia may indicate impaired maternal glucose control; in addition, this finding can be integrated with clinical examination in planning labor and delivery management.

Polyhydramnios (amniotic fluid index ≥26 cm or deepest vertical pocket ≥10 cm) may be associated with diabetes, with a variety of fetal anomalies, and with twin-twin transfusion syndrome; a minority of cases are idiopathic.

Multiple Gestation

Serial assessments of fetal growth in multiple gestation cannot be performed by physical examination. I recommend monthly sonograms for growth, from about 20 weeks onward. Growth discrepancy of 20% or more, or discrepancy in fluid volumes in same-sex twins, raises the possibility of twin-twin transfusion syndrome and marks the pregnancy for more intensive assessments.

Third-Trimester Bleeding

Ultrasound examination is highly accurate in determination of placental location and can be used to make the diagnosis of placenta previa. In the patient in whom placenta previa is excluded, the finding of a retroplacental lucency may support the clinical diagnosis of placental abruption. In patients with placenta previa, targeted sonographic evaluation can predict placenta accreta, increta, or percreta and be helpful in planning of surgical delivery.

Fetal Health

Ultrasound examination can also be used to assess the health of the fetus in utero. The biophysical profile is a sort of in utero Apgar score, which can be used as a means of antepartum fetal assessment. Doppler velocimetry of the umbilical arteries has proved to be helpful in management of some high-risk pregnancies; the finding of absent or reversed diastolic flow is an indication for delivery or intensive surveillance.

SUBSEQUENT PRENATAL VISITS

The first prenatal visit is usually scheduled shortly after a positive pregnancy test result. If the patient has already had a preconception visit, the baseline laboratory and clinical evaluation has already been performed; if not, it can be done at this time. If the patient is at risk for ectopic pregnancy, this can be excluded by means of an ultrasound examination performed at 5 to 6 weeks' gestation.

Subsequent visits in the uncomplicated pregnancy are scheduled at monthly intervals until 32 weeks, then every other week until 36 weeks, and then weekly until delivery. At each prenatal visit, the patient's weight, blood pressure, and urinary protein and glucose determinations are recorded. After 12 weeks, the fetal heart is auscultated. After 14 weeks, the fundal height is measured from the symphysis to the top of the uterus. Late in pregnancy, Leopold's maneuvers are used to assess fetal position, and examination of the cervix may be in order.

Weight Gain

There is a wide range of normal weight gain during pregnancy. For women who are underweight before the pregnancy, many gain 15 to 20 pounds or more by the 20th week of pregnancy; large women may gain substantially less. Most patients gain between 0.5 and 1 pound per week during the last 20 weeks of gestation. The frequency of poor pregnancy outcomes is increased in underweight women who do not show "catch-up" weight gain early in pregnancy, and in women of normal prepregnant weight but who have poor weight gain.

Accelerated weight gain may be due to edema, particularly in the third trimester, or simply to overeating. Poor weight gain is most often due to either morning sickness or self-imposed dietary restriction; particularly when the patient was slim before the pregnancy and has gained little weight by the 20th week, a dietary consultation may be in order. Fetal

TABLE 5. Weight Gain During Normal Pregnancy

Fetal Compartment	
Fetus	3500 gm
Amniotic fluid	500 gm
Placenta	500 gm
Total	4500 gm
Maternal Compartment	
Blood volume	2000 gm
Extravascular fluid	2000 gm
Uterine hypertrophy	1000 gm
Breast enlargement	500 gm
Total	5500 gm

and maternal components of weight gain are given in Table 5.

Concordance of the gestational dating and measurement of the uterus is used to screen for growth abnormalities. If the fundal size lags significantly behind gestational dating (3-cm discrepancy or greater, between 20 and 38 weeks' gestation), the differential diagnosis includes IUGR and decreased amniotic fluid; evaluation is by sonography. If the fundal height is significantly ahead of dates, multiple gestation, macrosomatia, and polyhydramnios may be the cause, and, again, ultrasound examination is indicated.

Fetal Activity

Fetal movement is first perceived by most multiparous patients between 16 and 18 weeks and by primiparous patients between 18 and 20 weeks. Beyond 26 weeks' gestation, maternal perception of fetal movement is the best screening tool for potential fetal jeopardy.

The normal fetus has a 20- to 60-minute sleep-wake cycle. Thus, the normal fetus should be moving for part of every hour. A simple and practical screen for fetal activity is "count to 10" charting. Starting at 26 weeks' gestation, the mother records daily the time the fetus takes to reach 10 kicks. Recording is done at a time when the fetus is usually active—early evening for most pregnancies. If the fetus does not reach 10 kicks within an hour, the mother comes in for fetal monitoring. Kick counting has been demonstrated to halve the rate of stillbirth in low-risk pregnancies.

The fetal heart is auscultated at each visit beyond 12 weeks' gestation. The baseline fetal heart rate is normally between 120 and 160 beats per minute; this declines from early gestation toward term. Occasional irregularities in the fetal heart rate are normal, just as occasional premature beats in the adult heart are normal. However, frequent "missed beats" suggest an abnormality of the cardiac conduction system and should be evaluated by fetal echocardiography.

Edema

Edema of the legs is common during late pregnancy. This is due to compression of the venous return from the legs by the gravid uterus as well as lowered plasma oncotic pressure. It improves with rest in the recumbent position and tends to recur late during the day. This edema can be reduced by having the patient either add a period of lateral recumbency to her schedule or spend a half-hour each day in a swimming pool. Edema of the hands or the face is pathologic and may be indicative of preeclampsia.

Blood Pressure

The blood pressure is measured at each prenatal visit. Normal blood pressure during pregnancy ranges from 90/50 to 130/80 mm Hg. Pressures in the first trimester of 130/80 mm Hg or more suggest mild chronic hypertension.

The blood pressure normally falls from prepregnant and first-trimester values to reach a a nadir during the late second trimester and then rises back to the prepregnant values near term. About 10% of patients during their first pregnancy develop pregnancy-induced hypertension, defined as a rise in the blood pressure of 30 mm Hg systolic and 15 mm Hg diastolic above first-trimester values. If the blood pressure rise is accompanied by proteinuria or generalized edema, the patient has preeclampsia. Preeclampsia, when it develops, resolves only after delivery and may present significant threats to both maternal and fetal health.

Urinary Glucose and Protein

At each prenatal visit, a dipstick determination of urinary protein and glucose levels is also performed.

During normal pregnancy, renal blood flow increases to such an extent that the capacity of the kidney to reabsorb filtered glucose may be exceeded, even in the presence of normal blood glucose levels. Thus, 1+ or 2+ glycosuria is common during pregnancy. Glycosuria in the 3+ or 4+ range may be indicative of hyperglycemia and is assessed by a blood glucose determination.

Urinary protein is also checked at each visit. Trace proteinuria is common and generally innocuous. Values of 1+ occasionally occur during normal pregnancy but may be indicative of early preeclampsia. Urinary protein dipstick determinations of 2+ or greater are always abnormal and mandate evaluation for preeclampsia and/or renal disease. As mentioned before, elevation in blood pressure, generalized edema, and proteinuria are the cardinal signs of preeclampsia.

COMMON COMPLAINTS

A variety of discomforts are reported by the normal pregnant patient. Many of these relate to physiologic changes and can be managed with reassurance and symptomatic treatment. In an occasional patient, the complaints are persistent or severe enough to require further intervention.

Morning sickness is nearly universal during the first trimester. Patients usually report a queasy or unsettled feeling to the stomach on arising. This may be accompanied by occasional or even daily vomiting, most often occurring early in the day. Small, dry carbohydrate feedings immediately on arising and holding off on intake of liquids until later in the day are usually effective in controlling these complaints. An antiemetic medication may occasionally be required, although given the medicolegal furor over alleged teratogenic effects of doxylamine (Bendectin), most obstetricians are reluctant to prescribe drugs for morning sickness.

Danger signs in morning sickness are steady weight loss of more than 10 pounds, the development of orthostatic symptoms suggestive of hypovolemia, or persistent ketonuria. Patients who are significantly dehydrated, or who are not responding to the measures described earlier, generally do well with intravenous hydration and placing the gut at rest for 24 to 48 hours. An occasional patient has severe and protracted nausea and vomiting, hyperemesis gravidarum. These patients usually require hospital admission, with vigorous replacement of vitamin, fluid, and electrolyte losses. If the nausea and vomiting persist, a careful evaluation of potential underlying causes should be undertaken; if no cause is found, nasogastric feedings or parenteral nutrition may be used to tide the patient over through the period of hyperemesis. Fortunately, the nausea and vomiting associated with pregnancy tend to resolve by 12 weeks of gestation.

Gastric reflux also occurs commonly during pregnancy, usually in the third trimester. With rising progesterone levels, the tone of the lower esophageal sphincter decreases. This, together with pressure on the stomach by the growing uterus, increases the tendency toward reflux. Some patients complain of a sour taste in the mouth; others actually notice regurgitation of food from the stomach back into the mouth. These symptoms may be controlled by means of smaller, more frequent meals. Reflux is most marked and most disturbing when the patient lies down. Elevating the head of the bed by 4 to 6 inches by placing wooden blocks or bricks underneath the bedposts is helpful; some patients need to sleep in a reclining chair, in a semiupright posture. If this is not effective, metoclopramide (Reglan), increases lower esophageal sphincter tone, accelerates gastric emptying, and often provides dramatic relief.

A general feeling of fatigue or loss of energy occurs in many pregnant women, particularly those who are active. This is usually due to the demands of the pregnancy asking mother to "slow down." However, patients who report severe limitation of activity need to be evaluated for cardiac or pulmonary disease.

Numbness and tingling of the medial aspect of the hand (thumb, index finger, and the middle half of the middle finger) occur in about 5% of pregnant women. This is due to compression of the median nerve in the carpal tunnel on the volar aspect of the wrist. The complaint is most pronounced in the dominant hand and is typically more severe at night and during the early morning hours, improving during the day. The diagnosis is usually apparent by history but may be confirmed on physical examination by the presence of Tinel's sign (a tingling or shocklike sensation in the affected areas on percussion of the median nerve) or the findings of sensory loss or wasting of the thenar muscles of the affected hand. Splinting at night, injection of the carpal tunnel with corticosteroids, or even surgical carpal tunnel release may be necessary during pregnancy. Symptoms should abate in 2 to 10 weeks after delivery.

Varicose veins are a common complaint, are more frequent in multigravid women, and tend to increase in severity with advancing gestation. Elastic support hose are used to control the associated discomfort. Because the varicosities are at least in part due to the compression of the venous return from the legs by the gravid uterus, surgical treatment of varicose veins is not recommended during pregnancy.

Leg cramps, particularly occurring at night, may be troublesome. The physiologic basis of these cramps is unclear. Most patients respond to calcium supplements. However, in a rare patient, the cramps may be so persistent or severe as to require medication.

LABORATORY TESTING LATER IN PREGNANCY

Glucose Screening

The hormonal changes of pregnancy, particularly the production by the placenta of human placental lactogen, make pregnancy a "diabetogenic" state. Elevated glucose levels during pregnancy have adverse effects on the fetus.

It is my routine to perform a 50-gram Glucola screening test at 26 to 28 weeks' gestation for all patients. One hour after the Glucola is taken, a blood sample to determine glucose level is drawn. A result of 130 mg per dL or less is normal; if the result is above 130 mg per dL, a 3-hour glucose tolerance test is done.

For patients at high risk (e.g., family history of diabetes, obese, or previous macrosomic infant), a Glucola screen is performed shortly after the first prenatal visit, and then either a subsequent Glucola screen or a full glucose tolerance test is done at 26 to 28 weeks.

The glucose tolerance test includes a fasting blood glucose determination, followed by a 100-gram oral glucose load. Then, blood glucose levels are determined at 1, 2, and 3 hours. The upper limits of normal for plasma glucose are fasting, 105 mg per dL or less; 1 hour, 190 mg per dL or less; 2 hours, 165 mg per dL or less; 3 hours, 145 mg per dL or less. If two or more values are abnormal on the 3-hour glucose tolerance test, the patient is diagnosed as having gestational diabetes and treated with education regarding diet and exercise and, if needed, insulin.

TABLE 6. **Group B Streptococcus Screening**

If the patient has had an infant with group B streptococcal sepsis, plan intrapartum antibiotic prophylaxis.*

If any urine culture is positive for group B streptococcus, treat and also plan intrapartum antibiotic prophylaxis.*

If the patient presents in preterm labor or with preterm rupture of the membranes, treat prophylactically pending results of group B streptococcal vaginal-rectal culture.

Culture the lower vagina and rectum at 35–38 wk in normal pregnancies. If the result is positive, plan intrapartum prophylaxis.*

Intrapartum prophylaxis

Ampicillin, 2 gm IV q 6 h

or

Penicillin, 5,000,000 U IV then 2,500,000 U IV q 4 h

or

Clindamycin (Cleocin), 900 mg IV q 8 h

Group B Streptococcus Screening

About 10% of pregnant women have colonization of the lower vagina and/or rectum with group B beta-hemolytic streptococci at the time of labor. Infants exposed to group B streptococcus at delivery are at risk for potentially life-threatening group B streptococcal sepsis, and this risk is all but eliminated by antepartum screening and intrapartum antibiotic prophylaxis. My policy is summarized in Table 6.

PRETERM BIRTH PREVENTION

Preterm birth, defined as delivery between weeks 20 and 36 of the pregnancy, is the single most important cause of neonatal morbidity and mortality. Although the outcomes of premature infants improve year by year, treatment in the newborn intensive care unit is expensive, and despite superb neonatal care, some infants born early will have serious or even lifelong health problems, including cerebral palsy due to prematurity.

Some preterm deliveries are medically indicated because of either a maternal health problem or deteriorating fetal condition. The majority of preterm births, however, are caused by preterm labor or preterm rupture of the membranes. One of the most important goals of prenatal care is to identify patients at high risk for preterm birth. All patients should be educated regarding signs and symptoms of preterm labor. The patient's awareness of preterm labor signs and symptoms is the best means to make the diagnosis before advanced cervical change. Therapy is most effective when preterm labor is diagnosed in its early stages!

Risk factors for preterm delivery include uterine anomalies (e.g., bicornuate uterus), multiple gestation, and history of a prior premature birth. Women at the extremes of reproductive age (age younger than 15 years or older than 35 years) are at higher risk than are women between 20 and 30 years. Women who smoke or use drugs are at higher risk than nonsmokers and non–drug users. Single women are at higher risk than married women of the same age and reproductive history. Women with major life stressors, even positive changes, appear to be at greater risk than women whose social situation is stable throughout the pregnancy. For women with identified risk factors, in addition to intensive preterm labor education, increased surveillance by means of more frequent prenatal visits and/or cervical examinations may be in order.

Bacterial vaginosis has been identified as a risk factor for preterm labor, but there is still controversy as to the potential impact of therapy. It seems reasonable to treat patients with an appropriate antibiotic, e.g., metronidazole or clindamycin cream, and observe as for other high-risk patients. Women who have a short cervix demonstrated by ultrasound examination (normal length is ≥3.5 cm) are also at increased risk for premature delivery and may benefit from diminished activity as well as frequent visits and heightened maternal awareness of signs and symptoms of preterm labor.

The presenting symptoms for preterm labor vary widely. Some women identify individual, discrete contractions. Others first recognize a low backache, a pelvic pressure sensation, an increase in vaginal discharge, or "menstrual cramps." I have found that educating patients regarding these signs and symptoms, and asking them to call and come in for evaluation if they experience these problems, increases the likelihood of early diagnosis of preterm labor, at the expense of an increased number of unscheduled visits.

In the patient with regular uterine activity who is suspected of being in premature labor, a variety of tocolytic drugs can be used to slow or stop contractions. In addition, in women at high risk for preterm delivery, the use of antenatal corticosteroids (dexamethasone or betamethasone) has been shown to accelerate fetal pulmonary maturation and improve newborn outcomes. Prophylaxis against group B streptococcal sepsis is also recommended (see Table 6).

The use of home uterine activity monitoring for high-risk patients has been controversial. Whereas home uterine activity monitoring may benefit selected patients, most of the randomized studies to date have not shown benefit. In my practice, home uterine activity monitoring is seldom used, except for patients with multiple gestation or documented to have an inability to perceive uterine activity.

ANTENATAL FETAL TESTING AND ASSESSING FETAL HEALTH

The overall rate of perinatal (fetal and newborn) mortality in the United States is about 12 per 1000 pregnancies. Stillbirth—death of the fetus before delivery—accounts for about two thirds of perinatal mortality and occurs in about 8 pregnancies per 1000.

Stillbirth may be caused by unpredictable events

TABLE 7. **Common Indications for Nonstress Tests**

Maternal

Hypertension requiring medication
Diabetes
Severe asthma
Symptomatic cardiac disease
Systemic lupus
Chronic renal impairment
Severe anemia
? Age ≥40 y

Obstetric

Preeclampsia
Intrauterine growth retardation or discordant twins
Prior stillbirth, unexplained
Decreased fetal movement
Postdate pregnancy (≥41 wk)
? All twins after 34 wk

such as auto accidents, abdominal trauma, umbilical cord accidents, or placental abruption. More commonly, however, the cause is one that is potentially detectable, such as chronic uteroplacental insufficiency or a fetal anomaly. For the general obstetric population, the best measure to diminish the rate of stillbirth is to instruct mothers regarding "kick counting" as described earlier. However, there are certain maternal and obstetric conditions that place the pregnancy at a markedly increased risk for chronic uteroplacental insufficiency and stillbirth (Table 7). For these patients, formal antenatal fetal testing is recommended.

Available tests for fetal health in utero include nonstress testing, contraction stress testing, biophysical profile, and Doppler velocimetry. A discussion of the pros and cons of each of the individual antenatal tests is beyond the scope of this article, and the antenatal testing protocols vary from institution to institution.

I use the nonstress test as the primary means for antepartum surveillance. Patients are monitored by means of an external Doppler device and tocodynamometer, on a twice-a-week basis for most high-risk conditions. The baseline fetal heart rate is recorded. The fetal heart rate tracing is examined for long-term variability, fetal heart rate decelerations, and fetal heart rate accelerations. If the heart rate tracing shows good long-term variability, and at least two accelerations 15 beats above baseline and lasting at least 15 seconds, within 30 minutes, the tracing is reactive. In the patient who is not specifically at risk for oligohydramnios (e.g., the patient with diabetes but no evidence of hypertension or vascular disease), a reactive nonstress test is an excellent predictor of fetal health until the next testing interval. In the patient who is at risk for oligohydramnios, the amniotic fluid volume is assessed in addition to the nonstress test. A diminished amniotic fluid volume (amniotic fluid index of <5 cm) is generally an indication for delivery at or near term and for hospitalization remote from term. Patients with mild variable decelerations on the nonstress test tracing, but with normal fluid volume, are monitored with twice-a-week testing. Patients who have a nonreactive nonstress test, moderate or severe variable decelerations, or late decelerations are usually delivered at or near term; remote from term, management is individualized. The use of antenatal testing as described before has been shown to dramatically reduce the rate of stillbirth; high-risk patients observed with a twice-a-week testing protocol have a stillbirth rate in the range of 0.6 to 1 per 1000, which is lower than the stillbirth rate for untested low-risk patients.

In any patient followed up with serial tests of fetal well-being, consideration must be given to the relative risks and benefits of delivery versus continued expectant management. For example, the patient with mild chronic hypertension at 36 weeks' gestation, with normal fetal growth and normal fluid volume, can be safely followed up with continued nonstress tests. A similar patient whose infant develops asymmetrical IUGR might be best managed by delivery rather than continued antenatal testing.

A special case, and a leading cause of perinatal mortality, is postdate pregnancy. For pregnancies dated on the basis of "certain" last menstrual period, about 10% will deliver at or beyond 42 weeks' gestation. For pregnancies dated by ultrasonography, about 3% will deliver beyond 42 weeks' gestation, and in the majority of these pregnancies, the infant will show stigmas of "dysmaturity"—loss of subcutaneous fat, diminished amniotic fluid volume, and meconium-stained skin and nails. The perinatal mortality rate rises slightly from 41 to 42 weeks' gestation, and the rise accelerates after 42 weeks' gestation. Therefore, for patients with a favorable cervix, I recommend delivery shortly after 40 weeks' gestation. If the cervix is unfavorable for labor induction, by 41 weeks the patient is offered the options of labor induction versus twice-a-week nonstress tests and amniotic fluid checks. I deliver patients regardless of the cervical examination by about 42 weeks' gestation, if the dating of the pregnancy is secure, because beyond that gestational age, the risks associated with postmaturity outweigh those of need for cesarean section for failed induction.

PRENATAL DETECTION OF BIRTH DEFECTS

About 1% of infants are born with a serious birth defect, and an additional 3% have a minor anomaly. Prenatal care includes screening for risk factors for birth defects, genetic counseling if indicated, sonography, and serum marker screening. For certain disorders, invasive prenatal diagnostic testing and molecular or cytogenetic studies are indicated. Detectable anomalies include chromosomal aneuploidy, metabolic defects, and many structural defects.

Cytogenetics and Molecular Genetics

For the patient who is at increased risk for chromosomal abnormalities or for any of the steadily in-creasing numbers of congenital diseases that can be diagnosed by biochemical or molecular genetic testing, genetic counseling and either chorionic villus sampling (CVS) or amniocentesis may be offered.

Amniocentesis has been the mainstay of chromosomal diagnosis for decades. After ultrasound examination to evaluate fetal and placental location, a sterile preparation of the abdomen is performed, a 20- or 22-gauge needle is introduced into the amniotic cavity under continuous ultrasound guidance, and fluid is withdrawn. Fetal fibroblasts from the amniotic fluid can be induced to proliferate in the laboratory, and after 7 to 10 days, chromosome preparations can be made or gene probe tests performed. Biochemical testing of the amniotic fluid can be useful in diagnosis of ventral wall and neural tube defects.

In the past, amniocentesis was usually performed at 15 to 20 weeks. However, with the use of ultrasonography in guiding the needle into the amniotic cavity, amniocentesis can be performed in many patients as early at 12 to 14 weeks' gestation. However, the attributable rate of fetal loss is about 1 per 200 after 15 weeks, and it is higher (1 per 50 to 100) for amniocentesis before 14 weeks.

CVS offers an earlier means of cytogenetic and molecular genetic fetal assessment. CVS is usually done at 10 to 12 weeks. A small amount of placental tissue is aspirated under direct ultrasound guidance, through either the transabdominal or transcervical approach. The sample of chorionic villi can be used for direct chromosome preparations, or cells can be grown in culture for gene probe or biochemical testing. The pregnancy loss rate in relation to CVS is similar to that from early amniocentesis.

Serum Marker Screening

The use of serum marker screening has proved to be an effective tool for identifying pregnancies at high risk for certain fetal anomalies and for downstream complications.

A maternal serum sample is drawn at 15 to 20 weeks' gestation, and the levels of alpha-fetoprotein (AFP), estriol, and hCG are determined.

An AFP level of greater than 2.5 multiples of the median occurs in about 2% of well-dated singletons; among these pregnancies are more than 95% of anencephalics, more than 80% of fetuses with neural tube defects, and more than 80% of fetuses with gastroschisis or omphalocele. In addition, a chromosomal abnormality is present in 0.5 to 1.0% of pregnancies with an elevated maternal serum AFP level.

The combination of maternal age, gestational age, and serum marker results can be used to calculate risk for Down syndrome. About 4% of well-dated singleton pregnancies in women younger than 35 years will have a calculated Down syndrome risk of 1 in 360 or greater; these women are offered genetic counseling, targeted sonography, and amniocentesis; if all accept amniocentesis, about 60% of fetuses with Down syndrome will be detected.

Maternal serum screening may be considered by

women age 35 years or older as an alternative to universal amniocentesis. At age 35 to 40 years, the calculated risk based on serum screening will be 1 in 360 or greater in about 25% of women, and 80 to 85% of Down syndrome cases will be detected if this 25% cohort accepts amniocentesis. The women age 35 years or older at delivery must understand that 15 to 20% of Down syndrome cases will be missed by serum marker screening!

Pregnancies with unexplained low hCG or elevated maternal serum AFP are at risk for placental abruption, fetal death, IUGR, preterm birth, and preeclampsia. To these patients, I recommend close clinical follow-up and consideration of a 32- to 34-week sonogram for growth.

Sonographic Assessment for Fetal Anomalies

If the patient's history places her at increased risk for fetal structural defects that can be identified by ultrasound examination, a targeted sonogram should be arranged. A partial listing of such defects is given in Table 8.

TABLE 8. **Anomalies That Are Detectable by Ultrasonography***

Cardiovascular System

Arrhythmias
Cardiomyopathy
Cardiosplenic syndromes
Double-outlet right ventricle
Ebstein's anomaly
Endocardial cushion defect
Hypoplastic left ventricle
Hypoplastic right ventricle
Pericardial tumors (teratoma)
Rhabdomyoma
Situs inversus
Tetralogy of Fallot
Transposition of the great arteries
Ventricular septal defect

Central Nervous System

Anencephaly, exencephaly
Agenesis of the corpus callosum
Choroid plexus cysts
Dandy-Walker malformation
Encephalocele
Holoprosencephaly
Hydranencephaly
Hydrocephalus
Intracranial neoplasm
Microcephaly
Open spina bifida
Porencephalic cyst
Toxoplasmosis

Craniofacial

Cleft lip
Cystic hygroma
Micrognathia

Gastrointestinal Tract

Cholelithiasis
Duodenal atresia
Gastroschisis
Hepatic calcifications
Meconium peritonitis
Omphalocele
Persistent right umbilical vein

Genitourinary System

Ambiguous genitalia
Bladder outlet obstruction
Ectopic ureterocele
Hydronephrosis
Hypospadias
Infantile polycystic kidneys
Multicystic dysplastic kidney
Ovarian cyst
Pelvic kidney
Renal agenesis

Extremities

Arthrogryposis
Clubfeet
Limb shortening
Polydactyly
Radial aplasia
Skeletal dysplasias

Thoracic

Cystic adenomatoid malformation
Diaphragmatic hernia
Hydrothorax, chylothorax
Pulmonary sequestration

*This is a partial listing of sonographically detectable defects. Each of these defects has been diagnosed at Sharp Perinatal Center in the past 5 years.

Whereas the American College of Obstetrics and Gynecology does not endorse routine sonography, I recommend a comprehensive sonogram to all patients for these reasons:

1. A compelling argument can be made for 16- to 20-week sonography for all pregnancies to confirm dates, determine placental location, diagnose twins, and improve accuracy of maternal serum marker screening.

2. Numerous studies have demonstrated that targeted, comprehensive sonographic assessment at 18 to 20 weeks' gestation, with use of high-resolution equipment and by an expert sonographer, results in diagnosis of more than 50% of major fetal anomalies, with few false-positive results. Such a screening program has cost/benefit considerations more favorable than maternal serum marker screening.

3. Given the potential benefits and the absence of risk, I believe that it is ethically indefensible *not* to offer a high-resolution sonogram (if need be, at the patient's own expense) to all pregnant women.

RECORD KEEPING

It is both sound medical practice and an essential medicolegal protection to clearly document care provided during the course of the pregnancy. Standardized prenatal record forms provide a compact, convenient, and legible format for record keeping. For patients with unusually complex medical histories, it may be worthwhile to dictate a narrative report or summary at or after the preconception or first prenatal visit. The same is true for patients developing serious pregnancy complications. A copy of the prenatal record is sent to the hospital's labor and delivery unit after the results of the prenatal laboratory studies have returned, and thereafter on a more or less monthly basis. If a patient needs to travel out of the area or plans to transfer care to another physician after about 20 weeks' gestation, a photocopy of the prenatal record is provided to her. In addition, for patients with unusual or complex medical histories or obstetric management plans, e.g., patients with serious maternal medical problems or carrying fetuses with identified anomalies, a typewritten summary of the delivery plan may be helpful. It is presently recommended that records from the pregnancy be stored for at least 7 years after delivery. In fact, if space permits, it may be prudent to keep these records for an even longer time.

FAMILY-ORIENTED CARE

In the face of the growing complexity of the technical aspects of obstetric care, it is easy to lose the human element in prenatal care. As discussed earlier, I have found it helpful to schedule an uninterrupted 30- to 60-minute visit for the initial examination. In addition, it is often helpful to plan on a longer than usual visit in the late third trimester, at which time the process of intake into the hospital maternity unit can be explained, labor signs and symptoms reviewed, and any questions or worries about the labor and delivery process answered. Patients who are attending childbirth classes often have lists of questions and can be encouraged to bring them to this visit. Specific questions that many patients have, but fail to ask, include issues regarding episiotomy, the likelihood that a cesarean section will be needed, and the availability and use of obstetric anesthesia, such as epidural anesthesia, on the labor and delivery unit.

Childbirth classes are offered by many hospitals and community organizations. The content and quality vary widely, and obstetrics care providers should be willing to help develop and monitor content for these courses. Our hospital sponsors excellent classes, and I recommend prepared childbirth courses most highly to my patients.

Couples should tour the hospital well in advance of delivery. Particularly for women delivering their first infant or who have had a complicated pregnancy, this visit can be most reassuring. In our maternity hospital, every attempt is made to provide a family-centered delivery experience, with large and private labor and delivery rooms, while preserving the safety precautions of in-house obstetricians, anesthesia, operating room staff, neonatologists, and a newborn intensive care unit.

ECTOPIC PREGNANCY

method of
PETER M. HORVATH, M.D.
Albany Medical College
Albany, New York

Ectopic pregnancy is a gestation that implants outside of the endometrial cavity. Most commonly, the ectopic site is in the ampullary portion of the fallopian tube; however, extratubal ectopic implantations may occur in the abdomen, ovary, or cervix. (The following discussion of management is largely limited to tubal ectopic pregnancies.) The true incidence of ectopic pregnancy is difficult to ascertain because early ectopic gestations may die and be absorbed without any maternal symptoms. Whereas the frequency of such "tubal abortion" is unknown, the incidence of clinically detectable ectopic pregnancy has increased nearly fivefold since 1970 in the United States. The most recent statistics suggest an incidence of 1.6% of reported pregnancies overall, with a 2.7% incidence in older (>35 years) women. Ectopic pregnancy is a major cause of maternal morbidity, and it accounts for 5 to 6% of all maternal deaths in the United States.

Numerous factors increase the risk for ectopic pregnancy (Table 1); the most important of these are related to abnormalities of the fallopian tube. Commonly, patients have a history of pelvic inflammatory disease, tubal or pelvic surgery, previous ectopic pregnancy, or adhesive disease associated with advanced stages of endometriosis. Less often, ectopic pregnancy may occur in patients without such risk factors, in morphologically normal fallopian tubes. The underlying etiologic factors are not well understood in these

TABLE 1. Incidence of Ectopic Pregnancy Related to Risk Factors

Risk Factors	Approximate Incidence (%)
General population	1–2
Pelvic inflammatory disease	10–15
Previous tubal surgery (reanastomosis, salpingolysis, neosalpingostomy, salpingotomy)	5–30
Previous ectopic pregnancy	10–15
Intrauterine device in place	4–9

cases, but two major hypotheses are (1) an abnormal endocrine milieu (secondary to ovulatory dysfunction or minimal endometriosis) may lead to abnormal tubal transport of the early embryo and (2) genetically abnormal embryos may be predisposed to abnormal nidation and may thus implant with greater frequency in ectopic locations.

HISTORY AND PHYSICAL EXAMINATION

Patients with ectopic pregnancy are generally encountered in two different clinical settings. In the emergency department, patients present with a wide range of abdominal and pelvic pain, often accompanied by vaginal bleeding. Various degrees of hemodynamic alterations are encountered, and the exact gestational age is more difficult to pinpoint and often more advanced. A second group are typically asymptomatic patients at high risk for developing ectopic pregnancy who are being managed expectantly and in a prospective fashion. By definition, these patients present earlier in the natural course of their disease and therefore offer the practitioner the greatest opportunity for clinical management options.

Ectopic pregnancy has been referred to as the "great masquerader" because its clinical presentation may mimic many abdominal and pelvic conditions. Clearly, women who present with late or ruptured ectopic gestations and who have surgical (acute) abdomens require emergency surgical intervention. On the other hand, women with early, unruptured ectopic gestations may present in protean ways. Abdominal pain, usually unilateral, is the most common complaint. Abnormal vaginal bleeding, syncopal symptoms, and a history of a missed or unusual menstrual period are also frequently reported. On examination, patients may have clear-cut peritoneal signs if intraperitoneal bleeding has occurred; however, they may have minimal or no abdominal signs if the pregnancy is unruptured. Adnexal tenderness and fullness as well as uterine softening and mild enlargement may be appreciated on pelvic examination. An occasional patient—even with an advanced ectopic gestation—may present with completely atypical features, complaining perhaps of nothing more than vague midline intermittent cramping and malaise. Abdominal and pelvic examinations may be completely unremarkable.

DIAGNOSTIC TESTING

The first step is, of course, to confirm or exclude the diagnosis of pregnancy. Commercially available urinary pregnancy tests that use monoclonal antibody technology may be used for screening. These urinary tests may have sensitivities in the range of 50 to 100 mIU of human chorionic gonadotropin (hCG) per mL. Serum pregnancy testing should be used in all symptomatic patients as well as in all patients in whom a reliable estimate of the date of conception cannot be made. With rare exception, and for practical clinical purposes, a negative result of serum β-hCG testing (<5 mIU per mL) excludes the diagnosis of ectopic pregnancy. A complete blood count is essential in the initial evaluation of ectopic pregnancy. Serial hemoglobin and hematocrit determinations may be used in preoperative monitoring. In addition, blood typing and determination of antibody status are mandatory.

In the woman with a positive serum pregnancy test result, the first thing to establish is whether she wishes to keep the pregnancy. If the patient is desirous of keeping her pregnancy, the next step is to try to establish the location and viability of the gestation.

With regard to viability (regardless of location), serial quantitative determinations of the β subunit of hCG (β-hCG) are extremely helpful in differentiating between normal and abnormal gestations. In normal pregnancy, β-hCG titers increase in a logarithmic fashion and are often said to double in approximately 48 hours. In fact, there is quite a bit of variation in this doubling time as it relates to gestational age: in very early gestations, the mean doubling time may be as little as 38 to 45 hours; in later gestations (>6 weeks), it may be as much as 96 hours or more. Further, there is great variation about the mean doubling time in different patients at the same gestational age. At the lower limits of normal, β-hCG values should rise by approximately 67% in 2 days in early pregnancy, or by 100% in 3 days. Failure to double in 72 hours suggests an abnormal gestation. In addition to ascertaining viability, serial β-hCG measurements corroborate information gained from transvaginal ultrasound imaging. Last, quantitative β-hCG titers obtained 12 to 24 hours after uterine curettage can accurately pinpoint the location of a pregnancy often more quickly and practically than histopathologic examination. Specifically, dropping titers after curettage are diagnostic of a nonviable intrauterine gestation; plateauing or rising levels are diagnostic of ectopic gestations (Figure 1).

An explanatory note of caution in ordering and interpreting serum β-hCG levels is in order. Two standards have been developed and are used in different hCG assays: the Second International Standard (2nd IS) and the Third International Standard (3rd IS), formerly known as the First International Reference Preparation.

Reported levels with the 2nd IS are approximately 50% lower than those with the 3rd IS. Clearly, one must know which standard is being used in the laboratory to make accurate clinical decisions. Values of β-hCG in the following discussion refer to the 3rd IS.

Whereas serial quantitative β-hCG testing may suggest an abnormal gestation by plateauing, decreasing, or inappropriately rising titers, the definitive diagnosis of ectopic pregnancy rests on demonstrating a pregnancy outside the uterine corpus. Noninvasive ultrasonographic imaging of the uterus and adnexae has become the mainstay of diagnosis. Endovaginal (transvaginal) imaging is clearly superior to the transabdominal route, allowing diagnosis of an intrauterine gestational sac (GS) 1 week earlier. The first structure that can be identified endovaginally is the GS. The true GS can be differentiated from the decidual reaction of a pseudo-GS by the double-lined, echo-dense ring that surrounds the former. All intrauterine pregnancies should have an identifiable GS by the middle to end of the fifth gestational week. The second structure to be identified is the yolk sac (YS). The YS can be detected early in the sixth gestational week. It should be round in cross-section and should measure at least 4 mm in diameter. The fetal pole becomes evident during the seventh gestational week adjacent to the YS. Fetal heart rate activity can routinely be detected in normal pregnancies by the middle of this week. Definitive diagnosis of a viable intrauterine pregnancy requires demonstration of fetal heart activity within the uterus. Intrauterine location of a pregnancy can be documented solely on the basis of an intrauterine GS, or preferably a YS. Demonstration of an intrauterine GS or YS without subsequent demonstration of a fetal pole is evidence of a blighted (intrauterine) pregnancy. When the quantitative β-hCG value (3rd IS) exceeds 2000 mIU per mL, virtually all intrauterine gestations should be identifiable. Nonvisualization of an intrauterine gestation indicates either an ectopic location or a recently completed abortion. With quantitative β-hCG values less than 2000 mIU per mL, the possibilities are a normal gestation that is too early to visualize, an abnormal gestation (intrauterine or ectopic), or a recently completed abortion.

For practical purposes, demonstration of an intrauterine gestation is usually considered adequate to exclude ectopic pregnancy because heterotopic pregnancy (coexistent ectopic and intrauterine) is rare (1 in 30,000). The possibility of heterotopic pregnancy should not be forgotten, especially in the patient who has undergone extensive fertility treatment, in particular the assisted reproductive technologies such as in vitro fertilization. Some estimate that the incidence of heterotopic pregnancy in this population may be as high as 1%. Careful ultrasonographic examination of the adnexae and cul-de-sac should be performed even when intrauterine pregnancy has been documented.

MANAGEMENT

The patient who presents to the emergency department with an acute abdomen, clear-cut peritoneal signs, and hemodynamic instability requires emergent laparotomy. The majority of these patients will have large ectopic pregnancies that have destroyed the fallopian tube and have ruptured or are actively bleeding; salpingectomy is indicated. In symptomatic but stable patients, or in asymptomatic high-risk patients being managed expectantly, diagnostic testing should be performed as outlined earlier.

Current standards employ surgery as the mainstay of treatment. Operative laparoscopy has replaced laparotomy in many (if not most) hospitals for management of all but the hemodynamically compromised patient with acute abdomen and hemoperitoneum. In patients desiring to maintain fertility potential, the standard procedure for tubal ectopic gestations is linear salpingostomy with removal of the pregnancy. A dilute (40%) solution of vasopressin is often injected on the antimesenteric border over the gestation. Incision may be made with scissors, an electrosurgical needle, harmonic scalpel, or laser, as equipment allows. Hemostasis is usually easily achieved with point cautery if needed. Very early (5- to 6-week) gestations may be more difficult to evacuate and may be at somewhat higher risk for persistent trophoblastic proliferation than slightly later gestations. Operative time is typically less than an hour and recovery is rapid. Larger ectopic gestations and some located in more proximal portions of the fallopian tube (isthmic) may require segmental resec-

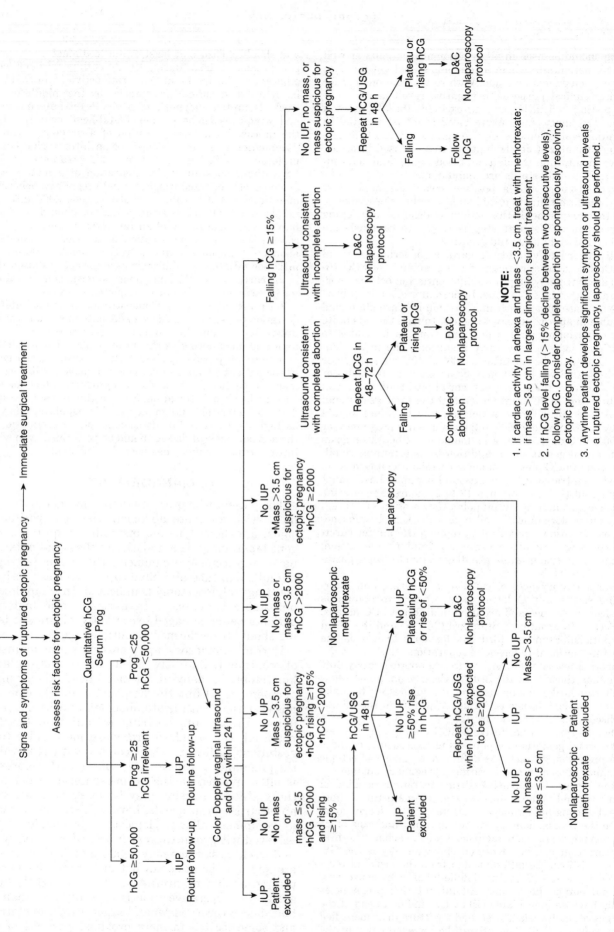

Figure 1. Ectopic pregnancy flow-chart algorithm. *Abbreviations:* hCG = human chorionic gonadotropin; Prog = progesterone; IUP = intrauterine pregnancy; USG = ultrasonography; D & C = dilatation and curettage. (Redrawn from Stovall TG, Ling FW: Ectopic pregnancy. Diagnostic and therapeutic algorithms minimizing surgical intervention. J Reprod Med 38:808–812, 1993.)

tion, which can also be done easily through a laparoscopic approach. Tubal repair, if necessary, is performed at a later time. Laparotomy is appropriate if instrumentation or operator experience is inadequate.

Although operative laparoscopy offers numerous advantages over laparotomy, including reductions in morbidity of patients and in health care costs, an even more exciting change in the management of early ectopic gestations has been the more widespread use of medical management options. A superb algorithm for the management of early ectopic pregnancy has been developed and popularized by Stovall and Ling (see Figure 1). Early diagnosis maximizes opportunities for alternative therapeutic options, in particular an option for medical management. The success of the algorithm outlined in Figure 1 is predicated on the following principles:

1. Symptomatic patients with surgical (acute) abdomens are treated by emergency surgery.
2. Quantitative serum β-hCG levels of greater than 2000 mIU per mL (3rd IS) in the absence of an intrauterine gestational sac are diagnostic of ectopic pregnancy. Medical or surgical management depends on whether an adnexal mass larger than 3.5 cm can be identified by ultrasonography and on clinical judgment. (Adnexal cardiac activity is a relative contraindication to medical management even with a smaller mass.)
3. Metabolism of hCG should yield a decrement of 15% of β-hCG titer in approximately 72 hours.
4. Ectopic pregnancies rarely rupture before 6.5 to 7 gestational weeks.

The medical (methotrexate) protocol of Stovall and Ling is outlined in Table 2. The dosage of methotrexate,* 50 mg per m² intramuscularly, is well tolerated and in my experience has virtually none of the side effects reported with the older multiple-dose (methotrexate–citrovorum rescue) protocols. Baseline liver function tests are obtained, but I have yet to have an occasion to follow these tests serially. Nomograms to calculate body surface area (m²) are available in most oncology textbooks. Patients must be cautioned to abstain from multivitamins (containing folic acid), alcohol, and sexual intercourse. Pelvic pain may increase in as many as 30 to 70% of patients with resolution of the pregnancy. Nonsteroidal analgesics may be offered. Time to resolution (quantitative β-hCG value of <5 mIU per mL) may be prolonged (2 to 7 weeks) in some patients, and they should be counseled appropriately.

With the appropriate application of algorithms, approximately 40% of patients can avoid initial surgical intervention; 85 to 95% of appropriately selected patients will complete therapy, with approximately 5% requiring a second dose of methotrexate. Tubal patency rates (by hysterosalpingography) are on the order of 80%, approximately the same as with conservative surgical approaches. Approximately 4% of

*Not FDA approved for this indication.

TABLE 2. **Single-Dose Methotrexate Protocol for Ectopic Pregnancy Treatment**

Day	Therapy
0*	hCG, D & C, CBC, AST, BUN, creatinine, blood type + Rh
1	MTX, hCG
4	hCG
7†	hCG

*In those patients not requiring D & C before MTX initiation (hCG >2000 mIU/mL [3rd IS] and no gestational sac on transvaginal ultrasound examination), day 0 and day 1 are combined.
†If <15% decline in hCG titer between days 4 and 7, give second dose of MTX 50 mg/m² on day 7. If ≥15% decline in hCG titer between days 4 and 7, monitor weekly until hCG is <15 mIU/mL.
Abbreviations: hCG = quantitative human chorionic gonadotropin-β subunit, mIU/mL; D & C = dilatation and curettage; CBC = complete blood count; AST = aspartate aminotransferase, units/L; BUN = blood urea nitrogen; MTX = intramuscular methotrexate, 50 mg/m².
From Stovall TG, Ling FW: Single-dose methotrexate: An expanded clinical trial. Am J Obstet Gynecol *168*:1759–1762, 1993.

patients undergoing conservative surgery will have a persistence of trophoblastic activity, and β-hCG levels will fail to show an appropriate decrement. If levels begin to rise postoperatively, a diagnosis of persistent ectopic pregnancy is suspected, and the patient should undergo salpingectomy. Alternatively, methotrexate therapy as outlined before may be considered in these patients. Another circumstance in which chemotherapy may be considered is in the treatment of nontubal ectopic gestations, such as abdominal, cervical, or ovarian ectopic pregnancy. Consultation with gynecologic subspecialists is certainly warranted in these difficult management situations.

Rh-negative women who are unsensitized to the D antigen should be given Rh immune globulin (RhoGAM) to prevent isoimmunization. At gestational ages of less than 13 weeks, 50 μg of D immune globulin should be given; women with older gestations should receive 300 μg.

VAGINAL BLEEDING IN LATE PREGNANCY

method of
MATT H. BACKER, Jr., M.D.
St. Louis University
St. Louis, Missouri
Naval Medical Center
San Diego, California

Vaginal bleeding in the third trimester (more than spotting or blood-tinged mucus) occurs in 4% of pregnancies, is a serious threat to mother and child, and requires immediate evaluation. The best outcome results when evaluation and treatment are done in a hospital offering continuous electronic fetal monitoring, ultrasound imaging, fetal maturity studies, hemogram and blood coagulation studies, and the ability to perform cesarean section 24 hours a day. Neonatal consultation and a high-risk nursery also improve the outcome. Management of this complication requires evaluation, stabilization, and definitive therapy.

EVALUATION

As soon as bleeding is reported, the physician responsible for delivery must determine (1) the volume of bleeding; (2) the estimated date of confinement and parity; (3) associated symptoms, such as pain, syncope, labor, or membrane rupture; and (4) risk factors—previous cesarean section, myomectomy, metroplasty, cerclage, condylomata, hypertension, trauma, drug use, or earlier bleeding.

The patient is met by the attending physician at the hospital, where these standing orders have been or should be initiated:

1. Assess the volume of hemorrhage (some units weigh pads).

2. Record vital signs every 5 minutes.

3. Examine the *abdomen* for fetal heart activity, fundal height, and uterine contractions and tonus (*no vaginal examinations*).

4. Gain venous access with an Intracath and begin infusion to keep the vein open with dextrose 5% in lactated Ringer's crystalloid.

5. Initiate fetal heart rate and uterine monitoring.

6. Send blood for complete blood count, type, and crossmatch and extra blood for coagulation studies if later needed. Tape another tube of blood without anticoagulant on the wall for clot observation; it should clot in 8 minutes and not lyse.

7. If the patient is in shock, begin blood replacement and insert a Foley catheter. (Crossmatched blood should exceed estimated loss by 2 units.)

8. Ultrasound examination for placental location and fetal size, presentation, and well-being or anomalies should be done by the most experienced person present.

At the bedside, the attending physician now considers the possible causes, which are usually placental or uterine in this order of occurrence:

1. Placental abruption, which is usually painful, occurs in 1% of pregnancies but accounts for 30% of third-trimester bleeding. It is mild in 50%, moderate in 25%, and severe in 25%, and it is still a killer with an overall fetal loss of 30% and maternal loss up to 5%.

2. Placenta previa, usually a painless bleeding, occurs in 0.5% of pregnancies and causes 20% of the hemorrhage of late pregnancy. With ideal care, fetal loss is less than 20% (mostly due to prematurity), and maternal mortality is less than 1%.

3. Vasa previa is a condition in which the umbilical vessels course through the membranes in advance of the presenting part. It occurs only once in 3000 pregnancies, but if unrecognized, it is lethal to the fetus.

4. Uterine causes include uterine rupture and cervical lesions; prior hysterotomy for cesarean section or myomectomy alerts one to this.

STABILIZATION

Blood loss must be replaced with whole blood (if available) or with packed cells. The hematocrit must be maintained at 30% and the urine output at 30 mL per hour (the "30/30" rule). If blood in the wall tube, in the bed, or around the venipuncture does not clot, prothrombin time, activated partial thromboplastin time, platelet count, fibrinogen, and fibrin split product determinations must be made.

Monitor strips are reviewed by the attending physician for fetal heart rate, for variability of decelerations, and for the pattern of uterine contractions. Leopold's maneuvers

should be attempted to determine the number, polarity, and lie of fetuses.

Repeated sonography should confirm the location of the placenta. Less useful in the diagnosis of abruption, some machines with high resolution can detect retroplacental hematomas.

Amniocentesis for fetal maturity is useful if delivery can be postponed.

Vaginal examination is contraindicated with ultrasound evidence of significant placenta previa. With a mild abruption or marginal previa suspected, cautious digital and speculum examinations may be done, but only with a "double setup" (in which immediate cesarean delivery can be done should heavy bleeding ensue). If cervical effacement and some dilatation are found, the fetus is sufficiently mature, and no placenta or fetal vessels are seen or felt, artificial rupture of the membranes is indicated, with the attachment of a scalp electrode for monitoring. With vasa previa, blood from the vagina will contain nucleated fetal red blood cells.

THERAPY

Abruptio Placentae

Abruptio placentae is variously treated, depending on the severity of the bleeding and the viability and maturity of the fetus. With mild abruption, no labor, and a healthy but immature infant, blood replacement and monitored observation should be attempted, with or without tocolysis. A distressed fetus must always be delivered by the most expeditious means because major hemorrhage may be hidden. With severe abruption and a viable fetus, rapid cesarean delivery is indicated. Fetal death implies separation of more than 50% of the placenta and blood loss in excess of 2 liters. With fetal death, vaginal delivery with transfusion can sometimes be accomplished if the cervix is favorable and the contraction pattern favorable. Oxytocin (Pitocin) may be used.

Patients in shock require central venous pressure or Swan-Ganz monitoring, and the possibility of disseminated intravascular coagulation should be anticipated. Coagulopathies may require fresh-frozen plasma (start with 4 units), platelet transfusion (start with 10 packs), and/or cryoprecipitate (4 units) for hypofibrinogenemia. Heparin and fibrinolysins should be avoided. Ten percent of these patients have another abruption in a subsequent pregnancy.

Postpartum hemorrhage may require bilateral hypogastric artery ligation or even hysterectomy.

Placenta Previa

Placenta previa is treated differently according to its location (the type or degree of previa), the amount of hemorrhage, and the maturity of the fetus. Although the first hemorrhage with a previa may be profuse, it kills the fetus less often than does the initial bleed with an abruption.

Total (central) placenta previa diagnosed after the 36th week of gestation is treated with blood replacement and prompt cesarean section. Bleeding of more than 2 liters in any 24-hour period also mandates section regardless of maturity. With lesser bleeding and an immature fetus, restricted observation in the hospital, with blood replacement that maintains the hematocrit above 30%, can be attempted.

Marginal placenta previa or the "low-lying placenta," confirmed by sonography and vaginal examination under double setup, can sometimes be successfully delivered vaginally. Even when this is accomplished, fetal morbidity is higher than with abdominal delivery.

Cesarean section for placenta previa should be of the low vertical type, preferably under general anesthesia. Breech and transverse presentations are more common, and incision through the placenta is bloody. Maternal death is rare, but postpartum hemorrhage may occur because of placenta accreta or failure of the lower uterine segment to contract.

Vasa Previa

Vasa previa, if recognized before fetal demise, is managed by abdominal delivery. Recurrent severe variable decelerations in labor associated with bleeding suggest this condition. The pulsating cord can sometimes be felt through a partially dilated cervix. An Apt test done on the fetal blood in the vagina will demonstrate fetal hemoglobin. Because the hemorrhage is fetal, the neonate may well require transfusion.

Uterine Rupture

Uterine rupture requires laparotomy and usually hysterectomy. Whereas the majority follow previous cesarean section, spontaneous rupture can occasionally be seen in the grand multipara, after hyperstimulation with oxytocin, or after intrauterine manipulation. Fetal mortality and maternal mortality are high (50% and 10%) if treatment is delayed.

Cervical Lesions

Cervical lesions rarely bleed for the first time in the third trimester, but both benign (condylomata) and malignant (carcinoma) lesions have been reported. These should be evident on speculum examination, and their treatment is that of the lesion. The "bloody show" seen in both term and premature labor is due to the laceration of small cervical vessels.

CONCLUSION

Although antepartum hemorrhage is still a formidable complication, successful management has been greatly improved by the ready availability of blood products and by ultrasonic imaging.

HYPERTENSIVE DISORDERS OF PREGNANCY

method of
BAHA M. SIBAI, M.D.
University of Tennessee, Memphis
Memphis, Tennessee

Hypertensive disorders are the most common medical complications of pregnancy with a reported incidence ranging between 5 and 10%. These disorders are the second leading cause of maternal death in the United States and a leading cause of perinatal mortality and morbidity worldwide. The clinical manifestations in some of these disorders are usually similar (e.g., hypertension, generalized edema, proteinuria, hematuria, renal insufficiency); however, they may result from different underlying causes (essential hypertension, gestational hypertension, preeclampsia, renal disease, or connective tissue disease). Hypertension is the hallmark for the diagnosis of these disorders. Therefore, in caring for pregnant women with hypertension, it is important to differentiate among gestational hypertension, chronic hypertension, preeclampsia, and silent renal disease (Table 1). In general, maternal and perinatal outcomes are usually good in those who have either mild essential chronic hypertension or gestational hypertension. In contrast, maternal and neonatal complications are increased among pregnant women who have secondary chronic hypertension, renal disease, or severe preeclampsia.

DEFINITIONS AND CLASSIFICATION

The terminology used to describe the hypertensive disorders of pregnancy and the definitions used to diagnose hypertension in pregnancy have been confusing and inconsistent. Some of these terms, such as pregnancy-induced hypertension, are vague and broad, whereas others, such as pregnancy-associated hypertension, are nonspecific. In addition, a variety of classifications have been proposed by the American College of Obstetricians and Gynecologists, the International Society for the Study of Hypertension in Pregnancy, and the Working Group on High Blood Pressure in Pregnancy. In general, all current definitions and classification schemes have certain pitfalls as they relate to clinical diagnosis and management.

An overall discussion of all hypertensive disorders of pregnancy is beyond the scope of this article. In this review, hypertensive disorders are divided into three major categories: chronic hypertension, gestational hypertension, and preeclampsia (see Table 1).

CHRONIC HYPERTENSION

The incidence of chronic hypertension in pregnancy ranges from 1 to 5%, depending on the woman's age, body mass index, and ethnic origin. In the majority of cases, the etiology is essential hypertension. However, consideration of additional, potentially correctable causes, such as renovascular disease, pheochromocytoma, coarctation of the aorta, or Cushing's syndrome, is extremely important.

TABLE 1. **Hypertensive Disorders of Pregnancy**

Clinical Findings	Chronic Hypertension	Gestational Hypertension	Preeclampsia	Renal Disease
Time of onset of hypertension	<20 wk	Usually after 33 wk	<20 wk	Usually before 20 wk
Degree of hypertension	Mild or severe	Mild	Mild or severe	Usually severe
Proteinuria*	Absent	Absent	Usually present	Usually severe
Serum urate >5.5 mg/dL (0.33 mmol/L)	Rare	Absent	Present in almost all cases	Variable
Hemoconcentration	Absent	Absent	Present in severe disease	Present in some conditions
Thrombocytopenia	Absent	Absent	Present in severe disease	May be present†
Serum creatinine ≥1.2 mg/dL	Absent	Absent	Rare	Usually present
Hepatic dysfunction	Absent	Absent	Present in severe disease	Absent

*Defined as ≥300 mg in a 24-h urine collection.
†Present in hemolytic-uremic syndrome and patients with lupus nephritis.

Diagnosis

The diagnosis of chronic hypertension during pregnancy is usually based on either a history of hypertension before pregnancy or blood pressure elevations to at least 140/90 mm Hg before 20 weeks' gestation. The diagnosis is more severe when definite evidence of hypertension is documented before conception, particularly when antihypertensive agents have been prescribed.

The diagnosis of chronic hypertension may be difficult in pregnant women in whom the blood pressure before pregnancy is not known. During normal pregnancy, blood pressure progressively decreases from the first trimester, reaching a nadir at 14 to 24 weeks' gestation, with a gradual return to prepregnancy levels during the third trimester. As a result of these physiologic changes in blood pressure during the second trimester, many women with actual chronic hypertension before pregnancy will have normal blood pressure readings before 20 weeks' gestation. The majority of these women subsequently develop increased blood pressure during the third trimester and thus will be erroneously diagnosed as having gestational hypertension or preeclampsia.

In the nonpregnant state, hypertension is classified as mild, moderate, severe, or very severe on the basis of either systolic or diastolic blood pressure readings. In pregnancy, it is easier to classify chronic hypertension into mild (systolic pressure between 140 and 159 mm Hg and/or diastolic pressure between 90 and 109 mm Hg) and severe (systolic pressure ≥160 mm Hg and/or diastolic pressure ≥110 mm Hg). In pregnancies complicated by chronic hypertension, perinatal outcome is adversely affected mostly because of superimposed preeclampsia. The diagnosis of superimposed preeclampsia should be made on the basis of exacerbated hypertension plus the development of either new-onset proteinuria (at least 1 gram per 24 hours) or elevated uric acid levels (at least 6 mg per dL) after 20 weeks' gestation. In women receiving antihypertensive drugs, this diagnosis can be made solely on the basis of new-onset proteinuria or elevated uric acid values criteria. In women with renal disease, proteinuria and elevated uric acid values may already be present from early in pregnancy. In such women, the diagnosis of superimposed preeclampsia may be difficult. I recommend establishing the diagnosis on the basis of onset of thrombocytopenia or symptoms such as persistent headaches, visual abnormalities, or epigastric pain.

Maternal and Fetal Risks

Pregnancies complicated by chronic hypertension are associated with increased maternal and perinatal risks, such as superimposed preeclampsia, abruptio placentae, fetal growth restriction, and preterm birth. The frequency of these complications is particularly increased in women with long-standing severe hypertension, in those with secondary hypertension, and in those with pre-existing cardiovascular or renal disease. In contrast, except for superimposed preeclampsia, these complications are rare in women with mild, uncomplicated essential chronic hypertension.

Management

Management of the patient with chronic hypertension should begin before conception to establish the etiology as well as the severity of the hypertension. Attention should be paid to the degree and duration of the hypertension, presence of associated medical disorders (cardiac, renal, diabetes, connective tissue disease), presence of target organ damage (left ventricular dysfunction, renal insufficiency, cerebrovascular disease), type and number of antihypertensive drugs required to control maternal blood pressure, and outcome in previous pregnancies. In addition, attention should be paid to maternal diet, social habits (drugs, alcohol, smoking), and activity. Based on this assessment, the patient is then classified as having low-risk hypertension (essential hypertension without associated medical disorders or target organ involvement) or high-risk hypertension (patients with severe hypertension and those with target organ damage or associated medical disorders). Patients with primary renal disease with renal insufficiency (serum creatinine concentration greater than 1.4 mg per dL) and hypertension and those with severe hypertension requiring multidrug therapy should be informed about the risks to the fetus and the potential for renal failure during pregnancy or post partum.

The use of angiotensin-converting enzyme drugs during pregnancy is associated with fetal growth restriction, oligohydramnios, neonatal renal failure, and neonatal death. In addition, chronic use of atenolol (Tenormin) during pregnancy has adverse effects on placental function and fetal growth. Therefore, women receiving such medications should be switched to different agents before conception. Some of the drugs that are believed relatively safe for use in pregnancy are listed in Table 2. In addition, the adverse effects of illicit drugs, alcohol, and smoking on maternal blood pressure as well as on the fetus should be emphasized, and the woman should be encouraged to discontinue their use before conception.

Early onset of prenatal care and careful antepartum supervision with proper fetal testing are the keys for a successful outcome of pregnant women with chronic hypertension. At the time of the first prenatal visit, it is important to determine gestational age and confirm an estimated date of confinement, which are important to monitor fetal growth and for timing of delivery. The majority of patients will have low-risk chronic hypertension and thus will have a favorable maternal and perinatal prognosis without the use of antihypertensive drugs. Fetal testing should include an ultrasound examination every 4 weeks to monitor fetal growth and amniotic fluid starting in the third trimester and nonstress testing starting at 34 to 36 weeks' gestation. The patient should be carefully monitored for the development of superimposed preeclampsia or abnormal fetal growth. The onset of either of these complications requires either hospitalization or frequent antenatal testing. Timing for delivery should be individualized according to each particular situation. Delivery is indicated at or beyond 37 weeks' gestation in those who develop either superimposed preeclampsia or abnormal fetal test result or growth, whereas pregnancy can usually continue until cervical ripening or until 41 weeks' gestation in women not requiring antihypertensive medications and who have normal fetal growth.

On the other hand, fetal and maternal morbidity and mortality are increased in pregnant women with high-risk chronic hypertension. Antihypertensive drugs are indicated in these women for long-term maternal benefit and to prevent the short-term risks of hypertensive crisis. In addition, these women require frequent prenatal evaluations (at least every 2 weeks) and may require multiple hospital admissions for the control of maternal blood pressure or for the management of associated medical disorders. Moreover, serial ultrasound examinations to monitor fetal growth and fetal testing (nonstress test and biophysical profile) should be started at 26 weeks' gestation and done more frequently than is described for the low-risk group.

Pharmacologic Treatment

The indications for and the benefits of antihypertensive drugs in the management of chronic hypertension in pregnancy remain unclear. Therefore, the decision to initiate drug therapy in a woman with chronic hypertension should take into account the severity of the hypertension, the response in maternal blood pressure during the second trimester, the potential risk of damage to target organs, and the presence or absence of pre-existing cardiovascular disease. My experience indicates that maternal blood pressure will spontaneously decrease to normotensive values during pregnancy in nearly 50% of women with mild uncomplicated chronic hypertension. In addition, the results of the largest prospective randomized trial conducted to date by me revealed no beneficial effects from antihypertensive

TABLE 2. **Drug Therapy for Hypertension in Pregnancy***

Drug	Daily Oral Dose	Indications and Comments
Methyldopa (Aldomet)	750–4000 mg in 3 or 4 divided doses	First drug of choice in chronic hypertension Safety to the fetus and long-term effects on the infant well studied
Labetalol (Normodyne, Trandate)	300–2400 mg in 3 or 4 divided doses	Second or an alternative drug in chronic hypertension Initial drug to treat severe hypertension in preeclampsia Limited data regarding long-term effects on infant
Nifedipine (Procardia)	40–120 mg in 4 divided doses	Second or an alternative drug in chronic hypertension Drug of choice to control blood pressure in severe preeclampsia both ante partum and post partum Limited data regarding long-term effects on infant
Thiazide diuretics (hydrochlorothiazide)	25–50 mg in 2 divided doses	Patients with salt-sensitive chronic hypertension and those with evidence of left ventricular diastolic dysfunction May cause plasma volume depletion To be discontinued if superimposed preeclampsia or poor fetal growth develops

*All other drugs that are used in nonpregnancy are either rarely indicated or contraindicated to treat hypertension in pregnancy.

drugs in the management of these pregnancies. It is my policy to discontinue or not to initiate antihypertensive drugs in all women with uncomplicated mild hypertension (low risk) at the time of their first prenatal visit. Only 15% of these women will subsequently require drug therapy because of exacerbated severe hypertension. Furthermore, antihypertensive drugs are continued or initiated in all women considered to have high-risk chronic hypertension and in those whose diastolic blood pressure at time of first prenatal visit is at least 105 mm Hg (Korotkoff's 5). The initial drug of choice is methyldopa because its safety during pregnancy has been documented in clinical trials and by long-term pediatric follow-up. The daily dosage and indications for drugs recommended for use during pregnancy are summarized in Table 2.

GESTATIONAL HYPERTENSION

Gestational hypertension is defined as the development of high blood pressure without other symptoms of preeclampsia after 20 weeks' gestation in a previously normotensive woman. Persistent elevation in blood pressure to at least 140/90 mm Hg on at least two separate occasions more than 4 hours apart is the hallmark for the diagnosis of this disorder. In clinical practice, the majority of women with hypertensive disorders of pregnancy fit this diagnosis. In some women, gestational hypertension may be only an early manifestation of preeclampsia, whereas in others it may be an early sign of unrecognized chronic hypertension. In general, this diagnosis is made late in the third trimester, during labor, or immediately post partum. As a result, pregnancy outcome in these women is invariably good without drug therapy. However, about 20% of these pregnancies may progress to preeclampsia and will be at slightly increased risk for fetal growth restriction (5 to 10%), abruptio placentae (0.6 to 0.8%), and eclampsia (development of convulsions, 0.1%). Thus, those who have a ripe cervix for induction (Bishop's cervical score ≥6) at 38 weeks' gestation or later should undergo induction of labor for delivery. For those remote from term (<37 weeks), management should include restricted activity with rest at home, close observation of maternal blood pressure and urine protein level, and instructions regarding symptoms of preeclampsia. Fetal evaluation with nonstress testing should begin at time of diagnosis and be repeated at weekly intervals.

PREECLAMPSIA

Preeclampsia has traditionally been defined as the occurrence of hypertension, edema, and proteinuria after 20 weeks' gestation in a previously normotensive woman. In general, preeclampsia is diagnosed in the presence of gestational hypertension plus proteinuria and/or hyperuricemia. It is classified as mild or severe primarily on the basis of the degree of elevation in blood pressure (similar to chronic hyper-

TABLE 3. **Clinical Findings Consistent with Severe Preeclampsia**

Severe hypertension plus proteinuria
Mild hypertension plus severe proteinuria (>5 gm/24 h)
Cerebral dysfunction
Persistent headaches or visual symptoms
Changes in mental status
Convulsions
Acute renal failure or oliguria
Thrombocytopenia (<1,000,000/mm³)
Documented microangiopathic hemolysis
Severe epigastric pain plus liver dysfunction
Onset of pulmonary edema

tension), the degree of proteinuria (above or below 5 grams in a 24-hour urine sample), or both. However, emphasis on either hypertension or proteinuria may minimize the clinical importance of other disturbances in various organ systems that make preeclampsia severe (Table 3).

Pathogenesis and Pathophysiology

Preeclampsia is a disorder of unknown etiology that is peculiar to human pregnancy. Many theories regarding its cause have been suggested in the past centuries, but none has withstood the test of time. One of the earliest abnormalities noted in women with preeclampsia is failure of the second wave of trophoblast invasion into the spiral arteries of the uterus. As a result of this defect in placentation, there is failure of the normal cardiovascular adaptations (increased plasma volume and reduced systemic vascular resistance) that are characteristic of normotensive pregnancies. In established preeclampsia, both cardiac output and plasma volume are reduced, whereas systemic vascular resistance is increased. These abnormalities are usually present in women with severe disease. These changes result in reduced perfusion of the placenta, kidneys, liver, and brain. In addition, endothelial dysfunction with resultant vasospasm, altered vascular permeability, activation of the coagulation systems, altered prostanoids ratio, and abnormal nitric oxide production are major pathophysiologic abnormalities.

Prevention

Prevention of preeclampsia requires knowledge of its etiology as well as the availability of methods for prediction of those at risk. Most of the available methods for prediction suffer from poor sensitivity and poor positive predictive values. As a result, most clinical trials on prevention have used patients with risk factors that increase the incidence for this disorder (Table 4). For many years, salt restriction and diuretic drugs have been used to prevent preeclampsia. The only randomized trial of a low-salt diet in pregnancy did not demonstrate such a benefit. In addition, a meta-analysis of nine randomized trials comprising more than 7000 subjects regarding the

TABLE 4. **Risk Factors for Preeclampsia**

Factor	Incidence (%)
Nulliparity	6–7
Obesity	10–15
Multifetal pregnancy	10–20
Family history of preeclampsia/eclampsia	15–25
Previous severe preeclampsia-eclampsia	20–50
Pre-existing hypertension or renal disease	15–30
Insulin-dependent diabetes mellitus	10–35
Hereditary coagulation defects	15–25
Antiphospholipid syndrome	15–20
Abnormal uterine Doppler velocimetry	15–40
Systolic/diastolic ratio >2.6	
Resistance index >0.58	
Presence of a notch	

use of diuretics in pregnancy revealed a decrease in the incidence of edema and hypertension but not in the incidence of preeclampsia. The results of a review of early studies in women at risk for preeclampsia suggested that low doses of aspirin (50 to 150 mg daily) reduced the incidence and severity of preeclampsia. However, several large multicenter and multinational randomized trials in nulliparous women and women at various degrees of risk for preeclampsia found no beneficial effects in the aspirin-treated women. In addition, a trial supported by the National Institute of Child Health and Development found no reduction in the incidence of preeclampsia with the administration of aspirin in women with chronic hypertension, multifetal gestation, previous history of preeclampsia, or insulin-dependent diabetes. At present, I do not recommend the use of aspirin for this purpose.

The results of epidemiologic studies suggested an inverse association between dietary calcium intake and the incidence of preeclampsia-eclampsia in certain populations. In addition, the results of few studies in high-risk women, a multicenter randomized trial of 1094 nulliparous women in Argentina, and a meta-analysis suggested that calcium supplementation (2 grams per day) from early in pregnancy can reduce the incidence of preeclampsia. However, the results of a large, randomized, double-blind trial in 4589 nulliparous women performed by the National Institute of Child Health and Development found no such benefit. Therefore, calcium supplementation should not be used to prevent preeclampsia.

Treatment

Early diagnosis, close medical supervision, and timely delivery are the key steps in the management of preeclampsia. The ultimate goals of treatment must always be safety of the mother first and then the delivery of a live infant who will not require intensive and prolonged neonatal care. Therefore, once the diagnosis is established, subsequent management should be based on the initial evaluation of maternal and fetal conditions. On the basis of the results of this evaluation, a decision is then made

regarding hospitalization, expectant management, or delivery. This decision should depend on one or more of the following: severity of the disease process, maternal condition and desire, gestational age, fetal status according to tests of fetal well-being, and presence of labor or rupture of membranes.

Mild Preeclampsia

Women with preeclampsia require close observation for early detection of sudden worsening of the disease process. Women with mild preeclampsia at term (≥37 weeks) should be considered for delivery, particularly if the cervix is favorable for induction or if they have labor or rupture of the membranes. Women who are remote from term can be managed expectantly provided that they receive close maternal and fetal evaluation. This evaluation should ideally be performed in the hospital if possible. However, outpatient management may be considered if compliance is expected to be good, symptoms are absent, hypertension and proteinuria are mild, and the result of fetal testing is normal. Regardless of the management strategy chosen, the woman should have evaluation of blood pressure, weight, urinary protein excretion, platelet count (two times per week), liver enzymes (two times per week), and symptoms of worsening preeclampsia, and she should be encouraged to have relative rest. In addition, the fetus should be monitored with serial ultrasound examinations for growth and quantity of amniotic fluid (every 3 weeks) and with the nonstress test (two times per week). During this management, the patient must be educated about immediate reporting of labor, vaginal bleeding, abdominal pain, and symptoms of worsening preeclampsia. If there is evidence of disease progression in either maternal or fetal conditions, hospitalization or delivery is then indicated.

The role and benefits of antihypertensive drugs in the management of mild preeclampsia are unclear. The results of 10 randomized trials revealed conflicting findings. Few of these trials revealed reduced frequency of progression to severe disease and premature delivery with drug therapy. However, the results of two large randomized trials conducted by me found no clear benefit to drug treatment in women with mild preeclampsia. Thus, I do not recommend drug therapy for these women.

Severe Preeclampsia

Severe preeclampsia may be rapidly progressive, resulting in sudden deterioration in the status of both mother and fetus; thus, prompt hospitalization is required. Prompt delivery is clearly indicated when there is imminent eclampsia, multiorgan dysfunction, or fetal distress or when fetal gestational age is 34 weeks or more. Early in gestation, however, prolongation of pregnancy with intensive monitoring at a tertiary care facility may be indicated to improve neonatal survival and reduce short-term and long-term neonatal morbidity. The benefits of this management have been documented in four studies. However, such management entails risks to both mother and fetus and thus requires extensive maternal counseling as well as daily evaluation of both maternal and fetal conditions. Women who have a sustained diastolic blood pressure of at least 110 mm Hg receive either labetalol and/or nifedipine in doses as described in Table 2. The aim of drug therapy is to keep the mean arterial pressure below 126 mm Hg (but not less than 105 mm Hg) and the diastolic pressure below 105 mm Hg (but not less than 90 mm Hg). These thresholds are important for both maternal and fetal safety.

HELLP Syndrome

Some patients with preeclampsia may develop laboratory evidence of hemolysis (H), elevated liver enzymes (EL), and low platelets (LP), characterized as the HELLP syndrome. Several of the signs, symptoms, and laboratory abnormalities that constitute this syndrome may be confused with similar findings that are usually present in a number of distinct medical and surgical disorders. This is particularly true when the manifestations develop remote from term. Diagnosis is often delayed, and management is usually complicated by inappropriate medical and surgical treatments. The typical patient is usually white and complains of epigastric or right upper quadrant pain with nausea, vomiting, diarrhea, or nonspecific viral syndrome–like symptoms. Some of the patients may complain of hematuria, bleeding from the gums, petechia or purpura, or jaundice. Hypertension or proteinuria may be slight or absent. These pregnancies are associated with substantial maternal and perinatal morbidity. Thus, the presence of this syndrome requires immediate hospitalization and consideration for delivery within 48 hours, depending on gestational age and maternal condition. These women also require close monitoring for at least 48 hours after delivery because of the risks for pulmonary edema, renal failure, and continued hemolysis and thrombocytopenia. Differential diagnosis for these women should include hemolytic-uremic syndrome, thrombotic thrombocytopenic, purpura, acute fatty liver of pregnancy, and exacerbation of lupus.

Intrapartum and Postpartum Management

Women with preeclampsia should have close observation during labor and delivery and post partum, with special attention to fluid intake and output, level of blood pressure, and cerebral symptoms. The primary objective of this management is to prevent cerebral complications (encephalopathy, convulsions, or hemorrhage), pulmonary edema, and renal failure. The threshold for treatment of blood pressure is a sustained diastolic blood pressure of 110 mm Hg or more. Other experts recommend mean arterial pressure greater than 125 mm Hg. The initial treatment of choice is hydralazine (Apresoline) given intravenously in 5- to 10-mg bolus doses to be repeated as needed every 20 minutes for up to a cumulative total of 25 to 30 mg. Alternative drugs could also include labetalol (20 to 40 mg) intravenous doses or nifedipine (10 to 20 mg) orally.

Women with preeclampsia have an increased risk for convulsions during labor. The risk is highest in women with severe preeclampsia remote from term, those with cerebral symptoms, and those with HELLP syndrome. Therefore, intravenous magnesium sulfate should be given prophylactically during labor and post partum to all women with preeclampsia. I recommend a loading dose of 6 grams for a period of 15 to 20 minutes, followed by a maintenance dose of 2 grams per hour to be administered during labor and for at least 12 hours post partum. The efficacy of magnesium sulfate in preventing and treating eclamptic convulsions has been proved in randomized trials.

Occasionally, preeclampsia may worsen after delivery or may develop for the first time within 1 week post partum. In addition, some women with the HELLP syndrome may continue to show deterioration in their laboratory findings and/or in renal function for several days post partum. Therefore, close maternal observation should continue beyond delivery. The use of invasive hemodynamic monitoring is rarely indicated in the management of women with severe preeclsia.

OBSTETRIC ANESTHESIA

method of
BRADLEY E. SMITH, M.D.
Vanderbilt University Medical Center
Nashville, Tennessee

In celebration of the 50th anniversary edition of *Conn's Current Therapy*, it is fitting to briefly review the progress of the practice of obstetric anesthesia since that first edition. In 1948, maternal mortality was approximately 15 per 10,000. Maternal mortality is now approximately 1 to 1.5 per 10,000 in the United States. Neonatal mortality was approximately 35 to 40 per 1000 live births and has now declined to well below 10 per 1000 live births in the United States. Although the forerunner of today's lumbar epidural analgesia for labor (caudle anesthesia) had been introduced by Robert Hingson in 1942, it was rarely used. "Saddle block" had only been introduced by John Adriani and John Parmley in 1946, and there was still great resistance to its use.

Inhalation anesthesia was the routine anesthetic for both vaginal and cesarean deliveries. The most frequent inhalation anesthetics were ether, ethylene, and cyclopropane, all of which were inflammable and explosive. Little wonder that aspiration of vomitus during inhalation anesthesia was the most frequent cause of maternal death due to anesthesia, and overall, anesthesia accounted for 3 to 10% of all maternal mortality. Today, inhalation anesthesia has almost disappeared in obstetrics, as have maternal deaths due to aspiration. Pain relief during prepartum labor was usually by the intramuscular route with morphine or meperidine and large doses of scopolamine. Delivery rooms were quiet because infants frequently did not cry robustly owing to the maternal sedation. Attention to the effects of maternal sedation was finally focused by Virginia Apgar in 1953 when she published her famous "Apgar score." However, the use of heavy medication and prominent use of general anesthesia continued into the 1970s and even 1980s.

Fifty years later, almost every obstetric hospital retains a qualified staff of highly skilled and trained anesthesia personnel who largely administer only regional blocks during obstetric labor. These highly trained personnel are required because regional anesthesia, despite its marvelous pain-relieving qualities, retains the potential to cause serious complications. These include maternal convulsions, total spinal block, hypotension, and rarely even paraplegia.

CHOICE OF ANESTHESIA AND ANALGESIA IN NORMAL PREGNANCIES

Pain Relief During Labor

Psychologic Management of Labor Pain

Grantly Dick Read had published his famous treatise entitled "Childbirth Without Fear" only 6 years before the first *Conn's Current Therapy*. His methods, along with related techniques such as natural childbirth, psychoprophylaxis, Lamaze, and medical hypnosis, were slow to gain popularity. Even today, psychologic preparation for labor is a great benefit to most pregnant patients and should not be neglected even when use of continuous epidural analgesia techniques is anticipated. Psychologic support helps the mother relax and better endure the discomfort and reduces the total quantity of necessary sedatives and pain relievers.

Sedative and Narcotic Management of Labor Pain

Heavy prepartum use of narcotic and sedative drugs has almost entirely disappeared from American obstetric practice owing to recognition of their detrimental effects on the infant. However, some centers still use small intravenous doses of these drugs in the prepartum period for reassurance and comfort. A popular method is the use of fentanyl (Sublimaze) 25 μg given intravenously by patient-controlled analgesia (PCA) pumps, with a 10-minute block out. Some use 6.25 mg of meperidine (Demerol) by the same method, and yet others may add 0.5 mg diazepam (Valium) at 1-hour intervals. Newborn respiratory depression may develop when these drugs are used.

Paracervical Block

Paracervical block, properly administered, delivers major pain relief during cervical dilatation and descent of the head, particularly in multiparous women. When used along with pudendal block, it may be sufficient pain relief for spontaneous or outlet forceps delivery. It is established by infiltration of approximately 10 mL of 1% lidocaine (Xylocaine) in the submucosal tissue of the cervix at 4 and 8 o'clock positions, with a delay between the injections. Careful fetal heart rate monitoring should be carried out during and immediately after each injection. A fetal heart rate of less than 100 along with fetal acidosis can develop immediately after this block. It is recommended that the block be abandoned immediately if fetal bradycardia develops. If fetal bradycardia does develop, alert, expectant waiting will usually be rewarded by return of the fetal heart rate to normal, but persistence of fetal bradycardia may indicate fetal deterioration or imminent fetal demise. However, the incidence of this serious complication is low. The use of bupivacaine (Marcaine) for this block has ceased in many centers because of suggestions that it may cause a higher incidence of fetal bradycardia.

Continuous Lumbar Epidural Analgesia During Labor

The general trend has been toward reduction in concentration of the local anesthetic used in this block. The addition of small doses of opioids in the epidural space improves pain relief and allows such small concentrations of local anesthetic to be used that little or no voluntary muscle paralysis occurs. There is some suggestion that epidural analgesia may slow labor, cause maternal fever, or increase the incidence of forceps or cesarean delivery. Nonetheless, epidural analgesia remains popular because it is effective.

Technique. A large epidural needle is inserted into the epidural space by any of a variety of techniques. A thin plastic catheter is then advanced about 3 cm beyond the needle tip. Immediately, a test to determine whether the catheter tip is epidural, intrathecal, or intravascular is carried out by injection of 3 mL of 1.5% lidocaine with 1:100,000 epinephrine. Signs of excitement, convulsions, respiratory impairment, or tachycardia may indicate intravascular placement, whereas the rapid onset of muscle weakness may indicate intrathecal placement. In the absence of these signs, an initial dose of local anesthetic can be given. One of several acceptable medication schemes is the use of a mixture of 8 to 10 mL of 0.25% bupivacaine and 5 μg per mL of sufentanil (Sufenta). Analgesia can usually be maintained with an infusion of 10 to 14 mL per hour of 0.125% bupivacaine with 5 μg per mL of sufentanil. Bolus doses of up to 4 mL each may be needed if the analgesic level is inadequate.

Combined Spinal-Epidural Analgesia During Labor

Combined spinal-epidural (CSE) analgesia is rapidly superseding the older epidural analgesia techniques for labor. In this method, "spinal" injection of opioids and local anesthesia combined with epidural analgesia vastly relieves early labor pain almost immediately and usually allows the laboring woman to walk about if she chooses.

Technique. CSE analgesia is also sometimes called the "double-needle technique." An epidural needle is initially inserted into the epidural space, followed by placement of a second thin intrathecal needle placed through the first needle. With the patient in the sitting position, many experts inject 10 μg of sufentanil or 25 μg of fentanyl along with 2.5 mg of bupivacaine and 0.2 mg of epinephrine diluted with preservative-free saline to a total volume of 2 to 3 mL of solution.

Anesthesia During Vaginal Delivery

Pudendal Block for Vaginal Delivery

Pudendal block is a useful option, particularly in multiparous women, to establish surgical anesthesia of the perineum. It has no effect on the course of labor and is administered by the obstetrician at the time of birth. Many women may be comfortable during episiotomy, vacuum extraction of the fetus, or even outlet forceps delivery. It is executed by placing 10 mL of 1% lidocaine on each pudendal nerve at the origin of the sacrosciatic ligament. Complications are possible with inadvertent administration of as little as 3 mL of 1% lidocaine into a vein or into a highly vascular area or 300 mg in the less vascular tissues.

Spinal Anesthesia (Saddle Block) for Vaginal Delivery

In the primiparous patient, saddle block anesthesia is usually administered when the infant's head is at about +2 to 3 station late in second stage, but it may be established earlier in the multiparous patient. Hypotension occurs in approximately 18% of patients who receive saddle block anesthetics, so blood pressure should be monitored carefully. Saddle block provides complete pain relief and pelvic relaxation for low forceps and midforceps delivery and fetal rotation or perineal surgery virtually without pain for the mother and does not affect uterine contractions.

Technique. After subarachnoid puncture with the smallest possible needle (25 to 27 gauge) (many now prefer the Sprotte design to avoid spinal headaches), a dose of about 0.5 mL of 0.75% bupivacaine in dextrose, diluted to 1.5 to 2 mL with cerebrospinal fluid, should produce anesthesia to about T-10, if the patient sits erect about 30 seconds after the injection. Some controversy has arisen of late concerning an alleged elevated incidence of radicular pain in the legs associated with the use of 5% lidocaine for this purpose. If lidocaine is to be used because of its more rapid onset, 0.8 to 1 mL (40 to 50 mg) of 5% lidocaine may be diluted to 3 mL with preservative-free 5% glucose.

Inhalation Analgesia for Vaginal Delivery

Inhalation of anesthetic vapors in concentrations too low to produce surgical anesthesia can be a safe and simple form of effective analgesia for vaginal delivery. This technique can allow the mother to remain conversant, alert, and cooperative and self-controlled without danger to the infant. Constant inhalation of 40 to 50% nitrous oxide and oxygen, 0.25 to 0.4% isoflurane (Forane), or 1 to 1.5% sevoflurane (Ultane) is effective in producing analgesia and am-

nesia in approximately 75% of patients. All of these agents demonstrate essentially no effects on the fetus at these low-dose concentrations.

General Anesthesia for Vaginal Delivery

General anesthesia is now almost never used in vaginal delivery except under special circumstances. When it is needed, the dose, depth, and duration of anesthesia before delivery should be minimized. Mixing of all intravenous and inhalational anesthetics with the fetal blood begins almost immediately after administration. Induction of general anesthesia (not "inhalation analgesia") usually calls for endotracheal intubation to avoid aspiration of gastric contents or loss of patency of the airway.

INHALATION ANESTHETIC AGENTS

These anesthetics pass the placenta immediately, and in anesthetic concentrations they can all produce significant respiratory and neurologic depression in the newborn. All but nitrous oxide can lead to postpartum uterine bleeding. Although they are of great help in certain obstetric complications (e.g., tetanic uterine contractions), their routine obstetric use is not recommended because of their ability to "make the infant sleepy." Inhalation of sevoflurane 4 to 6% in 100% oxygen, with reduction to 3 to 4% when stable anesthesia is reached, can result in surgical anesthesia in about 3 to 4 minutes but includes a danger of aspiration. More frequently, intravenous induction, a muscle paralysant, and endotracheal intubation are to be preferred.

THIOPENTAL

Thiopental may cause depression of newborn breathing. A dose of 3.5 mg of thiopental (Pentothal) per kg intravenously is commonly used. The shortest interval practical between induction and delivery of the infant is safest for the infant. High-risk or premature infants are even more susceptible to respiratory depression of the newborn.

KETAMINE

Although much slower in onset, intravenous ketamine (Ketalar) in small doses (up to 0.75 mg per kg) is recognized as a safe alternative to thiopental for induction in obstetrics. Both immediate newborn alertness and delayed newborn alertness appear better than with thiopental, and the blood pressure of both mother and newborn are better supported. However, neurologic complications and respiratory depression may be caused by ketamine doses greater than 0.75 mg per kg. Rare hallucinations may occur during emergence from ketamine, but they can be prevented or treated by 2 mg of intravenous diazepam.

PROPOFOL

This new induction agent is notable for its antinausea qualities and prompt, pleasant emergence. For either vaginal or cesarean delivery, induction with 1.5 to 2.5 mg of propofol (Diprivan) per kg intravenously is pleasant, appears to suppress hypertension due to endotracheal intubation, and is no more depressant on the fetus than thiopental.

Anesthesia During Cesarean Section

Major regional analgesia is favored for cesarean section today. The mother is alert and able to participate in and remember the birth, and serious respiratory depression of the infant caused by anesthetics, narcotics, and sedatives is avoided.

Technique of Epidural Block for Cesarean Section

After an infusion is started with a large intravenous catheter, 800 to 1500 mL of intravenous lactated Ringer's solution without dextrose (to avoid responsive neonatal hypoglycemia) is administered to help prevent hypotension. The epidural catheter is placed and tested for safety as outlined earlier. After the test dose, medication for cesarean section under epidural block could include 15 to 22 mL of bupivacaine 0.5% mixed with 100 μg of fentanyl, or 4 mg of morphine, administered in three divided doses. Later, if discomfort develops, 75% of the original dose of the same solution may be added about every hour, provided that a pinprick test verifies a safe block level. If some discomfort persists, intravenous analgesics and tranquilizers may be used in reduced doses.

Ketamine in doses of 5 to 10 mg intravenously is used by many experts as a supplemental analgesic-sedative during surgery, and it does not depress respiration in these small doses. However, narcotics and benzodiazepines synergize their respiratory depressant effects when used together, particularly during high regional block analgesia, and therefore extreme alertness for respiratory depression of the mother should always be exercised. Fentanyl in 25-μg intravenous boluses with midazolam (Versed) in 0.5-mg boluses is a common combination.

Technique of Spinal Anesthesia for Cesarean Section

Bupivacaine 0.75% in doses of 8 to 13 mg along with 20 μg of fentanyl or 0.2 mg of "spinal morphine" (Duramorph) mixed with 0.2 mL of 1:1000 fresh epinephrine is often used for subarachnoid block for cesarean section. After injection, the patient is placed supine with her head on a pillow, and the table is tilted 15 degrees to the left. A pillow, balloon, or wedge is placed under the right hip to displace the uterus away from the vena cava and aorta. Arterial blood pressure is monitored at least every 60 seconds. If the systolic pressure falls 30% below the preanesthesia level or below 100 mm Hg, the left uterine displacement is increased, the Trendelenburg position is steepened, the rate of intravenous infusion is increased, oxygen by face mask is administered, and 12.5 mg of ephedrine or 0.5 to 1 μg of phenylephrine per kg may be used.

Technique of General Anesthesia for Cesarean Section

Before anesthesia is induced, neutralization of acid stomach contents with 30 mL of oral sodium bicitrate (Bicitra) is useful. Some also administer 150 mg of intravenous ranitidine (Zantac) and/or 10 mg of intravenous metoclopramide (Reglan) to reduce production of stomach acid and to promote expulsion of acid into the duodenum. The dangers of aortocaval compression are present during general as well as regional anesthesia. The patient is placed on the operating table in left lateral recumbent position until the start of the skin preparation, then elevated to the left on a pillow, or the uterus should be manually deflected to the left during cesarean section under general as well as regional anesthesia.

Premedication is usually omitted because of its effect on the infant. An intravenous infusion is started with use of a large catheter. During "prepping," the patient is preoxygenated for 3 minutes. When the surgeon is ready, 0.6 mg of scopolamine (for amnesia and protection against vagal cardiovascular reflexes) and 0.3 mg of pancuronium are given about 3 minutes before induction followed by thiopental, 3.5 mg per kg, or ketamine, 0.75 mg per kg. After unconsciousness, intravenous succinylcholine (Anectine) 2 mg per kg followed by a continuous drip of 0.2% succinylcholine is added. Cricoid pressure should be instituted and maintained by someone other than the anesthetist as soon as consciousness is impaired. The trachea is intubated and ventilation is checked in both lungs with a stethoscope before the incision is permitted.

Even these limited doses of drugs may result in reduction of alertness or depression of the respirations of the newborn, and therefore preparations for newborn resuscitation should be made in advance. After tracheal intubation, many elect to administer only nitrous oxide 4 liters per minute and oxygen 4 liters per minute until the cord is clamped. In this case, the level of anesthesia can be deepened with thiopental and/or narcotics and/or potent inhalation agents immediately when the cord is clamped. The continuing use of succinylcholine drip (or pancuronium) should be monitored with a nerve block stimulator. Some experts advocate addition of a small dose of fentanyl, sufentanil, or alfentanil (Alfenta) and/or a limited concentration of a potent inhalation anesthetic agent before birth of the infant to reduce maternal stress response and the possibility of memory. However, the possibility of respiratory depression in the newborn after administration of these drugs cannot be disregarded.

POSTPARTUM PAIN CONTROL

Control of Postpartum Pain After Vaginal Delivery

The intensity of pain in the postpartum period after vaginal delivery is rarely as severe as in cesarean section. A variety of oral analgesic agents are commonly employed for this purpose (see later), and rarely, a few doses of common parenteral opioid agents are used. Oral and parenteral opioids or even milder oral analgesics such as oxycodone 5 mg and acetaminophen 325 mg orally (Percocet) every 6 hours, often in conjunction with antiprostaglandins (e.g., ibuprofen [Motrin] 400 mg orally every 6 hours), have become standard in treating this type of pain. Research has shown many deficiencies in this method, including "peaks and valleys" in the intensity of pain due to the varying blood levels achieved by intermittent intramuscular injection. On the other hand, this method is by far the least costly of all those that are described here and may be expedient and sufficient in many patients. In the occasional patient with a large episiotomy or perineal lacerations, it may be anticipated that the pain will be severe enough to warrant use of techniques described in conjunction with cesarean section.

Patient-Controlled Analgesia After Cesarean Section

Although the concept of PCA is more than 25 years old, its popularity has surged in the past few years. Numerous studies verify that eliminating the peaks and valleys of analgesia along with the undefinable psychologic comfort of knowing that the patient can instantly treat her own pain clearly results in overall administration of a lesser total dose of analgesic agent over any given time. Although many narcotics are in use for PCA, a typical basic plan for PCA might be an initial intravenous bolus of 2 mg of morphine followed by patient-controlled injections of 1 mg of morphine on demand no more frequently than every 10 minutes with a maximal total dose of 20 mg in any 4 hours. Unexpected apnea from the respiratory depressant effects of the opioids has been reported, but it is not as frequent as after intrathecal or epidural use of opioids. This should be anticipated by standing orders for stat intravenous injection of 200 μg of naloxone (Narcan) if the nurse suspects respiratory depression.

CHOICE OF ANESTHESIA AND ANALGESIA IN COMPLICATED PREGNANCIES

Forceps

Forceps are rarely used in modern obstetrics but still have some indications. During the use of forceps or vacuum extraction devices, a relaxed perineum and a quiet patient aid in preventing maternal vaginal lacerations and extension of the episiotomy and help minimize trauma to the infant's head. These conditions are provided by spinal and epidural blocks, which also allow the mother to participate in the birth.

Breech Presentation

Many experts advocate epidural analgesia for vaginal breech births. An alternative choice consists of

good psychic support supplemented by minimal narcotics and tranquilizers, a paracervical block in the first stage, and a quick induction of general endotracheal anesthesia, including succinylcholine, when the infant's umbilicus becomes visible.

Multiple Births

The second infant may be delivered under pudendal or local anesthesia in some cases. If the second infant is to be delivered by means of version and breech extraction, endotracheal general inhalation anesthesia may be used to relax the uterus, in which case preparations for active resuscitation of the infant should be made in advance.

Tetanic Contractions

Regional anesthesia does not relax the uterus. The older standard method of rapid relaxation of the uterus during tetanic contractions required endotracheal inhalation anesthesia. A new faster anesthetic, sevoflurane, at 3 to 4% is preferable to halothane (Fluothane), which may cause hypotension, or isoflurane, which is slower and may also cause hypotension. Intravenous "beta-stimulator" catecholamines do not work as completely or as rapidly. Intravenous nitroglycerin (in 100- to 300-μg boluses) may relax the uterus but often causes dangerous maternal hypotension.

Fetal Distress

When fetal distress exists, further depression of the newborn by potent anesthetics given to the mother should be avoided. Some experts advocate spinal anesthesia in fetal distress, but if it is used, no time should be wasted, nor should hypotension be tolerated.

Antepartum Hemorrhage

Sudden antepartum bleeding leading to maternal hypotension is detrimental to the fetus, and hypovolemia adds risk to the mother from anesthesia of any type. All forms of major regional block are frequently contraindicated in this emergency, because the resulting sudden sympathetic blockade paralyzes the compensatory mechanisms ordinarily required to maintain the mother's blood pressure during hemorrhage. Management by local anesthesia, pudendal block, or subanesthetic inhalation analgesia is recommended when applicable, but with all choices, maternal vascular volume should be restored as rapidly as possible with an appropriate fluid. Vasopressors should *not* be used in place of adequate volume replacement. Potent inhalation anesthetics are avoided because they may accentuate the hypotension caused by hypovolemia.

Pregnancy-Induced Hypertension (Toxemia of Pregnancy)

In a toxemic pregnancy, maternal liver and kidney function may be poor, convulsions may be encountered, severe maternal hypertension and increased sensitivity to vasopressors frequently exist, and the infant is often born prematurely and is undernourished. Some obstetricians still believe that hypotension develops more easily during epidural analgesia. Care should be taken to evaluate and correct the hypovolemia frequently seen in toxemia before any regional block is placed. In managing general anesthesia during toxemia, efforts to attenuate the hypertensive response to endotracheal intubation are important. For this, nitroglycerin 100 to 300 μg by intravenous bolus is sometimes used. Intravenous magnesium sulfate synergizes with anesthetic muscle relaxants and may contribute to newborn drug depression.

Prematurity

In premature newborns, respiratory and cardiovascular depression can result from pain or anesthetic drugs given to the mother. Continuous epidural analgesia is the method of choice during the first and second stages of labor. Saddle block is excellent for delivery but is not suitable for labor. Pudendal block is not dangerous in prematurity but does not relax the birth canal sufficiently to minimize head trauma to the premature infant.

Diabetes

Major regional analgesia is desirable when practical. Insulin and glucose control should be meticulous and should be monitored frequently during labor and the induction of anesthesia. Most experts restrict maternal intravenous glucose, which may stimulate insulin release by the infant, leading to hypoglycemia.

Cardiac Disease

Less than 2% of pregnant patients suffer from severe heart disease, which is less than half the incidence noted 40 years ago, but an increasing proportion of pregnant cardiac patients today suffer from complicated congenital heart defects. Continuous epidural analgesia is popular for patients with a wide variety of acquired or congenital heart lesions. Great caution should be exercised in regard to the potential of regional anesthesia to precipitate heart failure or intracardiac reversal of shunt by causing a sudden decrease in peripheral systemic resistance. There should be continuing consultation with the cardiologist.

Sickle Cell Disease

Sickle cell disease remains a grave threat to women with the SS hemoglobin configuration and to their infants. Although stasis in the peripheral vascular bed and possible coagulation problems at the needle site have been theoretical objections to the use of major regional analgesia in sickle cell disease, no objective evidence has ever been offered to support these theories. Inhalation anesthesia has not been followed by sickle cell crisis, and there are reports that it may protect against sickling for several hours.

COMPLICATIONS OF ANESTHESIA
Airway Obstruction

Less than 20 years ago, 11 obstetric patients were reported to have died in New York City in one 2-year period because of failure to achieve and maintain ventilation of the lungs during induction of general anesthesia for obstetric delivery. Before induction of general anesthesia, it is essential that the obstetrician and the anesthetist agree on the steps to be taken should intubation of the trachea prove impossible. These will vary according to the condition of the mother and the infant. This "failed intubation" protocol should be instituted skillfully.

Aspiration of Gastric Contents

Aspiration of stomach contents is a major hazard during heavy sedation, under general anesthesia, or even under major regional anesthesia. Until recently, reports from Great Britain demonstrated that 35% of all anesthetic-related obstetric deaths were directly caused by inhalation of stomach contents. However, aspiration of gastric contents is now reported to be fatal in less than 10% of aspirations by obstetric patients in reporting university hospitals. Treatment of aspiration pneumonia should be based on the principles of immediate establishment of airway and ventilation, suppression of transudation by positive end-expiratory intratracheal pressure, and careful monitoring for inadequate ventilation or the delayed development of bacterial pneumonia. Although steroid therapy after aspiration into the trachea has been advocated by many, evidence from animal research indicates that it is ineffective. The combination of ranitidine (Zantac) 150 mg and metoclopramide (Reglan) 10 mg given orally 90 minutes before surgery as prophylaxis against acid aspiration is helpful.

COMPLICATIONS OF SPINAL AND EPIDURAL ANESTHESIA
Hypotension and Circulatory Failure During Spinal or Epidural Anesthesia

Hypotension and circulatory failure may account for 34% of all maternal deaths due to anesthesia and are also a hazard to the fetus. The most frequent cause of maternal death is the aortocaval compression syndrome complicated by blockade of the sympathetic nervous system incidental to spinal or epidural anesthesia. This syndrome can be diagnosed by the presence of hypotension, dyspnea, and acute apprehension, often with tachycardia. It is treated by lifting the uterus to the left or placing the patient on her left side or tilting the patient to the left with a pillow. Further treatment of hypotension includes position change, vigorous fluid infusion, and, if necessary, a bolus injection of intravenous ephedrine 12.5 mg, or phenylephrine 0.5 to 1 μg per kg.

Seizures due to Local Anesthetics During Epidural Anesthesia

Convulsions due to local anesthetic drugs may account for about 11% of all disastrous complications of regional anesthesia. Unexpected neurologic events ranging from disorientation to tonic-clonic convulsions after the injection of a local anesthetic drug should be assumed to be due to the local anesthetic until proved otherwise, even in pregnant patients. Local anesthetic-induced convulsions are rarely due to allergy but most often result from elevated blood concentrations of the local anesthetic. Subarachnoid (spinal) anesthesia almost never results in convulsions because of the small dose of local anesthetic. With prompt therapy, lidocaine-induced convulsions have relatively benign neurologic and cardiovascular sequelae; however, seizures due to bupivacaine are much more ominous for cardiovascular collapse. Emergency treatment of local anesthetic convulsions consists of skillful support of cardiovascular function and prompt ventilation. The injection of a small bolus dose (100 mg of thiopental or 5 mg of diazepam) intravenously along with succinylcholine 40 to 80 mg followed by intermittent positive-pressure breathing is useful.

Subarachnoid Instillation of Local Anesthetic ("Total Spinal")

Unintended total spinal anesthesia is still a frequent problem during both intended spinal and epidural anesthesia and may occur in as many as 1 in every 1000 attempted epidural blocks. The epidural catheter can "migrate" into the subdural space from the epidural space some hours after original institution of the block, leading to a total spinal after a reinjection. When this occurs during establishment of spinal block, the duration of both respiratory and cardiovascular embarrassment can be expected to be relatively shorter than the planned duration of the intended subarachnoid block. Total spinal anesthesia resulting from subarachnoid injection of local anesthetic that was intended for the epidural space is a greater emergency because the dose of local anesthetic injected is usually much greater than is used for intentional spinal anesthesia. Patients experiencing this unfortunate situation should be adequately sedated immediately until the complete return of spontaneous vital functions. Respiratory and cardiovascular support usually prevents the otherwise fatal outcome of this complication.

Inadvertent Dural Puncture During Attempted Epidural Block

Even a skilled anesthetist may puncture the dura in up to 0.5 to 2% of attempts. A second attempt at an epidural in an adjacent interspace is routine in this event, but extreme care should be taken to administer and observe test doses at every subsequent injection into the epidural catheter. Because postpartum headaches occur in 25 to 75% of patients who have experienced inadvertent dural puncture by the epidural needle, immediate precautions against headache may be desirable. Immediate postpartum instillation of large volumes (up to 60 mL) of normal saline has been 75% successful in preventing headache. Persistent spinal headaches are usually eliminated by injections of autologous blood (10 mL) in the epidural space no sooner than the third postpartum day.

Hazards of Obstetric Anesthesia to the Newborn

Three main factors may contribute to anesthesia-related morbidity in newborns: (1) sedatives, analgesics, and anesthetics administered to the mother during labor; (2) trauma of labor and delivery; and (3) asphyxia due to impaired exchange of respiratory gases during labor and delivery. Obstetric factors such as toxins from amnionitis, muscle depression due to magnesium sulfate, and other factors cannot be disregarded. A newborn is more susceptible than an adult to anesthetic overdose because the undeveloped brain is more susceptible to these drugs. Modern practice attempts to minimize the use of prepartum sedatives by encouraging the use of psychologic techniques such as prepared childbirth, regional analgesia techniques, and concurrent use of synergistic but less depressant drugs.

POSTPARTUM CARE

method of
ALEXANDER A. REITER, M.D.
Baylor College of Medicine
Houston, Texas

The postpartum period or puerperium, or the so-called fourth trimester of pregnancy, begins after the delivery of the newborn and the placenta and empirically ends 6 weeks afterward.

At that time, most of the anatomic and physiologic changes that occurred during the pregnancy have reversed. The uterine involution is completed and ovulation may occur, especially in non–breast-feeding mothers. The hematologic, immunologic, and biochemical parameters return to the prepregnancy values. Some of the most dreadful obstetric complications, such as hemorrhage, eclamptic seizures, thromboembolic phenomena, and severe infections, may occur during the postpartum period. Immediate recognition and appropriate management of these complications are essential for intact maternal survival.

IMMEDIATE POSTPARTUM PERIOD

This is usually defined as the first 24 to 48 hours after the delivery and overlaps with the period of hospitalization.

Postpartum Hemorrhage

During the first 1 or 2 hours after the delivery, the vital signs are monitored every 30 minutes and the degree of vaginal bleeding is carefully assessed. Bleeding in excess of 500 mL in the first 12 hours after the delivery is considered abnormal. This is difficult to quantitate, however, and the diagnosis of postpartum hemorrhage is based on maternal hemodynamic changes, such as falling hemoglobin and hematocrit values, and the subjective assessment of the bleeding. The incidence of this complication is about 4%, and it accounts for about 10% of the non–abortion-related maternal mortality in the United States. Causes of postpartum hemorrhage include (1) uterine atony in about 50% of cases; (2) birth canal trauma in 20% of cases; (3) uterine rupture, uterine inversion from excessive umbilical cord traction, and placenta previa in 20% of cases; and (4) retained products of conception and coagulopathies in 10% of cases.

Aggressive management of postpartum hemorrhage is critical in limiting significant morbidity and decreasing the maternal mortality rates. Large-bore intravenous lines should be started immediately while blood products are made available. Clotting studies and baseline hemoglobin and hematocrit values are obtained; the patient's vital signs and urinary output are frequently monitored. The birth canal should be methodically inspected, and any source of bleeding should be repaired. If the source of bleeding is not identified, hemostatic sutures are applied over the entire bleeding area.

Birth canal hematomas can enlarge rapidly, causing intense pain (never to be overlooked in this situation) and significant hemodynamic changes that are disproportional to the amount of external bleeding. If atony is suspected, the uterus is externally massaged and pharmacologic agents that increase the uterine tonus are administered. (1) Oxytocin is usually administered intravenously at a concentration of 10 to 20 units in 1000 mL of a crystalloid solution, at a rate of about 200 mL per hour. Intravenous bolus administration of oxytocin should be avoided because it can cause hypotension and cardiac arrhythmia. (2) Ergot preparations, such as ergonovine maleate (Ergotrate) or methylergonovine (Methergine) 0.2 mg, can be administered intramuscularly in patients who do not respond to oxytocin. Ergot drugs cause more sustained uterine contractions that can last for several hours. They can cause hypertension and therefore are not used in patients with cardiac disease or high blood pressure. (3) Prostaglandin 15-methyl $F_{2\alpha}$ (Hemabate) 250 μg can be given intramuscularly every 30 to 60 minutes.

Surgical intervention is indicated when there is an anatomic uterine defect or if atony cannot be pharmacologically controlled. In this last case, the first step should be the postpartum curettage, meant to remove remnant products of conception. I recommend that this procedure be done under continuous ultrasound guidance (if available) to reduce the risk for uterine perforation. Radiographic embolization of the bleeding vessels or laparotomy with uterine and hypogastric artery ligation and hysterectomy are occasionally indicated in the most difficult cases of postpartum hemorrhage.

Infection

Puerperal febrile morbidity is usually defined as a temperature of 38°C or greater on two separate occasions, at least 4 hours apart, usually excluding the first 24 hours after delivery. Infectious causes of febrile morbidity include urinary tract infection, endometritis, parametritis, and thrombophlebitis. Other infections, such as wound infection, infected hematoma, pelvic cellulitis, and septic pelvic thrombophlebitis, develop later and are more common after cesarean section than after vaginal delivery. The diagnosis is made by careful physical examination, laboratory studies such as white blood cell count, blood cultures, urinary cultures, and transcervical cultures of the endometrial cavity. This last one is recommended if there is poor response to the initial empirical antimicrobial therapy.

Uterine infections are usually polymicrobial, involving both gram-positive and gram-negative aerobes and anaerobes. For this reason, one of the most common antimicrobial regimens includes ampicillin 2 grams every 6 hours and gentamicin 80 to 100 mg every 8 hours, titrated to peak and trough levels. Clindamycin 900 mg every 8 hours is occasionally added, especially if anaerobic infection is suspected.

Monotherapy with a broad-spectrum penicillin-like or cephalosporin-like agent has been shown to be effective in most of the cases. Parenteral therapy is usually continued for 24 hours after the patient is afebrile. Infected wounds or episiotomies need to be explored and drained. If pelvic thrombophlebitis is suspected, full heparinization should be initiated and continued for 7 to 10 days.

Excessive breast engorgement can occasionally cause *noninfectious* febrile morbidity that will usually respond to local ice packs, intense milk expression, and antipyretic analgesia.

Bladder Dysfunction

Urinary retention with bladder overdistention and inability to void spontaneously is a common complication of the early postpartum period.

This occurs because of two reasons: (1) the bladder's sensation and its capability to contract spontaneously are diminished by conduction anesthesia and by painful lesions in the genital tract, especially in the periurethral area; (2) the rate of accumulation of urine in the bladder after delivery is significantly increased by the mobilization of extracellular fluids accumulated during pregnancy and by the diuresis of the large volumes of intravenous fluids infused during labor.

If unable to void spontaneously, the parturient should be straight catheterized and the residual volume measured.

A Foley catheter should be left in place for 48 to 72 hours if serial catheterizations become necessary.

In the rare case that bladder function does not resume after 72 hours, the Foley catheter should be left in place for an additional period of 3 to 4 days.

Episiotomy

During the first few days after the delivery, the parturient may experience pain related to the episiotomy. This usually responds well to mild analgesics. Uncomplicated episiotomy usually heals within 2 to 4 weeks.

Extensive episiotomies, especially if complicated by laceration of the rectal sphincter, are usually more painful, and stronger analgesics and stool softeners are indicated. Ice packs to the perineum help reduce the edema and the discomfort during the first 24 hours after episiotomy repair. The perineum needs to be cleaned "front to back" and kept dry to facilitate the healing process.

Intense, prolonged perineal pain unresponsive to analgesics needs to be carefully evaluated for the possibility of hematoma or infection and abscess. Hemorrhoids (especially if thrombosed) can be another source of intense perineal pain.

Afterbirth Pain

The abdominal pain associated with the physiologic uterine contractions is usually more intense during breast-feeding. It can be treated with mild analgesics because it decreases in intensity by the third or fourth postpartum day. Significant, persistent lower abdominal pain, especially if it is associated with fever, suggests the possibility of endometritis or urinary tract infection.

Lactation

By the second postpartum day, a modest amount of colostrum can be expressed from the nipples. Colostrum is rich in proteins and minerals and has less sugar and fat than the milk. The major components of milk are proteins, lactose, water, and fat. Within 3 to 4 days from the delivery, the breasts can become engorged and cause discomfort. A well-managed breast-feeding program, such as every 3 hours alternating sides, should be enough to resolve the engorgement. If engorgement is associated with fever and localized redness and induration, mastitis needs to be considered and treated promptly with an antistaphylococcal agent.

Breast-feeding should be encouraged for the benefit of mother-child bonding and to satisfy most of the infant's initial nutritional needs. If suppression of lactation is desired, it can be achieved by applying breast binders and ice packs, using mild analgesics, and avoiding nipple stimulation. Bromocriptine (Parlodel), a dopamine-receptor agonist that was extensively used in the past, is no longer recommended for lactation suppression because of increased risk for maternal cerebrovascular accidents.

LATE POSTPARTUM PERIOD

This is arbitrarily defined as the time between the patient's discharge from the hospital and the 6 weeks postpartum visit.

Hospital Discharge

In the past, parturients were kept in the hospital for 3 days if they were primipara and for 2 days if multipara. Cesarean section patients were usually hospitalized for 4 to 5 days. Many patients are now routinely discharged 24 hours after vaginal delivery and 72 hours after cesarean section. However, the recommendation of the American College of Obstetricians and Gynecologists for 2 days of postpartum hospitalization has been made into law in some states and will probably be universally accepted. Early discharge from the hospital should be allowed only after the vaginal bleeding is carefully evaluated and the hematocrit is found to be stable. Other laboratory tests to be assessed before the discharge include the Rh factor (anti-Rh prophylaxis must be administered in the appropriate cases) and the rubella immune status so that rubella vaccine can be administered in susceptible cases.

Prenatal vitamins are recommended for another 4 to 6 weeks. Iron supplements are offered to iron-deficient, anemic patients.

Late Hemorrhage

Within 2 or 3 days after delivery, the decidua remaining in the uterus becomes differentiated into two layers. The superficial one becomes necrotic and is sloughed in the lochia. The basal layer, adjacent to the myometrium, which contains the fundi of endometrial glands, remains intact and is the source of new endometrium. The process of endometrial regeneration takes about 7 to 10 days, except at the placental site, where it is completely restored after about 6 weeks.

The vaginal bleeding (lochia rubra) decreases during the first 3 to 4 postpartum days and becomes pale and thinner (lochia serosa) between days 3 and 10. Then, it becomes thicker and white-yellow (lochia alba, because leukocytes replace erythrocytes), and this persists for about 3 to 5 weeks.

Abnormal vaginal bleeding late in the puerperium can be caused by retention of placental fragments or by subinvolution at the placental site (the formation of endometrium is defective). The first approach to control the bleeding should be medically directed, using either methylergonovine or prostaglandins as previously described. If the bleeding is not controlled by these means, surgical curettage is indicated.

Depression

Postpartum "blues" with symptoms such as anxiety, insomnia, irritability, loss of appetite, or fatigue can occur in up to 70% of the parturients. However, most of those symptoms resolve spontaneously within 10 to 15 days. In other cases, they resolve only after encouraging family support, rest, and occasional counseling.

More severe cases, especially those associated with previous psychologic problems, may necessitate psychiatric counseling and antidepressant or antipsychotic medications.

Activity

Normal physical activity can be resumed a couple of days after routine vaginal delivery and about 4 weeks after uncomplicated cesarean section. Sexual activity may be resumed when the bleeding has subsided, the birth canal lacerations have healed, and the perineum is comfortable. The libido is diminished in the postpartum period, however, most women return to their usual level of energy by 6 weeks post partum.

Contraception

Ovulation can occur at about 4 weeks after delivery in nonlactating women. Breast-feeding can delay the onset of ovulation but is a poor contraceptive choice. Combination oral contraceptive pills may be started as early as 2 to 3 weeks after delivery in both lactating and nonlactating women. An intrauterine contraceptive device can be inserted in selected patients after their first menses. Barrier contraception is a good alternative because of its ease of use and the additional protection against sexually transmitted diseases.

RESUSCITATION OF THE NEWBORN

method of
ALFRED L. GEST, M.D.
Baylor College of Medicine
Houston, Texas

As a preface to discussing neonatal resuscitation, I strongly encourage anyone involved with delivery room care of the newborn to take the provider portion of the Neonatal Resuscitation Program sponsored by the American Academy of Pediatrics and the American Heart Association. One of the goals of this program is to have at least one person skilled in neonatal resuscitation in attendance at every delivery, and an additional skilled person readily available, with the intent of improving perinatal morbidity and mortality. Although it may not be possible to prove that this program is achieving its intended purpose, it does present a logical, coordinated approach to neonatal resuscitation, and as such, I highly recommend it.

At birth, the newborn must make rapid cardiopulmonary adaptation for the transition from intrauterine to extrauterine life. An effective neonatal resuscitation ensures the accomplishment of a successful transition to postnatal life.

In utero, the placenta is the organ of respiration and the lungs are filled with fluid. Because the lung does not function to oxygenate the blood in utero, oxygenated blood from the placenta via the umbilical vein traverses the ductus venosus, enters the inferior vena cava, and empties into the right atrium. This blood is then shunted through the foramen ovale into the left side of the heart, which in turn distributes oxygenated blood to the brain and peripheral circulation. The right side of the heart primarily receives blood with a lower oxygen content, which is ejected into the pulmonary artery but is then diverted to the aorta rather than the high-resistance lungs diverted via the ductus arteriosus. This blood is then distributed to the placenta via the aorta and umbilical arteries to receive oxygen and nutrients and to release carbon dioxide and waste products.

As the newborn is delivered and takes the first few breaths, several changes occur that allow the lungs to become responsible for respiration. First, the lungs expand as they are filled with gas, and fetal lung fluid gradually leaves the alveoli by moving into the extra-alveolar interstitium, which is eventually cleared by lung lymphatic vessels. At the same time, the pulmonary vascular resistance decreases precipitously and pulmonary blood flow correspondingly increases. With occlusion of the umbilical cord, systemic vascular resistance increases. Even though the foramen ovale and ductus arteriosus remain anatomically open, the decrease in pulmonary vascular resistance and the increase in systemic vascular resistance effectively reverse the direction of blood flow through these two shunt pathways. Elevated pulmonary vascular resistance caused by hypoxia, acidosis, and hypothermia leads to right-to-left shunting through the foramen ovale and ductus arteriosus, thus prolonging the fetal circulatory pathways and impairing oxygen delivery. It is apparent that minimization of hypoxia, acidosis, and hypothermia at birth helps ensure a smooth transition to a normal postnatal circulation.

Fortunately, the first few breaths of most newborn infants are effective and allow the cardiopulmonary adaptations previously discussed to take place. However, some infants are asphyxiated in utero and are born with ineffective respiration or apnea, which leads to hypoxia and acidosis, making these adaptations difficult.

In animal studies, total asphyxia initially causes a short period of increased respiratory effort followed by apnea. This condition is known as primary apnea, and during this time spontaneous respiration can be restored by tactile stimulation. However, if asphyxia continues, the infant develops gasping respiration, the heart rate continues to decrease, and the blood pressure begins to fall. The infant then takes a last gasping breath (the "last gasp") and enters a period known as secondary apnea. Now the infant is unresponsive to stimulation, and only positive-pressure ventilation restores spontaneous respiration. The longer the delay in resuscitation, the longer it takes for spontaneous respiration to occur. Because the fetus may experience asphyxia in utero, he or she may undergo primary and secondary apnea in utero. Therefore, when the infant is born apneic, one cannot differentiate between primary and secondary apnea and one must assume that the infant is in secondary apnea and initiate positive-pressure ventilation.

PREPARATION

Preparation is the essential first step of effective neonatal resuscitation. Infants requiring resuscitation are often born in hospitals where most infants are healthy. This implies that when infants who do require treatment for neonatal respiratory depression are born, specialized neonatal expertise is not likely to be present. It is therefore essential to ensure that personnel adequately skilled in neonatal resuscitation be present at every delivery, whether or not perinatal problems are anticipated. At deliveries in which a normal, healthy infant is expected, one person (e.g., physician, nurse, respiratory therapist) who has the skills to perform a complete neonatal resuscitation must be present. If this person is also caring for the mother, another person who is capable of initiating and assisting with neonatal resuscitation must be present. It is inappropriate to have someone on call to provide neonatal resuscitation, as this may cause unnecessary delay. At high-risk deliveries in which neonatal asphyxia is likely, two persons not involved in the care of the mother must be readily available, and one of these two must be skilled in endotracheal intubation and the administration of medications.

Equipment needed for a complete resuscitation is listed in Table 1. This equipment should be present in every delivery area and routinely checked to ensure that it is all working properly. When the antepartum or intrapartum history suggests that an asphyxiated infant may be born, all equipment should be immediately accessible. One should quickly check to ensure that the radiant warmer is heating, that oxygen is flowing through the tubing, that suction is functioning properly, that the resuscitation bag and mask can provide an adequate seal and generate pressure, and that the laryngoscope light source is functional. Several minutes into the resuscitation of a cyanotic infant is not the time to realize that the valve to the oxygen source was never opened. For multiple gestations, a full complement of equipment and personnel is needed for each infant.

INITIAL STEPS OF RESUSCITATION

Although certain aspects of neonatal resuscitation make it unique, the basic ABCs (airway, breathing, circulation) of resuscitation in any age group still apply. Most infants respond to airway management and the initiation of positive-pressure ventilation if needed. Chest compressions and, in particular, medications are rarely necessary. This also applies to medically complicated infants such as those prenatally detected to have complex congenital heart disease or hydrops fetalis. The basic rules of neonatal resuscitation still apply, and one should not forget the ABCs in the excitement that sometimes accompanies a prenatally detected complex patient. As we

TABLE 1. Equipment and Supplies for Resuscitation

Environment
  Radiant warmer (with temperature probe)
  Blankets, towels (warm)
  Wall clock with sweep second hand
Suction
  Bulb syringe
  Suction catheters (No. 6, 8, 10 French)
  Regulated wall suction
  Meconium aspiration devices
Airway management
  Stethoscope
  Oxygen
  Flowmeter
  Oxygen tubing
  Infant resuscitation bag (with pressure-release
    valve and manometer)
  Masks (premature and infant sizes)
  Laryngoscope
  Size 0 and 1 laryngoscope blades
  Endotracheal tubes (2.5, 3.0, 3.5—all uncuffed)
  Stylets
Vascular access
  Umbilical catheters (No. 3.5 and 5 French)
  Umbilical catheterization tray
  Syringes (1, 3, 5, 10, 20, and 60 mL)
  Needles (various gauges from 25 to 18)
  Stopcocks
  Suture (3-0 or 4-0 silk)
  Sterile saline (10 mL)
  Intravenous catheters
  Intravenous tubing
  Umbilical tape
Medications
  Epinephrine (1:10,000)
  Naloxone hydrochloride (Narcan) (1 or 0.4 mg/mL)
  Intravenous solutions (normal saline, 10% dextrose)
  Sodium bicarbonate (4.2%, 0.5 mEq/mL)
  Albumin (5%)
  Sterile water
Miscellaneous
  Gloves (sterile and nonsterile)
  Masks, with eye shield
  Quick reference card for ages and weight

begin to discuss the individual steps of neonatal resuscitation, the importance of continuous evaluation of the patient to assist in the decision-making process before proceeding to the next step in neonatal resuscitation cannot be overemphasized.

One extremely important aspect of newborn resuscitation that is unique is the importance of temperature control. Simply keeping the newborn warm decreases morbidity. In fact, paying attention to temperature should come before the *A* in the ABCs.

Cold stress in the newborn leads to increased oxygen consumption and increased metabolic demand, which further complicate the resuscitation of the asphyxiated newborn. This is especially true in the very-low-birth-weight (VLBW) infant. The large surface area of the newborn relative to body mass and the newborn's poor insulating ability (decreased body fat, particularly in preterm infants) accelerate heat loss. Heat can be lost by four different mechanisms: evaporation, convection, radiation, and conduction. Evaporative heat loss is increased by failure to dry off amniotic fluid. This evaporative heat loss is exacerbated in VLBW infants whose skin lacks a well-developed, keratinized epidermal barrier. Convective heat loss occurs when ambient air temperature is less than the infant's skin temperature. Heat loss by radiation to cold objects in a delivery room is a major cause of thermal stress in newborns, and if the infant is placed on cool blankets or towels for resuscitation, heat loss by conduction can occur. Therefore, it is easy to see how quickly a newborn can lose heat and how important it is for the first steps of resuscitation to include ways to minimize this heat loss. This is easily accomplished by placing the newborn under a prewarmed towel or blanket. One must remember to remove the wet blanket or towel from the infant or evaporative heat loss will continue. Drying of the infant has an added benefit of providing gentle stimulation, which may aid in the onset of spontaneous respiration.

Equally important is not allowing the infant to become too warm. An infant must never be left on a radiant warmer on manual control for more than a few minutes before placing the warmer on servocontrol. One should make sure that the control temperature is properly set (approximately 36.5°C). It is important to know how the warmer and temperature probe work and to ensure proper functioning.

Establishment of an open airway is accomplished by placing the neonate on the back with the neck in a neutral to slightly extended position on a flat radiant warmer bed. The neck should not be hyperextended or flexed, and the warmer bed should not be in the Trendelenburg position, as was once recommended. If needed, a rolled blanket or towel may be placed under the shoulder, extending the head slightly. The newborn should now be in the best position to maintain an open airway.

When the infant has been correctly positioned, the mouth and nose should be quickly suctioned. The material in the mouth should be suctioned first to decrease the risk for aspiration should the infant gasp. A bulb syringe or mechanical suction device may be used. Deep suctioning of the esophagus and stomach or prolonged suctioning is contraindicated because it can produce a vagal response leading to apnea and bradycardia. Suctioning should be limited to 3 to 5 seconds. This time limit, in addition to the avoidance of deep suctioning, should lessen the risk of vagal-induced apnea or bradycardia. Unfortunately, prolonged and deep suctioning is a common, preventable mistake that often causes bradycardia and leads to additional interventions.

The next step is to provide tactile stimulation. The infant has already been dried and suctioned, which in many cases is sufficient tactile stimulation to initiate respiration. If not, there are two safe and appropriate ways to provide additional tactile stimulation: (1) briefly slapping or flicking the soles of the feet, and (2) rubbing the infant's back. Other actions such as slapping the infant's back or buttocks or blowing cool oxygen or air into the infant's face can result in unnecessary bruising and hypothermia. Tactile stimulation should not be prolonged. If there is no response to one or two flicks of the feet, it is not appropriate to then try to rub the infant's back. The time elapsed from placing the infant under the warmer to positioning, suctioning, and providing additional tactile stimulation should be no more than 15 to 20 seconds. During this period, the adequacy of respiration and the heart rate should be assessed. Because one must assume that apnea noted at birth must be secondary apnea, it is now time to proceed to positive-pressure ventilation.

The initial steps of warming, positioning, suctioning, and stimulation are applied in every newborn delivery. The remaining guidelines to resuscitation depend on evaluation of the infant while those initial steps of resuscitation are performed. Apgar scores are of little value to the pediatrician or neonatologist at the delivery. Continued need for resuscitation depends on three clinical signs: (1) respiratory effort, (2) heart rate, and (3) color. If the infant demonstrates a regular, effective breathing pattern after tactile stimulation, one should proceed to checking the heart rate. If the infant is gasping or apneic or has ineffective respiration, positive-pressure ventilation should be given. When respiratory effort has been evaluated and the appropriate action taken, if needed, the heart rate is monitored. If the heart rate is greater than 100, one should proceed to evaluate the infant's color. If the heart rate is less than 100, even if the infant has spontaneous respiration, one should proceed to positive-pressure ventilation. The heart rate can be monitored by auscultation or palpation of the pulse in the umbilical cord, although it is generally more prudent to auscultate, especially for the less experienced. Monitoring of the heart rate determines the extent of resuscitation, as discussed later. The infant's color should be evaluated next. Peripheral cyanosis (acrocyanosis) is common in the newborn, but central cyanosis is abnormal. Central cyanosis involves the entire body, including the mucous membranes. If central cyanosis is present in a newborn with adequate respiration and a heart rate greater than 100, free-flowing oxygen should be administered. Oxygen should be delivered at a flow rate of 5 liters per minute via an oxygen hose and held steadily (not waved back and forth) 0.5 inch from the infant's nares. This will deliver approximately 80% inspired oxygen to the infant. It is easier to deliver free-flow oxygen with the oxygen hose than to attempt to do it with the bag and mask. It will not work with all types of bag-and-mask setups. The infant should receive a high concentration of oxygen until the color becomes pink; then oxygen should be gradually withdrawn to the degree that the newborn can maintain a pink color.

MECONIUM-STAINED AMNIOTIC FLUID

Another situation unique to the resuscitation of the newborn is that of meconium-stained amniotic fluid. Thin, watery meconium-stained fluid has not been proved to contribute to increased perinatal morbidity, and specific management of these infants is probably unnecessary. However, thick and particulate meconium-stained amniotic fluid can lead to meconium aspiration syndrome, with or without persistent pulmonary hypertension. To minimize this risk, the infant's mouth, pharynx, and nose should be suctioned with a No. 10 French catheter by the obstetrician as the infant's head is delivered but before the shoulders are delivered. After delivery, the infant should be placed under a radiant warmer, and before drying, any remaining meconium should be suctioned from the hypopharynx. The trachea should then be suctioned under direct vision. This is best accomplished by intubating with an endotracheal tube and applying suction (no more than 100 mm Hg) to a special meconium aspiration device attached to the endotracheal tube as the tube is withdrawn. Passing a suction catheter through the endotracheal tube is inappropriate as it may be too small to suction particulate meconium. Reintubation followed by repeated suctioning should be performed until all meconium is removed, provided the infant's condition remains stable. Free-flow oxygen should be provided with all intubation attempts to minimize the risk of hypoxia. It is important to monitor the heart rate continuously, as positive-pressure ventilation may have to be initiated before all the meconium can be removed from the trachea. Gastric contents should be suctioned for meconium to prevent the possibility of later regurgitation and aspiration. However, this should be done only after resuscitation is completed and the infant's condition is stable.

POSITIVE-PRESSURE VENTILATION

Positive-pressure ventilation is the single most valuable therapeutic technique for resuscitating a newborn. Unfortunately, it is also the technique requiring the most skill and practice to apply correctly. Although an anesthesia bag may be used, it is a more difficult technique to master, and in my opinion it is not nearly as effective at delivering the higher pressures sometimes required to resuscitate a sick newborn. A self-inflating resuscitation bag is preferable and should be equipped with a face mask and oxygen reservoir that enable the bag to deliver a higher concentration of oxygen (90 to 100%). Without the oxygen reservoir, the self-inflating bag is unable to deliver a high concentration of oxygen. The flow of oxygen through the tubing should be increased to 8 to 10 liters per minute and be connected to the oxygen inlet on the resuscitation bag. The self-inflating bags have a pressure-release valve, commonly called a pop-off valve, that usually releases at 25 to 35 cm H_2O pressure. It is often necessary to occlude this pop-off valve to generate a sufficient amount of pressure to effectively ventilate a newborn's nonaerated lungs, especially with the first few breaths. With the pop-off valve occluded, care should be taken not to overventilate the newborn, as this may cause a pneumothorax. A pressure manometer should always be used in conjunction with the bag to prevent overdis-

tention of the lung. Masks come in different shapes and sizes, with or without cushioned rims. One should take care in positioning the mask so that it covers the chin, mouth, and nose, but not the eyes.

At the time of need for bag-and-mask ventilation, the infant should be in the correct position for an open airway with the neck in a neutral to slightly extended position. The ventilator stands in a position so as not to obstruct the view of the newborn's chest. The mask is placed over the infant's face and light downward pressure is applied while the edges of the mask are squeezed to form a seal between the mask and the face. Large amounts of downward pressure are not required. Constant re-evaluation is necessary to ensure that the seal is adequate and that chest expansion is occurring with each assisted ventilation. If chest expansion is inadequate, the most common problem is an inadequate seal. Second, the infant's airway could be blocked by improper positioning or occluded by secretions. It may be necessary to reposition the infant or suction the infant's mouth and nose. If a good seal is obtained and an airway is maintained, then increasing the pressure may be necessary to move the chest. Pressures of 20 to 40 cm H_2O are often required in infants with respiratory conditions that decrease lung compliance. The infant should be ventilated at a rate of 40 to 60 times per minute. After 15 to 30 seconds of effective bag-and-mask ventilation, the heart rate determines the next step of resuscitation. If the heart rate is greater than 100 and spontaneous, effective respiration has begun, one should gradually decrease bag-and-mask ventilation, provide free-flowing oxygen, and observe for the continuation of effective respiration. If the heart rate is 60 to 100 and increasing, one should continue bag-and-mask ventilation. If the heart rate is 60 to 100 and not increasing, one should reassess the adequacy of ventilation, and if the heart rate remains less than 80, one should begin chest compressions. If the heart rate is less than 60, one should again assess for the adequacy of ventilation and immediately begin chest compressions. The adequacy of the seal between the mask and the infant's face cannot be overly emphasized.

CHEST COMPRESSIONS

Chest compressions are performed on the lower third of the sternum, located between an imaginary line drawn between the nipples and the xiphoid process. One must avoid applying pressure directly over the xiphoid. There are two methods for compressing the chest: (1) the thumb method and (2) the two-finger method. The thumb technique involves encircling the infant's body with both hands and placing the thumbs on the sternum and the fingers under the infant. Extreme caution must be used in stabilizing the fingers under the back; flexing the fingers can injure the infant's spine. The thumbs are used to compress the sternum. The two-finger method uses the tips of the first two fingers or the middle and ring finger placed in a perpendicular position over the lower sternum. Only the fingertips rest on the chest, and pressure is applied directly downward. Obviously, long fingernails preclude the use of this method. The fingertips need to remain in contact with the sternum at all times, with no thumping of the sternum. One should use pressure sufficient to depress the sternum 0.5 to 0.75 inch. The Neonatal Resuscitation Program suggests interposing chest compressions with ventilation in a 3:1 ratio. This amounts to 90 compressions and 30 breaths per minute. Therefore, the ventilation rate during chest compressions is lower than the 40 to 60 range recommended when chest compressions are not being performed. The heart rate should be evaluated every 30 seconds and chest compressions continued until the heart rate is greater than 80.

ENDOTRACHEAL INTUBATION

Endotracheal intubation is indicated when prolonged positive-pressure ventilation is required or bag-and-mask ventilation is deemed ineffective. It is also indicated in the special circumstance of infants born with thick or particulate meconium in the amniotic fluid or in the case of congenital diaphragmatic hernia. Intubation is a skill that takes practice and that becomes easier to do with experience.

At least two people are required for endotracheal intubation. The second person prepares the tape for securing the tube in place, administers free-flow oxygen during the attempt, monitors the heart rate, limits the time of the attempt to no more than 20 seconds, assesses if the attempt is successful, helps determine the appropriateness of the position of the tube, and helps secure the tube in place. In preparation for intubation, the laryngoscope should be equipped with a No. 0 blade for premature infants and a No. 1 blade for full-term infants (although many skilled intubators find a No. 0 blade sufficient for full-term infants as well). One should double-check to see that the light source is functional. The proper-sized endotracheal tube is selected based on the infant's weight. A 2.5-mm (internal diameter) size is appropriate for infants less than 1.0 kg, a 3.0-mm size for infants weighing 1.0 to 2.0 kg, and a 3.5-mm size for infants weighing more than 2.0 kg. The use of a stylet is optional but is not really necessary. If a stylet is used, one should take care that the tip of the stylet does not protrude beyond the tip of the endotracheal tube and that the stylet is easily removable once in the tube. Mechanical suctioning (not to exceed 100 mm Hg) should be available as well as free-flow oxygen to provide a high concentration of oxygen during the procedure to minimize hypoxia. The resuscitation bag and mask should be kept at the bedside for use between intubation attempts and for connecting to the endotracheal tube after intubation is accomplished. The infant is placed in the proper position with the head midline and the neck slightly extended. The laryngoscope handle is held in the left hand, regardless of the handedness of the operator, and the blade is inserted between the tongue and palate until the tip of the blade rests in the vallecula. The glottis is visualized by lifting the entire blade in a direction parallel to the length of the laryngoscope handle. One should never use the laryngoscope like a lever, as in a "prying" or "can opener" type of maneuver. Once the glottis is in view, the endotracheal tube is inserted with the right hand until the vocal cord guideline (the heavy black line near the tip of the tube) is at the level of the vocal cords. Another guideline for positioning the endotracheal tube is to add 6 to the infant's weight in kilograms and then tape the endotracheal tube at that number of centimeters at the gum. One should hold the endotracheal tube securely until it is taped into position, listen for the presence of equal breath sounds bilaterally in the axillae, then obtain a chest radiograph of the infant. One should be sure to record the position at which the tube is taped, as this is useful for repositioning later and for determining whether the tube has inadvertently shifted in position.

Often one is so elated at successfully passing the tube that one fails to pay attention to the distance that it is inserted. Much harm can come from having an endotracheal tube inserted too far. If the endotracheal tube is inserted too far, it can rest in the right mainstem bronchus, causing poor oxygen and carbon dioxide exchange and overdistention of that lung segment, possibly leading to pulmonary interstitial emphysema and pneumothorax. In the premature infant, extra care should be taken to ensure good endotracheal tube placement, as the 6 plus weight in kilograms rule may be less reliable; the tube may need to be inserted less far. To ensure against esophageal intubation, one should listen for air entering the stomach and observe for gastric distention. Esophageal intubation usually becomes apparent as secretions enter the endotracheal tube and the patient does not respond clinically.

MEDICATIONS

Resuscitation medications are rarely needed in the newborn; adequate ventilation with 100% oxygen is usually sufficient, with adequate being the key. However, in the newborn whose heart rate remains less than 80 despite adequate ventilation with 100% oxygen and effective chest compressions for more than 30 seconds, or in the newborn with a heart rate of zero, medications should be administered. The initial medication in such a scenario is epinephrine. Epinephrine increases cardiac output by increasing the heart rate and myocardial contractility and increases blood pressure by causing peripheral vasoconstriction. It should be given rapidly and can be given intravenously or via endotracheal tube in a dose of 0.1 to 0.3 mL of the 1:10,000 solution per kg. The intravenous route is preferable as plasma concentrations via the endotracheal route are sometimes low. However, intravenous access has usually not been established when the first dose of epinephrine is required, so it may be preferable to give the higher recommended dose when administered via the endotracheal route. During this time, umbilical venous access can easily be established in any infant by inserting a catheter in the umbilical vein 2 or 3 cm so that the catheter tip is below the liver. The umbilical vein is the single, large, thin-walled vessel usually in the 12 o'clock position when looking at the infant with his or her head at the top. Thereafter, all medications are preferably given by this route. Epinephrine administration may be repeated every 5 minutes if the heart rate remains less than 100. (Epinephrine should never be given in the umbilical artery.)

If there is no response to epinephrine, one should suspect metabolic acidosis. This is also a good time to reassess ventilation and to double-check that 100% oxygen is being administered. In this case, sodium bicarbonate is indicated in a dose of 2 mEq per kg. It can be given only intravenously. Intracranial hemorrhage has been associated with the use of bicarbonate in animal studies. To reduce that risk, sodium bicarbonate in the commercially available 4.2% solution (0.5 mEq per mL) should be given slowly over a minimum of 2 minutes, not to exceed a rate of 1 mEq per kg per minute. Hypovolemia may be present in the newborn and is usually a known event (e.g., umbilical cord accidents, placenta previa) and is indicated by pallor and poor perfusion despite a normal pH and PO_2, and weak pulses despite a good heart rate. Hypovolemia must also be considered if there is no response to the administration of epinephrine and bicarbonate. A dose of 10 mL per kg of volume expander should be given intravenously, slowly. In the premature infant at risk for intracranial hemorrhage, this volume should always be given slowly over at least 30 minutes. However in the hypovolemic, asphyxiated full-term infant it may be necessary to administer the volume over 5 to 10 minutes. It is essential to monitor the heart rate and discontinue medications once the heart rate is greater than 100.

In the special instance of an infant born with respiratory depression to a mother who received narcotics within 4 hours of delivery, naloxone hydrochloride (Narcan), 0.1 mg per kg, given rapidly is indicated. In my experience this is a rare occurrence, and I find that naloxone is often given in unwarranted situations. It should be remembered that apnea can always be effectively controlled with bag-and-mask ventilation while the narcotic administration history is checked. When needed, naloxone may be given by endotracheal tube, intravenously, intramuscularly, or subcutaneously. It should not be given if the mother has a narcotic dependency, as this may precipitate withdrawal in the infant. The infant who receives naloxone should be observed, as the narcotic causing the respiratory depression may have a longer duration of action than the naloxone, whose duration of action is 1 to 4 hours.

Successful neonatal resuscitation requires communication between the resuscitation team and obstetric staff, advanced preparation, and skilled and knowledgeable personnel. The ability to resuscitate newborns should be available at all hospitals for every newborn delivery regardless of the presence of highly specialized perinatal services.

CARE OF THE HIGH-RISK NEONATE

method of
MICHAEL E. SPEER, M.D.
Methodist Hospital
Houston, Texas

Approximately 5% of infants require some degree of intervention during the neonatal period. The time of greatest need is after delivery. Although many of these infants are seen in the 10% of the obstetric population that is defined as high risk, a number of these infants are born after an uneventful pregnancy, labor, and delivery. Anticipation and preparation of these infants' medical requirements must be a constant. Proactive, not reactive, behavior should be the norm. To facilitate this initial care, many hospitals have established a resuscitation area either within the delivery room or in an immediately adjacent area that is completely equipped to meet the acute needs of the distressed neonate. Further, the personnel responsible for assessment and resuscitation of the infant should be certified through the Neonatal Resuscitation Program offered by the American Academy of Pediatrics and the American Hospital Association.

GENERAL CONSIDERATIONS

The concept of neonatal risk assessment and consideration of outcome can best be approached by the assessment of birth weight and gestational age. Most, although not all, neonatal illnesses (risk) may be predicted by the relationships inherent in these two measurements. Thus, the clinician must determine both the general and the specific risk to assign a diagnosis and a prognosis. Birth weight, usually measured at the time of birth or slightly thereafter, can be assessed within ± 10 grams. (Although many hospitals may still use an avoirdupois measuring system [pounds and ounces], calculations regarding the newborn infant are much easier and more accurate if the metric system is employed.) Gestational age is usually calculated from the maternal menstrual history, but in the absence of gestational age, important information may be calculated by a system that evaluates the physical and neurologic maturation of the infant (Figure 1). The establishment of risk can then be appraised by a combination of weight, gestational age, and weight for gestational age. For example, an infant weighing 1250 grams at birth who is born at 34 weeks' gestation has a markedly different mortality than an infant of the same birth weight born at 27 weeks' gestation. Thus, within particular weight and gestational age categories, divisions can be made that have relevance in predicting the incidence of certain types of problems (Table 1). Note that, e.g., all infants weighing less than 2500 grams are low birth weight, but only those less than 1000 grams are extremely low birth weight (ELBW).

Neonatal mortality (number of deaths before 28 days of age per 1000 live births) depends on birth weight and gestational age. In a tertiary care neonatal center, neonatal mortality approximates 60% in those infants born at 24

Neuromuscular Maturity

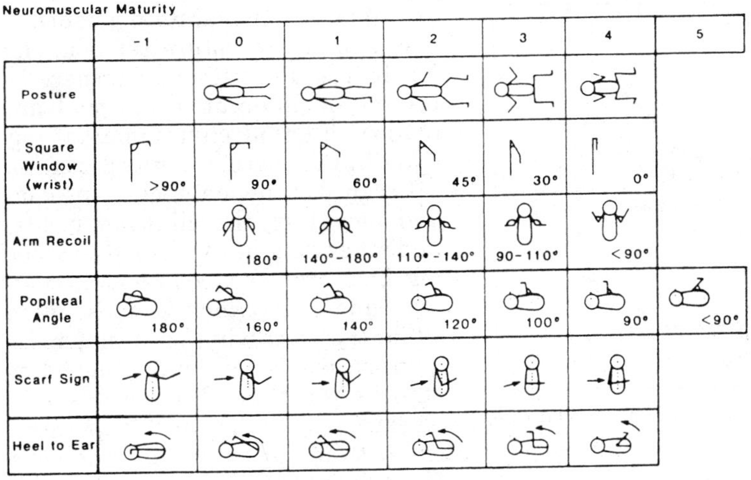

	-1	0	1	2	3	4	5
Posture							
Square Window (wrist)	>90°	90°	60°	45°	30°	0°	
Arm Recoil		180°	140°-180°	110°-140°	90°-110°	<90°	
Popliteal Angle	180°	160°	140°	120°	100°	90°	<90°
Scarf Sign							
Heel to Ear							

Physical Maturity

Skin	sticky friable transparent	gelatinous red, translucent	smooth pink, visible veins	superficial peeling &/or rash, few veins	cracking pale areas rare veins	parchment deep cracking no vessels	leathery cracked wrinkled
Lanugo	none	sparse	abundant	thinning	bald areas	mostly bald	
Plantar Surface	heel-toe 40-50 mm: -1 <40 mm: -2	>50mm no crease	faint red marks	anterior transverse crease only	creases ant. 2/3	creases over entire sole	
Breast	imperceptible	barely perceptible	flat areola no bud	stippled areola 1-2mm bud	raised areola 3-4mm bud	full areola 5-10mm bud	
Eye/Ear	lids fused loosely:-1 tightly:-2	lids open pinna flat stays folded	sl. curved pinna; soft; slow recoil	well-curved pinna; soft but ready recoil	formed &firm instant recoil	thick cartilage ear stiff	
Genitals male	scrotum flat, smooth	scrotum empty faint rugae	testes in upper canal rare rugae	testes descending few rugae	testes down good rugae	testes pendulous deep rugae	
Genitals female	clitoris prominent labia flat	prominent clitoris small labia minora	prominent clitoris enlarging minora	majora & minora equally prominent	majora large minora small	majora cover clitoris & minora	

Maturity Rating

score	weeks
-10	20
-5	22
0	24
5	26
10	28
15	30
20	32
25	34
30	36
35	38
40	40
45	42
50	44

Figure 1. Expanded New Ballard Score includes extremely premature infants and has been refined to improve accuracy in more mature infants. (From Ballard JL, Khoury JC, Wedig K, et al: New Ballard Score, expanded to include extremely premature infants. J Pediatr *119*:417–423, 1991.)

weeks' gestation; however, mortality in infants born at 29 weeks' gestation is only 5%.

The small infant, whether born prematurely or small for gestational age, has difficulty with temperature regulation and glucose homeostasis. In addition, infants who are very small for gestational age have a much increased risk of congenital malformations (18% in one large series of small-

TABLE 1. **Definitions of Low Birth Weight and Relationship of Gestational Age to Birth Weight**

Measure	Definition
Low birth weight (LBW)	<2500 gm
Very low birth weight (VLBW)	<1500 gm
Extremely low birth weight (ELBW)	<1000 gm
Large for gestational age (LGA)	Birth weight >90th percentile for gestation
Appropriate for gestational age (AGA)	Birth weight between 10th and 90th percentile for gestation
Small for gestational age (SGA)	Birth weight <10th percentile for gestation

for-gestational-age infants weighing between 1501 and 2500 grams). Infants with chromosomal anomalies (trisomy 13, trisomy 18, and trisomy 21) as well as those with various types of dwarfism are found among this category of infants. Large-for-gestational-age infants are more at risk for birth trauma and, if born to a mother with diabetes mellitus, for hypoglycemia, hypocalcemia, hyperbilirubinemia, and respiratory distress syndrome.

THE BASIS OF CARE

In recent years, much focus and energy have been on the technologic aspects of neonatal medicine, such as extracorporeal membrane oxygenation, mechanical ventilation, and in-line oxygen monitoring. Despite such advanced technology, the three basic principles of care that have greatly improved mortality and morbidity and form the cornerstones of modern neonatology are warmth, fluids, and nutrition.

The Zone of Thermal Neutrality

Pierre Budin in 1907 observed that if an infant's temperature remained between 32.5 and 33.5°C (90.5

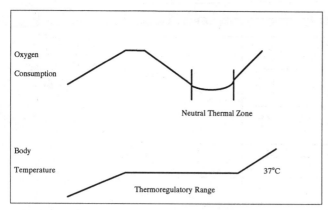

Figure 2. Relationship of thermal neutrality and oxygen consumption.

and 92.3°F), only 10% of the infants survived. On the other hand, if the infant's body temperature was maintained in the normal range between 36 and 37°C (96.8 and 98.6°F), 77% survived. He recommended an air temperature of 30°C (86°F) for the small, fully clothed infant. Unfortunately, his conclusions were not understood and were ignored for the first 50 years of this century. Implementation of these ideas was left to Silverman, who in 1964 demonstrated in low-birth-weight infants an improved survival from 68 to 84% merely by increasing the incubator temperature 3.7°C (4°F) (29.9 to 33.6°C [85 to 89°F]). Somewhat before Silverman's reports, Hill and Cross observed that oxygen consumption and rectal temperatures varied with the environmental temperature. Hill and Cross noted a set of thermal conditions at which heat production (measured as oxygen consumption) is minimal yet the core temperature is within the normal range. This zone of basal oxygen consumption is called the neutral thermal zone (Figure 2). Outside the neutral thermal zone, oxygen consumption rises over the remainder of the thermoregulatory range of the patient. Only when body cooling takes place does the oxygen consumption fall. Maintaining the infant within the neutral thermal environment also translates into better effective growth for the preterm infant, who otherwise would use caloric intake for temperature maintenance. For the term infant, the lower limit of the control range (that range of environmental temperatures at which body temperature can be kept constant by means of regulation) is between 20 and 23°C (68 and 73.4°F). This is far different from the lower adult limit of 0°C (32°F). For both preterm and term infants, the ability to regulate core temperature is intact; however, the control range before body heating and cooling take place is much narrower than that found in older infants, children, and adults. A corollary to this is that heat loss is controlled, to a large degree, by the amount of surface area in relationship to relative mass, whereas heat production and conservation are a function of mass (e.g., one piglet has a large surface area relative to mass; a group of piglets huddled together have a relatively small surface area in rela-

tion to mass). To maintain a neutral thermal environment, the temperature set point for servocontrolled incubators and radiant warmers is 36.5°C (96.1°F). Infants of different gestational and postnatal ages require different environmental temperatures to remain in the thermal neutral zone.

Because of the metabolic consequences of heat gain and heat loss, the clinician needs to have a clear understanding of the four basic mechanisms regarding heat transfer: *conduction, evaporation, irradiation,* and *convection.* As most infants are cared for while they are lying on a mattress, conductive heat gain or loss is minimal. Depending on the circumstances, the other three modes of heat transfer may be extremely important. Evaporative heat loss is critical both in any infant after delivery and in the very small immature infant in the hours and days after parturition. Each milliliter of evaporation that occurs results in 0.58 kcal of body heat loss. This type of heat loss can result in a significant fall in the body temperature of the newly born infant. Further, through evaporation, the premature infant nursed under a radiant warmer has insensible water losses of 3 to 5 mL per kg per hour. Therefore, the fluid and caloric consequences of this evaporative loss must be considered when designing fluid and nutritional therapy.

Irradiant heat loss or heat gain depends on the circumstances present. Shortwave radiant energy from the sun can penetrate Plexiglas walls of an incubator; long wavelength reradiation through the plastic wall cannot take place (greenhouse effect). Most radiant energy transfer is composed of longwave energy (Figure 3). Irradiant heat losses or gains also depend on gradients of temperature between objects, with movement of energy from the warm object to the cold object. Irradiant heat losses or gains are usually inconsequential unless objects surrounding the infant are significantly colder or hotter. If that is the case, radiant energy is lost or gained by the infant. If a barrier is placed between the two gradients, heat loss or gain is diminished as energy has to be conducted *through* the barrier before it can again undergo irradiant transfer (Figure 4). A radiant warmer maintains an infant's core temperature in a neutral thermal environment, replacing evaporative and convective heat losses.

Heat transfer by convection is common in the everyday environment. Air conditioners and hot air furnaces cool and heat by convection. A standard convection-heated incubator warms the infant's envi-

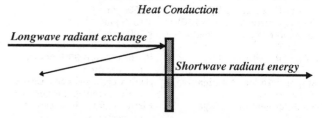

Figure 3. Behavior of short- and longwave radiant energy.

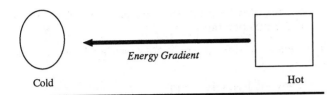

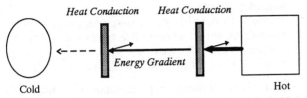

Figure 4. Reduction of heat loss utilizing barriers (shaded bars). ← = direction and magnitude of energy (heat) flux.

ronment by passing a stream of air through a heated coil. By maintaining an environment within the range of thermoneutrality, it lessens energy expenditure. In addition, the heated air warms the inner walls of the incubator and any barrier placed between the infant and the inner walls (see earlier). The main losses of heat energy in an incubator environment are evaporative. Evaporative loss, in turn, can be affected by the degree of humidity present. Less evaporation occurs with higher humidity. Also, irradiant heat losses may occur if the environment external to the incubator is unduly cold (air conditioned). Heat gain is unusual and has already been discussed (greenhouse effect).

Fluid and Electrolyte Homeostasis

The water content of the human infant decreases progressively from approximately 85% of body weight at 28 weeks' gestation to approximately 75% at term. This can be compared with the water content of the reference adult, which is 61%. The observed weight loss after delivery can be accounted for by the loss of water and sodium from the extracellular space. Fluid losses are increased in the premature infant because of the greater water content found in their skin and a thinner epidermis that results in increased skin permeability. Maintenance fluids should ideally represent those fluids that are equal to insensible water losses (skin and pulmonary) plus urinary and gastrointestinal losses. In general, insensible water losses account for 1 to 3 mL per kg per hour. The smaller amount is found in the term infant and those prema-

TABLE 3. Composition of Gastrointestinal Fluids (mEq/L)

Constituent	Gastric	Small Bowel
Na^+	130–140	100–140
K^+	10–15	10–30
Cl^-	140–155	50–60
HCO_3^-	0	50–75

ture infants weighing more than 1500 grams at birth cared for in an incubator. The larger losses are found in the smaller preterm infant cared for within an incubator and infants receiving phototherapy. Insensible losses experienced when the infant is cared for under a radiant warmer are approximately twice those experienced when the infant is nursed within an incubator. These insensible water losses range from 2 to 5 mL per kg per hour depending on the size and gestational age of the infant. Insensible water loss in an infant weighing less than 1250 grams cared for under a radiant warmer can be reduced by 25% with the use of a plastic heat shield.

A urinary flow of at least 2 mL per kg per hour is appropriate urinary output in an infant who is receiving a normal solute load (approximately 20 mOsm per 100 kcal metabolized) and who has normal renal concentrating ability (500 to 700 mOsm per liter). Thus, *maintenance* fluid requirements range between 70 and 170 mL per kg per day in the absence of abnormal gastrointestinal or evaporative losses (Table 2). Further, provision of approximately 150 mL of fluid per kg per day between the third and fifth day of life is necessary for adequate nutritional support. Abnormal losses from the gastrointestinal tract must be calculated as specific replacement above the normal fluid needs of the infant (Table 3).

When enteral feedings cannot be instituted, adequate fluid and electrolytes should be provided intravenously. Although in this regard the mainstay of current treatment is the administration of 10% dextrose in water, consideration should be given to providing full nutritional support as soon as is practical (see later). The electrolyte composition of fluid from skin and lungs, as well as urine, is normally hypotonic (20 to 40 mEq per liter). Electrolytes in the form of sodium and potassium chloride, therefore, are added to the intravenous maintenance fluids at the rate of 2 to 4 mEq per kg per day. Smaller and less mature infants have higher urinary losses, and sodium replacement may approach 4 mEq per kg per

TABLE 2. Fluid Requirements of the Newborn Infant with Normal Renal Function

Birth Weight (gm)	Estimated Insensible Water Loss (mL/kg/h)*	Water for Solute Excretion (2 mL/kg/h minimum)	Total Maintenance Fluid (mL/kg/d)
500–750	3–5	2	120–170
751–1000	3–4	2	120–150
1001–1500	2–3	2	100–120
>1501	1–2	2	70–100

*Dependent on the physical environment.

day. Measurement of levels of electrolytes, calcium, blood urea nitrogen, and creatinine in the first 24 hours of life generally reflects the maternal values. Consequently, obtaining these laboratory studies in the infant during this time is of limited value. The exception to this is found in the ELBW infant whose insensible water losses equal or exceed 120 mL per kg per day. In these infants, as the serum sodium level is an excellent indication of hydration status, a baseline sodium measurement at the time of birth and then every 6 hours thereafter allows better control of fluid management. In the enterally fed preterm infant whose birth weight is more than 1500 grams and who is clinically stable, the measurement of serum electrolyte levels may not be necessary. If this same infant is receiving only intravenous fluids, then the measurement of serum electrolyte levels can be performed once the infant has reached 48 hours of age. Assessment of renal function, unless clinically indicated, is usually not necessary. Thus, the clinical condition and age of the infant should dictate the frequency and type of laboratory evaluation. The more clinically unstable the infant is, the greater the number and frequency of any laboratory evaluations.

The serum calcium level at birth correlates with increasing gestational age. The lowest serum levels are found between 24 and 48 hours of life because of limited response of the parathyroid gland to hypocalcemia but are usually in excess of 7 mg per dL. Symptomatic hypocalcemia (a serum calcium level less than 7 mg per dL or an ionized calcium level less than 4.4 mg per dL [1.1 mmol per liter]) is unusual but may be present in the following circumstances: prematurity, infants of diabetic mothers, hypoxic ischemic encephalopathy, and intrauterine growth retardation. Treatment of symptomatic hypocalcemia can be achieved by slowly giving 100 mg of calcium gluconate per kg intravenously while monitoring the heart rate, followed by the continuous infusion of 250 to 500 mg of either calcium gluconate or calcium gluceptate per kg per day added to the usual daily intravenous fluids.

Fluid and electrolyte needs should be calculated separately and then combined to determine the final fluid composition.

Example. Intravenous fluid for a 3-day-old, 1000-gram hypocalcemic infant cared for under a radiant warmer.

1. Water requirements = 150 mL per kg per day
   Sodium and potassium requirements = 3 mEq per kg per day of each
   Calcium salt requirements = 300 mg per kg per day
2. 3 mEq of sodium and potassium per day = 2 mEq per 100 mL of intravenous fluid, at 150 mL per day
   300 grams of calcium gluceptate per day = 200 mg per 100 mL of intravenous fluid, at 150 mL per day
3. Fluid and electrolyte orders = D10W + 2 mEq of NaCl per 100 mL + 2 mEq of KCl per 100 mL +

200 mg of calcium gluceptate per 100 mL at a rate of 6.5 mL per hour

The goals of short-term intravascular fluid therapy are to

- Prevent hypoglycemia
- Limit negative fluid balance to 1 to 2% of birth weight per day
- Attempt to provide protein-sparing carbohydrate calories equal to or near the basal metabolic rate (approximately 50 kcal per kg per day), which is equal to 8 mg of glucose per kg per minute

All newborn infants, but particularly those born before 34 weeks' gestation, show evidence of impaired handling of water and solute loads. The neonatal kidney demonstrates a glomerular-tubular imbalance with glomerular predominance (i.e., the tubule is more functionally immature than the glomerulus, and the persistently low glomerular filtration rate per nephron is still excessive relative to the tubular functional capacity). The newborn is able to dilute urine maximally to osmolalities of 30 to 50 mOsm per liter and to concentrate urine maximally to 700 to 800 mOsm per liter (less than the 1200 mOsm per liter seen in children and adults). The renal threshold and/or proximal tubular reabsorption of several compounds is lower in the newborn kidney. Thus, substances such as bicarbonate, phosphate, sodium, amino acids, and glucose may be filtered at lower plasma values than in the older infant and child, and because of incomplete tubular reabsorption, urinary losses are increased. The incomplete ability of the distal tubule to regenerate bicarbonate and excrete hydrogen ions also plays a role in the observed lower serum bicarbonate levels found in the newborn infant. Thus, an anticipatory approach to fluid management is mandatory.

Nutrition

Nutritional support for the newborn infant has unfortunately been seriously neglected until relatively recently. Although it may not be necessary to provide complete nutritional support by the first or second day of life, the cumulative body of evidence strongly suggests that inadequate nutrition during the period of cellular proliferation of the central nervous system results in an irreversible deficit in the number of cells. In addition, inadequate intake of essential fatty acids results in biochemical evidence of deficiency within 48 hours.

Basal caloric needs to prevent tissue catabolism approximate 50 to 60 kcal per kg per day. Further, because of the immaturity of various enzymatic processes, some amino acids that are nonessential in the adult (e.g., tyrosine and cysteine) may be necessary in the premature infant. It has been shown that total protein intakes of less than 2 grams per kg per day are inadequate for appropriate growth. Thus, the administration of 10% dextrose at a rate calculated to provide a maintenance fluid intake of 70 mL per kg per day provides a maximal available caloric source of only 28 kcal. If 5% dextrose is used because of fears of hyperglycemia, such as often occurs in the infant weighing less than 1000 grams at birth, it would follow that even more catabolic activity will take place.

In light of these facts, it is important to address the caloric requirement of these infants as soon as possible after birth. If adequate enteral intake cannot be accomplished safely, parenteral nutrition should be started within 3 days of parturition (Table 4). Adequate amounts of protein (amino acids), carbohydrate (glucose), and fat (lipids) as well as appropriate vitamins and minerals (including trace elements) should be provided. Heparin, 1 unit per mL, is added to parenteral nutrition given by a central catheter. Intravenous lipid is provided concomitantly, beginning at 2 grams per kg of body weight per day, and advancing to a maximum of 4 grams per kg of body weight per day. Serum triglyceride levels are monitored while the amount of intravenous lipid is increased. At the recommended rates of administration (130 mL of total parenteral nutrition per kg per day and 20 mL of 20% lipid per kg per day), an infant receives nutrients on a per-kilogram basis as shown in Table 4.

Enteral feedings should be started as soon as the infant is stable. The metabolic needs of the preterm neonate of a gestational age of less than 34 weeks are best met by the use of fortified expressed breast milk or a specially prepared preterm formula. Fortified breast milk has the advantage of providing human milk protein and certain antimicrobial factors (lysozymes, IgM, and secretory IgA) as well as improved digestibility. The fortification is necessary, however, to give sufficient calories and adequate amounts of minerals for appropriate bone growth. Frequently, fluid volumes of 160 mL per kg per day or greater and the use of hind milk (increased fat content) are necessary to achieve adequate growth when fortified breast milk is used. The proprietary formulas provide increased amounts of protein, minerals (particularly calcium and phosphorus), and vitamins. They also have a whey/casein ratio of 60:40, similar to that of human milk, and a low osmolarity of less than 300 mOsm per liter. Whether human milk or a formula is chosen, feedings should be introduced slowly and advanced in an incremental fashion (20 to 25 mL per kg per day). When enteral feedings are used in conjunction with total parenteral nutrition and intravenous lipids, care must be taken not to exceed 60% of the total caloric intake as fat because of the risk of ketosis and acidosis. Given the less than optimal biologic value of soy protein, formulas using this protein should be avoided in the preterm neonate.

SPECIAL PROBLEMS

The following examples constitute special areas of the care of the high-risk infant that may dictate that the infant be transferred to a tertiary nursery environment. This is particularly true if 24-hour-a-day in-house physician management cannot be ensured.

Respiratory System

Hyaline Membrane Disease

Hyaline membrane disease (HMD), also known as respiratory distress syndrome, occurs in approximately 40,000 infants each year (14% of low-birth-weight infants) born in the United States. The incidence is inversely related to gestational age and approaches 80% in infants born at less than 28 weeks whose mothers have not received corticosteroids. The cause of HMD is a paucity of pulmonary surfactant at the alveolar air-liquid interface. This lack of surfactant results in increased intra-alveolar surface tension, decreased lung compliance, and increased work of breathing. At the end of exhalation, the radius of an alveolus decreases, and the pressure required to keep the alveolus expanded increases because of the relationship of pressure and surface tension, as illustrated by Laplace's law. Laplace's law

TABLE 4. **Total Parenteral Nutrition Formulation for the Preterm Neonate***

Neonatal TPN		Constituent Intake (/kg/d)†	Caloric Intake (kcal/kg/d)†
Component	*Amount (per 100 mL)*		
Dextrose	12.5 gm	16.25 gm of glucose	55.3
Amino acids	2.4 gm	3.12 gm of protein	11.4
KPO$_4$	1.5 mmol	4.00 gm of fat	40.0
NaCl	2.6 mEq		
MgSO$_4$	0.5 mEq		
KCl	0.2 mEq		
Calcium gluconate	1.5 mmol		
		150 mL of fluid	≈107 total
Cysteine	72 mg		
Trace elements‡	‡		
Vitamins per protocol	‡		

*TrophAmine is used as the amino acid source.
†See text.
‡Trace elements (i.e., zinc, copper, chromium, manganese, and selenium) and multivitamins must be added.
Abbreviation: TPN = total parenteral nutrition.

TABLE 5. **Relationship Between the Lecithin/Sphingomyelin Ratio and Phosphatidylglycerol and the Incidence of Hyaline Membrane Disease**

	L/S Ratio < 1	L/S Ratio > 2*	PG Present	L/S < 2; PG (−)	L/S > 2; PG (+)
Incidence of HMD (%)	100	<0.5	<0.5	>80	0

*See text.

Abbreviations: L/S = lecithin/sphingomyelin ratio; PG = phosphatidylglycerol.

states that the pressure P required to maintain an air space at a given radius of curvature r is equal to twice the surface tension T divided by the radius ($P = 2T/r$). Thus, the tendency of all alveoli is toward collapse unless surface tension can be reduced. This tendency is exacerbated by the highly compliant chest wall of the preterm infant.

Surfactant is produced by the type II alveolar epithelial cell beginning between 20 and 24 weeks of gestation. The degree of pulmonary maturity can be estimated in utero by measuring the components of pulmonary surfactant in the amniotic fluid. The most frequently measured parameters are the lecithin/sphingomyelin ratio (L/S ratio) and phosphatidylglycerol (PG). The relative risk of HMD can be predicted on the basis of the results of these tests (Table 5). With a mature lung, the L/S ratio is typically greater than 2 and the PG is positive. In the presence of maternal diabetes mellitus or Rh isoimmunization, the risk of HMD when the L/S ratio is between 2 and 3 is approximately 13%. The factors that contribute to either a relative increase or decrease in the risk of HMD are found in Table 6. The role of premature rupture of the fetal membranes affecting the incidence of HMD is controversial.

Surfactant replacement therapy has dramatically reduced the morbidity and mortality due to HMD. It may be given either prophylactically, shortly after delivery, or as treatment (rescue) once HMD has been diagnosed. Because the lack of naturally occurring surfactant results in progressive atelectasis and the need for pulmonary support, undue delay in surfactant administration may be detrimental to the patient. Prophylactic endotracheal intubation and administration of surfactant in infants of less than 31 weeks' gestation has been shown to be superior to rescue therapy and is recommended. Surfactant is most beneficial in the patient with HMD when given

for at least 2 doses, with a third dose optional. In the more mature newborn, intubation and surfactant replacement should be considered in any patient whose oxygen requirement equals or exceeds an FIO_2 of 0.5. This recommendation also applies to those patients who require oxygen because of neonatal pneumonia or massive aspiration syndrome, as both of these conditions are associated with increased surfactant consumption.

The benefits of maternal corticosteroids are incontrovertible, even if given for less than 24 hours before delivery. Not only is the relative risk of HMD decreased, but the incidence of symptomatic patent ductus arteriosus (PDA) and intraventricular hemorrhage is also diminished. Antenatal corticosteroids should be administered unless immediate delivery is anticipated.

As HMD is a transient, self-limited disease, treatment should be predicated on the maintenance of adequate oxygenation and ventilation through that time needed for the infant to produce adequate surfactant material (i.e., 48 to 72 hours after birth). Therapy, therefore, is directed toward increasing the Po_2 in poorly ventilated lung units, relieving hypoxic vasoconstriction, and reducing intrapulmonary right-to-left shunting. Although oxygen administration by hood may be effective in the milder forms of the disease, this form of therapy should be reserved for those infants who do not have significant oxygen requirements (i.e., $FIO_2 < 0.5$) and who can maintain a functional residual capacity by an expiratory grunt. Continuous positive airway pressure (CPAP) is most useful in larger infants (birth weight of >1500 grams and >31 weeks' gestation) who can maintain spontaneous ventilation without apnea. Although nasal CPAP can be used acutely, endotracheal CPAP allows the administration of exogenous surfactant and improved airway stabilization. Positive-pressure ventilatory support is indicated in those infants who have significant apnea (i.e., <31 weeks' gestation) or who cannot maintain adequate oxygenation with an FIO_2 of 1.00 and maximum CPAP (8 to 10 cm H_2O). Because of the short time constants that exist in patients with HMD, relatively rapid respiratory rates (60 per minute) and short inspiratory times (0.2 second) result in better oxygenation and significantly less air leak (e.g., pneumothorax, pneumopericardium) and bronchopulmonary dysplasia than slow rates and long inspiratory times. A moderate degree of respiratory acidosis (Pco_2 between 50 and 65 mm Hg) is not injurious to the patient in the absence of hypoxemia and is not an indication to increase mean airway pressure.

TABLE 6. **Factors That Increase or Decrease the Incidence of Hyaline Membrane Disease**

Increase Risk	Decrease Risk
Male sex	Pregnancy-induced hypertension
White race	Chronic maternal hypertension
Prematurity	Subacute placental abruption
Maternal diabetes (classes A, B, and C)	Maternal narcotic addiction
	Prenatal corticosteroids
Elective cesarean section	
Second-born twin	
Rh isoimmunization	
Family history of HMD	

TABLE 7. **Conditions Associated with Persistent Pulmonary Hypertension of the Neonate**

Pulmonary Maladaptation		Pulmonary Maldevelopment	
Transient	*Persistent*	*Maldevelopment*	*Underdevelopment*
Hypoxia	Meconium aspiration pneumonia	Intrauterine hypoxia	Diaphragmatic hernia
Hypothermia	Amniotic fluid aspiration	Meconium aspiration	Potter's syndrome
Hypoglycemia	Bacterial pneumonia	Fetal ductal closure	Alveolar capillary dysplasia
Polycythemia	Bacterial septicemia	Congenital heart disease	

High-frequency ventilation, including jet and oscillatory types, has not been shown to improve survival from HMD. Further, a meta-analysis of these techniques demonstrated a significant increase in the incidence of intraventricular hemorrhage (IVH). Therefore, these techniques should be considered to be experimental. Nitric oxide has shown promise in the treatment of persistent pulmonary hypertension of the neonate (PPHN), but not HMD. Liquid ventilation using a perfluorocarbon moiety holds promise but is highly experimental. Large infants (>34 weeks' gestation; birth weight of >2000 grams) in whom conventional mechanical ventilation and surfactant therapy fail may be candidates for extracorporeal membrane oxygenation.

Persistent Pulmonary Hypertension

High pulmonary vascular resistance (PVR) is the norm in utero. After delivery, pulmonary resistance abruptly falls, primarily in response to the presence of oxygen within the alveoli. In infants with PPHN, this decrease does not occur, and variable degrees of right-to-left shunting persist through the foramen ovale and ductus arteriosus. There are two categories of disorders of the pulmonary vascular bed that result in PPHN: maladaptation and maldevelopment (Table 7). Maladaptation refers to the situation in which the pulmonary vascular bed is structurally normal but PVR remains high after birth. The cause of the transient form is usually considered to be acute, and the response to therapy is usually rapid. Persistent vasoconstriction is associated with more severe causes such as bacterial septicemia in which mediators such as thromboxane are released that result in intense pulmonary vasoconstriction. Maldevelopment, on the other hand, refers to conditions in which the pulmonary vasculature is abnormal. One type of in utero maldevelopment results when the medial musculature of arterioles is hypertrophied and extends into normally nonmuscularized vessels. These conditions are associated with increased pulmonary blood flow, premature closure of the ductus arteriosus (maternal prostaglandin synthetase inhibitors such as aspirin or indomethacin), or increased systemic blood pressure (intrauterine hypoxia). The other form of maldevelopment occurs with pulmonary underdevelopment. These infants have elevated PVR due to a reduction in the total cross-sectional area of the lung. Two tests may be of benefit in deciding whether PPHN exists in a given patient: (1) in patients with PPHN, right-to-left shunting occurs

across the ductus arteriosus, and there is often an oxygen gradient between the arterial saturation found preductal (right arm) compared with the postductal saturation, and (2) increasing the fraction of inspired oxygen to an FIO_2 of 1.00 often increases the arterial PO_2, especially early in the hospital course. If arterial oxygenation cannot be improved either by increasing the FIO_2 or by other techniques (e.g., alkalosis, lowering PVR), the infant should be evaluated or re-evaluated for cyanotic congenital heart disease.

The goal of therapy in PPHN is twofold: increase oxygen delivery and decrease oxygen demand (Table 8). Oxygen demand can be decreased by ensuring that a neutral thermal environment exists and that the infant is sedated with either morphine sulfate (0.1 mg per kg per dose) or fentanyl as a continuous infusion of 1 to 5 μg per kg per minute. Paralysis (e.g., pancuronium bromide [Pavulon], 0.1 mg per kg per dose) is reserved for those infants requiring extremely high ventilator pressure. Careful ventilatory management, such as described for HMD, should be practiced so as to lessen the long-term effects of air leak. In severe forms of PPHN, consideration should be given to maintaining the arterial PO_2 in the 35 to 45 mm Hg range to decrease lung injury. Serial arterial lactate concentrations and the acid-base status should be carefully monitored. Worsening metabolic acidosis or a rising lactate level implies inadequate tissue delivery of oxygen. If optimal ventilatory care does not improve oxygenation, active attempts to lower PVR should be made. Data from the Nitric Oxide Collaborative Trial have demon-

TABLE 8. **Management of Persistent Pulmonary Hypertension: Increase Oxygen Delivery**

Cardiac output	Volume replacement and dopamine up to 20 μg/kg/min
Hemoglobin concentration	Maintain at ~15 gm/dL by transfusion of packed red blood cells
Oxygen saturation and arterial PO_2	1. Improve distribution of ventilation Surfactant replacement Positive end-expiratory pressure 2. Lower PVR Induced alkalosis: raise the pH to between 7.55 and 7.65 with combination of mild hyperventilation and sodium bicarbonate Drug therapy: nitroprusside (1–5 μg/kg/min); nitric oxide

strated a favorable effect in approximately 50% of patients with PPHN due to diseases *not* associated with underdevelopment of lung parenchyma. In a few patients, extracorporeal membrane oxygenation will be a necessary component of treatment.

Cardiac Disease

Congenital Heart Disease

Innocent heart murmurs or Still's murmurs occur in virtually all infants. These need *no* evaluation, once it is established that there are no constitutional symptoms and the murmur is transitory or episodic. True congenital heart disease, on the other hand, is a major health problem, although a relatively infrequent occurrence (eight infants with congenital heart disease per 1000 births). Approximately one third of all infants with congenital heart disease die within the first month of life. The most common acyanotic lesions are ventricular septal defects, atrial septal defects, and PDA. Many of these close spontaneously over the first days to months of life and are asymptomatic, except for the presence of a murmur. Patients with hypoplastic left heart syndrome usually present within the first week of life with symptoms of cardiovascular collapse and profound metabolic acidosis.

Cyanotic congenital heart disease may be thought of as the 5 T's: transposition of the great arteries, tetrology of Fallot, tricuspid atresia, total anomalous venous return, and truncus arteriosus (pulmonary valve atresia can be thought of as a pseudotruncus).

The hyperoxia test can be helpful in determining whether a given infant has cyanotic congenital heart disease or pulmonary disease. The infant is placed in a hood and 100% oxygen is administered. If the arterial Po_2 rises in excess of 150 mm Hg, cyanotic heart disease is unlikely. An important caveat must be stated: This test must be performed early in the evaluation of the cyanotic infant. If the physician delays unduly, many severe pulmonary conditions (e.g., HMD, PPHN) will not demonstrate a rise in arterial Po_2 with the administration of 100% oxygen.

Most of the more severe cardiac lesions depend on adequate ductal circulation to sustain appropriate pulmonary blood flow and systemic cardiac output (e.g., transposition of the great arteries, hypoplastic left heart syndrome). If a ductus-dependent lesion is suspected, administration of prostaglandin E_1 (alprostadil [Prostin VR Pediatric]), 0.05 to 0.1 µg per kg per minute initially and then titrated to a maintenance dose of 0.01 to 0.4 µg per kg per minute by a continuous intravenous infusion, should be started. The physician must be prepared to intubate and ventilate such patients, as apnea occurs in approximately 15% of infants treated with prostaglandin E_1 (particularly those below 2000 grams in birth weight).

PDA normally undergoes spontaneous physiologic closure by the third day of life. In the preterm infant, however, ductal closure is inversely related to gestational age. In neonates of less than 30 weeks' gestation or 1000 grams of birth weight, the incidence of nonclosure may be in excess of 75% even with the administration of indomethacin postnatally. In those symptomatic infants whose ductus remains patent after a trial of indomethacin, surgical ligation should be undertaken. An asymptomatic ductus does not need definitive (closure) treatment in the neonatal period. As noted, administration of corticosteroids to the mother to reduce the incidence and severity of HMD will result in a diminished number of clinically significant PDAs.

Evaluation of the patient with suspected congenital heart disease, in addition to the physical examination (with four extremity blood pressure measurements), includes chest radiographs and real-time color Doppler cardiac ultrasonography. Electrocardiography may be of benefit in instances of suspected tachyarrhythmia or heart block but is of limited utility in the immediate newborn period due to the presence of physiologic right ventricular hypertrophy.

Blood Pressure

Hypotension is an accompanying problem in many neonatal conditions. It is found frequently in association with hypovolemia, either real or functional (i.e., after acute blood loss or the "third spacing" of intravascular fluid). In the ELBW infant, hypotension is a frequent finding during the first several days of life. Speculation regarding the ability of the ELBW infant to properly maintain corticosteroid homeostasis has been raised by several authors. Moise and colleagues have shown that maternal administration of corticosteroids is associated with less need for blood pressure support (dopamine) during the first 48 hours of life. Further, increasing evidence suggests that refractory hypotension in the ELBW population is secondary to inadequate adrenal response to stress and responds to the administration of corticosteroid replacement therapy. This results in improved vascular tone and augmented cardiac contractility. Treatment of hypovolemia involves the replacement of colloid (e.g., 5% albumin, normal saline, fresh-frozen plasma, or red blood cells).

In the seriously ill neonate, increased capillary permeability is a frequent finding leading to edema formation after overaggressive use of volume replacement. Again, the adequacy of tissue perfusion, as measured by urine output and acid-base homeostasis, should take precedence over a given value of mean arterial blood pressure. Once an adequate vascular volume has been ensured, inotropic support with either dopamine (Intropin) or dobutamine (Dobutrex) therapy, 5 to 20 µg per kg per minute, can be started. There is little evidence that using these two agents in combination is any more efficacious that one alone, and the combination may be harmful if afterload resistance is increased in the face of poor myocardial contractility.

Gastrointestinal System

Necrotizing Enterocolitis

Necrotizing enterocolitis is the primary inflammatory bowel disease seen in the neonatal period. The incidence ranges between 3 and 5% of newborn infants admitted to intensive care units (1% overall) and affects preterm infants predominantly. Term infants, particularly those with diminished left ventricular stroke volume (e.g., hypoplastic left heart syndrome, coarctation) or severe hypoxic-ischemic insult in the perinatal period, are at risk. The cause is multifactorial, but common components include the presence of enteral feedings and impairment of mesenteric blood supply. Multiple pathogens (bacterial, fungal, and viral) have been associated with necrotizing enterocolitis, but the exact determining factor initiating the disease process is unknown. The most common presenting findings include apnea, feeding intolerance, and abdominal distention. Hematochezia is a frequent associated finding. Diagnosis is confirmed by (1) the finding of pneumatosis cystoides intestinalis on abdominal radiographs, or (2) subserosal gas at the time of surgery, or (3) the presence of typical microscopic findings. Thrombocytopenia is common and is an excellent laboratory marker to follow in determining response to treatment. Early recognition, aggressive fluid resuscitation, bowel decompression, and broad-spectrum antibiotic administration (e.g., ampicillin or vancomycin, and gentamicin or amikacin ± clindamycin) are of the utmost importance to ensure an optimal outcome. If perforation or abscess formation occurs, surgical intervention is necessary. Serial abdominal radiographs, particularly a left lateral decubitus film, obtained every 4 to 8 hours depending on the clinical condition of the patient, should be performed during the first several days of the illness to identify any free intra-abdominal air. Once a degree of clinical stability has ensued, total parenteral nutritional support, as outlined previously, is vital. The infant should be given nothing orally for a period of at least 10 to 14 days before any attempt at refeeding.

The mortality rate for necrotizing enterocolitis approaches 15% in most neonatal centers. Approximately 10 to 15% of surviving infants have intestinal strictures, but few have clinical symptoms of obstruction.

Jaundice

Bilirubin and biliverdin, the breakdown products of heme, are antioxidants. However, excessive levels of unconjugated bilirubin have been associated with encephalopathy. The difficulty lies in determining what bilirubin level in a given patient is potentially dangerous. The overall incidence of autopsy-proven kernicterus in premature infants has dramatically fallen in recent years. Some have suggested that the cessation of the use of benzyl alcohol–containing fluids in the nursery has contributed to this decline. Further, a Dutch report that examined 831 5-year-old children who had been born prematurely found no association between bilirubin values and neurologic outcome unless the infant had sustained an IVH. However, there is clearly a level of bilirubin at which demonstrated neurologic injury can occur, in both the preterm and the term infant. The clinical spectrum of bilirubin encephalopathy includes choreoathetoid cerebral palsy, hearing loss, and death.

Elevation of the serum bilirubin level resulting in jaundice (≥5 mg per dL) occurs in approximately 50% of full-term newborn infants and most preterm infants after the first day of life. Virtually all these infants have no underlying pathologic reason for the jaundice. This *physiologic jaundice* is due to a shortened red blood cell life span, relative hepatic cellular enzyme immaturity, and enterohepatic circulation caused by increased β-glucuronidase activity and decreased intestinal transit times due to small volumes of feeds and/or gut immaturity.

Jaundice that is present at birth, or occurring before 18 hours of life, is almost always due to hemolysis (glucose-6-phosphate dehydrogenase and ABO or Rh isoimmunization are the most frequent causes in the United States) and requires evaluation. Similarly, jaundice persisting beyond 2 to 3 weeks of age requires evaluation whether it is due to elevated conjugated or elevated unconjugated bilirubin. Jaundice that involves only the face and upper thorax requires no evaluation unless it is found at less than 24 hours of age or is persistent. The American Academy of Pediatrics has issued treatment recommendations for the term infant *without* hemolytic disease (Table 9). Note that phototherapy need not be started until the total serum bilirubin level exceeds 15 mg per dL. In the preterm infant or the infant with hemolytic disease, no absolute guidelines exist! The National Institute for Child Health and Development guidelines for the level of bilirubin at which exchange transfusion is recommended are shown in Table 10. Whether these guidelines represent optimal care is not known. Phototherapy can be administered by using either a special blue or green fluorescent light

TABLE 9. **Management of Hyperbilirubinemia in the Healthy Term Newborn**

Age in Hours	Total Serum Bilirubin Concentration (mg/dL [μmol/L])		
	Phototherapy	*Exchange Transfusion if Phototherapy Fails*	*Exchange Transfusion and Phototherapy*
≤24*			
25–48	≥15 [260]	≥20 [340]	≥25 [430]
48–72	≥18 [310]	≥25 [430]	≥30 [510]
>72	≥20 [340]	≥25 [340]	≥30 [510]

*Clinically apparent jaundice in the first 24 h of life should be evaluated separately from the recommendations in this table.

TABLE 10. **Bilirubin Levels and Exchange Transfusion Criteria:**
Level at Which Exchange Transfusion Is Recommended at Given Birth Weights

Infant Category	Bilirubin Levels (mg/dL) for Birth Weights of				
	<1250 Grams	1250–1499 Grams	1500–1999 Grams	2000–2499 Grams	>2500 Grams
Normal risk	13	15	17	18	20
High risk	10	13	15	17	18

or a quartz-halide light. If phototherapy is instituted with blue lights, there should be at least four special blue lamps coupled with two daylight lamps to decrease the discomfort and vertigo that may occur in the nursery staff. Whether fluorescent lights or quartz-halide lights are used, the equivalent of at least 10 to 12 watts per cm^2 per nm of irradiance must be available at the level of the mattress. Higher levels of irradiance provide little or no additional benefit; therefore, "double-bank" lights are usually not necessary if a single bank of lights provides appropriate irradiance. Enteral nutrition (formula or breast-feeding) or parenteral nutrition should be continued while phototherapy is administered.

Neurologic Disease

Intracranial Hemorrhage

Hemorrhage within the cranium is unusual in the term infant and has been associated with untoward events occurring during the process of parturition, although it may occur spontaneously, particularly in the case of subarachnoid bleeding. In the preterm infant of 31 completed weeks' gestation or less, the incidence of subependymal hemorrhage or IVH ranges between 20 and 30% of inborn infants cared for at tertiary care units. An incidence as high as 45% may occur in less skilled facilities or in outborn infants. The incidence and severity of hemorrhage are inversely related to the degree of prematurity, with ELBW infants having significantly more severe forms of IVH. Neurologic sequelae occur frequently in those infants with either intraparenchymal hemorrhage or acute hemorrhage associated with acute ventricular dilatation. For the milder forms of hemorrhage (i.e., subependymal or minimal bleeding into the ventricle without dilatation), the neurologic outcome is no different from that found in the preterm infant without hemorrhage. Spastic diplegia is the most common form of motor impairment in preterm infants. The cause of IVH is unknown but appears to be related in large part to wide swings in blood pressure and the presence of a perfusion-reperfusion injury involving the periventricular region of the premature infant's brain. Thus, measures designed to provide the least manipulation of the infant during the first 3 to 5 days of life have been shown to decrease the incidence of bleeding.

Seizures

The presence of seizures in the newborn period may portend significant sequelae later in life, but the prognosis depends on the cause of the seizure, not the seizure itself in most instances. An electroencephalogram should be obtained during the clinical symptoms thought to represent a seizure phenomenon if at all possible. Most episodes of subtle automatisms such as lip smacking, chewing, apnea, clonus, and tonic posturing are *not* electrographic seizures of cortical brain origin. In those infants who manifest seizure activity after a complicated delivery, most of these clinical findings are cortical release phenomena and not true seizures. Among the causes of neonatal seizures are hypoxic-ischemic encephalopathy, intracranial hemorrhage, infections, metabolic derangements, developmental brain anomalies, and drug withdrawal. Identification and treatment of the underlying condition are paramount to appropriate seizure control. Phenobarbital is the initial treatment of choice: 20 mg per kg as a loading dose, followed by 4 to 5 mg per kg per day maintenance therapy. (Up to 40 mg per kg can be given as a loading dose, but one must monitor for respiratory depression and apnea.) Phenytoin (Dilantin) can be added for better seizure control but has unpredictable absorption when given orally. Diazepam (Valium) and lorazepam (Ativan) are useful in the treatment of status epilepticus, but their short half-lives make them unacceptable for maintenance therapy.

Hypoxic-Ischemic Encephalopathy

There is little relationship between resultant neurologic sequelae, including cerebral palsy, and the events of birth. Further, the term "birth asphyxia" is imprecise and should not be used. The American Academy of Pediatrics and the American College of Obstetricians and Gynecologists have noted that a neonate who has had hypoxia in the immediate perinatal period that is severe enough to result in encephalopathy will demonstrate other evidence of injury including *all* of the following:

- Profound metabolic or mixed acidemia (pH of <7.00) on an umbilical cord arterial blood sample, if obtained
- Persistence of an Apgar score of 0 to 3 for longer than 5 minutes
- Neonatal neurologic sequelae (e.g., seizures, coma, hypotonia)
- Multiorgan system dysfunction (i.e., cardiovascular, gastrointestinal, hematologic, pulmonary, or renal system)

One third of infants who sustain the degree of hypoxia-ischemia sufficient to cause injury to the brain die. Apgar scores at 1 minute have no correlation with neurologic outcome, and low scores at 5 minutes have little bearing on outcome unless these low scores are persistent. The neurologic symptoms are apparent at the time of delivery. The symptoms may worsen in the succeeding 24 to 48 hours to the point of cortical brain death and brain stem dysfunction, or they may improve during a 5- to 7-day period. In those infants whose neurologic and electroencephalographic examinations become normal, neurologic sequelae are exceedingly unusual and most likely have another explanation than hypoxic-ischemic injury. Cerebral palsy resulting from hypoxic-ischemic encephalopathy is usually a spastic quadriplegia associated with severe mental retardation. The cause of other forms of cerebral palsy is unknown. It should be noted that pre-existing neurologic abnormalities may frequently result in neurologic depression of the infant at the time of delivery.

Treatment is directed toward adequate resuscitation of the infant at the time of delivery and support of those systems that are dysfunctional. Of primary importance is attention to those areas discussed previously regarding warmth, fluids, and nutritional support. Maintaining a heat-conserving environment while providing adequate caloric support with glucose is critical. Most infants who sustain a significant hypoxic-ischemic event, as defined previously, have release of arginine vasopressin (antidiuretic hormone) with subsequent retention of water from diminished urine production. Further, transient acute tubular necrosis is a frequent finding. Providing enough nutritional support to maintain a neutral nitrogen balance while ensuring fluid restriction to decrease the risk of hyponatremia and cerebral edema may be difficult. If an infant required intubation to maintain pulmonary function, biochemical and clinical monitoring that demonstrates recovery must take place before extubation is attempted.

Although head ultrasonography is useful in the preterm infant (to document IVH), computed tomography or magnetic resonance imaging is more useful in the term infant. If an assessment regarding the extent of neurologic injury is desired, magnetic resonance imaging or computed tomography performed at 2 to 4 weeks of age provides more information.

Infectious Disease

The frequency of septicemia in the newborn infant ranges between 1 and 5 per 1000 live births. Meningitis occurs at between 0.4 and 1 per 1000 live births. This high incidence of infection exists because of the relative immaturity of the newborn infant's immune system (Table 11).

Infection is acquired in three distinct ways: transplacental (maternal infection), intrapartum (vaginal flora), or post partum (nosocomial). Each of the three routes of acquisition implies different pathogens and thus different treatment regimens.

Infection (bacterial, viral, protozoan, spirochetal, or fungal) may present initially with virtually any

TABLE 11. Host Defense of the Newborn Compared with That of the Adult

Decreased humoral antibodies: IgG, IgM, IgA
Decreased polymorphonuclear phagocytes
Diminished phagocytosis
Decreased white blood cell killing
Decreased complement, opsonins, lysozymes
Diminished specific enzyme production

combination of abnormal clinical findings. These findings may be represented by merely poor feeding or may be a fulminant shock state. Aggressive evaluation and treatment are necessary as the mortality associated with infection ranges between 10 and 50%, depending on the gestational age of the infant and the severity of the presenting symptoms. The history and clinical examination should guide the intensity of the laboratory and radiographic evaluation and the urgency of starting therapy. For example, maternal chorioamnionitis associated with an asymptomatic term infant with normal vital signs does not require any additional laboratory evaluation other than a blood culture. On the other hand, fulminant septic shock requires evaluation of at least the following: acid-base balance, oxygenation, electrolyte levels, glucose levels, a complete blood and platelet count, and appropriate radiographs.

Blood and cerebrospinal fluid cultures are appropriate in most patients. Although a urine culture can be obtained in the infant evaluated for infection at the time of birth, primary urinary tract infection is unusual at this time. After the first 48 to 72 hours of life, however, a urine culture should be obtained, either by catheterization of the bladder or by suprapubic aspiration, in addition to cultures of blood and cerebrospinal fluid. Additional culture sites should be determined by the clinical findings. Surface cultures are not indicated.

Most maternally acquired bacterial pathogens (i.e., transplacental or vaginal flora) are sensitive to a combination of ampicillin (Omnipen, Polycillin, Principen) and gentamicin (Garamycin). Nosocomially acquired bacterial infection, however, includes resistant microorganisms such as methicillin-resistant *Staphylococcus aureus*. Thus, vancomycin (Vancocin) in combination with either a third-generation cephalosporin (e.g., cefotaxime [Claforan]) or an aminoglycoside (amikacin [Amikin], gentamicin) would be indicated. Because of the rapid emergence of resistant bacteria to the third-generation cephalosporins, many authors recommend that they be used only in narrowly defined circumstances such as gram-negative meningitis. The duration of treatment depends on the microorganism isolated and the site of infection. A total treatment time of 10 days for simple bacteremia, a minimum of 14 days for meningitis caused by a group B steptococci, and 21 days for gram-negative bacillary meningitis is recommended. Once a particular bacterium is isolated and antibiotic sensitivities are identified, treatment should be directed to the narrowest spectrum antibiotic possible.

Further, stopping antibiotic therapy as quickly as possible is advisable because of increasing concerns regarding the emergence of resistant bacteria (e.g., vancomycin-resistant enterococci). With currently available bacteriologic techniques (assuming appropriate blood inoculum), antibiotics should be stopped no later than 48 hours after negative cultures have been obtained. In a patient with clinical infection and negative cultures, treatment should be continued for the 10-day minimum. Because of possible ototoxicity and renal toxicity, peak and trough levels of vancomycin and the aminoglycosides (e.g., gentamicin, amikacin) should be determined when steady-state serum levels have occurred (i.e., before and after the fifth dose) in the patient with normal renal function. Treatment of viral, protozoan, or fungal disease is best carried out in consultation with or by a pediatric infectious disease specialist.

Ethical Issues

Neonatal Mortality

Although neonatal care has improved markedly in the last decade, the issues of when to resuscitate and when to cease support are very much with us. Parents must be involved in these major decisions, but a realization that parental wishes are not always medically appropriate has to be present. Frank and substantive discussions in ethically difficult situations, using the most recent outcome data, must be an ongoing activity of those persons who care for ill infants. It should be remembered that from a moral and ethical perspective, omission or commission of an act is equivalent (i.e., withdrawal of care versus not adding to the level of care). Just because "we can do something" does not mean that "we should do something." Parents deserve from their child's physician the best medical information and the best recommendation based on that information. Physicians are the ones to make the recommendation for withdrawal of care, when appropriate. We do not ask the parents to withdraw care! Further, this information must be conveyed in easily understandable English, not medical jargon.

An autopsy should be requested in most instances of fetal or neonatal death. Sixty percent of autopsies reveal information not known at the time of death. Some of this information indicates a problem of an inheritable nature that will have a bearing on future pregnancies. In addition, an autopsy allows the physician to help the parents in their progression through the grieving process.

Referral to a Tertiary Care Center

Maternal or neonatal transfer should occur whenever the infant's expected or present illness is beyond the capabilities of either the physician or the hospital. Even though a physician may have the necessary training to manage a given condition, if the proper facilities (personnel and equipment) are not available, the morbidity and cost of the infant's acute care

will rise. Further, as preterm and very ill term infants are at an increased risk for developmental disability, the planning and coordination of such children with special needs may be better carried out through the auspices of a tertiary care center, with the primary care being done in a "medical home."

NORMAL INFANT FEEDING

method of
WILLIAM J. KLISH, M.D.
Baylor College of Medicine
Houston, Texas

BREAST-FEEDING

Breast-feeding remains the optimal choice of infant feeding by all major societies and agencies, including the American Academy of Pediatrics and the World Health Organization. These groups base their recommendations on the strong scientific evidence of decreased infant mortality in developing countries and decreased morbidity in developed countries seen in exclusively breast-fed infants compared with those fed human milk substitutes. No commercially processed infant formula has been developed that reproduces the immunologic properties, nutrient bioavailability, digestibility, and trophic effects of human milk. Breast-feeding also offers psychologic and behavioral benefits to both mother and infant. The postpartum status of the mother is improved by hormones released during breast-feeding. Infant sucking induces the release of oxytocin, thereby accelerating the involution of the uterus. Exclusive breast-feeding resulting in frequent nipple stimulation can suppress ovulation. However, in developed countries, where more "structured" feeding schedules are practiced, suppression may not be sustaining and therefore not used as a form of birth control. Animal studies have demonstrated an increased threshold for maternal stress, presumably due to the hormones released during breast-feeding.

Physician's Role in Infant-Feeding Decision-Making

Prenatal visits should include discussion of infant-feeding issues. This provides the parents an opportunity to make an informed choice by gaining information. Allowing this open discussion of the facts helps diffuse guilt, because not knowing about or a lack of support from a physician for breast-feeding causes guilt. Studies have demonstrated that prenatal education and breast-feeding support from family and friends, especially the infant's father, are associated with the mother's choice of breast-feeding regardless of maternal age, ethnic group, educational level, or marital status. Prenatally, mothers are intensely focused on readiness for the birth experience; therefore, breast-feeding instruction and information need to be reviewed after delivery. The office and clinic environment can send a strong message to parents about the priorities of the clinician and staff. An office replete with formula advertisements in the form of posters, pads, and pencils gives a subtle message that may undermine any verbal lip service to breast-feeding. A thorough history and breast examination should be performed during the prenatal period. A history of previous breast surgery and previous breast-feeding experiences should be obtained. Previous breast surgery is not a contraindication to breast-feeding; however, the type of surgery (augmentation vs. reduction) and surgical technique used (periareolar vs. submammary) might affect lactation performance and must be considered during the progression of lactation. An assessment of nipple type allows early intervention when appropriate. Flat and inverted nipples are not always of concern because the infant latches on to the areola and not the nipple. Breast care beyond normal daily hygiene is not necessary. Practices such as "toughening of the nipples" are not recommended and can actually damage breast tissue.

Initiation of Breast-Feeding

Breast-feeding is enhanced by early initiation. It is ideal to place the infant at the breast immediately after birth. Test feedings of water are not necessary to assess sucking and swallowing. Subsequent feedings are usually sporadic, depending on the use of maternal medication during labor and delivery, but should not be more than 3 to 4 hours apart. Frequent feedings provide the necessary hormonal stimulation needed for the establishment of an adequate maternal milk volume. To allow adequate milk transfer to the infant, proper positioning and latch-on at the breast are important. This is facilitated with hands-on instruction provided by knowledgeable nursing or medical staff. Breast-feeding books and videos are helpful but should not be used as a replacement for supportive assistance. Hospital policies that support rooming-in options and avoidance of water and glucose feedings after breast-feeding send a clear message to breast-feeding mothers. Controlled studies have clearly demonstrated that infants who are given water, glucose water, or formula instead of human milk exclusively in the first week lose more weight, regain it more slowly, and have higher bilirubin levels and fewer stools.

Early feedings should not be timed to some predetermined duration. Each infant is individual in his or her feeding behavior and especially in the first few days may be too sleepy to nurse for long durations. Feeding durations may range from 3 to 20 minutes at each breast. Improper positioning and latch-on at the breast rather than the length of feeding are associated with the degree of nipple soreness. Both breasts are usually offered at each feeding; however, some infants may fall asleep before taking the second breast. An understanding that the fat content in the milk increases as the breast is emptied is further validation of the importance of not limiting the feeding duration. This change in milk fat content also explains why the infant can get an adequate volume and caloric intake by nursing one breast at a feeding.

Frequent feedings allowing time for complete breast emptying are associated with adequate maternal lactogenic hormone levels and increased milk volume. Most infants drive their mothers' milk volume by waking for 10 to 12 feedings in a 24-hour period. Some infants may sleep for one extended duration of 4 hours in a 24-hour period and as a result cluster those 10 or so feedings in a tighter period. Given these variations in infant behavior and the move to shorter hospital stays, instruction regarding breast-feeding should be kept simple and as uncomplicated as possible. Discharge information regarding breast-feeding should also emphasize what to expect in terms of breast changes with the increase in milk flow, frequency, and duration of feedings; and signs of adequate milk intake including stooling and urination patterns.

Early Breast-Feeding Management and Follow-up

With the change to shorter hospital stays after delivery, breast-feeding mothers are discharged with little instruction before the transition from colostrum to transitional and subsequent mature milk. Most mothers experience increased breast fullness during the first few days after delivery. However, a distinction should be made between breast fullness and engorgement. Breast fullness is a normal transitory state during which the breast tissue remains compressible, allowing the infant to suck efficiently and comfortably. Engorgement is caused by improper positioning as well as a delay or restriction in feeding frequency and duration. It presents as generalized swollen rigid tissue, resulting in a taut, shiny appearance of the breast. Given this tightness, the infant finds it difficult to grasp the breast, causing increased milk stasis and maternal discomfort. Prompt intervention is needed to promote milk flow and reduce swelling. An electric *intermittent* minimal pressure breast pump along with warm compresses may need to be used to facilitate milk flow. Providing the primipara mother with information on these breast changes, emphasizing the importance of frequent feedings, significantly reduces the chances of severe engorgement.

Another result of early hospital discharge is the loss of the opportunity by the physician to observe the establishment of successful breast-feeding. To compensate for this, a mechanism for early postpartum follow-up is essential to ensure breast-feeding success. A visit to the office on the third postpartum day allows the physician to assess the infant's positioning at the breast, passing of meconium stool, and urination patterns, and maternal breast changes. On postpartum day 6, a follow-up telephone call is helpful to document feeding frequency and duration, to check urine and stool frequency, and to offer support

TABLE 1. **Signs of Adequate Milk Intake in the Exclusively Breast-Fed Infant**

Nurses approximately 8–10 times/24 h; may have cluster feedings

Has at least six (paper) to eight (cloth) wet (pale yellow urine) diapers in 24 h

Has transition from meconium (tarry) to milk stool (yellow, seedy) by postpartum day 7; may have as many as 5–10 stools/d during the first month, less often after 4 wk

Has initial weight loss not exceeding 10% of birth weight

Regains birth weight by the second week of life, with an average weight gain of 30 gm/d thereafter

and information. This should be followed by a clinic (or home) visit at 2 weeks to check the infant's weight gain. Follow-up allows monitoring of the mother's and infant's progress and early intervention when necessary. Exclusively breast-fed infants receiving adequate milk intake usually follow the pattern described in Table 1.

Inadequate infant weight gain may be due to infant or maternal factors. An assessment of the breast-feeding mother-infant dyad is necessary to make a thorough assessment. Treating only one member of this dyad is not sufficient if breast-feeding is to be preserved. The most common cause of inadequate milk supply is improper instruction to the mother. Maternal stress and fatigue can result in a faulty milk ejection (letdown) reflex. When supplemental feeding is necessary, the mother should continue breast stimulation by mechanical breast pumping to maintain milk volume. If milk volume is maintained, exclusive breast-feeding can again resume once the infant's weight gain improves.

When mothers complain of sore nipples, the first step is to observe the infant latching on to the breast. Infants should latch on to the soft tissue of the areola, not the base of the nipple. For this reason, mothers with flat or even inverted nipples may not experience a problem with breast-feeding because the infant sucks the areola and not the nipple. If the physician is not experienced in observing breast-feeding, an experienced individual should be consulted.

Breast-Feeding and Maternal Employment

Many women return to work outside the home after delivery; in these cases continuation of breast-feeding is possible but requires some planning and support. Mothers have reported that maintenance of lactation is easier if the return to employment is delayed for a few months post partum. When that is not possible, a gradual return to full-time employment may facilitate the development of feeding and pumping schedules. The mother needs to express her milk during the work day to maintain hormonal levels and milk volume. A variety of electric and battery-operated breast pumps are available for purchase and rental. Expressed breast milk should be refrigerated and fed to the infant within 48 hours.

Glass or hard plastic is ideal for milk storage. When soft plastic bags are used, it is best to use two bags to prevent leakage during storage. Mothers should be informed that it is normal to see a decrease in expressed milk volume during a 5-day work week. Breast-feeding exclusively on the weekend restores the lowered volume.

Many companies have seen a decrease in employee absenteeism due to infant illness when mothers can continue breast-feeding. Some companies provide facilities to allow privacy while pumping. Enabling a mother to continue this breast-feeding relationship after her return to work outside the home makes the transition from full-time mother to working mother less stressful.

Maternal Fever

Maternal fever *is not* a contraindication to breast-feeding. The maternal ability to manufacture secretory IgA specific to the infection that her infant is exposed to and excrete it in her milk provides her infant with a unique and potent protection from infection. Cessation of breast-feeding during this time prevents this elegant protective cycle from occurring.

Contraindications to Breast-Feeding

Some Maternal Medications

Breast-feeding is contraindicated during maternal use of drugs of abuse (i.e., heroin, cocaine). There are few other drugs that are contraindicated during breast-feeding. Up-to-date references are important to keep current with recommendations. The *Physicians' Desk Reference* is a poor resource for information on the excretion of drugs in breast milk.

Breast Cancer

A mother with breast cancer should not nurse her infant to allow immediate definitive treatment. Prolactin levels remain quite high during lactation, and prolactin may advance mammary cancer.

Human Immunodeficiency Virus–Positive Mother

The Centers for Disease Control and Prevention and the Public Health Service recommend that women who test positive for human immunodeficiency virus (HIV) antibody should be counseled to avoid breast-feeding.

FORMULA FEEDING

Because not all mothers are able or willing to breast-feed their infants, substitute methods of infant feeding have always been available. The history of modern infant formulas began in 1849, when Baron Justus von Leibig recognized that all living tissue, including food, was composed of different proportions of carbohydrate, fat, and protein. This resulted in the first commercially available human milk substitute, Baron von Leibig's Soluble Food, which was available in the United States by 1869. The composition of infant formulas has evolved greatly during the past century as our understanding of nutrient requirements, absorptive physiology, and metabolic disturbances has advanced. A large array of routine and special-purpose infant formulas is currently available. To select the proper formulas for particular circumstances, it is necessary to understand the significance of the various nutrients constituting them.

Energy Content of Infant Formulas

Infant formulas contain energy in the form of carbohydrate and fat as well as protein, minerals, vitamins, and water in amounts sufficient to meet all the nutritional requirements of a healthy, growing infant. The energy content of a routine infant formula is 20 kcal per ounce. This caloric density was chosen because human milk contains an average of 20 kcal per ounce even though there are significant variations in the energy content of human milk depending on the stage of lactation. Formulas for premature infants usually contain 24 kcal per ounce because premature infants frequently have difficulty ingesting an adequate volume of formula. Occasionally, formula for premature infants is mixed to provide 27 to 30 kcal per ounce.

Carbohydrates in Infant Formulas

Lactose

Lactose is the most common sugar in infant formula. Because lactose is the disaccharide found in almost all mammalian milks, including human milk, it is the logical choice for the carbohydrate for routine infant feeding. Human milk contains approximately 7 grams of lactose per 100 mL (7%). Most infant formulas also contain 7% lactose.

Lactose is hydrolyzed on the brush border of the intestine by lactase, a disaccharidase enzyme, releasing the monosaccharides glucose and galactose, which are then absorbed. Lactase is present in a relatively small amount in comparison to the other disaccharidases. For every unit of lactase activity present on the intestinal brush border, there are 2 units of sucrase activity and approximately 6 to 8 units of maltase activity. For this reason, it is common to have lactose intolerance after acute gastroenteritis. Nonspecific injury to the intestinal mucosa affects lactase activity more significantly than that of the other more plentiful disaccharidases.

Because lactose is absorbed less efficiently than are other sugars such as sucrose or starch, some is allowed to enter the distal bowel. It is fermented there by intestinal bacteria, resulting in a slightly lower pH in the intestinal lumen. This change in the intestinal milieu appears to favor the growth of acidophilic bacteria such as lactobacillus at the expense of less favorable, pathogenic bacteria. The lower pH also appears to enhance the absorption of calcium and phosphorus from the distal small intestine.

Premature infants are born with less lactase than are full-term infants. Infants born at 30 to 34 weeks' gestation have intestinal lactase levels approximately 50% of the level in a full-term infant. Lactose is still an important component of the diet of the premature infant because of the benefits described. However, because of this limited lactose tolerance, formulas for premature infants contain lactose combined with other carbohydrates to decrease the lactose load.

Even though lactose intolerance is a well-recognized complication of acute gastroenteritis, it does not occur as often as one might expect. In a study of infants admitted to the hospital with acute diarrhea, only 13% developed significant clinical symptoms of lactose intolerance and required a change in formula. Almost all the infants who developed lactose intolerance recovered their ability to absorb lactose within 30 days. Most infants, therefore, do not need lactose restriction simply because they develop acute gastroenteritis. Infants who do develop secondary lactose intolerance and are switched to a lactose-free formula should be rechallenged with lactose within a month to determine recovery.

Sucrose

Sucrose-based formulas are indicated for the feeding of infants with lactose intolerance. These formulas should be used only when indicated because sucrose has a less favorable influence on the intestinal pH in the normal infant. Occasionally, infants are born with sucrase-isomaltase deficiency and cannot tolerate sucrose. These infants, however, should be able to tolerate lactose-containing formulas. Infants with significant generalized small bowel disease may malabsorb sucrose. For these infants, formulas are available with modified corn syrup solids or glucose polymers as the carbohydrate source.

Modified Starch and Emulsifiers

Under normal circumstances, starch is digested in the intestinal lumen by α-amylase secreted by the pancreas and salivary glands. This results in a mixture of maltose, isomaltose, and α–limit dextrins, which are low-molecular-weight starches (three to five glucose units). These products are then further hydrolyzed to glucose by maltase enzymes present on the intestinal brush border. The glucose formed is either absorbed directly or spilled back into the lumen of the intestine for distal absorption. An alternative pathway for the digestion of starch is through hydrolysis by glucoamylase, which is a brush border enzyme. Pancreatic amylase secretion is low in the newborn, so starch is digested largely by intestinal glucoamylase. Very few clinical situations have been documented, however, in which starch is not tolerated by the normal newborn.

Most infant formulas contain starch in one form or another. It may be present as an emulsifier in the form of tapioca or cornstarch or added to a formula for calories in the form of corn syrup solids. Several products that are derived from the hydrolysis of cornstarch are available commercially for use as a calorie additive to formulas.

An advantage of adding modified starch or glucose polymers to formulas as a source of calories is that they change the osmolality little because of their large molecular size. They are also readily absorbed because they are hydrolyzed by maltase, the most abundant disaccharidase. They are colorless, impart little sweetness, and have low viscosity, so they can be added in significant amounts without changing the physical characteristics of a formula. Whenever additives are put in formulas, care must be taken so that they do not dilute the other ingredients and result in nutrient imbalances. For example, a standard 20 kcal per ounce formula normally contains about 10% of its calories as protein. If this formula is fortified to 30 kcal per ounce by adding carbohydrate, the protein content drops to about 6.5% of the calories, which represents a marginal protein intake in a normal child.

Fat

Long Chain Triglycerides

Fat provides the major source of energy for growing infants. In human milk, about 50% of the energy is from fat, and in commercial formulas fat provides 40 to 50% of the energy. Most routine infant formulas contain vegetable oil as the source of fat. Cow milk contains much less essential fatty acid (linoleic acid) than does human milk. This initially led manufacturers of infant formulas to add vegetable oil to the skimmed cow milk base of their preparations. These oils continue to be used not only because of their essential fatty acid content, but also because they are better absorbed from the infant gut than butterfat.

Fatty acids essential for humans are the derivatives of 18:2n6 (omega-6) fatty acid, or linoleic acid. This acid cannot be made in mammalian tissue. Linoleic acid and its derivative 20:4n6 arachidonic acid are components of cell membranes but more importantly serve as precursors for prostaglandins. Essential fatty acid should provide at least 3% of the total caloric intake of an individual. Human milk contains about 7% of the calories as linoleic acid, depending on the maternal diet. Unmodified cow milk has only about 1%. Most commercial infant formulas contain more than 10%.

Some have suggested that fatty acids that are the derivatives of the omega-3 fatty acid linolenic acid be added to infant formulas. Data exist that imply that premature infants fed these fatty acids have increased visual acuity and perhaps enhanced intellectual achievement. However, if they are not added in an appropriate proportion to omega-6 fatty acids, growth retardation may result. Studies are ongoing to determine their appropriateness for infant formulas.

Fat is the most difficult component of food to digest and absorb because of its hydrophobic nature. A normal adult can absorb only about 95% of ingested fat. Infants are less efficient and sometimes absorb as little as 85% of the ingested fat. A sophisticated system for the absorption of long chain triglycerides exists. Ingested triglycerides are emulsified by bile salts. The small emulsion particles, or micelles, provide a large surface area for the action of pancreatic and human milk lipase. Lipase removes the two outer fatty acids from the glycerol backbone of the triglyceride, leaving the easily absorbed monoglyceride and the fatty acids. These pass into the mucosal cells of the small intestine, where they are reassembled into triglycerides, coated with a protein, and extruded as chylomicrons into the lymphatics of the small bowel. The longer the chain length of the fatty acids, the slower the absorption. The introduction of double bonds into the fatty acid enhances absorption.

Medium Chain Triglycerides

Medium chain triglycerides are absorbed more efficiently than are long chain triglycerides in normal infants. The addition of medium chain triglycerides to formula for premature infants enhances not only the absorption of fat but also the absorption of calcium and magnesium.

Most of the uniqueness associated with medium chain triglycerides is due to one physical property. Medium chain triglycerides are partially soluble in water because of the enhanced solubility of their fatty acids. At 20°C, 69 mg of octanoic acid (C_8) dissolves in 100 mL of H_2O compared with 0.7 mg of palmitic acid (C_{16}). Pancreatic lipase can also hydrolyze medium chain triglycerides more effectively than long chain triglycerides, resulting in more efficient digestion in situations in which the lipase level is decreased in the intestinal lumen. Once octanoic acid is released, it is so hydrophilic that it enhances the solubility of other triglycerides. This enhanced solubility allows more triglyceride to get to the intestinal mucosa, where brush border lipase can hydrolyze it to allow absorption. Because of this property, medium chain triglycerides can bypass the need for emulsification by bile acids. They are also not dependent on pancreatic lipase for hydrolysis because they can use brush border lipase. About half of the absorbed medium chain triglycerides are transported directly into the portal venous system rather than the lymphatics. Medical indications for the use of medium chain triglycerides are pancreatic insufficiency, hepatic insufficiency, and diseases that affect the lymphatics of the intestinal tract such as lymphangiectasia and perhaps severe congestive heart failure.

Medium chain triglycerides do have side effects, however. As early as 1968, when they were first being introduced, at least one publication warned that diarrhea could occur in patients fed medium chain triglycerides. If medium chain triglycerides are malabsorbed either because of overfeeding or intestinal mucosal disease, they enhance secretion in the distal small bowel, which results in diarrhea. This side effect is a risk of using medium chain triglycerides as a caloric supplement in infant formula. Some studies have implied that feeding medium chain triglycerides stimulates the resting metabolic rate, resulting in an increase in caloric requirements for an individual. If this proves to be true, the advantage of feeding this fat due to increased absorption would be offset by this increase in caloric requirements. Finally, medium chain triglycerides are more difficult to manufacture, so they are more expensive than long chain triglycerides.

Protein

Casein

Casein is a group of milk-specific proteins characterized by their low solubility at an acidic pH, resulting in curd formation, and by their ability to form complex micelles with calcium and phosphorus salts. There are four electrophoretic groups of casein that are represented in cow milk in the following portions: α (50 to 55%), β (30 to 35%), κ (15%), γ (5%). Genetic and species variation is present in each group. Human casein is more heterogeneous than is cow casein, and β-casein is predominant. Differences exist in the amino acid composition between human and bovine casein even within the electrophoretic groups, accounting for the slight differences in biologic value of the proteins.

Whey

Whey is the protein that remains in solution after casein has been precipitated by acid. It is a mixture of proteins that frequently have important biologic functions. The predominant whey protein in human milk is α-lactalbumin, which is involved in lactose synthesis. Lactoferrin is the second most abundant whey protein in human milk and is thought to play a role in iron absorption as well as in local host defense. Lysozyme, another whey protein, has antibacterial properties, and because it is resistant to digestive enzymes, it can pass intact through the infant's intestinal tract. Immunoglobulins composed principally of secretory IgA are present and impart local intestinal immunity to the infant fed human milk. β-Lactoglobulin is the predominant protein found in whey of bovine milk. Its function is unknown.

Whey-predominant formulas tend to mimic human milk more closely, making these formulas popular, particularly for the feeding of the premature infant. These have the advantage of being rapidly emptied from the stomach due to little curd formation. They appear to have virtually eliminated the problem of lactobezoars, which were seen occasionally in preterm infants in the past. They may sometimes be helpful in minimizing gastroesophageal reflux because they are emptied rapidly from the stomach.

Soy Proteins

Soy-based protein formulas, because they are lactose free, are primarily indicated for use in infants with lactose intolerance. They can also be fed to infants of strict vegetarians if the parents refuse to use products based on cow milk. Most soy formulas, however, are used for infants who are suspected of having cow milk protein intolerance. Soy-based formulas were introduced in the 1950s. Most prolonged diarrhea in infants seen during that period was thought to be due to cow milk protein intolerance. Many of these infants responded to feedings with soy protein formula, thus establishing this indication. Carbohydrate intolerance as a cause of chronic diarrhea was not well described until the 1960s. We now know that much of the chronic diarrhea seen in infancy is due to carbohydrate intolerance, and the cessation of diarrhea in many of the infants described in these early papers was probably due to the fact that soy formulas are lactose free. Infants who are known to be sensitive to cow milk protein should have soy protein introduced cautiously, because many of these infants are also intolerant to soy.

Soy protein formulas have also been used in the treatment of infantile colic because of the presumed intolerance to cow milk protein in this syndrome. Many of the studies of the use of soy protein formulas for this purpose are inconclusive, because defining a study population of infants with colic is difficult because of the lack of specific criteria for this syndrome.

A potential problem that could arise from the prolonged feeding of soy formula is bone demineralization. Phytic acid is a contaminant in the processing of soy protein and can form a complex with certain minerals such as calcium and zinc. This results in the decreased absorption of these minerals. The absence of lactose in soy formula is an additional factor that can interfere with calcium absorption. Most soy protein–based formulas have calcium added to help eliminate this problem. All soy products contain phytoestrogens in biologically significant amounts. Their importance in soy formula has yet to be determined.

Hydrolyzed Protein

Hydrolyzed cow milk protein is used in a group of infant formulas. These formulas are designed for use in infants who are intolerant to intact cow milk protein, but they are also helpful in infants who have a limited ability to absorb nutrients due to either a short gut or intestinal mucosal disease. The protein is hydrolyzed enzymatically, and most is broken down to free amino acids and small peptides. However, some products contain higher molecular weight peptides that are capable of antigenic expression. In infants with known protein hypersensitivity, it is important to select a product that contains little antigenic potential.

Because hydrolyzed protein in essence is predigested, it is absorbed efficiently in the proximal small intestine, hence its advantage in patients with the short-gut syndrome. Most products made with hydrolyzed protein have little residue, which results in a decrease in fecal production. This decrease is helpful in infants in whom fecal material might be a disadvantage, such as in perineal burns or rectal surgery. Hydrolyzed protein does not require pancre-

TABLE 2. **Standard Milk-Based Formulas**

Formula	Content (gm/100 mL)			Content (mg/100 mL)			Source		Osmolality (mOsm/kg of H$_2$O) and General Comments
	Pro	Fat	CHO	$\frac{Na}{K}$	$\frac{Ca}{P}$	Fe	CHO	Fat	
Similac (Ross) (20 kcal/30 mL)	1.5	3.6	7.1	$\frac{18}{70}$	$\frac{49}{37}$	1.2 (without iron 0.2)	Lactose	Coconut oil Soy oil	300 Whey/casein ratio is 18:82
Similac (ready to feed) (24 kcal/30 mL)	2.2	4.2	8.4	$\frac{27}{106}$	$\frac{72}{56}$	1.5 (low iron 0.2)	Lactose	Coconut oil Soy oil	380 Whey/casein ratio is 18:82 Available for hospital use only
Similac concentrate mixed to 24 kcal/oz	1.8	4.3	8.5	$\frac{22}{84}$	$\frac{59}{45}$	1.4	Lactose	Coconut oil Soy oil	360 Prepared from standard Similac concentrate Patient requires formula instruction before discharge
Similac (27 kcal/30 mL)	2.5	4.7	9.5	$\frac{31}{119}$	$\frac{82}{63}$	0.2	Lactose	Coconut oil Soy oil	410 Whey/casein ratio is 18:82; additional iron should be supplied
Enfamil (Mead Johnson) (20 kcal/30 mL)	1.5	3.8	6.9	$\frac{18}{72}$	$\frac{52}{35}$	1.3 (low iron 0.1)	Lactose	Palm olein Soy oil Coconut oil Sunflower oil	300 Whey/casein ratio is 60:40
Enfamil (24 kcal/oz)	1.8	4.5	8.2	$\frac{22}{86}$	$\frac{62}{42}$	1.5	Lactose	Palm olein Soy oil Coconut oil Sunflower oil	320 Whey/casein ratio is 60:40
Enfamil Concentrate mixed to 24 kcal/oz	1.8	4.4	8.5	$\frac{18}{86}$	$\frac{62}{42}$	1.6	Lactose	Palm olein Soy oil Coconut oil Sunflower oil	360 Whey/casein ratio is 60:40
Gerber	1.5	3.6	7.1	$\frac{22}{72}$	$\frac{50}{39}$	1.2 (low iron 0.3)	Lactose	Palm oil Soy oil Coconut oil Sunflower oil	320 Whey/casein ratio is 18:82
Good Start	1.6	3.4	7.3	$\frac{16}{65}$	$\frac{43}{24}$	1.0	Lactose Maltodextrins	Palm oil Soy oil Safflower oil Coconut oil	260 Partially hydrolyzed whey protein formula
Lacto-Free (Mead Johnson) (20 kcal/oz)	1.5	3.7	6.9	$\frac{20}{73}$	$\frac{55}{37}$	1.1	Corn syrup solids	Palm oil Soy oil Coconut oil Sunflower oil	200 Lactose-free milk protein isolate Whey/casein ratio is 20:80

Abbreviations: Pro = protein; CHO = carbohydrate.

atic enzymatic digestion before absorption, making these products helpful in treating infants with pancreatic insufficiency from diseases such as cystic fibrosis.

Formulas based on hydrolyzed protein do have several disadvantages, however. They tend to taste bad because of the presence of the sulfated amino acids, which tend to impart a sulfur-like flavor. The more complete the hydrolysis, the worse the flavor is. The osmolality of formulas prepared with hydrolyzed protein tends to be high, which may result in osmotic diarrhea if used improperly. They are also expensive.

Nucleotides

Adenosine, thymidine, guanine, and cytosine, the basic molecules that make up DNA, are present in various forms in human milk. There is some evidence that they may help modulate the immune response when added to infant formula. At least one prototype formula with nucleotides exists but has not yet been thoroughly tested in the United States.

Infant Formula Classification

Commercially available infant formulas fall into several categories, which include (1) formulas designed for the normal newborn infant (Table 2); (2) formulas designed for the infant with simple formula intolerances (Table 3); (3) special formulas for infants with complex absorptive disorders (Table 4); and (4) formulas for low-birth-weight infants (Table 5).

Formulas for premature infants differ from regular

TABLE 3. Soy-Based Formulas

Formula	Content (gm/100 mL)			Content (mg/100 mL)			Source		Osmolality (mOsm/kg of H₂O) and General Comments
	Pro	Fat	CHO	$\frac{Na}{K}$	$\frac{Ca}{P}$	Fe	CHO	Fat	
Isomil (Ross) (20 kcal/30 mL)	1.6	3.6	6.9	$\frac{29}{72}$	$\frac{70}{50}$	1.2	Corn syrup solids Sucrose	Soy oil Coconut oil	240 Soy protein isolate formula Lactose-free formula
Isomil SF (Ross) (20 kcal/30 mL)	1.8	3.6	6.7	$\frac{29}{73}$	$\frac{70}{50}$	1.2	Hydrolyzed cornstarch	Soy oil Coconut oil	180 Soy protein isolate formula Lactose and sucrose free
Isomil DF (20 kcal/30 mL)	1.8	3.6	6.7	$\frac{29}{72}$	$\frac{70}{50}$	1.2	Hydrolyzed cornstarch	Soy oil Coconut oil	180 Soy protein isolate formula Lactose and sucrose free, with fiber
ProSobee (Mead Johnson) (20 kcal/30 mL)	2.0	3.5	6.7	$\frac{24}{81}$	$\frac{63}{49}$	1.3	Corn syrup solids	Palm olein Coconut oil Soy oil Sunflower oil	200 Soy protein isolate formula Lactose and sucrose free
All-Soy (Carnation) (20 kcal/30 mL)	2.1	3.7	6.7	$\frac{28}{78}$	$\frac{68}{47}$	1.3	Sucrose Tapioca starch	Soy oil	206 Soy protein isolate formula Corn free Lactose free

Abbreviations: Pro = protein; CHO = carbohydrate.

TABLE 4. Specialized Formulas

Formula	Content (gm/100 mL)			Content (mg/100 mL)			Source		Osmolality (mOsm/kg of H₂O) and General Comments
	Pro	Fat	CHO	$\frac{Na}{K}$	$\frac{Ca}{P}$	Fe	CHO	Fat	
Alimentum (Ross) (20 kcal/30 mL)	1.9	3.8	6.8	$\frac{29}{79}$	$\frac{70}{50}$	1.2	Sucrose Modified tapioca starch	MCT oil Safflower oil Soy oil	370 For malabsorption problems Protein is casein hydrolysate with added amino acids 50% fat from MCT oil
Nutramigen (Mead Johnson) (20 kcal/30 mL)	1.9	2.6	8.9	$\frac{31}{73}$	$\frac{63}{42}$	1.3	Corn syrup solids	Corn oil Soy oil	320 For malabsorption problems Protein is casein hydrolysate with added amino acids
Pregestimil (Mead Johnson) (20 kcal/30 mL)	1.9	3.7	6.9	$\frac{26}{73}$	$\frac{62}{42}$	1.3	Corn syrup solids Modified corn starch Dextrose	MCT oil Corn oil Soy oil Safflower oil	300 For malabsorption problems Protein is casein hydrolysate with added amino acids 55% fat from MCT oil
Pregestimil (24 kcal/30 mL)	2.3	4.4	8.3	$\frac{31}{88}$	$\frac{74}{50}$	1.6	Same as Pregestimil 20	Same as Pregestimil 20	360 For malabsorption problems Patient needs formula instruction before discharge
Portagen (Mead Johnson) (20 kcal/30 mL)	2.3	3.2	7.7	$\frac{37}{83}$	$\frac{63}{47}$	1.3	Corn syrup solids Sucrose	MCT oil Corn oil	220 MCT formula for LCT intolerance Protein is sodium caseinate 87% MCT oil (long-term use not recommended because of low content of essential fatty acid)
Lofenalac (Mead Johnson) (20 kcal/30 mL)	2.2	2.6	8.7	$\frac{31}{68}$	$\frac{63}{47}$	1.3	Corn syrup solids Modified tapioca starch	Corn oil	360 Low phenylalanine formula used in treatment of PKU Protein is specially processed casein hydrolysate reduced in phenylalanine with other added amino acids
Phenyl-Free (Mead Johnson) (20 kcal/30 mL)	3.3	1.1	10.7	$\frac{66}{223}$	$\frac{83}{83}$	1.9	Sucrose Corn syrup solids Modified tapioca starch	Corn oil Coconut oil	790 Protein provided as amino acids without phenylalanine
Similac PM 60/40 (Ross) (20 kcal/30 mL)	1.5	3.8	6.9	$\frac{16}{58}$	$\frac{38}{19}$	0.15	Lactose	Soy oil Coconut oil	280 Low renal solute load Minerals comparable to human milk Lactalbumin/casein and calcium/phosphorus ratios comparable to human milk Low-iron formula

Abbreviations: Pro = protein; CHO = carbohydrate; MCT = medium chain triglyceride; LCT = long chain triglyceride; PKU = phenylketonuria.

TABLE 5. **Formulas Designed for Low-Birth-Weight Infants**

Formula	Content (gm/100 mL)			Content (mg/100 mL)			Source		Osmolality (mOsm/kg of H₂O) and General Comments
	Pro	Fat	CHO	Na / K	Ca / P	Fe	CHO	Fat	
Enfamil Premature, Iron-Fortified (Mead Johnson) (24 kcal/30 mL)	2.4	4.3	8.9	31 / 82	132 / 66	1.5* (low iron 0.2)	Corn syrup solids Lactose	Soy oil MCT oil Coconut oil	310 For low-birth-weight infants Available for hospital use only Whey/casein ratio is 60:40 40% fat from MCT oil
Similac Special Care, Iron-Fortified (Ross) (24 kcal/30 mL)	2.2	4.3	8.5	34 / 103	144 / 72	1.5* (low iron 0.3)	Lactose Hydrolyzed corn starch	MCT oil Soy oil Coconut oil	280 For low-birth-weight infants Available for hospital use only Whey/casein ratio is 60:40 50% fat from MCT oil Recommended vitamin D supplement 400 IU/d
Similac Special Care (Ross) (20 kcal/30 mL)	1.8	3.6	7.1	29 / 86	120 / 60	0.2	Lactose Hydrolyzed corn starch	MCT oil Soy oil Coconut oil	235 Available for hospital use only
Similac Natural Care (Ross) (24 kcal/30 mL)	2.2	4.3	8.5	34 / 103	168 / 84	0.3	Hydrolyzed cornstarch Lactose	MCT oil Soy oil Coconut oil	Designed to be mixed with human milk or to be fed alternately with human milk to low-birth-weight infants
Enfamil Human Milk Fortifier with EBM (Mead Johnson) @ 4 pkt/ 100 mL	1.7	3.5	9.0	30 / 70	116 / 59	<0.1	Glucose polymers Lactose	—	380 For low-birth-weight infants, or infants with volume restriction on EBM Available for hospital use only Whey/casein ratio is 60:40 Recommended mixture is 2 pkt of fortifier/100 mL of human milk for 24 h, afterward increased to 4 pkt/100 mL for full fortification Does not contain iron

*Also available as low-iron formula.

Abbreviations: Pro = protein; CHO = carbohydrate; MCT = medium chain triglyceride; EBM = expressed breast milk.

infant formulas in that they contain more calories and greater amounts of all nutrients including minerals such as sodium, potassium, calcium, and phosphorus. Most formulas for premature infants are whey predominant, the fat is a blend of medium and long chain triglycerides, and the formula contains a low concentration of lactose. These formulas are recommended for feeding to low-birth-weight newborns until they achieve a body weight of approximately 1.8 kg. The composition of these formulas differs markedly from that of human milk. When the very-low-birth-weight infant is fed human milk exclusively, the infant's needs for growth may not be met and certain nutrient deficiencies may develop. However, because human milk may provide immunologic protection, the use of a human milk fortifier supplements the nutrients deficient in human milk. In all infants other than the very-low-birth-weight infants, human milk remains the optimal feeding mixture.

INTRODUCTION TO SOLID FOODS

Solid foods can be introduced to infants at 4 to 6 months of age depending on development as well as social, cultural, and economic considerations. The feeding of solids before 4 months of age offers no nutritional or developmental benefits and may result in excessive weight gain. Until about 4 months of age, the feeding of solids by spoon is difficult because of the presence of the extrusion reflex. When food is placed on the anterior half of the tongue, this protective reflex causes the tongue to move forward, pushing food from the mouth. Caregivers attempt to stay ahead of this reflex by scraping the food from the chin and pushing it back in. There is no need to feed with a spoon until this reflex spontaneously disappears at 4 to 5 months of age. At 6 months of age, an infant's iron stores may be diminished, so the introduction of solids to supplement this nutrient is desirable.

When solid foods are introduced, single-ingredient foods should be selected and introduced one at a time in no less than 3-day intervals to permit the identification of food intolerances if present. Infant cereal is the optimal first supplemental food because it not only contains additional energy but is fortified with iron. Cereal should be fed by spoon and not added to the nursing bottle except for medically indicated reasons such as gastroesophageal reflux.

The order in which solid foods have traditionally been introduced has been cereal, fruit, yellow vegetables, green vegetables, meats, and desserts. There is no physiologic reason why this order of introduction is necessary. After cereals, the food that is introduced can be at the discretion of the parent.

Commercially prepared strained foods and those prepared at home are both acceptable. If infant foods are prepared at home, precaution should be taken to avoid highly seasoned food or food salted to adult taste. The salt content of commercially prepared U.S. baby food is low. Honey should not be fed to infants younger than 12 months, because of its association with infant botulism.

The amount of water needed by infants to replace their losses and provide for growth is available in both human milk and infant formula during the nursing period. Healthy infants require little or no supplemental water except in hot weather. When solid foods are introduced, additional water is required because the renal solute load is high in solid foods because of their higher protein and salt content. Infants should be offered water to allow an opportunity to fulfill fluid needs without an obligatory intake of extra calories. Fruit juice is not a good choice as a water substitute because fruit juices may introduce poor eating habits by emphasizing the sweet flavor. If placed in a bottle that an infant is allowed to drink from over prolonged periods, fruit juice increases the risk of nursing bottle caries.

Vitamin Supplements

Vitamin K is effective in preventing hemorrhagic disease of the newborn because it prevents or minimizes the postnatal decline of the vitamin K–dependent coagulation factors II, VII, IX, and X. Vitamin K is given as a single intramuscular dose of 0.5 to 1 mg or an oral dose of 1.0 to 2.0 mg. Large doses of water-soluble vitamin K analogues can produce hyperbilirubinemia.

Questions still exist about whether breast-fed infants require any vitamin or mineral supplements before the introduction of solid foods at 6 months of age. The vitamin D content of human milk is low, and rickets can occur in breast-fed infants who are deeply pigmented and have an inadequate exposure to sunlight. Therefore, vitamin D supplementation is recommended for these breast-fed infants at a dose of 400 IU per day. There is no evidence that vitamin A or E is needed for healthy breast-fed term infants.

Fluoride supplementation is not recommended until after 6 months of age.

DISEASES OF THE BREAST

method of
ROGER S. FOSTER, JR., M.D.
Emory University
Atlanta, Georgia

Breast cancer is the most important of all breast diseases. For the average woman, the cumulative probability of developing breast cancer by the age of 90 years is about 9%. Of the women who do develop breast cancer, 20 to 30% can be expected to die of breast cancer. Death from breast cancer currently reduces the life expectancy of the average woman in North America by approximately 0.5 year. The risk of death from breast cancer can be reduced by both earlier detection and effective primary treatment.

SCREENING FOR BREAST CANCER

In the screening of asymptomatic women for breast cancer, breast palpation and mammography are the two techniques of proven value. There are no convincing data to establish the worth of thermography, transillumination, or sonography as screening procedures.

Mammographic screening of asymptomatic women aged 50 to 74 years has been demonstrated in several controlled trials to reduce breast cancer deaths by about one third. The benefits of screening mammography for average-risk women younger than 50 years are less and are the subject of considerable debate. The density of normal breast tissue makes imaging more difficult in younger women, and faster tumor growth rates may make it more difficult to get a screening benefit, particularly if mammograms are performed at intervals longer than annually. Nevertheless, there is increasing evidence of a benefit from the screening of women aged 40 to 49 years. The American Cancer Society recommends that mammographic screening of average-risk women begin at the age of 40 years.

Factors that place a woman at increased risk for breast cancer include family history, early menarche, late menopause, nulliparity, first full-term pregnancy after the age of 30 years, and exposure to ionizing radiation. The two most important risk factors, however, are female sex and increased age. Less than 1% of all breast cancers occur in women younger than 30 years, 2% occur in women younger than 35 years, and 70% occur in women older than 50 years. No factors can define a set of women older than 40 years who are not at significant risk of breast cancer; therefore, breast cancer screening is important in all women. It is estimated that 5 to 10% of breast cancers in the United States occur in women who have inherited a strong genetic susceptibility. A positive family history of breast cancer is of particular significance when the patient's mother, aunt, or daughter has had breast cancer diagnosed before the age of 50 years or when a relative has had bilateral breast cancer.

Genetic screening for inherited mutations that put patients at high risk for breast cancer is becoming available. A decision to order such testing is complex. Genetic testing should not be ordered until there has been informed counseling of the patient about the many issues involved with genetic testing. These issues include the psychologic impact of the information on the individual tested, as well as on any relatives; how the information will be used in clinical management; and confidentiality of the information relative to potential health, disability, and life insurance and/or work place discrimination.

On the basis of currently available data, the breast cancer screening program that I recommend is as follows:

1. Women aged 20 to 39 years with no personal or significant family history of breast cancer: breast self-examination (BSE) monthly and clinical breast examination (CBE) every 2 to 3 years.
2. Women aged 40 to 49 years: BSE monthly, CBE yearly, and mammography yearly. For women younger than 50 years who decide to have mammographic screen-

ing, I advise annual mammograms, rather than every-other-year mammography, because of the more rapid growth rate and shorter time to reach a palpable size in younger women.

3. Women aged 50 to 65 years: BSE monthly, CBE yearly, and mammography every year.

4. Women aged 65 years and older: BSE monthly, CBE yearly, and mammography every 1 to 2 years. (Medicare guidelines permit payment for screening mammograms only every 2 years in the absence of symptoms or a personal history of breast cancer.)

5. Women aged 75 years and older: CBE yearly, monthly BSE if they are capable. Any mammography screening should be restricted to those in general good health with a long life expectancy, because the benefits of screening probably take 5 or more years to become evident.

6. Women with a strong family history of breast cancer, or of premenopausal breast cancer: BSE monthly, CBE yearly, and mammography yearly beginning at the age of 35 years.

7. Women who have been treated for one breast cancer should have yearly follow-up mammograms.

BENIGN BREAST PROBLEMS

The most important aspect of the management of benign breast problems is to exclude the possibility of malignancy.

Physiologic Nodulation and Fibrocystic Breast Disease

The breasts of premenopausal women undergo repeated cyclical hormonal stimulation, and physiologically induced breast nodulations (or lumpiness) develop in many women. Such nodulations typically increase during the premenstrual period and regress afterward. Accompanying symptoms are variable, but for some women there may be fairly severe premenstrual pain, swelling, and tenderness. The term "fibrocystic breast disease" for a condition that occurs to some degree in the majority of women is inappropriate and frightening. There is no increased risk for breast cancer associated with fibrocystic breast changes unless there are pathologic findings of epithelial proliferation, such as ductal or lobular hyperplasia (slightly increased risk) or atypical hyperplasia (moderately increased risk). Treatment of the patient with physiologic breast nodulation and moderate discomfort is careful physical examination (best performed during the postmenstrual interval) and reassurance, with the suggestion that analgesics such as aspirin be used if the symptoms interfere with physical or sexual activity.

The degree of breast nodulation is probably not related to the ingestion of methylxanthines (caffeine, theophylline, theobromine), but in some women the degree of breast tenderness may be related. For the rare patient whose problem does not respond to simple measures, there is a limited role for treatment with antiestrogen medication such as tamoxifen (Nolvadex); bromocriptine (Parlodel), which inhibits pituitary prolactin; or an impeded androgen such as danazol (Danocrine), which inhibits the release of pituitary gonadotropins. Attempts at treating these patients with subcutaneous mastectomies have resulted in symptomatic failures and complications, and such treatment is inappropriate.

Women with asymmetrical areas of breast nodulation may require additional investigation. Breast imaging may be obtained as appropriate for the patient's age: ultrasonography for women younger than 35 years and mammography with or without ultrasonography for older women. Fine-needle aspiration biopsy (to be described) of such areas occasionally demonstrates malignant cells even in the absence of a distinct mass or a mammographic or ultrasonographic abnormality. If the fine-needle aspiration biopsy demonstrates an adequate number of normal ductal cells, there is considerable reassurance that the area is benign, and open breast biopsy is not necessary.

Gross Cysts

In contrast to physiologic breast nodulations, true breast masses, which are distinguished as being discrete, dense, dominant, and different from the rest of the breast tissue, should receive surgical attention. Most palpable true breast masses are aspirated with a fine needle (e.g., 21 gauge). Gross cysts, which can occur in patients of any age but are most common in the 15 years before menopause, are completely evacuated, and the fluid is discarded if it is typical cyst fluid (tawny to grayish or dark green opalescent fluid). Cytologic examination and further evaluation of the patient are necessary if the fluid is bloody.

Fibroadenomas

Fibroadenomas are benign fibroepithelial neoplasms that occur most commonly in women younger than 30 years. Fibroadenomas tend to be quite firm, mobile, nontender, and well delineated, and some resistance to withdrawal of the needle occurs after attempted aspiration. Cytologic examination is obtained on material aspirated with a fine needle from any solid lesion in which malignancy is deemed a possibility. Fibroadenomas and other true discrete breast masses may be excised on an outpatient basis, usually with local anesthesia.

An alternative to removing benign breast masses is observation after a negative "triple test." A negative triple test consists of physical examination consistent with a benign lump, a breast image (ultrasonogram or mammogram) consistent with a benign lump, and a needle biopsy result consistent with a benign lump.

Nipple Discharges

Nipple discharge is of clinical significance only if it is spontaneous. Self-induced nipple discharges have no importance, and patients should be taught not to squeeze the nipples as part of BSE. Spontaneous serous and bloody discharges are most commonly caused by an intraductal papilloma, but mammographic evaluation followed by excision of the distal duct or ducts is necessary to rule out the possibility of a carcinoma. Nonlactational milky discharge should be evaluated with a test for serum prolactin because of the possibility of a pituitary adenoma.

Infection

Most of the infections that occur in other areas of the body can occur in the breast. Infections from *Staphylococcus aureus*, *Staphylococcus epidermidis*, and *Streptococcus* species are particularly common in lactating breasts, and if the lesion is cellulitis and not an abscess, it can usually be managed with antibiotics; breast-feeding can be continued during treatment. A nipple shield or breast pump may be used if a nipple fissure makes breast-feeding painful. If a breast abscess is present, the abscess should be drained. Alternative drainage techniques are needle aspiration, catheter drainage (e.g., placed under ultrasound guidance), or open surgical drainage. Recurrent periareolar abscess in nonlactating women is commonly caused by squamous metaplasia of the lactiferous ducts. Treatment is by surgical excision of the abnormal distal duct or ducts, usually after the acute process has been controlled by drainage of the abscess and antibiotics.

Noninfectious Breast Inflammations

Trauma to the breast can cause a breast mass that may mimic the clinical characteristics of carcinoma. Sometimes the clinical history and mammographic appearance are sufficiently convincing to permit management by observation only, but most commonly biopsy is required to exclude a malignancy.

Thrombosis of a superficial vein in the breast (Mondor's disease) can cause skin retraction that mimics the Cooper ligament retraction caused by a breast cancer. The linear cord of the thrombosed vein can usually be palpated. Sometimes the thrombosis occurs after a surgical procedure or after a blow to the breast, but frequently there is no evident cause. Once breast cancer has been excluded, no specific treatment is required.

Localized breast erythema of unknown cause occurs occasionally. The process may last days to months. Such patients need to be examined by an experienced clinician and may require a biopsy to exclude inflammatory carcinoma or infection.

COSMETIC SURGERY

Cosmetic surgery may be desired by women who have asymmetrically sized breasts, whose breasts have not developed to an acceptable size or have involuted after pregnancy, or whose breasts have developed to an abnormally large size. The augmentation mammoplasty operation involving the use of submusculofascial Silastic bag implant is relatively simple and usually provides good cosmetic results, but there has been controversy about safety. Reduc-

tion mammoplasty for excessively large and heavy breasts is a more complex procedure in which the breast is resized and the nipple-areolar complex is repositioned. When the volume of breast tissue is satisfactory but stretching of skin has led to marked ptosis, a mastopexy operation, in which excess skin is removed and the nipple-areolar complex is repositioned, can be performed.

PRIMARY BREAST CANCER

Diagnosis and Staging of Breast Cancer

The diagnosis of a palpable breast cancer can be established by fine-needle aspiration biopsy, by core-cutting needle biopsy, by open incisional biopsy, or by excisional biopsy. Fine-needle aspiration biopsy is of particular value because it can be performed as an office procedure. Although this procedure is conceptually a simple technique, the operator must be able to obtain an adequate sample, and the cytopathologist must be experienced in providing reliable interpretation. The diagnosis of nonpalpable breast cancers that are detectable only by mammography is made either by needle biopsy or by open biopsy. Open biopsy is performed after the area to be biopsied is localized by the mammographic placement of a needle at the site from which the specimen is to be taken. Fine-needle aspiration biopsy and core needle biopsy of mammographic lesions may be done with ultrasound guidance or with a stereotactic mammography technique.

Excisional biopsies of lesions known or suspected to be cancer should be performed as formal partial mastectomies—that is, a small margin of apparently normal breast tissue surrounding the lesion is also excised, and the pathologist paints the external surface with ink before sectioning—so that it can be established that there are tumor-free margins. If tumor-free margins are obtained and the patient's definitive treatment is to be partial mastectomy, no further resection of breast tissue is needed; the cosmetic results are better than when a second resection of breast tissue must be performed after an excisional biopsy.

The histologic type of breast cancer has a bearing on both the prognosis and the management. The most important distinction in terms of biologic behavior is between invasive breast cancer, which has a relatively high likelihood of systemic metastases, and noninvasive or in situ cancer, in which there should be no systemic metastases. Unfortunately, the noninvasive cancers are much less common than the invasive cancers; they are, however, being increasingly recognized with screening mammography.

The two different types of noninvasive breast cancer are (1) ductal carcinoma in situ (DCIS, or intraductal carcinoma), which usually involves only one breast, and (2) lobular carcinoma in situ (LCIS), sometimes referred to as lobular neoplasia, which commonly involves both breasts. With the passage of time, noninvasive intraductal carcinomas frequently, but not inevitably, develop into invasive cancer. A coexistent invasive carcinoma has been reported in about 20% of patients whose predominant lesion is a DCIS. In 15 to 20% of patients with small areas of DCIS who have undergone only a limited biopsy, invasive ductal carcinoma develops in the same site over a median interval of 10 years. In about 25% of patients with LCIS who have undergone only biopsy, invasive carcinoma develops over a median interval of 20 years and the risk is relatively even for both breasts and is not specifically related to the site at which the LCIS was biopsied.

Invasive ductal carcinoma is the most common type of invasive breast carcinoma, accounting for about 70% of these cancers. Invasive ductal carcinomas frequently cause a productive fibrosis, which is responsible for much of the hardness that is felt on palpation and the grittiness that is felt when the tumor is cut with a knife or entered with a needle. Lobular invasive carcinoma accounts for 5 to 10% of invasive cancers. The biologic behavior and prognosis of lobular carcinoma are similar to those of invasive ductal carcinoma. Medullary carcinomas account for 5% of invasive cancers, and it has been suggested that they carry a somewhat more favorable prognosis. Their biologic behavior is not much different from that of invasive ductal carcinoma. Colloid, tubular, adenocystic, and papillary carcinomas are relatively rare types and generally carry much better prognoses than do the more common types of invasive carcinoma.

Once a diagnosis or even strong presumptive diagnosis of breast cancer has been made, the clinical stage, or extent of disease, should be established. Clinical TNM (tumor, node, metastases) staging is based on the size of the primary cancer and any invasion of skin or underlying muscle or chest wall, clinical evidence of involvement of regional nodes (axillary, supraclavicular, or infraclavicular), and any evidence of more distant metastases. In addition to physical examination, the clinical evaluation of all patients with invasive breast cancer should include a chest radiograph and liver enzyme assays to screen for hepatic involvement. Routine bone scans, liver scans, and computed tomographic scans are not indicated unless the patient is symptomatic, has evidence of locally advanced disease on physical examination, or has an elevated liver enzyme level.

Pathologic staging of breast cancer is more definitive than clinical staging. For surgically operable invasive breast cancers, the presence or absence of histologically documented regional node metastases (axillary nodes) and the determination of the absolute number of nodes involved by metastases may provide the most important information for prognosis and for decision-making in relation to the use of systemic adjuvant chemotherapy. The levels of estrogen and of progesterone receptor proteins in the tumor provide additional prognostic and management information; high levels of receptor proteins indicate both a slightly more favorable prognosis and a greater likelihood of response to hormonal therapy when there are metastases.

Treatment

Local and/or Regional Treatment

The majority of patients are probably candidates for breast-conserving surgery; in the United States, however, the most common local and/or regional treatment for surgically operable carcinoma of the breast is total mastectomy and axillary dissection with preservation of the chest wall muscles (modified radical mastectomy). For most patients with stage I or II breast cancer, radiotherapy to the regional lymph nodes after mastectomy and axillary dissection does not improve survival and increases morbidity. Breast-conserving surgery (lumpectomy or partial mastectomy and radiotherapy) is increasingly being used.

In my practice, most patients with primary invasive cancers less than 4 to 5 cm in diameter are treated by partial (segmental) mastectomy followed by radiotherapy (5000 rad to the breast delivered through tangential ports with or without a radiation boost to the tumor bed); an axillary dissection is usually performed through a separation incision. This technique has been demonstrated by the National Surgical Adjuvant Breast Project studies and six other studies to provide 10-year survival rates similar to those obtained with modified radical mastectomy and to permit preservation of the breast in most of the patients. A small percentage of patients treated by partial mastectomy demonstrate recurrence of tumor in the breast and subsequently require a total mastectomy. In many patients older than 70 years, it is my practice to omit breast irradiation after partial mastectomy, as in-breast recurrence rates are much lower without irradiation than they would be in younger patients.

Most women whose disease is unsuited to partial mastectomy are offered either immediate or delayed breast reconstruction. In some patients, the breast is appropriately reconstructed with a submuscular tissue expander and a Silastic implant; many patients are better served by procedures that transfer the abdominal or latissimus dorsi muscle with overlying fat and skin.

Patients with noninvasive DCIS may present particular difficulties in relation to the amount of breast tissue that needs to be removed. In contrast to most invasive cancers, many intraductal carcinomas involve the breast so diffusely that they cannot be excised by partial mastectomy, and thus many women with these prognostically favorable tumors are treated by total mastectomy, which may be followed by reconstruction. Patients with localized intraductal carcinoma may be treated by a combination of partial mastectomy and breast irradiation, or occasionally partial mastectomy without irradiation.

Appropriate management of LCIS is even more poorly defined; because this disease is diffuse and bilateral, any management policy should be the same for both breasts. Most patients with LCIS are managed with a conservative policy of repeated physical and mammographic examinations; selected patients may elect bilateral total mastectomy and breast reconstruction.

Systemic Adjuvant Treatment

Although in 95% of patients the disease is apparently localized to the breast and regional nodes at the time of initial treatment, systemic metastases develop during a 10-year period in approximately one third of the patients receiving only local regional therapy (surgery with or without radiotherapy). In the era before systemic adjuvant therapy, 75% of the patients with metastases to the axillary nodes had recurrences and were dead at 10 years. Patients with palpable tumors but without axillary node metastases have a recurrence rate of more than 40% at 10 years. For axillary node–negative patients with invasive tumors 1 cm or less in diameter, which are frequently detected by screening mammography, 90% are expected to be free of recurrence at 10 years. For patients with noninvasive cancers, who should be recurrence free if resection is complete, the 10-year systemic recurrence rate is 1 to 2%, presumably because an invasive component was present and missed at pathologic diagnosis.

It has been shown that systemic adjuvant therapy can produce modest but quite meaningful reductions in recurrence and improvements in survival in both premenopausal and postmenopausal patients with breast cancer. Benefit has been seen in both node-positive patients and in those node-negative patients who are higher risk. The relative magnitude of the benefits of systemic adjuvant therapy are similar in high-risk and low-risk patients. Because a higher proportion of the low-risk patients are destined never to have a recurrence, the absolute benefits of systemic therapy are less for them. A larger proportion of the lower risk patients bear the cost and toxicity of treatment without benefit. Outside the context of a formal clinical trial, systemic adjuvant therapy is not recommended for patients with invasive tumors less than 1 cm in diameter or for patients with the smaller pure tubular, papillary, or colloid histologic findings, and it is not recommended for noninvasive cancers. Systemic adjuvant therapy is given to almost all patients with primary breast cancer with metastases to the regional nodes and to most patients with tumors 3 cm in diameter and larger.

Patients with node-negative tumors in the 1- to 3-cm range are problematic; overall, recurrences can be expected in approximately 30% of these patients. The ability to distinguish the majority of patients who will not benefit from chemotherapy from the minority who will is imperfect. Most patients with node-negative 1- to 3-cm cancer are treated with systemic adjuvant treatment.

When premenopausal patients are treated with systemic adjuvant therapy, a cytotoxic chemotherapy protocol is most often used. Postmenopausal patients whose breast cancer hormone receptor assays are negative also have improved survival rates with cytotoxic chemotherapy. Postmenopausal patients with hormone receptor–positive tumors are most commonly treated with the antiestrogen tamoxifen (Nolvadex). Many clinicians prescribe cytotoxic chemotherapy in addition to tamoxifen for postmenopausal women with receptor–positive tumors, particularly for higher risk patients.

METASTATIC BREAST CANCER

Metastatic breast cancer is rarely cured, which is the reason for the emphasis on systemic adjuvant therapy given at the time of diagnosis of the primary tumor. There has been an attempt to cure metastatic breast cancer in younger women with the use of intensive cytotoxic chemotherapy programs that require special support of the bone marrow through transplantation of bone marrow cells, peripheral blood progenitor cells, or both along with the administration of blood cell growth factors. The preliminary data from the uncontrolled reports are encouraging, but the favorable results may be related to the screening and the selection of patients rather than the treatment. The data from the controlled trials currently under way are not yet available.

The common sites for breast cancer metastases include bone, the liver, the lungs, the brain, and the chest wall. Although a limited number of patients remain free of disease after resection of solitary lung, brain, or cutaneous metastases, treatment of metastatic breast cancer is, for the most part, palliative. Therapy for metastatic breast cancer includes both cytotoxic chemotherapy and hormonal manipulations, as well as site-specific local therapy.

Patients with oncologic emergencies such as hypercalcemia, central nervous system metastases, unstable bone metastases, or pleural effusion need prompt therapy specific for the problem. Hypercalcemia usually responds to intravenous hydration and furosemide-induced diuresis. Brain and spinal cord metastases should be treated with high doses of corticosteroids, and immediate neurosurgical and radiotherapy consultations should be obtained. Patients with hip and leg pain should undergo bone scan and radiographic evaluations to determine whether lesions that may lead to pathologic fracture are present; impending fractures can be prevented by radiotherapy with or without insertion of a metal prosthesis as indicated. Large pleural effusions can be treated by insertion of a chest tube to evacuate the effusion, after which a sclerosing agent can be injected to create an adherence between the parietal and visceral pleura (pleurodesis).

About 50% of breast cancer patients are estrogen- or progesterone-receptor–positive. Hormonal manipulations are preferred over cytotoxic chemotherapy in many receptor-positive and receptor-unknown patients because the response durations tend to be longer and side effects are fewer. Older patients and patients with well-differentiated tumors are more likely to be receptor-positive. Initial hormonal therapies include antiestrogens, such as tamoxifen; progestational agents; and, for premenopausal patients, oophorectomy or agents that suppress pituitary gonadotrophins. The median duration of an endocrine response is about 12 to 18 months. After initial response to hormonal therapy and then further progression of disease, additional responses may be obtained by secondary hormonal manipulations. Patients whose disease is unsuited for hormonal manipulations or is no longer responsive are treated with combination cytotoxic chemotherapy. Response to current first-line combination chemotherapy occurs in 50 to 75% of patients, with a median duration response of 6 to 12 months. Response to second-line chemotherapy regimens tends to be less.

ENDOMETRIOSIS

method of
DEBORAH A. METZGER, Ph.D., M.D.
Reproductive Medicine Institute of Connecticut
Hartford, Connecticut
Yale University School of Medicine
New Haven, Connecticut

Endometriosis is a painful, chronic disease characterized by the growth of endometrial tissue outside the uterus. It most often affects the ovaries, fallopian tubes, ureter, peritoneum, bowel, bladder, and in rare cases, the lungs, cesarean section scars, appendectomy scars, and episiotomies. The disease was first described in the 1920s and today is believed to affect 5 to 15% of women of reproductive age.

It is important that we acknowledge the chronic, recurring nature of this disease and accept the fact that we are unable to prevent recurrences with any one treatment approach, be it surgery, hormones, or pregnancy. These women require and deserve long-term, integrated care aimed at preserving fertility, improving function, and preventing recurrences. We are limited in providing adequate treatment for these women because universal regimens for integrated medical and surgical treatment of endometriosis are lacking.

PATHOPHYSIOLOGY OF ENDOMETRIOSIS

Endometriosis is a progressive disease involving peritoneal implants, fibrosis, adhesions, and the formation of endometriomas. Although many theories have been proposed to explain the development of endometriosis, such as retrograde menstruation, metaplasia, or embryonic rests of müllerian tissue, the most popular and widely accepted theory is that of Sampson, who proposed that during menstruation, viable endometrial cells reflux through the fallopian tubes and implant on the surrounding pelvic structures. By a similar mechanism, viable endometrial cells may implant in open wounds or be transported to distant sites within vascular or lymphatic channels.

Although these theories may explain how endometriosis implants arise, none offer insight into why some women are predisposed and others are protected. Practically all menstruating women have retrograde menstruation and the appropriate hormonal milieu, yet the disease develops in only a few. Clinical and epidemiologic studies have suggested a familial predisposition. Another association has been postulated between the amount of retrograde menstruation and the functional status of the immune system. Several studies have demonstrated that women with a greater amount of retrograde menstruation, such as those with short cycle lengths, menorrhagia, or outflow obstruction, have a much higher chance of developing endometriosis. Intrauterine devices, which increase menstrual flow, are three times as likely to be associated with endometriosis, whereas oral contraceptives, which tend to decrease menstrual flow, are associated with a 50% reduction in the prevalence of endometriosis.

Regardless of how endometrial cells arrive in the abdomen, dysfunction of the immune system results in the inability to remove endometrial cells in a timely way, thus increasing the possibility of endometriosis development. Abnormalities of T lymphocyte cytotoxicity, B lymphocyte function, natural killer cell activity, and complement deposition have been observed in women with endometriosis. Clinical evidence of alterations in immune system function are twice as likely in women with endometriosis such as chronic yeast infections and environmental allergies, both of which are often associated with fatigue.

Once the endometrial cells have implanted on peritoneal surfaces, steroid hormones and growth factors provide support for growth and development of the lesions. Thus, the propensity to develop endometriosis is a balance among cell invasiveness, the immune system, the endocrine environment, and the number of endometrial cells that reach the peritoneal cavity.

Once implants of endometriosis develop, a multistep evolution of the disease that involves cyclical menstrual bleeding, an inflammatory reaction, scarring, fibrosis, and sequestration of implants takes place. Hormonal factors are of central importance in the pathogenesis of endometriosis. Like endometrium found in the uterine cavity, endometriosis implants respond to the fluctuating blood levels of ovarian hormones during the menstrual cycle. At the end of each menstrual cycle, endometriosis implants break down and bleed, causing pain and/or eliciting an inflammatory reaction with subsequent scarring, fibrosis, and adhesions of the affected tissues.

DIAGNOSIS

Endometriosis should be suspected in any patient with the triad of dysmenorrhea, dyspareunia, and infertility. However, it should be kept in mind that the symptoms of endometriosis may be quite variable and are for the most part determined by the areas of involvement. Although it occurs most frequently in the pelvis, endometriosis has been found in most areas of the body. After the pelvic organs, the next most commonly affected locations include the appendix, terminal ileum, cervix, perineum, abdominal scars, umbilicus, inguinal region, and ureter. Only rarely is endometriosis encountered on the diaphragm, extremities, pleura, lungs, gallbladder, spleen, stomach, or kidney.

Symptoms of pain tend to be most severe at the time of menstruation, although some women experience the most intense pain around the time of ovulation. The severity of symptoms does not always correlate with the extent of the disease, and not infrequently, patients with extensive disease exhibit minimal symptoms, whereas some with minimal disease may have marked symptoms. Patients with infertility may not exhibit any pain or significant dysmenorrhea.

The most common physical findings of pelvic endometriosis are generalized pelvic tenderness, nodular induration of the uterosacral ligaments, ovarian enlargement, and a fixed, retroverted uterus. Just as the symptoms of endometriosis can be quite variable depending on the tissues and organs involved, the pelvic findings may also be confused with other gynecologic disorders such as pelvic inflammatory disease, pelvic masses, and ectopic pregnancy.

A definitive diagnosis of endometriosis can be made only by direct visualization of the pelvis. Laparoscopy is the procedure of choice because it provides a panoramic view of the entire abdomen. Several classifications of the extent of disease involvement have been developed to determine the effects of therapy and prognosis for fertility. A significant limitation of all the classification systems has been the poor correlation between the extent of disease and pain symptoms. This apparent lack of correlation may be related to the morphologic and functional heterogeneity of implants, which change over time. Initial implants, which are petechial or clear vesicles, show the highest level of in vitro prostaglandin $F_{2\alpha}$ production, whereas more typical implants (blue, black, or brown) are the least active physiologically.

It has been suggested that there is a relationship between the characteristics of a patient's symptoms and the type of endometrial implant present. Characteristics such as the color, degree of fibrosis, depth, size, and location may determine the type of symptoms experienced. Moreover, a natural progression may occur in an individual implant with age, from superficial clear and red lesions to powder burn, diffusely fibrotic peritoneal implants. Adolescents are more likely to have nonpigmented and subtle lesions. Prostaglandin production is increased twofold in these "early" forms, possibly correlating with dysmenorrhea. Together, these findings describe a general progression from dysmenorrhea in younger women to pelvic pain and/or dyspareunia with the development of black, fibrotic lesions in older women. Thus, there is a need for a staging system that considers the variations in lesion type, location, depth, and size.

TREATMENT OF PAIN

The goals of treatment of endometriosis are to decrease pain, increase function, limit recurrence of disease, and maintain or enhance fertility. In planning therapy, one must consider many variables, such as the age of the patient, extent of disease, degree of symptoms, and desire for immediate or deferred fertility. Hormonal therapy, surgery, and expectant management have been used alone or in combination to treat endometriosis. When treatment is initiated only after patients become symptomatic, there often is a sense of failure and disappointment on the part of both physician and patient. For this reason it is important to acknowledge that endometriosis is a chronic condition requiring long-term solutions and a multidisciplinary approach.

The rationale behind treatment is based on the factors thought to be involved in the pathogenesis of endometriosis-related symptoms: retrograde menstruation, implants, estrogen, and the immune system. Optimal treatment of patients can be achieved by a three-pronged approach that includes (1) initial surgery to remove visible implants, (2) a 3- to 6-month course of hypoestrogenemia, followed by (3) extended amenorrhea to inhibit retrograde menstruation. Nonspecific enhancement of immune function can be achieved by attention to diet, exercise, and stress management. More specific immunotherapy can be offered to women with chronic yeast or environmental allergies, who may have significant fatigue. If this integrated approach is used, the vast majority of patients experience long-term pain relief with minimal chance of recurrence.

For patients with dysmenorrhea and/or mild pelvic pain as their presenting symptoms, initial treatment may consist of a 2- to 3-month trial of oral contraceptives and nonsteroidal anti-inflammatory agents. Patients who fail to obtain adequate relief, develop recurrence of symptoms while being treated conservatively, or have more severe pain require definitive diagnosis and aggressive treatment.

Surgical Management

Not surprisingly, many gynecologists have approached endometriosis as a surgical disease under the assumption that if all disease can be excised and proper anatomic relationships restored, the patient can be cured. However, it is now apparent that the initial pain relief experienced by the patient is often short-lived: symptoms may reoccur in 12 to 54% of all women within a year. Rather than serving as an indicator of a lack of efficacy, these data should focus our attention on what aspects of surgery may be important in achieving pain relief, particularly in the context of a multifaceted approach that includes postoperative hormonal suppression.

Localization of tenderness on physical examination generally corresponds to the location of the anatomic source(s) of pain, and for this reason, it is important to do a careful preoperative pelvic examination to map the areas of maximal tenderness.

Preoperative hormonal therapy has been advocated by some to lessen the need for extensive tissue dissection and to decrease the risk of postoperative adhesion formation. On the other hand, preoperative hormonal therapy makes the endometriosis less visible with the risk of leaving disease behind that may be reactivated with the resumption of menstruation. Although there have been no controlled studies to determine the best approach, whether or not a surgeon uses preoperative hormonal treatment should have no bearing on the overall approach to the treatment of endometriosis that is described here.

Traditionally, conservative resection of endometriosis was performed by laparotomy, but laparoscopic surgery is being used increasingly for all stages of disease. In addition to establishing a diagnosis of endometriosis, laparoscopy permits concurrent treatment. However, there is still a role for laparotomy in the treatment of endometriosis. Regardless of the route of surgery, there are general principles of surgical management of endometriosis that improve success.

Although it may appear obvious, endometriosis

cannot be treated unless it is recognized. Thorough intraoperative examination of the pelvis is essential with particular attention directed to the ovaries, anterior cul-de-sac, broad ligament under the ovaries, uterosacral ligaments, and posterior cul-de-sac.

For superficial implants, ablation of the implants is sufficient. However, for implants that demonstrate scarring, retraction, immobility of the peritoneum, or nodularity, wide local excision is necessary to remove the entire implant. Failure to excise deep-seated implants in the cul-de-sac, particularly where there is complete or partial obliteration of the cul-de-sac, may be responsible for rapid recurrence of symptoms after surgery. Moreover, these fibrotic implants do not respond particularly well to hormonal suppression. Bowel resection may be necessary in some cases. Endometriomas also respond poorly to hormonal suppression, and recurrence is common after surgical drainage. The endometrioma capsule must be removed to minimize recurrence.

Adhesion formation is common after surgery, and attention to minimizing adhesions helps maintain fertility and prevent subsequent pain due to adhesions. Although laparoscopic surgery appears to decrease the risk of adhesion reformation when compared with laparotomy, techniques to decrease adhesion formation should be a part of any surgical procedure. These include strict hemostasis, careful handling of the tissues, minimal use of suture, and use of high-power settings on electrocautery instruments and laser to minimize thermal damage and tissue necrosis. A variety of adhesion barriers are currently available (Interceed, Preclude, and Seprafilm), and many others are under development.

Finally, selected patients may benefit from adjunctive pain-relieving measures such as presacral neurectomy, uterosacral nerve transection, or uterine suspension.

Medical Management

The three commonly used classes of hormonal suppressive agents for endometriosis are progestins, danazol, and a gonadotropin-releasing hormone (GnRH) agonist (nafarelin [Synarel]). Although the mechanism of their actions differs, all these medications produce a hypoestrogenic environment, amenorrhea, and atrophy of intrauterine endometrium as well as endometriosis implants. All are equally effective; however, cost and tolerance of side effects may be the most important determinants in the selection of a specific agent.

Attention has focused on the GnRH agonists as a versatile method of ovarian suppression because of the ability to ameliorate many of the hypoestrogenic side effects of these medications with hormonal "add-back." Many different agents have been added to GnRH agonists to treat symptoms such as loss of bone density, hot flashes, and breakthrough bleeding. My preference is to use norethindrone acetate 2.5 mg daily during the entire duration of GnRH agonist treatment because it also suppresses ovarian func-

tion, prevents hot flashes, and minimizes loss of bone density without adding estrogen.

Women who have inadequate pain relief in the absence of bleeding may have sources of pain in addition to endometriosis. The commonly found problems coexisting with endometriosis include abdominal wall trigger points, hernias, interstitial cystitis, pelvic congestion, and irritable bowel syndrome.

Controlled studies show a high degree of efficacy of hormonal therapy when relief of pain and dysmenorrhea are used as end points. Although most women continue to experience significant relief of general pelvic pain and dyspareunia once the medications are stopped, dysmenorrhea invariably returns with the resumption of cyclic menses. Approximately 25 to 30% report recurrence of pelvic pain symptoms within 6 months of treatment. It is not clear whether recurrence is due to reactivation of residual disease or the acquisition of new implants. Women who are more likely to have recurrences include those with severe disease or large endometriomas.

Continuous Oral Contraceptives

Because pain and dysmenorrhea often recur within a few months of cessation of hormonal therapy, the continuation of amenorrhea with less expensive, more easily tolerated medications is desirable. Because the symptom that returns first is dysmenorrhea and retrograde menstruation appears to be a factor in the development and recurrence of endometriosis, it seems rational to prevent menstruation. There are several methods by which this can be achieved. First, suppression can be continued with GnRH agonists with hormonal add-back. This is an expensive approach and should be reserved for those patients resistant to other treatments. A second method is the use of depo medroxyprogesterone acetate (Depo-Provera) or high-dose oral medroxyprogesterone acetate (30 to 50 mg daily).* Although these are inexpensive, side effects and breakthrough bleeding may make them unacceptable to many patients. Finally, oral contraceptives (OCPs)† may be used to continue the hormonal suppression and symptom improvement initially achieved with GnRH agonists or other hormonal therapy. When taken continuously, i.e., only active pills are taken without a break for menses, OCPs are quite versatile, and current formulations minimize breakthrough bleeding and side effects. Treatment is continued until conception is desired or the patient reaches menopause.

Side effects, such as increased appetite, depression, and premenstrual syndrome symptoms can be minimized by starting with 35 μg of estrogen, low-progestin pills containing norethindrone (0.4 to 0.5 mg) or desogestrel. Although triphasic pills are popular, the variation in the estrogen and/or progestin dose makes it difficult to avoid breakthrough bleeding and dysmenorrhea. Therefore, only monophasic

---

*Exceeds dosage recommended by the manufacturer.
†Not FDA approved for this indication.

pills, taken at the same time each day, should be used. Younger women may require additional progestin to maintain ovarian suppression, and this can be accomplished by switching to a pill with a higher norethindrone content or by adding norethindrone to the current OCP (0.35 to 2.5 mg daily). Women who develop headaches taking OCPs containing 35 μg of estrogen can be switched to 20-μg pills. This regimen can be modified for smokers (while they are on a smoking cessation program) by prescribing norethindrone acetate (0.35 to 2.5 mg daily) and oral (0.5 to 1.0 mg twice daily) or transdermal estradiol* (0.375 to 0.1 mg once or twice weekly) to prevent headaches and breakthrough bleeding. If breakthrough bleeding and side effects of OCPs can be prevented or treated, the vast majority of patients with endometriosis achieve long-term pain relief.

Additional Treatment Approaches

Women with endometriosis want to know about their disease, and health care providers can encourage their patients by answering questions and supplying resources. Information is also available from the Endometriosis Association (8585 North 76th Place, Milwaukee, WI 53223; telephone, 414-355-2200). Many women also need help with emotional issues such as disability from constant or unpredictable pain, multiple unsuccessful attempts at treatment, unpleasant drug side effects, and relationship issues related to dyspareunia or an inability to have intercourse.

Women with endometriosis often describe a feeling of not being in control of their lives. Physicians and health care personnel can go a long way in restoring some of their loss of control by encouraging the patient to be a partner with the physician in determining the best course of treatment. Women with endometriosis should be encouraged to explore diet and nutritional alternatives, chiropractic, acupuncture, psychotherapy, physical therapy, pain clinics, and stress management to enhance their quality of life and allow them to regain a sense of control.

Recurrence of Symptoms or Inadequate Pain Relief

Recurrence of symptoms and inadequate pain relief are discouraging for both patient and physician. Listed here are some points to consider with these patients:

1. The diagnosis may be wrong, or endometriosis may be present in addition to another pain-producing abnormality—repeat a careful pelvic examination.

2. The focus of treatment may be on crisis management rather than long-term suppression of symptoms, i.e., prevention.

3. The patient may have an unrecognized chronic pain syndrome or pre-existing depression.

4. The patient may have endometriosis that is particularly sensitive to estrogen, even in the presence of progestins—use a progestin-only pill.

5. You or your patient may have unrealistic goals.

6. You may not like taking care of endometriosis/chronic pelvic pain patients.

7. The patient may have endometriosis that is resistant to treatment, or treatment options may be limited by side effects or intolerances.

8. Surgical excision may not have been done or was incomplete, i.e., fibrotic nodules were not excised.

HYSTERECTOMY

For patients with recurrent or intractable pain associated with endometriosis, hysterectomy remains the definitive treatment. For women who have been treated for infertility, removal of the uterus, tubes, and ovaries is a sensitive issue, and the premature recommendation of hysterectomy as the only treatment option will be met with resistance, emotional reaction to impending loss, and bereavement. It is important that the decision to proceed with a hysterectomy be made primarily by the patient, who, with support from her physician, needs to sort through her choice between the hope of children but continued pain versus control over her life. By making this important realization herself, she willingly relinquishes her uterus as opposed to having it taken from her. This difference in perception by the patient makes the postoperative recovery easier, although a mourning period is not unusual and should be acknowledged by the caregivers.

In young women remote from menopause, whether bilateral oophorectomy is mandatory to achieve a permanent cure remains controversial. The incidence of symptom recurrence after hysterectomy with ovarian conservation has been reported to be as low as 1% and as high as 85%. Namnoum and colleagues have shown that women who had ovarian conservation at the time of hysterectomy for endometriosis were 6.1 times more likely to develop recurrent pain and 8.1 times more likely to require reoperation than women who initially had oophorectomy and were given postoperative hormone replacement therapy. Moreover, the women with ovarian conservation had milder disease than those who underwent oophorectomy, and thus conservation of the ovaries was considered valid because of the apparent low risk of recurrence. Thus, ovarian conservation may not fulfill the goals of "definitive" therapy.

All visible endometrial tissue should be removed at the time of hysterectomy to prevent recurrence of symptoms due to fibrotic or deep nodules. Postoperative hormonal replacement can be commenced immediately after surgery and should include both estrogen and a progestin. The progestin attenuates the growth-promoting effects of estrogen and decreases the possibility of recurrent pain due to endometriosis. Alternatively, the patient can be treated with progestins alone for hypoestrogenic symptoms for 3 to 6

---

*Not FDA approved for this indication.

months, followed by either estrogen alone or combined, continuous estrogen and progestin.

Recurrence of pain after hysterectomy is not frequent, but when it does occur is discouraging to both patient and physician. The most common reasons for recurrence of pain include (1) reactivation of endometriosis in the setting of unopposed estrogen administration, (2) adhesions, (3) residual ovary, (4) ovarian remnant, and (5) reasons for pain unrelated to endometriosis.

TREATMENT OF INFERTILITY

At some point, nearly all women with endometriosis express concern about their future fertility. Often they are encouraged to get pregnant right away because it may be impossible later. However, with a well-planned approach, women with endometriosis have an excellent chance of conceiving when they are ready.

Pain and Infertility

Women with pain and infertility associated with endometriosis face several dilemmas: (1) the very treatments that provide other women with long-standing pain relief are contraindicated in women trying to conceive, (2) common fertility treatments, such as superovulation or in vitro fertilization (IVF), may hasten the return of endometriosis symptoms, (3) women attempting to conceive are reluctant to take medication in the luteal phase of the cycle, (4) dysmenorrhea and pelvic pain may progressively worsen as they have regular menses, and (5) these patients may require periodic surgical treatment that may further compromise fertility. Thus, there is an urgency to get pregnant before the pain symptoms become disabling.

Several approaches may augment fertility and minimize pain. First, a plan for fertility treatment should be mapped out in advance including a time allotment of 12 to 18 months, depending on the emotional, financial, and social needs of the couple. The proposed treatments should have an appropriate benefit/risk ratio. Aggressive treatment with superovulation and intrauterine insemination and/or IVF should be considered for all women, but particularly for those older than 35 years.

There are also options for management of dysmenorrhea that are compatible with conception. Primrose oil (omega-3 fatty acids), when taken daily, has been successfully used to significantly decrease dysmenorrhea. In addition, oral progesterone (200 mg three times daily) or progesterone suppositories may be started 2 days after the luteinizing hormone surge to decrease dysmenorrhea.

Pathophysiology of Infertility with Endometriosis

In spite of the apparent association of infertility and endometriosis, there is a paucity of evidence to identify the specific mechanism(s) of infertility due to this enigmatic disease. Three separate factors may play a role in infertility associated with endometriosis: implants, ovarian endometriomas, and adhesions. Each may contribute separately to a reduction in fertility by different mechanisms, which include alterations in immune system function, peritoneal fluid composition, anatomic relationships, and ovarian function. To confuse the issue even further, a high rate of additional infertility factors has been noted in these couples, including male factor, cervical factor, luteal phase defect, and tubal factor. In spite of this confusion, controlled studies suggest that the presence of endometriosis implants significantly compromises fertility potential.

The type of endometriosis that is encountered in women presenting with infertility is generally asymptomatic, and the indication for performing laparoscopy is as part of an infertility evaluation. For patients with endometriosis and infertility, it is important to stress the importance of a complete and thorough work-up of infertility factors. In many couples, endometriosis is not the only problem affecting their ability to conceive.

Surgical Treatment

Theoretically, the pregnancy rates after conservative surgery should be equivalent for each stage of disease, because the surgery is intended to excise all visible disease as well as correct anatomic distortion and lyse adhesions. When conservative resection of endometriosis is performed by laparotomy, pregnancy rates decline with disease severity. In contrast, when compared with expectant management of minimal and mild disease, laser laparoscopic treatment of endometriosis appears to have a fertility-enhancing effect significantly above that reported for other types of treatment, i.e., expectant management, hormonal therapy, or laparotomy. Indeed, for severe endometriosis, pregnancy rates after laser laparoscopy appear to be much better than those reported after laparotomy (65 vs. 40%). This discrepancy in pregnancy rates may be due to the greater risk of reformation of adhesions with laparotomy, particularly in more severe disease.

Other Fertility-Enhancing Treatments

For patients who fail to conceive after laparoscopic surgery, several fertility-enhancing regimens have demonstrated value. Repeated surgery may be of benefit by diminishing the amount of endometriosis that has recurred. Although the numbers are small and the surgical procedures were performed by laparotomy, the reported pregnancy rates of 25 to 40% are promising and may offer women who cannot or do not want to undergo advanced reproductive technologies as a treatment option.

Treatment with clomifene citrate and intrauterine insemination improves fecundity over periovulatory intercourse in couples with either unexplained infertility or surgically corrected endometriosis. Cycle fecundity rates as high as 9.5% have been reported. The efficacy of human menopausal gonadotropins and intrauterine insemination appears to be stage specific, with the cycle fecundity remaining fairly constant for stages I to III but dropping precipitously for stage IV (8.3, 11, 14.3, and 0%, respectively). This may reflect the fact that superovulation with intrauterine insemination is dependent on an intact ovum pickup mechanism that may be altered by adhesions in severe disease.

Gamete intrafallopian transfer allows the direct insertion of gametes into the fallopian tube, thus ensuring that the gametes reach the proper location. Pregnancy rates are comparable to those of women with other infertility diagnoses. Moreover, the laparoscopic retrieval of oocytes provides an opportunity to treat endometriosis under the same anesthesia without adversely affecting the probability of conception. Likewise, IVF offers opportunity for conception, particularly in women with tubal damage, in situations in which assessment of fertilizing capacity of the gametes is indicated and when other treatments have failed.

Treatments That Have No Efficacy in Enhancing Fertility

Recent studies have shown that hormonal treatment of mild and moderate endometriosis does not offer any advantage over expectant management for enhancing fertility. Moreover, the time during actual treatment delays conception, because all these hormonal agents are effective contraceptives. In addition, women are exposed to the risks and side effects of these hormonal agents without receiving any benefit. Thus, medical therapy has no place for enhancing conception in the treatment of endometriosis-associated infertility.

Few studies have reported pregnancy rates using preoperative or postoperative hormonal therapy, and fewer still have compared results with a control group. In spite of the paucity of published studies, some trends can be gleaned from these data. It appears that neither preoperative nor postoperative hormonal therapy is effective for the treatment of infertility associated with endometriosis.

DYSFUNCTIONAL UTERINE BLEEDING

method of
WILLIAM R. PHIPPS, M.D.
University of Rochester
Rochester, New York

PATHOPHYSIOLOGY AND ASPECTS OF PATIENTS' PRESENTATION

The term "dysfunctional uterine bleeding" (DUB) refers to abnormal uterine bleeding that is not a consequence of structural or systemic disease. Usually, DUB is related to anovulatory menstrual cycles. Women with ovulatory cycles may also have DUB, probably best specifically referred to as ovulatory DUB. Ovulatory DUB is thought to be a result of the effects of abnormal arachidonic acid metabolism on endometrial function.

The pathophysiology and optimal treatment of anovulatory DUB are best understood by comparison with the normal menstrual cycle. In the proliferative phase of the normal cycle, estrogen produced by the dominant follicle causes endometrial glands and stroma to proliferate. After ovulation, the corpus luteum produces large amounts of progesterone, in addition to estrogen, causing secretory changes in the endometrium. In the absence of pregnancy, degeneration of the corpus luteum is associated with the withdrawal of estrogen and progesterone, leading to a normal menses, an orderly and self-limited event that involves desquamation of the entire endometrium.

Unlike normal menstrual bleeding, anovulatory DUB involves exposure of the endometrium to estrogen unopposed by progesterone for relatively long periods. This prolonged exposure to estrogen leads to abnormally high and structurally unstable endometrium. The tissue is delicate and undergoes essentially spontaneous breakdown with associated bleeding. The process is not an orderly one, may go on more or less indefinitely, and involves different portions of the endometrium at different times.

The clinical picture of anovulatory DUB is one of irregular episodes of often painless bleeding occurring in an unpredictable fashion, with episodes ranging from a day of spotting to several weeks of continuous, heavy bleeding. Long periods of amenorrhea may or may not be interspersed among bleeding episodes. The cyclical symptoms of mittelschmerz and premenstrual molimina are absent. Patients particularly at risk include postmenarchal teenagers, perimenopausal women, and women with polycystic ovarian syndrome or obesity-related anovulation.

Women with ovulatory DUB in general present with menorrhagia, that is, heavy and/or prolonged menses occurring at regular intervals of 24 to 35 days. Monthly blood loss greater than 70 to 80 mL is considered abnormal and is often associated with iron deficiency anemia. As a practical matter, it is difficult to precisely quantify blood loss, and thus, decisions about both investigating and treating a patient for menorrhagia largely hinge on her subjective complaints.

DIAGNOSTIC CONSIDERATIONS

To make the diagnosis of DUB, other entities responsible for abnormal bleeding per vagina must first be excluded with reasonable certainty; these are shown in Table 1. A careful history and physical examination are, of course, essential. It is particularly important to establish the patient's ovulatory status, which may require basal body temperature charting, serum progesterone determinations, or endometrial sampling. It is important to realize that some patients with ovulatory DUB may be oligo-ovulatory and thus may have irregular and heavy menses. Decisions about what diagnostic studies should be performed need to be individualized, although most patients should at least have a complete blood count.

When a tentative diagnosis of anovulatory DUB is made, the decision about whether or not to do endometrial sampling before medical therapy depends primarily on the patient's risk for having endometrial hyperplasia or adenocarcinoma, two conditions that may also occur as a result of chronic anovulation. It is mandatory to rule out pregnancy with a serum or sensitive urine pregnancy test be-

TABLE 1. **Causes of Abnormal Vaginal Bleeding**

Dysfunctional Uterine Bleeding
Ovulatory DUB
Anovulatory DUB

Pelvic Malignancies
Endometrial adenocarcinoma
Uterine sarcoma
Cervical or vaginal carcinoma
Gestational trophoblastic neoplasia

Benign Anatomic Lesions
Endometrial hyperplasia
Uterine myoma(s) or adenomyosis
Endometrial or endocervical polyp(s)
Cervical or vaginal endometriosis
Vaginal adenosis
Müllerian anomalies associated with
    partial outflow obstruction

Inflammatory Processes
Endometritis
Cervicitis
Infectious or atrophic vaginitis

Pregnancy-Related Bleeding
Threatened abortion
Missed or incomplete abortion
Ectopic pregnancy
Molar pregnancy
Third-trimester or puerperal bleeding

Bleeding Diatheses
Platelet disorders
Anticoagulation therapy
Severe hepatic disease

Miscellaneous
Pelvic lacerations or trauma
Intrauterine device
Intravaginal foreign body
Drug-related causes
Hypothyroidism
Uterine sarcoidosis

fore such sampling, which can usually be accomplished in an office setting using a Pipelle endometrial suction curet or similar device.

When the tentative diagnosis is ovulatory DUB, it is particularly important to rule out not only endometrial hyperplasia or adenocarcinoma, but also other conditions that often manifest as menorrhagia. These include anatomic lesions, such as uterine submucosal myomas and endometrial polyps, as well as bleeding diatheses. Transvaginal ultrasonography may be useful in identifying anatomic lesions, particularly when coupled with sonohysterography, which involves instillation of fluid into the uterus so as to enhance ultrasonographic assessment of lesions protruding into the cavity. Diagnostic hysteroscopy can also be invaluable in this context. From a diagnostic standpoint, however, there is little if any place for traditional dilatation and curettage, except in conjunction with hysteroscopy.

TREATMENT

After initial diagnostic measures, attention is directed to therapeutic intervention. The first goal of DUB therapy is to stop the acute bleeding episode. Uterine curettage by itself may provide a substantial acute therapeutic effect, although in general, there is no reason not to start medical therapy immediately after endometrial sampling of any kind.

In most cases of anovulatory DUB, the bleeding can be stopped with the administration of a progestin. A typical progestin regimen is medroxyprogesterone acetate (Provera),* 10 to 20 mg orally once daily for 10 days. This agent usually stops the bleeding during the time it is being administered, followed by more or less orderly withdrawal bleeding starting immediately after it is discontinued. This sequence of events is similar to that during the secretory phase of the normal cycle. It is important to advise the patient at risk for pregnancy that occasionally, ovulation occurs as a result of progestin administration.

Another therapeutic option useful in stopping acute anovulatory DUB involves oral contraceptive pills (OCPs),† for example, having the patient take 2 to 4 low-dose (30 to 35 μg of estrogen) pills daily for 5 days. The bleeding should stop within 1 or 2 days, and as with progestin therapy, withdrawal bleeding is to be expected within a few days of the last pill. For the patient who has been bleeding heavily for a prolonged time and who has little residual endometrial tissue, it may be best to initially use high-dose estrogen therapy, for example, conjugated estrogens (Premarin),* 25 mg by intravenous bolus every 4 hours for 2 or 3 doses. The immediate improvement with such therapy is due more to a pharmacologic effect of estrogen on small-vessel hemostasis than to estrogen's ability to cause proliferation and healing of endometrial tissue. In general, once the bleeding has stopped in response to the Premarin, an OCP regimen should be started immediately.

Patients who are diagnosed as having anovulatory DUB, but show no response to the regimens previously described, require additional evaluation. This may consist of endometrial sampling if not previously performed, transvaginal ultrasonography, or hysteroscopy.

Once the acute episode of anovulatory DUB has been treated, attention is directed toward the possible need for long-term treatment. For the patient who is usually ovulatory, for whom it is thought that the bleeding episode just treated is unlikely to recur, a period of observation may be all that is necessary. On the other hand, some form of long-term therapy is indicated for patients in whom the anovulatory state responsible for the DUB is unlikely to abate spontaneously. The goals of this long-term therapy, which must include a progestin component, are to prevent recurrences of the unpredictable bleeding episodes, prevent endometrial hyperplasia, and lower the patient's risk for endometrial cancer. An iron supplement may be started at this time, if needed, as well.

Long-term treatment with OCPs† in the usual cyclical fashion is the best treatment for most patients with anovulatory DUB. Such therapy is particularly

---

*Exceeds dosage recommended by the manufacturer.
†Not FDA approved for this indication.

useful for those women who occasionally undergo spontaneous ovulation and need birth control, as well as those with polycystic ovarian syndrome, because of amelioration of the associated hyperandrogenism. Patients who are not candidates for OCP use may be treated with cyclical progestin treatment, for example, Provera, 10 mg orally once daily the first 10 to 14 days of each month. Anovulatory patients with DUB who desire pregnancy should, of course, have an appropriate hormonal evaluation followed by initiation of ovulation induction therapy.

Patients diagnosed as having ovulatory DUB are usually best treated in the long run with either OCPs* or a nonsteroidal anti-inflammatory drug regimen, such as ibuprofen,* 400 mg orally every 6 hours, starting on cycle day 1 and continuing through cessation of menses. Both of these treatments not only decrease the amount of bleeding but also address the often associated problem of dysmenorrhea. Another option is danazol,* 200 mg orally daily; most patients thus treated continue to experience regular menses, although side effects may be a problem. Still another option is the use of a progestin-releasing intrauterine device such as the Progestasert.*

At times, patients with either anovulatory or ovulatory DUB have a consistently poor response to the long-term medical options described, or unacceptable side effects. In that situation, consideration may be given to treatment with a long-acting gonadotropin-releasing hormone (GnRH) agonist,* to induce a menopause-like state. Long-term treatment with a GnRH agonist for most patients is problematic, however, largely because of the adverse effects on bone density. In general, patients with DUB failing to respond to the regimens described are best treated surgically, by either endometrial ablation or hysterectomy.

---

*Not FDA approved for this indication.

AMENORRHEA

method of
DAVID S. GUZICK, M.D., Ph.D.
*University of Rochester School of Medicine and
   Dentistry*
Rochester, New York

Amenorrhea, the absence of menstrual bleeding, is a common condition and a frequent reason that women of reproductive age seek health care. Many diverse conditions, such as congenital anatomic disorders of the female reproductive tract; endocrinopathies including hypothalamic, thyroid, and adrenal diseases; and chronic systemic illness, may manifest as amenorrhea. Although definitions of amenorrhea are not uniform, women who fail to menstruate by the age of 16 years in the presence of normal secondary sexual characteristics or by the age of 14 years in the absence of normal secondary sexual characteristics should be investigated. Furthermore, in a woman who has

previously been menstruating, 3 months of amenorrhea is considered abnormal and should be evaluated.

Traditionally, amenorrhea is classified as either primary (in women who have never menstruated) or secondary (in women who have previously menstruated for a variable time before the cessation of menses). However, some causes most commonly associated with primary amenorrhea (e.g., gonadal dysgenesis) may manifest as secondary amenorrhea, whereas others most commonly associated with secondary amenorrhea (e.g., hyperandrogenic anovulation) may manifest as incomplete puberty with primary amenorrhea. This article focuses on the diagnosis of patients with amenorrhea based on clinical presentation and the judicious use of laboratory testing. I attempt to provide a conceptual approach to the evaluation of amenorrhea that emphasizes clinical assessment. A careful history and physical examination alone guide the clinician to the appropriate major diagnostic categories; a judicious use of a small number of laboratory tests then leads to definitive diagnosis.

PRIMARY AMENORRHEA

It is common for reviews of the diagnostic assessment of primary amenorrhea to make heuristic use of flow-charts. I do some of that here but emphasize the initial categorization of individuals with primary amenorrhea according to four types of clinical presentation: sexual infantilism, congenital genital ambiguity, acquired virilization, and incomplete puberty. This categorization follows an approach developed by Paul MacDonald* in his teachings to house staff and fellows at the University of Texas, Southwestern Medical School. Using this classification system forces the clinician to think about the key features of a patient's clinical presentation; furthermore, once the patient is assigned to one of the four major categories, there is a laboratory test or clinical finding that distinguishes among the major diagnoses in the category. In this manner, the combination of clinical assessment and limited laboratory testing almost always guides the clinician to the likely diagnosis. If several options remain in a particular diagnostic grouping, additional laboratory tests can help discriminate between the possibilities.

This article emphasizes the clinical approach to the four broad categories of primary amenorrhea based on history, physical examination, and one or two diagnostic tests within each category. This approach completes the diagnostic evaluation for the vast majority of women presenting with primary amenorrhea. Less common causes are not reviewed in detail.

Sexual Infantilism

Sexual infantilism is characterized by the absence of secondary sexual development, corresponding to Tanner stage 1. This can be most readily assessed clinically by the absence of breast budding. However,

---

*I learned this approach as a fellow of Dr. MacDonald. However, responsibility for any errors of omission or commission remains with me.

- Characterized by no endogenous estrogen production
- Two possible defects:
  1) Inability of gonads to produce estrogen
  2) Failure of pituitary to secrete gonadotropin
- Evaluation: draw FSH; if elevated, examine patient for presence of uterus and obtain karyotype.

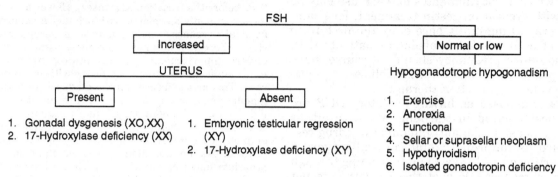

Figure 1. Sexual infantilism. *Abbreviation:* FSH = follicle-stimulating hormone.

breast development may have been induced by exogenous estrogen administration, because it is common for patients in this category to have been given oral contraceptives to induce cyclical withdrawal bleeding. In such cases, the clinician must, through the history, ascertain the status of secondary sexual characteristics at the time of initial presentation for primary amenorrhea, before the patient began exogenous estrogen therapy.

As indicated in Figure 1, the absence of secondary sexual characteristics is caused by the lack of endogenous estrogen production, due either to an inability of the ovaries to produce estrogen even when stimulated by gonadotropins or to a lack of adequate gonadotropin stimulation of normally responsive ovaries. Discrimination between these two possibilities can be readily accomplished by testing the serum follicle-stimulating hormone (FSH) level. An elevated FSH value (>30 mIU per mL) implies ovarian unresponsiveness, whereas a normal or low level of FSH implies a lack of ovarian stimulation. If the FSH value is elevated, the patient should be examined for the presence or absence of a uterus. The presence of a uterus is good (but not perfect) office-based evidence of the absence of a Y chromosome; a karyotype should be obtained for confirmation.

If a uterus is present, by far the most common cause of sexual infantilism is gonadal dysgenesis, which is also the most common cause of primary amenorrhea generally. Gonadal dysgenesis is characterized by "streak" gonads that do not contain any germinal elements. Patients with the classic form of gonadal dysgenesis, Turner's syndrome or 45,XO gonadal dysgenesis (O designates the absence of the second sex chromosome), generally present with short stature (<58 inches) and can display a variety of other characteristics, such as a webbed neck, a shieldlike chest with wide-set nipples, and shortening of the fourth or fifth digits. Other karyotypic variants are mosaicism, structural abnormalities of the second sex chromosome, and pure gonadal dysgenesis (i.e., XX or XY). In patients with pure XY

gonadal dysgenesis or mosaics with a Y chromosome, there is a risk of gonadal malignancies, i.e., dysgerminomas or gonadoblastomas; thus, it is generally recommended that the gonads be removed in such patients. Malignancy is a more common problem in congenital genital ambiguity or acquired virilization; however, such neoplasms in an XY individual presenting with sexual infantilism are rare.

Initiation of low-dose estrogen therapy (1 mg of oral estradiol-17β [Estrace] or 0.3 mg of conjugated equine estrogens [Premarin]) at 12 to 13 years of age in conjunction with a progestin (5 mg of medroxyprogesterone acetate [Provera]) promotes the development of secondary sexual characteristics and is associated with a growth spurt without an acceleration of bone age or a reduction in the final body height. The estrogen can be given each day, with the progestin added on the 1st through the 12th calendar days of each month. This regimen induces regular withdrawal bleeding, thus simulating normal menstrual cycles. Once the final height is achieved, an estrogen-progestin oral contraceptive can be used to prevent the long-term sequelae of hypoestrogenism without increasing the risk of endometrial hyperplasia or cancer.

Karyotypic females with 17α-hydroxylase deficiency present with sexual infantilism and primary amenorrhea (see Figure 1) due to negligible estrogen production from deficiencies of C_{21} and C_{19} steroids. Progesterone, 11-deoxycorticosterone, and corticosterone levels are elevated. Hypertension and hypokalemic alkalosis may be present. Treatment is aimed at providing the missing steroids. Sex steroids must be given to effect sexual development. In patients with absence of the uterus and elevated FSH level, 17α-hydroxylase deficiency with an XY karyotype or embryonic testicular regression may be the cause. Karyotypic males may present with disorders ranging from normal-appearing female external genitalia and a blind vaginal pouch to ambiguous genitalia or a small phallus with hypospadias (see next section).

Patients with primary amenorrhea, sexual infantilism, and a normal or low FSH level (see Figure 1) have hypogonadotropic hypogonadism by exclusion. Idiopathic and genetic forms of multiple pituitary hormone deficiency are also included in this group. Deficiency of pulsatile gonadotropin-releasing hormone (GnRH) may be caused by a congenital defect that is undetected until puberty as well as by trauma, tumors, vascular lesions, or inflammatory processes. Psychiatric and functional conditions can also suppress GnRH. Gonadotropin-deficient patients are usually of normal height for age when seen during adolescence, unlike patients with constitutional delay in growth and puberty.

Craniopharyngioma originating from the pituitary stalk is the most common tumor associated with sexual infantilism. The peak incidence occurs between 6 and 14 years of age. Patients often present with headache, visual changes, short stature, diabetes insipidus, and hypothyroidism. In addition to gonadotropin deficiency, there may be deficiency in thyroid-stimulating hormone (TSH), adrenocorticotropic hormone, growth hormone, and vasopressin. Computed tomography or magnetic resonance imaging (MRI) is useful for diagnosis. Surgical excision is typically required, and postoperative radiation therapy is often needed because of incomplete tumor resection. Other rare central nervous system tumors associated with sexual infantilism and primary amenorrhea are germinomas, astrocytomas, and hypothalamic or optic gliomas occurring independently or in conjunction with neurofibromatosis.

Functional gonadotropin deficiency, typically associated with secondary amenorrhea, may be associated with primary amenorrhea when there is severe systemic or chronic disease, malnutrition, hypothyroidism, anorexia nervosa, and extreme levels of exercise or psychogenic stress. Weight loss to less than 85% of ideal weight for height, due to either chronic disease or dieting, is associated with gonadotropin deficiency. Chronic renal disease in childhood may be associated with sexual infantilism, although normal gonadotropin secretion ensues after kidney transplant. A delay in puberty and subsequent menarche may be noted in patients with hypothyroidism; treatment with thyroxine can initiate puberty. Patients with anorexia nervosa may present with primary amenorrhea and sexual infantilism or delayed puberty in association with suppressed GnRH pulsatility and other neuroendocrine derangements. Psychotherapy, behavioral modification, and dietary modification are the mainstays of therapy. Exercise—particularly, vigorous training starting before puberty, such as in gymnastics and ballet dancing—may also be associated with low gonadotropin levels and primary amenorrhea or delayed sexual development. The underlying cause is unclear but may involve body composition and changes in neuroendocrine signals from the brain that promote fuel mobilization, redistribution, and utilization. Counseling concerning the risks of excessive exercise and the importance of adequate caloric intake is advisable.

Congenital Genital Ambiguity

The patient with congenital genital ambiguity often attracts medical attention at the time of birth. However, if the ambiguity is subtle, he or she may not be seen until a later age, when parental concern or amenorrhea brings the patient to a physician. Thus, a careful history of events surrounding delivery and subsequent pediatric examinations, as well as a detailed genital examination, is important. If a patient with primary amenorrhea is assigned to the category of congenital genital ambiguity, a disorder of fetal endocrinology is likely: either incomplete masculinization of a male fetus or virilization of a female fetus in utero (Figure 2). If a uterus is present, karyotyping differentiates between an XX individual with a probable enzyme deficiency and a patient with some variant of gonadal dysgenesis or true hermaphroditism (coexistence of ovarian and testicular tissue). Patients with an XX karyotype may be further categorized according to 17-hydroxyprogesterone level. An elevated 17-hydroxyprogesterone level indicates congenital adrenal hyperplasia, most commonly due to 21-hydroxylase deficiency. In patients with a normal 17-hydroxyprogesterone level, genital ambiguity may be due to in utero exposure to maternal androgens or a variant of gonadal dysgenesis. In patients with absence of the uterus and an XY karyotype, incomplete virilization due to androgen resistance such as testicular feminization is a possible cause. Testosterone enzyme defects and embryonic testicular regression are also possibilities.

Acquired Hirsutism and Virilization

Primary amenorrhea associated with acquired hirsutism or virilization and various degrees of genital and breast maturation but no genital ambiguity is an uncommon yet important presentation of primary amenorrhea, because it raises the possibility of a dysgenetic gonadal tumor. The karyotype differentiates between women with a likely dysgenetic gonadal tumor and those with either Cushing's syndrome or an ovarian or adrenal cause of the amenorrhea (Figure 3).

Incomplete Puberty

Patients with incomplete puberty are characterized by primary amenorrhea in a setting of normal secondary sexual characteristics (Figure 4). These patients can be divided into two categories: those with a müllerian abnormality and those with a normal uterus and vagina. In patients with a normal uterus, there are sometimes obstructive lesions due to a lack of normal vertical fusion of the down-growing müllerian duct and up-growing urogenital sinus during embryogenesis. Clinical presentation in affected patients includes primary amenorrhea, cyclical lower abdominal pain, and often a vaginal mass due to hematocolpos. Defects in vertical fusion may occur anywhere along the vagina. Correction of the problem involves excision of the obstructive septum.

- Characterized by abnormal androgen representation in utero
- Two possible problems:
  1) Incomplete masculinization of male fetus
  2) Virilization of female fetus
- Evaluation:

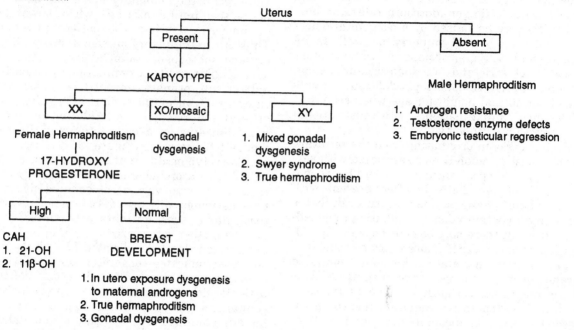

Figure 2. Congenital genital ambiguity. *Abbreviation:* CAH = congenital adrenal hyperplasia; OH = hydroxylase.

In patients without a uterus, müllerian agenesis (Mayer-Rokitansky-Küster-Hauser or Rokitansky's syndrome) or testicular feminization syndrome may be the cause of primary amenorrhea. Müllerian agenesis is the second most common cause of primary amenorrhea. Affected patients have a normal 46,XX karyotype but lack a uterus and vagina. Ultrasonography or MRI may be used to confirm the diagnosis. An intravenous urogram is indicated for evaluation because of the high incidence of renal anomalies (15 to 40%). Ovarian function is normal in these women,

but they are unable to carry a pregnancy because of the absence of a uterus. Ovarian stimulation, oocyte retrieval, fertilization in vitro, and transfer of embryos to a volunteer surrogate with a uterus offer a means of having a genetic offspring. A vagina can be created surgically or through progressive dilatation of the blind-ending vaginal pouch or dimple on the perineum. Patients often require extensive teaching and training about sexual functioning and their inability to carry a pregnancy.

Testicular feminization, or androgen resistance

- Characterized by primary amenorrhea in a setting of varying degrees of genital and breast maturation, no genital ambiguity, but acquired hirsutism or virilization.
- Evaluation:

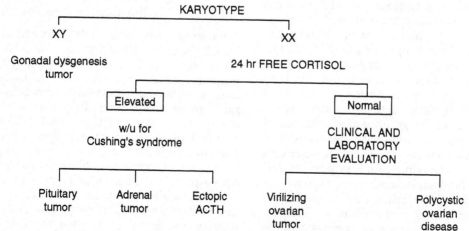

Figure 3. Acquired hirsutism or virilization. *Abbreviations:* w/u = work-up; ACTH = adrenocorticotropic hormone.

- Characterized by primary amenorrhea in a setting of genital and breast maturation and no genital ambiguity
- Can be conveniently divided into two categories: those with an associated abnormality of the uterus and /or vagina and those with a normal uterus and vagina.
- Evaluation:

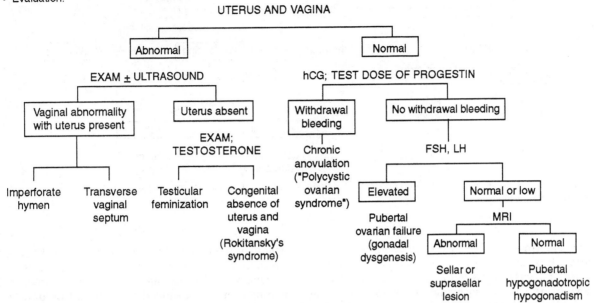

Figure 4. Incomplete puberty. *Abbreviations:* FSH = follicle-stimulating hormone; hCG = human chorionic gonadotropin; LH = luteinizing hormone; MRI = magnetic resonance imaging; exam = physical examination.

syndrome, is also characterized by primary amenorrhea, absence of a uterus, a blind-ending vaginal pouch, and a 46,XY karyotype. Although affected patients have normal breast development, pubic and axillary hair is scant. This disorder, either X-linked recessive or X-linked dominant, is due to a defect in the androgen receptor. In patients who present with an inguinal hernia and primary amenorrhea, complete androgen resistance should be suspected. These patients may be differentiated clinically from those with müllerian agenesis because of their paucity of pubic and axillary hair. An elevated serum testosterone level confirms the diagnosis. Breast development in these women probably results from a lack of suppression of breast tissue anlage by testosterone during fetal life, stimulation of breast tissue by estrogens derived from direct testicular secretion, and peripheral aromatization of testosterone to estrogens. Bilateral gonadectomy is essential after breast development because of the increased risk of malignancy in inguinal and abdominal testes.

The evaluation of women with a normal reproductive tract and primary amenorrhea is similar to the evaluation of those with secondary amenorrhea. Once pregnancy has been eliminated as an explanation, a progestin challenge (e.g., 10 mg of medroxyprogesterone acetate for 5 to 10 days) may be given as a clinically useful (although not perfect) test to differentiate the patient with normal estrogen levels from the patient with hypoestrogenism. Estrogen priming of the endometrium is required before progestin-induced withdrawal bleeding. In general, if withdrawal bleeding ensues, chronic anovulation or

polycystic ovarian syndrome is the most likely cause of the amenorrhea. The clinical presentation includes primary amenorrhea or, more typically, perimenarchal oligomenorrhea. Some evidence of androgen excess (e.g., hirsutism, acne) is typically present, and obesity is common (i.e., 60 to 70% of cases). In adolescent patients, low-dose oral contraceptives containing 30 to 35 μg of ethinyl estradiol may be prescribed to initiate and maintain cyclical menses. When fertility becomes desirable, ovulation can usually be induced with clomiphene citrate.

In patients who have no withdrawal bleeding in response to a progestin challenge, the serum FSH level should be measured. An elevated FSH value indicates pubertal ovarian failure or gonadal dysgenesis. Patients with gonadal dysgenesis who have some secondary sexual development are usually mosaics, i.e., have a 45,XO/XX karyotype. Treatment is as previously described, i.e., estrogen-progestin therapy. If gonadotropin levels are normal or low, MRI is indicated to investigate the possibility of a sellar or suprasellar lesion such as craniopharyngioma or germinoma. Normal MRI results suggest pubertal hypogonadotropic hypogonadism. Further evaluation and management follow guidelines previously given for sexual infantilism.

SECONDARY AMENORRHEA

Women with secondary amenorrhea (Figure 5) should be evaluated for physiologic causes, including pregnancy, lactation, and premature menopause. Once these causes have been excluded, the possibility

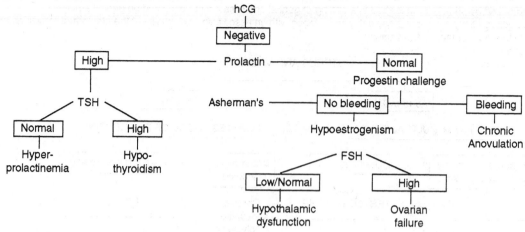

Figure 5. Secondary amenorrhea. *Abbreviations:* FSH = follicle-stimulating hormone; hCG = human chorionic gonadotropin; TSH = thyroid-stimulating hormone.

of hyperprolactinemia should be assessed. A progestin challenge is sometimes used in women with secondary amenorrhea to differentiate between those with normal and those with low estrogen levels, although a clinical history and physical examination can generally accomplish the same goal.

Acquired abnormalities of the outflow tract associated with normal estrogen levels and secondary amenorrhea, assessed by the lack of withdrawal bleeding and/or physical examination, include Asherman's syndrome and, rarely, cervical stenosis. Women with Asherman's syndrome or intrauterine adhesions have either amenorrhea or hypomenorrhea. Most patients give a history of dilatation and curettage or of previous uterine surgery, such as metroplasty, myomectomy, or cesarean section. Severe pelvic infections, such as tuberculosis and schistosomiasis, are rare causes of Asherman's syndrome. The hysterosalpingogram reveals multiple filling defects or, less commonly, obliteration of the uterine cavity. Hysteroscopic lysis of intrauterine adhesions is the preferred method of treatment, after which 90% of patients resume normal menses. Cervical stenosis due to a surgical procedure such as conization for cervical neoplasia can be a cause of secondary amenorrhea.

Prolactin, the primary hormone controlling lactation, is secreted by the lactotrophs of the anterior pituitary and is under inhibition by dopaminergic neurons in the hypothalamus. An elevated prolactin level in nonpregnant women is a common cause of secondary amenorrhea. Many factors are associated with abnormal prolactin secretion, including breast manipulation during examination, stress, a host of medications (such as estrogens, antidopaminergic drugs, and opioids), prolactinomas, and destructive lesions of the hypothalamus. Hyperprolactinemia may also be associated with chronic renal failure, hypothyroidism, and ectopic production by bronchogenic tumors.

In women presenting with secondary amenorrhea, the serum prolactin concentration should be assessed regardless of the presence or absence of galactorrhea, because about one third of women with hyperprolactinemia do not have galactorrhea. Because of the myriad causes of an elevated prolactin level (>20 ng per mL), a second blood test should be done to confirm the diagnosis, preferably at midmorning with the patient in the fasting state. The TSH level should be measured to investigate the possibility of primary hypothyroidism as a cause of amenorrhea and galactorrhea due to stimulation of the lactotrophs by excess thyrotropin-releasing hormone secretion. Hyperprolactinemia in the patient with a normal TSH level might prompt evaluation of the pituitary by MRI or computed tomography. Even mild elevations of prolactin levels may be associated with pituitary adenomas, although the natural history of microadenomas (i.e., <1 cm) is typically benign.

Whether or not the patient has an adenoma, her amenorrhea should be treated medically, because hypoestrogenism increases the risk of osteoporosis. A dopamine agonist, such as bromocriptine (Parlodel), 2.5 mg per day increasing by increments of 2.5 mg at 2-week intervals if necessary, should normalize the prolactin level and prompt resumption of regular cyclical menses. Bromocriptine treatment should be taken at night to avoid postural hypotension. Patients unable to tolerate oral bromocriptine because of gastrointestinal side effects may take it intravaginally. Women who become pregnant during bromocriptine treatment may discontinue its use once pregnancy is diagnosed, although the agent is not associated with an increased risk of fetal malformations. Patients in whom medical management fails, particularly those with macroadenomas, may require surgical intervention or, rarely, radiation therapy.

Women in whom a progestin challenge induces withdrawal bleeding may be classified as having chronic anovulation with estrogen present. Polycystic ovarian syndrome is the most common cause of secondary amenorrhea in this setting. Women frequently present with chronic anovulation beginning at menarche, with evidence of androgen excess. Hyperinsulinemia is common. Obesity is stereotypic but is not a necessary characteristic. Treatment depends on the reproductive goals of the patient. If pregnancy is not desired, low-dose oral contraceptives may be prescribed. Patients desiring fertility usually ovulate in response to clomiphene citrate (Clomid, Serophene), 50 mg administered daily from days 3 to 7 or 5 to 9 of the menstrual cycle. Dosage may be increased by increments of 50 mg up to 200 mg per day; approximately 75 to 80% of patients so treated ovulate. In those who show no response to clomiphene, gonadotropins or laparoscopic ovarian drilling may be used.

Other rare causes of secondary amenorrhea with normal estrogen levels are thyroid disorders, adult-onset adrenal hyperplasia, Cushing's disease, and ovarian and adrenal tumors.

Women with a normal outflow tract in whom withdrawal bleeding does not occur after a progestin challenge are hypoestrogenic. Determining gonadotropin levels allows further subclassification. Those with FSH levels greater than 30 mIU per mL have hypergonadotropic hypogonadism or gonadal failure, whereas those with low or normal values have hypothalamic-pituitary dysfunction secondary to weight loss, stress, exercise, anorexia nervosa, hypothalamic or pituitary tumors, or isolated gonadotropin deficiency. As noted previously, these causes may also be associated with primary amenorrhea. In hypothalamic amenorrhea, suppression of GnRH secretion is responsible for low or decreased gonadotropin levels and resultant hypoestrogenism. Counseling often corrects the disorder, with the resumption of menstrual cyclicity. However, in patients with persistent amenorrhea, the administration of pulsatile GnRH or of gonadotropins may be utilized for ovulation induction if pregnancy is desired. Oral contraceptives* or estrogen-progestin treatment is indicated to maintain normal bone density in women not interested in fertility.

Exercise amenorrhea is similarly the result of reduced GnRH pulse frequency. Reduction in the amount of exercise often corrects the amenorrhea. However, pulsatile GnRH or gonadotropin therapy may also be necessary to induce ovulation. Hormone replacement therapy to prevent bone loss is indicated if the patient declines to alter her exercise program. Simple weight loss in anorexia nervosa does not explain the amenorrhea in affected patients. Absence or diminution of luteinizing hormone response to GnRH has been a consistent finding. Psychiatric counseling is necessary because of the potentially life-threatening nature of this disorder. Hormone replacement therapy should be administered until sufficient weight gain allows a return of cyclical menses.

Women with hypergonadotropic hypergonadism include some patients with gonadal dysgenesis who may menstruate for a variable time before ovarian failure. A woman who presents with secondary amenorrhea before the age of 30 years should undergo a karyotyping to rule out the presence of a Y chromosome, because of the risk of gonadal malignancy. Treatment should be aimed at correcting the hypoestrogenism with hormone replacement or oral contraceptives. Most women with gonadal dysgenesis are infertile, although pregnancies have been reported in women with 46,XX/45,XO karyotype. Normal pregnancy and delivery may be accomplished with donor eggs, in vitro fertilization, endometrial synchronism, and early support of the pregnancy with exogenous estrogen and progesterone.

Amenorrhea and elevated gonadotropin levels in a woman younger than 40 years are considered premature ovarian failure. Causes include ovarian failure secondary to chemotherapy, pelvic irradiation, and ovarian surgery as well as genetic or autoimmune causes. In the transition to ovarian failure, follicular depletion may not be complete, and spontaneous ovulation and pregnancy may occasionally occur. Karyotyping and thyroid and adrenal evaluation, including specific endocrine antibody testing, should be performed. Complications of estrogen deficiency may be prevented by hormone replacement therapy. In patients desiring pregnancy, the use of donor oocytes with synchronization of the endometrium has resulted in pregnancy rates of 30 to 50%.

DYSMENORRHEA

method of
RONALD M. NELSON, M.D.
White Memorial Medical Center
Los Angeles, California

Dysmenorrhea is a common menstrual symptom. A majority of women (70%) experience pain during menstruation at some time during their reproductive years. For many, this pain is a tolerated burden of menstruation, and medical attention is not frequently sought. They will rely on simple analgesics for relief. In about 25%, however, the pain is significant enough to require professional assistance. Severe dysmenorrhea with incapacitation and a loss of normal daily activity is experienced by 10 to 15%.

Dysmenorrhea is classified as primary or secondary. Primary dysmenorrhea occurs in the absence of pelvic pathology, whereas secondary dysmenorrhea is associated with underlying pelvic disease or abnormality.

The etiology and pathophysiology underlying dysmenorrhea have been well established. As a result, rational and effective medical therapy has dramatically improved the long-term management of women with this disorder.

PRIMARY DYSMENORRHEA

Primary dysmenorrhea almost invariably occurs with ovulatory cycles. Adolescent females make up a large proportion of women with primary dysmenorrhea. The menstrual pain usually begins some 6 to 12 months after menarche, coinciding with the onset of ovulation cycles. The prevalence of primary dysmenorrhea declines with advancing age, vaginal deliveries, and oral contraceptive use.

The pain usually begins with the onset of menstrual flow but may precede it by several hours. Typically lasting from

---

*Not FDA approved for this indication.

several hours to 1 to 2 days, the pain seldom persists for more than 2 to 3 days. Systemic complaints (nausea, vomiting, diarrhea, and headaches) frequently accompany the menstrual pain.

It is well established that primary dysmenorrhea is caused by increased production and concentration of prostaglandin $F_{2\alpha}$ in the endometrium during the luteal and menstrual phases of the cycle. Analysis of secretory endometrium, endometrial washings, and menstrual fluid has demonstrated significantly higher levels of prostaglandin in women with dysmenorrhea. These findings correlate well with the observation of hypercontractility of uterine muscle during menses in dysmenorrhea. The inhibition of prostaglandin production by prostaglandin synthetase inhibitors has been shown to lower the endometrial concentration of prostaglandin and to be quite effective in relieving the symptom of dysmenorrhea.

SECONDARY DYSMENORRHEA

Menstrual pain associated with detectable pelvic pathology is secondary dysmenorrhea. It is more frequently seen in the older woman and is often associated with endometriosis, leiomyomata, adenomyosis, pelvic infection, and use of intrauterine devices. Secondary dysmenorrhea in the adolescent may be caused by congenital obstructive defects of the genital tract.

For therapeutic reasons, it is important to distinguish between primary and secondary dysmenorrhea. Primary dysmenorrhea is approached more commonly with conservative medical management, whereas secondary dysmenorrhea is more commonly treated surgically. The pain of secondary dysmenorrhea usually occurs in older women, worsens with time, and may not be restricted to the menses. Dyspareunia is a common associated complaint.

A detailed history and pelvic examination are usually sufficient to distinguish between primary and secondary dysmenorrhea. Laboratory tests are generally of little value. A pelvic ultrasound examination and/or diagnostic laparoscopy should be considered when pelvic pathology is suspected or there is no response to conservative medical management.

MEDICAL MANAGEMENT OF PRIMARY DYSMENORRHEA

The two medical approaches that have been most successful in the treatment of primary dysmenorrhea are the inhibition of ovulation with oral contraceptives* and the inhibition of prostaglandin production with prostaglandin synthetase inhibitors. The choice between these approaches depends on whether the patient desires oral contraception for birth control and whether there may be a contraindication to the use of either approach.

Inhibition of Ovulation

Combined oral contraceptives would be the treatment of first choice if the patient desires birth control. Oral contraceptives produce a marked reduction in the concentration of prostaglandin in the menstrual fluid and result in a considerable decrease

---

*Not FDA approved for this indication.

TABLE 1. **Treatment of Dysmenorrhea with Prostaglandin Synthetase Inhibitors**

| Generic Name | Trade Name | Dosage | |
		Strength (mg)	Frequency
Naproxen sodium	Aleve	220	q 8 h
	Anaprox	275	q 6 h
	Anaprox DS	550	q 12 h
	Naprelan	1000	Daily
Naproxen	Naprosyn	250–500	q 12 h
Ibuprofen	Motrin	400	q 4–6 h
	Ibu	400	q 4–6 h
Ketoprofen	Orudis	50–75	q 6–8 h
Mefenamic acid	Ponstel	500	Initial
		250	q 6 h
Diclofenac potassium	Cataflam	50	q 8 h

in uterine muscle contractility. With combined oral contraceptives, most women find relief from primary dysmenorrhea. If there is an incomplete response to oral contraceptives, a prostaglandin synthetase inhibitor can be added.

Ovulation may be inhibited with danazol (Danocrine)* and gonadotropin-releasing hormone agonist.* Although extremely effective, they have limited application for primary dysmenorrhea. Either approach is expensive, associated with significant side effects, and not recommended for long-term therapy.

Prostaglandin Synthetase Inhibitors

If oral contraception is not acceptable, the drug of choice for treatment of primary dysmenorrhea is a prostaglandin synthetase inhibitor. Nonsteroidal anti-inflammatory agents have proved to be extremely effective prostaglandin inhibitors. Commonly used agents approved for management of dysmenorrhea are listed in Table 1. They are rapidly absorbed and act quickly in reducing prostaglandin concentration in the endometrium. The effect is so rapid that treatment before the onset of menstruation is usually unnecessary. The rate of overall effectiveness in relieving pain ranges from 70 to 90%.

Side effects associated with these nonsteroidal anti-inflammatory agents are generally relatively mild. The most common symptoms are heartburn, nausea, dizziness, visual disturbances, bronchospasm, and allergic reactions. The medications are usually well tolerated because of the short duration of therapy required. Contraindications to these drugs include a history of previous ulcer disease and bronchospastic reactions to ingestion of aspirin or aspirin-like drugs.

SURGICAL MANAGEMENT

Surgical approaches in the management of primary dysmenorrhea are rarely indicated. Presacral

---

*Not FDA approved for this indication.

neurectomy is not indicated in the absence of pelvic pathology. There has been an enthusiasm for transection of the uterosacral ligaments at the time of diagnostic laparoscopy for refractory dysmenorrhea. This approach remains controversial and should not be recommended until further controlled studies have documented its usefulness and long-term effectiveness.

Treatment of secondary dysmenorrhea is directed toward the underlying cause. In most instances, medical management is less successful, except when the dysmenorrhea is associated with use of an intrauterine device.

PREMENSTRUAL SYNDROME

method of
JOSEPH F. MORTOLA, M.D.
Cook County Hospital
Chicago, Illinois

Advances in elucidating the pathophysiology of premenstrual syndrome (PMS) have permitted the development of sound pharmacologic interventions for this previously treatment-resistant disorder. The earlier high failure rates of medical therapy for PMS can largely be attributed to improper diagnosis of the syndrome, overinclusion of patients with poorly characterized symptoms in controlled clinical trials, and underutilization of rigorous experimental methodology in studies of the efficacy of various therapies. Although no medications are currently approved by the Food and Drug Administration for the treatment of PMS, extensive, well-designed studies have been conducted that can guide the clinician's treatment of the disorder. As a result, less proven nonpharmacologic modalities such as dietary modification, exercise regimens, and psychotherapy are more quickly supplanted by the use of medication. Before initiation of treatment, however, accurate diagnosis is required, particularly because PMS often mimics other disorders, including depression, anxiety disorders, and thyroid disease.

DIAGNOSIS

The prevalence of PMS is estimated to be 2.5% in women of reproductive age. Although prevalence rates of up to 80% have been reported, this figure is attributable to the inclusion of a large number of women with normal premenstrual symptoms, referred to as molimina, in the PMS population. Currently, diagnostic criteria are available that permit a more accurate assessment of women in need of medical intervention because of disabling disruption of social, vocational, and avocational performance (Table 1). Even with such strict diagnostic criteria, however, PMS is among the most common disorders in reproductive-age women.

Although more than 150 symptoms have been ascribed to PMS, careful statistical analysis in well-selected populations reveals the symptom constellation to be much more specific and well-defined. Only a specific group of symptoms occurs exclusively in the luteal phase of the menstrual cycle with sufficient frequency to merit inclusion in the syndrome. The most common of these symptoms are

TABLE 1. Diagnostic Criteria for Premenstrual Syndrome

1. Presence by self-report of at least one of the following somatic *and* affective symptoms during the 5 d before menses in each of the three prior menstrual cycles:

Affective	Somatic
Depression	Breast tenderness
Angry outbursts	Abdominal bloating
Irritability	Headache
Anxiety	Swelling
Confusion	
Social withdrawal	

2. Relief of the above symptoms within 4 d of the onset of menses, without recurrence until at least cycle day 12
3. Presence of the symptoms in the absence of any pharmacologic therapy, hormone ingestion, or drug or alcohol use
4. Reproducibility of the symptoms during two cycles of prospective recording
5. Presence of identifiable dysfunction in social or economic performance by one of the following criteria:
   Marital or relationship discord confirmed by partner
   Difficulties in parenting
   Poor work or school performance; poor attendance or tardiness
   Increased social isolation
   Legal difficulties
   Suicidal ideation
   Seeking of medical attention for somatic symptoms

From Mortola JF, Girton L, Yen SS: Depressive episodes in premenstrual syndrome. Am J Obstet Gynecol *161*:1682–1687, 1989.

fatigue (92% of women with PMS), irritability (91%), depression (85%), breast tenderness, and bloated sensations in the abdomen or extremities. Appetite disturbance restricted to the luteal phase of the cycle is seen in 75% of women with PMS and is usually experienced as increased food cravings, particularly for carbohydrates. The other commonly noted behavioral symptoms are mood lability with alternating sadness and anger (81%), oversensitivity to trivial environmental events (69%), crying spells (65%), social withdrawal (65%), and difficulty concentrating (47%). Common physical symptoms also include acne (71%) and gastrointestinal upset (48%). Although less often observed, vasomotor flushes (18%), heart palpitations (13%), and dizziness (13%) occur more frequently in women with PMS than in women who do not suffer from the syndrome.

None of the symptoms of PMS is unique to the disorder, and even presentation of the entire constellation of symptoms is less important in establishing the diagnosis than is the timing of the symptoms' occurrence with respect to the menstrual cycle. From the fourth day of menses until at least cycle day 12, symptoms, if they occur at all, are sporadic and no more common than would be expected in the general population. This criterion for the relatively symptom-free interval is applicable to most reproductive-age women, although women with menstrual cycles that are typically shorter than 26 days may have the onset of symptoms slightly earlier than day 12. The importance of prospectively documenting symptoms in establishing the diagnosis of PMS has been demonstrated in numerous studies. Validated symptom inventories such as the Calendar of Premenstrual Experiences (University of California, San Diego) are the most reliable methods of establishing the diagnosis (Figure 1). Prospective recording over the course of two menstrual cycles is optimal to ensure reproducibility in the timing of symptoms. Scores on such inventories should reveal at least a twofold increase in total

Name _____ Month/Year _____ Age _____ Unit # _____

Begin your calendar on the *first* day of your menstrual cycle. Enter the calendar date below the cycle day. Day 1 is your *first* day of bleeding. Shade the box above the cycle day if you have bleeding. ■ Put an X for spotting. ☒

If more than one symptom is listed in a category, i.e., nausea, diarrhea, constipation, you do not need to experience all of these. Rate the most disturbing of the symptoms on the 1-3 scale.

Weight: Weigh yourself before breakfast. Record weight in the box below date.

Symptoms: Indicate the severity of your symptoms by using the scale below. Rate each symptom at about the same time each evening.

     0 = **None** (symptom not present)   2 = **Moderate** (interferes with normal activities)

     1 = **Mild** (noticeable but not troublesome)   3 = **Severe** (intolerable, unable to perform normal activities)

Other Symptoms: If there are other symptoms you experience, list and indicate severity.

Medications: List any medications taken. Put an X on the corresponding day(s).

Bleeding																																									
Cycle Day	1	2	3	4	5	6	7	8	9	10	11	12	13	14	15	16	17	18	19	20	21	22	23	24	25	26	27	28	29	30	31	32	33	34	35	36	37	38	39	40
Date																																									
Weight																																									
SYMPTOMS																																									
Acne																																									
Bloatedness																																									
Breast tenderness																																									
Dizziness																																									
Fatigue																																									
Headache																																									
Hot flashes																																									
Nausea, diarrhea, constipation																																									
Palpitations																																									
Swelling (hands, ankles, breast)																																									
Angry outbursts, arguments, violent tendencies																																									
Anxiety, tension, nervousness																																									
Confusion, difficulty concentrating																																									
Crying easily																																									
Depression																																									
Food cravings (sweets, salts)																																									
Forgetfulness																																									
Irritability																																									
Increased appetite																																									
Mood swings																																									
Overly sensitive																																									
Wish to be alone																																									
Other Symptoms																																									
1. _____																																									
2. _____																																									
Medications																																									
1. _____																																									
2. _____																																									

Figure 1. Calendar of Premenstrual Experiences (COPE). (© University of California, San Diego; Department of Reproductive Medicine, Division of Reproductive Endocrinology.)

symptom severity during the last week of the menstrual cycle in comparison with the second week.

In addition to the type of symptoms and their timing, several other criteria should be fulfilled to accurately diagnose PMS. These include the identifiable presence of socioeconomic difficulties and the absence of pharmacologic therapy with hormonal agents such as oral contraceptives.

DIFFERENTIAL DIAGNOSIS

The differential diagnosis of PMS includes a rather large number of medical and psychiatric disorders. Fortunately, the majority of these can be easily excluded by use of a prospective symptom calendar, history and physical examination, and simple laboratory investigation. In a study of 263 women presenting with the complaint of PMS, the use of oral contraceptives was found to confound the diagnosis in 10.6%. Early menopause was found in 10.2%. The most common disorders were depression and anxiety disorders which were observed in 30.5%. These were easily identified from the absence of a symptom-free interval through either self-reporting or prospective recording. Eating disorders were observed in 5.3%, and substance abuse disorders in 3.8%. Medical conditions, the most common of which were diabetes and thyroid disease, were found in 8.6%. Menstrual cycle irregularities were obtained by history in 16.6%. Because of the medical conditions and perimenopausal conditions that may present as PMS, laboratory evaluation should include serum glucose, thyroid-stimulating hormone, and follicle-stimulating hormone measurements.

PATHOPHYSIOLOGY

PMS is a psychoneuroendocrine disorder that has been the subject of considerable scientific investigation. There is extensive evidence that the pathophysiologic basis of PMS is primarily the result of changes in central nervous system neurotransmitter economy that are induced by cyclical fluctuations in ovarian steroid (estrogen and progesterone) levels. There is currently a basis for implicating adrenergic, opioid, γ-aminobutyric acid, and serotonin systems in the behavioral manifestations as well as the physical manifestations of PMS. Each of these neurotransmitter systems has been demonstrated to be influenced by estrogen and/or progesterone. The reason that women show different degrees of sensitivity to these ovarian steroid–induced neurotransmitter alterations, however, remains unknown. It is more likely that these differences in susceptibility are biologically endowed than that they are the result of environmental contingencies.

TREATMENT

Selective Serotonin Reuptake Inhibitors

Selective serotonin reuptake inhibitors (SSRIs)* are the first-line pharmacologic intervention for PMS. SSRIs act with relative specificity on the serotonergic system and hence differ from the majority of antidepressants, which have simultaneous effects on several neurotransmitter systems. Unlike SSRIs, classic antidepressants are remarkably ineffective in the treatment of PMS; in fact, they show even less efficacy in some studies than placebo. This finding is

---

*Not FDA approved for this indication.

consistent with data that PMS and depression have distinct neuroendocrine manifestations.

Fluoxetine (Prozac) is the SSRI that has been most studied in PMS. It has been demonstrated in independent, double-blind, placebo-controlled studies to have a success rate of 90% in the 85% of patients who can tolerate the medication, yielding an overall response rate of 75%. The clinical demonstration of the efficacy of SSRIs in PMS is supported by the finding of differences in serotonin markers in women with PMS and fluctuations of serotonin levels during the menstrual cycle. The effective dose of fluoxetine is 20 mg daily. It is best taken in the morning, because it is generally an activating drug. In a minority of patients, it is sedating, and these individuals are best treated with an evening or bedtime regimen. Although it is safe to prescribe 60 to 80 mg per day in single or divided doses, the vast majority of patients respond to a 20-mg dose. In a Canadian multicenter study, no significant rise in the response rate was noted at doses above 20 mg, although the incidence of side effects was greater at higher doses. Widely publicized reports of an increased risk of suicidal or homicidal behavior in patients who are taking fluoxetine have been refuted in careful studies. Nonetheless, acceptance of the drug by patients continues to be a problem. Reassurance that the earlier reports are unsubstantiated is often required. One small study suggested that fluoxetine administration in patients with PMS may be limited to the luteal phase. In clinical practice, the medication is started on day 14 of the menstrual cycle and continued until day 2 of the following cycle. This is a desirable method of initiating therapy, because smaller total monthly doses are required. Not infrequently, patients are unable to tolerate a full 20-mg dose of fluoxetine with either luteal-phase-only administration or full-cycle administration. In these patients, doses as small as 5 mg per day should be prescribed initially. Fluoxetine is available in a convenient elixir form for this purpose. In addition to fluoxetine, clinical trials have demonstrated the efficacy of other SSRIs, including sertraline (Zoloft) and paroxetine (Paxil). No studies demonstrate the superiority of one agent in the SSRI class over others. However, because the elimination rate of fluoxetine is considerably longer than that of other SSRIs, there is a theoretical reason to use this agent as the first-line drug in patients in whom SSRI administration is limited to the luteal phase.

Approximately 15% of patients taking SSRIs experience side effects of sufficient severity or discomfort to warrant discontinuation of the drug. The most commonly reported side effects are agitation or insomnia, gastrointestinal disturbance, headache, and sexual dysfunction, which may include loss of libido, impotence, and anorgasmia. Each of these occurs with sufficient severity to require discontinuation of treatment in approximately 5% of patients. A higher percentage of patients experiences these symptoms to lesser degrees.

The most commonly observed side effect of SSRIs is headache, which occurs in up to 20% of patients.

Often the headaches resolve during the first 2 weeks of therapy. A variety of gastrointestinal complaints have been noted in up to 15% of patients taking fluoxetine. These most commonly include nausea and diarrhea. Approximately 9% of patients using fluoxetine report marked anorexia. In patients with PMS, this has not been noted to a degree that warrants discontinuation of the drug. Rarely, hematologic disturbances, including anemia and thrombocytopenia, as well as alterations in liver enzymes have been observed in patients taking SSRIs. These effects do not occur with sufficient frequency to mandate routine monitoring of asymptomatic patients.

The incidence of a decline in libido during treatment with SSRIs is reported to be approximately 2% in studies of depressed patients. However, this figure may be falsely low because of the already decreased libido that usually accompanies depression. In nondepressed patients, it appears that decreased libido is more commonly noted, particularly in women with PMS.

Although large doses of SSRIs given to animals have not been associated with birth defects, human studies are not yet conclusive. The use of fluoxetine in pregnant or breast-feeding patients should therefore be discouraged. Contraception is recommended for patients with PMS treated with SSRIs.

Benzodiazepines

At least two double-blind studies have demonstrated the efficacy of alprazolam (Xanax)* in the treatment of PMS. The usual dose is 0.25 mg four times a day during the luteal phase of the cycle. Occasionally, higher doses, 0.5 mg up to four times a day, are required. Although efficacy has been demonstrated at these doses, clinically, many patients report significant improvement when the medication is taken during the luteal phase on an as-needed basis.

The side effect of greatest concern is alprazolam's addictive potential. This has prompted a number of clinicians to substitute other benzodiazepines for alprazolam in the treatment of PMS. Although there is a sound theoretical rationale to posit that other benzodiazepines may have an efficacy similar to that of alprazolam on the basis of their biochemical similarity, this has not been demonstrated in controlled studies. Moreover, although alprazolam may be more addictive than some other benzodiazepines, all agents in this class carry a substantial risk of addiction. For this reason, the use of benzodiazepines in PMS should be carefully restricted to luteal phase administration in reliable patients. Addiction to alprazolam has not been reported when the agent is restricted to use during this prescribed interval.

Withdrawal symptoms similar to those observed with barbiturates have been noted on discontinuation of alprazolam prescribed on a daily basis. These can range from mild anxiety, dysphoria, and/or insomnia to more severe manifestations, such as muscle cramps, nausea, perspiration, and tremor. Withdrawal seizures have also been reported. Patients with underlying seizure disorders are not candidates for alprazolam because of the repeated alteration in the seizure threshold induced by the cyclical initiation and discontinuation of the drug.

In addition to addiction, three other side effects of alprazolam are commonly observed. Drowsiness occurs in up to 40% of patients. This symptom sometimes resolves after a period of weeks on the medication. Lowering the dose and using a more frequent dosing schedule are often successful in relieving this side effect. Approximately 5% of individuals taking alprazolam have hypotension. Lightheadedness has also been reported in a similar number of individuals. Discontinuation of therapy is uncommonly required in individuals experiencing the latter two side effects. A number of more idiosyncratic symptoms have been reported in patients taking alprazolam. Among the most disturbing of these is paradoxical agitation, which usually resolves only with stopping of the drug.

Administration of alprazolam has not been demonstrated to be safe in pregnancy and has been reported to cause lethargy in the infants of nursing mothers. Women taking this agent for PMS should be instructed to use reliable methods of birth control.

Gonadotropin-Releasing Hormone Agonists*

In 1984, Muse and colleagues published the first results demonstrating a dramatic reduction of symptoms in women with PMS using daily injections of a gonadotropin-releasing hormone (GnRH) agonist. Since that time, several other reports using different GnRH agonists have confirmed these results. GnRH agonists cause pituitary desensitization to native GnRH, which is thought to be the result of internalization of the GnRH receptor. Depending on the potency of the agonist, the desensitization phase (termed down-regulation) requires 7 to 21 days. Once down-regulation has been established, it persists for as long as the agonist is administered. During down-regulation, secretion of luteinizing hormone and follicle-stimulating hormone by the pituitary is substantially reduced. As a result, there is insufficient stimulation of the ovary for normal sex steroid production. Circulating estrogen levels are therefore in the postmenopausal range, and progesterone levels are similarly low.

The daily subcutaneous injection form of GnRH agonists is cumbersome for the patient. Administration of GnRH analogues may be associated with localized pain and irritation at the injection site. However, depot formulations of the compounds have become available. These are administered as monthly intramuscular injections. A nasal spray has also been formulated that is available for two- or three-times-a-day use. Although the nasal spray is less uncom-

---

*Not FDA approved for this indication.

*Not FDA approved for this indication.

fortable than subcutaneous administration, absorption may be somewhat more erratic, and compliance of the patient becomes a greater concern.

In women, the side effect profile of GnRH agonists is largely the result of hypoestrogenism. Most women taking the medication experience significant hot flashes. These are generally classic postmenopausal hot flashes that last for minutes and tend to be more pronounced on the upper torso and face. The hot flashes tend to be most bothersome at the initiation of the down-regulation phase. In some women, they continue to be highly disturbing, but in others, their perceived severity decreases over weeks to months.

The acute menopausal syndrome includes emotional lability and insomnia in addition to hot flashes. In general, these symptoms tend to be less disturbing than the symptoms of severe PMS.

The long-term use of GnRH analogues is limited by the effects of chronic hypoestrogenism. The most pronounced of these is osteoporosis. As a result, use of GnRH analogues is limited to a period of 6 months unless accompanied by serial bone densitometry to demonstrate maintenance of bone integrity. There is also concern regarding the long-term consequences of negating the putative protective effect of estrogen on cardiovascular disease in women. Large epidemiologic studies are required to quantify this risk. Other symptoms of menopause, although not posing health risks, are also of concern in the use of GnRH analogues. These include vaginal dryness, an increase in urinary tract symptoms, and a decrease in skin collagen content.

Given the association between breast and gynecologic cancers and ovarian function, there is a potential protective effect of long-term GnRH agonist administration that may lower the risk of breast, ovarian, and endometrial carcinoma. Proof of this possible effect also awaits large-scale epidemiologic studies.

To reverse the potential side effects of GnRH agonist administration, low-dose estrogen and progestin replacement therapy, similar to that used in postmenopausal women, has been advocated. Because almost all the short- and long-term side effects of the therapy are the result of hypoestrogenism, this approach is based on a sound rationale. There is substantial evidence to suggest that such "add-back" therapy may maintain the majority of the beneficial effects of GnRH agonists on the symptoms of PMS.

TREATMENTS OF UNPROVEN EFFICACY

Progesterone*

In the past, progesterone given in the form of vaginal or rectal suppositories was widely prescribed for PMS. This practice was based on uncontrolled studies. Progesterone has now been shown to be no more effective than placebo in treating PMS symptoms.

Moreover, there is evidence that both the physical and the emotional symptoms of PMS may be progesterone induced. Thus, administration of progesterone commonly results in increased breast tenderness, bloating of the abdomen and extremities, and emotional lability. The use of progesterone in the treatment of PMS cannot be advocated.

Oral Contraceptives*

The success of treating PMS with oral contraceptive agents has not been consistent. For the most part, the side effects of oral contraceptive agents, including mood effects (particularly depression), water retention, and appetite changes, are precisely those that women with PMS experience. There appears to be a small percentage of women for whom oral contraceptives provide a hormonal milieu preferable to their endogenous estrogen and progesterone. In general, however, these agents are not effective in the treatment of PMS.

Vitamin B₆*

At least one placebo-controlled study of vitamin B_6 in PMS showed efficacy, although other studies failed to replicate these results. The efficacy of vitamin B_6 therapy in the syndrome is therefore controversial. At high doses (>600 mg per day), vitamin B_6 therapy has been associated with peripheral neuropathy. If this therapy is tried in PMS, patients must be cautioned against excess dosages.

Diet and Dietary Supplements

Multiple dietary supplements have been attempted in PMS, including magnesium, linoleic acid in the form of evening primrose oil, and multivitamin regimens. None of these has proved effective in treating PMS. Dietary restriction, such as the elimination of caffeine and chocolate, has not been demonstrated to be effective in PMS either. One well-controlled study has shown that a carbohydrate-enriched, tryptophan-supplemented powdered drink Escape, was effective in relieving PMS symptoms. Confirmatory studies are required before this treatment can be advocated.

DRUGS USED FOR SPECIFIC INDICATIONS

Premenstrual Migraines and Danazol

Although several reports have indicated the efficacy of danazol (Danocrine)* in PMS, since the advent of GnRH analogues, its use has been largely restricted to the treatment of premenstrual migraines. Danazol is a derivative of the synthetic androgen 17-α-ethinyl testosterone. As such, it possesses significant androgenic properties. Administration of danazol results in amenorrhea in a

---

*Not FDA approved for this indication.

*Not FDA approved for this indication.

majority of women. The objective of therapy is to obtain the beneficial effects that occur secondary to this amenorrhea. The usual dose is 600 to 800 mg per day in divided doses. The side effect profile of danazol is considerable and is the result of both its androgenic activity and its antiestrogen properties. Acne and weight gain are commonly reported. Decreased breast size is a particularly disturbing complaint for many women. More rarely, overtly masculinizing side effects are noted, including deepening of the voice and clitoromegaly. Fluid retention with danazol therapy is particularly disturbing to women with PMS.

The antiestrogenic side effects, although better tolerated by most women than the androgenic effects, can be quite bothersome. These are the same side effects observed with GnRH analogues and include hot flashes, vaginal dryness, and emotional lability. Although the osteoporosis that accompanies GnRH agonist therapy is less of a concern with danazol, the effects on lipid profiles are more worrisome. They are due to the combined adverse effects of hypoestrogenism and hyperandrogenism. For this reason, the use of danazol should be accompanied by monitoring of lipid profiles.

Danazol is contraindicated during pregnancy because of in utero female pseudohermaphroditism. There have also been reports of hepatotoxicity, signified by increased liver function tests, with danazol therapy. Therefore, liver function studies should be monitored periodically in patients taking this drug. Taken together, approximately 80% of women using danazol experience side effects.

On the basis of the benefit/risk ratio, danazol is a poor choice for most patients with PMS. Overall, it has many more side effects than GnRH analogues. Danazol may be somewhat more effective, however, in treating premenstrual migraines than are GnRH analogues. But because there are conventional, effective antimigraine medications with fewer side effects than those of danazol, this agent should not be considered a first-line agent even for premenstrual migraines.

Water Retention and Diuretics

Of the diuretics that have been used in PMS, spironolactone (Aldactone) has achieved the greatest popularity. This is largely the result of specific properties of this agent that are uniquely suited to hormonally based disorders. Spironolactone is an aldosterone inhibitor. As such, it has considerable structural similarity to steroid hormones. Because of its steroidal properties and diuretic effects, spironolactone showed promise as an effective agent in the treatment of PMS. It was hypothesized that the inhibition of steroidogenesis seen with this agent might also improve hormonally related mood changes as well as the physical symptoms of breast tenderness, water retention, and weight gain that accompany PMS. Overall, the results achieved with spironolactone

have been disappointing, and it appears to be a mildly helpful agent at best. Nonetheless, because of its antisteroidal properties, it remains the diuretic most often chosen in the treatment of the water retention symptoms of PMS.

Because of its aldosterone antagonist activity, spironolactone is a potassium-sparing diuretic. Patients should therefore be warned against taking potassium supplements while using this medication. Hypotensive effects are rarely observed in healthy young women.

Spironolactone has been associated with a number of side effects in women. They occur rarely, but when they do occur, gastrointestinal symptoms are the most common. Central nervous system side effects, including drowsiness, lethargy, headache, and mental confusion, also occasionally occur. Because of spironolactone's inhibition of steroid synthesis, irregular menses are not uncommon in patients taking this agent daily.

Many of the side effects of spironolactone have been noted with long-term daily administration. In general, adverse reactions are fewer when use is limited to the luteal phase of the cycle. Because spironolactone is now used primarily to treat the water retention symptoms of PMS, therapy can be limited to short-term administration—usually for 7 to 10 days in the luteal phase of the cycle. Many of the agents that are most effective in treating overall PMS symptoms, particularly the mood and appetite disturbances, are less effective in relieving the water retention symptoms of bloating and breast tenderness. In these cases, spironolactone provides a relatively safe adjunctive therapy.

Other diuretics have also been tried in PMS, with variable success in alleviating the water retention symptoms. For the most part, these are reserved for patients in whom spironolactone has failed or has caused significant side effects. The most commonly used class of diuretics after spironolactone is the thiazides. Thiazide diuretics are often combined with an antikaliuretic agent such as triamterene. Even with these preparations, however, hypokalemia remains the major concern. Not uncommonly, diuretics are abused by women who become highly concerned about their weight. Particularly in women with PMS who are concerned about bloating, cautions about the overuse of diuretics should be stressed.

In addition to hypokalemia, thiazide diuretics are occasionally associated with anaphylactic responses, hematologic and central nervous system disturbances, and serious cardiac arrhythmias. Fortunately, these are rare events.

Overall, the side effect profile is better and the dosage tolerance range is higher with spironolactone than with thiazide diuretics. For this reason, as well as the potential for some beneficial effects exerted by its antisteroid properties, spironolactone remains the diuretic of choice for PMS. The use of more potent diuretics or high-dose thiazides in patients with PMS should be discouraged.

MENOPAUSE

method of
DANIEL R. MISHELL, JR., M.D.
*University of Southern California School of
Medicine and Women's and Children's
Hospital*
Los Angeles, California

The mean age of menopause is about 51 years, with a normal distribution curve and 95% confidence limits between ages 45 and 55. The average life expectancy for a woman in the United States is about 78 years, so about one third of a woman's life is spent postmenopausally. This time of life should be considered an estrogen deficiency state, and improvement in both the quality and the quantity of life can be obtained with the use of estrogen replacement during the postmenopausal years.

GENITOURINARY EFFECTS

Atrophy in the genitourinary tract can produce symptoms of atrophic vaginitis with itching, burning, dyspareunia, and possible vaginal bleeding. Local estrogen therapy rapidly relieves these symptoms, but because vaginal administration of estrogen results in irregular systemic absorption, estrogen is best administered systemically for long-term prevention of vaginal atrophy as well as osteoporosis. Estrogen deficiency may also cause uterine prolapse as the supporting ligaments lose their tonicity. In addition, cystocele and rectocele may develop as a result of estrogen deficiency. These changes can be prevented or alleviated by administering estrogen. The trigone of the bladder and the urethra are embryologically derived from estrogen-dependent tissue, and postmenopausal estrogen deficiency causes atrophy of these structures, producing symptoms of urinary urgency, incontinence, dysuria, and urinary frequency. Because of atrophy of collagen in the periurethral fascia, urinary stress incontinence can also occur. If these symptoms develop postmenopausally, estrogen replacement alleviates the problem in a high percentage of women.

CENTRAL NERVOUS SYSTEM CHANGES

The pathognomonic symptom of the menopause is the hot flush or flash, which is caused by a decrease in circulating estrogen levels. The best treatment for the hot flush is estrogen, which has been shown to alleviate symptoms better than placebo. It is best to administer the estrogen at bedtime to prevent the hot flushes that can interfere with sleep. The usual initial dosage is 0.625 mg of conjugated estrogen (Premarin) or estropipate (Ogen), 1 mg of estradiol (Estrace), or 0.05 mg of transdermal estradiol (Vivelle, Climara), although higher doses may be necessary, especially for a woman whose ovaries have been removed premenopausally. For women with contraindications to estrogen therapy—specifically, cancer of the breast or endometrium—other medications that are effective in treating hot flushes include oral medroxyprogesterone acetate (Provera), in a dosage of 20 mg per day. Hot flushes can also be relieved by a single injection of medroxyprogesterone acetate (Depo-Provera),*† 150 mg given once every 3 months. In addition, clonidine (Catapres)* in a dosage of 150 μg per day can also reduce the incidence of hot flushes more than placebo.

Symptoms such as anxiety, depression, irritability, and fatigue increase after the menopause, but it has not been demonstrated that estrogen replacement significantly relieves these symptoms more than placebo in women who do not have hot flushes that interfere with their sleep. Studies indicate that estrogen users may be less likely to develop Alzheimer's disease. Because urinary incontinence and dementia are the two major reasons that women are admitted to long-term care facilities, estrogen replacement may enable women to remain in a self-care environment.

Studies have shown that postmenopausal estrogen users have a significantly thicker skin and a greater amount of collagen in the dermis than postmenopausal women who do not use estrogen. Thus, systemic estrogen use can retard the wrinkling and thinning of the skin that occur postmenopausally. Estrogen replacement also reduces the incidence of tooth loss in postmenopausal women.

OSTEOPOROSIS

Postmenopausal osteoporosis affects about 25% of women but is uncommon in black individuals and in obese women. Thin white and Asian women lose about 1 to 2% of bone mass each year after the menopause. Bone loss is more rapid in trabecular bone, which is found mainly in the thoracic spine and distal radius, than in cortical bone, which is present in the axial skeleton. If postmenopausal osteoporosis occurs, the incidence of fractures in the spine and distal radius begins to increase about age 60 years and continues to increase significantly thereafter. The incidence of fractures of the neck of the femur, made up mainly of cortical bone, usually starts to rise at about age 70 years and increase at a logarithmic rate thereafter.

Estrogen therapy reduces the bone loss associated with postmenopausal osteoporosis and thus decreases the fracture rate in women, prolonging their productive life span as well as providing great savings in health care costs. Supplemental calcium therapy and weight-bearing exercise are ancillary measures that by themselves, i.e., without estrogen, retard but do not prevent postmenopausal bone loss. The following factors are known to increase the risk of osteoporosis: (1) white or Asian race, (2) reduced weight for height, (3) early spontaneous menopause

---

*Not FDA approved for this indication.

†This use of Depo-Provera is not listed in the manufacturer's official directive.

or early surgical menopause, (4) family history of osteoporosis, (5) diet low in calcium intake, high in caffeine intake, or high in alcohol intake, (6) cigarette smoking, and (7) sedentary lifestyle. Routine screening by dual-energy x-ray absorptiometry or measurement of urinary collagen cross-link assays is not cost-effective and is not recommended to determine whether osteoporosis is developing postmenopausally, unless the decision whether or not to use estrogen replacement depends on whether bone is being lost.

Osteoporosis is associated with an increased rate of bone resorption, and the administration of estrogen returns the resorption rate to normal. Numerous prospective and retrospective epidemiologic studies have shown that estrogen therapy reduces the amount of postmenopausal bone loss: when estrogen is discontinued, the rate of bone loss rapidly increases to the same rate as that occurring immediately postmenopausally. Therefore, estrogen replacement therapy should be initiated soon after menopause occurs and should be maintained as long as a woman is ambulatory, to reduce the incidence of hip fractures after age 70 years. The minimal daily dosage of estrogen needed to prevent osteoporosis is 0.625 mg of conjugated equine estrogen (Premarin), 0.625 of estropipate (Ogen, Ortho-Est), 0.05 mg of micronized estradiol (Estrace), or 0.05 mg of transdermal estradiol (Vivelle, Climara). It is recommended that in addition to estrogen, about 1000 mg calcium should be ingested daily, and weight-bearing exercise such as walking should be encouraged. Supplemental use of vitamin D may be beneficial in geographic areas without frequent exposure to sunlight.

CARDIOVASCULAR EFFECTS

Because estrogen replacement regimens have a minimal effect on liver globulins, postmenopausal estrogen users do not have higher mean blood pressure values than women not ingesting estrogen. It is safe to provide estrogen replacement for postmeno-

pausal women with or without pre-existing hypertension. Because natural estrogens do not produce a hypercoagulable state, postmenopausal women with or without a previous history of thrombophlebitis probably do not have an increased incidence of thrombophlebitis with estrogen replacement therapy. However, some studies indicate that estrogen replacement slightly increases the rate of pulmonary embolism. Use of estrogen replacement has been shown, in numerous retrospective as well as prospective epidemiologic studies, to reduce the risk of myocardial infarction by about 50%. Estrogen replacement also reduces the risk of stroke death by about 30%. Oral estrogen raises levels of the cardioprotective high-density lipoprotein cholesterol as well as directly increasing coronary artery blood flow. The substantial reduction in the rate of myocardial infarction, the major cause of mortality in women, is a major beneficial effect of estrogen. Age-adjusted data from several studies indicate that mortality from all causes is significantly lower in estrogen users than in nonusers (Table 1).

NEOPLASTIC EFFECTS

Six meta-analyses, each combining the data from several epidemiologic studies, have shown that there is no significantly increased risk of breast cancer in women using estrogen replacement therapy compared with nonusers. Several epidemiologic studies investigating the relation of estrogen use and breast cancer have shown a higher risk of breast cancer in current but not previous postmenopausal estrogen users, who have used the estrogen for 5 years or longer, whereas several other studies have reported no changes in risk of breast cancer in current or recent long-term users of estrogen replacement. Because none of these studies is a randomized clinical trial and all are observational studies, the increased risk of breast cancer noted only in current but not past long-term users in some but not other studies is most probably due to detection bias. This statement

TABLE 1. **Age-Specific All-Cause Mortality Rates and Rate Ratios**

Age (y)	Mortality Rate/1000 Person-Years		Mortality Rate Ratio	95% Confidence Interval
	Estrogen Nonuser (N = 222)	Estrogen User (N = 232)		
50–59	2.1 (1/478)*	6.2 (3/485)*	2.96	0.31–28.43
60–69	7.3 (14/1930)	6.1 (12/1973)	0.84	0.39–1.81
70–79	34.7 (57/1641)	16.7 (30/1793)	0.48	0.31–0.75
≥80	47.5 (15/316)	22.0 (8/364)	0.46	0.20–1.09
Total	19.6 (87/4365)	11.2 (53/4615)	0.56†	0.40–0.79†

*Number of deaths per person-years of observation shown in parentheses.
†Age-adjusted relative risk using the Mantel-Haenszel method.
From Ettinger B, Friedman GD, Bush T, Quesenberry CDP Jr: Reduced mortality associated with long-term postmenopausal estrogen therapy. Reprinted with permission from The American College of Obstetricians and Gynecologists (Obstetrics and Gynecology, 1996, Vol 87, Pages 6–12).

is strengthened by the observation that the 5-year survival rate for breast cancer is significantly higher among estrogen users than among nonusers. Because estrogen can stimulate the growth of a nonpalpable breast cancer, it is advisable that all women have mammograms before initiation of estrogen therapy. If no tumor is found, the woman should be informed that oral estrogen use will not increase the risk of developing breast cancer.

There is a significantly increased risk of developing endometrial cancer in postmenopausal women who are ingesting estrogen without progestins. This risk increases with longer duration of estrogen use as well as with higher dosage. The endometrial cancer that develops in estrogen users is usually well-differentiated and is usually cured by performing a simple hysterectomy. This increased risk of developing endometrial carcinoma in women receiving estrogen replacement can be prevented by also administering progestins. The duration of progestin therapy is more important than the dosage, and it is now recommended that the progestin be administered for at least 12 days per month. To avoid the nuisance of withdrawal bleeding that occurs with the intermittent use of progestin, it is now recommended that in most women, the progestin be given in small doses daily with the estrogen.

The addition of progestin to the estrogen therapy acts synergistically to cause a slight increase in bone density. However, progestins reverse some of the beneficial effects of estrogen on serum lipids and thus should not be given to women without a uterus. Nearly all epidemiologic studies investigating the use of progestins with estrogen and the risk of breast cancer have shown no protective effects. Therefore, a beneficial effect of progestin on breast cancer risk has not been substantiated.

TREATMENT REGIMENS

The treatment regimen most commonly used in the United States is the administration of 0.625 mg of conjugated estrogen or estropipate or 1 mg of estradiol orally given daily. If the uterus is present, a progestin is usually given. In the sequential regimen, 5 to 10 mg of medroxyprogesterone acetate is added daily for the first 10 to 12 days each month. With this regimen, about 80% of women have regular withdrawal bleeding, an annoying problem that decreases patients' compliance.

It is not necessary, however, to induce withdrawal bleeding and slough the endometrium to reduce the risk of endometrial cancer. A continuous regimen in which the estrogen is given daily together with a small dose of oral progestin, such as 2.5 mg of medroxyprogesterone acetate, reduces the chance of developing uterine bleeding as well as avoiding a week without treatment, during which symptoms may appear. Data from several studies indicate that beyond a few months after initiating therapy, most women do not bleed with this regimen, and the endometrium usually remains atrophic. A routine pretreatment endometrial biopsy is unnecessary, as it is not cost-effective, and routine annual endometrial biopsies are not necessary unless breakthrough bleeding occurs. For women who do bleed, if a sonogram of the uterus reveals the endometrial thickness to be less than 5 mm, a biopsy is probably unnecessary, because the endometrium is nearly always atrophic.

CONCLUSION

Estrogen replacement therapy is indicated for nearly all postmenopausal women because of its numerous beneficial effects. Contraindications to estrogen replacement are uncommon. They include a history of breast cancer, recent history of endometrial cancer, active liver disease, and the presence of thrombophlebitis. A previous history of thrombophlebitis is not an absolute contraindication for estrogen replacement, nor are hypertension and diabetes mellitus.

VULVOVAGINITIS

method of
SEBASTIAN FARO, M.D., PH.D.
Rush–Presbyterian–St. Luke's Medical Center
Chicago, Illinois

The most common gynecologic complaint addressed by the physician rendering ambulatory care to the female patient is vulvovaginitis, which may be due to an allergic reaction, infection, or lack of hormones. The three most common causes of vaginitis are bacteria, *Candida albicans,* and *Trichomonas vaginalis.* Although a variety of bacteria may cause vaginitis, the two most common types of bacterial vaginitis are *Gardnerella vaginalis* infection and anaerobic vaginitis (bacterial vaginosis). The latter is a polymicrobial infection due to an overgrowth of anaerobic bacteria but may also involve *G. vaginalis.* In addition to *T. vaginalis,* other parasites may cause vulvovaginitis.

Vulvovaginitis due to a lack of estrogen is referred to as atrophic vaginitis, whereas inflammation due to the application of an external irritant is referred to as contact vulvovaginitis. The differentiation of microbial and nonmicrobial vulvovaginitis can be established by performing colposcopically directed biopsy of the vulva and a macroscopic as well as a microscopic examination of the vaginal discharge. The vaginal discharge reflects the status of the lower genital tract environment. In an asymptomatic or healthy or normal vagina, the discharge has a pH of 3.2 to 4.5, is white to slate gray, and does not have an odor. Microscopic examination reveals squamous epithelial cells that are estrogenized and not covered with bacteria, thus obliterating the nucleus and cell membranes. There is not an abundance of white blood cells (WBCs). The bacteria seen in the surrounding milieu are usually not clumped together and consist mainly of bacilli.

The examination of a patient complaining of vaginal burning, discomfort, dyspareunia, or abnormal vaginal discharge should begin with a detailed history. It is often helpful to show the patient a photograph or diagram of the vulva, vestibule, introitus, and vagina, then ask her to indicate on the diagram where her symptoms are located. Frequently, the patient states she has vaginal itching when in reality the inflammation is localized to the introitus. Questions should be asked as to whether or not she douches; if so, how often, and with which agent? Does the douching agent contain perfume? Is the patient utilizing a new soap or a new laundry detergent? Questions should be asked regarding her sexual habits. Is she using a new form of birth control? For example, has she begun to use a spermicidal cream or jelly or a coital lubricant? Does she practice cunnilingus, which may result in excessive moisture on the vulva and clitoris, thus resulting in maceration of the tissue and inflammation?

CONTACT VAGINITIS

Patients with contact vaginitis present with complaints of itching or burning that involves the vulva but usually does not involve the vagina. The vagina is involved only if the inflammatory agent is introduced into the vagina. The tissues appear erythematous and excoriated. Inspection of the vulva with the aid of a colposcope does not reveal any discrete lesions. The vagina commonly has a normal pH, unless the patient has been douching repeatedly with either an acidic or an alkaline solution.

Elimination of the suspected agent often results in resolution of the symptoms. In some instances, a topical steroid ointment or cream may be required. The patient should be advised to apply the cream lightly and rub it into the affected area thoroughly. It should not be applied for longer than 10 days, because prolonged administration of a topical steroid may result in thinning of the tissues, and thus in continuing symptoms.

ATROPHIC VAGINITIS

Postmenopausal patients not receiving estrogen replacement therapy often develop atrophic vaginitis. The hallmark of this condition is regression of the genital structures; the labia become less prominent, the vaginal mucosa becomes smooth owing to the loss of the rugae, and the epithelium thins. The pink color gives way to a pale pink to white. The pH often is above 4.5 and may be as high as 7.5. There is a change in the bacterial flora, with the lactobacilli no longer being dominant. The patient commonly complains of burning, dyspareunia, and vaginal spotting. In addition, the patient may complain of urinary incontinence and burning when she urinates. The latter complaint is due to the passage of urine over the atrophic tissue.

Pelvic examination reveals the vulva to be smooth with loss of definition of the external genitalia, especially loss of the labia minora. The vagina is as described previously. The vaginal discharge is scant and appears gray. The pH is between 5.0 and 7.5. Microscopic examination of the discharge reveals few epithelial cells; those present tend to be elliptical to round and are referred to as parabasal cells. The bacteria tend to be few in number, and numerous WBCs may be present. If a specimen of the vaginal discharge is cultured for aerobes and anaerobes, there will be a noticeable decrease in or absence of lactobacilli as well as an increase in anaerobic colonization. It is important to remember that the same presentation is found in patients who have had a total hysterectomy with bilateral salpingo-oophorectomy.

It is extremely important in patients with vaginal bleeding or spotting that the origin of the bleeding be determined. The etiology of the bleeding should be established before estrogen therapy is instituted. If the patient has a uterus, an endometrial biopsy should be performed. Other possible sites of origin are the lower urinary tract and rectum, which should be investigated.

Treatment for this condition is not systemic or topical antibiotics but hormonal replacement. This can be accomplished by applying topical estrogen cream or oral estrogen or a combination of both. If topical estrogen cream is utilized after the acute phase has been corrected, the patient may require a maintenance program of once-weekly or as-needed use of the estrogen cream.

MICROBIAL VAGINITIS

The physician attempting to treat the patient with complaints of vaginal itching, burning, or discomfort must be familiar with the normal status of the healthy or asymptomatic vagina. The symptomatic vagina has a pH of greater than 4.5 and usually above 5. The discharge is usually a cream color, green, yellow, or dirty gray. The odor is usually offensive and described as fishlike or foul (fetid). The discharge is frequently frothy, that is, it appears to contain air bubbles. The amount of discharge may vary from scant to copious, depending on the phase of the menstrual cycle, the concentration of estrogen and progesterone influencing the vagina, and the number of growing microbes present.

The lower genital tract has an endogenous microflora made up primarily of aerobic and anaerobic bacteria. The predominant bacterium of an asymptomatic vagina is *Lactobacillus*. This bacterium may play a pivotal role in maintaining the equilibrium of the healthy vagina by maintaining a pH of 3.8 to 4.2 through the production of lactic acid. This pH is not favorable to the growth of other more pathogenic bacteria, such as the facultative and obligate anaerobes. In addition, it is theorized that the ability of lactobacilli to produce hydrogen peroxide may also play a role in suppressing the growth of anaerobic bacteria. Thus, when a patient is found to have vaginitis, the pH is often above 5 and there is a marked reduction in the number of lactobacilli.

Before examining the patient, the physician should ask questions focusing on factors that may influence the normal vaginal environment. The patient should attempt to describe the characteristics of the initial episode and how the episodes have changed over time. Has she used antibiotics? Have they been used for maintenance or therapeutic indications? Does the patient douche? If so, how often and with what agent? Questions regarding sexual habits should be asked. How many sexual partners does she have? Does she know whether her partner has sexual contact with others? Does she practice cunnilingus, fellatio, or rectal intercourse? The patient should be asked to localize her symptoms, that is, are they located at the opening of the vagina or in the vagina proper? Finally, she should be asked to characterize her discharge with regard to color, consistency, and odor.

HUMAN PAPILLOMAVIRUS VESTIBULITIS

The examination should begin with the external genitalia. Attention should be paid to the medial aspect of the labia minora and majora, especially the area of the vestibule and introitus. Patients often complain of itching or burning and dyspareunia in this area. Examination often reveals a horseshoe-shaped area of erythema, which is commonly painful or tender to palpation. Examination under magnification reveals the presence of glistening papules. Application of 5% acetic acid turns this epithelium white, which is characteristic of human papillomavirus (HPV) infection. It is best to refer the patient for further evaluation to a gynecologist specializing in infections of the genital tract. Colposcopically directed biopsies are required to establish a diagnosis. Treatment is usually initiated with laser ablation of this area followed by intravaginal application of 5-fluorouracil cream. The patient should undergo colposcopic examinations of the vulva, vagina, and cervix every 3 to 4 months for the next 2 years to determine whether there is a recurrence. The patient's partner requires a similar examination to determine whether there are HPV lesions present on his penis.

YEAST VAGINITIS

Typically, yeast favors a pH of 4.5 or lower, but not always. WBCs are usually present, and the number of free-floating bacteria is usually reduced. The discharge is white and tends to be pasty but may be liquid. Classically, the discharge is cottage cheese–like and clings to vaginal epithelium. The microscopic picture may be that of elliptical yeast cells, budding cells, cells with germ tubes present, or long strands of pseudohyphae. These different forms of the yeast can easily be seen when the vaginal discharge is mixed with potassium hydroxide (KOH). It is not necessary to culture routinely for yeast, except when the patient's symptoms suggest a yeast infection but no fungal forms are seen microscopically.

Atypically, the patient may have a vaginal pH above 4.5 and there may be an increase in the number of bacteria seen in a wet preparation of the vaginal discharge. The physician should rely on a wet preparation mixed with KOH to rule out the presence of yeast.

Initial treatment should be with an intravaginal cream, ointment, or suppository such as clotrimazole (Lotrimin, Gyne-Lotrimin, Mycelex G), miconazole (Monistat), terconazole (Terazol), or nystatin. These are all beneficial in treating yeast vulvovaginitis. There are different dosing regimens ranging from a single dose to 3-day and 7-day courses. A patient with an initial infection may do well with a short treatment schedule if the precipitating factors can be established. Patients with recurrent infection require longer treatment regimens and the possible use of maintenance therapy. Some patients benefit from gentian violet applied as a vaginal paint or tampon. In addition, consideration should be given to examination and treatment of the patient's sexual partner. Ketoconazole (Nizoral) has been used in single doses of 400 mg with good results. However, hepatic and renal toxicities have been reported, and use of ketoconazole for vaginal yeast infection has not been encouraged.

BACTERIAL VAGINOSIS

The vagina houses a complex ecosystem. One component consists of a large number and variety of bacteria. The endogenous bacterial flora comprises gram-positive and gram-negative aerobic, facultative, and obligate anaerobes. The bacteriology of a healthy vaginal ecosystem is dominated by *Lactobacillus acidophilus*. This bacterium appears to exert its influence by maintaining the pH between 3.8 and 4.2, resulting in the suppression of the potentially pathogenic bacteria. This pH range also favors the growth of lactobacilli as well as other commensal bacteria, such as *Corynebacterium*, diphtheroids, and other nondescript streptococci.

These bacteria, as well as others, may act synergistically with one another, whereas others, such as lactobacilli and facultative and obligate anaerobes, may act antagonistically. Some strains, such as *L. acidophilus*, produce hydrogen peroxide, which is toxic to anaerobic bacteria; because they lack the enzyme catalase, anaerobic bacteria cannot convert hydrogen peroxide to oxygen and water. Other mechanisms by which bacteria, such as lactobacilli, inhibit the growth of other bacteria are the production and secretion of lysozyme and bacteriocins. It is important to note that the equilibrium of the vaginal ecosystem is extremely delicate and can easily be disrupted. Once the equilibrium is significantly disturbed, the growth of lactobacilli is retarded. This, in turn, may result in a decrease in the hydrogen ion concentration or an increase in pH. The alteration in pH causes a further decline in the growth of lactobacilli and greater growth of the potentially pathogenic bacteria.

The initial insult or factor that begins the change in the ecosystem is not known. However, if this alteration favors the growth of *G. vaginalis*, a further decrease in hydrogen ion concentration occurs. When the pH reaches a value of 5 or greater, facultative anaerobic bacterial growth occurs. Growth of *G. vagi-*

TABLE 1. **Characteristics of the Vaginal Ecosystem**

Characteristic	Healthy Ecosystem	Bacterial Vaginosis
Discharge	White to slate gray	Dirty gray
pH	3.8 to 4.2	>4.5
Clue cells	Absent	Present
WBCs	Rare	Rare
Whiff test	Negative	Positive

nalis and the facultative anaerobes results in a progressive decrease in the oxygen concentration, favoring growth of obligate anaerobic bacteria. This causes the condition known as bacterial vaginosis (BV). Another organism that can alter the ecosystem in a similar manner is *T. vaginalis*. This protozoan favors a more alkaline pH (>4.5), which favors growth of the facultative and obligate anaerobic bacteria.

BV is characterized by a vaginal pH greater than 4.5, the presence of clue cells, and a fishlike odor. This odor is typically manifested when a drop of vaginal discharge is mixed with a drop of concentrated KOH, releasing catecholamines (whiff test). The patient may also complain of a copious, dirty gray vaginal discharge with a foul or fishy odor. This odor may also be noted by the patient's sexual partner. However, approximately 50% of patients with BV are asymptomatic and are diagnosed because they are being examined for another reason.

BV is not an infection but should be viewed as a disturbance in the vaginal ecosystem. This disturbance in the endogenous vaginal microflora is significant, because it has been linked to postpartum endometritis, posthysterectomy pelvic infection, and preterm labor. Therefore, many obstetrician-gynecologists recommend that pregnant and preoperative patients be screened for BV. The differences between a healthy vaginal ecosystem and BV are listed in Table 1.

The color of the vaginal discharge is not a reliable characteristic with regard to establishing a diagnosis. However, any color other than white or slate gray should be considered abnormal. The key characteristics that can be utilized during the pelvic examination to assist in establishing an accurate diagnosis are pH, the presence of a fishlike odor when the vaginal discharge is mixed with KOH and the presence of clue cells.

The pH can be determined easily and inexpensively by placing a ColorpHast pH strip on the lateral vaginal wall and comparing the wall's color with the accompanying chart. A pH lower than 4.5 essentially rules out the presence of BV. A pH higher than 4.5 does not establish, but is strongly suggestive of, the diagnosis of BV. A microscopic examination of the vaginal discharge must be performed to determine whether clue cells are present and whether there is an absence of a dominant bacterial morphotype. Evaluation of the vaginal discharge can be of assistance in differentiating among a variety of causes of vaginitis (Table 2). Although the conditions are presented as pure entities in Table 2, it should be understood that any of these conditions can be present simultaneously. The noticeable presence of WBCs (>5 per high-power field) indicates that an inflammatory response has been triggered. Women with pure BV do not have WBCs in their vaginal discharge.

A specimen of the vaginal discharge should be collected by swabbing the lateral vaginal wall with a cotton-tipped applicator. The applicator is immersed in 2 to 3 mL of normal saline and vigorously agitated to dilute the specimen. A drop of the resulting solution should be placed on a glass slide, covered with a glass coverslip, and examined with the assistance of 40× magnification.

The microscopic picture of BV is characterized by the presence of numerous individual free-floating bacteria, the absence of a dominant bacterial morphotype, the presence of clue cells, and the relative absence of WBCs. Clue cells are defined as squamous epithelial cells that have numerous bacteria adherent to their cytoplasmic membrane. If a Gram stain is performed, clue cells are seen to have gram-negative bacteria adherent to the cytoplasmic membrane. This is characteristic of *G. vaginalis* infection. The whiff test is performed by placing a drop of vaginal discharge on a glass slide and mixing in a drop of concentrated KOH; if there is a significant concentration of anaerobic bacteria present, a fishlike odor is detected.

Typically, in uncomplicated BV, WBCs are not present in the vaginal discharge. The presence of an obvious leukorrhea should alert the physician to the possible existence of an associated condition, i.e., a sexually transmitted disease (STD). The frequency of recurrent BV is linked to the frequency of sexual

TABLE 2. **Evaluation of the Vaginal Ecosystem**

Characteristic	Healthy	Bacterial Vaginosis*	Trichomoniasis*	Candidiasis
pH	3.8–4.2	≥5	≥5	<5
Squamous cells	Estrogenized	Clue cells +	Clue cells ±	Estrogenized
KOH (whiff test)	Negative	Fishlike odor +	Fishlike odor ±	No odor
KOH preparation		Destruction of all cellular constituents		Hyphae remain
Dominant bacterial morphotype	Bacilli	None	None	Bacilli
WBCs	Rare	Rare	Positive	Positive

*The + indicates present; ± indicates present or absent.

intercourse. Patients who experience recurrent episodes of BV should be queried as to their sexual practices. The presence of vaginal leukorrhea should alert the physician to the possible existence of pelvic inflammatory disease (PID). Therefore, the patient presenting with BV and leukorrhea should be evaluated for PID, trichomoniasis, cervical gonorrhea, and chlamydial infection.

Individuals found to be positive for an STD should also be evaluated for syphilis, hepatitis B, and human immunodeficiency virus. If there is strong suspicion that gonorrhea or chlamydia (or both) is present, appropriate treatment should be instituted. In the patient found to be culture-positive for the gonococcus and/or chlamydia, cultures should be repeated within 1 to 2 weeks after completion of therapy. She should also be encouraged to refrain from sexual intercourse during this period. If this is not possible or practical, the patient should insist that her partner wear a condom. Patients treated for PID should be re-evaluated within 72 hours after beginning antibiotic therapy to determine whether there has been a positive response. Patients failing to demonstrate improvement should be re-evaluated for having either more advanced PID or other pelvic diseases.

Patients found to have BV may be treated with one of the regimens listed in Table 3.

The patient should be re-evaluated 7 and 30 days after the completion of therapy to ensure that the condition has resolved. She should be advised to either refrain from intercourse or have her partner wear a condom. This practice should continue throughout the follow-up period.

Individuals who have recurrent or persistent BV should be treated as described earlier and, when found to be free of BV, should be considered for maintenance therapy. There are no good data available with regard to maintenance therapy, but two factors that may contribute to recurrent BV are (1) the vaginal ecosystem is cleared of clue cells, and there is now a high-density mixture of bacteria, but noticeable lactobacilli are lacking, and (2) the vaginal pH remains above 4.5. A patient with both these factors is likely to have a relapse in a short time, and unless the pH is restored to a range of 3.8 to 4.2, lactobacilli will not resume a place of dominance in the vaginal ecosystem. Thus, a healthy vaginal ecosystem will not become re-established, and the BV cycle is likely to begin again.

Unfortunately, there are no specific medications or treatments for restoring the vaginal pH to a range of 3.8 to 4.2. However, acid gel can be administered twice daily for 10 to 14 days in an attempt to lower the pH of the vagina. One week after the completion of therapy, the patient should be re-evaluated to determine whether a healthy vaginal ecosystem has been restored. Failure of the patient to respond to therapy is an indication for referral to a specialist with an interest in vulvovaginal disease.

PARASITIC VULVOVAGINITIS

The most common agent of parasitic genital infection is *T. vaginalis*. Other common but less frequent parasites are *Phthirus pubis*, *Sarcoptes scabiei*, and *Enterobius vermicularis*.

P. pubis, commonly referred to as "the crabs," is one of three species of lice that infect humans; the others are *Pediculus humanus corporis*, the body louse, and *Pediculus humanus capitis*, the head louse. Lice are transmitted by person-to-person contact. Although the pubic louse is most commonly transmitted via sexual contact, cases have been documented in which transmission has occurred from toilet seats, bed linen, and infected loose hairs. The incidence of infection is highest among individuals with gonorrhea and syphilis. The affected patient presents with itching, evidence of excoriation, erythema, irritation, and inflammation. Patients who have a large number of bites may even develop a mild elevation in body temperature, malaise, and irritability.

The diagnosis is established by taking a detailed history and carefully examining the patient. The adult crab louse and nits (eggs) can be seen by the naked eye. A simple magnifying glass facilitates examining the pubic area. The pubic lice may appear as scabs; however, when the scab is removed and examined microscopically, the crab louse becomes easy to identify. If no adults are present, the eggs or nits can be identified.

Treatment must be effective against both the adult lice and the nits. The partner of the infected patient must also be examined, as should other household members. Several agents are available, including preparations with pyrethrins and piperonyl butoxide (RID [liquid and shampoo]; Triple X Kit [liquid and shampoo]; and Barc [liquid]), lindane (Kwell [lotion, shampoo, and cream]), crotamiton (Eurax [cream and lotion]), 20% benzyl benzoate, and 10% sulfur ointment. The pediculicide should remain in contact with the infected area for at least 1 hour to be ovicidal. Kwell is probably the most commonly used pediculicide. The proper use of this agent requires the patient to shower before applying the Kwell (1% γ-benzene hexachloride), which then remains on the body surface for 8 hours. This process should be followed for three applications of Kwell, and each 8-hour application is followed by a shower. The patient should wash thoroughly with soap and water to remove the Kwell. After the final shower, no further treatment should be necessary.

TABLE 3. **Antibiotic Regimens for the Treatment of Bacterial Vaginosis**

Clindamycin (Cleocin) vaginal cream, 2%, one applicator administered intravaginally, qhs × 7 nights

Metronidazole vaginal gel (MetroGel), 0.75%, one applicator bid × 7 d

Metronidazole (Flagyl), 250 mg orally tid × 7 d or 375 mg orally bid × 7 d

Clindamycin (Cleocin), 300 mg orally tid × 7 d

Amoxicillin-clavulanate (Augmentin), 500 mg orally tid × 7 d

Kwell is absorbed, especially if the skin has been severely excoriated, and may cause neurotoxicity. This agent should not be used on children or pregnant women.

The patient's clothing and fomites should also be treated for adult lice and nits. Clothes should be washed in hot water (125°F), and nonwashable items should be dry cleaned; either process will kill adult lice, nymphs, or nits. Inanimate or nonwashable items that cannot be processed by dry cleaning can be treated with disinfectants containing pyrethrin and piperonyl butoxide.

Sarcoptes scabiei is the causative agent of scabies, which is transmitted via close personal contact. The organism is transmitted by sexual and nonsexual contact. The hands and feet are initially infected. The female breast may have lesions resembling those of Paget's disease. Infection may occur in skin folds such as the umbilicus, the groin, and where the buttocks meet the thigh. The characteristic lesion is a burrow. Most sites are erythematous and excoriated, as is most commonly seen in the web between the fingers.

The infection can be diagnosed by taking skin scrapings and examining them microscopically for the presence of the mite. Other diagnostic modalities are needle extraction of a mite from a burrow; epidermal shave biopsy of a burrow or papule; covering the burrow with ink and wiping with alcohol (if a mite is present, it will be stained by the ink); scraping the burrow, mixing the scrapings with mineral oil, and examining microscopically; punch biopsy; and placing topical tetracycline on the infected area, and wiping, and then examining under ultraviolet light for fluorescence.

Treatment of scabies is best accomplished with topical agents such as 1% γ-benzene hexachloride (lindane cream or lotion, Kwell, or Scabene), crotamiton (Eurax), or sulfur.

DISEASE CAUSED BY *TRICHOMONAS VAGINALIS*

T. vaginalis is a protozoan with five flagella, four located anteriorly and one located in an undulating membrane. The organism has the ability to adhere to epithelial cells. The hallmark of *T. vaginalis* infection is vaginal discharge, which may vary in color from a dirty gray to a yellow-green. The discharge appears frothy owing to the presence of gas bubbles. The pH of the discharge is usually greater than 5. The patient may complain of dyspareunia, dysuria, pruritus, and a foul vaginal odor. She also may note an exacerbation of symptoms shortly after her menses.

Pelvic examination may reveal the vulva to be erythematous, slightly edematous, and excoriated. Petechiae may be present on the cervix and vaginal walls. A urine specimen may also reveal the presence of trichomonads. One or two drops of the vaginal discharge mixed with 1 to 2 mL of normal saline and examined microscopically typically shows numerous bacteria, WBCs, and mobile trichomonads. However, if no protozoans are seen, it would be beneficial to inoculate a medium designed for the growth of *T. vaginalis* (e.g., Diamond's medium), because this is a more sensitive method of detecting *T. vaginalis* than microscopic examination of vaginal discharge.

Treatment should be instituted with metronidazole, 250 mg given orally three times daily for 7 days or 375 mg orally twice a day for 7 days. I prefer this regimen over intravaginal suppositories, because the organism commonly infects extravaginal sites, such as the bladder, urethra, or periurethral glands. I have found that the single 2-gram dose is not well tolerated by the patient because of gastric upset. The male partner should be treated to achieve a cure in the female patient. Condoms should be utilized during the treatment period. The patient should be reexamined to determine whether the organism has been eradicated and the vaginal environment restored to a healthy state.

CONCLUSION

Patients who present to the physician with vulvovaginitis of microbial etiology should be considered to have an STD. Consideration should be given to obtaining a culture specimen to test for the presence of *Neisseria gonorrhoeae* and *Chlamydia trachomatis*. In addition, serologic study for syphilis should be performed. These recommendations should be followed especially for the patient who is between the ages of 15 and 30 years, unmarried, and sexually active.

TOXIC SHOCK SYNDROME

method of
P. JOAN CHESNEY, M.D., C.M.
University of Tennessee, Memphis and LeBonheur Children's Medical Center Memphis, Tennessee

Toxic shock syndrome (TSS) is fatal in 3 to 5% of cases, usually as a result of irreversible respiratory failure, refractory cardiac arrhythmias, or severe bleeding. Such deaths can potentially be prevented by early recognition, early and intensive monitoring, and treatment of each of the well-described multisystem components of this disease. Some of the sequelae are probably toxin mediated, but most appear to be related to the severity and duration of hypotension and are therefore potentially preventable.

PATHOGENESIS

TSS appears to be mediated by a toxin or toxins produced by certain strains of *Staphylococcus aureus*. As with other bacterial toxin–mediated diseases, the bacteria themselves are usually present in a single focus and often only in relatively small numbers. With few exceptions, blood, urine, and cerebrospinal fluid cultures are negative. Positive cultures are obtained from the focus of infection.

Typically, surgical wounds or a site of infection is associated with minimal or no inflammatory reaction. Thus, numerous case reports suggest that in a patient with TSS, all recent surgical wounds and any suspected sites should be opened, cultured, and irrigated even if no clinical evidence of inflammation is apparent.

The toxins mediating this syndrome and their mechanisms of action are not yet defined with certainty. Toxic shock syndrome toxin type 1 (TSST-1), a protein of 24,000 daltons, is a valuable marker for the *S. aureus* strains isolated from 95% of menstrually associated cases of TSS. In nonmenstrual TSS, as few as 63% of *S. aureus* isolates produce TSST-1. This finding suggests the likely involvement of other unidentified toxins, such as the staphylococcal enterotoxins, particularly in nonmenstrual cases.

TSST-1 and the staphylococcal enterotoxins are potent T cell mitogens. As superantigens, they bind simultaneously to the antigen-processing cell and the T lymphocyte receptor. The resulting rapid production, release, and circulation of monokines and lymphokines are thought to be responsible for the rapid onset and multisystem manifestations of TSS. Monoclonal antibodies to both TSST-1 and tumor necrosis factor have provided protection in animal models of TSS.

The two most important pathophysiologic effects of the toxin(s) and cytokine mediators in this syndrome are a decrease in peripheral venous tone and extensive capillary leakage of intravascular fluid into the interstitial spaces. This results in a rapidly progressive hypovolemia. In addition to the ensuing poor tissue perfusion, the toxin or mediators appear to have direct toxic effects on the myocardium, kidneys, lungs, liver, muscles, lymphoid tissue, and, possibly, the central and peripheral nervous systems. Hence, the three most important, immediate principles of management are rapid restoration of the intravascular volume, inactivation and/or elimination of the toxin, and drainage and treatment of the focus of infection.

RECURRENCES

Without therapy, up to 65% of women who develop their initial episode of TSS during menses will experience at least one more episode during subsequent menses. Subsequent episodes may be mild or severe. Recurrences may also occur in patients with nonmenstrual TSS. Women who develop TSS with menses take many months to develop antibody to TSST-1. Patients with nonmenstrual TSS generally develop antibody soon after their illness.

MANAGEMENT

Table 1 outlines the principles of management of TSS.

Monitoring

Immediate and appropriate monitoring for early recognition of the well-described acute complications resulting from multisystem organ damage should be established in all hospitalized patients.

Antimicrobials

Antimicrobials are indicated to eradicate organisms from the infected site, to treat the rare patient

TABLE 1. **Principles of Management of Toxic Shock Syndrome**

Locate focus of infection

  Obtain cultures of blood and focus of infection
  Drain and débride if accessible
  Irrigate extensively
  Remove any foreign bodies if possible

Rapidly restore intravascular volume

Start parenteral antimicrobial therapy

  Eradicate the organism
    Use bactericidal antibiotic inhibiting cell wall formation, e.g., β-lactamase–resistant antistaphylococcal antibiotic
    Give maximal doses for age
  Stop protein synthesis
    Stop synthesis of toxin, enzyme, cytokine
    Alternatives include clindamycin (Cleocin) and azithromycin (Zithromax)

Consider immune globulin intravenous (IGIV) for restricted situations

  Disease refractory to initial aggressive fluid support and vasopressors
  Focus of infection inaccessible to drainage
  Persistent oliguria in spite of extensive fluid replacement and pulmonary edema

Consider methylprednisolone for patients unresponsive to IGIV

Practice anticipatory and aggressive management of multisystem organ failure (see Table 2)

with positive blood or urine cultures, and to prevent recurrences.

TSS-associated strains of *S. aureus* are usually resistant to penicillin and ampicillin but sensitive to the β-lactamase–resistant (BLR) penicillins. Toxin-producing methicillin-resistant *S. aureus* (MRSA) associated with TSS has rarely been identified. Therefore, vancomycin should be considered only if the patient is considered to be at increased risk for MRSA infection. For patients allergic to penicillin, vancomycin hydrochloride (Vancocin) or clindamycin hydrochloride (Cleocin) is the drug of first choice. A BLR penicillin is administered at a maximal intravenous dose appropriate for the patient's age until the patient is afebrile and has not required pressor agents for 2 to 3 days. At that time, an oral BLR penicillin is administered, 50 to 100 mg per kg per day every 6 hours, not to exceed 4 grams.

In the late logarithmic phase of bacterial growth, when toxin production is maximal, inhibitors of cell wall formation, such as β-lactam antibiotics, may not be as effective at killing bacteria and thereby stopping toxin production. On the other hand, protein synthesis inhibitors may act immediately to inhibit the synthesis of toxins(s) and, potentially, of other proteins, including cytokines. At concentrations well below those required to inhibit bacterial growth, clindamycin, azithromycin (Zithromax), and gentamicin almost completely block TSST-1 production in vitro. Additional preliminary results suggest a potential benefit for the addition of clindamycin to the β-lactam drug for the therapy of TSS. As no controlled trials of clindamycin use for TSS have been performed, the individual physician must decide whether to add clindamycin. It may be used at 25 mg per kg per day not to exceed 2 to 4 grams per day.

Combined intravenous and oral therapy should total 10 to 14 days. In bacteremic patients, the possibility of additional therapy for endocarditis or other complications should be considered.

Methylprednisolone

A retrospective study demonstrated that a short course of methylprednisolone (Solu-Medrol) or dexamethasone (Decadron) was associated with a reduction in the duration of fever and severity of disease if given early enough. As well, steroids appeared to be beneficial in an animal model. Steroids should probably be reserved for the severely ill patient unresponsive to antibiotics and fluid resuscitation.

Removal of Foreign Bodies and Drainage

Of equal importance to antimicrobial selection is identification of the infected focus, removal of all foreign bodies (e.g., tampons, gauze packing, sutures, prostheses), and drainage, irrigation, and culture of the suspected focus. The correct techniques for removing and/or eradicating toxins are not known, because the tissue distribution, sites, and mechanisms for inactivation of TSST-1, the staphylococcal enterotoxins, and other unidentified toxins are not yet known.

Supportive Management

Severely ill patients need to be cared for in an intensive care setting so that myocardial dysfunction, hemodynamic derangements, pulmonary edema, adult respiratory distress syndrome, acute renal failure, encephalopathy, and disseminated intravascular coagulation, if present, can be appropriately monitored and treated.

Aggressive management of hypovolemic TSS patients is crucial (Table 2). The most important aspect of the nonspecific symptomatic therapy is fluid replacement. The rapid restoration of intravascular volume to achieve adequate tissue perfusion should be accomplished immediately. Because of the ongoing capillary leak syndrome, the fluid replacement required to maintain organ perfusion may far exceed the amount of fluid calculated to be necessary on the basis of normal replacement and fluid deficit volumes. Thus, some adults have required 12 liters of fluid in the first 24 hours in addition to vasopressors to stabilize the circulating blood pressure. Edema is inevitable as a result of the continued vascular capillary fluid leak. Close monitoring in an intensive care unit determines when the correct intravascular volume has been achieved. Peripheral edema and pleural and pericardial effusions can sequester massive volumes of fluid. Once the patient's blood pressure is stable, the judicious use of diuretics helps to mobilize fluid.

TABLE 2. **Supportive and Symptomatic Therapy for Complications of Toxic Shock Syndrome**

Hypovolemia and Hypotension

Initial Therapy
1. Oxygen, intubation, PEEP.
2. Large-bore intravascular catheter.
3. Rapid administration of 20–40 mL/kg of crystalloid over 1 h to stabilize BP and achieve urine output of ≥2 mL/kg/h.

If No Response After 1 h
1. Transfer to ICU.
2. Continue crystalloid at 20 mL/kg/h; may require many times maintenance doses to restore BP.
3. Establish CVP line.
4. Correct electrolyte, calcium, and acid-base status.

If No Response After 2–4 h
1. Place pulmonary artery Swan-Ganz and arterial catheters.
2. Establish status of myocardium and lungs.
3. Consider use of dopamine hydrochloride (dopamine HCl) or dobutamine hydrochloride (Dobutrex) for myocardial dysfunction.
4. Appropriately treat myocardial dysfunction if needed.
5. Look for sources of bleeding.
6. Consider IGIV 400 mg given over several hours.

If BP Remains Unstable After 12–24 h
1. Look for continued source of toxin production.
2. Consider other techniques for toxin removal (see text).
3. Consider methylprednisolone sodium succinate (Solu-Medrol), 30 mg/kg q 6 h for 2 doses.

Adult Respiratory Distress Syndrome

Anticipate ARDS.

Electrolyte and Acid-Base Status

Correct initial hyponatremia and acidosis.

Hypocalcemia

Anticipate hypocalcemia and tetany.
Maintain physiologic levels of calcium.

Acute Renal Failure

Avoid nephrotoxic drugs.
Monitor and dialyze if necessary.

Thrombocytopenia and Disseminated Intravascular Coagulation

Give fresh-frozen plasma and platelets if needed.

Edema, Pericardial and Pleural Effusion

Maintain adequate intravascular volume before using diuretic to mobilize extravascular fluid.

Hypoferrinemia and Anemia

Give no treatment unless there is blood loss.

Hepatic Dysfunction

Avoid drugs conjugated in the liver.

Central Nervous System Dysfunction

Anticipate irrational behavior, seizures.

Abbreviations: BP = blood pressure; CVP = central venous pressure; DIC = disseminated intravascular coagulation; ICU = intensive care unit; PEEP = positive end-expiratory pressure; ARDS = adult respiratory distress syndrome.

Numerous reports have documented the initial hemodynamic changes to be a markedly decreased systemic vascular resistance, decreased mean arterial pressure, and increased cardiac output. In some patients, however, after an initial phase of increased cardiac output, myocardial contractility decreases, presumably owing to a toxin-mediated cardiomyopathy. This results in a decreased cardiac output, increased pulmonary artery wedge pressure, and increased central venous pressure. This stage of myocardial dysfunction may not be readily apparent from the nonspecific electrocardiogram findings but will be quickly recognized from increased central venous and pulmonary artery wedge pressure readings, a lowered cardiac index, and an abnormal echocardiogram. Early recognition of myocardial failure and potential arrhythmias should lead to changes in management, such as decreasing the amount of fluid volume administered and considering afterload reduction, a subject beyond the scope of this discussion. Whereas dopamine (Intropin) may be effective in the early stages, before myocardial dysfunction develops, dobutamine (Dobutrex) or a combination of the two agents is preferable when myocardial damage has been demonstrated.

Immune Globulin Intravenous

The absence of antibody to the toxin(s) responsible for TSS may be important in the pathogenesis and course of the disease. Absence or low titers of antibody to TSST-1 are found in almost all patients at the onset of menstrual TSS. Acquisition of antibody to TSST-1 in control populations is age related, with more than 88% of individuals 20 years or older having high titers of antibody. The failure to develop antibody after menstrual TSS appears to correlate with an ongoing risk of recurrent disease.

High levels of antibody to TSST-1 and to the staphylococcal enterotoxins are present in intravenous immune globulin (immune globulin intravenous [IGIV]) preparations. In vitro, these antibodies inhibit the production and/or release of cytokines by antigen-processing cells and lymphocytes. In a rabbit model of TSS, human IGIV given at the time of administration of toxin or organism prevented TSS. When IGIV was given up to 29 hours after TSST-1 administration, the increase in survival among the IGIV-treated animals was still significant. No adverse reactions were noted in the IGIV-treated animals, and there was no evidence of disease mediated by the formation of antigen-antibody complexes. The mechanism of action of these antibodies is unknown but may be the result of impaired binding of the toxins to cellular receptors.

Consideration should be given to the administration of IGIV to patients severely ill with TSS. Anecdotal case reports have indicated a beneficial effect. However, until more information is available, and because IGIV is expensive and most patients respond rapidly once therapy is initiated, most investigators would reserve administration of IGIV for patients with an inaccessible focus of infection and/or for those whose condition continues to deteriorate. The amount most often used is 400 mg per kg given as a single dose over several hours. This dose results in a serum antibody titer of 1:100 or greater, higher than the titer that appears to provide immunity to TSST-1.

The potential risks and benefits of this form of therapy must be considered for each patient. It is possible that early administration of IGIV could blunt the immune response to TSST-1 or other toxins and increase the risk of a recurrent episode. Other side effects related to IGIV use are an aseptic meningitis syndrome associated with fever, headache, nausea, and vomiting as well as the acute onset of rigors, bronchospasm, hypotension, cyanosis, vascular collapse, and decreased renal function.

Miscellaneous Considerations

Anecdotal case reports suggest that if an unstable blood pressure persists despite aggressive management, and if an unsuspected site of infection with continued toxin production cannot be found, techniques that might remove toxins from the blood, such as plasmapheresis or hemodialysis, might be useful. These forms of therapy have not been studied and should be considered investigational.

One patient with TSS due to S. aureus infection of a herniorrhaphy incision did not recover for 5 days despite aggressive resuscitation and intravenous nafcillin (Nafcil) administration, until povidone-iodine (Betadine) irrigation and soaks of a well-drained, normal-appearing but still infected wound were instituted. Saline irrigations and povidone-iodine irrigations and soaks of infected foci, including the vagina, should be considered as additional means of eradicating the source of toxin. Povidone-iodine is readily absorbed from the vagina after only a 2-minute application, leading to 5- to 15-fold increases in serum total iodine and inorganic iodide concentrations within 15 minutes. This finding should be noted when this form of therapy is considered.

Other multisystem manifestations commonly present in hospitalized patients with TSS are listed in Table 2. Each complication should be managed according to standard guidelines. The anticipation and early recognition of these complications are of great importance. Although hypocalcemic tetany is uncommon, hypocalcemia that appears to be mediated by a toxin-induced, calcitonin-like molecule is common and may be life-threatening. Maintaining physiologic calcium concentrations may be important.

The hypoferrinemia, most often incidentally detected on routine blood chemistry panels, is a physiologic response to acute inflammation and need not be treated.

PREVENTION

Adequate therapy of the initial episode of TSS is the cornerstone of the prevention of recurrences. Administering a BLR penicillin during the acute illness and discontinuing tampon use decrease the recurrence rate to less than 5% in menses-associated cases. Women may remain susceptible to TSS until they have developed anti–TSST-1 antibody. Serum antibody levels to TSST-1 could be monitored, and tampon use can be cautiously resumed once a significant titer has been achieved. Such individuals may also continue to be at risk as long as they are colonized with TSST-1–producing strains of *S. aureus* and have no antibody to TSST-1. Thus, repeating vaginal cultures several months after the initial episode may be of help in identifying persistent carriers. Aside from continuing to avoid tampon use, optimal management of such carriers is not known but, after BLR antibiotics have been tried without success, might include a course of an oral antibiotic such as rifampin (Rifadin)* to eliminate cervicovaginal *S. aureus* carriage.

The patterns of tampon use that will minimize the risk of menstrual TSS are unclear. Use of superabsorbent tampons clearly increases the risk of TSS, and such tampons can now be identified by the consumer from the manufacturer's absorbency labels. The use of pads at night and removal of tampons when symptoms suggestive of TSS develop are two recommendations with which most investigators would concur. The optimal frequency for changing tampons to minimize risk is not clear.

For women who have had TSS with menses, post partum, or with a vaginal infection or contraceptive use, tampon use should be discontinued until antibody to TSST-1 is present. Women using intravaginal contraceptive devices should be informed of their slightly increased risk of TSS. Physicians should instruct their patients to use tampons judiciously.

As a result of the unexpected and potentially severe consequences of TSS, issues regarding surgical prophylaxis to prevent postoperative TSS have been raised. Most investigators consider the low risk of postoperative TSS comparable to that of a severe antimicrobial reaction. For short, clean procedures, perioperative prophylaxis to prevent TSS is not indicated.

---

*Not FDA approved for this indication.

CHLAMYDIA TRACHOMATIS

method of
SEBASTIAN FARO, M.D., PH.D.
*Rush–Presbyterian–St. Luke's Medical Center
Chicago, Illinois*

Chlamydia trachomatis is a true bacterial parasite that requires ATP to carry on its metabolic processes and reproduction. This species is responsible for trachoma and two major sexually transmitted diseases (STDs), lymphogranuloma venereum and infection of the lower and upper genital tract. Serovars L1, L2, and L3 are responsible for lymphogranuloma venereum, whereas serovars A through K are responsible for infection of the lower and upper genital tract. The latter infection includes urethritis, Bartholin's gland abscess, cervicitis, endometritis, and salpingitis. These serovars have also been implicated as a possible cause of preterm labor, premature rupture of amniotic membranes, septic abortion, and postpartum endometritis.

The significance of *C. trachomatis* is not due to the infections it causes but to the sequelae secondary to salpingitis, namely, damage to the fallopian tubes. This, in turn, leads

TABLE 1. Historical Risk Factors for Contracting *Chlamydia trachomatis* Infection

Multiple sexual partners
History of sexually transmitted disease (STD)
Having a partner with an STD
First sexual intercourse at an early age
History of having used an intrauterine device
Previously treated for pelvic inflammatory disease
Recent onset of
　Postcoital bleeding or spotting
　Dyspareunia
　Vague lower abdominal pain
　Irregular uterine bleeding
　Breakthrough bleeding with use of oral contraceptive pills

to partial damage of the endothelial cells, which inhibits migration of a fertilized ovum and results in ectopic pregnancy. Damage could also be complete, in that conception cannot take place and infertility results. Because infection is usually asymptomatic, this bacterium often goes undetected. Therefore, it is important for the physician and other health care providers to consider the presence of this infection in their patients of reproductive age.

Some investigators urge screening of all patients of reproductive age for the presence of *C. trachomatis*. However, this practice would likely have a poor yield and would not be cost-effective. It would be better to obtain a detailed history to determine whether a patient is at risk for contracting an STD (Table 1). This determination is extremely important, because it alerts the physician to look for clues to the presence of an STD.

DIAGNOSIS

During the pelvic examination, the physician should examine the vaginal discharge microscopically to determine whether the patient has a leukorrhea and/or trichomoniasis. The presence of leukorrhea may suggest that the patient has pelvic inflammatory disease (PID), but this finding is not pathognomic of salpingitis. The presence of trichomoniasis indicates that the patient is at risk for other STDs. There is a tendency for an STD to travel in the company of other STDs; for example, *Neisseria gonorrhoeae* and *C. trachomatis* are found to co-infect the same person in approximately 60% of cases when one organism has already been found.

Another physical clue to possible infection with *C. trachomatis* is the presence of endocervical mucopus. This characteristic is usually detected by placing a Dacron-tipped applicator into the endocervical canal and rotating it full circle for approximately 30 seconds. A purulent exudate on the tip of the applicator is highly suggestive of the presence of *C. trachomatis*. The specimen should be processed for the isolation and identification of *C. trachomatis* by one of the following methods: culture, fluorescent antibody-antigen detection, DNA or RNA probes, antibody-antigen detection (enzyme-linked immunosorbent assay), or polymerase chain reaction. The specimen should also be processed for the detection of *N. gonorrhoeae* and should be gram stained. The presence of white blood cells and the absence of bacteria would suggest, and would be compatible with, *C. trachomatis* infection. The presence of white blood cells containing gram-negative diplococci is highly suggestive of infection with *N. gonorrhoeae*.

Other physical clues are a cervix that bleeds briskly when gently touched with a cotton- or Dacron-tipped applicator, pain on palpation, and movement of the cervix and uterus. Pain may also be elicited when the adnexae are palpated. The patient may complain of dysuria and/or urinary frequency. A urinalysis may reveal the presence of pyuria and the absence of bacteria. This result should prompt the physician to obtain a urethral specimen for the isolation of *C. trachomatis* and *N. gonorrhoeae*.

TREATMENT

Individuals found to have evidence of chlamydial infection should start on appropriate treatment. A test in which the answer cannot be obtained within 30 minutes is too long to wait to begin treatment. Remember: infection of the genital tract is typically asymptomatic, and therefore, discovery is based solely on the investigational procedures of the physician. Because the infection may have been in place for a prolonged time, it may already have ascended to the upper genital tract. Any further delay may result in increased damage to the fallopian tubes. Administration of appropriate treatment should commence immediately. If cultures do not support the diagnosis, treatment can be stopped.

Patients who are found to have positive cultures should be counseled as to the significance of such an infection—specifically, for the possibility of the patient's potential risk for infertility associated with the number of episodes of PID experienced by the patient. Individuals who experience a single episode of PID have a 13% risk of being infertile, two episodes are associated with a 35% risk, and those who have had three episodes of PID have approximately a 75% risk of infertility.

Treatment of urethritis is based on whether the gonococcus is present. In the absence of the gonococcus, treatment is directed against *C. trachomatis* (23 to 55% of cases), *Ureaplasma urealyticum* (20 to 40%), or *Trichomonas vaginalis* (2 to 4%). Treatment regimens for chlamydial infection in the absence of other STDs are listed in Table 2.

Patients whose symptoms persist should return for re-evaluation to determine whether (1) they complied with treatment by taking their medicine and (2) they refrained from sexual intercourse to avoid reinfection. A second swab specimen should also be obtained, not only to determine whether reinfection has occurred but also to see whether *T. vaginalis* is present. If trichomonads are detected, the patient should be treated with metronidazole (Flagyl), 250 mg orally, three times daily for 7 days. If the patient

TABLE 2. Treatment Regimens for Uncomplicated Chlamydial Infection

Doxycycline (Vibramycin), 100 mg orally bid × 7 d
Erythromycin base, 500 mg orally qid × 7 d
Erythromycin ethylsuccinate, 800 mg orally qid × 7 d
Erythromycin base, 250 mg orally qid × 14 d
Erythromycin ethylsuccinate, 400 mg orally qid × 14 d
Azithromycin (Zithromax), 1 gm orally in a single dose
Amoxicillin, 500 mg orally tid × 7 d
Amoxicillin-clavulanate (Augmentin), 500 mg orally tid × 7 d

TABLE 3. Oral Antibiotic Regimens for the Treatment of Ambulatory Patients with a Diagnosis of Endometritis and/or Salpingitis

Metronidazole (Flagyl), 500 mg bid × 7 d, *plus* ofloxacin, 300 mg bid × 7 d
Clindamycin (Cleocin), 300 mg tid × 7 d, *plus* ofloxacin, 300 mg bid × 7 d
Amoxicillin-clavulanate (Augmentin), 500 mg tid × 7 d

does not have trichomoniasis and was treated with doxycycline, a second course of doxycycline could be instituted or one of the alternative choices listed in Table 2 could be chosen.

Patients with endocervical mucopus should be treated as being infected with both *C. trachomatis* and *N. gonorrhoeae*. It is difficult to determine the appropriate treatment regimen in such cases, because it is not known whether the infection is confined to the cervix or has begun to ascend to the upper genital tract. If there is no evidence or suggestion of upper tract involvement, standard treatment with ceftriaxone (Rocephin), 125 mg once intramuscularly, and doxycycline, 100 mg orally twice daily for 7 days, is acceptable. Individuals whose infection is confined to the cervix can be treated with ceftriaxone, 125 mg once intramuscularly, and azithromycin, 1 gram in a single dose. The patient should be advised not to engage in sexual intercourse during the management phase and should be educated on prevention of reinfection. The patient's partner, and anyone else she has had sexual contact with, must be treated as well.

The patient with endometritis should have an endometrial biopsy, and the specimen should be divided into two portions. One specimen should be sent for the isolation and identification of *N. gonorrhoeae*, *C. trachomatis*, and aerobic, facultative, and obligate anaerobic bacteria. The other specimen should be processed for histologic evaluation. The presence of plasma cells strongly suggests that the infection has involved the fallopian tubes. Treatment for this level of infection is best carried out with a broad combination of agents (Table 3).

Ofloxacin has been demonstrated to be as effective as ceftriaxone for the treatment of gonorrhea, and as effective as doxycycline for treating chlamydial infection. The combination of an anaerobic agent such as metronidazole or clindamycin with ofloxacin offers a regimen with activity against the non–sexually transmitted agents that are endogenous to the lower genital tract and may be involved in the infectious process. Another potentially useful agent (not yet approved by the Food and Drug Administration) is trovafloxacin, a fluoroquinolone. This agent has activity against both the gonococcus and chlamydiae as well as the gram-negative and gram-positive facultative and obligate anaerobic bacteria.

Patients suspected of having PID and requiring hospitalization must also receive antibiotic regimens that are effective against the commonly involved

TABLE 4. **Parenteral Antibiotic Regimens for the Treatment of Hospitalized Patients with a Diagnosis of Pelvic Inflammatory Disease**

Cefoxitin (Mefoxin), 2 gm intravenously q 8 h,
   plus doxycycline, 100 mg (may be given orally) q 12 h
Cefotetan (Cefotan), 2 gm q 12 h,
   plus doxycycline, 100 mg q 12 h
Ceftizoxime (Cefizox), 2 gm q 8 h,
   plus doxycycline, 100 mg q 12 h
Ampicillin-sulbactam (Unasyn), 3 gm q 6 h
Piperacillin-tazobactam (Zosyn), 3.375 gm q 6 h
Metronidazole (Flagyl), 500 mg q 8 h,
   plus ofloxacin, 300 mg, 12 h
Clindamycin (Cleocin), 900 mg q 8 h
   plus gentamicin, 2 mg/kg of body weight (loading dose),
   followed by 1.5 mg/kg administered q 8 h
Ofloxacin (Floxin), 300 mg q 8 h
Trovafloxacin (not yet approved by the FDA), 200 mg q 24 h

STDs as well as the aerobic, facultative, and obligate anaerobic bacteria. The hospitalized patient can receive any one of the regimens listed in Table 4.

The pregnant patient with cervical infection can be treated with azithromycin, 1 gram orally in a single dose. She should *not* receive doxycycline or quinolones. The Centers for Disease Control and Prevention recommends erythromycin; however, this antibiotic is not well tolerated by pregnant women. An alternative is amoxicillin, 500 mg orally three times daily for 7 days; this agent is not effective against penicillinase-producing *N. gonorrhoeae* but is effective against non–penicillinase-producing strains.

The patient who is found to be positive for an STD should also be screened for hepatitis B, human immunodeficiency virus (HIV) infection, and syphilis. Pregnant patients found to be positive for gonorrhea and chlamydia should be screened in each trimester for reinfection as well as for syphilis, hepatitis B, and HIV infection.

Patients treated for uncomplicated PID typically show response to antibiotic therapy within 48 hours. Patients not improving after 48 hours of antibiotic therapy should be re-evaluated to determine whether the infection has progressed, e.g., to a tubo-ovarian abscess.

The partner of a patient known to have an STD should be referred to a physician who specializes in the treatment of STDs. This is essential in controlling the spread of the diseases. It is important to educate both the patient and her partner as to the method of transmission and the significant morbidity associated with *C. trachomatis* infection.

PELVIC INFLAMMATORY DISEASE

method of
SHERWOOD C. LYNN, JR., M.D.
College of Medicine, University of South Alabama
Mobile, Alabama

The term "pelvic inflammatory disease" (PID) originated with the description of the effects of the ascending infection of the fallopian tubes with *Neisseria gonorrhoeae*. Despite the term's being used synonymously with salpingitis or acute salpingitis, these designations might well understate the degree of pelvic involvement. PID describes the acute inflammation of the serosal surfaces of the uterus, oviducts, ovaries, broad ligaments, bladder, rectum, and pelvic side walls. It is, inherent in its definition, pelvic peritonitis. The term chronic PID has been used in the past to describe the sequelae of the acute infection but should be reserved for the true chronic nature of PID associated with tuberculosis, actinomycosis, and perhaps *Chlamydia trachomatis* infection. Finally, PID is more commonly used in reference to sexually transmitted infections rather than surgically related infections such as septic abortion or post–cesarean section endometritis, myometritis, and/or parametritis.

Of the nation's estimated 12 million annual cases of sexually transmitted diseases (STDs), more than 8% have advanced to PID by the time of identification. This diagnosis is responsible for 2 to 3 million clinic visits and more than a quarter million hospitalizations per year. In addition, as many as 150,000 surgical procedures are performed on patients carrying this diagnosis per year. To the estimated $3.5 billion in direct and indirect medical costs must be added the psychosocial impact of infertility, ectopic pregnancy, and chronic pelvic pain. One fourth of women who have PID are destined to experience subsequent problems, including a 10% risk for infertility (20% after a second and 50% after a third episode), a 6- to 10-fold increase in ectopic pregnancy, and a 15 to 20% risk for chronic pelvic pain.

ETIOLOGY

PID is the result of infection of the upper genital tract by an ascending infection of the vagina and cervix. The offending organism gains access from the penis or ejaculate, perhaps adherent to sperm or even trichomonads, and sequentially invades the mucosa of the endometrium and endosalpinx. This invasion incites an inflammatory response that involves the submucosa, then the muscularis, and finally the serosa. Whereas 99% of cases are caused by ascending infection, the remainder are related to appendiceal rupture, other intraperitoneal abscess, hematogenous spread, and lymphatic spread. Approximately 85% of cases are spontaneous, but 15% are associated with instrumentation of the uterus, e.g., endometrial biopsy, dilatation and curettage, intrauterine contraceptive device (IUCD) insertion, and hysterosalpingography.

Although PID is polymicrobial, the upper tract infection has historically been defined by lower tract culture. *N. gonorrhoeae* remains a significant initiating organism. Up to 6% of sexually active women of reproductive age will have positive cervical cultures, and 10 to 20% of these women with "gonococcal cervicitis" will develop PID. Of women with the clinical picture of PID who have positive cervical cultures, only 22% will have *N. gonorrhoeae* isolated as the sole organism from the peritoneum. In 78% of cases, it will be found in combination with other organisms or not at all. It is a gram-negative diplococcus requiring a carbon dioxide–enriched culture environment. It produces a rapid and intense inflammatory response associated with dramatic cellular and tissue destruction in the tube. Piliated and nonpiliated strains elaborate a lipopolysaccharide that acts as both a chemotactic agent for polymorphonuclear leukocytes and a toxin that desquamates the ciliated tubal mucosal cells. Many of the recent isolates produce β-lactamase, rendering the penicillins ineffective for treatment.

As a result of new detection techniques, *C. trachomatis* has been shown to surpass the gonococcus as the primary cause of STD. The clinical entity produced by this organism is much more insidious and results in less tissue damage than that caused by the gonococcus. As an obligate intracellular parasite, the elementary body attaches to specific receptors on the columnar cells, inducing phagocytosis. The elementary body then transforms into the reticulate body, which uses the host synthetic mechanism to reproduce itself. The reticulate body then reorganizes into the elementary body, which fills and finally ruptures the cell 48 to 72 hours after phagocytosis. Perhaps because of the protected intracellular reproductive mechanism, much of the tissue damage is induced by antigen-antibody complexes.

Haemophilus influenzae has been cultured from cervix and tube in laparoscopically proven salpingitis usually associated with pyosalpinx. It appears that this organism ascends to the upper genital tract and destroys the involved tissue similarly to *N. gonorrhoeae*. Whether mycoplasmas incite PID is controversial. *Mycoplasma pneumoniae*, *Mycoplasma hominis*, and *Ureaplasma urealyticum* have been isolated from patients with documented PID. Although colonization of the lower genital tract with *M. hominis* and *U. urealyticum* frequently occurs at birth, it tends to clear with age. However, these organisms are not cultured from the normal upper genital tract. Nonetheless, experimental evidence from primate research indicates that mycoplasmas do produce a mild inflammatory reaction in the oviduct. Many other organisms have been isolated from the endocervix, endometrium, tubes, and cul-de-sac, largely dependent on the point in the disease process at which cultures are taken. Cultures for the aerobic nonhemolytic streptococci, *Escherichia coli*, group B streptococci, coagulase-negative staphylococci, anaerobic *Bacteroides* species, *Peptococcus*, *Veillonella*, and *Peptostreptococcus* have been reported from simultaneous samples taken for various isolates and may or may not confirm *N. gonorrhoeae* and/or *Chlamydia*. *Actinomyces israelii* may rarely be the causal agent when there is an IUCD in utero, and *Mycobacterium tuberculosis* may prove to be the agent in a more chronic clinical picture and may be hematogenously spread to the pelvis from other sites in the body. Finally, there have been several reports of an association of PID with herpesviruses and cytomegaloviruses, a relationship that needs further study.

RISK FACTORS

Women between the ages of 16 and 25 years with multiple sexual partners and whose initial sexual encounter occurs at an early age are at particularly high risk for PID. Black and other nonwhite women are at higher risk than whites are, although white teenagers are at ever increasing risk. Women who have experienced a previous episode of PID are at an increased risk. Instrumentation of the endometrial cavity, e.g., endometrial biopsy, dilatation and curettage, and insertion of an IUCD, is a risk factor. Whereas hormonal contraception may provide protection against *N. gonorrhoeae* by rendering the cervical mucus progestational, it may produce ectopy of the cervix, which may increase the risk for chlamydial infection. Barrier contraceptive methods, especially if used with spermicidal agents that may also be bactericidal, should be most protective. Although early data reported a causal relationship of PID to IUCD use, stratification of these data by age has failed to confirm the original interpretation. The data do demonstrate, however, the extremely high risk of young women

with multiple sexual partners who also use this method of birth control. Isthmic tubal ligation blocks the channel of bacterial spread, thus dramatically reducing the risk for PID.

DIAGNOSIS

The most common symptom of PID is lower abdominal and pelvic pain of relatively short duration, usually within 7 days of menses. There are usually other associated symptoms that must be elicited, including a purulent vaginal discharge, abnormal bleeding, dysuria, nausea, vomiting, tenesmus, and fever. Upper abdominal pain is a relatively late symptom and may represent Fitz-Hugh–Curtis syndrome. Gonococcal PID is generally rapid in its course, whereas chlamydial PID is more insidious. Superinfection or co-infection with other organisms is common.

Although not all patients will be febrile, all must have low abdominal, adnexal, and cervical motion tenderness. Many will exhibit rebound tenderness to the lower abdomen. Right upper quadrant tenderness should be carefully assessed and, if present, should generate consideration of hospitalization for therapy. A speculum examination usually demonstrates a purulent cervicovaginal discharge and cervical motion tenderness. Bimanual examination confirms cervical, uterine, and adnexal tenderness with bilateral parametrial fullness, although a definite mass may not be palpable. The sensation of a full or bulging cul-de-sac may also be appreciated without palpating a definite mass.

Confirmation of the clinical diagnosis is obtained by DNA probe for the gonococcus and chlamydiae and by Gram's stain of the cervical mucus. The Gram stain is a rapid means of demonstrating the gonococcus as gram-negative, intracellular diplococci. I also obtain a complete blood count, erythrocyte sedimentation rate, β-human chorionic gonadotropin (β-hCG) level, and urinalysis. Liver function studies should be obtained as indicated. Endometrial biopsy showing leukocytic infiltration has been demonstrated to aid in the diagnosis, but I do not routinely use this test, reserving it for those patients with questionable signs and symptoms. Although transvaginal ultrasound imaging is obtained routinely in the emergency department, it is not frequently helpful and, in fact, may be misleading. It has been useful only in defining suspected pelvic abscesses.

Those patients with minimal symptoms of short duration and physical findings are treated as outpatients with follow-up examinations within 72 hours. Inpatient therapy is indicated for uncertain diagnosis, severe illness including nausea and vomiting, upper abdominal disease, and failed outpatient management. I also think that evidence or even suspicion of an inflammatory mass is sufficient grounds for admission. I admit all patients with human immunodeficiency virus (HIV) infection who present with symptoms consistent with PID, despite the apparent severity, because of the risk for abscess formation. A number of situations not necessarily related to strict medical guidelines argue for hospitalization, e.g., unpredictable compliance, especially with adolescents, and uncertain follow-up.

TREATMENT

Treatment of PID is directed at rapid resolution of symptoms reflecting improvement of the inflammation and its resultant sequelae. Because of the expense of hospitalization, many patients are treated in offices, clinics, and emergency departments. Table 1 provides the 1993 recommendations of the Centers for Disease Control and Prevention (CDC) for outpatient treatment. I routinely give ceftriaxone (Rocephin), 250 mg intramuscularly, and add doxycycline (Vibramycin), 100 mg orally twice daily, for 14 days to complete the antichlamydial therapy. In patients who cannot tolerate tetracyclines, erythromycin, 500 mg orally four times daily, is added to the ceftriaxone. Because of several early, outpatient failures and the emergence of resistant strains, I have abandoned the ofloxacin-clindamycin regimen. Outpatients failing to respond to therapy within 3 days are admitted for parenteral antibiotic therapy.

Additional criteria for admission and inpatient therapy identified at the initial evaluation include high fever or leukocytosis, upper peritoneal signs, an adnexal mass, an IUCD in utero, or an uncertain diagnosis including potential surgical emergencies. Table 2 provides the 1993 CDC recommendations for inpatient therapy. For the patients with minimal criteria for admission, I usually initiate treatment with a second- or third-generation cephalosporin and doxycycline, e.g., cefotetan (Cefotan), 2 grams, and doxycycline, 100 mg, intravenously twice daily. However, in patients who have advanced disease, are outpatient treatment failures, or have HIV infections, I generally use triple therapy consisting of ampicillin, 2 grams every 6 hours, clindamycin, 900 mg every 8 hours, and gentamicin, 2 mg per kg loading dose then 1.5 mg per kg maintenance dose every 8 hours, all intravenously. If there is not a rapid response to therapy, I move toward invasive diagnostic modalities, including laparoscopy, which may be helpful in establishing a diagnosis. It is used in conjunction with serial β-hCG determinations to diagnose and treat PID in the presence of ectopic pregnancy and to treat appendicitis. Even in those cases that have ultrasound confirmation of an inflammatory mass, laparoscopy has proved helpful in abscess drainage.

I routinely treat for 2 days beyond resolution of

TABLE 1. 1993 Centers for Disease Control and Prevention Guidelines for Ambulatory Management of Acute Pelvic Inflammatory Disease

Regimen A

Cefoxitin (Mefoxin), 2 gm IM, plus probenecid, 1 gm PO in a single dose concurrently, or ceftriaxone (Rocephin), 250 mg IM, or other parenteral third-generation cephalosporin (e.g., ceftizoxime [Cefizox] or cefotaxime [Claforan])

plus

Doxycycline (Vibramycin), 100 mg PO bid for 14 d

Regimen B

Ofloxacin (Floxin), 400 mg PO bid for 14 d

plus

Clindamycin (Cleocin), 450 mg PO qid, or metronidazole, 500 mg PO bid for 14 d

From the Centers for Disease Control and Prevention: 1993 Sexually transmitted diseases treatment guidelines. MMWR Morb Mortal Wkly Rep 42(RR-14):78–80, 1993.

TABLE 2. 1993 Centers for Disease Control and Prevention Guidelines for Inpatient Management of Acute Pelvic Inflammatory Disease

Regimen A

Cefoxitin (Mefoxin), 2 gm IV q 6 h, or cefotetan (Cefotan), 2 gm q 12 h

plus

Doxycycline (Vibramycin), 100 mg IV or PO q 12 h

This regimen should be given for at least 48 h after the patient improves clinically. Doxycycline, 100 mg PO bid, is then continued for a total of 14 d.

Regimen B

Clindamycin (Cleocin), 900 mg IV q 8 h

plus

Gentamicin (Garamycin), loading dose IV or IM (2 mg/kg body weight) followed by a maintenance dose (1.5 mg/kg) q 8 h

This regimen should be given for at least 48 h after the patient improves clinically. Doxycycline 100 mg PO bid or clindamycin 450 mg PO qid is given to complete a total of 14 d of therapy. Clindamycin provides more effective anaerobic coverage for abscesses but has not been determined to be effective against *Chlamydia trachomatis*.

From the Centers for Disease Control and Prevention: 1993 Sexually transmitted diseases treatment guidelines. MMWR Morb Mortal Wkly Rep 42(RR-14):78–80, 1993.

clinical symptoms, then discharge on doxycycline (100 mg orally twice daily) to complete 2 weeks of tetracycline therapy. My patients are seen back in the office in 10 days to 2 weeks. If there is any evidence of a persistent mass at that time, tetracycline is continued and discussion of possible surgical intervention is initiated. It should be stressed that every effort is made to identify and treat the sexual partners of these patients.

UTERINE LEIOMYOMAS

method of
JOHN A. ROCK, M.D.
Emory University School of Medicine
Atlanta, Georgia

Uterine leiomyomas are the most common pelvic neoplasm in women. The incidence of uterine leiomyoma is reported to be approximately 20% in women older than 30 years; however, postmortem examinations of women suggest a somewhat higher incidence, as do diagnostic laparoscopies for the assessment of infertility, pregnancy wastage, and pelvic pain. Because of their incidence and their impact on women's health and quality of life, these uterine tumors are of great importance. Leiomyomas are the most common indication for hysterectomy. About 30% of all hysterectomies are performed for leiomyomas. Abnormal uterine bleeding, abdominal pelvic pain, and abdominal pelvic organ dysfunction (urinary frequency, constipation) are symptoms often associated with enlarging leiomyomas. Alternatively, altered reproductive capacity (infertility, pregnancy wastage, premature delivery) has been related to uterine leiomyoma, but a cause-and-effect relationship is less clear.

PATHOPHYSIOLOGY

Studies have demonstrated that many uterine leiomyomas are cytogenetically abnormal. They are monoclonal proliferations of connective tissue and smooth muscle cells. Chromosomes 7, 12, and 14 have been found to be most frequently involved in leiomyoma and include both translocations and deletions. Many other chromosomes, including the X chromosome, have also been implicated. The concept that most human tumors, including uterine leiomyoma, are cytogenetically abnormal clones is rapidly gaining acceptance. This theory suggests that uterine leiomyomas are composed of genetically abnormal clones of cells derived from a single progenitor that has undergone mutation. The mutation results in cells that respond abnormally to one or more growth factors, causing tumor cell growth, whereas adjacent normal myometrial cells, without mutation, replicate in a conditioned and normal fashion. Other studies indicate that a number of growth factors, including insulin-like growth factors and their binding proteins, play a modulating role in uterine leiomyoma growth. It is also possible that epidermal growth factor as well as others also modulates leiomyoma growth, with some growth factors stimulated by estrogen and others by progestins. This variable modulation concept may explain why some uterine leiomyomas respond more dramatically than others to gonadotropin-releasing hormone agonist (GnRHa).

Uterine leiomyomas generally occur in one of three anatomic locations: (1) intramural (occurring in the midportion of the myometrium), (2) subserosal (projecting outwardly into the pelvic cavity), or (3) submucosal (projecting into the uterine cavity). Subserosal leiomyomas may grow into the broad ligament or other adjacent structures. Both subserosal and submucosal leiomyomas may also become pedunculated. Some subserosal leiomyomas have become detached from their uterine surface and reattached to other tissues and/or organs in the abdominal cavity. These migratory tumors are referred to as parasitic leiomyomas.

Approximately 80% of uterine leiomyomas are multiple. The most common histologic changes of uterine leiomyomas are degeneration, hemorrhage, and ulceration. These changes may occur in up to two thirds of all uterine leiomyomas. Degenerative changes include (1) hyaline degeneration, (2) hydropic (edema) degeneration, (3) red (infarction) degeneration, (4) calcific degeneration, (5) myxomatous degeneration, and (6) fatty degeneration. Whether myomas also degenerate into leiomyosarcomas (LMS) or whether LMS develop spontaneously remains controversial. Most data favor a malignant degeneration process. Such a malignant degeneration of uterine leiomyoma to LMS occurs in approximately 0.5% of all leiomyomas. In either case, uterine LMS accounts for only 1.3% of all uterine malignant neoplasms. The histologic difference between leiomyomas and LMS is based on the numbers of mitoses per high-power field and the presence of atypia seen on histologic examination. Tumors with fewer than 5 mitoses per 10 high-power field examinations and no atypia are considered to be benign.

Adenomyosis is sometimes confused with uterine leiomyoma because of similar presenting symptoms and physical findings. Differentiation of the two pathologic processes has historically been based on histologic examination. However, magnetic resonance imaging in some patients appears to have the ability to make a presurgical differentiation. Such a distinction is important, because adenomyosis usually involves the entire uterus. Although the surgeon may resect an adenomyoma, the disease process continues within the uterine musculature.

SYMPTOMS

Although a majority of leiomyomas are asymptomatic, approximately 33% do present with symptoms. These symptoms include abnormal uterine bleeding, pelvic pain and/or pressure, and reproductive abnormalities (infertility, pregnancy wastage, and preterm labor).

DIAGNOSIS

The diagnosis of uterine leiomyoma is made primarily by physical examination. However, the patient's history and imaging techniques may be supportive as well as diagnostic. Leiomyomas are suspected when, on bimanual examination, the uterus is found to be enlarged, irregular in outline, firm, and nontender. Imaging techniques useful when the physical examination fails to provide a clear diagnosis include pelvic ultrasonography, magnetic resonance imaging, and/or computed tomography. Of these imaging techniques, pelvic ultrasonography is both effective and least expensive and therefore preferred. If adenomyosis must also be ruled out, MRI has proved to be effective. Hysterosalpingograms may be useful in the diagnosis of intracavitary disease. The diagnosis of uterine leiomyoma is also frequently made in asymptomatic patients undergoing laparoscopy or laparotomy for other pelvic disorders.

The evaluation of a patient with uterine leiomyoma should attempt to accurately determine the number, location, and size of each uterine tumor. The total uterine leiomyoma size has traditionally been estimated on the basis of equivalent gestational size. Imaging techniques now allow the assessment of uterine volume, which may prove to be far more accurate in observing patients.

Additional studies of importance in assessing uterine leiomyoma include (1) hematocrit or hemoglobin and (2) coagulation studies (fibrinogen, prothrombin time, bleeding time), in patients with abnormal uterine bleeding; and/or (3) endometrial biopsy, in patients at risk for endometrial hyperplasia. Surgical diagnostic procedures (laparoscopy, hysteroscopy) are occasionally required to accurately assess the location, number, and size of the uterine tumor. In general, however, imaging techniques such as ultrasonography may provide this information (Table 1).

MANAGEMENT

Management of uterine leiomyoma depends on (1) symptoms resulting from the tumor, (2) size and number of tumors, (3) the patient's desire to maintain reproductive function, and (4) the patient's age. Active management (medical or surgical) is not generally recommended for uterine leiomyoma less than the equivalent of a 12 weeks' gestational size with minimal or no symptoms. As the composite uterine volume increases above this size or if rapid growth occurs or if symptoms of abnormal uterine bleeding, significant pelvic pain, or reproductive function disorders occur that are likely to be related to the tumors, then active management should be considered.

Treatment for uterine leiomyoma may be divided into two general options: expectant management or

TABLE 1. **Evaluation of Uterine Leiomyoma**

Abdominal-pelvic examination
Imaging procedures (when physical examination is inconclusive)
  Ultrasonography
  Magnetic resonance imaging
  Computed tomography
Hematologic studies (with abnormal bleeding)
  Hemoglobin or hematocrit
  Coagulation bleeding studies
    Prothrombin time
    Bleeding time
    Fibrinogen platelets
Histologic studies (with abnormal bleeding)
  Endometrial biopsy
  Curettage
Adjuvant procedures (when tumor size affects other pelvic organ
    function)
  Intravenous pyelogram
  Barium enema study
Adjuvant procedures (when diagnosis is unclear with above
    testing)
  Hysteroscopy
  Laparoscopy
  Sonohysterography
  Hysterogram

active management. Active management may include medical or surgical options (Table 2).

Expectant management is the treatment of choice in patients with minimal or controllable symptoms (menorrhagia, metrorrhagia) whose tumors are stable in size or are noted to be only slow growing after 2 years of observation. Interval examinations should be every 6 months for 2 years and then yearly thereafter unless significant changes occur during this period. The abnormal uterine bleeding may be controlled with nonsteroidal anti-inflammatory drugs, progestins, or low-dose oral contraceptives (Table 3).

Medical management of uterine leiomyoma is based on the finding that estrogens generally stimulate uterine growth. GnRHa suppresses pituitary gonadotropin release, which in turn suppresses ovarian estrogen production. The resulting hypoestrogenemia is associated with a reduction in uterine volume of

TABLE 2. **Management Options for Treating Uterine Leiomyoma**

Expectant management
  Uterine size less than the equivalent of 12-wk gestation
  Minimal or controllable symptoms
Medical management
  GnRHa suppression
  GnRHa suppression with estrogen-progestin add-back
Surgical management
  Hysteroscopic excision of submucous or pedunculated
    leiomyoma
  Laparoscopic excision or destruction of subserous
    leiomyoma
  Laparotomy with myomectomy
  Hysterectomy (abdominal or vaginal)
Combined medical-surgical management
  Preoperative GnRHa suppression
  Conservative or definitive surgery

TABLE 3. **Expectant Management of Leiomyoma**

Initial abdominal-pelvic examination followed by repeated
  examinations every 6 mo for 2 y, then yearly
Symptom Control
Abnormal Uterine Bleeding

Nonsteroidal anti-inflammatory drugs*
  Ibuprofen (Motrin), 400 mg PO q 4 h beginning with earliest
    onset of bleeding
  Naproxen sodium (Anaprox), 550 mg PO initially, then 275 mg
    PO q 6 h beginning with earliest onset of bleeding
  Mefenamic acid (Ponstel), 500 mg PO initially, then 250 mg
    PO q 6 h beginning with earliest onset of bleeding
Progestins
  Medroxyprogesterone acetate (Provera), 10 mg PO daily × 14
    d each month, starting cycle day 12
  Norethindrone (Micronor),* 0.35 mg PO daily × 14 d each
    month, starting cycle day 12
  Norgestrel (Ovrette),* 0.075 mg PO daily × 14 d each month,
    starting cycle day 12 or daily without break
Oral contraceptive agents
  Norgestrel and ethinyl estradiol (Ovral),* 1 tablet daily for 21
    of 28 d
  Desogestrel and ethinyl estradiol (Ortho-Cept),* 1 tablet daily
    for 21 of 28 d
  Norethindrone and mestranol (Norinyl 1 + 50),* 1 tablet daily
    for 21 of 28 d

Abdominal Pelvic Pain

Nonsteroidal anti-inflammatory drugs as just listed

*Not FDA approved for this indication.

approximately 40%. This reduction is usually more prominent in leiomyomas in which the uterine composite size is greater than 12 weeks' gestation. The effect of GnRHa is maximal at approximately 3 months of therapy, with little or no additional size reduction beyond this time. After cessation of GnRHa therapy, rapid regrowth of tumors back to pretreatment size is most commonly observed. Therefore, this management option is generally recommended only as a presurgical adjuvant or in patients with pending menopause. Postmenopausal patients receiving hormone replacement therapy will occasionally remanifest their myoma symptoms. This is not common because the dose of hormone replacement therapy is much lower than the body's endogenous hormone production. If this occurs, the patient's hormone regimen may need to be "customized" to suppress her myoma symptoms. Longer management with GnRHa is reported to be beneficial with use of "add-back" therapy after the first 12 weeks of GnRHa administration (Table 4). GnRHa therapy should not be used alone for more than 6 months because a prolonged hypoestrogenic state may result in significant bone loss.

Surgical management includes four separate operative options: (1) laparoscopic excision or destruction of leiomyoma, (2) hysteroscopic resection of pedunculated or broad-based submucous leiomyoma, (3) laparotomy with myomectomy, and (4) hysterectomy (Table 5). The decision to use a surgical approach should be based on the adverse effects that the leiomyomas have on the patient's quality of life. Symptomatic patients (abnormal uterine bleeding, abdominal pel-

TABLE 4. Medical Management of Leiomyoma

Uterine leiomyoma size reduction through ovarian estrogen suppression
    Submucous leiomyoma >2 cm
    Subserous leiomyoma greater than equivalent 12-wk gestation size
GnRHa ovarian estrogen suppression
    Leuprolide acetate (Lupron Depot), 3.75 mg IM monthly × 3 mo
    Nafarelin acetate (Synarel),* 200 μg intranasally bid × 3 mo
    Goserelin acetate (Zoladex),* 3.6 mg SC monthly × 3 mo
GnRHa ovarian estrogen suppression with estrogen-progestin add-back†
    3 mo of one of the above GnRHa followed by
    Continued GnRHa, plus
        Conjugated estrogens (Premarin), 0.625 mg PO qd
        Medroxyprogesterone acetate (Provera), 2.5 mg PO qd

*Not FDA approved for this indication.
†GnRHa with add-back does not have FDA approval for medical management of uterine leiomyoma; however, sufficient research and clinical data support its merit in leiomyoma management.

vic pain, reproductive disorders) are candidates for surgical intervention if the symptoms can be reasonably related to the leiomyoma. Laparoscopic excision of pedunculated leiomyoma or coagulation of the leiomyoma by laser or electrical current has enjoyed some success; however, these approaches are applicable only to the small, subserous leiomyoma. With the advances in laparoscopic technique, removal of larger intramural myomas has been reported. This procedure has the benefit of decreased postoperative pain and quicker postoperative recovery. Laparoscopic myomectomy requires laparoscopic suturing expertise. The myometrium needs to be carefully reapproximated and hemostasis achieved. Antepartum uterine incision dehiscence has been reported after laparoscopic myomectomy. Thus, careful observation during pregnancy should be recommended for the patient who wishes to conceive after laparoscopic myomectomy.

Hysteroscopic resection of submucous leiomyoma offers a less extensive surgical approach to uterine cavitary lesions when the tumors are thought to be related to abnormal uterine bleeding or reproductive disorders. It is recommended that these surgical procedures be preceded by GnRHa suppression for a 3-month period to reduce the size of the tumor (particularly with tumors larger than 2 cm) as well as to reduce blood loss during the procedure. However, approximately 20% of patients require additional surgery after hysteroscopic resection of leiomyoma.

Laparotomy with myomectomy may be considered for the patient who meets the American College of Obstetricians and Gynecologists (ACOG) criteria for myomectomy (Table 6) or who is desirous of maintaining her reproductive capacity, presents with symptoms requiring surgical intervention, or is unresponsive to expectant management. GnRHa suppression for a 3-month period has proved to be beneficial in reducing tumor volume and operative bleeding in patients whose leiomyomas have a composite size of greater than 12 weeks' gestation. GnRHa suppression may also be used preoperatively to improve a patient's hematocrit by decreasing uterine bleeding. It should be kept in mind that approximately 25% of patients who have undergone a myomectomy will later require another surgical procedure, because the recurrence rate is approximately 50% in patients with multiple leiomyomas.

Hysterectomy may be considered in symptomatic

TABLE 5. Surgical Management of Leiomyoma

Hysteroscopic excision of submucous or pedunculated leiomyoma
    <2 cm without GnRHa ovarian estrogen suppression
    >2 cm with GnRHa ovarian estrogen suppression
    20% of cases require additional management at a later date
Laparoscopic excision-destruction of subserous or pedunculated leiomyoma
    Excision limited by size of leiomyoma
    Destruction of leiomyoma by laser or bipolar electrocautery
    Because of potential complications, this procedure is still considered investigational
Laparotomy with myomectomy
    For patients who fail to conceive or who experience recurrent pregnancy wastage in whom the leiomyoma would appear to be a contributing cause
    For patients who wish to preserve reproductive capacity (see Table 6)
Hysterectomy (abdominal or vaginal)
    For patients with
        >12-wk gestation equivalent size uterus
        Rapidly growing leiomyoma
        Excessive abnormal uterine bleeding unresponsive to conservative management
        Abdominal and/or pelvic pain unresponsive to conservative management
    Abdominal hysterectomy the preferred route except in smaller symptomatic leiomyoma
    Retention of ovaries in premenopausal patients (see Table 7)

TABLE 6. American College of Obstetricians and Gynecologists Criteria for Myomectomy

Procedure: Myomectomy*
Indication: Leiomyomas in infertility patients, as a probable factor in failure to conceive or in recurrent pregnancy loss

Confirmation of indication: In the presence of failure to conceive or recurrent pregnancy loss:
1. Presence of leiomyomas of sufficient size or specific location to be a probable factor
2. No more likely explanation exists for the failure to conceive or recurrent pregnancy loss

Actions prior to procedure:
1. Evaluate other causes of male and female infertility or recurrent pregnancy loss
2. Evaluate the endometrial cavity and fallopian tubes, e.g., hysterosalpingogram
3. Document discussion that complexity of disease process may require hysterectomy

Unless otherwise stated, each numbered item must be present.

*Evaluation of the quality of care provided with this procedure, when performed for the indication listed, will be possible through assessment of ongoing or repetitive patterns of care ("trending").
Modified from the American College of Obstetricians and Gynecologists: Uterine leiomyomata. Technical Bulletin No. 192. Washington, DC, © ACOG, May 1994.

Procedure: Hysterectomy, abdominal or vaginal*

Indication: Leiomyomas

Confirmation of indication: Presence of 1 or 2 or 3
1. Asymptomatic leiomyomas of such size that they are palpable abdominally and are a concern to the patient
2. Excessive uterine bleeding evidenced by either of the following:
   a. Profuse bleeding with flooding or clots or repetitive periods lasting for more than 8 days
   b. Anemia due to acute or chronic blood loss
3. Pelvic discomfort caused by myomas (a or b or c)
   a. Acute and severe
   b. Chronic lower abdominal or low back pressure
   c. Bladder pressure with urinary frequency not due to urinary tract infection

Actions prior to procedure:
1. Confirm the absence of cervical malignancy
2. Eliminate anovulation and other causes of abnormal bleeding
3. When abnormal bleeding is present, confirm the absence of endometrial malignancy
4. Assess surgical risk from anemia and need for treatment
5. Consider patient's medical and psychologic risks concerning hysterectomy

Contraindication:
1. Desire to maintain fertility, in which case myomectomy should be considered
2. Asymptomatic leiomyomas of size less than 12 weeks' gestation determined by physical examination or ultrasound examination

Unless otherwise stated, each numbered and lettered item (except contraindications) must be present.

*Evaluation of the quality of care provided with this procedure, when performed for indications 2 and 3, will be possible through assessment of ongoing or repetitive patterns of care ("trending").

Modified from the American College of Obstetricians and Gynecologists: Uterine leiomyomata. Technical Bulletin No. 192. Washington, DC, © ACOG, May 1994.

patients who are uninterested in further reproductive function provided that the ACOG criteria for hysterectomy for leiomyoma are met (Table 7).

CANCER OF THE ENDOMETRIUM

method of
ANDREW BERCHUCK, M.D.
Duke University Medical Center
Durham, North Carolina

Endometrial cancer is the most common gynecologic malignant neoplasm in the United States, and the median age at presentation is 60 years. The majority of cases are diagnosed when endometrial biopsy is performed to investigate the cause of abnormal uterine bleeding. Because most endometrial adenocarcinomas are confined to the uterus at diagnosis, hysterectomy is the cornerstone of therapy, and 70 to 80% of patients with this disease are cured.

PRIMARY THERAPY

Most patients are suitable candidates for primary surgical therapy, but in cases in which surgery is considered unacceptably risky, curative treatment can often be accomplished with radiation therapy. For patients with cancer confined to the uterus, the cure rate with radiation therapy is only about 50 to 60%, compared with 80 to 90% with surgery. Patients in whom neither surgery nor radiation can be accomplished are best treated with progestin therapy. Many patients respond well to progestin therapy with megestrol acetate (Megace) 40 to 80 mg orally twice daily, as evidenced by cessation of bleeding, and progestin therapy may be curative in some cases.

Because many women with endometrial cancer are obese and have accompanying medical conditions such as diabetes mellitus and hypertension, a careful preoperative evaluation should be performed. Medical problems should be optimized before surgery in hopes of avoiding perioperative complications. In addition to a history and physical examination and routine preoperative blood tests, a chest radiograph is performed to exclude the presence of lung metastases. Additional radiographic studies and other diagnostic procedures should be employed selectively in the minority of patients who have signs or symptoms of metastatic disease.

Thrombophlebitis leading to pulmonary embolus is the most common cause of death after surgery for endometrial cancer. Therefore, either minidose heparin (5000 to 8000 units subcutaneously every 8 hours, starting the evening before surgery) or intermittent pneumatic compression devices are used for prophylaxis. In addition, because the vagina is heavily colonized by bacteria, prophylactic antibiotics such as cefazolin (Ancef) 1 gram intravenously every 6 hours are administered perioperatively (4 doses total starting 1 hour before surgery) to decrease the frequency of pelvic infection. Finally, before surgery, the patient's bowel is prepared with oral magnesium citrate and enemas.

The majority of endometrial adenocarcinomas can be cured by performing abdominal hysterectomy and removal of the fallopian tubes and ovaries. Surgical exploration is performed through a midline lower abdominal incision to allow access to the upper abdomen. The abdominal organs are carefully palpated, with special attention paid to the omentum and peritoneal surfaces. After exploration, a self-retaining retractor is placed in the incision and the bowel is packed into the upper abdomen. Approximately 100 mL of normal saline is instilled into the pelvis, aspirated, and submitted for cytologic examination. Extrafascial hysterectomy and bilateral salpingo-oophorectomy are then performed. After the specimen has been extirpated, the uterus is opened and the cavity is inspected. The location of the cancer and gross depth of invasion into the uterine wall are noted. In many cases, frozen section is performed to define the depth of invasion intraoperatively. In addition, a sample of tumor is submitted for determination of estrogen- and progesterone-receptor levels.

The majority of endometrial adenocarcinomas are either well or moderately differentiated, and these cancers are usually confined to the inner part of the uterine wall. Because minimally invasive cancers have a low incidence of occult metastases, further staging beyond gross inspection and palpation is not usually productive. If the cancer is poorly differentiated or is noted to invade into the outer half of the uterine wall or to involve the cervix, however, further surgical staging is performed. This includes sampling of the regional lymph nodes in the pelvic and aortic areas, which are the most common sites of occult metastases. Approximately 10% of apparent early-stage cases are found to have occult lymph node metastases. In addition, 5 to 10% of patients with endometrial cancer will be found to have visible extrauterine disease at surgical exploration. The most common sites of grossly apparent metastases are the ovaries, peritoneal surfaces, and lymph nodes. In these cases, attempts are usually made to remove the extrauterine metastases.

Most patients with endometrial cancer have stage I or II disease that appears to be confined to the uterus (Table 1), and survival rates for this group are excellent with surgery alone. Because 10 to 20% of these patients will develop recurrent cancer, adjuvant therapy is often prescribed for patients at high risk for recurrence. External pelvic radiation has been employed frequently as adjuvant therapy, but an unequivocal survival benefit has not been demonstrated. In the past, as many as 30 to 40% of patients with early-stage disease have been considered candidates for adjuvant pelvic radiation on the basis of prognostic factors such as poor histologic grade, deep myometrial invasion, and cervical involvement. More recently, selective lymph node sampling has been used to identify patients who actually have evidence of early metastatic disease and are likely to benefit from adjuvant radiation. With

use of this selection process, only 10 to 20% of patients receive pelvic radiation. In addition, if aortic lymph nodes are involved, the radiation field can be tailored to include this area, which is not part of the standard pelvic field. Thus, with surgical staging, more patients are spared the potential morbidity of radiation, whereas radiation fields can be planned accurately for patients who are most likely to benefit from adjuvant therapy.

Approximately 10 to 15% of patients with early-stage endometrial cancer are found to have malignant cells in pelvic peritoneal washings obtained at laparotomy. Most series have shown that a positive result on cytologic examination is associated with an increased risk for recurrence even when there is no other evidence of metastatic disease. When a positive cytologic result is the only evidence of extrauterine spread, I have instilled radioactive phosphorus P 32 intraperitoneally 5 to 7 days postoperatively using a small plastic catheter that is inserted at the time of surgery. Survival of these patients has been better than that of a historical control group. When both positive cytologic results and lymph node metastases are found, I do not combine ^{32}P and external radiation, however, because an unacceptably high proportion of patients treated in this fashion subsequently have developed small bowel obstruction.

TREATMENT OF RECURRENT DISEASE

Although postsurgical surveillance has not been proved to improve outcome in patients who have undergone treatment for early-stage endometrial cancer, I continue to encourage patients to return for periodic examinations. Eighty-five percent of patients who develop recurrence do so within 3 years of primary therapy. Patients are seen every 4 months for the first 2 years and every 6 months the third through fifth years. Detection of recurrences in the vagina is the primary focus of my examination, because approximately half of patients with localized vaginal recurrence can be salvaged with radiation and/or surgery. A chest radiograph is ordered on a yearly basis to detect recurrent disease in the lungs, but the utility of this practice is dubious because pulmonary metastases cannot be treated effectively.

Endometrial cancer initially recurs locally in the pelvis in 50% of patients, at distant sites in 25% of patients, and both locally and at distant sites in 25% of patients. A significant proportion of pelvic recurrences are confined to the vagina and can be cured with radiation therapy. Other pelvic recurrences are also usually treated with radiation, but salvage rates are much poorer. Treatment of distant metastases is either with progestin therapy or cytotoxic chemotherapy. Approximately 25% of patients with metastatic disease will have a significant response to progestins such as megestrol acetate (40 to 80 mg orally twice daily), and some of these responses are prolonged. A favorable response to progestins usually occurs in well-differentiated cancers

TABLE 1. **International Federation of Gynecology and Obstetrics (FIGO) Staging of Endometrial Carcinoma***

Stage I: Confined to the Uterus
IA No myometrial invasion
IB Inner half myometrial invasion
IC Outer half myometrial invasion

Stage II: Cervical Involvement
IIA Endocervical gland involvement
IIB Cervical stromal invasion

Stage III
IIIA Positive peritoneal cytology result, adnexal metastases, uterine serosal involvement
IIIB Vaginal metastases
IIIC Pelvic or aortic lymph node metastases

Stage IV
IVA Bladder or rectal involvement
IVB Distant metastases

*Note: Within each stage, the histologic grade also is recorded (G1 = well differentiated, G2 = moderately differentiated, G3 = poorly differentiated).

that express steroid receptors. I use the receptor status of the tumor to determine whether progestin therapy is appropriate. If tumor from the site of recurrence cannot be obtained to measure estrogen- and progesterone-receptor levels, I use the receptor status of the primary tumor to guide therapy.

Patients with metastatic or recurrent cancers that do not express steroid receptors are treated with cytotoxic chemotherapy. The most frequent regimen employed includes doxorubicin (Adriamycin)* 50 mg per m² intravenously and cisplatin (Platinol)* 50 mg per m² intravenously administered every 3 weeks. Although a substantial proportion of patients have objective responses, few are cured. Thus, although cure rates are excellent after surgery in patients with early-stage disease, further improvement in survival for patients with endometrial cancer awaits the development of effective treatment for metastatic disease.

---

*Not FDA approved for this indication.

CARCINOMA OF THE UTERINE CERVIX

method of
MAUREEN A. JARRELL, M.D.

Wendover Ob/Gyn & Infertility, Incorporated
Greensboro, North Carolina

Invasive cervical carcinoma is the third most common gynecologic malignant neoplasm in the United States with a frequency of occurrence of 10 in 100,000 women, resulting in 4800 deaths per year. Squamous carcinoma of the cervix, which comprises more than 95% of these cases, is known to be a sexually transmissible disease. The association between this cancer and the sexual promiscuity of the patient and her male partners is clear. Early age at first coitus, multiple sexual contacts, male partners who have had multiple contacts, and smoking history contribute to the risk. Immunosuppression, transplantation, chemotherapy, or human immunodeficiency virus infection may increase this risk. Cervical screening with the Papanicolaou (Pap) smear can prevent the development of invasive disease by detecting the precursor lesions, cervical intraepithelial neoplasia (CIN). Invasive cervical carcinoma is a major cause of morbidity and death throughout the world, especially in areas where Pap smear screening is not available.

ETIOLOGY

Human papillomavirus (HPV) has been shown to be important in the development of cervical cancer. Most cervical cancers and precursor lesions contain HPV DNA. Several types of HPV may infect the human cervix with an incidence as high as 40% in some populations. These viral types vary in their ability to integrate into the host DNA. HPV can be separated into two groups. Low-risk types (6, 11) most commonly result in condyloma or mildly dysplastic cervical changes (CIN I). Low-risk viruses rarely progress to high-grade lesions. High-risk HPV subtypes (16, 18, 33, 35) are most commonly associated with higher grades of precursor lesion (CIN II and III) and are thought

to represent the major risk for the development of carcinoma. These high-risk viruses produce proteins that are capable of inactivating host tumor suppressor proteins.

DIAGNOSIS

The squamocolumnar junction or transformation zone of the cervix is the site where neoplastic cervical changes begin. This is the area sampled by the Pap smear. Evidence that Pap smear screening decreases the incidence of invasive cervical cancer is compelling. In most cases, there is a long interval between the development of a precursor lesion and the growth of invasive cancer. Therefore, despite the limitations of sampling errors, there are usually many opportunities to intercept the progression of the disease. Annual screening should begin at 18 years of age or at the beginning of sexual contact. Longer screening intervals may be indicated after three consecutive negative screens in a patient who is thought to be of low risk.

When taken correctly, the Pap smear includes a sampling of the exocervix and endocervix. Examiners should take care to avoid air drying of the specimen. A smear in which endocervical cells are absent indicates that the zone of highest risk was not sampled, and this smear should be repeated.

The Bethesda classification of Pap smears is currently the most commonly used in the United States. This classification includes a statement regarding the adequacy of the smear obtained. It recognizes two categories of cellular abnormality, low-grade and high-grade squamous intraepithelial neoplasia. Although low-grade squamous intraepithelial neoplasia may regress spontaneously, some lesions are more aggressive. All patients with squamous intraepithelial neoplasia should be referred for colposcopic evaluation. The Bethesda classification also includes "atypical cells of uncertain significance." The management of this category of lesion is controversial because 20% may be associated with high-grade lesions. Some experts recommend determination of HPV subtype by assays such as the hybrid capture assay (Digene Diagnostics, Beltsville, MD), which detects low-risk and high-risk viral infection. Usefulness of this assay awaits further study.

Diagnosis of a precursor lesion is made only after histologic confirmation. Any time a cervical lesion is visible, a biopsy should be obtained regardless of the results of the Pap smear. Most precursor lesions, however, can be seen only with the aid of a colposcope. This device allows a low-power magnification of the cervix and should include a search for the squamocolumnar junction. Application of a dilute solution of acetic acid helps identify areas of mucosal abnormality, allowing directed biopsies. Endocervical curettage is also recommended.

TREATMENT OF THE PRECURSOR LESION

Colposcopic examination not only helps in the diagnosis of precursor lesions but also helps to select those early lesions that are likely to regress spontaneously. CIN I lesions require no treatment but can be observed conservatively in the patient who is compliant. High-grade lesions must be treated to prevent progression. Most lesions can be treated successfully in the office with cryotherapy or loop excision of the transformation zone.

TABLE 1. **International Federation of Gynecology and Obstetrics Staging of Cervical Carcinoma**

Preinvasive Carcinoma

Stage	0	Carcinoma in situ; intraepithelial carcinoma

Invasive Carcinoma

Stage	I	Carcinoma confined to cervix (extension to corpus should be disregarded)
	IA	Preclinical carcinoma
		IA1 Minimal microscopically evident stromal invasion (early stromal invasion)
		IA2 Lesions detected microscopically that can be measured; upper limits of measurement not be deeper than 5 mm from base of epithelium (surface or glandular), second dimension, horizontal spread, not to exceed 7 mm; larger lesions staged as IB
	IB	All other stage I lesions
Stage	II	Carcinoma extends beyond cervix onto either vagina or parametrium but not to lower third of vagina and not to pelvic wall
	IIA	No obvious parametrial involvement
	IIB	Obvious parametrial involvement
Stage	III	Carcinoma extends either to lower third of vagina or to pelvic wall; if hydronephrosis or nonfunctioning kidney, unless known to be due to another cause, must allocate to stage IIIB
	IIIA	Involvement of lower third of vagina; no extension to pelvic wall
	IIIB	Extension to pelvic wall or hydronephrosis or nonfunctioning kidney
Stage	IV	Carcinoma extends beyond true pelvis or involves mucosa of bladder or rectum; if bullous edema, assignment to stage IV not permitted
	IVA	Spread to bladder or rectum
	IVB	Spread to distant organs

INVASIVE DISEASE

The most common symptom of cervical carcinoma is abnormal vaginal bleeding. Bleeding may be associated with sexual intercourse. Heavy vaginal discharge may also be a symptom. Staging of cervical carcinoma is primarily based on clinical examination. The stage may be modified by the findings of the physical examination, chest radiograph, skeletal survey, intravenous pyelogram, cystoscopy, and sigmoidoscopy. The stage is not modified by imaging scans or by operative findings. Table 1 shows the current international staging for invasive carcinoma of the cervix. When available, information gathered from imaging studies may alter the choice of treatment regardless of the assigned clinical stage. At times, a barium enema examination may be added to the work-up of patients who are to be treated with radiation therapy. In these patients, knowledge of diverticular or other colon disease before pelvic irradiation may help in the assessment of rectal bleeding or other complications.

Treatment

Stage IA

Diagnosis of stage IA carcinoma of the cervix is most often made by cone biopsy. The diagnosis of microinvasive disease identifies patients who have invasive disease but a negligible risk for metastases. The Society of Gynecologic Oncologists defines this stage to be tumors with 3 mm or less stromal invasion and no vascular space involvement. For the patient who desires future childbearing, treatment may be limited to cone biopsy, if all margins are negative and the endocervical curettage above the level of the cone biopsy shows no evidence of disease. Patients who have completed childbearing should be treated with simple hysterectomy. When medical compromise prohibits surgery, this stage of disease may be treated with radiation therapy in the form of implants (brachytherapy).

Stages IB and IIA

Carcinomas of the cervix that are confined to the cervix or upper vagina can be treated with radical hysterectomy with pelvic lymphadenectomy, radiation therapy, or a combination of the two. Radiation therapy and radical surgery are equally effective treatments for this stage of disease, offering 5-year survival rates exceeding 85%. Surgical therapy allows preservation of ovarian and vaginal function and avoids the long-term side effects of radiation therapy. The operation is best performed on young women with small exophytic tumors. The operative procedure begins with a thorough abdominal exploration and para-aortic lymph node biopsies to determine the extent of disease. When this exploration is satisfactory for complete resection, the operation is performed. Radical hysterectomy differs from simple hysterectomy in that the parametria, the uterosacral ligaments, and a cuff of upper vagina are excised en bloc with the uterus and cervix. Patients with negative pelvic lymph nodes and clear surgical margins have a survival rate of 80 to 90% and do not require radiation therapy. When metastatic disease to the pelvic lymph nodes is found or tumor margins are positive, the survival rate drops to 45%; for these patients, adjuvant pelvic radiation therapy may decrease the risk for local recurrence.

Radiation therapy is sometimes used as the only treatment for stage IB and IIA disease. It is always the treatment of choice when the patient is elderly or medically compromised or when the initial surgical exploration shows that the tumor has spread beyond the cervix. In these cases, external megavoltage radiation therapy is combined with brachytherapy. In young patients, when radiation treatment is anticipated, one or both ovaries may be moved out of the pelvis to avoid radiation castration.

Large bulky stage IB cervical tumors may fail treatment with either surgery or radiation therapy. In these tumors, simple hysterectomy often follows external radiation therapy. In some patients, chemotherapy may be added to the treatment plan.

Stages IIB, III, and IV

Patients with advanced stages of cervical carcinoma are treated with radiation therapy. Body imaging scans are extremely valuable in treatment planning for these patients. A large necrotic carcinoma may give rise to reactive lymph nodes in the absence of metastatic spread. Guided fine-needle aspiration of suspicious findings should be used to confirm the presence or absence of metastatic disease. When disease is spread to the para-aortic region, radiation treatment fields may be extended to include these areas, and this will result in an increase in long-term survival in some patients.

External radiation therapy delivers uniform doses to the entire pelvis, including the pelvic lymph nodes, and is administered first in the treatment sequence to shrink the tumor volume. Radiation implants deliver high-energy doses to the cervix and surrounding areas and are delivered after external therapy.

High failure rates in the treatment of advanced cervical carcinoma are caused by the bulk of tumor and spread of disease outside the treatment field. Chemotherapy given in association with radiation therapy may alter the course of systemic spread of the disease and increase local control.

PREGNANCY

Patients in whom invasive cervical carcinoma is diagnosed at the time of pregnancy present difficult management problems. Within each stage of disease, survival is similar to that of nonpregnant women. Disease management is generally the same during pregnancy, with the added consideration of the fetus. Decisions that require interrupting the pregnancy before treatment, or delaying the treatment until the fetus is viable, are highly stressful to the patient and physician. It is important that this diagnosis be made as early as possible during the pregnancy; therefore, visualization of the cervix and Pap smear are recommended at all first antepartum visits. Abnormal Pap smears are evaluated by colposcopy and, when necessary, by cervical biopsy. In these patients, examination is aided by the natural eversion of the endocervix during pregnancy. Cone biopsy should be avoided in the first trimester.

RECURRENT DISEASE

Patients with cervical carcinoma are observed closely for recurrent disease because in some patients, a central pelvic recurrence can still be cured with radiation or exenterative surgery. Most recurrent disease will appear within the first 2 years of follow-up. Recurrences are generally found by Pap smear, by transvaginal or transrectal fine-needle aspiration of suspicious nodules, or by body imaging techniques. Symptoms of recurrence may be pelvic pain or lower extremity edema. Ureteral obstruction may occur because of central disease or spread to para-aortic lymph nodes. When patients have recurrence, disease is often found at multiple sites. If solitary recurrences outside the pelvis are found, they can be treated with surgical excision or radiation therapy. Patients with unresectable pelvic disease or widespread distant disease may be treated

with platinum-based chemotherapy. This modality of treatment is often compromised by bone marrow suppression due to previous radiation therapy or decreased renal function resulting from ureteral compromise. Although chemotherapy has been shown to reduce the bulk of disease when it is used as the primary treatment, no survival benefit has ever been shown for recurrent disease. Response rates are approximately 20%. Pain management can be a most difficult problem for the patient with recurrent cervical cancer. Invasion of bone and nerve tracks is common. Some success has been obtained with implanted epidural catheters, allowing the benefit of pain relief without central nervous system suppression.

TUMORS OF THE VULVA

method of
RAYMOND H. KAUFMAN, M.D.
Baylor College of Medicine
Houston, Texas

Both benign and malignant neoplasms are found on the vulva. Careful inspection of the vulva and vagina is still the best means of recognizing the disease processes involving this area. The colposcope can be of some help in carefully examining the vulvar tissues; however, the use of a hand magnifying glass (2× to 4×) will usually suffice. Office vulvar biopsies should be liberally performed because in many instances, a specific diagnosis is based on the findings of the biopsy. The Keyes cutaneous dermal punch biopsy instrument allows the clinician to obtain an adequate specimen for evaluation. A 4-mm punch usually suffices for providing a tissue specimen. After the biopsy sample is obtained, the tissue specimen should be oriented on a small piece of filter paper or paper towel before it is placed into the fixative. This allows proper sectioning of the specimen, avoiding tangential cuts and occasionally an erroneous diagnosis. Washing the vulva with 4 to 5% acetic acid frequently highlights mucosal lesions such as intraepithelial neoplasia, which often turns acetowhite after the application of the solution. This change is also often seen in the presence of human papillomavirus (HPV) infection involving the vulvar tissues. Toluidine blue staining of the vulva has been used in the past to highlight the lesions of intraepithelial and invasive carcinoma; however, this has proved to be of little practical use in the diagnosis of malignant vulvar neoplasms.

BENIGN TUMORS OF THE VULVA

A wide spectrum of benign solid and cystic tumors involve the vulva. These tumors can easily be subclassified on the basis of the tissue of origin, embryologic derivation, morphologic findings, or gross appearance. I subdivide the benign tumors of the vulva into solid and cystic tumors. They are classified in Table 1.

If a tumor is not causing the patient discomfort and the diagnosis is apparent on the basis of gross inspection, it can be left alone. However, if the clini-

TABLE 1. **Benign Tumors of the Vulva: Classification**

Benign Solid Tumors
Epidermal origin
  Condyloma acuminatum
  Molluscum contagiosum
  Acrochordon
  Seborrheic keratosis
  Nevus
Epidermal appendage origin
  Hidradenoma
  Sebaceous adenoma
  Basal cell carcinoma
Mesodermal origin
  Fibroma
  Lipoma
  Neurofibroma
  Leiomyoma
  Granular cell myoblastoma
  Hemangioma
  Pyogenic granuloma
  Lymphangioma
  Angiomyxoma
Bartholin's and vestibular gland origin
  Adenofibroma
  Mucus adenoma
Urethral origin
  Caruncle
  Prolapse of the urethral mucosa
Benign Cystic Tumors
Epidermal origin
  Epidermal inclusion cysts
  Pilonidal cysts
Epidermal appendage origin
  Sebaceous cysts
  Hidradenoma
  Fox-Fordyce disease
  Syringoma
Embryonic remnant origin
  Mesonephric (Gartner's) cysts
  Paramesonephric (müllerian) cysts
  Urogenital sinus cysts
  Cysts of canal of Nuck (hydrocele)
  Adenosis
  Cysts of supernumerary mammary glands
  Dermoid cysts
Bartholin's gland origin
  Duct cysts
  Abscess
Urethral and paraurethral origin
  Paraurethral (Skene's duct) cysts
  Urethral diverticula
Miscellaneous origin
  Endometriosis
  Cystic lymphangioma
  Liquefied hematoma

Adapted from Kaufman RH, Faro S (eds): Benign Diseases of the Vulva and Vagina, 4th ed. St. Louis, Mosby–Year Book, 1994, pp 168, 268.

cian is not absolutely sure of the problem, a biopsy should be performed.

Benign Solid Tumors

The most common of the benign solid tumors affecting the vulva are the acrochordon (often called fibroepithelial polyp), fibroma, lipoma, neurofibroma, granular cell tumor, and solid tumors arising in the Bartholin and vestibular glands. When the diagnosis is in doubt or the tumor is causing discomfort, the tumor should be widely excised either in the office with the use of local anesthesia or in the hospital while the patient is under general anesthesia. Wide local excision with primary closure of the defect is all that is required.

Benign Cystic Tumors

The most common cystic tumors involving the vulva are the epidermal inclusion cyst and developmental cysts of urogenital sinus, paramesonephric duct, mesonephric duct, and Bartholin's duct. Once again, if the clinician is confident of the diagnosis and the patient is asymptomatic, these can be left untreated. If the diagnosis is in doubt or if the patient has symptoms related to the mass, a local excision is usually adequate therapy.

The hidradenoma is often a confusing tumor for clinicians as well as pathologists. It is not uncommonly confused with a primary or metastatic adenocarcinoma of the vulva. The distinction is made on the basis of the characteristic pattern of the tumor as well as the absence of nuclear atypia and multilayering of cells. This tumor is easily removed in the office by local excision with use of local anesthesia.

Bartholin's duct cyst and abscess are seen in approximately 2% of new gynecologic patients. The cysts arise within the duct system of the Bartholin gland. Occlusion of the duct usually occurs near the opening of the main duct into the vestibule. Most cysts involve only the main duct and thus are unilocular, although occasionally one or more loculi lie deep in the main cyst. The majority of patients with small Bartholin's duct cysts are asymptomatic. If the cyst becomes enlarged, discomfort and pressure may be experienced by the patient, as may discomfort during coitus and walking. Treatment under these circumstances is best managed by marsupialization. The incision for marsupialization should be made medially enough so that the new orifice of the duct is located close to the original opening of the Bartholin duct into the vestibule. An incision 4 to 6 cm in length is made extending through the wall of the cyst. After evacuation of the contents, the lining of the cyst is sewn to the mucosal and skin surfaces with interrupted fine, absorbable sutures.

An acute Bartholin abscess may arise primarily or may occur in the presence of a previous Bartholin duct cyst. Culture of the contents of an abscess reveals a wide spectrum of organisms. The chief symptoms of a Bartholin abscess consist of pain and tenderness over the affected gland. The rapidity of development and the extent of involvement depend on the size of an infected cyst and the virulence of the infectious agent. Objective signs include unilateral swelling over the site of the affected gland, redness of the overlying skin, and frequently edema of the surrounding labia. An acute Bartholin abscess usually requires surgical therapy, but local application of heat in the form of hot, wet dressings or sitz baths may promote spontaneous drainage within 72 hours. If treatment is begun early enough with a broad-spectrum antibiotic, formation of an abscess can occasionally be prevented. Incision and drainage of the abscess can be accomplished in the physician's office. Marsupialization of the abscess by the use of a Word catheter, an inflatable bulb-tipped closed catheter, is effective treatment. The catheter is inserted into the abscess cavity after a small stab incision is made into the abscess close to the hymenal ring, and the contents of the abscess are evacuated. After the catheter is inserted, the balloon is inflated with 2 mL of saline. The distal end of the catheter is then tucked into the vagina. The catheter should be left in place for at least 4 to 6 weeks, after which time the balloon is deflated and the catheter is removed. The patient rarely notes the presence of the catheter and may engage in sexual activity without disturbing it.

MALIGNANT NEOPLASMS OF THE VULVA

Both intraepithelial and invasive neoplasms are found on the vulva. The International Society for the Study of Vulvar Diseases has classified intraepithelial neoplastic disorders of the vulvar skin and mucosa as follows:

1. Squamous (may include HPV changes)
   A. Vulvar intraepithelial neoplasia (VIN)-1 (mild dysplasia)
   B. VIN-2 (moderate dysplasia)
   C. VIN-3 (severe dysplasia; carcinoma in situ
2. Other
   A. Paget's disease
   B. Melanoma, level 1

The incidence rate of VIN-3 has nearly doubled between 1973 to 1976 and 1985 to 1987 (Sturgeon and colleagues). During this same period, however, the incidence rate of invasive carcinoma remained stable. Sturgeon and colleagues reported that the incidence of VIN-3 increased from 1.1 to 2.1 cases per 100,000 women-years. The largest increase occurred in white women younger than 35 years. The peak incidence of in situ carcinoma decreased in time from women older than 54 years to women between the ages of 35 and 54 years. Several possible factors may explain the increased incidence of this disease and its occurrence at a younger age. Heightened awareness of neoplasia on the part of the physician plays some role in its more frequent diagnosis. Associated with this factor is an increasing tendency to perform biopsies on questionable lesions. A third factor is the increased occurrence of viral infections involving the lower genital tract. The association of HPV with the development of lower genital tract neoplasia is now well accepted. Whereas most condylomata acuminata of the lower genital tract are associated with infection by HPV-6 and HPV-11, vulvar squamous cell carcinoma of the vulva is most often associated with HPV type 16. However, it has been postulated that possibly two forms of invasive squamous cell carcinoma of the vulva are seen. One is observed most often in younger women whose lesions morphologically resemble changes seen with intraepithelial neoplasia, who smoke, and whose tumors have a high association with HPV infection. The other type of cancer is seen more often in older women with a more well differentiated type of squamous cell carcinoma, who do not smoke, and whose lesions are infrequently associated with HPV infection.

The diagnosis of VIN must be established by biopsy before treatment is undertaken. The lesions are often multifocal, and if this is the case, several biopsy specimens should be taken from different sites to establish that the lesion is in fact intraepithelial and not invasive.

Treatment of VIN-3

Opinion regarding management of intraepithelial squamous cell carcinoma of the vulva has changed radically during the past 2 decades. The treatment should be individualized on the basis of location and extent of the lesion. Both wide local excision and laser surgery are appropriate under proper circumstances. Hatch has recommended treatment triage on the basis of the location and size of lesions:

Mucosal lesions
　Laser epidermis to papillary dermis
Hair-bearing lesions
　Less than 1 cm in diameter: laser to reticular dermis
　More than 1 cm in diameter: excise

If wide local excision is chosen as a method of treatment, the entire lesion should be surgically removed, taking with it at least 0.5 to 1 cm of normal tissue. Frozen sections should be taken from the distal margins of the excised tissue to be certain that there is no residual disease. If disease is noted along the margins of the excised tissue, further skin and mucosa should be removed until the margins are free of disease. Recurrence of disease is related to the presence or absence of free margins. When extensive VIN-3 is present, wide local excision may consist of performance of a wide superficial skinning vulvectomy. The skin and a small amount of subcutaneous tissue are removed, leaving the bulk of the vulvar structures intact. The defect can often be closed primarily, but it will occasionally be necessary to use a skin graft to adequately cover the denuded vulvar surfaces. If the disease extends into the anal canal, it is necessary to remove the anal mucosa up to the level of the pectinate line. The rectal mucosa can then be undermined and pulled down to cover the defect.

The use of the carbon dioxide laser in treating VIN is becoming increasingly popular. It is an excellent tool for the treatment of this disease, especially disease that is localized. Before this approach is used, however, an occult invasive carcinoma must be excluded by adequate biopsies. Lesions demonstrating thickening of the tissues or those that appear ulcerated are best treated by excision rather than by the laser. When the laser is used, the lesion and a surrounding 0.5 to 1 cm of normal tissue should be ablated down to a depth of 1 to 3 mm depending on the location of the lesion. On skin surfaces, the ablation should be carried down to a depth of 3 mm to remove any possible disease that has extended down into the superficial skin appendages. A depth of destruction to 1 mm is adequate on mucosal surfaces.

I prefer not to use the carbon dioxide laser in treating extensive VIN. Attempts to remove the entire lesion in one session prove to be time-consuming, uncomfortable for the patient, and associated with significant postoperative discomfort.

The primary complications observed after laser therapy to the vulva are pain, bleeding, and discharge. Usually, the degree of pain is related to the area of the vulva treated and to the depth of treatment. The pain usually becomes most severe 4 to 5 days after therapy and may persist for another 5 to 10 days. The use of analgesics and warm sitz baths is of value in alleviating the symptoms.

Paget's disease of the vulva requires surgical treatment (wide local excision) similar to that for squamous cell carcinoma in situ. An underlying adnexal carcinoma may be found in a small number of patients, and if this proves to be the case, more radical treatment will be required. Intraepidermal migration of Paget's cells often occurs; thus, an adequate margin of normal-appearing tissue must be removed. When the disease involves large areas of the vulva, a wide superficial vulvectomy can be performed. This is carried out in the form of a skinning vulvectomy with removal of the skin and underlying adnexal structures, leaving the subcutaneous fat in place. If an underlying adnexal or invasive carcinoma is found, a second procedure consisting of a more extensive vulvectomy and inguinal-femoral lymphadenectomy should be performed.

INVASIVE MALIGNANT NEOPLASMS OF THE VULVA

Invasive malignant vulvar tumors are classified in Table 2. The most common of the malignant tumors is squamous cell carcinoma with an annual incidence of 1.5 cases per 100,000. This most often presents as a raised granular tumor on the vulva but may also be seen as a thickened white plaque, or granular ulceration. Invasive squamous cell carcinoma is often seen in association with lichen sclerosus, which in the past led to the concept that lichen sclerosus was a precursor of invasive carcinoma. However, the likelihood that an individual with lichen sclerosus will ultimately develop invasive carcinoma of the vulva is less than 5%. HPV infection (especially HPV-16) may also be associated with invasive squamous cell carcinoma of the vulva. In addition to the presence of a mass, the patient symptomatically often complains of pruritus, bleeding from the vulva, discharge, and occasionally pain. The diagnosis is established on the basis of a biopsy.

TABLE 2. **Malignant Tumors of the Vulva: Classification**

Epithelial tumors of the skin and mucosa
  Squamous cell origin
    Squamous cell carcinoma
    Verrucous carcinoma
  Basal cell carcinoma
  Melanoma
  Adenocarcinoma
    Paget's disease
    Skin appendage
Malignant tumors of the urethra
Bartholin's gland carcinoma
  Squamous cell carcinoma
  Adenocarcinoma
  Adenoid cystic carcinoma
  Adenosquamous carcinoma
  Transitional cell carcinoma
Carcinoma and sarcoma of ectopic breast tissue
Soft tissue sarcomas
  Embryonal rhabdomyosarcoma
  Leiomyosarcoma
  Malignant fibrous histiocytoma
  Epithelial sarcoma

Treatment

Treatment to a large extent depends on the stage of disease. Also of importance is an understanding of the method of spread of vulvar carcinoma. This is by direct extension and through the lymphatics to the ipsilateral inguinal and femoral lymph nodes. From here, the cancer may spread to the contralateral groin nodes and/or to the deep pelvic lymph nodes.

Surgical staging also plays a role in the decision as to appropriate therapy. The International Federation of Gynecology and Obstetrics (FIGO) staging system for carcinoma of the vulva is surgically accomplished and is as follows:

Stage 0: Carcinoma in situ; intraepithelial carcinoma

Stage I: Tumor confined to the vulva and/or perineum—2 cm or less in greatest dimension, nodes are negative

Stage II: Tumor confined to the vulva and/or perineum—more than 2 cm in greatest dimension, nodes are negative

Stage III: Tumor of any size with
1. Adjacent spread to the lower urethra and/or the vagina, or the anus, and/or
2. Unilateral regional lymph node metastasis

Stage IVA: Tumor invades any of the following: upper urethra, bladder mucosa, rectal mucosa, pelvic bone, and/or bilateral regional node metastasis

Stage IVB: Any distant metastasis including pelvic lymph nodes

Before treatment is planned, the patient should be carefully evaluated for the presence of distant metastasis, although this is highly unlikely in a stage I or II lesion. Certainly, a preoperative chest radiograph, bone scan, and computed tomographic scan of the pelvis looking for enlarged lymph nodes should be performed, especially in those individuals with suspected stage III and IV disease.

Whereas radical vulvectomy with bilateral femoral-inguinal lymph node dissection was in the past considered the standard of care for all invasive carcinomas of the vulva, this is no longer true today. Treatment is individualized and based on the knowledge of the natural spread of vulvar carcinoma.

Stage I Carcinoma

With a tumor localized to one side of the vulva, a partial deep vulvectomy with ipsilateral groin node dissection is considered adequate treatment. This allows preservation of much of the normal vulvar anatomy and is also associated with less postoperative morbidity than is radical vulvectomy. In excising the tumor, at least a 2 to 3 cm margin of normal skin should be removed surrounding the tumor, and the subcutaneous fat should be excised down to the fascia. A groin dissection should be performed through a separate incision. If there is no evidence of spread to the groin lymph nodes, no further therapy is required. If, however, positive nodes are found, then contralateral lymph nodes should be removed or the contralateral groin should be treated with external beam radiotherapy. The deep pelvic nodes should also receive external beam therapy as well. In the presence of a midline lesion, a bilateral inguinal-femoral lymph node dissection should be performed. After surgical excision of the lesion and groin lymph nodes, suction drainage should be left in place until the drainage has decreased to a minimal amount.

Levenbach and colleagues have suggested injecting isosulfan blue solution (0.5 mL) into the tumor margin before the lymph node dissection. The dye is transported by lymphatic vessels to the lymph nodes, turning them a deep blue. This allows the easy identification of the sentinel node. Frozen sections can then be taken, and if no tumor is identified, it is not necessary to remove the deep nodes.

Stage II Disease

Depending on the size of the tumor, an operative procedure similar to that recommended for stage I disease can be carried out for stage II disease. Occasionally, however, when the lesion is of sufficient size, it will be necessary to perform a complete deep vulvectomy to remove the entire tumor along with an adequate margin of normal tissue. When this is done, the inguinal and femoral lymph nodes are removed through separate groin incisions. To close a large defect, it is often necessary to swing skin flaps with attached subcutaneous fat to cover the defect.

Stage III Disease

Stage III disease that has spread to the lower urethra and vagina is also treated by vulvectomy with removal of the lower portion of the urethra and/or vagina to allow at least a 2-cm margin of normal tissue. When the anus is involved with the tumor,

it may be necessary to perform a vulvectomy with abdominoperineal resection while removing the anus. Bilateral inguinal and femoral lymph nodes should be removed through separate groin incisions. It is occasionally necessary to use a full-thickness skin flap using the gracilis muscle to cover a large vulvar defect that cannot be covered by a "rhomboid" flap.

The use of radiotherapy may decrease the size of a large, bulky lesion to the point at which a less radical excision is required.

Stage IV Disease

Therapy for stage IV vulvar carcinoma must be individualized. Depending on whether there is evidence of distant metastasis, local palliative excision and/or radiation therapy is used. In the absence of distant metastasis, the patients are managed as described for stage III disease.

VERRUCOUS CARCINOMA

Verrucous carcinoma, often called condyloma of Buschke-Löwenstein, presents as a large, irregular cauliflower-like lesion. It locally invades the vulvar tissue without metastasis occurring. Like condylomata acuminata, it has been found to be associated with HPV-6. A biopsy usually confirms the diagnosis. The lesion can usually be easily distinguished from invasive squamous cell carcinoma in that large, broad areas of relatively well differentiated squamous cells are noted to be "pushing" down into the dermis rather than infiltrating into it.

Treatment

The treatment of verrucous carcinoma consists of wide local excision. Rarely is it necessary to consider performing a groin lymph node dissection. Only if enlarged, suspicious lymph nodes are palpated should a groin dissection be performed. Radiation therapy is contraindicated in the management of this tumor because doing so frequently transforms it into an aggressive neoplasm that may metastasize.

BASAL CELL CARCINOMA

Basal cell carcinoma usually arises as a solitary, ulcerated lesion with raised, round, pearly edges. If left untreated, this lesion will continue to destructively invade the vulvar tissues. Only rarely does basal cell carcinoma metastasize.

Treatment

Treatment consists of wide local excision of the neoplasm. It is not necessary to perform a regional lymph node dissection because spread to the lymph nodes is extremely rare.

MELANOMA

Melanoma occurs as a primary vulvar lesion uncommonly. When it does occur, however, early diagno-

TABLE 3. **Methods for Microstaging Melanoma**

Clark's Levels	Breslow's Levels (Modified)
1. Intraepithelial	<0.76 mm
2. Into papillary dermis	0.76–1.49 mm
3. Fills papillary dermis	1.50–2.49 mm
4. Into reticular dermis	2.50–3.99 mm
5. Into subcutaneous fat	≥4 mm

sis is mandatory if cure is to be achieved. Prognosis is directly related to the depth of invasion of the tumor. Several methods for microstaging melanoma have been proposed. The staging systems of Clark and of Breslow are most commonly used by the pathologist. They are listed in Table 3.

The diagnosis is established on the basis of biopsy. The microstaging is finally determined after excision of the neoplasm.

Treatment

Level 1 and 2 melanomas have an extremely good prognosis. Melanoma that extends into the subcutaneous fat carries with it an almost hopeless outlook.

Tumors invading less than 1 mm can be treated by wide local excision, removing the underlying subcutaneous fat. When the level of invasion is deeper than 1 mm, a wide radical excision of the neoplasm is recommended along with ipsilateral inguinal-femoral lymph node removal. The lymph node dissection is more prognostic than therapeutic because once spread to the regional lymph nodes has occurred, the prognosis is extremely poor regardless of additional adjunctive therapy that is attempted.

BARTHOLIN'S GLAND CARCINOMA

The diagnosis of Bartholin's gland carcinoma is established when the neoplasm is localized to the region of the Bartholin gland and histologic evidence of Bartholin's gland structures is contiguous to the tumor. In addition, the skin overlying the neoplasm should be intact. Suspicion of a malignant neoplasm of the Bartholin gland should be aroused when the postmenopausal woman suddenly develops what is thought to be a Bartholin duct abscess or cyst. Another finding that should arouse suspicion is the presence of a solid mass developing in this region.

Treatment

Bartholin's gland carcinomas are managed in a manner similar to invasive squamous cell carcinoma of the vulva.

SOFT TISSUE SARCOMA

Soft tissue sarcomas are extremely rare. They usually present as rapidly growing solid tumors. The diagnosis is made on the basis of biopsy or histologic examination of the surgical specimen. Therapy consists primarily of wide local excision. Radiotherapy is of little use in the management of most vulvar sarcomas.

CONTRACEPTION

method of
PAULA J. ADAMS HILLARD, M.D.
University of Cincinnati
Cincinnati, Ohio

The voluntary control of fertility through the use of effective contraception is a relatively modern development with important implications for individuals, couples, and societies. In the United States, data about fertility and contraception are available through the National Surveys of Family Growth, conducted periodically by the National Center for Health Statistics. In 1990, there were approximately 58 million women of reproductive age (defined as 15 to 44 years). About 60% of them were using some reversible method of contraception. Others were not at risk for pregnancy because of pregnancy, sterilization, or abstinence. Eighty-eight percent of all women at risk for conception were using a method of contraception; 12% were not using contraception.

The most frequently used method of contraception was female sterilization, used by 18% of U.S. women; oral contraceptives were used by 17%, condoms by 11%, and male sterilization by 8%. Of note, the contraceptive options (and available national data) in 1990 differ somewhat from those available today: the implantable subdermal levonorgestrel system, depot medroxyprogesterone acetate, and female condoms are now available, and the contraceptive sponge is no longer available.

Data from the National Survey of Family Growth also revealed that in 1988, nearly 40% of births were unintended. Estimates factoring in pregnancies that ended in abortion placed the percentage of unintended pregnancies at 57%. An estimated 53% of these pregnancies occurred among the 10% of women using no method of contraception. The remaining 47% (1.7 million pregnancies in 1988) occurred in women who were using a method of contraception. All methods of contraception can fail to prevent pregnancy.

Contraceptive efficacy depends on both the inherent effectiveness of the method itself and correct, consistent, and ongoing use of the method. The inherent or theoretical effectiveness of a method is difficult if not impossible to ascertain. The failure rates of contraceptive methods during actual use or among typical users have been shown to be higher than the estimated rates for perfect use. In addition, under-reporting of abortion leads to underestimates of contraceptive failure. Analysis of data from the 1988 National Survey of Family Growth, corrected for under-reporting of abortion, revealed the following failure rates for reversible methods of contraception: oral contraceptives, 8%; condoms, 15%; diaphragm, 16%; periodic abstinence, 26%; spermicides alone, 25%.

The failure rate of a method during actual use depends on a number of factors, such as the user's age, experience in using the method, and motivation to prevent pregnancy. The motivation to use contraception effectively varies, depending on the intent of contraception: to postpone pregnancy, to space births, or to avoid pregnancy. These factors result in variations in the percentage of incorrect or inconsistent use of a given method and thus variations in the failure rate among typical users.

The United States has the notoriety of having the highest rate of adolescent pregnancy in the developed world. This is in spite of comparable levels of sexual activity; adolescents in the United States are *not* more likely to be sexually active than are teens in other countries. In addition to high levels of adolescent pregnancy, approximately half of the pregnancies in adolescents are terminated in abortion, leading to high abortion rates in the United States compared with other developed countries. The lowest rates of adolescent pregnancy and abortion occur in Japan and the Netherlands. In Japan, cultural and societal norms encourage the postponement of sexual involvement by adolescents. In the Netherlands, responsible sexual activity is encouraged through comprehensive sexuality education and the facilitated access to contraceptive care.

Although adolescent pregnancy is a clear social problem in the United States, adolescents are not responsible for even the majority of unintended or nonmarital births, nor are adolescents responsible for the majority of abortions that occur in the United States. Adolescents account for only 21% of unintended pregnancies, 31% of nonmarital births, and 23% of abortions in the United States. Whereas adolescent pregnancy remains a significant problem for both individual women and society, the problems of unintended pregnancy, nonmarital births, and abortions are significant issues for the United States as a whole.

HORMONAL METHODS

Combination oral contraceptives have a failure rate with perfect use of 0.1% and a failure rate among typical users of 3 to 8%. The highest failure rates occur among adolescents, many of whom frequently miss pills and use the pills in an on-again, off-again manner. The most commonly used pills in the United States today contain 35 μg of ethinyl estradiol and various doses and formulations of progestins; both hormones are present in doses that are many times lower than combination pills that were available in the 1960s and 1970s. The lowest doses are generally preferable to minimize potential hormonal effects or risks. Current pill formulations are available in monophasic or multiphasic dosing regimens and in 21- or 28-day packaging (with 21 hormonally active pills and 7 placebos). The pills act by inhibiting gonadotropin secretion and thus inhibiting ovulation. In addition, the progestin component has contraceptive effects on the cervical mucus and endometrium.

Strong precautions for the prescription of oral contraceptives include pregnancy, undiagnosed vaginal bleeding, active liver disease, estrogen-dependent malignant neoplasia, history of stroke, and coronary artery disease. Smokers older than 35 years have an increased risk for cardiovascular morbidity and mortality, including risk for myocardial infarction, and thus use of the pill is contraindicated. Caution and individualization should be used before prescribing pills for women with migraine headaches with aura, hypertension, diabetes mellitus, and other com-

plicated medical conditions. In these situations, the risks of pregnancy should also be weighed carefully against the risks of contraceptive methods.

Potential serious risks for women who take combination oral contraceptives include an increased risk for venous thrombosis and embolism (approximately 15 to 30 per 100,000 pill users compared with approximately 60 per 100,000 women-years with pregnancy and 5 per 100,000 nonusers). Cohort studies have not shown an increased risk for breast cancer. Some case-control studies have shown an increased relative risk for early, premenopausal breast cancer; other studies have shown no increased risk.

Side effects that are not medically serious but sometimes bothersome can have an impact on compliance and should be discussed before prescribing. Breakthrough bleeding occurs in 5 to 30% of first cycles; nausea, breast tenderness, weight gain, and mood changes are infrequent but should be discussed in an effort to provide preventive guidance and minimize early discontinuation.

Noncontraceptive benefits of oral contraceptives include improved cycle control, decreased menstrual flow and dysmenorrhea, decreased risk for symptomatic pelvic inflammatory disease (PID), decreased risk for benign breast disease, and improved acne. The use of oral contraceptives provides clear protection against both ovarian and endometrial cancer, as demonstrated in multiple studies.

Progestin-only contraceptive pills (minipills) have a perfect-use failure rate of 0.5% with failure rates among typical users of 3 to 10%. The contraceptive action of progestin-only pills is due primarily to the effect on the endometrium and cervical mucus; ovulation is not consistently suppressed. Minipills are dependent on consistent use. Food and Drug Administration labeling states precautions that are identical to those for combination pills; however, a review of the medical literature and data does not substantiate all of these warnings. Common side effects include menstrual irregularities. Situations in which minipills are appropriate include women with contraindications to estrogen use or breast-feeding women.

Depot medroxyprogesterone acetate (Depo-Provera) given as 150 mg intramuscularly every 12 weeks is a long-acting contraceptive method that is now approved for use in the United States. Its failure rate is low, 0.3%, and it is relatively nondependent on compliance. It acts by blocking the luteinizing hormone surge and thus inhibiting ovulation. Its primary advantage is that it is coitus independent, and thus compliance is less an issue than with oral contraceptives. However, the method requires a schedule of follow-up every 12 weeks, an interval that may be difficult to remember. Another advantage of this method is that of privacy; the method can be used discreetly.

Abnormal menstrual bleeding occurs commonly; however, after 1 year of use, more than 50% of users become amenorrheic. This may be an advantage for many women; however, amenorrhea cannot be predicted. Weight gain of 3 to 5 pounds per year is common. Decreases in bone density have been noted in long-term users of this method, although the magnitude of this risk is not well established. Use of depot medroxyprogesterone acetate can result in a delay of 6 to 9 months in the return of fertility. Epidemiologic studies have found that there is no increased risk for infertility after discontinuation of this method.

Subdermal levonorgestrel implants (Norplant) consist of six Silastic capsules containing levonorgestrel. These rods are implanted subdermally in the upper, inner arm and provide contraception for 5 years. The failure rate is low, 0.2% and is not dependent on compliance. Luteinizing hormone levels are suppressed, and only one third of cycles are ovulatory. Both the endometrium and cervical mucus are affected by the levonorgestrel, with resultant contraceptive effects. Abnormal menstrual bleeding, including irregular or prolonged bleeding as well as amenorrhea, occurs frequently—in at least 80% of users in the first year. The implants must be surgically removed, and if they have been improperly inserted, removal can be difficult. Weight gain, acne, changes in hair growth, depression, and functional ovarian cysts may occur. Although the initial cost is relatively high, this method is cost-effective if it is used for several years. Careful preinsertion counseling and the availability of clinicians to address the patient's concerns during use are helpful in supporting ongoing use.

BARRIER METHODS

Barrier methods include the male and female condom, diaphragm, and cervical cap. The vaginal contraceptive sponge is no longer available. Some of these methods are used in combination with chemical spermicides, which can also be delivered in vehicles such as foam, cream, jelly, film, or vaginal suppository. Currently available spermicides include nonoxynol 9 and octoxynol 9. Failure rates for barrier methods and spermicides range from 2% (perfect use of condoms) to 21% (typical use of spermicides alone). Spermicides act by disrupting cell membranes (surfactants); barriers may act mechanically by blocking entry of sperm into the cervix and as a vehicle for spermicides.

Spermicides require application 10 to 30 minutes before intercourse and remain effective for variable intervals up to 8 hours. Anatomy may preclude fit of diaphragm or cervical cap; these two methods require fitting and are available only by prescription. Diaphragms increase the risk for urinary tract infections. Allergic reactions to latex, the spermicide itself, or the base vehicle may occur in 1 to 5%. Barriers and spermicide methods provide protection (about a 50% reduction) from sexually transmitted diseases (STDs) and PID, with a protective effect on the risk for tubal infertility and ectopic pregnancy. The fact that they are nonhormonal is considered an advantage for some individuals. Spermicides and condoms are available without a prescription and are relatively inexpensive, depending on frequency of use. These methods are extremely compliance dependent; most failures are due to nonuse or incorrect use.

The condom is being used increasingly as a contraceptive method; in addition, it is being used in combination with hormonal or other methods in an effort to decrease the risk for STDs. Data derived from the use of condoms in heterosexual couples who are serodiscordant for human immunodeficiency virus infection indicate that the consistent use of condoms results in low rates of infection.

OTHER METHODS

The intrauterine device (IUD) is an infrequently used method of contraception in the United States that is widely used in other developed countries worldwide. In the 1970s, the Dalkon Shield IUD was widely used; its use was subsequently found to be associated with an increased risk for PID and septic incomplete abortions. The legacy of this IUD led to the view that all IUDs are dangerous. Other IUDs, including the copper-7, were withdrawn from the market as the result of corporate business decisions.

Subsequently, two modern IUDs have become available, the TCu-380A and a progesterone-releasing device. Studies provided reassurance that except in the first few weeks after insertion, there is not an increased risk for infection. The primary mechanism of action of the IUD is in the production of an intrauterine environment that is spermicidal; the device is not an abortifacient. The IUD has been found to protect against ectopic as well as intrauterine pregnancies, suggesting extrauterine effects as well.

The copper T is effective for 10 years; the progesterone-containing device must be replaced yearly. The failure rate is less than 1% for the copper device and approximately 2% for the progesterone device. The most important precaution or contraindication for IUD use relates to sexual behaviors that place an individual at increased risk for STDs. Individuals who are not in a mutually monogamous sexual relationship should probably choose alternative contraceptive methods. Excessive menstrual bleeding or anomalies of the uterine cavity may be relative contraindications. When used for 10 years, the IUD is cost-effective.

Periodic abstinence, also termed fertility awareness, natural family planning, or rhythm method, includes various methods of estimating timing of ovulation and the avoidance of intercourse during and around this time. A number of specific methods have been described and include the cervical mucus method, symptothermal method, calendar or rhythm method, or combinations of these. These methods take into account the period of viability of sperm in the female genital tract (2 to 7 days) and the viability of the ovum (about 1 to 3 days), with abstinence required during the time of fertility. The failure rates are highly variable, ranging from 1 to 26%, and the method requires great commitment, cooperation, and communication from both partners. The method has been described as being unforgiving of imperfect use.

Women with irregular cycles or vaginal or cervical infections experience difficulty with this method. The advantages of the method include the fact that it is nonhormonal and fits certain religious teachings and beliefs.

Emergency contraception refers to the use of a method of contraception after unprotected intercourse, whether as a result of rape, coercion, contraceptive failure (condom slipping or breaking, cervical cap dislodged), or unplanned coitus.

The most widely used method of emergency contraception (also referred to as postcoital contraception or morning-after pills) involves the use of combination oral contraceptive pills containing 50 μg of ethinyl estradiol plus 0.5 mg of levonorgestrel (Ovral). Two of these pills are taken within 72 hours of unprotected intercourse; two additional pills are then taken 12 hours later. This regimen is associated with nausea and vomiting in a significant percentage of patients; thus, an antiemetic should also be prescribed. The regimen is effective in preventing at least 75% of pregnancies that would otherwise have occurred. It has been estimated that the use of emergency contraception could prevent 2.3 million unintended pregnancies and 1 million abortions annually in the United States.

Although emergency contraception should be considered for use *only* in emergencies and not as a routine ongoing contraceptive method, this option should be discussed with every individual who requests contraception, because lack of knowledge about the availability of emergency contraception is a significant drawback to its use.

Other methods that have been used as emergency contraception include the insertion of a copper-containing IUD, high-dose progestins, and other hormonal options. The efficacy of these methods is not well established; thus, the use of combination oral contraceptives as described before (the Yuzpe regimen) should be considered the primary option for emergency contraception in the United States.

Psychiatric Disorders

ALCOHOLISM

method of
STEPHEN M. JURD, M.B., B.S.
*Royal North Shore Hospital and University of
   Sydney
Sydney, New South Wales, Australia*

In a substantial proportion of all patients presenting for medical treatment, alcohol is a causal factor or a coexisting health risk. One of every six patients in family practice and one of five in hospital practice is at risk. Community statistics indicate that lifelong prevalence of alcohol abuse among men is in the range of 19 to 30%. Usual estimates of point prevalence of serious drinking problems (alcohol dependence) range from 3 to 5% of the adult male population. Women have approximately half the risk of men.

THE PHYSICIAN'S ROLE

There is no doubt that much alcohol-related illness goes undiagnosed. Therefore, the physician's principal role is that of case identification and provision of information to the patient. The usual situation is that neither physician nor patient has considered behavioral change as a health strategy. The next stage depends on the severity of the presenting problem and the patient's willingness to accept treatment.

LEVELS OF SEVERITY

There are essentially three levels of severity that require clinical attention: hazardous, harmful, and dependent drinking. The first two levels have been defined from epidemiologic studies that have indicated an increased risk for a variety of disorders once these limits are exceeded. A standard drink is a 1-ounce (30-mL) shot of whiskey, a 2-ounce (60-mL) glass of fortified wine, a 4-ounce (120-mL) glass of table wine, and a 10-ounce (300-mL) glass of beer.

Women are more sensitive to the effects of alcohol than are men. There are three reasons for this: women are, overall, smaller than men; women have a lower percentage lean body mass (alcohol is poorly distributed to adipose tissue); and women have lower levels of gastric alcohol dehydrogenase. For these reasons, women have higher blood levels per standard drink consumed.

Hazardous Drinking

Drinking more than four standard drinks (40 grams of alcohol) daily in men or more than two standard drinks (20 grams of alcohol) a day in women confers a significant risk for alcohol-related problems. To maintain low-risk drinking, there should be two or three alcohol-free days each week and no episodes of drinking more than six drinks on one occasion.

Harmful Drinking

This exists when known alcohol-related harm, such as any of the problems listed in Table 1, occurs in the presence of hazardous drinking.

Alcohol Dependence Syndrome

This syndrome is a complex biopsychosocial disorder that has internationally accepted major features:

1. Subjective awareness of compulsion to drink, usually manifested by multiple attempts to control, cut down, or abstain
2. Stereotyped, narrowed pattern of drinking, i.e., the drinking predicts the social life rather than vice versa
3. Increased importance of drinking over other activities, eroding work, family, and personal responsibilities
4. Pharmacologic tolerance resulting in an increased capacity to drink without showing signs of intoxication
5. Repeated withdrawal symptoms (e.g., nausea, tremor, irritability, and anxiety, especially in the morning)
6. Relieving or preventing withdrawal by drinking
7. Reinstatement of pathologic drinking after a period of abstinence

These features, as in any syndrome, tend to predict each other's presence, but not always. In general, the presence of three features is required for a diagnosis of alcohol dependence syndrome, although the presence of any feature is relevant. Dependence ranges from the mildest degree to the most severe. Severe dependence is usually complicated by multiple problems. The presence of dependence does not mean that affected individuals will experience serious withdrawal, but the more severe the dependence, the more likely it is that clinically significant withdrawal will occur.

ALCOHOL-RELATED PROBLEMS

An attempt to summarize the many complications of excessive drinking is made in Table 1. The ubiquity of excessive drinking means that many of these problems present in relative isolation, leading alcohol to be considered the modern "great imitator" of other diseases.

FAMILY PROBLEMS

Every problem drinker seriously affects the lives of at least four other people. The family disruption may result in the development of psychiatric symptoms in family members. Domestic violence commonly coexists with alcohol problems and cannot be managed without dealing with the alcohol problem. Some family members are assisted by Al-Anon, a self-help group for relatives of problem drinkers. This group is available to families regardless of whether the drinker accepts treatment.

TABLE 1. **Alcohol-Related Problems**

Trauma	Psychiatric Problems	Neurologic Problems
Motor vehicle accidents	Suicide	Peripheral neuropathy
Falls	Parasuicide	Subdural hematoma
Fractures	Depression	Wernicke-Korsakoff psychosis
Head injuries	Paranoia	**Muscle Problems**
Drownings	Dementia	Myopathy
Domestic fires	Alcohol withdrawal delirium	Rhabdomyolysis
Social Problems	Anxiety	**Hematologic Disorders**
Financial problems	Phobias	Macrocytosis
Marital conflict	Panic attacks	Anemia
Absenteeism	**Gastrointestinal Disorders**	Thrombocytopenia
Unemployment	Gastritis	Leukopenia
Drunk driving	Ulcers	**Metabolic Disorders**
Convictions	Reflux esophagitis	Obesity
Assault	Esophageal varices	Gout
Homicide	Diarrhea	Hyperlipidemia
Domestic violence	Vomiting	Diabetes
Indirect Presentations*	Fatty liver	Impotence
Spouse	Mallory-Weiss syndrome	Gynecomastia
Injury	Cirrhosis	**Obstetric Problems**
Depression	Pancreatitis	Low birth weight
Psychosomatic illness	**Cardiovascular Problems**	Fetal alcohol syndrome
Children	Hypertension	Second-trimester abortion
Abuse	Arrhythmias	**Oncologic Problems**
Depression	**Respiratory Problems**	Oropharyngeal cancers
Anxiety	Lung abscess	Esophageal cancers
School refusal	Sleep apnea	
	Tuberculosis	

*Indirect presentations occur when family members display problems consequent to the drinking of their relative.

DIAGNOSIS

The high frequency of alcohol problems in clinical practice and the low diagnosis rate indicate a need for a much higher index of suspicion. Meticulous assessment is required wherever one of the problems listed in Table 1 presents.

History of Alcohol Use

An attitude of nonjudgmental acceptance of heavy drinking as a common human behavior should pervade all history-taking efforts. One technique that emerges from this attitude is the "top-high" technique, in which one deliberately overestimates the amount consumed and places the onus of denial on the patient, for example, "I bet you could drink two bottles of whiskey in a day." A variant of this technique can be used in taking a daily drinking estimate by asking whether a patient has the first drink of the day before or after breakfast! This having been ascertained, the clinician builds up a picture of the typical drinking that occurs in a day. This eventually allows the clinician to estimate how many standard drinks (10 grams of alcohol) are consumed during an average day. The perceived benefits and the social setting of the drinking should also be elicited.

Physical Examination

During the physical examination, the physician looks for the following signs:

1. Signs of trauma
2. Signs of liver disease—tender hepatomegaly, spider nevi, secondary lunulae, palmar erythema, bruising, parotid enlargement, ascites

3. Conjunctival injection, facial telangiectasia, tongue and hand tremors
4. Hypertension, obesity
5. Withdrawal features, commonly anxiety, sweating, and tachycardia
6. Evidence of intoxication—alcohol on the breath, ataxia, disinhibition

Clinical Investigations

These are used to confirm the suspected diagnosis. Because all tests have a low sensitivity, negative test results cannot exclude alcohol problems.

1. Liver function tests show some abnormality in about 50% of cases; the γ-glutamyltransferase measurement is the most sensitive.
2. The mean corpuscular volume is elevated.
3. Blood alcohol levels may be detected, especially in emergencies. Apparent sobriety with a substantial blood alcohol level may clarify the situation.
4. Screening devices such as the Alcohol Use Disorders Identification Test (AUDIT)* can assist in identifying individuals who need more detailed assessment. This instrument is in the public domain and does not require permission for reproduction. Each question is scored on a scale of 0 to 4, the left column scoring 0, the right column 4. A score below 8 indicates nonhazardous drinking. A score of 8 to 15 indicates hazardous or harmful drinking. A score above 15 indicates probable dependence.

*See Jurd S: Alcohol-related problems. *In* Rakel RE (ed): Conn's Current Therapy 1995. Philadelphia, WB Saunders Co, 1995, p 1039.

TREATMENT

Brief Intervention

After a thorough assessment as just outlined, patients whose alcohol use is hazardous or harmful but not dependent should receive a brief (10- to 15-minute) intervention along the following lines.

Feedback. Explain why alcohol is relevant to the patient, providing details about any abnormal test results and never explaining away minor abnormalities if they fit the clinical situation. Indicate to patients who have no clinically apparent harm how their drinking behavior puts them at risk.

Listen. Pay careful attention to the way in which the patient responds to the information provided. Defensiveness may interfere with communication and requires clarification, without argument.

Outline Benefits. Provide an account of the future prospects, outlining the benefits to the patient if drinking behavior is altered.

Set Goals. Inform the patient of the limits of low-risk drinking. If harm is manifest, a brief (1- to 3-month) period of abstinence may be indicated.

Set Strategies. Provide suggestions about altering behaviors, e.g., start with a nonalcoholic drink, avoid heavy drinking parties, resurrect an old hobby, engage in physical fitness activities, alternate alcoholic and nonalcoholic drinks, avoid buying rounds of drinks.

Evaluate. Encourage each patient to return for a review of his or her progress with attempts at behavioral change. Exceeding the drinking goals set should not be seen as a failure but as part of a learning process.

If clinically significant medical problems are present, closer follow-up is indicated, with regular monitoring of any abnormal test results. Despite all efforts by clinicians, some people who are dependent will not disclose their symptoms, so prolonged inability to change drinking behavior should indicate a need to consider a diagnosis of alcohol dependence.

ALCOHOL DEPENDENCE

If patients are physically dependent, they will experience some withdrawal symptoms. These can be a potent stimulant to return to drinking. An inpatient detoxification program is often necessary to allow the patient to withdraw safely from alcohol. Sedatives such as chlordiazepoxide (Librium) or diazepam (Valium) may occasionally ease withdrawal, but great care should be taken to taper the dose to ensure that the sedative is stopped before discharge. At least relative malnutrition is the rule in alcohol dependence, so multivitamins, particularly vitamin B_1 (thiamine), should be prescribed.

Regular contact with the clinician, especially early in the abstinence period, can be helpful, as can referral to a counselor skilled in drug and alcohol problems. Difficulties with personal relationships and family situations commonly require attention. Patients with more severe or complicated problems or continual relapses may benefit from an inpatient rehabilitation program. These exist in a variety of forms, and the clinician should attempt to match the patient to the appropriate program.

The seventh feature of alcohol dependence is a return to pathologic use after a period of abstinence. The more severe the dependence, the more inevitable the return to damaging drinking habits. Under these circumstances, the only solution is lifelong total abstinence. This is a tall order for those who value alcohol highly and is why members of Alcoholics Anonymous (AA) say they do it "one day at a time." AA is a worldwide self-help organization founded in 1935 in Akron, Ohio, that has more than 1.5 million members. It is based on spiritual principles and encourages altruistic endeavor but makes no demands of its members apart from a desire to stay sober. AA can be an invaluable source of support for patients who espouse abstinence as a goal.

LONG-TERM FOLLOW-UP

It is rare for patients to change ingrained habits without a struggle. Maintenance of a nonjudgmental stance and positive expectations despite a relapse are useful. Patients often learn from a relapse and are better able to pursue complete recovery. Experience indicates that even the most profoundly damaged patients can attain long-term sobriety.

DRUG ABUSE

method of
MARK S. GOLD, M.D.
University of Florida Brain Institute
Gainesville, Florida

Drug use and addiction have been called the nation's number one public health problem. Cigarette smoking and dependence constitute the single most common preventable cause of death in the United States. Overall, the prevalence of alcoholism in the United States is 16%, of drug addiction 8%, and of alcohol plus another drug of abuse 30 to 84%. So prevalent are drug problems that it would be difficult to imagine insulting a patient by asking about tobacco, alcohol, and other drugs. All patients from children to adults should be evaluated for tobacco status, drinking, drug use, and dependence at each visit. Breath, urine, and serum tests are underused by physicians, as is interviewing of spouse, friends, and employer. Drugs produce numerous medical problems and complaints that are commonly treated by physicians. However, only recently have physicians begun to identify and vigorously treat the causative problem.

In the past, physicians perceived addition as self-afflicted. Whereas first use is voluntary, drug addiction is involuntary. Addiction is characterized by overwhelming loss of control, obsessive drug ruminations, and compulsive use independent of dire consequences. Drugs are taken for their positive specific brain rewarding effects. Therefore, addiction is a disease of the brain. Opiates are targeted at the brain's endogenous opioid systems, marijuana at the brain's endogenous cannabinoid systems, benzodiazepines and alcohol at the brain's γ-aminobutyric acid (GABA) receptor complex, cocaine at the brain's dopamine reuptake transporter. Ultimately, all drugs attempt to gain rapid access to the areas of the brain that produce intense pleasure and reward. These hard-wired dopamine brain reward circuits can be stimulated in research studies and accessed and stimulated by drugs of abuse. Drugs of abuse have important local effects but are targeted at brain regions normally activated by food or sex.

Cocaine, for example, has important local effects whether it is smoked or sniffed, causing profound changes in pulmonary function or causing nasal ulceration, sinusitis, hoarseness, and perforation. However, no one uses cocaine for its effects on the lung or the nose. First use of heroin is generally associated with nausea and vomiting. Side effects and toxicity are tolerated for as long as the user receives the desired brain reinforcement from the drug. Even a clear understanding of drug risks does not prevent use. Alcohol- and drug-related impairment of physicians is ample evidence for the lack of relative power of medical facts and education. How many times did we marvel or shake our heads when seeing a patient using portable oxygen or after lung surgery for cancer who quickly resumed smoking? The risks of crack smoking or intravenous self-administration are similarly minimized and ignored because of the power and importance of brain reward.

Scientific progress has provided us with a working neuroanatomy for drug reinforcement, models for drug use and relapse, and new treatments. Millions of different chemicals exist, but fewer than 25 of these are voluntarily self-administered by animals and abused by humans. Widely diverse chemicals such as opiates, cocaine, ethanol, nicotine, and all other known abused drugs enhance endogenous brain reward mechanisms, increase dopamine cell firing rate, and increase dopamine release at critical brain pleasure and reward sites. Treatment models have evolved from a primary focus on detoxification as the sine qua non of treating addiction. Advances in treatment have given physicians confidence that medical therapies for addictions work and have cost-effective outcomes similar to those for other chronic medical diseases such as hypertension, inflammatory bowel diseases, diabetes, and asthma.

DETOXIFICATION

Most physicians evaluate and treat patients addicted to tobacco, alcohol, and opiates. A good history, examination, blood and/or urine testing, and understanding of the natural history of dependence and withdrawal make treatment decisions easier. If detoxification is regarded by itself, as a stand-alone treatment, then it is not effective. Detoxification is not a treatment of addiction but rather a first step in a long process of neuroadaptive and behavioral change. Detoxification is meant to help an addict safely withdraw from chronic drug self-administration with a modicum of withdrawal symptoms and distress. Detoxification also provides an opportunity for physicians to evaluate and treat addicts for their myriad medical and dental complications. Targets for treatment include the drug dependence; relapse; behavioral, family, and social problems; diseases masked by the drug use; and diseases acquired by the addict.

Current detoxification protocols are short term and targeted at acute abstinence. Protracted withdrawal complaints that are prolonged and clearly not limited to the immediate effects of drug absence are recognied for many drugs (Table 1).

ALCOHOL DEPENDENCE

Diagnosis

Many Americans drink alcoholic beverages; pathologic attachment to alcohol and dependence are much less common. Alcohol abuse and dependence have an annual prevalence of approximately 8% of adults in the United States. Alcoholic individuals have a variety of specific alcohol preferences from beer and wine to vodka. Which alcoholic beverage is consumed is not as relevant as the drinker's response to the so-called CAGE questionnaire (attempts to cut down on drinking, being annoyed by criticism about drinking, feeling guilty about drinking, and using alcohol as an eye opener). Diagnostic issues are explained in detail in the preceding article.

The CAGE and other standardized screening questionnaires have been proposed to help physicians identify alcohol abuse and dependence before a conviction for driving under the influence or tragic consequence. Physicians have detected alcoholism by further investigation of patients with abnormal γ-glutamyltransferase activity; increases in alanine aminotransferase, aspartate aminotransferase, and γ-glutamyltransferase; fractures; sleep disorders; gastrointestinal complaints; depression; accidents; and family, job, and other social problems. Evidence suggests that a new and simple blood test, carbohydrate-deficient transferrin (CDT), may be the most useful biologic marker for excessive alcohol consumption. CDT has also been used by researchers to independently monitor the alcoholic patient during treatment to detect a relapse.

Risk

For both men and women, the majority of the variation in risk for lifetime alcohol dependence and abuse is attributable to genetic factors. The risk for alcohol dependence is increased in both the sons and the daughters of alcoholic men and women. Alcohol dependence can be seen on both sides of the family, with alcoholism risk about four times higher in the children of alcoholic individuals than in control

TABLE 1. **Tobacco and Other Withdrawal Syndromes**

Acute Abstinence	Nicotine	Cocaine	Alcohol	Heroin
Onset	10 h	1–12 h	6–24 h	4–6 h
Peak	1–3 d	1 wk	3–7 d	2–3 d
Duration	3–4 wk	3 mo	1–2 wk	2 wk
Detoxification	Patch		Benzodiazepines	Methadone
Treatment	Gum	?	Carbamazepine	Clonidine

ALCOHOLISM

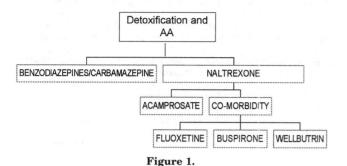

Figure 1.

subjects. Lack of "normal" response to drinking and the ability to consume large amounts of alcoholic beverages without the typical impairment may also be predictive markers for alcoholism risk.

Relapse Prevention

Assessment and treatment of withdrawal are described in the preceding article. Like all other drugs of abuse, alcohol is self-administered by animals and humans, produces a rush or high, and enhances brain reward by increasing the release of dopamine in the nucleus accumbens. However, alcohol accomplishes this increase by an overall increase in GABA action. Alcohol and benzodiazepines used for detoxification share many important features and can be substituted for each other. Benzodiazepines do not help once detoxification is completed. New treatments for alcoholic patients include opiate antagonists like naltrexone (ReVia) and acamprosate,* which block alcohol's free access to brain reward and alter the typical high produced by drinking. Whereas loss of health, loved ones, and employment may not be adequate punishment or incentive to stop drinking, interfering with alcohol's brain rewarding effects works well. Naltrexone reduces craving for alcohol, blunts anticipatory or "happy hour" anticipation of alcohol reward, and stops a slip from becoming a binge. In general, after successful detoxification, I treat alcoholic patients with daily 12-step Alcoholics Anonymous (AA) meetings and 50 mg of naltrexone each morning. I have begun to offer treatment that fits nicely with the standard 90 AA meetings in 90 days by adding 90 naltrexone in 90 days. Thereafter, I re-evaluate the patient's naltrexone, but the patient continues to participate and, it is hoped, progress in the 12-step recovery program. Adding naltrexone to any existing alcoholism treatment program improves the program by reducing relapse by 50% (Figure 1).

Addiction is a chronic illness much like diabetes or hypertension. Relapse should be considered no more a failure than a high glucose level could be considered treatment failure by an endocrinologist. Considering addiction a moral failure is as ridiculous as

*Not available in the United States.

Table 2. **Benzodiazepines: Top 200 Prescriptions**

1977	1989	1995
1. Diazepam	4. Alprazolam	10. Alprazolam
13. Flurazepam	24. Triazolam	31. Lorazepam
17. Chlordiazepoxide	42. Diazepam	48. Clonazepam
	64. Lorazepam	57. Diazepam
	97. Clonazepam	

considering overweight, cardiovascular disease, cancer of all forms, or diabetes the result of moral failure.

BENZODIAZEPINES

Benzodiazepines are widely used. Nearly 10% of the entire U.S. population has had some short-term use in the past 12 months. Benzodiazepines remain important, effective, useful, and widely prescribed medications (Tables 2 and 3).

In my experience, benzodiazepine abuse is rare. Daily use occurs in 1 to 2% of patients. When abuse occurs, it is found in patients who have taken high doses of benzodiazepines for long periods, who have alcohol or another drug dependency, or who have a strong family history for alcoholism. Benzodiazepine withdrawal is typically treated by careful assessment of the level of dependence, stabilization, substitution, and taper. Stabilize the patient with an equivalent dose of diazepam (Valium) or chlordiazepoxide (Librium) three or four times daily. Taper at a rate that corresponds to the elimination half-life of the drug of addiction. Slower taper is generally better. Outpatient protocols with a diazepam taper of 5 mg per week and inpatient protocols with 5% reduction a day have been proposed, yet this is an area that is more of an art than a science. Individual differences, observations of the patient's responses to treatment, and protection of the patient who desires a rapid detoxification and release are important considerations.

OPIATES

The opiate withdrawal syndrome shares a number of signs and symptoms with alcohol withdrawal and nicotine withdrawal. The role of the largest cluster of noradrenergic neurons in the brain, the pontine locus caeruleus (LC), has been implicated in the wide

Table 3. **Benzodiazepines: Conversion Table**

Benzodiazepine Medication	Dose Equivalence (mg)
Alprazolam (Xanax)	0.5–1.0
Chlordiazepoxide (Librium)	25–50
Clonazepam (Klonopin)	1–2
Clorazepate (Tranxene)	15
Diazepam (Valium)	10
Lorazepam (Ativan)	2
Oxazepam (Serax)	10
Triazolam (Halcion)	0.25–0.50

variety of behaviors produced by opiate withdrawal. LC neurons, which possess a high density of mu and kappa opiate receptors, are inhibited by opiates. However, during spontaneous or precipitated withdrawal, the LC firing increases. LC activity correlates with overt hypertension, tachycardia, nervousness, and other opiate withdrawal behavior. LC hyperactivity can be suppressed and withdrawal treated by opiates and the alpha$_2$-adrenergic antihypertensive clonidine (Catapres), which decrease LC activity. Surgical destruction of the LC eliminates all aspects of opiate withdrawal, but self-administration of opiates continues unabated. This dramatic finding again supports the dissociation of the brain's neuroadaptive response to chronic drug administration, producing physiologic withdrawal signs and symptoms, drug seeking, and self-administration. Dopaminergic, cholinergic, and glutaminergic factors are also important in opiate action and withdrawal.

Opiate withdrawal is generally easy to recognize and not fatal. Confirmation may be supplied by administering the narcotic antagonist naloxone and provoking withdrawal. Treatment errors tend to be made in the direction of overtreatment or over-replacement with opiates on the basis of the patient's reports of use or observation of signs or symptoms.

Withdrawal generally begins 2 to 8 hours after the last parenteral dose or 6 to 12 hours after the last oral dose or in 1 to 2 days if the patient is maintained with methadone. Opiate withdrawal has a flulike presentation, with eyes watering, nose running, sweating, fever, bone pain, anorexia, stomach cramps, and yawning; autonomic symptoms emerge as symptoms peak at 48 to 72 hours. Withdrawal generally begins with grade 0 and continues through grades 3 or 4 if untreated. Some patients report little more than a flulike illness, and others report the delusion that they are going to die (Table 4).

Ideally the patient can be examined, stabilized, and evaluated for a detoxification. The acute withdrawal syndrome is time limited, ending within 10 days of the last dose. Opiates have been the standard opiate addiction detoxification treatment. They have been safe and effective. However, the use of methadone in outpatient and neonatal detoxification has been challenged by discovery of the effectiveness of the alpha$_2$-adrenergic agonist clonidine. Clonidine has the advantage of being a nonaddicting, nonopiate treatment given to the addict after withdrawal be-

TABLE 4. Acute Opiate Withdrawal

Grade 0 Anxiety, craving for opiates
Grade 1 Yawning, perspiration, lacrimation, rhinorrhea, panic, drive for opiates
Grade 2 Mydriasis, gooseflesh, tremors, hot and cold flashes, chills, drive for opiates
Grade 3 Hypertension, increased pulse, increased respiration, increased temperature, nausea, restlessness, aches, cramps
Grade 4 Vomiting, diarrhea, ejaculation, fear of death being imminent

TABLE 5. Characteristics of Opioid Dependence

Opiate stabilization and medical evaluation for detoxification safety and efficacy
Detoxification: methadone, buprenorphine, clonidine, lofexidine
Opiate maintenance: methadone, *l*-acetyl-α-methadol (LAAM), buprenorphine
Rapid detoxification: naloxone-precipitated withdrawal reversed by clonidine followed by naltrexone maintenance
Opiate antagonist maintenance: naltrexone (ReVia 100 mg Monday and Wednesday, 150 mg Friday)
12-step fellowship: Narcotics Anonymous
Therapeutic communities/long-term drug-free treatment: Daytop Villages, Phoenix House

gins. Although it is difficult to standardize, I have used 17 μg per kg per day in divided doses for the first 4 or 5 days of withdrawal treatment. Thereafter, the dose is tapered to zero by day 14. The patient would typically be treated with 0.1 to 0.2 mg four times daily with doses as needed and doses withheld depending on symptoms and blood pressure. Methadone has the advantage of reversal of all withdrawal symptoms. Clonidine induces hypotension, which can be accentuated by a patient's concurrent drug use. Dose adjustments are common during a clonidine detoxification as the physician correlates hypotension and other side effects with the patient's withdrawal signs and symptoms. Clonidine detoxification has been coupled with the long-acting opiate antagonist naltrexone and has been given as part of an accelerated detoxification–relapse prevention treatment protocol. The use of clonidine followed by naltrexone and 12-step treatment programs has been successful for physicians and other health professionals. The mixed opioid agonist-antagonist buprenorphine (Buprenex) has been used in detoxification with success (Table 5).

As discussed for alcoholism, detoxification is not treatment and should not be confused with addiction. For heroin addicts, maintenance treatment with a long-acting opiate such as methadone, *l*-acetyl-α-methadol (LAAM),* or buprenorphine can be regarded as a success when the patient is abstinent from all illegal drugs and demonstrates markedly improved functioning in all other areas of life. Similarly, 12-step fellowships, long-term drug-free residential treatment centers, and naltrexone maintenance have successfully treated addicts who wish to remain opiate free.

SMOKING: TOBACCO AND MARIJUANA

Tobacco

Most experts respect the pathologic attachment between the cigarette and the smoker-addict and expect this relationship to be as illogical and difficult to break as any other addiction. Smoking is an intensely addicting illness. A typical smoker who inhales 30 cigarettes a day and takes 10 puffs per

---

*Not available in the United States.

cigarette and has done this for 20 years smokes at least 240 times a day or 87,600 times a year and in toto has smoked at least 1,752,000 times before coming for treatment. Because inhalation is an extremely powerful route of drug self-administration, more similar to intravenous use than to oral, compelling brain reward and pathologic attachment are more likely. Addiction to cigarettes has made tobacco use the number one cause of preventable death, killing at least 400,000 Americans per year, three times as many as all other addicting drugs combined. Tobacco-nicotine is the addicting drug that is reported to have the poorest rate of treatment success, but these data may simply reflect the fact that a variety of effective treatment options are not available. For example, maintenance with a nicotine patch or gum is not generally a treatment option. Treatment options do not generally include residential treatment or medications that make behavioral relapse prevention more effective. Tobacco addiction is trivialized by equating it with nicotine dependence and equating treatment with nicotine detoxification.

Withdrawal complaints, although troubling, are not life-threatening. Nicotine withdrawal includes irritability, confusion, agitation, insomnia, concentration problems, lethargy, yawning, and craving—all reversed by smoking. The standard approach to cigarette smoking addiction, often referred to as nicotine dependence, is detoxification and abstinence with social prohibitions. Of all the cigarette smoking patients presenting for treatment, only 20 to 30% have not resumed smoking within a year. Most of the smokers who have quit have quit without formal treatment. However, the success rate is less than 5% for unaided quit attempts. Physicians should ask all patients about their use of tobacco products; advise all patients to stop; and assist their efforts with materials, a quit date, and nicotine detoxification using nicotine replacement with the "gum" or "patch." Both the nicotine gum and patch are available without a prescription in the United States. Nicotine skin patches are generally preferred because they are well tolerated, topical, inconspicuous, passive, and initially successful in up to 30% of patients.

Gum. Nicotine replacement and detoxification are frequently prescribed by physicians as part of a smoking cessation program. A meta-analysis on efficacy of nicotine replacement therapies in smoking cessation from nearly 18,000 subjects from all randomized trials of nicotine gum, patches, sprays,* and inhalers* has strongly suggested that all of the currently available forms of nicotine replacement are effective therapies to aid smoking cessation. The first generally available nicotine replacement was nicotine polacrilex (Nicorette), a gum resin laden with nicotine. Because it is chewed, it helps satisfy the oral aspects of smoking. In addition, the initial "burst" of nicotine simulates that of a cigarette. It has the advantages of being convenient to carry, easy to titrate, and controlled by the patient, and it also

allows the patient some oral satisfaction. Many people experience side effects associated with chewing of the gum such as mouth soreness, hiccups, dyspepsia, jaw ache, and impaired absorption when it is taken with orange juice, citrus candies, coffee, or other acidic beverages. Most of these side effects are only mildly bothersome and can be alleviated with proper "parking" technique. This includes the gum's being chewed slowly until a peppery taste emerges and then placed between the cheek and gum to allow drug absorption. Also, because many foods and beverages interfere with absorption, nothing should be placed in the mouth 15 minutes before use or while chewing the gum. The 4-mg gum and the patch appear to be equal in efficacy at smoking cessation, and the combination has been used with intractable patients. Most commonly, patients do not chew enough pieces per day to achieve maximal benefit from use. Encourage use on a fixed schedule *for 1 to 3 months*. Some patients transfer nicotine dependency from cigarettes to the gum.

Patch. The transdermal nicotine patch, sold under the trade names Nicoderm, Habitrol, ProStep, and Nicotrol, has several advantages over the gum. The patch is applied once a day and then allowed to work. The patch is unobtrusive and provides steady-state, not bolus, nicotine. Smokers frequently complain that the patch does not feel like smoking. Fifty percent of users will have a localized rash that is usually mild and self-limited. Suggesting the application of hydrocortisone cream (5%) to the area or rotating patch sites may ameliorate such local reactions. Less than 5% of patients discontinue use because of this reaction. They should know that the goal of treatment is detoxification. After detoxification, motivational enhancement can help the patient to begin the process of lifestyle change. It is also important to emphasize to all patients that they should abstain from smoking while using the patch. Concurrent smoking may lead to nicotine toxicity.

Spray and Inhaler. Nicotine nasal spray delivering 0.5 mg of nicotine in each nostril has been shown to reverse nicotine abstinence, especially in highly dependent patients. The nicotine nasal spray and nicotine vapor inhaler may be available for physicians to prescribe in a short time. As in alcohol and opiate withdrawal, clonidine has been used to reverse the autonomic signs and symptoms seen in cigarette smoking discontinuation or nicotine abstinence.

Treatment: Maintaining Abstinence

Tobacco smoking–nicotine dependence is a good model for all the other addictions. Many smokers are co-morbid for alcohol and other drug dependencies. Studies have shown that 85% of alcoholic individuals smoke cigarettes, and the majority of cocaine, opiate, and other addicts smoke. Smoking recovery rates are similar to those of other drug dependencies. This association is useful for physicians; if they ask all patients at all visits about their tobacco use status, they will know whom to ask the most vigorous questions about alcohol and other drug use. Identifying

---

*Not available in the United States.

and treating co-morbid illnesses improve outcomes. Smokers are addicted to the drug nicotine; benefit from the central antidepressant effects of nicotine and tobacco smoke; report stimulant effects; derive satisfaction from holding cigarettes and inhaling; and are attached to this image, rituals associated with use, and other associations from sights and smells to brands. Smoking and inhalation allow rapid absorption from the lungs and access to the brain, producing stimulant-like effects similar in many ways to those of cocaine. The patch and the gum and other nicotine preparations have little in common with smoking, which almost instantly delivers to the brain a bolus of nicotine and a large variety of other psychoactive substances and approximately 4000 chemical compounds.

Because nicotine detoxification is limited in efficacy, antidepressants such as fluoxetine (Prozac)* and bupropion (Wellbutrin)* have been studied and reported. Both of these traditional antidepressants reduce dropouts and improve abstinence rates of detoxified smokers. Data using positron emission technology have demonstrated that nicotine administration is not equal in all ways to smoking tobacco. Smoking cigarettes induces a change in brain monoamine oxidase activity, which suggests that smokers are getting significant antidepressant effects from smoking. These data help explain the resistance to treatment and multiple failures that are commonplace among smokers. Many cigarette smokers, like alcoholics and opiate addicts, have a protracted abstinence syndrome often lasting for a year or more. Finding an antidepressant effect of cigarette smoke may also explain the withdrawal boredom and depression, the high prevalence of depressives, and family history positive for depression among smokers. I have tried naltrexone in cigarette smoking abstinence and believe that naltrexone decreases detoxification dropouts and relapse (Figure 2).

Marijuana

Marijuana, our most commonly used illicit drug, is the major illicit drug of abuse for young people. Tetrahydrocannabinol (THC) is the principal psychoactive ingredient in marijuana and, like all other addicting drugs, is self-administered in animals and humans. The higher the THC content, the more users prefer and choose it over marijuana with less THC. Daily marijuana use has increased to the point that it exceeds daily alcohol use in some surveys of high-school seniors. Throughout the United States, students are presenting for addiction treatment complaining of loss of control of their marijuana use, inability to stop despite health and life consequences, and an overall feeling that they are hooked. College students who smoke marijuana regularly have residual neuropsychologic effects that carry over past acute intoxication and supervised abstinence. Test results for attention, verbal fluency, executive func-

*Not FDA approved for this indication.

CIGARETTE SMOKING

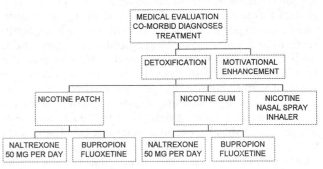

Figure 2.

tioning, and new word learning were significantly impaired by marijuana. Clinicians are evaluating and treating more patients who describe themselves as marijuana dependent. The synthesis of novel THC antagonists will allow us to treat toxicity and overdoses but also will allow us to identify those patients who are physiologically dependent on marijuana in the same way that naloxone (Narcan) can be used to provoke opiate withdrawal.

Smoking Marijuana Versus Ingestion

Much controversy exists regarding what marijuana is and what it does. Simplistic comparisons are made between dronabinol (Marinol), the oral form of THC, and inhalation of cannabis, the most common way that marijuana is used today. Δ^9-THC produces antinociception, catalepsy, anticonvulsive activity, hypothermia, hyperexcitability, and depression of motor activity through interaction with cannabinoid receptors that occur naturally in our brain. Although many similarities exist between THC and marijuana effects, differences exist as well. Marijuana can be ingested orally, but the most common model of marijuana self-administration is by smoking and inhalation. This smoke contains more than 150 compounds in addition to the major psychoactive component, Δ^9-THC. Many of the cannabinoids and other complex organic compounds found in marijuana smoke appear to have psychoactive properties; other components have yet to be tested for long- or short-term safety in animals and humans. In humans, marijuana use begins with the volatilized THC produced by the burning of the cigarette and is followed by deep inhalation. The marijuana is then rapidly absorbed from the lungs, which allows THC, major metabolites, and other smoke constituents to spread throughout the body and brain. Marijuana and tobacco smoke are similar; the primary difference between the two is that marijuana smoke contains cannabinoids and tobacco smoke contains nicotine. The effects of marijuana smoking are similar to the effects of tobacco smoking. Chronic marijuana smoking results in mild airway obstruction, decreased exercise tolerance, chronic cough, bronchitis, and dependence. Whereas both marijuana and tobacco increase the number of inflammatory cells in the lung, they differentially affect the activation of these inflammatory cells, possibly leading to differential effects on lung injury and physiologic consequences, including altered alveolar epithelial permeability. Lung function decreases more significantly with concurrent use of tobacco cigarettes. Psychiatric changes, visual distortions, and perceptual problems are special problems for the marijuana-intoxicated driver or worker. Motor performance is further compromised by the drug's specific affinity for THC receptors in the cerebellum. Marijuana use is clearly related to driving impairment.

The discovery of a G protein–coupled cannabinoid receptor together with the identification of the putative endogenous cannabinoid ligand anandamide led to the discovery of our endogenous cannabinoid neural system. This system is the subject of intensive neuroscientific and pharmacologic investigation. New medical treatments that can modulate pain sensitivity appear to be a likely outcome. Two subtypes of cannabinoid receptors, CB1 and CB2, have been described. Anandamide is a brain constituent that binds to CB1 and parallels Δ^9-THC in its interactions with the brain's cannabinoid receptors. Addiction research in this area may lead to the discovery of CB-mediated therapeutic applications including analgesia, attenuation of nausea and vomiting, appetite stimulation, memory disorders, decreased intestinal motility of diarrhea, decreased bronchial constriction of asthma, antirheumatic and antipyretic actions, and treatment of convulsive disorders. In addition to cannabinoid agonists, antagonists have been synthesized. In one report, precipitated withdrawal was clearly demonstrated by use of a selective antagonist in rats chronically treated with Δ^9-THC.

OVERDOSE

Treatment of Overdose

Individuals with overdose of narcotic analgesics such as heroin, morphine, or methadone typically present to emergency departments with respiratory depression, pinpoint pupils, and central nervous system depression. Convulsions are not generally observed with the exception of propoxyphene (Darvon), codeine, and meperidine (Demerol). Narcotic overdose is a common problem and an increasingly reported cause of poison-related death. Treatment in this setting is focused on reversal of opiate access to opioid receptors and thus reversal of central nervous system depression, respiratory depression and other hypotension, bradycardia, and other mu-opioid agonist effects. After airway, breathing, and circulation have been established, I give 5 ampules of 0.4-gram naloxone, the short-acting opiate antagonist, intravenously as a bolus, repeated every 2 to 3 minutes until 10 mg has been given. Naloxone is short acting, and the patient should be treated with two thirds of the dose necessary to reverse the overdose given every

hour until the opiates are no longer a threat. Opiate withdrawal symptoms provoked by naloxone are not life-threatening. Repeated administration of naloxone produces less and less withdrawal response, fewer and fewer withdrawal symptoms.

Persons with overdose of cocaine, amphetamine, marijuana, phencyclidine hydrochloride (PCP), barbiturates, lysergic acid diethylamide (LSD), and a variety of other substances from flunitrazepam to Ecstasy (see later) commonly present in emergency departments and are treated symptomatically. Management of overdose and toxic reactions to opiates, barbiturates, alcohol, benzodiazepines, and other drugs is usually focused on airway, breathing, and circulation. Thereafter, oxygen, 50% dextrose, naloxone, and 100 mg of intravenous thiamine are given, depending on the clinical presentation. Local poison control centers are valuable resources when a patient is intoxicated with a substance or substances of abuse and presents in an emergency setting. Many physicians are trained in clinical toxicology, a field with identification and treatment of patients poisoned with drugs and other chemicals.

Benzodiazepines

If the specific drug overdose and treatment protocol are well known, the emergency may be handled differently. Although it is safe with a large margin of clinical safety in a benzodiazepine overdose, the typical procedure is emesis induction, gastric lavage, evaluation for concurrent drug taking, observation, and support. Flumazenil (Romazicon) may be given when the patient has respiratory depression or coma, and it is given after the risk for withdrawal seizure or panic is considered. The smallest amount of flumazenil is typically given as a bolus of 0.2 mg during 30 seconds with additional doses given at a rate of 0.2 mg per minute. The total dose is usually less than 1 mg, although 0.2 to 5.0 mg is the typical range.

Cocaine

Toxic reactions to cocaine have been described in intravenous cocaine users, crack smokers, and those who use cocaine and alcohol together. Cocaine increases blood pressure acutely but increases intracerebral blood pressure much more than anticipated on the basis of standard blood pressure monitoring. It produces vasoconstriction and vasospasm. Cocaine also causes hyperpyrexia, epileptic seizures, myocardial infarction, ischemic strokes, and transient ischemic accidents. When used with alcohol, cocaine produces cocaethylene in the body of the user. Cocaethylene is much like cocaine but longer lasting and associated with many cocaine overdoses. Cocaethylene is neurotoxic, hepatotoxic, and cardiotoxic. Cocaine is metabolized largely by plasma cholinesterase to benzoylecgonine, which is inactive and found in urine for up to 2 to 3 days after use. Increasing the availability of metabolic enzymes is one avenue for cocaine overdose and cocaine treatment research.

No specific treatment for cocaine overdose, toxicity, withdrawal, or relapse prevention exists (Table 6).

MDMA

MDMA (3,4-methylenedioxymethamphetamine; also called Ecstasy) has been a common cause of emergency visits among young people, especially those people who have been attending a "rave" or all-night dance. Decreased appetite, restlessness, anxiety, panic, depression, nystagmus, motor tics, hyperpyrexia, dehydration, and exhaustion have been reported as emergency presentations. Dehydration and hyperpyrexia have been the major causes of death reported after MDMA was taken and provided the energy and motivation to dance all night in a poorly ventilated hot environment without appropriate hunger and thirst cues. MDMA has toxic effects on the raphe nucleus and causes a prolonged decrease in available brain serotonin. This effect has been linked to persistent panic, obsessive-compulsive features, and depression in certain users.

Marijuana

There are no specific medical therapies to treat overdoses or specifically reverse the effects of marijuana. Overdose is not generally a problem for users of marijuana alone, but marijuana's inhibition of the vomiting reflex has been reported to be important in problem drinking and ethanol overdose. The identification and localization of the cannabinoid receptor in the brain have greatly advanced our knowledge of the molecular mechanism of marijuana. The paucity of receptors in the brain stem could possibly explain why high doses of marijuana do not lethally suppress cardiovascular and respiratory function.

Lysergic Acid Diethylamide

At least 1 in 10 adolescents tries LSD before high-school graduation. LSD is colorless and odorless. It is generally sold impregnated on a blotting paper,

TABLE 6. Amphetamine, Cocaine, MDMA

The more dopamine reuptake transporter binding, the greater self-administration.

Animals self-administer cocaine to increase and then maintain extracellular dopamine levels in reward or pleasure areas.

Cocaine self-administration is highly valued and all animals will exert an extraordinary amount of work, accept considerable punishment and frustration for the opportunity to self-administer the drug.

Unlimited access to stimulants is more likely to end in death.

Amphetamine, like cocaine, produces robust increases in extracellular dopamine in the nucleus accumbens; when total stimulant availability is limited, they are used in binges, without satiety.

MDMA has amphetamine-like effects on dopamine levels but also has toxic effects on serotonin cell bodies.

Abbreviation: MDMA = 3,4-methylenedioxymethamphetamine.

stamp, or cube. LSD is well absorbed orally from the gastrointestinal tract and other mucous membranes; peak LSD levels occur within 60 minutes after ingestion. LSD is slowly eliminated in the urine, and detection of metabolites may be possible for 3 or 4 days. Patients may say that they have taken LSD and in fact they have taken some other drug or poison. When possible, it is a good idea to talk to another person who shared the drug or used from the same batch at the same time. It is always ideal when dealing with a patient with a psychiatric emergency believed to be due to a toxin or drug to try to recover the offending drug. Sending a friend back to retrieve the drug for analysis is a good idea, which, together with stored blood and urine, can provide a definitive diagnosis. A dose of 50 μg produces LSD-related psychotomimetic effects mainly through specific interactions with serotonergic systems in the brain. Effects in humans can be reported with 1 μg within 1 hour of ingestion lasting up to 6 hours. Sympathetic stimulation with increased heart rate and respiration and some cholinergic effects with lacrimation, salivation, and nausea are reported while the user is describing marked alterations in visual perceptions. These changes may include delusions of persecution and grandiosity with hallucinations, alteration of body image, changes in hearing, synesthesia (seeing smells, hearing colors), magnification of touch, and distortion of time. LSD flashbacks, parts of the previous LSD experience, may be a problem and occur in many ex-users. These flashbacks may be triggered by marijuana smoking or other drug use. Emotions and emotional responses become intensified, labile, and difficult to control. LSD is a potent agonist at the 5-hydroxytryptamine (5-HT) 1A autoreceptors, thus accounting for its direct inhibitory effect on raphe neurons. Buspirone (Buspar) has similar effects and is an anxiolytic without producing hallucinations. LSD's interaction with the 5-HT$_2$ receptors is highly correlated with hallucinogenicity. LSD, mescaline, and other phenethylamine hallucinogens have been related to 5-HT$_2$ receptor stimulation of cortical interneurons. LSD emergencies are treated by providing the patient with a secure environment, reducing sensory stimulation, giving benzodiazepine if necessary for extreme anxiety and panic, and providing reassurance and positive feedback. Clozapine (Clozaril) or risperidone (Risperdal) is used for prolonged adverse psychedelic reactions to hallucinogens.

Flunitrazepam

Flunitrazepam (Rohypnol or "roofies") has been described by some as the "Quaalude of the 90s." Flunitrazepam is taken to produce a sense of relaxation, calm, and well-being. It is commonly taken with LSD to reduce adverse effects. Emergency visits reported to be related to flunitrazepam include prolonged headache, amnesic episodes, nightmares, rape, and the emergence of a variety of unintended behaviors. Psychomotor impairment is reported to persist for 12 hours after a 2-mg dose. Whereas loss of memory for a day or an entire weekend has been reported anecdotally for flunitrazepam, many of the unexpected disinhibiting effects are attributable to the drug and concurrent use of alcohol.

ADDICTION

Abuse, withdrawal, and emergency department presentations or consequences are not addiction. Addiction has two central features. The first is the loss of control over the use of addicting substances characterized by continued use despite adverse consequences of that use (the unmanageability of substance use and therefore of life itself). The addict will report a persistent desire or many unsuccessful attempts to cut down or control use. The second central feature of addiction is the denial of the use of alcohol and/or other intoxicating drugs and the denial of the consequences of that use (dishonesty). Use continues despite clear knowledge of physical or psychologic problems caused by the drug. The third feature is that the substance is often taken in larger amounts or for longer times than intended and occupies a great deal of time and energy. Obtaining the substance, hiding use, using, and recovering from its effects become the addict's life. Tolerance and withdrawal are not necessary for addiction to exist.

Addiction is more likely to occur if the host is at high risk and there is rapid brain access to potent rewarding drugs of abuse such as cocaine and opiates and smoking of marijuana and/or nicotine. This feature has tended to make smoking similar to injecting the drug with a needle in terms of rapidity of brain access and reward and thus addiction liability. Study of laboratory animals has allowed us to identify the events necessary for drug reinforcement. Rats, monkeys, and humans self-administer all drugs of abuse for their positive effects. The reinforcing effects of addictive drugs are not dependent on effects of physical dependence or withdrawal. The reinforcing effects can be demonstrated in animals from good and bad "homes," abused or neglected, and in all monkeys, rodents, or humans independent of most social variables. Dopaminergic neurons that originate in the ventral tegmental area and terminate in the forebrain, especially the nucleus accumbens, are thought to be the neuroanatomic basis for drug abuse and drug addiction (Table 7).

Cocaine, amphetamine, and opiates produce a rapid and profound brain rewarding effect that we are not prepared for on the basis of the typical neural function or evolution. The power and persistence of this reward cause rapid changes in behavior and brain. Everything associated with the drug use event becomes powerfully conditioned and able to stimulate the brain, like seeing the drug before use. Loss of control is a central part of all addiction theory. As important as loss of control is, it is a mystery. Compulsive use does not necessarily mean high volume or even repetitive use. Attachment to the drug and simple calculations of dose, frequency, and duration provide more than either measure alone. This com-

TABLE 7. **Drugs Are Taken for Brain Reward**

Substances that are self-administered by laboratory animals are the same ones that humans use and abuse.

Opiates, cocaine, amphetamine, anesthetics, barbiturates, and other drugs of abuse produce a high, stimulate their own taking, and enhance brain reward.

Animals will self-administer drugs of abuse in the absence of tolerance, physical dependence, withdrawal, or any prior history of use. Brain lesions that eliminate withdrawal do not interfere with drug taking.

Substances that can be abused enhance dopamine release in reward circuits projecting from the ventral tegmental area to the nucleus accumbens.

Specific lesions of the dopamine-rich ventral tegmental area or nucleus accumbens eliminate cocaine and amphetamine self-administration. The greater the lesion, the more the disruption.

pulsion to find and use the drug becomes embedded within the addict's motivational hierarchy even to the extent that it supplants or suppresses the motivational aspects of natural reinforcers such as social interactions, love, work, eating, drinking, and sexual behavior. This critical effect, called motivational toxicity, is well known to us in the classic compulsive use of cocaine by laboratory animals in which they ignore opportunities to feed, drink, and copulate in favor of cocaine self-administration. Use continues in the absence of drug-induced euphoria as the addict uses drugs to remain "normal."

ADDICTION AND THE BRAIN: A COCAINE VACCINE ON THE HORIZON?

The target of all drugs of abuse is the brain, and treatment needs to consider that the target has been altered by years of potent drugs. No one drinks for the effects of alcohol on the gastric mucosa, nor do individuals sniff cocaine for effects on the nasal septum or smoke for effects on the lung. Changes in brain are both acute and prolonged and in some patients may be permanent. Advances involving in vivo voltammeter and microdialysis make it possible to monitor the synaptic levels of brain dopamine in the nucleus accumbens of freely moving animals. These studies show that drugs of abuse are so powerful in changing behavior and reprogramming the animal or human subject because they produce more powerful increases in dopamine than any natural rewards, even sex or food. These potent actions in the primitive motivational circuits of the brain evolved and were fixed long before the first occurrence of addiction. The susceptibility of lower animals to drug dependence is a function of prior use, dose, and route of administration as well as of the drug itself. If the drug can get to the primitive mesotelencephalic dopamine reward system in the brain of an animal or a human being, it can cause the organism to pay attention and attribute species-specific survival significance to the drug self-administration event. Cocaine and other psychostimulants are more likely to be used to death than are other rewarding drugs of abuse, but lesions of the mesolimbic dopamine pathway can eliminate cocaine taking.

Considerable research directed at identifying the systems of the brain that relate to the intense addictive properties of cocaine has confirmed the central role of brain dopamine systems in cocaine addiction. Acutely, cocaine increases extracellular dopamine in the nucleus accumbens. Abstinence after chronic cocaine use is associated with a marked and persistent decrease in the brain's dopamine transporter, decreased cerebral blood flow, and decreased brain glucose metabolism. Parkinsonism and hyperprolactinemia have also been reported and related to cocaine-induced dopamine depletion. Long-lasting pleasure system dysfunction has been reported and related to modification of the mesolimbic dopamine neurons by cocaine. Animals without dopamine reuptake transporters do not respond to cocaine either biochemically or behaviorally. Dopamine systems in general and cocaine's dopamine transporter binding site in particular are necessary for cocaine to produce its psychostimulant effects. Molecular cloning has identified a single gene encoding the dopamine transporter and explaining the binding of cocaine to the carrier protein. Anticocaine antibodies targeted at cocaine reinforcement sites on the dopamine transporter may yield a cocaine vaccine. Catalytic antibodies to cocaine facilitate the breakdown of cocaine to inactive ecgonine methyl ester and benzoic acid. Developing bovine and other cholinesterases may provide us with new cocaine-metabolizing agents for overdose treatment. A number of cocaine vaccines are intensively being studied at present.

PREVENTION

Early Detection

Early recognition may allow one to simply advise a person to stop using or suggest that the person read some materials or attend an educational group. The alcoholic individual, early in the course of the illness, makes a series of decisions about relationships, family, and work that are part of a pathologic attachment to alcohol, which is accompanied by a reprioritization. The earlier the person's abuse or dependence is identified, the less there is to repair.

Co-morbidity

Alcoholics have co-morbid medical disorders such as hepatitis or cirrhosis; personality disorders such as antisocial personality disorder; other drug use and nicotine dependence; and a number of psychiatric disorders, from major depression and bipolar illness to eating disorders and anxiety disorders. Pharmacologic treatment of the co-morbid disorder is absolutely essential in preventing alcohol relapse and in preventing suicide of the male, depressed alcoholic. Co-morbid medical, neurologic, psychiatric, and other illnesses are common for all drug-dependent patients. Successful identification and treatment can improve addiction treatment outcomes.

CONCLUSION

Drug addiction is a brain disease, and new treatments are being tested that help prevent relapse, reverse changes induced by the drugs, and even prevent reintoxication. This newer view of addiction as a brain disease, which is rooted in the biology of motivation or reward, can yield important new approaches for treatment. The application of these new treatments requires a re-education of treatment professionals so that patients with addiction can benefit from combined treatment in the same way that depressed patients are treated—medications plus psychiatric therapy are better than either alone. Naltrexone has been shown to improve treatment outcome. Addiction is a lifelong chronic relapsing illness for which there is no specific cure. The possibility of creating new pharmacologic agents or vaccines to specifically target and short-circuit the addiction is on the horizon, portending the addition of powerful new medical treatments to already well-established behavioral treatments. Treatment should be individualized as much as possible and still retain the essential ingredients shown to be effective during the last decade.

ANXIETY

method of
ANDREW W. GODDARD, M.D.
Yale University School of Medicine
New Haven, Connecticut

Anxiety and fear are normal human emotions that facilitate adaptive coping to stressful or dangerous environments. After appropriate management or cessation of the stressor, fear responses generally subside rapidly. The physician becomes suspicious of pathologic forms of anxiety when there is exaggerated intensity and duration of normal stress responses or when the patient presents with cardinal symptoms of a specific anxiety disorder, such as a spontaneous panic attack, a phobia, an obsession, or a flashback. In approaching the assessment of the anxious patient, it is necessary to rule out an anxiety disorder due to a medical condition or substance use (e.g., thyrotoxicosis, caffeinism, alcohol withdrawal) and medical conditions that may masquerade as a clinical anxiety disorder (e.g., cardiac arrhythmias, seizure disorders, asthma). The clinician should also look carefully for co-morbid conditions, especially major depression and substance abuse. This article describes four common anxiety disorders (panic disorder is covered in a subsequent article) and their medical management. As a general rule, medications should be offered as part of a treatment plan that includes cognitive-behavioral (stress management) psychotherapies.

GENERALIZED ANXIETY DISORDER

Generalized anxiety disorder (GAD) is a common (lifetime prevalence 5%) anxiety disorder, the essential feature of which is chronic persistent anxiety for a period of more than 6 months. Patients usually are worrying excessively about a number of issues in their lives, report being unable to control the worrying, and are experiencing distress and impairment due to their symptoms. To meet DSM-IV (*Diagnostic and Statistical Manual of Mental Disorders*, Fourth Edition, American Psychiatric Association) criteria for GAD, patients also need to have three of six associated symptoms including restlessness, fatigue, difficulty concentrating, irritability, muscle tension, and sleep disturbance. The illness tends to develop during adolescence and early adulthood, running a chronic course thereafter. Symptoms tend to be exacerbated by stressful life events. There is some evidence that GAD is a familial condition related to major depression, although this finding awaits confirmation.

Several classes of medication are useful in the control of GAD symptoms. The partial serotonin 1A receptor agonist buspirone (BuSpar) is a safe first-line treatment. Although there is still controversy about whether buspirone is as effective as the benzodiazepines (BZDs) for GAD, its longer term use is not complicated by discontinuation or withdrawal syndromes. Patients are commenced on a regimen of 5 mg three times daily (tid) for 1 week and then increased to 10 mg tid, which is the average dose required. Therapeutic responses start to occur after 2 weeks of treatment. A maximal dose for buspirone is 60 mg per day. The main side effects early in treatment include dizziness, headaches, nausea, and sedation. Historically, the BZDs have been the mainstay of pharmacotherapy for GAD. These agents work rapidly, are safe, and are mostly inexpensive. Approximately 60 to 70% of patients will have a fair to good therapeutic response to a BZD trial. These agents are generally contraindicated in patients with a history of substance abuse. They should be considered a second-line choice for GAD because of the issue of physiologic dependence with chronic administration. Diazepam (Valium) 5 mg tid is a typical regimen. High-potency BZDs, such as lorazepam (Ativan) 1 mg tid or alprazolam (Xanax) 0.5 mg tid or four times a day, may also be used. The main early side effects of the BZDs include sedation, memory impairment, and ataxia. Patients should be warned about operating heavy machinery and about interaction with other sedative agents such as alcohol. The sedative effects of the BZDs should be tolerated after 1 to 2 weeks of therapy.

Antidepressants are indicated in GAD patients who have failed to respond to buspirone or BZD tri-

als. The tricyclic imipramine (Tofranil)* is the best studied of these, with well-controlled trials demonstrating efficacy and tolerability comparable to diazepam. Imipramine can be started at a dose of 25 mg at bedtime and increased by 25 mg per week until a target dose of 150 to 200 mg per day is reached. Patients should be cautioned about anticholinergic side effects, stimulation reactions (which can be seen with most antidepressants), and postural hypotension. Carbohydrate craving and weight gain are longer term side effects. If imipramine is poorly tolerated, other antidepressants worth trying include trazodone (Desyrel),* clomipramine (Anafranil),* the selective serotonin reuptake inhibitors (SSRIs),* and the newer antidepressants venlafaxine (Effexor)* and nefazodone (Serzone).* The duration of medical treatment for GAD exacerbations is generally 4 to 6 months at which time patients should be tapered from their medicines.

SOCIAL PHOBIA

Social phobia is an anxiety disorder characterized by intense anxiety before and during situations involving social interaction or task performance in front of others with consequent avoidance of these situations. A central feature of the patient's experience is a pervasive fear of negative criticism from others during social contact (see DSM-IV for details). The lifetime prevalence rates of social phobia in the general community range from 3 to 13%. Two subtypes of social phobia are recognized clinically, the specific or performance subtype and the generalized subtype. The specific subtype is not unlike other specific phobias (e.g., animal or height phobias). It is usually confined to one or two situations such as public speaking, writing in front of others, eating in front of others, or using public restrooms. By contrast, patients with generalized social phobia are much more impaired because they are fearful of most kinds of social contact.

The pharmacologic treatment of social phobia depends on the subtype. For the specific subtype, medication is used as an adjunct to cognitive-behavioral therapy. As-needed administration of a BZD or a beta blocker, or both, 30 to 60 minutes before a performance situation can be useful early in treatment. Of the BZDs, it is important to select an agent with a rapid onset of action such as diazepam 5 mg, alprazolam 0.5 mg, or lorazepam 0.5 to 1.0 mg. Of the beta blockers, atenolol (Tenormin) 25 to 50 mg orally is preferred because it is cardioselective and has poor central nervous system penetrance. Patients should take a test dose of these medications before using them in situations. Patients with generalized social phobia respond favorably to treatment with an SSRI (sertraline [Zoloft],* fluoxetine [Prozac],* fluvoxamine [Luvox],* or paroxetine [Paxil]*) or the monoamine oxidase inhibitor phenelzine (Nardil).* Tricyclic antidepressants are not particularly useful.

---

*Not FDA approved for this indication.

These patients may take 8 to 12 weeks to derive therapeutic benefit. After stabilization, a maintenance treatment period of at least 6 months is reasonable before a trial of taper. Typical effective dose ranges for the SSRIs are fluoxetine 20 to 80 mg per day, sertraline 50 to 200 mg per day, paroxetine 20 to 60 mg per day,* and fluvoxamine 150 to 300 mg per day. The effective dose range for phenelzine is 60 to 90 mg per day. With SSRIs, patients should be counseled about gastrointestinal, overstimulation, and sexual side effects. The last, however, may be advantageous to social phobics with sexual performance anxiety. Patients receiving phenelzine need to be advised about the necessity of adhering to a low-tyramine diet. Sedation, anticholinergic side effects, and postural hypotension are common with phenelzine. There are some data supporting the use of the BZD clonazepam (Klonopin)† in generalized social phobia. Clonazepam 0.5 mg tid orally is a typical starting regimen. Buspirone may also be a treatment option for patients who fail to respond to or are unsuitable for the protocols mentioned.

OBSESSIVE-COMPULSIVE DISORDER

Obsessive-compulsive disorder (OCD) is another common (lifetime prevalence 2.5%) anxiety disorder that causes a range of disability and runs a chronic course when it is untreated. Patients become symptomatic (as with most anxiety disorders) in the teenage and young adult years, although childhood onset is not uncommon. The cardinal symptoms of the disorder are obsessions and/or compulsions. Obsessions are unwanted, repetitive thoughts that are not a part of the patient's usual thinking. The obsessions often concern issues such as contamination, illness, violence, sexually inappropriate behavior, religion, and superstition. Compulsions are repetitive, voluntary behaviors that the patient has an overwhelming urge to enact. They often occur in response to obsessions and are designed to neutralize the obsession in some way. For example, compulsive hand washing is often an attempt to deal with contamination obsessions.

The treatment results with modern pharmacotherapy are only fair, with approximately 50% of all patients having satisfactory treatment responses. OCD symptoms respond preferentially to SSRI antidepressants and clomipramine (Anafranil), which is a nonselective serotonin reuptake blocker. Clomipramine, fluoxetine, fluvoxamine, and sertraline are approved by the Food and Drug Administration as antiobsessional medications. The conduct of SSRI therapy in OCD is similar to that described for social phobia. Clomipramine is a tricyclic antidepressant and hence carries an appreciable side effect burden as mentioned previously. In addition, sedation can be pronounced, even at low doses, and is a common cause of treatment noncompliance. Seizures are a significant risk above 250 mg per day. Patients can be started with 25 mg at bedtime and increased by 25 mg every 3 days until a target dose of 150 mg per day is reached. As with the SSRIs, it is important to wait 8 to 12 weeks at an effective dose to obtain therapeutic benefits. OCD patients with a history of Tourette's syndrome or motor tic disorder may benefit from the addition of a low dose of a neuroleptic agent such as haloperidol (Haldol) 0.5 to 1 mg at bedtime.

POST-TRAUMATIC STRESS DISORDER

Traumatic life events can lead to the anxiety syndrome of post-traumatic stress disorder (PTSD). In DSM-IV, a trauma is defined as an event or situation that poses a threat to life or a risk for serious injury to self or others. After exposure to the event, the individual's emotional response should include horror, helplessness, and intense fear. Some examples of traumatic events would be combat exposure, natural disasters, violent personal assault, and severe automobile accidents. Other diagnostic features are the presence of re-experiencing symptoms such as nightmares, flashbacks, or intrusive memories; the presence of avoidance of trauma-related cues and numbing of general responsiveness; and the presence of signs and symptoms of increased arousal. The syndrome must persist for more than a month to qualify for PTSD. Lifetime prevalence rates vary from 1 to 14%. Approximately one third of patients who develop acute PTSD will go on to develop chronic illness (lasting 3 months or more).

The management of PTSD depends on the duration of the clinical syndrome. Acute PTSD may be managed by debriefing, crisis counseling, peer and family support, and short-term pharmacotherapy with BZDs. The medical management of chronic PTSD is challenging because many patients in this phase of illness are treatment resistant. There is some evidence that antidepressants provide relief from re-experiencing symptoms. Amitriptyline (Elavil),* imipramine, phenelzine,* and fluoxetine* have some utility. Fluoxetine is thought to be of benefit for civilians with PTSD but not for combat-exposed veterans. BZDs are used sparingly for long-term treatment, particularly in populations of veterans, in whom substance abuse may be a prominent complication. However, they may provide short-term relief from hyperarousal symptoms such as irritability, increased startle, hypervigilance, and sleep disturbance.

*Not FDA approved for this indication.

BULIMIA NERVOSA

method of
B. TIMOTHY WALSH, M.D.
*Columbia University College of Physicians and
   Surgeons*
New York, New York

Bulimia nervosa refers to an eating disorder whose salient characteristic is frequent episodes of binge-eating,

---

*Exceeds dosage recommended by the manufacturer.
†Not FDA approved for this indication.

usually followed by self-induced vomiting. Whereas various patterns of excessive food intake have been noted for centuries, this syndrome was formally recognized and defined only about 15 years ago. Bulimia nervosa occurs primarily among young women, and epidemiologic studies suggest that between 1 and 3% of the young adult female population of the United States may suffer from this disorder. Although patients with bulimia nervosa recognize that their eating behavior is grossly abnormal and are typically concerned about their lack of control over eating, they are usually also ashamed of the disturbance and may come to medical attention only inadvertently or with great reluctance.

DIAGNOSIS

Diagnostic criteria for bulimia nervosa are presented in Table 1. The essential behavioral characteristic of this syndrome is the presence of recurrent episodes of binge-eating followed by inappropriate compensatory behavior to avoid weight gain. Many patients with bulimia nervosa consume impressive amounts of food during binges, ranging from 1000 to several thousand calories per episode. The current criteria require a minimal frequency of two episodes of binge-eating per week for at least 3 months for patients to qualify for the diagnosis. Although patients may plan their eating binges, once the eating has begun, they feel a limited amount of control over their eating behavior, and it is this sense of loss of control that is particularly distressing. Patients with bulimia nervosa regularly engage in activities intended to prevent the weight gain that would otherwise result from the binge-eating. Self-induced vomiting is the compensatory technique most frequently employed, occurring in 90% of patients with bulimia nervosa seen in eating disorder clinics. Other commonly employed techniques are the abuse of laxatives, diuretics, and diet pills; vigorous exercise; and severe food restriction when not binge-eating. Patients with bulimia nervosa are intensely concerned with their shape and weight and often base their self-esteem primarily on how much they weigh.

If the patient provides a full history, the diagnosis of bulimia nervosa is usually not difficult. However, because of the shame and embarrassment associated with this illness, patients, particularly when they visit their general physician, may not be forthcoming. Therefore, the physi-

cian should consider the diagnosis of bulimia nervosa in young women who express an intense desire to lose weight, who request prescriptions for diet pills or diuretics, or who exhibit some of the physical signs or symptoms or the laboratory abnormalities noted later. In such cases, the physician should gently but directly inquire about the occurrence of binge-eating and whether the patient has ever had the need to resort to the use of self-induced vomiting or the misuse of laxatives or diuretics out of fear of gaining weight.

For patients with bulimia nervosa of several years' duration, treatment by one of the established methods described later is indicated and should be initiated as soon as the diagnosis is established. However, the physician should also be aware that there are probably many individuals with mild variants of bulimia nervosa, for example, young people who, for a few months, binge-eat and occasionally induce vomiting. Although definitive information is not available, it is possible that brief interventions and counseling based on the approaches described later, perhaps augmented by recently developed self-help guides, may be sufficient to prevent such behavioral problems from progressing into full-blown bulimia nervosa.

CLINICAL CHARACTERISTICS

Most patients with bulimia nervosa are women in their late teens to mid-twenties. Most have had the disorder for several years before presenting for treatment and report that episodes of binge-eating occur five or more times weekly. The patients who present to clinics for treatment are usually of normal body weight, and about one quarter have past histories of anorexia nervosa. In the current diagnostic nomenclature, the diagnosis of bulimia nervosa cannot be applied to individuals who simultaneously meet criteria for anorexia nervosa. Therefore, individuals with anorexia nervosa who regularly engage in binge-eating and purging should be given the diagnosis of anorexia nervosa, binge-eating/purging type, not the diagnosis of bulimia nervosa, and treatment should be focused on anorexia nervosa.

The occurrence of binge-eating among the obese has recently attracted attention. Recurrent binge-eating appears to afflict a significant fraction of obese individuals presenting for weight loss treatment, but bulimia nervosa is uncommon, because most obese individuals with binge-

---

TABLE 1. **Diagnostic Criteria for Bulimia Nervosa**

A. Recurrent episodes of binge-eating. An episode of binge-eating is characterized by both of the following:
   (1) Eating, in a discrete period of time (e.g., within any 2-hour period), an amount of food that is definitely larger than most people would eat during a similar period of time and under similar circumstances.
   (2) A sense of lack of control over eating during the episode (e.g., a feeling that one cannot stop eating or control what or how much one is eating).
B. Recurrent inappropriate compensatory behavior in order to prevent weight gain, such as self-induced vomiting; misuse of laxatives, diuretics, enemas, or other medications; fasting; or excessive exercise.
C. The binge-eating and inappropriate compensatory behaviors both occur, on average, at least twice a week for 3 months.
D. Self-evaluation is unduly influenced by body shape and weight.
E. The disturbance does not occur exclusively during episodes of anorexia nervosa.

Specify type

Purging Type: during the current episode of bulimia nervosa, the person has regularly engaged in self-induced vomiting or the misuse of laxatives, diuretics, or enemas.

Nonpurging Type: during the current episode of bulimia nervosa, the person has used other inappropriate compensatory behaviors, such as fasting or excessive exercise, but has not regularly engaged in self-induced vomiting or the misuse of laxatives, diuretics, or enemas.

Reprinted with permission from the Diagnostic and Statistical Manual of Mental Disorders, Fourth Edition. Copyright 1994 American Psychiatric Association.

eating do not regularly engage in the inappropriate compensatory behaviors required for this diagnosis. (It has been suggested that the term binge-eating disorder be applied to obese or normal-weight individuals with recurrent binge-eating who do not engage in inappropriate compensatory behavior.)

PHYSICAL SIGNS AND COMPLICATIONS

There are no physical signs that are invariably present among patients with bulimia nervosa. However, in some individuals, the behavior may result in physical abnormalities that may be noted during physical examination and may alert the physician to the presence of this syndrome.

Significant dental problems have been reported in patients with bulimia nervosa, particularly among those who repeatedly induce vomiting. The lingual surfaces of the upper anterior teeth may become eroded and more sensitive to changes in temperature. As the biting edges deteriorate, the teeth may also take on a moth-eaten appearance. These dental problems appear to be caused by the repeated exposure of the teeth to stomach acid, gradually leading to decalcification and erosion of the lingual surfaces.

Some patients with bulimia nervosa, again primarily those who induce vomiting, develop painless bilateral salivary gland enlargement that is occasionally striking. The glandular enlargement appears to be due to hypertrophy, not to inflammatory cell infiltration, and usually diminishes if eating behavior normalizes.

Patients who induce vomiting by stimulating the gag reflex occasionally develop calluses on the dorsal surface of their hands, known as Russell's sign. The frequency of severe gastrointestinal complications in bulimia nervosa is low. Nonetheless, life-threatening complications have been reported, including esophageal tears and gastric rupture after binge-eating. There is a higher frequency of menstrual disturbance among women with bulimia nervosa compared with their peers, although it is not clear what features of the illness, such as the abnormal eating patterns or weight fluctuations, are responsible for these reproductive disturbances.

Some patients with bulimia nervosa resort to the use of syrup of ipecac to induce vomiting, and some such patients may be vulnerable to the development of myopathy because of toxic effects of absorbed emetine.

LABORATORY ABNORMALITIES

Patients who induce vomiting or abuse laxatives or diuretics are prone to develop the expected fluid and electrolyte disturbances. A significant fraction of patients who repeatedly induce vomiting develop hypokalemic alkalosis, which can occasionally be profound.

About one quarter of patients with bulimia nervosa have elevation of serum amylase values, which is largely of salivary origin and, presumably, is a reflection of the binge-eating and vomiting. A moderate elevation of the total amylase value in an otherwise healthy young person may therefore suggest the presence of bulimia nervosa.

ASSOCIATED PSYCHOLOGIC DISTURBANCES

It is now amply documented that patients with bulimia nervosa frequently exhibit disturbances of mood, typically a fluctuating level of depression accompanied by significant anxiety. It remains unclear to what degree such mood disturbances should be viewed as etiologic factors in the development of bulimia and to what degree as the result of a significant behavioral problem. However, it is important for the physician to inquire about the presence of depression.

Many patients with bulimia nervosa have current or past histories of drug abuse, particularly alcohol and stimulants that may initially have been used for weight reduction. In addition, patients may abuse, in large quantities, over-the-counter appetite suppressants and laxatives.

TREATMENT

In the last 15 years, two major treatment interventions have been developed for bulimia nervosa. One is a form of psychologic treatment, referred to as cognitive-behavioral therapy, and the second is the use of antidepressant medication. Both forms of treatment appear to be effective for many patients with bulimia nervosa, but definitive guidelines are not currently available to predict which patients respond preferentially to which form of treatment. Cognitive-behavioral therapy has the advantage of being time limited, usually requiring between 2 and 5 months, and, of course, does not entail the risk of medication side effects. On the other hand, this form of treatment is best conducted by therapists with specific training and experience, and it requires a serious commitment of time and energy from the patient. The use of antidepressant medication is more straightforward for most physicians; its major disadvantages are the risk of side effects and lack of certainty about how long antidepressant medication needs to be continued in patients who respond to it.

The cognitive-behavioral psychotherapy that has been developed for bulimia nervosa focuses specifically on the disturbed eating behavior. This form of treatment is pragmatic and relatively atheoretical—it does not assume any deep-seated psychologic causation for the eating disturbance. Rather, it focuses on the abnormal behavior and on maladaptive patterns of thinking that appear to perpetuate the eating disorder. Typically, patients in this form of therapy meet with the therapist once or twice a week for the first month of treatment. The patient is required to record the details of episodes of binge-eating, both the foods consumed and the environmental and emotional circumstances. The therapist helps the patient first to identify the factors that appear to trigger episodes of binge-eating and then to devise alternative coping methods. For example, most patients with bulimia nervosa are intensely and overly concerned with their weight and believe that the consumption of a "normal" diet will produce uncontrolled and unacceptable weight gain. They therefore frequently attempt to rigidly restrict their caloric intake and expect to remain in perfect control of their diet at all times. The constant caloric deprivation and psychologic pressure appear to set the stage for binge-eating, particularly at times of emotional stress. Cognitive-behavioral treatment attempts to educate the patient about the importance of maintaining caloric intake, to clarify the distortions of thinking, and to develop a more flexible and realistic approach to eating. The therapist in cognitive-behavioral treatment is active and directive, and in these ways, such therapy differs substantially from traditional psychoanalytic forms of psychotherapy.

There are now compelling data to suggest that many patients with bulimia nervosa have impressive and lasting responses to cognitive-behavioral treatment. This form of treatment is best delivered by a mental health practitioner with experience with cognitive-behavioral techniques and specifically with their application to patients with eating disorders. Self-help manuals based on the cognitive-behavioral approach have been published, and preliminary work suggests that their use may be of substantial benefit. Such manuals may provide access to cognitive-behavioral strategies in environments where experienced clinicians are unavailable.

The second major treatment modality for patients with bulimia nervosa is the use of antidepressant medication. The association between mood disturbance and bulimia nervosa has prompted more than a dozen double-blind, placebo-controlled trials, which have demonstrated conclusively that antidepressant medication, at least in the short term, is more effective than placebo in the treatment of bulimia nervosa. Most classes of antidepressant medication have been demonstrated to be effective. There have been no direct "head-to-head" trials comparing one antidepressant with another, and most antidepressants appear to have similar "antibulimic" efficacy. The choice of an antidepressant is therefore governed primarily by the frequency of side effects and by the risk for untoward reactions, and in these regards, the newer antidepressants, especially the selective serotonin reuptake inhibitors (SSRIs), are generally preferable.

Among the SSRIs, only fluoxetine (Prozac) has been rigorously studied in bulimia nervosa. Whereas a dose of 20 mg per day of fluoxetine is sufficient for the treatment of most patients with depression, 60 mg per day appears to be required for effective treatment of bulimia nervosa. Treatment with fluoxetine can be begun at 20 mg per day and quickly increased to 60 mg per day. For many patients, the response is rapid, with a clear decrease in binge-eating occurring 1 to 2 weeks after the initiation of fluoxetine. However, it is wise to continue fluoxetine for at least 4 weeks before concluding that a patient has failed to respond. Fluoxetine is usually well tolerated by patients with bulimia nervosa; common side effects include nausea, insomnia, and mild nervousness. Rarely, patients may develop a serious allergic reaction with features of serum sickness; the appearance of a rash should therefore prompt immediate consideration of discontinuing the fluoxetine.

The pharmacologic management of patients who fail to respond to fluoxetine is not well defined and is complicated by the long half-life of fluoxetine and by its inhibition of components of the cytochrome P-450 enzyme system. One strategy is to add a small dose (25 mg per day) of the tricyclic antidepressant desipramine (Norpramin)* to fluoxetine. Because of

*Not FDA approved for this indication.

fluoxetine's inhibition of the metabolism of desipramine, it is advisable to monitor plasma levels of desipramine. Because tricyclic antidepressants prolong cardiac conduction and can be dangerous in individuals with conduction disease, an electrocardiogram should be obtained before treatment with desipramine is initiated. If no improvement is apparent within 2 weeks, fluoxetine should be discontinued and a full trial of desipramine undertaken. The dose can be gradually increased to 150 to 250 mg per day, depending on side effects and on plasma level, which should be above 150 ng per mL but below 500 ng per mL. Because of the slow elimination of fluoxetine, the plasma desipramine level should be monitored periodically (e.g., every 2 weeks) until steady state is achieved.

Additional pharmacologic interventions include the use of other antidepressants (except bupropion [Wellbutrin], which has been associated with the occurrence of seizures in patients with bulimia nervosa) and, possibly, medications that are employed for weight loss, such as fenfluramine (Pondimin)* and phentermine (Fastin, Ionamin).* Such agents must be employed with caution because their effectiveness in bulimia nervosa is not established and weight loss in this population occasionally precipitates the development of anorexia nervosa. Although only rarely necessary, hospitalization should be considered for patients who have failed to respond to both structured forms of psychotherapy and antidepressant medication on an outpatient basis as well as for patients with severe or unstable medical complications.

*Not FDA approved for this indication.

DELIRIUM

method of
STUART C. YUDOFSKY, M.D.
Baylor College of Medicine
Houston, Texas

Delirium is a transient, organically induced change in mental status in which consciousness, thinking, mood, and behavior are affected. Disturbances in perception, in language, in the sleep-wake cycle, and in autonomic functioning are also common in this condition. The onset of delirium is usually abrupt, and—unusual for psychiatric disorders—the severity of the symptoms commonly fluctuates widely in a 24-hour period. During such fluctuations, the patient can temporarily become calm and lucid, which may lead to the false clinical conclusion that the condition and its underlying causes have been effectively treated. The duration of an episode of delirium is generally brief, persisting hours to weeks, with the symptoms worse at night and in unfamiliar, sensory-deprived environments, such as hospital intensive care units. Table 1 summarizes the common clinical features of delirium.

TABLE 1. **Clinical Features of Delirium**

Impaired Consciousness

Hypoactive state: reduced alertness, poor attention, distractibility, poor concentration, apathy, somnolence
Hyperactive state: hypervigilance, hyperattentiveness to irrelevant stimuli

Disorganized Thinking

Confused, rambling, incoherent, and irrelevant speech; bewilderment
Delusional: often fearful of being harmed or in danger; distrustful of unfamiliar people and settings

Altered Perception

Hallucinations: visual, auditory, and tactile
Illusions, including misrepresentations of visual, auditory, and tactile stimuli that lead to delusional fears

Behavioral and Motor Changes

Hypoactive state: lethargy, social withdrawal, disinterest, low levels of motivation; sluggish perseverative actions, reduced reflexes, hypotonic musculature
Hyperactive state: restlessness, uncooperative, oppositional; increased reflexes, myoclonus, hypertonic musculature, tremor

Memory Impairment

Poor registration and retention of new information; deficits in immediate recall; hazy recollections of past events

Disorientation

Disoriented to person, time, and place

Disturbed Affect

Hypoactive state: blunted emotional response, depressed, tearful, apathetic
Hyperactive state: anxious, fearful, apprehensive, irritable, rageful
(Note that affect is characteristically labile, involving fluctuations from hypoactive and hyperactive states.)

Autonomic Dysfunction

Flushing, sweating, tachycardia, mydriasis, palpitations, hypertension, fever, diarrhea, incontinence
Pallor, anhidrosis, bradycardia, hypotension, miosis, hypothermia, constipation, and urinary retention

Disturbed Sleep

Alterations in sleep-wake cycle, with restlessness and insomnia in the evenings and with daytime drowsiness

EPIDEMIOLOGY

It is likely that delirium is the most common and serious psychiatric syndrome that occurs among patients in the general hospital setting. Approximately 18% of general hospital patients develop delirium during their hospital stays, and fatality rates, depending on the population studied, range from 15 to 65%. Delirium occurs commonly across the entire life cycle, including in infants and children as well as among the elderly. At highest risk for delirium are people with pre-existing neurologic, metabolic, or oncologic disorders; people with multiple medical illnesses; those who are taking many types of medications; and those who abuse alcohol or psychoactive substances.

ETIOLOGY

Virtually any illness, medication, abused substance, or toxin that directly or indirectly affects the brain can lead to delirium. Table 2 summarizes the disorders and Table 3 the medications that most commonly lead to this syndrome.

EVALUATION AND DIAGNOSIS

History

The evaluation of delirium is directed toward discovering the medical condition or conditions that underlie the syndrome through careful history and physical examination, which, in turn, direct the types of laboratory tests that should be ordered. It is imperative to secure a comprehensive psychosocial history that includes information about the patient's pre-existing personality, temperament, psychiatric conditions, interpersonal relationships, and occu-

pational and family environments, because these factors may provide useful data about the causes and clinical manifestations of the delirium. An example would be a delirious patient with a history of multiple fights while intoxicated with alcohol. This information might direct the clinician to evaluate the patient for traumatic brain injury, for liver disease, and for the acute and withdrawal effects of alcohol and other substances of abuse as well as to alert the nursing staff about the high potential for agitated or aggressive behavior.

Laboratory Testing

When the underlying cause of delirium is unclear from the history and physical examination, the following diagnostic tests should be considered: complete blood count; blood chemistries including electrolytes, blood urea nitrogen, liver function tests, creatinine, and glucose; thyroid function tests; blood and/or urine screening for alcohol, drugs, heavy metals, or poisons; electrocardiogram; chest radiograph; and electroencephalogram (EEG). The classic EEG pattern for delirium is generalized slowing in both the hypoactive and the hyperactive presentations. However, in delirium associated with alcohol or barbiturate intoxication or with alcohol withdrawal—including delirium tremens—high-voltage, fast-wave activity may occur. Advances in EEG technology that include quantitative EEG and spectral analysis techniques have increased the diagnostic sensitivity of the test. Special tests of patients suspected of having delirium may be indicated by initial history, physical examination, and screening test results. These commonly include lumbar puncture, arterial blood gas analysis, blood cultures, computed tomographic brain scan, or magnetic resonance imaging. Finally, careful docu-

TABLE 2. **Common Causes of Delirium**

Infectious

Virtually any bacterial or viral infection that leads to systemic illness and/or encephalitis, meningitis, or abscess
Common causes: meningococcus, syphilis, streptococcus, tuberculosis, and acquired immune deficiency syndrome

Metabolic

Fluid and electrolyte imbalance, acid-base imbalance; renal failure, uremia; hepatic failure; anemias, vitamin deficiencies, endocrinopathies

Central Nervous System

Seizures, stroke, traumatic brain injury, tumors, autoimmune-inflammatory disorders, degenerative diseases, hydrocephalus

Withdrawal States

Alcohol, barbiturates, benzodiazepines, sedative hypnotics, analgesics, opiates

Cardiopulmonary

Shock, hypoxia, myocardial infarction, congestive heart failure, hypotension, hypertensive encephalopathy, respiratory failure

Toxic or Heavy Metal

Pesticides; industrial solvents, lead, mercury, and manganese

Medications and Drugs

Virtually any substance of abuse, particularly cocaine, amphetamines, phencyclidine, lysergic acid diethylamide (LSD), alcohol, marijuana, opiates, barbiturates, in both toxic and withdrawal states
For medications associated with delirium, see Table 3

Miscellaneous

Intense or unusual environmental stimuli; sensory deprivation; postoperative conditions; temperature dysregulation

---

mentation in the medical record of a patient's mental status during evaluation and treatment stages is helpful to record the pattern of delirium as well as to assess whether the syndrome is improving with treatment.

Physical Examination

In diagnosing medical conditions that underlie delirium, all aspects of the comprehensive physical examination can, and often do, provide vital information. Careful observation of the patient, both during episodes of delirious agitation and confusion and during calm periods, cannot be overemphasized. For example, in the case of the aforementioned patient with alcohol dependency and traumatic brain injury, observation of the skin would have revealed abrasions around the knuckles, bruising about the face, and swelling of the scalp from recent fighting; diaphoretic wetness of the skin from the autonomic dysfunction of alcohol withdrawal; and petechiae and asterixis from the associated liver disorder.

TREATMENT

The first principle in the treatment of delirium is the precise diagnosis and rapid reversal, where possible, of the medical condition that underlies the disorder. For example, if the delirium is secondary to a toxic dose of a medication (e.g., lithium) or an abused substance (e.g., methamphetamine), discontinuation of the drug and, if required, procedures to remove the substance from the patient's system (e.g., dialysis) are the first steps of treatment. Similarly, if the delirium stems from acute, life-threatening illnesses such as bacterial encephalopathy, subarachnoid bleeding, or metabolic acidosis, rapid diagnosis and focused treatment are critical.

The second aspect of care is the simultaneous treatment of the symptoms of delirium. Should the patient exhibit psychosis such as visual hallucinations, paranoid thoughts, and/or manic affects, an antipsychotic medication is indicated. In the hospital setting, haloperidol (Haldol) is most frequently used for this purpose because of its reduced anticholinergic properties and fewer cardiovascular side effects compared with other neuroleptics. Haloperidol may also be administered to the patient orally, intramuscularly, and intravenously. For the frail or elderly patient, initiate treatment with low doses such as 0.5 mg orally or intramuscularly twice per day and at bedtime. Substantially higher doses (e.g., 4 mg every 6 hours while awake) may be required for younger and stronger patients. New-generation antipsychotic drugs including risperidone (Risperdal) 0.5 to 2 mg two times a day and olanzapine (Zyprexa) 5 to 10 mg once a day are gaining increased use in the treatment of delirium because of their advantage of not having extrapyramidal side effects. When the patient with delirium also exhibits irritability, agitation, or oppositional behaviors, acute sedation may be required. The two categories of medications most commonly used for this purpose are antipsychotic drugs, in the dose regimen described before, and benzodiazepines. Lorazepam (Ativan), a benzodiazepine, may be used by itself or in combination with haloperidol for severely agitated patients with delirium. Initiate lorazepam with a test dose of 1 mg (orally, intramuscularly, or intravenously) and observe the ensuing level of sedation and calmness during the next 45 minutes. If little change has occurred, add 2 mg every hour until behavioral control is achieved. Thereafter, use the time between administration of the medication and the return of the agitation to gauge the frequency of dosing. Note that lorazepam is an excellent medication to treat the agitation associated with de-

TABLE 3. **Medications Causing Delirium**

Analgesics	**Anticonvulsants**	**Drug Withdrawal**
Meperidine	Phenobarbital	Alcohol
Opiates	Phenytoin	Barbiturates
Pentazocine	Valproic acid	Benzodiazepines
Salicylates	**Anti-inflammatory Drugs**	**Sedative Hypnotics**
Antibiotics	ACTH	Barbiturates
Acyclovir, ganciclovir	Corticosteroids	Benzodiazepines
Aminoglycosides	Ibuprofen	Glutethimide
Amodiaquine*	Indomethacin	**Sympathomimetics**
Amphotericin B	Naproxen	Aminophylline
Cephalexin	Phenylbutazone	Amphetamines
Cephalosporins	Steroids	Cocaine
Chloramphenicol	**Antineoplastic Drugs**	Ephedrine
Chloroquine	Aminoglutethimide	Epinephrine
Ethambutol	Asparaginase	Phenylephrine
Gentamicin	Decarbazine	Phenylpropanolamine
Interferon	5-Fluorouracil	Theophylline
Sulfonamides	Hexamethylenamine	**Miscellaneous Drugs**
Tetracycline	Methotrexate (high dose)	Baclofen
Ticarcillin	Tamoxifen	Bromides
Vancomycin	Vinblastine	Chlorpropamide
Anticholinergic Drugs	Vincristine	Cimetidine
Antihistamines (e.g., chlorpheniramine)	**Antiparkinsonian Drugs**	Disulfiram
Antispasmodics	Amantadine	Ergotamines
Atropine/homatropine	Bromocriptine	Lithium
Belladonna alkaloids	Carbidopa	Metrizamide
Benztropine	Levodopa	Metronidazole
Biperiden	**Antituberculous Drugs**	Phenelzine
Diphenhydramine	Isoniazid	Podophyllin (by absorption)
Phenothiazines (especially thioridazine)	Rifampin	Procarbazine
Promethazine	**Cardiac Drugs**	Propylthiouracil
Scopolamine	Beta blockers (e.g., propranolol)	Quinacrine
Tricyclic antidepressants (especially amitriptyline)	Captopril	Ranitidine
Trihexyphenidyl	Clonidine	Timolol ophthalmic
	Digitalis	
	Disopyramide	
	Lidocaine	
	Mexiletine	
	Methyldopa	
	Quinidine	
	Procainamide	
	Tocainide	

*Not available in the United States.

Reprinted from Wise MG, Gray KF: Delirium, dementia, and amnestic disorders. *In* Hales RE, Yudofsky SC (eds): American Psychiatric Press Textbook of Neuropsychiatry, 2nd ed. Washington, DC, American Psychiatric Press, 1994.

lirium because of its multiple routes of administration, because of its intermediate-range half-life, and because it can be used in patients with liver disease. To avoid potentially disabling side effects, both antipsychotic drugs and benzodiazepines should be tapered, usually in 3 to 4 days, as soon as the delirium subsides.

Concurrent with the treatment of the underlying causes and the symptomatic manifestations of delirium are psychosocial and environmental interventions. These include encouraging (1) regular and frequent interactions with trusted relatives and friends of the patient; (2) repeated reassurance and support from the medical staff; (3) reorientation of the patient with use of clocks, calendars, secured windows, and radio and television news programs; (4) reduction of distracting stimuli such as loud noises and bright lights; and (5) removal from the patient's immediate environment of dangerous and frightening objects, such as sharp knives, containers with hot liquids, and the like. The physician should devote adequate time to communicate with the family members and endeavor to answer their questions about the meaning and duration of delirium. This communication is especially important because the patient, on recovery, is likely to be amnestic for much of the course of the delirium and will question family members about such. Similarly, on resolution of the patient's delirium, the physician should explain to the patient the meaning of what has occurred in the context of preventing future episodes of delirium as well as to allay fears about and misinterpretations of the event.

MOOD DISORDERS

method of
DAVID L. DUNNER, M.D.
University of Washington
Seattle, Washington

Mood disorders are prevalent among community samples and in general practice settings. Studies suggest that at least 3 to 10% of the general population will experience a significant mood disorder in their lifetime and that 15 to 30% of patients seen in primary care settings have a mood disorder. Unfortunately, considerable misdiagnosis and undertreatment of mood disorders occur in primary care settings. Mood disorders are associated with both physical and psychosocial dysfunction. About 15% of patients with depression die as a result of suicide. The economic cost of depression in the United States was estimated in 1990 at more than $40 billion annually. This figure included both direct and indirect costs. In spite of the finding that patients with mood disorders are misdiagnosed and undertreated in primary care settings, depression is relatively easy to diagnose and newer treatments are enhancing compliance, with the result that treatment is being (increasingly) more effective. In this chapter, I review the types of mood disorders and discuss their treatment.

DEFINITIONS

The key to the diagnosis of all mood disorders is the *Diagnostic and Statistical Manual of Mental Disorders*, Fourth Edition (DSM-IV) definition of major depressive episode. Symptoms and behaviors of a major depressive episode include depressed mood, decreased interest in usual activities (anhedonia), weight loss or weight gain, oversleeping or undersleeping, psychomotor agitation or retardation, fatigue or loss of energy, feelings of worthlessness or guilt, difficulty concentrating, and suicidal thoughts. If five of these symptoms (including depressed mood or anhedonia) are present nearly every day for 2 weeks or longer, the condition is termed a major depressive episode. If there is no other exclusionary condition, the diagnosis is major depressive disorder, which can be classified as single episode, recurrent, chronic (lasting 2 years or more), or in partial remission and in terms of severity (mild, moderate, severe), with psychotic features, with melancholic features, with catatonic features, with atypical features (not meeting criteria for melancholic features and presence of mood reactivity, weight gain, hypersomnia, leaden paralysis, and interpersonal rejection sensitivity), with postpartum onset (if the disorder begins within 4 weeks postpartum), and with seasonal pattern (regular occurrence of onsets and offsets of symptoms at particular times of the year). Major depressive disorder affects women more frequently than men. The initial episode can be at any age, and the disorder is recurrent in almost half of cases.

If the symptoms of major depressive episode are present sporadically more days than not (but not every day in 2-week intervals) for 2 years or more, the condition would be termed dysthymic disorder. The DSM-IV criteria for dysthymic disorder are at variance with this definition, but all patients I have studied who met criteria for dysthymic disorder also met this definition. Dysthymic disorder is a persistent condition with age at onset frequently in childhood or adolescence. Dysthymic disorder can be compli-cated by single or recurrent episodes of major depressive disorder (so-called double depression).

If the depressive disorder is associated with manic episodes (a week or longer of symptoms including elated or irritable mood, grandiosity, decreased need for sleep, racing thoughts, distractibility, increase in activity, and impulsive behavior) that cause severe disruption in psychosocial function or result in hospitalization, bipolar I disorder is classified. Bipolar I disorder affects women and men equally. The onset is generally after puberty, and first episodes after 40 years of age are unusual. The course of the disorder is generally marked by recurrent manic and major depressive episodes.

If the symptoms of a manic episode are mild and last for 4 days or more and are *not* socially incapacitating, the condition is diagnosed as hypomanic episode. Bipolar II disorder is diagnosed if there are one or more hypomanic episodes and major depressive episodes. Patients with bipolar II disorder usually present with histories of recurrent depression. Hypomanic episodes are usually productive periods, and patients do not consider them a sign of illness. The depressions can be severe, and suicide attempts and death from suicide are common.

Cyclothymic disorder, mixed bipolar I disorder, and rapid cycling all present instances of frequent mood alterations of manic or hypomanic and depressive symptoms. In cyclothymic disorder, the mood disorder persists for 2 years or more, the highs are too brief to meet criteria for hypomanic episode (less than 4 days), and the depressions are too brief to meet criteria for major depressive episode (less than 2 weeks). In general, cyclothymic disorder is a condition seen among outpatients. Mixed bipolar I disorder is a manic (severe) condition with symptoms of manic episode and symptoms of a major depressive episode present every day for at least a 1-week period. Rapid cycling is a longitudinal course modifier that can be applied to patients with bipolar I or bipolar II disorder if there are four or more hypomanic, manic, mixed, or major depressive episodes in a 1-year period. Rapid cycling patients are much more likely to be women than men and may have histories of thyroid dysfunction. They show a poorer response to lithium maintenance therapy than do non–rapid cycling bipolar patients.

If a depressive syndrome occurs in the context of a significant life event, adjustment disorder with depressed mood is diagnosed. However, if the symptoms persist to meet criteria for major depressive episode, then major depressive disorder is the appropriate diagnosis.

Uncomplicated bereavement is also characterized by the symptoms of major depressive episode. However, if depressive symptoms persist for more than 2 months or are severe, a diagnosis of major depressive disorder is made.

A mood disorder occurring in the context of a medical condition that might cause the symptoms (such as hypothyroidism or other endocrine dysfunction, cancer of the pancreas or other malignant neoplasm) is classified as mood disorder due to a general medical condition. A mood disorder that might be related to substance use (e.g., amphetamines, cocaine) or use of medication (e.g., antihypertensives) is classified as substance-induced mood disorder. Both mood disorder due to a general medical condition and substance-induced mood disorder can be specified as depression-like, major depression–like, with manic features, or with mixed features, depending on presenting symptoms. Interestingly, if a patient develops a hypomanic or manic episode while being treated for depression with an antidepressant, the condition is technically not rediagnosed as bipolar but instead is termed major depressive disorder with antidepressant-induced hypomania. It is my view that such patients do, indeed, have bipolar disorder and should be treated accordingly.

Mood disorders that do not meet criteria for any of the preceding conditions are diagnosed with a residual category not otherwise specified (NOS). A listing of NOS disorders thought to merit further study before their inclusion in the DSM system is provided in the Appendix of the DSM-IV. Some of these conditions, such as recurrent brief depression, are listed in the *International Statistical Classification of Diseases and Related Health Problems*, 10th revision (ICD-10).

Mood disorders due to a general medical condition and substance-induced mood disorders are examples of co-morbidity (having two or more conditions simultaneously). Mood disorders can complicate other psychiatric conditions (such as panic disorder and Axis II personality disorders), and other psychiatric conditions can complicate the course of mood disorders. Co-morbidity is a common clinical situation and has treatment implications. Patients with multiple disorders are more difficult to treat than are patients with a single disorder. One approach to co-morbidity is to establish which disorder is "primary" (came first) and try to treat the primary disorder in hopes that the co-morbid condition will abate. In some instances (e.g., obsessive-compulsive disorder with "secondary" major depressive disorder), the treatment might be a serotonergic antidepressant. In other conditions (e.g., primary major depressive disorder with secondary alcoholism), treatment of both the primary and secondary disorder may need to be considered independently.

Most patients with depressive mood states also experience anxiety, and anxiety can be the chief complaint for patients best diagnosed as depressed. The differentiation of generalized anxiety disorder from major depressive disorder can pose difficulties, especially in primary care settings, and result in inappropriate treatment with benzodiazepines rather than with antidepressants. In general, anxiety disorders have their onset before age 35 years, are chronic, and are usually accompanied by panic attacks. Major depressive disorder can have an early or late age at onset and is frequently episodic. The diagnosis of major depressive disorder alone and not major depressive disorder and generalized anxiety disorder is made for those patients who meet criteria for both conditions.

TREATMENT OF MOOD DISORDERS

Treatment of a patient with a mood disorder depends on the phase of illness being treated (acute, chronic, or recurrent depression or acute or recurrent mania), its severity, and whether the condition is a bipolar or unipolar condition. The components of treatment are varied and include pharmacotherapy; psychotherapies that have been developed for the treatment of depression; and physical therapies, such as electroconvulsive treatment and bright light therapy.

Pharmacotherapy

All medications approved for the treatment of depression show equal efficacy (Table 1). About 70% of depressed outpatients respond at 4 to 6 weeks of treatment once an effective dose is achieved. Because medications show equal efficacy, I recommend that the first choice of an antidepressant be based on side effects and tolerability. Selective serotonin reuptake inhibitors (SSRIs) are the preferred first-choice treatment of depression. SSRIs show efficacy equal to that of other antidepressants but lower dropout rates because of side effects, especially compared with tricyclic antidepressants (TCAs). TCAs are unsafe in overdose situations, and 1.5 grams of a TCA can be lethal in overdose. SSRIs and other newer medications are generally safe in overdose. TCAs have cardiovascular effects and a broad side effect profile related to their lack of receptor specificity.

Selective Serotonin Reuptake Inhibitors

SSRIs are thought to be effective by increasing serotonin at the postsynaptic nerve ending by blocking the reuptake of serotonin into the presynaptic nerve. Other mechanisms have also been suggested, but all involve effects on serotonergic nerve transmission.

The SSRIs approved in the United States for treatment of depression include fluoxetine (Prozac), sertraline (Zoloft), and paroxetine (Paxil). Fluvoxamine (Luvox) is approved for treatment of obsessive-compulsive disorder. These medications are more similar to each other than dissimilar in terms of side effects. The common side effects of SSRIs include gastrointestinal disturbances, mostly nausea and occasionally diarrhea; occasional insomnia (about 15% of patients); occasional sedation (about 15% of patients); and sexual dysfunction (ejaculatory disturbances in men and delayed orgasm and decreased sexual desire in women). Drug interactions with the cytochrome P-450IID6 enzyme system can occur, and coadministration of TCAs with SSRIs can result in elevated TCA blood levels. Sertraline and fluvoxamine also significantly inhibit the cytochrome P-450IIIA4 system.

SSRIs are given once daily, usually in the morning, and the gastrointestinal side effects seem to be prevented by taking SSRIs with a large glass of water with a meal. If the patient develops sedation, the medication can be switched to bedtime. If, when taking an SSRI, the patient develops treatment-emergent insomnia, I would recommend the addition of a sedative agent. Abrupt discontinuation of sertraline and paroxetine has been associated with a syndrome characterized by anxiety, insomnia, gastrointestinal symptoms, and agitation. Tapering of these compounds is advised. Concomitant use of SSRIs with monoamine oxidase inhibitors (MAOIs) has resulted in severe drug interactions and fatality. SSRIs show a broad spectrum of clinical activity and are effective in the treatment of obsessive-compulsive disorder, panic disorder, bulimia nervosa, and social phobia as well as depression.

Fluoxetine is usually administered as 20 mg once daily. The need for dose titration is less than for other SSRIs. In depressed patients with excessive anxiety, elderly patients, and depressed patients with secondary panic attacks, beginning at 10 mg or even 5 mg can be beneficial. Doses above 60 mg in general do not enhance antidepressant response. Fluoxetine

TABLE 1. **Antidepressants**

Drug	Adult Therapeutic Dose Range (mg/d)	Dosing	Relative Need for Dose Titration	Safety in Overdose	Notable Side Effects
Fluoxetine (Prozac)	20–60	qd	Low	Yes	
Sertraline (Zoloft)	50–200	qd	Moderate	Yes	
Paroxetine (Paxil)	20–50	qd	Low	Yes	
Fluvoxamine (Luvox)*	50–200	qd	Moderate	Yes	
Venlafaxine (Effexor)	75–450†	bid	High	Yes	Hypertension
Nefazodone (Serzone)	300–600	bid	Moderate	Yes	
Mirtazapine (Remeron)	15–60	qd	Moderate	Yes	
Trazodone (Desyrel)	150–600	qd to bid	Moderate	Yes	Priapism (males)
Bupropion (Wellbutrin)	225–450	bid to tid	Moderate	Yes	Seizure
Amitriptyline (Elavil)	75–300	qd	High	No	
Imipramine (Tofranil)	75–300	qd	High	No	
Doxepin (Sinequan)	75–300	qd	High	No	
Nortriptyline (Pamelor)	50–200	qd	High	No	
Desipramine (Norpramin)	50–200	qd	High	No	
Protriptyline (Vivactil)	20–60	qd	High	No	
Trimipramine (Surmontil)	75–300	qd	High	No	
Clomipramine (Anafranil)*	75–300	qd	High	No	Seizure
Maprotiline (Ludiomil)	100–225	qd	High	No	Seizure
Amoxapine (Asendin)	100–600	qd	High	Yes	Dopamine-blocking effects

*Approved treatment of obsessive-compulsive disorder and not currently approved in the United States for treatment of depressive disorder.
†Exceeds dosage recommended by the manufacturer.

has a long half-life (72 hours) and an active metabolite (norfluoxetine) with a longer (7-day) half-life. This property may be an advantage in the noncompliant depressed patient and in instances when long-term treatment is indicated. Also, discontinuation side effects are unusual. A long half-life can be a disadvantage in situations calling for rapid drug discontinuation, as in the instance of a depressed patient with an unstable medical condition or when switching to an MAOI is the next treatment sequence.

Sertraline can be associated with more treatment-emergent diarrhea than the other SSRIs. The beginning dose is usually 50 mg, and dose titration is required more frequently with sertraline than with other SSRIs. The dose range is up to 200 mg daily. Beginning with lower doses in anxious patients, patients with panic disorder, or the elderly is usually advised. Sertraline has a short half-life (24 hours) and an active metabolite (norsertraline) that has a 72-hour half-life.

Paroxetine is usually administered in 20-mg doses. The need for titration is intermediate for paroxetine compared with fluoxetine and sertraline. Paroxetine has a short half-life (24 hours) and no active metabolite. Discontinuation side effects are seen more frequently with abrupt discontinuation of paroxetine than with the other SSRIs. The dose range for paroxetine is 20 to 50 mg, and half this dose is recommended as a starting dose for elderly patients or patients with panic disorder.

Fluvoxamine is usually begun at 50 mg with dose increments to 150 or 200 mg per day. Fluvoxamine is not approved in the United States for treatment of depression but rather is approved for treatment of obsessive-compulsive disorder. This medication, however, has been used worldwide for the treatment of depressive conditions. Fluvoxamine inhibits a number of cytochrome P-450 enzymes, particularly cytochrome P-450IIIA4, and concomitant administration of terfenadine (Seldane), astemizole (Hismanal), triazolam (Halcion), alprazolam (Xanax), and cisapride (Propulsid) are to be avoided.

Newer Medications

Venlafaxine (Effexor) is a serotonin and norepinephrine reuptake inhibitor that shares side effects of SSRIs (such as gastrointestinal side effects and sexual dysfunction) and can also cause hypertension in some patients. Hypertension is usually dose related above 225 mg per day and occurs in a small percentage of patients, but blood pressure monitoring is usually advised while patients are taking this drug. I recommend starting at very low doses of venlafaxine (usually half of a 37.5-mg pill per day) and increasing that dose every 3 days as tolerated to a starting plateau of 150 mg per day; waiting at that dose for about 3 weeks to determine whether there is a clinical effect and, if not, increasing to 300 mg per day; waiting another 3 weeks and then titrating to 450 mg* per day for an additional 3 or 4 weeks to determine whether there is a response. In general, venlafaxine is quite useful in depressed patients who are treatment resistant to other antidepressant agents. Venlafaxine is metabolized by the cytochrome P-450IID6 enzyme system. It is possible that at

*Exceeds dosage recommended by the manufacturer.

higher doses there may be inhibition of cytochrome P-450IID6, but coprescription of a TCA during treatment with venlafaxine would appear illogical. Discontinuation side effects similar to those of sertraline and paroxetine have been observed.

Nefazodone (Serzone) has a serotonin reuptake effect and also down-regulates serotonin type 2 (5-HT$_2$) receptors. Nefazodone effects on the noradrenergic system are weak. Priapism associated with trazodone, a related compound, is not observed with nefazodone. Somnolence is a major side effect, and nefazodone seems to lack the sexual dysfunction effects associated with the SSRIs. Dose titration is required. The usual starting dose is 100 mg twice daily, and I aim for 300 mg per day as an initial dose level. Doses can be increased to 600 mg per day in divided doses. Nefazodone is an inhibitor of the cytochrome P-450IIIA4 enzyme system.

Mirtazapine (Remeron) is the latest medication to be added to the list of antidepressants in the United States. This medication is given at bedtime in starting doses of 15 mg with dose increments to 45 or 60 mg. It is sedating as a result of its histamine-receptor blockade. Mirtazapine blocks 5-HT$_2$ and 5-HT$_3$ receptors; thus, nausea is less frequently seen with mirtazapine than with SSRIs, and sexual dysfunction should be a rarely experienced side effect. Sedation and weight gain (related to histamine$_1$-receptor blockade) seem to the most prominent side effects of mirtazapine. Two cases of agranulocytosis with mirtazapine were reported in clinical trials. No effects on the cytochrome P-450 enzyme system have been reported.

Tricyclic Antidepressants

The TCAs are generally divided into the secondary and tertiary amines. The tertiary amine tricyclics (imipramine, doxepin, and amitriptyline) tend to have more sedating side effects than the secondary amine tricyclics (nortriptyline and desipramine), which are not activating as had previously been thought but are actually less sedating than the tertiary amine TCAs. Two other TCAs, protriptyline and trimipramine, are less frequently used. Clomipramine (a TCA) is marketed in the United States for treatment of obsessive-compulsive disorder but is also used in Europe for the treatment of mood disorders.

Amitriptyline (Elavil and others), imipramine (Tofranil and others), and doxepin (Sinequan) are generally given in single daily dosing at bedtime. Dose titration of these compounds is required, and usual starting doses are 50 mg with dose titration upward, as tolerated, to 300 mg per day. In the elderly, beginning at lower doses, i.e., 5 or 10 mg, may be preferable. For the secondary amine TCAs desipramine (Norpramin) and nortriptyline (Pamelor), starting doses are generally in the same range, with maximal doses of about 200 mg per day. Blood level monitoring of nortriptyline has been suggested as relevant for depressed inpatients, with a blood level range of 50 to 150 ng per mL reflecting optimal plasma levels.

Higher and lower blood levels than this "therapeutic window" are associated with lessened therapeutic response. Determination of this blood level response range in outpatients is lacking, however. Trimipramine (Surmontil) dosing is similar to that of desipramine. Protriptyline (Vivactil) is a more potent compound, and beginning doses are about 10 mg per day, with maximal doses in the range of 30 to 40 mg per day.

The side effects of TCAs are multiple and are a result of the effects of TCAs on numerous receptors. Anticholinergic side effects include dry mouth, blurring of vision, constipation, urinary retention, increased sweating, and increased heart rate. Antihistaminic effects include sedation and weight gain, and alpha-adrenergic effects include blood pressure changes. These medications have quinidine-like effects on cardiac rhythms. Seizures and cardiac dysrhythmias occur in overdose situations. Approximately 7000 TCA overdose deaths occur in the United States annually.

I have found TCAs, especially the more sedating ones (amitriptyline, imipramine, or doxepin) useful should a male patient have treatment-emergent insomnia when being treated with an SSRI. In women, I prefer to use trazodone for this sedating effect. (I do not recommend trazodone for men because of the potential for the occurrence of priapism.) In patients who have chronic pain and depression, combined treatment with an SSRI and a TCA may be optimal. Blood levels of TCAs can be elevated when they are coadministered with SSRIs, and thus blood level monitoring of the TCA might be useful.

Heterocyclics

No classification of antidepressant is entirely satisfactory, but in general what are called the heterocyclic antidepressants (to differentiate them from the TCAs) might include four compounds. Maprotiline (Ludiomil) is similar to TCAs, tends to be noradrenergic in terms of its biologic function rather than serotonergic, and has efficacy similar to that of desipramine. It also has a higher seizure rate than desipramine, and I generally do not recommend its use for this reason because other medications are available. Amoxapine (Asendin) has a tetracyclic structure and is metabolized to a compound that has dopamine-blocking effects. Thus, amoxapine can be associated with Parkinson-like side effects and the possibility of developing a tardive dyskinesia syndrome. Although one would think that amoxapine might be an ideal drug for the treatment of patients with psychotic depression (because its dopamine-blocking effects would be important for antipsychotic efficacy), the use of an antidepressant plus an antipsychotic generally would be preferred because the dose of each medication could be better controlled. I also do not recommend amoxapine for the treatment of depressed patients.

Trazodone (Desyrel) has serotonergic effects, particularly down-regulation of postsynaptic 5-HT$_2$ receptors. Trazodone is safe in overdose. The major difficulty with trazodone as noted before is the possibility of development of priapism in male patients. Thus, I do not recommend that trazodone be used as a first-line treatment for depressed male patients. The use of trazodone has probably increased considerably in the past few years as a sedative medication in depressed women who are taking SSRIs and who develop treatment-emergent insomnia. Doses of 50 to 150 mg per day are common in primary care settings. Higher doses, up to 400 to 600 mg per day, are sometimes used in psychiatric practice. Sedation is a common side effect.

Bupropion (Wellbutrin) is a noradrenergic receptor blockade medication that is activating. Its major dangerous side effect involves seizures, and the risk for seizures can be increased if the patient has a prior seizure history, a history of head trauma or loss of consciousness, a family history of seizures, or a personal history of bulimia or if the patient takes bupropion at too high of a single dose (above 200 mg) or increases the dose above 450 mg per day. Given these caveats, bupropion is effective and is widely prescribed by psychiatrists although less so by primary care physicians. It should be used in multiple daily dosing two or three times a day and doses increased toward 450 mg per day. Insomnia is a frequent side effect.

Monoamine Oxidase Inhibitors

The MAOIs have food and drug interactions that can result in hypertensive crises. MAOIs are not recommended if the patient has recently taken an antidepressant (2-week washout period is recommended; 5 weeks for fluoxetine), and patients should be drug free for 2 weeks after stopping an MAOI before using another antidepressant. A low-tyramine diet is recommended. The MAOIs in general cause side effects such as sedation and weight gain. Phenelzine (Nardil) is quite effective for the treatment of not only major depression but also panic disorder. The initial dose is 45 mg (15 mg three times daily [tid]), and 60 to 90 mg is the usual antidepressant dose range. Tranylcypromine (Parnate) may be quite effective for the treatment of bipolar depression and tends to be less sedating than phenelzine. The usual starting dose is 30 mg (10 mg tid), and doses in the range of 60 to 90 mg are common.

Sustained-Release Preparations

Several sustained-release preparations are being studied, and some are likely to be approved for use by the Food and Drug Administration by the time of publication of this volume. The advantages of sustained-release preparations include less frequent dosing (and thus increasing compliance of the patient) and alleviation of side effects associated with rapid discontinuation. Sustained-release preparations of bupropion, venlafaxine, and paroxetine have been studied, and sustained-release bupropion has been approved.

Psychotherapy

A number of psychotherapies have been developed and studied for the treatment of depressive conditions. Two in particular, interpersonal psychotherapy (IPT) and cognitive-behavioral psychotherapy (CBT), have been shown in controlled studies of depressed outpatients to be effective, especially in milder cases of depression. Treatment manuals for IPT and CBT have been developed to guide the therapeutic process. These psychotherapies tend to be brief (16 to 20 sessions) and are administered once or twice a week. The use of other psychotherapies in depressed patients may be effective, but the data demonstrating efficacy for other treatments are generally lacking from controlled treatment trials.

Cognitive-Behavioral Psychotherapy

CBT was developed by Beck and associates and relies on the observation that depressed patients frequently have negative thoughts (cognitions). The treatments are generally effected by having patients examine these negative thoughts in view of current ongoing behavior. Homework assignments are given, and the emphasis is on current activities. A form of CBT has been developed for the treatment of chronically depressed outpatients.

Interpersonal Psychotherapy

IPT was developed by Klerman and colleagues and is a therapy more psychoanalytic than CBT in its framework, involving emphasis on how depressed patients interact with other individuals and their explorations of early childhood experiences. The emphasis of IPT is largely on current life events.

Physical Treatments

Electroconvulsive therapy (ECT) is an effective treatment of severe depression, depression with psychotic features, and depression with catatonic features. ECT can also be effective for treatment of acute manic conditions. The treatments are generally administered in a hospital setting, although outpatient office-based treatments can be used at times. The procedure involves anesthesia of the patient, providing succinylcholine for muscle relaxation, and administration of a small electrical current (bitemporally or unilaterally), which will induce a brief (30-second or so) convulsion. The tonic-clonic nature of this convulsion is modified by the actions of the succinylcholine. The patient awakens from the treatment usually within 20 minutes and may be confused for some parts of the day. Treatments are usually administered 3 days a week; in general, treatments are administered until the patient improves, and then a few additional treatments are given. If the treatment is successful, the patient should then be maintained with an antidepressant to reduce the risk for relapse. A space-occupying mass in the brain is a contraindication to ECT. I generally do not advise ECT during

TABLE 2. **Treatment Guidelines for Major Depressive Episode**

Severity	Course		
	First Episode	*Chronic*	*Recurrent*
Mild	Psychotherapy	Psychotherapy; antidepressant pharmacotherapy if poor response	Antidepressant pharmacotherapy and psychotherapy
Moderate	Antidepressant pharmacotherapy	Antidepressant pharmacotherapy plus psychotherapy	Antidepressant pharmacotherapy plus psychotherapy
Severe	Antidepressant pharmacotherapy or ECT	ECT or antidepressant; add psychotherapy when improved	ECT or antidepressant; add psychotherapy when improved

Abbreviation: ECT = electroconvulsive therapy.

concomitant lithium administration because cases of neurotoxicity have been reported in such patients.

An experimental ECT-like treatment, repetitive transcranial magnetic stimulation, is being studied. The procedure has been successfully used in depressed outpatients. No seizures occur during the procedure, and there is less confusion than with ECT. This procedure is currently being studied for its antidepressant efficacy and safety.

Bright Light Treatment

Bright light treatment is effective for depressed patients with seasonal pattern (seasonal affective disorder or winter depression). The treatment usually involves administration of bright lights in the morning hours; several light application devices have been recommended. The light box is a 2500- or 10,000-lux device that patients are advised to sit in front of with their eyes open for 2 hours or half an hour, respectively. The dawn simulator is a rheostat-like device attached to bedroom lights, and the technique involves gradually increasing light intensity in the bedroom in the early morning hours until full lights are on at the time of awakening. A light visor has also been suggested as a technique to provide light treatment.

TREATMENT OF SPECIFIC MOOD DISORDERS

Major Depressive Disorder

Treatment of the first episode of a major depressive disorder should take into account the differential diagnosis of this condition (a number of medical conditions such as endocrine dysfunction, tumors, and central nervous system lesions are associated with depression). Thus, there is need for a medical and laboratory evaluation. Treatment might proceed according to the principles outlined in Table 2. Severity can be assessed through patient-rated scales, such as the Beck Depression Inventory, or by the clinician through scales such as the Hamilton Rating Scale for Depression (HAM-D). In general, if the HAM-D result is in the mild range and the disorder is acute, I would recommend the use of psychologic therapies such as IPT or CBT. These therapies are effective for

the treatment of patients with mild depressive states.

If the disorder is of moderate severity, I would recommend beginning treatment with an SSRI. The rationale for using pharmacotherapy for moderate depression is based on research studies that show that as the presenting depression is more severe, psychotherapy is less effective and medication is relatively more effective. If the presenting condition is chronic (i.e., 2 years or more), I would recommend treatment with both medication and psychotherapy. If the presenting condition is recurrent, I would also recommend treatment with an SSRI combined with psychotherapy, the idea being that medication is used on a long-term basis to prevent recurrence, and "booster sessions" of psychotherapy may be necessary for the mild recurrences that are likely to occur.

If the presenting depression is severe, complicated with catatonic features or with psychosis, or is treatment resistant, I would recommend hospitalization and ECT. ECT is usually considered after pharmacotherapy has been provided and has failed.

The duration of initial treatment should be at least 6 to 8 weeks to determine whether there is a response, meaning 6 to 8 weeks after an adequate treatment dose has been achieved. If there is a satisfactory response, the medication should be continued at the same dose for an additional 4 to 6 months. If there is a history of recurrent depression, I would recommend continued pharmacotherapy for at least 5 years at the dose that achieved remission in the 6- to 8-week period.

If the patient does not respond to the initial treatment (treatment resistant) or has side effects of this treatment (treatment intolerant), one could choose from a wide variety of treatment options. These might include augmentation with another medication, such as buspirone (BuSpar) 5 to 10 mg tid, lithium, or thyroid hormone (triiodothyronine being preferable in unipolar patients to thyroxine); adding pindolol (Visken)* 2.5 mg tid to patients treated with fluoxetine or paroxetine; adding a more noradrenergic acting compound to the SSRI, such as bupropion beginning with doses of 75 mg per day and increasing to 150 mg per day in divided doses; or switching to a

*Not FDA approved for this indication.

different compound, either a different SSRI or one of the newer medications that might have a different mechanism of action.

Because dysthymic disorder is a mood disorder of long-standing duration, I would suggest initiating treatment as one would for mild or moderate chronic major depression, i.e., psychotherapy plus pharmacotherapy. Duration of treatment for dysthymic disorder or chronic major depressive disorder is not established by research studies, but I recommend at least 1 year of pharmacotherapy at an effective dose.

Bipolar Disorders

In general, the treatment of a bipolar disorder is to administer a mood-stabilizing medication for long-term maintenance therapy. The three mood-stabilizing medications that have demonstrated success include lithium carbonate, valproic acid (Depakene),* and carbamazepine (Tegretol).* The setting where one begins treatment will determine which of these medications might be used as a first-choice drug and what other medications might be employed. For example, if one is treating an acutely manic patient in a hospital setting, treatment usually begins with a sedating compound that might be given intramuscularly, such as haloperidol or lorazepam, or both, followed by administration of a mood stabilizer. I prefer to use lithium carbonate for a never-treated first-episode manic patient and would begin with low doses, 300 mg at bedtime, and increase the dose 300 mg every day, with frequent (every-other-day) blood level monitoring of lithium levels. Therapeutic lithium levels for acute mania are 1.0 to 1.5 mEq per liter. An alternative would be to use rapid loading of valproate, up to 20 mg per kg, which has been shown to be an effective way of administering valproic acid acutely, or to begin with lower doses of carbamazepine or valproic acid and increase the dose more slowly. For acute mania, therapeutic blood levels are 50 to 125 μg per mL for valproic acid and 6 to 12 μg per mL for carbamazepine. In general, I prefer to increase doses slower in acutely manic patients because the issue of long-term tolerability is paramount, and if patients experience undue side effects early in treatment, they are apt not to take the medication for long-term maintenance. I realize that hospital stays are well below what is necessary to treat a manic patient and there is considerable pressure to try to discharge patients earlier and earlier because of limits on hospital stays. However, with bipolar disorder, it would seem that the issue is less important to get the patient out of the hospital acutely than to prevent return of the patient to the hospital, which is likely to happen if the patient is inadequately treated or if the patient rejects a maintenance medication that could be effective for preventing recurrences. The plan for acute mania is to get the patient stabilized and discharged and then to slowly taper the non–mood stabilizer medication (the benzodiazepine and/or the psychotic medication) and to watch for the development of a depressive phase after the manic phase. Maintenance blood levels for lithium are 0.5 to 0.8 mEq per liter.

For a bipolar II patient, hypomania is usually not reported as a disorder because such individuals are often productive during these times, but they will present with depression. Thus, taking the history of a depressed patient for the presence of hypomania is important. For the depressed bipolar II patient, I would begin treatment with a mood stabilizer and then add an antidepressant. The treatment for the depressed phase of bipolar I or bipolar II depression should be approached with caution because one is concerned about the tendency of pharmacotherapy to switch patients from depression to mania or hypomania. The SSRIs, venlafaxine, bupropion, and tranylcypromine may tend to cycle bipolar depressed patients to mania and hypomania less frequently than the TCAs and are preferred.

One form of bipolar disorder, rapid cycling, is more difficult to treat and less lithium responsive to maintenance therapy. I recommend a treatment plan involving structure of one's days, education regarding the illness, noting moods on a daily calendar, and having maintenance therapy with combinations of treatment such as lithium plus valproate or lithium plus carbamazepine. The addition of thyroxine has been noted to be helpful. Thyroid abnormalities have been reported in women with rapid cycling disorders, and monitoring thyroid function with thyroid-stimulating hormone levels is important.

Depression due to a General Medical Condition

The treatment of a patient with a general medical condition and depression requires some knowledge of the possibility of drug interactions that might be involved in the application of such treatment. Depending on the type of medical disorder, it may be appropriate to rely only on psychotherapy and in other cases to provide antidepressant medication. Interestingly, stimulants (methylphenidate [Ritalin]*) have been shown to be effective in the treatment of a number of medical conditions associated with depression, such as acquired immune deficiency syndrome plus depression. As a general rule, one should not withhold treatment of depression because the patient has a medical condition that may be "causing" the mood disorder.

Substance-Induced Depression

The treatment of this type of co-morbid disorder is quite difficult because, in general, the first goal of treatment is to eliminate the use of the substance that is associated with the depressive state. In cases in which the substance is alcohol or an illegal substance such as marijuana, cocaine, or amphetamine,

---

*Not FDA approved for this indication.

*Not FDA approved for this indication.

there is often considerable difficulty in getting the patient to stop using the offending agent. In general, antidepressants are less effective if the patient is abusing substances. On the other hand, I have had excellent results in many depressed individuals who have stopped using substances, in which case the decisions about how to treat the depressive disorder rely on the course of the depressive disorder, previous history, family history, and ongoing medical situations. I recommend the use of urine toxicology screens to monitor patients who have substance abuse histories and who are coming in for treatment of an ongoing mood disorder. If the substance is a medication, treatment should include changing to an alternative treatment (such as from propranolol to atenolol).

Other Mood Disorders

Treatment of adjustment disorder with depressed mood usually involves supportive psychotherapy. Depressive symptoms are usually not persistent or sufficiently severe in quality to merit use of antidepressant medication. However, if the symptoms persist or become more severe, the diagnosis can be changed to major depressive disorder. Uncomplicated bereavement usually requires little intervention. Sometimes the use of sedatives to improve sleep on a temporary basis can be of some benefit, along with supportive measures for the individual and other family members who have recently experienced the loss.

Considerable research is ongoing regarding the treatment of milder depressed states that have not been accepted into the DSM nomenclature but instead are in the Appendix of DSM-IV. One such condition is mixed anxiety depressive disorder. This condition is allegedly common in primary care settings and is defined as patients whose depression is generally mild and who do not meet DSM-IV criteria for generalized anxiety disorder, major depressive disorder, or dysthymic disorder. The identification of such patients sufficient to provide adequate numbers for research is an ongoing effort. Whether such patients are best treated with brief psychotherapy, pharmacotherapy, or both and how long to treat such patients are current research issues. Whether such patients exist in the numbers that have been claimed for their prevalence is also problematic. In general, I would recommend that if the primary care clinician identifies a patient with depression, the patient should be treated with medication if the depression has been ongoing for at least several weeks.

Seasonal Pattern

Patients with seasonal pattern are those who experience a depressive episode usually beginning in the fall or winter of the year and whose depressions remit usually toward spring. Such patients may have a diagnosis of major depressive disorder, recurrent, or bipolar I or bipolar II disorder. If the patients have a bipolar disorder, they should be treated with a mood-stabilizing medication and treatment should proceed for the depressed phase. If the patient has major depressive disorder, recurrent and is mildly depressed, treatment of the winter depression with bright light therapy can be effective. Patients with seasonal pattern have, by definition, recurrent depression. I believe it is important to consider maintenance pharmacotherapy in their long-term management.

Atypical Depression

Studies show that the response of patients with atypical depression to TCAs (imipramine) is poorer than their response to phenelzine. SSRI treatment may also be associated with better treatment outcome.

Co-morbidity

For patients who have co-morbid excessive anxiety, panic attacks, panic disorder, obsessional features or obsessive-compulsive disorder, social phobia, or bulimia nervosa, the choice of an SSRI as first-line treatment seems well founded because SSRIs are generally approved for the treatment of a number of such psychiatric conditions in addition to their use in uncomplicated depression. Use of an SSRI is also recommended if the co-morbid disorder (such as panic disorder, bulimia nervosa, or obsessive-compulsive disorder) antecedes the mood disorder (the mood disorder is secondary) or the mood disorder begins before the complicating co-morbid features develop (the mood disorder is primary) and the co-morbid condition is secondary.

SCHIZOPHRENIA

method of
STEPHEN R. MARDER, M.D.
*West Los Angeles Veterans Affairs Medical
    Center and University of California, Los
    Angeles School of Medicine*
Los Angeles, California

Schizophrenia is a severe psychiatric disorder that is characterized by psychotic symptoms, such as hallucinations and delusions, and impairments in social and vocational adjustment. It affects approximately 1% of the world population. In the United States, 25% of hospital-bed days and 20% of Social Security benefit days are devoted to patients with schizophrenia. This illness usually has its onset in the late teenage years or the twenties, but it may emerge during childhood and at any point during adulthood. Although the cause or causes of schizophrenia have not been identified, it has become evident that this disorder is associated with abnormalities in the structure and function of the brain.

Individuals with schizophrenia demonstrate remarkable differences in the severity of their illness and the nature of their psychopathology. Moreover, psychopathology in an individual will vary according to the phase of the illness. For these reasons, it is difficult to describe a treatment strategy that can be applied to all individuals with schizophrenia. Rather, the treatment plan will depend on the patient's symptomatic presentation and the phase of the illness.

Psychopathology in schizophrenia can be classified into three dimensions: psychotic, negative, and disorganized. Psychotic symptoms include hallucinations, ideas of reference, and delusions. These are symptoms that tend to result in hospitalization and to disrupt the lives of patients. Negative symptoms include decreased motivation, emotional blunting, and impoverished speech and thought. These symptoms are associated with the social and vocational impairments in schizophrenia. Disorganized symptoms include disorganized speech and behavior as well as impairments in attention and information processing. These symptoms are also associated with the social and vocational impairments in schizophrenia.

Schizophrenia can be conceptualized as having three phases, each with its own clinical characteristics and each with its own treatment strategies. The acute stage is characterized by psychotic symptoms that require clinical attention. These symptoms may represent a first psychotic episode or a relapse in an individual who had previously been ill. The goals of treatment are to control disturbed behaviors and to alleviate acute symptoms. The majority of patients will recover from an acute episode and enter a stabilization period during which acute symptoms have been controlled, but patients remain at risk for relapse if treatment is interrupted or if the patient is exposed to stress. The goals of treatment are to minimize the likelihood of relapse and to assist patients in their return to community life. The third stage is the stable phase when the illness is in a relative stage of remission. The goals during this phase are to prevent psychotic relapse and to assist patients in improving their level of functioning. The goals of each strategy are unlikely to be reached with only a single treatment modality. Rather, the optimal treatment of schizophrenia requires a creative combining of psychosocial and pharmacologic strategies.

TREATMENT DURING THE ACUTE PHASE

Who Should Be Treated?

Nearly all acute episodes of schizophrenia will be managed with antipsychotic medications. Antipsychotics are effective for treating nearly all of the symptoms associated with schizophrenia. It is common for antipsychotics to result in substantial improvement, or even remission of positive symptoms, while negative and disorganized symptoms are minimally affected and continue to impair the patient's social recovery. Approximately 60 to 70% of drug-treated patients with acute schizophrenia will achieve a complete remission or experience only mild symptoms; the remaining 30 to 40% will continue to experience different levels of psychotic symptoms. These findings are from studies that took place before the introduction of newer antipsychotics including clozapine (Clozaril), risperidone (Risperdal), and olanzapine (Zyprexa). It is likely that the remission rate would be somewhat higher if trials with these other agents were included.

Choice of an Antipsychotic

Once a decision is made to initiate pharmacotherapy, the clinician is faced with a number of choices including the route of administration, the choice of drug, and the dosage (Table 1). The decision regarding route of administration is usually straightforward. Under most conditions, patients should be treated with an oral antipsychotic. Most antipsychotic drugs have half-lives that permit a single daily dose. Short-acting intramuscular drugs are useful when the patient refuses oral dosing and when a rapid onset is helpful. Intramuscular administration of most antipsychotics results in peak plasma levels in about 30 minutes with clinical effects emerging within 15 to 30 minutes. Most orally administered dopamine receptor antagonists (DAs) result in a peak plasma level in 1 to 4 hours after administration.

Antipsychotics can also be administered as long-acting injectable compounds. These drugs differ from short-acting compounds in that they have a gradual onset of action and are eliminated slowly. As a result, these drugs are helpful for long-term maintenance therapy but not for acute treatment. The reason is that clinicians are unable to titrate dose against side effects or clinical effects because the onset of clinical effects may occur weeks or months after a drug or dosage change.

Antipsychotics can be categorized in two groups: the older conventional antipsychotics, which have also been called DAs; and the newer second-generation drugs, which have been called serotonin dopamine antagonists (SDAs). This chapter uses the terms DA and SDA, which refers to the theory that the antipsychotic effects of DAs result from the blockade of D_2 receptors and the SDAs differ in having effects related to a balance of D_2 and 5-hydroxytryptamine 2A receptor antagonism. The DAs are further categorized as being low, mid, or high potency, with the higher potency drugs having a greater affinity for D_2 receptors and a greater tendency to cause extrapyramidal side effects (EPS). Low-potency drugs are less likely to cause EPS but more likely to cause postural hypotension, sedation, and anticholinergic effects.

In selecting between these groups, the most important advantage of the SDAs is that they cause considerably less EPS than DAs do. This is an important advantage because EPS (which include akathisia, with subjective and objective restlessness; parkinsonism, with rigidity, gait disturbance, and tremor; and dystonia, with abrupt-onset, sometimes bizarre muscle spasms affecting mainly the musculature of the head and neck) are usually the most serious side effects associated with antipsychotics. For example, with clozapine, olanzapine, and sertindole,* EPS almost never occur, whereas with risperidone, EPS can usually be avoided at doses that are effective for treating psychosis. SDAs may also be more effective than conventional drugs for managing

---

*Not yet approved for use in the United States.

TABLE 1. **Selected Antipsychotic Drugs for Schizophrenia**

Drug	Routes of Administration	Usual Daily Oral Dose (mg)	Sedation	Autonomic	EPS
Phenothiazines					
Chlorpromazine (Thorazine)	Oral, IM	200–600	+ + +	+ + +	+ +
Fluphenazine (Prolixin)	Oral, IM, depot	2–20	+	+	+ + +
Trifluoperazine (Stelazine)	Oral, IM	5–30	+ +	+	+ + +
Perphenazine (Trilafon)	Oral, IM	8–64	+ +	+	+ + +
Thioridazine (Mellaril)	Oral	200–600	+ + +	+ + +	+ +
Butyrophenone					
Haloperidol (Haldol)	Oral, IM, depot	5–20	+	+	+ + +
Thioxanthene					
Thiothixene (Navane)	Oral, IM	5–30	+	+	+ + +
Dihydroindolone					
Molindone (Moban)	Oral	20–100	+ +	+	+ +
Dibenzoxazepine					
Loxapine (Loxitane)	Oral, IM	20–100	+ +	+	+ +
Arylpiperidylindole					
Sertindole*	Oral	12–24	+	+ +	0?
Thienobenzodiazepine					
Olanzapine (Zyprexa)	Oral	7.5–25†	+	+ +	0?
Benzisoxazole					
Risperidone (Risperdal)	Oral	2–16	+	+ +	+
Dibenzodiazepine					
Clozapine (Clozaril)	Oral	150–900	+ + +	+ + +	0?

*Not yet approved for use in the United States.
†Exceeds dosage recommended by the manufacturer.
Abbreviation: EPS = extrapyramidal side effects; + = mild; + + = moderate; + + + = severe.

negative and cognitive symptoms. Clozapine, the first SDA, has been demonstrated to be effective for patients who respond poorly to DAs, and there is evidence that the other SDAs may share this advantage. The disadvantages of SDAs include their cost—which is much greater than the cost of DAs—and their lack of availability in short- or long-acting injectable forms.

Choosing among the SDAs is a problem because these agents have not been adequately compared with one another. As mentioned previously, clozapine is not viewed as a first-line agent because of its tendency to cause agranulocytosis in about 1% of patients. It also causes sedation, anticholinergic effects, seizures, and postural hypotension. Other side effects of the SDAs include weight gain for all of these agents; male ejaculatory side effects in risperidone, sertindole, and perhaps olanzapine; and mild sedation with olanzapine. Sertindole causes a dose-dependent increase in the QT_C interval of the electrocardiogram. Thus far, it is unclear if sertindole is associated with an increased risk for ventricular tachyarrhythmias.

If the long-term plan includes the use of long-acting depot antipsychotic, the short-acting form of the depot drug—haloperidol or fluphenazine in the United States—is the logical choice. If the patient will be managed with an oral antipsychotic, the clinician should consider prior drug responses if this information is available. Patients who had uncomfort-

able side effects or an inadequate response—in terms of positive, negative, or cognitive symptoms—while receiving a DA may be candidates for an SDA. All of the SDAs, with the exception of clozapine, should be considered first-line agents.

Dosage Selection

Finding the optimal dosage of an antipsychotic can be a difficult challenge, particularly with the DAs. Titrating dosage against clinical response is usually not possible because there is a delay of days or even weeks between the time a drug and dose are selected and the patient's therapeutic response. If the clinician is dissatisfied with the clinical response and raises the dose during the first weeks of treatment, it is possible that the dose will be higher than the minimally effective dose. This can be a substantial problem for high-potency DAs because EPS often occur at the doses that are needed to treat psychotic symptoms. As a result, the appropriate dosing strategy is to select a dose on the basis of the patient's prior drug responses or, if this is not possible, to prescribe a dose that has been demonstrated to be effective in groups of patients. After the patient is started at this dose, the patient and clinician wait until the patient responds or develops side effects. An adequate trial on an antipsychotic is probably 6 to 8 weeks, although if a patient has failed to demonstrate any improvement by 4 weeks, the likelihood of a clinical response is relatively low.

Dosage comparison studies provide guidance to clinicians who are making decisions regarding the doses of DAs for most patients with schizophrenia. Doses below 300 mg of chlorpromazine (or 5 mg of fluphenazine or haloperidol) are likely to be too low for many psychotic patients. At the same time, doses above 1000 mg of chlorpromazine (or 20 mg of haloperidol or fluphenazine) are seldom necessary and may lead to substantial side effects. In other words, most patients will respond to doses between 5 and 20 mg of fluphenazine or haloperidol or equivalent amounts of another DA. Children and elderly patients should be treated with much lower doses. Among the SDAs, clozapine dose is the most difficult to determine. Although most patients respond to doses between 300 and 600 mg daily, the dose is often determined by the amount of sedation and orthostatic hypotension that the patient is able to tolerate. Because the other SDAs have relatively mild side effects, finding an effective dose that is not associated with severe side effects is less difficult.

Managing Poor Responders

A substantial proportion of patients with schizophrenia—estimated in different studies as 25 to 40% of individuals—will fail to demonstrate an adequate response to an antipsychotic. Patients do not fall neatly into the categories of responders and nonresponders. Nearly every patient with schizophrenia will improve to some extent when he or she receives an antipsychotic. Among the DAs, a poor response to one agent usually predicts an inadequate response to all of the DAs. Thus, the introduction of the SDAs, particularly clozapine, provides new alternatives for these patients.

A number of well-designed studies indicate that about 60% of patients who are refractory to DA will be substantially improved after a 6-month trial with clozapine. Although there is some evidence that refractory patients also respond to risperidone, the evidence is only preliminary at this writing. Olanzapine and sertindole are currently being evaluated in refractory patients.

Although the evidence that olanzapine, risperidone, and sertindole are effective for patients who respond poorly to DAs is not adequate, it is reasonable to administer a trial of one or more of these agents before patients are prescribed clozapine. The reason is that clozapine can be a difficult medication for many patients. This is partly due to the need for weekly blood monitoring while the patient is receiving this agent and also due to other side effects including sedation, hypotension, weight gain, and seizures.

TREATMENT DURING THE STABILIZATION AND STABLE PHASE

After recovery from an acute psychotic episode, patients with schizophrenia enter a stabilization phase during which they remain vulnerable to relapse if their medications are reduced rapidly or if they are exposed to stress. During this phase, it is important for clinicians to carefully monitor medication compliance and to maintain patients with an antipsychotic dose that is similar to the dose that was effective in treating the acute episode. If the long-term treatment plan includes management with a long-acting depot antipsychotic, patients should be gradually changed from an oral to a depot agent during a 3- to 4-month period. During this phase, it may also be helpful for clinicians to meet with families and to emphasize that patients are more vulnerable to relapse when they are exposed to environments that are high in hostility and criticism.

After this stabilization period, most patients will enter a stable or maintenance phase in which symptoms are minimal. Antipsychotics are effective in reducing the risk for relapse in patients during this phase. Although studies differ depending on the population, approximately 70% of stable patients who are changed to a placebo will relapse each year, whereas only about 30% of patients receiving an antipsychotic will relapse. Clinicians are often tempted to discontinue medications in patients who have been well and stable for prolonged periods. Unfortunately, these patients also have high relapse rates when their medications are discontinued. These findings support the practice of maintaining patients with antipsychotics after they have recovered from a psychotic episode.

Most patients who have had more than one episode of schizophrenic psychosis should be maintained with an antipsychotic for at least 5 years of maintenance and often indefinitely. Relapse rates for first-episode patients are somewhat lower than rates for patients who have had multiple episodes. A reasonable strategy for most first-episode patients is to continue drugs for at least a year after an episode with consideration of dosage reduction or observation off drugs during the following year.

Psychosocial Treatment

Most patients will benefit from a combination of drug and psychosocial treatments. A substantial body of evidence indicates that certain types of individual psychotherapy, vocational rehabilitation, family therapy, and social skills training can improve the social adjustment of individuals with schizophrenia. These treatments are most effective during the outpatient phase of treatment when psychotic thought processes and impairments in information processing are less likely to interfere with psychosocial treatments. One of the important advantages of newer drugs is that their decreased side effects, management of negative and cognitive symptoms, and acceptance by patients will result in patients' being more active participants in psychosocial treatments.

PANIC DISORDER

method of
JACK M. GORMAN, M.D.

Columbia University College of Physicians and
Surgeons
New York, New York

Panic disorder is a common and debilitating illness, affecting approximately 2 to 3% of the population and defined by the occurrence of spontaneous panic attacks. Although the illness is severe and associated with considerable morbidity, it has been the focus of vigorous scientific research during the past 2 decades, and promising advances have been made toward the development of effective treatment strategies to control symptoms and improve clinical course.

The core clinical feature of panic disorder is the spontaneous panic attack, a rapid crescendo of intense fear lasting approximately 10 to 30 minutes and occurring with several somatic and cognitive symptoms. The patient experiences a sudden, massive outburst of autonomic activity with palpitations, shortness of breath, chest pain, trembling, diaphoresis, dizziness, and paresthesias. In addition, patients fear that they will die, go crazy, or lose control of themselves. The experience of panic is exceptionally frightening; patients often believe that they are having a heart attack, stroke, or other medical emergency. A spontaneous panic attack by definition occurs "out of the blue," without any environmental or situational trigger. Panic attacks are common events that are also seen in a number of medical and psychiatric conditions as well as in a significant portion of the general population. However, for the diagnosis of panic disorder to be made, the patient must experience recurrent, unexpected panic attacks; after an attack, the patient has at least a 1-month period of fearing the occurrence or consequences of another attack. This persistent fear is known as anticipatory anxiety. Panic disorder usually begins in late adolescence to early adulthood and is two to three times more likely to affect women than men.

Closely associated with panic disorder is the development of phobic avoidance, in which the patient's fear of experiencing future attacks leads to an avoidance of places or situations in which a panic attack has occurred previously, such as while driving a car, riding the subway, or being inside an elevator. This avoidance can then generalize to other situations and become so severe that the patient may be globally incapacitated, unable even to venture out of the house unless accompanied by a close friend or relative. This extreme form of avoidant behavior is known as agoraphobia and occurs in an estimated 50 to 60% of patients with panic disorder as a significant complication of the illness.

Panic disorder creates numerous impairments in lifestyle, and patients often find it inordinately difficult to function in regular work and social environments. Also, because intense physical symptoms predominate the clinical picture, panic disorder patients routinely seek help from various medical specialists and are frequent users of medical emergency departments. It is necessary for the clinician to inquire about co-morbid psychiatric illnesses, because panic patients are at serious risk for the development of major depression and have an elevated attempted suicide rate. Furthermore, patients with panic disorder have a propensity toward self-medication with alcohol and nonprescription sedative hypnotics; the presence of a co-morbid substance use disorder thus needs to be ruled out because this may preclude the use of certain treatments, particularly the benzodiazepines, in this population.

DIFFERENTIAL DIAGNOSIS

Panic disorder has been referred to as the "great masquerader" because the vast array of intense somatic symptoms that characterize the illness can mimic a host of medical and psychiatric conditions. The clinician must be careful to rule out, through proper history, physical examination, and laboratory evaluation, any possible organic etiology of the panic symptoms. A number of conditions need to be excluded, as shown in Table 1.

TREATMENT

Successful treatment of panic disorder targets the spontaneous panic attack. Once the panic attacks are blocked, anticipatory anxiety decreases with a subsequent reduction in phobic avoidance. Proper treatment involves use of specific pharmacologic therapy as well as cognitive-behavioral psychotherapeutic intervention. A good treatment strategy must be tailored to the needs of the individual patient and may involve drug treatment alone, cognitive-behavioral therapy (CBT) alone, or a combination of the two modalities.

Pharmacotherapy

Antidepressants

Antidepressants have long been known to block the spontaneous panic attack and induce clinical remission in most patients. The major advance in recent years in the treatment of panic disorder has been the advent of the selective serotonin reuptake inhibitors (SSRIs) and their recognition as powerful

TABLE 1. **Common Organic Causes of
Panic Symptoms**

Condition	Diagnostic Considerations
Endocrine	
Hypothyroidism	Thyroid function studies
Hyperthyroidism	Thyroid function studies
Hyperparathyroidism	Serum calcium determination
Pheochromocytoma	24-h urine collection for catecholamine metabolites
Cardiovascular	
Acute myocardial infarction	Electrocardiography
Cardiac arrhythmias	Consider 24-h monitor
Mitral valve prolapse	Echocardiography
Neurologic	
Temporal lobe epilepsy	Electroencephalography
Vestibular disorders	Referral to ear, nose, and throat specialist or neurologist
Substance Withdrawal	
Alcohol, barbiturate, opiate	Urine and serum toxicology
Acute Intoxication	
Amphetamines, cocaine	Urine and serum toxicology

TABLE 2. **Medication Regimens for Panic Disorder**

Medication	Initial Dose	Target Dose
SSRIs		
Fluoxetine (Prozac)	5–10 mg/d	20–40 mg/d
Paroxetine (Paxil)	10 mg/d	20–40 mg/d
Sertraline (Zoloft)	25 mg/d	50–200 mg/d
Fluvoxamine (Luvox)	25 mg/d	75–100 mg/d
TCAs		
Imipramine (Tofranil)	10 mg/d	100–300 mg/d
Nortriptyline (Pamelor)	10 mg/d	50–150 ng/mL (BL)
Clomipramine (Anafranil)	10 mg/d	50–200 mg/d
Desipramine (Norpramin)	10 mg/d	100–300 mg/d
MAOIs		
Phenelzine (Nardil)	15 mg/d	45–90 mg/d
Benzodiazepines		
Alprazolam (Xanax)	0.25–0.5 mg tid	2–6 mg total/d
Lorazepam (Ativan)	0.5 mg tid	1–2 mg total/d
Clonazepam (Klonopin)	0.25–0.5 mg bid	1–3 mg total/d

Abbreviations: SSRIs = selective serotonin reuptake inhibitors; TCAs = tricyclic antidepressants; MAOIs = monoamine oxidase inhibitors; BL = blood level.

antipanic drugs. The SSRIs act preferentially at serotonin receptors, blocking reuptake and enhancing availability of this neurotransmitter, and should now be considered the first-line treatment of panic disorder. Currently available SSRIs include fluoxetine (Prozac), paroxetine (Paxil), sertraline (Zoloft), and fluvoxamine (Luvox). These medications possess distinct advantages compared with the traditional antidepressants in that they maintain a much more favorable side effect profile while achieving comparable and often greater efficacy. SSRIs have little anticholinergic activity and are less likely to produce dry mouth, blurred vision, constipation, and urinary hesitancy. In addition, SSRIs have no significant cardiovascular effects and will not usually alter blood pressure or cardiac rhythm. Other problem side effects such as weight gain and sedation are uncommon, and these medications are also relatively safe when taken in overdose. It is imperative that SSRIs be initiated at low doses because there is a risk for exacerbating anxiety and causing jitteriness early in treatment. Titration to higher doses should then be done gradually and cautiously. Dosages are shown in Table 2. Apart from the initial stimulatory effects, SSRIs can cause gastrointestinal distress, headache, sleep disturbance, sexual dysfunction, and hypomania. SSRIs typically exert their antipanic effects after 4 weeks, with continued improvement evident through the first 3 months of drug treatment.

The tricyclic antidepressants (TCAs)* also have the ability to block spontaneous panic and, before the introduction of the SSRIs, represented the standard pharmacologic treatment of panic disorder. If a trial of one or more SSRIs proves ineffective in a particular patient, implementation of a TCA is the next consideration in the treatment strategy. TCAs such as imipramine (Tofranil), nortriptyline (Pamelor), desipramine (Norpramin), and clomipramine (Anafranil) are inexpensive, highly effective medications and achieve panic blockade in approximately 80% of patients. Unfortunately, they cause a number of deleterious side effects, including those associated with a high degree of cholinergic blockade. They also adversely affect the cardiovascular system, with resultant tachycardia, orthostatic hypotension, and cardiac conduction delays. Weight gain and sedation also occur and can affect the patient's compliance. TCAs are potentially lethal in overdose. Panic patients are sensitive to the effects of TCAs, and it is important that the starting dose be low and gradually increased to therapeutic levels. Typical dosages are shown in Table 2. Therapeutic effects are generally seen after approximately 8 to 12 weeks of treatment.

The monoamine oxidase inhibitors (MAOIs),* such as phenelzine (Nardil), are the third class of antidepressants with marked antipanic activity. The major disadvantage of MAOIs is their risk for producing a hypertensive crisis owing to inhibition of monoamine metabolism. To prevent this medical emergency, patients are required to follow a special tyramine-free diet. In addition, several medications, including most sympathomimetic amines, antihistamines, and meperidine, are contraindicated. Other side effects include orthostatic hypotension, weight gain, and sedation. Because of these limiting factors, MAOIs are used in panic disorder as third-line agents for patients refractory to the other available treatments.

Benzodiazepines

Therapeutic response to antidepressant treatment usually takes a minimum of 4 weeks or longer; however, it is often necessary to achieve antipanic effects more quickly. High-potency benzodiazepines such as alprazolam (Xanax), clonazepam (Klonopin), and lorazepam (Ativan) all have been shown to block spontaneous panic as well as ameliorate anticipatory anxiety and are able to produce their effects within the first week of treatment. These medications are thus extremely effective for rapid anxiolysis during the initiation phase of antidepressant therapy and can later be used intermittently to abort episodes of acute panic. Benzodiazepines are also useful for patients who have contraindications to using antidepressants or who cannot tolerate the unwanted side effects of those drugs. Sedation is the main side effect of the benzodiazepines, with ataxia, memory disturbance, and paradoxical disinhibition occurring infrequently. The major disadvantage of chronic benzodiazepine use is the likelihood of physiologic dependency. This can result in a serious withdrawal syndrome if the drug is abruptly discontinued, characterized by rebound anxiety, insomnia, and an increased risk for

*Not FDA approved for this indication.

*Not FDA approved for this indication.

seizures. Slow, gradual tapering of the benzodiaze-pine dosage is thus recommended for all patients. Usual dosages are shown in Table 2.

Cognitive-Behavioral Therapy

Although psychotropic medications have been the mainstay of treatment of panic disorder, recent evidence shows that CBT is also a highly effective treatment. CBT for panic disorder involves four main components: (1) breathing retraining to decrease the tendency to hyperventilate; (2) cognitive restructuring to block catastrophic, anxiety-producing and distorted thoughts; (3) interoceptive deconditioning to desensitize the patient to somatic sensations; and (4) exposure training to reduce phobic avoidance. A usual course of CBT lasts approximately 3 months, and research is revealing that the combination of medication plus CBT may be more effective in treating panic than either modality alone.

Physical and Chemical Injuries

BURNS

method of
DAVID N. HERNDON, M.D.
Shriners Burns Institute
Galveston, Texas

Injuries from thermal, chemical, or electrical burn affect more than 1.2 million people per year in the United States alone. Most burns are classified as minor and can be treated on an outpatient basis; however, nearly 5% are categorized as moderate to severe and often require hospitalization. A moderate burn injury is a burn over 15 to 25% of the total body surface area (TBSA) that is less than 10% full-thickness burn and does not involve the eyes, ears, face, hands, feet, or perineum. In children, smaller burns are considered more severe, and a burn over 10 to 20% of the TBSA that is less than 10% full-thickness burn is a moderate injury. Patients with moderate burns can be managed either in a burn center or at a community hospital by physicians with experience in burn care.

Major burn injuries are defined as burns covering more than 25% of the TBSA in adults and 20% of the TBSA in children, or any full-thickness burn over more than 10% of the TBSA. All significant injuries of the eyes, ears, face, hands, feet, or perineum are considered major burns. Patients with these injuries should be treated at specialized burn centers. Regardless of burn size and distribution, inhalation injury, electrical burns, burns with associated trauma, and burns in high-risk patients are difficult to manage and should be treated in a burn unit (Table 1).

During the last 2 decades, burn mortality rates have decreased owing to new treatment modalities derived from ongoing research. In 1952, a 50% TBSA burn was associated with a 50% mortality rate. Today, a young healthy person can be expected to survive almost any size burn, even in the presence of complicating conditions such as inhalation injury and other trauma. A better understanding of burn pathophysiology, resuscitation, early wound closure, metabolic changes, nutritional support, and infection control have all contributed to the increase in long-term survival of severely burned patients.

Because of the major improvements in survival of burned patients, the newer challenges that remain in burn care involve associated issues, such as better pain control, prevention of hypertrophic scarring, and efficient rehabilitation for full return to occupation and vocation. Effective control of scarring could lead to better cosmetic and functional outcome, and application of therapeutic techniques in splinting and exercise should improve the ability of burned patients to return to normal activities and employment.

INITIAL EVALUATION

The treatment of burn injuries begins at the scene by controlling the burning process and removing the caustic agent. For flame burns, the patient should be placed on the ground and either rolled into or covered with fire-resistant material. After the flame has been extinguished, all remaining embers are removed that could deepen the wound, such as charred clothing. The patient is then covered with dry sheets and blankets to retain heat, because hypothermia often becomes a problem immediately after burn. Every effort should be made to keep the patient warm. With chemical burns, all contaminated clothing should be removed immediately and the exposed area profusely irrigated with copious quantities of water or saline. Care should be taken in rinsing the exposed and contaminated areas to direct water flow away from the uninjured areas. A chemically burned person should never be submerged for decontamination, because doing so may carry the noxious chemical to noncontaminated areas and thus spread the injury.

As with all traumatic injuries, airway patency is of primary importance. In cases in which there is a possible inhalation injury, 100% oxygen should be administered by face mask. At the slightest indication of impending airway obstruction, such as development of stridor or tachypnea, prophylactic intubation should be performed. Smoke inhalation may cause severe upper airway hyperemia and edema and can lead to significant hypoxemia. If possible, the patient should be placed on an oxygen saturation monitor; however, normal readings should be interpreted with caution, because the presence of carbon monoxide in the blood can falsely elevate oxygen saturation. Carbon monoxide, which has an affinity for hemoglobin of 280 times that of oxygen, is present in most smoke. Because it also binds to hemoglobin, the carbon dioxide is measured as oxygen by oxygen saturation monitors. The treatment for carbon monoxide inhalation is 100% oxygen, which decreases the half-life of carbon monoxide from 4 hours with room air to 45 minutes. If there is any question, endotracheal intubation with 100% oxygen is the safest course. In severe burns to the face and oropharynx, endotracheal intubation may be impossible, and emergent cricothyroidotomy may be required.

Once the airway is established, intravenous fluid therapy is the next priority. Fluids should be admin-

TABLE 1. **Definition of Severity of Burn**

Factor	Mild		Moderate		Severe	
	Adult	*Child*	*Adult*	*Child*	*Adult*	*Child*
TBSA burn (%)	<15	<10	15–25	10–20	>25	>20
TBSA full-thickness burn (%)	0		<10		>10	
Affected body area					Eyes, ears, face, hands, feet, perineum	
Associated conditions					Inhalation injury, electrical burn, other trauma, high-risk patient	

Abbreviation: TBSA = total body surface area.

istered primarily by peripheral large-bore intravenous catheters, which are safely secured by suture ligation as soon as possible in the evaluation of the patient, because it has been shown that delays in resuscitation will adversely affect outcome. In patients whose age, associated injury, or medical condition may complicate resuscitation, central venous catheters may be inserted before placement landmarks are obscured by edema; however, peripheral access should be attained first to begin resuscitation. If necessary, catheters can be placed through burned skin. Venous cutdowns for the saphenous vein in the ankle or groin are indicated if necessary. In patients with moderate and severe burns and older patients with smaller burns and co-morbid conditions urethral catheters should routinely be placed to monitor resuscitation.

Once the airway is secure and fluid resuscitation has begun, attention to associated conditions should proceed at a more deliberate pace. Severe burn injury can cause alterations in gastrointestinal tract function. Nasogastric tubes should be placed initially in patients with moderate and severe burns for gastric decompression and later for feeding. Early alimentation, at 6 to 8 hours after burn, has been shown to diminish the hypermetabolic response and maintain intestinal integrity. Occasionally, the placement of duodenal feeding tubes is necessary to achieve this goal because of gastric ileus. Initial laboratory examinations should include hemoglobin and hematocrit, electrolytes, serum osmolarity, blood urea nitrogen and creatinine, and arterial blood gas analysis for moderate and severe burns. Routine electrocardiographic monitoring and frequent temperature determinations should also be performed.

An initial, rapid examination of the burn wounds is made, which includes an assessment of distal pulses and tissue compartment pressures. Full-thickness injuries produce a nonyielding eschar that does not expand with increasing edema. Thus, generalized swelling that occurs in burn injury and under burned skin increases tissue pressures and diminishes venous return, impeding circulation in an affected extremity. With circumferential burns, diminished pulse or absence of a pulse with a normal measured central blood pressure indicates the need for immedi-ate escharotomies. Measured tissue pressures exceeding 40 mm Hg also should prompt intervention. If vascular compromise has been prolonged, reperfusion after an escharotomy may cause a reactive hyperemia in the underlying muscles, which can lead to edema formation in the muscle compartment and may necessitate fasciotomies. Systemic acidosis may occur in conjunction with acute release of the by-products of anaerobic metabolism by escharotomies and fasciotomies. The most common complications of escharotomy are hypovolemia and anemia from bleeding, which can be avoided by using careful technique.

A coordinated treatment plan is essential if the burn patient has evidence of other traumatic injury. Physicians distracted by the burn may miss associated injuries. Failure to respond to calculated amounts of resuscitation volume should increase an already high level of suspicion for another associated injury. Initial burn treatment may be superseded if the trauma is severe enough to warrant surgical intervention; however, a burn center should be quickly notified so that a timely burn treatment protocol can be established. To prepare a patient for transfer to a burn unit, the airway must be evaluated, intravenous access must be guaranteed, and the burn wounds should be covered with dry dressings without ointments or creams, to avoid further heat loss and enable the wounds to be treated with biologic dressings if indicated.

FLUID RESUSCITATION

The first step in effective resuscitation is a rapid clinical assessment of the extent and depth of the burn injury, a determination of the presence or absence of an inhalation injury, and evaluation for other traumatic injuries. An accurate estimation of the area and depth of the burn is essential. The commonly used "rule of nines" provides a quick assessment of the TBSA burned for adults. In children, however, it can overestimate burn size, because the head makes up a relatively larger area in proportion to other areas, especially in infants (Table 2). Age-appropriate diagrams or Lund and Browder charts can be used to definitively quantify burn size. The

TABLE 2. **Estimation of Body Surface Area**

| Body Area | Percentage of Total Body Surface Area | |
	Adult	Child
Head and neck	9	18
Anterior torso	18	18
Posterior torso	18	18
Arm	9	9
Leg	18	14
Perineum	1	1

size of the palm of the patient's hand is approximately 1% TBSA and can be a useful guide to quantitate a noncontinuous or splattered burn distribution.

Once the surface area of the burn is established, appropriate fluid resuscitation is initiated. Tissue perfusion must be preserved to prevent hypoperfusion. Burn shock is caused by edema, transvascular fluid shifts, and massively increased evaporative volume losses. The maximal amount of edema occurs 8 to 12 hours after injury in small burns and up to 24 to 48 hours after injury in large burns. The prime goal of fluid resuscitation is to support the patient through this period. Multiple resuscitation formulas have been used with success. The Parkland or Baxter formula is the most commonly used; it recommends 2 to 4 mL per kg per % TBSA burn of lactated Ringer's solution in the first 24 hours after burn, with half being given in the first 8 hours and the remainder given in the next 16 hours. This formula is effective for the initial calculations for adults but will underestimate the evaporative fluid loss in children. The resuscitation in children should be based on body surface area instead of weight and should begin with 5000 mL per m² TBSA burn + 2000 mL per m² TBSA of lactated Ringer's solution with 5% dextrose in water in the first 24 hours, again divided, with half given in the first 8 hours and the remainder given in the next 16 hours. Children, especially infants, have relatively small glycogen stores and should be given lactated Ringer's solution with 5% dextrose in water to avoid hypoglycemia in the early stages of resuscitation.

Smoke inhalation injury is suspected if the patient presents with clinical features such as facial burns, carbonaceous sputum, or a history of injury in a closed space. Smoke inhalation can also be assumed if carboxyhemoglobin levels are elevated immediately after burn or if an injury is diagnosed with the aid of fiberoptic bronchoscopy and/or xenon 133 ventilation-perfusion scintigraphy. A thorough examination for fractures, organ damage, and other injuries should proceed simultaneously with resuscitation. Delays in resuscitation can increase the amount of fluid needed for adequate resuscitation by 30%, and patients with smoke inhalation injury can require up to 33% more fluid volume.

Once resuscitation has been initiated, the patient must be monitored constantly for the effectiveness of resuscitation efforts. All formulas are only guidelines

to fluid replacement, and the adequacy of resuscitation must be measured and frequent changes made in the infusion rates to avoid under-resuscitation or over-resuscitation. Urine output of 0.5 to 1.0 mL per kg per hour is a good clinical indicator of vital organ perfusion and can be used to guide therapy. If any question arises during the early course, invasive cardiac monitoring may be indicated to optimize fluid therapy. During the first 24 hours, a severely burned patient can also develop a high serum glucose level with glycosuria, causing an osmotic diuresis and making frequent glucose measurements necessary.

Hypertonic salt solutions are used by some to resuscitate burn patients; however, studies have not been able to demonstrate decreased fluid requirements or decreased percent weight gain with use of hypertonic saline rather than lactated Ringer's solution. In fact, the dramatic and rapid increases in blood pressure after infusion of hypertonic saline have been suggested to do more harm than good. Hyperchloremic acidosis is a real potential effect of hypertonic saline that could adversely potentiate the pre-existing metabolic acidosis of hypovolemic shock. For these reasons, it is not currently recommended in the treatment of burns, but it could be used in other formulations in the future after further research.

All the resuscitation formulas currently used adequately resuscitate patients, so renal failure has ceased to be a major cause of death in burns. However, burned patients who are adequately volume repleted can still have compromised perfusion of vital organs such as the gut. Burn injury is known to decrease mesenteric blood flow and mucosal integrity despite the normalization of central venous pressure and cardiac output. In experimental burn models, blood flow to the gut decreases by approximately 40% despite adequate urine production and cardiac output. A decrease in mucosal integrity can cause an increase in gut permeability, which allows bacteria to translocate into the mesenteric lymph nodes and seed distant organs.

WOUND CARE

Current therapy for burn wound care can be divided into three stages—assessment, management, and rehabilitation. The assessment stage involves determination of the extent of injury on the basis of the depth and size of the wound and the overall condition of the patient. Accurate evaluation of burn depth is essential in development of a successful treatment plan. Second-degree burns heal within 3 weeks with conservative management using topical antimicrobials and usually do not exhibit hypertrophic scarring or cause functional impairment. However, burns that take more than 3 weeks to heal often cause unsightly hypertrophic scarring, provide only a thin, tenuous epithelial cover for months, and can result in limitations from burn scar contracture.

Burn wound depth is generally assessed by an experienced examiner from the characteristics of the wound. First-degree burns are erythematous and painful and have an intact skin barrier. Blisters are characteristic of superficial second-degree burns that involve only the papillary dermis. After removal of the blisters, the wound is pink, wet, and hypersensitive to touch. Burns that extend into the reticular dermis are deep second-degree burns that blister; however, the surface is usually a mottled pink and white, capillary refill is slow or absent, and the wound is less sensitive to pinprick than the surrounding normal skin. Charred full-thickness third-degree burns are leathery, firm, and insensate owing to destruction of nerve endings. Full-thickness burns that are not charred may appear similar to deep second-degree burns. They are often mottled and do not blanch with pressure. Immersion scald burns may be full-thickness burns that have a red appearance and can give the impression of a second-degree injury; however, on closer inspection, they do not blanch with pressure and are insensate.

It must be pointed out that assessment by examination can be difficult because of the dynamic characteristics of some partial-thickness burns. Some burns that appear superficial on day 1 may appear deep on day 3. Because the evaluation of burn depth is essential to effective management, numerous devices and techniques have been developed to evaluate burn depth. Burn wound biopsy, vital dyes, ultrasonography, fluorescein fluorometry, thermography, light reflectance, magnetic resonance imaging, and laser Doppler flowmetry have all been used with varying success to determine burn depth. Laser Doppler flowmetry and light reflectance have shown some promise; however, these technologies are still being refined and are not standard in everyday clinical use.

Once the extent of burn injury is established, an individualized management plan should be instituted. After the burn wound has been cleaned and débrided, an appropriate burn dressing is placed. A burn dressing should serve three principal functions. First, it must protect the damaged epithelium and provide splinting action to maintain the desired position of function. Second, the dressing should be occlusive to reduce evaporative heat loss and minimize cold stress. Finally, the dressing should provide comfort. Superficial dermal burns are quite sensitive to air currents, and large wounds will drain over time. A good burn wound dressing eliminates exposure to air currents and absorbs wound secretions.

Both biologic and synthetic dressings can be used for second-degree burns. Cutaneous allograft of harvested cadaver skin is an effective biologic dressing that has been shown to prevent evaporative water loss, reduce pain, and decrease the density of bacteria on the wound surface. Porcine xenograft is also effective, is more readily available, and is easy to apply, but it does not control bacterial proliferation as well as allograft. Synthetic dressings have also been used to cover superficial burns but do not have the antimicrobial properties of biologic dressings and should not be applied to burns in which wound contamination is suspected.

Topical antimicrobial agents are used to limit bacterial proliferation and fungal colonization in burn wounds. The three most commonly used topical antimicrobials are mafenide acetate (Sulfamylon), silver sulfadiazine (Silvadene), and 0.5% silver nitrate solution. Nystatin can be added to Silvadene to reduce the incidence of invasive candidal growth. The ultimate goal of topical antimicrobial therapy is to prevent invasive infection until the burn wound re-epithelializes or can be excised and grafted.

An aggressive approach to burn wound excision is the standard of current third-degree burn care. Early excision of the entire wound with closure at the first operation in large burns (greater than 30% TBSA third-degree burn) has been shown to reduce mortality. All surgical excisions, however, must be customized to the individual patient. Tangential excision by sequentially shaving the eschar from the burned area until a viable tissue plane is achieved gives better cosmetic results and is rapid and effective, although significant hemorrhage from the dermis or deeper tissue may occur. Tourniquets are used to reduce blood loss during tangential excision of the extremities, but this technique is still controversial owing to the difficulty in differentiating viable from nonviable tissue. In patients with deep full-thickness wounds who will not tolerate significant blood losses or multiple transfusions, fascial excision with electrocautery is indicated to minimize blood loss.

Once the burn wound is excised, rapid wound closure is essential. In small burns—less than 30% TBSA—good wound closure can be obtained with split-thickness skin grafts taken at $8/1000$ inch from normal skin areas. With massive burns—more than 50% TBSA—skin graft donor sites are limited, and complete closure after total excision is achieved by a combination of autograft and allograft or a synthetic wound covering. In large wounds, autograft can be meshed 4:1 and overlaid with nonexpanded meshed cadaver skin. This technique allows a larger body surface area to be covered with limited amount of split-thickness autograft. Repeated grafting is required in large burns, with sequential harvesting of limited donor sites until the entire burn wound is closed with autologous skin.

CRITICAL CARE SUPPORT

Once a patient with a large burn has been resuscitated and the wounds are covered, support of organ dysfunction and the hypermetabolic response becomes paramount. Particular attention is directed at the lungs, nutrition, and metabolic support. Lung injury from smoke inhalation or release of toxic mediators from the burn may necessitate a course of ventilatory support. Every effort should be made to wean patients from the ventilator early, if possible, because conventional mechanical ventilation with high tidal volumes and low respiratory rates can cause an increase in interstitial edema and barotrauma in previously compromised lungs.

Pressure-controlled ventilation has improved care,

although the rates of ventilator-associated complications are still high. High-frequency oscillatory ventilation is a new technique that uses subtidal volumes delivered in a progressive stepwise fashion until a preset oscillatory equilibrium is reached. This technique aids in reducing pulmonary barotrauma and, through vibratory air movement, clears airway casts and markedly improves ventilation at lower mean airway pressures. The initial response to toxic smoke inhalation is the sloughing off of the ciliated cells lining the airways that, in combination with exudate-containing fibrinogen, form casts that can block the tracheobronchial tree after injury. This new mode of ventilation may improve the clearance of debris and thereby, pulmonary toilet.

Metabolic rates in patients with severe burns (more than 40% TBSA) are 100 to 150% above their basal rates. These patients have increased energy and protein requirements that must be satisfied to prevent impaired wound healing, cellular dysfunction, and decreased resistance to infection. Early enteral feedings have been shown to reduce levels of catabolic hormones, improve nitrogen balance, maintain gut mucosal integrity, lower the incidence of diarrhea, and decrease hospital stay. Total parental nutrition in burn patients has been associated with metabolic and immunologic complications, and its use is limited to supporting patients with severe gastrointestinal dysfunction.

The Curreri formula is used most often to calculate caloric and protein needs in adult patients (Table 3). Children have a higher body surface area relative to weight and are at a higher risk for developing protein-calorie malnutrition, because they have relatively less body fat and muscle mass than adults. For these reasons, a formula based on body surface area, such as the Galveston formula, is more accurate (see Table 3). In burn patients, the composition of enteral tube feedings should consist of 40 to 70% carbohydrate, 10 to 20% fat, and 1 to 2 grams of protein per kg per day. Vitamin and mineral supplementation is recommended, particularly vitamins A and C and zinc. Decreased fat content and the addition of fatty acids found in fish oil may also be recommended in the future.

The level of metabolic alteration experienced by burn patients is directly related to the extent of the injury. The decrease in cardiac output and metabolic rate initially occurring has been referred to as the "ebb phase." After successful resuscitation, cardiac output returns to normal and then increases above normal levels, with a simultaneous increase in resting energy expenditure; this has been referred to as the "flow phase" of the hypermetabolic response. Severe burn injury can drive the metabolic rate to twice normal, but the rate increase can be blunted to 40 to 60% above normal with the use of bulky dressings and higher ambient temperatures. A true reset in central temperature to around 38.6°C occurs between the 5th and 15th days after burn injury and

TABLE 3. **Estimations of Caloric Needs in Burns**

Formula	Age (y)	Daily Requirements		
Curreri	16–59	25 kcal/kg	+	40 kcal/% burn
	>60	20 kcal/kg	+	65 kcal/% burn
Galveston	0–1	2100 kcal/m²	+	1000 kcal/m² burn
	1–11	1800 kcal/m²	+	1300 kcal/m² burn
	12–18	1500 kcal/m²	+	1500 kcal/m² burn

remains elevated for up to 2 months in burns covering more than 60% TBSA. This reset is due to the direct stimulation of the hypothalamus by inflammatory mediators and various cytokines. When attempts are made to decrease the core temperature by cooling or by use of antipyretics, the patient produces heat by increasing the metabolic rate to compensate.

There is a massive release of amino acids from the lean muscle mass that consists primarily of glutamine, with free concentrations falling by 50% after severe injury. This release is a result of greater transport of amino acids out of the cells as well as increased proteolysis. Effectors of this response are likely to be increases in glucocorticoids and decreases in anabolic hormones such as growth hormone and insulin-like growth factor. Growth hormone treatment in burns has been shown to improve protein metabolism as well as to shorten donor site healing times and length of hospital stay.

Postburn hypermetabolism is also characterized by rises in heart rate and lipolysis. Beta-blocking agents such as propranolol (Inderal) can lower the heart rate and reduce the left ventricular work and rate pressure product as well as decrease peripheral lipolysis. The administration of propranolol (0.5 mg per kg) in a child with a 60% burn causes only a 20% decrease in heart rate. Pharmacologic manipulation in conjunction with adequate nutrition and early burn wound closure may be beneficial in the treatment of the severely burned patient.

REHABILITATION

Once complete closure of the burn wound is achieved, the treatment emphasis changes from wound management to rehabilitation. Better control of burn scar may be obtained by application of pressure garments to healed skin grafts as well as healed deep second-degree burns. The routine use of pressure garments appears to reorient collagen strands so that scars become smoother and flatter and mature more quickly. Pressure garments and plastic molds for the face and neck have been found to reduce the incidence of scar contracture. Early splinting in combination with pressure garments reduces the formation of joint contractures that limit rehabilitation. The mainstay of treatment, however, is frequent and vigorous occupational and physical therapy beginning immediately after skin closure.

MOUNTAIN SICKNESS

method of
JONATHAN R. BROOME, M.B., B.S.
Alverstoke, Hampshire,
United Kingdom

As elevation above sea level increases, barometric pressure decreases, and the partial pressure of inspired oxygen available for transport from lungs to tissues is reduced. Hemoglobin desaturation and tissue hypoxia occur increasingly with altitude and are aggravated by the extra metabolic demands of physical exertion.

In mountainous regions, indigenous peoples show physiologic adaptation to the relative environmental hypoxia; this permits permanent residence up to about 4000 m above sea level, with some temporary settlements even higher. Given time, visitors to altitude also acclimatize, but up to 50% of lowland people who ascend too rapidly to altitudes over 2500 to 3000 m suffer acute mountain sickness (AMS) of varying severity. Short stays of 1 to 2 hours at altitude rarely produce symptoms in healthy people, but subacute mountain sickness may occur in both infants and adults from lowland regions who ascend to and remain for weeks or months at high elevations. Chronic mountain sickness (CMS) is a disease of adulthood among indigenous highland dwellers. This article summarizes the clinical features of these conditions, together with the main preventive and therapeutic measures.

ACUTE MOUNTAIN SICKNESS

AMS may be a "benign" self-limiting condition or may progress to a serious, potentially fatal disorder with features of high-altitude pulmonary edema (HAPE) and high-altitude cerebral edema (HACE).

Benign Acute Mountain Sickness

More than 95% of AMS sufferers develop headache, usually frontal, within 6 to 8 hours of arrival at altitude. Other common manifestations, in order of decreasing frequency, are sleep disturbance with vivid dreams and periodic sleep apnea; anorexia, nausea, and vomiting; fatigue and lassitude; and transient dizziness. Clinical signs may include periorbital or peripheral edema, a few scattered inspiratory crackles on chest auscultation, and flame-shaped retinal hemorrhages (usually asymptomatic).

Management

With avoidance of further ascent, rest, and maintenance of hydration, most symptoms of benign AMS resolve spontaneously in 2 to 5 days. Specific treatment with oral ibuprofen, 400 mg every 8 hours, is effective for altitude headache, and the carbonic anhydrase inhibitor acetazolamide (Diamox), 250 mg every 8 hours orally, has been shown to improve the general symptoms of AMS (although side effects such as diuresis, peripheral paresthesias, and gastrointestinal upset, may be poorly tolerated). Dexamethasone, 8 mg orally followed by 4 mg every 6 hours, may also provide symptomatic relief in those unable to tolerate acetazolamide. If mild symptoms of AMS either fail to resolve or progress to HAPE or HACE, *urgent descent is the cornerstone of management*; all other measures are secondary.

High-Altitude Pulmonary Edema

HAPE occurs in less than 2.5% of people ascending to 3500 to 4200 m. There is often a history of vigorous exercise in otherwise healthy but unacclimatized people who have ascended too rapidly; victims are frequently climbers or skiers. Highland dwellers who return to altitude after a period at low level are also at risk. Features of HAPE often manifest during the second night after ascent. They can also develop rapidly during exertion in the first few days. Symptoms of benign AMS may precede or accompany the development of HAPE. Typical early symptoms are profound breathlessness on physical effort and disproportionately long recovery time. Dyspnea at rest develops. Cough, sometimes associated with chest pain, is initially nonproductive but progresses to expectoration of white, then later blood-tinged, frothy sputum. Features of HACE may coexist, and victims may be confused and lack insight into the severity of their condition. If untreated, the respiratory distress progressively worsens, and death from massive pulmonary edema may occur within hours.

Early clinical signs include resting tachycardia, tachypnea, and central cyanosis on exertion. Auscultation reveals lung crackles, which may initially be confined to the right middle zone but become bilateral, generalized, and increasingly coarse as the condition develops. Slight fever is common. A right ventricular heave may be palpable, but signs of heart failure are absent (the etiology is controversial but probably involves patchy hypoxic pulmonary vasoconstriction with high pulmonary artery pressure that causes stress failure of pulmonary capillaries).

The diagnosis is usually made clinically, but chest radiographs show asymmetrical patchy shadowing in both lung fields, often with sparing of the costophrenic angles. The electrocardiogram may suggest right-sided heart strain, with right axis deviation, peaked P waves, and T wave changes in the right chest leads.

Management

Early recognition of inappropriate dyspnea should prompt immediate descent to a lower elevation; a reduction in altitude of only a few hundred meters can produce remarkable functional recovery. If the prevailing environmental conditions delay descent, the victim should be kept warm, and several therapeutic options may be used to "buy time" until evacuation is possible. Oxygen administration is lifesaving and produces symptomatic relief in most cases. The percentage of inspired oxygen achievable depends on the type of mask available: flow rates should be high initially; then, as symptoms improve, flow can be reduced. In a well-equipped medical facility at moderate altitudes, treatment with rest and oxygen alone may be successful.

In an emergency, simulated descent of 1500 m or more can be achieved by use of a lightweight (6.6 kg), portable hyperbaric bag (Gamow or Certec) that can be pressurized above ambient pressure with the victim inside. Pressurization is achieved and maintained by a manual or mechanical pump; newer versions allow supplemental oxygen administration and carbon dioxide removal. Hyperbaric bags have been shown to be effective for relieving symptoms of HAPE and benign AMS; however, the victim may suffer relapse on being removed from the bag, and use of hyperbaria should be regarded as a temporizing measure until actual descent to a lower attitude is possible.

Drug therapy may be combined with oxygen administration or hyperbaria. The calcium channel blocker nifedipine (Procardia), has been used successfully to reduce pulmonary vascular resistance and pulmonary artery pressure; an initial dose of 10 mg sublingually is followed by 20 mg every 6 hours of a slow-release oral preparation. Morphine sulfate has provided symptomatic relief in doses of 10 to 30 mg intravenously, but the dose must be carefully titrated to avoid undue respiratory depression, and morphine is contraindicated in the presence of HACE. Use of diuretics is no longer recommended, because they may aggravate pre-existing fluid depletion. If pulmonary infection cannot be ruled out, administration of broad-spectrum antibiotics is prudent. It is important to stress that these measures are adjuncts to but not substitutes for descent.

High-Altitude Cerebral Edema

The incidence of HACE is slightly less than that of HAPE, but features of the two conditions commonly coexist. The precise pathophysiologic mechanism is unclear, but HACE may be seen as a progression of the symptoms of benign AMS: headache with photophobia, and nausea and vomiting may increase in severity as cerebral edema worsens. With rising intracranial pressure, lethargy, weakness, incoordination, visual disturbance, and progressive deterioration in higher mental function and consciousness level occur. If untreated, victims can lapse into coma and die within hours.

Physical signs of HACE include progressive ataxia that may become truncal, and upper motoneuron signs of exaggerated tendon reflexes and extensor plantar responses. Retinal hemorrhages are a poor discriminator, because they may be seen in both benign AMS and HACE; papilledema is a late finding. Cyanosis, dyspnea, and the clinical features of HAPE are commonly present.

Management

For HACE, as with HAPE, the diagnosis is largely clinical, and urgent descent is the treatment of choice. Oxygen and hyperbaria may be used if immediate descent is not possible, but the response to these measures is less rapid than with HAPE. Dexamethasone, 8 mg intravenously followed by 4 mg,

every 6 hours intravenously or orally, has been shown to produce clinical improvement in HACE and is an effective adjunct to descent.

Prediction and Prevention of Acute Mountain Sickness

There is wide individual variation of and no reliable way to prejudge individual susceptibility to AMS; age, sex, build, fitness, and physiologic measures, such as hypoxic ventilatory response at sea level, are not useful predictive factors. The combination of a strong gag reflex, dizziness after 1 minute of hyperventilation, and short breath-hold time have been related to susceptibility to AMS, but these findings require confirmation. Persons who have experienced AMS are at greater risk of recurrence on re-exposure to altitude.

General preventive considerations, such as (1) ensuring adequate warm clothing, appropriate physical fitness, sufficient fluid intake; (2) a high-carbohydrate, low-fat diet; and (3) avoidance of sleeping tablets or sedative drugs are all prudent measures for those venturing into the mountains. Above altitudes of about 2500 m, however, the key to prevention of AMS is to allow time for acclimation through gradual ascent. Modest exercise is encouraged during the first few days at altitude, but severe exertion should be avoided. The adage "climb high, sleep low" is sound advice, and to acclimate to altitudes above 3000 m, the daily increase in sleeping altitude should not exceed 300 to 500 m, with a second night spent at the same altitude every 3 to 4 days. Unfortunately, visitors to altitude often have inflexible itineraries, and group pressures may endanger susceptible individuals.

For those known to be susceptible or for whom adequate acclimation is not possible, drug prophylaxis is an option. Oral acetazolamide, 250 mg twice daily (or 500 mg of a slow-release preparation daily), started 2 days before ascent, appears to speed acclimation and provides good (but not infallible) protection against AMS. Treatment may normally be stopped after 4 to 5 days at altitude, although continued use of this agent may reduce physical deterioration in climbing groups remaining at high altitude for longer periods. Intolerance of acetazolamide's side effects may limit its use in some people, and it is contraindicated in persons allergic to sulfonamides. Oral dexamethasone, 4 mg every 12 hours, is an effective alternative, but symptoms of AMS may occur if the drug is stopped at altitude, and its prolonged use is limited by potential steroid side effects. Nifedipine, 20 mg every 8 hours, has been reported as giving effective prophylaxis against HAPE in persons previously affected.

SUBACUTE MOUNTAIN SICKNESS

A condition termed subacute mountain sickness has been described in infants of the Han race who were born in mainland China and whose families later moved to a highland region (3600 m) in Tibet. A similar syndrome in adults has been reported in Indian army personnel serving in the western Himalayas (at about 6000 m). Both infants and adults presented with marked peripheral edema and severe, right ventricular failure, probably secondary to pulmonary arterial hypertension; there were no features of pulmonary edema. Susceptible infants were fatally afflicted after a mean of some 9 weeks at altitude; polycythemia was absent. Autopsy findings were of right-sided heart hypertrophy and dilatation with medial hypertrophy and muscularization of pulmonary arterioles. In adults, severe edema and dyspnea developed after about 10 weeks at altitude; signs of congestive cardiac failure were accompanied by papilledema and polycythemia. Investigations showed biochemical evidence of sodium and water retention; pulmonary arterial hypertension with right ventricular hypertrophy and dilatation were confirmed.

Management

All symptoms in adults resolved spontaneously without specific treatment within 2 weeks of descent. Timely descent is recommended for both infant and adult cases.

CHRONIC MOUNTAIN SICKNESS (MONGE'S DISEASE)

CMS is most common among men in Andean populations resident above about 3300 m, but it also occurs in other highland regions of the world. Marked polycythemia that is disproportionately high for the altitude is characteristic; values for other cellular blood elements are normal. The excessive erythropoiesis is stimulated by chronic hypoxia, perhaps aggravated by a combination of hypoventilation (which worsens with age), cigarette smoking, and chronic lower respiratory tract infection.

Symptoms, which often develop insidiously, include reduced exercise tolerance as well as nonspecific neuropsychiatric complaints such as headaches, irritability, lassitude, insomnia, mental slowness, and depression. Symptoms resolve if the sufferer descends to sea level but return on reascent. Signs are variable but include deep cyanosis of the lips and wine red mucosae, congested conjunctivae, venous dilatation of extremities, finger clubbing, and signs of right ventricular hypertrophy.

Management

Permanent descent to sea level is usually curative but is often impractical for social reasons. Periodic venisection improves symptoms and lowers hematocrit in most patients; values should be reduced to a level within 2 standard deviations of the population mean for the altitude. The relative immunity of women to CMS has led to the prolonged use of the female hormone analogue medroxyprogesterone acetate to act as a respiratory stimulant. This agent may reduce hemoglobin levels, but dose-related side effects such as loss of libido can be troublesome.

DISTURBANCES DUE TO COLD

method of
DANIEL F. DANZL, M.D.
University of Louisville
Louisville, Kentucky

ACCIDENTAL HYPOTHERMIA

Accidental hypothermia occurs when the body's core temperature unintentionally drops below 35°C. At this temperature, the compensatory physiologic responses to conserve heat begin to fail. Primary hypothermia results from exposure in previously healthy patients, but the mortality is much higher when diseases or injuries result in secondary hypothermia, which is often under-reported. Cold-induced tragedies continue to afflict both military and civilian populations. Urban indoor and outdoor settings produce the most cases in the United States.

Pathophysiology

Humans are unable to generate sufficient heat to maintain thermoneutrality under a variety of conditions (Table 1). Significant cold exposure normally activates the preoptic anterior hypothalamus, which orchestrates thermoregulation. Physiologic responses to the cold include shivering thermogenesis as well as endocrinologic and autonomic nervous system activities. Adaptive behavioral responses include donning of more clothing and seeking a heat source. Radiation normally accounts for 55 to 65% of the heat loss. Conductive losses increase up to 5 times in wet clothing and 23 times in water. Compensatory responses to heat loss through radiation, conduction, convection, evaporation, and respiration eventually fail. As the core temperature continues to fall, the patient becomes poikilothermic and cools to the ambient temperature.

Each organ system is affected uniquely. Cerebral metabolism is depressed 6 to 7% per 1°C. Cerebrovascular autoregulation remains intact until below 25°C, which helps maintain cortical blood flow. The electroencephalographic activity is clearly not prognostic and silences around 19 to 20°C. The lowest temperature for a neurologically intact survivor of accidental hypothermia is 15.2°C, and of induced hypothermia, 9°C.

Cardiovascular effects are often pronounced. After the initial tachycardia, there is progressive bradycardia. The heart rate drops to half its normal rate at 28°C. Hypothermia also progressively depresses the mean arterial pressure and cardiac index. Core temperature "afterdrop" refers to the continual decline in core temperature after removal from the cold. This phenomenon results from temperature equilibration

TABLE 1. **Factors Predisposing to Hypothermia or Frostbite**

Physiologic

Decreased Heat Production

Age extremes (infants, elderly)
Prior cold injury
Dehydration or malnutrition
Overexertion
Endocrinologic insufficiency
Trauma (multisystem or extremity)
Physical conditioning
Diaphoresis or hyperhidrosis
Hypoxia

Impaired Thermoregulation

Central nervous system trauma, disease
Spinal cord injury
Pharmacologic or toxicologic agents
Metabolic disorders
Sepsis

Psychologic

Mental status or attitude
Fear or panic
Peer pressure
Fatigue
Intense concentration on tasks
Hunger
Intoxicants

Environmental

Heat loss (conductive, evaporative, radiative, convective)
Ambient temperature or humidity
Duration of exposure
Wind chill factor
Altitude ± associated conditions
Quantity of exposed surface area

Increased Heat Loss

Vascular diseases
Shock
Poor acclimatization or conditioning
Dermatologic malfunction
Burns
Emergent resuscitations

Mechanical

Inadequate insulation
Constricting or wet clothing or boots
Immobility or cramped positioning

and reversal of circulatory arteriovenous shunting in the extremities.

All atrial arrhythmias are commonly encountered, have a slow ventricular response, and should be considered innocent. The clinical significance of ventricular arrhythmias is more difficult to assess, because suppressed pre-existent ectopy may reappear during rewarming. The decreased ventricular fibrillation threshold is a real hazard below 28°C. Cardiac cycle prolongation is pronounced, as reflected in the corrected QT interval. A J wave, or Osborn hypothermic hump, may be present at the junction of the QRS complex and ST segment.

Respiratory stimulation is followed by a progressive reduction in respiratory minute volume, which reflects the metabolic depression. Carbon dioxide production falls 50% for each 8°C drop in temperature. Although renal blood flow declines, there is a large initial paradoxical osmolar diuresis. Vasoconstriction in the extremities expands the capacitance vessels, temporarily producing a central hypervolemia.

Clinical Presentation

Historical circumstances suggest the diagnosis when exposure is obvious. More subtle presentations predominate in urban settings. As a result, the clinician may misfocus on a solitary diagnosis of a medical, toxicologic, neurologic, traumatic, or psychiatric emergency. Symptoms are often vague, and physical findings nonspecific or deceptive. For example, if tachycardia is disproportionate for the temperature, one should consider a secondary cause of hypothermia, such as hypoglycemia, hypovolemia, or a drug overdose. Persistent hyperventilation suggests a central nervous system (CNS) lesion or an organic acidosis, such as lactic acidosis or diabetic ketoacidosis. A cold-induced ileus and rectal spasm mimic and mask an acute abdomen. When the level of consciousness is inconsistent with the temperature, an overdose or CNS trauma or infection should be suspected. Hypothermic areflexia can also obscure a spinal cord injury. Lastly, temporary psychiatric sequelae during hypothermia include maladaptive behavior such as paradoxical undressing, which is the inappropriate removal of clothes in response to a cold stress.

Treatment

Hypothermia is confirmed with a core temperature (e.g., rectal, esophageal, tympanic) measurement, preferably from two sites. Further heat loss should be gently prevented, and cardiac monitoring initiated. Hypothermia adversely affects tissue oxygenation by numerous mechanisms, including the leftward shift of the oxyhemoglobin dissociation curve. Most patients are significantly dehydrated and will benefit from a bolus crystalloid administration.

Routine hematologic evaluations should include arterial blood gases uncorrected for temperature. An uncorrected pH of 7.4 and P_{CO_2} of 40 mm Hg reflect acid-base balance at any temperature. The hematocrit also increases 2% per 1°C drop in temperature, which can mask anemia. Leukopenia does not imply the absence of infection, because bone marrow suppression and white blood cell sequestration are common. Unfortunately, there is no safe predictor of the electrolyte status. For example, hyperkalemic electrocardiogram changes are obscured by hypothermia. Hypokalemia is more common in chronic hypothermia. Lastly, cold induces a renal glycosuria, which does not exclude hypoglycemia.

A full clotting screen is necessary, because cold hemagglutination and coagulation are aberrant. Platelet function is impaired. Cold also directly inhibits the enzymatic reactions of the coagulation cascade. This in vivo coagulopathy is not reflected by a deceptively normal prothrombin time, partial thromboplastin time, or International Normalized Ratio; these tests are performed at 37°C in the laboratory.

Rewarming Strategies

Choosing passive versus active rewarming is the key clinical decision. Passive external rewarming is noninvasive and ideal for mild cases in previously healthy patients. The patient should simply be covered with insulating materials. Active rewarming should be considered in the following situations: core temperature below 32°C, age extremes, CNS dysfunction, endocrine insufficiency, and cardiovascular instability.

Active external rewarming can be accomplished with heating blankets, radiant heat sources, and immersion. There is a potential for thermal injury to vasoconstricted skin with electric blankets. There are reservations about externally heating the extremities. Limiting heat application to the trunk minimizes many of the physiologic concerns with these techniques. For example, heating the extremities after the occurrence of the diuresis and fluid sequestration common to chronic hypothermia causes a core temperature afterdrop.

There are many techniques for delivering direct heat internally. Active core rewarming options include inhalation of heated, humidified oxygen; intravenous fluids and irrigation of the peritoneum, thorax, or gastrointestinal tract; hemodialysis; extracorporeal rewarming; and diathermy. Airway rewarming (40 to 45°C) with a mask or endotracheal tube is a valuable adjunct in all cases, because the access is simple. Preoxygenation and gentle technique prevent intubation arrhythmias. The inhalation eliminates respiratory heat loss. During massive volume resuscitations, heated intravenous fluid and blood are helpful adjuncts. Countercurrent heat exchangers are the most efficient method for heating and delivering the fluid.

Peritoneal lavage is another option for severely hypothermic patients. Peritoneal dialysate at 40 to 45°C delivered by two catheters with outflow suction efficiently transfers heat. Thoracostomy tube irrigation with warm saline is also valuable. The sterile saline is warmed to 42°C, infused anteriorly, and then continuously drained from the efferent midaxillary tube. Finally, irrigation of the gastrointestinal tract is of limited value and should be reserved for use in combination with all available techniques in patients with cardiac arrest.

Extracorporeal rewarming is potentially indicated in patients with cardiac arrest, completely frozen extremities, or severe rhabdomyolysis. The standard circuit uses a mechanical pump with an oxygenator and heat exchanger. Other options are continuous arteriovenous, venovenous, and hemodialysis rewarming. Cardiopulmonary resuscitation is indicated unless (1) a do-not-resuscitate status is documented and verified, (2) obviously lethal injuries are present, (3) chest wall depression is impossible, (4) any signs of life are present, or (5) rescuers are endangered by evacuation delays or altered triage conditions.

The misdiagnosis of a cardiac arrest should be avoided. Palpation of peripheral pulses is difficult when an extreme bradycardia is coupled with peripheral vasoconstriction. The examiner should take a full minute to check for a central pulse, especially if no cardiac monitor is available. After one attempt to defibrillate with 2 watt-seconds per kg, active rewarming should be continued past 32°C. Successful re-establishment of flow below that temperature is rare.

Resuscitation pharmacology usually reflects substandard therapeutic activity while the patient is cold, which progresses to toxicity after rewarming. Drug protein binding increases, and metabolism and excretion are impaired. Manipulation of the vasoconstricted and depressed cardiovascular system must be avoided. Bretylium (Bretylol) is the only effective antiarrhythmic agent at low temperatures. During ventricular fibrillation, 10 mg per kg should be infused. The empirical use of levothyroxine and corticosteroids is hazardous.

Because hypothermia is a great masquerader, no rigid treatment protocol can be suggested. Clinical treatment should be predicated on the duration and extent of temperature depression and the severity of the predisposing factors. The caveat "No one is dead until he or she is warm and dead" is evolving. Indicators of grave prognosis include evidence of cell lysis (hyperkalemia over 10 mEq per L), intravascular thrombosis (fibrinogen value below 50 mg per dL), and ammonia levels above 250 mmol per L.

PERIPHERAL COLD INJURIES

Peripheral local cold injuries include freezing and nonfreezing syndromes. Frostbite is the most common freezing injury. Trench foot and immersion foot are nonfreezing injuries resulting from exposure to wet cold. Nonfreezing injury after exposure to dry cold is called chilblain (pernio). With a cold stress, the core temperature is maintained at the expense of vasospasticity and shunting, which prevent heat distribution to the extremities.

Pathophysiology

A unique aspect of peripheral cold injury is the pathogenesis of the freezing injury cascade. Tissue is initially damaged by the freeze-thaw insult and subsequently by progressive dermal ischemia. Before freezing, tissue cooling increases the viscosity of the vascular contents as the microvasculature constricts.

The freeze-thaw sequence begins during extracellular fluid crystallization. Water exits the cell, causing intracellular dehydration, hyperosmolality, cellular shrinkage, and collapse. Arachidonic acid breakdown products are then released from underlying damaged tissue into the vesicle fluid. Both prostaglandin $F_{2\alpha}$ and thromboxane A_2 produce platelet aggregation, leukocyte immobilization, and vasoconstriction. Endothelial cells are quite sensitive to cold injury, and the microvasculature distorts and clogs.

After tissue thawing, there is progressive edema formation for 48 to 72 hours. Subsequent thrombosis and early superficial necrosis develop. This tissue eventually mummifies and demarcates, often more than 60 to 90 days later, hence the surgical aphorism, "Frostbite in January, amputate in July."

The incidence and severity of peripheral cold injury are determined by the duration and intensity of cutaneous cold exposure. Factors predisposing to peripheral cold injuries are listed in Table 1.

Clinical Presentation

The initial presentation of frostbite is often deceptively benign. Unlike in burns, classification of frostbite by degrees is often prognostically inaccurate and therapeutically misleading. The physical findings present 24 to 72 hours after completion of rewarming are more reliably used to classify frostbite. Superficial or mild frostbite does not entail eventual tissue loss, but deep or severe frostbite does. "Frostnip" is a superficial cold insult producing transient numbness or tingling that resolves after rewarming.

All patients with frostbite have some initial sensory deficiency in light touch, pain, or temperature. Acral areas and distal extremities are the usual insensate sites. Patients also complain of being clumsy or having a "chunk of wood" sensation in the extremity.

Deep frostbite may initially appear to be deceptively benign. However, tissues remaining frozen can appear mottled, violaceous, pale yellow, or waxy. Favorable presenting signs are warmth, normal color, and some sensation. If the subcutaneous tissue is soft and pliable or the dermis can be rolled over the bony prominences, the injury may be superficial.

Rapid rewarming produces an initial hyperemia, even in severe cares. A residual violaceous hue is ominous. Early formation of clear, large blebs is a more favorable sign than smaller, dark, hemorrhagic blebs, which imply cold damage to the subdermal vascular plexus.

Chilblain is a form of dry cold injury often developing after repetitive exposures. These "cold sores" typically involve facial areas and the dorsa of the hands and feet. Young females, especially those with a history of Raynaud's phenomenon, are at risk. Persistent vasospasticity and vasculitis result in pruritus, erythema, and mild edema. Plaques, blue nodules, and ulcerations eventually develop. Treatment of perniosis is difficult; the physician should consider using nifedipine (Procardia) at a dose of 20 to 60 mg daily.

Immersion (trench) foot is produced by prolonged exposure to wet cold at above-freezing temperatures. Feet often appear erythematous, edematous, or cyanotic. The bullae are indistinguishable from those seen in frostbite. However, this vesiculation proceeds to ulceration and liquefaction gangrene. In milder cases, hyperhidrosis, cold sensitivity, and painful ambulation persist for years.

Warm water immersion foot affects the soles of the feet and results from waterlogging of the thick stratum corneum. This commonly occurs in individuals wearing wet shoes for prolonged periods owing to a lack of shelter.

Ancillary diagnostic adjuncts continue to be investigated for peripheral cold injuries. Doppler ultrasound, digital plethysmography, scintigraphy, routine radiography, and angiography do not consistently predict tissue loss at presentation. Delayed studies may guide subsequent therapy.

Treatment

Mills popularized rapid immersion rewarming after extensive experience with severe Alaskan frostbite cases. Before thawing, frozen parts should not be exposed to dry heat sources. Tissue refreezing is also disastrous; as an extreme example, it is preferable to ambulate to safety on frozen extremities. A treatment protocol is summarized in Table 2.

A circulating tank is ideal for the extremities, but a large container suffices for the hands and feet. Care should be taken to avoid thermal injury, which occurs if the water temperature exceeds 42°C. A common error is premature termination of rewarming, because the establishment of reperfusion is quite painful. Rewarming may take up to 1 hour.

Extreme caution should be exercised in treating patients with completely frozen extremities, because they are invariably hypothermic. Thawing produces significant core temperature, fluid, and electrolyte fluxes. Persistent cyanosis after a complete thaw should suggest raised fascial compartment pressures.

Management of frostbite vesicles also varies. Some physicians initially leave large, clear blisters intact; however, sterile aspiration or débridement seems preferable. The débridement of hemorrhagic vesicles can extend the injury by allowing secondary desiccation of deep dermal layers. There are two strategies to inhibit prostaglandins. Topical aloe vera (Dermaide) is a specific thromboxane inhibitor. Systemi-

---

TABLE 2. **Treatment of Frostbite**

Before Thawing
1. Stabilize core temperature.
2. Address medical or surgical conditions.
3. Protect and do not massage frozen part.
4. Avoid partial thawing and refreezing.
5. Extricate from environment.

Thaw
1. Provide parenteral analgesia and hydration.
2. Rapidly rewarm entire part in 38–40°C circulating water until distal flush (thermometer monitoring).
3. Requires 10–60 min with gentle motion of part by the patient without friction massage.

After Thawing
1. For clear vesicles—aspirate if intact; débride if broken.
2. For hemorrhagic vesicles—do not débride; may aspirate.
3. Apply topical aloe vera (Dermaide) q 6 hs.
4. Use ibuprofen, 400 mg orally q 12 h (12 mg/kg/d).
5. Administer tetanus and streptococcal prophylaxis.
6. Elevate part in protective cradle.
7. Use whirlpool hydrotherapy two or three times daily (37°C).
8. Avoid vasoconstrictors, including nicotine.

cally, ibuprofen is preferable to the salicylates. Ibuprofen produces fibrinolysis in addition to limiting the accumulation of inflammatory mediators.

Multiple experimental antithrombotic and vasodilatory treatment regimens have been proposed. There is no conclusive evidence of enhanced tissue salvage from administration of dextran, heparin, steroids, nonsteroidal anti-inflammatory agents, dimethylsulfoxide (DMSO),* nonionic detergents, dipyridamole (Persantine), calcium channel blockers, or hyperbaric oxygen. Pentoxifylline (Trental), 400 mg given orally every 8 hours, may facilitate small-vessel perfusion.

A long-acting alpha blocker, phenoxybenzamine (Dibenzyline),* 10 mg per day up to 60 mg per day, may decrease the refractory vasospasm during the clinical course in selected patients. Aggressive hydration is essential to minimize orthostatic hypotension. Sympathectomy, both medical (e.g., intra-arterial reserpine*) and surgical, can relieve painful vasospasm and decrease edema but has not been demonstrated to enhance tissue salvage.

Sequelae

Residual neuropathic symptoms are common and result from abnormal sympathetic tone and neuronal damage. Dermatologic findings include lymphedema, ulcerations, hair and nail deformities, and epidermoid or squamous carcinomas. Occult musculoskeletal injuries are the most pronounced in children. Premature epiphyseal fusion and fragmentation are another concern. Amputation decisions should be deferred unless there is supervening sepsis or gangrene. The ultimate tissue salvage after a spontaneous slough usually far exceeds the most optimistic initial estimates.

---

*Not FDA approved for this indication.

DISTURBANCES DUE TO HEAT

method of
PETER HANSON, M.Sc., M.D.
University of Wisconsin Clinical Science Center
Madison, Wisconsin

Heat illness represents a continuum of morbid responses to heat exposure in which fluid and electrolyte balance, cardiovascular regulation, and central nervous system function are progressively impaired. Heat illnesses occur most commonly in athletes, military recruits, and outdoor workers who perform sustained activity in warm, humid environments. Episodic heat illness is also associated with seasonal heat waves; it commonly affects elderly persons, the homeless population, and patients taking medications with anticholinergic activity. During the 1995 Chicago heat wave, for example, patients living alone or confined to bed with medical problems were at highest risk for heat-related death.

Table 1 summarizes the clinical findings for various heat illnesses.

HEAT SYNCOPE

Heat syncope usually occurs in the setting of heat exposure and orthostatic stress such as standing in military formation. Another cause is inappropriate use of whirlpool and sauna baths, especially after exercise or ingestion of alcohol. Cutaneous vasodilatation, the absence of muscle venous pump activity, and moderate fluid loss due to sweating all contribute to reduced central venous return and low ventricular filling volumes. Syncope is probably mediated by activation of ventricular stretch receptors due to inadequate filling, causing vagal reflex bradycardia and loss of sympathetic vasomotor tone (Bezold-Jarisch reflex).

Treatment

Treatment of heat syncope is supportive: vital signs should be monitored closely, and the airway protected from tongue obstruction or emesis. Venous return is initially enhanced by raising of the lower extremities and cooling of the skin. Volume repletion may be required if orthostatic intolerance persists (see later). Victims of heat syncope should be questioned about the possible role of drugs or alcohol or a history of recurrent orthostatic intolerance, which may indicate autonomic dysfunction.

HEAT CRAMPS

Involuntary, painful fasciculations or contractures of skeletal muscle, heat cramps occur in the setting of excessive sweat losses in unacclimatized athletes or outdoor workers. The exact mechanism of heat cramps is unresolved, although most clinical and experimental evidence points to depletion of body sodium and chloride stores or dilutional hyponatremia due to the excessive intake of salt-free water. Other electrolyte abnormalities may also be involved (e.g., of calcium, potassium).

Treatment

Rapid replenishment of serum sodium using oral (0.1% NaCl solution) or intravenous (normal saline) fluids is usually successful in terminating heat cramps.

HEAT EXHAUSTION

Heat exhaustion is a syndrome of progressive intravascular volume depletion due to sustained sweat loss with inadequate fluid replacement that typically occurs in athletes (e.g., football players, runners) who are inadequately acclimatized. However, heat exhaustion is also common in a variety of outdoor occupations that require sustained moderate activity in warm weather. Symptoms include progressive fatigue, weakness, nausea, dizziness, and near-syncope when attempting to stand or walk. Rectal temperature is moderately increased (38 to 39.5°C), the skin is cool and vasoconstricted, and active sweating is

TABLE 1. **Usual Clinical Findings in Heat Illness**

Parameter	Heat Exhaustion	Heat Stroke
Level of consciousness	Mild confusion Presyncope on standing	Marked alteration Delirium, coma
Skin findings	Vasoconstricted—cool Active sweating	Vasodilated—warm Dry or sweating
Rectal temperature	38–40°C	>42°C
Cardiovascular features		
Heart rate	Heart rate 90–120 bpm	>120 bpm
Systemic blood pressure	Usually <110 mm Hg with marked orthostatic drop of >20 mm Hg	Varies—low if in shock Low vascular resistance

Laboratory studies	Hemoconcentration
	Variable serum electrolytes
	Mild increase in muscle enzymes
		Multisystem abnormalities
		  ↑ Muscle, hepatic enzymes
		  ↑ Uric acid, lactate, K⁺
		  ↓ Glucose
		  ↓ Coagulation factors
		  ↓ Platelets
		  + Myoglobinuria
		  + Hemoglobinuria

Abbreviations: ↑ = increased; ↓ = decreased; + = positive appearance in urine.

usually present. In the supine position, the heart rate is mildly elevated, the arterial blood pressure is in the low-normal or hypotensive range, and the jugular venous pressure is not visible. With orthostatic stress (standing), there is a marked decrease in blood pressure, with systolic values falling to below 90 mm Hg. Laboratory studies reveal hemoconcentration, variable electrolyte patterns (due to combined effects of electrolyte losses and hemoconcentration), and increased urine specific gravity.

Treatment

Initial treatment is similar to that for heat syncope, but with added emphasis on active cooling and intravascular volume repletion using oral or intravenous electrolyte fluids. If intravenous fluids are required, half-normal or quarter-normal saline may be more appropriate, because such solutions approximate the sodium concentration of sweat in unacclimatized persons. Intravenous glucose and water (D5W) should be used with caution, because hyponatremia may occur with excessive hypotonic fluid replacement. Administration of intravenous fluid therapy should be guided by stabilization of vital signs and normalization of orthostatic hypotension, serum electrolyte values, and urine output. Extensive laboratory work is usually unnecessary unless there is evidence of concomitant hyperthermia, as discussed in the next section.

Table 2 summarizes the treatment of heat illnesses.

HEAT STROKE

Heat stroke is a critical extension of the heat exhaustion syndrome that may manifest in either a

TABLE 2. **Treatment of Heat Illnesses**

Illness	Evaluation and Therapy	Additional Considerations
Heat syncope	Elevate legs, restore venous return and vasomotor tone Fluid replacement and cooling of skin as needed	Possible drug effects Baroreflex disorders (if recurrent)
Heat cramps	Rest Oral or IV sodium chloride	Increase salt intake Limit salt-free water intake
Heat exhaustion	Monitor vital signs, rectal temperature Fluid replacement PO or IV to restore orthostatic blood pressure and urine output	Laboratory studies (complete blood count, electrolytes, blood urea nitrogen, creatinine, urinalysis) for severe hypotension or suspected prior hyperthermia

Heat stroke	Treat as multisystem injury
	Continuous vital signs monitoring
	Immediate cooling to <39°C (avoid body immersion)
	Comprehensive baseline laboratory studies (see text)
	Initiate diuresis with mannitol or loop diuretic
	Fluid replacement as needed to maintain blood pressure and urine output
	Judicious use of vasopressors, inotropic agents if needed
		Watch for
		  Rhabdomyolysis
		  Renal failure (acute tubular necrosis)
		  Hepatic failure
		  Disseminated intravascular coagulation
		  Hypoglycemia

classic or an exertional form. Classic heat stroke occurs during prolonged heat exposure, resulting in progressive dehydration, hyperthermia, and eventual cessation of sweating. Exertional heat stroke occurs over a shorter time and is associated with combined effects of heat exposure and high-intensity exercise. Active sweating is usually present but is inadequate to maintain effective cooling.

In both forms of heat stroke, there is marked central nervous system impairment, ranging from delirium to coma and convulsions. The rectal temperature exceeds 42°C but may be lower after transport to a medical facility. The skin is warm and flushed, unless circulatory collapse has occurred. There is moderate to severe tachycardia, and blood pressure values vary according to cardiac function and vasomotor tone.

Treatment

Emergency treatment of heat stroke requires a multisystem management approach. Immediate cooling of body temperature is essential. Immersion in an ice bath has been used in some military training centers, but it is now discouraged because intense reflex cutaneous vasoconstriction due to the ice bath may actually inhibit heat loss. Alternative methods that are highly effective include local "spot" application of ice packs to the neck, axillae, and groin (which are areas of vascular countercurrent exchange) and spraying of the skin with tepid water while fanning vigorously to promote evaporative cooling. Rectal temperature must be monitored continuously. Active cooling efforts should be discontinued when body temperature falls to 39°C. Consciousness usually returns at this point.

Insertion of large-bore intravenous catheter lines and use of a Foley catheter are also essential. The hemodynamic state resembles a low vascular resistance circulatory failure, and definitive cardiovascular support may require insertion of a pulmonary artery catheter to facilitate the judicious use of vasopressors (dopamine or norepinephrine) and intravenous fluids (saline). Fluid therapy should be administered in small boluses of 250 to 500 mL to avoid cerebral or pulmonary edema. Urine output should be monitored carefully, and intravenous mannitol (Osmitrol), 25 to 50 grams, or furosemide (Lasix), 40 to 80 mg, should be administered to initiate diuresis.

Comprehensive laboratory studies should be ordered, including complete blood count with platelet count, liver function panel, creatinine kinase, measurement, coagulation panel, and evaluation of glucose, lactate, electrolytes, calcium, uric acid, blood urea nitrogen, creatinine, and arterial blood gases. The urine should be tested for presence of hemoglobin and/or myoglobin.

Major complications of heat stroke are hypoglycemia, metabolic acidosis, renal failure due to acute tubular necrosis, rhabdomyolysis, disseminated intravascular coagulation syndrome, and hepatic failure. Some studies suggest that occult endotoxemia, originating from increased gastrointestinal perme-

ability, may play an additional role in the clinical manifestations of heat stroke syndrome. Patients with documented or suspected heat stroke should always be admitted for observation, because complications may not develop for 24 to 48 hours. Some studies have indicated that victims of exertional heat stroke may exhibit abnormal thermoregulatory responses to exercise and may remain at risk for repeated episodes of heat illness during heat exposure and exercise.

SPIDER BITES AND SCORPION STINGS

method of
JOSEPH G. PHANEUF, M.D.
Kaiser Permanente Medical Center
Hayward, California
University of California, San Francisco
San Francisco, California

SPIDER BITES

The misdiagnosis of spider bites is quite common. A review of 600 spider bites in Southern California during a 30-year period revealed that only 10% were probably caused by spiders. Approximately 80% were determined to be caused by other arthropods, and 10% by disease states, such as erythema nodosum and erythema migrans.

The misdiagnosis of brown recluse spider bite is especially common. A necrotic skin lesion is not necessarily the result of a brown recluse spider bite. Several other spiders commonly found in the United States, including *Chiracanthium* (sac spider), *Argiope* (orb weaver), *Phidippus* (jumping spider), *Lycosa* (wolf spider), and *Tegenaria* (funnel web spider), have been reported to cause local skin necrosis. Bites from other arthropods, such as ticks and kissing bugs, can also occasionally cause local skin necrosis. Disease states that can cause local skin necrosis include diabetic ulcer, infected herpes simplex, trauma, factitious ulceration, local thrombosis, and drug reactions.

Brown Recluse Spider
(*Loxosceles reclusa*)

L. reclusa, known as the brown recluse or fiddle-back spider, has a leg span of 1 to 5 cm and may be recognized from the dark, violin-shaped marking on the dorsal cephalothorax. This marking may be faint or absent, depending on the species and time of last molting. At present, there are 13 species of *Loxosceles* in the United States.

The spider's natural habitat, especially in the southern United States, is outdoors, where it resides under rocks, woodpiles, and debris. However, it is a common house spider in the Midwest, where it can be found in closets, storage boxes, basements, and attics.

Brown Recluse Spider Bites (Loxoscelism)

L. reclusa is a common spider in the Mississippi river valley, but most well-documented *L. reclusa* bites occur in Missouri, Oklahoma, Arkansas, Kansas, Tennessee, and Texas.

The brown recluse spider prefers to avoid human contact and hunts for food at night, so patients are usually bitten while sleeping or when putting on shoes or clothing left in the spider's territory. Bites usually occur during the spring, summer, or early fall.

Bites of any *Loxosceles* species can cause local necrosis, but the main species responsible for necrotic bites in the United States is *L. reclusa*.

Nonetheless, most bites of *L. reclusa* do not result in skin necrosis and instead are insignificant, are frequently painless, and heal rapidly without complications. Bites rarely cause hemolysis. The varied clinical presentation depends on the amount and concentration of venom at time of the bite as well as on the patient's immune response to the venom. Severe dermatonecrosis is more likely to occur if a bite occurs where there is abundant fatty tissue, such as the abdomen, buttocks, and thighs.

A clinically significant bite is usually a solitary necrotic skin lesion 0.5 to 2.0 cm in diameter. If necrosis is present at multiple sites and the patient is very toxic, other causes should be sought, such as emboli, vasculitis, and septicemia. A necrotizing bacterial infection should be suspected if the affected area is large, fluctuant, and rapidly enlarging.

Patients with a clinically significant reaction to a brown recluse spider bite develop considerable pain and erythema at the bite site, which then rapidly progresses, within several hours, to a dusky cyanosis. A halo or ring of pallor due to vasoconstriction is commonly noted around the cyanotic bite site, with reactive erythema peripheral to the halo. Within 48 hours, a hemorrhagic blister may develop, and within 1 week, a small area of necrosis may be evident. The bite site may be eccentrically shaped, as determined by gravitational spread of the venom.

A mild systemic reaction may manifest as fever, general malaise, nausea, and arthralgias. Generalized toxic erythema or urticaria may also occur and is usually not associated with hemolysis. Intravascular hemolysis may occur, but it rarely progresses to disseminated intravascular coagulation (DIC) and renal failure. Clinically significant hemolysis from a brown recluse spider bite is more common in young children. If systemic reaction is suspected, serial urinalyses and hematologic evaluation should be done.

Treatment

For almost all brown recluse spider bites, only conservative treatment, consisting of local wound care, pain medication if indicated, and tetanus toxoid injection if due, is needed. Elevating an affected extremity and cooling the bite site increase the patient's comfort. Unnecessary treatment for local necrosis includes use of antivenin, hyperbaric oxygen, and vasodilator and steroid agents. Dapsone is often recommended, although it is not approved by the Food and Drug Administration for this use. However, because almost all bites heal uneventfully with conservative treatment, no evidence exists that dapsone will change the final outcome. Dapsone can cause severe hemolysis or the dapsone hypersensitivity syndrome. If clinically significant hemolysis should occur, whether dapsone or venom is the cause of hemolysis may be difficult to determine.

Early, wide excision of the bite is not indicated. Surgery within the first 2 weeks may result in dehiscence or otherwise could be disabling or disfiguring. For those rare bites that have not healed uneventfully after 1 to 2 months, repair by plastic surgery may be necessary.

Mild systemic reactions, such as toxic erythema and urticarial eruptions (without hemolysis), are self-limited. For those rare patients in whom clinically significant hemolysis develops, hospitalization is indicated to monitor for DIC and renal failure. Simple hydration may be the best treatment for severe anemia, because transfused blood may react with the venom and worsen hemolysis. The venom is rapidly inactivated in tissue. Therefore, the overall strategy is to help the patient survive DIC and renal failure, which are usually of short duration and reversible.

Prevention

Brown recluse spiders are insensitive to residual pesticides, and chemical treatment is not likely to rid a house of spiders. Good insect control in the home may reduce the total number of brown recluse spiders by decreasing their food supply. Sealing the home by installing weather stripping, especially at door openings, may provide some benefit. The best preventive measure is shaking out shoes, clothing, and linens before using them.

Black Widow Spider (*Latrodectus mactans*)

Immature black widow spiders have multicolored stripes of yellow, white, black, and orange configured in a chevron pattern on the dorsal side of the abdomen. Mature female spiders are glossy black with an abdomen about 6 mm in width and 15 mm in length, and a leg spread of 40 mm. The ventral side of the abdomen always has a red marking, which may consist of two red triangles or the typical hourglass-shaped red marking. The black widow spider is commonly found outdoors in barns, garages, and storerooms. This spider may spin its web just outside homes, where outdoor lighting attracts insects. Most bites occur in the summer or fall.

Four species of *Latrodectus* are found in the United States. *L. mactans* is most commonly found in the eastern states; *Latrodectus hesperus* is found in the western states. Serious black widow spider bites are more common in western states such as Arizona and California.

Black Widow Spider Bites

Envenomation by *L. mactans* or *L. hesperus* may cause mild to severe pain in several muscle groups within 30 minutes to 3 hours after the bite. The bite itself is commonly felt as a pinprick sensation. The skin shows little or no reaction at the bite site. *Latrodectus* venom is a neurotoxin that stimulates release of acetylcholine and epinephrine as well as of other neurotransmitters. Deep musculoskeletal pain is the main symptom in severe envenomation. The pain may mimic that seen in acute abdominal pain or renal colic. However, the presence of pain in several muscle groups should help in the differential diagnosis. Anxiety, hypertension, and tachycardia are also commonly seen with severe envenomation.

Treatment

Only analgesic agents and application of an ice pack at the bite site may be required in mild cases. Intravenous narcotic agents may be required to treat severe pain. Calcium gluconate is usually not helpful. Black widow spider antivenin (antivenin *L. mactans*, equine origin) is the most effective treatment and makes the patient pain free in about 1 hour. Serum sickness is uncommon with this product. Because antivenin can cause anaphylaxis, serum sickness, or a hypersensitivity reaction, it should be used only for patients with severe intractable pain in whom the benefits clearly outweigh the risks. When a patient is taking a beta-blocking agent, antivenin is usually contraindicated, because beta-adrenergic blockade complicates treatment of anaphylaxis. Beta-blocking agents also seem to predispose patients to anaphylaxis from any cause.

SCORPION STINGS

Bark Scorpion (*Centruroides exilicauda*)

C. exilicauda is a small, slender scorpion about 2 inches long. The body color varies from straw yellow to dark yellow-brown. The common name, bark scorpion, comes from its habit of climbing trees and resting under loose bark. The scorpions also commonly hide on the ground under rocks, wood, and debris. Bark scorpions feed on insects at night and rest in cool moist spots during the day, including inside shoes and clothing.

Scorpions are not aggressive but will sting if disturbed. Most scorpions found in the United States inflict stings, which usually cause local burning pain, occasional swelling, and no systemic symptoms, but *C. exilicauda* has a neurotoxic venom that can cause a life-threatening crisis. The species is found mainly in Arizona, but parts of Texas, New Mexico, Nevada, and small areas of California also have colonies of this scorpion.

Bark Scorpion Stings

Most stings by *C. exilicauda* result in severe pain at the sting site and only local paresthesias. Adults are stung more often than children; however, children are more likely to have a serious reaction and require intensive supportive care. Severe envenomation may result in tachycardia, hypertension, restlessness, roving eye movements, hypersalivation, respiratory distress, muscle twitching, and flailing of extremities. Uncontrollable jerking of the extremities and thrashing about may be mistaken for seizures or hysteria.

Treatment

For most stings that cause local pain and paresthesias, only analgesic agents, local application of an ice pack, and tetanus toxoid when indicated are necessary. Treatments that are not effective include corticosteroids, antihistamines, atropine, epinephrine, and calcium.

The treatment of severe envenomation is controversial. All experts agree that maintenance of a clear airway is the primary objective, especially in children. Some physicians use antivenin (available to licensed physicians only in Arizona), which controls symptoms in about an hour. Other physicians rarely use antivenin, and instead monitor patients in an intensive care unit and may use midazolam (Versed) to treat symptoms. Caution is advisable, however, because use of sedative or hypnotic agents in an attempt to control abnormal movements may compromise respiration and may cause apnea.

ACKNOWLEDGMENTS

Franklin Ennik, M.A., formerly of the Vector-Borne Disease Section, California State Department of Health Services, Berkeley, California, provided entomologic consultation. The Medical Editing Department, Kaiser Foundation Research Institute, provided editorial assistance.

SNAKE VENOM POISONING

method of
FINDLAY E. RUSSELL, M.D., Ph.D.
University of Arizona Health Sciences
Tucson, Arizona

In the United States, approximately 45,000 snakebites occur each year. Of these, about 8000 are inflicted by venomous snakes, and 6700 are duly reported. In 1980, the 20 species of rattlesnakes (*Crotalus* species, *Sistrurus* species) accounted for 61% of all snake venom poisoning cases; copperheads (*Agkistrodon contortrix* subspecies), 21%; cottonmouths (*Agkistrodon piscivorus* subspecies), 9%; unidentified species, 8%; coral snakes (*Micrurus fulvius* and *Micruroides*), less than 1%; and exotic snakes, approximately 0.3%. Six to 12 deaths are attributed to snake venom poisoning each year. Most of these can be assigned to four categories: untreated, undertreated, or mistreated cases; patients younger than 4 years; patients older than 70 years, with some debilitating disease; and members of religious sects who handle venomous snakes as part of their religious ceremonies.

The largest number of bites by venomous snakes is inflicted by the western diamondback rattlesnake *Crotalus atrox*, although the eastern diamondback *Crotalus adamanteus* must be considered the more dangerous. The time from bite to arrival at a medical facility varies considerably from state to state and usually reflects transit time. In California, the average time is 33 minutes, whereas some patients are seen as early as 20 minutes and others not for 3 to 4 hours; in Idaho, it is 75 minutes. The average time from bite to antivenom administration at 12 medical centers in endemic snakebite areas during 1993 was 54 minutes.

Of 800 bites by native North American snakes I have treated or seen between 1951 and 1994, 24% did not end in envenomation (dry bites); 16% were so trivial as not to require specific treatment; 28% were minimal envenomations; 20% were moderate envenomations; and 12% were severe poisonings. Most of the copperhead bites caused minor envenomation, but most of the bites by the eastern diamondback rattlesnake were either moderate or severe. Bites by the timber rattlesnake *Crotalus horridus horridus*, the Southern Pacific rattlesnake *Crotalus viridis helleri*, and the western diamondback rattlesnake *C. atrox* also tended to cause moderate or severe envenomation. Most bites occurred between 9 AM and 6 PM, with the largest number between 3 and 6 PM. Ninety-five percent of bites were on an extremity.

CLASSIFICATION OF POISONING IN CROTALID BITES

The extent of poisoning is based on the following evaluation of clinical manifestations.

Minimal envenomation: Swelling, erythema, and ecchymosis are usually limited to the immediate area of the bite site. Systemic symptoms and signs are absent or minimal. Coagulation parameters are normal. No other significant laboratory abnormalities are found.

Moderate envenomation: Swelling, erythema, and ecchymosis are present, may involve most of the involved extremity, and spread slowly. Systemic symptoms and signs are present but not life-threatening; they include weakness, nausea, vomiting, oral paresthesias or unusual taste, mild hypotension (systolic blood pressure [SBP] of >80 mm Hg), tachycardia, and tachypnea. Coagulation parameters may be abnormal, but no clinically significant bleeding is present. There are no severe abnormalities in other laboratory tests.

Severe envenomation: Swelling and ecchymosis involve the extremity and spread rapidly. Systemic symptoms and signs are markedly abnormal, including nausea and vomiting, changes in mental status, hypotension (SBP of <80 mm Hg), severe tachycardia, and tachypnea or other respiratory compromise. Coagulation parameters are abnormal, with serious bleeding or threat of spontaneous bleeding. Prothrombin time and partial thromboplastin time show severe disruption or are unmeasurable. Fibrinogen is undetectable, and the platelet count is less than 20,000 cells per mm³. Severe abnormalities of other laboratory values may be present.

Some envenomations can also be categorized as *trivial*, that is, the injury requires no more treatment than cleansing the wound, applying a dressing, and giving the appro-

priate antitetanus agent. Finally, about one quarter of all crotalid bites do not end in envenomation.

CLINICAL MANIFESTATIONS

Table 1 lists the most significant findings in rattlesnake venom poisoning in the United States.

Local Findings

The evidence of envenomation usually appears locally, before systemic symptoms are detected. Pain or paresthesia is usually the initial complaint, and in many instances, the pain is out of proportion to that caused by an uncomplicated traumatic injury. In most crotalid venom poisoning cases I have seen, some pain was evident within 5 minutes of the bite. In bites by some *Crotalus* species, however, only minor pain is present, and the patient may complain of numbness about the wound. In most moderate or severe poisonings, pain increases with time, not only because of the effects of the venom but also because of the pressure of the swelling. Pain is most severe after bites by *C. adamanteus* and *C. atrox* and is much less after poisonings by *Crotalus cerastes*, *Crotalus scutulatus*, and *A. contortrix*. Early on, a bluish discoloration or ecchymosis may develop around the bite area.

TABLE 1. **Symptoms and Signs of Bites by Rattlesnakes in the United States**

Symptom or Sign	Frequency per 100 Cases
Fang marks	100
Swelling and edema	74
Pain	65
Ecchymosis	51
Vesiculations	40
Changes in pulse rate	60
Weakness	72
Sweating and/or chill	64
Numbness or tingling of tongue and mouth, scalp, or feet	63
Faintness or dizziness	57
Nausea, vomiting, or both	48
Changes in blood pressure	46
Change in body temperature	31
Swelling of regional lymph nodes	40
Fasciculations	41
Increased blood clotting time	39
Formation of spherical red blood cells	18
Tingling or numbness of affected part	42
Necrosis	27
Changes in respiratory rate	40
Decreased hemoglobin value	37
Abnormal electrocardiogram	26
Cyanosis	16
Hematemesis, hematuria, or melena	15
Glycosuria	20
Proteinuria	16
Unconsciousness	12
Thirst	34
Increased salivation	20
Swollen eyelids	2
Retinal hemorrhage	2
Blurred vision	12
Convulsions	1
Muscular contractions	6
Increased blood platelets	4
Decreased blood platelets	42

Some swelling and edema are usually present soon after a crotalid envenomation, sometimes within 10 minutes. They are most severe after envenomations by *C. adamanteus, C. atrox, C. horridus horridus,* and *C. viridis helleri* and are least severe after bites by *C. cerastes, C. scutulatus, A. contortrix,* and *Sistrurus* species. Swelling and edema are negligible after bites by coral snakes. I have never seen a rattlesnake envenomation in which diagnosable swelling has not been observed within 30 minutes; it often occurs within 15 minutes. Swelling may be minimal at those times, and progressing to severity only some hours later. Induration is common in many cases of crotalid envenomation, and skin temperature is often altered. Vesiculations may occur after bites by some species of rattlesnakes.

Systemic Findings

Weakness, sweating, and chills are common in moderate to severe envenomations. Changes in taste (metallic, rubbery, or minty taste, or tingling about the mouth) are common after envenomation by *C. viridis helleri, C. adamanteus,* and *C. horridus horridus,* but relatively uncommon after *C. atrox* bites. Patients have told me that they experienced these paresthesias within minutes of an envenomation. Fasciculations about the face are sometimes seen after rattlesnake bites. Nausea occurs in a few minimal envenomations, and nausea and vomiting are often seen in moderate poisonings and in most severe cases. Spontaneous bleeding is common in severe poisonings but uncommon in moderate envenomations, and it is generally absent in minimal envenomations. Necrosis, kidney, heart, and other tissue changes are seen in some moderate and severe cases.

MEDICAL TREATMENT

Pit Viper (Rattlesnake, Cottonmouth, and Copperhead) Bites

1. Evaluate the patient's status and preadmission treatment.
2. Determine concomitant drug or alcohol use.
3. If a tourniquet has inadvertently been placed, apply one or two less constricting band(s) proximal to them, start intravenous (IV) infusion of a crystalloid solution, and remove the tourniquet slowly.
4. Start IV infusion of a crystalloid solution (e.g., lactated Ringer's solution or NaCl). If shock or severe bleeding is present, consider colloid solutions, plasma, or whole blood.
5. Consider use of antivenom (see number 11).
6. Cleanse the wound with soap and water.
7. Loosely immobilize the part in a functional position just below heart level.
8. When the patient is stable, give an appropriate analgesic, if indicated.
9. Administer a mild sedative if necessary.
10. Give an appropriate antitetanus agent if indicated.
11. Give antivenom (Antivenin [Crotalidae] Polyvalent [ACP]):
    a. No ACP is indicated in trivial or dry bites.
    b. Follow package instructions.
    c. Check the patient's allergy history.
    d. Skin test only if horse serum ACP is indicated, and keep a shock cart with epinephrine at the bedside.
    e. If the skin test is positive and ACP is deemed necessary, request consultation through the regional poison control center.
    f. Dilute ACP in 500 mL of crystalloid solution, and start an IV infusion at a slow rate, increasing after the first 10 minutes if there is no reaction. The amount of fluid should be adjusted to the size of the patient and normal fluid input and output.
    g. For *minimal* envenomation, give 5 to 8 vials; for *moderate* envenomation, 8 to 13 vials; for *severe* envenomation, 14 to 30 or more vials.
    h. Attempt to give the total dose during the first 4 to 6 hours.
    i. Use of antivenom after 30 hours may be limited to reversal of coagulopathy.
    j. Determination of the dosage of ACP should include evaluation of all symptoms, signs, and laboratory findings.
    k. Measure the circumference of the involved part just above the bite and at 10 and 20 cm proximal to this point, and at all three places on the other extremity for comparison.
    l. Make and record the circumference readings every 15 minutes during ACP administration and every 1 to 2 hours thereafter to document edema.

General Recommendations

1. Observe every patient for a minimum of 6 hours, even if there are no presenting symptoms or signs.
2. Do not leave the patient unattended.
3. Do not delay immediate or vigorous treatment, if indicated.
4. Do not use ice or other cold applications.
5. Do not apply a tourniquet.
6. Do not use steroids, except for hypersensitivity reactions to antivenom.
7. Parenteral fluids are usually adequate for hypotension. Vasopressor agents should be used as only short-term agents in the presence of shock.
8. Do not use heparin for coagulopathies.
9. Do not explore surgically for assessment of severity.
10. Excisional therapy is not recommended.
11. Do not consider fasciotomy unless there is *sustained* objective evidence of true compartment syndrome, in which case a surgical consultation should be obtained. Despite the usual presence of subcutaneous edema in viper bites, vascular compromise is rarely documented.

Coral Snake Bites

1. Follow the supportive procedures outlined for pit viper bites, except for antivenom.

2. To give antivenom for eastern coral snake (*M. fulvius*) bites:
   a. Follow package instructions.
   b. Skin test only if antivenom is indicated. Keep epinephrine at the bedside.
   c. If the skin test is positive and antivenom is deemed necessary, request consultation through the regional poison control center.
3. Administer antivenom for North American coral snake (*M. fulvius*) bites IV in a continuous drip:
   a. If there are definite punctures, 3 to 5 vials in diluent (e.g., 250 to 500 mL of saline) should be given as early as possible, without waiting for the appearance of symptoms or signs of envenomation.
   b. If symptoms or signs develop, 3 to 5 more vials should be administered, and more if indicated.
4. There is no antivenom for the Arizona coral snake (*Micruroides euryxanthus*). Treatment is supportive; rarely are these bites serious.

DISCUSSION

The treatment of snake venom poisoning in the United States has improved markedly in the past 40 years. Mortality and morbidity have been drastically reduced. The wide distribution and use of antivenom since about 1954 have reduced the fatality rate from approximately 3 to 5% to less than 0.2%, although it is considered that some of the earlier deaths might be attributable to secondary infections or other complicating factors. In the 1078 cases of crotalid venom poisoning detailed in 1980, the death rate was 2.6% for patients who did not receive antivenom, but it was only 0.28% for patients who did. Further evidence of improved treatment is reflected by the length of hospital stay. In 1965, the average snake venom–poisoned patient spent 6.4 days in the seven hospitals studied where five or more patients were treated. Today, the average hospital stay for antivenom-treated patients is 2.9 days, and for those not receiving antivenom, about 5.3 days. The stay for those having a fasciotomy without receiving antivenom is about 9.8 hospital days, which includes subsequent follow-up visits for complications.

In spite of the efficacy of the current antivenom used in the United States, the high incidence of both immediate and delayed reactions to horse serum, from which it is derived, is of considerable concern to physicians treating snake venom poisoning. Approximately 75% of antivenom-treated patients have some sort of a delayed reaction to horse serum. In most of these cases, the reactions are minor: feeling of warmth (particularly of the face), minimal temperature elevation, and anxiety. This group constituted about 20% in one series of patients. Another 15% had transient reactions, consisting of malaise, pruritus, urticaria, elevated body temperature, and nausea. All of these cases responded to diphenhydramine hydrochloride, which is given to patients on discharge from many hospitals. Less than 5% of the patients returned to a medical facility to obtain more definitive treatment for a serious horse serum reaction. About 3 to 5% of my patients have experienced immediate horse serum reactions or anaphylaxis, although some physicians note a higher incidence. My opinion, which is based on consultations relating to immediate horse serum reactions, is that many of the referred cases appear to have involved a rapid, often bolus, injection of the antiserum.

Clinical experiences with a new affinity column–purified ovine antivenom (CroTab, Therapeutic Antibodies, Nashville, TN) appear to indicate that it is a safer product than the one currently employed, and animal studies show that it is more efficacious.

HAZARDOUS MARINE ANIMALS
method of
PAUL S. AUERBACH, M.D., M.S.
Stanford University School of Medicine
Stanford, California

The expanses of ocean that cover the earth are the greatest wilderness. Seventy-one percent of the earth's surface is composed of ocean, the volume of which exceeds 325 million cubic miles. Within the undersea realm exists four fifths of all living organisms. Some aquatic microorganisms, plants, and animals can be hazardous to humans. It is the purpose of this chapter to describe treatment for marine envenomations.

Naturally occurring aquatic zootoxins are designated oral toxins (poisonous to eat; they include bacterial poisons and products of decomposition), parenteral toxins (venom produced in specialized glands and injected mechanically [spine, needle, fang, fin, and dart]), and crinotoxins (venom produced in specialized glands and administered as slime, mucus, or gastric secretion).

FIRST AID

The physician should adhere to fundamental principles of medical rescue. Simultaneous with any specific interventions directed against a particular venom or poison, the rescuer must be certain that the victim maintains a patent airway, breathes spontaneously or assisted, and is supported by an adequate blood pressure. Because marine envenomations may afflict a scuba diver, the rescuer should anticipate near-drowning, immersion hypothermia, decompression sickness, or arterial air embolism. Conversely, any victim rescued from the ocean should be thoroughly examined for external signs of a bite, puncture, or sting.

Anaphylaxis

An envenomation or administration of antivenin can elicit an allergic reaction. The signs and symptoms of anaphylaxis may occur within minutes of exposure and include hypotension, bronchospasm, tongue and lip swelling, laryngeal edema, pulmonary edema, seizures, cardiac arrhythmia, pruritus, urticaria, angioedema, rhinitis, conjunctivitis, nausea, vomiting, diarrhea, abdominal pain, gastrointestinal bleeding, and syncope. Most severe allergic reactions occur within 15 to 30 minutes of envenomation, and nearly all occur within 6 hours. Fatalities are related to airway obstruction or hypotension. Acute elevated pulmonary vascular resistance may contribute to hypotension that results from generalized arterial vasodilatation.

Decisive treatment should be instituted at the first indication of hypersensitivity:

1. Maintain the airway and administer oxygen.

2. Obtain intravenous access and administer crystalloid to achieve a systolic blood pressure of 90 mm Hg in an adult. If the reaction is severe or the victim is older than 45 years, apply a cardiac monitor.

3. Administer epinephrine. Begin with administration of aqueous epinephrine 1:1000 subcutaneously in the deltoid region. The dose for adults is 0.3 to 0.5 mL and that for children, 0.01 mL per kg. If the reaction is sustained, the initial dose may be repeated in 15 to 20 minutes. Aerosolized aqueous epinephrine is not adequate to abort systemic anaphylaxis. If the reaction is limited to pruritus and urticaria, there is no wheezing or facial swelling, and the victim is older than 45 years, administer an antihistamine and reserve epinephrine for a worsened condition.

If the reaction is life-threatening and there is no response to subcutaneous epinephrine, administer epinephrine intravenously. An adult should receive a 0.1-mg bolus of 1:1000 aqueous epinephrine (0.1 mL) diluted in 10 mL of normal saline (final dilution 1:100,000) infused over 10 minutes (10 μg per minute). A mixture for continuous infusion is prepared by adding 1 mg of 1:1000 aqueous epinephrine (1 mL) to 250 mL of normal saline to create a concentration of 4 μg per 1 mL. This infusion should be started at 1 μg per minute (15 minidrops per minute) and increased to 4 to 5 μg per minute if the clinical response is inadequate. In children and infants, the starting dose is 0.1 μg per minute up to a maximum of 1.5 μg per kg per minute, noting that infusion rates in excess of 0.5 μg per kg per minute may be associated with cardiac ischemia and arrhythmias.

4. Relieve bronchospasm. Widely employed bronchodilators for inhalation are albuterol (Ventolin, Proventil), 0.5 mL, or metaproterenol (Alupent, Metaprel), 0.3 mL in 2.5 mL of normal saline administered by hand-held nebulizer. If a liquid beta$_2$-sympathomimetic agent is not available, micronized versions may be administered by a hand-held metered dose inhaler with spacer. Inhaled ipatropium may be added in refractory cases.

5. Administer an antihistamine. A mild reaction may be managed with diphenhydramine HCl (Benadryl), 50 to 75 mg intravenously (IV), intramuscularly (IM), or orally (PO). The dose for children is 1 mg per kg. Nonsedating antihistamines, such as terfenadine (Seldane), 60 mg PO, or cimetidine (Tagamet), 300 mg, are adjuncts.

6. Administer a corticosteroid. If the reaction is severe or prolonged, or if the victim is regularly medicated with corticosteroids, administer hydrocortisone (Solu-Cortef), 200 to 300 mg, methylprednisolone (Solu-Medrol), 50 to 75 mg, or dexamethasone, 10 to 25 mg IV, with a 7- to 14-day oral taper to follow. The parenteral dose of hydrocortisone for children is 2.5 mg per kg. If therapy is initiated by mouth, administer prednisone 50 to 60 mg for adults and 1 mg per kg for children.

BACTERIOLOGY OF THE AQUATIC ENVIRONMENT

Wounds acquired in the aquatic environment are soaked in natural source water and sometimes contaminated with sediment. Penetration of the skin by spines or the razor-sharp edges of coral may inoculate pathogenic organisms, leading to a wound that heals slowly and with marked soft tissue inflammation. Such a wound may become infected and be refractory to standard antimicrobial therapy. Indolent or extensive soft tissue infections develop in the normal or immunocompromised host. A clinician faced with a serious infection after an aquatic injury frequently needs to administer antibiotics before definitive laboratory identification of pathogenic organisms.

Ocean water provides a saline milieu for microbes. Although the greatest number and diversity of bacteria are found near the ocean surface, diverse bacteria and fungi are found in marine silts, sediments, and sand. Marine bacteria are generally halophilic, heterotrophic, motile, and gram-negative rod forms. Growth requirements vary from species to species with respect to utilization of organic carbon and nitrogen sources, requirements for various amino acids, vitamins and cofactors, sodium, potassium, magnesium, phosphate, sulfate, chloride, and calcium. Most marine bacteria are facultative anaerobes, which are able to thrive in oxygen-rich environments. Few are obligatory aerobes or anaerobes. Some marine bacteria are highly proteolytic.

Numerous bacteria, microalgae, protozoans, fungi, yeasts, and viruses have been identified in or cultured from seawater, marine sediments, and marine life and from marine-acquired or marine-contaminated infected wounds or body fluids of septic victims (Table 1). In the setting of wound infection or sepsis, the clinician should alert the laboratory that a marine-acquired organism may be present, because special culture and identification techniques may be indicated.

The objectives for the management of infections from marine microorganisms are to recognize the clinical condition, culture the organism, and provide antimicrobial therapy. Management of marine-acquired infections should include therapy against *Vibrio* species. Third-generation cephalosporins (cefoperazone, cefotaxime, or ceftazidime) provide excellent coverage; first- and second-generation products (cefazolin, cephalothin, cephapirin, cefamandole, cefo-

TABLE 1. **Bacterial and Fungal Species Isolated from Marine Water, Sediments, Marine Animals, and Marine-Acquired Wounds**

Achromobacter	Pasteurella multocida
Acinetobacter lwoffi	Propionibacterium acnes
Actinomyces	Proteus mirabilis
Aerobacter aerogenes	Proteus vulgaris
Aeromonas hydrophila	Providencia stuartii
Aeromonas sobria	Pseudomonas aeruginosa
Alcaligenes faecalis	Pseudomonas beijerinckii
Alteromonas espejiana	Pseudomonas cepacia
Alteromonas haloplanktis	Pseudomonas iridescens
Alteromonas macleodii	Pseudomonas maltophilia
Alteromonas undina	Pseudomonas marinoglutinosa
Bacillus cereus	Pseudomonas nigrifaciens
Bacillus subtilis	Pseudomonas putrefaciens
Bacteroides fragilis	Pseudomonas stutzeri
Branhamella catarrhalis	Salmonella enteritidis
Chromobacterium violaceum	Serratia
Citrobacter	Staphylococcus aureus
Clostridium botulinum	Staphylococcus citreus
Clostridium perfringens	Staphylococcus epidermidis
Clostridium tetani	Streptococcus
Corynebacterium	Vibrio alginolyticus
Deleya venustus	Vibrio carchariae
Edwardsiella tarda	Vibrio cholerae
Enterobacter aerogenes	Vibrio damsela
Erysipelothrix rhusiopathiae	Vibrio fluvialis
Escherichia coli	Vibrio furnissii
Flavobacterium	Vibrio harveyi
Fusarium solani	Vibrio hollisae
Klebsiella pneumoniae	Vibrio mimicus
Legionella pneumophila	Vibrio parahaemolyticus
Micrococcus sedentarius	Vibrio pelagius II
Micrococcus tegragenus	Vibrio splendidus I
Mycobacterium marinum	Vibrio vulnificus
Neisseria catarrhalis	

nicid, ceforanide,* or cefoxitin) appear to be less effective in vitro. Imipenem-cilastatin (Primaxin) is efficacious against gram-negative marine bacteria, as are trimethoprim-sulfamethoxazole (Bactrim, Septra), tetracycline, azlocillin (Azlin), mezlocillin (Mezlin), and piperacillin (Pipracil). Gentamicin, tobramycin (Nebcin), and chloramphenicol have tested favorably against Pseudomonas putrefaciens and Vibrio strains. Nonfermentative bacteria (such as Alteromonas, Pseudomonas, and Deleya species) appear to be sensitive to most antibiotics.

There is no advantage to quantitative wound culture before the appearance of a wound infection. Pending a prospective evaluation of prophylactic antibiotics in the management of marine wounds, the following recommendations are based on the indolent nature and malignant potential of soft tissue infections caused by Vibrio species:

1. Minor abrasions or lacerations (e.g., coral cuts or superficial sea urchin puncture wounds) do not require the administration of prophylactic antibiotics in the normal host. Persons who have a chronic disease (e.g., diabetes, hemophilia, or thalassemia) or are immunologically impaired (e.g., leukemia, acquired immune deficiency syndrome, undergoing che-

motherapy or prolonged corticosteroid therapy), or who suffer from serious liver disease (e.g., hepatitis, cirrhosis, or hemochromatosis), particularly those with elevated serum iron levels, should immediately after the injury be given oral ciprofloxacin (Cipro), trimethoprim-sulfamethoxazole, or tetracycline therapy, as these persons appear to have an increased risk for serious wound infection and bacteremia. Preliminary experience suggests that cefuroxime (Zinacef) may be a useful alternative. Penicillin, ampicillin, and erythromycin are not acceptable alternatives. Norfloxacin (Noroxin) may be less efficacious against certain vibrios. Other quinolones (ofloxacin, enoxacin, pefloxacin,* fleroxacin,* lomefloxacin) have not been extensively tested against Vibrio, so although they may be reliable alternatives, this awaits definitive evaluation. The appearance of an infection indicates the need for prompt antibiotic therapy. If an infection develops, antibiotic coverage should be chosen that will be efficacious against Staphylococcus and Streptococcus, as these are still the most common perpetrators of infection. In general, the fluoroquinolones, which are particularly effective for treating gram-negative bacillary infections, may become less and less useful against resistant staphylococci.

2. Serious injuries from an infection perspective include large, deep puncture wounds or a retained foreign body. Examples are stingray spine wounds, deep sea urchin punctures, scorpaenid spine envenomations that enter a joint space, and full-thickness coral cuts. If the victim requires hospitalization and surgery for standard wound management, recommended antibiotics include gentamicin, tobramycin, amikacin, trimethoprim-sulfamethoxazole, cefoperazone, cefotaxime, ceftazidime, or chloramphenicol. There may be an increased tendency to seizures in patients who simultaneously receive imipenem or ciprofloxacin and theophylline.

If the victim is managed as an outpatient, the drugs of choice to cover Vibrio are ciprofloxacin, trimethoprim-sulfamethoxazole, or tetracycline. Cefuroxime (Ceftin, Zinacef), is an alternative. It is a clinical decision whether or not oral therapy should be preceded by a single intravenous or intramuscular loading dose of a similar or different antibiotic, commonly an aminoglycoside.

3. Infected wounds should be cultured for aerobes and anaerobes. Pending culture and sensitivity results, the patient should be managed with antibiotics as described previously. A person who has been wounded in a marine environment and who develops rapidly progressive cellulitis and/or myositis should be suspected of suffering from Vibrio parahaemolyticus or Vibrio vulnificus infection, particularly in the presence of chronic liver disease. If a wound infection is minor and has the appearance of a classic erysipeloid reaction (Erysipelothrix rhusiopathiae), penicillin, cephalexin, or erythromycin should be administered.

---

*Not available in the United States.

*Investigational drug in the United States.

STONY CORALS

True (stony) corals exist in colonies that possess calcareous outer skeletons with pointed horns and/or razor-sharp edges. Snorkelers and divers frequently handle or brush against these living reefs, inflicting superficial cuts and abrasions on the extremities. Coral cuts are probably the most common injuries sustained under water. The initial reaction to a coral cut is stinging pain, erythema, and pruritus, most commonly on the forearms, elbows, and knees. Divers without gloves frequently receive cuts to the hands. A break in the skin may be surrounded within minutes by an erythematous wheal that fades in 1 to 2 hours. "Coral poisoning" describes these red, raised welts and local pruritus. Low-grade fever may be present and does not necessarily indicate an infection. With or without prompt treatment, this may progress to cellulitis with ulceration and tissue sloughing. These wounds heal slowly (3 to 6 weeks) and result in prolonged morbidity. In an extreme case, the victim develops cellulitis with lymphangitis, reactive bursitis, local ulceration, and wound necrosis.

Coral cuts should be promptly and vigorously scrubbed with soap and water, then irrigated copiously with a forceful stream of freshwater or normal saline to remove all foreign particles. It is occasionally helpful to use hydrogen peroxide to bubble out "coral dust." Any fragments that remain can become embedded and increase the risk for an indolent infection or foreign body granuloma. If stinging is a major symptom, there may be an element of envenomation by nematocysts. A brief rinse with diluted acetic acid (vinegar) or isopropyl alcohol 20% may diminish the discomfort (after the initial pain from contact with the open wound). If a coral-induced laceration is severe, it should be closed with adhesive strips rather than sutures if possible; preferably, it should be débrided for 3 to 4 days and closed in a delayed fashion.

There are a number of approaches to take with regard to wound care. The first (preferred) is to apply twice-daily sterile wet-to-dry dressings, using saline or a dilute antiseptic (povidone-iodine solution, 1 to 5%). Alternatively, a nontoxic topical antibiotic ointment (bacitracin or polymyxin B–bacitracin–neomycin [Neosporin]) may be used sparingly, the wound covered with a nonadherent dressing (Telfa), and secondary infections dealt with as they arise. A less often utilized approach is to apply a full-strength antiseptic solution, followed by a powdered topical antibiotic, such as tetracycline powder.* No method has been supported by a prospective trial.

Despite best efforts, the wound may heal slowly, with moderate to severe soft tissue inflammation and ulcer formation. All devitalized tissue should be débrided regularly using sharp dissection. This should be continued until a bed of healthy granulation tissue is formed. Wounds that appear infected should be cultured and treated with antibiotics as previously discussed.

The patient who demonstrates malaise, nausea, and low-grade fever may be suffering from a systemic form of coral poisoning or be manifesting early signs of a wound infection. It is prudent at this point to search for a localized infection, procure a wound culture(s) or biopsy as indicated, and initiate antibiotic therapy pending confirmation of the organisms. If the patient is started with antibiotic therapy and does not respond, a supplemental trial of systemic corticosteroids (prednisone 60 mg tapered over 2 weeks) is not unreasonable. In the absence of an overt infection, the natural course of the affliction is spontaneous improvement during a 4- to 12-week period.

SPONGES

Sponges are composed of elastic "skeletons" embedded with spicules of silicon dioxide or calcium carbonate. Two general syndromes, with minor variations, are induced by contact. The first is a pruritic dermatitis similar to plant-induced allergic dermatitis. A typical offender is the friable fire sponge *Tedania ignis*.

Within a few hours after skin contact, the reactions are characterized by itching and burning, which may progress to local joint swelling, soft tissue edema, vesiculation, and stiffness, particularly if small pieces of broken sponge are retained in the skin near the interphalangeal or metacarpophalangeal joints. The skin may become mottled or purpuric. Untreated, mild reactions subside within 3 to 7 days. With large skin surface area involvement, the victim may complain of fever, chills, malaise, dizziness, nausea, muscle cramps, and formication. Bullae may become purulent. Systemic erythema multiforme or an anaphylactoid reaction may develop 7 to 14 days after a severe exposure. In severe cases, surface desquamation of the skin may follow in 10 days to 2 months. No medical intervention can retard this process. Recurrent eczema and persistent arthralgias are rare complications.

The second syndrome is an irritant dermatitis and follows the penetration of small spicules into the skin. Most sponges have spicules; "toxic" sponges may possess toxins that enter microtraumatic lesions caused by the spicules.

Because it is usually impossible to distinguish clinically between the allergic and spicule-induced reactions, it is safest to treat for both. The skin should be gently dried. Spicules should be removed, if possible, using adhesive tape or a facial peel. As soon as possible, dilute (5%) acetic acid (vinegar) soaks for 10 to 30 minutes three or four times daily should be applied to all affected areas. Although topical steroid lotions may help to relieve the secondary inflammation, they are of no value as an initial decontaminant. If they precede the vinegar soak, they may worsen the primary reaction. Delayed primary therapy or inadequate decontamination may result in the persistence of bullae, which may become purulent and require months to heal. Erythema multiforme may require

---

*Not available in the United States.

the administration of systemic corticosteroids, beginning with a moderately high dose (prednisone 60 to 100 mg) tapered over 2 to 3 weeks. Other anecdotal remedies for the management of sponge envenomation that have been suggested without demonstration of efficacy include antiseptic dressings, broad-spectrum antibiotics, methdilazine (Tacaryl), pyribenzamine, phenobarbital, diphenhydramine, promethazine hydrochloride, and topical carbolic oil* or zinc oxide cream.

After the initial decontamination, a mild emollient cream or steroid preparation may be applied to the skin. If the allergic component is severe, particularly if there is weeping, crusting, and vesiculation, systemic corticosteroids (prednisone 60 to 80 mg, tapered over 2 weeks) may be beneficial. Severe itching may be controlled with an antihistamine. Frequent wound checks are important, because some patients develop significant infections.

Sponge-diver's disease is a stinging syndrome related to contact with the tentacles of anemones that attach to the base of a sponge. Treatment should include that for coelenterate envenomation.

COELENTERATES

Coelenterates are an enormous group, comprising approximately 10,000 species, at least 100 of which are dangerous to humans. Coelenterates hazardous to humans possess venom-charged stinging cells called nematocysts and include feather hydroids, fire coral, the Portuguese man-of-war, Indo-Pacific jellyfish, soft corals, and anemones. Seabather's eruption, commonly misnomered "sea lice," refers to a dermatitis that involves predominately covered areas of the body and has been postulated to be caused by larvae of the thimble jellyfish *Linuche unguiculata* or the sea anemone *Edwardsiella lineata*. The larger jellyfish include the Portuguese man-of-war *Physalia physalis,* the deadly box jellyfish *Chironex fleckeri,* and the sea wasp *Chiropsalmus quadrumanus.* These creatures are armed with some of the most potent venoms in existence. An adult *Chironex* carries enough venom (in excess of 10 mL) to kill three adults. Sea nettles are considerably less lethal animals and can be found in both temperate and tropical waters, particularly in the Chesapeake Bay.

There is considerable phylogenetic relationship among all stinging species, such that the clinical features of the coelenterate syndrome are fairly constant, with a spectrum of severity.

Mild Envenomation

The stings caused by the hydroids and hydroid corals, along with lesser envenomations by jellyfish and anemones, result predominantly in skin irritation. There is usually an immediate pricking or stinging sensation, accompanied by pruritus, paresthesias, burning, throbbing, and radiation of the pain

centrally from the extremities to the groin, abdomen, and axillae. The area involved by the nematocysts becomes red-brown-purple, often in a linear whiplike fashion, corresponding to "tentacle prints." Other features are blistering, local edema, and wheal formation, as well as violaceous petechial hemorrhages. The papular inflammatory rash is strictly confined to the areas of contact and may persist for up to 10 days. Areas of body hair appear to be somewhat more protected (from contact) than hairless areas. Seabather's eruption is manifest as a papular rash beneath bathing suit–covered areas.

If an envenomation is slightly more severe, then the aforementioned symptoms, which are evident in the first few hours, can progress over a course of days to local necrosis, skin ulceration, and secondary infection. This is particularly true of certain anemone stings.

Untreated, the minor to moderate skin disorder resolves in 1 to 2 weeks, with occasional residual hyperpigmentation for 1 to 2 months. Rubbing can cause lichenification. Local hyperhidrosis, fat atrophy, and contracture may occur. Permanent scarring may result. Persistent papules or plaques at the sites of contact may be accompanied by localized arthritis and joint effusion. Granuloma annulare, which is usually both a sporadic and a familial inflammatory dermatosis, has been associated with a *Physalia utriculus* envenomation.

Moderate and Severe Envenomation

The prime offenders in this group are the anemones, *Physalia* species, and Indo-Pacific jellyfish. The skin manifestations are compounded by the onset of systemic symptoms, which may appear immediately or be delayed by several hours:

1. Neurologic—malaise, headache, aphonia, diminished touch and temperature sensation, vertigo, ataxia, spastic or flaccid paralysis, mononeuritis multiplex, parasympathetic dysautonomia, plexopathy, radial-ulnar-median nerve palsies, delirium, loss of consciousness, convulsions, coma, and death
2. Cardiovascular—anaphylaxis, hemolysis, hypotension, small-artery spasm, bradyarrhythmias (including electromechanical dissociation and asystole), tachyarrhythmias, congestive heart failure, and ventricular fibrillation
3. Respiratory—rhinitis, bronchospasm, laryngeal edema, dyspnea, cyanosis, pulmonary edema, and respiratory failure
4. Musculoskeletal and rheumatologic—abdominal rigidity, diffuse myalgia and muscle cramps, muscle spasm, fat atrophy, arthralgias, reactive arthritis (seronegative symmetrical synovitis with pitting edema), and thoracolumbar pain
5. Gastrointestinal—nausea, vomiting, diarrhea, dysphagia, hypersalivation, and thirst
6. Ocular—conjunctivitis, chemosis, corneal ulcers, iridocyclitis, elevated intraocular pressure, synechiae, iris depigmentation, chronic unilateral glaucoma, and lacrimation

*Not available in the United States.

7. Other—acute renal failure, chills, fever, and nightmares

The extreme example of envenomation occurs with *Chironex fleckeri,* the dreaded box jellyfish. The sting is immediately intensely painful, and the victim usually struggles purposefully for only a minute or two before collapse. The toxic skin reaction may be quite intense, with rapid formation of wheals, vesicles, and a darkened reddish brown or purple whiplike flare pattern with stripes of 8 to 10 mm in width. With major stings, skin blistering occurs within 6 hours, with superficial necrosis in 12 to 18 hours. On occasion, a pathognomonic "frosted" appearance with transverse cross-hatched pattern may be present. *Physalia* and anemone stings, although extremely painful, are rarely fatal. Death after *Physalia* stings has been attributed to anaphylaxis, primary respiratory failure, or cardiac arrhythmia.

A person recently stung by *P. physalis* may develop recurrent cutaneous eruptions for 2 to 3 weeks after the initial episode, without repeated exposure to the animal. This may take the form of lichenification, hyperhidrosis, angioedema, vesicles, large bullae, nodules that resemble erythema nodosum, granuloma annulare, or a more classic linear urticarial eruption. Acute regional vascular insufficiency of the upper extremity has been reported after jellyfish envenomation. It can be manifested by acral ischemia, signs and symptoms of compartment syndrome, and massive edema.

Treatment

Therapy is directed at stabilizing major systemic decompensation, opposing the venom's multiple effects, and alleviating pain. Generally, only severe *Physalia* or toxic jellyfish stings result in rapid decompensation. In both cases, supportive care is based on the presenting signs and symptoms. Hypotension should be managed with the prompt intravenous administration of crystalloid, such as lactated Ringer's solution. This must be done in concert with detoxification of any nematocysts (particularly those of *Chironex* or *Chiropsalmus*) that are still attached to the victim, to limit the perpetuation of envenomation. Hypotension is usually limited to very young or elderly victims who suffer severe and multiple stings, and it is worsened by fluid depletion that accompanies protracted vomiting. Hypertension is an occasional side effect of a jellyfish envenomation, such as that of *Carukia barnesi.* Excessive catecholamine stimulation is one putative cause, which has prompted clinical intervention with phentolamine (Regitine), an alpha-adrenergic blocking agent (5 mg IV as an initial dose). Bronchospasm may be managed as an allergic component. If the victim is in respiratory distress with wheezing, shortness of breath, or heart failure, pulse oximetry or arterial blood gas measurement may be used to guide supplemental oxygen administration. Seizures are generally self-limited but should be treated with intravenous diazepam (Valium) for 24 to 48 hours, after which they rarely recur.

All victims with a systemic component should be observed for a period of at least 6 to 8 hours, as rebound phenomena after successful treatment are not uncommon. All elder victims should yield an electrocardiogram and be observed on a cardiac monitor, with frequent checks for arrhythmias. Urinalysis demonstrates the presence or absence of hemoglobinuria, indicating hemolysis after the putative attachment of *Physalia* venom to red blood cell membrane glycoprotein sites. If this is the case, the urine should be alkalinized with bicarbonate to prevent the precipitation of pigment in the renal tubules, while a moderate diuresis (30 to 50 mL per hour) is maintained with a loop diuretic (such as furosemide) or mannitol (0.25 gram per kg IV every 8 to 12 hours). In rare instances of acute progressive renal failure, peritoneal dialysis or hemodialysis may be necessary.

If there are signs of distal ischemia or an impending compartment syndrome, standard diagnostic and therapeutic measures apply. These include Doppler ultrasonography and/or angiography for diagnosis, regional thrombolysis for acutely occluded blood vessels, and measurement of intracompartmental tissue pressures to guide fasciotomy. Reversible regional sympathetic blockade may be efficacious if vasospasm is a dominant clinical feature. However, the vasospasm associated with a jellyfish envenomation may be severe and prolonged and refractory to regional sympathectomy and intra-arterial reserpine therapy.

A small child may pick up tentacle fragments on the beach and place them into his or her mouth, resulting in rapid intraoral swelling and potential airway obstruction, particularly in the presence of exceptional hypersensitivity. In such cases, an endotracheal tube should be placed before edema precludes visualization of the vocal cords. In no case should any liquid be placed in the mouth if the airway is not protected.

C. fleckeri produces the only coelenterate venom for which there is a specific antidote. If the reaction is severe, *Chironex* antivenin* should be administered IV as soon as possible. The IM route is less preferred. The antivenin is supplied in ampules of 20,000 units. The dose is 1 ampule (diluted 1:5 to 1:10 in isotonic crystalloid; dilution with water is not recommended) administered IV over 5 minutes, or 3 ampules IM. Although the antivenin is prepared by hyperimmunizing sheep, the risk of anaphylaxis or serum sickness should be assumed to be the same as for equine hyperimmune globulin preparations. In addition to its lifesaving properties, the early administration of antivenin may markedly reduce pain and decrease subsequent skin scarring. Antivenin administration may be repeated once or twice every 2 to 4 hours until there is no further worsening of the reaction (skin discoloration, pain, or systemic effects). A large sting in an adult may require the initial

---

*Not available in the United States.

administration of 2 ampules. The antivenin may also be used to neutralize the effects of a *Chiropsalmus* envenomation. The antivenin should be stored in a refrigerator at 2 to 10°C and must not be frozen. Concomitant administration of a corticosteroid (hydrocortisone 200 mg IV) is often recommended for its anti-inflammatory activity but is no substitute for the administration of antivenin.

Often, pain can be controlled by treating the dermatitis. However, if pain is excruciating and there is no contraindication (head injury, altered mental status, respiratory depression, allergy, profound hypotension), the administration of narcotics is often indicated. Severe muscle spasm may respond to 10% calcium gluconate (5 to 10 mL IV slow push), diazepam (5 to 10 mg IV), or methocarbamol (1 gram, no faster than 100 mg per minute through a widely patent IV line).

Coelenterate Dermatitis

If a person is stung by a coelenterate, the following steps should be taken:

1. In the case of a known or suspected box jellyfish envenomation, the victim must be rapidly assessed for the adequacy of breathing and supported with an airway and artificial ventilation if necessary. The victim should be moved as little as possible. It is absolutely essential to immediately apply acetic acid 5% (vinegar) liberally ("flood" the skin) to any adherent tentacles before any attempt is made to remove them, to paralyze the nematocysts and avoid worsening the envenomation. One should not expect significant pain relief from this maneuver. Although most nematocysts cannot penetrate the thickened skin of the human palm, the rescuer should pay particular attention to his or her own skin protection. If acetic acid is not available, aluminum sulfate–surfactant (Stingose) may be used in substitution, although its efficacy has not been well demonstrated for a *Chironex* envenomation. Isopropyl alcohol 40 to 70% should be used as a last resort. A number of authors recommend that alcohol not be used, based upon in vitro observation of inefficacy and nematocyst discharge after the application of this detoxicant.

2. For other coelenterate envenomations, the wound should be immediately rinsed with seawater, *not with freshwater.* The wound should not be rubbed with a towel or clothing to remove adherent tentacles. Freshwater and abrasion stimulate any nematocysts that have not already fired. The gross tentacles should be removed with forceps or a well-gloved hand.

Commercial (chemical) cold packs applied over a dry cloth have been shown to be effective when applied to mild to moderate *Physalia* stings. Whether or not the direct application of ice to envenomed skin and the resulting freshwater melt stimulates the discharge of nematocysts has not been determined.

Applications of hot packs or gentle rinses with hot water are not recommended, as they may worsen the envenomation or in repeated applications lead to lymphangitis. However, beach patrol members who have been stung by jellyfish (presumably Portuguese man-of-war) report that an immediate hot shower with a forceful stream of water relieves the pain. This observation implies that a forceful jet of water that might dislodge tentacle fragments and nematocysts can supercede the deleterious effects of freshwater (hypotonic) that lead to nematocyst discharge.

3. Acetic acid (vinegar) 5% is the treatment of choice to inactivate the toxin. An alternative is isopropyl alcohol (40 to 70%). Baking soda has been recommended for sea nettle envenomations. Perfume, aftershave lotion, or high-proof liquor are less efficacious and may be detrimental. The detoxicant should be applied continuously for at least 30 minutes or until there is no further pain. Other substances reputed to be effective as alternatives are organic solvents such as formalin, ether, and gasoline (all to be condemned); dilute ammonium hydroxide; olive oil; sugar; urine; and papain (papaya latex [juice] or unseasoned meat tenderizer).

4. No systemic drugs are of verifiable use. Ephedrine, atropine, calcium, methysergide, and hydrocortisone have all been touted at one time or another, but there is no proof that they help. Antihistamines may be useful if there is a significant allergic component. The administration of epinephrine is appropriate only in the setting of anaphylaxis.

5. Immersing the area into hot water is generally not recommended, as the hypotonic solution causes nematocysts to fire.

6. Once the wound has been soaked with vinegar or alcohol, the remaining nematocysts must be removed. The easiest way to do this is to apply shaving cream or a paste of baking soda (after first removing residual vinegar), flour, or talc and to shave the area with a razor or reasonable facsimile. If sophisticated facilities are not available, the nematocysts should be removed by making a sand or mud paste with seawater and using this to help scrape the victim's skin with a sharp-edged shell or piece of wood. The rescuer must take care not to become envenomed; bare hands must be frequently rinsed.

7. Local anesthetic ointments (lidocaine HCl, 2.5%) or sprays (benzocaine, 14%) or mild steroid lotions (hydrocortisone 1%) may be soothing. Calamine with 1% menthol has been recommended for seabather's eruption.

8. Patients should receive standard antitetanus prophylaxis.

9. There is no need for prophylactic antibiotic therapy. The wounds should be checked for infection at 3 and 7 days after injury. Any ulcerating lesions should be cleaned three times a day and covered with a thin layer of nonsensitizing antiseptic ointment. A jellyfish sting to the cornea may cause a foreign body sensation, photophobia, and decreased (or "hazy") vision. Ophthalmologic examination reveals hyperemic sclera, chemosis, and irregularity of the corneal epithelium with stromal edema. Depending on the extent of the wound, the anterior chamber may demon-

strate the inflammatory response of iridocyclitis ("flare" with or without cells). The patient should be referred to an ophthalmologist, who may prescribe a steroid-containing eye medication such as prednisolone acetate 1% with hyoscine 0.25%. It is not recommended that any traditional skin detoxicant be applied directly to the cornea, as it is likely to worsen the tissue injury.

Delayed Reaction

A delayed reaction in areas of skin contact similar in appearance to erythema nodosum may be accompanied by fever, weakness, arthralgias, painful joint swelling and effusions. This may recur multiple times over the course of 1 to 2 months. The treatment is a 10- to 14-day taper of prednisone, starting with 50 to 80 mg. This may need to be prolonged or repeated with each flare of the reaction.

Persistent Hyperpigmentation

Postinflammatory hyperpigmentation is common after the stings of many jellyfish and other lesser coelenterates. A solution of hydroquinone 1.8% in a glycol-alcohol base (70% ethyl alcohol, n-propylene glycol mixed at a 3:2 ratio) twice a day as a topical agent for 3 to 5 weeks has been used successfully to treat hyperpigmentation that followed a *Pelagia noctiluca* sting.

ECHINODERMATA

Sea Urchins

The spines of sea urchins are often quite brittle and break off easily in the flesh, lodging deeply and making removal difficult. Pedicellariae are small and delicate seizing organs attached to the stalks scattered among the spines. The outer surface of each jaw is covered by a large venom gland, which is triggered to contract with the jaw on contact.

Venomous spines inflict immediate and intensely painful stings. The pain is initially characterized by burning, which rapidly evolves into severe local muscle aching with visible erythema and swelling of the skin surrounding the puncture site(s). Frequently, a spine lodges in the victim. Some sea urchin (e.g., *Diadema setosum* or *Strongylocentrotus purpuratus*) spines contain purplish dye, which may give a false impression of spines left in the skin. If a spine enters into a joint, it may rapidly induce severe synovitis. If multiple spines have penetrated the skin, particularly if they are deeply embedded, the victim may rapidly develop systemic symptoms, which include nausea, vomiting, paresthesias, numbness and muscular paralysis, abdominal pain, syncope, hypotension, and respiratory distress. The presence of a frank neuropathy may indicate that the spine has lodged in contact with a peripheral nerve. The pain from multiple stings may be sufficient to cause delir-

ium. Secondary infections and indolent ulceration are common.

The stings of pedicellariae are often of greater magnitude, causing immediate intense and radiating pain, local edema and hemorrhage, malaise, weakness, paresthesias, hypesthesia, arthralgias, aphonia, dizziness, syncope, generalized muscular paralysis, respiratory distress, hypotension, and, rarely, death. In some cases, the pain may disappear within the first hour, whereas the localized muscular weakness or paralysis persists for up to 6 hours.

The envenomed body part should immediately be immersed in nonscalding hot water (upper limit 113°F, or 45°C) to tolerance for 30 to 90 minutes in an attempt to achieve pain relief. Any pedicellariae that are still attached to the skin must be removed by applying a shaving foam and gently scraping with a razor. Embedded spines should be removed with care, as they are easily fractured. If the spines are removed and black or purplish discoloration surrounds the wound, this is often merely spine dye and of no consequence. Although some thin venomous spines may be absorbed within 24 hours to 3 weeks, it is best to remove those that are easily reached and leave the remainder for dissolution. All thick calcium carbonate spines should be removed because of the risk for infection, a foreign body encaseation granuloma, or a dermoid inclusion cyst. External percussion to achieve fragmentation may prove disastrous if a chronic inflammatory process is initiated in sensitive tissue of the hand or foot. If the spines have acutely entered into joints or are closely aligned to neurovascular structures, the surgeon should take advantage of an operating microscope to remove all spine fragments. The extraction should be performed as soon as possible after the injury. If the spine has entered into an interphalangeal joint, the finger should be splinted until the spine is removed to limit fragmentation and further penetration. This may also control the fusiform finger swelling that is commonly noted after a puncture in the vicinity of the middle or proximal interphalangeal joint. It is inappropriate to rummage about in a hand wound in the emergency department, virtually looking for a needle in a haystack. If there is a question about whether a spine is present, soft tissue density radiographic techniques (magnetic resonance imaging or mammography is best) for a radiopaque foreign body may be diagnostic. Although the calcium carbonate is relatively inert, it is accompanied by slime, bacteria, and organic epidermal debris. Therefore, secondary infections are common, and deep puncture wounds are an indication for prophylactic antibiotics.

Some sea urchin spines are phagocytosed in the soft tissues and ultimately dissolve. The granulomas caused by retained sea urchin spine fragments generally appear as flesh-colored or dye-colored surface or subcuticular nodules 2 to 12 months after the initial injury. In thin-skinned areas, they are erythematous and rubbery, painless, and infrequently umbilicated. In thicker skinned areas (palms and soles, knees) that are frequently abraded, they develop a keratinized appearance. Although necrosis and microabscess formation may be evident microscopically, suppuration is unusual. If a spine cannot be removed and forms a nidus for cyst or granuloma formation, the lesion may be removed surgically. Intralesional injection with a corticosteroid (triamcinolone hexacetonide [Aristospan] 5 mg per mL) is less efficacious but may be successful. Systemic anti-inflammatory drugs may be minimally helpful but are not a substitute for removal of the spine. A diffuse delayed reaction, consisting of cyanotic induration, fusiform swelling in the digits, and focal phalangeal bone erosion, may be treated with systemic corticosteroids and antibiotics.

Starfish

The carnivorous *Acanthaster planci* is a particularly venomous species. The sharp, rigid, and venomous aboral spines of this animal may grow to 4 to 6 cm and can penetrate the hardiest of diving gloves. As a spine enters the skin, it carries venom into the wound, with immediate pain, copious bleeding, and mild edema. The pain is generally moderate and self-limited, with remission during a period of 0.5 to 3 hours. The wound may become dusky or discolored. Multiple puncture wounds may result in acute systemic reactions, which include paresthesias, nausea, vomiting, lymphadenopathy, and muscular paralysis. If a spine fragment is retained, a granulomatous lesion akin to that from a sea urchin puncture wound may develop. A victim who has been previously sensitized may suffer a prolonged (weeks) reaction consisting of local edema and pruritus. Treatment is similar to that for a sea urchin puncture. Because of the stout nature of the spines, it is rare to retain a fragment.

STINGRAYS

The stingrays are the most commonly incriminated group of fishes involved in human envenomations. The venom organ consists of one to four venomous stings on the dorsum of an elongate, whiplike caudal appendage. Stingray "attacks" are purely defensive gestures that occur when an unwary human handles, corners, or steps on a camouflaged creature while wading in shallow waters. The tail of the ray reflexly whips upward and accurately thrusts the caudal spine(s) into the victim, producing a puncture wound or jagged laceration. The integumentary sheath covering the spine is ruptured, and venom is released into the wound, along with mucus, pieces of the sheath, and fragments of the spine. On occasion, the entire spine tip is broken off and remains in the wound.

Because of the retrorse serrated teeth and powerful strikes, significant lacerations can result. Secondary bacterial infection is common. Osteomyelitis may occur if the bone is penetrated. The lower extremities, particularly the ankle and foot, are involved most often. The envenomation causes immediate local intense pain, edema, and variable bleeding. The pain may radiate centrally, peaks at 30 to 60 minutes, and may last for up to 48 hours. The wound is initially dusky or cyanotic and rapidly progresses to erythema and hemorrhagic discoloration, with rapid fat and muscle hemorrhage and necrosis. If discoloration around the wound edge is not immediately apparent, within 2 hours it will often extend several centimeters from the wound. Minor stings may simulate bacterial cellulitis. Systemic manifestations include weakness, nausea, vomiting, diarrhea, diaphoresis, vertigo, tachycardia, headache, syncope, seizures, inguinal or axillary pain, muscle cramps, fasciculations, generalized edema (with truncal wounds), paralysis, hypotension, arrhythmias, and death.

The success of therapy is largely related to the rapidity with which it is undertaken. Treatment is directed at combating the effects of the venom, alleviating pain, and preventing infection. The wound should be irrigated immediately with whatever cold diluent is at hand. If sterile saline or water is not available, tap water may be used. This removes some venom and mucus, provides mild anesthesia, and induces local vasoconstriction, possibly retarding the absorption of the toxin. In a rapid primary exploration of the wound, any visible pieces of the spine or integumentary sheath should be removed. Local suction, if applied in the first 15 to 30 minutes, may be of some value (this is controversial), as may a proximal constriction band (also controversial) that occludes only superficial venous and lymphatic return. This should be released for 90 seconds every 10 minutes to prevent ischemia.

As soon as possible, the wound should be soaked in nonscalding hot water to tolerance (upper limit 113°F, or 45°C) for 30 to 90 minutes. This attenuates some of the thermolabile components of the protein venom and relieves pain. There is no indication for the addition of ammonia, magnesium sulfate, potassium permanganate, or formalin to the soaking solution. In this circumstance, they are toxic to tissue and/or they obscure visualization of the wound. During the hot-water soak, the wound should be explored and débrided of any readily visible pieces of the sting's integumentary sheath, which would continue envenomation. Cryotherapy is disastrous, and there are no data to support the use of antihistamines or steroids.

Pain control should be initiated during the first débridement or soaking period. Narcotics may be necessary. Local infiltration of the wound with 1 to 2% lidocaine (Xylocaine) without epinephrine may be quite useful.

After the soaking procedure, the wound should be prepared in a sterile fashion, re-explored, and thoroughly débrided. Wounds should be packed open for delayed primary closure or sutured loosely around adequate drainage. Prophylactic antibiotic therapy is recommended because of the high incidence of ulceration, necrosis, and secondary infection. A victim who is to be treated and released should be observed for a period of at least 3 to 4 hours for systemic side effects.

Wounds that are not properly débrided or explored and cleansed of foreign material may fester for weeks or months. It is not at all uncommon for such wounds to appear infected, when in reality what exists is a chronic draining ulcer initiated by persistent retained organic matter. After time, exploration may reveal erosion of adjacent soft tissue structures and the formation of an epidermal inclusion cyst or other related foreign body reaction. As with other marine-acquired wounds, indolent infection should prompt a search for unusual microorganisms.

SCORPION FISH

Distributed in tropical and less commonly in temperate oceans, several hundred species of scorpion fishes are divided into three groups typified by different genera on the basis of venom organ structure: (1) *Pterois* (zebra fish, lionfish, and butterfly cod), (2) *Scorpaena* (scorpion fish, bullrout, and sculpin), and (3) *Synanceja* (stonefish). Some species bury themselves in the sand, and most dangerous types lie motionless on the bottom. The venom organs consist of 12 to 13 (of 18) dorsal, 2 pelvic, and 3 anal spines, with associated venom glands. Stonefish venom has been likened in potency to cobra venom.

When any of these fish is removed from the water, handled, stepped on, or otherwise threatened, it reflexly erects the spinous dorsal fin and flares out the armed gill covers and the pectoral and anal fins. If provoked while still in the water, it will actually attack. The venom is injected by a direct puncture wound through the skin, which tears the sheath and may fracture the spine, in a manner analogous to that of a stingray envenomation.

Pain is immediate and intense, with radiation centrally. Untreated, the pain peaks at 60 to 90 minutes and persists for 6 to 12 hours. In the case of the stonefish, the pain may be severe enough to cause delirium and may persist at high levels for days. The wound and surrounding area are initially ischemic and then cyanotic, with more broadly surrounding areas of erythema, edema, and warmth. Vesicles may form. Rapid tissue sloughing and close surrounding areas of cellulitis, with anesthesia adjacent to peripheral hypesthesia, may be present within 48 hours. Systemic effects include anxiety, headache, tremors, maculopapular rash, nausea, vomiting, diarrhea, abdominal pain, diaphoresis, pallor, restlessness, delirium, seizures, limb paralysis, peripheral neuritis or neuropathy, lymphangitis, arthritis, fever, hypertension, respiratory distress, bradycardia, tachycardia, atrioventricular block, ventricular fibrillation, congestive heart failure, pericarditis, hypotension, syncope, and death. Pulmonary edema is a bona fide sequel. Resulting death in humans, which is extremely rare, usually occurs within the first 6 to 8 hours. The wound is indolent and may require months to heal, only to leave a cutaneous granuloma or marked tissue defect, particularly after a second-

ary infection or deep abscess. Mild pain may persist for days to weeks. After successful therapy, paresthesias or numbness in the affected extremity may persist for a few weeks.

First aid and emergency therapy are identical to those for a stingray envenomation. A stonefish antivenin* is manufactured by the Commonwealth Serum Laboratories, Melbourne, Australia. In cases of severe systemic reactions from stings of *Synanceja* species, and rarely from other scorpion fish, it is administered IV. The antivenin is supplied in ampules containing 2 mL (2000 units) of hyperimmune horse serum, with 1 mL capable of neutralizing 10 mg of dried venom. After skin testing to estimate the risk for an anaphylactic reaction to equine sera, the antivenin should be diluted in 50 to 100 mL of normal saline and administered slowly IV. Although the product may be given IM predilution, this route is not recommended in serious envenomations, as absorption may be erratic. As a rough estimate, 1 vial should neutralize one or two significant stings (punctures).

OCTOPUSES

Octopuses and cuttlefish are usually harmless and retiring. Octopus bites are rare but can result in severe envenomations. Fatalities have been reported from the bites of the Australian blue-ringed (or "spotted") octopuses, *Octopus (Hapalochlaena) maculosus* and *O. (H.) lunulata*. These small creatures, which rarely exceed 20 cm in length with tentacles extended, are found throughout the Indo-Pacific area (Australia, New Zealand, New Guinea, Japan) in rock pools, under discarded objects and shells, and in shallow waters, posing a threat to curious children, tidepool visitors, fossickers, and unwary divers.

The venom apparatus of the octopus consists of the anterior and posterior salivary glands, salivary ducts, buccal mass, and beak. This complex, concealed by the tentacles, is fronted by two parrot-like, powerful and chitinous jaws (beak), which bite and tear with great force at food held by the suckers. The venom, normally released into the water to subdue crabs, may be injected into the victim with great force through the dermis down to the muscle fascia. The toxin contains at least one fraction identical to tetrodotoxin, which blocks peripheral nerve conduction by interfering with sodium conductance in excitable membranes. This paralytic agent rapidly produces neuromuscular blockade, notably of the phrenic nerve supply to the diaphragm, without any apparent direct cardiotoxicity. It has been estimated that enough venom may be present in one adult (25-gram) octopus to paralyze 10 adult humans.

Most victims are bitten on the hand or arm as they handle the creature. An octopus bite usually consists of two small puncture wounds produced by the chitinous jaws. The bite goes unnoticed or causes only a small amount of discomfort, described as a minor

---

*Not available in the United States.

ache, slight stinging, or pulsating sensation. Occasionally, the site is initially numb, followed in 5 to 10 minutes by discomfort that may spread to involve the entire limb, persisting for up to 6 hours. Local urticarial reactions occur variably, and profuse bleeding at the site is attributed to a local anticoagulant effect. Within 30 minutes, there are considerable erythema, swelling, tenderness, heat, and pruritus. By far the most common local tissue reaction is the absence of symptoms, a small spot of blood, or a tiny blanched area. Within 10 to 15 minutes of the bite, the patient notices oral and facial numbness, rapidly followed by systemic progression. Voluntary and involuntary muscles are involved, and the illness may rapidly progress to total flaccid paralysis and respiratory failure. Other symptoms include perioral and intraoral anesthesia (classically, numbness of the lips and tongue), diplopia, blurred vision, aphonia, dysphagia, ataxia, myoclonus, weakness, a sense of detachment, nausea, vomiting, peripheral neuropathy, flaccid muscular paralysis, and respiratory failure that may lead to death. Ataxia of cerebellar configuration may occur after an envenomation that does not progress to frank paralysis. The victim may collapse from weakness and remain awake, so long as oxygenation can be maintained. When breathing is disturbed, respiratory assistance may allow the victim to remain mentally alert, although paralyzed. Cardiac arrest is probably a complication of the anoxic episode.

First aid at the scene should include the pressure-immobilization technique. If practicable by virtue of location of the sting, a cloth or gauze pad of approximate dimensions 6 to 8 cm by 6 to 8 cm by 2 to 3 cm (thickness) should be placed directly over the sting and held firmly in place by a circumferential bandage 15 to 18 cm wide applied at lymphatic-venous occlusive pressure. The arterial circulation should not be occluded, as determined by the detection of arterial pulsations and proper capillary refill. One hypothesis holds that the pressure-immobilization technique devascularizes the area immediately below the pad and prevents the distribution of venom into the general circulation. The limb is then splinted in the position of function. The splint and bandage should be released after the victim has been brought to proper medical attention and the rescuer is prepared to provide systemic support.

Treatment is based on the symptoms and is supportive. Prompt mechanical respiratory assistance has by far the greatest influence on the outcome. Respiratory demise should be anticipated early, and the rescuer should be prepared to provide artificial ventilation, including endotracheal intubation and the application of a mechanical ventilator. The duration of the intense clinical venom effect is 4 to 10 hours, after which the victim who has not suffered an episode of significant hypoxia shows rapid signs of improvement. If there is no period of hypoxia, mentation may remain normal. Complete recovery may require 2 to 4 days. Residua are uncommon and are related to anoxia rather than venom effects.

Management of the bite wound is controversial. Some clinicians recommend wide circular excision of the bite wound down to the deep fascia, with primary closure or immediate full-thickness free skin grafts, whereas others advocate observation and a nonsurgical approach. Because the local tissue reaction is not a significant cause of morbidity, excision is putatively recommended to remove any sequestered venom.

SEA SNAKES

Sea snakes are probably the most abundant reptiles on earth. The snakes are distributed in the tropical and warm temperate Pacific and Indian oceans, with the highest number of envenomations occurring along the coast of Southeast Asia, in the Persian Gulf, and in the Malay Archipelago.

The well-developed venom apparatus consists of 2 to 4 hollow maxillary fangs and a pair of associated venom glands. Fortunately, because the fangs are short and easily dislodged from their sockets, most bites do not result in significant systemic envenomation. The protein venom is quite toxic and includes stable peripheral neurotoxins more potent than those of terrestrial snakes. *Enhydrina schistosa* is considered to be the most dangerous sea snake. *E. schistosa* is the most widely distributed sea snake in the Arabian Sea.

Bites are usually the result of accidental handling of snakes snared in the nets of fishermen, or of wading and accidentally stepping on a snake. Nearly all bites involve the extremities. Initially, a sea snake bite does not cause great pain and may resemble no more than a pinprick. Fang marks are characterized by multiple pinhead-sized hypodermic-like puncture wounds, usually 1 to 4, but potentially up to 20. In some cases, particularly if a superficial injury has been perpetrated through the arm or leg of a neoprene wet suit, the fang marks may be difficult to visualize, because of the lack of a localized reaction.

The onset of symptoms can be as rapid as 5 minutes or as long as 8 hours after the bite. Characteristic symptoms include painful muscle movement, lower extremity paralysis, arthralgias, trismus, blurred vision, dysphagia, drowsiness, vomiting, and ptosis. Neurotoxic symptoms are rapid in onset and usually appear within 2 to 3 hours. If symptoms do not develop within 6 to 8 hours, there has been no envenomation.

The first complaint may be one of euphoria, malaise, or anxiety. Over 30 to 60 minutes, classic muscle aching and stiffness (particularly of the bitten extremity and neck muscles) develop, along with a "thick tongue" and sialorrhea, indicative of speech and swallowing dysfunction. Within 3 to 6 hours, moderate to severe pain is noted with passive movements of the neck, trunk, and limbs. Ascending flaccid or spastic paralysis follows shortly, beginning in the lower extremities, and deep tendon reflexes diminish and may disappear after an initial period of spastic hyper-reactivity. Nausea, vomiting, myoclonus, muscle spasm, ophthalmoplegia, ptosis, dilated and poorly reactive pupils, facial paralysis, trismus, and the pulmonary aspiration of gastric contents are frequent complications. Occasionally, bilateral painless swelling of the parotid glands develops.

Severe envenomations are marked by progressively intense symptoms within the first 2 symptom hours. Patients become cool and cyanotic, begin to lose vision, and may lapse into coma. Failing vision is reported to be a preterminal symptom. If peripheral paralysis predominates, the victim may remain conscious if hypoxia is avoided. Leukocytosis may exceed 20,000 white blood cells per mm^3; elevated plasma creatine kinase levels are variable. An elevated aspartate aminotransferase level reflects hepatic injury. Pathognomonic myoglobinuria becomes evident about 3 to 6 hours after the bite and may be accompanied by albuminuria and hemoglobinuria.

Cerebrospinal fluid is normal. Respiratory distress and bulbar paralysis, pulmonary aspiration-related hypoxia, electrolyte disturbances (predominately hyperkalemia), and acute renal failure (attributed in part to myonecrosis and pigment load) all contribute to the ultimate demise, which can occur hours to days after the untreated bite. Preterminal hypertension may occur. The mortality is 25% in patients who do not receive antivenin and 3% overall.

The bitten limb should be immobilized and maintained in a dependent position while the victim is kept as quiet as possible. The pressure-immobilization technique for venom sequestration described previously for blue-ringed octopus bite should be applied.

Incision and suction therapy for snakebite is highly controversial. It should be employed only under the

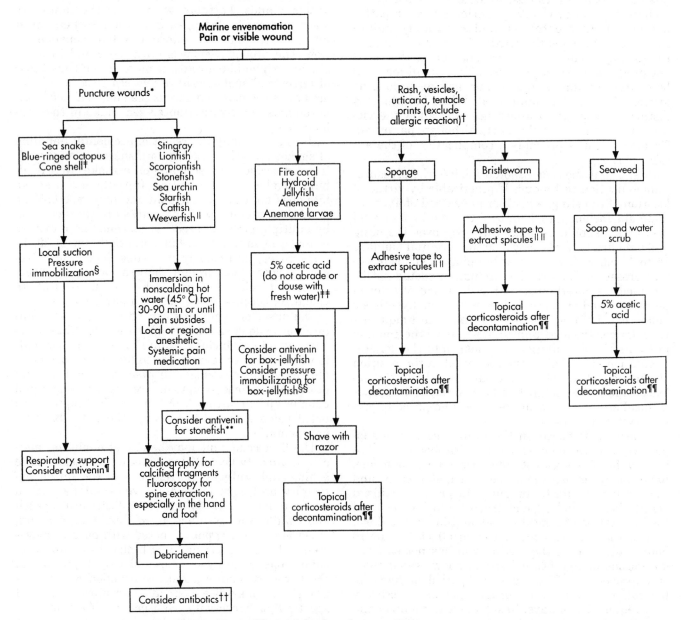

Figure 1 *See legend on opposite page*

following conditions: a mechanical suction extractor device is not available; the victim is seen within 5 minutes of the bite; the victim is elderly, chronically ill, or less than 32 kg in body weight; the snake is positively identified as venomous; clear puncture marks are seen; the pressure-immobilization technique cannot be employed; and antivenin will be unavailable for 2 hours. Two longitudinal parallel incisions should be made directly through the fang marks for a length of 5 mm to a depth of 5 to 10 mm. Cruciate incisions are improper. Suction is better applied with a rubber suction cup or commercial plunger-type venom extraction device; the mouth should be used only as a last resort, as the introduction of mouth flora into the wound creates a contaminated human bite situation. Suction should be applied continuously for 30 to 60 minutes. A rescuer with denuded intraoral mucous membranes should take care to rapidly spit out the mixture of blood and venom. There is little clinical enthusiasm for the perpetuation of incision and suction therapy, which may soon be relegated to therapeutic history.

With any evidence of envenomation, polyvalent sea snake antivenin* should be administered after appropriate skin testing for equine serum hypersensitivity. If this is not available, tiger snake antivenin* should be used. The administration of antivenin should begin as soon as possible and is most effective

---

*Not available in the United States.

if initiated within 8 hours of the bite. The minimal effective adult dosage is 1 ampule (1000 units), which neutralizes 10 mg of *E. schistosa* venom. Depending on the severity of the envenomation, 3000 to 10,000 units (3 to 10 ampules) may be required. The proper administration of antivenin is clearly described on the antivenin package insert.

Sea snake envenomation may induce severe physiologic derangements that require intensive medical management. Urine output and measured renal function should be closely monitored, as hemolysis and rhabdomyolysis release hemoglobin and myoglobin pigments into the circulation, which precipitates acute renal failure. If hemoglobinuria or myoglobinuria are detected, the urine should be alkalinized with sodium bicarbonate and diuresis promoted with a loop diuretic (furosemide) and/or mannitol. Acute renal failure may necessitate a period of peritoneal dialysis or hemodialysis. Hemodialysis offers an alternative therapy that may be successful if antivenin is not available.

Respiratory failure should be anticipated as paralysis overwhelms the victim. Endotracheal intubation and mechanical ventilation may be required until antivenin adequately neutralizes the venom effects. Serum electrolyte levels should be measured regularly to guide the administration of fluids and electrolyte supplements. Hyperkalemia related to rhabdomyolysis and renal dysfunction must be promptly recognized and treated.

Figure 1. Algorithmic approach to marine envenomation.

*A gaping laceration, particularly of the lower extremity, with cyanotic edges suggests a stingray wound. Multiple punctures in an erratic pattern with or without purple discoloration or retained fragments are typical of a sea urchin sting. One to eight (usually two) fang marks are usually present after a sea snake bite. A single ischemic puncture wound with an erythematous halo and rapid swelling suggests scorpion fish envenomation. Blisters often accompany a lionfish sting. Painless punctures with paralysis suggest the bite of a blue-ringed octopus; the site of a cone shell sting is punctate, painful, and ischemic in appearance.

†Wheal and flare reactions are nonspecific. Rapid (within 24 hours) onset of skin necrosis suggests an anemone sting. "Tentacle prints" with cross-hatching or a frosted appearance are pathognomonic for box jellyfish *(Chironex fleckeri)* envenomation. Ocular or intraoral lesions may be caused by fragmented hydroids or coelenterate tentacles. An allergic reaction must be treated promptly.

‡Sea snake venom causes weakness, respiratory paralysis, myoglobinuria, myalgias, blurred vision, vomiting, and dysphagia. The blue-ringed octopus injects tetrodotoxin, which causes rapid neuromuscular paralysis.

§If *immediately* available (which is rarely the case), local suction can be applied without incision using a plunger device, such as The Extractor (Sawyer Products, Safety Harbor, FL). As soon as possible, venom should be sequestered locally with a proximal venous-lymphatic occlusive band of constriction or (preferably) the pressure-immobilization technique, in which a cloth pad is compressed directly over the wound by an elastic wrap that should encompass the entire extremity at a pressure of 9.33 kPa (70 mm Hg) or less. A splint is then applied. Incision and suction are not recommended.

¶Early ventilatory support has the greatest influence on outcome. The minimal initial dose of sea snake antivenin is 1 to 3 vials; up to 10 vials may be required.

‖The wounds range from large lacerations (stingrays) to minute punctures (stonefish). Persistent pain after immersion in hot water suggests a stonefish sting or a retained fragment of spine. The puncture site can be identified by forcefully injecting 1 to 2% lidocaine or another local anesthetic agent without epinephrine near the wound and observing the egress of fluid. Do not attempt to crush the spines of sea urchins if they are present in the wound. Spine dye from already-extracted sea urchin spines disappears (is absorbed) in 24 to 36 hours.

**The initial dose of stonefish antivenin is 1 vial per two puncture wounds.

††The antibiotics chosen should cover *Staphylococcus, Streptococcus,* and microbes of marine origin, such as *Vibrio.*

‡‡Acetic acid 5% (vinegar) is a good all-purpose decontaminant and is mandated for the sting from a box jellyfish. Alternatives, depending on the geographic region and indigenous jellyfish species, include isopropyl alcohol, bicarbonate (baking soda), ammonia, and preparations containing these agents.

§§The initial dose of box jellyfish antivenin is 1 ampule intravenously or 3 ampules intramuscularly.

¶¶If inflammation is severe, steroids should be given systemically (beginning with at least 60 to 100 mg of prednisone or its equivalent) and the dose tapered over a period of 10 to 14 days.

‖‖An alternative is to apply and remove a thin layer of rubber cement or commercial facial peel materials followed by topical soaks of 30 mL of 5% acetic acid (vinegar) diluted in 1 liter of water for 15 to 30 minutes several times a day until the lesions begin to resolve. Anticipate surface desquamation in 3 to 6 weeks.

(Adapted from Auerbach PS [ed]: Wilderness Medicine: Management of Wilderness and Environmental Emergencies, 3rd ed. St Louis, Mosby–Year Book, 1995, pp 1368–1369.)

If there is no early evidence of envenomation, the victim should be observed for 8 hours before discharge from the hospital.

SUMMARY

A summary algorithmic approach to marine envenomation can be taken when the causative agent cannot be positively identified (Figure 1).

ACUTE POISONINGS

method of
HOWARD C. MOFENSON, M.D.,
THOMAS R. CARACCIO, Pharm.D., and
JOSEPH GREENSHER, M.D.
*Long Island Regional Poison Control Center
East Meadow, New York*

COMMON ABBREVIATIONS

AC	=	activated charcoal
ABG	=	arterial blood gas
ALT	=	alanine aminotransferase
AMA	=	against medical advice
AST	=	aspartate aminotransferase
AV	=	atrioventricular
BUN	=	blood urea nitrogen
CDC	=	Centers for Disease Control and Prevention
CK	=	creatine kinase
CNS	=	central nervous system
ECG	=	electrocardiogram
EEG	=	electroencephalogram
FDA	=	Food and Drug Administration
GABA	=	γ-aminobutyric acid
GI	=	gastrointestinal
G6PD	=	glucose-6-phosphate dehydrogenase
HIV	=	human immunodeficiency virus
ICU	=	intensive care unit
IM	=	intramuscular
IV	=	intravenous
MAO	=	monoamine oxidase
MDAC	=	multiple-dose activated charcoal
NAC	=	*N*-acetylcysteine
NIOSH	=	National Institute for Occupational Safety and Health
OSHA	=	Occupational Safety and Health Administration
$Paco_2$	=	arterial carbon dioxide tension
Pao_2	=	arterial oxygen tension
PEEP	=	positive end-expiratory pressure
pK_a	=	negative logarithm of dissociation constant
WBC	=	white blood cell

MEDICAL TOXICOLOGY (INGESTIONS, INHALATIONS, DERMAL AND OCULAR ABSORPTIONS)

Epidemiology

An estimated 5 million potentially toxic exposures occur each year in the United States. Poisoning is responsible for almost 12,000 deaths (including those caused by carbon monoxide) and more than 200,000 hospitalizations.

Poisoning accounts for 2 to 5% of pediatric hospital admissions, 10% of adult admissions, 5% of hospital admissions in the elderly population (older than 65 years), and 5% of ambulance calls. In one urban hospital, drug-related emergencies accounted for 38% of the emergency department visits. One evaluation of a medical intensive care unit (ICU) and step-down unit in a 3-month period indicated that 19.7% of admissions were for poisonings.

The largest number of fatalities resulting from poisoning are caused by carbon monoxide (CO). Most occur before arrival at the hospital. The mortality resulting from CO poisoning decreased from 600 deaths in 1989 to 500 in 1991. The other principal toxicologic fatalities in 1994 were due to gases and fumes, asthma therapies, automotive products, chemicals, hydrocarbons, antihistamines, and cleaning substances. Less than 1% of overdose cases reaching the hospitals result in fatality. However, patients presenting in a deep coma to medical care facilities have a fatality rate of 13 to 35%. The largest single cause of coma of inapparent etiology is drug poisoning.

Pharmaceutical preparations are involved in 40% of poisonings. The number one pharmaceutical toxic exposure is to acetaminophen. The leading pharmaceuticals causing fatalities in 1994 were the analgesics, antidepressants, sedative hypnotics or antipsychotic drugs, stimulants and street drugs, cardiovascular agents, and alcohols.

The severity of the manifestations of acute poisoning exposures varies greatly with the intent of the victim.

Nonintentional (accidental poisoning) exposures make up 60 to 65% of all poisoning exposures. The majority are acute, occur in children younger than 5 years, occur in the home, and result in no or minor toxicity. Many are ingestions of relatively nontoxic substances that require minimal medical care.

Intentional (suicidal poisoning) exposures constitute 10 to 15% of exposures and may require the highest standards of medical and nursing care and the use of sophisticated equipment for recovery. Intentional ingestions are often of multiple substances and frequently include ethanol, acetaminophen, and aspirin. Suicides make up 60 to 90% of the reported fatalities. About 25% of suicides are attempted with drugs. Sixty percent of patients who take a drug overdose use their own medication and 15% use drugs prescribed for close relatives. The majority of drug-related suicide attempts involve a central nervous system (CNS) depressant, and coma management is vital to the treatment.

Assessment and Maintenance of Vital Functions

The initial assessment of all medical emergencies follows the principles of basic and advanced cardiac

TABLE 1. **Important Measurements and Vital Signs**

| Age | BSA (m²) | Weight (kg) | Height (cm) | Pulse (bpm), Resting | Blood Pressure | | | RR (rpm) |
| | | | | | Hypotension | Hypertension | | |
						SIGNIFICANT	SEVERE	
NB	0.19	3.5	50	70–190	<40/60	>96	>106	30–60
1–6 mo	0.30	4–7	50–65	80–160	<45/70	>104	>110	30–50
6 mo–1 y	0.38	7–10	65–75	80–160	<45/70	>104	>110	20–40
1–2 y	0.50–0.55	10–12	75–85	80–140	<47/74	>74/112	>82/118	20–40
3–5 y	0.54–0.68	15–20	90–108	80–120	<52/80	>76/116	>84/124	20–40
6–9 y	0.68–0.85	20–28	122–133	75–115	<60/90	>82/122	>86/130	16–25
10–12 y	1.00–1.07	30–40	138–147	70–110	<60/90	>82/126	>90/134	16–25
13–15 y	1.07–1.22	42–50	152–160	60–100	<60/90	>86/136	<92/144	16–20
16–18 y	1.30–1.60	53–60	160–170	60–100	<60/90	>92/142	>98/150	12–16
Adult	1.40–1.70	60–70	160–170	60–100	<60/90	>90/140	>120/210	10–16

Abbreviations: BSA = body surface area; bpm = beats per minute; rpm = respirations per minute; RR = respiratory rate; NB = newborn.

Data from Nadas A: Pediatric Cardiology, 3rd ed. Philadelphia, WB Saunders Co, 1976; Blumer JL (ed): A Practice Guide to Pediatric Intensive Care. St Louis: CV Mosby 1990; AAP and ACEP Respiratory Distress in APLS Pediatric Emergency Medicine Course, 1993, p 5; Second Task Force on blood pressure control in children—1987. Pediatrics 79:1, 1987; Linakis JG: Hypertension. Fliesher GR, Ludwig S (eds): Textbook of Pediatric Emergency Medicine, 3rd ed. Baltimore, Williams & Wilkins, 1993, p 249.

life support. Determine the adequacy of the patient's airway, degree of ventilation, and circulatory status. Establish and maintain the vital functions. Vital signs should be measured frequently and should include body core temperature. Evaluation of vital functions should include not only rate numbers but also effective function (e.g., respiratory rate and depth and air exchange) (Table 1).

Assess the level of consciousness by immediate AVPU signs (alert, responds to verbal stimuli, responds to painful stimuli, and unconscious). If the patient is unconscious, assess the severity by the Reed classification (Table 2) or the Glasgow Coma Scale (Table 3).

If the patient is comatose, administer 100% oxygen; establish vascular access; obtain blood for pertinent laboratory studies; administer glucose, thiamine, and naloxone (Narcan); and consider intubation to protect the airway. Pertinent laboratory studies include arterial blood gases (ABGs), electrocardiography (ECG), glucose, electrolytes, renal and liver tests, and for all intentional ingestions the acetaminophen plasma concentration (APC). Consider radiography of the chest and abdomen.

The severity of a stimulant's effects can also be assessed (Table 4). The assessment should be recorded to follow the trend.

Exposure: Completely expose the patient by removing clothes and other items that interfere with a full evaluation. Look for clues to etiology in the clothes, including the hat and shoes.

Prevention of Toxin Absorption and Reduction of Local Damage

Routes

Poisoning exposure routes include ingestion (80%), dermal (7%), ophthalmologic (5%), inhalation (5%), insect bites and stings (2.7%), and parenteral injections (0.3%). The effect of the toxin may be local, systemic, or both.

Local effects (skin, eyes, mucosa of respiratory or gastrointestinal [GI] tract) occur where contact is made with the poisonous substance. Local effects are nonspecific chemical reactions that depend on the chemical properties (e.g., pH), concentration, contact time, and type of exposed surface.

TABLE 2. **Classification of the Level of Consciousness**

Stage	Status	Conscious Level	Pain Response	Reflexes Response	Respiration	Circulation
0	Lethargic, able to answer questions and follow commands	Asleep	Arousable	Intact	Normal	Normal
I	Responsive to pain, brain stem and deep tendon reflexes intact	Comatose	Withdraws	Intact	Normal	Normal
II	Unresponsive to pain	Comatose	None	Intact	Normal	Normal
III	Unresponsive to pain, most reflexes absent, respiratory depression	Comatose	None	Absent	Depressed	Normal
IV	Unresponsive to pain, all reflexes absent, cardiovascular and respiratory depression	Comatose	None	Absent	Cyanosis	Shock

Modified from Reed CE, Driggs MF, Foote CC: Acute barbiturate intoxication: A study of 300 cases based on a physiologic system of classification of the severity of the intoxication. Ann Intern Med 37:290, 1952.

TABLE 3. **Glasgow Coma Scale**

Scale	Adult Response	Score	Pediatric (0–1 y)*
Eye opening	Spontaneous	4	Spontaneous
	To verbal command	3	To shout
	To pain	2	To pain
	None	1	No response
Motor response			
To verbal command	Obeys	6	
To painful stimuli	Localized pain	5	Localized pain
	Flexion withdrawal	4	Flexion withdrawal
	Decorticate flexion	3	Decorticate flexion
	Decerebrate extension	2	Decerebrate extension
	None	1	None
Verbal response, adult	Oriented and converses	5	Cries, smiles, coos
	Disoriented but converses	4	Cries or screams
	Inappropriate words	3	Inappropriate
	Incomprehensible sounds	2	Grunts
	None	1	Gives no response
Verbal response, child	Oriented	5	
	Words or babbles	4	
	Vocal sounds	3	
	Cries or moans to stimuli	2	
	None	1	

*From Seidel J: Preparing for pediatric emergencies. Pediatr Rev 16:466–472, 1995.
Modified from Teasdale G, Jennett B: Assessment of coma and impaired consciousness. Lancet 2:81–84, 1974; and Simpson D, Reilly P: Pediatric coma scale. Lancet 2:450, 1982.

Systemic effects occur when the poison is absorbed into the body and depend on the dose, the distribution, and the functional reserve of the organ systems. Complications resulting from shock, hypoxia, chronic exposure, and existing illness may also influence systemic toxicity.

Delayed Toxic Action

Most pharmaceuticals are absorbed within 90 minutes. However, the patient with exposure to a potential toxin may be asymptomatic at the time of presentation for several reasons: the substance may be nontoxic, an insufficient amount of the toxin may have been involved, or a sufficient amount may not yet have been absorbed or metabolized to produce toxicity.

Absorption may be significantly delayed for several reasons:

1. A drug with anticholinergic properties is involved (e.g., antihistamines, belladonna alkaloids, diphenoxylate with atropine [Lomotil], phenothiazines [PTZs], and cyclic antidepressants).
2. Sustained-release and enteric-coated preparations, which have delayed and prolonged absorption, are involved.
3. Concretions may form (e.g., salicylates, iron, glutethimide, and meprobamate) that can delay absorption and prolong the action.

Substances must be metabolized to a toxic metabolite or time is required to produce a toxic effect on the organ system (e.g., acetaminophen, *Amanita phalloides* mushrooms, acetonitrile, carbon tetrachloride, colchicine, digoxin, ethylene glycol, heavy metals, methanol, methylene chloride, monoamine oxidase inhibitors [MAOIs], oral hypoglycemic agents, parathion, and paraquat).

Decontamination

Decontamination procedures should be considered for an asymptomatic patient if the patient has been exposed to potentially toxic substances in toxic amounts.

Ocular exposure should be treated immediately with water or saline irrigation for 15 to 20 minutes with the eyelids fully retracted. Do not use neutralizing chemicals. All caustic and corrosive injuries should be evaluated with fluorescein dye and by an ophthalmologist.

Dermal exposure is treated immediately with copious irrigation (not forceful flushing) for 30 minutes. Shampooing the hair; cleansing fingernails, navel, and perineum; and irrigating the eyes are necessary in an extensive exposure. The clothes should be specially bagged and may have to be discarded. Leather goods can be irreversibly contaminated and must be abandoned. Caustic (alkali) exposures can require hours of irrigation. Dermal absorption can occur with, for example, pesticides, hydrocarbons, and cyanide.

TABLE 4. **Classification of the Severity of Stimulant**

Severity	Manifestations
Grade 1	Diaphoresis, hyper-reflexia, irritability mydriasis, tremors
Grade 2	Confusion, fever, hyperactivity, hypertension, tachycardia, tachypnea
Grade 3	Delirium, mania, hyperpyrexia, tachydysrhythmia
Grade 4	Coma, convulsions, cardiovascular collapse

Modified with permission from Espelin DE, Done AK: Amphetamine poisoning. Effectiveness of chlorpromazine. N Engl J Med 278:1361–1365, 1968. Copyright 1968 Massachusetts Medical Society. All rights reserved.

Injection exposures to drugs and toxins can involve envenomation. Cold packs and tourniquets should not be used, and incision is generally not recommended. Venom extractors may be used within minutes of envenomation, and proximal lymphatic constricting bands or elastic wraps may be used to delay lymphatic flow and immobilize the extremity.

Inhalation exposure to toxic substances is managed by immediately removing the victim from the contaminated environment, by protected rescuers if necessary.

GI exposure is the most common route of poisoning. GI decontamination may be done by gastric emptying (induction of emesis, gastric lavage), adsorption by administering single or multiple doses of activated charcoal (AC), or whole-bowel irrigation. No procedure is routine; the procedure should be individualized on the basis of the patient's age, properties of the substance ingested, and time since the ingestion. If no attempt is made to decontaminate the patient, the reason should be clearly documented on the medical record (e.g., time elapsed, past peak of action, ineffectiveness, or risk of procedure).

Gastric Emptying Procedures. The procedure used is influenced by the patient's age and the procedure's effectiveness (the size of the orogastric tube used in a small child may not be large enough for adequate lavage, e.g., with iron tablets), time of ingestion (gastric emptying is usually ineffective more than 1 hour after ingestion), clinical status (asymptomatic time of peak effect has elapsed or the patient's condition is too unstable), formulation of substance ingested (regular release, sustained release, enteric coated), amount ingested, caustic action, and rapidity of onset of CNS depression or stimulation (convulsions). Most studies show that only 30% (19 to 62%) of ingested toxins are removed by gastric emptying under optimal conditions. It has not been demonstrated that the procedure improved the outcome.

A mnemonic for gathering information is SATS: substance, amount and age, time of ingestion, and symptoms.

Attempt to obtain ample information about the patient. A mnemonic for this is AMPLE: A, for age and allergies; M, for available medications; P, for past medical history including pregnancy or psychiatric illnesses, substance abuse, or intentional ingestions; L, for time of last meal, which may influence absorption and the onset and peak action; and E, for events leading to the present condition. The intent should be determined.

Consult the regional poison control center for the exact ingredients and the latest management. The first-aid information on the labels of products is notoriously inaccurate, and product ingredients change.

Syrup of Ipecac–Induced Emesis. This is most useful for young children with a recent witnessed ingestion of a known agent. To be effective, vomiting should be induced immediately at the site (in the home). The poison control center should be called before emesis is induced.

Contraindications or situations in which induction of emesis is inappropriate include the following:

1. Caustic ingestions.
2. Loss of airway protective reflexes. This can occur with substances that can produce rapid onset of CNS depression (e.g., ethanol, short-acting [SA] benzodiazepines (BZPs), SA barbiturates, SA nonbarbiturate sedative hypnotics, SA opioids, tricyclic antidepressants) or convulsions (e.g., beta blockers, camphor, calcium channel blockers, chloroquine, codeine, isoniazid, mefenamic acid, nicotine, propoxyphene, phencyclidine, organophosphate insecticides, strychnine, and cyclic antidepressants).
3. Ingestion of high-viscosity petroleum distillates (e.g., gasoline, lighter fluid, kerosene).
4. Significant vomiting before presentation or hematemesis.
5. Age younger than 6 months (no established dose, safety, or efficacy).
6. Foreign bodies (ineffective, may aspirate).
7. Clinical conditions: pregnancy, neurologic impairment, hemodynamic instability, increased intracranial pressure, and hypertension.
8. Delay in presentation (more than 1 hour after ingestion).

There may be interference with administration of AC or oral antidotes. The patient cannot tolerate oral intake for a mean of 2 to 3 hours after ipecac-induced emesis.

The dose of syrup of ipecac (SI) for the 6- to 9-month-old infant is 5 mL; for the 9- to 12-month-old, 10 mL; and for the 1- to 12-year-old, 15 mL. For children older than 12 years and adults, the dose is 30 mL. The dose may be repeated once if the child does not vomit in 15 to 20 minutes. The vomitus should be inspected for remnants of pills or toxic substances, and the appearance and odor should be documented. When SI is not available, 30 mL of mild dishwashing soap (not electric dishwasher detergent) may be used, although it is less effective.

Complications are rare but include aspiration, protracted vomiting, rarely cardiac toxicity with long-term abuse, pneumothorax, gastric rupture, diaphragmatic hernia, intracranial hemorrhage, and Mallory-Weiss tears.

Gastric Aspiration and Lavage. The contraindications are similar to those for ipecac-induced emesis. The procedure can be accomplished after the insertion of an endotracheal tube in CNS depression or controlled convulsions. The patient should be placed with the head down and lower than the hips in a left lateral decubitus position. The location of the tube should be confirmed by radiography, if necessary, and suctioning should be available.

Contraindications to gastric aspiration and lavage include the following:

1. Caustic ingestions (risk of esophageal perforation)
2. Uncontrolled convulsions, because of the danger of aspiration and injury during the procedure

3. High-viscosity petroleum distillate products

4. CNS depression or absent protective airway reflexes, which require insertion of an endotracheal tube to protect against aspiration

5. Significant cardiac dysrhythmias, which should be controlled

6. Significant emesis before presentation or hematemesis

7. Delay in presentation (more than 1 hour after ingestion)

The best results with gastric aspiration and lavage are obtained with the largest possible orogastric tube that can reasonably be passed (nasogastric tubes are not large enough except for liquid ingestions). For adults, use a large-bore orogastric Lavacuator hose or a No. 42 French Ewald tube. For children, use a No. 22 to No. 28 French orogastric-type tube, but this is usually ineffective with solid ingestions (e.g., iron tablets).

The amount of fluid used varies with the patient's age and size. In general, aliquots of 50 to 100 mL per lavage are used for adults and 5 mL per kg up to 50 to 100 mL per lavage for children. Larger amounts of fluid may force the toxin past the pylorus. Many physicians add AC after the initial aspiration as a marker and many instill AC before removing the tube. Lavage fluid is 0.89% saline.

Complications are rare and may include respiratory depression, aspiration pneumonitis, cardiac dysrhythmias caused by increased vagal tone (e.g., beta-adrenergic blockers, calcium channel blockers, digoxin overdoses), esophageal-gastric tears and perforation, electrolyte imbalance in young children, laryngospasm, and mediastinitis.

Activated Charcoal. Oral AC adsorbs the toxin on its surface before GI absorption and interrupts enterogastric and enterohepatic circulation of toxic metabolites. AC is a stool marker, indicating that the toxin has passed through the GI tract.

AC does not effectively adsorb small molecules or molecules lacking carbon as listed in Table 5. AC adsorption may be diminished by the concurrent presence of ethanol, milk, cocoa powder, and ice cream.

There are a few relative contraindications to the use of AC:

TABLE 5. Substances Poorly Adsorbed by Activated Charcoal

C—Caustics and corrosives, cyanide*
H—Heavy metals (arsenic, iron, lead, lithium, mercury)
A—Alcohols (ethanol, methanol, isopropyl) and glycols (ethylene glycol)
R—Rapid onset or absorption of cyanide and strychnine
C—Chlorine and iodine
O—Others insoluble in water (substances in tablet form)
A—Aliphatic and poorly absorbed hydrocarbons (petroleum distillates)
L—Laxatives, sodium, magnesium, potassium

*If cyanide is ingested, AC is given in large doses; 1 gm of AC adsorbs 35 mg of cyanide.

1. It should not be given before, concomitantly with, or shortly after oral antidotes unless it has been proved not to interfere significantly with their effectiveness. It does not interfere with the effectiveness of N-acetylcysteine (NAC) in acetaminophen overdose (although there is up to a 39% reduction in NAC) and it may contribute to vomiting.

2. It does not effectively adsorb caustics and corrosives, may produce vomiting or cling to the mucosa, and may falsely appear as a burn at endoscopy.

3. It should not be given if the patient is comatose without securing the airway.

4. It should not be given if there are no bowel sounds (may form concretions or perforation).

The dose of activated charcoal is 1 gram per kg per dose orally, with a minimum of 15 grams. Optimal dosage has not been established. Ideal therapy allegedly requires a 10:1 ratio of AC to toxin. The usual initial adult dose is 60 to 100 grams and the dose for children is 15 to 30 grams. It is administered orally as a slurry mixed with water or by nasogastric or orogastric tube. Caution: Be sure the tube is in the stomach. AC is usually administered initially with a cathartic in adults. Cathartics are not necessary in children.

MULTIPLE-DOSE ACTIVATED CHARCOAL. Repeated dosing with AC decreases the half-life and increases the clearance of phenobarbital, dapsone, salicylate, quinidine, theophylline, and carbamazepine. With multiple-dose AC (MDAC), subsequent cathartics should be given every 24 hours, not with each dose. No controlled studies have demonstrated that MDAC or cathartics alter the clinical course of an intoxication. The MDAC dose varies from 0.25 to 0.50 gram per kg every 1 to 4 hours, and continuous nasogastric tube infusion of 0.25 to 0.5 gram per kg per hour has been used to decrease vomiting.

GI dialysis involves the diffusion of the toxin from the higher concentration in the serum of the mesenteric vessels to the lower levels in the GI tract mucosal cells and subsequently into the GI lumen, where the concentration has been lowered by adsorption by the intraluminal AC.

Complications of AC have been reported in at least a dozen cases. There are many cases of unreported pulmonary aspirations and "charcoal" lungs, intestinal obstruction (three cases reported), empyema after esophageal perforation, and hypermagnesemia and hypernatremia, which have been associated with repeated concurrent doses of AC and saline cathartics.

Catharsis. This is used to hasten the elimination of any remaining toxin in the GI tract. There have been no studies demonstrating the effectiveness of a cathartic used alone. AC and cathartic were more effective than AC alone in managing slow-release theophylline overdose. However, a cathartic with AC was less effective than AC alone in salicylate poisoning. A study using AC alone and magnesium citrate indicated no benefit when the cathartic was administered.

Cathartics are relatively contraindicated in the following circumstances:

1. Ileus as indicated by absence of bowel sounds
2. Intestinal obstruction or evidence of intestinal perforation
3. Cases with pre-existing electrolyte disturbances
4. Magnesium salts contraindicated in renal impairment
5. Sodium salts in heart failure or diseases requiring sodium restriction

Magnesium sulfate or sodium sulfate is administered in doses of 250 mg per kg per dose as 20% solutions. The adult dose is 30 grams. Sorbitol is given at 2.8 mL per kg to a maximum of 200 mL of a 70% solution in adults. Sorbitol should not be used for children. It is best to avoid cathartics for pediatric patients because hyponatremia, hypocalcemia, hyperphosphatemia, and death have occurred.

Whole-Bowel Irrigation. In whole-bowel irrigation, bowel-cleansing solutions of polyethylene glycol (PEG) with balanced electrolytes are used to avoid changes in body weight or electrolytes.

Indications (not approved by the Food and Drug Administration [FDA]): Whole-bowel irrigation may be indicated with ingestions of substances that are poorly adsorbed by AC, such as iron and other heavy metals, lithium, and sustained-release preparations. The procedure has been studied and used successfully in iron overdose when abdominal radiographs revealed incomplete emptying of excess iron. There are additional implications in other ingestions, as in body packing of illicit drugs (e.g., cocaine and heroin). The procedure is to administer, orally or by nasogastric tube, the solution (GoLYTELY or Colyte), at 0.5 liter per hour in children younger than 5 years and 2 liters per hour in adolescents and adults for 5 hours. The end point is reached when the rectal effluent is clear or radiopaque materials can no longer be seen in the GI tract on abdominal radiographs.

Contraindications: These measures should not be used if extensive hematemesis, ileus, or signs of bowel obstruction, perforation, or peritonitis are present.

Animal experiments in which PEG was added to AC indicated that AC-salicylate and AC-theophylline combinations resulted in decreased adsorption and desorption of salicylate and theophylline and no therapeutic benefit over AC alone. Polyethylene solutions are bound by AC in vitro, which decreases the efficacy of AC.

Dilution. Dilutional treatment is indicated for the immediate management of caustic and corrosive poisonings but is otherwise not useful. Administration of large quantities of diluting fluid—above 30 mL in children and 250 mL in adults—may produce vomiting, reexposing the vital tissues to the effects of local damage, and possible aspiration.

Neutralization. Neutralization has not been proved to be safe or effective.

Endoscopy and Surgery. Surgery has been required in the management of body packer's obstruction, intestinal ischemia produced by cocaine ingestion, and local caustic action of iron.

Common Toxicologic Presentations

Table 6 shows the common toxicologic presentations and their most frequent toxicologic and medical etiologies. A mnemonic for miosis is VCPOOP: valproic acid, clonidine, phencyclidine, organophosphates, opioids, phenothiazines. A mnemonic for mydriasis is SHAW: sympathomimetic, hallucinogens, anticholinergic, withdrawal.

Differential Diagnosis of Poisons on the Basis of Central Nervous System Manifestations

Neurologic parameters help in classifying and assessing the need for supportive treatment and provide diagnostic clues to the etiology. See Tables 7 through 10.

Guidelines for In-Hospital Disposition

Classification as a high-risk patient depends on clinical judgment. Any patient with the need for cardiorespiratory support or persistent altered mental status for 3 hours or more should be considered for intensive care.

Guidelines for admitting patients older than 14 years to an ICU, after 2 to 3 hours in the emergency department, include the following:

1. Need for intubation
2. Seizures
3. Unresponsiveness to verbal stimuli
4. Arterial carbon dioxide partial pressure greater than 45 mm Hg
5. Cardiac conduction or rhythm disturbances (any rhythm except sinus arrhythmia)
6. Close monitoring of vital signs during antidotal therapy or elimination procedures
7. Need for continuous monitoring
8. QRS complex greater than 0.10 second in tricyclic antidepressant poisoning
9. Systolic blood pressure less than 80 mm Hg
10. Grade 3 or 4 stimulation or depression (see Tables 2, 3, and 4)
11. Hypoxia, hypercarbia, acid-base disturbance, metabolic abnormalities
12. Extremes of temperature
13. Progressive deterioration or significant underlying medical disorders

Use of Antidotes

Antidotes are available for only a relatively small number of poisons. An available antidote should be administered only after the vital functions have been established. Table 11 lists the toxins for which antidotes are available. Table 12 summarizes the commonly used antidotes, their indications, and methods of administration. Consult the regional poison control center for further information on these antidotes.

Text continued on page 1196

TABLE 6. **Common Clinical Presentations and Etiologies of Poisonings**

Clinical Presentation	Toxic Agents	Medical Diseases
Acidosis, metabolic	Alcohols and glycols Cyanide Iron Isoniazid Metformin Salicylates Toluene	Diabetes mellitus Convulsions GI losses Inborn errors of metabolism Lactic acidosis Shock Starvation Renal tubular acidosis Uremia
Bradycardia	Beta-adrenergic blockers Calcium channel blockers Central alpha agonists Cholinergic agents CNS depressants Digitalis (acute) Lithium Opioids Organophosphate insecticides Phenylpropanolamine (reflex) Quinidine Tricyclic or cyclic antidepressants	Increased ICP Structural heart lesions Conduction defects Hypothermia Sleep Athletes at rest Jaundice Stokes-Adams syndrome Carotid sinus syndrome Hypothyroidism
Bradypnea, hypoventilation, apnea	Botulism Cholinergic drugs Clonidine CNS depressants Colchicine Elapidae envenomation (coral, cobra) Ethanol Neuromuscular blockers Nicotine Organophosphate insecticides Paralytic agents (in shellfish, tetrodotoxin) Paralytic plants (poison hemlock) Sedative hypnotics Ticks	Vascular CNS disorders Neuromuscular disorders Guillain-Barré syndrome Myasthenia gravis Poliomyelitis Amyotrophic lateral sclerosis Muscle disorders Muscular dystrophy Polymyositis, dermatomyositis Myotonia Electrolyte abnormalities Hypokalemia Hypophosphatemia Familial paralysis
Coma	Alcohols Barbiturates Benzodiazepines Carbon monoxide Gases and fumes Neuroleptics Opioids Sedative hypnotics Tricyclic or cyclic antidepressants	Anoxia Diabetic ketoacidosis and nonketotic hyperosmolar coma Encephalopathies Epilepsy, postictal CVA Electrolyte disturbances Hepatic encephalopathy Hypertensive encephalopathy Infections (meningitis, brain abscess) Hypoglycemia Metabolic disorders Shock (septic, cardiogenic) Trauma Uremia
Convulsions	Alcohols or glycols Camphor Carbon monoxide Cyanide Heavy metals (lead, lithium) Hypoglycemia agents Isoniazid Mushroom (*Gyromitra*) Opioids (propoxyphene, meperidine) Phenothiazines Salicylates Strychnine Sympathomimetics (cocaine, amphetamines, PCP) Theophylline Tricyclic or cyclic antidepressants Withdrawal	Anoxia Febrile (child) Infections Metabolic or endocrine (hypoglycemia, hyponatremia, hypocalcemia, inborn metabolic) disorders Neoplastic Traumatic Vascular (CVA) Idiopathic epilepsy

TABLE 6. **Common Clinical Presentations and Etiologies of Poisonings** *Continued*

Clinical Presentation	Toxic Agents	Medical Diseases
Dysrhythmias	Anticholinergic agents Antidysrhythmic agents Antihypertensive agents Beta-adrenergic blockers Calcium channel blockers Chloral hydrate Chloroquine Digitalis Lithium Neuroleptics Nonsedating antihistamines (terfenadine, astemizole) Opioids (propoxyphene) Sympathomimetics (cocaine, amphetamine, PCP, phenylpropanolamine, theophylline) Tricyclic antidepressants	Electrolyte disturbances Hereditary (e.g., prolonged QT interval) Hypoxia Idiopathic Myocarditis Myocardial infarction Sick sinus syndrome Uremia
Hypertension	Anticholinergic (T)* Clonidine (R) Hallucinogens (T) Lead encephalopathy (B) Licorice MAOI overdose and interaction Phenylephrine (R) Phenylpropanolamine (R) Sympathomimetics (T) (amphetamine, cocaine, PCP, theophylline) Thyroid (T) Vitamine A excess (B) Withdrawal (T)	Aldosteronism (primary) Acute porphyria Carcinoid syndromes Coarctation of aorta Congenital adrenal hyperplasia Essential hypertension Hyperthyroidism Increased intracranial pressure Pheochromocytoma Psychologic causes or anxiety Renal disease
Hypotension	Antihypertensive agents (T) Arsenic (T) Barbiturates (T) Beta-adrenergic blockers (B) Calcium channel blockers (B) Carbon monoxide (T) Caustics (T) Clonidine (B) Cyanide (T) Cyclic antidepressants (T) Digitalis (acute B, chronic T) Disulfiram reaction (T) Ethanol Heavy metals Iron (T) Opioids (B) Organophosphate insecticides (B) MAOI (T) Neuroleptics (T) Nitrites Sedative hypnotics (T) Theophylline (T) Vasodilators (nitrites) (T)	Adrenal insufficiency Anaphylaxis Anoxia Burns Cardiac causes (dysrhythmias, myopathypericardial disease, aortic aneurysm) Fluid sequestration (ascites, bowel obstruction) GI losses Heart failure Hemorrhage Hypothermia Hypovolemia or dehydration Sepsis Shock of any cause Spinal cord dysfunction
Hyperthermia (see Temperature Disturbances)		
Hypothermia	Alpha-adrenergic antagonists Barbiturates Benzodiazepines Beta-adrenergic antagonists Carbon monoxide Ethanol Hypoglycemic agents Nitrites Opioids Phenothiazines Sedative hypnotics†	Adrenal insufficiency Cold blood or IV fluids Diabetic ketoacidosis Environmental Hypoglycemia Hypothalamic lesions Hypothyroidism Shock Spinal cord transection Uremia

Table continued on following page

TABLE 6. **Common Clinical Presentations and Etiologies of Poisonings** *Continued*

Clinical Presentation	Toxic Agents	Medical Diseases
Miosis	Clonidine Imidazoles Organophosphates Opioids (all except those in the following list) PCP Phenothiazines Cholinergic medications	Pontine lesions Aging Iritis Posterior synechiae Neurosyphilis
Mydriasis	Anticholinergic agents Botulism (delayed) Ethanol Hallucinogens Methanol (delayed) Opioids (meperidine, dextromethorphan, diphenoxylate [Lomotil]) Sedative hypnotics† Sympathomimetics Withdrawal	Midbrain lesions Ocular trauma Cranial trauma Increased intracranial pressure
Organic brain syndrome (toxic psychosis)	Anticholinergic agents Ethanol Digitalis Hallucinogens Inhalants (solvents) Stimulants (cocaine, amphetamines, PCP) Withdrawal	Infections Metabolic disorders Psychosis
Pulmonary edema	Cardiac: antidysrhythmics, beta-adrenergic antagonists, calcium channel blockers, cyclic antidepressants Noncardiac: barbiturates, hydrocarbon aspiration, opioids, organophosphates, salicylates, toxic gases Irritant gases: smoke, chlorine inhalation Neurogenic: sympathomimetics	Aspiration Fluid overload Heart failure Hypoxia Near-drowning Shock
Tachycardia	Alcohols and glycols (early) Anticholinergics Antihistamines CNS stimulants Digitalis (chronic) Hallucinogens Nitrates and nitrites PCP Phenothiazines Plants Salicylates Sedative hypnotics (early)† Sympathomimetics (amphetamines, cocaine, theophylline) Thyroid Tricyclic or cyclic antidepressants Withdrawal	Fever Hyperthermia Hyperthyroidism Hypovolemia Shock Dysrhythmia PAT, atrial dysrhythmias Electrolyte imbalance Anxiety Carditis Heart failure
Tachypnea and hyperventilation	Acidosis (ethanol ketoacidosis, ethylene glycol, methanol, phenformin) Carbon monoxide CNS stimulants (camphor) Cyanide Dinitrophenol Salicylates Sympathomimetics (amphetamines, cocaine, theophylline) Withdrawal Inhaled gases Irritant gases	Temperature elevation Compensation metabolic acidosis Pneumonitis Other pulmonary conditions Heart failure Other cardiac conditions

TABLE 6. **Common Clinical Presentations and Etiologies of Poisonings** *Continued*

Clinical Presentation	Toxic Agents	Medical Diseases
Torsades de pointes	Amantadine (Symmetrel) Arsenic Antidysrhythmic agents IA, IB, IC, III Cocaine Erythromycin Fluoride Haloperidol (Haldol) Itraconazole (Sporanox) Maprotiline (Ludiomil) Nonsedating antihistamines (terfenadine, astemizole) Organophosphates Pentamidine Phenothiazines (e.g., thioridazine) Sotalol (Betapace) Thallium	Congenital long QT syndromes (Romano-Ward; Jervell and Lange-Nielsen) Electrolyte derangement ($\downarrow$ magnesium, $\downarrow$ calcium) Coronary artery disease
Wheezing	Aspirin Beta blockers (bronchospasm) Cholinergic medications Cholinergic mushroom Irritant gases: chlorine, smoke, occupational hypersensitivity	Bronchospasm asthma Cardiac asthma Foreign body Cystic fibrosis Pneumonia Anaphylaxis Carcinoid

*T = tachycardia; B = bradycardia; R = reflex bradycardia initially.

†Includes barbiturates and benzodiazepines.

Abbreviations: GI = gastrointestinal; CNS = central nervous system; CVA = cerebrovascular accident; MAOI = monoamine oxidase inhibitor; PAT = paroxysmal atrial tachycardia; ICP = intracranial pressure; PCP = phencyclidine; IV = intravenous; PAT = paroxysmal atrial tachycardia.

TABLE 7. **Central Nervous System Depressants***

General Manifestations	CNS Depressants
Bradycardia Bradypnea† Shallow respirations Hypotension Hypothermia Flaccid coma Miosis Hypoactive bowel sounds Frozen addict syndrome§	Alcohols and glycols (S-H) Anticonvulsants (S-H) Antidysrhythmics (S-H) Antihypertensives (S-H) Barbiturates (S-H) Benzodiazepines (S-H)‡ Butyrophenones (Syly) Beta-adrenergic blockers (Syly) Calcium channel blockers (Syly) Digitalis (Syly) Opioids (O)‖¶ Lithium (mixed) Muscle relaxants Phenothiazines (Syly) Nonbarbiturate, benzodiazepine sedative hypnotic (S-H)‖ (chloral hydrate, glutethimide, methaqualone, methyprylone, ethchlorvynol, bromide) Tricyclic antidepressants late (Syly)

*Central nervous system depressants are cholinergics (C), opioids (O) and sedative hypnotics (S-H), sympatholytic agents (Syly). The hallmarks are lethargy, sedation, stupor, and coma.

†Barbiturates may produce an initial tachycardia.

‡Benzodiazepines rarely produce coma that interferes with cardiorespiratory functions.

§The "frozen addict" syndrome is due to a neurotoxin resulting from improper synthesis of an analogue of meperidine. Its manifestations are similar to those of the permanent type of parkinsonism.

‖Convulsions are produced by codeine, propoxyphene (Darvon), meperidine (Demerol), glutethimide, phenothiazines, methaqualone, and tricyclic or cyclic antidepressants.

¶Pulmonary edema is common with opioids and sedative hypnotics.

TABLE 8. **Central Nervous System Stimulants***

General Manifestations	CNS Stimulants
Tachycardia Tachypnea and dysrhythmias Hypertension Convulsions Spastic coma‡ Toxic psychosis Mydriasis (reactive) Agitation and restlessness Moist skin Tremors	Amphetamines (Sy) Anticholinergics (Ach)† Cocaine (Sy) Camphor (mixed) Ergot alkaloids (Sy) Isoniazid (mixed) Lithium (mixed) Lysergic acid diethylamine (LSD) (H) Hallucinogens (H) Mescaline and synthetic analogues Metals (arsenic, lead, mercury) Methylphenidate (Ritalin) (Sy) Monoamine oxidase inhibitors (Sy) Pemoline (Cylert) (Sy) Phencyclidine (H)§ Salicylates (mixed) Strychnine (mixed) Sympathomimetics (Sy) (phenylpropanolamine, theophylline, caffeine, thyroid) Withdrawal from ethanol, beta-adrenergic blockers, clonidine, opioids, sedative hypnotics (W)

*The CNS stimulants are anticholinergics (Ach), hallucinogens (H), sympathomimetics (Sy), and withdrawal (W). The hallmarks of CNS stimulants are convulsions and hyperactivity.

†Anticholinergics produce dry skin and mucosa and decreased bowel sounds.

‡Flaccid coma eventually develops after seizures.

§Phencyclidine may produce miosis.

Enhancement of Elimination

The medical methods for elimination of absorbed toxic substances are diuresis, dialysis, hemoperfusion, exchange transfusion, plasmapheresis, enzyme induction, and inhibition. Methods of increasing urinary excretion of toxic chemicals and drugs have been studied extensively, but the other modalities have not been well evaluated.

In general, these methods are needed in only a minority of instances and should be reserved for life-threatening circumstances or when a definite benefit is anticipated.

Diuresis

Diuresis increases the renal clearance of compounds that are eliminated primarily by the renal route, are significantly reabsorbed in the renal tubules, and have a small volume of distribution (Vd) and low protein binding (PB). The risks of diuresis are fluid overload, with cerebral and pulmonary edema, and disturbances in acid-base and electrolyte balances. Failure to produce diuresis may imply renal failure. At present, the only effective diuresis used in the management of the poisoned patient is alkaline diuresis. Diuretics have been administered to maintain the diuresis.

Although acid diuresis may enhance the elimination of weak bases (e.g., amphetamines, fenfluramine [Pondimin], quinidine, phencyclidine, strychnine), it is not recommended because of adverse effects of metabolic acidosis with rhabdomyolysis (e.g., precipitation of myoglobin), cardiotoxicity, and lack of proven clinical effectiveness. Alkalinization with or without diuresis with sodium bicarbonate (NaHCO$_3$) at 1 to 2 mEq per kg in 15 mL of D5W per kg may be used in the therapy of weak acid intoxications, such as with salicylates (severe salicylate poisoning

TABLE 9. Hallucinogens*

General Manifestations	Hallucinogens
Tachycardia and dysrhythmias	Amphetamines
Tachypnea	Anticholinergics
Hypertension	Carbon monoxide
Hallucinations, usually visual	Cardiac glycosides
Disorientation	Cocaine
Panic reaction	Ethanol
Toxic psychosis	Hydrocarbon inhalation (abuse)
Moist skin	Hydrocarbon inhalation (occupational)
Mydriasis (reactive)	Lysergic acid diethylamide
Hyperthermia	Marijuana
Flashbacks	Mescaline (peyote)
	Mescaline-amphetamine hybrids†
	Metals (chronic mercury, arsenic)
	Mushrooms (psilocybin)
	Phencyclidine
	Plants (morning glory seeds, nutmeg)

*There is considerable overlap in this category; however, the major hallmark manifestation is hallucinations.

†The mescaline-amphetamine hybrids are methylene dioxymethamphetamine (MDMA, Ecstasy, Adam) and methylene dioxyamphetamine (MDA, Eve), which have been associated with deaths.

TABLE 10. Autonomic Nervous System

General Manifestations	Agents
Anticholinergic	
Tachycardia, dysrhythmias rare	Antihistamines
Tachypnea	Antispasmodic GI preparations
Hypertension (mild)	Antiparkinsonian preparations
Hyperthermia	Atropine
Hallucinations	Cyclobenzaprine (Flexeril)
Mydriasis (unreactive)	Mydriatic ophthalmologic agents
Flushed skin	Over-the-counter sleep agents
Dry skin and mouth	Plants (*Datura* species), mushrooms
Hypoactive bowel sounds	Phenothiazines (early)
Urinary retention	Scopolamine
Lilliputian hallucinations	Tricyclic or cyclic antidepressants (early)
Cholinergic	
Bradycardia (muscarinic)	Bethanechol
Tachycardia (nicotinic effect)	Carbamate insecticides (carbaryl)
Miosis (muscarinic)	Edrophonium
Diarrhea (muscarinic)	Organophosphate insecticides (malathion, parathion)
Hypertension (variable)	Parasympathetic agents (physostigmine, pyridostigmine)
Hyperactive bowel sounds	Toxic mushrooms (*Amanita muscaria*, *Clitocybe* species)
Excess urination (muscarinic)	
Excess salivation (muscarinic)	
Lacrimation (muscarinic)	
Bronchospasm (muscarinic)	
Muscle fasciculations (nicotinic)	
Paralysis (nicotinic)	

can require hemodialysis, which avoids complications of fluid overload), long-acting barbiturates (LABs) (e.g., phenobarbital), 2,4-dichlorophenoxyacetic acid, chlorpropamide, methotrexate, and methanol. Additional boluses of 0.5 mEq per kg can be administered to maintain alkalinization, but avoid blood pH values higher than 7.55. Many clinicians use the alkalinization without the diuresis because of the danger of fluid overload. Hemodynamic status, fluids, blood gases and electrolytes, and glucose must be closely monitored during these procedures. See NaHCO$_3$ in Table 12. Saline diuresis, but not forced diuresis, is used in lithium intoxications.

Dialysis

Dialysis is an extrarenal means of removing certain substances from the body and can substitute for the kidney when renal failure occurs. Dialysis is not the first measure instituted; however, it may be lifesaving later in the course of a severe intoxication. It is needed in only a minority of intoxicated patients.

Peritoneal dialysis utilizes the peritoneum as the membrane for dialysis. It is only 1/20 as effective as hemodialysis. It is easier to use and less hazardous to the patient but also less effective in removing the toxin; thus, it is seldom used except for small infants.

TABLE 11. **Common Poisons and Their Recommended Antidotes**

Toxin	Antidote
Acetaminophen (in many analgesics)	*N*-Acetylcysteine
Anticholinergics (antihistamines, plants, GI medications)	Physostigmine (use with caution)
Anticoagulants (in rodenticides)	Vitamin K$_1$
Antimony (ant paste)	Dimercaprol (BAL), penicillamine
Arsenic (ant traps)	Dimercaprol (BAL), penicillamine
Benzodiazepines	Flumazenil (Romazicon)
Beta blockers	Glucagon
Bismuth (GI medication)	Dimercaprol (BAL)
Botulism	Botulism antitoxin
Calcium channel blockers	Atropine
Carbamate insecticide	Calcium gluconate
Carbon monoxide	100% oxygen, hyperbaric oxygen
Chloroquine (Aralen) (antimalarial)	Diazepam (Valium)
Cyanide (fruit stone seeds, nitroprusside for hypertension, plastic fires, metal polishes)	Lilly cyanide kit, contains amyl nitrite, sodium nitrite, sodium thiosulfate Investigative vitamin B$_{12a}$
Digoxin, digitoxin in plants	Fragment antibody (Digibind)
Ethylene glycol (antifreeze)	Ethanol
Fluoride (rodenticides)	Calcium gluconate
Gold (antirheumatoid)	Dimercaprol (BAL)
Gyromitra mushrooms	Pyridoxine
Hydralazine (antihypertensive)	Pyridoxine
Hydrofluoric acid (etching glass)	Local calcium gluconate jelly Soak in magnesium sulfate
Iron (dietary supplements)	Deferoxamine (Desferal)
Isoniazid (antituberculous)	Pyridoxine
Lead (old paints and plaster, dust)	Calcium disodium edetate (EDTA) Dimercaprol (BAL), dimercaptosuccinic acid (DMSA, succimer)
Mercury (fungicides, thermometers)	Dimercaprol (BAL), penicillamine, DMSA
Methanol (antifreeze, dry gas)	Ethanol
Nitrites, dyes (methemoglobinemia)	Methylene blue
Opioids	Naloxone (Narcan)
Organophosphate insecticides	Atropine, pralidoxime
Phencyclidine (abused, "angel dust")	Ammonium chloride *not* recommended
Phenobarbital	Sodium bicarbonate
Phenothiazine (dystonic reaction)	Diphenhydramine (Benadryl)
Phenylurea rodenticide (Vacor)	Nicotinamide
Salicylate	Sodium bicarbonate
Snake bite venom	Antivenom
Spider bite venom, *Latrodectus* (black widow)	Antivenom
Tricyclic and cyclic antidepressants	Sodium bicarbonate
Withdrawal	
Opioids	Methadone, clonidine
Barbiturates	Phenobarbital
Benzodiazepines	Diazepam
Ethanol	Benzodiazepines
Other sedative hypnotics	Phenobarbital or diazepam

Abbreviations: GI = gastrointestinal; BAL = British antilewisite; EDTA = ethylenediaminetetra-acetic acid.

Hemodialysis is the most effective means of dialysis but requires experience with sophisticated equipment. Blood is circulated past a semipermeable membrane by an extracorporeal method. Substances are removed by diffusion down a concentration gradient. Anticoagulation with heparin is necessary.

Hemodialysis is contraindicated when (1) the substance is not dialyzable, (2) effective antidotes are available, (3) hemodynamic instability (e.g., shock) is present, and (4) coagulopathy is present because heparinization is required.

The patient-related criteria for dialysis are (1) anticipated prolonged coma and the likelihood of complications, (2) renal compromise (toxin excreted or metabolized by kidneys and dialyzable chelating agents in heavy metal poisoning), (3) laboratory confirmation of lethal blood concentration, (4) lethal-dose poisoning with an agent with delayed toxicity or known to be metabolized into a more toxic metabolite (e.g., ethylene glycol, methanol), and (5) hepatic impairment when the agent is metabolized by the liver and clinical deterioration occurs despite optimal supportive medical management.

Dialyzable substances diffuse easily across the dialysis membrane and have the following characteristics: (1) a small molecular weight (less than 500 and preferably less than 350); (2) a Vd of less than 1 liter per kg; (3) low PB, less than 50%; (4) high water solubility (low lipid solubility); and (5) high plasma concentration and a toxicity that correlates reasonably with the plasma concentration (Tables 13 and 14).

Hemodialysis also has a role in correcting disturbances that are not amenable to appropriate medical

Text continued on page 1204

TABLE 12. **Initial Doses of Antidotes for Common Poisonings**

Antidote	Use	Dose	Route	Adverse Reactions (AR) and Comments
N-Acetylcysteine (NAC, Mucomyst). Stock level to treat 70-kg adult for 24 h: seven vials, 20%, 30 mL.	Acetaminophen, carbon tetrachloride (experimental).	140 mg/kg loading, followed by 70 mg/kg q 4 h for 17 doses.	PO	Nausea, vomiting. Dilute to 5% with sweet juice or flat cola.
Atropine. Stock level to treat 70-kg adult for 24 h: 1 gm (1 mg/mL in 1 or 10 mL).	Organophosphate and carbamate pesticides.	*Child:* 0.02–0.05 mg/kg repeated q 5–10 min to maximum of 2 mg as necessary until cessation of secretions. *Adult:* 1–2 mg q 5–10 min as necessary. Dilute in 1–2 mL of 0.89% saline for endotracheal instillation. *IV infusion dose:* Place 8 mg of atropine in 100 mL of D5W or saline. Concentration = 0.08 mg/mL. Dose range = 0.02–0.08 mg/kg/h or 0.25–1 mL/kg/h. Severe poisoning may require supplemental doses of IV atropine intermittently in doses of 1–5 mg until drying of secretions occurs.	IV or ET	Tachycardia, dry mouth, blurred vision, and urinary retention. Ensure adequate ventilation before administration.
Calcium chloride (10%). Stock level to treat 70-kg adult for 24 h: 5–10 vials, 1 gm (1.35 mEq/mL).	Hypocalcemia, fluoride, calcium channel blockers.	0.1–0.2 mL/kg (10–20 mg/kg) slow push q 10 min up to maximum of 10 mL (1 gm). Because calcium response lasts 15 min, some patients may require continuous infusion of 0.2 mL/kg/h up to maximum of 10 mL/h during monitoring for dysrhythmias and hypotension.	IV	Administer slowly with BP and ECG monitoring and have magnesium available to reverse calcium effects. **AR:** Tissue irritation, hypotension, dysrhythmias resulting from rapid injection. Contraindications: Digitalis glycoside intoxication.
Calcium gluconate (10%). Stock level to treat 70-kg adult for 24 h: 5–10 vials, 1 gm (0.45 mEq/mL).	Hypocalcemia, fluoride, calcium channel blockers, hydrofluoric acid, black widow envenomation.	0.3–0.4 mL/kg (30–40 mg/kg) slow push; repeat as needed up to maximum dose of 10–20 mL (1–2 gm).	IV	Same comments as calcium chloride.
Calcium gluconate gel. Stock level: 3.5 gm.	Hydrofluoric acid.	2.5 gm of USP powder added to 100 mL of water-soluble lubricating jelly (e.g., K-Y Jelly or Lubifax) (or 3.5 gm into 150 mL). Some use 6 gm of calcium carbonate in 100 gm of lubricant. Place injured hand in surgical glove filled with gel. Apply q 4 h. If pain persists, calcium gluconate injection may be needed (following).	Dermal	Powder is available from Spectrum Pharmaceutical Company in California: 1-800-772-8786. Commercial preparation of calcium gluconate gel is available from Pharmascience in Montreal, Quebec: 514-340-1114.
Infiltration of calcium gluconate.	Hydrofluoric acid.	Dose: Infiltrate each square cm of affected dermis or subcutaneous tissue with about 0.5 mL of 10% calcium gluconate using a 30-gauge needle. Repeat as needed to control pain.	Infiltrate	
Cyanide antidote kit. Stock level to treat 70-kg adult for 24 h: two Lilly Cyanide Antidote kits.	Cyanide; hydrogen sulfide (nitrites are given only; do not use sodium thiosulfate for hydrogen sulfide). Individual portions of the kit can be used in certain circumstances (consult PCC).	Amyl nitrite: 1 crushable ampule for 30 s of every minute. Use new ampule q 3 min. May omit step if venous access is established.	Inhalation	If methemoglobinemia occurs, do not use methylene blue to correct this because it releases cyanide.

Antidote (stock)	Indications	Dose	Route	Comments / Adverse Reactions
Cyanide antidote kit. Stock level to treat 70-kg adult for 24 h: two Lilly Cyanide Antidote kits.	Cyanide; hydrogen sulfide (nitrites are given only; do not use sodium thiosulfate for hydrogen sulfide). Individual portions of the kit can be used in certain circumstances (consult PCC). Do not use sodium thiosulfate for hydrogen sulfide. Individual portions of the kit can be used in certain circumstances (consult PCC).	Sodium nitrite: *Child:* 0.33 mL/kg 3% solution if hemoglobin level is not known, otherwise follow tables with product. *Adult:* up to 300 mg (10 mL). Dilute nitrite in 100 mL of 0.9% saline, administer slowly at 5 mL/min. Slow infusion if fall in BP. Sodium thiosulfate: *Child:* 1.6 mL/kg 25% solution, may be repeated q 30–60 min to a maximum of 12.5 gm or 50 mL in *adult.* Administer over 20 min.	IV	If methemoglobinemia occurs, do not use methylene blue to correct this because it releases cyanide. Nausea, dizziness, headache. Tachycardia, muscle rigidity, and bronchospasm (rapid administration).
Dantrolene, sodium (Dantrium). Stock level to treat 70-kg adult for 24 h: 700 mg in 35 vials (20 mg per vial).	Malignant hyperthermia.	2–3 mg/kg IV rapidly. Repeat loading dose q 10 min, if necessary up to a maximal total dose of 10 mg/kg. When temperature and heart rate decrease, slow the infusion to 1–2 mg/kg q 6 h for 24–48 h until all evidence of malignant hyperthermia syndrome has subsided. Follow with oral doses of 1–2 mg/kg qid for 24 h as necessary.	IV or PO	Available as 20-mg lyophilized dantrolene powder for reconstitution, which contains 3 gm of mannitol and sodium hydroxide in 70-mL vials. Mix with 60 mL of sterile distilled water without a bacteriostatic agent and protect from light. Use within 6 h after reconstituted. **AR:** Hepatotoxicity occurs with cumulative dose of 10 mg/kg; thrombophlebitis (best given in central line).
Deferoxamine (DFO, Desferal). Stock level to treat 70-kg adult for 24 h: 12 vials (50 mg per ampule).	Iron (100 mg of DFO binds 8.5–9.3 mg of iron).	IV infusion of 15 mg/kg/h (3 mL/kg/h in 100 mL D5W), maximum of 6 gm/d. Rates of >45 mg/kg/h if conc > 1000 μg/dL.	Preferred IV; avoid therapy >24 h	Hypotension (minimized by avoiding rapid infusion rates). DFO challenge test (50 mg/kg) is unreliable if negative. **AR:** Confusion, somnolence, coma, hypotension.
Diazepam (Valium). Roche. Stock level to treat 70-kg adult for 24 h: 200 mg.	Any intoxication that provokes seizures when specific therapy is not available, for example, amphetamines, PCP, barbiturate and alcohol withdrawal, chloroquine poisoning.	*Adult:* 5–10 mg (maximum of 20 mg) at a rate of 5 mg/min until seizure is controlled. May be repeated two or three times. *Child:* 0.1–0.3 mg/kg up to 10 mg slowly over 2 min.	IV	Intramuscular absorption is erratic. Establish airway and administer 100% oxygen and glucose.
Digoxin-specific Fab antibodies (Digibind). Stock level to treat 70-kg adult for 24 h: 20 vials.	Digoxin, digitoxin, oleander tea with the following: (1) imminent cardiac arrest or shock, (2) hyperkalemia of >5.0 mEq/L, (3) serum digoxin of >10 ng/mL (adult) or >5 ng/mL (child) at 8–12 h after ingestion in adults, (4) digitalis delirium, (5) ingestion of more than 10 mg in adult or 4 mg in child, (6) bradycardia or second- or third-degree heart block unresponsive to atropine, (7) life-threatening digitoxin or oleander poisoning.	1. *Amount (total mg) ingested known* multiplied by bioavailability (0.8) = body burden. The body burden divided by 0.6 (0.6 mg of digoxin is bound by one vial of 40 mg of Fab) = number of vials needed. 2. *If amount is unknown but the steady-state serum concentration is known in ng/mL.* Digoxin: ng/mL × (5.6 L/kg Vd) × (wt kg) = μg body burden. Body burden divided by 1000 = mg body burden/0.6 = number of vials needed. Digitoxin: ng/mL × (0.56 L/kg Vd) × (wt kg) = body burden. Body burden divided by 1000 = mg body burden/0.6 = number of vials needed. 3. *If the amount is not known,* it is administered in life-threatening situations as 10 vials (400 mg) IV in saline over 30 min in adults. If cardiac arrest is imminent, administer 20 vials (adult) as a bolus.	IV	Administer by infusion over 30 min through a 0.22-μm filter. If cardiac arrest is imminent, may administer by bolus injection. Consult PCC for more details. Allergic reactions (rare), return of condition being treated with digitalis glycoside.

Table continued on following page

TABLE 12. **Initial Doses of Antidotes for Common Poisonings** *Continued*

Antidote	Use	Dose	Route	Adverse Reactions (AR) and Comments
Dimercaprol (BAL in oil). Stock level to treat 70-kg adult for 24 h: 1200 mg (four ampules, 100 mg/mL 10% in oil in 3-mL ampule).	Chelating agent for arsenic, mercury, lead, antimony, bismuth, chromium, copper, gold, nickel, tungsten, and zinc.	3–5 mg/kg q 4 h, usually for 5–10 d.	Deep IM	Local infection site pain and sterile abscess, nausea, vomiting, fever, salivation, hypertension, and nephrotoxicity (alkalinize urine). Fatal dose, 20–40 mg/kg. **AR:** Dry mouth, drowsiness.
Diphenhydramine (Benadryl). Antiparkinsonian action. Stock level to treat 70-kg adult for 24 h: five vials (10 mg/mL, 10 mL each).	Used to treat extrapyramidal symptoms and dystonia induced by phenothiazines, phencyclidine, and related drugs.	*Child:* 1–2 mg/kg IV slowly over 5 min up to maximum of 50 mg, followed by 5 mg/kg per 24 h orally divided q 6 h in children up to 300 mg per 24 h. *Adult:* 50 mg IV followed by 50 mg PO qid for 5–7 d. Note: Symptoms abate within 2–5 min after IV administration.	IV and PO	
Ethanol (ethyl alcohol). Stock level to treat 70-kg adult for 24 h: three bottles 10% (1 L each).	Methanol, ethylene glycol.	10 mL/kg loading dose concurrently with 1.4 mL/kg (average) infusion of 10% ethanol. (Consult PCC for more details.)	IV	Nausea, vomiting, sedation. Use 0.22-μm filter if preparing from bulk 100% ethanol.
Flumazenil (RoMazicon). Stock level to treat 70-kg adult for 24 h: 10 vials (0.1 mg/mL, 10 mL).	Benzodiazepines.	Administer 0.2 mg (2 mL) over 30 s. (Pediatric dose not established, 0.01 mg/kg.) Wait 3 min for a response. If desired consciousness is not achieved administer 0.3 mg (3 mL) over 30 s. Wait 3 min for response. If desired consciousness is not achieved administer 0.5 mg (5 mL) over 30 s at 60-s intervals up to a maximal cumulative dose of 3 mg (30 mL) (1 mg in children). Because effects last only 1–5 h, if there is a response monitor carefully over next 6 h for resedation. If multiple repeated doses, consider a continuous infusion of 0.2–1 mg/h.	IV	It is not recommended to improve ventilation. Its role in CNS depression needs to be clarified. It should not be used routinely in comatose patients. It is *contraindicated* in cyclic antidepressant intoxications, stimulant overdose, long-term benzodiazepine use (may precipitate life-threatening withdrawal), if benzodiazepines are used to control seizures, in head trauma. **AR:** Nausea, vomiting, facial flushing, agitation, headache, dizziness, seizures, and death. Uncommon.
Folic acid (Folvite). Stock level to treat 70-kg adult for 24 h: two 100-mg vials.	Methanol or ethylene glycol (investigational).	1 mg/kg up to 50 mg q 4 h for 6 doses.	IV	
Glucagon. Stock level to treat 70-kg adult for 24 h: 100 mg (10 vials, 10 units).	Beta blockers, calcium channel blockers, hypoglycemic agents.	*Adult:* 5–10 mg, then infuse 1–5 mg/h. *Child:* 0.05–0.1 mg/kg, then infuse 0.07 mg/kg/h. Large doses up to 100 mg per 24 h have been used.	IV	Hyperglycemia, nausea, and vomiting. Dissolve in D5W, not in 0.9% saline. Do not use diluent in package because of possible phenol toxicity.
Magnesium sulfate. Stock level to treat 70-kg adult for 24 h: approximately 25 gm (50 mL of 50% or 200 mL of 12.5%).	Torsades de pointes.	*Adult:* 2 gm (20 mL of 20%) over 20 min. If no response in 10 min, repeat and follow by continuous infusion 1 gm/h. *Child:* 25–50 mg/kg initially, maintenance with 30–60 mg/kg per 24 h (0.25–0.50 mEq/kg per 24 h) up to 1000 mg per 24 h. (Dose not studied in controlled fashion.)	IV	Use with caution if there is renal impairment.
Methylene blue. Stock level to treat 70-kg adult for 24 h: five ampules (10 mg per 10 mL).	Methemoglobinemia.	0.1–0.2 mL/kg of 1% solution, slow infusion, may be repeated q 30–60 min.	IV	Nausea, vomiting, headache, dizziness.

Drug	Indication	Route	Dose	Comments / AR
Nalmefene (Revex). Stock level: not established.	Narcotic antagonist.	IV, IM, SC	The dose for opioid overdose as bolus in adults is 0.5–1 mg q 2 min up to a total of 2 mg IV. May also be given IM or SC. In patients with renal failure, administer over 1 min. In postoperative opioid depression reversal IV 0.1–0.5 µg/kg every 2 min as needed and may repeat up to a total dose of 1 µg/kg.	Role in comatose patients and opioid overdose is not clear. It is 16 times more potent than naloxone and duration of action is up to 8 h (half-life 10.8 h compared with naloxone, 1 h). Clinical trials in more than 1750 patients have not shown significant adverse reactions.
Naloxone (Narcan). Stock level to treat 70-kg adult for 24 h: 3 vials (1 mg/mL, 10 mL).	Comatose patient; ineffective ventilation or adult respiratory rate <12 rpm; opioids.	IV, ET	In suspected overdose administer IV 0.1 mg/kg in a child younger than 5 y up to 2 mg. In older children and adults administer 2 mg q 2 min up to a total of 10–20 mg. Can also be administered into the ET. If no response by 10 mg, a pure opioid intoxication is unlikely. If opioid abuse is suspected, restraints should be in place before administration, initial dose 0.1 mg to avoid withdrawal and violent behavior. The initial dose is then doubled every minute progressively to a total of 10 mg. A continuous infusion has been advocated because many opioids outlast the short half-life.	Larger doses of naloxone may be required for more poorly antagonized synthetic opioid drugs: buprenorphine, codeine, dextromethorphan, fentanyl, pentazocine, propoxyphene, diphenoxylate, nalbuphine, new potent designer drugs, or long-acting opioids such as methadone. **Complications:** Although naloxone is safe and effective, there are rare reports of complications (less than 1%) of pulmonary edema, seizures, hypertension, cardiac arrest, and sudden death. The infusions are titrated to avoid respiratory depression and opioid withdrawal manifestations. Tapering of infusions can be attempted after 12 h and when the patient's condition has been stabilized.
Physostigmine (Anti-lirium). Stock level to treat 70-kg adult for 24 h: 10 ampules (2 mL each).	Anticholinergic agents (not routinely used, indicated only if life-threatening complications).	IV	*Child:* 0.02 mg/kg slow push to maximum of 2 mg q 30–60 min. *Adult:* 1–2 mg q 5 min to maximum of 6 mg.	**AR:** Bradycardia, asystole, seizures, bronchospasm, vomiting, headaches. Do not use for cyclic antidepressants.
Pralidoxime (2-PAM, Protopam). Stock level to treat 70-kg adult for 24 h: 12 vials (1 gm per 20 mL).	Organophosphates.	IV	*Child ≤ 12 y:* 25–50 mg/kg maximal (4 mg/kg/min); *older than 12 y:* 1–2 gm per dose in 250 mL of 0.89% saline over 5–10 min. Maximal 200 mg/min. Repeat q 6–12 h for 24–48 h. Maximal adult dose 12 gm/d. Alternative: Main infusion 1 gm in 100 mL of 0.9% saline at 5–20 mg/kg/h (0.5–12 mL/kg/h) up to maximal 500 mg/h or 50 mL/h. Titrate to desired response. End point is absence of fasciculations and return of muscle strength.	Nausea, dizziness, headache. Tachycardia, muscle rigidity, and bronchospasm (rapid administration).

Table continued on following page

TABLE 12. **Initial Doses of Antidotes for Common Poisonings** *Continued*

Antidote	Use	Dose	Route	Adverse Reactions (AR) and Comments
Pyridoxine (vitamin B₆). Stock level to treat 70-kg adult for 24 h: four ampules (50 mg in 5-mL or 250 mg in 25-mL vial).	Seizures caused by isoniazid or *Gyromitra* mushrooms; ethylene glycol (investigational).	Isoniazid (INH): *Unknown amount ingested*: 5 gm (70 mg/kg) in 50 mL of D5W over 5 min with diazepam 0.3 mg/kg IV at rate of 1 mg/min in child or 10 mg per dose at rate up to 5 mg/min in adults. Use different site (synergism). May repeat q 5–20 min until seizure controlled. Up to 375 mg/kg has been given (52 gm). *Known amount ingested*: 1 gm for each gram of INH ingested over 5 min with diazepam (dose above). *Gyromitra* mushrooms: 25 mg/kg for child or 2–5 gm for adult over 15–30 min to maximum of 20 gm.	IV	After seizure is controlled, administer remainder of pyridoxine at 1 gm per 1 gm of INH or total 5 gm as infusion over 60 min. **AR:** Uncommon; do not administer in same bottle as sodium bicarbonate. For *Gyromitra* mushrooms, some use 25 mg/kg/PO early when mushroom is suspected.
Sodium bicarbonate (NaHCO₃). Stock level to treat 70-kg adult for 24 h: 10 ampules or syringes (500 mEq).	Tricyclic antidepressant (TCA) cardiotoxicity (wide QRS >0.10 s, ventricular tachycardia, severe conduction disturbances); metabolic acidosis; phenothiazine cardiotoxicity.	Ethylene glycol: 100 mg daily. 1–2 mEq/kg undiluted as a bolus. If no effect on cardiotoxicity, repeat twice a few minutes apart. An infusion of NaHCO₃ may follow to keep blood pH at 7.5–7.55 but not higher.	IV	Monitor serum sodium and potassium and blood pH because fatal alkalemia and hypernatremia have been reported. Continuous infusion of bicarbonate by itself is of limited usefulness in setting of TCA intoxication because of delayed onset. Prophylactic NaHCO₃ has not been encouraged.

Sodium bicarbonate (NaHCO₃). Stock level to treat 70-kg adult for 24 h: 10 ampules or syringes (500 mEq).	*Salicylate:* To keep blood pH 7.5–7.55 (not >7.55) and urine pH 7.5–8.0. Alkalinization is recommended if salicylate concentration > 40 mg/dL in acute poisoning and at lower levels if symptomatic in chronic intoxication. 2 mEq/kg raises blood pH 0.1 unit. *Adult* with clear physical signs and laboratory findings of acute moderate or severe salicylism: bolus 1–2 mEq/kg followed by infusion of 100–150 mEq NaHCO₃ added to 1 L of 5% dextrose at rate of 200–300 mL/h. *Child:* Bolus same as adult followed by 1–2 mEq/kg in infusion of 20 mL/kg/h 5% dextrose in 0.45% saline. Add potassium when patient voids. Rate and amount of the initial infusion, if patient is volume depleted: 1 h to achieve urine output of 2 mL/kg/h and urine pH of 7–8. In mild cases without acidosis and with urine pH of >6, administer 5% dextrose in 0.9% saline with 50 mEq/L or 1 mEq/kg NaHCO₃ as maintenance to replace ongoing renal losses. If acidemia and pH < 7.2, add 2 mEq/kg as loading dose followed by 2 mEq/kg q 3–4 h to keep pH at 7.5–7.55. If acidemia, recommend isotonic NaHCO₃, three ampules to 1 L of D5W at 10–15 mL/kg/h or sufficient to produce normal urine flow and a urine pH of 7.5 or higher.	IV	Monitor both urine pH and blood pH. Do not use urine pH alone to assess the need for alkalinization because of the paradoxical aciduria that may occur. Adjust the urine pH to 7.5–8 by (NaHCO₃) infusion. After urine output established add potassium, 40 mEq/L.
Sodium bicarbonate (NaHCO₃). Stock level to treat 70-kg adult for 24 h: 10 ampules or syringes (500 mEq).	*Long-acting barbiturates:* phenobarbital, mephobarbital (Mebaral), metharbital (Gemonil), primidone (Mysoline). Note: Alkalinization is not effective for the shorter and intermediate barbiturates.	IV	2 mEq/kg during the first hour or 100 mEq in 1 L of D5W with 40 mEq/L potassium at rate of 100 mL/h in adults. Adequate potassium is necessary to accomplish alkalinization. Additional NaHCO₃ and potassium chloride may be needed. Adjust the urine pH to 7.5–8 by (NaHCO₃) infusion.

Abbreviations: ET = endotracheal tube; BP = blood pressure; USP = U.S. Pharmacopeia; PCC = poison control center; PCP = phencyclidine; rpm = respirations per minute.

TABLE 13. Considerations for Hemodialysis or Hemoperfusion

Serious Ingestions

Immediately notify the nephrologist. Compounds that are ingested in potentially lethal doses in which rapid removal may improve the prognosis include

Amatoxins from *Amanita phalloides* mushroom: any amount with symptoms

Arsenic trioxide: 120 mg in adults

Ethylene glycol: 1.4 mL/kg 100% solution or equivalent

Methanol: 6 mL/kg 100% solution or equivalent

Paraquat: 1.5 gm in adults

Diquat: 1.5 gm in adults

Mercuric chloride: 1.0 gm in adults

Dialyzable Substances

Alcohol*	Isoniazid
Ammonia	Lithium*
Amphetamines	Meprobamate
Anilines	Paraldehyde
Antibiotics	Potassium*
Barbiturates (long-acting)*	Procainamide
Boric acid	Quinidine
Bromides*	Quinine*
Calcium	Salicylates*
Chloral hydrate*	Strychnine
Fluorides	Thiocyanates
Iodides	

Nondialyzable Substances

Anticholinergics	Glutethimide
Antidepressants (cyclic and monoamine oxidase inhibitors)	Hallucinogens
	Methyprylon (Noludar)†
Barbiturates (short-acting)	Methaqualone†
Benzodiazepines	Opioids including heroin
Digitalis and related drugs	Phenothiazine
Ethchlorvynol	Phenytoin

*Most useful.
†Controversial.

management. These are easily remembered by the "vowel" mnemonic:

A = refractory acid-base disturbances.

E = refractory electrolyte disturbances.

I = intoxication with dialyzable substances (e.g., ethanol,* ethylene glycol,* isopropyl alcohol,* methanol,* lithium,* salicylates,* and theophylline). Dialysis is rarely indicated with aminoglycosides, carbamazepine, phenobarbital, and phenytoin.

O = overhydration.

U = uremia (renal failure).

Complications of dialysis include hemorrhage, thrombosis, air embolism, hypotension, infections, electrolyte imbalance, thrombocytopenia, and removal of therapeutic medications.

Hemoperfusion

Hemoperfusion is the parenteral form of oral AC. Heparinization is necessary. The patient's blood is routed extracorporeally through an outflow arterial catheter and then through a filter adsorbing cartridge (charcoal or resin) and returned through a venous catheter. High flow rates (e.g., 300 mL per

*Toxins for which hemodialysis is preferred to hemoperfusion.

minute) through the filter are used to maximize the efficient use of the filter. Cartridges must be changed every 4 hours. Blood glucose, electrolytes, calcium, albumin, complete blood count (CBC), platelets, and serum and urine osmolarity must be carefully monitored. This procedure has extended extracorporeal removal to a large range of substances that were formerly either poorly dialyzable or nondialyzable. It is not limited by molecular weight, water solubility, or protein binding. However, hemoperfusion is limited by a Vd greater than 400 liters, plasma concentration, and rate of flow through the filter. AC cartridges are primarily used for hemoperfusion in the United States. Analysis of studies using hemodialysis and hemoperfusion indicates that they do not reduce morbidity or mortality substantially except in certain cases (e.g., with theophylline). Hemoperfusion may be recommended in combination with hemodialysis (e.g., for paraquat, electrolyte disturbances).

The contraindications are similar to those for hemodialysis.

The patient-related criteria for hemoperfusion are (1) anticipated prolonged coma and the likelihood of complications, (2) laboratory confirmation of lethal blood concentrations, (3) lethal-dose poisoning with an agent with delayed toxicity or known to be metabolized into a more toxic metabolite, and (4) hepatic impairment when an agent is metabolized by the liver and there is clinical deterioration despite optimal supportive medical management.

Limited data are available to determine which toxins are best treated with hemoperfusion. However, hemoperfusion has proved useful in glutethimide intoxication, barbiturate overdose even with SA barbiturates (SABs), carbamazepine, phenytoin, theophylline intoxication, and chlorophenothane (DDT). See Tables 13 and 14.

Complications include hemorrhage, thrombocytopenia, hypotension, infection, leukopenia, depressed phagocytic activity of granulocytes, decreased immunoglobulin levels, hypoglycemia, hypothermia, hypocalcemia, pulmonary edema, and air and charcoal embolism.

Plasmapheresis

Plasmapheresis consists of removal of a volume of blood. All the extracted components are returned to the blood except the plasma, which is replaced with a colloidal protein solution. Clinical data related to guidelines and efficacy in toxicology are limited. Centrifugal and membrane separators of cellular elements are used. Plasmapheresis can be as effective as hemodialysis or hemoperfusion for toxins with high protein binding and may be useful for toxins not filtered by hemodialysis and hemoperfusion. It has been used in certain diseases such as myeloma, idiopathic thrombocytopenia, systemic lupus erythematosus, rheumatoid arthritis, and myasthenia gravis.

Use of plasmapheresis has been reported anecdotally in the following intoxications: propranolol (re-

TABLE 14. **Plasma Concentrations Above Which Removal by Extracorporeal Measures Can Be Indicated***

Drug	Plasma Concentration	Protein Binding (%)	Vd (L/kg)	Method of Choice†
Amanitin	Not available	25	1.0	HP
Ethanol	500–700 mg/dL	0	0.3	HD
Ethchlorvynol	150 µg/mL	35–50	3–4	HP
Ethylene glycol	25–50 µg/mL	0	0.6	HD
Glutethimide	100 µg/mL	50	2.7	HP
Isopropyl alcohol	400 mg/dL	0	0.7	HD
Lithium	4 mEq/L	0	0.7	HD
Meprobamate	100 µg/mL	0	NA	HP
Methanol	50 mg/dL	0	0.7	HD
Methaqualone	40 µg/dL	20–60	6.0	HP
Other barbiturates	50 µg/dL	50	0–1	HP
Paraquat	0.1 mg/dL	Poor	2.8	HP > HD
Phenobarbital	100 µg/dL	50	0.9	HP > HD
Salicylates	80–100 mg/dL	90	0.2	HD > HP
Theophylline		0	0.5	
Chronic	40–60 µg/mL			HP
Acute	80–100 µg/mL			HP
Trichloroethanol	250 µg/mL	70	0.6	HP

*In mixed or chronic drug overdoses, extracorporeal measures may be considered at lower drug concentrations.
†HP = hemoperfusion; HD = hemodialysis; HP > HD = hemoperfusion preferred over hemodialysis.
Modified from Winchester JF: Active methods for detoxification. *In* Haddad LM, Winchester JF (eds): Clinical Management of Poisoning and Drug Overdose, 2nd ed. Philadelphia, WB Saunders Co, 1990, pp 148–167; Balsam L, Cortitsidis GN, Fienfeld DA: Role of hemodialysis and hemoperfusion in the treatment of intoxications. Contemp Manage Crit Care 61–71, 1990.

moved 30%); levothyroxine (removed 30%); salicylate (removed 10%); and digoxin, phenobarbital, prednisolone, and tobramycin (removed less than 10%). Complications include infection, allergic reactions including anaphylaxis, hemorrhagic disorders, thrombocytopenia, embolus and thrombus, hyper- and hypovolemia, dysrhythmias, syncope, tetany, paresthesia, pneumothorax, adult respiratory distress syndrome, and seizures.

Supportive Care, Observation, and Therapy of Complications

The Comatose Patient or Patient with Altered Mental Status

If airway protective reflexes are absent, endotracheal intubation is indicated. If respirations are ineffective, ventilate with 100% oxygen. If a cyanotic patient fails to respond to oxygen, consider methemoglobinemia. Perform a reagent strip test for blood glucose to detect hypoglycemia and send the specimen to the laboratory for confirmation.

Glucose. Administer glucose if the glucose reagent strip visually reads less than 150 mg per dL. Venous rather than capillary blood should be used for the reagent strip if the patient is in shock or is hypotensive.

Hypoglycemia accompanies many poisonings, including those with ethanol (especially in children), clonidine (Catapres), insulin, organophosphates, salicylates, sulfonylureas, and the fruit or seed of a Jamaican plant called akee. If hypoglycemia is present or suspected, administer glucose immediately as an intravenous (IV) bolus in the following doses: neonate, 10% glucose (5 mL per kg); child, 25% glucose

at 0.25 gram per kg (2 mL per kg); and adults, 50% glucose at 0.5 gram per kg (1 mL per kg).

Large amounts of glucose given rapidly to nondiabetic patients may cause transient reactive hypoglycemia and hyperkalemia and may accentuate damage in ischemic cerebrovascular and cardiac tissue. If focal neurologic signs are present, it may be prudent to withhold glucose, because hypoglycemia rarely causes focal signs (<10%).

Thiamine. This agent is administered to avoid precipitating the thiamine deficiency encephalopathy (Wernicke-Korsakoff syndrome) in alcohol abusers and in malnourished patients. The overall incidence of thiamine deficiency in ethanol abusers is 12%. Thiamine at 100 mg IV should be administered around the time of the glucose administration but not necessarily before the glucose, because it is more important to correct the hypoglycemia. The clinician should be prepared to manage anaphylaxis associated with thiamine, but it is extremely rare.

Naloxone. This reverses CNS and respiratory depression, miosis, bradycardia, and decreased GI peristalsis caused by opioids acting through mu, kappa, and delta receptors. It also affects endogenous opioid peptides (endorphins and enkephalins), which accounts for the variable responses reported in intoxications with ethanol, BZPs, clonidine, captopril (Capoten), and valproic acid and in spinal cord injuries. There is a high sensitivity for predicting a response if pinpoint pupils and circumstantial evidence of opioid abuse (e.g., track marks) are present.

In suspected overdose in a child younger than 5 years, administer IV naloxone 0.1 mg per kg up to 2 mg; in older children and adults administer 2 mg every 2 minutes for 5 doses up to a total of 10 mg. Naloxone can also be administered into an endotracheal tube. If there is no response by 10 mg, pure opioid intoxication is unlikely. If opioid abuse is suspected, restraints should be in place before the administration of naloxone, and it is recommended that the initial dose be 0.1 to 0.2 mg to avoid withdrawal and violent behavior. The initial dose is then doubled every minute progressively to a total of 10 mg. Naloxone may unmask concomitant sympathomimetic intoxication as well as withdrawal.

Larger doses of naloxone may be required for more poorly antagonized synthetic opioid drugs: buprenorphine (Buprenex), codeine, dextromethorphan, fentanyl, pentazocine (Talwin), propoxyphene (Darvon), diphenoxylate, nalbuphine (Nubain), new potent "designer" drugs, or long-acting opioids such as methadone.

Indications for a continuous infusion include a second dose for recurrent respiratory depression, exposure to poorly antagonized opioids, a large overdose, and decreased opioid metabolism (e.g., impaired liver function). A continuous infusion has been advocated because many opioids outlast the short half-life ($t_{1/2}$) of naloxone (30 to 60 minutes). The naloxone infusion hourly rate is equal to the effective dose required to produce a response (improvement in ventilation and arousal). An additional dose may be required in 15 to 30 mintues as a bolus. The infusions are titrated to avoid respiratory depression and manifestations of opioid withdrawal. Tapering of infusions can be attempted after 12 hours and when the patient's condition has been stabilized.

Complications: Although naloxone is safe and effective, there are rare (less than 1%) reports of complications of pulmonary edema, seizures, hypertension, cardiac arrest, and sudden death.

Role Not Clarified

NALMEFENE (Revex). This long-acting parenteral opioid antagonist, approved by the FDA, is undergoing investigation but its role for comatose patients and in opioid overdose is not clear. It is 16 times more potent than naloxone and its duration of action is up to 8 hours ($t_{1/2}$ of 10.8 hours, compared with 1 hour for naloxone).

FLUMAZENIL (Romazicon). This agent is a pure competitive BZP antagonist. It has been demonstrated to be safe and effective for BZP-induced sedation. It is not recommended to improve ventilation. Its role in CNS depression needs to be clarified. It should not be used routinely for comatose patients and is not an essential ingredient of the coma therapeutic regimen. It is contraindicated in cyclic antidepressant intoxications, in stimulant overdose, in long-term BZP use (may precipitate life-threatening withdrawal), if BZPs are used to control seizures, and in head trauma. There have been reports of seizures, dysrhythmias, and death.

Convulsions

Convulsions may be the direct effect of the toxin or secondary to hypoxia or other metabolic or electrolyte disturbances.

Specific therapy should be administered, for example, 100% oxygen for CO, calcium for ethylene glycol–produced hypocalcemia, IV glucose for intoxications that induce hypoglycemia, and pyridoxine and diazepam for isoniazid seizures and *Gyromitra* mushroom toxicity. Seizures in patients receiving lithium, salicylates, and theophylline may indicate toxic concentrations in the brain that require hemodialysis or hemoperfusion.

As anticonvulsants, diazepam and lorazepam are the agents of choice, but recurrent or persistent seizures require phenobarbital and possibly neuromuscular blockers (as adjuncts), pentobarbital coma, or general anesthesia. Rapid IV injection of propylene glycol, the vehicle in BZP and phenytoin IV preparations, may cause dysrhythmias, hypotension, apnea, and shock. Therefore, inject slowly (Table 15), administer with cardiac and blood pressure monitoring, and be prepared with ventilatory support to treat apnea. The patient should be monitored throughout the infusion and until 60 minutes after its completion. The propylene glycol vehicle may add to the toxicity in ethylene glycol intoxications. PEG, the vehicle for lorazepam, can be nephrotoxic when used long term. See Table 15 for anticonvulsant doses in children. Table 16 gives the treatment of status epilepticus.

BZPs enhance the activity of γ-aminobutyric acid (GABA), the major inhibitory neurotransmitter. Respiratory depression and hypotension occur in about 10% of patients.

Diazepam enters the brain rapidly and acts within seconds, but its duration of action is only 20 to 30 minutes. Administer BZPs directly or as close to the IV puncture site as possible to avoid adherence to tubing. They should be administered slowly. See Tables 15 and 16.

Lorazepam (Ativan) is a BZP but has a slower onset of action (2 to 3 minutes compared with seconds) and a longer duration of action (2 to 12 hours compared with 20 to 30 minutes) than diazepam. See Tables 15 and 16.

Midazolam (Versed) depresses all levels of the CNS through increased action of GABA. The $t_{1/2}$ is 2 to 4 hours and the duration of sedation is 30 minutes to 2 hours, although its effects may last for 10 hours or more after infusion. The dosage is 0.05 to 0.1 mg per kg IV, with a maximum of 2.5 mg per dose over 2 minutes. Respiratory arrest may occur if it is given rapidly or in excessive doses. Although not approved by the FDA, it has been used safely and effectively in status epilepticus refractory to standard anticonvulsants.

Phenytoin stabilizes neuronal membranes and reduces sodium influx and calcium passage through the membranes. Phenytoin is effective as a single agent in termination of 56 to 80% of seizures, but with toxic and metabolic disturbances this rate falls to 40%. Phenytoin does not enhance the activity of GABA and therefore is not effective against cocaine, isoniazid, *Gyromitra* mushroom, and theophylline intoxications that interfere with GABA. Dilute in

TABLE 15. **Common Anticonvulsant Therapy**

Agent	Dose	Maximal Rate	Duration of Action
Children			
Diazepam IV	Initial 0.3 mg/kg Repeat 10–15 min Maximum 5 mg <5 y Maximum 10 mg >5 y	1 mg/min	20–30 min
Phenytoin IV	15–20 mg/kg Maximum 30 mg/kg or 25 mg/min	1 mg/kg/min	6 h
Phenobarbital IV	10–20 mg/kg Maximum 40 mg/kg or 30 mg/min	1 mg/kg/min	6–8 h
Lorazepam IV	Initial 0.05–0.1 mg/kg Repeat 0.05 mg/kg	1 mg/min	2–12 h
Adults			
Diazepam IV	Initial 5–10 mg Repeat 10–15 min Maximum 30 mg	5 mg/min	20–30 min
Phenytoin	Initial 20 mg/kg Maximum 30 mg/kg	50 mg/min*	6 h
Phenobarbital	Initial 20 mg/kg Maximum 1200 mg	100 mg/min	6–8 h
Lorazepam	Initial 2–10 mg Repeat 10–15 min Maximum 10 mg	2 mg/min	2–12 h

*For adults with cardiopulmonary disease, administer less than 25 mg/min.

0.89% saline (not glucose, which causes crystallization) to a concentration of 10 mg per mL. A 0.22-μm filter should be placed on the IV line. Phenytoin acts within 20 minutes. Determine a phenytoin level 30 to 60 minutes after administration.

Phenobarbital interferes with the transmission of impulses from the thalamus to the cortex by enhancing the effect of GABA. A loading dose 20 mg per kg gives a serum level of 20 μg per mL. The disadvantage of phenobarbital is its slow absorption by the brain parenchyma; 10 to 20 minutes is required for its anticonvulsive effects. It also has a long $t_{1/2}$ of

TABLE 16. **Management of Status Epilepticus**

Time	Procedure
0–5 min, immediate measures	1. Assess cardiorespiratory function; implement appropriate life support. 2. Take history, and perform neurologic and physical examination. 3. Continuously monitor vital signs; notify personnel for potential endotracheal intubation. 4. Obtain blood specimens for anticonvulsant drug levels, glucose, BUN, creatinine, calcium, magnesium, electrolytes, complete blood count, metabolic screen, drug screen, arterial blood gases. Obtain EEG if possible.
6–9 min, initial treatment	5. Start IV infusion. If hypoglycemia confirmed or blood glucose determination unavailable, administer to adult 50 mL of 50% (25 gm) glucose, 100 mg of thiamine, 1–2 gm of magnesium to alcoholic or malnourished patients (child: 2 mL/kg 25% glucose).
10–45 min	6. For adult, infuse diazepam, 0.15–0.25 mg/kg, up to 30 mg total not faster than 5 mg/min (child: 0.1–1.0 mg/kg up to 5 mg) or infuse lorazepam, 0.1 mg/kg, up to 10 mg total not faster than 2 mg/min (child: 0.05–0.5 mg/kg, range 1–4 mg). 7. For adult, begin infusion of phenytoin, 18–20 mg/kg, not faster than 50 mg/min (child: 18–20 mg/kg not faster than 1 mg/kg/min or 25 mg/min). This may take 20–40 min total; carefully monitor ECG, respiration, and blood pressure. If patients are receiving phenytoin, give 9 mg/kg. 8. If seizures persist, give additional phenytoin, 5 mg/kg, not faster than 50 mg/min (child: 1 mg/kg/min) and, if needed, another 5 mg/kg until a maximum of 30 mg/kg has been given.
46–60 min, refractory	9. If seizures persist, intubate and ventilate; for adult, administer phenobarbital, 20 mg/kg, not faster than 100 mg/min IV (child: 20 mg/kg not faster than 1 mg/kg/min).
>1 h	10. If seizures persist, administer pentobarbital anesthesia, 5 mg/kg at 25 mg/min, followed by 0.5–3 kg/h; or general anesthesia with isoflurane should be implemented (anesthesiology assistance required); or propofol (Diprivan) anesthesia (anesthiology assistance required); or midazolam, for adult 5–10 mg bolus not faster than 4 mg/min followed by 0.05–0.4 mg/kg/h. Neuromuscular blockers, if needed; they are adjuncts, not anticonvulsants.

Abbreviations: BUN = blood urea nitrogen; EEG = electroencephalogram; ECG = electrocardiogram.
Data from Watson C: Status epilepticus. Clinical features, pathophysiology, and treatment. West J Med *156*:558–559, 1991; Jagonda A, Riggio S: Refractory status epilepticus in adults. Ann Emerg Med *22*:1337–1348, 1993; and Cascarino GB: Generalized convulsive status epilepticus. Mayo Clin Proc *71*:787–792, 1996.

50 to 100 hours and alters the mental status for prolonged periods. It is the drug of choice for barbiturate withdrawal. Determine the serum phenobarbital concentration 30 to 60 minutes after administration.

Neuromuscular blockers or general anesthesia: If anticonvulsants fail to control seizures within 1 hour after their onset, the patient may require neuromuscular blockade and assisted ventilation. Refractory convulsions may be managed by general anesthesia with halothane. These agents are not anticonvulsants and require electroencephalographic (EEG) monitoring for nonmotor brain seizure activity.

Pentobarbital anesthesia requires intubation, ventilatory support, hemodynamic monitoring, preferably with a Swan-Ganz catheter, and continuous EEG monitoring. The loading dose is 5 mg per kg at an infusion rate of 25 mg per kg per minute, followed by maintenance at 2.5 mg per kg per hour to achieve an EEG that shows a suppression-burst pattern. Recurrent seizures are treated with a 50-mg bolus followed by an increase in the maintenance infusion to 0.5 mg per kg per hour. Tapering is recommended after 12 to 24 hours of EEG control at a rate of 0.5 to 1 mg per kg per hour every 4 to 6 hours.

Status epilepticus refers to a seizure episode that lasts for more than 30 minutes or a series of seizures when the victim does not regain consciousness between seizures. After 90 minutes of seizure activity, CNS neuron damage occurs, electrolyte abnormalities develop, lactic acidosis develops within 30 minutes (it normalizes within 1 hour after the seizures cease), and convulsions become more difficult to control.

Substances that cause refractory seizures include alcohol, amphetamines, amoxapine (Asendin), cocaine, isoniazid, lead (chronic lead encephalopathy), and theophylline.

Complications of prolonged seizures include hypoxia, hypoglycemia, hyperthermia, hypotension, dysrhythmias, rhabdomyolysis and myoglobinemia, pulmonary and cerebral edema, and disseminated intravascular coagulation. In addition, leukemoid reactions and cerebrospinal fluid (CSF) pleocytosis develop.

The treatment of status epilepticus is outlined in Table 16.

Pulmonary Edema

Pulmonary edema complicating poisoning may be cardiac or noncardiac. See Table 6 for causes of pulmonary edema.

In cardiogenic etiologies, left atrial pressure and pulmonary capillary hydrostatic pressure are increased. This is accompanied by congestive heart failure. Fluid overload during forced diuresis may be a factor, particularly if the intoxicants have an antidiuretic effect (e.g., opioids, barbiturates, and salicylates). Some toxic agents produce increased pulmonary capillary permeability, and other agents may cause a massive sympathetic discharge resulting in neurogenic pulmonary edema (e.g., opioids and sali-

cylates). The management consists of fluid administration monitored by a Swan-Ganz catheter, administration of diuretics, use of vasopressors with afterload reduction, and use of inotropic agents and oxygen. If renal failure is present, hemodialysis may be necessary.

The noncardiac type of pulmonary edema occurs with inhaled toxins, such as ammonia, chlorine, and oxides of nitrogen, or with drugs, such as salicylates, opioids, paraquat, and IV ethchlorvynol (Placidyl). This type does not respond to cardiac support measures and requires oxygen with intensive respiratory management, using mechanical ventilation with positive end-expiratory pressure (PEEP) if necessary.

Hypotension and Circulatory Shock

Hypotension and circulatory shock may be caused by heart failure resulting from myocardial depression, hypovolemia (fluid loss or venous pooling), decrease in peripheral vasculature resistance (adrenergic blockage), or loss of vasomotor tone caused by CNS depression. See Table 6 for causes of hypotension.

Management consists of correction of hypoxia, volume expansion, correction of acidosis, rewarming in hypothermia, correction of electrolyte disturbances, and treatment of dysrhythmias producing hypotension and vasopressors, if necessary.

Vasopressors may be considered earlier if there is danger of fluid overload. Dopamine infused at 2 to 20 µg per kg per minute is the vasopressor usually chosen. However, for agents producing alpha-receptor blockage that are antidopaminogenic (e.g., PTZs and tricyclic antidepressants), norepinephrine, an alpha agonist, is preferable and is infused at 4 to 8 µg per minute in adults (0.1 to 1.0 µg per kg per minute in children) titrated every 5 to 10 minutes to the desired effect. Epinephrine infusion at 1 µg per kg per minute titrated to the desired response may also be used. Vasopressors may be used in combination. Norepinephrine and epinephrine are the choice in severe hypotension.

Treat the cardiac dysrhythmias that contribute to hypotension and poor perfusion (usually with rates lower than 40 per minute or above 180 per minute in adults). Treat a wide QRS interval immediately with an NaHCO$_3$ bolus. Table 17 shows specific agents for cardiotoxic intoxications.

Hypothermic hypotension does not respond to fluids but does respond to warming. In hypothermia with a body temperature of 32°C (90°F), a systolic blood pressure of 70 to 90 mm Hg would be expected.

Cerebral Edema

Cerebral edema or increased intracranial pressure in intoxicated patients is produced by hypoxia, hypercapnia, hypotension, hypoglycemia, and drug-impaired capillary integrity. Computed tomography (CT) may aid in diagnosis. Cerebral edema is managed by attempting to control cerebral blood volume to maintain mean arterial pressure (MAP) between 60 and 90 mm Hg and cerebral perfusion pressure

TABLE 17. **Specific Therapy for Cardiotoxic Ingestions**

Toxic Ingestion	Specific Therapy	Vasopressor
Beta-adrenergic antagonist	Glucagon	Epinephrine
	Amrinone (Inocor) Isoproterenol	Dobutamine
Calcium channel blocker	Calcium	Dopamine
	Glucagon	Dobutamine
	Sodium bicarbonate Amrinone	Isoproterenol
Alpha-adrenergic antagonist	Norepinephrine or phenothiazine	Phenylephrine
Cyclic antidepressants	Sodium bicarbonate	Norepinephrine Phenylephrine
Cholinergic agents	Atropine	Dopamine
Opioids	Naloxone	Dopamine
Magnesium	Calcium	Dopamine

between 50 and 70 mm Hg. The cerebral perfusion pressure is calculated as the difference between the MAP and the intracranial pressure. Inappropriate secretion of antidiuretic hormone may play a role in some poisonings, including those involving acetylsalicylic acid, barbiturates, carbamazepine (Tegretol), chlorpropamide (Diabinese), indomethacin (Indocin), opioids (especially morphine), sympathomimetics, tolbutamide (Orinase), and tricyclic antidepressants.

Management consists of correction of the ABGs, metabolic abnormalities, and blood pressure. Monitor intake and output, urine specific gravity, patient's daily weight, serum electrolytes, blood urea nitrogen (BUN), creatinine, hemoglobin, and hematocrit and obtain a chest radiograph. Perform head CT. Assessment by a neurosurgeon is advised; intracranial pressure monitors are helpful but have complications.

If the sodium value is low enough to produce major CNS symptoms, the serum sodium level should be raised 5 to 10 mEq per liter to correct symptoms. Administer furosemide (Lasix) at 0.25 to 0.5 mg per kg and concentrated sodium chloride (6 mEq per kg raises the serum sodium value by 10 mEq per liter).

The increased intracranial pressure may be reduced by giving 20% mannitol, 0.5 to 1.0 gram per kg (100 grams in 500 mL of D5W, infused over a 30-minute period, acts in minutes and peaks in 90 minutes).

Hyperventilation to a carbon dioxide tension (P_{CO_2}) of 25 mm Hg (not below 25) reduces intracranial pressure within 2 to 30 minutes. Hypocapnia produces pH-mediated cerebrovascular vasoconstriction that decreases the cerebral blood flow 5% for each millimeter fall in P_{CO_2}. However, respiratory support with PEEP raises the intracranial pressure.

The head should be elevated 30 degrees if the vital signs are stable.

Fluid administration to correct dehydration and for daily maintenance should be minimized.

Most current studies have demonstrated no improvement in functional outcome in head injury with high-dose corticosteroids, but they reduce edema around a tumor or abscess.

Pentobarbital, loading dose 5 to 30 mg per kg IV, is given to stabilize the membranes, to decrease neuronal metabolism, and to suppress bursts as seen on the EEG.

Hypertension

Hypertension in a young person is more significant than that in a chronically hypertensive individual. Hypertension associated with poisonings is initially transient and does not require therapy. However, an emergency hypertensive crisis, although rare, can develop during alcohol withdrawal, cocaine and other sympathomimetic drug overdose, opioid withdrawal, MAOI drug and food interaction and overdose, and sudden discontinuation of antihypertensive therapy.

Acute emergency hypertensive crisis is defined as a diastolic blood pressure greater than 120 to 130 mm Hg or, more important, is associated with target organ damage. Manifestations of target organ damage are classified as cardiac (pulmonary edema, myocardial ischemia or infarction), CNS (mental status changes, coma, convulsions or cerebrovascular accident), renal (hematuria, azotemia), and retinopathy (papilledema, hemorrhages).

Acute emergency hypertensive crisis is managed with nitroprusside, 10 µg per kg per minute for no longer than 10 minutes and then 0.3 to 2 µg per kg per minute (maximal dose 2 µg per kg per minute). Therapy at higher rates or for more than 48 to 72 hours or renal insufficiency may cause accumulation of thiocyanate, a toxic metabolite, and the thiocyanate level should be determined at 48 hours of therapy. Thiocyanate poisoning (paresthesia, tinnitus, blurred vision, and delirium) is treated with 25% sodium thiosulfate, 1.65 mL per kg, without sodium nitrite and without waiting for laboratory confirmation. Diazoxide or longer acting antihypertensives are usually not recommended because they have a prolonged duration of action. See Table 18.

If focal neurologic signs are present, do not treat mild or moderate hypertension and perform CT.

Dysrhythmias

Cardiac dysrhythmias can occur with poisoning. A wide QT interval occurs with PTZs, and a wide QRS

TABLE 18. **Antihypertensive Drugs for Emergency Use**

Drug	Adult Dose	Pediatric Dose
Nitroprusside	0.3–2 mg/kg/min; 10 µg/kg/min can be given for 10 min initially.	Same.
Phentolamine	2.5–5 mg IV slowly.	0.02–0.1 mg/kg IV slowly.
Labetalol	20 mg IV q 10 min.	0.5 mg/kg IV followed by 0.25 mg/kg q 2 h.
Diazoxide	1–3 mg/kg IV, maximum of 150 mg IV q 5–15 min until desired effect; repeat q 4–24 h.	Same.

complex occurs with tricyclic antidepressants, quinine, or quinidine overdose. Digitalis, cocaine, cyanide, propranolol, theophylline, and amphetamines are among the more frequent toxic causes of dysrhythmias. Normalization of metabolic disturbances and adequate oxygenation correct many of the dysrhythmias; antidysrhythmic drugs or a cardiac pacemaker or cardioversion may be required in other cases.

Life-threatening hemodynamically unstable ventricular dysrhythmias should receive DC conversion. Synchronized DC conversion should be used with caution in digitalis intoxication because of the tendency to produce ventricular fibrillation. This is an indication for Fab. If DC conversion is used in digitalis intoxications, start with the lowest electrical dose.

For less urgent ventricular tachycardia, IV lidocaine at 1 to 3 mg per kg with ECG and blood pressure monitoring may be used.

Tricyclic antidepressant overdose with evidence of cardiac toxicity such as wide QRS tachycardia should be treated with a bolus of $NaHCO_3$ at 2 mEq per kg IV.

Primary therapy for torsades de pointes consists of magnesium sulfate, 2 grams slowly IV as a 20% solution over 1 minute, followed by an infusion of 1 gram per hour. In children the dose is 25 to 50 mg per kg. Overdrive pacing may also be used. If hemodynamic compromise is present, use DC conversion. Avoid class I and class III antidysrhythmic agents. See Table 6 for etiologies and Table 12 for dosages.

Unstable bradycardia and second- and third-degree heart blocks should be managed in an emergency with a transvenous or external pacemaker. For less urgent but unstable patients with bradycardia (syncope, hypotension) treat with atropine at 0.01 to 0.03 mg/kg IV (minimum, 0.1 mg) or isoproterenol at 1 to 10 μg per minute IV. Hypothermia with a body temperature of 32 to 35°C (90 to 95°F) is associated with bradycardia with a heart rate of 40 to 50 beats per minute, which becomes normal on rewarming.

Unexplained cardiac arrest in a young person warrants examination for drugs hidden in the bowel, vagina, or rectum (in body packers or body stuffers).

Specific antidotal therapy and vasopressors for cardiac toxicity are listed in Table 17.

Renal Failure

Renal failure may be due to tubular necrosis as a result of hypotension, hypoxia, or a direct effect of the poison (e.g., salicylate, paraquat, acetaminophen, carbon tetrachloride) or heavy metals on the tubular cells. With hemoglobinuria or myoglobinuria, hemoglobin or myoglobin may precipitate in the renal tubules and produce renal failure.

The mechanisms of renal damage by toxin include

Acute tubular necrosis, which is due to prolonged ischemia, nephrotoxic agents, heavy metals, aminoglycosides (act on proximal tubules), and radiographic contrast media (patients older than 65 years, those with diabetes mellitus)

Drug-induced acute interstitial nephritis (e.g., penicillins, sulfonamides, nonsteroidal anti-inflammatory drugs [NSAIDs])

Inter-renal deposition of pigment (myoglobinuria often associated with rhabdomyolysis, hemoglobinuria)

Any significant hypotension or ischemia caused by a toxin

Rhabdomyolysis

Rhabdomyolysis (muscle necrosis) occurs with prolonged immobilization on a hard surface, violent muscle activity, prolonged convulsions, myositis, and some metabolic myopathies. Destruction of the muscle membrane causes lysis or leakage of the muscle cytoplasmic constituents including myoglobin. Rhabdomyolysis has more than 150 causes but occurs most frequently with intoxications by amphetamines, ethanol, heroin, cocaine, and phencyclidine.

Myoglobinemia and myoglobinuria may occur with or without rhabdomyolysis. The creatine kinase level is often higher than 10,000 units. Rhabdomyolysis may result in myoglobinemia, in which myoglobin can precipitate in the renal tubules and cause renal failure, compartment syndrome, disseminated intravascular coagulation, and metabolic abnormalities.

Management of myoglobinuria consists of fluid diuresis to produce a urine output of 3 to 5 mL per kg per hour or 200 to 350 mL per hour and administration of furosemide at 2 to 5 mg per kg up to 200 mg in adults and mannitol, 0.5 gram per kg of a 20% solution (25 grams in adults), over 30 minutes, if necessary. Alkalization of the urine to pH greater than 7.0 by adding $NaHCO_3$ to IV fluids is controversial but should be considered if acidosis is present or if there are high levels of potassium. Correct and monitor any associated electrolyte abnormalities, metabolic acidosis, and hyperthermia.

Acute Hepatic Failure

Acute fulminant hepatic failure is a clinical syndrome resulting from massive necrosis of liver cells leading to encephalopathy and severe impairment of hepatic function. The encephalopathy is usually present and prior liver disease is usually absent. The condition is potentially reversible. Acute hepatic encephalopathy is a universal feature of acute hepatic failure (AHF). It is abrupt and usually starts within 5 to 7 days of massive hepatic failure. Cerebral edema occurs in 75 to 80% of those whose condition progresses to coma and is the leading cause of death. The most frequent cause is infectious. Other frequent causes include hepatotoxic drugs. The mechanisms of toxin-induced hepatotoxicity are as follows:

1. Direct hepatocellular damage by phallotoxins binding to hepatocyte membranes (e.g., *A. phalloides*)
2. Metabolic conversion of acetaminophen to a hepatotoxic intermediate metabolite (*N*-acetyl-*p*-benzoquinonimine [NAPQI])

3. A vascular disturbance such as hepatic vein thrombosis (pyrrolizidine alkaloids)

The clinical and morphologic presentations are

1. Acute hepatitis: methyldopa, isoniazid, phenytoin, NSAIDs, lovastatin
2. Cholestasis: androgens, oral contraceptives, erythromycin estolate, metronidazole (Flagyl), chlorpropamide, chlorpromazine, increased alkaline phosphatase and bilirubin
3. Hepatic necrosis: acetaminophen, carbon tetrachloride, *A. phalloides,* yellow phosphorus
4. Chronic hepatitis: methyldopa, arsenic, isoniazid, halothane

The laboratory and clinical evidence does not become apparent until at least 24 to 36 hours after exposure to the toxin. If the hepatic damage is severe, the bilirubin and prothrombin time continue to worsen after 2 to 3 days. Metabolic acidosis and hypoglycemia are signs of poor prognosis.

Vasodilators of the microcirculation of the liver (e.g., NAC) may affect nitric oxide–induced control of vascular tone and increase oxygen delivery to the liver. Many patients appear to benefit from NAC as an antidote for acetaminophen (APAP) toxicity. In addition, NAC prolongs survival, allowing orthotopic liver transplantation (OLT) in patients with APAP toxicity and in patients with AHF of other toxic and nontoxic causes. Hepatotoxicity is aggravated in chronic alcoholics and patients chronically receiving enzyme inducer drugs such as anticonvulsants.

Criteria for OLT in fulminant liver failure are listed in Table 19. Mortality is greater than 80% and

TABLE 19. **Criteria for Predicting Death and the Need for Liver Transplantation**

Cause	Criteria
Acetaminophen poisoning	pH < 7.3 regardless of grade of encephalopathy* or prothrombin time > 100 s
	Serum creatinine > 3.4 mg/dL (300 µmol/L) or > 2 mg/dL
	In patients with grade 3 or 4 encephalopathy Bilirubin > 20 mg/dL
All other causes	Prothrombin time > 100 s (regardless of grade of encephalopathy) or any three of the following (regardless of grade of encephalopathy):
	Age younger than 10 y or older than 40 y
	Liver failure caused by non-A, non-B hepatitis or halothane-induced hepatitis, or idiosyncratic drug reaction
	Duration of jaundice before onset of encephalopathy >7 d or >2 d
	Prothrombin time > 50 s
	Bilirubin > 17.5 mg/dL (300 µmol/L)

*Encephalopathy classification: grade 1 = confused or altered mood; grade 2 = inappropriate behavior or drowsiness (mild obtundation); grade 3 = stuporous but arrestable, markedly confused behavior; grade 4 = coma with or without decerebrate posturing unresponsive to painful stimuli.

Modified from O'Grady JG, Alexander GJM, Hayllar KM, Williams R: Early indicators of prognosis in fulminant hepatic failure. Gastroenterology 97:439–445, 1989; and Caraceni P, Van Thiel DH: Acute liver failure. Lancet 345(8943):163–169, 1995. © by The Lancet Ltd, 1995.

with OLT is 60 to 80%. This indicates 20% unnecessary OLT. The mortality in lesser grade encephalopathy is only 20%.

Temperature Disturbances

Although the most frequent cause of temperature elevation in toxicologic emergencies is infection (usually secondary to aspiration pneumonia), elevations are often not associated with the prostaglandin mechanisms of fever. See Table 6 for etiologies of temperature elevation.

Hyperthermia in toxicologic emergencies is due to excess muscle activity, hypermetabolic state, interferences with oxidative phosphorylation, and impaired dissipation of heat. It occurs in anticholinergic, sympathomimetic overdoses (cocaine) and ethanol withdrawal. Toxicologic temperature elevations require external cooling measures, control of excess muscular activity such as convulsions, and, in malignant hyperthermia, dantrolene and bromocriptine. Antipyretics are not useful in these cases.

Hyperthermia syndromes involve life-threatening elevations of temperature. The syndromes are characterized by altered mental state, rigidity, metabolic acidosis, and temperature elevation, except in the serotonin syndrome.

The neuroleptic malignant syndrome is an idiosyncratic reaction of patients receiving neuroleptic medications (PTZs and butyrophenones).

Malignant hyperthermia (MH) is associated with drug interactions (e.g., when synthetic opioids [e.g., meperidine] or tricyclic antidepressants are administered to patients receiving MAOIs.

The serotonin syndrome may occur with or without hyperthermia. It occurs in patients receiving MAOIs who take serotonergic drugs (meperidine, clomipramine) or serotonin inhibitors (fluoxetine [Prozac], sertraline [Zoloft], paroxetine [Panil]) without a drug-free interval of at least 5 weeks.

Management of hyperthermia:

1. Immediately discontinue the offending agent. Hyperventilate with 100% humidified cooled oxygen at high gas flow rates, at least 10 liters per minute.
2. A BZP is required to allow the patient to tolerate the cooling measures, such as an ice bath. It reduces motor activity and muscle tone and protects the patient from seizures (e.g., with cocaine, amphetamines).
3. Correct acid-base and electrolyte disturbances. Hyperkalemia is common and, if life-threatening, should be treated with hyperventilation, calcium bicarbonate, and intravenous glucose and insulin. If it is refractory, hemodialysis may be necessary.
4. Simultaneously, actively cool the patient (e.g., with intravenous cold saline, not lactated Ringer's); lavage the stomach, bladder, and rectum with cold saline; and use a hypothermic blanket. Monitor the core body temperature.
5. Dysrhythmias usually respond to treatment of acidosis and hyperkalemia. Antidysrhythmic agents may be used if needed, with the exception of calcium

channel blockers (which may cause hyperkalemia and cardiovascular collapse).

6. Determine and monitor ABGs, creatine kinase, electrolytes and calcium, clotting, core temperature, serum and urine myoglobin, and urine output. Consider monitoring with a central line.

7. Dantrolene sodium, a phenytoin derivative, inhibits calcium release from the sarcoplasmic reticulum, resulting in decreased muscle contraction.

Dantrolene (acts peripherally) with dopamine agonists, bromocriptine mesylate, or amantadine hydrochloride (Symmetrel) (acts centrally) has been reported to be successful in combination with cooling and good supportive measures in MH. Dantrolene does not reverse the rigidity or psychomotor disturbances resulting from the central dopamine blockade and is therefore often used in combination with bromocriptine.

The dose is 2 to 3 mg per kg IV as a bolus and then 1 mg per kg per minute with incremental increases (average dose 2 to 5 mg per kg). Repeat the loading dose every 10 minutes (maximal total dose 10 mg per kg) or until the signs of MH (e.g., tachycardia, rigidity, increased end-tidal carbon dioxide, and temperature elevation) are controlled. Hepatotoxicity occurs at doses higher than 10 mg per kg. To prevent recurrence, administer 1 mg per kg every 6 hours for 24 to 48 hours after the episode. After that, oral dantrolene is used at 1 mg per kg every 6 hours for 24 hours as necessary. Watch for thrombophlebitis after dantrolene administration. The drug is best administered into a central vein.

8. Bromocriptine mesylate at 2.5 to 10 mg orally or through a nasogastric tube three times a day or amantadine at 100 mg twice a day has been used; there are no scientific data concerning their efficacy but they seem theoretically reasonable. They are to be used with dantrolene.

Hypothermia means a temperature below 95°F (35°C). It may occur when an overdose (e.g., of a CNS depressant) interferes with physiologic responses (vasoconstriction, muscle activity) when the victim is exposed to a cool environment. Hypothermia is frequently associated with hypoglycemia. See Table 6 for the etiology.

The management depends on body temperature and hemodynamic stability. Administer glucose if the patient is hypoglycemic. In severe hypothermia, there may be bradycardia with a heart rate of 40 to 50 beats per minute, and hypotension (70 to 90 mm Hg systolic) should not be vigorously treated or fluid overload may occur. Management consists of rewarming.

1. Body temperatures of 32 to 35°C (89.6 to 95°F) with stable hemodynamics are managed by increasing the body's heat production with gradual external rewarming at 1°C per hour, for example, by wrapping in insulated material such as blankets, offering warm liquids if the patient is alert, and providing a warm environment.

2. Body temperatures of 30 to 32°C (86 to 89.6°F) with stable hemodynamics require transfer of heat to the patient, for example, with heated blankets, warmed intravenous solutions (D5W 0.9% saline warmed to 37 to 43°C), and warmed humidified oxygen. Cardiac monitoring should be carried out.

3. Body temperatures of 30 to 32°C (86 to 89.6°F) with unstable hemodynamics require the initiation of active core rewarming in addition to the preceding measures, for example, with heated humidified oxygen (42 to 45°C), a warming bath (40 to 41°C), and heated GI irrigation (gastric lavage and colonic enemas). Monitor vital signs.

4. Body temperatures below 30°C (86°F) require rapid rewarming by invasive procedures because of the danger of ventricular fibrillation; for example, use peritoneal lavage with heated dialysate (40 to 42°C), extracorporeal blood rewarming, thoracotomy, and mediastinal lavage with heated fluids. Vital signs require close monitoring.

The Agitated, Violent, and Psychotic Victim

Violence is aggressive assault or combativeness. Agitation is uncontrollable restlessness or excessive excitability. Psychosis is a mental derangement that may cause violence or aggression. These patients may harm themselves and others. See Table 3 for a classification of the severity of stimulant manifestations.

The causes of violence may be psychiatric, situational frustration, and organic diseases. Most patients labeled as violent are schizophrenic, especially of the paranoid type (30 to 40%). Organic violent behavior usually occurs in patients older than 40 years without a previous psychiatric history. The patients are disoriented, lethargic, or stuporous and have visual hallucinations or illusions and abnormal vital signs. No patient with physical restraints should be placed on a gurney. Physical restraints should not be used for psychiatric patients.

Drugs and chemicals may produce violence or precipitate violent psychosis in a patient with an underlying psychiatric disorder. Agents with which this occurs most frequently include amphetamines, anticholinergics (scopolamine, jimsonweed), cocaine, ethanol (intoxication, intolerance, and withdrawal), hallucinogens, phencyclidine, sedative hypnotics (intoxication or withdrawal), and occupational chemicals including sulfides and mercury.

Differential diagnosis requires exclusion of hypoxia, hypoglycemia, electrolyte disturbances, and metabolic and endocrine disorders. In one review, hypoglycemia accounted for 9% of violent patients. The diaphoretic violent patient usually has an organic cause of the disorder (e.g., hypoglycemia, sepsis, withdrawal, heatstroke, myocardial infarction, or pulmonary edema).

If physical restraints are needed, record the reason (e.g., to facilitate evaluation or because there is a psychiatric or personality disorder or a need to administer medication to prevent harm to the patient and/or others). Physical restraints should be monitored frequently (at least every 15 minutes, and the monitoring should be documented) to prevent neurovascular sequelae and avoid rhabdomyolysis. Figure 1 shows a seclusion and restraint record.

Pharmacologic restraints include haloperidol and other agents and rapid tranquilization. Haloperidol (Haldol) produces competitive blockade of the postsynaptic dopamine receptors, depresses the cortex and hypothalamus, and has strong alpha-adrenergic and anticholinergic blocking activity. Do not use the long-acting decanoate salt of haloperidol.

The dose of haloperidol for young adults varies from 0.5 to 5 mg orally three times a day or 2 to 5 mg intramuscularly (IM) every 4 to 8 hours, as needed. The doses may be increased rapidly. For prompt control use 5 to 10 mg and repeat every 30 to 60 minutes for 8 doses. The maximal oral daily dose is 100 mg or the IM dose 0.1 mg per kg per day. If parenteral administration is used, change to the oral route as soon as possible. Doses higher than 10 mg do not increase effectiveness. The initial dose for the elderly patient should be decreased to 0.5 to 2.0 mg.

The side effects of haloperidol are primarily dystonic reactions, although the neuroleptic malignant syndrome has been described after a single dose. Avoid haloperidol in the presence of pregnancy, lactation, lithium (encephalopathic interaction), phencyclidine intoxication, withdrawal syndromes, and intoxications with drugs with anticholinergic properties. Haloperidol and PTZs both have undesirable anticholinergic and alpha-blocking effects.

Alternatives are lorazepam, thiothixene (Navane), fluphenazine (Prolixin), and droperidol (causes hypotension). Chlorpromazine is not advised because of its alpha-adrenergic blocking effects, which causes orthostatic hypotension.

When rapid tranquilization is used, explain to the patient that the medication will have a calming effect. A combination of antipsychotic medication with lorazepam is more effective than antipsychotic medication alone. Core psychotic symptoms do not respond to a few doses but require weeks of therapy. See Table 20.

Most patients respond to a combination of haloperidol at 5 mg IM or thiothixene (Navane) at 10 mg and lorazepam at 5 mg IM in the same syringe. The medication is administered hourly. Most patients respond to 1 to 3 doses. The use of antipsychotic medications IV in the emergency department has not been well studied. The dosage should be reduced to half for patients older than 65 years.

Investigational Procedures Used in Toxicologic Emergencies

Extracorporeal membrane oxygenation has been considered for shock in tricyclic antidepressant and quinidine poisoning.

Intra-aortic balloon counterpulsation has been considered for poisoning caused by beta-adrenergic blockers, calcium channel blockers, and medications

Name of Patient _____ Chart # _____

Date _____ Seclusion Time in _____ Time out _____

Physician order obtained Dr. _____ Date _____

Limbs circle 1 2 3 4   Time in _____ Time out _____ Date _____

The following measures to alter the patient's behavior have failed

[ ] Patient has been removed from stimuli

[ ] Patient has been encouraged to express feeling in usual manner

[ ] Staff has been assigned to listen to patient

[ ] Patient has been offered noncompetitive tasks to complete

[ ] Patient has been medicated

[ ] Other Specify _____

Reason for seclusion and restraint explained to patient.

_____

Behavior necessitating restraint _____

_____

Vital signs on admission to seclusion P _____ R _____ Temp _____ BP _____ Time _____

Name of physician (write clearly) _____

Nurse _____

Date	Time	Seclusion	VS	Bath	Fluids	Food	Limb	Circu-	Range	Staff
		Room	q 15	Room	(cc)		RA LA	lation	of	sign.
			min				RL LL		motion	
							Waist			

Figure 1. Seclusion and restraint record.

TABLE 20. **Rapid Tranquilization
of the Violent Patient**

Type	Tranquilization*
Schizophrenia, mania, or other psychosis	Lorazepam 2–4 mg IM combined with haloperidol 5 mg IM or thiothixene 10 mg IM or Thiothixene 10 mg IM or 20 mg concentrate or Haloperidol 5 mg IM or 10 mg concentrate or Loxapine 10 mg IM or 25 mg concentrate PO
Personality disorder	Lorazepam 1–2 mg PO q 1–2 h or 2–4 mg (0.5 mg/kg) IM q 1–2 h
Alcohol withdrawal	
Agitation, tremors, abnormal VS	Chlordiazepoxide 25–50 mg PO q 4–6 h
Older than 65 y, liver disease	Lorazepam 2 mg PO q 2 h
Extreme agitation	Lorazepam 2–4 mg IM q h RT if not controlled
Cocaine or amphetamine	Mild to moderate agitation, thiothixene 10 mg PO q 8 h Severe agitation, thiothixene 10 mg IM or 20 mg concentrate or haloperidol 5 mg IM or 10 mg concentrate
Phencyclidine	
Mild hyperactivity, tension, anxiety, excitement	Diazepam 10–30 mg PO or Lorazepam 2–4 mg IM (0.05 mg/kg)
Severe agitation, excitement, hallucinations, bizarre behavior	Haloperidol 5–10 mg IM q 30–60 min

*All doses given q 30–60 min, half the dose for those older than 65 y.
Abbreviations: VS = vital signs; RT = rapid tranquilization.
Modified from Dubin WR, Weiss KJ: Handbook of Psychiatric Emergencies. Springhouse, PA, Springhouse Corp, 1991, p 31.

that cause a temporary decrease in coronary perfusion.

Surfactant has been considered for potential use in hydrocarbon aspiration and inhalation injuries and in near-drowning. In a study of aspirated hydrocarbons in animals it was found to be detrimental.

Transplantation of lungs has been tried unsuccessfully for paraquat poisoning.

Nondepolarizing neuromuscular blocking agents have produced prolonged paralysis when used in combination in a patient receiving corticosteroids.

Laboratory and Radiographic Studies

Initially, obtain an ECG for dysrhythmias or conduction delays (resulting from cardiotoxic medications); a chest radiograph for aspiration pneumonia (if there is a history of loss of consciousness, unarousable state, vomiting) and noncardiac pulmonary edema; and electrolyte and glucose concentrations in the blood. Calculate the anion gap (AG), and obtain acid-base and ABG profiles (if respiratory distress or altered mental status) and serum osmolality assay.

See Table 21 for appropriate testing on the basis of clinical toxicologic presentation. All laboratory specimens should be carefully labeled, timed, and dated. For potential legal cases a "chain of custody" must be established. Assessment of the laboratory studies may give a clue to the etiologic agent.

Electrolyte, Acid-Base, and Osmolality Disturbances

Evaluate and correct electrolyte and acid-base disturbances. Metabolic acidosis (low pH with a low arterial P_{CO_2} [Pa_{CO_2}] and low HCO_3^-) with an increased AG is seen with many agents in overdose.

Metabolic Acidosis and the Anion Gap. The AG is an estimate of the anions other than chloride and HCO_3^- necessary to counterbalance the positive charge of sodium. The AG gives a clue to the etiology, compensation, and complications.

The AG is calculated from the standard serum electrolytes by subtracting the total carbon dioxide (reflects the actual measured HCO_3^-) and chloride from the sodium: $Na^+ - (Cl^- + HCO_3^-) = AG$. Potassium is usually not used in the calculation because it may be hemolyzed and is an intracellular cation. The lack of an AG does not exclude a toxic etiology.

The normal gap was found to be 8 to 12 mEq per liter by flame photometry. However, a lower normal AG of 7 ± 4 mEq per liter has been determined by newer techniques (e.g., ion-selective electrodes or coulometric titration). Some studies have found the AG to be relatively insensitive for determining the presence of toxins.

It is important to recognize the AG toxins salicylates, methanol, and ethylene glycol because they have specific antidotes and hemodialysis is effective in management.

A list of the etiologies of increased AG, decreased

TABLE 21. **Conditions of the Patient
and Appropriate Tests**

Condition	Tests
Comatose	Toxicologic tests (acetaminophen, sedative hypnotic, ethanol, opioids, benzodiazepine) Glucose, ammonia, CT, CSF analysis
Respiratory toxin	Spirometry, arterial blood gases, chest radiography, monitor O_2 saturation
Cardiac toxin	ECG 12 lead and monitoring, echocardiogram, serial cardiac enzymes, hemodynamic monitoring
Hepatic toxin	Enzymes (AST, ALT, GGT), ammonia, albumin, bilirubin, glucose, PT, PTT, amylase
Nephrotoxin	BUN, creatinine, electrolytes (Na^+, K^+, Mg^{2+}, Ca^{2+}, PO_4^{3-}), serum and urine osmolarity, 24-h urine for heavy metals, creatine kinase, serum and urine myoglobin, urinalysis, and urinary sodium
Bleeding	Platelets, PT, PTT, bleeding time, fibrin split products, fibrinogen type and match blood

Abbreviations: CT = computed tomography; CSF = cerebrospinal fluid; AST = aspartate aminotransferase; ALT = alanine aminotransferase; GGT = γ-glutamyltransferase; PT = prothrombin time; PTT = partial thromboplastin time.

TABLE 22. **Etiologies of Metabolic Acidosis**

No Gap Hyperchloremic	Increased Gap Normochloremic	Decreased Gap
Acidifying agents	Methanol	Laboratory error†
Adrenal insufficiency	Uremia*	Intoxication (Br, Li)
Anhydrase inhibitors	Diabetic ketoacidosis*	Protein abnormal
Fistula	Paraldehyde,* phenformin	Sodium low
Osteotomies	Isoniazid	
Obstructive uropathies	Iron	
Renal tubular acidosis	Lactic acidosis†	
Diarrhea, uncomplicated*	Ethanol,* ethylene glycol*	
Dilutional	Salicylates, starvation, solvents	
Sulfamylon		

*Indicates hyperosmolar situation. Studies have found that the anion gap may be relatively insensitive for determining the presence of toxins.
†Lactic acidosis caused by carbon monoxide, cyanide, hydrogen sulfide, hypoxia, ibuprofen, iron, isoniazid, ischemia, phenformin, salicylates, seizures, or theophylline.

AG, or no AG is shown in Table 22. The most common cause of a decreased AG is laboratory error. Lactic acidosis produces the largest AG and can result from any poisoning that causes hypoxia, hypoglycemia, or convulsions.

Other blood chemistry derangements that suggest certain intoxications are shown in Table 23.

Serum Osmolal Gaps. The serum osmolality is a measure of the number of molecules of solute per kilogram of solvent, or mOsm per kg of water. The osmolarity is solute per liter of solution, or mOsm per liter of water at a specified temperature. Osmolarity is usually a calculated value and osmolality is usually a measured value. They are considered interchangeable when 1 liter equals 1 kilogram. The normal serum osmolality is 280 to 290 mOsm per kg. Serum for the freezing point osmolarity measurement and serum electrolyte specimens for calculation should be drawn simultaneously.

The serum osmolal gap is defined as the difference between the measured osmolality determined by the freezing point method and the calculated osmolarity determined as follows: the serum sodium value multiplied by 2 plus the BUN divided by 3 (0.1 molecular weight [MW] of BUN), plus the blood glucose value divided by 20 (0.1 MW of glucose). This gap estimate is usually within 10 mOsm of the simultaneously measured serum osmolality. Ethanol, if present, may be included in the equation to eliminate its influence on the osmolality; the ethanol concentration divided by 4.6 (0.1 of ethanol MW) is added to the equation. See Table 24.

Calculated mOsm =

$$2Na^+ + \frac{BUN}{3}_{(mg/dL)} + \frac{blood\ glucose}{20}_{(mg/dL)} + \frac{ethanol}{4.6}_{(mg/dL)}$$

The osmolal gap is valid for a hemodynamically intact individual; it is not valid in shock and the postmortem state. Metabolic disorders such as hyperglycemia, uremia, and dehydration increase the osmolarity but usually do not cause gaps greater than 10 mOsm per kg.

A gap greater than 10 mOsm per kg suggests that unidentified osmolal-acting substances are present: acetone, ethanol, ethylene glycol, ethchlorvynol, glycerin, isopropyl alcohol, isoniazid, ethanol, mannitol, methanol, NaHCO$_3$ (1 mEq per kg raises osmolality 2 mOsm per liter), and trichloroethane. Alcohols and glycols should be sought when the degree of obtundation exceeds that expected from the blood ethanol concentration (BEC) or when other clinical conditions exist, such as visual loss (methanol), metabolic acidosis (methanol and ethylene glycol), and renal failure (ethylene glycol).

A falsely elevated osmolal gap may be produced by other low-molecular-weight un-ionized substances (acetone, dextran, dimethyl sulfoxide, diuretics, ethyl ether, mannitol, sorbitol, trichloroethane), diabetic ketoacidosis, hyperlipidemia, and unmeasured electrolytes (e.g., magnesium).

False-negative results occur when a normal osmolal gap may be reported in the presence of alcohol or glycol poisoning if the parent compound is already

TABLE 23. **Blood Chemistry Derangements in Toxicology**

Derangement	Toxin or Disease
Acetonemia without acidosis	Acetone or isopropyl alcohol
Hypomagnesemia	Ethanol, digitalis
Hypocalcemia	Ethylene glycol, oxalate, fluoride
Hyperkalemia	Beta blockers, acute digitalis, renal failure
Hypokalemia	Diuretics, salicylism, sympathomimetics, theophylline, corticosteroids, chronic digitalis
Hyperglycemia	Diazoxide, glucagon, iron, isoniazid, organophosphate insecticides, phenylurea insecticides, phenytoin, salicylates, sympathomimetic agents, thyroid, vasopressors
Hypoglycemia	Beta blockers, ethanol, insulin, isoniazid, oral hypoglycemic agents, salicylates
Elevated CK	Amphetamines, ethanol, cocaine, phencyclidine
Elevated creatinine and normal BUN	Isopropyl alcohol, diabetic ketoacidosis

Abbreviation: CK = creatine kinase.

TABLE 24. **Alcohols and Glycols**

Alcohol or Glycol	1 mg/dL in Blood Raises Osmolality mOsm/L by	Molecular Weight	Conversion Factor*
Ethanol	0.228	40	4.6
Methanol	0.327	32	3.2
Ethylene glycol	0.190	62	6.2
Isopropanol	0.176	60	6.0
Acetone	0.182	58	5.8
Propylene glycol	Not available	72	7.2

*Example: methanol osmolality. Subtract the calculated osmolarity from the measured serum osmolality (freezing point method) = osmolar gap × 3.2 (0.1 molecular weight) = estimated serum methanol concentration.

metabolized. This can occur when the osmolal gap is measured after a significant time has elapsed since ingestion. In alcohol and glycol intoxications, an early osmolar gap is due to the relatively nontoxic parent drug and delayed metabolic acidosis and an AG is due to the more toxic metabolites.

The serum concentration mg per dL = mOsm gap × MW of substance divided by 10. See Table 24.

Radiographic Studies

Chest and neck radiographs are obtained for pathologic conditions such as aspiration pneumonia and pulmonary edema, for foreign bodies, and to determine the location of the endotracheal tube.

Abdominal radiographs are obtained to detect radiopaque substances. The mnemonic for radiopaque substances seen on abdominal radiographs is CHIPES: C, chlorides and chloral hydrate; H, heavy metals (arsenic, barium, iron, lead, mercury, zinc); I, iodide; P, Play Doh, Pepto-Bismol, phenothiazine (inconsistent); E, enteric-coated tablets; S, sodium, potassium, and other elements in tablet form (bismuth, calcium, potassium) and solvents containing chlorides (e.g., carbon tetrachloride).

Toxicologic Studies

In the average toxicologic laboratory, false-negatives occur at a rate of 10 to 30% and false-positives at a rate of 0 to 10%. Table 25 lists test interactions that should be considered.

The predictive value of the positive screen is about 90%. A negative toxicology screen does not exclude poisoning. The negative predictive value of toxicologic screening is about 70%. For example, the following BZPs may not be detected by routine screening tests for BZP: alprazolam (Xanax), clonazepam (Klonopin), temazepam (Restoril), and triazolam (Halcion).

The "toxic" urine screen is a qualitative urine test for several common drugs, usually substances of abuse (cocaine and metabolites, opioids, amphetamines, BZPs, barbiturates, and phencyclidine). These tests are usually available within 2 to 6 hours. Because these tests may vary in different hospitals and communities, the physician should determine exactly which substances are included in the toxic urine screen of his or her laboratory.

It is always advisable to determine the plasma acetaminophen level in any intentional overdose situation, as there are no clinical manifestations to guide the decision about treatment except the plasma acetaminophen level more than 4 hours after ingestion. For best results, the treatment should be started within 8 hours.

Ethylene glycol, red blood cell cholinesterase, and serum cyanide assays are not readily available.

For certain ingestions quantitative blood levels should be obtained at specific times after ingestion to avoid spurious low values in the distribution phase that result from incomplete absorption. Table 26 lists the times after ingestion when the quantitative tests should be obtained (the elimination phase). It is always wise to obtain serial quantitative tests to follow the trend because the peak may be delayed.

The detection time is the number of days after intake of a substance during which an individual would be expected to excrete detectable levels of the substance or metabolite in urine. In general, urine detection is possible for 1 to 3 days after cocaine exposure, 2 to 4 days after heroin (monoacetylmorphine is diagnostic of heroin use but is detectable for only 12 hours after use), and 2 to 4 days after phencyclidine; if use is chronic, double the time.

Nontoxic Ingestions (Table 27)

Criteria for nontoxic ingestion are as follows:

1. There is absolute identification of the product.
2. There is absolute assurance that a single product was ingested.
3. There is assurance that there is no signal word from the Consumer Product Safety Commission on the container's label.
4. The amount ingested is known to a good approximation.
5. It is possible to call back at frequent intervals to determine whether symptoms have developed.
6. The exposed individual is free of symptoms.
7. If the exposed individual is younger than 1 year or older than 6 years, a satisfactory explanation of the circumstances is necessary to exclude chemical maltreatment by the caretaker in the former case and to exclude a "cry for help" indicating an intolerable home situation in the latter case.

TABLE 25. **Interferences with Common Toxicologic Testing**

Drug or Toxin	Method*	Factors Causing False-Positives or Interferences
Acetaminophen	SC	Salicylate, methylsalicylate (can increase level 10% in µg/mL), phenol, salicylamide, bilirubin, renal failure (each 1 mg/dL increase in creatinine = 30 µg/mL acetaminophen)
	GC	Phenacetin
	HPLC	Cephalosporins, sulfonamides
	IA	Phenacetin
Amphetamines (*d*-amphetamines)	GC	Other volatile stimulant amines, meperidine metabolites, antihistamine metabolites
	IA	Phenylpropanolamine, ephedrine, fenfluramine, isometheptene, isoxsuprine, phentermine, phenmetrazine, doxepin,† labetalol, *l*-amphetamine in Vicks inhalers, ranitidine, ritodrine, benzathine penicillin‡ (FPIA)
	TLC	See amines just listed
Barbiturates	IA	NSAIDs produce false-negatives
Benzodiazepines	IA	Oxazepam, temazepam, alprazolam; NSAIDs produce false-negatives
Chloride	SC	Bromide (0.8 mEq of Cl = 1 mEq of Br)
Cocaine	IA	"Coca teas" (benzoylecgonine)
	TLC	Urochromes and endogenous acids
Creatinine	SC	Ketoacidosis may increase creatinine up to 2–3 mg/dL in end-point assays, cephalosporins, creatinine with rhabdomyolysis
Digoxin	IA	Endogenous digoxin-like naturetic substances in newborn (1 ng/mL), renal failure (1 ng/mL), cross-reacting metabolites in renal failure (2 ng/mL), pregnancy, liver disease, oleander and other plant glycosides, digoxin-binding antibody (Fab)
Ethanol	SC	Other alcohols, ketones (by oxidation methods); isopropanol (by enzyme methods); *Candida albicans* and *Proteus*, ethanol production
Ethylene glycol	SC	Other glycols, propylene glycol in IV phenytoin, diazepam and others, triglycerides
	GC	Propylene glycol: falsely lowers value by interfering with internal standard
Iron	SC	Deferoxamine falsely lowers TIBC 15%; lavender-topped Vacutainer has EDTA, binds and lowers iron
Isopropanol	GC	Isopropanol in skin disinfectants may produce elevations in blood concentration up to 40 mg/dL but usually trivial
Lithium	Any method	Green-topped Vacutainer (heparin) tube with lithium may elevate lithium 6–8 mEq/L
Marijuana	IA	Passive inhalation of marijuana smoke can produce a urine level of marijuana metabolites of 20 µg/ml
11-Nor-9-carboxyltetra-hydrocannabinol	TLC	Melanin, steroids, methadone, antihistamines
Methemoglobinemia	SC	Sulfhemoglobinemia (10% cross + by co-oximeter), methylene blue (2 mg/kg transient false + 15% methemoglobin level) hyperlipidemia (triglyceride 6000 = methemoglobin 28.6%)
Opioids (morphine or codeine)	IA	Cross-reactive with hydrocodone, hydromorphine, oxycodone, 6-monoacetylmorphine, two poppy seed bagels for 16 h, one lemon poppy seed muffin, Vick's Formula 44
	TLC	Hydrocodone, dextromethorphan
Osmolarity	Any	Lavender-topped Vacutainer tubes (EDTA) 15 mOsm/L, gray-topped Vacutainer tubes (fluoride-oxalate) 150 mOsm/L, blue-topped Vacutainer tubes (citrate) 10 mOsm/L
		Falsely normal if vapor pressure methods used
Phencyclidine, dextromethorphan	IA	Phencyclidine analogues, phenothiazines, diphenhydramine, antihistamines, methadone, meperidine
Salicylates	SC	Phenothiazines, acetaminophen, ketosis, salicylamide, diflunisal, accumulated salicylate metabolites in renal failure (10% increased)
		Decreased or altered salicylate by bilirubin; phenylketones
	GC	Methylsalicylate, eucalyptol, theophylline
	HPLC	Antibiotics, theophylline
Theophylline	SC	Diazepam, caffeine, accumulated theophylline metabolites in renal failure
	HPLC	Acetazolamide, cephalosporins, endogenous xanthines and accumulated theophylline metabolites in renal failure
	IA	Caffeine, accumulated theophylline metabolites in renal failure

*All assays within a methologic group are not equivalent. Performance depends on the specific brand or formulation.

†Doxepin gives unconfirmed amphetamine by Abbot Adx test. The test is negative if not confirmed by thin-layer chromatography (Merigen KS, Browning R, Kellerman A: Doxepin causing false-positive urine test for amphetamine. Ann Emerg Med 22:1370, 1993).

‡Benzathine salt of phenoxypenicillin with Syva EMIT I polyclonal assay (Berthier M, Bonneau D, Mura P, et al: Benzathine as a cause for a false-positive test result for amphetamines. J Pediatr 127:669–670, 1995).

Abbreviations: SC = spectrochemical; GC = gas chromatography (interferences more common with older methods); HPLC = high-performance liquid chromatography; IA = immunoassay; TLC = thin-layer chromatography; FPIA = fluorescent polarization immunoassay; NSAIDs = nonsteroidal anti-inflammatory drugs; TIBC = total iron-binding capacity; EDTA = ethylenediaminetetra-acetic acid.

Adapted from Olsen KR: Poisoning & Drug Overdose, 2nd ed. Norwalk, CT, Appleton & Lange, 1994, pp 37–38.

TABLE 26. **Substances with Which Quantitative Blood Values May Be Necessary***

Substance	Specimen	Time After Ingestion to Obtain Specimen	Toxic Concentration
Acetaminophen (see "Acetaminophen" section)	Serum	>4 h	>150 µg/mL at 4 h
Carboxyhemoglobin	Blood	Stat	Extrapolate
Carbamazepine	Serum	Stat	>12 µg/mL
Digoxin	Serum	6–8 h	>2 ng/mL adult, >4 ng/mL child
Ethanol	Serum	0.5–1 h	>80 mg/dL (800 µg/mL)
Ethylene glycol	Serum	0.5–1 h	>20 mg/dL (200 µg/mL)
Iron			
Liquid	Serum	2 h	>350 µg/dL (3.5 µg/mL)
Tablet	Serum	4 h	>350 µg/dL (3.5 µg/mL)
Isopropanol	Serum	0.5–1 h	>50 mg/dL (500 µg/mL)
Lithium	Serum	8–12 h	>1.5 mEq/L
Methanol	Serum	0.5–1 h	>20 mg/dL (200 µg/mL)
Methemoglobin	Blood	Stat	>30%
Paraquat	Plasma	8 h	>1 µg/mL within 24 h
Phenobarbital	Serum	Stat	>40 µg/mL
Phenytoin	Serum	1–2 h	>20 µg/mL
Primidone	Serum	Stat	>12 µg/mL
Salicylate	Serum	After 6 h	>30 mg/dL (300 µg/mL)
Theophylline	Serum		
Liquid	Serum	1 h	>20 µg/mL
Regular tablet	Serum	1–3 h	>20 µg/mL
Slow release	Serum	3–10 h	>20 µg/mL

*Note that serial levels are needed to follow the trend in all cases. Because of delayed peak times, a single blood or plasma level is not sufficient to exclude intoxication.

COMMON POISONS

Acetaminophen (*N*-acetyl-*p*-aminophenol [APAP], Tylenol, called paracetamol in the United Kingdom). *Toxic mechanism:* At therapeutic doses of APAP, less than 5% is metabolized by cytochrome P-450IIE1 to a toxic reactive oxidizing metabolite, *N*-acetyl-*p*-benzoquinonimine (NAPQI). In overdose, sufficient glutathione is not available to reduce the excess NAPQI into a nontoxic conjugate and it forms covalent bonds with hepatic intracellular proteins to produce centrilobular necrosis and by a similar mechanism renal damage. *Toxic dose:* The therapeutic dose is 10 to 15 mg per kg per dose with a maximum of 5 doses per 24 hours and a maximal total daily dose of 2.5 grams. The acute single toxic dose is greater than 140 mg per kg, possibly greater than 200 mg per kg in child. Factors affecting the cytochrome P-450 enzymes (enzyme inducers such as anticonvulsants [barbiturates, phenytoin], isoniazid, alcoholism) and factors that decrease glutathione stores (e.g., alcoholism, malnutrition, and human immunodeficiency virus [HIV]) contribute to the toxicity of APAP. Chronic alcoholics who ingest APAP at 3 to 4 grams per day for a few days can have depleted glutathione stores and require NAC therapy at 50% below hepatotoxic blood APAP levels on the nomogram. *Kinetics:* Onset of action occurs in 0.5 to 1 hour, the peak plasma concentration occurs in 20 to 90 minutes but usually 2 to 4 hours after an overdose, and the duration is 4 to 6 hours. The Vd is 0.9 liter per kg. PB is low, less than 50% (albumin); $t_{1/2}$ is 1 to 3 hours. The route of elimination is hepatic metabolism to an inactive nontoxic glucuronide conjugate and inactive nontoxic sulfate metabolite by two saturable pathways, and less than 5% is metabolized to the reactive metabolite NAPQI. In children younger than 6 years, metabolic elimination occurs to a greater degree by conjugation with the sulfate pathway, which may be hepatoprotective. *Manifestations:* The four phases of the intoxication's clinical course may overlap, and the absence of a phase does not exclude toxicity. Phase I occurs within 0.5 to 24 hours after ingestion and may consist of a few hours of malaise, diaphoresis, nausea, and vomiting or there may be no symptoms. CNS depression or coma is not a feature. Phase II occurs 24 to 48 hours after ingestion and is a period of diminished symptoms. The liver enzymes aspartate aminotransferase (AST) (earliest) and alanine aminotransferase (ALT) may increase as early as 4 hours or as late as 36 hours after ingestion. Phase III occurs in 48 to 96 hours, with peak liver function abnormalities at 72 to 96 hours. The degree of elevation of the hepatic enzyme values does not correlate with outcome. Recovery starts in about 4 days unless hepatic failure develops. Less than 1% of patients develop fulminant hepatotoxicity. Phase IV occurs in 4 to 14 days with hepatic enzyme abnormalities reaching resolution. If extensive liver damage has occurred, sepsis and disseminated intravascular coagulation may ensue. Death can occur at 7 to 14 days. Transient renal failure may develop at 5 to 7 days with or without evidence of hepatic damage. Rare cases of myocarditis and pancreatitis have been reported. *Management:* (1) GI decontamination: Emesis may be useful within 30 minutes. However, it may interfere with the retention of activated charcoal (AC) and NAC. Gastric lavage is not necessary if AC is administered early.

TABLE 27. **Substances Usually Nontoxic When Ingested (Unless Ingested in Very Large Quantity)**

Abrasives	Lipstick
Acne preparations	Lubricants
Adhesives	Lysol disinfectant spray (70% ethanol), not the
A and D ointment	bowl cleaner
Air fresheners	Magic Marker
Ajax cleanser	Makeup (eye, liquid facial)
Aluminum foil	Mascara (domestic)
Antacids	Massengil disposable douches
Antibiotic ointments	Matches (book type, three books)
Antiperspirants	Mineral oil (unless aspirated)
Ashes (wood, fireplace)	Miracle-Gro plant food
Automobile wax	Newspaper
Baby products, cosmetics	Nutrasweet
Baby wipes	PAAS easter egg dyes (after 1980)
Ballpoint pen inks	Paints (indoor latex acrylic)
Bath oil (castor oil and perfume)	Paste, library type
Bathtub floating toys	Pencil lead (graphite)
Battery (conventional, if bitten)	Perfumes*
Bleach, less than 5%	Preparation H suppository or ointment
Body conditioners	Saccharin
Bubble bath soaps (detergents)	Sachets (essential oils)
Calamine lotion	Shampoo (liquid)
Clotrimazole (Lotrimin) cream	Shaving creams and lotions
Dehumidifying packets (silica or charcoal)	Shoe polish
Deodorants (spray and refrigerator)	Silica gel
Deodorants (underarm)	Silly Putty
Detergents (phosphate type, anionic)	Soaps and soap products
Dishwashing liquid soap (not automatic electric	Soil
dishwasher)—Mr. Clean, Dawn, Joy, Tide, Wisk	Spackles
Disposable diapers—not aspirated	Starch
Easter egg dyes	Sunscreen and suntan preparations
Erasers	Sweetening agents (saccharin, aspartame)
Etch A Sketch	Teething rings (fluid may have unsterile water
Eye makeup: pencil, shadow, mascara	and bacteria)
Fabric softener	Thermometers (mercury, alcohol)
Felt-tipped markers and pens	Toilet water*
Fertilizer (nitrogen, phosphoric acid, and potash, no	Toothpaste (even with fluoride)
insecticide or herbicides)	Vaseline
Fingernail polish	Vitamins (even with fluoride)
Finger paint	Warfarin (single dose, <0.5%)
Lanolin	Water color paint
Latex paint	Windex glass cleaner with ammonia
Laxatives	

*May contain high amounts of ethanol.

Studies have indicated that AC is useful within 4 hours after ingestion. MDAC has not been well studied. AC does adsorb NAC if they are given together, but this is not clinically important. However, if AC must be given along with NAC, separate the administration of AC from that of NAC by 1 to 2 hours to avoid vomiting. Use saline sulfate cathartic in adults because it can enhance the activity of the sulfate metabolic pathway, which may be hepatoprotective. (2) NAC (Table 28; also see Table 12). NAC, a deriva-

tive of the amino acid cysteine, acts as a sulfhydryl donor for glutathione synthesis and may enhance the nontoxic sulfation pathway, resulting in conjugation of NAPQI. Oral NAC should be administered within the first 8 hours after a toxic amount of APAP has been ingested. NAC may be started while the results of the blood tests for the acetaminophen plasma concentration (APC) are awaited, but there is no advantage to giving it before 8 hours. If the APC more than 4 hours after ingestion is above the lower line on

TABLE 28. **Protocol for *N*-Acetylcysteine Administration**

Route	Loading Dose	Maintenance Dose	Course Duration (h)	FDA Approval
Oral	140 mg/kg	70 mg/kg q 4 h	72	Yes
Intravenous (England, Canada)	150 mg/kg over 15 min	50 mg/kg over 4 h followed by 100 mg/kg over 16 h	20	No
Intravenous (investigational in United States)	140 mg/kg	70 mg/kg q 4 h	48	No

the modified Rumack-Matthew nomogram (Figure 2), continue the full 17-dose maintenance course. Repeated blood specimens should be obtained 4 hours after the initial level if it is greater than 20 μg per mL because of unexpected delays in the peak caused by food and coingestants. An IV preparation (see Table 28) has been used in Europe and Canada for about 20 years but is not approved in the United States (studies are in progress). There have been a few anaphylactoid reactions and deaths with the IV route. *Variations in therapy:* (a) In patients with chronic alcoholism it is recommended that NAC be administered at 50% below the lower toxic line on the nomogram. (b) If emesis occurs within 1 hour after NAC administration, the dose should be repeated. To avoid emesis, use the proper dilution from 20 to 5% NAC, and serve in a palatable vehicle in a covered container with a straw. If this is unsuccess-

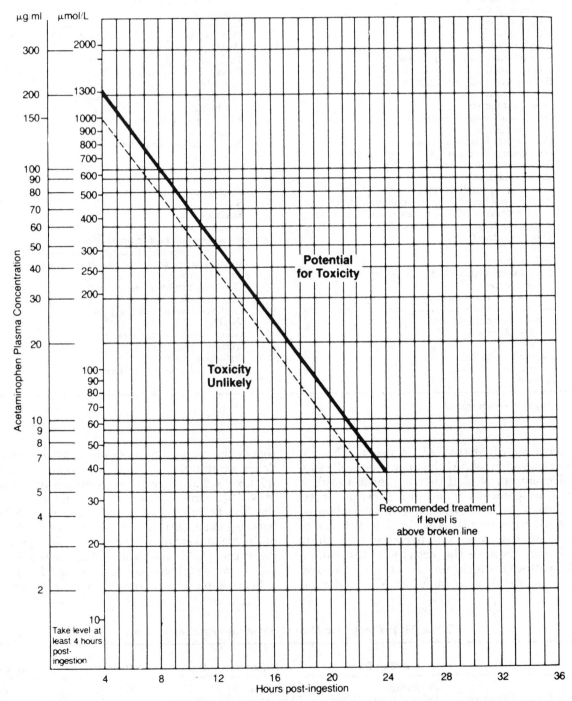

Figure 2. Nomogram for acetaminophen intoxication. Start *N*-acetylcysteine therapy if levels and time coordinates are above the lower line on the nomogram. Continue and complete therapy even if subsequent values fall below the toxic zone. The nomogram is useful only in acute, single ingestions. Levels in serum drawn before 4 hours may not represent peak levels. (From Rumack BH, Matthew H: Acetaminophen poisoning and toxicity. Reproduced by permission of Pediatrics, Vol 55, Page 871, Figure 2, Copyright 1975.)

ful, administer through a nasogastric tube or a fluoroscopically placed nasoduodenal tube by a slow drip over 30 to 60 minutes. Antiemetics may be used if necessary: metoclopramide (Reglan) at 10 mg per dose IV a half-hour before NAC (child: 0.1 mg per kg with a maximum of 0.5 mg per kg per day) or as a last resort ondansetron (Zofran) at 32 mg (0.15 mg per kg) by infusion over 15 minutes and repeat for 3 doses if necessary. The side effects of ondansetron are anaphylaxis and increases in liver enzyme values. (c) Some investigators recommend variable durations of NAC therapy, stopping the therapy if the APC becomes nondetectable in serial determinations and the liver enzymes (ALT and AST) remain normal after 36 hours. (d) Time of administration: There is a loss of efficacy if NAC is initiated more than 8 to 10 hours after ingestion, but the loss is not complete and NAC may be initiated 36 or more hours after ingestion. Late treatment (after 24 hours) has been shown to decrease the morbidity and mortality in fulminant liver failure caused by acetaminophen and other etiologic agents. (e) Extended-relief caplet (ER is embossed on the caplet) contains 325 mg of immediate-release and 325 mg of delayed-release formulations. A single serum APAP determination 4 hours after ingestion can underestimate the dose because the extended-release formulation can yield secondary delayed peaks. In overdoses of extended-release formulation, it is recommended that additional APAP levels at 4-hour intervals after the initial level be obtained. If any peak is in the toxic zone, initiate therapy. (3) Pregnancy: It is recommended that pregnant patients with toxic plasma concentrations of APAP be treated with NAC to prevent hepatotoxicity in both fetus and mother. The available data suggest no teratogenicity caused by NAC or APAP. (4) Chronic intoxication: Indications for NAC therapy are a history of 3 to 4 grams for several days, elevated liver enzyme values (AST and ALT), and chronic alcoholism or use of chronic enzyme inducers. (5) Specific support care may be needed to treat liver failure, pancreatitis, transient renal failure, and myocarditis. (6) Liver transplantation has a definite but limited role in acute APAP overdose. According to a retrospective analysis, a continuing rise in the prothrombin time (4 day peak, 180 seconds), pH less than 7.3 (2 days after overdose), serum creatinine greater than 3.3 mg per dL, severe hepatic encephalopathy, and a disturbed coagulation factor VII/V ratio of more than 30% suggest a poor prognosis and may be indicators for hepatology consultation for consideration of OLT. (7) Extracorporeal measures are not expected to be of benefit. *Laboratory investigations:* The therapeutic reference range is 10 to 20 μg per mL. For toxic levels see the nomogram in Figure 2. Appropriate reliable methods for analysis are radioimmunoassay, high-performance liquid chromatography (HPLC), and gas chromatography. Spectroscopic assays often give falsely elevated values. Cross-reactions: bilirubin, salicylate, salicylamide, difunisal, phenols, and methyldopa increase the APAP level. Each 1 mg per dL increase in creatinine

increases the APAP plasma level 30 μg per mL. Monitor: If a toxic APAP level is present, monitor the liver profile (including AST, ALT, bilirubin, prothrombin time), serum amylase, blood glucose, CBC, platelet count, phosphate, electrolytes, bicarbonate, ECG, and urinalysis. *Disposition:* All cases of intentional ingestion require a serum APAP level obtained 4 hours or more after ingestion. Patients who ingest more than 140 mg per kg should receive therapy within 8 hours after ingestion or until the results of the APC determination 4 hours after ingestion are known.

Amphetamines (illicit methamphetamine ["ice"], diet pills, various trade names). *Analogues:* 3,4-methylenedioxymethamphetamine (MDMA; known as Ecstasy, XTC, Adam) and 3,4-methylenedioxyamphetamine (MDEA; known as Eve). Other similar stimulants are phenylpropanolamine and cocaine. *Toxic mechanism:* Amphetamines have a direct CNS stimulant effect and a sympathetic nervous system effect by releasing catecholamines from alpha- and beta-adrenergic nerve terminals but inhibiting their reuptake. Phenylpropanolamine stimulates only the beta-adrenergic receptors. *Toxic dose:* Child, 1 mg per kg dextroamphetamine; adult, 5 mg per kg. A dose of 12 mg per kg has been reported to be lethal. *Kinetics:* Amphetamine is a weak base with a pK_a of 8 to 10. Onset of action is in 30 to 60 minutes. Peak effects occur at 2 to 4 hours. The $t_{1/2}$ is pH dependent; it is 8 to 10 hours with acidic urine (pH less than 6.0) and 16 to 31 hours with alkaline urine (pH greater than 7.5). The Vd is 2 to 3 liters per kg. Elimination is 60% hepatic to a hydroxylated metabolite that may be responsible for psychotic effects. Excretion by the kidney is 30 to 40% at alkaline urine pH and 50 to 70% at acidic urine pH. *Manifestations:* Effects are seen within 30 to 60 minutes after ingestion. Restlessness, irritation and agitation, tremors and hyper-reflexia, and auditory and visual hallucinations occur. Dilated but reactive pupils, cardiac dysrhythmias (supraventricular and ventricular), tachycardia, and hyperpyrexia may precede seizures, convulsions, hypertension, paranoia, violence, intracranial hemorrhage, rhabdomyolysis, myoglobinuria, psychosis, and self-destructive behavior. Paranoid psychosis and cerebral vasculitis occur with chronic abuse. *Management* (similar to that for cocaine): (1) Provide supportive care: blood pressure and cardiac thermal monitoring and seizure precautions. Diazepam (see Table 12). (2) GI decontamination: Administer AC and MDAC. (3) Treat anxiety, agitation, and convulsions with diazepam. If diazepam fails to control seizures, use neuromuscular blockers and monitor the EEG for nonmotor seizures. Avoid neuroleptics (PTZs and butyrophenone), which can lower the seizure threshold. (4) Cardiovascular disturbances: Hypertension and tachycardia are usually transient and can be managed by titration of diazepam. Nitroprusside may be used for hypertensive crisis; use a maximal infusion rate of 10 μg per kg per minute for 10 minutes, followed by 0.3 to 2 μg per kg per minute. Myocardial ischemia is managed by oxygen, vascular access, BZPs, and nitroglycerin. Aspirin and thrombolysis are not routinely recommended because of the danger of intracranial hemorrhage. Delayed hypotension can be treated with fluids and vasopressors if needed. Life-threatening tachydysrhythmias may respond to an alpha blocker (e.g., phentolamine at 5 mg IV for adults and 0.1 mg per kg IV for children) and a short-acting beta blocker (esmolol at 500 μg per kg IV over 1 minute for adults and 300 to 500 μg per kg over 1 minute for children). Ventricular dysrhythmias may respond to lidocaine or, in a severely hemodynamically compromised patient, immediate synchronized electrical cardioversion. (5) Treat rhabdomyolysis and myoglobinuria with fluids, alkaline diuresis, and diuretics. (6) Treat hyperthermia with external cooling and cool 100% humidified oxygen. (7) If focal neurologic symptoms are present, consider a diagnosis of a cerebrovascular accident and perform CT of the head. (8) Treat paranoid ideation and threatening behavior with rapid tranquilization. (See the earlier discussion of violent patients.) (9) Observe for suicidal depression, which may follow intoxication and may require suicidal precautions. (10) Extracorporeal measures are of no benefit. *Laboratory investigations:* Monitor: ECG and cardiac monitoring, ABGs and oxygen saturation, electrolytes, blood glucose, BUN, creatinine, creatine kinase and cardiac fraction (if chest pain), and liver profile; evaluate for rhabdomyolysis and check urine for myoglobin, cocaine and metabolites, and other substances of abuse. The peak plasma concentration is 10 to 50 ng per mL 1 to 2 hours after ingestion of 10 to 25 mg. The toxic plasma concentration is 200 ng per mL. Cross-reactions occur with amphetamine derivatives (e.g., methylenedioxyamphetamine derivative [MDA], Ecstasy), brompheniramine, chlorpromazine, ephedrine, phenylpropanolamine, phentermine, phenmetrazine, ranitidine, and Vicks Inhaler (*l*-desoxyephedrine) and may give false-positive results. *Disposition:* Symptomatic patients should be observed in a monitored unit until the symptoms resolve and then observed for a short time after resolution for relapse.

Anticholinergic Agents. Drugs with anticholinergic properties include antihistamines (H₁ blockers); neuroleptics (PTZs); tricyclic antidepressants; antiparkinsonism drugs (trihexyphenidyl [Artane], benztropine [Cogentin]); over-the-counter sleep, cold, and hay fever medicines (methapyrilene); ophthalmic products (atropine); products of common plants including jimsonweed (*Datura stramonium*), deadly nightshade (*Atropa belladonna*), and henbane (*Hyoscyamus niger*); and antispasmodic agents for the bowel (atropine derivatives). *Toxic mechanism:* By competitive inhibition, anticholinergic agents block the action of acetylcholine on postsynaptic cholinergic receptor sites. The mechanism involves primarily the peripheral and CNS muscarinic receptors. *Toxic dose:* Toxic amounts of atropine are 0.05 mg per kg in a child and greater than 2 mg in adults. The minimal estimated lethal dose of atropine is greater than 10 mg in adults and greater than 2 mg in

2-year-old children. Other synthetic anticholinergic agents are less toxic, with the fatal dose varying from 10 to 100 mg. *Kinetics:* The onset of action with IV administration occurs in 2 to 4 minutes; peak effects on salivation after an IV or IM dose occur in 30 to 60 minutes. The onset after ingestion is in 30 to 60 minutes, peak action occurs in 1 to 3 hours, and the duration is 4 to 6 hours, but symptoms are prolonged with overdose or sustained-release preparations. *Manifestations:* Anticholinergic signs: hyperpyrexia ("hot as a hare"), mydriasis ("blind as a bat"), flushing of skin ("red as a beet"), dry mucosa and skin ("dry as a bone"), "Lilliputian-type" hallucinations and delirium ("mad as a hatter"), coma, dysphagia, tachycardia, moderate hypertension, and rarely convulsions and urine retention. *Management:* (1) If respiratory failure occurs, use intubation and assisted ventilation. (2) For GI decontamination, use caution with emesis in a diphenhydramine overdose because of rapid onset of action and seizures. Use AC if bowel sounds are present; MDAC is not recommended. (3) Control seizures with BZPs (diazepam or lorazepam). (4) Physostigmine (see Table 12) is not routine and is reserved for life-threatening anticholinergic effects refractory to conventional treatments. It should be administered with adequate monitoring and resuscitative equipment available. Avoid if a tricyclic antidepressant is present. (5) Relieve urine retention by catheterization to avoid reabsorption. (6) If cardiac dysrhythmias are present, treat supraventricular tachycardia only if unstable. Control ventricular dysrhythmias with lidocaine or cardioversion. (7) Control hyperpyrexia by external cooling. (8) Hemodialysis and hemoperfusion are not effective. *Laboratory investigations:* These include ABGs (in respiratory depression), electrolytes, glucose, and ECG monitoring. Anticholinergic drugs and plants are not routinely included in screens for substances of abuse. *Disposition:* Symptomatic patients should be observed in a monitored unit until the symptoms resolve and then observed for a short time after resolution for relapse.

Antihistamines (H₁-receptor antagonists). Antihistamines include the H₁-blocker "sedating anticholinergic" type. A single adult dose includes (1) ethanolamines: diphenhydramine (Benadryl) 25 to 50 mg, child 1 mg per kg; dimenhydrinate (Dramamine) 50 mg; and clemastine (Tavist) 1.34 to 2.68 mg; (2) ethylenediamines: tripelennamine (Pyribenzamine) 25 to 50 mg, child 1 mg per kg; (3) alkylamines: chlorpheniramine (Chlor-Trimeton) 4 to 8 mg, child 0.9 mg per kg; brompheniramine (Dimetane) 4 to 8 mg, child 0.125 mg per kg; (4) piperazines: cyclizine (Marezine) 50 mg, hydroxyzine (Atarax) 50 to 100 mg, child 0.6 mg per kg; meclizine (Antivert) 50 to 100 mg; and (5) phenothiazine (Phenergan) 12.5 to 25 mg, child 0.1 mg per kg.

THE H₁-BLOCKER SEDATING ANTIHISTAMINES. Many of these agents are used in combination with other medication, such as acetaminophen, aspirin, codeine, dextromethorphan, ephedrine, phenylephrine, phenylpropanolamine, and pseudoephedrine. *Toxic mechanism:* H₁ sedating type antihistamines produce blockade of cholinergic muscarinic receptors (anticholinergic action) and depress or stimulate the CNS; in large overdoses, some have a cardiac membrane-depressant effect (e.g., diphenhydramine) and cause alpha-adrenergic receptor blockade (e.g., promethazine). *Toxic dose:* For diphenhydramine, the estimated toxic oral amount in a child is 15 mg per kg and the potential lethal amount is 25 mg per kg. In an adult the potential lethal amount is 2.8 grams. Ingestion of five times the single dose of an antihistamine is toxic. *Kinetics.* Onset is in 15 to 30 minutes to 1 hour, peak occurs in 1 to 4 hours; PB is 75 to 80%; Vd is 3.3 to 6.8 liters per kg; and $t_{1/2}$ is 3 to 10 hours. Elimination is 98% hepatic by N-demethylation. Interactions with erythromycin, ketoconazole (Nizoral), and derivatives produce excessive blood levels and ventricular dysrhythmias. *Manifestations:* Exaggerated anticholinergic effects, jaundice (cyproheptadine), coma, seizures, dystonia (diphenhydramine), rhabdomyolysis (doxylamine), and in large doses cardiotoxic effects (diphenhydramine). *Management and Disposition* (see "Anticholinergic Agents"): NaHCO₃ at 1 to 2 mEq per kg IV may be useful for myocardial depression and QRS prolongation.

THE NONSEDATING SINGLE-DAILY-DOSE ANTIHISTAMINES. Single adult doses include terfenadine (Seldane) 10 mg; astemizole (Hismanal) 10 mg, child 0.6 mg per kg; loratadine (Claritin) 10 mg; fexofenadine (Allegra) 60 mg. *Toxic mechanism:* They produce peripheral H₁ blockade and do not possess anticholinergic and sedating actions. They can produce prolonged QT intervals and torsades de pointes if blood levels are elevated because of impaired hepatic function, or interactions with enzyme-inhibiting drugs (cimetidine, ketoconazole and derivatives, or macrolide antibiotics). Loratadine and fexofenadine have not been reported to have these drug interactions. *Toxic dose:* An adult with an overdose of 3360 mg of terfenadine developed ventricular tachycardia and fibrillation that responded to lidocaine and defibrillation; a 1500-mg overdose produced hypotension. Cases of delayed serious dysrhythmias (torsades de pointes) have been reported with more than 200 mg of astemizole. *Kinetics:* Onset occurs in 1 hour, peak effects occur in 4 to 6 hours, and duration is greater than 24 hours. More than 90% protein bound. Plasma $t_{1/2}$ is 3.5 hours. Metabolism is in the GI tract and liver. Only 1% is excreted unchanged, 60% in feces and 40% in urine. The chemical structure of these medications prevents entry into the CNS. *Manifestations:* Overdose produces headache, nausea, confusion, and serious dysrhythmias (e.g., torsades de pointes). *Management:* (1) Obtain an ECG and establish cardiac monitoring. Treat dysrhythmias with standard agents. Torsades de pointes is best treated with magnesium sulfate at 4 grams or 40 mL of a 10% solution IV over 10 to 20 minutes (see Table 12) and countershock if the patient fails to respond. (2) GI decontamination with AC is advised. *Disposition:* All children who ingest nonsedating antihistamines or adults who ingest

more than the therapeutic maximal dose require close cardiac monitoring for torsades de pointes for at least 24 hours. Patients receiving concurrent macrolide antibiotics or ketoconazole should not continue to take these while receiving terfenadine or astemizole. Medical evaluation is required for chronic use of this combination.

Barbiturates. Barbiturates are used as sedatives, anesthetic agents, and anticonvulsants. *Toxic mechanism:* Barbiturates are GABA agonists (increase chloride flow and inhibit depolarization). They enhance the CNS depressant effect and depress the cardiovascular system. *Toxic dose:* (1) The short-acting barbiturates (SABs) (including the intermediate-acting agents) and their hypnotic doses are amobarbital (Amytal) 100 to 200 mg, aprobarbital (Alurate) 50 to 100 mg, butabarbital (Butisol) 50 to 100 mg, butalbital (Sandoptal) 100 to 200 mg, pentobarbital (Nembutal) 100 to 200 mg, and secobarbital (Seconal) 100 to 200 mg. They cause toxicity at lower doses than long-acting barbiturates (LABs) and have a minimal toxic dose of 6 mg per kg; the fatal adult dose is 3 to 6 grams. (2) The LABs include mephobarbital (Mebaral) 50 to 100 mg and phenobarbital (Luminal) 100 to 200 mg. These have a minimal toxic dose greater than 10 mg per kg; the fatal adult dose is 6 to 10 grams. A general rule is that an amount 5 times the hypnotic dose is toxic and 10 times the hypnotic dose is potentially fatal. Methohexital and thiopental are ultra-short-acting (USA) parenteral preparations and are not discussed. *Kinetics:* They are enzyme inducers. (1) SABs are highly lipid soluble, penetrate the brain readily, and have shorter elimination times. Onset is in 10 to 30 minutes, the peak occurs in 1 to 2 hours, the duration is 3 to 8 hours. The Vd is 0.8 to 1.5 liters per kg. The pK_a is about 8. Mean $t_{1/2}$ varies from 8 to 48 hours. (2) LABs have longer elimination times and may be used as anticonvulsants. Onset is in 20 to 60 minutes, the peak occurs in 1 to 6 hours or in an overdose 10 hours, and the duration is greater than 8 to 12 hours. The Vd is 0.8 liter per kg. The pK_a of phenobarbital is 7.2 and alkalinization of urine promotes its excretion. The $t_{1/2}$ is 11 to 120 hours. *Manifestations:* In mild intoxication, the initial symptoms resemble those of alcohol intoxication and include ataxia, slurred speech, and depressed cognition. Severe intoxication causes slow respirations, coma, and loss of reflexes (except pupillary light reflex). Hypotension (venodilatation), hypothermia, and hypoglycemia occur and death is by respiratory arrest. Bullous skin lesions ("barb burns") over pressure points may be present. Barbiturates can precipitate an attack of acute intermittent porphyria. *Management:* (1) Establish and maintain the vital functions. Intense supportive care including intubation and assisted ventilation should dominate the management. All stuporous and comatose patients should have glucose, thiamine, and naloxone IV and be admitted to the intensive care unit (ICU). (2) GI decontamination: Avoid emesis, especially in SAB ingestions. AC with a single-dose cathartic, followed by MDAC (0.5

gram per kg) every 2 to 4 hours, has been shown to reduce the serum $t_{1/2}$ of phenobarbital by 50% but its effect on the clinical course is undetermined. (3) Fluid management: Administer fluids to correct dehydration and hypotension. Vasopressors may be necessary to correct severe hypotension and hemodynamic monitoring may be needed. Observe carefully for fluid overload. (4) Alkalinization (ion trapping) is used for phenobarbital (pK_a 7.2) but not for SABs. $NaHCO_3$, 1 to 2 mEq per kg IV in 500 mL of 5% dextrose for adults or 10 to 15 mL per kg for children during the first hour, followed by sufficient bicarbonate to keep the urine pH at 7.5 to 8.0, enhances excretion of phenobarbital and shortens the $t_{1/2}$ by 50% (see Table 12). Diuresis is not advocated because of the danger of cerebral or pulmonary edema. (5) Hemodialysis shortens the $t_{1/2}$ to 8 to 14 hours and charcoal hemoperfusion shortens the $t_{1/2}$ to 6 to 8 hours. Both may be effective for both LABs and SABs. If the patient does not respond to supportive measures or if the phenobarbital plasma concentration is greater than 150 µg per mL, both procedures may be tried to shorten the $t_{1/2}$. (6) Treat any bullae as a local second-degree skin burn. (7) Treat hypothermia. *Laboratory investigations:* Most barbiturates are detected by routine drug screens and can be measured in most hospital laboratories. Monitor barbiturate levels, ABGs, a toxicology screen including acetaminophen and ethanol, glucose, electrolytes, BUN, creatinine, creatine kinase, and urine pH. Minimal toxic plasma levels are greater than 10 µg per mL for SABs and greater than 40 µg per mL for LABs. Fatal levels are 30 µg per mL for SABs and greater than 80 to 150 µg per mL for LABs. SABs and LABs can be detected in urine 24 to 72 hours after ingestion and LABs up to 7 days. *Disposition:* All comatose patients should be admitted to the ICU. Awake and oriented patients with an overdose of an SAB should be observed for at least 6 asymptomatic hours and those with an overdose of an LAB for at least 12 asymptomatic hours. In an intentional overdose, psychiatric clearance is needed before discharge. Chronic use can lead to tolerance, physical dependence, and withdrawal and requires follow-up.

Benzodiazepines. BZPs are used as anxiolytics, sedatives, and relaxants. *Toxic mechanism:* GABA agonists produce CNS depression and increase chloride flow, inhibiting depolarization. *Toxic dose:* In the elderly the therapeutic dose should be reduced 50%. BZPs have an additive effect with other CNS depressants. (1) For long-acting (LA) BZPs ($t_{1/2}$ greater than 24 hours), the maximal therapeutic doses are chlordiazepoxide (Librium) 50 mg, clorazepate (Tranxene) 30 mg, clonazepam (Klonopin) 20 mg, diazepam (Valium) 10 mg or 0.2 mg per kg for children, flurazepam (Dalmane) 30 mg, and prazepam (Centrex) 20 mg. (2) Short-acting (SA) BZPs ($t_{1/2}$ 10 to 24 hours) include alprazolam (Xanax) 0.5 mg and lorazepam (Ativan) 4 mg or 0.05 mg per kg for children, which act similarly to the LABZPs. (3) The BZPs that are USA ($t_{1/2}$ less than 10 hours) are more toxic and include temazepam (Restoril) 30 mg, triazolam (Halcion) 0.5

mg, midazolam (Versed) 0.2 mg per kg, and oxazepam (Serax) 30 mg. (4) In overdoses: LABZPs: 10 to 20 times the therapeutic dose (greater than 1500 mg of diazepam or 2000 mg of chlordiazepoxide) has been ingested with mild coma without respiratory depression. Fatalities are rare, and most patients recover within 24 to 36 hours after overdose with LABZPs and SABZPs. Asymptomatic nonintentional overdoses of less than five times the therapeutic dose may be observed. USABZPs have produced respiratory arrest and coma within 1 hour after 5 mg of triazolam and death with ingestion of as little as 10 mg. Midazolam and diazepam administered by rapid IV injection have produced respiratory arrest. *Kinetics:* Onset of CNS depression is usually in 30 to 120 minutes, and the peak usually occurs within 1 to 3 hours with the oral route. The Vd is 0.26 to 6 liters per kg (LABZP, 1.1 liter per kg). PB is 70 to 99%. *Manifestations:* Ataxia, slurred speech, and CNS depression. Deep coma leading to respiratory depression suggests the presence of SABZPs or a search for other causes. *Management:* (1) GI decontamination: Emesis should be avoided. Gastric lavage (within 1 hour) and AC are advised if the ingestion was recent. (2) Supportive treatment should be provided but intubation and assisted ventilation are rarely required. (3) Flumazenil (see Table 12) is a specific BZP receptor antagonist that blocks chloride flow and inhibitor neurotransmitters. It reverses sedative effects of BZPs, zolpidem (Ambien), and endogenous BZPs associated with hepatic encephalopathy. It is not recommended to reverse BZP-induced hypoventilation. It should be used with caution in overdoses if there is possible BZP dependence (can precipitate life-threatening withdrawal), if a cyclic antidepressant is suspected, or if the patient has a known seizure disorder. *Laboratory investigations:* Most BZPs can be detected in urinary drug screens. Quantitative blood levels are not useful. The BZPs usually not detected in urinary screens include alprazolam, clonazepam, flunitrazepam,* lorazepam, lormetazepam,* midazolam, oxazepam, temazepam, and triazolam. BZPs may not be detected if the dose is less than 10 mg, elimination is rapid, or there are different or no metabolites. Cross-reactions occur with NSAIDs (tolmetin, naproxen, etodolac, and fenoprofen). *Disposition:* If the patient is comatose, admit to the ICU. If the overdose was intentional, psychiatric clearance is needed before discharge. Chronic use can lead to tolerance, physical dependence, and withdrawal.

Beta-Adrenergic Blockers (beta blockers). Beta blockers are used in the treatment of hypertension and a number of systemic and ophthalmologic disorders. Lipid-soluble drugs have CNS effects, active metabolites, a longer duration of action, and interactions with other drugs (e.g., propranolol). Cardioselectivity is lost in overdoses. Intrinsic partial agonist agents (e.g., pindolol) may initially produce tachycardia and hypertension. A cardiac membrane depressive effect (quinidine-like) occurs with overdose but not therapeutic doses (e.g., metoprolol, sotalol).

*Not available in the United States.

The alpha-blocking effect is weak (e.g., labetalol). Properties of beta blockers include the factors listed in Table 29. *Toxic mechanism:* Beta blockers compete with the catecholamines for receptor sites and block receptor action in the bronchi and the vascular smooth muscle and myocardium. *Toxic dose:* Ingestions of more than twice the maximal recommended daily therapeutic dose are considered toxic (Table 30). Ingestion of propranolol at 1 mg per kg by a child may produce hypoglycemia. Fatalities have been reported in adults with 7.5 grams of metoprolol. The most toxic agent is sotalol and the least toxic atenolol. *Kinetics:* Regular release usually causes symptoms within 2 hours. Propranolol's onset of action is in 20 to 30 minutes; the peak is at 1 to 4 hours but may be delayed with coingestants and sustained-release preparations. The duration is 4 to 6 hours but in overdoses may be 24 to 48 hours and longer with the sustained-release type. With sustained-release preparations the onset may be delayed 6 hours and the peak 12 to 16 hours; the duration may be 24 to 48 hours. The regular preparation with the longest $t_{1/2}$ is nadolol (12 to 24 hours) and with the shortest is esmolol (5 to 10 minutes). The PB is

TABLE 29. **Pharmacologic and Toxic Properties of Beta Blockers***

Name	Dose	Lipid Solubility	Intrinsic Sympathomimetic Activity (Partial Agonist)	Membrane-Stabilizing Effect	Cardiac Selectivity (Beta Selective)	Alpha Blocker
Acebutolol (Sectral)	Maximal daily dose 800 mg, therapeutic plasma level 200–2000 ng/mL	Moderate	+	+	+	+
Alprenolol†	Maximal daily dose 800 mg, therapeutic plasma level 50–200 ng/mL	Moderate	2+	+	−	−
Atenolol (Tenormin)	Maximal daily dose 100 mg, therapeutic plasma level 200–500 ng/mL	Low	−	−	2+	−
Betaxolol (Kerlone)	Maximal daily dose 20 mg, therapeutic plasma level NA	Low	+	−	+	−
Carteolol (Cartrol)	Maximal daily dose 10 mg, therapeutic plasma level NA	No	+	−	−	−
Esmolol (Brevibloc) Class II antidysrhythmic, IV only		Low	−	−	+	−
Labetalol (Trandate)	Maximal daily dose 800 mg, therapeutic plasma level 50–500 ng/mL	Low	+	±	−	+
Levobunolol (eye drops 0.25% and 0.5%)	Maximal daily dose 20 mg, therapeutic plasma level NA	No	−	−	−	−
Metoprolol (Lopressor)	Maximal daily dose 450 mg, therapeutic plasma level 50–100 ng/mL	Moderate	−	−	2+	−
Nadolol (Corgard)	Maximal daily dose 320 mg, therapeutic plasma level 20–400 ng/mL	Low	−	−	−	−
Oxyprenolol†	Maximal daily dose 480 mg, therapeutic plasma level 80–100 ng/mL	Moderate	2+	+	−	−
Pindolol (Visken)	Maximal daily dose 60 mg, therapeutic plasma level 50–150 ng/mL	Moderate	3+	±	−	−
Propranolol (Inderal) (class II antidysrhythmic)	Maximal daily dose 360 mg, therapeutic plasma level 50–100 ng/mL	High	−	2+	−	−
Sotalol (Betapace) (class III antidysrhythmic)	Maximal daily dose 480 mg, therapeutic plasma level 500–4000 ng/mL	Low	−	−	−	−
Timolol (Blocadren)	Maximal daily dose 60 mg, therapeutic plasma level 5–10 ng/mL	Low	−	±	−	−

*− indicates no effect; + indicates mild effect; 2+ indicates moderate effect; 3+ indicates severe effect; ± indicates no effect or mild effect; NA indicates not available.
†Not available in the United States.

TABLE 30. **Carbon Monoxide Exposure and Possible Manifestations**

CO in Atmosphere (%)	Duration of Exposure (h)	COHb Saturation (%)	Manifestations
<0.0035 (35 ppm)	Indefinite	3.5	None
0.005–0.01 (50–100 ppm)	Indefinite	5	Slight headache, decreased exercise tolerance
Up to 0.01 (100 ppm)	Indefinite	10	Slight headache, dyspnea on vigorous exertion, may impair driving skills
0.01–0.02 (100–200 ppm)	Indefinite	10–20	Moderate dyspnea on exertion; throbbing, temporal headache
0.02–0.03 (200–300 ppm)	5–6	20–30	Severe headache, syncope, dizziness, visual changes, weakness, nausea, vomiting, altered judgment
0.04–0.06 (400–600 ppm)	4–5	30–40	Vertigo, ataxia, blurred vision, confusion, loss of consciousness
0.07–0.10 (700–1000 ppm)	3–4	40–50	Confusion, tachycardia, tachypnea, coma, convulsions
0.11–0.15 (1100–1500 ppm)	1.5–3	50–60	Cheyne-Stokes respiration, coma, convulsions, shock, apnea
0.16–0.30 (1600–3000 ppm)	1.0–1.5	60–70	Coma, convulsions, respiratory and heart failure, death
>0.40 (>4000 ppm)	Few minutes		Death

Abbreviation: COHb = carboxyhemoglobin.

variable, 5 to 93%. The Vd is 1 to 5.6 liters per kg. Atenolol, nadolol, and sotalol have enterohepatic recirculation. *Manifestations:* See toxic properties and Table 30. Lipid-soluble agents produce coma and seizures. Bradycardia and hypotension are the major symptoms and may lead to cardiogenic shock. Intrinsic partial agonists may initially cause tachycardia and hypertension. Bronchospasm may occur in patients with reactive airway disease with any beta blocker because the selectivity is lost in overdoses. ECG changes include atrioventricular (AV) conduction delay and frank asystole. Membrane-depressant effects produce prolonged QRS and QT intervals which may result in torsades de pointes. Sotalol produces a prolonged QT. Hypoglycemia (blocking of catecholamine counter-regulatory mechanisms) and hyperkalemia may occur, especially in children. *Management:* (1) Establish and maintain vital functions. Establish vascular access, a baseline ECG, and continuous cardiac and blood pressure monitoring. Have a pacemaker available. Hypotension is treated with fluids initially, although it usually does not respond. Frequently, glucagon and cardiac pacing are needed. Cardiology consultation should be sought. (2) GI decontamination is done initially with AC and a single-dose cathartic. MDAC is recommended for symptomatic patients with ingestions of beta blockers with enterohepatic recirculation or sustained release (no data). Gastric lavage is done if it is less than 1 hour after ingestion. If gastric lavage is done, use prelavage atropine (0.02 mg per kg for a child and 0.5 mg for an adult) and cardiac monitoring. Whole-bowel irrigation should be considered in large overdoses with sustained-release preparations (no studies). (3) Cardiovascular disturbances: Obtain cardiac consultation. Class IA (procainamide, quinidine) and class III (bretylium) antidysrhythmic agents are not recommended. Bradycardia in asymptomatic hemodynamically stable patients requires no therapy. It is not predictive of the future course. If the patient is unstable (has hypotension or high-degree AV block), use atropine at 0.02 mg per kg up to 2 mg in adults,

glucagon, and a pacemaker. In ventricular tachycardia use overdrive pacing. A wide QRS interval may respond to NaHCO$_3$ (see Table 12). Torsades de pointes (associated with sotalol) may respond to magnesium sulfate (see Table 12) and overdrive pacing. Prophylactic magnesium for a prolonged QT interval has been suggested but there are no data. Do not use epinephrine, because an unopposed alpha effect may occur. Hypotension and myocardial depression are managed by correction of dysrhythmias, Trendelenburg's position, fluids, glucagon, and/or amrinone (Inocor). Hemodynamic monitoring may be needed to manage fluid therapy. Glucagon (see Table 12) is the initial drug of choice. It works through adenylate cyclase and bypasses catecholamine receptors, so it is not affected by beta blockers. It increases cardiac contractility and heart rate. It is given as an IV bolus of 5 to 10 mg* over 1 minute, followed by continuous infusion at 1 to 5 mg per hour (children, 0.15 mg per kg followed by 0.05 to 0.1 mg per kg per hour). In large doses and in infusion therapy use D5W, sterile water, or saline as the diluent to reconstitute glucagon in place of the 0.2% phenol diluent provided with some drugs. Effects are seen within minutes. It can be used with other agents such as amrinone. Amrinone inhibits the enzyme phosphodiesterase, which metabolizes cyclic AMP. Administer a bolus of 0.15 to 2 mg per kg (0.15 to 0.4 mL per kg) IV followed by infusion of 5 to 10 µg per kg per minute. (4) Treat hypoglycemia with IV glucose and emergency hyperkalemia with calcium (avoid if digoxin is present), bicarbonate, and glucose. (5) Control convulsions with diazepam or phenobarbital. (6) If bronchospasm is present, give beta$_2$ nebulized bronchodilators and aminophylline. (7) Extraordinary measures include intra-aortic balloon pump support. (8) Extracorporeal measures: Hemodialysis for atenolol, acebutalol, nadolol, and sotalol (low Vd, low PB) may be helpful, particularly with evidence of renal failure. It is not effective for propranolol, metoprolol, and timolol. (9)

---

*Exceeds dosage recommended by the manufacturer.

Investigational: Prenalterol has successfully reversed both bradycardia and hypotension (it is not available in the United States). *Laboratory investigations:* Measurement of blood levels is not readily available or useful. (For propranolol the toxic level is greater than 2 ng per mL.) Monitor: ECG and cardiac monitoring, blood glucose and electrolytes, BUN, creatinine, and ABGs if respiratory symptoms are present. *Disposition:* Asymptomatic patients with a history of overdose require a baseline ECG and continuous cardiac monitoring for at least 6 hours with regular-release preparations and for 24 hours with sustained-release preparations. Symptomatic patients should be observed with cardiac monitoring for 24 hours. If seizures, abnormal rhythm, or vital signs indicate, admit to the ICU.

Calcium Channel Blockers. These agents are used in the treatment of effort angina, supraventricular tachycardia, and hypertension. *Toxic mechanism:* Calcium channel blockers reduce the influx of calcium through the slow channels in membranes of the myocardium, the AV nodes, and vascular smooth muscles and result in peripheral, systemic, and coronary vasodilatation, impaired cardiac conduction, and depression of cardiac contractility. All calcium channel blockers have vasodilatory action, but only bepridil, diltiazem, and verapamil depress myocardial contractility and cause an AV block. *Toxic dose:* Any ingested amount greater than the maximal daily dose has the potential of being severely toxic. The maximal oral daily doses are amlodipine (Norvasc) 10 mg; bepridil (Vascor) 400 mg; diltiazem (Cardizem) 360 mg, toxic dose greater than 2 grams, child 6 mg per kg; felodipine (Plendil) 10 mg; isradipine (DynaCirc) 20 mg; nicardipine (Cardene) 120 mg; nifedipine (Procardia) 120 mg, child 0.9 mg per kg per day; nimodipine (Nimotop) 360 mg; nitrendipine (Baypress)* 80 mg; and verapamil (Calan) 480 mg, child 4 to 8 mg per kg. *Kinetics:* Onset of action of regular-release preparations varies: verapamil, 60 to 120 minutes; nifedipine, 20 minutes; diltiazem, 15 minutes after ingestion. The peak effect for verapamil is at 2 to 4 hours, nifedipine 60 to 90 minutes, and diltiazem 30 to 60 minutes; however, the peak action may be delayed for 6 to 8 hours. The duration is up to 36 hours. With sustained-release preparations the onset is usually at 4 hours but may be delayed; the peak effect is at 12 to 24 hours; and concretions and prolonged toxicity can develop. The $t_{1/2}$ for hepatic elimination varies from 3 to 7 hours. The Vd varies from 3 to 7 liters per kg. *Manifestations:* Hypotension, bradycardia, and conduction disturbances occur 30 minutes to 5 hours after ingestion. A prolonged PR interval is an early and constant finding and may occur at therapeutic doses. Torsades de pointes has been reported. All degrees of blocks may occur and may be delayed 12 to 16 hours. Lactic acidosis may be present. It does not affect intraventricular conduction, so the QRS interval is usually not affected. Hypocalcemia is rarely present.

---

*Not available in the United States.

Hyperglycemia may be present because of calcium-dependent insulin release. Mental status changes, headaches, seizures, hemiparesis, and CNS depression may occur. Calcium channel blockers may precipitate respiratory failure in Duchenne's muscular dystrophy. *Management:* (1) Establish and maintain vital functions. Obtain a baseline ECG and have continuous cardiac and blood pressure monitoring. A pacemaker should be available. Cardiac consultation should be sought. (2) GI decontamination: AC is recommended and MDAC may be useful (no data). If a large sustained-release preparation is involved, consider MDAC for 48 to 72 hours and whole-bowel irrigation, but the effectiveness has not been investigated. (3) If the patient is symptomatic, obtain immediate cardiac consultation because a pacemaker and hemodynamic monitoring may be needed. (4) If a heart block occurs, atropine is rarely effective and isoproterenol may produce vasodilatation. Consider the use of a pacemaker early. (5) Treat hypotension and bradycardia with positioning, fluids, and calcium gluconate or calcium chloride, glucagon, amrinone, and ventricular pacing. Calcium gluconate or calcium chloride (see Table 12): Avoid calcium salts if digoxin is present. Calcium usually reverses depressed myocardial contractility but may not reverse nodal depression or peripheral vasodilatation. Calcium chloride is used as a 10% solution at 0.1 to 0.2 mL per kg up to 10 mL in an adult or calcium gluconate as a 10% solution at 0.3 to 0.4 mL per kg up to 20 mL in an adult. Administer IV over 5 to 10 minutes. Monitor for dysrhythmias, hypotension, and serum calcium. The aim is to increase the calcium value 4 mg per dL to a maximum of 13 mg per dL. The calcium response lasts 15 minutes and may require repeated doses or a continuous calcium gluconate infusion (0.2 mL per kg per hour up to a maximum of 10 mL per hour). If calcium fails, try glucagon (see Table 12) for its positive inotropic or chronotropic effect or both. Amrinone, an inotropic agent, may reverse calcium channel blockers. The effective dose is 0.15 to 2 mg per kg (0.15 to 0.4 mL per kg) by IV bolus followed by infusion of 5 to 10 µg per kg per minute. (6) Hypotension: Fluids, norepinephrine, and epinephrine may be required for hypotension. Amrinone and glucagon have been tried alone and in combination. Dobutamine and dopamine are often ineffective. (7) Extracorporeal measures (e.g., hemodialysis and charcoal hemoperfusion) are not considered useful. (8) Patients receiving digitalis and calcium channel blockers run the risk of digitalis toxicity because calcium channel blockers increase digitalis levels. (9) Extraordinary measures such as the intra-aortic balloon pump and cardiopulmonary bypass have been used successfully. (10) Hyperglycemia does not require insulin therapy. *Laboratory investigations:* Specific drug levels are not easily available and are not useful. Monitor blood glucose, electrolytes, calcium, ABGs, pulse oximetry, creatinine, BUN, hemodynamics, ECG, and cardiac function. *Disposition:* Monitor for regular-release preparations for at least 6 hours and for sustained-release preparations for 24 hours after alleged ingestion. For intentional overdose, psychiatric clearance is needed. Symptomatic patients should be admitted to the ICU.

Carbon Monoxide. CO is an odorless, colorless gas produced by incomplete combustion; it is an in vivo metabolic breakdown product of methylene chloride used in paint removers. *Toxic mechanism:* The affinity of CO for hemoglobin is 240 times greater than that of oxygen; it shifts the oxygen dissociation curve to the left, which impairs hemoglobin release of oxygen to tissues, and inhibits the cytochrome oxidase system. *Toxic dose and manifestations:* See Table 30. CO exposure and manifestations: Exposure to 0.5% for a few minutes is lethal. Contrary to popular belief, the skin rarely shows a cherry red color in the living patient. Sequelae correlate with the level of consciousness at presentation. ECG abnormalities may be noted. Creatine kinase is often elevated; rhabdomyolysis and myoglobinuria may occur. The carboxyhemoglobin (COHb) expresses as a percentage the extent to which CO has bound with the total hemoglobin. This may be misleading in the anemic patient. The patient's presentation is more reliable than the COHb level. The manifestations listed for each level are in addition to those already listed at the preceding level. Note that 0.01% = 100 ppm. A level greater than 40% is usually associated with obvious intoxication. The COHb may not correlate reliably with the severity of the intoxication, and linking symptoms to specific levels of COHb is frequently inaccurate. *Kinetics:* The natural metabolism of the body produces small amounts of COHb, less than 2% for nonsmokers and 5 to 9% for smokers. CO is rapidly absorbed through the lungs. The rate of absorption is directly related to alveolar ventilation. Elimination occurs through the lungs. The $t_{1/2}$ of COHb in room air (21% oxygen) is 5 to 6 hours; in 100% oxygen, 90 minutes; in hyperbaric oxygen at 3 atmospheres oxygen, 20 to 30 minutes. *Management:* (1) Adequately protect the rescuer. Remove the patient from the contaminated area. Establish vital functions. (2) The mainstay of treatment is 100% oxygen via a non-rebreathing mask with an oxygen reservoir or endotracheal tube. Give 100% oxygen to all patients until the COHb level is 2% or less. Assisted ventilation may be necessary. (3) Monitor ABGs and COHb. Determine the present COHb level and extrapolate to the COHb level at the time of exposure using the $t_{1/2}$ of COHb in different percentages of ambient oxygen (see kinetics just discussed). Note: A near-normal COHb level does not exclude significant CO poisoning, especially if measured several hours after the termination of exposure or if oxygen has been administered before obtaining the sample. (4) The exposed pregnant woman should be kept in 100% oxygen for several hours after the COHb level is almost zero because COHb concentrates in the fetus and oxygen is needed longer to ensure elimination of CO from the fetal circulation. Monitor the fetus. CO and hypoxia are teratogenic. (5) Metabolic acidosis should be treated with sodium bicarbonate only if the pH is below 7.2 after correc-tion of hypoxia and adequate ventilation. Acidosis shifts the oxygen dissociation curve to the right and facilitates oxygen delivery to the tissues. (6) Use of the hyperbaric oxygen (HBO) chamber: The decision must be made on the basis of availability of a hyperbaric chamber, the ability to handle other acute emergencies that may coexist, extrapolated COHb, and the severity of the poisoning. The standard of care for persons exposed to CO has yet to be determined, but most authorities recommend HBO with any of the following guidelines: (a) if the HBO is not readily available, a COHb greater than 40%; if the HBO is readily available, COHb greater than 25%; (b) if the patient is unconscious or has a history of loss of consciousness or seizures; (c) if cardiovascular dysfunction (clinical ischemic chest pain or ECG evidence of ischemia) is present; (d) if there is metabolic acidosis; (e) if symptoms persist despite 100% oxygen therapy; (f) if there is an initial COHb greater than 15% in a child, in a patient with cardiovascular disease, or in a pregnant woman; or (g) if there are signs of maternal or fetal distress regardless of COHb level. Infants and fetuses are a special problem because fetal hemoglobin has greater affinity for CO than adult hemoglobin. A neurologic-cognitive examination has been used to help determine which patients with low CO levels should receive more aggressive therapy. Testing should include the following: general orientation memory testing (address, phone number, date of birth, present date) and cognitive testing (serial 7s, digit span, forward and backward spelling of three-letter and four-letter words). Patients with delayed neurologic sequelae or recurrent symptoms for up to 3 weeks may benefit from HBO treatment. (7) Treat seizures and cerebral edema. *Laboratory investigations:* ABGs may show metabolic acidosis and normal oxygen tension. If there is significant poisoning, monitor the ABGs, electrolytes, blood glucose, serum creatine kinase and cardiac enzymes, renal function, and liver function. Obtain a urinalysis and test for myoglobinuria. Obtain a chest radiograph if there has been smoke inhalation or the patient is considered for HBO chamber. ECG monitoring is needed especially if the patient is older than 40 years, has a cardiac history, or has moderate to severe symptoms. Determine the blood ethanol level and conduct toxicology studies on the basis of symptoms and circumstances. Monitor COHb during and at the end of therapy. The pulse oximeter has two wavelengths and overestimates oxyhemoglobin saturation in CO poisoning. The true oxygen saturation is determined by blood gas analysis measuring the oxygen bound to hemoglobin. The co-oximeter measures four wavelengths and separates out COHb and the other hemoglobin-binding agents from oxyhemoglobin. Fetal hemoglobin has a greater affinity for CO than does adult hemoglobin and the COHb may be falsely elevated as much as 4% in young infants. *Disposition:* Patients with no or mild symptoms (less than 5 minutes) who become asymptomatic after a few hours of oxygen therapy and have a CO level below 10%, a normal physical examination, a normal neurologic-cognitive examination, and normal arterial gas parameters may be discharged but instructed to return if there are any signs of neurologic dysfunction. Patients with CO poisoning requiring treatment need follow-up neuropsychiatric examinations.

Caustics and Corrosives. The U.S. Consumer Products Safety Commission labeling recommendations on containers for acids and alkalis indicate the potential for producing serious damage: caution (weak irritant), warning (strong irritant), danger (corrosive). Some common acids with corrosive potential are acetic acid (>50%), calcium oxide, formic acid, glycolic acid (>10%), hydrochloric acid (>10%), mercuric chloride, nitric acid (>5%), oxalic acid (>10%), phosphoric acid (>60%), sulfuric acid (battery acid) (>10%), zinc chloride (>10%), and zinc sulfate (>50%). Some common alkalis with corrosive potential include ammonia (>5%), calcium carbide, calcium hydroxide (dry), potassium hydroxide (lye) (>1%), and sodium hydroxide (lye) (>1%). *Toxic mechanism:* Acids produce mucosal coagulation necrosis and an eschar and may be systemically absorbed, but with the exception of hydrofluoric acid they do not penetrate deeply. Injury to the gastric mucosa is more likely, although specific sites of injury for acids and alkalis are not clearly defined. Alkalis produce liquefaction necrosis and saponification and penetrate deeply. The esophageal mucosa is more likely to be damaged. Oropharyngeal and esophageal damage by solids is more frequent than by liquids. Liquids produce superficial, circumferential burns and gastric damage. *Toxic dose:* The toxicity is determined by concentration, contact time, and pH. Significant injury is more likely at pH values less than 2 or greater than 12, stricture at pH 14, prolonged contact time, and large volumes. *Manifestations:* The absence of oral burns does not exclude the possibility of esophageal or gastric damage. General clinical findings include stridor; dysphagia; drooling; oropharyngeal, retrosternal, and epigastric pain; and ocular and oral burns. Alkali burns are yellow, soapy, frothy lesions. Acid burns are gray-white and later form an eschar. Abdominal tenderness and guarding may be present if there is perforation. *Management:* Bring the container; the substance must be identified and the pH of the substance, vomitus, tears, and saliva tested. *Ingestion, ocular, and dermal management:* (1) Prehospital and initial hospital management. If ingestion occurs, all GI decontamination procedures are contraindicated except for immediate rinsing, removal of the substance from the mouth, and then dilution with small amounts (sips) of milk or water. Check for ocular and dermal involvement. Contraindications to oral dilution are dysphagia, respiratory distress, obtundation, and shock. If ocular involvement occurs, immediately irrigate with tepid water for at least 30 minutes, perform fluoroscein staining of the eye, and consult an ophthalmologist. If dermal involvement occurs, immediately remove contaminated clothes and irrigate the skin with tepid water for at least 15 minutes. Consult with a burn specialist. (2) For acid ingestion, some authorities advocate a small flexible nasogastric tube and aspiration within 30 minutes after ingestion. (3) The patient should receive only IV fluids after dilution until endoscopic consultation is obtained. (4) Endoscopy is valuable for predicting damage and the risk of stricture. The indications are controversial, with some authorities recommending it in all caustic ingestions regardless of symptoms, whereas others are selective, using clinical features such as vomiting, stridor, and drooling and oral or facial lesions as criteria. Endoscopy is indicated for all symptomatic patients or those with intentional ingestions. Endoscopy may be done immediately if the patient is symptomatic but is usually done 12 to 48 hours after ingestion. After 72 hours there is increased risk of perforation. (5) Corticosteroids may be ineffective and are considered mainly for second-degree circumferential burns. If used, start hydrocortisone sodium succinate IV at 10 to 20 mg per kg per day within 48 hours and change to oral prednisolone at 2 mg per kg per day. Continue prednisolone for 3 weeks and then taper the dose. (6) Provide tetanus prophylaxis. Antibiotics are not useful prophylactically. (7) An esophagogram is not useful in the first few days and may interfere with endoscopic evaluation; later it may be used to assess the severity of damage. (8) Investigative therapy includes agents to inhibit collagen formation and intraluminal stents. (9) Esophageal and gastric outlet dilatation may be needed if there is evidence of stricture. Bougienage of the esophagus has, however, been associated with brain abscess. Interposition of the colon may be necessary if dilatation fails to provide a passage of adequate size. *Inhalation management* requires immediate removal from the environment, administration of humid supplemental oxygen, and observation for airway obstruction and noncardiac pulmonary edema. Obtain radiographic and ABG evaluation when appropriate. Intubation and respiratory support may be required. Certain caustics produce systemic disturbances; formaldehyde causes metabolic acidosis; hydrofluoric acid, hypocalcemia and renal damage; oxalic acid, hypocalcemia; phenol, hepatic and renal damage; and pitric acid, renal injury. *Laboratory investigations:* If acid has been ingested, determine the acid-base balance and electrolytes. If there are pulmonary symptoms, use chest radiography, ABGs, and pulse oximetry. *Disposition:* Infants and small children should be medically evaluated and observed. Admit all symptomatic patients. Admit to the ICU if there are severe symptoms or danger of airway compromise. After endoscopy, if there is no damage, the patient may be discharged when oral feedings are tolerated. Intentional exposures require psychiatric evaluation before discharge.

Cocaine (benzoylmethylecgonine). Cocaine is derived from the leaves of *Erythroxylon coca* and *Truxillo coca*. A body packer is one who conceals many small packages of cocaine contraband in the GI tract or other areas for illicit transport. A body stuffer spontaneously ingests substances for the purpose of hiding evidence. *Toxic mechanism:* Cocaine directly stimulates CNS presynaptic sympathetic neurons to release catecholamines and acetylcholine, blocks presynaptic reuptake of the catecholamines, blocks the sodium channels along neuronal membranes, and increases platelet aggregation. Long-term use depletes the CNS of dopamine. *Toxic dose:* The maximal mucosal local anesthetic therapeutic dose is 200 mg or 2 mL of 10% solution. Psychoactive effects occur at 50 to 95 mg; cardiac and CNS effects occur at 1 mg per kg. The potential fatal dose is 1200 mg intranasally, but death has occurred with 20 mg parenterally. *Kinetics:* See Table 31. Cocaine is well absorbed by all routes including nasal insufflation and oral, dermal, and inhalation routes. It is metabolized by plasma and liver cholinesterase to the inactive metabolites ecgonine methyl ester and benzoylecgonine. Plasma pseudocholinesterase is congenitally deficient in 3% of the population and decreased in fetuses, in young infants, in elderly persons, in pregnancy, and in liver disease. Individuals with this enzyme deficit are at increased risk for life-threatening cocaine toxicity. The PB is 8.7%; the Vd, 1.2 to 1.9 liters per kg; 10% is excreted unchanged. Cocaine and ethanol undergo liver synthesis to form cocaethylene, a metabolite with a $t_{1/2}$ three times longer than that of cocaine. This metabolite may account for some of cocaine's cardiotoxicity and appears to be more lethal than cocaine or ethanol alone. *Manifestations:* (1) CNS: euphoria, hyperactivity, agitation, convulsions, intracranial hemorrhage; (2) eye-ear-nose-throat: mydriasis, septal perforation; (3) cardiovascular: cardiac dysrhythmias, hypertension and hypotension (severe overdose), chest pain (occurs frequently but only 5.8% have true myocardial ischemia and infarction); (4) hyperthermia (vasoconstriction, increased metabolism); (5) GI: ischemic bowel perforation if ingested; (6) rhabdomyolysis, myoglobinuria, and renal failure; (7) premature labor and abruptio placentae; (8) in prolonged toxicity suspect body cavity packing; (9) mortality resulting from cerebrovascular accidents, coronary artery spasm and myocardial injury, and lethal dysrhythmias. *Management:* (1) Supportive care: blood pressure, cardiac, thermal monitoring and seizure precautions. Diazepam is the choice for treatment of cocaine toxicity with agitation, seizures, dysrhythmias; the dose is 10 to 30 mg IV at 2.5 mg per minute for adults and 0.2 to 0.5 mg per kg at 1 mg per minute up to 10 mg for a child. (2) GI decontamination: If cocaine was ingested, administer AC.

MDAC may adsorb cocaine leakage from body stuffers or body packers. Whole-bowel irrigation with PEG solution has been used in body packers and stuffers if the contraband is in a firm container. If packages are not visible on an abdominal radiograph, a contrast study and/or ultrasonography can help to confirm successful passage. PEG may desorb the cocaine from AC. Cocaine in the nasal passage can be removed with an applicator dipped in a non–water-soluble product (lubricating jelly). (3) In body packers and stuffers, secure venous access and have drugs readily available to treat life-threatening manifestations until contraband is passed in the stool. Surgical removal may be indicated if a packet does not pass the pylorus, in a symptomatic body packer, or in intestinal obstruction. (4) Cardiovascular disturbances: Hypertension and tachycardia are usually transient and can be managed by careful titration of diazepam. Nitroprusside may be used for hypertensive crisis. Myocardial ischemia is managed by oxygen, vascular access, BZPs, and nitroglycerin. Aspirin and thrombolysis are not routinely recommended because of danger of intracranial hemorrhage. Dysrhythmias are usually supraventricular tachycardias and do not require specific management. Adenosine is ineffective. Life-threatening tachydysrhythmias may respond to phentolamine, 5 mg IV bolus adult, 0.1 mg per kg child, at 5- to 10-minute intervals. Phentolamine also relieves coronary artery spasm and myocardial ischemia. Electrical synchronized cardioversion should be considered for hemodynamically unstable dysrhythmias. Lidocaine is not recommended initially but may be used after 3 hours for ventricular tachycardia. Wide complex QRS ventricular tachycardia may be treated with $NaHCO_3$ at 2 mEq per kg as a bolus. Beta-adrenergic blockers are not recommended. (5) Treat anxiety, agitation, and convulsions with diazepam. If diazepam fails to control seizures, use neuromuscular blockers and monitor the EEG for nonmotor seizures. (6) Hyperthermia: Administer external cooling and cool humidified 100% oxygen. Neuromuscular paralysis to control seizures reduces temperature. Dantrolene and antipyretics are not recommended. (7) Treat rhabdomyolysis and myoglobinuria with fluids, alkaline diuresis, and diuretics. (8) If the patient is pregnant, monitor the fetus and observe for spontaneous abortion. (9) Treat paranoid ideation and threatening behavior with rapid tranquilization. (See the earlier section on violent patients.) Observe for suicidal de-

TABLE 31. **Different Routes and Kinetics of Cocaine**

Type	Route	$t_{1/2}$ (min)	Onset	Peak (min)	Duration (min)
Cocaine leaf	Oral, chew		20–30 min	45–90	240–360
Hydrochloride	Insufflation	78	1–3 min	5–10	60–90
	Ingested	54	20–30 min	50–90	Sustained
	Intravenous	36	30–120 s	5–11	60–90
Freebase, crack	Smoked	—	5–10 s	5–11	Up to 20
Coca paste	Smoked	—	Unknown		

pression that may follow intoxication and may require suicidal precautions. (10) If focal neurologic manifestations are present, consider cerebrovascular accident and perform CT. (11) Extracorporeal measures are of no benefit. *Laboratory investigations:* Monitor: ECG and cardiac monitoring, ABGs and oxygen saturation, electrolytes, blood glucose, BUN, creatinine, creatine kinase and cardiac function if chest pain, liver profile, rhabdomyolysis and urine for myoglobin, urine for cocaine and metabolites and other substances of abuse, abdominal radiography or ultrasonography for body packers. A urine sample collected more than 12 hours after cocaine intake contains little or no cocaine. If cocaine is present, it has been used within the past 12 hours. Cocaine's metabolite benzoylecgonine may be detected within 4 hours after a single nasal insufflation and up to 48 to 114 hours after use. Intravenous drug users should have HIV and hepatitis virus testing. Cross-reactions with herbal teas, lidocaine, and droperidol may give false-positive results with some laboratory methods. *Disposition:* Patients with mild intoxication or a brief seizure that does not require treatment who become asymptomatic may be discharged after 6 hours with appropriate psychosocial follow-up. If there are cardiac or cerebral ischemia manifestations, monitor in the ICU. Body packers and stuffers require ICU care until passage of the contraband.

Cyanide. Some sources of cyanide: (1) Hydrogen cyanide (HCN) is a by-product of burning plastic and wools and is produced in residential fires and salts in ore extraction. (2) Nitriles, such as acetonitrile (artificial nail removers), are metabolized in the body to produce cyanide. (3) Cyanogenic glycosides in the seeds of fruit stones (as amygdalin in apricots, peaches, apples) in the presence of intestinal β-glucosidase form cyanide (the seeds are harmful only if the capsule is broken). (4) Sodium nitroprusside, the antihypertensive vasodilator, contains five cyanide groups. *Toxic mechanism:* Cyanide blocks the cellular electron transport mechanism and cellular respiration by inhibiting the mitochondrial ferricytochrome oxidase system and other enzymes. This results in cellular hypoxia and lactic acidosis. *Toxic dose:* The ingestion of 1 mg per kg or 50 mg of HCN can produce death within 15 minutes. The lethal dose of potassium cyanide is 200 mg. Five to 10 mL of 84% acetonitrile is lethal. The permissible exposure limit for volatile HCN is 10 ppm, and 300 ppm is fatal in minutes. *Kinetics:* Cyanide is rapidly absorbed by all routes. In the stomach it forms hydrocyanic acid. The PB is 60%; the Vd, 1.5 liters per kg. Cyanide is detoxified by metabolism in the liver via the mitochondrial endogenous thiosulfate-rhodanese pathway, which catalyzes the transfer of sulfur to cyanide to form irreversibly the less toxic thiocyanate, which is excreted in the urine. The $t_{1/2}$ for cyanide elimination from the blood is 1.2 hours. Cyanide is also detoxified by reacting with hydroxocobalamin (vitamin B_{12a}) to form cyanocobalamin (vitamin B_{12}). Elimination is through the lungs. *Manifestations:* HCN has the distinctive odor of bitter almonds (odor of

silver polish). The clinical findings are flushing, hypertension, headache, hyperpnea, seizures, stupor, cardiac dysrhythmias, and pulmonary edema. Cyanosis is absent or appears late. Various ECG abnormalities may be present. *Management:* (1) Protect rescuers and attendants. Immediately administer 100% oxygen and continue during and after the administration of the antidote. If cyanide is inhaled, remove the patient from the contaminated atmosphere. Attendants should not administer mouth-to-mouth resuscitation. (2) Cyanide antidote kit (see Table 12): The clinician must decide whether to use any or all components of the kit. The mechanism of action of the antidote kit is to form methemoglobin (MetHb), which has a greater affinity for cyanide than the cytochrome oxidase system and forms cyanomethemoglobin. The cyanide is transferred from MetHb by sodium thiosulfate, which provides a sulfur atom that is converted by the rhodanese-catalyzed enzyme reaction (thiosulfate sulfurtransferase) to convert cyanide into the relatively nontoxic sodium thiocyanate, which is excreted by the kidney. Procedure for using the antidote kit: Step 1, amyl nitrite inhalant Perles, is only a temporizing measure (forms only 2 to 5% MetHb) and can be omitted if venous access is established. Administer 100% oxygen and the inhalant for 30 seconds of every minute. Use new Perle every 3 minutes. Step 2, sodium nitrite ampule, is not necessary in poisonings associated with residential fires, smoke inhalation, nitroprusside, or acetonitrile. It is administered IV to produce MetHb of 20 to 30% at 35 to 70 minutes after administration. For adults, 10 mL of a 3% solution of sodium nitrite (child, 0.33 mL per kg of 3% solution) is diluted to 100 mL with 0.9% saline and administered slowly IV at 5 mL per minute. If hypotension develops, slow the infusion. Step 3, sodium thiosulfate, is useful alone in smoke inhalation, nitroprusside toxicity, and acetonitrile toxicity and should not be used at all in hydrogen sulfide poisoning. For adults, administer 12.5 grams of sodium thiosulfate or 50 mL of 25% solution (child, 1.65 mL per kg of 25% solution) IV over 10 to 20 minutes. If cyanide-related symptoms recur, repeat antidotes in 30 minutes as half of the initial dose. The dosage regimen for children on the package insert must be carefully followed. One hour after antidotes are administered, the MetHb level should be obtained and should not exceed 20%. Methylene blue should not be used to reverse excessive MetHb. (3) GI decontamination after oral ingestion by gastric lavage and AC is recommended but is not too effective (1 gram binds only 35 mg of cyanide). (4) Treat seizures with IV diazepam. Correct acidosis with $NaHCO_3$ if it does not resolve rapidly with therapy. (5) Treat metabolic acidosis with $NaHCO_3$. (6) There is no role for the HBO chamber, hemodialysis, or hemoperfusion. (7) Other antidotes: In France, hydroxocobalamin (vitamin B_{12a}) is used (it exchanges its hydroxyl with free cyanide to form cyanocobalamin). It has proved effective when given immediately after exposure in large doses of 4 grams (50 mg per kg) or 50 times the amount of cyanide in the exposure with 8 grams of sodium thiosulfate (it has FDA orphan drug approval). *Laboratory investigations:* Obtain and monitor ABGs, oxygen saturation, blood lactate (takes 0.5 hour), blood cyanide (takes hours), hemoglobin, blood glucose, and electrolytes. Lactic acidemia, decreases in the arterial-venous oxygen difference, and bright red venous blood occur. If smoke inhalation is the possible source of exposure, obtain COHb and MetHb concentrations. The cyanide level in whole blood for a smoker is less than 0.5 µg per mL; in flushing and tachycardia, 0.5 to 1.0 µg per mL; in obtundation, 1.0 to 2.5 µg per mL; and in coma and death, greater than 2.5 µg per mL. *Disposition:* Asymptomatic patients should be observed for a minimum of 6 hours. Patients who ingest nitrile compounds must be observed for 24 hours. Patients requiring antidote administration should be admitted to the ICU.

Digitalis. Cardiac glycosides are found in cardiac medication, common plants, and the skin of *Bufo* species of toad. More than 1 to 3 mg may be found in a few leaves of oleander or foxglove. *Toxic mechanism:* Cardiac glycosides inhibit the enzyme Na$^+$,K$^+$-ATPase, leading to intracellular potassium loss, increased intracellular sodium producing phase 4 depolarization, increased automaticity, and ectopy. Increased intracellular calcium and potentiation of contractility occur. Pacemaker cells are inhibited and the refractory period is prolonged, leading to AV blocks. Vagal tone is increased. *Toxic dose:* The digoxin total digitalizing dose is 0.75 to 1.25 mg or 10 to 15 µg per kg in those older than 10 years and 40 to 50 µg per kg in those younger than 2 years; 30 to 40 µg per kg at 2 to 10 years of age produces a therapeutic serum concentration of 0.6 to 2.0 ng per mL. The acute single toxic dose is more than 0.07 mg per kg or more than 2 to 3 mg in adults; however, 2 mg in a child or 4 mg in an adult usually produces mild toxicity. Serious and fatal overdoses are greater than 4 mg in a child and greater than 10 mg in an adult. Digoxin clinical toxicity is usually associated with serum digoxin levels of 3.5 ng per mL or more in adults. Patients at greatest risk of overdose include those with cardiac disease, electrolyte abnormalities (low potassium, low magesium, low thyroxine, high calcium), or renal impairment and those receiving amiodarone, quinidine, erythromycin, tetracycline, calcium channel blockers, and beta blockers. *Kinetics:* Digoxin is a metabolite of digitoxin. Digoxin's oral onset occurs within 1 to 2 hours, peak levels at 2 to 3 hours, and peak effects at 3 to 4 hours; the duration is 3 to 4 days. In overdose, the typical onset is at 30 minutes with peak effects in 3 to 12 hours. The IV onset is in 5 to 30 minutes, the peak level occurs immediately, and the peak effect occurs at 1.5 to 3 hours. Elimination is 60 to 80% renal. The Vd is 5 to 6 liters per kg. The cardiac/plasma ratio is 30:1. The elimination $t_{1/2}$ is 30 to 50 hours. After an acute ingestion overdose, the serum concentration does not reflect the tissue concentration for at least 6 hours or more, and steady state is reached 12 to 16 hours after the last dose. *Manifesta-*

tions: These may be delayed 9 to 18 hours. (1) GI effects: nausea and vomiting are always present in acute ingestion and may occur in chronic ingestion. (2) Cardiovascular effects: The "digitalis effect" on the ECG consists of scooped ST segments and PR prolongation. In overdose, any dysrhythmia or block is possible but none is characteristic. Bradycardia occurs in acute overdose with healthy hearts, tachycardia with existing heart disease or chronic overdose. Ventricular tachycardia is seen only in severe poisoning. (3) CNS effects are headaches, visual disturbances, and colored-halo vision. (4) Potassium disturbances: Hyperkalemia is a predictor of serum digoxin concentrations greater than 10 ng per mL and of 50% mortality without treatment. If serum potassium was less than 5.0 mEq per liter, all survived; if 5 to 5.5 mEq per liter, 50% survived; and if greater than 5.5 mEq per liter, all died. Hypokalemia is commonly seen with chronic intoxication. Patients with normal digitalis levels may have toxicity in the presence of hypokalemia. (5) Chronic intoxications are more likely to produce scotoma, color perception disturbances, yellow vision, halos, delirium, hallucinations or psychosis, tachycardia, and hypokalemia. *Management:* Obtain a cardiac consultation and have a pacemaker readily available. (1) GI decontamination: Use caution with vagal stimulation, and avoid emesis and gastric lavage. Administer AC; if a nasogastric tube is required for AC, consider pretreatment with atropine (0.02 mg per kg for a child and 0.5 mg for an adult). MDAC may interrupt enterohepatic recirculation of digitoxin and adsorb active metabolites. (2) Digoxin-specific antibody fragment (Fab, Digibind) 40 mg binds with 0.6 mg of digoxin and is then excreted through the kidneys. It decreases digoxin 50-fold. (See Table 12.) Indications: Life-threatening hemodynamically unstable dysrhythmias (ventricular dysrhythmias or rapid deterioration of clinical findings); ingestions greater than 4 mg in a child and 10 mg in an adult; serum potassium greater than 5.0 mEq per liter produced by cardiac glycoside toxicity; serum digoxin toxicity (more than 10 ng per mL in adults or more than 5 ng per mL in children) 6 to 8 hours after acute ingestion; unstable severe bradycardia or second- or third-degree blocks unresponsive to atropine; digitalis delirium and thrombocytopenia responds; useful in treatment of life-threatening digitoxin and oleander poisoning. Empirical digoxin-specific Fab fragment therapy may be administered as a bolus through a 22-µm filter if there is a critical emergency. If less urgent, administer over 30 minutes. The empirical dose is 10 vials for adults and 5 vials for children.

Calculation of dose: The amount (total mg) known to have been ingested multiplied by 80% bioavailability (0.8) = body burden. If the agent was given as liquid capsules or IV, do not multiply by 0.8. The body burden divided by 0.6 (0.6 mg of digoxin is bound by 1 vial of 40 mg of Fab) = number of vials needed. If the amount is unknown but the steady-state serum concentration is known, for digoxin:

Digoxin (ng/mL) × (5.6 L/kg Vd) × (weight, kg)
    = µg body burden

Body burden/1000 = mg body burden

Body burden/0.6 = number of vials needed

For digitoxin:

Digitoxin (ng/mL) × (0.56 L/kg Vd) × (weight, kg)
    = body burden

Body burden/1000 = mg body burden

Body burden/0.6 = number of vials needed

(3) Antidysrhythmic agents and a pacemaker should be used only if Fab therapy fails. The onset of action is within 30 minutes. Complications of Fab therapy are mainly related to withdrawal of digoxin and worsening heart failure and include hypokalemia, decreased glucose (if low glycogen stores), and allergic reactions (rare). Digitalis administered after Fab therapy is bound and may be inactivated for 5 to 7 days. (4) For ventricular tachydysrhythmias, correct electrolyte disturbances and administer lidocaine or phenytoin. For torsades de pointes, administer 20 mL of 20% magnesium sulfate IV given slowly over 20 minutes, or 25 to 50 mg per kg in a child, and titrate to control the dysrhythmia. Discontinue magnesium if hypotension, heart block, or decreased deep tendon reflexes occur. Magnesium is used with caution if renal impairment is present. Ventricular pacing should be reserved for patients who fail to respond to Fab. (5) Do not use antidysrhythmics of classes IA, IC, II, and IV and agents that increase conduction time (e.g., procainamide, bretylium, diltiazem, and beta blockers). Class IB drugs can be used. (6) Cardioversion is used with caution; start at a setting of 5 to 10 joules and pretreat with lidocaine, if possible, because it may precipitate ventricular fibrillation or asystole. (7) Treat unstable bradycardia and second-degree and third-degree AV block with atropine. If the patient is unresponsive, use Fab. A pacemaker should be available if the patient fails to respond. Avoid isoproterenol, which causes dysrhythmias. (8) Electrolyte disturbances: Potassium disturbances are due to a shift, not a change in total body potassium. Treat hyperkalemia (>5.0 mEq per liter) with Fab only. Never use calcium, and do not use insulin or glucose. Do not use sodium bicarbonate concomitantly with Fab because it may produce severe life-threatening hypokalemia. Sodium polystyrene sulfonate (Kayexalate) should not be used. Treat hypokalemia with caution because it may be cardioprotective. (9) Extracorporeal procedures are ineffective. Hemodialysis is used for severe or refractory hyperkalemia. *Laboratory investigations:* Monitor baseline ECG and continuous cardiac function and blood glucose, electrolytes, calcium, magnesium, BUN, and creatinine determinations. Measure initial digoxin levels more than 6 hours after inges-

tion because earlier values do not reflect the tissue distribution. Obtain free (unbound) serum digoxin concentrations after Fab therapy because the free (unbound) digoxin decreases and reflects the true level. Cross-reactions: An endogenous digoxin-like substance cross-reacts in most common immunoassays (not with HPLC) and values as high as 4.1 ng per mL have been reported in newborns, in patients with chronic renal failure or abnormal immunoglobulins, and in the third trimester of pregnancy. *Disposition:* Consult with a poison control center and cardiologist experienced with digoxin-specific Fab fragments. All patients with significant dysrhythmias, symptoms, an elevated serum digoxin concentration, or elevated serum potassium level should be admitted to the ICU. Fab fragments and pacemaker therapy should be readily available. Asymptomatic patients with nontoxic levels should have studies repeated in 12 hours.

Ethanol (grain alcohol). See Table 32. *Toxic mechanism:* Ethanol has a CNS hypnotic and anesthetic effect by a variety of mechanisms, including membrane fluidity and effect on the GABA system. It promotes cutaneous vasodilatation (contributes to hypothermia), stimulates secretion of gastric juice (gastritis), inhibits secretion of the antidiuretic hormone, inhibits gluconeogenesis (hypoglycemia), and influences fat metabolism (lipidemia). *Toxic dose:* 1 mL per kg of absolute or 100% ethanol or 200 proof ethanol (proof defines alcohol concentration in beverages) results in a blood ethanol concentration (BEC) of 100 mg per dL. The potential fatal dose is 3 grams per kg for children or 6 grams per kg for adults. Children frequently have hypoglycemia at a BEC greater than 50 mg per dL. *Kinetics:* Onset of action occurs 30 to 60 minutes after ingestion, peak action is at 90 minutes on an empty stomach, and the Vd is 0.6 liter per kg. The major route (>90%) of elimination is by hepatic oxidative metabolism. The first step involves the enzyme alcohol dehydrogenase (ADH), which converts ethanol to acetaldehyde. The kinetics in this step are zero order at a constant rate (regardless of the level) of 12 to 20 mg per dL per hour (12 to 15 mg per dL per hour in nonalcoholic drinkers, 15 mg per dL per hour in social drinkers, 30 to 50 mg per dL per hour in alcoholics, and in children 28 mg per dL per hour). At a low BEC (less than 30 mg per dL), the metabolism is by first-order kinetics. In the second step of metabolism the acetaldehyde is metabolized by acetaldehyde dehydrogenase to acetic acid. In subsequent steps, acetic acid is metabolized via the Krebs citric acid cycle to carbon dioxide and water. The enzyme steps are dependent on nicotinamide adenine dinucleotide, which interferes with gluconeogenesis. Only 2 to 10% of ethanol is excreted unchanged by the kidneys. Estimation of BEC or amount ingested (SG indicates specific gravity):

$$\text{BEC (mg/dL)} = \frac{\text{amount ingested (mL)} \times \% \text{ ethanol in product} \times \text{SG (0.79)}}{\text{Vd (0.6 L/kg)} \times \text{body weight (kg)}}$$

TABLE 32. **Summary of Alcohol and Glycol Features***

Feature	Methanol	Isopropanol	Ethanol	Ethylene Glycol
Principal uses	Gas line Antifreeze Sterno Windshield wiper deicer	Solvent Jewelry cleaner Rubbing	Beverage Solvent	Antifreeze Deicer
Odor	None	None	Yes	None
Specific gravity	0.719	0.785	0.789	1.12
Fatal dose	1 mL/kg, 100%	3 mL/kg, 100%	5 mL/kg, 100%	1.4 mL/kg
Hepatic enzyme	Alcohol dehydrogenase	Alcohol dehydrogenase	Alcohol and acetaldehyde dehydrogenases	Alcohol dehydrogenase
Toxic metabolite	Formate, formaldehyde	Acetone	Acetaldehyde	Glyoxylic acid, oxalate
Drunkenness	±	2+	2+	1+
Metabolic change		Hyperglycemia	Hypoglycemia	Hypocalcemia
Metabolic acidosis	4+	0	1+	2+
Anion gap	4+	±	2+	4+
Ketosis	Ketobutyric	Acetone	Hydroxybutyric	None
GI tract	Pancreatitis	Hemorrhagic gastritis	Gastritis	
Visual	Blindness, pink optic disk			
Crystalluria	0	0	0	+
Pulmonary edema				+
Renal failure				+
MW	32	60	46	62
Osmolality†	0.337	0.176	0.228	0.190

*0 indicates no effect; + indicates mild effect; ± indicates no effect or mild effect; 2+ indicates moderate effect; 3+ indicates severe effect.

†1 mL/dL of substances raises the freezing point osmolarity of serum. The validity of the correlation of osmolality with blood concentrations has been questioned. Inebriation index: methanol < ethanol < ethylene glycol < isopropanol.

Abbreviation: MW = molecular weight.

Dose (amount ingested) =

$$\frac{\text{BEC (mg/dL)} \times \text{Vd (0.6)} \times \text{body weight (kg)}}{\% \text{ ethanol} \times \text{SG (0.79)}}$$

Manifestations: See Table 33. (1) Acute: BECs over 30 mg per dL produce euphoria; over 50 mg per dL, incoordination and intoxication; over 100 mg per dL, ataxia; over 300 mg per dL, stupor; and over 500 mg per dL, coma. Levels of 500 to 700 mg per dL may be fatal. Children frequently have hypoglycemia at a BEC above 50 mg per dL. (2) Chronic alcoholic patients tolerate a higher BEC, and correlation with manifestation is not valid. A rapid interview for alcoholism uses the CAGE questions: C, Have you felt the need to cut down? A, Have others annoyed you by criticizing your drinking? G, Have you felt guilty about your drinking? E, Have you ever had a morning eye-opening drink to steady your nerves or get rid of a hangover? Two affirmative answers indicate probable alcoholism. *Management:* Inquire about trauma and disulfiram use. (1) Protect from aspiration and hypoxia. Establish and maintain vital functions. The patient may require intubation and assisted ventilation. (2) GI decontamination plays no role. (3) If the patient is comatose, administer IV 50% glucose at 1 mL per kg in adults and 25% glucose at 2 mL per kg in children. Thiamine, 100 mg IV, is administered if the patient has a history of chronic alcoholism, malnutrition, or suspected eating disorders and to prevent Wernicke-Korsakoff syndrome. Naloxone has produced a partial inconsistent response and is not recommended for known alcoholic

TABLE 33. **Clinical Signs in the Intolerant Ethanol Drinker**

Ethanol (mg/dL)	Blood (µg/mL)	Concentration* (mmol/L)	Manifestations† in Nonalcoholics
>25	>250	>5.4	Euphoria
>47	>470	>10.2	Mild incoordination, sensory and motor impairment
>50	>500	>10.8	Increased risk of motor vehicle accidents
>100	>1000	>21.7	Ataxia (legal toxic level in many localities)
>150	>1500	>32.5	Moderate incoordination, slow reaction time
>200	>2000	>43.4	Drowsiness and confusion
>300	>3000	>65.1	Severe incoordination, stupor, blurred vision
>500	>5000	>108.5	Flaccid coma, respiratory failure, hypotension; may be fatal

*Ethanol concentrations are sometimes reported as percents. Note that mg% is not equivalent to mg/dL because ethanol weighs less than water (specific gravity 0.79). A 1% ethanol concentration is 790 mg/dL and 0.1% is 79 mg/dL.

†There is a great variation in individual behavior at particular blood ethanol levels. Behavior is dependent on tolerance and other factors.

CNS depressants. (4) General supportive care: Administer fluids to correct hydration and hypotension; correct electrolyte abnormalities and acid-base imbalance. Vasopressors and plasma expanders may be necessary to correct severe hypotension. Hypomagnesemia is frequently present in chronic alcoholics. In hypomagnesemia administer a loading dose of 2 grams of a 10% magnesium sulfate IV solution over 5 minutes in the ICU with blood pressure and cardiac monitoring and have 10% calcium chloride on hand in case of overdose. Follow with constant infusion of 6 grams of 10% magnesium sulfate over 3 to 4 hours. Be cautious with magnesium if renal failure is present. (5) Hypothermic patients should be warmed. See general treatment of poisoning. (6) Hemodialysis may be used in severe cases when conventional therapy is ineffective (rarely needed). (7) Treat repeated or prolonged seizures with diazepam. Brief "rum fits" do not require long-term anticonvulsant therapy. Repeated seizures or focal neurologic findings may warrant skull radiographs, lumbar puncture, and CT of the head, depending on the clinical findings. (8) Treat withdrawal with hydration and large doses of chlordiazepoxide (50 to 100 mg) or diazepam (2 to 10 mg) IV; these may be repeated in 2 to 4 hours. Large doses of BZPs may be required for delirium tremors. Withdrawal can occur in the presence of an elevated BEC and can be fatal if untreated. *Laboratory investigations:* The BEC should be specifically requested and followed. (Gas chromatography or a Breathalyzer test gives rapid reliable results if there is no belching or vomiting; enzymatic methods do not differentiate between the alcohols.) Monitor ABGs, electrolytes, and glucose; determine anion and osmolar gaps (measure by freezing point depression, not vapor pressure); and check for ketosis. See discussion of general management. The AG increases 1 mg per kg for each 4.5 mg per dL BEC. Obtain a chest radiograph to determine whether aspiration pneumonia is present. Obtain renal and liver function tests and bilirubin levels. *Disposition:* Clinical severity (e.g., intubation, assisted ventilation, aspiration pneumonia) should determine the level of hospital care needed. Young children with significant accidental exposure to alcohol (calculated to reach a BEC of 50 mg per dL) should have BEC obtained and blood glucose levels monitored for hypoglycemia frequently for 4 hours after ingestion. Patients with acute ethanol intoxication seldom require admission unless a complication is present. However, intoxicated patients should not be discharged until they are fully functional (can walk, talk, and think independently), have had suicide potential evaluated, have a proper disposition environment, and have a sober escort. Extended liability means that a physician can be held liable for subsequent injuries or death of an intoxicated patient who has been allowed to sign out against medical advice (AMA). No patient can sign out AMA with an altered mental status.

Ethylene Glycol. Ethylene glycol is found in solvents, windshield deicer, antifreeze (95%), and air-conditioning units and has contaminated imported wines. Ethylene glycol is a sweet-tasting, colorless, water-soluble liquid with a sweet aromatic aroma. *Toxic mechanism:* Ethylene glycol is oxidized by ADH to glycolaldehyde and then is metabolized to glycolic acid and glyoxylic acid. Glyoxylic acid is metabolized to oxalic acid. Ethylene glycol metabolites are metabolized via pyridoxine-dependent pathways to glycine, benzoic acid, and hippuric acid and by thiamine- and magnesium-dependent pathways to α-hydroxyketoadipic acid. The metabolites of ethylene glycol produce a profound metabolic acidosis, increased AG, hypocalcemia, deposition of oxalate crystals in tissues, and renal damage. *Toxic dose:* The ingestion of 0.1 mL of 100% ethylene glycol per kg can result in a toxic serum ethylene glycol concentration (SEGC) of 20 mg per dL, a level that requires ethanol therapy, the antidote. Ingestion of 3.0 mL of 100% solution by a 10-kg child or 30 mL of 100% ethylene glycol by an adult produces an SEGC of 50 mg per dL (8.1 mmol per liter), a concentration that requires hemodialysis. The fatal amount is 1.4 mL of 100% solution per kg. *Kinetics:* Absorption by dermal, inhalation, and ingestion routes. Ethylene glycol is rapidly absorbed from the GI tract. Onset is in 30 minutes to 12 hours, and the peak level usually occurs at 2 hours. Without ethanol the $t_{1/2}$ is 3 to 8 hours, with ethanol 17 hours, with hemodialysis 2.5 hours. The Vd is 0.65 to 0.8 liter per kg. For metabolism, see the toxic mechanism discussion. Renal clearance is 3.2 mL per kg per minute. About 20 to 50% is excreted unchanged in the urine. Equations for calculating SEGC and amount ingested:

Calculation of SEGC:

$$0.12 \text{ mL/kg of } 100\% = \text{SEGC } 10 \text{ mg/dL}$$

$$\text{SEGC (mg/dL)} = \frac{\text{amount ingested (mL)} \times \% \text{ EG} \times \text{SG (1.12)}}{0.65 \text{ L/kg (Vd)} \times \text{weight (kg)}}$$

$$\text{Amount ingested (mL)} = \frac{\text{SEGC (mg/dL)} \times 0.65 \text{ L/kg} \times \text{weight (kg)}}{\% \text{ EG} \times \text{SG EG (1.12)}}$$

Manifestations: Phase I: The onset is 30 minutes to 12 hours after ingestion or longer with concomitant ethanol ingestion. The patient acts inebriated at an SEGC of 50 to 100 mg per dL. Hypocalcemia, tetany, and calcium oxalate and hippuric acid crystals in the urine may be observed within 4 to 8 hours but are not always present. Early, before metabolism of ethylene glycol, an osmolal gap may be present. Later, the metabolites of ethylene glycol produce changes starting 4 to 12 hours after ingestion, including an AG, metabolic acidosis, coma, convulsions, cardiac disturbances, and pulmonary and cerebral edema. Oral mucosa and urine fluoresce under Wood's light if "antifreeze" ethylene glycol has been ingested. Phase II: After 12 to 36 hours, cardiopulmonary deterioration occurs with pulmonary edema and congestive heart failure. Phase III: This occurs in 36 to 72 hours; oliguric renal failure resulting from oxalate crystal deposition and from tubular necrosis predominates and pulmonary edema occurs. Phase IV: Neurologic sequelae occur 6 to 10 days after ingestion. They include facial diplegia, hearing loss, bilateral visual disturbances, elevated CSF pressure with or without elevated protein and pleocytosis, vomiting, hyper-reflexia, dysphagia, and ataxia. *Management:* (1) Establish and maintain the vital functions. Protect the airway and use assisted ventilation, if necessary. (2) GI decontamination has a limited role, with only gastric lavage within 30 to 60 minutes after ingestion. AC is not effective. (3) Obtain baseline serum electrolytes and calcium, glucose, ABGs, ethanol, SEGC (difficult to obtain, often takes more than 48 hours), and methanol concentrations. In the first few hours determine the measured serum osmolality and compare it with the calculated osmolarity (see "Serum Osmolal Gaps"). (4) If seizures occur, exclude hypocalcemia and treat with IV diazepam. If hypocalcemic seizures occur, treat with 10 to 20 mL of 10% calcium gluconate (0.2 to 0.3 mL per kg for children) slowly IV and repeat as needed. (See Table 12.) (5) Correct metabolic acidosis with sodium bicarbonate IV. (6) Ethanol therapy (see Table 12): The enzyme ADH has 10 times greater affinity for ethanol than ethylene glycol. Therefore, ethanol blocks the metabolism of ethylene glycol at BECs of 100 to 150 mg per dL. Initiate therapy if there is a history of ingestion of 100% ethylene glycol at 0.1 mL per kg, the SEGC is more than 20 mg per dL, there is an osmolar gap not accounted for by other alcohols or factors (e.g., hyperlipidemia) (see "Serum Osmolal Gaps"), there is metabolic acidosis with an increased AG, there are oxalate crystals in the urine or positive antifreeze fluorescence of urine, and while awaiting hemodialysis. Ethanol should be administered IV (the oral route is less reliable) to produce a BEC of 100 to 150 mg per dL. The loading dose is derived from the formula 1 mL of 100% ethanol per kg = a BEC of 100 mg per dL (which protects against metabolism of ethylene glycol). Therefore, 10 mL of 10% ethanol is administered IV concomitantly with a maintenance dose of 10% ethanol of 2.0 mL per kg per hour (alcoholic), 0.83 mL per kg per hour (nondrinker), or 1.4 mL per kg per hour (social drinker). Increase infusion rate of 10% ethanol to 2 to 3.5 mL per kg per hour when the patient is receiving hemodialysis. (7) Hemodialysis: Obtain nephrology consultation. Early hemodialysis is indicated if the ingestion was potentially fatal, if the SEGC is more than 50 mg per dL (some recommend at levels of more than 25 mg per dL), if severe acidosis or electrolyte abnormalities occur despite conventional therapy, or if congestive heart failure or renal failure is present. Hemodialysis reduces the ethylene glycol $t_{1/2}$ from 17 hours with ethanol therapy to 3 hours. Continue therapy (ethanol and hemodialysis) until the SEGC is less than 10 mg per dL or undetectable, the glycolate level is undetectable, the acidosis has cleared, there are no mental disturbances, the creatinine level is normal, and the urine output is adequate. This may require 2 to 5 days. (8) Adjunct therapy: Thiamine (100 mg per day [children 50 mg] slowly over 5 minutes IV or IM and repeated every 6 hours) and pyridoxine (50 mg IV or IM every 6 hours) have been recommended until intoxication is resolved but have not been extensively studied. Folate may be given at 50 mg IV (child, 1 mg per kg)* every 4 hours for 6 doses. (9) Therapy with 4-methylpyrazole orally at 15 mg per kg followed by 5 mg per kg in 12 hours and then 10 mg per kg every 12 hours until levels of the toxin are not detectable, which blocks ADH without causing inebriation, is being investigated. *Laboratory investigations:* Monitor blood glucose, electrolytes, urinalysis (look for oxalate ["envelope"] and monohydrate ["hemp seed"] crystals and for urine fluorescence), and ABGs. Obtain ethylene glycol and ethanol levels, plasma osmolarity (use freezing point depression method), calcium, BUN, and creatinine. An SEGC of 20 mg per dL is toxic (ethylene glycol levels are difficult to obtain). If possible, obtain a glycolate level. Fluorescence: The oral mucosa and urine (do not put in a glass tube) fluoresce under Wood's light if antifreeze ethylene glycol is present. Cross-reactions: propylene glycol, a vehicle in many liquids and IV medications (phenytoin, diazepam), other glycols, and triglycerides may produce spurious ethylene glycol levels. *Disposition:* All patients who ingest significant amounts of ethylene glycol should be referred to the emergency department. If the SEGC cannot be obtained, follow up for 12 hours, monitoring the osmolal gap, acid-base parameters, and electrolytes to exclude development of metabolic acidosis with an AG.

Hydrocarbons. The lower the viscosity and surface tension or the greater the volatility, the greater the risk of aspiration. Volatile substance abuse has resulted in the "sudden sniffing's death syndrome," most likely caused by dysrhythmias. *Toxicologic classification and toxic mechanism:* All systemically absorbed hydrocarbons can lower the threshold of the myocardium to dysrhythmias produced by endogenous and exogenous catecholamines. (1) Petroleum distillates are aliphatic hydrocarbons. Toxic dose: A few drops aspirated produce chemical pneumonitis but are poorly absorbed from the GI tract and produce no systemic toxicity by this route. Examples are gasoline, kerosene charcoal lighter fluid, mineral spirits (Stoddard's solvent), and petroleum naphtha. (2) Aromatic HCs are six-carbon ringed structures that produce CNS depression and in chronic abuse may have multiple organ effects. Examples are benzene (chronically produces leukemia), toluene, styrene, and xylene. The ingested seriously toxic dose is 20 to 50 mL in an adult. (3) Halogenated hydrocarbons are aliphatic hydrocarbons with one or more halogen substitutions (Cl, Br, Fl, or I). They are highly volatile and abused as inhalants. They are well absorbed from the GI tract, produce CNS depression, and have metabolites that can damage the liver and kidneys. Examples are methylene chloride (may be converted to CO in the body), dichloroethylene

---

*Exceeds dosage recommended by the manufacturer.

(also causes a disulfiram [Antabuse] reaction ["degreaser's flush"] when associated with consumption of ethanol), and 1,1,1-trichloroethane (Glamorene Spot Remover, Scotchgard, typewriter correction fluid) (acute lethal oral dose 0.5 to 5 mL per kg). (4) Dangerous additives to the hydrocarbons include those in the mnemonic CHAMP: C, camphor (demothing agent); H, halogenated hydrocarbons; A, aromatic hydrocarbons; M, metals (heavy); and P, pesticides. These may warrant gastric emptying with a small-bore nasogastric lavage tube. (5) Heavy hydrocarbons have high viscosity, low volatility, and minimal GI absorption, so gastric decontamination is not necessary. Examples are asphalt (tar), machine oil, motor oil (lubricating oil, engine oil), home heating oil, and petroleum jelly (mineral oil). (7) Mineral seal oil (e.g., signal oil), found in furniture polishes, is a low-viscosity, low-volatility oil with minimal absorption that never warrants gastric decontamination. It can produce severe pneumonia if aspirated. *Management of hydrocarbon ingestion:* (1) Asymptomatic patients who ingested small amounts of petroleum distillates may be observed at home by reliable caretakers for development of signs of aspiration (cough, wheezing, tachypnea, and dyspnea) with telephone contact for 4 to 6 hours. (2) Inhalation of any hydrocarbon vapors in a closed space can produce intoxication. Remove the victim from the environment, and administer oxygen and respiratory support. (3) GI decontamination is not advised in hydrocarbon ingestions that usually do not cause systemic toxicity (petroleum distillates, heavy hydrocarbons, mineral seal oil). For hydrocarbons that cause systemic toxicity in small amounts (aromatic hydrocarbons, halogenated hydrocarbons) pass a small-bore nasogastric tube (these substances are liquids) and aspirate if appropriate time has not elapsed (absorption with aromatic and halogenated hydrocarbons is complete in 1 to 2 hours) and spontaneous vomiting has not occurred. Patients with altered mental status should have the airway protected because of concern over uncontrolled vomiting. Although some toxicologists advocate ipecac-induced emesis under medical supervision instead of small-bore nasogastric gastric lavage, we do not. AC is suggested, but there are no scientific data concerning its effectiveness and it may produce vomiting. AC may, however, be useful for adsorbing toxic additives or coingestants. (4) The symptomatic patient who is coughing, gagging, choking, and wheezing on arrival has probably already aspirated. Offer supportive respiratory care, maintain the airway, provide assisted ventilation, offer supplemental oxygen with monitoring of pulse oximetry, measure ABGs, obtain a chest radiograph and ECG, and admit to the ICU. A chest radiograph for aspiration may be positive as early as 30 minutes and almost all are positive within 6 hours. If bronchospasm occurs, administer nebulized beta-adrenergic agonist and IV aminophylline if necessary. Avoid epinephrine because of susceptibility to dysrhythmias. If cyanosis is present that does not respond to oxygen and the PaO$_2$ is normal, suspect methemoglobinemia

that may require therapy with methylene blue (see Table 12). Corticosteroids and prophylactic antimicrobial agents have not been shown to be beneficial. (Fever or leukocytosis may be produced by the chemical pneumonitis itself.) It is not necessary to surgically treat pneumatoceles that develop because they usually resolve. Most infiltrations resolve spontaneously in 1 week except for lipoid pneumonia, which may last up to 6 weeks. Dysrhythmias may require alpha- and beta-adrenergic antagonists or cardioversion. (5) There is no role for enhanced elimination procedures. (6) Methylene chloride is metabolized in several hours to CO. See the section on treatment of CO poisoning. Give 100% oxygen, and monitor serial COHb levels, ECG, and pulse oximetry. (7) Halogenated hydrocarbons are hepatorenal toxins; therefore, monitor hepatorenal function. *N*-Acetylcysteine therapy may be useful if there is evidence of hepatic damage. (8) Investigational: Surfactant has been used for hydrocarbon aspiration in an animal study of aspirated hydrocarbons and was found to be detrimental. Extracorporeal membrane oxygenation has been used successfully for a few patients with life-threatening respiratory failure. *Laboratory investigations:* Monitor ECG continuously; ABGs; liver, pulmonary, and renal function; serum electrolytes; and serial chest radiographs. *Disposition:* Asymptomatic patients with small ingestions of petroleum distillates can be managed at home. Symptomatic patients with an abnormal chest radiograph, oxygen saturation, or ABGs should be admitted. If the patient becomes asymptomatic, oxygenation is normal, and repeated radiographs are normal, the patient can be discharged.

Iron. There are more than 100 over-the-counter iron preparations for supplementation and treatment of iron deficiency anemia. *Toxic mechanism:* Toxicity depends on the amount of elemental (free) iron available in various salts (gluconate 12%, sulfate 20%, fumarate 33%, lactate 19%, chloride 21% of elemental iron), not the amount of the salt. Locally, iron is corrosive and may cause fluid loss, hypovolemic shock, and perforation. Excessive free iron in the blood is directly toxic to the vasculature and leads to the release of vasoactive substances, which produce vasodilatation. In overdose, iron deposits injure mitochondria in liver, the kidneys, and the myocardium. The exact mechanism of cellular damage is not clear. *Toxic dose:* The therapeutic dose of elemental iron is 6 mg per kg per day. Elemental iron at 20 to 40 mg per kg per dose may produce mild self-limited GI symptoms, a dose of 40 to 60 mg per kg produces moderate toxicity, more than 60 mg per kg produces severe toxicity and is potentially lethal, and more than 180 mg per kg is usually fatal without treatment. Children's chewable vitamins with iron have from 12 to 18 mg of elemental iron per tablet or 0.6 mL of liquid drops. These preparations rarely produce toxicity unless extremely large quantities are ingested. Calculation of the amount of elemental iron ingested:

Elemental iron (mg/kg) =

$$\frac{\text{number of tablets ingested} \times \%\ \text{elemental iron}}{\text{body weight (kg)}}$$

Kinetics: Absorption occurs chiefly in the upper small intestine, usually with iron in the ferrous ($+2$) state absorbed into the mucosal cells, where it is oxidized to the ferric ($+3$) state and bound to ferritin. Iron is slowly released from ferritin into the plasma to become bound to transferrin and transported to specific tissues for production of hemoglobin (70%), myoglobin (5%), and cytochrome. About 25% of iron is stored in the liver and spleen. In overdoses, larger amounts of iron are absorbed because of direct mucosal corrosion. There is no mechanism for elimination of iron (elimination 1 to 2 mg per day) except through bile, sweat, and blood loss. *Manifestations:* Serious toxicity is unlikely if the patient remains asymptomatic for 6 hours, has a normal white blood cell count and glucose, and has a negative abdominal radiograph. Iron intoxication usually follows a biphasic course. A phase may be omitted entirely. Phase I: GI mucosal injury occurs 30 minutes to 12 hours after ingestion. Vomiting starts 30 minutes to 1 hour after ingestion and is persistent. Hematemesis and bloody diarrhea, abdominal cramps, fever, hyperglycemia, and leukocytosis occur. Enteric-coated tablets may pass through the stomach without causing symptoms. Acidosis and shock can occur within 6 to 12 hours. Phase II is a latent period of apparent improvement over 8 to 12 hours after ingestion. Phase III is the systemic toxicity phase (12 to 48 hours after ingestion) with cardiovascular collapse and severe metabolic acidosis. Phase IV (2 to 4 days after ingestion) is characterized by hepatic injury associated with jaundice, elevated liver enzymes, prolonged prothrombin time, and kidney injury with proteinuria and hematuria. Pulmonary edema, disseminated intravascular coagulation, and *Yersinia enterocolitica* sepsis can occur. In phase V (4 to 8 weeks after ingestion), sequelae of the pyloric outlet or intestinal stricture may cause obstruction or anemia secondary to blood loss. *Management:* (1) GI decontamination: Induce emesis immediately in ingestions of elemental iron greater than 40 mg per kg if the child has not already vomited. Gastric lavage with 0.9% saline is less effective than emesis because of the large size of the tablets but may be useful if chewed tablets and liquid preparations are involved. AC is ineffective. Obtain an abdominal radiograph after emesis or lavage to determine the success of gastric emptying procedures. Children's chewable vitamins and liquid iron are not radiopaque. If radiopaque iron is still present, consider whole-bowel irrigation with PEG solution (see the section on evaluation and general management). (2) In extreme cases, removal by endoscopy or surgery was necessary because coalesced iron tablets produced hemorrhagic infarction in the bowel and perforation peritonitis. (3) Deferoxamine (DFO) (see Table 12): About 100 mg of DFO binds only 8.5 to 9.35 mg of free iron in the serum in transit. The DFO

infusion (the IV route is preferred) should not exceed 15 mg per kg per hour or 6 grams daily but higher rates (up to 45 mg per kg per hour) and larger daily amounts have been administered and tolerated in extreme cases of iron poisoning (greater than 1000 µg per dL). The deferoxamine-iron complex is hemodialyzable if renal failure develops. Indications for chelation therapy are any of the following: serious clinical intoxication (severe vomiting and diarrhea [often bloody], severe abdominal pain, metabolic acidosis, hypotension, or shock); symptoms that persist or progress to more serious toxicity; estimate of elemental iron ingestion that is quite high and presence of symptoms; serum iron (SI) greater than 500 µg per dL. Chelation should be performed as early as possible, within 12 to 18 hours, to be effective. Start the infusion slowly and gradually increase to avoid hypotension. Successful chelation results in a urine color change from a positive vin rosé color to a normal color. Adult respiratory distress syndrome has developed in patients with high doses of DFO for several days; therefore, avoid prolonged infusions over 24 hours. The end points of treatment are absence of symptoms and clearing of the urine that was originally a positive vin rosé color. In a diagnostic chelation test, deferoxamine, 50 mg per kg in children or 1 gram in adults IM, produces a vin rosé color (ferroxime-iron complex) of the urine within 3 hours. This is not a reliable test for elevated SI levels; however, obtain a baseline urine sample for comparison with subsequent specimens. (4) Supportive therapy: IV bicarbonate may be needed to correct the metabolic acidosis. Hypotension and shock treatment may require fluid volume expansion, vasopressors, and blood transfusions. Attempt to keep the urine output at more than 2 mL per kg per hour. Coagulation abnormalities and overt bleeding require blood products and vitamin K. (5) Pregnant patients are treated similarly to any others with iron poisoning. (6) Extracorporeal measures: Hemodialysis and hemoperfusion are not effective. Exchange transfusion has been used in single cases of massive poisonings in children. *Laboratory investigations:* Iron poisoning produces AG metabolic acidosis. Monitor the CBCs, blood glucose, SI, stools and vomitus for occult blood, electrolytes, acid-base balance, urinalysis and urine output, liver function tests, BUN, and creatinine. If GI bleeding occurs, obtain the blood type and match blood. SI measured at the proper time correlates with the clinical findings. The lavender top Vacutainer tube contains EDTA, which falsely lowers the SI. Obtain the SI before administering deferoxamine. SI levels at 2 to 6 hours less than 350 µg per dL predict an asymptomatic course; levels of 350 to 500 µg per dL are usually associated with mild GI symptoms; levels above 500 µg per dL predict a 20% risk of shock and serious iron intoxication with phase III manifestations. A follow-up SI after 6 hours may not be elevated even in severe poisoning; however, an SI at 8 to 12 hours is useful for excluding delayed absorption from a bezoar or sustained-release preparation. The total iron-binding capacity is not a necessary study. Abdominal radiographs can visualize adult iron tablet preparations before they dissolve. A negative radiograph does not exclude iron poisoning. Iron sepsis: Patients who develop high fevers and signs of sepsis after iron overdose should have blood and stool cultures checked for *Y. enterocolitica. Disposition:* Observe the patient who is asymptomatic or has minimal symptoms for persistence and progression of symptoms or development of signs of toxicity (GI bleeding, acidosis, shock, altered mental state). A patient with mild self-limited GI symptoms who becomes asymptomatic or has no signs of toxicity for 6 hours is unlikely to have a serious intoxication and can be discharged after psychiatric clearance, if needed. Patients with moderate or severe toxicity should be in the ICU.

Isoniazid (isonicotinic acid hydrazide, INH, Nydrazid). INH is a hydrazide derivative of vitamin B_3 (nicotinamide) used as an antituberculosis drug. *Toxic mechanism:* INH produces pyridoxine deficiency by doubling the excretion of pyridoxine (vitamin B_6) and by inhibiting the interaction of pyridoxal 5-phosphate (the active form of pyridoxine) with L-glutamic acid decarboxylase to form GABA, the major CNS neurotransmitter inhibitor, resulting in seizures and coma. INH blocks the conversion of lactate to pyruvate, resulting in profound lactic acidosis. *Toxic dose:* The therapeutic dose is 5 to 10 mg per kg (maximum of 300 mg) daily. A single acute dose of 15 mg per kg lowers the seizure threshold, 35 to 40 mg per kg produces spontaneous convulsions, more than 80 mg produces severe toxicity, and 200 mg per kg is an obligatory convulsant. The malnourished, those with a previous seizure disorder or alcoholism, and slow acetylators are more susceptible to INH toxicity. In chronic intoxication, 10 mg per kg per day produces hepatitis in 10 to 20% of patients but doses of 3 to 5 mg per kg per day affect less than 2%. *Kinetics:* Rapid absorption from intestine occurs in 30 to 60 minutes, onset is in 30 to 120 minutes with a peak 5 to 8 μg per mL within 1 to 2 hours. The Vd is 0.6 liter per kg; PB is minimal. Elimination is by liver acetylation to a hepatotoxic metabolite, acetylisoniazid, which is then hydrolyzed to isonicotinic acid. Slow acetylators show a $t_{1/2}$ of 140 to 300 minutes (mean 5 hours) and eliminate 10 to 15% unchanged in the urine. Most (45 to 75%) whites and 50% of African blacks are slow acetylators and with chronic use (without pyridoxine supplements) may develop peripheral neuropathy. Fast acetylators show a $t_{1/2}$ of 35 to 110 minutes (mean 80 minutes) and excrete 25 to 30% unchanged in the urine. About 90% of Asians and patients with diabetes mellitus are fast acetylators and may develop hepatitis with chronic use. In overdose and hepatic disease, the serum $t_{1/2}$ may increase. INH inhibits the metabolism of phenytoin, diazepam, phenobarbital, carbamazepine, and prednisone. These drugs also interfere with the metabolism of INH. Ethanol may decrease the INH $t_{1/2}$ but increase its toxicity. *Manifestations:* Within 30 to 60 minutes, nausea, vomiting, slurred speech, dizziness, visual disturbances, and ataxia are present. Within 30 to 120 minutes, the major clinical triad of severe overdose develops: (1) refractory convulsions (90% of overdose patients have one or more seizures), (2) coma, and (3) resistant severe AG lactic acidosis (secondary to convulsions), and metabolic blocks with pH often 6.8. Acidosis occurs after seizures. *Management:* (1) Control seizures: Administer pyridoxine, 1 gram for each gram of isoniazid ingested (see Table 12). If the dose ingested is unknown, give at least 5 grams (70 mg per kg) of pyridoxine IV. Pyridoxine is administered in 50 mL of D5W or 0.9% saline over 5 minutes IV. Do not administer in the same bottle as $NaHCO_3$. Repeat IV pyridoxine every 5 to 20 minutes until seizures are controlled. Total doses of pyridoxine up to 52 grams have been safely administered. However, patients given 132 and 183 grams of pyridoxine have developed a persistent crippling sensory neuropathy. Some authorities recommend prophylactic pyridoxine if there is a history of ingestion of 80 mg per kg. Administer diazepam concomitantly with pyridoxine but at a different site. They work synergistically. Administer diazepam IV at 0.3 mg per kg slowly at rate of 1 mg per minute in children or 10 mg per dose slowly at rate of 5 mg per minute in adults. After the seizures are controlled, administer the remainder of the pyridoxine (1 gram per gram of INH) or total dose of 5 grams as an infusion drip over 60 minutes. Do not use phenobarbital (it increases INH metabolism to toxic metabolites) or phenytoin (it interferes with INH metabolism and is not effective). (2) In asymptomatic patients or patients without seizures, pyridoxine should be considered prophylactically in gram-for-gram doses with large overdoses (80 mg per kg per dose or more) of INH (although there are no studies). (3) In comatose patients, pyridoxine administration may result in rapid regaining of consciousness. (4) Correction of the acidosis and correction of the seizures may occur spontaneously with pyridoxine administration. Administer $NaHCO_3$ if acidosis persists. (5) GI decontamination: After the patient is stabilized, or if the patient is asymptomatic, gastric lavage may be performed after recent (less than 1 hour) ingestion with protection of the airway, if necessary. AC may be administered. (6) Hemodialysis is rarely needed because of antidotal therapy and the short half-life but may be used as an adjunct for uncontrollable acidosis and seizures. Hemoperfusion has not been adequately evaluated. Diuresis is ineffective. *Laboratory investigations:* INH produces AG metabolic acidosis. Therapeutic levels are 5 to 8 μg per mL and acute toxic levels are more than 20 μg per mL. Monitor the blood glucose (often hyperglycemia), electrolytes (often hyperkalemia), bicarbonate, ABGs, liver function tests (elevations occur with chronic exposure), BUN, and creatinine. *Disposition:* Asymptomatic or mildly symptomatic patients who become asymptomatic may be observed in the emergency department for 4 to 6 hours. Larger amounts of INH may warrant pyridoxine and longer periods of observation. Those with intentional ingestions require psychiatric evaluation before discharge. Patients with convulsions or coma should be admitted to the ICU.

Isopropanol (IP or rubbing alcohol, solvents, lacquer thinner). Coma has occurred in children sponged for fever with isopropanol. See Table 32. *Toxic mechanism:* Isopropanol is a gastric irritant. It is metabolized to acetone, a CNS and myocardial depressant. It inhibits gluconeogenesis. Normal propyl alcohol is related to isopropanol but is more toxic. *Toxic dose:* The toxic dose is 0.5 to 1 mg of 70% isopropanol per kg (1 mL of 70% isopropanol per kg produces a blood isopropyl alcohol concentration [BIPC] of 70 mg per dL). The CNS depressant effect is twice that of ethanol. *Kinetics:* Onset is within 30 to 60 minutes and the peak at 1 hour after ingestion. Elimination is renal. Isopropyl alcohol is metabolized to acetone. The Vd is 0.6 liter per kg. The BIPC and amount ingested can be estimated by using equations in ethanol kinetics and specific gravity of 0.785:

$$\text{BIPC (mg/dL)} =$$

$$\frac{\substack{\text{amount ingested (mL)} \times \% \text{ isopropyl alcohol} \\ \text{in product} \times \text{SG (0.79)}}}{\text{Vd (0.6 L/kg)} \times \text{body weight (kg)}}$$

$$\text{Dose (amount ingested)} =$$

$$\frac{\text{BIPC (mg/dL)} \times \text{Vd (0.6 L/kg)} \times \text{body weight (kg)}}{\% \text{ ethanol} \times \text{SG (0.79)}}$$

Manifestations: Ethanol-like inebriation with an acetone odor of the breath, gastritis occasionally with hematemesis, acetonuria, and acetonemia without systemic acidosis are seen. CNS depression: lethargy at 50 to 100 mg per dL, comatose at 150 to 200 mg per dL, potentially fatal in adults at more than 240 mg per dL. Hypoglycemia and seizures may occur. *Management:* (1) Protect the airway with intubation and administer assisted ventilation if necessary. If the patient is hypoglycemic, administer glucose. Supportive treatment is similar to that for ethanol. (2) GI decontamination has no role. (3) Hemodialysis in life-threatening overdose is rarely needed. Consult a nephrologist if the BIPC is greater than 250 mg per dL. *Laboratory investigation:* Monitor isopropyl alcohol levels, acetone, glucose, and ABGs. The osmolal gap increases 1 mOsm per 5.9 mg per dL of isopropyl alcohol and 1 mOsm per 5.5 mg per dL of acetone. Absence of excess acetone in the blood (normal, 0.3 to 2 mg per dL) within 30 to 60 minutes or excess acetone in the urine within 3 hours excludes the possibility of significant isopropanol exposure. *Disposition:* Symptomatic patients with concentrations greater than 100 mg per dL require at least 24 hours of close observation for resolution and should be admitted. If the patient is hypoglycemic, hypotensive, or comatose, admit to the ICU.

Lead. Lead is an environmental toxin. Acute lead intoxication is rare and is usually caused by inhalation of lead, resulting in severe intoxication and often death. It may be produced by burning lead batteries or using a heat gun to remove lead paint. It also results from exposure to high concentrations of organic lead (e.g., tetraethyl lead). Chronic lead poisoning occurs most often in children 6 months to 6 years of age who are exposed in their environment and in adults in certain occupations. See Table 34. In the United States, the incidence of children 1 to 5 years of age with a venous blood lead VBPb level greater than 10 μg per dL decreased from 88.2% in a survey of 1976 to 1980 to 8.9% in survey of 1988 to 1991 as a result of measures to reduce lead in the environment, particularly by reducing leaded gasoline. However, an estimated 1.7 million children between 1 and 5 years old have blood lead levels greater than 10 μg per dL and more than 1 million workers in over 100 different occupations are exposed to lead. *Toxic dose in chronic lead poisoning:* An intake of more than 5 μg per kg per day in children or more than 150 μg per day in adults can give a positive lead balance. In 1991, the Centers for Disease Control and Prevention (CDC) recommended routine screening for children. The CDC recommended a VBPb or a capillary blood lead determination for all children. In children a VBPb greater than 10 μg per dL was determined by the CDC to be a threshold of concern (it was 25 μg per dL in 1985). The average VBPb in the United States is 4 μg per dL. In occupational exposure (see Table 34) a VBPb greater than 40 μg per dL is indicative of increased lead absorption in adults. *Toxic mechanism:* Lead affects the sulfhydryl enzyme systems of the proteins, the immature CNS, the enzymes of heme synthesis, vitamin D conversion, the kidneys, the bones, and growth. Lead alters the tertiary structure of cell proteins, denaturing them and causing death. Risk factors are mouthing behavior of infants and children and excessive oral behavior (pica), living in the inner city, a poorly maintained home, and poor nutrition (e.g., low calcium and iron). The CDC questionnaire was recommended at every pediatric visit. See Table 35. If any answers to the CDC questionnaire are positive, obtain a blood screening test for lead. However, studies have suggested that to be more accurate in identifying lead exposure the questionnaire would have to be modified for each community because it has had poor sensitivity (40%) and specificity (60%). *Sources of*

TABLE 34. **Occupations Associated with Lead Exposure**

Lead production or smelting	Demolition of ships and bridges
Production of illicit whiskey	Battery manufacturing
Brass, copper, and lead foundries	Machining or grinding lead alloys
Radiator repair	Welding of old painted metals
Scrap handling	Thermal paint stripping of old buildings
Sanding of old paint	Ceramic glaze and pottery mixing
Lead soldering	
Cable stripping	
Instructor or janitor at firing range	

Modified from Rempel D: The lead-exposed worker. JAMA *262*:532–534, 1989. Copyright 1989, American Medical Association.

TABLE 35. **CDC Questionnaire: Priority Groups for Lead Screening**

1. Children 6–72 mo old (was 12–36 mo) who live in or are frequent visitors to older deteriorated housing built before 1960
2. Children 6–72 mo old who live in housing built before 1960 with recent, ongoing, or planned renovation or remodeling
3. Children 6–72 mo old who are siblings, housemates, or playmates of children with known lead poisoning
4. Children 6–72 mo old whose parents or other household members participate in a lead-related industry or hobby
5. Children 6–72 mo old who live near active lead smelters, battery recycling plants, or other industries likely to result in atmospheric lead release

lead (Table 36): (1) The primary source of lead is deteriorating lead-based paint, which forms leaded dust. Lead concentrations in indoor paint were not reduced to safer levels (0.06%) until 1978. Lead can also be produced by improper interior or exterior home renovation (scraping or demolition). (2) The use of leaded gasoline (limited in 1973) resulted in residues from leaded motor vehicle emissions. Lead persists in the soil near major highways and deteriorating homes and buildings. Vegetables grown in contaminated soil may contain lead. (3) Oil refineries and lead-processing smelters are sources. (4) Food cans produced in Mexico contain lead solder (95% do not in the United States). (5) Lead pipes (until 1950) and pipes with lead solder (until 1986) deliver lead-containing drinking water (calcium deposits, however, may offer some protection). Water at the consumer's tap should have a lead level less than 15 ppb. See Table 37. (6) Occupational exposure (see Table 34): Occupational Safety and Health Administration (OSHA) standards require employers to provide showering and clothes changing facilities for personnel working with lead; however, businesses with less than 25 employees are exempt from regulation. The OSHA lead standard of 1978 set a limit of 60 μg per dL for occupational exposure to lead. At a blood lead level of 60 μg per dL, a worker should be removed from lead exposure and not allowed back until the level is below 40 μg per dL. Many authorities feel that this level should be lower. The lead residue on workers' clothes may represent a hazard to their families. Others occupationally exposed to lead include plumbers, pipefitters, lead miners, auto repairers, shipbuilders, printers, steel welders and

TABLE 36. **Product Lead Content (%) by Dry Weight**

Product	Lead (%)	Product	Lead (%)
Plastic additives	2.0	Construction material	0.1
Priming inks	2.0	Fertilizers	0.1
Plumbing fixtures	2.0	Toys and recreational games	0.1
Solder	0.6	Curtain weights	0.1
Pesticides	0.1	Fishing weights	0.1
Stained glass came	0.1	Glazes, enamels, frits	0.06
Wine bottle foils	0.1	Paint	0.06

TABLE 37. **Agency Regulations and Recommendations for Lead Content**

Agency	Specimen	Level	Comments
CDC	Blood, child	10 μg/dL	Investigate community
OSHA	Blood, adult	60 μg/dL	Medical removal from work
OSHA	Air	50 μg/m³	PEL
	Air	0.75 mg/m³	Tetraethyl or tetramethyl
ACGIH	Air	150 μg/m³	TWA
EPA	Air	1.5 μg/m³	3-mo average
EPA	Water	15 μg/L (ppb)	5 ppb circulating
EPA	Food	100 μg/d	Advisory
FDA	Wine	300 ppm	Plan to reduce 200 ppm
EPA	Soil and dust	50 ppm	
CPSC	Paint	600 ppm (0.06%)	By dry weight

Abbreviations: CDC = Centers for Disease Control and Prevention; OSHA = Occupational Safety and Health Administration; ACGIH = American Conference of Governmental Industrial Hygienists; EPA = Environmental Protection Agency; FDA = Food and Drug Administration; CPSC = Consumer Products Safety Commission; PEL = permissible exposure limit (highest level over 8-h workday; TWA = time-weighted average (air concentration for 8-h workday and 40-h workweek).

cutters, construction workers, and those in rubber product manufacturing. (7) Leaded pots to make molds, "kusmusha" tea. (8) Hobbies (see Table 38) associated with lead exposure: making stained glass windows, lead fish sinkers, or curtain weights, especially if ingested and retained; imported pottery with ceramic glaze can leach large amounts of lead into acids (e.g., citrus fruit juices). (9) Some "traditional" folk remedies or cosmetics that contain lead: "Azarcon por empacho" ("Maria Louisa," 90 to 95% lead trioxide), a bright orange powder (Hispanic culture, especially Mexican, for digestive problems and diarrhea); "Greta" (4 to 90% lead), a yellow powder for "empacho" ("empacho" refers to a variety of GI symptoms; Hispanic cultures, especially Mexican); "Payloo-ah," an orange-red powder for rash and fever (Southeast Asian cultures, especially northern Laos Hmong immigrants); "Alkohl" (Al-kohl, kohl, suma,

TABLE 38. **Hobbies Associated with Lead Exposure**

Casting of ammunition
Collecting antique pewter
Collecting or painting lead toys (i.e., soldiers and figures)
Ceramics or glazed pottery
Refinishing furniture
Making fishing weights
Home renovation
Jewelry making (lead solder)
Glassblowing lead glass
Bronze casting
Print making and other fine arts (when lead white, flake white, chrome yellow pigments are involved)
Liquor distillation
Hunting and target shooting
Painting
Car and boat repair
Burning lead-painted wood
Making stained lead glass
Copper enameling

5 to 92% lead), a black powder (Middle Eastern, African, and Asian cultures as cosmetic and umbilical stump astringent); "Farouk," an orange granular powder with lead (Saudi Arabian); "Bint Al Zahab" to treat colic (Saudi Arabian); "Surma" (23 to 26% lead), a black powder used in India as a cosmetic and to improve eyesight; "Bali goli," a round black bean that is dissolved in "grippe water" (used by Asian and Indian cultures to aid digestion). (10) Substance abuse: The synthesis of amphetamines includes lead acetate, which may not be removed before use. Lead poisoning as a result of sniffing organic lead gasoline has been reported. *Kinetics:* Absorption of lead is 10 to 15% of the ingested dose in adults; in children up to 40% is absorbed, especially when iron deficiency anemia is present. Inhalation absorption is rapid and complete. The Vd in blood (0.9% of total body burden) is 95% in red blood cells; the $t_{1/2}$ is 35 to 40 days; $t_{1/2}$ in soft tissue, 45 days; and $t_{1/2}$ in bone (99% of the lead), 28 years. Lead is eliminated via the stool (80 to 90%); kidneys (10%; 80 μg per day); and hair, nails, sweat, and saliva. Organic lead is metabolized in the liver to inorganic lead; 9% is excreted in the urine per day. Lead passes through the placenta to the fetus and is present in breast milk. *Manifestations:* See Table 39. Adverse health effects include (1) Hematologic: Lead inhibits δ-aminolevulinic acid dehydratase early in the synthesis of heme (which has been associated with CNS symptoms) and ferrochelatase (which transfers iron to ferritin for iron incorporation into protoporphyrin to produce heme); anemia is a late finding. Decreased heme synthesis starts at more than 40 μg per dL. Basophilic stippling occurs in 20% of those with severe lead poison-

ing. (2) Neurologic: segmental demyelination and peripheral neuropathy, usually of motor type (wrist and ankle drop), occur in workers. A VBPb greater than 70 μg per dL (usually greater than 100 μg per dL) produces encephalopathy in children (symptom mnemonic is PAINT: P, persistent forceful vomiting and papilledema; A, ataxia; I, intermittent stupor and lucidity; N, neurologic coma and refractory convulsions; T, tired and lethargic). Decreased cognitive abilities have been associated with a VBPb higher than 10 μg per dL, behavior problems, decreased attention span, and learning abilities. IQ scores may begin to decrease at 15 μg per dL. In adults, peripheral neuropathies and "lead gum lines" at the dental border of the gingiva occur. Encephalopathy is rare in adults. (3) Renal nephropathy with damaged capillaries and glomeruli is seen at VBPb greater than 80 μg per dL, but renal damage and hypertension have been observed with low VBPb levels. Lead reduces excretion of uric acid, and high-level exposure is associated with hyperuricemia and "saturnine gout," Fanconi's syndrome (aminoaciduria and renal tubular acidosis), and tubular fibrosis. A linear association between hypertension and 30 μg per dL has been reported. (4) Reproductive effects include spontaneous abortion, transient delay in development (catch-up age 5 to 6 years), a decreased sperm count, and abnormal sperm morphology. Lead is transmitted across the placenta in 75 to 100% of cases and is teratogenic. (5) Metabolic: Decreased cytochrome P-450 (alters metabolism of medication and endogenously produced substances), decreased activation of cortisol, and decreased growth caused by interference with vitamin conversion (25-hydroxyvitamin D to

TABLE 39. **Summary of Lead-Induced Health Effects in Adults and Children**

Blood Lead Level (μg/dL)	Age Group (Adult or Child)	Health Effect
>100	Adult	Encephalopathic signs and symptoms
>80	Adult	Anemia
	Child	Encephalopathy
		Chronic nephropathy (e.g., aminoaciduria)
>70	Adult	Clinically evident peripheral neuropathy
	Child	Colic and other GI symptoms
>60	Adult	Female reproductive effects
		CNS disturbances and symptoms (i.e., sleep disturbances, mood changes, memory and concentration problems, headaches)
>50	Adult	Decreased hemoglobin production
		Decreased performance on neurobehavioral tests
		Altered testicular function
		GI symptoms (i.e., abdominal pain, constipation, diarrhea, nausea, anorexia)
	Child	Peripheral neuropathy
>40	Adult	Decreased peripheral nerve conduction
		Hypertension, age 40–59 y
		Chronic neuropathy
>25	Adult	Elevated erythrocyte protoporphyrin in males
15–25	Adult	Elevated erythrocyte protoporphyrin in females
	Child	Decreased intelligence and growth
>10	Fetus/child	Preterm delivery
		Impaired learning
		Reduced birth weight
		Impaired mental ability

Abbreviations: GI = gastrointestinal; CNS = central nervous system.
From Implementation of the Lead Contamination Control Act of 1988. MMWR Morb Mortal Wkly Rep *41*:288–290, 1992.

1,25-dihydroxyvitamin D) have been seen at VBPb of 20 to 30 μg per dL. (6) Other abnormalities of thyroid, cardiac, and hepatic function occur in adults. Abdominal colic is seen in children with a level greater than 50 μg per dL. *Management:* The basis of treatment is removal of the source. Cases of poisoning in children should be reported to the local health department and cases of occupational poisoning to OSHA. Control the exposure by identifying and abating source, improving housekeeping by wet mopping and using a high-phosphate detergent solution, allowing cold water to run for 2 minutes before using it for drinking, and planting shrubbery in contaminated soil to keep children away. (1) GI decontamination: Lead does not bind to AC. Do not delay chelation therapy for complete GI decontamination in severe cases. Whole-bowel irrigation has been used before treatment. Some authorities recommend abdominal radiography followed by GI decontamination, if necessary, before switching to oral therapy. (2) Supportive care includes measures to deal with refractory seizures (continue antidotal therapy, diazepam, and possibly neuromuscular blockers), hepatic and renal failure, and intravascular hemolysis. Treat seizures with diazepam, followed by neuromuscular blockers if needed. (3) Chelation therapy is used for children with levels above 45 μg per dL and adults with levels above 80 μg per dL or at lower levels with a positive lead mobilization test. See Table 40. Dimercaprol (BAL, British antilewisite) is a peanut oil–based dithiol (two sulfhydryl molecules) that combines with one atom of lead to form a heterocyclic stable ring complex. It is usually reserved for cases in which VBPb is above 70 μg per dL. It chelates red blood cell–bound lead and enhances its elimination through the urine and bile. It crosses the blood-brain barrier. About 50% of patients have adverse reactions including a bad metallic taste in the mouth, pain at the injection site, sterile abscesses, and fever. Edetate calcium disodium (ethylene diaminetetra-acetic acid, CaNa₂EDTA, Versenate) is a water-soluble chelator given IM (with 0.5% procaine) or IV. The calcium in the compound is displaced by divalent and trivalent heavy metals, which form a soluble complex that is stable at physiologic pH (but not at acid pH) and enhances clearance in the urine. It is usually administered IV, especially in severe cases. It must not be administered until adequate urine flow is established. It may redistribute lead to the brain; therefore BAL is started at VBPb levels exceeding 55 μg per dL in children and 100 μg per dL in adults. Phlebitis occurs at concentrations above 0.5 mg per mL. Alkalinization of the urine may be helpful (see Table 12). CaNa₂EDTA should not be confused with sodium EDTA (disodium edetate), which is used to treat hypercalcemia; inadvertent use may produce severe hypocalcemia. Succimer (dimercaptosuccinic acid, DMSA, Chemet), a derivative of BAL, is an oral agent approved by the FDA in 1991 for chelation in children with a VBPb above 45 μg per dL. The recommended dose is 10 mg per kg every 8 hours for 5 days, then every 12 hours for 14 days (see Table 12). DMSA is under investigation to determine its role for children with VBPb less than 45 μg per dL. Although not approved for adults, it has been used in the same dosage. Monitor the CBC, liver transaminases, and urinalysis for toxicity. D-Penicillamine is given at 20 to 40 mg per kg per day, not to exceed 1 gram per day. It is an oral chelator used to enhance the urinary elimination of lead; it is not FDA approved and has a 10% adverse reaction rate. Succimer is preferred. D-Penicillamine is used in adults with minimal symptoms but high VBPb levels. A VBPb above 70 μg per dL or clinical symptoms suggesting encephalopathy in children indicate a potential life-threatening emergency. Management should be accomplished in a medical center with a pediatric ICU by a multidisciplinary team including a critical care specialist, toxicologist, neurologist, and neurosurgeon with careful monitoring of neurologic parameters, fluid status, and intracranial pressure if necessary. These patients need close monitoring for hemodynamic instability. Adequate hydration should be maintained to ensure renal excretion of lead. Monitor fluids, renal and hepatic function, and electrolytes. While waiting for adequate urine flow, therapy

TABLE 40. **Pharmacologic Chelation Therapy for Lead Poisoning**

Drug	Route	Dose	Duration	Precautions	Monitor
Dimercaprol (BAL in oil)	IM	3–5 mg/kg q 4–6 h	3–5 d	G6PD deficiency Concurrent iron therapy	AST and ALT
CaNa₂EDTA (Calcium Disodium Versenate)	IM or IV	50 mg/kg/d	5 d	Inadequate fluid intake Renal impairment	Urinalysis BUN Creatinine
D-Penicillamine (Cuprimine)	PO	10 mg/kg/d, increase 30 mg/kg over 2 wk	6–20 wk	Penicillin allergy Concurrent iron therapy Lead exposure Renal impairment	Urinalysis BUN Creatinine CBC
2,3-Dimercaptosuccinic acid (DMSA; succimer)	PO	10 mg/kg per dose tid for 5 d 10 mg/kg per dose bid for 14 d	19 d	AST and ALT Concurrent iron therapy G6PD deficiency Lead exposure	AST and ALT

Abbreviations: BAL = British antilewisite; G6PD = glucose-6-phosphate dehydrogenase; AST = aspartate aminotransferase; ALT = alanine aminotransferase; BUN = blood urea nitrogen; CBC = complete blood count; EDTA = ethylenediaminetetra-acetic acid.

should be initiated with intramuscular dimercaprol (BAL) only (25 mg per kg per day divided into 6 doses). Four hours later, a combination of a second dose of BAL IM with CaNa$_2$EDTA (50 mg per kg per day) IV as a single dose infused over several hours or as a continuous infusion is given. The double therapy is continued until VBPb is less than 40 μg per dL. Therapy is continued for 72 hours and followed by one of two alternatives: either parenteral therapy with the two drugs (CaNa$_2$EDTA and BAL) for 5 days or continued therapy with CaNa$_2$EDTA alone if there is a good response and VBPb is below 40 μg per dL. If a report on VBPb has not been obtained, continue therapy with both BAL and EDTA for 5 days. In patients with lead encephalopathy, parenteral chelation should be continued with both drugs until the patient is clinically stable before changing therapy. Mannitol and dexamethasone can reduce the cerebral edema, but removal of the lead is essential and their role in lead encephalopathy is not clear. Avoid surgical decompression to reduce cerebral edema. If BAL and CaNa$_2$EDTA are used together, a minimum of 2 days with no treatment should elapse before considering another 5-day course of therapy. Repeat the 5-day course with CaNa$_2$EDTA alone if the blood lead level remains above 40 μg per dL or in combination with BAL if it is above 70 μg per dL. If a third course is required, unless there are compelling reasons, wait at least 5 to 7 days before administering. Continue chelation therapy at all costs. After chelation therapy, a period of equilibration of 10 to 14 days should be allowed and repeated determinations of VBPb concentrations should be obtained. If the patient is stable enough for oral intake, oral succimer at 30 mg per kg per day in three divided doses for 5 days followed by 20 mg per kg per day in two divided doses for 14 days has been suggested, but data are limited. Continue therapy until VBPb is less than 20 μg per dL in children or 40 μg per dL in adults. Chelators combined with lead are hemodialyzable in the event of renal failure. *Laboratory investigations:* (1) A classification of blood lead concentrations in children is given in Table 41. (2) The lead mobilization test is used to determine the chelatable pool of lead. It consists of the administration of 25 mg per kg in children or 1 gram in adults as a single dose deeply IM with 0.5% procaine diluted 1:1 or as an infusion. Empty the bladder and collect the urine for 24 hours (3 days if there is renal impairment). A modified 8-hour collection may be obtained. If the ratio of micrograms of lead excreted in the urine to the milligrams of CaNa$_2$EDTA administered is greater than 0.6, it represents an increased lead body burden, and therapeutic chelation is indicated. However, many consider this test of little importance in making the decision about chelation. The use of x-ray fluorescence of bone as an alternative to determine the lead burden is being tested. (3) Evaluate the CBC, serum ferritin, VBPb levels, erythrocyte protoporphyrin (greater than 35 μg per dL indicates lead poisoning as well as iron deficiency and other causes), electrolytes, serum calcium and phosphorus,

TABLE 41. **Classification of Blood Lead Concentrations in Children**

Blood Lead (μg/dL)	Classification	Recommended Interventions
<9	I	None
10–14	IIa	Community intervention Repeat blood lead determination in 3 mo
15–19	IIb	Individual case management Environmental counseling Nutritional counseling Repeat blood lead determination in 3 mo
20–44	III	Medical referral Environmental inspection and/or abatement Nutritional counseling Repeat blood lead determination in 3 mo
45–69	IV	Environmental inspection and/or abatement Nutritional counseling Pharmacologic therapy: succimer oral or CaNa$_2$EDTA parenteral Repeat q 2 wk for 6–8 wk, monthly for 4–6 mo
>70	V	Hospitalization in intensive care unit Environmental inspection and/or abatement Pharmacologic therapy: dimercaprol IM alone initially, then dimercaprol IM and CaNa$_2$EDTA together; repeat every week

urine, BUN, and creatinine. Abdominal and long bone radiographs are not routine but may be useful in certain circumstances for identifying radiopaque material in bowel and lead lines in proximal tibia (these occur after prolonged exposure in association with VBPb above 50 μg per dL). Serial VBPb measurements are obtained on days 3 and 5 during treatment, 7 days after chelation therapy, then every 1 to 2 weeks for 8 weeks, and then every month for 6 months. Stop the IV infusion at least 1 hour before obtaining blood for lead determination. (4) Neuropsychologic tests are difficult to perform in young children but should be considered at the end of treatment, especially to determine auditory dysfunction. *Disposition:* All patients with levels above 70 μg per dL or who are symptomatic should be admitted. If a child is hospitalized, all lead hazards must be removed before allowing the child to return home. The source must be eliminated by environmental and occupational investigations. The local health department should be involved in dealing with children with lead poisoning and OSHA with occupational lead poisoning. Consultation with the poison control center and/or an experienced toxicologist is necessary when using chelation therapy. Follow-up VBPb concentrations should be obtained within 1 to 2 weeks and followed every 2 weeks for 8 weeks and then monthly for 6 months if the patient required chelation therapy. All patients with VBPb values above 10 μg per dL should be followed up at least every 3 months until 2VBPb is 10 μg per dL or 3VBPb is <15 μg per dL.

Lithium (Li, Eskalith, Lithane). Lithium is an A-1 alkali metal whose primary use is in the treatment of bipolar psychiatric disorders. Most intoxications are chronic overdoses. One gram of lithium carbonate contains 189 mg of lithium, a regular tablet 300 mg or 8.12 mEq, and a sustained-release preparation 450 mg or 12.18 mEq. *Toxic mechanism:* The brain is the primary target organ of toxicity but the mechanism is unclear. Lithium may interfere with physiologic functions by acting as a substitute for cellular cations (sodium and potassium), depressing neural excitation and synaptic transmission. *Toxic dose:* A lithium dose of 1 mEq per kg (40 mg per kg) results in a serum lithium concentration of about 1.2 mEq per liter. The therapeutic serum lithium concentration in acute mania is 0.6 to 1.2 mEq per liter and for maintenance 0.5 to 0.8 mEq per liter. Serum lithium levels are usually obtained 12 hours after the last dose. The toxic dose is determined by clinical manifestations and serum levels after the distribution phase. Acute ingestion of twenty 300-mg tablets (300 mg increases the serum lithium concentration by 0.2 to 0.4 mEq per liter) in adults and may produce serious intoxication. Chronic intoxication is produced by any state that increases lithium reabsorption. Risk factors that predispose to chronic lithium toxicity are febrile illness, impaired renal function, hyponatremia, advanced age, lithium-induced diabetes insipidus, dehydration, vomiting and diarrheal illness, concomitant drugs (thiazide and spironolactone diuretics, NSAIDs, salicylates, angiotensin-converting enzyme inhibitors [captopril], and selective serotonin reuptake inhibitors [SSRIs] [e.g., fluoxetine and antipsychotic drugs]). *Kinetics:* GI absorption is rapid and peaks in 2 to 4 hours after regular-release preparations, and complete absorption occurs by 6 to 8 hours. Absorption may be delayed 6 to 12 hours after sustained-release preparations. The onset of toxicity may occur at 1 to 4 hours after acute overdose but is usually delayed because lithium enters the brain slowly. The Vd is 0.5 to 0.9 liter per kg. Lithium is not protein bound. The $t_{1/2}$ after a single dose is 9 to 13 hours; at steady state it may be 30 to 58 hours. The renal handling of lithium is similar to that of sodium, by glomerular filtration and reabsorption (80%) by the proximal renal tubules. Adequate sodium must be present to prevent lithium reabsorption. More than 90% of lithium is excreted by the kidney unchanged; 30 to 60% within 6 to 12 hours. Alkalinization of the urine increases clearance. *Manifestations:* One should distinguish among side effects, acute, acute on chronic therapy, and chronic intoxications. Chronic is the most common and dangerous type of intoxication. (1) Side effects of lithium include fine tremor, GI upset, hypothyroidism, polyuria and frank diabetes insipidus, dermatologic manifestations, and cardiac conduction deficits. Lithium is teratogenic. (2) Toxic effects: Patients with acute poisoning may be asymptomatic with an early high serum lithium concentration of 9

mEq per liter and deteriorate as the serum level falls 50% and lithium is distributed to the brain and the other tissues. The onset of nausea and vomiting may occur within 1 to 4 hours, but the systemic manifestations are usually delayed several more hours. It may take as long as 3 to 5 days for serious symptoms to develop. Acute toxicity is manifested by neurologic findings including weakness, fasciculations, altered mental state, myoclonus, hyper-reflexia, rigidity, coma, and convulsions with limbs in hyperextension. Cardiovascular effects are nonspecific and occur at therapeutic doses, flat T or inverted T waves, AV block, and prolonged QT interval. Lithium is not a primary cardiotoxin. Cardiogenic shock is secondary to CNS toxicity. Chronic intoxication is associated with manifestations at lower serum lithium concentrations. There is some correlation with manifestations especially at higher serum lithium concentrations. See Table 42. Permanent neurologic sequelae can result from lithium intoxication. *Management:* (1) Establish and maintain vital functions. Institute seizure precautions and treat seizures, hypotension, and dysrhythmias. Restore normothermia. (2) Evaluation: Examine for rigidity and signs of hyper-reflexia, hydration, renal function (BUN, creatinine), and electrolytes, especially sodium. Inquire about use of diuretics and other drugs that increase the serum lithium concentrations and discontinue them. If the patient is receiving chronic therapy, discontinue the lithium. Obtain serial serum lithium concentrations every 4 hours until the concentration peaks and there is a downward trend toward an almost therapeutic range, especially with sustained-release prep-

TABLE 42. **Classification of Severity of Chronic Lithium Intoxication**

Classification	Manifestations	Blood Concentration (mEq/L) in Chronic Intoxication*
Subacute or pretoxic	Apathy, fine tremor, vomiting and diarrhea, weakness	<1.2
Mild intoxication	Lethargy, drowsiness; hypertonia, hyper-reflexia; muscle rigidity, dysarthria; ataxia, apathy, nystagmus	1.2–2.5
Moderate intoxication	Impaired consciousness; severe fasciculations; coarse tremor, severe ataxia; myoclonus, paresthesias; diabetes insipidus, electro-cardiographic changes; renal tubular acidosis; paralysis, blurred vision	2.5–3.5
Severe intoxication	Muscle twitching, coma; severe myoclonic jerking; cardiac dysrhythmias; seizures, spasticity, shock	>3.5

*Plasma lithium concentrations (not an absolute correlation).
Modified from El-Mallakh RS: Treatment of acute lithium toxicity. Vet Hum Toxicol 26:31–35, 1984.

arations. Monitor vital signs including temperature and ECG and conduct serial neurologic examinations including mental status and urine output. Obtain a nephrology consultation if there is a chronic and elevated serum lithium level (above 2.5 mEq per liter), a large ingestion, or altered mental state. (3) Fluid and electrolyte therapy: An IV line should be established and hydration and electrolyte balance restored. Determine the serum sodium level before administration of 0.89% saline fluid in chronic overdoses because hypernatremia may be present as a result of diabetes insipidus. Although current evidence indicates that an initial 0.89% saline infusion (200 mL per hour) enhances excretion of lithium, once hydration, output, and normonatremia are established administer 0.45% saline and slow the infusion (100 mL per hour). (4) GI decontamination: Gastric lavage is useful only after recent acute ingestion and is not necessary after chronic intoxication. AC is ineffective. With slow-release preparations, whole-bowel irrigation may be useful but this has not been proved. Sodium polystyrene sulfonate (Kayexalate), an ion exchange resin, at 15 to 50 grams orally every 4 to 6 hours may be useful in preventing absorption and in enhancing the removal in acute massive overdoses, but it is difficult to administer. The data are based on a few uncontrolled studies. (5) Hemodialysis is the most efficient method of removing lithium from the vascular compartment. It is the treatment of choice for severe intoxications with an altered mental state and seizures and in anuric patients. Long runs are used until the serum lithium level is below 1 mEq per liter because of extensive re-equilibration. Monitor the serum lithium level every 4 hours after dialysis for rebound. Repeated and prolonged hemodialysis may be necessary. Expect a lag in neurologic recovery. *Laboratory investigations:* Monitor: CBC (lithium causes significant leukocytosis), renal dysfunction, thyroid dysfunction (chronic intoxication), ECG, and electrolytes. Determine the serum lithium concentrations every 4 hours until there is a downward trend near the therapeutic range. The levels do not always correlate with the manifestations but are more predictive in severe intoxications. A value above 3.0 mEq per liter with chronic intoxication and altered mental state indicates severe toxicity. Patients with a value above 9 mEq per liter after an acute overdose may be asymptomatic. Cross-reactions: The green-top Vacutainer specimen tube containing heparin spuriously elevates the serum lithium value 6 to 8 mEq per liter. *Disposition:* An acute asymptomatic lithium overdose cannot be medically cleared on the basis of a single lithium level. Patients should be admitted if they have any neurologic manifestations (altered mental status, hyper-reflexia, stiffness, or tremor). Patients should be admitted to the ICU if they are dehydrated, have renal impairment, or have a high or rising lithium level.

Methanol (wood alcohol). The concentration of methanol in Sterno fuel is 4% (it also contains ethanol), in windshield washer fluid 30%, and in gas line antifreeze 100%. *Toxic mechanism:* Methanol is metabolized by hepatic ADH to formaldehyde and formate. Formate produces tissue hypoxia, metabolic lactic acidosis, and retinal damage. Formate is converted by folate-dependent enzymes to carbon dioxide. *Toxic dose:* The minimal toxic amount is approximately 100 mg per kg. One tablespoonful (15 mL) of 40% methanol was lethal for a 2-year-old child and can cause blindness in an adult. The fatal oral dose is 30 to 240 mL of 100% methanol (20 to 150 grams). The toxic blood methanol concentration (BMC) is above 20 mg per dL, the very serious toxicity and potentially fatal level greater than 50 mg per dL. The blood methanol concentration and amount ingested can be estimated using the following equations and a specific gravity of 0.719.

$$BMC\ (mg/dL) =$$

$$\frac{amount\ ingested\ (mL) \times \%\ methanol\ in\ product \times SG\ (0.719)}{Vd\ (0.6\ L/kg) \times body\ weight\ (kg)}$$

$$Dose\ (amount\ ingested) =$$

$$\frac{BMC\ (mg\ per\ dL) \times Vd\ (0.6\ L/kg) \times body\ weight\ (kg)}{\%\ ethanol \times SG\ (0.719)}$$

Kinetics: Onset can start within 1 hour but is typically delayed 12 to 18 hours by metabolism to toxic metabolites. It may be delayed longer if ethanol is ingested concomitantly. Onset may be up to 72 hours in infants. The peak blood methanol concentration occurs at 1 hour. The Vd is 0.6 liter per kg (total body water); $t_{1/2}$ is 8 hours (with ethanol blocking it is 30 to 35 hours and with hemodialysis 2.5 hours). For metabolism see the section on toxic mechanism. Elimination is renal. *Manifestations:* Slow metabolism may delay onset for 12 to 18 hours in adults or longer if ethanol is ingested concomitantly. Methanol may produce inebriation, a formadehyde odor on the breath, hyperemia of the optic disk, violent abdominal colic, "snow" vision, blindness, and shock. Later, worsening acidosis, hypoglycemia, and multiple organ failure develop; death results from complications of intractable acidosis and cerebral edema. Methanol produces an osmolal gap (early) and its metabolite formate produces AG metabolic acidosis (later). Absence of an osmolar gap or AG does not always exclude methanol intoxication. *Management:* (1) Protect the airway by intubation to prevent aspiration and administer assisted ventilation as needed. Administer 100% oxygen if needed. Consult with a nephrologist early regarding the need for hemodialysis. (2) GI decontamination procedures have no role. (3) Treat metabolic acidosis vigorously with sodium bicarbonate at 2 to 3 mEq per kg IV. Large amounts may be needed. (4) Ethanol therapy and hemodialysis (see Table 12): Classically, ethanol therapy was started if the blood methanol concentration was above 20 mg per dL and hemodialysis was added if the concentration was above 50 mg per dL, but values less than 25 mg per dL are currently used as an indication for hemodialysis. Ethanol therapy: ADH has 100 times greater affinity for ethanol than methanol. Therefore, ethanol blocks the metabolism of methanol at a blood methanol concentration of 100 to 150 mg per dL. Initiate therapy to block metabolism if there is a history of ingestion of 0.4 mL of 100% methanol per kg, the blood methanol level is above 20 mg per dL or the patient has an osmolar gap that is not accounted for, or the patient is symptomatic or acidotic with an increased AG and/or hyperemia of the optic disk. (See Table 12.) Hemodialysis increases the clearance of both methanol and formate 10-fold over renal clearance. Continue to monitor methanol levels and/or formate levels every 4 hours after the procedure for rebound. Toxicologists and nephrologists have recommended early hemodialysis at blood methanol levels greater than 25 mg per dL because it significantly shortens the course of the intoxication and provides better outcomes. Other indications for early hemodialysis are significant metabolic acidosis, electrolyte abnormalities despite conventional therapy, and the presence of visual or mental symptoms. A serum formate level greater than 20 mg per dL has also been used as a criterion for hemodialysis. If hemodialysis is used, increase the infusion rate of 10% ethanol to 2.0 to 3.5 mL per kg per hour. Obtain the BEC and glucose every 2 hours. Continue therapy with both ethanol and hemodialysis until a blood methanol level is undetectable, there is no acidosis, and there are no mental or visual disturbances. This may require 2 to 5 days. (5) Treat hypoglycemia with IV glucose. (6) A bolus of folinic acid and folic acid has been used successfully in animal investigations to enhance formate metabolism to carbon dioxide and water. Administer leucovorin (Wellcovorin) at 1 mg per kg up to 50 mg IV every 4 hours for several days. (7) 4-Methylpyrazole inhibits ADH and is being investigated for use in methanol and ethylene glycol poisoning (see dosage under ethylene glycol management). It is not yet approved in the United States. (8) Obtain ophthalmologic consultation initially and at follow-up. *Laboratory investigations:* Methanol is detected on drug screens if specified. Monitor methanol and ethanol levels every 4 hours, electrolytes, glucose, BUN, creatinine, amylase, and ABGs. Formate levels correlate more closely than blood methanol levels with severity of intoxication and should be obtained if possible. If methanol levels are not available, the osmolal gap × 3.2 can be used to estimate the blood methanol levels in mg per dL. *Disposition:* All patients who ingest significant amounts of methanol should be referred to the emergency department for evaluation and blood methanol concentration. Ophthalmologic follow-up of all intoxications should be arranged.

Monoamine Oxidase Inhibitors. MAOIs include MAO-A inhibitors, the hydrazine phenelzine sulfate (Nardil; dose 60 to 90 mg per day), isocarboxazid (Marplan; 10 to 30 mg per day), and the nonhydrazine tranylcypromine (Parnate; 20 to 40 mg per day). The MAO-B inhibitor selegiline (deprenyl, Eldepryl; 10 mg per day), an antiparkinsonism agent, does not have toxicity similar to that of MAO-A and is not discussed. MAOIs are used to treat severe depression. *Toxic mechanism:* MAO enzymes are responsible for the oxidative deamination of both endogenous and exogenous catecholamines. MAO-A in the intestinal wall also metabolizes tyramine in food. MAOIs permanently inhibit MAO enzymes until a new enzyme is synthesized 14 days or longer. The toxicity results from the accumulation, potentiation, and prolongation of the catecholamine action followed by profound hypotension and cardiovascular collapse. *Toxic dose:* Toxicity begins at 2 to 3 mg per kg and fatalities occur at 4 to 6 mg per kg. Death has occurred after a single dose of tranylcypromine of 170 mg in an adult. *Kinetics:* Structurally, MAOIs are related to amphetamines and catecholamines. The hydrazine peak level occurs at 1 to 2 hours; elimination is by hepatic acetylation metabolism and excretion of inactive metabolites in the urine. The nonhydrazine peak level is at 1 to 4 hours, and elimination is by hepatic metabolism to active amphetamine-like metabolites. The onset of symptoms in overdoses is delayed 6 to 24 hours after ingestion, peak activity occurs at 8 to 12 hours, and the duration is 72 hours or longer. Peak MAO inhibition occurs in 5 to 10 days and lasts as long as 5 weeks. *Manifestations:* (1) Acute ingestion overdose: Phase I consists of an adrenergic crisis in which onset is delayed for 6 to 24 hours and the peak may not be reached until 24 hours. Manifestations start as hyperthermia, tachycardia, tachypnea, dysarthria, transient hypertension, hyper-reflexia, and CNS stimulation. Phase II consists of neuromuscular excitation and sympathetic hyperactivity with increased temperature (above 104°F [40°C]), agitation, hyperactivity, confusion, fasciculations, twitching, tremor, masseter spasm, muscle rigidity, acidosis, and electrolyte abnormalities. Seizures and dystonic reactions may occur. The pupils are mydriatic, sometimes nonreactive, with a "Ping-Pong gaze." Phase III, CNS depression and cardiovascular collapse, occurs in severe overdose as the catecholamines are depleted. Symptoms usually resolve within 5 days but may last 2 weeks. Phase IV consists of secondary complications: rhabdomyolysis, cardiac dysrhythmias, multiple organ failure, and coagulopathies. (2) Biogenic interactions usually occur while therapeutic doses of MAOIs are given or shortly after they are discontinued, before the new MAO enzyme is synthesized. The onset occurs within 30 to 60 minutes after exposure. The following substances have been implicated: indirect-acting sympathomimetics (e.g., amphetamines); serotonergic drugs, opioids (e.g., meperidine, dextromethorphan), tricyclic antidepressants, and SSRIs (fluoxetine, sertraline, paroxetine); and tyramine-containing foods (wine, beer, avocados, cheese, caviar, chocolate, chicken liver) and L-tryptophan. SSRIs should not be started for at least 5 weeks after MAOIs have been discontinued. In mild cases, usually caused by foods, headache and hypertension develop and last for several hours. In severe cases, malignant hypertension and malignant hyperthermia syndromes consisting of hypertension or hyperthermia, altered mental state, skeletal muscle rigidity, shivering (often beginning in the masseter muscle), and seizures may occur. The serotonin syndrome, which may be due to inhibition of serotonin metabolism, has clinical findings similar to those in malignant hyperthermia and may occur with or without hyperthermia or hypertension. (3) Clinical findings in chronic toxicity include tremors, hyperhidrosis, agitation, hallucinations, confusion, and seizures and can be confused with withdrawal syndromes. *Management:* (1) MAOI overdose: GI decontamination with ipecac-induced emesis should not be used because it may aggravate the food-MAOI interaction hypertension. Use gastric lavage and AC or AC alone. If the patient is admitted to the hospital and is well enough to eat, order a nontyramine diet. Extreme agitation and seizures can be controlled with BZPs and barbiturates. Phenytoin is ineffective. Nondepolarizing neuromuscular blockers (not depolarizing succinylcholine) may be needed in severe cases of hyperthermia and rigidity. If there is severe hypertension (catecholamine mediated), use phentolamine, a parenteral alpha blocking agent, at 3 to 5 mg intravenously or labetalol, a combination of an alpha blocking agent and beta blocker, as a 20-mg IV bolus. If malignant hypertension with rigidity is present, use SA nitroprusside and BZP. Hypertension is often followed by severe hypotension, which should be managed with fluid and vasopressors. Caution: Vasopressor therapy should be administered at lower doses than usual because of an exaggerated pharmacologic response. Norepinephrine is preferred to dopamine, which requires release of intracellular amines. Cardiac dysrhythmias are treated with standard therapy but are often refractory, and cardioversion and pacemakers may be needed. For malignant hyperthermia, administer dantrolene (see Table 12), a nonspecific peripheral skeletal relaxing agent, which inhibits the release of calcium from the sarcoplasm. Dantrolene is reconstituted with 60 mL of sterile water without bacteriostatic agents; do not use glass equipment, protect from light, and use within 6 hours. The loading dose is 2 to 3 mg per kg IV as a bolus and is repeated until the signs of malignant hyperthermia (tachycardia, rigidity, increased end-tidal carbon dioxide, and temperature) are controlled. The maximal total dose is 10 mg per kg to avoid hepatotoxicity. When malignant hyperthermia subsides, give 1 mg per kg IV every 6 hours for 24 to 48 hours; then give 1 mg per kg orally every 6 hours for 24 hours to prevent recurrence. There is a danger of thrombophlebitis after peripheral dantrolene, and it should be administered through a central line if possible. In addition, provide external cooling and correct metabolic acidosis and electrolyte disturbances. BZP can be used for sedation. Dantrolene does not reverse central dopamine blockade; therefore, give bromocriptine mesylate at 2.5 to 10 mg orally or through a nasogastric tube three times a day. Treat rhabdomyolysis and myoglobinuria with fluid diuresis, furosemide, and alkalinization. Hemo-

dialysis and hemoperfusion are of no proven value. (2) Biogenic amine interactions are managed symptomatically similar to overdose. For the serotonin syndrome, cyproheptadine, a serotonin blocker, may be given at 4 mg orally every hour for 3 doses or methysergide (Sansert) at 2 mg orally every 6 hours for 3 doses, but their efficacy is not proved. *Laboratory investigations:* Monitor ECG, cardiac parameters, creatine kinase, ABGs, pulse oximetry, electrolytes, blood glucose, and acid-base balance. *Disposition:* All patients who ingest more than 2 mg per kg should be admitted to the hospital for 24 hours of observation and monitoring in the ICU because the life-threatening manifestations may be delayed. Patients with drug or dietary interactions that are mild may not require admission if symptoms subside within 4 to 6 hours and they remain asymptomatic. Patients with symptoms that persist or require active intervention should be admitted to the ICU.

Opioids (narcotic opiates). Opioids are used for analgesia, as antitussives, and as antidiarrheal agents and are illicit agents (heroin, opium) used in substance abuse. Tolerance, physical dependence, and withdrawal may develop. *Toxic mechanism:* At least four main opioid receptors have been identified. Mu is considered the most important for central analgesia and depression. Kappa and delta are predominant in spinal analgesia. The sigma receptors may mediate dysphoria. Death is due to dose-dependent CNS respiratory depression or is secondary to apnea, pulmonary aspiration, or noncardiac pulmonary edema. The mechanism of noncardiac pulmonary edema is unknown. *Toxic dose:* This depends on the specific drug, route of administration, and degree of tolerance. For therapeutic and toxic doses, see Table 43. In children, respiratory depression has been produced by 10 mg of morphine or methadone, 75 mg of meperidine, and 12.5 mg of diphenoxylate. Infants younger than 3 months are more susceptible to respiratory depression. Reduce the dose 50%. *Kinetics:* Oral onset of the analgesic effect of morphine is at 10 to 15 minutes; the effect peaks in 1 hour and the duration is 4 to 6 hours, but with sustained-release preparations (e.g., MS Contin) the duration is 8 to 12 hours. Opioids are 90% metabolized in the liver by hepatic conjugation and 90% excreted in the urine as inactive compounds. The Vd is 1 to 4 liters per kg; PB, 35 to 75%. The typical plasma $t_{1/2}$ of opiates is 2 to 5 hours, but that of methadone is 24 to 36 hours. Morphine metabolites include morphine-3-glucuronide (M3G) (inactive) and morphine-6-glucuronide (M6G) (active) and normorphine (active). Meperidine is rapidly hydrolyzed by tissue esterases into the active metabolite, normeperidine, which has twice the convulsant activity of meperidine. Heroin (diacetylmorphine) is deacetylated within minutes to the metabolite 6-monacetylmorphine (6MAM), which is diagnostic of heroin use, and morphine. Propoxyphene (Darvon) has a rapid onset, and death has occurred within 15 to 30 minutes after a massive overdose. Propoxyphene is metabolized to norpropoxyphene, an active metabolite with convulsive, car-

TABLE 43. **Doses, Onset, and Duration of Action of Common Opioids**

Drug	Adult Oral Dose	Child Oral Dose	Onset of Action (min)	Duration of Action (h)	Adult Fatal Dose
Camphored tincture of opium (0.4 mg/mL), paregoric	25 mL	0.25–0.50 mL/kg	15–30	4–5	NA
Codeine	30–180 mg (> mg/kg is toxic in a child, above 200 mg in adult; >5 mg/kg fatal in a child)	0.5–1 mg/kg	15–30	4–6	800 mg
Dextromethorphan	15 mg 10 mg/kg is toxic	0.25 mg/kg	15–30	3–6	NA
Diacetylmorphine (heroin)	60 mg Street heroin is less than 10% pure	NA	15–30	3–4	100 mg
Diphenoxylate (Lomotil)	5–10 mg 7.5 mg is toxic in a child, 300 mg is toxic in adult	NA	120–240	14	300 mg
Fentanyl (Sublimaze, Duragesic transdermal)	0.1–0.2 mg	0.001–0.002 mg/kg	7–8 IM	0.5–2	1.0 mg
Hydrocodone (Hycodan, Vicodin)	5–30 mg	0.15 mg/kg	30	3–4	100 mg
Hydromorphone (Dilaudid)	4 mg	0.1 mg/kg	15–30	3–4	100 mg
Meperidine (Demerol)	100 mg	1–1.5 mg/kg	10–45	3–4	350 mg
Methadone (Dolophine)	10 mg	0.1 mg/kg	30–60	4–12	120 mg
Morphine	10–60 mg Oral dose is six times parenteral dose; MS Contin (sustained-release)	0.1–0.2 mg/kg	<20	4–6	200 mg
Oxycodone (Percodan)	5 mg	NA	15–30	4–5	NA
Pentazocine (Talwin)	50–100 mg	NA	15–30	3–4	NA
Propoxyphene (Darvon)	65–100 mg 100 mg hydrochloride = 65 mg of napsylate, toxic at 10 mg/kg	NA	30–60	2–4	700 mg

Abbreviation: NA = not available.

diac dysrhythmic, and heart block properties. Symptoms of diphenoxylate (Lomotil) appear within 1 to 4 hours. It is metabolized into the active metabolite difenoxin, which is five times more active as a recurrent respiratory depressant. Death has been reported in children after a single tablet. *Manifestations:* (1) Initial or mild intoxication produces miosis, a dull face, drowsiness, partial ptosis, and "nodding" (head drops to chest and then bobs up). Larger amounts produce the classic triad of miotic pupils (exceptions follow), respiratory depression, and depressed level of consciousness (flaccid coma). The blood pressure, pulse, and bowel sounds are decreased. (2) Dilated pupils do not exclude opioid intoxication. Some exceptions to miosis include dextromethorphan (paralyzes iris), fentanyl, meperidine, and diphenoxylate (rarely). Physiologic disturbances including acidosis, hypoglycemia, hypoxia, and postictal state or a coingestant may also produce mydriasis. (3) Usually the muscles are flaccid, but increased muscle tone may be produced by meperidine and fentanyl (chest rigidity). (4) Seizures are rare but can occur with codeine, meperidine, propoxyphene, and dextromethorphan. Hallucinations and agitation have been reported. (5) Pruritus and urticaria caused by histamine release of some opioids or by sulfites may be present. (6) Noncardiac pulmonary edema often occurs after resuscitation and naloxone administration, especially with IV abuse. (7) Cardiac effects include vasodilatation and hypotension. A heart murmur in one who is addicted to an IV drug suggests endocarditis. Propoxyphene can produce delayed cardiac dysrhythmias. (8) Fentanyl is 100 times more potent than morphine and can cause chest wall muscle rigidity. Some of its derivatives are 2000 times more potent than morphine. *Management:* (1) Supportive care, particularly an endotracheal tube and assisted ventilation. Temporary ventilation may be provided bag-valve-mask with 100% oxygen. Begin cardiac monitoring; establish IV access; and obtain specimens for ABG, glucose, electrolyte, BUN, creatinine, CBC, coagulation profile, and liver function determinations, a toxicology screen, and urinalysis. (2) GI decontamination: Do not induce emesis. Administer AC if bowel sounds are present. Cathartics may be used because of opioid-induced decreased GI mobility and constipation. (3) Naloxone (Narcan) (see Table 12): If addiction is suspected, restrain the patient first; then administer 0.1 mg and double the dose every 2 minutes until the patient responds or 10 to 20 mg has been given. If addiction is not suspected, give 2 mg every 2 to 3 minutes to total of 10 to 20 mg. It is essential to determine whether there is a complete response to naloxone (mydriasis, improvement in ventilation) because it is a diagnostic therapeutic test. A continuous naloxone infusion may be appropriate using the "response dose" every hour. Repeated doses of naloxone may be necessary because the effects of many opioids can last much longer than that of naloxone (30 to 60 minutes). Methadone may require a naloxone infusion for 24 to 48 hours. Half of the response dose may have to be repeated in 15 to 20 minutes, after starting the infusion. Acute iatrogenic withdrawal on administration of naloxone to a dependent patient should not be treated with morphine or other opioids. Naloxone's effects are limited to 30 to 60 minutes (shorter than those of most opioids) and withdrawal subsides in a short time. (4) Nalmefene (Revex), an FDA-approved long-acting (4 to 8 hours) pure opioid antagonist, is being investigated but its role in acute intoxication is unclear. It may have a role in place of naloxone infusion but could produce prolonged withdrawal. (5) Noncardiac pulmonary edema does not respond to naloxone and the patient requires intubation, assisted ventilation, PEEP, and hemodynamic monitoring. Fluids should be given cautiously in opioid overdose because they stimulate antidiuretic hormone. (6) If the patient is comatose, give 50% glucose (3 to 4% of comatose opioid overdose patients have hypoglycemia) and thiamine before naloxone. If the patient has seizures unresponsive to naloxone, administer diazepam and examine for other metabolic (hypoglycemia, electrolyte disturbances) and structural disturbances. (7) Hypotension is rare and should direct a search for another etiology. (8) If the patient is agitated, exclude hypoxia and hypoglycemia before considering opioid withdrawal. (9) Complications to consider include urine retention, constipation, rhabdomyolysis, myoglobinuria, hypoglycemia, and withdrawal. *Laboratory investigations:* For overdoses, monitor ABGs, blood glucose, and electrolytes; obtain chest radiographs and an ECG. For drug abusers, consider testing for hepatitis B, syphilis, and HIV antibody (HIV testing usually requires consent). Blood opioid concentrations are not useful. They confirm the diagnosis (morphine therapeutic 65 to 80 ng per mL, toxic greater than 200 ng per mL) but are not useful for making a therapeutic decision. Cross-reactions can occur with Vicks Formula 44, poppy seeds on bagels, and other opioids (codeine and heroin are metabolized to morphine). Naloxone at 4 mg IV was not associated with a positive enzyme multiple immunoassay technique (EMIT) urine screen at 60 minutes, 6 hours, or 48 hours. *Disposition:* If a patient responds to IV naloxone, careful observation for relapse and the development of pulmonary edema is required with cardiac and respiratory monitoring for 6 to 12 hours. Patients requiring repeated doses of naloxone or an infusion or who develop pulmonary edema require ICU admission and cannot be discharged from the ICU until they are symptom free for 12 hours. IV complications are expected to be present within 20 minutes after injection, and discharge after 4 symptom-free hours has been recommended. Adults with oral overdose have a delayed onset of toxicity and require observation for 6 hours. Children with oral opioid overdose should be admitted to the hospital for 24 hours of observation because of delayed toxicity. Restrain the patient who attempts to sign out AMA after treatment with naloxone, at least until psychiatric evaluation.

Organophosphates and Carbamates. Sources of cholinergic intoxication are insecticides, medications (carbamates), and some mushrooms. Examples of organophosphate (OP) insecticides are malathion (Cythion; low toxicity, median lethal dose [LD_{50}] 2800 mg per kg), chlorpyrifos (Dursban; moderate toxicity, LD_{50} 250 mg per kg), and parathion (high toxicity, LD_{50} 2 mg per kg); carbamate insecticides are carbaryl (Sevin; low toxicity, LD_{50} 500 mg per kg), propoxur (Baygon; moderate toxicity, LD_{50} 95 mg per kg), and aldicarb (Temik; high toxicity, LD_{50} 0.9 mg per kg). Carbamate medicinals include neostigmine and physostigmine (Antilirium). Cholinergic compounds also include the dreaded "G" nerve war weapons Tubun (GA), Sarin (GB), Soman (GB), and VX. *Toxic mechanism:* (1) OPs phosphorylate the active site on red blood cell acetylcholinesterase and pseudocholinesterase in the serum (3% of the general population has a deficiency) and other organs, causing irreversible inhibition. There are two types of OP action: direct action by the parent compound (e.g., tetraethyl pyrophosphate) and indirect action by the toxic metabolite (e.g., paraoxon or malaoxon). (2) Carbamates (esters of carbonic acid) cause reversible carbamylation of the active site of the enzymes. When a critical amount of cholinesterase is inhibited more than 50% from baseline, acetylcholine accumulates, causing transient stimulation of conduction and soon after paralysis of conduction, through cholinergic synapses and sympathetic terminals (muscarinic effect), the somatic nerves, the autonomic ganglia (nicotinic effect), and CNS synapses. (3) Major differences of the carbamates from OPs: Carbamate toxicity is less and the duration is shorter; carbamates rarely produce overt CNS effects (poor CNS penetration); with carbamates the acetylcholinesterase returns to normal rapidly, so blood values are not useful even in confirming the diagnosis; with carbamates, pralidoxime, the enzyme regenerator, may not be necessary in the management of mild intoxication (e.g., carbaryl), but atropine is required. *Toxic dose:* Parathion's minimal lethal dose is 2 mg in children and 10 to 20 mg in adults. The lethal dose of malathion is greater than 1375 mg per kg (it is 1000 times less toxic than parathion) and that of chlorpyrifos is 25 grams, and they are unlikely to cause death. *Kinetics:* Absorption is by all routes. The onset of acute ingestion toxicity occurs as early as 3 hours, usually before 12 hours, and always before 24 hours. Lipid-soluble agents absorbed by the dermal route (e.g., fenthion) may have a delayed onset of more than 24 hours. Inhalation toxicity occurs immediately after exposure. Massive ingestion can produce intoxication within minutes. The effects of the thions (e.g., parathion, malathion) are delayed because they undergo hepatic microsomal oxidative metabolism to their toxic metabolites, oxons (e.g., paraoxon, malaoxon). The $t_{1/2}$ of malathion is 2.89 hours and of parathion is 2.1 days.

The metabolites are eliminated in the urine, and the presence of p-nitrophenol in the urine is a clue up to 48 hours after exposure. *Manifestations:* Many OPs produce a garlic odor on the breath, from the gastric contents, or from the container. Diaphoresis, excessive salivation, miosis, and muscle twitching are helpful clues. (1) Early, a cholinergic (muscarinic) crisis develops and consists of parasympathetic nervous system activity. DUMBELS is a mnemonic for the manifestations of defecation, cramps, and increased bowel mobility; urinary incontinence; miosis (mydriasis may occur in 20%); bronchospasm and bronchorrhea; excess secretion; lacrimation; and seizures. Bradycardia, pulmonary edema, and hypotension may be present. (2) Later, sympathetic and nicotinic effects occur consisting of muscle weakness and fasciculation (eyelid twitching is often present), adrenal stimulation and hyperglycemia, tachycardia, cramps in muscles, and hypertension (mnemonic MATCH). Finally, paralysis of the skeletal muscles ensues. (3) CNS effects are headache, blurred vision, anxiety, ataxia, delirium and toxic psychosis, convulsions, coma, and respiratory depression. Cranial nerve palsies have been noted. Delayed hallucinations may occur. (4) Delayed respiratory paralysis and neurologic and neurobehavioral disorders have been described after certain OPs or dermal exposure. The "intermediate" syndrome consists of paralysis of proximal and respiratory muscles developing 24 to 96 hours after the successful treatment of OP poisoning. A delayed distal polyneuropathy has been described with certain OPs (e.g., tri-o-cresyl phosphate [TOCP], bromoleptophos, methomidophous). (5) Complications include aspiration, pulmonary edema, and adult respiratory distress syndrome. *Management:* (1) Protect health care personnel with protective clothing (masks, gloves, gowns, goggles, and respiratory equipment or hazardous material suits as necessary). General decontamination consists of isolation, bagging, and disposal of contaminated clothing and other articles. Establish and maintain vital functions. Institute cardiac and oxygen saturation monitoring. Intubation and assisted ventilation may be needed. Suction secretions until atropinization drying is achieved. (2) Specific decontamination: Dermal: Prompt removal of clothing and cleansing of all affected areas of skin, hair, and eyes. Ocular: irrigation with copious amounts of tepid water or 0.9% saline for at least 15 minutes. GI: if ingestion is recent, use gastric lavage with airway protection, if necessary, and administer AC. (3) Antidotes: Atropine sulfate (see Table 12) is both a diagnostic and a therapeutic agent. Atropine counteracts the muscarinic effects but is only partially effective for the CNS effects (seizures and coma). Use preservative-free atropine (no benzyl alcohol). If the patient is symptomatic (bradycardia or bronchorrhea), administer a test dose of 0.02 mg per kg for a child or 1 mg for an adult IV. If there are no signs of atropinization (tachycardia, drying of secretions, and mydriasis), immediately administer atropine at 0.05 mg per kg for a child or 2 mg for an adult every 5 to 10 minutes as needed to

dry the secretions and clear the lungs. Beneficial effects are seen within 1 to 4 minutes and the maximal effect in 8 minutes. The average dose in the first 24 hours is 40 mg, but 1000 mg or more has been required in severe cases. Glycopyrrolate (Robinul) may be used if atropine is not available. Maintain the maximal dose for 12 to 24 hours; then taper it and observe for relapse. Poisoning, especially with lipophilic agents (e.g., fenthion, chlorfenthion), may require weeks of atropine therapy. The alternative is a continuous infusion of 8 mg of atropine in 100 mL of 0.9% saline at rate of 0.02 to 0.08 mg per kg per hour (0.25 to 1.0 mL per kg per hour) with additional 1- to 5-mg boluses as needed to dry the secretions. Pralidoxime chloride (2-PAM) has antinicotinic, antimuscarinic, and possibly CNS effects. It may require a reduction in the dose of atropine (see Table 12). It acts to reactivate the phosphorylated cholinesterases by binding the phosphate moiety on the esteritic site and displacing it. It should be given early before "aging" of the phosphate bond produces tighter binding. However, reports indicate that 2-PAM is beneficial even several days after the poisoning. Improvement is seen within 10 to 40 minutes. The initial dose of 2-PAM is 1 to 2 grams in 250 mL of 0.89% saline over 5 to 10 minutes for a maximum of 200 mg per minute (adults) or 25 to 50 mg per kg for a maximum of 4 mg per kg per minute (children younger than 12 years). Repeat every 6 to 12 hours for several days. An alternative is a continuous infusion of 1 gram in 100 mL of 0.89% saline at 5 to 20 mg per kg per hour (0.5 to 12 mL per kg per hour) up to 500 mg per hour and titrate to the desired response. The maximal adult daily dose is 12 grams. Cardiac monitoring and blood pressure monitoring are advised during and for several hours after the infusion. The end point is absence of fasciculations and return of muscle strength. (4) Contraindicated drugs: Do not use morphine, aminophylline, barbiturates, opioids, phenothiazine, reserpine-like drugs, parasympathomimetics, or succinylcholine. (5) Noncardiac pulmonary edema may require respiratory support. (6) Seizures may respond to atropine and 2-PAM, but the effect is not consistent and anticonvulsants may be required. (7) Cardiac dysrhythmias may require electrical cardioversion or antidysrhythmic therapy if the patient is hemodynamically unstable. (8) Extracorporeal procedures are of no proven value. *Laboratory investigations:* Monitor chest radiograph, blood glucose (nonketotic hyperglycemia occurs frequently), ABGs, pulse oximetry, ECG, blood coagulation status, liver function, hyperamylasemia (pancreatitis has been reported), and the urine for the metabolite alkyl phosphate p-nitrophenol. Draw blood for red blood cell cholinesterase determination before giving pralidoxime. In mild poisoning, this value is 20 to 50% of normal; in moderate poisoning, 10 to 20% of normal; and in severe poisoning, 10% of normal (more than 90% depressed). A postexposure rise of 10 to 15% in the cholinesterase determined in at least 10 to 14 days confirms the diagnosis. *Disposition:* Asymptomatic patients with a normal examination after 6 to 8 hours of observation may be discharged. If intentional poisoning occurred, psychiatric clearance is required for discharge. Symptomatic patients should be admitted to the ICU. Observation of patients with milder carbamate poisoning, even those requiring atropine, for 6 to 8 hours without symptoms may be sufficient to exclude significant toxicity. If work place exposure occurred, notify OSHA.

Phencyclidine (PCP, "angel dust," "peace pill," "hog"). PCP is an arylcyclohexylamine related to ketamine and chemically related to the PTZs. It is a "dissociative" anesthetic that has been banned in the United States since 1979 and is now an illicit substance, with at least 38 analogues. It is inexpensively manufactured by "kitchen" chemists and is mislabeled as other hallucinogens. Improperly synthesized PCP may release cyanide when heated or smoked and can cause explosions. *Toxic mechanism:* PCP action is complex and not completely understood. It inhibits neurotransmitters and causes loss of pain sensation without depressing the CNS respiratory status. It stimulates alpha-adrenergic receptors and may act as a "false" neurotransmitter. The effects are sympathomimetic, cholinergic, and cerebellar. *Toxic dose:* The usual dose in joints is 100 to 400 mg weight; joints or leaf mixture, 0.24 to 7.9%, 1 mg per 150 leaves; tablets, 5 mg (usual street dose). CNS effects at 1 to 6 mg produce hallucinations and euphoria; 6 to 10 mg produces toxic psychosis and sympathetic stimulation, 10 to 25 mg produces severe toxicity, and more than 100 mg has resulted in fatality. *Kinetics:* PCP is a lipophilic weak base with a pK_a of 8.5 to 9.5. It is rapidly absorbed when smoked and snorted, poorly absorbed from the acid stomach, and rapidly absorbed from the alkaline media of the small intestine. It is secreted enterogastrically and is reabsorbed in the small intestine. The onset of action when it is smoked is at 2 to 5 minutes, with a peak in 15 to 30 minutes. The onset is at 30 to 60 minutes when it is taken orally and immediate when it is taken IV. Most adverse reactions in overdose begin within 1 to 2 hours. Its duration of action at low doses is 4 to 6 hours, and normality returns in 24 hours; in large overdoses fluctuating coma may last 6 to 10 days. The $t_{1/2}$ is 1 hour (in overdose, 11 to 89 hours). The Vd is 6.2 liters per kg and the PB is 70%. It is eliminated by gastric secretion, liver metabolism, and 10% urinary excretion of conjugates and free PCP. Renal excretion may be increased 50% with urinary acidification. PCP concentrates in brain and adipose tissue. *Manifestations:* The classic picture is one of bursts of horizontal, vertical, and rotary nystagmus, which is a clue (occurs in 50%); miosis; hypertension; and fluctuating altered mental state. There is a wide spectrum of clinical presentations. (1) Mild intoxication: A dose of 1 to 6 mg produces drunken and bizarre behavior, agitation, rotary nystagmus, and blank stare. Violent behavior and sensory anesthesia make these patients insensitive to pain, self-destructive, and dangerous. Most are communicative within 1 to 2 hours, are alert and ori-

ented in 6 to 8 hours, and recover completely in 24 to 48 hours. (2) Moderate intoxication: A dose of 6 to 10 mg produces excess salivation, hypertension, hyperthermia, muscle rigidity, myoclonus, and catatonia. Recovery of consciousness occurs in 24 to 48 hours and complete recovery in 1 week. (3) Severe intoxication: A dose of 10 to 25 mg results in opisthotonus, decerebrate rigidity, convulsions, prolonged fluctuating coma, and respiratory failure. This category involves a high rate of medical complications. Recovery of consciousness occurs in 24 to 48 hours, with complete normality in 1 month. (4) Medical complications include apnea, aspiration pneumonia, cardiac arrest, hypertensive encephalopathy, hyperthermia, intracerebral hemorrhage, psychosis, rhabdomyolysis and myoglobinuria, and seizures. Loss of memory and flashbacks last for months. PCP-induced depression and suicide have been reported. (5) Fatalities occur with ingestions greater than 100 mg and with serum levels higher than 100 to 250 ng per mL. *Management:* Observe for violent, self-destructive, bizarre behavior and paranoid schizophrenia. Patients should be placed in a low sensory environment and dangerous objects removed from the area. (1) GI decontamination is not effective because PCP is rapidly absorbed from the intestines. Avoid overtreating mild intoxication. Administer AC initially and MDAC every 4 hours because PCP is secreted into the stomach even if it is smoked or snorted. Continuous gastric suction is not routine but may be useful (with protection of the airway) in severe toxicity (stupor or coma) because the drug is secreted into the gastric juice. (2) Protect patients from harming themselves or others. Physical restraints may be necessary, but use them sparingly and for the shortest time possible because they increase the risk of rhabdomyolysis. Avoid metal restraints such as handcuffs. For behavioral disorders and toxic psychosis, diazepam is the agent of choice. Pharmacologic intervention includes diazepam at 10 to 30 mg orally or 2 to 5 mg IV initially; titrate upward to 10 mg, but up to 30 mg may be required. See the section on management of the violent patient. The "talk down" technique is usually ineffective and dangerous. Avoid PTZs and butyrophenones in the acute phase because they lower the convulsive threshold; however, they may be needed later for psychosis. Haloperidol (Haldol) administration has been reported to produce catatonia. (3) Seizures and muscle spasm control are managed with diazepam at 2.5 mg, up to 10 mg. (4) Hyperthermia (temperature above 38.5°C [101.3°F]) is treated with external cooling measures. (5) Hypertension is usually transient and does not require treatment. In an emergent hypertensive crisis (blood pressure above 200/115 mm Hg) use nitroprusside, 0.3 to 2 µg per kg per minute. The maximal infusion rate is 10 µg per kg per minute for only 10 minutes. (6) Acid ion trapping diuresis is not recommended because of the danger of myoglobin precipitation in the renal tubules. (7) Rhabdomyolysis and myoglobinuria are treated by correcting volume depletion and ensuring a urine output of at least

2 mL per kg per hour. Alkalinization is controversial because of PCP reabsorption. (8) Hemodialysis is beneficial if renal failure occurs; otherwise the extracorporeal procedures are not beneficial. *Laboratory investigations:* Marked elevation of the creatine kinase level may be a clue to PCP intoxication. Values greater than 20,000 units have been reported. Monitor urinalysis and test urine for myoglobin with *o*-toluidine blood reagent strip. A 3+ or 4+ test result and less than 10 red blood cells per high-power field on microscopic examination suggest myoglobinuria. Measure for PCP in the gastric juice, where it is concentrated 10 to 50 times higher than in blood or urine. Monitor blood for creatine kinase, uric acid (an early clue to rhabdomyolysis), BUN, creatinine, electrolytes (hyperkalemia), blood glucose (20% of intoxications involve hypoglycemia), urine output, liver function tests, ECG, and ABGs if there are any respiratory manifestations. PCP blood concentrations are not helpful. A level of 10 ng per mL produces excitation, 30 to 100 ng per mL coma, and greater than 100 ng per mL seizures and fatalities. PCP may be detected in the urine of the average user for 10 to 14 days or up to 3 weeks after the last dose. With chronic use it can be detected for more than 1 month. The analogue of PCP may not test positive for PCP in the urine. Cross-reactions: bleach and dextromethorphan may cause false-positive urine test results on immunoassay, doxylamine a false-positive result on gas chromatography. *Disposition:* All patients with coma, delirium, catatonia, violent behavior, aspiration pneumonia, sustained hypertension (blood pressure above 200/115 mm Hg), and significant rhabdomyolysis should be admitted to the ICU until they are asymptomatic for at least 24 hours. If patients with mild intoxication are mentally and neurologically stable and become asymptomatic (except for nystagmus) for 4 hours, they may be discharged in the company of a responsible adult. All patients must be assessed for risk of suicide before discharge. Drug counseling and psychiatric follow-up should be arranged. Warn patients that episodes of disorientation and depression may continue intermittently for 4 weeks or more.

Phenothiazines and Nonphenothiazines (neuroleptics). *Toxic mechanism:* Neuroleptics have complex mechanisms of toxicity including (1) block of the postsynaptic dopamine receptors, (2) block of peripheral and central alpha-adrenergic receptors, (3) block of cholinergic muscarinic receptors, (4) a quinidine-like antidysrhythmic and myocardial depressant effect in large overdose, (5) a lowered convulsive threshold, and (6) an effect on hypothalamic temperature regulation. See Table 44. *Toxic dose:* Extrapyramidal reactions, anticholinergic effects, and orthostatic hypotension may occur at therapeutic doses. See Table 44 for therapeutic doses. The toxic amount is not established, but the maximal daily therapeutic dose may result in significant side effects, and twice this amount is potentially fatal. Chlorpromazine (Thorazine), the prototype, may produce serious hypotension and CNS depression at doses above 200 mg (17

mg per kg) in children and 3 to 5 grams in adults. Fatalities have been reported after 2.5 grams of loxapine and mesoridazine and 1.5 grams of thioridazine. *Kinetics:* These agents are lipophilic and have unpredictable GI absorption. Peak levels occur 2 to 6 hours after ingestion and have enterohepatic recirculation. The mean serum $t_{1/2}$ in phase 1 is 1 to 2 hours and the biphasic $t_{1/2}$ is 20 to 40 hours. The PB is 92 to 98%. Chlorpromazine has oral onset at 30 to 60 minutes, peak at 2 to 4 hours, and a duration of 4 to 6 hours. With sustained-release preparations, the onset is at 30 to 60 minutes and the duration is 6 to 12 hours. The PB is 95%; the Vd, 10 to 40 liters per kg. Elimination is by hepatic metabolism, which results in multiple metabolites (some are active). Metabolites may be detected in urine months after chronic therapy. Only 1 to 3% is excreted unchanged in the urine. *Manifestations:* (1) PTZ overdose effects. Anticholinergic symptoms may be present early but are not life-threatening. Miosis is usually present (80%) if the PTZ has strong alpha-adrenergic blocking effect (e.g., chlorpromazine), but if there is strong anticholinergic activity mydriasis may occur. Agitation and delirium rapidly progress to coma. Major problems are cardiac toxicity and hypotension. The cardiotoxic effects are seen more commonly with thioridazine and its metabolite mesoridazine. These agents have produced the largest number of fatalities in PTZ overdoses. Cardiac conduction disturbances include prolonged PR, QRS, and QT_C intervals; U and T wave abnormalities; and ventricular dysrhythmias including torsades de pointes. Seizures occur mainly in patients with convulsive disorders or with loxapine. Sudden death in children and adults has been reported. (2) Idiosyncratic dystonic reactions are most common with the piperidine group. The reaction is not dose dependent and consists of opisthotonos, torticollis, orolingual dyskinesia, and oculogyric crisis (painful upward gaze). It occurs more frequently in children and women. (3) Neuroleptic malignant syndrome occurs in patients receiving chronic therapy and is characterized by hyperthermia, muscle rigidity, autonomic dysfunction, and altered mental state. One case has been reported with acute overdose. (4) The loxapine syndrome consists of seizures, rhabdomyolysis, and renal failure. *Management:* (1) Establish and maintain the vital functions. All patients with overdose require venous access, 12-lead ECG (to measure intervals), cardiac and respiratory monitoring, and seizure precautions. Monitor core temperature to detect a poikilothermic effect. The comatose patient may require intubation and assisted ventilation, 100% oxygen, IV glucose, naloxone, and 100 mg of thiamine. (2) GI decontamination: Emesis is not recommended. Gastric lavage may be useful but is not necessary if AC or a cathartic is administered promptly. MDAC has not been scientifically proved beneficial. A radiograph of the abdomen may be useful, if the PTZ is radiopaque. Haloperidol and trifluoperazine are most likely to be radiopaque. Whole-bowel irrigation may be useful when a large number of pills are visualized on a

TABLE 44. **Phenothiazine Daily Doses and Properties: Comparison of the Effects of Neuroleptics***

Compound	Antipsychotic	Anticholinergic	Extrapyramidal	Hypotensive and Cardiotoxic	Sedative
Phenothiazine					
Aliphatic†	1+	3+	2+	**2+**	3+
Chlorpromazine (Thorazine, 20–50 mg adult dose, range 20–2000 mg per 24 h)					
Promethazine (Phenergan 25–50 mg adult dose, range 25–200 mg per 24 h)					
Piperazine‡	3+	1+	3+	1+	1+
Fluphenazine (Prolixin 2.5–10 mg adult dose, range 2.5–20 mg per 24 h)					
Perphenazine (Trilafon 4–16 mg adult dose, range 10–30 mg per 24 h)					
Prochlorperazine (Compazine 5–10 mg adult dose, range 15–40 mg per 24 h)					
Trifluoperazine (Stelazine 2–5 mg adult dose, range 1–40 mg per 24 h)					
Piperidine†	1+	2+	1+	3+	3+
Mesoridazine (Serentil 25–100 mg adult dose, range 150–400 mg per 24 h)					
Thioridazine (Mellaril 25–100 mg adult dose, range 150–300 mg per 24 h)					
Nonphenothiazine					
Butyrophenone‡	3+	1+	3+	1+	1+
Haloperidol (Haldol 0.5–5.0 mg adult dose, range 1–100 mg per 24 h)					
Dibenzoxazepine‡	3+	1+	3+	1+	2+
Loxapine (Loxitane 10–50 mg adult dose, range 60–100 mg per 24 h)					
Dihydroindolone‡	3+	1+	3+	1+	1+
Molindone (Moban 5–25 mg adult dose, range 50–225 mg per 24 h)					
Thioxanthenes‡	3+	1+	3+	3+	1+
Thiothixene (Navane 2–15 mg adult dose, range 5–80 mg per 24 h)					
Chlorprothixene (Taractan 5–60 mg adult dose, range 75–200 mg per 24 h)					

*1+ indicates very low activity; 2+, moderate activity; 3+, very high activity. **Bold** indicates major effect. Equivalent doses: 100 mg of chlorpromazine, thioridazine = 50 mg of mesoridazine = 15 mg of loxapine, prochlorperazine = 10 mg of molindone, perphenazine = 5 mg of thiothixene = 2 mg of fluphenazine, haloperidol.
†Low antipsychotic potency.
‡High antipsychotic potency.

radiograph or sustained-release preparations are involved, but it has not been scientifically investigated for PTZ. (3) Treat convulsions with diazepam or lorazepam. A loxapine overdose may result in status epilepticus. If nondepolarizing neuromuscular blockade is required, use pancuronium (Pavulon) or vecuronium (Norcuron) (not succinylcholine [Anectine], which may cause malignant hyperthermia), and monitor the EEG during paralysis. (4) Dysrhythmias: Monitor with serial ECG. Treat unstable rhythms with electrical cardioversion. AVOID class IA antidysrhythmic drugs (procainamide, quinidine, and disopyramide). Hypokalemia predisposes to dysrhythmias and should be corrected aggressively. Supraventricular tachycardia with hemodynamic instability is treated with electrical cardioversion. The role of adenosine has not been defined. Avoid calcium channel blockers and beta blockers. QRS interval prolongation is treated with $NaHCO_3$ at 1 to 2 mEq per kg by IV bolus over a few minutes. Torsades de pointes is treated with 2 grams of a 20% magnesium sulfate solution IV over 2 to 3 minutes; if there is no response in 10 minutes, repeat and follow by a continuous infusion of 5 to 10 mg per minute or give as infusion of 50 mg per minute for 2 hours followed by 30 mg per minute for 90 minutes twice a day for several days, as needed. The dose in children is 25 to 50 mg per kg initially with a maintenance dose of 30 to 60 mg per kg per 24 hours (0.25 to 0.50 mEq per kg per 24 hours) up to 1000 mg per 24 hours. Monitor serum magnesium: Ventricular tachydysrhythmias: If the patient is stable, use lidocaine. If unstable, use electrical cardioversion. Heart blocks with hemodynamic instability should be managed with temporary cardiac pacing. (5) Hypotension is treated with the Trendelenburg position, 0.89% saline, and, if refractory or there is danger of fluid overload, administration of vasopressors. The vasopressor of choice is the alpha-adrenergic agonist norepinephrine (0.1 to 0.2 μg per gram per minute and titrated to response). Epinephrine and dopamine should not be used because beta-receptor stimulation in the presence of alpha-receptor blockade may provoke dysrhythmias and PTZs are antidopaminergic.

(6) Treat hypothermia or hyperthermia with external warming or cooling measures. Do not use antipyretic drugs. (7) Management of the neuroleptic malignant syndrome includes discontinuing the offending agent, aggressively reducing the temperature with passive and active cooling measures, correcting electrolyte and metabolic imbalances, and using dantrolene sodium (see Table 12 and the section on malignant hyperthermia syndrome management). The loading dose is 2 to 3 mg per kg IV as a bolus, and the loading dose is repeated until the signs of the syndrome (tachycardia, rigidity, and temperature) are controlled. The maximal total dose is 10 mg per kg. (8) Idiosyncratic dystonic reaction can be treated with diphenhydramine at 1 to 2 mg per kg per dose IV over 5 minutes up to a maximum of 50 mg IV; a response is noted within 2 to 5 minutes. Follow with oral doses for 5 to 7 days to prevent recurrence. (9) Extracorporeal measures (hemodialysis, hemoperfusion) are not effective in enhancing removal of these agents. *Laboratory investigations:* Monitor ABGs, renal and hepatic function, electrolytes, blood glucose, and creatine kinase and myoglobinemia in neuroleptic malignant syndrome. Most of these agents are detected by routine screens. A positive ferric chloride test of the urine occurs if there is a sufficient blood level; however, it is not specific (salicylates and phenolic compounds also give a positive result). Quantitative serum levels are not useful in management. Cross-reactions with EMIT tests occur with cyclic antidepressants. PTZs give false-negative pregnancy urine test results using human chorionic gonadotropin as the indicator and false-positive test results for urinary porphyrins, the indirect Coombs' test, urobilinogen, and amylase. *Disposition:* Asymptomatic patients should be observed for at least 6 hours after gastric decontamination. Symptomatic patients with cardiotoxicity, hypotension, or convulsions should be admitted to the ICU and monitored for 48 hours.

Salicylates (acetylsalicylic acid, aspirin, salicylic acid). *Toxic mechanism:* The primary toxic mechanisms include (1) direct stimulation of the medullary chemoreceptor trigger zone and respiratory center; (2) uncoupling of oxidative phosphorylation; (3) inhibition of the Krebs cycle enzymes; (4) inhibition of vitamin K–dependent and –independent clotting factors; (5) alteration of platelet function; and (6) inhibition of prostaglandin synthesis. *Toxic dose:* Acute mild intoxication occurs at a dose of 150 to 200 mg per kg (tinnitus, dizziness), moderate intoxication at 200 to 300 mg per kg, and severe intoxication at 300 to 500 mg per kg (CNS manifestations). An acute salicylate plasma concentration (SPC) higher than 30 mg per dL (usually over 40 mg per dL) may be associated with clinical toxicity. Chronic intoxication occurs at ingestions of more than 100 mg per kg per day for more than 2 days because of cumulative kinetics. Methyl salicylate (oil of wintergreen) is the most toxic form of salicylate; 1 mL of 98% methyl salicylate contains 1.4 grams of salicylate. Fatalities occurred with ingestion of 1 teaspoonful in a child

and 1 ounce in adults. It is found in topical ointments and liniments (18 to 30%). *Kinetics:* Acetylsalicylic acid is a weak acid with a pK_a of 3.5 and salicylic acid has a pK_a of 3.0. Salicylic acid is absorbed from the stomach and small bowel and dermally. Onset of action is within 30 minutes. Methyl salicylate and effervescent tablets are absorbed more rapidly. An SPC is detectable within 15 minutes after ingestion and the peak occurs in 30 to 120 minutes but may be delayed 6 to 12 hours in large overdoses, in overdoses with enteric-coated and sustained-release preparations, and if concretions develop. The therapeutic duration of action is 3 to 4 hours but is markedly prolonged in an overdose. The $t_{1/2}$ of salicylic acid is 3 hours after a 300-mg dose, 6 hours after a 1-gram overdose, and over 10 hours after a 10-gram overdose. The Vd is 0.13 liter per kg for salicylic acid but increases as the SPC increases. PB is up to 90% for salicylic acid at pH 7.4 at a therapeutic SPC, 75% at an SPC above 40 mg per dL, 50% at an SPC of 70 mg per dL, and 30% at an SPC of 120 mg per dL. Elimination includes Michaelis-Menten hepatic metabolism by three saturable pathways: (1) glycine conjugation to salicyluric acid (75%), (2) saturable glucuronyltransferase to salicyl phenol glucuronide (10%), and (3) salicyl aryl glucuronide (4%). Nonsaturable pathways involve hydrolysis to gentisic acid (<1%), and 10% is excreted unchanged. Acidosis increases the severity by increasing the nonionized salicylate that can move into the brain cells. In kidneys the un-ionized salicylic acid undergoes glomerular filtration and the ionized portion undergoes secretion in proximal tubules and passive reabsorption in the distal tubules. Renal excretion of salicylate is enhanced by alkaline urine. *Manifestations:* Ingestion of concentrated topical salicylic acid preparations (e.g., Compound W) can cause caustic mucosal injury to the GI tract. Consider occult salicylate overdose in any patient with an unexplained acid-base disturbance. Acute overdose: (1) Minimal symptoms, tinnitus, dizziness, and deafness, may occur at a high therapeutic SPC of 20 to 30 mg per dL. Nausea and vomiting may occur immediately as a result of local gastric irritation. (2) Phase I consists of mild manifestations (1 to 12 hours after ingestion at a 6-hour SPC of 45 to 70 mg per dL). Nausea and vomiting followed by hyperventilation are usually present within 3 to 8 hours after acute overdose. Hyperventilation with an increase in both rate (tachypnea) and depth (hyperpnea) is present but may be subtle. It results in a mild respiratory alkalosis (serum pH greater than 7.4 and urine pH greater than 6.0). Some patients may have lethargy, vertigo, headache, and confusion. Diaphoresis is prominent. (3) Phase II involves moderate manifestations (12 to 24 hours after ingestion at a 6-hour SPC of 70 to 100 mg per dL). Serious metabolic disturbances including a marked respiratory alkalosis, followed by AG metabolic acidosis, and dehydration occur. The pH may be normal, elevated, or depressed, with a urine pH less than 6.0. Other metabolic disturbances may include hypoglycemia or hyperglycemia, hypokalemia, decreased ionized calcium, and increased BUN, creatinine, and lactate. Mental disturbances (confusion, disorientation, hallucinations) may occur. Hypotension and convulsions have been reported. (4) Phase III involves severe intoxication (more than 24 hours at a 6-hour SPC of 100 to 130 mg per dL). In addition to the preceding clinical findings, coma and seizures develop and indicate severe intoxication. Pulmonary edema may occur. Metabolic disturbances include metabolic acidemia (pH less than 7.4) and aciduria (pH less than 6.0). In adults, alkalosis may persist until terminal respiratory failure. (5) In children younger than 4 years, a metabolic or mixed metabolic acidosis and respiratory alkalosis develop within 4 to 6 hours because these children have less respiratory reserve and accumulate lactate and other organic acids. Hypoglycemia is more common in children. (6) Fatalities occur at a 6-hour SPC greater than 130 to 150 mg per dL and result from CNS depression, cardiovascular collapse, electrolyte imbalance, and cerebral edema. Chronic salicylism is more serious than acute intoxication, and the 6-hour SPC does not correlate with the manifestations. It usually occurs with therapeutic errors in young children or the elderly with underlying illness, and the diagnosis is delayed because it is not recognized. Noncardiac pulmonary edema is a frequent complication in the elderly. Mortality is about 25%. Chronic salicylate poisoning in children may mimic Reye's syndrome. It is associated with exaggerated CNS findings (hallucinations, delirium, dementia, memory loss, papilledema, bizarre behavior, agitation, encephalopathy, seizures, and coma). Hemorrhagic manifestations, renal failure, and pulmonary and cerebral edema may occur. The metabolic picture is that of hypoglycemia and mixed acid-base derangements. A chronic SPC higher than 60 mg per dL with metabolic acidosis and an altered mental state is extremely serious. *Management:* Treatment is started on the basis of clinical and metabolic findings, not on the basis of salicylate levels. Continuous monitoring of the urine pH is essential for successful alkalinization treatment. Always obtain an acetaminophen plasma level. (1) Establish and maintain vital functions. If the mental state is altered, administer glucose, naloxone, and thiamine in standard doses. Depending on the severity, the initial studies include an immediate and a 6-hour postingestion SPC, ECG and cardiac monitoring, pulse oximetry, urine assays (analysis, pH, specific gravity, and ferric chloride test), chest radiography, ABGs, blood glucose, electrolytes and AG calculation, calcium (ionized), magnesium, renal and liver profiles, and prothrombin time. Test gastric contents and stool for occult blood. Bismuth and magnesium salicylate preparations may be radiopaque on radiographs. Consult a nephrologist for moderate, severe, or chronic intoxication. (2) GI decontamination: Gastric lavage and AC are useful (each gram of AC binds 550 mg of salicylic acid) if a toxic dose was ingested up to 12 hours before because of factors with salicylism that delay absorption, such as food, enteric-coated tablets, pylorospasm, concretions, and

coingestants. "It's never too late to aspirate salicylate." MDAC effectively reduces the $t_{1/2}$ and should be administered every 4 hours. Concretions may occur with massive (usually greater than 300 mg per kg) ingestions, and if blood levels fail to decline, prompt contrast radiography of the stomach may reveal concretions that must be removed by repeated lavage, whole-bowel irrigation, endoscopy, or gastrostomy. (3) Fluids and electrolytes (Table 45): Shock: Establish perfusion and vascular volume with 5% dextrose in 0.89% saline; then proceed with correction of dehydration and alkalinization. Fluids and bicarbonate: In acute moderate or severe salicylism (see Table 45), adults should receive a bolus of 1 to 2 mEq per kg of $NaHCO_3$ followed by an infusion of 100 to 150 mEq of $NaHCO_3$ added to 500 to 1000 mL of 5% dextrose and administered over 60 minutes. Children should receive a bolus of 1 to 2 mEq of $NaHCO_3$ per kg followed by an infusion of 1 to 2 mEq per kg added to 20 mL per kg of 5% dextrose administered over 60 minutes. Add potassium to the IV infusion after the patient voids. Attempt to achieve a target urine output of more than 2 mL per kg per hour and a target urine pH of more than 7. The initial infusion is followed by subsequent infusions (two to three times normal maintenance) of 200 to 300 mL per hour in adults or 10 mL per kg per hour in children. If the patient is acidotic and the serum pH is less than 7.15, an additional 1 to 2 mEq per kg $NaHCO_3$ is given over 1 to 2 hours, and persistent acidosis may require $NaHCO_3$ at 1 to 2 mEq per kg every 2 hours. Adjust the infusion rate, the amount of bicarbonate, and the electrolytes to correct serum abnormalities and to maintain the targeted urine output and urinary pH. Most authorities believe that the diuresis is not as important as the alkalinization or MDAC. Carefully monitor for fluid overload in those at risk of pulmonary and cerebral edema (e.g., the elderly) and because of inappropriate secretion of antidiuretic hormone. In patients with mild intoxication who are not acidotic and whose urine pH is greater than 6, administer 5% dextrose in 0.45% saline with $NaHCO_3$ at 50 mEq per liter or 1 mEq per kg as maintenance to replace ongoing renal losses. (4) Alkalinization: $NaHCO_3$ is administered to produce a serum pH of 7.4 to 7.5 and urine pH above 7. Carbonic anhydrase inhibitors (e.g., acetazolamide [Diamox]) should not be used. If the patient is acidotic, additional bicarbonate may be required. About 2 mEq per kg raises the blood pH by 0.1. In children, alkalinization may be a difficult problem because of the organic acid production and hypokalemia. Hypokalemic and fluid-depleted patients cannot undergo adequate alkalinization. Alkalinization is usually discontinued in asymptomatic patients with an SPC below 30 to 40 mg per dL but is continued in symptomatic patients regardless of the SPC. A decreased serum bicarbonate with a normal or high blood pH indicates respiratory alkalosis predominating over metabolic acidosis, and the bicarbonate should be administered cautiously. An alkalemia (pH of 7.40 to 7.50) is not a contraindication to

TABLE 45. **Fluid and Electrolyte Treatment of Salicylate Poisoning**

Type of Salicylism	Metabolic Disturbance	Blood pH	Urine pH	Hydrating Solution	Amount of NaHCO$_3$ (mEq/L)	Amount of Potassium (mEq/L)
Mild	Respiratory alkalosis	>7.4	>6.0	5% dextrose 0.45% saline	50 (adult) 1 mEq/kg (child)	20
Moderate						
Chronic	Respiratory alkalosis	>7.4	<6.0	D5W	100 (adult) 1–2 mEq/kg (child)	40
Child younger than 4 y	Metabolic acidosis	<7.4				
Severe						
Chronic	Metabolic acidosis	<7.4	<6.0	D5W	150 (adult) 2 mEq/kg (child)	60
Child younger than 4 y	Respiratory alkalosis					
CNS depressant coingestant	Respiratory acidosis	<7.4	<6.0	D5W	100–150*	60

*Correct hypoventilation.

Modified from Linden CH, Rumack BH: The legitimate analgesics, aspirin and acetaminophen. *In* Hansen W Jr (ed): Toxic Emergencies. Churchill Livingstone, New York, 1984, p 118.

bicarbonate therapy because these patients have a significant base deficit in spite of the elevated blood pH. (5) Potassium is added (20 to 40 mEq per liter) to the infusion after the patient voids. In severe, late, and chronic salicylism, potassium at 60 mEq per liter may be needed. When the serum potassium level is below 4.0 mEq per liter, add 10 mEq per liter over the first hour. If the patient has hypokalemia (less than 3 mEq per liter), flat T waves, and U waves, administer 0.25 to 0.5 mEq per kg up to 10 mEq per hour. Administer potassium with ECG monitoring. Recheck the serum potassium value after each rapidly administered dose. A paradoxical urine acidosis (alkaline serum pH and acidic urine pH) indicates that potassium is probably needed. (6) Convulsions: Treat with diazepam or lorazepam, but exclude hypoglycemia, low ionized calcium, cerebral edema, or hemorrhage with CT. If tetany develops, discontinue the NaHCO$_3$ therapy and administer 10% calcium gluconate at 0.1 to 0.2 mL per kg. (7) Pulmonary edema management consists of fluid restriction, high forced inspiratory oxygen (FIO$_2$), mechanical ventilation, and PEEP. (8) Cerebral edema management consists of fluid restriction, elevation of the head, hyperventilation, osmotic diuresis, and dexamethasone. (9) Administer vitamin K$_1$ parenterally to correct an increased prothrombin time of more than 20 seconds and coagulation abnormalities. If there is active bleeding, administer fresh plasma and platelets as needed. (10) Hyperpyrexia is managed by external cooling measures, not antipyretics. (11) Hemodialysis is the method of choice for removing salicylates because it corrects the acid-base, electrolyte, and fluid disturbances as well. Indications for hemodialysis include acute poisoning with an SPC greater than 100 to 130 mg per dL without improvement after 6 hours of appropriate therapy; chronic poisoning with cardiopulmonary disease and an SPC as low as 40 mg per dL with refractory acidosis, severe CNS manifestations (coma and seizures), and progressive deterioration, especially in the elderly; impairment of vital organs of elimination; clinical deterioration in spite of good supportive care, repeated doses of

AC, and alkalinization; and severe refractory acid-base or electrolyte disturbances despite appropriate corrective measures. *Laboratory investigations:* In all intentional salicylate overdoses, the acetaminophen plasma level should be determined after 4 hours. (1) Continuously monitor ECG, urine output, urine pH, and specific gravity. Every 2 to 4 hours in severe intoxication monitor SPC, glucose (in salicylism, CNS hypoglycemia may be present despite a normal serum glucose level), electrolytes, ionized calcium, magnesium, and phosphorus, AG, ABGs, and pulse oximetry. Daily, monitor BUN, creatinine, liver function tests, and prothrombin time. (2) In the ferric chloride test, 1 mL of boiled urine containing 2 or 3 drops of 10% ferric chloride turns purple if salicylates are present. This is a nonspecific test and is positive for ketones (if the sample is not boiled), PTZs, and phenolic compounds in urine. (3) The SPC: The therapeutic value is less than 10 mg per dL for analgesia and 15 to 30 mg per dL for an anti-inflammatory effect. Mild toxicity occurs at values above 30 mg per dL (tinnitus, dizziness), severe toxicity above 80 mg per dL (CNS changes). Cross-reaction: Diflunisal (Dolobid) results in a falsely high SPC. The Done nomogram (Figure 3) has been used as a predictor of the expected severity after an acute single ingestion. The nomogram is not useful for chronic intoxications; for enteric-coated aspirin; or for methyl salicylate, phenyl salicylate, or homomethyl salicylate intoxications. The blood sample for use with the Done nomogram should be obtained 6 hours or more after ingestion. *Disposition:* There are limitations of SPCs, and patients are treated on the basis of clinical and laboratory findings. Patients who are asymptomatic should be monitored for a minimum of 6 hours and longer if enteric-coated tablets, a massive overdose, or suspicion of concretions is involved. Those who remain asymptomatic with an SPC below 35 mg per dL may be discharged after psychiatric evaluation, if indicated. Patients with chronic salicylate intoxication, acidosis, and an altered mental state should be admitted to the ICU. Patients with acute ingestion, an SPC below 60 mg per dL, and mild symptoms may

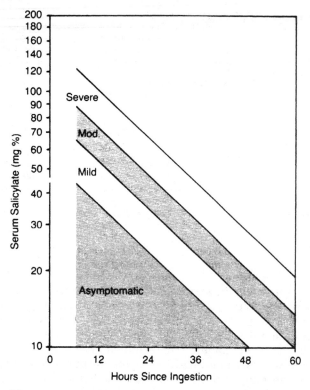

Figure 3. The Done nomogram for salicylate intoxication. For limitations of use, see *Laboratory Investigations*. (Redrawn from Done A: Salicylate intoxication: Significance of measurements of salicylate in blood in cases of acute ingestion. Reproduced by permission of Pediatrics, Vol 26, Page 800, Figure 3, Copyright 1960.)

be able to be treated in the emergency department. Patients with moderate or severe intoxications should be admitted to the ICU.

Theophylline. Theophylline is a methylxanthine alkaloid similar to caffeine and theobromine. Aminophylline is 80% theophylline. It is used in the acute treatment of asthma, pulmonary edema, chronic obstructive pulmonary disease, and neonatal apnea. *Toxic mechanism:* The proposed mechanisms of action include phosphodiesterase inhibition, adenosine receptor antagonism, inhibition of prostaglandins, and increases in serum catecholamines. Theophylline stimulates the CNS, respiratory, and emetic centers and reduces the seizure threshold; has positive cardiac inotropic and chronotropic effects; acts as a diuretic; relaxes smooth muscle and causes peripheral vasodilatation but cerebral vasoconstriction; increases gastric secretions and GI mobility; and increases lipolysis, glycogenolysis, and gluconeogenesis. *Toxic dose:* A single dose of 1 mg per kg produces a theophylline plasma concentration (TPC) of approximately 2 μg per mL. The therapeutic range is usually 10 to 20 μg per mL. An acute, single dose above 10 mg per kg yields mild toxicity; above 20 mg per kg, moderate toxicity; and above 50 mg per kg, serious, possibly fatal toxicity. Fatalities occur at lower doses in chronic toxicity, especially with risk factors (see

kinetics). Equation to estimate the theophylline blood concentration:

$$\text{TPC} = \frac{\text{dose (mg ingested)}}{\text{weight (kg)} \times \text{Vd (0.45 L/kg)}}$$

Kinetics: The pK_a is 9.5. Absorption from stomach and upper small intestine is complete and rapid with onset in 30 to 60 minutes. Peak TPC levels occur within 1 to 2 hours after ingestion of liquid preparations, 2 to 4 hours after regular tablets, and 7 to 24 hours after slow-release formulations. The Vd is 0.3 to 0.7 liter per kg. The PB is 40 to 60% in adults, mainly to albumin, and with low albumin free active theophylline is increased. Elimination is 90% by hepatic metabolism to the active metabolite 2-methylxanthine. The $t_{1/2}$ is 3.5 hours in a child and 4 to 6 hours in an adult. It is shorter in smokers and those taking enzyme inducer drugs. Elimination: Only 8 to 10% is excreted unchanged in the urine. Risk factors that produce a longer $t_{1/2}$ include age younger than 6 months or older than 60 years, enzyme inhibitor drugs (e.g., calcium channel blockers, oral contraceptives), H_2 blockers (e.g., cimetidine), ciprofloxacin (Cipro), erythromycin and macrolide antibiotics, isoniazid, illness (persistent temperature above 102°F [38.5°C]), viral illness, liver impairment, heart failure, chronic obstructive pulmonary disease, and influenza vaccine. *Manifestations:* Acute toxicity generally correlates with blood levels; chronic toxicity does not. See Table 46. (1) Acute single regular-release overdose (see Table 46): Vomiting and occasionally hematemesis occur at a low TPC. CNS stimulation results in restlessness, muscle tremors, and protracted tonic-clonic seizures, but coma is rare. Convulsions are a sign of severe toxicity and are usually

TABLE 46. **Theophylline Blood Concentrations and Acute Toxicity**

Plasma Concentration (μg/mL)	Toxicity Degree	Manifestations
8–10	None	Bronchodilatation
10–20	Mild	Therapeutic range: nausea, vomiting, nervousness, respiratory alkalosis, tachycardia
15–25		Mild manifestations of toxicity in 35%
20–40	Moderate	GI complaints and CNS stimulation
		Transient hypertension, tachypnea, tachycardia
		Some manifestations of toxicity in 80%
>60	Severe	Convulsions, dysrhythmias Hypokalemia, hyperglycemia
>100		Ventricular dysrhythmias, protracted convulsions, hypotension, acid-base abnormalities

Abbreviations: GI = gastrointestinal; CNS = central nervous system.

preceded by GI symptoms (except with sustained-release and chronic intoxications). Cardiovascular disturbances include cardiac dysrhythmias (supraventricular tachycardia) and transient hypertension with mild overdoses but hypotension and ventricular dysrhythmias with severe intoxications. Rhabdomyolysis and renal failure are occasionally seen. Children tolerate higher serum levels, and cardiac dysrhythmias and seizures occur at a TPC greater than 100 µg per mL. Metabolic disturbances, including hyperglycemia, pronounced hypokalemia, hypocalcemia, hypomagnesemia, hypophosphatemia, increased serum amylase, and elevation of uric acid, may occur. (2) Chronic intoxication occurs when multiple doses of theophylline are taken over 24 hours or when an interacting drug or illness interferes with theophylline metabolism. It is more serious and difficult to treat than acute intoxication. Cardiac dysrhythmias and convulsions may occur at a TPC of 40 to 60 µg per mL, and there is no correlation with TPC. The seizures occur without warning and are protracted, are repetitive, and may produce status epilepticus. Vomiting and typical metabolic disturbances do not occur. (3) Differences in slow-release preparations: Few or no GI symptoms occur; peak concentrations and convulsions may be delayed up to 12 to 24 hours after ingestion and convulsions occur without warning. *Management:* (1) Establish and maintain vital functions. If coma, convulsions, and vomiting occur, intubate immediately. Obtain the TPC, repeat the TPC determination every 2 to 4 hours to determine peak absorption, and consider a theophylline bezoar if the TPC fails to decline. Consult a nephrologist about charcoal hemoperfusion. (2) GI decontamination in acute overdose: Do not induce emesis. Gastric lavage can be done less than 1 hour after ingestion but may not be necessary if AC is available. AC is the choice for decontamination. Administer 1 gram per kg to all patients and follow with MDAC at 0.5 gram per kg every 2 to 4 hours until the TPC is less than 20 µg per mL. MDAC is effective in acute, chronic, and IV overdoses. AC shortens the $t_{1/2}$ by about 50%. AC may be indicated up to 24 hours after ingestion. Whole-bowel irrigation with a polyethylene-electrolyte solution orally or via nasogastric tube has been recommended for consideration for massive overdose, possible concretions, and slow-release preparations but its value is unproved. Whole-bowel irrigation may cause theophylline to be desorbed from AC. If intractable vomiting occurs, administer an antiemetic, metoclopramide (Reglan; 0.1 mg per kg adult dose), droperidol (Inapsine; 2.5 to 10 mg IV), or ondansetron (Zofran; 8 to 32 mg IV). The last, however, inhibits metabolism of theophylline. (3) Control convulsions with lorazepam or diazepam and phenobarbital. Phenytoin is ineffective. The convulsions in chronic intoxication are often refractory and may require, in addition to anticonvulsants, neuromuscular paralyzing agents, sedation, assisted ventilation, and EEG monitoring. (4) Hypotension is treated with fluids and vasopressors, if necessary. Norepinephrine at 0.05 µg per kg per minute is preferred over dopamine as the vasopressor. (5) Dysrhythmias: Supraventricular tachycardia with hemodynamic instability requires cardioversion. Low-dose beta blockers may be used but not for patients with reactive airway disease or hypotension. Adenosine is ineffective. For ventricular dysrhythmias, correct electrolyte disturbances. Lidocaine is the treatment of choice but has the potential to cause seizures at toxic concentrations. Cardioversion may be needed. (6) Hematemesis is managed with sucralfate (Carafate) at 1 gram four times daily and/or aluminum hydroxide–magnesium hydroxide (Maalox Therapeutic Concentrate) at 30 mL every 2 hours and blood replacement, if necessary. H_2 histamine blockers that are enzyme inhibitors are not used. (7) Correct fluid and metabolic disturbances. Hyperglycemia does not require insulin therapy. Hypokalemia should be corrected cautiously, as it may reflect largely an intracellular shift and not total body loss. Usually, adding 40 mEq of potassium to a liter of fluid suffices. Monitor the serum potassium value closely. (8) Charcoal hemoperfusion is the management of choice for serious intoxications. Hemoperfusion can increase the clearance two- to threefold over hemodialysis, but hemodialysis can be used if hemoperfusion is not available. Criteria are life-threatening events such as convulsions or dysrhythmias; intractable vomiting refractory to antiemetics; acute intoxications with TPC greater than 80 to 100 µg per mL, greater than 70 µg per mL 4 hours after an overdose with a slow-release formulation, or greater than 40 to 60 µg per mL in chronic intoxication; and acute or chronic overdoses with TPC above 40 µg per mL, especially if the patient has risk factors that lengthen the $t_{1/2}$ (see the discussion of kinetics). *Laboratory investigations:* Monitor vital signs, pulse oximetry, ABGs, hemoglobin, hematocrit (for GI hemorrhage), ECG and cardiac parameters, renal and hepatic function, electrolytes, blood glucose, acid-base balance, and serum albumin. Test gastric contents and stools for occult blood. The TPC should be determined after ingestion of liquid preparations within 1 to 2 hours, regular-release formulations within 2 to 4 hours, and slow-release formulations at 4 hours. Check the serum albumin level (a decrease in albumin level may cause manifestations of toxicity despite a normal TPC). A single TPC determination may be misleading; therefore, repeat the TPC measurement every 2 to 4 hours to determine the trend until a declining trend is reached and then monitor every 4 to 6 hours until the TPC is below 20 µg per mL. *Disposition:* Patients with mild symptoms and a TPC lower than 20 µg per mL may be treated in the emergency department and discharged when asymptomatic for a few hours. Admit anyone with an acute ingestion with a TPC above 35 µg per mL to a monitored bed with seizure precautions and suicide precautions if needed. If there are neurologic or cardiotoxic effects or the TPC is above 50 µg per mL, admit the patient to the ICU. An overdose of a slow-release preparation, regardless of symptoms or initial TPC, requires admission, monitoring, AC, and MDAC. In patients receiving chronic therapy, toxicity may occur at a lower TPC, and these patients should not be discharged until they are asymptomatic for several hours.

Tricyclic and Cyclic Antidepressants. Traditionally, tricyclic antidepressants have been an important cause of pharmaceutical overdose fatalities (more than 100 in 1992). The mortality has been reduced from 15% in the 1970s to less than 1% in the 1990s through a better understanding of their pathophysiology and improvements in management. See Table 47. *Toxic mechanism:* The major mechanisms of toxicity of the tricyclic antidepressants are central and peripheral anticholinergic effects, peripheral alpha-adrenergic blockade, quinidine-like cardiac membrane-stabilizing action blocking the fast inward sodium channels, and inhibition of synaptic neurotransmitter reuptake in the CNS presynaptic neurons. The tetracyclic, monocyclic aminoketone dibenzoxazepine possesses convulsive activity and less cardiac toxicity in overdoses. Triazolopyridine has less serious cardiac and CNS toxicity. *Toxic dose:* The therapeutic dose of imipramine is 1.5 to 5 mg per kg; a dose of less than 3 to 5 mg per kg may be mildly toxic; 10 to 20 mg per kg may be life-threatening, although doses of less than 20 mg per kg have produced few fatalities; more than 30 mg per kg is asso-

ciated with 30% mortality; and at doses higher than 70 mg per kg survival is rare. Doses of 375 mg in a child and as little as 500 to 750 mg in an adult have been fatal. In adults, 5 times the maximal daily dose is toxic and 10 times the maximal daily dose is potentially fatal. Major overdose symptoms are associated with plasma concentrations above 1 µg per mL (1000 ng per mL). Relative dosage equivalents are amitriptyline 100 mg = amoxapine 125 mg = desipramine 75 mg = doxepin 100 mg = imipramine 75 mg = maprotiline 75 mg = nortriptyline 50 mg = trazodone 200 mg. See Table 47. *Kinetics:* Cyclic antidepressants are lipophilic. They are rapidly absorbed from the alkaline small intestine, but absorption may be prolonged and delayed in massive overdose owing to anticholinergic action. Onset varies from less than 1 hour (30 to 40 minutes) rarely to 12 hours. The peak serum levels are reached in 2 to 8 hours, and the peak effect is in 6 hours but may be delayed 12 hours because of erratic absorption. The clinical effects correlate poorly with plasma levels. Cyclic antidepressants are highly protein bound to plasma glycoproteins (98% at a pH 7.5 and 90% at pH 7.0); the Vd is 10 to 50 liters per kg. The $t_{1/2}$ varies from 10 hours for imipramine to 81 hours for amitriptyline and 100 hours for nortriptyline. The active metabo-

TABLE 47. **Cyclic Antidepressants: Daily Doses and Major Properties***

Generic Name	Adult Daily Dose (mg)	Therapeutic Range (ng/mL)	Half-life (h)	Toxicity Antichol	CNS	Cardiac
Tricyclic Antidepressants: Major Toxicity Is Cardiac						
Tertiary amines demethylated into secondary active amine metabolites						
Amitriptyline (Elavil)	75–300	120–250	31–46	3+	3+	3+
Imipramine (Tofranil)	75–300	125–250	9–24	3+	3+	2+
Doxepin (Sinequan)	75–300	30–150	8–24	3+	3+	2+
Trimipramine (Surmontil)	75–200	10–240	16–18	3+	3+	2+
Secondary amines metabolized into inactive metabolites						
Nortriptyline (Pamelor)†	75–150	50–150	18–93	2+	3+	3+
Desipramine (Norpramin)	75–200	75–160	14–62	1+	3+	3+
Protriptyline (Vivactil)	20–60	70–250	54–198	2+	3+	3+
Newer Cyclic Antidepressants						
Tetracyclic agent produces a high incidence of cardiovascular disturbances and seizures						
Maprotiline (Ludiomil)	75–300	—	30–60	1+	2+	3+
Trizolopyridine, a noncyclic agent, produces less serious cardiac and CNS toxicity						
Trazodone (Desyrel)	50–600	700	4–7	1+	1+	1+
Monocyclic aminoketone produces seizures in doses >600 mg						
Bupropion (Wellbutrin)	200–400	—	8–24	1+	3+	1+
Dibenzazepine						
Clomipramine (Anafranil)	100–250	200–500	21–32	2+	2+	2+
Dibenoxazepine produces syndrome of convulsions, rhabdomyolysis, and renal failure						
Amoxapine (Asendin)	150–300	200–500	6–10	1+	3+	2+

*Other drugs with similar structures are cyclobenzaprine (Flexeril), a muscle relaxant (similar to amitriptyline) and carbamazepine (Tegretol), an anticonvulsant (similar to imipramine); however, they cause less cardiac toxicity. 1+ indicates mild effect; 2+ indicates moderate effect; 3+ indicates severe effect.

†Not available in the United States.

Abbreviations: Antichol = anticholinergic effect; CNS = central nervous system effect (primarily seizures); Cardiac = cardiac effect.

lites have considerable $t_{1/2}$ values. Elimination is by hepatic metabolism. The tertiary amines are metabolized into active demethylated secondary amine metabolites. The active secondary amine metabolites undergo 15% enterohepatic recirculation and are metabolized over a period of days into nonactive metabolites. The intestinal bacterial flora may reconstitute the active metabolites. Only 3% of an ingested dose is excreted in the urine unchanged. *Manifestations:* On arrival, alert, oriented patients may suddenly become comatose, have a seizure, develop hemodynamically unstable dysrhythmias within minutes, and die. Most patients with severe toxicity develop symptoms within 1 to 2 hours but onset may be delayed 6 hours after an overdose. (1) Small overdoses produce early anticholinergic effects, agitation, and transient hypertension, which are not life-threatening. (2) Large overdoses produce depression of CNS and myocardium, convulsions, and hypotension. Death usually occurs within the first 2 to 6 hours after ingestion. (3) ECG screening tools for TCA: QRS greater than 0.10 second, expect seizures, and QRS greater than 0.16 second, 50% developed ventricular dysrhythmias (20% of these life-threatening) and seizures; a terminal 40 milliseconds of the QRS axis greater than 120 degrees in the right frontal plane; an R wave greater than 3 mm by the right arm lead. The quinidine cardiac membrane-stabilizing effect produces depression of myocardium, conduction, and ECG changes. The peripheral alpha-adrenergic blockade produces hypotension. *Management:* (1) Establish and maintain vital functions. Even if the patient is asymptomatic, establish IV access, monitor vital signs and neurologic status, obtain a baseline 12-lead ECG, and continue cardiac monitoring for at least 6 hours from admission or 8 to 12 hours after ingestion. Measure the QRS interval every 15 minutes. (2) GI decontamination: Do not induce emesis, and omit gastric lavage if AC is available. If the mental state is altered, protect the airway. AC with cathartic at 1 gram per kg is recommended immediately and repeated once (0.5 mg per kg) in 4 hours without a cathartic. A clinical benefit of MDAC has not been demonstrated. (3) Control seizures. Alkalinization does not control seizures; use diazepam or lorazepam. Status epilepticus (amoxapine) may require high-dose barbiturates or neuromuscular blockers with IV diazepam. If this is not successful, use paralysis by short nondepolarizing neuromuscular blockers such as vecuronium, intubation, and assisted ventilation. A bolus of NaHCO$_3$ is recommended as an adjunct to correct the acidosis produced by the seizures. (4) Cardiovascular management: NaHCO$_3$ (see Table 12): administer 1 to 2 mEq per kg undiluted as a bolus and repeated twice a few minutes apart, if needed, for sodium loading and alkalinization, which increases PB. The sodium loading overcomes the sodium channel blockage and is more important than the alkalinization, which increases the PB from 90 to 98%. Indications include a QRS complex greater than 0.12 second, ventricular tachycardia, severe conduction disturbances, meta-

bolic acidosis, coma, and seizures. An infusion of NaHCO$_3$ may follow to keep the blood pH at 7.5 to 7.55. The continuous infusion by itself is of limited usefulness for controlling dysrhythmias because of its delayed onset of action. Bolus therapy is given as needed. Hyperventilation alone has been recommended, but the pH elevation is not so instantaneous and there is compensatory renal excretion of bicarbonate; therefore, it is not recommended. The combination of hyperventilation and NaHCO$_3$ has produced fatal alkalemia and is not recommended. Monitor the serum potassium (the sudden increase in blood pH can aggravate or precipitate hypokalemia), serum sodium, ionized calcium (hypocalcemia may occur with alkalinization), and blood pH. (5) Specific cardiovascular complications should be treated as follows: Hypotension with norepinephrine, a predominantly alpha-adrenergic drug, is preferred to dopamine. Hypertension that occurs early rarely requires treatment. Sinus tachycardia usually does not require treatment. Supraventricular tachycardia with hemodynamic instability requires synchronized electrical cardioversion, starting at 0.25 to 1.0 watt-second per kg, after sedation. Ventricular tachycardia that persists after alkalinization requires IV lidocaine or countershock if the patient is hemodynamically unstable. Ventricular fibrillation should be treated with defibrillation. Torsades de pointes is treated with 20% magnesium sulfate solution IV, 2 grams over 2 to 3 minutes, followed by a continuous infusion of 1.5 mL of 10% solution or 5 to 10 mg per minute (see Table 12). For bradydysrhythmias, atropine is contraindicated because of the anticholinergic activity. Isoproterenol at 0.1 μg per kg per minute with caution may produce hypotension. If the patient is hemodynamically unstable, use a pacemaker. (6) Extraordinary measures such as intraaortic balloon pump and cardiopulmonary bypass have been successful. (7) Investigational: Fab fragments specific for tricyclic antidepressants have been successful in animals. Prophylactic NaHCO$_3$ to prevent dysrhythmias is being investigated. (8) Contraindicated: Physostigmine has produced asystole. Flumazenil has produced seizures. *Laboratory investigations:* Monitor: If altered mental status or ECG abnormalities are present, obtain ABGs, ECG monitoring, chest radiography, blood glucose, serum electrolytes, calcium, magnesium, BUN and creatinine, liver profile, creatine kinase, and urine output; in severe cases, hemodynamic monitoring is indicated. Levels of the tricyclic and cyclic antidepressants below 300 ng per mL are therapeutic, levels above 500 ng per mL indicate toxicity, and levels above 1000 ng per mL indicate serious poisoning and are associated with QRS widening. *Disposition:* Admit to the ICU for 12 to 24 hours any patient with an antidepressant overdose who meets any of the following criteria: ECG abnormalities except sinus tachycardia, altered mental state, seizures, respiratory depression, and hypotension. Caution: in 25% of fatal cases the patients were alert and awake at presentation. Low-risk patients are those who do not have the preceding symptoms at 6 hours after ingestion, those who present with minor transient manifestations such as sinus tachycardia and subsequently become and remain asymptomatic for a 6-hour period, and asymptomatic patients who remain asymptomatic for 6 hours. These patients may be discharged if the ECG remains normal and they have normal bowel sounds, have AC repeated once, and undergo psychiatric counseling. Children younger than 6 years with nonintentional (accidental) exposures should be referred to the emergency department for monitoring, observation, and AC.

Section 18

Appendices and Index

REFERENCE INTERVALS FOR THE INTERPRETATION OF LABORATORY TESTS

method of
WILLIAM Z. BORER, M.D.
Thomas Jefferson University Hospital
Philadelphia, Pennsylvania

Most of the tests performed in a clinical laboratory are quantitative in nature. That is, the amount of a substance present in blood or serum is measured and reported in terms of concentration, activity (e.g., enzyme activity), or counts (e.g., blood cell counts). The laboratory must provide reference values to assist the clinician in the interpretation of laboratory results. These reference ranges specify the physiologic quantities of substance (concentrations, activities, or counts) to be expected in healthy individuals. Deviation above or below the reference range may be associated with a disease process, and the severity of the disease process may be associated with the magnitude of the deviation. Unfortunately, there is rarely a sharp demarcation between physiologic and pathologic values, and the transition between these two is often gradual as the disease process progresses.

The terms "normal" and "abnormal" have been used to describe the laboratory values that fall inside or outside the reference range, respectively. Use of these terms is now discouraged because it is virtually impossible to define normality and because normal may be confused with the statistical term "gaussian." Reference ranges are established from statistical studies in groups of healthy volunteers. Although these study subjects must be free of disease, they may have lifestyles or habits that result in subtle variations in their laboratory values. Examples of

these variables include diet, body mass, exercise, and geographic location. Age and sex may also affect reference values. When the data from a large cohort of healthy subjects fit a gaussian distribution, the usual statistical approach is to define the reference limits as two standard deviations above and below the mean. By definition, the reference range excludes the highest and the lowest 2.5% of the population. Nongaussian distributions are handled by different statistical methods, but the result is similar in that the reference range is defined by the central 95% of the population. In other words, the odds are 1 in 20 that a healthy individual will have a laboratory result that falls outside the reference range. If 12 laboratory tests are performed, the odds increase to about 1 in 2 that at least one of the results is outside the reference range. This means that all healthy

TABLE 1. **Base SI Units**

Property	Base Unit	Symbol
Length	meter	m
Mass	kilogram	kg
Amount of substance	mole	mol
Time	second	s
Thermodynamic temperature	kelvin	K
Electric current	ampere	A
Luminous intensity	candela	cd
Catalytic amount	katal	kat

TABLE 2. **Derived SI Units and Non-SI Units Retained for Use with the SI**

Property	Unit	Symbol
Area	square meter	m^2
Volume	cubic meter	m^3
	liter	L
Mass concentration	kilogram/ cubic meter	kg/m^3
	gram/liter	gm/L
Substance concentration	mole/cubic meter	mol/m^3
	mole/liter	mol/L
Temperature	degree Celsius	$°C = K - 273.15$

TABLE 3. **Standard Prefixes**

Prefix	Multiplication Factor	Symbol
yocto	10^{-24}	y
zepto	10^{-21}	z
atto	10^{-18}	a
femto	10^{-15}	f
pico	10^{-12}	p
nano	10^{-9}	n
micro	10^{-6}	μ
milli	10^{-3}	m
centi	10^{-2}	c
deci	10^{-1}	d
deca	10^{1}	da
hecto	10^{2}	h
kilo	10^{3}	k
mega	10^{6}	M
giga	10^{9}	G
tera	10^{12}	T

individuals are likely to have a few laboratory results that are unexpected. The clinician must then integrate the data with other clinical information such as the history and physical examination to arrive at the appropriate clinical decision. The reference range for many tests (especially enzyme and immunochemical measurements) will vary with the method used. It is important that each laboratory establish reference ranges appropriate for the methods it employs.

SI UNITS

During the 1980s, a concerted effort was made to introduce SI units (le Système International d'Unités). The rationale for conversion to SI units is sound. Laboratory data are scientifically more informative when the units are based on molar concentration rather than mass concentration. For example, the conversion of glucose to lactate and pyruvate or the binding of a drug to albumin is more easily understood in units of molar concentration. Another example is illustrated as follows:

Conventional Units
1.0 gram of hemoglobin
Combines with 1.37 mL of oxygen
Contains 3.4 mg of iron
Forms 34.9 mg of bilirubin
SI Units
4.0 mmol of hemoglobin
Combines with 4.0 mmol of oxygen
Contains 4.0 mmol of iron
Forms 4.0 mmol of bilirubin

The use of SI units would also enhance the standardization of nomenclature to facilitate global communication of medical and scientific information. The units, symbols, and prefixes employed in the International System are shown in Tables 1, 2, and 3.

Unfortunately, problems have arisen with the implementation of SI units in the United States. Their introduction in 1987 prompted many medical journals to report laboratory values in both SI and conventional units in anticipation of complete conversion to SI units in the early 1990s. The lack of a coordinated effort toward this goal has forced a retrenchment on the issue. Physicians continue to think and practice using laboratory results expressed in conventional units, and few if any American hospitals or clinical laboratories exclusively use SI units. It is not likely that complete conversion to SI units will occur in the foreseeable future, yet most medical journals will probably continue to publish both sets of units. For this reason, the tables of reference ranges in this appendix are given in both conventional units and SI units.

References

Drug Evaluations Annual. Chicago, American Medical Association, 1994.

Bick RL (ed): Hematology—Clinical and Laboratory Practice. St Louis, Mosby–Year Book, 1993.

Borer WZ: Selection and Use of Laboratory Tests. *In* Applied Laboratory Medicine. Philadelphia, WB Saunders Co, 1992, pp 1–5.

Campion EW: A retreat from SI units. N Engl J Med *327*:49, 1992.

Friedman RB, Young DS: Effects of Disease on Clinical Laboratory Tests, 3rd ed. Washington, DC, AACC Press, 1997.

Henry JB: Clinical Diagnosis and Management by Laboratory Methods, 19th ed. Philadelphia, WB Saunders Co, 1996.

Hicks JM, Young DS: DORA '97–'99: Directory of Rare Analyses. Washington, DC, AACC Press, 1997.

Jacobs DS, Demott WR, Grady HJ, et al: Laboratory Test Handbook, 4th ed. Baltimore, Williams & Wilkins Co, 1996.

Kaplan LA, Pesce AJ: Clinical Chemistry—Theory, Analysis, and Correlation, 3rd ed. St Louis, CV Mosby, 1996.

Kjeldsberg CR, Knight JA: Body Fluids—Laboratory Examination of Amniotic, Cerebrospinal, Seminal, Serous and Synovial Fluids, 3rd ed. Chicago, ASCP Press, 1993.

Laposata M: SI Unit Conversion Guide. Boston, NEJM Books, 1992.

Scully RE, Mc Neely WF, Mark EJ, Mc Neely BU: Normal reference laboratory values. N Engl J Med *327*:718–724, 1992.

Speicher CE: The Right Test—A Physician's Guide to Laboratory Medicine, 2nd ed. Philadelphia, WB Saunders Co, 1993.

Tietz NW (ed): Clinical Guide to Laboratory Tests, 3rd ed. Philadelphia, WB Saunders Co, 1995.

Wallach J: Interpretation of Diagnostic Tests—A Synopsis of Laboratory Medicine, 6th ed. Boston, Little, Brown, 1996.

Young DS: Implementation of SI units for clinical laboratory data. Ann Intern Med *106*:114–129, 1987.

Young DS: Determination and validation of reference intervals. Arch Pathol Lab Med *116*:704–709, 1992.

Young DS: Effects of Drugs on Clinical Laboratory Tests, 4th ed. Washington, DC, AACC Press, 1995.

TABLES OF REFERENCE VALUES

Some of the values included in the tables have been established by the clinical laboratories at Thomas Jefferson University Hospital, Philadelphia, Pennsylvania, and have not been published elsewhere. Other values have been compiled from the sources cited. These tables are provided for information and educational purposes only. They are intended to complement data derived from other sources including the medical history and physical examination. Users must exercise individual judgment when employing the information provided in this appendix.

Reference Values for Hematology

Test	Conventional Units	SI Units
Acid hemolysis (Ham test)	No hemolysis	No hemolysis
Alkaline phosphatase, leukocyte	Total score 14–100	Total score 14–100
Cell counts		
Erythrocytes		
Males	4.6–6.2 million/mm³	4.6–6.2 × 10¹²/L
Females	4.2–5.4 million/mm³	4.2–5.4 × 10¹²/L
Children (varies with age)	4.5–5.1 million/mm³	4.5–5.1 × 10¹²/L

Reference Values for Hematology *Continued*

Test	Conventional Units	SI Units
Leukocytes, total	4,500–11,000/mm³	4.5–11.0 × 10⁹/L
Leukocytes, differential counts*		
Myelocytes	0%	0/L
Band neutrophils	3–5%	150–400 × 10⁶/L
Segmented neutrophils	54–62%	3,000–5,800 × 10⁶/L
Lymphocytes	25–33%	1,500–3,000 × 10⁶/L
Monocytes	3–7%	300–500 × 10⁶/L
Eosinophils	1–3%	50–250 × 10⁶/L
Basophils	0–1%	15–50 × 10⁶/L
Platelets	150,000–400,000/mm³	150–400 × 10⁹/L
Reticulocytes	25,000–75,000/mm³	25–75 × 10⁹/L
	(0.5–1.5% of erythrocytes)	
Coagulation tests		
Bleeding time (template)	2.75–8.0 min	2.75–8.0 min
Coagulation time (glass tube)	5–15 min	5–15 min
D dimer	<0.5 μm/mL	<0.5 mg/L
Factor VIII and other coagulation factors	50–150% of normal	0.5–1.5 of normal
Fibrin split products (Thrombo-Wellco test)	<10 μg/mL	<10 mg/L
Fibrinogen	200–400 mg/dL	2.0–4.0 gm/L
Partial thromboplastin time (PTT)	20–35 s	20–35 s
Prothrombin time (PT)	12.0–14.0 s	12.0–14.0 s
Coombs' test		
Direct	Negative	Negative
Indirect	Negative	Negative
Corpuscular values of erythrocytes		
Mean corpuscular hemoglobin (MCH)	26–34 pg/cell	26–34 pg/cell
Mean corpuscular volume (MCV)	80–96 μm³	80–96 fL
Mean corpuscular hemoglobin concentration (MCHC)	32–36 gm/dL	320–360 gm/L
Erythrocyte sedimentation rate (ESR)		
Wintrobe		
Males	0–5 mm/h	0–5 mm/h
Females	0–15 mm/h	0–15 mm/h
Westergren		
Males	0–15 mm/h	0–15 mm/h
Females	0–20 mm/h	0–20 mm/h
Haptoglobin	20–165 mg/dL	0.20–1.65 gm/L
Hematocrit		
Males	40–54 mL/dL	0.40–0.54
Females	37–47 mL/dL	0.37–0.47
Newborns	49–54 mL/dL	0.49–0.54
Children (varies with age)	35–49 mL/dL	0.35–0.49
Hemoglobin		
Males	13.0–18.0 gm/dL	8.1–11.2 mmol/L
Females	12.0–16.0 gm/dL	7.4–9.9 mmol/L
Newborn	16.5–19.5 gm/dL	10.2–12.1 mmol/L
Children (varies with age)	11.2–16.5 gm/dL	7.0–10.2 mmol/L
Hemoglobin, fetal	<1.0% of total	<0.01 of total
Hemoglobin A₁c	3–5% of total	0.03–0.05 of total
Hemoglobin A₂	1.5–3.0% of total	0.015–0.03 of total
Hemoglobin, plasma	0.0–5.0 mg/dL	0.0–3.2 μmol/L
Methemoglobin	30–130 mg/dL	19–80 μmol/L

*Conventional units are percentages; SI units are absolute counts.

Reference Values* for Clinical Chemistry (Blood, Serum, and Plasma)

Analyte	Conventional Units	SI Units
Acetoacetate plus acetone		
Qualitative	Negative	Negative
Quantitative	0.3–2.0 mg/dL	30–200 μmol/L
Acid phosphatase, serum (thymolphthalein monophosphate substrate)	0.1–0.6 U/L	0.1–0.6 U/L
ACTH (see Corticotropin)		
Alanine aminotransferase (ALT, SGPT), serum	1–45 U/L	1–45 U/L
Albumin, serum	3.3–5.2 gm/dL	33–52 gm/L
Aldolase, serum	0.0–7.0 U/L	0.0–7.0 U/L
Aldosterone, plasma		
Standing	5–30 ng/dL	140–830 pmol/L
Recumbent	3–10 ng/dL	80–275 pmol/L

Table continued on following page

Reference Values* for Clinical Chemistry (Blood, Serum, and Plasma) *Continued*

Analyte	Conventional Units	SI Units
Alkaline phosphatase (ALP), serum		
Adult	35–150 U/L	35–150 U/L
Adolescent	100–500 U/L	100–500 U/L
Child	100–350 U/L	100–350 U/L
Ammonia nitrogen, plasma	10–50 µmol/L	10–50 µmol/L
Amylase, serum	25–125 U/L	25–125 U/L
Anion gap, serum, calculated	8–16 mEq/L	8–16 mmol/L
Ascorbic acid, blood	0.4–1.5 mg/dL	23–85 µmol/L
Aspartate aminotransferase (AST, SGOT), serum	1–36 U/L	1–36 U/L
Base excess, arterial blood, calculated	0 ± 2 mEq/L	0 ± 2 mmol/L
Bicarbonate		
Venous plasma	23–29 mEq/L	23–29 mmol/L
Arterial blood	21–27 mEq/L	21–27 mmol/L
Bile acids, serum	0.3–3.0 mg/dL	0.8–7.6 µmol/L
Bilirubin, serum		
Conjugated	0.1–0.4 mg/dL	1.7–6.8 µmol/L
Total	0.3–1.1 mg/dL	5.1–19.0 µmol/L
Calcium, serum	8.4–10.6 mg/dL	2.10–2.65 mmol/L
Calcium, ionized, serum	4.25–5.25 mg/dL	1.05–1.30 mmol/L
Carbon dioxide, total, serum or plasma	24–31 mEq/L	24–31 mmol/L
Carbon dioxide tension (PCO_2), blood	35–45 mm Hg	35–45 mm Hg
β-Carotene, serum	60–260 µg/dL	1.1–8.6 µmol/L
Ceruloplasmin, serum	23–44 mg/dL	230–440 mg/L
Chloride, serum or plasma	96–106 mEq/L	96–106 mmol/L
Cholesterol, serum or EDTA plasma		
Desirable range	<200 mg/dL	<5.20 mmol/L
LDL cholesterol	60–180 mg/dL	1.55–4.65 mmol/L
HDL cholesterol	30–80 mg/dL	0.80–2.05 mmol/L
Copper	70–140 µg/dL	11–22 µmol/L
Corticotropin (ACTH), plasma, 8:00 AM	10–80 pg/mL	2–18 pmol/L
Cortisol, plasma		
8:00 AM	6–23 µg/dL	170–630 nmol/L
4:00 PM	3–15 µg/dL	80–410 nmol/L
10:00 PM	<50% of 8:00 AM value	<50% of 8:00 AM value
Creatine, serum		
Males	0.2–0.5 mg/dL	15–40 µmol/L
Females	0.3–0.9 mg/dL	25–70 µmol/L
Creatine kinase (CK), serum		
Males	55–170 U/L	55–170 U/L
Females	30–135 U/L	30–135 U/L
Creatine kinase MB isoenzyme, serum	<5% of total CK activity	<5% of total CK activity
	<5% ng/mL by immunoassay	<5% ng/mL by immunoassay
Creatinine, serum	0.6–1.2 mg/dL	50–110 µmol/L
Estradiol-17β, adult		
Males	10–65 pg/mL	35–240 pmol/L
Females		
Follicular	30–100 pg/mL	110–370 pmol/L
Ovulatory	200–400 pg/mL	730–1470 pmol/L
Luteal	50–140 pg/mL	180–510 pmol/L
Ferritin, serum	20–200 ng/mL	20–200 µg/L
Fibrinogen, plasma	200–400 mg/dL	2.0–4.0 gm/L
Folate, serum	3–18 ng/mL	6.8–41 nmol/L
erythrocytes	145–540 ng/mL	330–1220 nmol/L
Follicle-stimulating hormone (FSH), plasma		
Males	4–25 mU/mL	4–25 U/L
Females, premenopausal	4–30 mU/mL	4–30 U/L
Females, postmenopausal	40–250 mU/mL	40–250 U/L
Gastrin, fasting, serum	0–100 pg/mL	0–100 mg/L
Glucose, fasting, plasma or serum	70–115 mg/dL	3.9–6.4 nmol/L
γ-Glutamyltransferase (GGT), serum	5–40 U/L	5–40 U/L
Growth hormone (hGH), plasma, adult, fasting	0–6 ng/mL	0–6 µg/L
Haptoglobin, serum	20–165 mg/dL	0.20–1.65 gm/L
Immunoglobulins, serum (see Immunologic Procedures)		
Iron, serum	75–175 µg/dL	13–31 µmol/L
Iron-binding capacity, serum		
Total	250–410 µg/dL	45–73 µmol/L
Saturation	20–55%	0.20–0.55
Lactate		
Venous whole blood	5.0–20.0 mg/dL	0.6–2.2 mmol/L
Arterial whole blood	5.0–15.0 mg/dL	0.6–1.7 mmol/L
Lactate dehydrogenase (LD), serum	110–220 U/L	110–220 U/L

Reference Values* for Clinical Chemistry (Blood, Serum, and Plasma) *Continued*

Analyte	Conventional Units	SI Units
Lipase, serum	10–140 U/L	10–140 U/L
Lutropin (LH), serum		
Males	1–9 U/L	1–9 U/L
Females		
Follicular phase	2–10 U/L	2–10 U/L
Midcycle peak	15–65 U/L	15–65 U/L
Luteal phase	1–12 U/L	1–12 U/L
Postmenopausal	12–65 U/L	12–65 U/L
Magnesium, serum	1.3–2.1 mg/dL	0.65–1.05 mmol/L
Osmolality	275–295 mOsm/kg water	275–295 mOsm/kg water
Oxygen, blood, arterial, room air		
Partial pressure (PaO₂)	80–100 mm Hg	80–100 mm Hg
Saturation (SaO₂)	95–98%	95–98%
pH, arterial blood	7.35–7.45	7.35–7.45
Phosphate, inorganic, serum		
Adult	3.0–4.5 mg/dL	1.0–1.5 mmol/L
Child	4.0–7.0 mg/dL	1.3–2.3 mmol/L
Potassium		
Serum	3.5–5.0 mEq/L	3.5–5.0 mmol/L
Plasma	3.5–4.5 mEq/L	3.5–4.5 mmol/L
Progesterone, serum, adult		
Males	0.0–0.4 ng/mL	0.0–1.3 mmol/L
Females		
Follicular phase	0.1–1.5 ng/mL	0.3–4.8 mmol/L
Luteal phase	2.5–28.0 ng/mL	8.0–89.0 mmol/L
Prolactin, serum		
Males	1.0–15.0 ng/mL	1.0–15.0 µg/L
Females	1.0–20.0 ng/mL	1.0–20.0 µg/L
Protein, serum, electrophoresis		
Total	6.0–8.0 gm/dL	60–80 gm/L
Albumin	3.5–5.5 gm/dL	35–55 gm/L
Globulins		
Alpha₁	0.2–0.4 gm/dL	2.0–4.0 gm/L
Alpha₂	0.5–0.9 gm/dL	5.0–9.0 gm/L
Beta	0.6–1.1 gm/dL	6.0–11.0 gm/L
Gamma	0.7–1.7 gm/dL	7.0–17.0 gm/L
Pyruvate, blood	0.3–0.9 mg/dL	0.03–0.10 mmol/L
Rheumatoid factor	0.0–30.0 IU/mL	0.0–30.0 kIU/L
Sodium, serum or plasma	135–145 mEq/L	135–145 mmol/L
Testosterone, plasma		
Males, adult	300–1200 ng/dL	10.4–41.6 nmol/L
Females, adult	20–75 ng/dL	0.7–2.6 nmol/L
Pregnant females	40–200 ng/dL	1.4–6.9 nmol/L
Thyroglobulin	3–42 ng/mL	3–42 µg/L
Thyrotropin (hTSH), serum	0.4–4.8 µIU/mL	0.4–4.8 mIU/L
Thyrotropin-releasing hormone (TRH)	5–60 pg/mL	5–60 ng/L
Thyroxine (FT₄), free, serum	0.9–2.1 ng/dL	12–27 pmol/L
Thyroxine (T₄), serum	4.5–12.0 µg/dL	58–154 nmol/L
Thyroxine-binding globulin (TBG)	15.0–34.0 µg/mL	15.0–34.0 mg/L
Transferrin	250–430 mg/dL	2.5–4.3 gm/L
Triglycerides, serum, after 12-h fast	40–150 mg/dL	0.4–1.5 gm/L
Triiodothyronine (T₃), serum	70–190 ng/dL	1.1–2.9 nmol/L
Triiodothyronine uptake, resin (T₃RU)	25–38%	0.25–0.38
Urate		
Males	2.5–8.0 mg/dL	150–480 µmol/L
Females	2.2–7.0 mg/dL	130–420 µmol/L
Urea, serum or plasma	24–49 mg/dL	4.0–8.2 nmol/L
Urea nitrogen, serum or plasma	11–23 mg/dL	8.0–16.4 nmol/L
Viscosity, serum	1.4–1.8 × water	1.4–1.8 × water
Vitamin A, serum	20–80 µg/dL	0.70–2.80 µmol/L
Vitamin B₁₂, serum	180–900 pg/mL	133–664 pmol/L

*Reference values may vary depending on the method and sample source used.

Reference Values for Therapeutic Drug Monitoring (Serum)

Analyte	Therapeutic Range	Toxic Concentrations	Proprietary Names
Analgesics			
Acetaminophen	10–20 µg/mL	>250 µg/mL	Tylenol
			Datril
Salicylate	100–250 µg/mL	>300 µg/mL	Aspirin
			Bufferin
Antibiotics			
Amikacin	25–30 µg/mL	Peak >35 µg/mL	Amikin
		Trough >10 µg/mL	
Gentamicin	5–10 µg/mL	Peak >10 µg/mL	Garamycin
		Trough >2 µg/mL	
Tobramycin	5–10 µg/mL	Peak >10 µg/mL	Nebcin
		Trough >2 µg/mL	
Vancomycin	5–35 µg/mL	Peak >40 µg/mL	Vancocin
		Trough >10 µg/mL	
Anticonvulsants			
Carbamazepine	5–12 µg/mL	>15 µg/mL	Tegretol
Ethosuximide	40–100 µg/mL	>150 µg/mL	Zarontin
Phenobarbital	15–40 µg/mL	40–100 ng/mL (varies widely)	Luminal
Phenytoin	10–20 µg/mL	>20 µg/mL	Dilantin
Primidone	5–12 µg/mL	>15 µg/mL	Mysoline
Valproic acid	50–100 µg/mL	>100 µg/mL	Depakene
Antineoplastics and Immunosuppressives			
Cyclosporine	50–400 ng/mL	>400 ng/mL	Sandimmune
Methotrexate, high dose, 48 h	Variable	>1 µmol/L 48 h after dose	
Tacrolimus (FK-506), whole blood	3–10 µg/L	>15 µg/L	Prograf
Bronchodilators and Respiratory Stimulants			
Caffeine	3–15 ng/mL	>30 ng/mL	
Theophylline (aminophylline)	10–20 µg/mL	>20 µg/mL	Elixophyllin
			Quibron
			Theo-Dur
			Slo-bid
Cardiovascular Drugs			
Amiodarone (obtain specimen more than 8 h after last dose)	1.0–2.0 µg/mL	>2.0 µg/mL	Cordarone
Digitoxin (obtain specimen 12–24 h after last dose)	15–25 ng/mL	>35 ng/mL	Crystodigin
Digoxin (obtain specimen more than 6 h after last dose)	0.8–2.0 ng/mL	>2.4 ng/mL	Lanoxin
Disopyramide	2–5 µg/mL	>7 µg/mL	Norpace
Flecainide	0.2–1.0 ng/mL	>1 ng/mL	Tambocor
Lidocaine	1.5–5.0 µg/mL	>6 µg/mL	Xylocaine
Mexiletine	0.7–2.0 ng/mL	>2 ng/mL	Mexitil
Procainamide	4–10 µg/mL	>12 µg/mL	Pronestyl
Procainamide plus NAPA	8–30 µg/mL	>30 µg/mL	
Propranolol	50–100 ng/mL	Variable	Inderal
Quinidine	2–5 µg/mL	>6 µg/mL	Cardioquin
			Quinaglute
Tocainide	4–10 ng/mL	>10 ng/mL	Tonocard
Psychopharmacologic Drugs			
Amitriptyline	120–150 ng/mL	>500 ng/mL	Elavil
			Triavil
Bupropion	25–100 ng/mL	Not applicable	Wellbutrin
Desipramine	150–300 ng/mL	>500 ng/mL	Norpramin
			Pertofrane
Imipramine	125–250 ng/mL	>400 ng/mL	Tofranil
			Janimine
Lithium (obtain specimen 12 h after last dose)	0.6–1.5 mEq/L	>1.5 mEq/L	Lithobid
Nortriptyline	50–150 ng/mL	>500 ng/mL	Aventyl
			Pamelor

Reference Values* for Clinical Chemistry (Urine)

Analyte	Conventional Units	SI Units
Acetone and acetoacetate, qualitative	Negative	Negative
Albumin		
Qualitative	Negative	Negative
Quantitative	10–100 mg/24 h	0.15–1.5 µmol/d
Aldosterone	3–20 µg/24 h	8.3–55 nmol/d
δ-Aminolevulinic acid (δ-ALA)	1.3–7.0 mg/24 h	10–53 µmol/d
Amylase	<17 U/h	<17 U/h
Amylase/creatinine clearance ratio	0.01–0.04	0.01–0.04
Bilirubin, qualitative	Negative	Negative
Calcium (regular diet)	<250 mg/24 h	<6.3 nmol/d
Catecholamines		
Epinephrine	<10 µg/24 h	<55 nmol/d
Norepinephrine	<100 µg/24 h	<590 nmol/d
Total free catecholamines	4–126 µg/24 h	24–745 nmol/d
Total metanephrines	0.1–1.6 mg/24 h	0.5–8.1 µmol/d
Chloride (varies with intake)	110–250 mEq/24 h	110–250 mmol/d
Copper	0–50 µg/24 h	0.0–0.80 µmol/d
Cortisol, free	10–100 µg/24 h	27.6–276 nmol/d
Creatine		
Males	0–40 mg/24 h	0.0–0.30 mmol/d
Females	0–80 mg/24 h	0.0–0.60 mmol/d
Creatinine	15–25 mg/kg/24 h	0.13–0.22 mmol/kg/d
Creatinine clearance (endogenous)		
Males	110–150 mL/min/1.73 m²	110–150 mL/min/1.73 m²
Females	105–132 mL/min/1.73 m²	105–132 mL/min/1.73 m²
Cystine or cysteine	Negative	Negative
Dehydroepiandrosterone		
Males	0.2–2.0 mg/24 h	0.7–6.9 µmol/d
Females	0.2–1.8 mg/24 h	0.7–6.2 µmol/d
Estrogens, total		
Males	4–25 µg/24 h	14–90 nmol/d
Females	5–100 µg/24 h	18–360 nmol/d
Glucose (as reducing substance)	<250 mg/24 h	<250 mg/d
Hemoglobin and myoglobin, qualitative	Negative	Negative
Homogentisic acid, qualitative	Negative	Negative
17-Hydroxycorticosteroids		
Males	3–9 mg/24 h	8.3–25 µmol/d
Females	2–8 mg/24 h	5.5–22 µmol/d
5-Hydroxyindoleacetic acid		
Qualitative	Negative	Negative
Quantitative	2–6 mg/24 h	10–31 µmol/d
17-Ketogenic steroids		
Males	5–23 mg/24 h	17–80 µmol/d
Females	3–15 mg/24 h	10–52 µmol/d
17-Ketosteroids		
Males	8–22 mg/24 h	28–76 µmol/d
Females	6–15 mg/24 h	21–52 µmol/d
Magnesium	6–10 mEq/24 h	3–5 mmol/d
Metanephrines	0.05–1.2 ng/mg creatinine	0.03–0.70 mmol/mmol creatinine
Osmolality	38–1400 mOsm/kg water	38–1400 mOsm/kg water
pH	4.6–8.0	4.6–8.0
Phenylpyruvic acid, qualitative	Negative	Negative
Phosphate	0.4–1.3 gm/24 h	13–42 mmol/d
Porphobilinogen		
Qualitative	Negative	Negative
Quantitative	<2 mg/24 h	<9 µmol/d
Porphyrins		
Coproporphyrin	50–250 µg/24 h	77–380 nmol/d
Uroporphyrin	10–30 µg/24 h	12–36 nmol/d
Potassium	25–125 mEq/24 h	25–125 mmol/d
Pregnanediol		
Males	0.0–1.9 mg/24 h	0.0–6.0 µmol/d
Females		
Proliferative phase	0.0–2.6 mg/24 h	0.0–8.0 µmol/d
Luteal phase	2.6–10.6 mg/24 h	8–33 µmol/d
Postmenopausal	0.2–1.0 mg/24 h	0.6–3.1 µmol/d
Pregnanetriol	0.0–2.5 mg/24 h	0.0–7.4 µmol/d

Table continued on following page

Reference Values* for Clinical Chemistry (Urine) *Continued*

Analyte	Conventional Units	SI Units
Protein, total		
Qualitative	Negative	Negative
Quantitative	10–150 mg/24 h	10–150 mg/d
Protein/creatinine ratio	<0.2	<0.2
Sodium (regular diet)	60–260 mEq/24 h	60–260 mmol/d
Specific gravity		
Random specimen	1.003–1.030	1.003–1.030
24-h collection	1.015–1.025	1.015–1.025
Urate (regular diet)	250–750 mg/24 h	1.5–4.4 mmol/d
Urobilinogen	0.5–4.0 mg/24 h	0.6–6.8 μmol/d
Vanillylmandelic acid (VMA)	1.0–8.0 mg/24 h	5–40 μmol/d

*Reference values may vary depending on the method used.

Reference Values for Toxic Substances

Analyte	Conventional Units	SI Units
Arsenic, urine	<130 μg/24 h	<1.7 μmol/d
Bromides, serum, inorganic	<100 mg/dL	<10 mmol/L
Toxic symptoms	140–1000 mg/dL	14–100 mmol/L
Carboxyhemoglobin, blood	*% Saturation*	*Saturation*
Urban environment	<5%	<0.05
Smokers	<12%	<0.12
Symptoms		
Headache	>15%	>0.15
Nausea and vomiting	>25%	>0.25
Potentially lethal	>50%	>0.50
Ethanol, blood	<0.05 mg/dL	<1.0 mmol/L
	<0.005%	
Intoxication	>100 mg/dL	>22 mmol/L
	>0.1	
Marked intoxication	300–400 mg/dL	65–87 mmol/L
	0.3–0.4%	
Alcoholic stupor	400–500 mg/dL	87–109 mmol/L
	0.4–0.5%	
Coma	>500 mg/dL	>109 mmol/L
	>0.5%	
Lead, blood		
Adults	<25 μg/dL	<1.2 μmol/L
Children	<15 μg/dL	<0.7 μmol/L
Lead, urine	<80 μg/24 h	<0.4 μmol/d
Mercury, urine	<30 μg/24 h	<150 nmol/d

Reference Values for Cerebrospinal Fluid

Test	Conventional Units	SI Units
Cells	<5/mm³, all mononuclear	<5 × 10⁶/L, all mononuclear
Protein electrophoresis	Albumin predominant	Albumin predominant
Glucose	50–75 mg/dL (20 mg/dL less than in serum)	2.8–4.2 mmol/L (1.1 mmol less than in serum)
IgG		
Children <14 y	<8% of total protein	<0.08 of total protein
Adults	<14% of total protein	<0.14 of total protein
IgG index	0.3–0.6	0.3–0.6
$\left(\dfrac{\text{CSF/serum IgG ratio}}{\text{CSF/serum albumin ratio}}\right)$		
Oligoclonal banding on electrophoresis	Absent	Absent
Pressure, opening	70–180 mm H₂O	70–180 mm H₂O
Protein, total	15–45 mg/dL	150–450 mg/L

Reference Values for Tests of Gastrointestinal Function

Test	Conventional Units	Test	Conventional Units
Bentiromide	6-h urinary arylamine excretion >57% excludes pancreatic insufficiency	Maximum (after histamine or pentagastrin)	
β-Carotene, serum	60–250 ng/dL	Males	9.0–48.0 mmol/h
Fecal fat estimation		Females	6.0–31.0 mmol/h
Qualitative	No fat globules seen by high-power microscope	Ratio: basal/maximum	
		Males	0.0–0.31
Quantitative	<6 gm/24 h (>95% coefficient of fat absorption)	Females	0.0–0.29
		Secretin test, pancreatic fluid	
Gastric acid output		Volume	>1.8 mL/kg/h
Basal		Bicarbonate	>80 mEq/L
Males	0.0–10.5 mmol/h	D-Xylose absorption test, urine	>20% of ingested dose excreted in 5 h
Females	0.0–5.6 mmol/h		

Reference Values for Immunologic Procedures

Test	Conventional Units	SI Units
Complement, serum		
C3	85–175 mg/dL	0.85–1.75 gm/L
C4	15–45 mg/dL	150–450 mg/L
Total hemolytic (CH₅₀)	150–250 U/mL	150–250 U/mL
Immunoglobulins, serum, adult		
IgG	640–1350 mg/dL	6.4–13.5 gm/L
IgA	70–310 mg/dL	0.70–3.1 gm/L
IgM	90–350 mg/dL	0.90–3.5 gm/L
IgD	0.0–6.0 mg/dL	0.0–60 mg/L
IgE	0.0–430 ng/dL	0.0–430 µg/L

Lymphocyte Subsets, Whole Blood, Heparinized

Antigen	Cell Type	Percentage	Absolute Cell Count
CD3	Total T cells	56–77%	860–1880
CD19	Total B cells	7–17%	140–370
CD3 and CD4	Helper-inducer cells	32–54%	550–1190
CD3 and CD8	Suppressor-cytotoxic cells	24–37%	430–1060
CD3 and DR	Activated T cells	5–14%	70–310
CD2	E rosette T cells	73–87%	1040–2160
CD16 and CD56	Natural killer (NK) cells	8–22%	130–500

Helper/suppressor ratio: 0.8–1.8

Reference Values for Semen Analysis

Test	Conventional Units	SI Units
Volume	2–5 mL	2–5 mL
Liquefaction	Complete in 15 min	Complete in 15 min
pH	7.2–8.0	7.2–8.0
Leukocytes	Occasional or absent	Occasional or absent
Spermatozoa		
Count	60–150 × 10⁶/mL	60–150 × 10⁶/mL
Motility	>80% motile	>0.80 motile
Morphology	80–90% normal forms	>0.80–0.90 normal forms
Fructose	>150 mg/dL	>8.33 mmol/L

DRUGS APPROVED IN 1996

method of
PAULA PIETRUCHA-DILANCHIAN, PHARM.D.
National Institutional Pharmacy Services
Houston, Texas

Generic Name	Trade Name (Manufacturer)	Dosage Form	Strength	Average Dosage Range	FDA Rating	Approved Use	Approval Date	Classification
Adapalene	Differin (Galderma)	Gel	0.10%	Apply daily	1-S	Acne vulgaris	Feb 96	Topical acne product
Albendazole	Albenza (Smith Kline Beecham)	Tablet	200 mg	400 mg bid or 15 mg/kg/d in divided doses (maximum, 800 mg/d)	1-P, V	Treatment of neurocysticercosis, hydatid disease	Jun 96	Anthelmintic
Amlexanox	Aphthasol (Block Drug Co)	Paste	5%	Apply qid	1-P	Treatment of signs and symptoms of aphthous ulcers in immunocompetent individuals	Dec 96	Misc
Anagrelide	Agrylin (Roberts)	Capsule	0.5 mg 1 mg	0.5 mg PO qid; maximum, 10 mg/d	1-P	Essential thrombocytopenia	Mar 97	Antiplatelet
Atorvastatin calcium	Lipitor (Parke-Davis)	Tablet	10 mg 20 mg 40 mg	10–80 mg/d PO	1-P	Treatment of dyslipidemias	Dec 96	Antihyperlipidemic agent
Azelastine hydrochloride	Astelin (Wallace)	Spray	137 μg/spray	2 sprays each nostril bid	1-S	Treatment of seasonal allergic rhinitis	Dec 96	Antihistamine
Betaine anhydrous	Cystadane (Orphan Medical)	Powder	1 gm/1.7 mL	3 gm bid/20 gm maximum	1-P	Treatment of patients with homocystinuria	Oct 96	Misc
Brimonidine tartrate	Alphagan (Allergan)	Solution	0.20%	1 drop in affected eye tid	1-S	Lowers IOP in open-angle glaucoma and ocular hypertension	Sep 96	Glaucoma agent
Butenafine hydrochloride	Mentax (Penederm)	Cream	1%	Apply daily for 4 wk	1-S	Treatment of interdigital tinea pedis	Oct 96	Antifungal
Cabergoline	Dostinex (Pharmacia & Upjohn)	Tablet	0.5 mg	0.25–1 mg PO twice a week	1-S	Treatment of hyperprolactinemic disorders	Dec 96	Misc
Cefepime	Maxipime (Bristol-Myers Squibb)	Injectable	500 mg 1 gm 2 gm	0.5–2 gm q 12 h IV/IM	1-S	UTI, skin infections, pneumonia	Jan 96	Antibiotic: cephalosporin
Cidofovir	Vistide (Gilead Sciences)	Injectable	75 mg/mL	5 mg/kg q week IV × 2 wk, then 5 mg/kg q 2 wk; administer with probenecid and saline hydration	1-S	CMV retinitis in patients with AIDS	Jun 96	Antiviral
Danaproid sodium	Orgaran (Organon)	Injectable	750 U/0.6 mL	750 U SC bid	1-S	Prophylaxis of postoperative DVT in patients undergoing elective hip replacement surgery	Dec 96	LMWH

Generic name	Brand name (manufacturer)	Form	Strength	Dosage	Code	Indication	Approved	Category
Docetaxel	Taxotere (Rhône-Poulenc Rorer)	Injectable	20 mg / 80 mg	60–100 mg/m² IV q 3 wk	1-P, H	Treatment of patients with locally advanced metastatic breast cancer who have progressed or relapsed during standard therapy	May 96	Antineoplastic
Donepezil hydrochloride	Aricept (Eisai/Pfizer)	Tablet	5 mg / 10 mg	5–10 mg/d PO	1-P	Treatment of mild to moderate dementia of the Alzheimer's type	Nov 96	Alzheimer's treatment: cholinesterase inhibitor
Fexofenadine hydrochloride	Allegra (Hoechst Marion Roussel)	Capsule	60 mg	60 mg bid PO	1-S	Treatment of symptoms associated with seasonal allergic rhinitis	Jul 96	Antihistamine—nonsedating
Fosfomycin tromethamine	Monurol (Forest Pharmaceuticals)	Powder	3 gm	3 gm 1 time PO	1-S	Uncomplicated UTI in women due to Escherichia coli and Enterococcus faecalis	Dec 96	Antibiotic
Fosphenytoin sodium	Cerebyx (Parke-Davis)	Injection	75 mg/mL	Loading dose: 10–20 mg PE/kg IM or IV; Maintenance dose: 4–6 mg PE/kg/d	1-S	Treatment of epilepsy	Aug 96	Anticonvulsant
Gemcitabine hydrochloride	Gemzar (Eli Lilly)	Injectable	20 mg/mL	1000 mg/m² IV every week up to 7 wk as indicated	1-P	Treatment of advanced or metastatic adenocarcinoma of the pancreas	May 96	Antineoplastic
Glatiramer acetate	Copaxone (Teva Pharmaceuticals)	Injectable	10 mg/mL	20 mg/d SC	1-S	Reduction of relapsing-remitting multiple sclerosis	Dec 96	Misc
Imiquimod	Aldara (3M)	Cream	5%	Apply three times a week	1-S	Genital and perianal warts	Feb 97	Misc
Indinavir sulfate	Crixivan (Merck)	Capsule	200 mg / 400 mg	800 mg PO q 8 h	1-P, H	Treatment of HIV infection in adults	Mar 96	Antiviral
Insulin lispro	Humalog (Lilly)	Injectable	100 U/mL	As directed	1-S	Treatment of insulin-dependent diabetes mellitus	Jun 96	Antidiabetic: insulin
Irinotecan hydrochloride	Camptosar (Pharmacia & Upjohn)	Injectable	20 mg/mL	125 mg/m² IV × 4 wk, adjust thereafter	1-P	Palliative treatment of squamous cell carcinoma, lymphomas, testicular carcinoma	Jun 96	Antineoplastic
Ivermectin	Stromectol (Merck)	Tablet	6 mg	150–200 µg/kg one-time PO dose	1-P	Treatment of strongyloidiasis and onchocerciasis	Nov 96	Anthelmintic
Latanoprost	Xalatan (Pharmacia)	Drops	0.005%	1 drop in affected eye daily (PM)	1-P	Reduction of IOP in patients with open-angle glaucoma and ocular hypertension	Jun 96	Glaucoma agent
Levofloxacin	Levaquin (McNeil)	Tablet / Injectable	500 mg / 500 mg	500 mg/d	1-S	Sinusitis, chronic bronchitis, pneumonia, skin infections, UTI, pyelonephritis	Dec 96	Antibiotic: fluoroquinolone

Table continued on following page

Generic Name	Trade Name (Manufacturer)	Dosage Form	Strength	Average Dosage Range	FDA Rating	Approved Use	Approval Date	Classification
Meropenem	Merrem IV (Zeneca)	Injectable	500 mg 1 gm	1–2 gm q 8 h IV	1-S	Intra-abdominal infection, pediatric bacterial meningitis	Jun 96	Antibiotic: carbapenem
Midodrine hydrochloride	ProAmatine (Roberts)	Tablet	2.5 mg 5 mg	10 mg tid PO	1-P	Treatment of symptomatic orthostatic hypotension	Sep 96	Vasopressor
Miglitol	Glyset (Bayer Corp)	Tablet	25 mg 50 mg 100 mg	25–100 mg PO tid	1-S	Adjunct to diet or diet plus sulfonylurea therapy to improve control in patients with NIDDM	Dec 96	Antidiabetic: α-glucosidase inhibitor
Minoxidil Mirtazapine	Rogaine (Upjohn) Remeron (Organon)	Solution Tablet	20 mg/mL 15 mg 30 mg	1 mL bid 15 mg/d (PM) PO	Rx to OTC 1-S	Treatment of alopecia Treatment of depression	Feb 96 Jun 96	Misc Antidepressant
Nelfinavir	Viracept (Agouron)	Tablet Powder	250 mg 50 mg/gm	750 mg PO tid with nucleoside analogue	1-P	HIV infection	Mar 97	Antiviral
Nevirapine	Viramune (Roxane)	Tablet	200 mg	200 mg/d PO × 14 d, then bid in combination with nucleoside analogue retroviral	1-P	Treatment of AIDS	Jun 96	Antiviral
Nicotine transdermal system	Nicoderm (Marion Merrell Dow)	Transdermal system	21 mg/d 14 mg/d 7 mg/d	Titrated	Rx to OTC	Aid to smoking cessation	Feb 96	Smoking deterrent
Nicotine polacrilex	Nicorette Gum (Marion Merrell Dow)	Chewing gum	2 mg 4 mg	2-mg gum: 30 pieces maximum 4-mg gum: 20 pieces maximum	Rx to OTC	Aid to smoking cessation	Feb 96	Smoking deterrent
Nilutamide	Nilandron (Hoechst Marion Roussel)	Tablet	50 mg	300 mg/d PO for 30 d, then 150 mg/d	1-S	Metastatic prostate cancer	Sep 96	Antiandrogen
Olanzapine	Zyprexa (Eli Lilly)	Tablet	5 mg 7.5 mg 10 mg	5–10 mg/d PO	1-S	Management of psychotic disorders	Sep 96	Antipsychotic
Olopatadine hydrochloride	Patanol (Alcon Laboratories)	Drops	0.10%	1–2 drops in affected eye bid (at 6- to 8-h intervals)	1-S	Temporary prevention of itching of the eye due to allergic conjunctivitis	Dec 96	Antihistamine

Generic name	Brand (Manufacturer)	Form	Strength	Dosage	Rating	Indication	Date	Class
Penciclovir	Denavir (SmithKline Beecham)	Cream	10 mg/gm	Apply q 2 h while awake for 4 d	1-S	Treatment of herpes labialis	Sep 96	Antiviral
Pentosan polysulfate sodium	Elmiron (Baker Norton)	Capsule	100 mg	100 mg PO tid	1-S	Relief of bladder pain or discomfort associated with interstitial cystitis	Sep 96	Urinary tract analgesic
Ranitidine bismuth citrate	Tritec (Glaxo Wellcome)	Tablet	400 mg	400 mg PO bid for 28 d	Not rated at time of publication	Healing or prevention of duodenal ulcer relapse due to *Helicobacter pylori* when used in conjunction with clarithromycin	Aug 96	*H. pylori* agent
Remifentanil hydrochloride	Ultiva (Glaxo)	Injectable	3 mL / 5 mL / 10 mL	0.025–0.2 µg/kg/min	1-S	Induction or maintenance of general anesthesia; analgesic component of anesthesia care	Jul 96	Anesthetic
Risperidone	Risperdal (Janssen)	Tablet	1 mg / 2 mg / 3 mg / 4 mg	1–3 mg PO bid	1-S	Management of psychotic disorders	Jun 96	Antipsychotic
Ritonavir	Norvir (Abbott)	Capsule / Solution	100 mg / 80 mg/mL	600 mg PO bid	1-P, H	Treatment of HIV infection in combination with nucleoside analogue or as monotherapy	Mar 96	Antiviral
Ropivacaine hydrochloride	Naropin (Astra)	Injectable	2 mg/mL / 5 mg/mL / 7.5 mg/mL / 10 mg/mL	5–200 mg, dose procedure dependent	1-S	Production of local or regional anesthesia for surgery, for postoperative pain management and obstetric procedures	Sep 96	Anesthetic
Sparfloxacin	Zagam (Rhône-Poulenc Rorer)	Tablet	200 mg	400 mg PO loading dose, then 200 mg daily total 10 d	1-S	Community-acquired pneumonia, acute bacterial exacerbations of chronic bronchitis, acute maxillary sinusitis	Dec 96	Antibiotic: fluoroquinolone
Tiludronate	Skelid (Sanofi Winthrop)	Tablet	240 mg	400 mg PO daily	1-S	Paget's disease	Mar 97	Bisphosphonate

Table continued on following page

Generic Name	Trade Name (Manufacturer)	Dosage Form	Strength	Average Dosage Range	FDA Rating	Approved Use	Approval Date	Classification
Tizanidine hydrochloride	Zanaflex (Athena Neurosciences)	Tablet	4 mg	4–36 mg/d PO	1-S	Acute or intermittent management of increased muscle tone associated with spasticity	Nov 96	Antispasmodic
Topiramate	Topamax (McNeil)	Tablet	25 mg 100 mg 200 mg	400 mg/d PO in 2 divided doses	1-S	Adjunctive treatment of partial-onset seizures in adults	Dec 96	Antiepileptic
Trandolapril	Mavik (Knoll Pharmaceutical)	Tablet	1 mg 2 mg 4 mg	1–4 mg/d PO	1-S	Treatment of hypertension	Apr 96	Antihypertensive: ACE inhibitor
Troglitazone	Rezulin (Warner-Lambert)	Tablet	200 mg 400 mg	200–600 mg/d PO	1-S	NIDDM	Jan 97	Antidiabetic: thiazolidinedione
Valsartan	Diovan (Ciba-Geigy)	Capsule	80 mg 160 mg	80–320 mg/d PO	1-S	Treatment of hypertension	Dec 96	Antihypertensive
Zafirlukast	Accolate (Zeneca)	Tablet	20 mg	20 mg PO bid	1-S	Prophylaxis and chronic treatment of asthma in adults and children 12 y and older	Sep 96	Leukotriene receptor antagonist
Zileuton	Zyflo (Abbott)	Tablet	600 mg	600 mg PO qid	1-S	Prophylaxis and chronic treatment of asthma in adults and children 12 y and older	Dec 96	Leukotriene pathway inhibitor

Abbreviations: 1 = new molecular entity; S = standard drug review; P = priority review drug; V = designated orphan drug; H = accelerated approval; Rx = prescription; OTC = over-the-counter; qd = every day; bid = twice daily; tid = three times daily; qid = four times daily; Misc = miscellaneous; IOP = intraocular pressure; CMV = cytomegalovirus; UTI = urinary tract infection; AIDS = acquired immune deficiency syndrome; DVT = deep venous thrombosis; LMWH = low-molecular-weight heparin; PE = phenytoin sodium equivalents; HIV = human immunodeficiency virus; NIDDM = non-insulin-dependent diabetes mellitus; ACE = angiotensin-converting enzyme.

NOMOGRAM FOR THE DETERMINATION OF BODY SURFACE AREA OF CHILDREN AND ADULTS

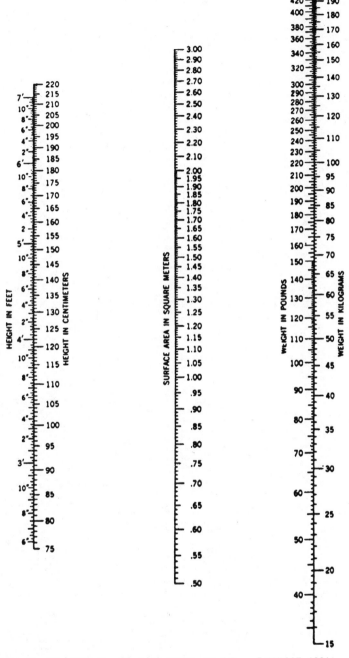

From Boothby WM, Sandiford RB: Boston Med Surg J *185*:337, 1921.

Index

Note: Page numbers in *italics* refer to illustrations; page numbers followed by t refer to tables.

1279

ISBN 0-7216-7223-X

90071